'OLOMEW'S AND TH' ROYAL LONL
)L C' 'DICINE A' 'TIS'

Greenfield's
Neuropathology

Greenfield's Neuropathology

SEVENTH EDITION

EDITED BY

David I Graham MBBCh PhD FRCPath FMedSci

*Professor of Neuropathology, University of Glasgow
and Institute of Neurological Sciences, Glasgow, UK*

Peter L Lantos MD PhD DSc FRCPath FMedSci

*Professor of Neuropathology, Institute of Psychiatry,
University of London, UK*

ARNOLD

A member of the Hodder Headline Group
LONDON · NEW YORK · NEW DELHI

First published in Great Britain 1958
Second edition 1963
Third edition 1976
Fourth edition 1984
Fifth edition 1992
Sixth edition 1997
Seventh edition published in 2002
by Arnold, a member of the Hodder Headline Group,
338 Euston Road, London NW1 3BH

http://www.arnoldpublishers.com

Distributed in the United States of America by Oxford University Press Inc.,
198 Madison Avenue, New York, NY 10016
Oxford is a registered trademark of Oxford University Press

Whilst the advice and information in this book are believed to be true and
accurate at the date of going to press, neither the authors nor the publisher
can accept any legal responsibility or liability for any errors or omissions
that may be made.

In particular (but without limiting the generality of the preceding
disclaimer) every effort has been made to check drug dosages;
however, it is still possible that errors have been missed. Furthermore,
dosage schedules are constantly being revised and new side-effects
recognized. For these reasons the reader is strongly urged to consult
the drug companies' printed instructions before administering any
of the drugs recommended in this book.

British Library Cataloguing in Publication Data
A catalogue record for this book is available from the British Library

Library of Congress Cataloging-in-Publication Data
A catalog record for this book is available from the Library of Congress

ISBN 0 340 74231 3

1   2   3   4   5   6   7   8   9   10

Publisher: Georgina Bentliff
Development Editor: Tim Wale
Production Editor: James Rabson
Production Controller: Bryan Eccleshall
Cover Design: Terry Griffiths

Produced and typeset by Gray Publishing, Tunbridge Wells, Kent
Printed and bound in Italy by Giunti

What do you think of this book? Or any other Arnold title?
Please send your comments to feedback.arnold@hodder.co.uk

Contents of Volume I

Chapter 6: Vascular diseases   281

Hannu Kalimo, Markku Kaste and Matti Haltia

Chapter 7: Malformations   357

Brian N. Harding and Andrew J. Copp

Chapter 8: Metabolic and neurodegenerative diseases of childhood   485

Brian N. Harding and Robert Surtees

Chapter 9: Perinatal neuropathology   519

*Hannah C. Kinney and Dawna
Duncan Armstrong*

Chapter 10: Nutritional and metabolic disorders   607

Clive Harper and Roger Butterworth

Chapter 11: Lysosomal diseases   653

Kinuko Suzuki and Kunihiko Suzuki

Chapter 12: Peroxisomal and mitochondrial disorders   737

James M. Powers and Darryl C. De Vivo

Chapter 13: Neurotoxicology   799

Doyle Graham and Thomas J. Montine

Chapter 14: Trauma   823

David I. Graham, Tom A. Gennarelli and
Tracy K. McIntosh

Chapter 15: Epilepsy   899

Mrinalini Honavar and Brian S. Meldrum

Chapter 16: Ophthalmic neuropathology 943

Philip J. Luthert and Susan Lightman

Chapter 17: Hypothalamus and pituitary 983

*Eva Horvath, Bernd W. Scheithauer,
Kalman Kovacs and Ricardo V. Lloyd*

Chapter 18: Regional neuropathology: diseases of the spinal cord and vertebral column   **1063**

Umberto De Girolami, Matthew P. Frosch and Charles H. Tator

Contents of Volume II

Chapter 1: Viral diseases   1

Seth Love and Clayton A. Wiley

Chapter 2: Parasitic and fungal diseases   107

Gareth Turner and Francesco Scaravilli

Chapter 3: Bacterial infections of the central nervous system   151

Françoise Gray and Jean-Michel Alonso

Chapter 8: Demyelinating diseases 471

*John W. Prineas, W. Ian McDonald and
Robin J.M. Franklin*

Chapter 9: Peripheral nerves

*Peter J. Dyck, P. James B. Dyck, Caterina Giannini,
Zarife Sahenk, Anthony J. Windebank and
JaNean Engelstad*

Contributors

Jean-Michel Alonso MD PhD
Chef de Laboratoire
Unite des Neisseria
Centre de Reference des Meningocoques
Institut Pasteur
Paris, France

Dawna Duncan Armstrong MD
Professor of Pathology and Pediatrics
Department of Pathology, Baylor College of Medicine
Texas Children's Hospital
Houston, TX, USA

Roland N Auer MD PhD
Professor of Pathology and Clinical Neuroscience
Health Sciences Centre
University of Calgary
Alberta, Canada

Martin Berry MD DSc FRCPath
Professor of Anatomy
GKT School of Biomedical Sciences
Neural Damage and Repair
Centre for Neuroscience
London, UK

William F Blakemore BVSc ScD MRCVS FRCPath
Professor of Neuropathology
Department of Clinical Veterinary Medicine
University of Cambridge
Cambridge, UK

Arthur M Butt PhD MPhil
Reader in Physiology
Division of Physiology
Centre for Neuroscience
King's College
London, UK

Roger Butterworth PhD DSc
Director, Neuroscience Research Unit
University Montreal, Hopital St-Luc
Montreal, Canada

Andrew J Copp MB BS MA DPhil
Neural Development Unit
Institute of Child Health
London, UK

Tim J Crow MD
University Department of Psychiatry
Warneford Hospital
Oxford, UK

William JK Cumming MD
Withington Hospital
Manchester, UK

Stephen J DeArmond MD PhD
Professor of Pathology (Neuropathology)
Department of Pathology and
The Institute for Neurodegenerative Diseases
University of California
San Francisco, CA, USA

Umberto De Girolami MD
Professor of Pathology
Harvard Medical School
Director, Division of Neuropathology
Brigham and Women's Hospital and
Children's Hospital Boston
Boston, MA, USA

Darryl C De Vivo MD
Sidney Carter Professor of Neurology
Professor of Pediatrics
Director, Pediatric Neurology, Emeritus
Associate Chairman (Neurology) for Pediatric
Neurosciences
Director, Colleen Giblin Research Laboratories
Columbia-Presbyterian Medical Center
The Neurological Institute
New York, NY, USA

P James B Dyck MD
Assistant Professor of Neurology
Department of Neurology
Mayo Clinic
Rochester, MN, USA

Peter J Dyck MD
Professor of Neurology
Department of Neurology
Mayo Clinic
Rochester, MN, USA

David W Ellison MD PhD MA MSc MRCP MRCPath
Reader in Neuro-oncological Pathology
University of Newcastle
Consultant Neuropathologist, Newcastle General Hospital
Cancer Research Unit, Medical School
University of Newcastle
Newcastle upon Tyne, UK

JaNeen Engelstad HT
Histology Technician
Department of Neurology
Mayo Clinic
Rochester, MN, USA

Margaret M Esiri DM FRCPath
Professor of Neuropathology
Consultant in Neuropathology
Neuropathology Department
Radcliffe Infirmary
Oxford, UK

Robin JM Franklin BSc BVetMed PhD MRCVS MRCPath
Department of Clinical Veterinary Medicine
University of Cambridge
Cambridge, UK

Matthew P Frosch MD PhD
C.S. Kubik Laboratory for Neuropathology
Department of Pathology
Massachusetts General Hospital
Boston, MA, USA

Thomas A Gennarelli MD FACS
Professor and Chair
Department of Neurosurgery
Medical College of Wisconsin
Milwaukee, WI, USA

Caterina Giannini MD PhD
Assistant Professor of Pathology
Department of Pathology
Mayo Clinic
Rochester, MN, USA

Manuel B Graeber MD PhD MRCPath
Professor of Neuropathology
Honorary Consultant, Hammersmith Hospitals NHS Trust
Chair, Department of Neuropathology
Division of Neuroscience and Psychological Medicine
Imperial College Faculty of Medicine
London, UK

David I Graham MBBCh PhD FRCPath FMedSci
Professor of Neuropathology
Department of Neuropathology
Institute of Neurological Sciences
Southern General Hospital
Glasgow, UK

Doyle Graham MD
Professor, Department of Pathology
Vanderbilt University School of Medicine
Nashville, TN, USA

Françoise Gray MD
Professor, Service d'Anatomie Pathologique
Neuropathologie, Hôpital Raymond Poincaré
Garches, France

Matti Haltia MD DMSc
Professor of Neuropathology
Department of Pathology
University of Helsinki
Helsinki, Finland

Brian N Harding MA DPhil BM BCh FRCPath
Consultant Histopathologist
Honorary Senior Lecturer
Department of Histopathology
Hospital for Sick Children
Great Ormond Street
London, UK

Clive Harper MD FRCPA
Professor of Neuropathology
Department of Pathology, University of Sydney
NSW, Australia

Mrinalini Honavar MD FRCPath
Director of Anatomic Pathology
Hospital Pedro Hispano
Matosinhos, Portugal
Consultant Neuropathologist
Institute of Psychiatry
London, UK

Eva Horvath PhD
Associate Professor of Pathology
Department of Pathology
St Michael's Hospital
Toronto, Ontario, Canada

Bradley T Hyman MD PhD
Professor of Neurology and Neurosciences
Harvard Medical School
Massachusetts General Hospital
Boston, MA, USA

James W Ironside BMSc MB ChB FRCPath FRCPEdin
Professor of Clinical Neuropathology
Honorary Consultant in Neuropathology
Neuropathology Laboratory
Department of Pathology
University of Edinburgh
Western General Hospital
Edinburgh, UK

Hannu Kalimo MD DMSc
Senior Consultant and Professor of Neuropathology
Department of Pathology
Turku University Hospital
Turku, Finland

Markku Kaste MD PhD
Professor of Neurology
Department of Neurology
University of Helsinki
Helsinki, Finland

Hannah C Kinney MD
Neuropathologist
Department of Pathology
Children's Hospital
Boston, MA, USA

Paul Kleihues MD
Professor and Director
International Agency for Research on Cancer
Lyon, France

Kalman Kovacs MD PhD
Professor of Pathology
Department of Pathology
St Michael's Hospital
Toronto, Ontario, Canada

Hans A Kretzschmar MD
Professor and Director
Institute of Neuropathology
Head, Creutzfeldt–Jakob Surveillance Unit, Germany
University of Munich
Munich, Germany

Georg W Kreutzberg MD
Max-Planck-Institute für Neurobiologie
Martinsried, Germany

Peter L Lantos MD PhD DSc FRCPath FMedSci
Professor of Neuropathology
Department of Neuropatholgy
Institute of Psychiatry
London, UK

Nigel Leigh BSc MB BS PhD FRCP
Professor of Clinical Neurology
Neuroscience Unit
Department of Neurology
London, UK

Susan Lightman FRCP FRCP Phth PhD
Head of Department
Professor of Clinical Ophthalmology
Department of Clinical Ophthalmology
Institute of Ophthalmology
University College London
London, UK

Ricardo V Lloyd MD PhD
Professor, Mayo Medical School
Mayo Clinic
Rochester, MN, USA

David N Louis MD
Department of Pathology/Neuropathology
Massachusetts General Hospital
Boston, MA, USA

Seth Love MBBCh (cam laude) PhD FRCP MRCP FRCPath MRCPath
Professor, Neuropathology
Institute of Clinical Sciences
Frenchay Hospital
Bristol, UK

James S Lowe DM FRCPath
Professor, Neuropathology
University Hospital, Queen's Medical Centre
Nottingham, UK

Philip J Luthert BSc FRCP FRCPath FRCOphth
Professor, Department of Pathology
Institute of Ophthalmology
University College London
London, UK

Mike Mahon BSc
Department of Biological Sciences
University of Manchester
Manchester, UK

W Ian McDonald PhD FRACP FRCP
Professor, Institute of Neurology
London, UK

Tracy K McIntosh MD
Professor, Head Injury Center
Vice-Chairman for Research
Department of Neurosurgery
University of Philadelphia
Philadelphia, PA, USA

Brian S Meldrum MB BChir PhD DSc
Emeritus Professor
GKT School of Biomedical Sciences
King's College London
London, UK

Suzanne S Mirra MD
Professor and Chair, Department of Pathology
State University of New York
Downstate Medical Center
New York, USA

Thomas J Montine MD PhD
Alvord Professor of Neuropathology
Director of Neuropathology
University of Washington
Seattle, WA, USA

Hugh Perry BSc DPhil
Professor of Experimental Neuropathology
CNS Inflammatory Group
School of Biological Science
Biomedical Science Building
University of Southampton
Southampton, UK

John D Pickard MChir FMedSci
Professor of Neurosurgery
Academic Neurosurgery Unit
University of Cambridge
Addenbrooke's Hospital, Cambridge, UK

James M Powers MD
Professor of Pathology
Department of Pathology
University of Rochester Medical Center
Rochester, NY, USA

John W Prineas MB BS FRCP
Professor, Royal Prince Alfred Hospital and the University
of Sydney
Institute of Clinical Neurosciences
The University of Sydney
NSW, Australia

Stanley B Prusiner MD
Professor of Neurology and Biochemistry
Institute of Neurodegenerative Diseases
University of California
San Francisco, CA, USA

Marc K Rosenblum MD
Chief, Neuropathology and Autopsy Service
Memorial Sloan-Kettering Cancer Center
Professor of Pathology
Weill Medical College of Cornell University
New York, USA

Zarife Sahenk MD PhD
Professor, Neurology
Neuromuscular Center
The Ohio State University
Columbus, OH, USA

Francesco Scaravilli MD PhD DSc FRCPath
Professor of Neuropathology
Division of Neuropathology
Institute of Neurology
University College London
London, UK

Bernd W Scheithauer MD
Professor, Department of Laboratory Medicine and
Pathology, Mayo Clinic
Rochester, MN, USA

Constantino Sotelo MD
Head of INSERM Unit 106
Batiment de Pédiatrie
Hôpital de la Salpêtriere
Paris, France
Chair of Developmental Neurobiology
Profesor Remedios Caro Almela
Institute of Neurosciences
Miguel Hernandez University
San Juan de Alicante, Spain

Robert Surtees MA BM PhD FRCPCH FRCP
Reader in Paediatric Neurology
Institute of Child Health
University College London
London, UK

Garnette R Sutherland BSc MD FRCSC
Department of Clinical Neurosciences
Head, Division of Neurosurgery
University of Calgary
Alberta, Canada

Kunihiko Suzuki MD
Neuroscience Center
Departments of Neurology and Psychiatry
University of North Carolina School of Medicine
Chapel Hill, NC, USA

Kinuko Suzuki MD
Department of Pathology and Laboratory Medicine
University of North Carolina School of Medicine
Chapel Hill, NC, USA

Charles H Tator CM MD PhD FRCSC
Professor and Past Chair of Neurosurgery
University of Toronto, Division of Neurosurgery
Toronto Western Hospital
Toronto, Ontario, Canada

Antoine Triller MD DSc
Director of Research
Biologie Cellulaire de la Synapse
INSERM CJF 94-10
Ecole Normale Superieure
Paris, France

Gareth Turner DPhil MRCPath
Clinical Lecturer in Histopathology
Nuffield Department of Clinical Laboratory Sciences
The John Radcliffe Hospital
Oxford, UK

Roy O Weller BSc PhD MD FRCPath
Neuropathology, Division of Clinical Neurosciences
University of Southampton School of Medicine
Southampton General Hospital
Southampton, UK

Clayton A Wiley MD PhD
Professor
Department of Pathology
University of Pittsburgh, PA, USA

Graham P Wilkin MSc PhD
Reader in Neurobiology
Biological Sciences
Imperial College
London, UK

Anthony J Windebank BM BCh FRCP
Professor of Neurology
Mayo Clinic
Rochester, MN, USA

Foreword

In 1605 the great English scholar, Sir Francis Bacon, published his magnificent work, 'The Advancement and Proficiencie of Learning', in which he laid down the prerequisites for, and the barriers to, the learning process in the sciences. Nearly 400 years later his words remain almost as relevant as they were then, and continue to provide insight and wisdom. He noted that in the same way that the precious commodity of water would be lost if not gathered into receptacles such as cisterns and conduits, so the 'liquor of Knowledge … would soon perish and vanish, if it were not conserved in Books. Traditions, Conferences, and in Places purposely designed to that end, as Universities, Colledges, Schools, where it may have fixt stations and Power and Ability of uniting and improving itself.'

When Godwin Greenfield first published his *Pathology of the Nervous System*, later to become *Greenfield's Neuropathology*, it was one of the first books to collect in one work the accumulated knowledge of a growing discipline. It was also published in an era when the printed word reigned supreme, and represented the only means of permanent transmission of information. In the early days of this new millennium, books no longer represent the only way of communicating and preserving knowledge. However, despite dire predictions by some of the demise of the printed word in the modern era, book publishing remains a thriving endeavour, and students at all stages of their careers remain enthusiastic readers of books. The introduction of the Internet and online publishing has provided alternatives to learning, and for a book to succeed against such competition it has to be relevant and meaningful, and perhaps be of an even higher standard than previously.

The publication of a new edition of any book is always an occasion for excitement and anticipation. For those familiar with the previous editions it is an opportunity to note improvements and advancements in a familiar setting, whereas for those who will be reading it for the first time, it is their guarantee of modernity. When the revision is of a work that is the standard in the discipline, the expectations are even higher. Readers expect the new edition to maintain the standards that made the book a classic in the first instance, and this places an even greater burden of responsibility on the editors and authors. New

editions are absolutely required to turn a textbook into a living organism with a continuous life of its own. Bacon laid down requirements for these, when he called for 'new Editions of Authors, with corrected impressions, more faithful Translations, more profitable Glosses, and more diligent Annotations.' Could the modern reader ask anything more of the editors of this new edition of *Greenfield*, than the provision of new authors, correction of previously held misinterpretations, faithful distillation of the literature, better figures and illustrations, and accurate and up-to-date references?

When Professors Graham and Lantos took over the editorship of the sixth edition they completely rejuvenated a textbook, which, while being the best comprehensive source in the field of neuropathology, had generally maintained the same format through many editions. Previous editors had done a fine job of modernizing the classic which Blackwood, McMenemy, Meyer and Norman had taken over from Greenfield, but the book had become less accessible and easy to read. The sixth edition maintained the high standards of scholarly discussion, comprehensiveness, and good illustrations. However, with this edition came a new format, great expansion of material, and a very well laid out style. The individual entities were easily found, while being well placed in the overall context of conceptual disease. Discussion of each subject also followed logical progression, with information on Clinical Behaviour, Pathology and Basic Sciences being easily accessible. In addition, although previous editions had been very cognizant of the neuropathological traditions of Europe and the Western hemisphere, the book remained a British endeavour. One of the great strengths of the sixth edition was the inclusion of a wide selection of international experts as authors. In many respects this reflects the internationalization of science and the greater ease of communication and sharing of information in the twenty-first century, but it also reflects the commitment of the editors to obtain the very finest authors, wherever they may reside. The result was a fresh new look at the discipline, which was a major factor in making the book so successful.

It is now more than 5 years since the previous edition, and, given the pace of change and discovery in the field, it is very timely to have a new edition. With this new edition, we may well ask how the Editors have responded to Bacon's charge. First, they have in general kept the format which has proved highly successful in the past, and which garnered wide praise. There are two new chapters, reflecting not only growth and expansion of knowledge in these fields, but also a need to emphasize the conceptual importance of these subjects on their own. One of these is a new chapter on the Metabolic and Neurodegenerative Diseases of Childhood, and the other is a separate chapter on Peroxisomal and Mitochondrial Diseases. In addition, the previous chapter on the Pathology of Schizophrenia, now with completely new authors, has wisely been expanded to cover the Pathology of Psychiatric Diseases. These will be most helpful to the reader. Of the remaining 26 chapters, there have been major changes in authorship in six, as well as less radical changes in a further 11. A brief look at the list of authors will reassure even the most critical of readers that the very highest quality of contributions has been assured. The inclusion of a strong international cast of authors has been continued, and there are a significant number of neurologists and neurosurgeons.

Bacon warned of certain 'Peccant Humors in Learning', among which he cautioned against the 'extreme affection of two extremities, Antiquity and Novelty'. By these he meant that the scholar should beware of rejecting either new ideas or old ones in a blanket fashion without thought. In the pages of this edition the reader will find the familiar, which has stood the tests of time and scrutiny, as well as new ideas waiting to be validated or rejected.

A medical text has, above all, to be of use to the practitioner. Books, knowledge and practice are intertwined. As William Osler wrote: 'To study the phenomena of disease without books is to sail an uncharted sea, while to study books without patients is not to go to sea at all'. The range of diseases seen by neuropathologists, neurologists and neurosurgeons has become enormous. With advances in therapeutic options and the imperative for genetic counselling in diseases previously considered unmanageable, the need for accuracy of diagnosis, and an ability to understand and interpret the complexity of classification and delineation of subgroups, are now essential parts of daily practice. This new edition contains a wealth of clinical and taxonomic information, and the format makes the access to this information simple. The importance of correlating clinical information with pathological findings is a common theme throughout, and in chapters such as the dementing diseases and movement disorders plays a major role. In addition, the enormous advances in modern imaging techniques have ushered in a new era of what will, one day, be living gross pathology. It remains up to the neuropathologist to assist in refining these studies and the current volume is replete with relevant images. It is essential for the modern neuropathologist to be familiar with these images. In diseases such as multiple sclerosis, magnetic resonance imaging techniques are often essential in guiding the pathologist to areas that would be missed in the gross examination. For all these reasons, and above all, for the adherence to the high standards of neuropathological description of disease that have always characterized this book, this edition will continue to be the Bible and day-to-day companion of the practising neuropathologist.

The late Lucien Rubinstein used to tell his trainees that neuropathology was like a string quartet, the highest form of art. By this he meant that the discipline consisted of different threads woven together to form a subject of complex beauty. These threads are basic neurosciences, general and specific neuropathological processes, and clinical disease and syndromes. It is of course interesting that in the past, each of these elements has been the domain of specialists who were not neuropathologists. Thus, the seminal pathological discoveries of Alzheimer's disease were described by a neurologist/psychiatrist, the lesions of multiple sclerosis were described by Charcot, a neurologist, while Harvey Cushing, a neurosurgeon, described the pathology of brain tumours. At the same time, fundamental principles of neuropathology, such as those dealing with growth, degeneration and regeneration, were enunciated by Ramon y Cajal, a basic neuroscientist. It is exciting to see how the emerging techniques of neuroscience have found their way into diagnostic, and experimental and clinical investigative studies. The tools of basic neuroscience, such as modern molecular biology, cytogenetics, transgenic animal work, molecular chemistry, confocal and *in situ* microscopy, and sophisticated imaging, are now standard in diagnostic and research neuropathology laboratories around the world. This edition is filled with the results of this work.

There are still many gaps in neuropathological knowledge. A glance at any of the major texts in basic neuroscience and in neurology will highlight the prevalence and importance of the study of normal higher functions such as cognition, learning, sleep and consciousness, as well as their clinical manifestations and consequences in disease. With some exceptions such as the dementias and the more obvious gross causes of changes in consciousness, the classical neuropathologist often does not have much to contribute to the discussion. However, this remains an exciting area for collaborative studies with molecular and chemical imagers, as well as with researchers studying these processes with transgenic and other molecular techniques. Let us hope that by the time of the next edition advances in these areas will have progressed sufficiently to be included.

To whom is this book addressed? It will be read assiduously by students and practitioners in the discipline of neuropathology, but I believe that it is essential reading for neurologists, neurosurgeons and neuroradiologists, and for any others interested in the dysfunctional nervous system. In an era where so much of how we understand the *normal* nervous system is accomplished by the study of the *abnormal,* it should also be highly valued by basic neuroscientists.

I believe that readers of this edition will find that the book remains true to Greenfield's original mandate, which was to provide a comprehensive review of the discipline. At the same time with this new edition, the editors have continued and improved on their own fine tradition. I would also like to think that Sir Francis Bacon would have approved strongly of this book. He felt that authors should be recognized. Addressing his patron King James he wrote, perhaps somewhat hopefully, that 'the Remuneration and Designation of writers concerning those parts of Knowledge [are] works and Acts wherein the Merit of many renowned Princes and other illustrious Persons hath been famed, towards the State of Learning.' I do not know whether the editors and authors of this edition will be recognized and rewarded by the monarch of the realm, but they will surely be thanked and applauded by all their readers.

Samuel K. Ludwin
Professor of Pathology (Neuropathology)
Queens University, Kingston, Canada
President, International Society of Neuropathology.

Preface

The invitation to be an editor of *Greenfield's Neuropathology* is both an honour and a privilege. At the same time it is a commitment that has required a decade to produce two editions. When first approached in 1993 we recognized the need to develop a strategic vision of neuropathology in order to ensure the continuing viability of what we believed to be the most widely read international text of neuropathology. The much changed sixth edition was published in 1997 and now the seventh edition is complete. We have been greatly helped in the task by the very positive feedback of the sixth edition for which we are grateful, and by the awareness that in order for the new edition to continue to meet the needs of its readers it would have to incorporate technical advances and a modern, twenty-first century approach including molecular genetics. The associated CD-ROM is another step in this direction.

Ever conscious of the need to maintain a balance between classical morphology of disease, and molecular and cellular neurobiology, the seventh edition has undergone considerable change not so much in format and style, but of content and its overall length has increased by 10–15%. The changes in part reflect not only the complexity of diseases of the nervous system and muscle, but also the major roles played by neuroimaging, and neuroscience in their investigation and diagnosis with the ultimate aim of a better understanding of the processes involved and better targeted therapy. Some chapters have been extensively re-written and updated again with the primary aim of providing not only a reference source of generally accepted fact, but also exciting recent developments in clinical neuroscience. We hope this has been achieved.

Although content is of the essence, we have not forgotten the need to present the new edition in a way appropriate to the standing of the book. Therefore, the two-volume format has continued with an increased number of colour illustrations, line diagrams and tables. Some black and white figures remain again reminding us that colour is not necessarily always the best presentation.

The reality of producing *Greenfield's* reflects an enormous amount of time and effort by all the contributions and those at Arnold in the development and production team. To the authors we owe nothing but gratitude given they are all busy practitioners with increasing professional and administrative commitments. The team at Arnold has cajoled, persuaded and motivated us to the extent that by and large the book is on schedule. Our particular thanks go to Georgina Bentliff, Director of Medical and Health Science Publishing, to Tim Wale, Senior Development Editor, James Watson, Health Sciences Marketing Manager and James Rabson, Editorial Production Manager, and Lesley Gray and her team at Gray Publishing whose constant support and help have encouraged us along the way to completion. Last, but not least, neither of us could have reached this point without the unstinting 'back-up' and support of our secretaries Mrs Marisa Hughes, Ms Irene Hart and Ms Anthea Hawley.

Finally, we can honestly say that we have read the text from start to finish. We have learned much and feel greatly enriched by the knowledge within this text. We hope that you the reader will find the help and advice you seek, and *Greenfield's* will become a companion in your work.

We have been humbled by the experience, but dare to think that in a small way we have also contributed to what, we hope, will remain as the text in neuropathology. And now we can hand over the onerous, but rewarding task of editors to the next generation with a sense of optimism in the future of the book.

D.I. Graham
P.L. Lantos

Abbreviations

AAG	allergic angiitis and granulomatosis	BDNF	brain derived neurotrophic factor
AAV	adeno-associated virus	bFGF	basic fibroblast growth factor
ACN	acute retinal necrosis	BFNC	benign familial neonatal convulsions
ACh	acetylcholine	BMAA	β-N-methylamino-L-alanine
AChE	acetylcholinesterase	BOAA	β-N-oxalylamino-L-alanine
AChR	acetylcholine receptor	BP	blood pressure
ACTH	adrenocorticotrophic hormone	BrDU	5-bromo-2'-deoxyuridine
AD	Alzheimer's disease	BS-1	*Bandeiraea (Griffinia) simplicifolia*
ADC	apparent diffusion coefficient		agglutinin
ADCA	autosomal dominant cerebellar ataxia	BSE	bovine spongiform encephalopathy
ADH	antidiuretic hormone	CAA	cerebral amyloid angiopathy
ADNFLE	autosomal dominant nocturnal frontal	CADASIL	cerebral autosomal dominant
	lobe epilepsy		arteriopathy with subcortical infarcts
ADP	adenosine diphosphate		and leucoencephalopathy
ADTN	2-amino-6,7-dihydroxytetralin	CAEV	caprine arthritis encephalitis virus
AETT	actyl-ethyl-tetramethyl tetralin	CAII	carbonic anhydrase II
AFP	α-fetoprotein	CALT	conjunctival associated lymphoid tissue
AGE	advanced glycation endproducts	CAM	cell adhesion molecule
AgNOR	silver staining of the nucleolar organizer	CAT	choline acetyl transferase
	region	CBD	corticobasal degeneration
AIDS	acquired immunodeficiency syndrome	CBF	cerebral blood flow
AION	anterior ischaemic optic neuropathy	CCK	cholecystokinin
Al	aluminium	CDG	carbohydrate deficient glycoprotein
ALD	adrenoleucodystrophy	CEA	carcinoembryonic antigen
ALL	acute lymphocytic leukaemia	CERAD	Consortium to Establish a Registry for
ALS	amyotropic lateral sclerosis		Alzheimer's Disease
AMAN	acute motor axonal neuropathy	CESD	cholesterol ester storage disease
AMC	arthrogryposis multiplex congenita	CGH	comparative genomic hybridization
AMD	age-related muscular degeneration	CGRP	calcitonin gene-related peptide
AMP	adenosine monophosphate	CI	cerebral infarction
AMPA	α-amino-3-hydroxy-5-methyl-4-isoxazole	CIDP	chronic inflammatory demyelinating
	propionic acid		polyneuropathy
AMSAN	acute motor and sensory axonal	CJD	Creutzfeldt–Jakob disease
	neuropathy	CLBD	cortical Lewy body disease
ANCA	antineutrophil cytoplasmic	CLIP	corticotrophin-like intermediate lobe
	autoantibodies		peptide
ANOR	analysis of nucleolar organizer region	CME	cystoid maculoid oedema
3-AP	3-acetylpyridine	CMRglc	cerebral metabolic rate of glucose
aPL	antiphospholipid		consumption
apoE	apolipoprotein E	CMR$_{o2}$	cerebral metabolic rate of oxygen
APP	amyloid precursor protein		consumption
APV	2-amino-5-phosphovaleric (acid)	CMT	Charcot–Marie–Tooth (disease)
ARC	AIDS-related complex	CMV	cytomegalovirus
ARIA	acetylcholine receptor inducing activity	CNEM	concentric needle electromyography
A-T	ataxia-telangiectasia	CNPase	2',3'-cyclic nucleotide-3'-
ATP	adenosine triphosphate		phosphodiesterase
AVED	ataxia with isolated vitamin E deficiency	CNQX	6-cyano-7-nitroquinoxaline-2,3-dione
AVM	arteriovenous malformation	CNS	central nervous system
βA4	β-amyloid peptide	CNTF	ciliary neurotrophic factor
BAL	British anti-Lewisite	CoA	coenzyme A
βAPP	β-amyloid precursor protein	COD-MD	cerebro-ocular dysplasia muscular
BBB	blood–brain barrier		dystrophy

CPAP	continual positive airways pressure
CPB	cardiopulmonary bypass
CPK	creatine phosphokinase
CPM	central pontine myelinolysis
CPP	cerebral perfusion pressure
CPT	carnitine palmitoyltransferase
CRABP	cellular retinoic acid binding protein
CRBP	cellular retinol binding protein
CRH	corticotrophin releasing hormone
CROP	cerebro-rhino-ocular-phycomycosis
CS	carbon sulfide
CSD	cat scratch disease
CSF	cerebrospinal fluid
CT	computed tomography
CTG	cytosine–thymine–guanine
CVB	cerebrovascular bed
CVS	chorionic villus sample
CVT	cerebral venous thrombosis
Cx	connexin
D	distal
DA	dopamine
DAG	dystrophin associated glycoprotein
DAI	diffuse axonal injury
ddC	dideoxycytidine
ddI	dideoxyinosine
DEC	diethylcarbamazine
DFP	diisopropyl fluorophosphate
DHAPAT	dihydroxyacetone-phosphate acyltransferase
DHCA	deep hypothermic circulatory arrest
DHP	dihydropyridine
DIC	disseminated intravascular coagulation
DIDMOAD	diabetes insipidus, diabetes mellitus, optic atrophy, deafness
DMBA	dimethylbenz[a]anthracene
DMPS	2,3-dimercaptopropane-sulfonate
DNA	deoxyribonucleic acid
DNT	dysembryoplastic neuroepithelial tumour
DOPAC	dihydroxyphenylacetic acid
DRD	dopa-responsive dystonia
DRG	dorsal root ganglion
DRPLA	dentatorubropallidoluysian atrophy
DWI	diffusion-weighted imaging
EA	episodic ataxia
EAA	excitatory amino acid
EAAR	excitatory amino acid receptors
EAE	experimental autoimmune encephalomyelitis
EAN	experimental allergic neuritis
EBNA	Epstein–Barr nuclear antigen
EBV	Epstein–Barr virus
ECASS	European Co-operative Acute Stroke Study
ECG	electrocardiogram
ECM	extracellular matrix
ECMO	extracorporeal membrane oxygenation
ECT	emission computed tomography
EEG	electroencephalogram
E-face	extracellular surface
EGF	epidermal growth factor
EGFR	epidermal growth factor receptor
EGL	external granular layer
EIAV	equine infectious anaemia virus
EMA	epithelial membrane antigen
EMG	electromyogram
EMS	eosinophilia-myalgia syndrome
ENU	ethylnitrosourea
EOFAD	early onset familial Alzheimer's disease

EPMR	epilepsy with mental retardation
ERG	electroretinogram
ESR	erythrocyte sedimentation rate
F-actin	actin filaments
FAD	flavin adenine dinucleotide
FAE	fetal alcohol effects
FAP	familial adenomatosis polyposis
FAS	fetal alcohol syndrome
FBD	familial British dementia
FCI	focal cerebral ischaemia
FFI	fatal familial insomnia
FGF	fibroblast growth factor
FISH	fluorescence *in situ* hybridization
FITC	fluorescein isothiocyanate
FIV	feline immunodeficiency virus
FSE	fast spin echo (imaging)
FSH	follicle stimulating hormone
FSH dystrophy	facioscapulohumeral dystrophy
FTA-ABS	fluorescent treponemal antibody absorption test
G-actin	globular actin
GABA	γ-aminobutyric acid
GAD	glutamic acid decarboxylase
GAE	granulomatous amoebic encephalitis
GAG	glycosaminoglycans
GAL-C	galactocerebroside
GCA	giant cell arteritis
GCI	global cerebral ischaemia
GDNF	glial cell derived neurotrophic factor
GEFS	generalized epilepsy with febrile seizures
GFAP	glial fibrillary acidic protein
GH	growth hormone
GHRH	growth hormone releasing hormone
GluR3	glutamate receptor protein 3
GLUT	glucose transporter
GlyR	glycine receptor
GM-CSF	granulocyte-macrophage colony-stimulating factor
GnRH	gonadotrophin hormone releasing hormone
GROD	granular osmiophilic deposits
GSS	Gerstmann–Sträussler–Scheinker (disease)
GTSF	glioblastoma-derived T cell suppressor factor
HAART	highly active antiretroviral therapy
HAM	HTLV-1 associated myelopathy
HARD+E	hydrocephalus, agyria, retinal dysplasia, encephalocele
HC	Huntington's chorea
HCG	human chorionic gonadotrophin
HCHWA	hereditary cerebral haemorrhage with amyloidosis
HCHWA-D	hereditary cerebral haemorrhage with amyloid angiopathy of the Dutch type
2,5-HD	2,5-hexanedione
HD	Huntington's disease
HDL	high density lipoproteins
H&E	haematoxylin and eosin
HGH	human growth hormone
5-HIAA	5-hydroxyindoleacetic acid
HIB	*Haemophilus influenzae* Pitman type B
h-IBM	hereditary inclusion body myositis
HIV	human immunodeficiency virus
HIV-1	human immunodeficiency virus type 1
HLA-DR	human leucocyte antigen DR
HMG	hydromethylglutaryl
HMG-CoA	3-hydroxy-3-methylglutaryl-coenzyme A
HMSN	hereditary motor and sensory neuropathy

HNE	4-hydroxy-2-nonenal		LTR	long terminal repeat
HNPCC	hereditary non-polyposis colon cancer		MABP	myelin-associated basic protein
HNPP	hereditary neuropathy with liability to pressure palsies		mAChR	muscarinic acetylcholine receptor
HPF	high power fields		MAG	myelin associated glycoprotein
HRP	horseradish peroxidase		MALT	mucosal associated lymphoid tissue
HSAN	hereditary sensory and autonomic neuropathy		MAM	methylazoxymethanol acetate
			MAP	microtubule associated protein
HSD	Hallervorden–Spatz disease		MAO	monoamine oxidase
HSP	heat shock protein		MASA	mental retardation, adducted thumbs, shuffling gait and aphasia
HSV	herpes simplex virus			
5-HT	5-hydroxytryptamine (serotonin)		MBK	methyl N-butyl ketone
5-HTR	serotonin receptor		MBP	myelin basic protein
HTLV-I	human T lymphotropic virus I		MCA	middle cerebral artery
HVA	homovanillic acid		MCAD	medium chain acyl-CoA dehydrogenase
HZV	herpes zoster-varicella		MCB	membraneous cytoplasmic bodies
IBM	inclusion body myositis		MCP	multicatalytic protease
IBO	ibotenic acid		M-CSF	macrophage colony-stimulating factor
ICA	internal carotid artery		MDA	malondialdehyde
ICAM	intercellular adhesion molecules		MDMA	3,4-methylenedioxymethamphetamine
ICD-O	International Classification of Disease – Oncology		MDM2	murine double minute 2
			ME	methionine-enkephalin
ICH	intracerebral haemorrhage		MELAS	mitochondrial encephalomyopathy, lactic acidosis, stroke-like episodes
ICP	intracranial pressure			
IDPN	β,β'-iminodipropionitrile		MERRF	myoclonus epilepsy with ragged red fibres
IEG	immediate early gene			
IFN	interferon		MFB	Marchiafava–Bignami (disease)
IGF	insulin-like growth factor		MGC	multinucleated giant cell
IGF-I	insulin-like growth factor I		MGluR	metabotropic glutamate receptor
IgM	immunoglobulin M		MGUS	monoclonal gammopathies of undetermined significance
IL	interleukin			
IML	intravascular malignant lymphomatosis		MHC	major histocompatibility complex
INH	isonicotinic acid hydrazide		MHC I, II	major histocompatibility complex (classes I, II)
ION	ischaemic optic neuropathy			
IP	intramembrane particle		MLD	metachromatic leucodystrophy
IP₃R	1,4,5-triphosphate receptor		MND	motor neuron disease
IRBP	interphotereceptor retinoid binding protein		MNGIE	myoneurogastrointestinal disorder and encephalopathy
			MNU	methylnitrosourea
IRMA	intraretinal microvascular abnormalities		MO	myelin oligodendrocyte
ISEL	in situ end labelling		MOG	myelin oligodendrocyte glycoprotein
IUGR	intrautenine growth restricted or retarded		MOSP	MO specific protein
			MPNSTs	malignant peripheral nerve sheath tumours
IVH	intraventricular haemorrhage			
JCV	JC virus		MPP+	1-methyl-4-phenylpyridinium
JME	juvenile myoclonic epilepsy		MPS	mucopolysaccharidosis
KA	kainate		MPT	mitochondrial permeability translation
LA	lupus anticoagulant		MPTP	N-methyl-4-phenyl-1,2,3,6-tetrahydropyridine
LAMP	limbic system associated membrane protein			
			MR	magnetic resonance
LAT	latency associated transcript		MRI	magnetic resonance imaging
LCAD	long chain acyl-CoA dehydrogenase		mRNA	messenger ribonucleic acid
LCMV	lymphocytic choriomeningitis virus		MRS	magnetic resonance spectroscopy
LDH	lactate dehydrogenase		MS	multiple sclerosis
LDL	low density lipoproteins		MSA	multiple system atrophy
LFA	leucocyte function associated		MSH	melanocyte stimulating hormone
LFB	Luxol-fast-blue		MSI	microsatellite instability
LG	limb girdle		MT	microtubule
LH	leuteinizing hormone		MW	microwave
LHON	Leber's hereditary optic atrophy		NA	noradrenaline
LHRH	luteinizing hormone releasing hormone		nAChR	nicotinic muscular acetylcholine receptor
LI	labelling index		NAD	neuroaxonal dystrophy
LMN	lower motor neuron		NAD	neonatal adrenoleucodystrophy
LMP	latent membrane protein		NAD	nicotinamide adenine dinucleotide
LOH	loss of heterozygosity		NADH-TR	nicotinamide adenine dinucleotide tetrazolium reductase
LPV	lymphotropic papova virus			
LT	leukotrienes		NADP	nicotinamide adenine dinucleotide phosphate
LTD	long-term depression			
LTP	long-term potentiation		NAIP	neuronal apoptosis inhibitory protein

NALD	neonatal adrenoleucodystrophy
NARP	neurogenic weakness, ataxia and retinitis pigmentosa
NBCCS	nevoid basal cell carcinoma syndrome
NBQX	2,3-dihydroxy-6-nitro-7-sulfamoylbenzo(f)-quinoxaline
NC	normal control
NCAM	nerve cell adhesion molecule
NCI	National Cancer Institute
NCI	neuronal cytoplasmic inclusions
NCL	neuronal ceroid lipofuscinosis
NF	neurofibromatosis
NF	neurofilament
NFH	heavy component of neurofilament
NFL	light component of neurofilament
NFM	medium component of neurofilament
NFP	neurofilament protein
NGF	nerve growth factor
NIH	National Institutes of Health
NINDS	National Institute of Neurological Disorders and Stroke
NMDA	N-methyl-D-aspartate
NO	nitric oxide
NOS	nitric oxide synthase
NREM	non-rapid eye movement
NT	neurotensin
NT3	neurotrophin-3
NTD	neural tube defects
O4	mouse monoclonal antibody (IgM)
OA	opiate abuse
OAT	ornithine amino-transferase
OEF	oxygen extraction fraction
OPCA	olivopontoccrebellar atrophy
OPIDN	organophosphate-induced delayed neuropathy
ORF	open reading frame
OTC	ornithine transcarbamylase
PA	perinodal astrocyte
PAC	platelet-activating factor
PACNS	primary angiitis of the central nervous system
PAH	polycyclic aromatic hydrocarbons
PAM	primary amoebic meningoencephalitis
PAN	perchloric acid naphthoquinone
PAN	polyarteritis [panarteritis] nodosa
PANCH	pituitary adenoma-neuronal choristoma
PAS	periodic acid-Schiff
PBP	progressive bulbar palsy
PC	phosphatidyl choline
PCO_2	carbon dioxide tension
PCNA	proliferating cell nuclear antigen
PCNSL	primary central nervous system lymphoma
PCR	polymerase chain reaction
PD	Parkinson's disease
PDGF	platelet derived growth factor
PDH	pyruvate dehydrogenase
PDP	presynaptic dense projection
PE	phosphatidyl ethanolamine
PEP	postencephalitic parkinsonism
PET	positron emission tomography
P-face	protoplasmic surface
PGL-I	phenolic glycolipid I
PHF	paired helical filaments
PI	perfusion MRI
PKU	phenylketonuria
PLAP	placental alkaline phosphatase
PLP	proteolipid protein

PLS	primary lateral sclerosis
PMA	progressive muscular atrophy
PML	progressive multifocal leucoencephalopathy
PMN	polymorphonuclear
PMP	peripheral myelin protein
PNET	primitive neuroectodermal tumour
PNMT	human N-methyltransferase
PNS	peripheral nervous system
PNU	N-3-pyridylmethyl-N'-p-nitrophenyl urea
PO_2	partial pressure for oxygen
POMC	pro-opiomelanocortin
PORN	progressive outer retinal necrosis
PPD	purified protein derivative
PPP	pentose phosphate pathway
PRL	prolactin
PrP	prion protein
PSD	postsynaptic differentiation
PSE	portal–systemic encephalopathy
PSP	progressive supranuclear palsy
pSS	primary Sjögren's syndrome
PTA	phosphotungstic acid
PTAH	phosphotungstic acid haematoxylin
PTBR	peripheral-type benzodiazepinc receptor
PTH	parathyroid hormone
PTL	perinated telencephalic leukoencephalopathy
PVC	polyvinyl chloride
PVL	periventricular leucomalacia
PVR	proliferative vitreoretinopathy
QUIS	quisqualic acid
RA	retinoic acid
RAR	retinoic acid receptor
RBC	red blood cells
RCA–1	ricinus communis agglutinin–1
rCBF	regional cerebral blood flow
REAL	Revised European-American Lymphoma (classification)
REM	rapid eye movement
RER	rough endoplasmic reticulum
RF	radiofrequency
RIA	radioimmunoassay
RNA	ribonucleic acid
RPE	retinal pigment epithelium
RSV	Rous sarcoma virus
RT-PCR	reverse transcription–polymerase chain reaction
PXR	retinoid X receptors
SAADH	syndrome of appropriate antidiuretic hormone secretion
SACE	serum angiotensin converting enzyme
SAF	filamentous animal virus
SAH	subarachnoid haemorrhage
SAM	substrate adhesion molecule
S_aO_2	arterial oxygen saturation
SAP	sphingolipid activator protein
SCA	spinocerebellar ataxia
SCa	slow component a
SCAD	short chain acyl-CoA dehydrogenase deficiency
SCAMP	secretory carrier membrane protein
SCARMD	severe childhood autosomal recessive muscular dystrophy
SCb	slow component b
SCZ	schizophrenia
SDH	subdural haematoma
SER	smooth endoplasmic reticulum
SFEMG	single fibre electromyography

SFP	Sorsby's fundus dystrophy
SGA	small for gestational age
SHH	sonic hedgehog
SIADH	syndrome of inappropriate antidiuretic hormone
s-IBM	sporadic inclusion body myositis
SIDS	sudden infant death syndrome
SIV	simian immunodeficiency virus
SLE	systemic lupus erythematosus
SMA	spinal muscular atrophy
SMN	survival motor neuron
SMON	subacute myelopathy, optic and peripheral neuropathy
SMPN	sensorimotor peripheral neuropathy
SMTM	sulcus medianus telencephali medii
SNAP	soluble NSF attachment protein
SOD	superoxide dismutase
SP	scapuloperoneal
SPARC	secreted protein acidic and rich in cysteine
SPECT	single photon emission computed tomography
SPEO	chronic progressive external ophthalmoplegia
S-PNET	supratentorial primitive neuroepithelial tumours
SSPE	subacute sclerosing panencephalitis
SSV	small synaptic vesicles
SRIF	somatotropin release inhibitory factor
SUPED	sudden unexpected death in epilepsy
SUR	sulforylurea receptor
SVZ	subventricular zone
T_3	triiodothyronine
T_4	tetraiodothyronine
TA	takayasus arthritis
TB	tuberculosis
TBI	traumatic brain injury
TCA	tricarboxylic acid
TEL	triethyl lead
TET	triethyl tin
Tg	transgenic
TGF	transforming growth factor
TGN	trans-Golgi network
TIA	transient ischaemic attack
TIPS	transjugular intrahepatic portal-sytemic shunts
TK	thymidine kinase

TL	tomato lectin
TLD	total length of disease
TLE	temporal lobe epilepsy
TMEV	Theiler's murine encephalomyelitis
TML	trimethyl lead
TMT	trimethyl tin
TNF	tumour necrosis factor
TOCP	triorthocresylphosphate
TPHA	Treponema pallidum haemagglutination assay
TPP	thiamine pyrophosphate
TRH	thyroid releasing hormone
TSC	tuberous sclerosis complex
TSH	thyroid stimulating hormone
TSP	tropical spastic paraparesis
TTP	thrombotic thrombocytopenic purpura
TTR	transthyretin
TUNEL	terminal transferase mediated nick-end labelling
UEA-I	Ulex europaeus I agglutinin
UMN	upper motor neurons
UV	ultraviolet
VA	vertebral artery
VAMP	vesicle associated protein
VAS	vesicle attachment site
VCAM	vascular cell adhesion molecule
VCF	velo–cardial–facial
VEC-DIC	video-enhanced contrast differential interface contrast
VEGF	vascular endothelial growth factor
VEP	visual evoked potentials
VHL	Von Hippel–Lindau (disease)
VIP	vasoactive intestinal peptide
VLCFA	very long chain fatty acids
VLDL	very low density lipoproteins
VLM	visceral larva migrans
VPA	valproic acid
VSCC	voltage-sensitive calcium channels
VWF	von Willebrand factor
VZ	ventricular zone
VZV	varicella-zoster virus
WBC	white blood cell
WHO	World Health Organization
WKS	Wernicke–Kossakoff syndrome
wt	wild type
YAC	yeast artificial chromosome

Volume I

The central neuron

CONSTANTINO SOTELO AND ANTOINE TRILLER

INTRODUCTION

The brain can be considered as an information-processing device at the interface between the body and the exterior world, made up of individual units, the nerve cells or neurons, which are derivatives of the embryonic ectoderm. Based on its origin and its types of morphological connections, the nervous system has been compared to an epithelium, where the cells are packed close together leaving a narrow intervening extracellular space and isolated from the blood vessels by a basal lamina. Neurons, although sharing many features with other cells, are unique, since they have been differentiated for communication: receiving, processing and transmitting information.

LIFE HISTORY OF THE NEURON: THE ORIGIN OF THE NEURON AND ITS MATURATION

Neuronal proliferation and cell migration, together with neuronal differentiation and axonogenesis, are the principal stages which, proceeding with defined kinetics, result in the formation of projection maps and synaptogenesis. The maturation of neuronal connections is attained mainly by activity-dependent mechanisms that involve competition between cells and regressive processes. Some of these processes culminate in developmental (or programmed) cell death.[191,324]

Neuronal proliferation during development

It is generally accepted that the generation of neurons takes place at certain stages of development, and that neuronal proliferative activity is practically lacking in the adult brain.[227] Therefore, neurons belong to the category of static, 'non-renewing' epithelial tissue.[240] The vast majority of neurons arise from the ventricular zone (VZ), formed by a pseudostratified epithelium, surrounding the ventricles. The nuclei of precursor cells undergo interkinetic migration.[358] Deoxyribonucleic acid (DNA) synthesis takes place in the outer part of the VZ, whereas mitosis occurs at its inner surface, generating a to-and-fro movement of the nuclei, which might allow regionally different cytoplasmic factors to enter the nucleus and regulate differential gene activity.[191] External factors (growth factors)[61,348] and intrinsic regulatory mechanisms or genetic factors regulate the cell cycle through their encoded proteins (cyclins, maturation promotion factor, etc.).

The cerebellum offers an optimal material to study cellular and molecular mechanisms regulating neuronal proliferation, because cerebellar granule cells, which are by far the most numerous neuronal population of the entire central nervous system (CNS), arise solely from a precise region of the neural tube and proliferate late during development. The precursors of granule cells first appear in the upper half of the rhombic lip. During the second half of intrauterine development, these precursors follow a tangential migration in the ventrodorsal direction over the surface of the cerebellar plate and, a few days before birth, they cover the entire cerebellar surface (in rats and mice), forming a secondary neuroepithelium, called the external granular layer (EGL). Neuronal precursors in the EGL proliferate extensively during the first weeks of postnatal life to produce the granule cells. That proliferation of granule cell precursors is dependent on Purkinje cells was first noticed more than 20 years ago, with the analysis of cerebellar phenotypes of mice affected by spontaneous mutations. For instance, in the reeler mutant, Purkinje cells do not complete their migration and remain far from the EGL. Under these conditions the number of granule cells generated is extremely reduced.[263] More direct evidence has been obtained with transgenic mice, in which expression of the transgene provoked the early postnatal death of Purkinje cells. In these cases, there was a blockade in cerebellar development, with proliferation arresting in the EGL and production of very few granule cells.[103,385]

The molecular nature of the Purkinje cell factor that acts as a mitogen controlling the proliferation of EGL cells has been identified recently. This factor is Sonic hedgehog (Shh), which is secreted by Purkinje cells, while the proteins involved in the Shh signalling pathway (Patched and Gli) are produced by the granule cell precursors.[75,467] In man, mutations in the patched gene have been implicated in the aetiology of sporadic medulloblastomas. Thus, since Patched (a Shh-binding protein) functions as an antagonist of Shh, the inability to arrest Shh signalling in EGL cells could favour the formation of medulloblastomas.

The number of cells generated from a particular portion of the VZ is very important and depends on three parameters: the size of the precursor pool, the duration of each cell cycle and the number of cell divisions for each progenitor cell. At present it is not known what regulates progenitor number or the number of their cell divisions. The best known parameter is the duration of the cell cycle. The advent of the autoradiographic method with tritiated thymidine[276] and of the immunocytochemical method using 5-bromo-2′-deoxyuridine (BrdU)[297,421] has been instrumental for the precise determination of cell-cycle kinetics. In general, the neuroblastic cell cycle lasts for a period that does not differ much from that of other classes of somatic cells, and changes as development proceeds. In early embryonic life, with rapidly proliferating cells, it is much shorter (8–12 h) than later on in development (25–30 h). The accuracy obtained with the available methods is excellent. For instance, the lengths of the sequential phases of the cell cycle have been determined in the neocortical proliferative zone of the 14-day-old mouse embryo (E14).[385] The G_1-phase, or intermitotic stage, lasts for 9.3 h. Postmitotic neurons are permanently arrested in this phase when they leave the cycle and, consequently, they are diploid cells. The S-phase, corresponding to the period of DNA synthesis, lasts for 15.1 h and the following phase or premitotic gap (G_2-phase) lasts for 3.8 h. Finally, the M-phase, during which cell division occurs, has a relatively short duration of 2 h compared with the duration of the whole cell cycle. Subtle changes in the duration of the cell cycle have major consequences for the final size of many neuronal populations. Thus, in some mutations (e.g. the splotch mutant mouse)[474] or in some experimental conditions, there is a lengthening of the cell cycle with corresponding severe alterations of the maturing brain and abnormally low numbers of neurons.

As development proceeds, the following new proliferative sites are generated by precursor cells that have migrated from specific regions of the VZ:

- The subventricular zone overlying the anterior wall of the lateral ventricle: These precursor cells start to divide locally and, while dividing, migrate into the olfactory bulb.[258]
- The upper half of the rhombic lip in the cerebellar neuroepithelium bordering the IVth ventricle provides the EGL[7] (see above).
- The primitive neuroepithelial cells of the lateral ventricles near the hippocampal formation: these migrate through the fimbria into the hippocampus, where they form the cell mass at the internal border of the dentate gyrus.[8]

All of these extraventricular proliferation sites share several common features. They almost solely generate small interneurons (microneurons of Altman): granule and periglomerular cells of the olfactory bulb, granule cells of the cerebellar cortex, and granule cells of the dentate gyrus. Moreover, they have a late proliferation period, which in the rat starts perinatally, when the ventricular neuroepithelium ceases proliferation, and extends into postnatal life.

Neuronal proliferation in adult nervous system: the neural stem cells

Although it is generally accepted that neuronal proliferation occurs at precise developmental periods, a few exceptions are known: (1) the continuous turnover of sensory neurons in the olfactory mucosa (originating from the olfactory placode;[148] (2) the generation of granule cells in the hippocampal dentate gyrus, which at a very slow pace continuously increases the number of these neurons,[21] even in the human brain;[97] and (3) the forebrain subventricular zone (SVZ: the extraventricular region at the origin of olfactory bulb neurons during ontogeny) of the adult mouse. Through well-designed homochronous and homotopic grafting experiments, in which donor SVZ was taken from adult transgenic mice carrying the neuron-specific enolase/lacZ hybrid gene (all neurons express β-galactosidase activity), and grafted in the SVZ region of adult wild-type recipients, Lois and Alvarez-Buylla[252] showed that lacZ expressing cells were present in the graft site and the ipsilateral olfactory bulb. In the latter region, labelled neurons were identified as granule and periglomerular cells.

NEURONAL STEM CELLS

The occurrence of neurogenesis in the adult brain, although known since the 1960s,[8] has created great expectations in the past few years. Experiments in vitro, initiated by Reynolds and Weiss,[341] have shown that in the forebrain of adult rodents there are cells that, under the stimulation with high concentrations of mitogens [epidermal growth factor (EGF), fibroblast growth factor-2 (FGF-2)], are able to proliferate and expand. Moreover, after withdrawal of the mitogens or the use of molecular strategies to orientate their differentiation, these cells can generate all three major neural cell types of the CNS: neurons, astrocytes and oligodendrocytes. Thus, these blastic cells have the two properties (self-renewal capacity and multipotency) which characterize stem cells.[281] The fast progress made in the field has provided evidence that neural stem cells occur in embryonic and adult CNS, not only in experimental animals but also in the adult human brain.[199] Moreover, neural stem cells have been immortalized by transfecting an oncogene to generate stable clones of cell lines with stem cell properties.[384] Several groups have recently shown that neural stem cells *in vivo*, after experimental transplantation into immature[52] or lesioned adult CNS,[420] can generate mature neurons and glial cells. The transplanted cells showed some degree of integration into the host's neural networks. These results emphasize the great interest of neural stem cell strategy for brain repair. Stem cells appear to migrate to damaged regions of the brain and, through local differentiation cues, to acquire the phenotypes of the missing cells, replacing them in the lesioned areas.

One of the key problems for a more complete understanding of the functional role of quiescent neural stem cells is their identification in the adult CNS. It is well established that stem cells are not broadly dispersed throughout the CNS but confined to a limited number of locations.[124,281] In adult, small laboratory rodents, cells with stem-cell properties after *in vitro* expansion with mitogens, and formation of floating cell aggregates or neurospheres (clonal neural cells in several developmental phases), have been obtained from tissue taken from periventricular regions, particularly around the lateral ventricles, and from the subgranular layer of the hippocampal dentate gyrus. More recently, neural stem cells have been also obtained from tissue taken from the cerebral cortex and spinal cord. The common feature for most of these cells is their location in ventricular and/or periventricular areas, regions which correspond to the remnants of the ventricular and subventricular zones of the developing CNS, where neuronal proliferation occurs.[124]

The lack of reliable markers for neural stem cells (nestin and Notch-1 are the most used ones) has made it difficult to identify these cells in the adult CNS. Studies in the forebrain, particularly in the rostral migratory stream, an expansion of the subventricular zone linking the anterior horn of the lateral ventricle with the olfactory bulb, have revealed the occurrence of neural stem cells within this structure.[86] This and other early investigations suggest that neural stem cells are located in the subventricular zone. However, the fact that the spinal cord, which also provides cells with stem-cell properties, is devoid of subventricular zone, prompted Frisen and his collaborators[199] to search for other sources of neural stem

cells, and they found solid evidence that a subpopulation of ependymal cells (about 5%) from the adult brain and spinal cord are neural stem cells. Ependymal cells *in vitro* are multipotent and have self-renewal capacity. Moreover, they divide *in vivo* to give rise to subventricular zone cells which generate olfactory bulb interneurons. Finally, in response to a spinal cord lesion, they only generate astrocytes that contribute to the formation of the glial scar. Despite these important results, the problem of neural stem-cell identification is not completely solved. The group of Alvarez-Buylla[253] reported that cells in the subventricular zone, labelled with glial fibrillary acidic protein (GFAP, an astrocytic marker), have stem-cell properties and generate olfactory bulb neurons.

Both ependymal cells and apposed astrocytes have, thus, been reported as neural stem cells. Owing to the close anatomical relations of the two cell types, the possibility of some cellular contamination in these experiments remains open. Another possibility is that both cell types are indeed stem cells. In this case, it becomes urgent to determine whether both classes of neural stem cell share some common lineage, or whether there are two independent populations of stem cells in the adult CNS. Nevertheless, knowledge of neural stem cells has not elucidated their role in the adult CNS. Although stem cells do not bring about the spontaneous repair of the brain, they at least participate in the formation of glial scars in the spinal cord.[199] By contrast, neural stem cells, particularly those in the subgranular layer of the hippocampal dentate gyrus, seem to participate in the processes of learning and memory. Increases in the number and complexity of hippocampal connections (neurons are added through the dentate gyrus) could provide the required morphological substratum for learning and memory functions. Thus, neural stem cells might not represent vestiges of evolution as previously suggested but would enable the adult hippocampal circuit to have the plastic capability required for high brain functions.[124] More knowledge is required about neural stem cell identity and markers, and about molecular ways to orientate their phenotypic differentiation,[458] before applying the neuronal stem-cell transplantation strategy as a therapeutic approach to neurodegenerative diseases and/or to CNS lesions.

Neuronal cell migration

Newly generated neurons need to move, sometimes for long distances, along specific pathways to reach their final destination. This movement (neuronal cell migration) is a distinct cellular process, which is essential for the establishment of the normal organization of the central and peripheral nervous systems. Thus, migration starts with a process of 'sorting out' of the young postmitotic neurons from the ventricular neuroepithelium, and proceeds along specific pathways following a precise spatiotemporal order.[173,331,380]

GLIAL-GUIDED NEURONAL MIGRATION

The analysis of the migratory behaviour of cerebellar granule cells by Ramon y Cajal[334] and his student. Terrazas[431] initiated modern thinking on possible mechanisms and pathways involved in neuronal migration. Cerebellar granule cells arise from a secondary neuroepithelium, the external granular layer. This germinative zone is composed of a superficial region where mitosis occurs, and a deeper region containing young postmitotic neurons. These neurons begin to differentiate by extending processes parallel to the long axis of the folia (horizontal polarity). The transition between the latter and a new phase of 'vertical polarity' is marked by the emergence of a new protoplasmic expansion, provided with a growth cone, which descends vertically from the basal pole of the cell body towards the white matter. The nucleus begins to descend within the vertical expansion once it penetrates the nascent molecular layer. Granule cell migration is the result of a double process: the elongation of a descending protoplasmic segment, and the subsequent intracellular displacement or emigration of the nucleus within this vertically orientated segment. The study of the inflections of the axon of the migrating granule cells allowed Terrazas[431] to conclude that the vertically descending expansion of these neurons follows the cleavage planes of lesser resistance, guided by either capillaries or glial cells, or both.

Rakic,[330] in his detailed electron microscopical study of granule cell migration across the molecular layer of the cerebellum of non-human primates, reported that each descending expansion (the leading process) maintains an intimate contact with the vertically orientated Bergmann fibres, their migratory axes. These observations were extended to other migrating neurons, particularly in the developing neocortex (Fig. 1.1a). Rakic's descriptions, indicating the need for specific surface membrane interactions between migrating neurons and radial glial fibres, gave rise to the concept of glial-guided migration.

MOLECULAR MECHANISMS IN GLIAL-GUIDED NEURONAL CELL MIGRATION

Migration in the CNS is a complex process, which implies the mediation of multiple receptor systems for each of the subsequent steps that, starting with a surface recognition phenomenon, and through differential adhesion and transmembrane signalling, will end with cell motility. Rakic et al.[332] presented an extensive overview of the presumptive molecular events taking place along these steps (Fig. 1.1b). These are reviewed below.

Recognition and induction of radial glial scaffold

The affinity of most of the migrating neurons for the surface of radial glial fibres strongly indicates that premigratory neurons must identify specific classes of transiently expressed molecules, displayed at the plasma membrane of the glial axis.

Although the precise nature of these identity molecules remains unknown, the molecular mechanisms involved could provide the young premigratory neurons with a glial specification programme to generate radial glial scaffolds. This phenotypic specification is characterized by the transient expression of markers, including nestin, brain lipid-binding protein (BLBP), the antigens recognized by the monoclonal antibodies (mAbs) RC1 and RC2, and the D4 antisera[390] that unmask the radial glial properties required for supporting neuronal migration. Using co-cultures of premigratory neurons and glial cells, it has been shown that the induction of the radial glial phenotype is mediated by neuronal–glial interactions.[160] In vivo studies, using either cerebellar transplants in adult pcd mutant mice,[398] or grafting neocortical Cajal-Retzius cells into adult wild-type mouse cerebella (Fig. 1.2),[390] have demonstrated that mature astrocytes can be transformed into juvenile radial glia, expressing transiently radial glial markers. Cajal-Retzius cells are the earliest generated cortical neurons and the first to mature. They are pioneer neurons, have a sub-pial location and disappear by apoptosis at postnatal ages. The role of Cajal-Retzius cells in neuronal migration has been emphasized by the molecular cloning of the reeler mutation. This gene, named reelin, encodes for a large extracellular protein, the Reelin, first expressed in the neocortex by Cajal-Retzius cells (Fig. 1.2)[4,78] and secreted in the marginal zone. Since the phenotype of the reeler mouse is characterized by an impaired migration and a failure of the correct layering of the telencephalic and cerebellar cortices, Reelin has been considered to be the essential protein for correct radial glial migration. Thus, Reelin could regulate cell-to-cell interactions critical for cell allocation (it could play the role of a stop signal or an adhesive molecule). It is known that Reelin acts through the conjunction of two membrane receptors of the low-density lipoprotein receptor (LDLR) superfamily: VLDLR and ApoER2.[391,443] Both receptors can bind disabled (mDab1) on their cytoplasmic tails, and mDab1 is known to be a key step for the Reelin signalling pathway. The use of in vitro diffusible test assays (Cajal-Retzius cells separated by a semipermeable membrane from cerebellar slices taken from P5 mice) has shown that the inductive effects of these cells are mediated by diffusible factors (Fig. 1.2). However, Reelin by itself is not able to induce the radial glial phenotype. Thus, it appears that the effect of Reelin is indirect and that other factors are required for the induction of radial glial scaffolds.[391]

The nature of such diffusible signals is beginning to be revealed. Indirect evidence strongly suggests that neuregulin (a member of the epidermal growth factor family) and its membrane receptor erbB4 are involved in the cerebellar induction of the radial glial scaffolds for granule cell migration.[344] Migrating granule cells, as well as their EGL precursors, express neuregulin and Bergmann fibres express erbB4 in the postnatal cerebellum. Moreover, when the glial erbB4 receptors are blocked, granule cells fail to induce the radial glial phenotype, whereas

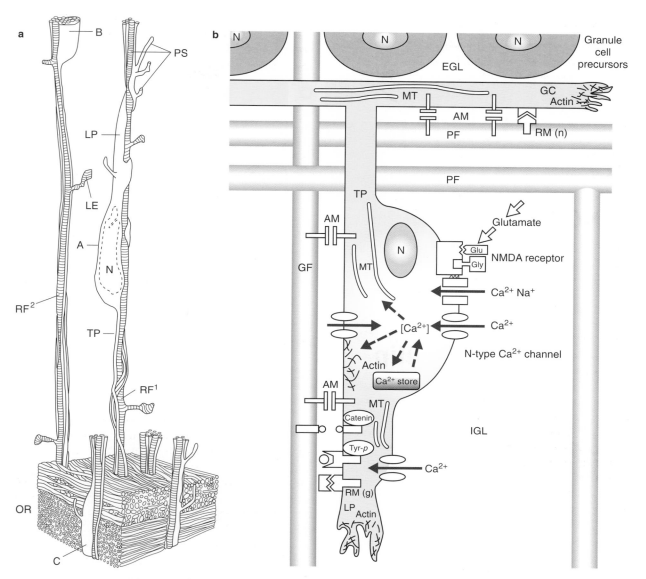

Figure 1.1 *Glial-guided migration. (a) Three-dimensional reconstruction of migrating neurons, obtained from micrographs of semi-serial sections of the occipital lobe. The lower portion of the diagram contains uniform, parallel fibres of the optic radiation (OR) and the remainder is occupied by more irregularly disposed fibre systems; the border between the two systems is easily recognized. Except for the lower portion of the figure, most of these fibres are deleted from the diagram to expose the radial fibres (striped vertical shafts, RF) to the migrating cells A, B and C. The soma of migrating cell A, with its nucleus (N) and voluminous leading process (LP), is situated within the reconstructed space, except for the terminal part of the attenuated trailing process and the tip of the vertical ascending pseudopodium. LE: lamellate expansions; PS: pseudopodia. (b) Model of cascade of molecular events that could take place during the morphogenetic transformation and migration of postmitotic granule cells in the developing cerebellar cortex. After their last mitotic division in the external granular layer (EGL), postmitotic granule cells elaborate two horizontal neurites that grow preferentially along already formed parallel neuronal fibres (PFs). Subsequently, a single descending neurite emanating from the cell soma follows the contours of the Bergmann glial fibre (GF) as it crosses the expanding molecular layer. Eventually, the cell nucleus (N) and the surrounding cytoplasm are translocated within the descending leading process into the internal granular layer (IGL). The developing granule cell provides an opportunity to examine the role of the various molecules that may be engaged in recognition, adhesion, transmembrane signalling and motility underlying directed neuronal migration. AM: homotypic adhesion molecule; GC: growth cone; Glu: glutamate; Gly: glycine; LP: leading process; MT: microtubule; TP: trailing process; RM(g): gliophilic recognition molecule; RM(n): neurophilic recognition molecule; Tyr-P: tyrosine phosphorylation. Reproduced by permission from (a) Brustle et al.[52] and (b) Rakic et al.[332]*

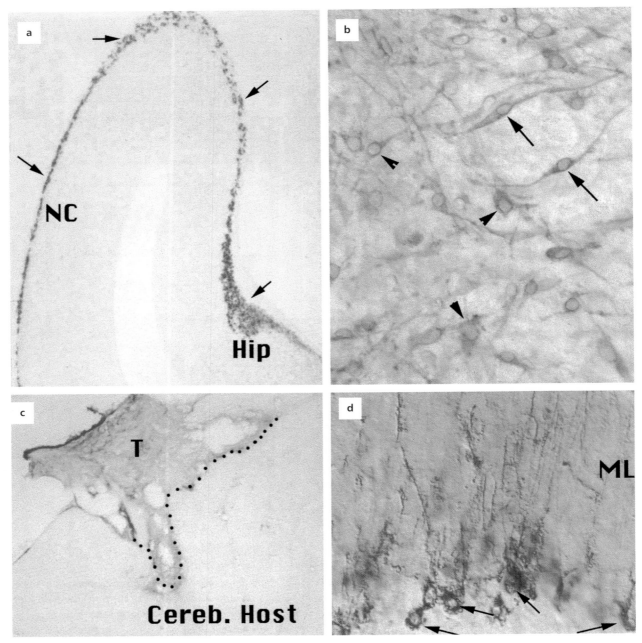

Figure 1.2 *Influence of embryonic Cajal-Retzius cells in the acquisition of the radial glial phenotype. (a) Frontal section of the fore-brain of a 15-day-old mouse embryo (E15), in situ hydridization with a molecular probe to visualize reelin mRNA. The transcripts are expressed in the marginal zone of the neocortex (NC) and hippocampus (Hip), in cells belonging to the Cajal-Retzius transient population of cells (arrows). (b) Induction of radial glial phenotype, revealed with mAb RC2, in an in vitro diffusible test assay. A cerebellar slice, taken from a P5 mouse, was cocultured for 10 days with the marginal zone (Cajal-Retzius cells' enriched material) of an E15 mouse neocortex. Both explants were separated by a semipermeable membrane. In these cerebellar slices, contrary to controls in which none of the cells was RC2 positive, many cells became RC2 positive. Some were monopolar or had short processes (arrowheads), whereas some others were bipolar (arrows) resembling radial glial cells. (c, d) In vivo induction of radial glial phenotype by Cajal-Retzius cells in the adult cerebellum In the control experiment (c), the host cerebellum (Cereb. Host) remained RC2 negative 7 days after transplantation of a graft devoid of Cajal-Retzius cells (the ventricular zone of a E15 cerebral cortex, T), which itself exhibited some RC2 immunoreactivity (T). In contrast, 7 days after the transplantation of the marginal zone (grafts enriched in Cajal-Retzius cells) (d), in the regions of the molecular layer (ML) overlaid by the grafted cells, RC2-immunostained Bergmann fibres (arrows) occurred, as the result of the inductive activity of the Cajal-Retzius cells. Reproduced by permission from (a) Alcantara et al.[4] and (b–d) Soriano et al.[390]*

activation of the receptor with soluble neuregulin mimics the effects of neurono-glial interactions in the induction of radial glial formation.

Adhesion

The gliophilic affinity also indicates that cell–cell adhesion molecules are involved in some of the mechanisms leading to correct neuronal migration. Such molecules must participate in neuronoglial interactions which are adhesive in nature. Most of the molecules belong to one of the following four main families: the cadherin superfamily, the integrin family, the immunoglobulin superfamily and the components of the extracellular matrix. The involvement of cell adhesion and extracellular matrix molecules in neural migration has been investigated in an *in vitro* model of isolated cerebellar folia. Blocking antibodies have been tested on granule cell migration for various adhesion molecules, neuron-glia cell adhesion molecule (L1/Ng-CAM), neural cell adhesion molecule (NCAM)[65,245] or for extracellular matrix molecules,[65] and all of them provoked a partial suppression of granule cell migration.

Molecular biology provides a way to prevent the expression of adhesion molecules, and to analyse further their function. For instance, knockout experiments by homologous recombination have been produced for the genes coding for NCAM[72] and tenascin.[354] Homozygous null mutant mice, although showing a complete loss of NCAM or tenascin immunoreactivity, did not exhibit qualitative alterations in neuron position. The failure to obtain abnormal migratory phenotypes in these mutants does not mean that NCAM and/or tenascin are not involved in the molecular mechanisms leading to neuronal cell migration.

A different approach was used by Galileo *et al.*[127] who, with recombinant retroviral vectors, delivered the antisense sequence for the β_1 integrin messenger ribonucleic acid (mRNA) and the *Escherichia coli lacZ* gene to small groups of clonally related neurons of the chick optic tectum. These vectors were injected into the alar mesencephalic plate of 3-day-old embryos (the primordium of the optic tectum, at the beginning of neurogenesis). The analysis of clones of lacZ-positive cells, migrating along radial glial fibres 3–9 days later, showed that the β_1 integrin sequences in the antisense orientation did not alter neuronal proliferation but blocked the migration of postmitotic neurons, which remained accumulated in the ventricular zone. Galileo *et al.*[127] concluded that the defect affects the migrating cells rather than the antisense-bearing radial glial cells and, therefore, that β_1 integrins are needed by tectal cells for their radial migration.

Transmembrane signalling

Adhesion receptors are also involved in transmembrane signalling, since they are able to provoke a diverse number of intracellular events involving second messengers, G-proteins and calcium.[332] Calcium is a universal candidate for transmembrane signalling, and variations in intracellular Ca^{2+} concentration have multiple roles, including the assembly and activation of cytoskeletal proteins needed for cell mobility. Recent studies by Rakic *et al.*[332] have addressed the questions of which Ca^{2+} channels regulate the levels of intracellular Ca^{2+} in migrating neurons, and how these channels are modulated. These studies used cerebellar slices, obtained from 10-day-old mice and maintained *in vitro*. In these slices, the movement of migrating granule cells was followed with laser scanning confocal microscopy, after application of the carbocyanine fluorescent dye DiI. The blockade of N-type Ca^{2+} channels by ω-conotoxin slows down the rate of granule cell migration, whereas the blockade of L- and T-Ca^{2+} channels is ineffective (Fig. 1.1b). More importantly, in order to assess the regulatory mechanisms underlying this Ca^{2+}-dependent process, these investigators examined the role of ionotropic receptors in granule cell migration. The blockade of non-*N*-methyl-D-asparate (NMDA) glutamate receptors and γ-aminobutyric acid-A (GABA$_A$) and GABA$_B$ receptors with specific antagonists has no effect on the distance covered by migrating granule cells. In contrast, the blockade of NMDA receptors with 2D(−)-2-amino-5-phosphovaleric acid (*D-AP*5) or dizo-cilpine maleate (MK-801) significantly reduces the mean distance of granule cell displacement, curtailing their migration. These results strongly suggest that NMDA receptors may play an early role in the regulation of Ca^{2+}-dependent granule cell migration. These results are represented schematically in Fig. 1.1b.

OTHER TYPES OF NEURONAL MIGRATION: TANGENTIAL MIGRATION

Morphological studies on migratory pathways of some non-cortical, neuronal populations have provided evidence that glial-guided migration is not the only way for neurons to reach their adult position. In some cases, the migration follows not a radial axis to the proliferative zone, as in glial-guided migration, but a tangential direction.

Circumferential migration

This is the case, for instance, for neurons of the brainstem precerebellar nuclei: the inferior olivary nucleus,[45] the lateral reticular nucleus[44] and the basal pontine nuclei.[328] In these structures, neurons originate in the caudal half of the rhombic lip, located dorsally at the lateral edge of the rhombencephalon, and migrate ventrally, away from their cerebellar target, by circumnavigating the ventrolateral aspect of the medulla oblongata and the pons, to settle in ventral positions (Fig. 1.3). These long migratory pathways, at the surface of the brainstem, are orientated almost perpendicular to the radial glial axes, preventing them from being involved in a guidance process. During their migration, neurons form compact rows of cells and move

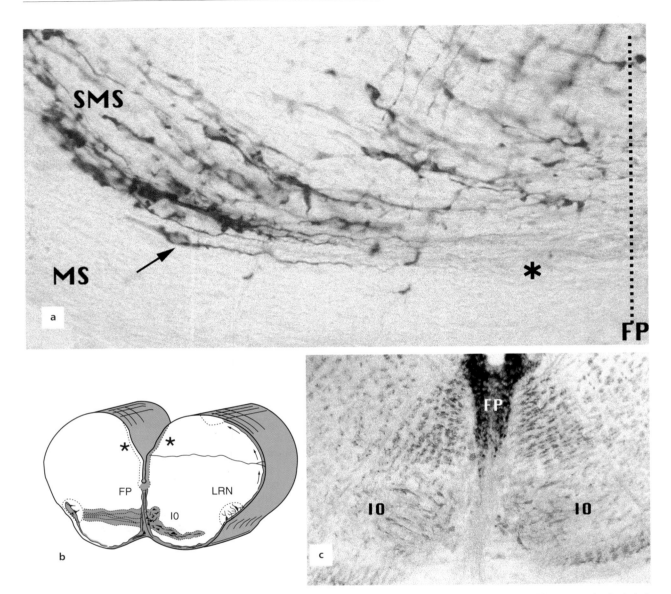

Figure 1.3 *Circumferential neurophilic migration of precerebellar neurons in the brainstem, frontal views. (a) Neurons in the inferior olivary nucleus, retrogradely filled after in vitro HRP injection in an E15 rat embryo. At this stage, migrating neurons have still not reached the final olivary domain (asterisk) and are migrating along the submarginal migratory stream (SMS), whereas the marginal stream (MS), under the pial surface, is free of migrating inferior olivary neurons. The migrating neurons are bipolar (arrow), with the leading processes (to the right) which give origin to the axons, crossing the midline through the floor plate (FP). (b) Schematic representation of the neurophilic migration of precerebellar neurons of the brainstem. Neurons originate in the lower rhombic lips (asterisks), and along either the marginal (red) or submarginal (green) migratory streams, reaching their contralateral (the lateral reticular nucleus, LRN) or ipsilateral (inferior olive, IO, locations, respectively). At the central midline, the floor plate (FP), stops the migrating IO neurons but allows the passage of LRN neurons. (c) Frontal section of an E13 mouse embryo, illustrating the ventral aspect of the caudal brainstem, double labelled with anti-calbindin antibodies and in situ hybridization with a molecular probe to visualize netrin1 mRNA. At this age, calbindin-positive cells have finished their circumferential migration and have reached the IO domain, remaining at both sides of the FP. The netrin1 transcripts (blue) are expressed at high levels by the perikarya of the floor plate cells, whereas their fibrous processes are free of transcripts. Reproduced by permission from (a, b) Bourrat and Sotelo[45] and Bloch-Gallego et al.[38]*

within their leading processes, their future axons. The leading processes of the migrating neurons cross the ventral midline through the floor plate. The behaviour of the cell bodies, following their nuclear translocation, varies according to the neuronal population: they stop without crossing the floor plate if they belong to inferior olivary (Fig. 1.3) and pontine nuclei, whereas they cross the floor plate if they belong to lateral reticular and external cuneate nuclei. This type of tangential migration has been named neurophilic, to differentiate it from gliophilic or glial-guided migration.[328] These names recognize the affinities of the growth cones of the leading processes for axonal or radial glial membranes, substrates along which they respectively move.

Tangential migration in the cerebral cortex

The hypothesis that neuronal migration and layer allocation in the neocortex is solely the result of glial-guided migration (radial unit hypothesis of Rakic) has been challenged by several investigators working on cell lineage analysis, who found dispersion of neuronal clones across the cerebral cortex.[460] Examination of clonal allocation in chimeric mice[427] and Lac Z expression in a transgenic mouse line[391] has provided evidence that not all but the majority of the neuronal clones remain restricted within radial columns in the neocortex and allocortex. Thus, the predominant mode of cell distribution in the cerebral cortex is both radial and clonally related. Nevertheless, some cortical neurons (less than 20%) do not follow a glial-guided migration. Using tracing experiments, marking cells with carbocyanines, it has been shown that cells in the embryonic lateral ganglionic eminence are able to cross the corticostriatal boundary to migrate tangentially into the developing neocortex,[81] and that such cells belong to a subpopulation of GABAergic cortical interneurons.[10] The expression of the transcription factors *Dlx-1* and *Dlx-2* (homeobox containing genes) is initially confined to the proliferative zone of the basal ganglia primordia (ganglionic eminence) and later in development it appears in tangentially migrating GABAergic interneurons of the cerebral cortex, suggesting that these transcription factors are required for their migration. The study of the phenotype of mice with a mutation in both *Dlx-1* and *Dlx-2* genes has not shown detectable cell migration from the basal ganglia primordia to the neocortex, which also has far fewer GABAergic interneurons.[10] Recent experimental findings, using carbocyanine cell tracing, have located the origin of these tangentially migrating cortical neurons to the medial ganglionic eminence. The migrating young neurons cross the lateral ganglionic eminence, reach the pial surface and, underneath, move tangentially towards the most dorsal regions of the developing neocortex.[239] Many of these neurons appear to differentiate into preplate neurons (Cajal-Retzius and subplaque neurons). The substrates used for migration have not been elucidated. Initially, they may use glial fibres,[81] followed by moving along plexuses of tangentially arranged axons, which are already present in the preplate.[452] Thus, this type of neuronal migration can be considered as a subclass of neurophilic migration.

Chain migration: the rostral migratory stream

Neuronal precursors giving rise to olfactory bulb interneurons are generated in the subventricular zone around the walls of the lateral ventricles. These cells, as demonstrated with transplantation experiments (Fig. 1.4),

reach the olfactory bulb along a tangentially orientated migratory pathway. This type of migration is characterized by specific features that give it its uniqueness: (1) the migrating cells are not young postmitotic neurons but blastic cells; (2) the generation and migration of these cells are not confined to the developmental period but lasts for almost the entire life of the animals; (3) during their tangential migration the cells do not follow radial glial axes; and (4) they migrate along a restricted region of the forebrain, named the rostral migratory stream, which corresponds to the subependymal zone spanning the wall of the anterior horn of the lateral ventricle and the virtual olfactory ventricle. The analysis of the cellular and molecular composition of the rostral migratory stream has disclosed that it is essentially composed of cells with neuronal and astrocytic phenotypes (Fig. 1.5). Neuronal cell precursors (the most numerous ones) migrate together, forming continuous cellular strands of migratory cells (chain migration). These chains of dividing cells move inside channels or tunnels formed by processes of a special subpopulation of astrocytes (Fig. 1.5).[195,254] The neuronal cells express the embryonic form of polysialic neural cell adhesion molecule (PSA-NCAM) (Fig. 1.4), and the astrocytes are tenascin-C positive.[195] Genetic deletion of the NCAM or neuramidase removal of PSA disrupts the configuration of the rostral migratory stream, reducing the number and speed of the migrating cells, without arresting entirely their migration.[64,184,307]

With *in vitro* explants of the subventricular zone, mixed with Matrigel and treated with mAb.7B11 (which recognizes a cell-surface antigen expressed by astrocytes) followed by complement-mediated lysis,[472] it was possible to study the chain migration of subventricular cells in the absence of their astrocytic channels. The results show that individual neuronal precursors migrate along the chains following a saltatory type of moving behaviour. Chain migration has, therefore, been considered as a unique type of migration, since the neural precursors can migrate along each other in the absence of other cell types.[472]

Using a different *in vitro* approach, neurosphere cell culture originating from neural stem cells occurring in the subventricular zone, it has been shown that the homotypic migration of the chain migration can be inhibited by blocking the $\alpha_6\beta_1$ integrin.[192] Despite the peculiarities of the three types of neuronal tangential migration, it is possible that migrating cells in all three types use the surface of other neuronal cells as substrate for migration. In this instance, all tangential migrations would belong to the generic class of neurophilic migration.

THE CONCEPT OF 'PASSIVE GENERIC GUIDANCE' IN NEURONAL MIGRATION

In vitro studies have revealed most of our present knowledge on mechanisms implied in gliophilic neuronal migration. The dynamics of granule cell motion along Bergmann fibres was analysed by Hatten *et al.*[162] in a

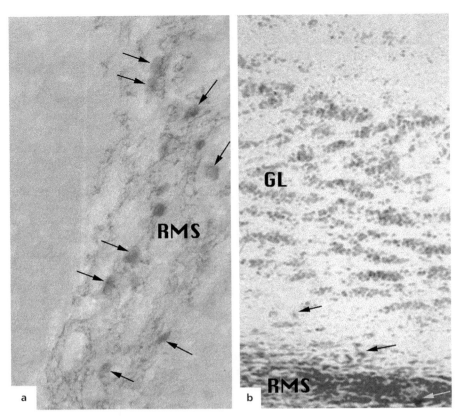

Figure 1.4 *Neurophilic migration in the rostral migratory stream (RMS) of the adult mouse, 7 days after homochronic and homo-topic transplantation. Wild-type mice were grafted, in the anterior horn of the lateral ventricle, with subventricular cells taken from a transgenic mouse line expressing lacZ in many neuronal cell lines, particularly in those migrating along the RMS and providing interneurons to the olfactory bulb. Frontal sections were treated with the Xgal technique to visualize β-galactosidase activity (blue cells), and immunostained with either (a) an anti-polysialic acid antibody labelling PSA-NCAM or (b) neutral red. Grafted neurons (arrows) are exclusively present along the RMS, at places containing the intrinsic neuronal cells composing the PSA-NCAM-positive migrating cellular chains (a). Seven days after grafting, the cells have reached the olfactory bulb (arrows in b), where they have left the RMS, to migrate radially towards the peripheral layers of the olfactory bulb through the internal granular layer (GL). (a) Reproduced by permission from Jankovski and Sotelo.[195]*

microculture system, using video-enhanced contrast dif-ferential interface contrast microscopy (VEC-DIC). The motion of the granule cell body along its glial guide is saltatory, with an average speed of 20–60 μm/h, and asyn-chronous with that of the continuous movement at the growing tip of the leading processes.

The *in vitro* approach has generated the important con-cept of 'passive generic guidance', proposed by Hatten[161] to explain her results on migration of hippocampal or cerebellar neurons along glial axes from the heterotopic region. In these experiments, hippocampal cells follow the normal stereotyped neuron–glia relationship when they move along cerebellar glia, and the same also applies to cerebellar cells on hippocampal glial axes. This 'passive generic' way of guidance has been recently corroborated in an experimental *in vivo* model: embryonic Purkinje cells, which do not use Bergmann fibres for their migra-tion (these fibres appear too late in fetal development), but use other radial glial cells, are capable of radial migra-tion along host Bergmann fibres, when transplanted into

the cerebellum of adult *pcd* mutant mice (devoid of Purk-inje cells).[398] This abnormal migration strongly suggests that a common mechanism must exist in the cerebellum for guiding neurons to their appropriate position.

However, although the mechanisms implied in neuro-nal migration are not fully understood, the occurrence of restricted migratory pathways suggests that migration is under the control of specific cues. In addition, the hetero-geneity of migratory pathways and substrates followed by migrating neurons, some of them sharing their origin in the same germinal matrix, indicates that distinct classes of migrating neurons respond differently to nearby cues. Thus, the concept of passive generic guidance requires important limitations. The most obvious one is that neu-rons normally following a glial-guided migration would be unable to migrate along a neurophilic pathway. To this aim, Jankovski and Sotelo[195] have carried out heterochronic and heterotopic transplantations (postnatal cerebellar pre-cursor cells into the adult rostral migratory stream) and have shown that young neurons that normally migrate

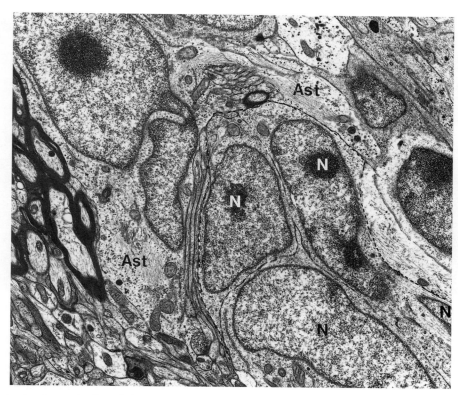

Figure 1.5 *Ultrastructural organization of the rostral migratory stream in the adult mouse forebrain. Parasagittal section illustrating one neuronal migratory chain, consisting of four, immature, densely packed cells of neuronal lineage (N), surrounded (dotted lines) by a large astrocyte (Ast) and numerous astrocytic processes. The astrocytes form relatively large tunnels, through which the neuronal elements of the RMS migrate from the subventricular zone to the olfactory bulb.*

along glial axes (cerebellar granule cells) are not able to migrate along the rostral migratory stream, and die at the transplantation sites. In contrast, precursors of cerebellar molecular layer interneurons (stellate and basket cells) which, like the subventricular cells, are able to migrate when proliferating and do not use glial axes, do migrate along the rostral migratory stream. Thus, neuronal migration is under the control of specific guiding cues.

CHEMOTACTIC CUES AND NEURONAL MIGRATION

One constant feature of neuronal migration is its unidirectional nature. In both glial-guided and tangential migrations, migrating neurons move only in one direction, although in transplantation experiments migration can occur in both directions.[195,398] Moreover, *in vitro* experiments with cocultures of postnatal cerebellar explants and embryonic Cajal-Retzius cells[390] showed that the Cajal-Retzius cells adjacent to the surface of cerebellar slices reverse the direction of migration, as if these pioneer neurons exert an attractive influence on migrating granule cells. A repulsive factor derived from the septum has been proven to participate in the migration of neuronal precursors along the rostral migratory stream.[183] Taken together, these data suggest that migrating neurons can move in both directions but that the potential for bidirectional migration is large-

ly restricted by tissue-dependent cues, which could act at a distance. Thus, it seems that chemotactic molecules of both chemoattractive and chemorepellant actions regulate the direction of the migrating neurons.

The chemical nature of the chemotactic molecules governing the directionality of migrating neurons has been revealed recently, particularly in tangentially migrating neurons. Thus, precerebellar neurons generated in the rhombic lip are influenced in their circumferential migration by netrin-1. Indeed, the analysis of these neurons in mice deficient in expression of netrin-1 has shown that basilar pontine neurons are missing,[370] and only less than 15% of inferior olivary neurons reach their ventromedial position.[38] Moreover, the spatiotemporal patterns of expression of netrin-1 (produced by the floor plate) (Fig. 1.3c) and its receptors [deleted in colorectal cancer (DCC) unc5H2, unc5H3 and neogenin] is consistent with a putative role of this diffusible molecule in attracting migrating precerebellar neurons in the developing embryos.[5,38] The full demonstration of the role of netrin-1 in tangential migration was obtained by coculturing, in collagen gel, rhombic lip explants of different embryonic ages with EBNA cells transfected with the netrin-1 gene. Under these conditions, both the leading processes of the migrating neurons and their translocating nuclei are attracted by the secreted netrin-1 molecules (Fig. 1.6).[5,481]

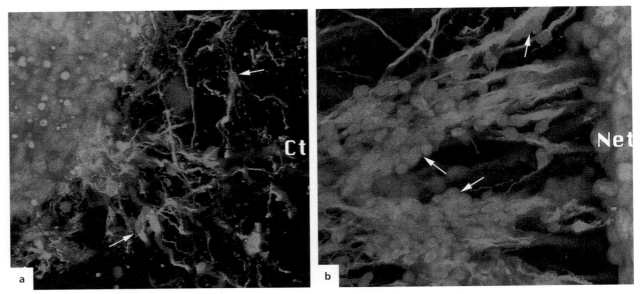

Figure 1.6 *Chemotropic influences on neurophilic migration: chemoattraction of precerebellar neurons towards netrin1-producing cells. These two micrographs illustrate an in vitro experiment in which small explants taken from the lower rhombic lip of an E14 mouse embryo have been cocultured at a distance with aggregates of EBNA-293 control (Ct in a) or stably transfected cells with a netrin1-c-myc expression vector (Net in b), and maintained in vitro for 48 h. Confocal images of the neuronal processes immunostained with anti-β-tubulin III antibodies (green) and the cell nuclei stained with ethidium bromide (red). Note that in the absence of netrin1 (a) few cells leave the explant. These cells (arrows) exhibit random orientations and have only moved as single cells for short distances. Conversely, in the presence of netrin1 (b), many cells leave the explant and form long chains of migrating cells (arrows) orientated to the source of netrin1. Reproduced by permission from Alcantara et al.*[5]

Similar types of *in vitro* study have provided direct evidence that neuronal precursors moving along the rostral migratory stream, and related young interneurons in their way from the medial ganglionic eminence to the cerebral cortex, are repelled by Slit-2 protein.[182,476,486] Since, in early embryonic life (E12 in the mouse) Slit-2 is expressed in the septal area,[291] this protein may be the repellant factor derived from the septum and implicated in guiding neuronal precursors during their migration to the olfactory bulb. These studies have revealed that netrin-1 and Slit-2, two secreted proteins known by their key role in axon guidance,[50] are also involved in guiding neuronal migration. Thus, it can be concluded that common molecular mechanisms are controlling guidance and directing neuronal cell migration.

Neuronal cell migration and neuropathology

The knowledge acquired during recent years about the cellular and molecular mechanisms subserving proper migration of neurons is of paramount importance in neuropathology. Alterations in neuronal cell migration participate in well-known cortical malformations such as lissencephaly and polymicrogyria. Discrete morphological alterations of acquired dysplasias are made more evident with modern, non-invasive imaging techniques. These more subtle anatomical defects, some of which are associated with mental retardation[329] and oth-

ers with epilepsy,[142] also result from small changes in neuronal position. Neurological diseases can also be extremely useful to basic neuroscience by offering optimal material for further studies of molecular mechanisms of cell migration. For example, in Kallmann's syndrome, a combination of hypogonadotropic hypogonadism with anosmia, the migration of luteinizing hormone-releasing hormone (LHRH) cells and the production of neuroepithelial olfactory cells are altered, which is manifested by the absence of olfactory nerves and the prevention of the entry of LHRH cells into the brain. A candidate gene, *KAL*, for X-linked Kallmann's syndrome has been cloned.[241] The gene encodes for a 680 amino acid protein, with a peptide signal but lacking a membrane anchoring domain. The interest in this protein is the presence of a conserved motif, shared by some proteins of the extracellular matrix (fibronectin) and by many cell adhesion molecules, which is compatible with a role for the KAL protein in the process of neuronal cell migration.

In glial-guided and neurophilic migration, the nucleus and surrounding soma of the migrating neurons move within the leading process, which has the properties of a growing neurite. This nuclear displacement or nucleokinesis appears to rely on microtubule-related transport. The identification of the human gene *LIS1* that, when mutated, is responsible for the Miller–Dieker syndrome and isolated lissencephaly sequence, has shed light on part of the molecular mechanisms implied in nucleokinesis.

LIS1 encodes the β-subunits of platelet-activating factor acetylhydrolase Ib (PAF-AHIB).[255,461] *LIS1* gene seems to control microtubule dynamics by reducing microtubule catastrophe events.[356] *LIS1* is highly conserved through phylogenesis, and is the homologue of the *NUDF* gene in *Aspergillus nidulans*. NUDS protein, required for nuclear migration in this filamentous fungus, is involved in a dynein-mediated process.[283] Thus, it has been proposed that such a dynein-mediated process is required for the nuclear translocation within the leading process in neuronal migration.[282] This point is important because the main difference between guided axonal growth and neuronal migration is that the translocation of the nucleus within the growing process occurs only in neuronal migration.

DEVELOPMENTAL OR PROGRAMMED NEURONAL CELL DEATH

Developmental or programmed neuronal cell death will be reviewed in Chapters 3 and 7 of this Volume.

THE NEURON AS A POLARIZED CELL

Despite the variability in shapes and sizes of neurons, three basic neuronal compartments can be easily recognized in most nerve cells: the dendrites, the soma and the axon with its terminal ramification. As postulated by the law of dynamic polarization,[374] these structurally different compartments fulfil specific functions, subserving the key role of neurons in transmitting information.

Soma, dendrite and axon: the three neuronal compartments

The soma or cell body is formed by the nucleus and its surrounding cytoplasm. It is the genetic and metabolic centre of the neuron. Its shape varies from ovoid to multipolar and in higher vertebrates its size ranges from less than 10 μm to about 40 μm. The soma issues two types of neurites, most often several dendrites and one axon.

The dendrites are elongations of the soma, and the primary or stem dendrites give rise to numerous branches that form the dendritic field, a tree-like structure covering a three-dimensional space (Fig. 1.7). Its membrane, together with that of the soma, is specialized in receiving inputs from other neuronal cells. The organization of the dendritic ramification, well seen with the Golgi method, can be extremely variable. It is one of the major features used to classify and identify neurons. A simple classification is based on the number of stem dendrites (monopolar to multipolar), and examples of neuronal types are illustrated in Fig. 1.7.

A single axon originates at a particular region of the soma or of a primary dendrite named the axon hillock (Fig. 1.7). It is prolonged by a thin portion of the axon, known as the initial segment, which enlarges to become the axon *per se*. Its size is variable and ranges from 0.1 to 20 μm in diameter, and from less than 10 μm to 1 m or more in length. The action potential is generated at the level of the initial segment and propagated along the axon. The conduction velocity depends on the diameter of the axon and upon the extent of myelination. Distally, the axon divides into a terminal ramification which ends in swellings, the presynaptic terminals, which subserve the transmission of synaptic information (see, for instance, the Purkinje cell in Fig. 1.7d).

THE NEURONAL CELL BODY

The cell body contains a large nucleus surrounded by the cytoplasm, which contains many organelles (Fig. 1.8a). The most important task of the soma is the maintenance of the neuron, its membranous composition and structural organization. All of the organelles described below serve the same function as those present in any other eukaryotic cells.[315]

Nucleus

In general, nerve cells have a large central nucleus which in small neurons, such as the granule cells of the cerebellum, can occupy most of the volume of the cell body, with only a small rim of surrounding cytoplasm. With light microscopy the appearance of the nucleus in a large neuron is generally clear, while in smaller neurons, it is often speckled with dots, being identical to that seen in other small cells such as the lymphocyte. It can be spherical, ellipsoid or polyhedric with rounded edges or deep foldings (Fig. 1.8a). In the large neurons of the Deiters' nucleus, they are generally spherical, while in other portions of the lateral vestibular nucleus, they may have an irregular shape with deep indentations. The ultrastructure of the nucleus and its limiting membrane is not different from that of other eukaryotic cells,[315] except for two features which appear characteristic of some neuronal nuclei: Barr corpuscles and nuclear inclusions.

Barr corpuscle or sex chromatin

The single and large nucleolus, which characterizes the neuronal nucleus, is generally free of any surrounding heterochromatin. In the female of most mammalian species, including man, Feulgen staining reveals a compact mass of chromatin, about 1 μm in diameter, apparently associated with the nucleolus and closely apposed to the inner face of the nuclear membrane.[18] This sexual dimorphism has been explained by considering that the Barr corpuscle (the compact mass of perinucleolar chromatin) is one of the two X chromosomes.

Nuclear inclusions

Nuclear inclusions are of varying frequency, depending on the neuronal cell type and the species. Two types of

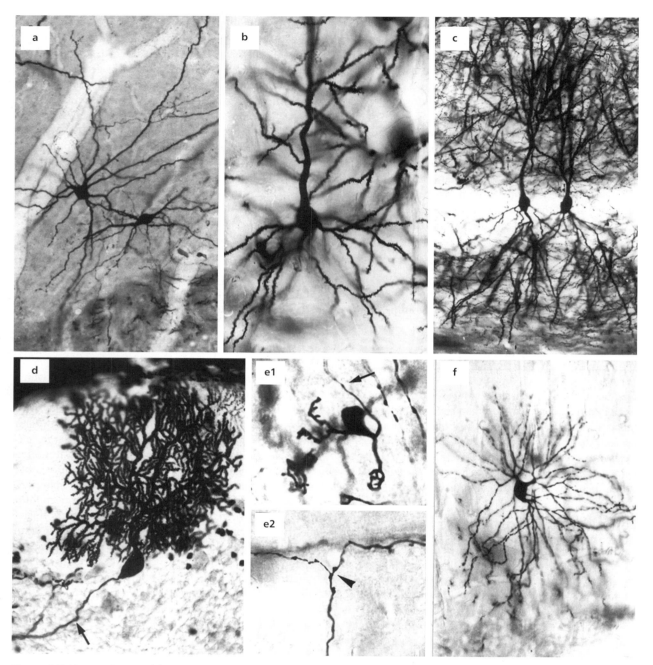

Figure 1.7 *Neuronal types. (a) Motor neuron in ventral horn of the spinal cord. (b) Pyramidal cell in layer V of the neocortex. (c) Pyramidal cell in the hippocampal CA1 region. (d) Cerebellar Purkinje cell and its axons (arrow). (e) Granular cell in the cerebellum. (e1) Soma and dendritic digits; the axon (arrow) emerges from a dendrite. (e2) The ascending axon divides (arrowhead) in the molecular layer and forms a parallel fibre. (f) Stellate cell from the molecular layer of the cerebellum. (a,b,c,e,f) Golgi impregnation; (d) extracellular injection of HRP. Invaginations of the nucleus are filled with a basophilic substance resembling that of a Nissl body. These indentations can be so deep as to assume the appearance of intranuclear inclusions.*

inclusion have been characterized with electron microscopy: rods and sheaths of filaments. There is usually a single rod per nucleus and they are formed of bundles of filaments, each of which is of approximately 7 nm in width. They are enriched in proteins, contain only a few lipids and are devoid of DNA and RNA.[209] The other type of inclusion is sheaths of filaments, each of which is about

7 nm wide, formed by two parallel arrays which have a combed aspect (Fig. 1.8e). The thickness of each array ranges from 40 to 180 nm, and the angle between the axis of the filaments varies from 40 to 80 nm, resulting in a paracrystalline structure. Nuclear inclusions seem to be age dependent,[106] and although their number can increase in certain conditions, they do not signify abnormality.

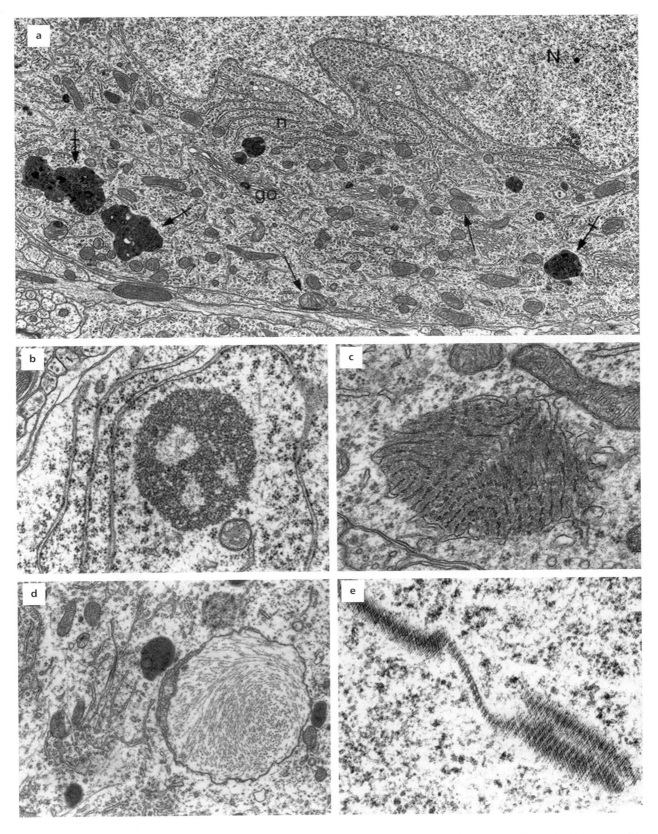

Figure 1.8 *Neuronal organelles and inclusions.* (**a**) *Electron micrograph of a rat Purkinje cell soma; note the indented nucleus (N), the Nissl body (n), Golgi complexes (go), mitochondria (arrows) and lipofuscin granules (crossed arrows).* (**b**) *Nucleosome in a neuron of area postrema.* (**c**) *Laminated inclusion body in a neuron of the medial cerebellar nucleus.* (**d**) *Neurofibrillary body in a neuron of the lateral vestibular nucleus.* (**e**) *Paracrystalline nuclear inclusion in the lateral vestibular nucleus.*

Nissl bodies

In material stained with basic dyes such as toluidine blue, cresyl violet or methyl blue, the Nissl bodies appear as highly basophilic, discontinuous, rhomboidal structures of various sizes. There is no specific relationship between the size of the neuron and that of the Nissl bodies, and in large neurons Nissl bodies are small and scattered in the cytoplasm.[403] Nissl bodies can be also present in large dendrites, but are absent from the somatic region giving rise to the axon hillock.

Nissl bodies are composed of granular or rough endoplasmic reticulum displaying a particular organization (Fig. 1.8a).[315] In motor neurons, for example, the Nissl body is formed by parallel arrays of the rough reticulum, with a space of 0.2–0.5 μm between each cistern. The external faces of the cisterns are covered with ribosomes, and between them free ribosomes or ribosomes forming rosettes are also present (Fig. 1.8a). Their shapes are highly subject to both post-mortem and fixation conditions.

Smooth or agranular reticulum

The cisterns comprising the agranular reticulum are in continuity with those of the rough reticulum, and are defined by the absence of associated ribosomes. In most neurons, the agranular reticulum constitutes the majority of the reticulum, and consists of tubular and cisternal structures with complex branching patterns. Frequently, the agranular reticulum extends beneath the plasma membrane, thus forming the hypolemmal cistern, a specific feature of Purkinje cells.[202] The smooth reticulum is found in the soma and in the dendrite, but unlike the rough endoplasmic reticulum (RER), it is also present in the axon.

Golgi apparatus

This organelle, found in all cell types,[94] is composed of five to seven parallel cisterns separated by a few micrometres and by a complex arrangement of smooth and coated vesicles (Fig. 1.8a). At their ends the cisterns are dilated and vesicles bud from them. In contrast to the reticulum, there is no direct connection between the Golgi cisterns. In general, the Golgi apparatus is curved, the convex and concave sides being the external and internal Golgi, respectively. They are usually multiple and scattered within neurons to form the Golgi complex, which lies roughly half way between the nucleus and the plasma membrane. The Golgi complex is heterogeneous and its chemical composition varies from the external to the internal side. As a consequence, the cisterns have different cytochemical properties depending on their localization and reflecting their function, with a *cis*-Golgi (osmiophilic) and a *trans*-Golgi (osmiophobic) compartment. Coated and smooth vesicles between the cisterns ensure the transport from one stack to another. The Golgi apparatus, facilitating the post-translational modifications of proteins, is a dynamic organelle.[315]

Mitochondria

Most cell functions depend on energy provided by mitochondria. These are membrane-bound, sausage-shaped organelles. In transverse section (Fig. 1.8a), they are about 0.1–0.2 μm wide and 0.5–1 μm long, but can reach 20 μm or more. In some instances, branched mitochondria can be observed. Mitochondria are present in all of the neuronal compartments, soma, dendrites and axons, and the most elongated ones are often found in the neurites. As in other cells, microcinematography has shown that they are constantly moving within the neuron.

Multivesicular bodies, lysosomes and lipofuscin granules

The multivesicular bodies, initially described in neurons by Palay and Palade,[308] are membrane-bound spherical structures which contain a variable number of spherical or ellipsoidal vesicles, embedded in a matrix of varying electron density. They can be found in any neuronal compartment, but most often in the dendrites or close to the Golgi apparatus. Early experiments with cationic ferritin or horseradish peroxidase (HRP)[116] have shown that these organelles are associated with the endocytotic pathway. In the retina, the multivesicular bodies were shown to be involved directly in the degradation of synaptic vesicles by the demonstration of synaptic vesicle antigen within them.[365]

The lysosomes, first identified by De Duve[83] are in dynamic relationship with the Golgi apparatus and the plasma membrane. These 0.3–0.5 nm vesicles are spherical or ovoid, membrane bound, and filled with a thin, granular, electron-dense material. Their size and shape are variable, and lysosomes of 1–2 μm are often encountered. The largest can be elongated, resembling mitochondria. During ageing and in some pathological conditions, the number of lysosomes can increase, and they can become more heterogeneous in shape. Both the multivesicular bodies and the lysosomes are directly involved in membrane trafficking and recycling.

The lipofuscin granules are also membrane bound (Fig. 1.8a), with a diameter between 1 and 2.5 μm. They are extremely electron dense with one or two clear vacuoles at the periphery. They are easy to visualize with a Sudan black B stain or a periodic acid–Schiff reaction, and by fluorescence microscopy, and they have a characteristic green–yellow autofluorescence. Their number increases with ageing, and they are then better stained by the Nile blue or the ferric-ferrocyanide method.

Cilia, centrioles and cytoplasmic inclusions

In neurons, the cilia have a 9 + 0 (peripheral and central doublets) microtubular arrangement, with a 8 + 1 towards the end of the cilia. In other cell types the tubular arrangement is 9 + 1.[102] It must be stressed here that the 9 + 1 and the 9 + 0 structure correspond to motile and non-motile cilia, respectively. The basal body at the origin of the cilia has a 9 + 0 triplet structure and, perpendicular to it, there is an associated centriole which also has a 9 + 0 arrangement. Other centrioles can occasionally be detected in the cytoplasm.

Many forms of inclusion have been described in the cytoplasm of apparently normal neurons.[168] The laminated body is irregular in shape, and appears as alternating dark and light zones arranged like a fingerprint (Fig. 1.8c). The dark zones are formed by a sheet of parallel tubes with a regular 70–100-nm space between them and are embedded in a semi-dense matrix (the light zones). At their periphery, these are connected with the endoplasmic reticulum. Another inclusion is the lamellar body composed by the stacking of cisternae derived from the agranular reticulum (see section on dendrites, below). Several other types of inclusion which are also frequently found seem to involve elements of the neuronal cytoskeleton (Fig. 1.8d).[403]

THE DENDRITES

Dendrites constitute the main receptive surface of the neuron. Synaptic potentials are propagated to the soma and, if their summation reaches threshold values of depolarization, an action potential is generated in the axon. For years, dendritic propagation of synaptic potentials was thought to occur passively. The finding of high-density voltage-gated Na$^+$ channels in the dendrites of some neurons (neocortical pyramidal cells), together with the discovery that action potentials, after being triggered in the axon, are able to propagate back into the dendritic tree, have dramatically changed our views on dendritic physiology. Dendrites act as two-way pathways, which may convey the activity level of the neuron to dendritic synapses and induce local changes most probably involved in some forms of synaptic plasticity,[409] a concept that was initially developed by Llinas.[250]

Dendrites can be distinguished from axons by morphological criteria (Fig. 1.7). Dendrites are multiple and unmyelinated, branch at acute angles and taper distally. Axons are single and frequently myelinated, branch at obtuse angles and terminate in small varicosities, the synaptic boutons, on dendrites and cell bodies of other neurons.

Ultrastructure of dendritic cytoplasm

Dendrites are natural extensions of neuronal cell bodies, making it very difficult to trace a precise boundary between the cell bodies and their proximal dendritic processes. Stem dendrites contain all cytoplasmic organelles (Fig. 1.9a). Only when the diameter of the dendrite begins to diminish do dendritic organelles become elongated and aligned parallel to the long dendritic axis, as if they were being funnelled into the core of the dendrite (Fig. 1.9b). Simultaneously with this change in ori-

entation, there is a drastic reduction in the number of Nissl bodies with increasing distance from the soma. Since one of the main criteria to differentiate dendritic from axonal profiles is the presence of ribosomes in dendrites, their sparse occurrence in distal segments is one important reason for the difficulties in identifying distal dendritic profiles.

In contrast, the agranular endoplasmic reticulum, rare in stem dendrites, becomes more abundant with increasing distance from the soma, and is a constant feature of dendritic spines (see below). In cerebellar Purkinje cells (Fig. 1.9b), the numerous cisterns can either form a loose meshwork with a predominantly longitudinal orientation that spreads all over the dendritic branches or contribute to the hypolemmal cistern.[310] Occasionally, there is a hypertrophic production of agranular endoplasmic reticulum, in the cell body and in the dendrites which forms 'lamellar bodies'. They consist of stacks of somewhat dilated cisterns (some of them in continuity with granular endoplasmic reticular profiles), separated from each other by dense particles. The 'lamellar bodies' have been considered as a change in the arrangement of the endoplasmic reticulum provoked by hypoxia during fixation.[394] The agranular endoplasmic reticulum in Purkinje cells has attracted interest in recent years owing to the work of De Camilli and collaborators.[422] These authors have localized the inositol 1,4,5-triphosphate receptor (IP$_3$R) in this organelle. The IP$_3$R is an intracellular Ca^{2+} channel gated by IP$_3$ that mediates the rise in intracytoplasmic Ca^{2+} induced by this second messenger. Although of a ubiquitous distribution, this receptor is present in exceptionally high levels in Purkinje cell bodies and dendrites (type I of the IP$_3$R), which to a much lesser extent also contain the ryanodine receptor. Immunocytochemical visualization of the IP$_3$R with colloidal gold has shown that this receptor is particularly distributed over the agranular endoplasmic reticulum. Concerning the dendrites, the IP$_3$R is present in the cisterns of the loose meshwork, the hypolemmal cisterna, the cisterns in the spines and the cisternal stacks. The latter are considered to reflect an adaptive fast response to hypoxic conditions by the IP$_3$R-rich endoplasmic reticulum of these neurons.

Dendritic spines

Spines are short, about 2 μm, protrusions that cover the surface of dendritic trees of many classes of neuron, particularly pyramidal and Purkinje cells. They vary in shape (slender, stubby, mushroom shaped) and are composed of a neck, joined by a narrow stalk to a more or less dilated head, which commonly is the site receiving the synaptic input. These structures greatly increase the receptive area for synaptic transmission.

Several biophysical models have been developed to test the range of possible specific functions of spines in neurotransmission. Owing to the anatomical configuration, the resistance of the spine head membrane is much greater

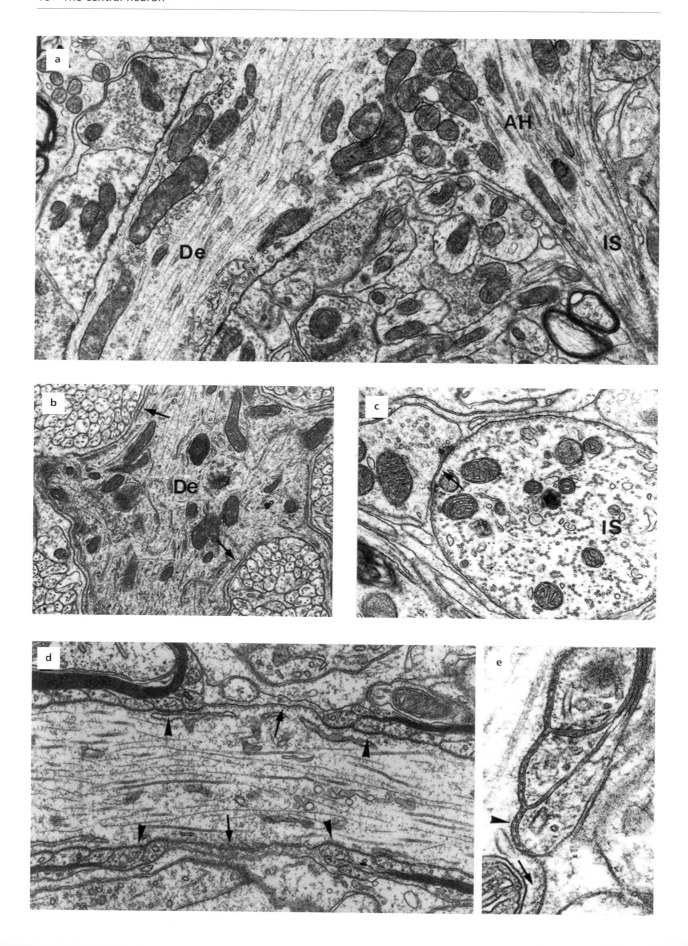

than the resistance in the spine stalk; thus, little centrifugal current can flow from the dendritic segment through the spine (the spine head remains isopotential). Conversely, the input resistance of the parent dendrite is usually small so that centripetal current can flow from the spine to the dendrite. In a way, spines can be viewed as devices specifically designed to inject current into the parent dendrite.

Since slight changes in spine morphology can have important functional consequences, spines have been considered as one of the strategic targets of many of the synaptic adaptive processes, and they are assumed to be the smallest units in neuronal integration and the primary sites of synaptic plasticity in the brain.[110] Thus, changes in spine morphology have been investigated in many cases of neuronal plasticity, including the initiation of hippocampal long-term potentiation (LTP). Using local superfusion techniques combined with two-photon laser-scanning microscopy, which allows fluorescence imaging of specific regions of postsynaptic dendrites, it has been shown that changes in spines are associated with hippocampal LTP.[96] Induction of long-lasting functional enhancement of synapses in area CA1 provokes the generation of new spines. This spine growth is produced neither by short-lasting functional enhancement nor by blocking LTP.

Apart from the postsynaptic differentiations, spines appear as almost empty bags filled with a fluffy material. Ribosomes are often present at the base of the spine, sometimes associated with the cisterns of endoplamic reticulum. The only dendritic organelle that constantly enters the spines is the agranular endoplasmic reticulum, which contributes to the formation of the spine apparatus and which is the site of the IP$_3$R, regulating the concentration of intracytosolic Ca^{2+}. The spine cytoskeleton[172,236] lacks microtubules and neurofilaments, but contains 8-nm filaments which have been identified as actin by their characteristic 5-nm banding pattern.

Recent work by the group of Matus,[201] using *in situ* hybridization with specific probes, has shown that β- and γ-isoforms of actin (cytoplasmic actins, normally expressed in neurons) are expressed at high levels by spine-bearing neurons. Moreover, transfection of epitope-tagged actin isoforms in hippocampal primary cultures has demonstrated that β- and γ-actins are the only isoforms to be selectively targeted to spines. In contrast, if other complementary DNAs (cDNAs) encoding for microtubule components [including tubulin and microtubule-associated protein-2 (MAP-2)] are used for transfecting the hippocampal neurons, the synthesized proteins remain confined to the dendritic shafts, without entering the spines. To determine whether the high expression of actin-cytoplasmic isoforms in spines is correlated with some specific function, for instance spine motility, spines were made fluorescent by transfecting either actin tagged with green fluorescent protein (GFP)[110] or simply GFP.[93] Spine motility was revealed in both primary cultures and slices, in hippocampal and cortical pyramidal cells as well as in cerebellar Purkinje cells. Visible changes occurred within seconds and all types of denditric protrusions (filopodia and spines) were highly dynamic. The motility ceased when neurons were treated with cytochalasin, which blocks actin polymerization, but the blockage of neuronal activity did not change the spine motility. Finally, spines reduce their motility with increasing age of the neurons. This interesting observation provides a molecular basis for structural plasticity and a new mechanism for synaptic plasticity.

→ THE AXONS

The axon corresponds to the single process that, emerging from the soma or occasionally from a dendrite, conducts inputs centrifugally towards the axon terminal. This unique process is smooth and thin, with almost uniform calibre all along its length and few branches. In most projecting neurons, the axons are covered by myelin sheaths. As the axon emerges, it becomes physiologically and structurally divisible into distinct regions, which are the axon hillock, the axon initial segment, the axon proper and the axon terminal, with a high degree of regional differentiation.[315]

Axon hillock, initial segment and nodal segment

By light microscopy the axon hillock is easily recognized by the absence of basophilic material (i.e. the Nissl substance). Frequently, the hillock is a conical region between the neuronal cell body and the initial segment, with the narrow end at the origin of the latter. Occasionally it emerges from a dendrite (Fig. 1.9a). Ultrastructurally, the axon hillock contains little granular endoplasmic reticulum free ribosomes, mitochondria and microtubules (MTs) as well as neurofilaments on their way from the perikaryon to the initial segment (Fig. 1.9a). The axon hillock and the initial segment contain sheaves of parallel arrays of MTs, which collect in the broad portion of the hillock and extend into the axon until the beginning of the myelin sheath, where they disperse. The MTs appear to be bound together by dense material distributed like bridges at irregular intervals along their length.[311,403]

Figure 1.9 *Cytological features of neuronal processes. (a) Axon hillock (AH) and initial segment (IS) of an axon emerging from a dendrite (De) of a giant cell of Deiters in the lateral vestibular nucleus. (b) Purkinje cell dendrite (De). Note the microtubules and the hypolemmal cisterna (arrows). (c) Transverse section of the initial segment of an axon in the lateral vestibular nucleus. Note the absence of undercoating at the axo-axonal synapse (arrow). (d) Node of Ranvier in a spinal cord axon. The undercoating (arrows) is only present at the nodal axolemma, between the myelin loops (arrowheads) present at the paranodal segments. (e) Higher magnification illustrating the undercoating (arrow) and glio-axonal contact (arrowhead).*

The initial segment of the axon is unlike any other known neuronal process. It arises from the summit of the axon hillock and terminates at the first heminode of Ranvier. Its whole extent measures between 20 and 35 μm in length and about 2 μm in diameter. Three distinct features characterize the initial segment (Fig. 1.9c):

- A dense layer of fine granular material undercoating the plasma membrane, in which an electron-light layer, 7.5 nm wide, can be observed containing electron-dense granulations almost regularly spaced, followed by a thin electron-dense lamina from which electron-dense triangular tufts (spiral filaments) protrude. This undercoating makes the axolemma appear thicker than the nearby neuronal or glial plasma membranes.
- Fascicles of MTs are suspended within the axoplasmic matrix, similar to those present in the axon hillock. MTs within the fascicles are bound together by thin cross-bars or arms.
- Although the axon hillock and the beginning of the axon fail to stain with basic dyes, clusters and rosettes of polyribosomes do occur at those levels of the axon. They are more frequent in the axon hillock and progressively diminish throughout the length of the initial segment, to disappear completely at the first heminode of Ranvier.

The initial segment is the trigger zone where the temporal pattern of impulses is established. Therefore, it must be a region with a considerably higher density of sodium channels than in the somatodendritic membrane or in the remaining axonal membrane (with the exception of the node of Ranvier, where the axon is thought to have similar electrical properties and a similarly high density of sodium channels). Thus, it is of interest to compare the ultrastructure of the initial segment with that of the axon at the nodal zone. Of the three features of the initial segment only one is also present at the node of Ranvier: the dense granular layer undercoating the inner aspect of the axolemma (Fig. 1.9d, e). This morphological and functional similarity suggests that the surface specialization is in some way related to the supposed high density of sodium channels. Evidence for the local differentiation of axonal membranes at the initial segment and the nodal zone has been provided using ferric ion and ferrocyanide to stain central nervous tissue following aldehyde fixation. With this staining, electron-dense aggregates of stain have been localized in the nodal region, whereas internodal and paranodal regions of the axolemma are free of staining. Moreover, the initial segments of axons are also densely stained, whereas the axolemma of the axon hillock remains unstained.[465] Use of the freeze-fracture method also has revealed differences in intramembrane particle (IP) density in the nodal zone axolemma. Hence, analysis of unmyelinated axons has disclosed a uniform membrane structure, with an IP density in the extracellular surface (E-face) of 145–300/μm^2. Conversely, in the nodal region of myelinated axons this density is greatly increased (~1300/μm^2), whereas the density is much lower in internodal/paranodal membranes.

The axon beyond the initial segment

The axoplasm contains all neuronal organelles, with the exception of Golgi apparatus, ribosomes and Nissl substance. Unlike in dendrites, neurofilaments are more numerous than microtubules. The latter, being constantly present in axons, are unevenly distributed, being most numerous in the vicinity of mitochondria and beneath the axonal membrane. The number of microtubules per surface unit of axoplasm is inversely proportional to the cross-sectional area of the axon. Hence, they are more closely packed in small axons, where neurofilaments are scanty, than in large axons, where neurofilaments are numerous.[312,315]

Protein targeting in the neuron

The biogenesis and maintenance of neuronal shape, connectivity and membranous composition through life imply that the nerve cell targets newly synthesized molecules to the appropriate compartments, and also recycles them specifically. While those for axonal conduction (such as channels) have to be sent towards the axon, those for transmission have to be routed down to the terminal arborization.

Biochemical polarization of the neuron

Our knowledge of the targeting of proteins in axons and dendrites is based mainly on *in vitro* approaches. After plating, nerve cells extend neurites with the plus-ends of the microtubules pointing towards the periphery[15] (axonal characteristic), and MAP-2, a dendritic marker, is present in all processes.[88] Secretory granules accumulate at the tip of the neurites together with endosomes and endoplasmic reticulum markers such as the Bip protein.[70] At this stage, the tips of neurites are comparable with the growing edges of non-polarized cells such as fibroblasts. Two major components, growth-associated protein of M_r 43 000 (GAP-43) and PP60c-src, which are associated with the plasma membrane, are found in these growth cones.[70]

At later stages of culture the cytoskeleton differentiates. The resulting polarity is comparable with that seen in the adult. The GAP-43 protein disappears from the tip of all neurites except from that of the axon, and synaptic proteins such as synapsin and synaptoporin move out from the neuronal soma towards the axonal growth cone.[70] At the same time, MAP-2 protein becomes progressively associated with dendrites. Indeed, in the adult *in vivo*, many other molecules are specifically expressed in axons and dendrites.

The mechanisms that lead to the heterogeneity of the distribution of cytoskeletal and membranous proteins are not fully understood. They may involve the specific targeting, retention and stabilization of proteins, and exclusion or targeting of mRNAs.

TRANSPORT AND TARGETING OF GLYCOSYLATED PROTEINS

Specific channels and receptors are glycosylated proteins which must accumulate at appropriate locations of the neuronal membrane. The general synthetic pathway for membranous proteins is the same in all eukaryotes. In brief, mRNAs are translated at the level of the RER, and peptides are subsequently transferred to the Golgi and then to the plasma membrane through the trans-Golgi network (TGN). However, the traffic to the final plasma membrane destination is rather complex. The mechanisms involve not only tags that specify the final destination, but also sorting and propelling along the cytoskeletal elements, regulation of vesicular transport and final fusion with the acceptor membrane. This routing is counteracted by pathways in the opposite direction, and recycling involves early endosomes, late endosomes and then lysosomes. These pathways are interconnected by cross-roads and the resulting maps characterize the cell types.[383]

The cargo from one organelle to another is carried by vesicles or tubular structures.[351] Schematically, membranes bud from a donor compartment, and then fuse with an acceptor one.[351] The intracellular fusion events use similar mechanisms with related molecules in all eukaryotes, and it is striking that the docking and fusion machinery is also comparable with that involved in synaptic vesicle exocytosis[109] (see below).

In the donor compartment, selective budding and selective retention may occur, and the choice of the membrane proteins involved results from specific sequences in their cytoplasmic domains. These stretches of proteins are recognized by cytoplasmic machinery such as clathrin or the clathrin-like vesicular coat.[229] Selective budding through coated vesicles is frequently observed from the Golgi to the TGN or from the plasma membrane. Proteins which are not selectively retained or selectively removed from the donor organelle are transferred via non-coated vesicles to the acceptor compartment.[204,351]

CELL POLARITY IN NEURONS COMPARED WITH NON-NEURONAL CELLS

After viral infection of neuronal cells *in vitro*, the haemaglutinin glycoproteins of the Fowel virus preferentially accumulate at the axonal membrane, while glycoproteins of the vesicular stomatitis virus or the Semliki Forest virus are transported towards the somatodendritic compartment.[89] These results helped to formulate a hypothesis that axonal and somatodendritic domains are different in terms of cellular traffic, a theory which still holds. Indeed, this fundamental concept is supported by the comparison of the cellular distribution of many membrane proteins of hippocampal neurons kept in culture

with Madin Darby Canine Kidney (MDCK) cells.[70] For example, the basolateral targeting signals of polyimmunoglobulin receptor of the low-density lipoprotein do mediate targeting to the somatodendritic compartment.[197] However, in other cases, this comparison between the polarity of epithelial cells and neurons has been challenged. Proteins with the glycophosphatidylinositol apical targeting signals are sent to both axons and dendrites.[70,197] Furthermore, many neuronal transmembrane proteins have targeting patterns that cannot be reconciled with this theory, including the β-amyloid precursor protein[150,433] and G-protein-coupled receptors.[475] An analysis of the targeting of metabotropic glutamate receptors (mGluR)[415] indicates that, unlike in epithelial cells, the targeting signal is found to be in the cytoplasmic tail of mGluR, indicating that neurons may use a cytoplasmic sorting signal, probably with a microtubule-based transport.[53] mGluRs normally found in the somatodendritic compartment are sorted to dendritic vesicles and targeted to this compartment, while presynaptic ones are found in both the somatodendritic and axonal compartments. This led to the notion that the final axonal localization may result from selective degradation in dendrites and stabilization in axons. This concept emphasizes the role of differential turnover and stabilization as mechanisms accounting for membrane heterogeneity.

RAB PROTEINS AND CELL POLARITY

The Rab proteins are *Ras*-like GTPases, also known as the small G-proteins. More than 30 members of the Rab family have been identified.[383] These molecules move from the donor to the acceptor compartment where docking takes place, and they are detected all along the exocytotic and endocytotic pathways. It was initially proposed that these molecules could be cues for correct targeting, but it now seems that they are switches for vesicular fusion.[109,143,204] The Rab proteins are specific for the organelle–organelle (e.g. reticulum-*cis*-Golgi) segments and for specific cellular compartments (e.g. apical vs basolateral). These specificities are similar in neurons and in other polarized epithelial cells.[383] Some Rab proteins are involved in specific neuronal functions such as the regulated vesicular exocytosis at axon terminals,[111,112] including Rab3a, which plays a key role in neurotransmitter release.[135,137,296]

SEGREGATION OF mRNA

The notion that dendritic transport of mRNA might exist in neurons comes from the observation that polyribosomes are selectively associated with dendritic spines within the dentate gyrus of the rat hippocampal formation.[414] The observation that the number of polyribosomes can be enhanced during reinnervation following denervation or during synaptogenesis[219] led to the suggestion that these polyribosomes may be involved in local synthesis and therefore contribute to the genesis and plasticity of the mosaic structure of the postsynaptic membrane.

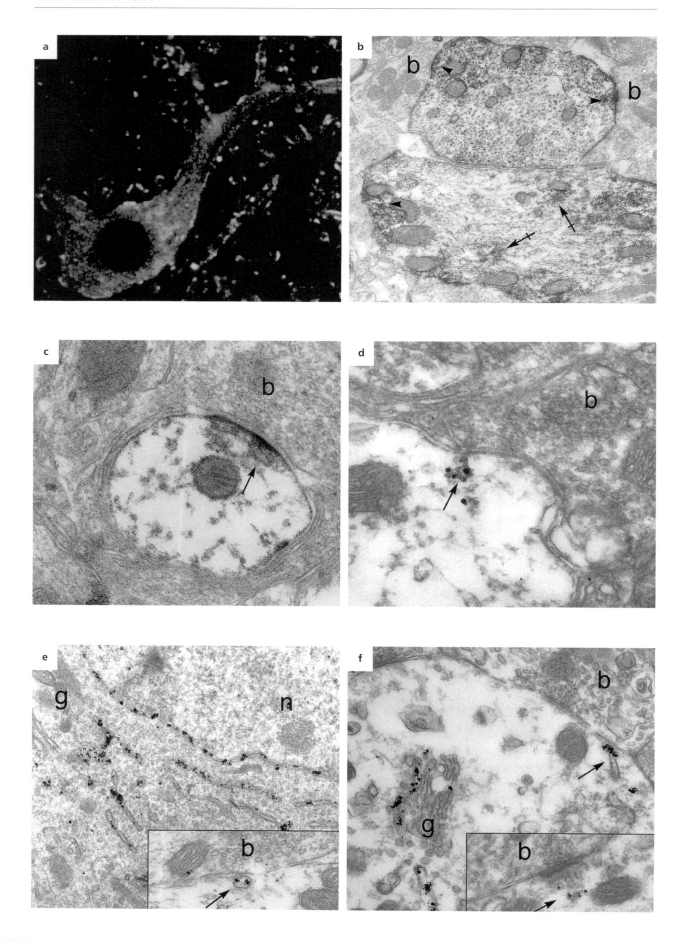

Differential subcellular distribution of mRNAs has been reported in the CNS. In the hippocampus and cerebral cortex, the mRNA of MAP-2 (a dendritic cytoskeletal molecule) can be detected in the neuropil, and therefore in dendrites. This partition of transcripts contrasts with that observed for mRNAs coding for other microtubule-associated proteins or for β-tubulin, which predominate in the soma.[51] Another interesting differential distribution pattern has been described for the transcripts of the α- and the β-subunits of the calcium/calmodulin-dependent protein kinase. The former were detected in the neuropil of the hippocampus and in layer I of the cortex of the frontal lobe, while the latter were only found in somata. This observation suggests that the two subunits are not translated in the same compartment.

One of the most challenging questions concerning the cell biology of synapses is how thousands of signals, which notify minute changes occurring at each postsynaptic differentiation and arising from a large number of synapses, can be treated somatically and subsequently induce a synaptic change on dendrites hundred of micrometres away. Indeed, subsynaptic mRNAs could encode neurotransmitter receptors. In the spinal cord, where glycinergic inhibition predominates, the α-subunit of the glycine receptor was found to be associated with subsynaptic cisternae. The glycine receptors accumulate in front of boutons with inhibitory function.[440] It could be assumed that these subsynaptic mRNAs might participate in the local subsynaptic synthesis of the glycine receptor (Fig. 1.10a).[326] Other mRNAs encoding for neurotransmitter receptors were found in dendrites, such as some subunits of the ionotropic (GluR[280] or NR[134]) or the metabotropic (mGluR[34]) glutamate receptors.

Recent data indicate that new receptors can be inserted into the postsynaptic membrane after physiological stimulation.[325] These receptors can either be inserted from a ready-to-use subsynaptic pool[261,298] or be translated from subsynaptic mRNAs.[130,325,326,413] These two processes are not exclusive, and the subsynaptic pool of receptors could either result from a targeting from the soma or be synthesized *in situ* from localized mRNAs. Convergent evidence supports the hypothesis of a restricted translation of proteins from perisynaptically located mRNAs.

mRNAs encoding secreted or transmembrane proteins were also found in dendrites. This is the case for the brain-derived neurotrophic factor (BDNF) and its receptor the TrkB receptor, the mRNAs of which were found to be transported distally in dendrites following synaptic activation.[435] This activity-dependent transport may underlie a subsynaptic protein synthesis of BDNF and TrkB. The former, which can be secreted by dendrites, and the latter, which is expressed in the dendritic membrane,[37] are probably involved in the modulation of synaptic transmission and in LTP in the hippocampus.[272]

A dendritic and subsynaptic synthesis and membrane insertion/secretion of protein imply the existence of competent cellular machinery. The existence of subsynaptic cisternae and polyribosomes was demonstrated a long time ago; however, it is only recently[130] that dendritic translational and secretion machinery was characterized with immunocytochemistry and electron microscopy (Fig. 1.10b–f). Some subsynaptic cisternae exhibit the features of RER, while others have immunoreactivities that are characteristic of the *cis-*, medial or *trans-*Golgi. Indeed, several biochemical studies had shown that translation[437] and glycosylation could occur in dendrites.[438]

The relation that may exist between activity and mRNA transport and/or protein synthesis has been challenged for the glutamate receptor. A direct implication of NMDA receptors and Ca^{2+} in local protein synthesis of calcium/calmodulin-dependent protein kinase II (CaMKII) was recently demonstrated in synaptosomes.[325,359] Entry of Ca^{2+} might also regulate mRNA transport to dendrites via calcium-sensitive RNA-binding proteins.[268]

The processes that underlie the transport of mRNA are not fully understood. RNAs move along microtubules as macromolecular particles, also referred to as granules.[3] Several constituents of these particles have been identified in different cell types (for references see Ref. 206). Some of them allow the movements of particles, other ensure the recognition of the RNAs to be transported, while others belong to the pathway of translation. Together with the cellular translation and secretion machinery, they are referred to as being the *trans-*acting factors. The localization of given mRNAs results from the interaction between transacting factors, the cytoskeleton

Figure 1.10 *Presence of glycine mRNA and of a secretory machinery under synapses.* **(a)** *Simultaneous detection of α$_1$-GlyR subunit mRNAs (red) and α-GlyR subunit proteins (green) in a spinal cord neuron. mRNAs are detected as granules within the dendritic cytoplasm and are accumulated under the dendritic membrane and near dendritic branch points.* **(b–d)** *Dendritic localization of α1-GlyR* **(b, d)** *and α$_2$-GlyR* **(d)** *GlyR subunit mRNAs labelled by* in situ *hybridization and revealed by HRP* **(b, c)** *or nanogold* **(d)** *methods.* **(b)** *Cross-sections of two adjacent dendrites with mRNAs detected within the dendroplasm (crossed arrows) and under dendritic membrane (arrowheads) in front of synaptic boutons* **(b)**. **(c, d)** *α-GlyR subunit mRNAs associated with cisternae (arrows) in front of synaptic boutons.* **(e, f)** *Immunolabelling of cisternae belonging to the secretory apparatus. The luminal side of the nuclear envelope (nucleus: n) and the endoplasmic reticulum cisternae is labelled for Bip, a reticulum resident protein* **(e)**. *Note that the Golgi apparatus (g) is devoid of signal. Bip immunoreactivity is present in the luminal side of a subsynaptic cisternae (inset, arrow). Cross-section of a proximal dendrite* **(f)** *containing a Golgi apparatus (g) whose trans-side is labelled with antigen-TGN38-associated gold particles that also labels a subsynaptic cisterna (arrow). Subset of subsynaptic cisternae (arrow) is also decorated with gold particles associated with Rab-1 antigens (inset, arrows). Reproduced by permission from Gardiol et al.[130] and Racca et al.[326]*

and targeting *cis*-acting sequence of the mRNA. In neurons, these dendritic targeting sequences are often located in the 3'UTR regions of mRNAs (e.g. CaMKIII-α,[271] Arc,[459] MAP-2[35]). The 3'UTR sequences are complex boxes which not only interact with transacting factors, but also are involved in the regulation of the stability and translation of mRNAs (for references see Ref. 82).

NEURONAL CYTOSKELETON

The cytoskeleton is the essential element that, through its static and dynamic properties, not only supports neuronal shapes but also plays an essential role in generating and maintaining the regional compartmentation.[55] Indeed, the neuronal cytoskeleton serves the dendritic and axonal transport systems that are so necessary for the continuous and targeted supply of materials to these processes, thus providing a mechanism for the chemical communication between the nucleus and perikaryon, and the most distal regions of neuronal processes.

The cytoskeleton can be defined as a well-organized lattice composed of a filamentous microtrabecular meshwork that forms a highly cross-linked gel, filling the entire volume of the neuron. Progress in morphological visualization, protein purification and gene cloning has expanded our knowledge of the chemical composition and the organization of its filamentous elements.

Neurons contain three major classes of cytoskeletal elements: MTs, neurofilaments and microfilaments, interconnected by protein bridges (side-arms). In the axon, there are two specialized regions. Immediately beneath the axolemma lies the membrane or cortical cytoskeleton, composed of a meshwork of actin filaments, fodrin-brain spectrin polymers and associated proteins. Deeper in the axoplasm neurofilaments and MTs form a cytoskeletal core of two overlapping networks, cross-linked by numerous side-arms.

Microtubules and microtubular domains

Tubulins

MTs in axons, as in other cells, are hollow tubes with an outer diameter of about 25 nm, and a wall formed by 13 globular subunits. They consist of tubulin molecules that, when extracted from the brain, appear as a dimer of about 100 kDa, and comprise about 20% of the total soluble protein. Each dimer is composed of two polypeptides, α-tubulin and β-tubulin. When these molecules assemble into MTs, the dimers line up, forming rows of protofilaments (the β-tubulin of one dimer joined to the α-tubulin of the next). In general, 13 of these protofilaments become arranged side by side, forming the MT wall. Analyses with optical and X-ray diffraction methods have shown that the protofilaments are not aligned in register but are staggered, producing a spiral. Thus, the assembly of tubulin into MTs resembles that of actin into filaments.

Owing to the specific orientation of their subunit arrangement, MTs are polarized polymers, and one end grows faster (the plus-end) than the other (the minus-end). Under precise conditions, free tubulin can be added to the outside of MTs to form curved protofilaments that, in cross-section, appear as hooks. This feature has been used to determine the direction of the MT polarity. When the hooks point clockwise, they identify the minus-ends, whereas counterclockwise orientation occurs at the plus-ends. Using this criterion, it has been established that MTs in axons are uniformly polarized. Their minus-ends are directed towards the perikaryon where MTs are nucleated from the centrosome (microtubular organizing centre), and their plus-ends point towards the distal axonal termination.[16] It is known that, in dividing cells, centrosomes play a key role in the organization of mitotic spindles, and that pericentriolar material contains a ring-like microtubule-nucleating protein composed among others by γ-tubulin (the nucleating protein). In neurons, γ-tubulin is not detectable in axons or dendrites, being exclusively present in cell bodies, in association with the centrosome. Blocking of γ-tubulin with specific antibodies stops the formation of new MTs. Hence, it has been assumed that the centrosome is the only generator of MTs in neurons, including axonal and dendritic MTs.[14]

Microtubule-associated proteins

When MTs are purified *in vitro*, the resulting product consists mainly of α- and β-tubulin and, in addition, several polypeptides, termed collectively microtubule-associated proteins (MAPs). The most prominent MAPs of brain MTs are high molecular weight proteins known as MAP-1 (350 kDa) and MAP-2 (280 kDa), and a group of closely related proteins with a much lower molecular mass, termed tau proteins (50–70 kDa). All these proteins are thought to be involved in the assembly and stabilization of MTs,[14] as well as in the interactions of MTs with membrane-bound organelles and other components of the cytoskeleton. Eight or so well-characterized high molecular weight brain MAPs are known (MAP-1A–C, MAP-2A–C, MAP-3, MAP-4, MAP-5) and, with the exception of MAP-4, which is glia specific, the other forms are present in neurons; MAP-2 differs from the other neuronal MAPs because it is mostly expressed in dendrites (Fig. 1.11a, b, d) where MTs are abundant (Fig. 1.11c).[270]

Tau proteins, another major component of the MAPs, constitute a series of proteins appearing as closely spaced bands on polyacrylamide gels. Immunocytochemical studies in adult brain have provided evidence that tau proteins are far more abundant in axons than in dendrites, providing a means to differentiate axons from dendrites. Recent knockout experiments of the tau gene in the mouse have shown that axonal growth is not impaired in cultured neurons. However, in small-calibre axons, MT stability is decreased and MT organization is altered. In these mice, there was an overexpression of MAP-1A which could com-

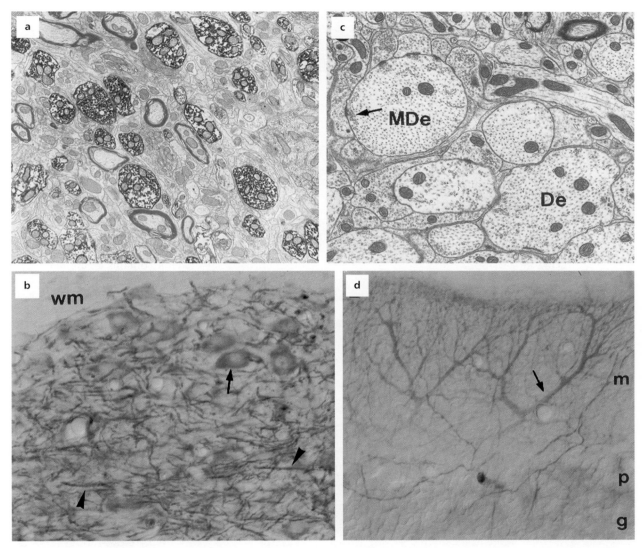

Figure 1.11 *Dendritic microtubules. (**a**, **b**) MAP-2 immunochemistry in the fastigial nucleus. (**a**) Immunoperoxidase reaction product covering dendritic profiles. (**b**) Slight and heavy staining of the neuronal cell bodies (arrow) and dendritic profiles (arrowheads), respectively, and lack of labelling of the white matter (wm). (**c**) Olfactory bulb illustrating dendritic profiles (De). Note the disposition of regularly spaced microtubules. One of the dendrites belonging to a mitral cell (MDe) establishes synaptic connections with granule cell dendritic gemmules (arrow). (**d**) MAP-2 staining of a Purkinje cell dendrite (arrow); m, p and g: molecular, Purkinje cell and granular layers, respectively.*

pensate somewhat for the absence of tau proteins, at least in large-calibre axons which appeared normal.[156]

Axonal microtubular domains

With the exception of MAP-2 and MAP-4, all of the other proteins associated with MTs constitute the axonal microtubular domains; MTs are not abundant in axons. They appear as small bundles intermixed with a broad meshwork of neurofilaments. In rats intoxicated with β-β-iminodipropionitrile (IDPN)[171] MTs are segregated from neurofilaments to form the central core of the axon. In the axon, MTs form large bundles, appear coated with numerous, single or anastomosed, fine strands of different sizes and contain granular material. This extensive meshwork of side-arms either cross-links MTs with each other or interconnects MTs with membrane-bound organelles; MAP-1A, MAP-1B and tau proteins are the main components of axonal side-arms cross-linking MTs with each other.

Neurofilaments and neurofilament domains

Neurofilaments have been known for more than 100 years, mostly because of their intense argyrophilia (Fig. 1.12a). These are the elementary organelles forming what were formerly termed neurofibrils.

Neurofilaments are neuron-specific intermediate filaments (class IV) of 8–10 nm in diameter and many micrometres long, which fill most of the axoplasm. In

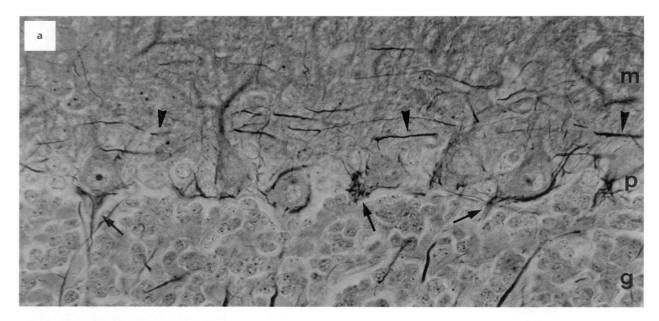

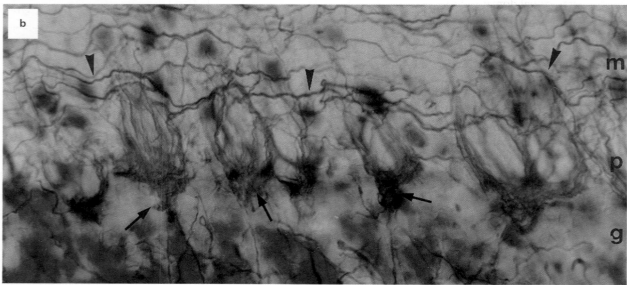

Figure 1.12 *Axonal neurofilaments. (a) Cajal reduced silver staining of the cerebellum. (b) Immunostaining with a monoclonal anti-body which recognizes phosphorylated neurofilaments (NFH) in a transgenic mouse line expressing β-galactosidase reaction in all neurons except for the Purkinje cells. In (a) and (b) the arrows point to the pinceau formations of basket cell axons around initial segments of Purkinje cell axons, and the arrowheads mark the transversally orientated basket axons; m, p and g: molecular, Purkinje cell and granular layers, respectively.*

contrast to MTs and actin filaments (F-actin), they are stable polymers with a low turnover. Neurofilaments are assembled in the perikaryon and move down the axon with little change, until the axon terminals, where they are degraded very rapidly (inhibition of proteolysis produces neurofilament rings in nerve terminals). This metabolic stability favours their role in the mechanical stability of axons and, therefore, in the cytoarchitecture of axonal branches, suggesting that neurofilaments are directly involved in the modulation of the axon calibre.

When protein analysis of the material conveyed by the slowest axonal transport was undertaken, five polypeptides constituted 70% of this material: two were the tubulins, and three others were the protein subunits of adult neurofilaments, light (NFL, 68 kDa), medium (NFM, 160 kDa) and heavy (NFH, 200 kDa). The three subunits, as all intermediary filament proteins, have a conserved central amino acid domain involved in the formation of coiled structures. In order to understand the molecular architecture of neurofilaments, *in vitro* reassembly experiments were carried out. The NFL subunits are able to assemble into homopolymeric 10 nm filaments, while NFM and NFH require coassembly with NFL for the formation of neurofilaments.[171] Furthermore, immunocytochemistry with antibodies against the three neurofilament proteins, in material prepared with the rapid freeze and deep etch method, has revealed the localization of each constituent of the triplet: anti-NFL uniformly decorated the neurofilament central core but not the side-arms. Anti-NFM also decorated the core, but less uniformly, and occasionally the stems of the side-arms. Anti-NFH, in contrast, decorated not the core but the side-arms. Thus, NFL is a component of the central core, whereas NFM and NFH are components of the side-arms cross-linking one neurofilament with another. Antibodies against one or several of the neurofilament triplets are excellent tools to visualize neurons, particularly their axons (Fig. 1.12b), which are more extensively stained than after silver impregnation (Fig. 1.12a, b).

Subaxolemmal or 'cortical' cytoskeleton: microfilaments

Immediately beneath the axolemma (about 100 nm), there is a peripheral axonal domain mostly occupied by complex networks of 6–8-nm filaments that link the axolemma to the central axonal core of neurofilaments and MTs. The chemical identity of this peripheral meshwork of filaments has been determined with histochemical methods: since a large portion of these filaments stained with phalloidin (a specific ligand of actin filaments) most of them correspond to F-actin. Hence, the subaxolemmal cytoskeleton is mainly composed of microfilament proteins.[171] Actin is a highly conserved protein with the property of self-assembly. Globular actin (G-actin) subunits constitute a cytoplasmic pool in dynamic equilibrium with polymerized F-actin. The latter, like MTs, are polarized structures with a growing end (the plus-end) and an opposite end (the minus-end) where subunits can be lost. The number of actin filaments is under strict cellular regulation: actin filaments can be assembled and disassembled in response to physiological signals. The dynamic equilibrium is reached at a critical concentration, when the number of subunits added to the plus-ends accounts for that lost at the minus-ends. This process, known as 'treadmilling', needs energy derived from adenosine triphosphate (ADP) and is similar to that observed in MTs.

Actin binding proteins

The functional importance of the process of actin assembly has prompted the investigation of factors involved in this process, and several actin binding proteins have been found in neurons. Some of them (profilin, gelsolin, actin depolymerizing factor, cofilin, villin, CAP90, BAM40) are needed as the assembly regulating proteins of actin filaments. Another protein, tropomyosin, is the major stabilizing and co-assembling protein of F-actin. Other important functional proteins are those that can cross-link actin filaments with each other: fimbrin and fascin, which are tight bundling proteins, and brain spectrin, which cross-links F-actin into a loose network. Brain spectrin in axons (α) is termed fodrin, while in dendrites (αβ) it is referred to as spectrin. Another important group of proteins comprises those that anchor F-actin to the plasma membrane: α- and β-ankyrins, talin and vinculin. Hence, the number of known actin binding proteins in neurons is rather large.[17]

Axonal transport

Distal dendritic branches and the entire axon, since they do not have polyribosomes, are excluded from protein synthesis. These two neuronal compartments depend solely upon the perikaryon for their proteins, creating an essential challenge to the general metabolic machinery of the neuron.

ANTEROGRADE AXONAL TRANSPORT

Weiss and Hiscoe[468] reported that nerve fibres proximal to a constriction became swollen, whereas those distally narrowed, as if a proximodistal motion of a semi-solid axoplasmic column of material was moving down the axon. Furthermore, after removal of the constriction, the accumulated material resumed its somatofugal movement at a rate of 1–2 mm/day (rate of regeneration of peripheral axons). Despite the local injury of the constriction, these experiments revealed the occurrence of a slow transport of materials in somatofugal direction ('slow axonal transport'). The application of radioactive tracers to the study of axonal transport[91] has revealed the occurrence of a rapid phase that takes place at a rate of 100–400 mm/day. The utilization of cell fractionation and biochemical analysis has made it possible to determine more accurately the transport kinetics of proteins and organelles, and five groups of average transport velocities were recognized. The first three groups (group I, 70–400 mm/day; group II, 20–70 mm/day; and group III, 4–20 mm/day) encompass the fast phase of axonal transport, and the last two groups (group IV, 1–4 mm/day; group V, 0.2–1.2 mm/day) the slow phase. The interest in this subdivision is due to the fact that the proteins conveyed in each transport group are theoretically different, and those in the same group must share the affinity for the transport mechanism as well as the carrier. It is known that neurofilament proteins and tubulins are conveyed by group V transport, whereas other cytoskeletal proteins, particularly actin, and certain glycolytic enzymes, including neuron-specific enolase, creatine kinase and aldolase, are conveyed by group IV transport. Moreover, these two groups of the slow phase carry about 80% of all the proteins leaving the perikaryon, and are aimed at retrieving cytoskeletal elements, providing the axon with structural support and with intra-axonal domains to direct the transport of proteins and membrane-bound organelles through the axoplasm.

These proteins move at the same rate as radiolabelled neurofilaments normally move along the axon. The three

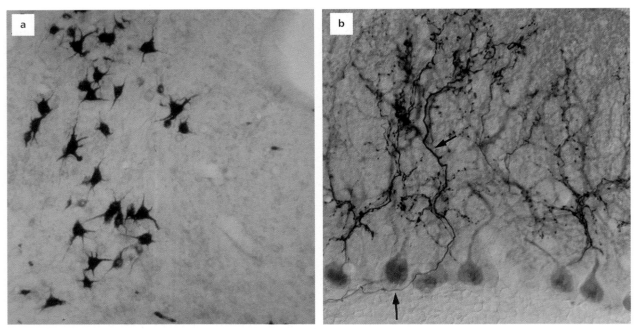

Figure 1.13 *Retrograde and anterograde axonal transport as markers of neuronal projections. (a) Lateral vestibular neurons retrogradely labelled after intraspinal injection of HRP. (b) Double labelling of the cerebellar cortex. The dark climbing fibres (arrows) exhibiting a Golgi-like staining have been labelled after injection of biocytin aminodextran in the contralateral inferior olive. The Purkinje cells are labelled with an anticalbindin antibody.*

groups of fast axonal transport mainly convey plasma membrane proteins such as Na^+ and K^+-ATPases, acetylcholinesterase and membrane-bound organelles, such as mitochondria, multivesicular bodies and secretory vesicles, including components of the synaptic vesicle membrane. Hence, almost one-third of the proteins flowing down the axon by the fast phase are targeted to axon terminals, and most of them will be employed in exocytosis during synaptic transmission. The physiological properties of this fast phase have been extremely useful for tracing connections in the brain (Fig. 1.13b).

SLOW AXONAL TRANSPORT: MICROTUBULAR PROTEIN TRANSPORT AND ASSEMBLY

Study in the 1980s, using pulse-labelling of cytoskeletal proteins with radioactive tracers, provided evidence that these proteins move down the axon as a discrete wave, suggesting that they are assembled in the perikaryon and transported in the form of intact sliding polymers (the polymer sliding model). Later on, experiments focusing on sites of MT assembly in the axon, using fluorescent photobleach recovery after laser beam irradiation, generated a different explanation: MTs in the axon are dynamic structures, and tubulins synthesized in the perikaryon can move as small oligomers (dimers) to be assembled into MTs.[50] This issue became even more controversial with the utilization of 'caged-fluorescein'-labelled tubulin, which permits the fluorescent labelling of a segment of axonal MTs and directly visualizes their transport and turnover. The results obtained varied

according to the material under examination[170] and are still a matter of debate.[295]

RETROGRADE AXONAL TRANSPORT

The early examination of living neurons (cell cultures) with phase-contrast microscopy has revealed that intra-axonal particles have bidirectional movements. The observation that the uptake of protein tracers (HRP) by axon terminals labels the cell bodies of origin (Fig. 1.13a) provided direct evidence in favour of a somatopetal axonal transport, termed retrograde transport.[230] Although there is a non-specific uptake of exogenous tracer molecules by the plasma membrane of the neuron, probably facilitated by the positive charge of these molecules, neuroactive molecules enter the axon via selective mechanisms, involving micropinocytosis through ligand receptor binding specificity. Tetanus toxin is taken up by all nerve fibres, as if receptor-like molecules for this toxin were present in all neurons. Treatment of axons with neuroaminidase suppresses the uptake of tetanus toxin, suggesting that gangliosides in the axonal membrane are involved. Neurotropic viruses are also transported by retrograde transport, including poliomyelitis, rabies and herpex simplex viruses, and their uptake is dependent on the axonal presence of specific receptors. Nerve growth factor (NGF) and other neurotrophins are also taken up by receptor-mediated endocytosis at axon terminals in a very specific manner. The view that neurons are sensitive to specific neurotrophins has allowed the elaboration of the concept that materials with trophic function are synthesized in and secreted from target cells (neurons or effector cells), incorporated by axon terminals and carried to the perikarya by retrograde transport. It is, therefore, possible that defects in this kind of axonal transport could be the cause of some neurodegenerative diseases, even if neurotrophins are normally produced by target cells. Hence, various materials can be taken up by distal axon terminals, some of them being essential signals for neuron survival.

The rate of retrograde transport differs with different materials. Thus, the retrograde transport of acetylcholinesterase was evaluated at a rate of 125 mm/day, whereas that of viruses has been estimated to be at about 60 mm/day. In any case, retrograde axonal transport only occurs at a fast rate. In addition to mitochondria that have bidirectional transport, the materials conveyed by retrograde axonal transport travel in large membrane-bound organelles, such as endosomes and autophagic vacuoles. Thus, while the fast anterograde transport conveys membrane-bound organelles involved in the exocytotic pathway, retrograde transport carries those involved in the endocytotic pathway, since the main mechanism of axonal uptake is micropinocytosis. The conjunction of anterograde and retrograde axonal transport provides a powerful means for transneuronal traffic. Materials and messengers can be secreted by postsynaptic elements and taken up by presynaptic ones, being conveyed thereafter towards the perikaryon (retrograde transneuronal transport). Conversely, such messengers can be released from presynaptic terminals and, without immediate function on the postsynaptic membrane, can be taken up by the postsynaptic neuron through an endocytotic mechanism (anterograde transneuronal transport). The occurrence of both types of transneuronal transport is of interest for tracing pathways in the CNS but, more importantly, it is a main factor in pathology. For instance, this is the mechanism for the entry and dissemination of viral particles through peripheral nerves, or for neurotoxicity (tetanus toxin, drugs such as the antineoplastic antibiotic doxorubicin, or even lead).

MICROTUBULES AS RAILS FOR FAST AXONAL TRANSPORT

Microtubules form small bundles in the axoplasm, where they are much less numerous than neurofilaments. Despite their low density, it is known that depolymerization of MTs with colchicine or other antimitotic drugs, or by cooling, arrests fast axonal transport. It was therefore considered that, similar to all cells, the movement of organelles along the axon resulted from an MT-based transport. The introduction, early in the 1980s, of the VEC-DIC, has made it possible to visualize the movement of single organelles along individual MTs.[48] Many of these organelles move bidirectionally and quickly (several micrometres per second). In the squeezed axoplasm of the squid giant axon, deprived of axolemma and separated from the cell body, the process of axonal transport is not affected. This discovery has provided a powerful model to

analyse not only morphologically, but also biochemically and pharmacologically, the mechanisms underlying fast anterograde and retrograde axonal transport.

KINESIN AS A MICROTUBULE-BASED MOTOR INVOLVED IN FAST ANTEROGRADE TRANSPORT

When the search for molecular motors or translocators started, two such molecules were already known in other classes of cell movement. One was myosin and the other flagellar dynein. Both molecules are mechanochemical proteins with ATPase activity, which can be distinguished pharmacologically by their differential susceptibility to ATPase inhibitors. The application of a non-hydrolysable analogue of ATP, adenylylimidodiphosphate, to squeezed squid axoplasm tightly binds organelles to MTs and thus limits their movements. Since AMP-PNP was a weak competitive inhibitor of myosin and flagellar dynein, it became clear that neither of these two mechanochemical ATPases was involved in fast axonal transport.

In 1985, two independent groups[170,230] purified a novel neuronal force-generating protein. One group obtained a 115-kDa polypeptide from the squid optic lobe, while the other purified a 130-kDa polypeptide from the chick brain. This novel protein was termed kinesin, and is involved in the movements of intra-axonal organelles. Since the velocity of kinesin ranges from 0.1 to 10 μm/s, it is involved in fast axonal transport.[169] Kinesins are holoenzymes of relatively small molecular mass (500 kDa or even less) which contain one to four copies of a principal polypeptide with a motor domain. The latter is responsible for the ATP-dependent force generation along MTs.[139] Kinesins are composed of head and tail domains, and it is the tail domain which provides the kinesin with its specificity to bind their cargoes, whereas the head domain binds to MTs. Recent molecular biology studies,[169] have shown that there are many classes of kinesins, indicating that the mammalian genome is able to encode 50–100 different kinesins, which have been grouped into three main classes:

- Kinesin-I, also known as true kinesin, is composed of heavy-chain (KHC) and light-chain (KLC) subunits. In mammals, there are three different KHC subunits (KIF-5A–C) and at least three other KLC subunits (KLC-1–3). Of these six subunits, KIF-5A and KIF-5C are exclusively expressed in neurons, and KLC-1 expression is also prominent in neurons. Hence, the expression of several KHC and KLC and their combination leads to the occurrence of six or more kinesin-I forms in neurons.
- Kinesin-II is found in three forms in the mouse (KIF-3A–C), but their role in neurons is poorly understood despite their occurrence in axons.
- UNC104: this family (homologue in the mouse of KIF-1A) is the motor of a subset of synaptic vesicles. Mice with an inactivated *KIF1A* gene, being deficient in synaptic vesicles, exhibit sensory and motor deficits, and die shortly after birth.

The large number of existing kinesins strongly indicates that they are motors specialized for different cargoes. It is known that members of kinesin-I class can bind to different membranous structures, such as synaptic vesicles, Golgi vesicles, mitochondria and lysosomes.[139] Nevertheless, the concept that every different membranous structure transported by the fast axonal flow requires a specific kinesin has been challenged by recent results obtained with hippocampal neuronal cultures transfected with a fusion construct of VAMP (synaptobrevin, a synaptic vesicle protein) and green fluorescent protein[2] which appear as fluorescent puncta or packets. Each punctum moves from the cell body to the axon terminals at 0.5 μm/s as in MT-based transport. However, each punctum was too large to be a single synaptic vesicle and contained many synaptic vesicles, together with calcium channels and soluble proteins of the endocytotic machinery used by axon terminals. Ultrastructural analysis of these puncta showed that they consist of large, dense-core synaptic vesicles and irregularly shaped tubular profiles, but lack small agranular synaptic vesicles. These results suggest that major cytoplasmic and membrane-associated protein precursors of the presynaptic active zones are assembled into prefabricated 'prototerminals'. If these results are corroborated, they indicate that many presynaptic proteins are assembled in the cell bodies early in their biogenesis and sorting pathways, and are transported together along the axons, probably using one single kinesin.

CYTOPLASMIC DYNEIN AND KINESIN AS PRESUMPTIVE RETROGRADE MOTORS

During the process of isolation of kinesin from bovine brain, several polypeptides also with binding properties to MTs and releasing ATP were obtained. One of these polypeptides was recognized as being MAP-1C. This was later identified as a two-headed cytoplasmic dynein (C-dynein), a different molecule from flagellar dynein, present in organisms without motile cilia. *In vitro*, C-dynein generates minus-end directed forces along MTs, that is, with a polarity opposite to that of kinesin. Although C-dynein has been proposed as a translocator for retrograde transport, this function may not be exclusive and it has also been implicated in slow phase transport.[48,171] It is now known that mammals have multiple C-dynein heavy-chain genes.[139] In addition to C-dynein, neurons express a class of kinesins, the KIF-C2, thought to generate minus-end directed forces. KIF-C2 occurs in dendrites and axons, and could contribute to retrograde axonal transport.

DENDRITIC TRANSPORT: DIFFERENCES TO AXONAL TRANSPORT

The polarization of the neuron, and the differences in composition of dendritic and axonal compartments, make it obvious that there are important differences in the quality of the transported materials, as well as in the underlying mechanisms. Since MTs are also the rails for dendritic transport (which is inhibited by drugs that depolymerize MTs), one important reason for a distinct dendritic transport emerges from the known differences between dendritic and axonal cytoskeleton. In dendrites MTs prevail, whereas neurofilaments are less abundant, and MAP-2 is constantly associated with dendritic MTs, while tau is practically absent. In axons MTs are uniformly orientated (minus-ends close to the perikaryon and plus-ends orientated towards the axon terminals), while in dendrites roughly half of them are orientated with the plus-ends directed towards the cell body and the remaining ones have their plus-ends orientated towards the distal dendritic terminations. Hence, these differences, particularly the presence of MTs of opposite polarity, have been considered as responsible for the compartmentation and polarity of the neurons. If MTs are the rails for organelle transport, their dendritic features would be enough to explain, for instance, the presence of polyribosomes and Golgi elements in dendrites and their absence in axons. Examples taken from other cell systems have provided some clues in favour of such an explanation.[167,473]

THE SYNAPSE: HISTORICAL BACKGROUND

To achieve their fundamental task of conveying encoded information, neurons need to communicate among themselves, or with effector cells (secretory cells, muscle fibres). This communication takes place at specific sites, at which the plasma membranes of the two interacting cells are juxtaposed. These zones are not sites of protoplasmic continuity but are sites of 'nerve cell articulations',[334] which were termed synapses by Sherrington. These are polarized structures that determine the direction of the impulse traffic which, through their valve-like property, drive the impulse in only one direction, from the presynaptic to the postsynaptic element.

The discovery in the middle of the nineteenth century that flow of electric current was involved in nerve conduction and muscle contraction generated the idea that communication between neurons was electrically mediated.[401] The general concept of chemical messengers in the transmission of synaptic information mainly emerged from the works of Loewi[251] and Dale *et al.*,[76] who were able to demonstrate that acetylcholine (ACh) was a neurotransmitter in the peripheral nervous system. Studies during the 1950s using intracellular recordings resulted in the demonstration of the chemical nature of synaptic transmission and the abandonment of the electrical transmission theory, which was considered a rare form of synaptic mediation almost exclusively observed in phylogenetically primitive forms.[401]

Today it is clearly demonstrated that fast- and short-term interactions between neurons can be mediated by chemical messengers (chemical synaptic transmission), as well as by passive spread of electrical impulses (electrotonic coupling or electrical synaptic transmission). Special emphasis will be placed on the fact that chemical and electrical transmission do not exclude each other, since in precise morphological situations both operate between the same two neurons, probably exerting cooperative action to modulate synaptic effectiveness.

CHEMICAL SYNAPSES

The functional requirements of a chemical synapse are:

- fast emission of chemical messengers triggered by an action potential of the presynaptic element
- rapid diffusion of the neurotransmitter ensuring a transient high concentration in the narrow space between nerve cells
- interaction with receptors responsible for the transduction of the chemical message.

These requirements are fulfilled by the particular structural and chemical organization of the elements forming the synaptic junction, which appears as an organelle shared between two cells specialized in activity regulated cell–cell communication.

Light microscopy of silver impregnated material was unable to give details of synaptic structure, and it was only with the advent of electron microscopy in the early 1950s that the features of its constituents could be revealed. The discontinuity between nerve cells was then definitively established by showing that presynaptic and postsynaptic elements are membrane bound.[315] Electron microscopy in combination with immunocytochemistry, and uptake experiments, could identify the neurotransmitters contained in synapses. More than 50 molecules have been found to be neuroactive in synaptic chemical communication. Among them are the classical neurotransmitters, amino acids (glutamate, GABA, glycine, taurine), monoamines [noradrenaline (NA), dopamine (DA), serotonin (5-HT)], ACh and the expanding group of neuropeptides. With the advance of molecular cloning, sequencing and subsequent development of antibodies, receptors can now be also localized on the neuronal membrane.

The morphological counterpart of a chemical synapse is the synaptic organelle or synaptic complex formed by the presynaptic element, the postsynaptic component and the synaptic cleft or intracellular space separating them (Fig. 1.14a). The structural characteristics of these elements allowed a classification of synapses and permitted an attempt to correlate structure with inhibitory or excitatory function (see the following section).

The presynaptic element

The cytological constituents of the presynaptic bouton include mitochondria, profiles of the smooth endoplasmic reticulum, cytoskeletal components, synaptic vesicles and a dense material abutting the presynaptic membrane.

PRESYNAPTIC MEMBRANE

A great advance in the study of the structural composition of plasma membranes has been achieved with the introduction of freeze fracture. With this method, plasma membranes are cleaved at the middle of their lipid bilayers; while their globular proteins are skirted, remaining in one or the other of the artificially created membrane halves. These appear as rounded particles of various sizes, called intramembrane particles (IPs).

This method does not allow examination of the true inner and outer surfaces of the plasma membrane, but of the external side of the created inner protoplasmic leaflet (P-face), and the internal side of the extracellular leaflet (E-face). These two faces are complementary, meaning that when one IP protrudes in the P-face there must be a corresponding pit in the E-face, and vice versa. Freeze fracture, by appraising the patterns of IPs' disposition at various functional regions of the neuronal plasma membrane, has helped to disclose regional differences, particularly in synaptic membranes, providing a way to correlate functional variations with structural heterogeneity.

With cryofracture of the presynaptic membrane, some large (8–10 nm) IPs are present on the E-face, and complementary dimples are detected on the P-face.[315] Freeze-etched preparations also revealed the presence of crater-like depressions in the presynaptic element. The depressions corresponded to the empty spaces between the presynaptic dense projections, and hence these holes were named the vesicle attachment sites (VAS),[317] or synaptopores. Although this has been a matter of debate, they probably correspond to the opening of vesicles captured during exocytosis. In addition, large particles, found at the presynaptic membrane in the vicinity of VAS, may correspond to calcium channels and contribute to the osmiophilia of the presynaptic differentiation. The presynaptic membrane, together with the presynaptic vesicular grid, correspond to the 'active zone' defined by Couteaux[69] at the neuromuscular junction.

PRESYNAPTIC DIFFERENTIATION

In his pioneering study, Gray[146] used phosphotungstic acid (PTA) to demonstrate the presence of electron-dense protrusions attached to the presynaptic membrane. These structures (Fig. 1.14a, b), known as the presynaptic dense projections (PDPs), are triangular with a height of 60–80 nm and spaced centre to centre at about 100 nm. The free access to the plasma membrane between the PDPs ranges from 20 to 50 nm. If by chance the section is parallel to the plane of the presynaptic membrane, one can see that the PDPs are disposed in a trigonal array. The presynaptic apparatus has also been extensively studied.[315,318] The PDPs are joined by filamentous crossbridges, with the synaptic vesicles nestling in the free space

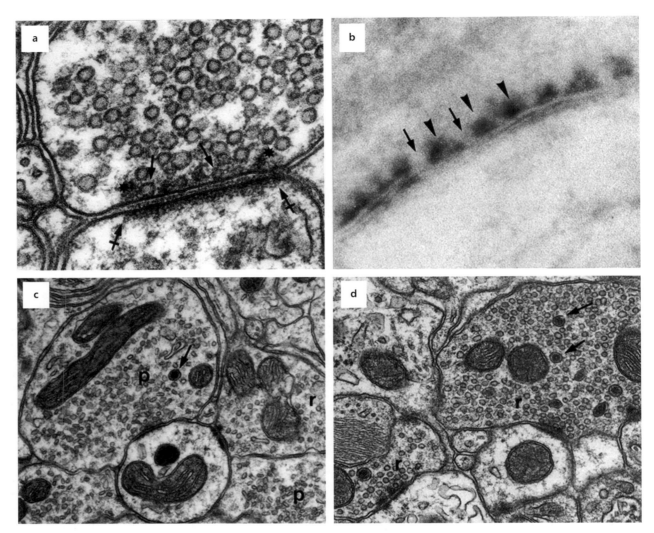

Figure 1.14 *Ultrastructural features of synaptic complexes. (**a**) Asymmetrical synapses between a parallel fibre and a Purkinje cell dendritic spine. Presynaptic vesicles (arrows) nestle between the presynaptic dense projections. The two most lateral are indicated by asterisks. The postsynaptic membrane is underlined by an electron-dense differentiation, the limits of which are indicated by crossed arrows. Note the fuzzy electron-dense discontinuous line in the synaptic cleft. (**b**) Synaptic complex within the spinal cord, specifically stained with an ethanolic solution of phosphotungstic acid. The presynaptic dense projections (arrowheads) delineate spaces (arrows) in which the presynaptic vesicles (not stained here) are present. (**c, d**) Pleomorphic (p) and round (r) vesicles containing boutons within the inferior olive establish symmetrical and asymmetrical synapses, respectively. Note the presence of large, dense-core vesicles (arrows).*

between them. The assemblage of the vesicles and the hexagonal array of PDPs are referred to as the presynaptic vesicular grid. The improved PTA staining,[39,146] allowing exclusive staining of the synaptic complex, has been used to count synapses and measure the size of the presynaptic complex during development and ageing.[30] Using semi-thin (0.5-mm thick) sections and electron microscopy (Fig. 1.14b), the presynaptic apparatus can be easily visualized in its full extent.[457] With this method the cellular organization of this structural element at the surface of an identified neuron has been determined.[441] In these studies, as in others,[457] the size (i.e. the number of PDPs) and the shape of the presynaptic grids as well as their number per bouton have been shown to be variable.

These observations correlate with physiological data,[226] and have led to the hypothesis that a single active zone behaves in an all-or-none manner, allowing the release of the content of at most one vesicle when the ending is active.

The PDPs are most probably a fixation artefact since quick freezing followed by freeze substitution fails to reveal this structure.[235] It has been suggested that PDPs could result from the precipitation induced by fixation of cytoskeletal networks associated with vesicles[172] and of molecules involved in the mobilization, docking and fusion of the presynaptic vesicles with the axonal plasma membrane.[194] The hexagonal distribution would then result from the accumulation of these molecules between the packed vesicles which are adjacent to the presynaptic membrane. Consequently, the presynaptic grid should reflect the number of vesicles that are lying close enough to the membrane to be potentially ready for exocytosis.

SYNAPTIC VESICLES

Synaptic vesicles are thought to contain neurotransmitters, and it is believed that the fusion of these vesicles to the axolemma, and the subsequent release of their content, is at the origin of the quantal release.[231,315]

Small clear vesicles or agranular vesicles

The diameter of small clear synaptic vesicles (SSVs) ranges between 40 and 60 nm, and they are present at various distances from the presynaptic membrane (Fig. 1.14a). Their shape depends upon the conditions of preservation. When OsO_4 and $KMnO_4$ are used as the primary fixative, or after aldehyde fixation and freeze fracture; the vesicles are always spherical.[394] When aldehydes are used as primary fixative, some presynaptic boutons have spherical vesicles while they are flattened in others (Fig. 1.14c, d).[447] It has been suggested that the osmolarity of the fixative could be a determinant of vesicular shape.[450] However, other experiments are not compatible with the notion that vesicles are simple osmometers: the sensitivity of vesicles to fixative depends upon the type of terminal.[315] With rapid freezing, in the absence of any fixatives, it has been demonstrated in the anteroventral cochlear nucleus of the rat that the actual shape of all these vesicles is spherical.[429]

The composition of the membrane of SSV has been intensively studied in the past few years[194,315] as a result of their paramount importance in neurotransmission. Recently, large numbers of proteins which are involved in the interactions of the synaptic vesicle with the cytoskeleton or with the presynaptic membrane have been identified (see section on synaptic release, below).

Dense-core vesicles

Vesicles with an electron-dense core are also present within endings. These can be classified according to their size. Small, dense-core vesicles have a diameter between 40 and 85 nm, and large vesicles range from 100 to 150 nm (Fig. 1.14c, d).

The small, dense-core vesicles which contain 20 nm dense osmiophilic granules can be separated into smaller (45–55 nm) and larger (75–85 nm) populations. These were first described in the autonomic nervous system and are generally associated with monoamines.[85] Initial work, using electron microscopy and autoradiography, demonstrated that tritiated noradrenaline was in the endings of the pineal gland which included small, dense-core vesicles. Later, dense-core vesicles were found in the majority of endings labelled with antibodies against dopamine-β-hydroxylase or directly against noradrenaline and serotonin (5-HT).[315]

The larger dense-core vesicles (100–150 nm) are generally thought to contain neuropeptides, since they resemble vesicles found in neurosecretory fibres in the hypophysis.[315] This type of vesicle is always intermingled with small clear vesicles (Fig. 1.14c, d). Direct evidence of the presence of peptides in large dense-core vesicles is scarce, but examples include somatostatin[114,416] and neurotensin.[434] It must be stressed that the dense-core vesicles are dispersed in the endings among the SSV, always at a distance from the active zone (for definition see below), thus excluding the possibility that the peptide could be released at the synaptic complex. However, it has been shown in the trigeminal nucleus of the rat that large, dense-core vesicle can undergo exocytosis at structurally non-specialized areas, outside the presynaptic active zone.[485]

The synaptic cleft

The intercellular space between the presynaptic and the postsynaptic elements of the central synapse is narrower than that of the neuromuscular junction and ranges between 15 and 30 nm. It is the least studied part of the synaptic complex. This space is obviously a point of adhesion since presynaptic and postsynaptic membranes remain attached during the preparation of synaptosomes. This critical point of contact is structurally organized[315] and is partially filled by an electron-dense material (Fig. 1.14a) which is most important at asymmetrical synapses (see section below). Thin filaments can occasionally be seen bridging the gap using electron microscopy[453] or unfixed rapidly frozen material which was subsequently deeply etched or freeze substituted.[187] Cytochemical and enzymic approaches[315] indicate that glycoproteins are components of the cleft. Staining with ruthenium red suggests the presence of glycosaminoglycans. Further, a decrease in the staining following treatment with neuraminidase indicates the presence of sialic residues. These families of molecules are constituents of the glycocalyx seen around most eukaryotic cells. The constituent molecules of the synaptic cleft have not been identified and it can be speculated that those involved in cell adhesion should play a key role in this region. The structural features of the cleft suggest that it is not isotropic and is not a free space for the diffusion of neurotransmitters.

The postsynaptic element

POSTSYNAPTIC MEMBRANE

The specialized structures capable of receiving and decoding synaptic information are located in the postsynaptic membrane, facing the presynaptic active zone. The functional heterogeneity of neuronal membranes assumes a structural heterogeneity (the mosaic concept of the neuronal membrane organization). Nevertheless, ultrastructural examination of postsynaptic membranes is rather disappointing: the same three-layered membrane structure, the unit membrane, binds the cytoplasm of the postsynaptic element at junctional as well as at nonjunctional sites, only distinct cytoplasmic differentiations mark the postsynaptic membrane, allowing its identification. Hence, from the early descriptions, postsynaptic differentiations (PSDs) appeared as a layer of electron-dense filamentous material (postsynaptic web) (Fig. 1.14a), corresponding to the electron-dense specializations in the presynaptic membrane and with the stained extracellular material in the synaptic cleft, together forming the synaptic complex.[309]

With the freeze fracture method, there was a common feature in the postsynaptic membranes of excitatory synapses: IPs, ranging in size from 6 to 20 nm and protuding into the E-face, aggregate into macular plates matched by an array of complementary pits in the P-face (Fig. 1.15a). Importantly, such a type of pattern distribution has never been encountered in postsynaptic membranes of symmetrical synapses,[157] supposed to be of inhibitory nature.

POSTSYNAPTIC DIFFERENTIATIONS

Substructure of PSDs

In standard electron micrographs, postsynaptic membranes are coated by a more or less prominent band of electron-dense cytoplasmic material (Fig. 1.14a). This band, by its apparent homogeneity, contrasts with the more complex disposition of presynaptic dense material in presynaptic vesicular grids. However, with high-resolution electron microscopy the fuzzy PSDs can occa-

sionally reveal a substructural organization, in which granular material seems to be embedded in a fine filamentous network.

Landis *et al.*[236] have studied, with this technical approach, the substructure of PSDs in a homogeneous synaptic population, that of the parallel fibre Purkinje cell dendritic spine in the molecular layer of the mouse cerebellum. Postsynaptic differentiations consist of a meshwork of thin filaments with adherent, heterogeneous globular particles. The thin protein filaments appear to be inserted into or in apposition to the true inner surface of the post synaptic membrane, and could correspond to the anchoring proteins of receptors. Distributed throughout the spine cytoplasm, actin-like microfilaments and thinner filaments, probably of brain spectrin, are arranged parallel to the stalk of the spine, with their tips entering the PSD.[172]

Chemical composition of PSDs

Since the 1970s, new subcellular fractionation methods have been developed for the isolation of PSDs from synaptosomal fractions. Protein analysis of the PSD fraction has revealed the occurrence of at least 15 major protein bands and ten minor bands.[205] Among the most abundant proteins in PSDs are cytoskeletal proteins, such as tubulin, actin and fodrin. The presence of these proteins reinforces the idea that PSDs are microspecialized zones of submembranous cytoskeleton.

The use of modern biochemistry and molecular biology (protein microsequencing and molecular cloning) has opened a new view of PSD protein composition. Hence, in the last few years two new and important components of PSDs have been identified: dynamin (for membrane

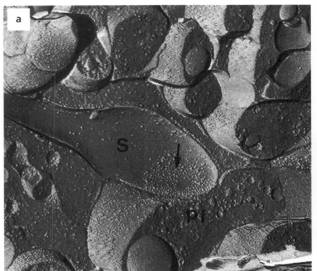
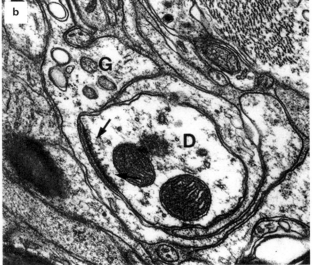

Figure 1.15 *Postsynaptic differentiation. (a) Freeze fracture of a Purkinje cell spine (s) in contact with a parallel fibre (pf). Note that E-face of the postsynaptic membrane contains clusters of large intramembranous particles (arrow). (b) Small dendrite (D) within the gracile nucleus covered by an astrocytic process (G) 6 months after dorsal root transection. Note that the postsynaptic differentiation (arrows) and the synaptic cleft material remain intact in the absence of a presynaptic element.*

endocytosis) and PSD-95 (for signalling mechanisms sensitive to changes in the GTP/GDP ratio).[205]

PSDs as valuable markers of postsynaptic surfaces

As a constituent of postsynaptic membranes, PSDs have been helpful in classifying synaptic junctions as asymmetrical or symmetrical (see section below) and in analysing some mechanisms involved in the development and fate of postsynaptic membranes. Indeed, the presence of PSDs in abnormal development[392] and their maintenance after degeneration of their presynaptic partners[396] have marked new views on the biology of postsynaptic membranes. The fate of PSDs after anterograde degeneration of presynaptic axon terminals is diverse. In a few systems, the entire postsynaptic zone is phagocytosed together with the degenerative debris of the presynaptic axon, while in others PSDs can persist after the complete removal of the necrotic presynaptic axon (Fig. 1.15b).[395] The frequent persistence of PSDs, despite the absence of synaptic function, is much in favour of their stability in central neurons.

Other subsynaptic organelles in addition to PSDs

The spine apparatus and the subsynaptic bodies are the two organelles that deserve to be considered as postsynaptic organelles.[315]

Spine apparatus

This consists of two or more flattened or distended sacs of smooth endoplasmic reticulum separated from each other by narrow plates of dense material (20 nm thick). The sacs are in continuity with the long cisternae of smooth endoplasmic reticulum in the cytoplasm of the parent dendrite. Their occasional occurrence in spines outside cerebral cortices and hippocampus testifies that they are not specific to spines of forebrain neurons. Although the functional significance of spine apparatuses remains unknown, the observations on IP_3R localization in Purkinje cell spines suggest that these organelles may be involved in the regulation of intracytoplasmic Ca^{2+} levels after postsynaptic activation.[424] This hypothetical function fits with results of Ca^{2+} content in Purkinje cell dendritic spines, a finding which indicates that one of the possible functions of the cisternal stacks is to sequester free Ca^{2+} entering the spine through ligand-gated or voltage-gated channels during synaptic transmission.[12]

Subsynaptic bodies

First described by Taxi[430] in the sympathetic ganglia of the frog, these consist of an electron-dense plate of cytoplasmic material 20–30 nm thick, situated 25–60 nm beneath and being shorter than the PSD. In the mammalian brain they are discontinuous, formed by a row of symmetrically spaced dense particles.[394] A special local-ization of subsynaptic bodies has been described primarily in the interpeduncular and habenular nuclei, in the neck of a spine or in a small dendritic profile sandwiched by twin axon terminals ('crest synapses').

Synaptic taxonomy

The 'synaptic junction' or 'synaptic complex', with its triadic configuration, is the structural correlate of chemically transmitting synapses. From the earliest ultrastructural studies, morphologists have made an effort to select some parameters of these triads upon which to establish a classification that could provide a better understanding concerning the organization and function of central interneuronal connections. At least four different taxonomies have been elaborated.

TYPES OF SYNAPSE ACCORDING TO THE ARRANGEMENT OF THE SYNAPTIC COMPLEXES

The first attempt to classify synaptic contacts in the cerebral cortex was made by Gray[145] who, on the basis of their junctional features, described two types. In type I synapses, presynaptic and postsynaptic membranes bear noticeable cytoplasmic densities, particularly a very prominent PSD (Fig. 1.14a). They also possess a widened synaptic cleft of 20–30 nm. In type II synapses, the synaptic cleft is narrower at about 15 nm and the PSD is much less pronounced (Fig. 1.14c). Gray completed his description by associating type I synapses with dendritic spines, and type II with neuronal cell bodies, whereas dendritic shafts can receive both types of synaptic contact. Later studies in non-cortical structures have not fully corroborated Gray's classification because it became clear that, in the CNS, type I and type II synapses are the extreme cases of a continuum of differentiation and that all of the intermediate forms can be encountered.

Type I and type II synapses were renamed by Colonnier[67] almost 10 years later. Based upon the configuration, Colonnier termed type I contacts asymmetrical synapses and type II contacts symmetrical synapses. Despite the inappropriateness of this new nomenclature (the functional polarity of the synapses always implicates structural asymmetry), it has been commonly used.

TYPES OF SYNAPSE ACCORDING TO THE SHAPE OF SYNAPTIC VESICLES IN PRESYNAPTIC ELEMENTS AND THEIR ASSOCIATION WITH SYNAPTIC COMPLEXES: FUNCTIONAL CORRELATION

The most commonly found synaptic vesicles in central axon terminals are the SSVs, which appear as rounded (Fig. 1.14a) or flattened (Fig. 1.14c) structures in aldehyde-fixed material (see section on the synaptic vesicles, above). This artefactual change in shape caused by aldehyde fixation is useful, because it permits identification of precise populations of axon terminals (Fig. 1.14c, d).

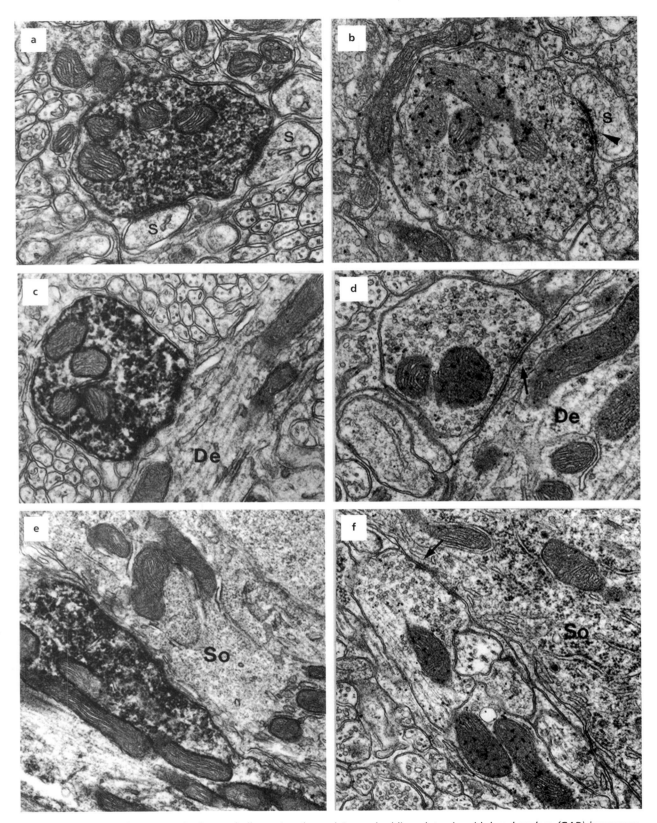

Figure 1.16 *GABAergic synapses in the cerebellar cortex. (a, c, e) Pre-embedding glutamic acid decarboxylase (GAD) immunocytochemistry. (b, d, f) Post-embedding immunodetection of GABA. (a, b) Stellate axon terminals synapsing on Purkinje cell spines (s) with an asymmetrical synaptic complex. (c, d) Stellate axon terminals synapsing on a Purkinje cell dendritic shaft (De) with a symmetrical synaptic complex. (e, f) Basket axons synapsing on a Purkinje cell soma with a symmetrical synaptic complex. Arrows and arrowheads: symmetrical and asymmetrical synapses, respectively.*

Moreover, in cortical structures where the correlation between the excitatory or the inhibitory nature of axon terminals and their ultrastructural identification can be made, it has been shown that excitatory synapses (for instance, cerebellar climbing, mossy and parallel fibres) are formed by boutons containing spherical vesicles and, conversely, those of inhibitory function (basket, stellate and Golgi cell axons) are filled with pleomorphic vesicles.[310] These observations prompted some morphologists to consider that rounded vesicles store excitatory neurotransmitters (i.e. glutamate) while flattened vesicles store inhibitory ones (i.e. GABA, glycine). This relation between functional dichotomy (excitation, inhibition) and structural dichotomy of SSVs (rounded, flattened) has been further consolidated by the high frequency of coincidences between one type of vesicular shape and one type of synaptic junction. Thus, most asymmetrical synapses contain rounded vesicles, whereas most symmetrical ones are filled with flattened vesicles.

This correlation, although quantitatively proven in some cortical areas, cannot be safely generalized to the entire CNS. Indeed, the number of exceptions has progressively increased as immunocytochemistry is applied to analyse the neurotransmitter content of SSVs.[400] The introduction of immunocytochemical methods with antibodies against neurotransmitters (Fig. 1.16b, d, f), their synthetic enzymes (Fig. 1.16a, c, e) and their receptors (see Fig. 1.24) will provide answers to each specific situation. This approach has revealed that while most axon terminals containing GABA establish symmetrical synapses (Fig. 1.16c–f), some of them form asymmetrical synapses on dendritic shafts and even spines (Fig. 1.16a, b).

TYPES OF SYNAPSE ACCORDING TO THE NEURONAL ELEMENTS INVOLVED

Conventional synapses

In a 'model neuron' the presynaptic elements of chemical synapses must necessarily be axons, and the postsynaptic ones either dendrites or somata. This is, indeed, what happens in the vast majority of central synapses. Therefore, axo-dendritic and axo-somatic synapses are also known as conventional synapses. The axo-dendritic synapses can be subdivided into two categories according to the dendritic region (spines or shafts) operating as postsynaptic partners. From these conventional synapses, those on spines are asymmetrical (Fig. 1.14a), while those on dendritic shafts and on somata can be both asymmetrical and symmetrical (Fig. 1.14c, d).

Unconventional synapses

Using the accepted morphological criterion of the 'synaptic complex', it became rapidly evident that neurons can become 'effector' or 'receptor' according to the neuronal system under examination. Although the relative number of such unconventional synapses is low, all possible combinations have been observed in the mammalian CNS: axo-axonal, dendro-dendritic, dendro-somatic, dendro-axonal, somato-dendritic, somato-somatic and somato-axonal.[312,315] From this diversity, the axo-axonal and the dendro-dentritic types (Fig. 1.17a, b), the most often encountered unconventional synapses, require further comments.

Axo-axonal synapses

These have been observed in two distinct situations, when the presynaptic axon terminal is synapsing either on another axon terminal or on an axon initial segment. The former was first reported by Gray[144] in the dorsal horn of the spinal cord, where they may provide the morphological basis for presynaptic inhibition (Fig. 1.17a). The latter are commonly present in many projection neurons in cortical areas (cerebellar Purkinje cells, neocortical and hippocampal pyramidal cells).

Dendro-dendritic synapses

Ramon y Cajal's suggestion[334] that synaptic transmission in axonless neurons, such as retinal amacrine cells and olfactory granule cells, could occur through presynaptic dendrites was first demonstrated on granule cells. These dendritic terminals or gemmules synapse on mitral cell dendrites (Fig. 1.17b) and are of inhibitory action.[333] It is accepted today that neurons having an axon in many regions of the CNS may have presynaptic properties at both axonal and dendritic levels. Furthermore, most of these unconventional synapses are established by local-circuit neurons.[393] The existence of all of these unconventional synapses has opened new views on different possibilities of information proceeding by local microcircuits, which may not even involve the whole neuronal entity.[366]

TYPES OF SYNAPSE ACCORDING TO THE COMPLEXITY OF THE ARRANGEMENT OF SYNAPTIC PARTNERS: SIMPLE AND SPECIALIZED SYNAPSES

All of the synaptic types described above have the common characteristic of simple geometry (Fig. 1.14a). All show the classical structure and belong to simple synapses. In addition, in a few situations, the geometry involved in the arrangement of synaptic partners is much more intricate; these are known as specialized synapses.[147,286,337,373,402,406]

Reciprocal synapses

These have been reported in the olfactory bulb,[333] and refer to a special arrangement of dendro-dendritic and somato-dendritic synapses. Reciprocal synapses are formed by adjacent regions of the same synaptic interface, in which two closely related synaptic complexes are polarized in opposite directions (Fig. 1.17b). They generally occur between granule cell gemmules and mitral cell bodies or

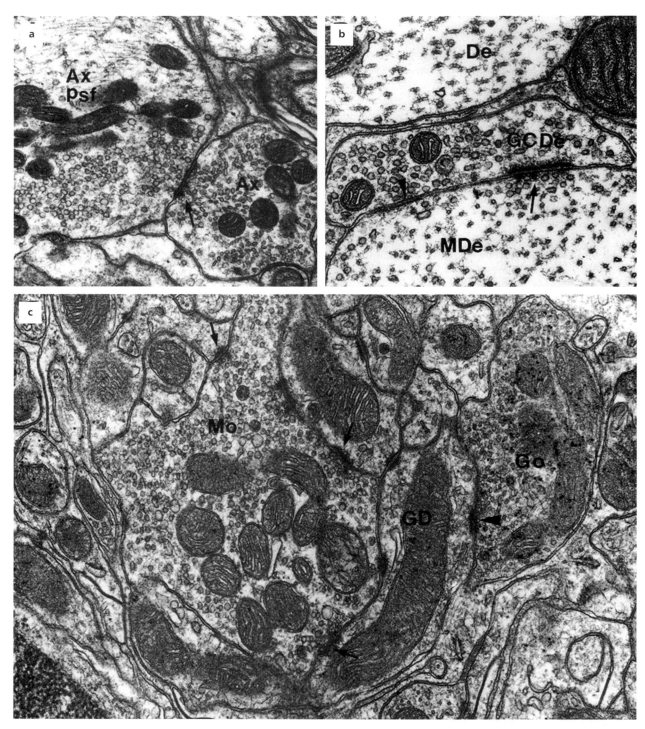

Figure 1.17 *Examples of non-conventional chemical synapses. (a) Axo-axonal synapse between a pleomorphic vesicle containing axon (Ax) and a primary sensory fibre (psf) with round vesicles in the nucleus gracilis of a cat. Note the symmetrical synaptic complex (arrow). (b) Reciprocal synapses between a mitral cell dendrite (MDe) and a granule cell dendrite (GCDe). Note the asymmetrical (arrow) and symmetrical (arrowhead) synaptic complexes. (c) Glomerular organization in the cerebellar granular layer. A central mossy fibre rosette (Mo) is synapsing on granule cell dendrites (arrows), and a peripheral Golgi cell axon (Go) establishes a synaptic contact with a granule cell dendrite (GD). The colloidal gold labelling above background corresponds to the immunodetection of GABA.*

dendrites. Immunocytochemistry with antibodies against glutamic acid decarboxylase (GAD), the GABA-synthesizing enzyme, indicates an inhibitory nature of the synaptic contacts from granule to mitral cells.[373]

Synaptic ribbons

This specialized type of synaptic organization was first described in the outer plexiform layer of the retina, between photoreceptors and dendrites of horizontal and bipolar cells. Furthermore, they have also been reported in neurons outside the retina, particularly in auditory and vestibular hair cells, and in electric fish electroreceptors. Cone pedicle synapses have been studied in rats[147] and in non-human primates.[337] The most peculiar feature in this complex synaptic arrangement is the occurrence of an electron-dense lamella bisecting the synaptic ridge and providing its plane of symmetry. This lamella or synaptic ribbon is almost completely surrounded by a halo of SSVs, aligned in rows and connected to the ribbon by filamentous arms.

Complex axo-axonal synaptic relations on axon initial segments

Only two examples of these specialized synaptic relations are known. One concerns the vortex-like axonal arrangement of descending basket cell axons around the initial segment of the cerebellar Purkinje cell axons, known as the 'pinceau formation'.[310,315] The second example is the axon-cap of the goldfish Mauthner cell.[286,406]

Glomerular synaptic arrangements

The term glomerulus was introduced at the end of the nineteenth century to designate intricate areas of globular appearance in the neuropil, supposed to be regions of complex neuronal interactions. Two glomerular arrangements were described, one in the cerebellar cortex (where mossy fibre rosettes synapse on granule cell dendritic digits; Fig. 1.17c), and the other in the olfactory bulb (where axon terminals of primary olfactory fibres synapse on dendritic tufts of mitral and tufted cells). The electron-microscopical examination of these two glomerular zones has corroborated their complex synaptic organization, and their demarcation from nearby neuropil by their partial encapsulation by astrocytic processes.[312,315]

Ultrastructural analysis of the brain has revealed the occurrence of somewhat similar complex synaptic arrangements in many other areas of the CNS: the substantia gelatinosa of the spinal cord and the descending trigeminal nucleus, the cranial sensory nuclei, the thalamic motor and sensory nuclei, the red nucleus and the inferior olive.[315] In almost all of them, there is a central axon contacting peripheral dendritic profiles through asymmetrical synapses, and a third component (a presynaptic axon or dendrite) which establishes symmetrical synapses on either the dendritic profiles, the central axon

or both. The only exception to this organization is the inferior olivary glomerulus, composed of a central core of small dendritic elements, termed dendritic protrusions, covered by a peripheral ring of axon terminals, and enwrapped by astrocytic processes.[402]

Synaptic release

Synaptic vesicles are involved in regulated secretory pathways through calcium-dependent exocytosis like other vesicles in many other systems. They are closely related to the vesicular systems involved in the constitutive recycling of membranes.[273]

BIOGENESIS OF THE SYNAPTIC VESICLES

There are two main pathways for the generation of vesicles. The first originates at the level of the TGN, for secretory proteins, and is referred to as the classic, regulated secretory pathway. Classic regulated secretory pathways exist in most specialized cells including exocrine and endocrine cells. In neurons, they are responsible for the exocytosis of neuropeptides contained in dense-core vesicles.[54] In addition to this classic pathway, another highly specialized vesicular system exists: that of the SSVs.[273] These vesicles are directly involved in local endocytosis and exocytosis at the periphery of the cell. The biogenesis of SSVs can only be understood if their cycle is considered in relation to other vesicular pathways.[273]

The total number of quanta to be released after a prolonged period of stimulation of isolated nerve–muscle preparation by far exceeds the number of available vesicles, indicating that the terminal is capable of producing such vesicles.[273] Experimental evidence indicates that SSVs are only generated at the nerve ending and not in the TGN, and that their constituents are transported down the axon. In cultured hippocampal neurons synaptophysin and other SSV proteins are not co-localized at the level of the soma where they are synthesized and post-translationally modified. Following treatment with brefeldin A, a molecule which induces the fusion of the TGN with early endosomes, synaptophysin was found within these fused organelles, while other vesicular proteins such as SV2 and synaptotagmin were not.[285] Hence, this experiment indicates that SSVs, with their complement of transmembrane proteins, are assembled at a distance from the TGN. Thus, schematically, membrane proteins of SSV are first transported by classic secretory pathways from the TGN to the plasma membrane of the terminal ending. Subsequently, the membrane is recycled through coated pits and coated vesicles to early endosomes, from which SSVs would then be generated.[273,339] This circuit for the assembly of synaptic vesicles was first proposed by Miller and Heuser.[278]

The formation and assembly of the molecular components of the synaptic vesicles require a complex machinery (for review see Ref. 155). The formation of a vesicle results from a budding from the plasma membrane of the synaptic terminal bouton or intracellular structures followed by separation of the invaginated structure. These processes are related to vesicular recycling (see below) and are mediated by a distinct set of molecules. The clathrin and the adaptor protein 2 (AP2) are involved in the budding process at the plasma membrane and plasma membrane-derived invaginations,[141,363,375] while the adaptor protein 3 (AP3) is responsible for budding at early endosomes.[101] The dynamin, a GTPase involved in the recycling of synaptic molecules, its associated lipid-modifying enzyme (SH3P4) and amphiphysine are all implicated in the fission step with or without the Clathrin/AP2 complex[343,379] (see also references in Ref. 155). It has been recently proposed that the function of dynamin could be to recruit additional molecules involved in the separation of the nascent vesicle from the plasma membrane.[213,371] This would lead to a modification of the lipid composition, thus allowing the separation of the forming vesicle from the negatively curved portion of the omega structure.[364]

Little is known of how the presynaptic machinery for the synaptic vesicle biogenesis and the presynaptic active zone are assembled during synaptogenesis, or how this structure is maintained in mature synapses. The current assumption is that all of the molecular components would be targeted specifically towards the presynaptic terminal bouton (see references in Ref. 349), but this hypothesis has been recently challenged by a combined video- and electron-microscopic study,[2] revealing that the presynaptic active zone components, including the presynaptic vesicles, were 'pre-assembled' and transported (0.5 μm/s) in the axon by means of a 'saltatory' movement with resting periods of 0.5–4.5 min.

CYTOLOGY OF NEUROTRANSMITTER RELEASE

The fusion of synaptic vesicles with the presynaptic membrane, and the extrusion of vesicular packages of transmitter, following an exocytotic process, are thought to be at the origin of quantal transmitter release.[203] Morphometric analysis at the neuromuscular junction indicates that, in a physiological situation, the vesicular membrane would completely coalesce with the presynaptic plasmalemma.[164] Examination of nerve endings with freeze fracture[164] showed transverse ridges with rows of particles on the P-face of the presynaptic membrane of motor end-plates. These structures were immediately associated with the presynaptic active zones previously described with standard electron microscopy.[69] All along these structures, dimples of various sizes were observed. They correspond to craters of vesicular openings caught at various stages of the exocytotic process, corresponding to the neck of omega-shaped structures. Comparable figures for synaptic vesicle openings were also found in the CNS (Fig. 1.18a).

CYTOLOGY OF VESICULAR RECYCLING

During normal activity, a motor ending does not swell, thus the added membrane during exocytosis has to be recycled. Ultrastructural observations following the uptake of HRP from the extracellular space during neuronal activity suggest that recycling should occur at the periphery of the active zone via clathrin-coated vesicles which would subsequently fuse with early endosomes (Fig. 1.18b).[273] This hypothesis is substantiated by the fact that synaptic markers are found in vesicular profiles that may correspond to early endosomes, and in coated vesicles. According to an alternative sequence of events, synaptic vesicles open briefly, do not flatten in the presynaptic membrane and are immediately recycled into the cytoplasm.[439] This apparent discrepancy may be explained by an earlier experiment analysing membrane recovery at different time points after stimulation, showing that both types of membrane recycling could occur.[278] Optical imaging now allows the study of recycling dynamics of the exocytotic and endocytotic cycle.[33,352]

The 'kiss-and-run' theory of neurotransmitter release postulates that the vesicle interacts with the presynaptic membrane transiently, and does not flatten in the presynaptic plasmalemma (Fig. 1.18b, model 1). This is a modern version of the previously proposed model.[439]

Two different sets of molecules (see above) are responsible for the recycling events occurring outside active zones. This process involves budding followed by fission, while the 'kiss-and-run' events correspond only to fission of vesicles. A clathrin/dynamin-mediated process is responsible for the budding–fission at the edge of the synapse.[73,123,423] A dynamin machinery is accountable for the retrieval of synaptic vesicle at the active zone.[6,362,464] The two pathways have different kinetics and may serve different functions:[222,234] the intra-active zone fission ('kiss-and-run') and the extra-active zone (budding–fission) may correspond to the recycling of the readily releasable and reserve pools of synaptic vesicles, respectively. These two mechanisms which coexist at synapses differ in their Ca^{2+}/Mg^{2+} sensitivity.[222]

PROTEINS INVOLVED IN SYNAPTIC RELEASE

The sequence of mechanical events leading to the extrusion of vesicular contents is still not fully understood. Analysis of the molecules involved in the exocytotic process has revealed that the machinery responsible for synaptic docking, activation and fusion is comparable to that of other forms of regulated secretion.[109,193] However, the speed of coupling between activity and opening of the synaptic vesicle suggests that additional elements are involved.

The proteins associated with synaptic vesicles are always present, independently of their neurotransmitter content. Two types of molecule (shown schematically in Fig. 1.19a) necessary for exocytosis are associated with synaptic vesicles or presynaptic plasmalemma. They include integral and peripheral membrane proteins, the latter either

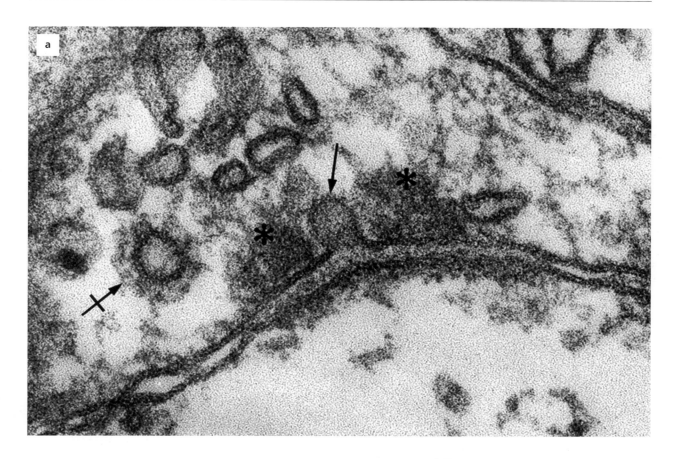

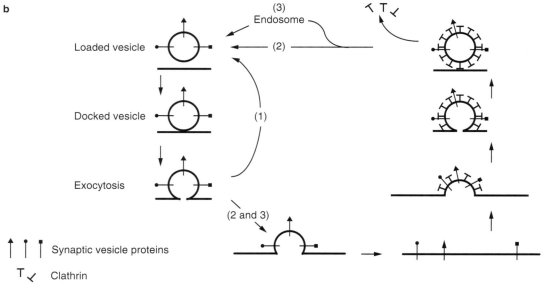

Figure 1.18 *Exocytosis and recycling at central synapses. (a) Synaptic vesicle (arrow) undergoing exocytosis between two presynaptic dense projections (asterisks). Note the presence of a coated vesicle (crossed arrow). (b) Schematic representation of possible recycling pathways in the nerve terminal. A neurotransmitter-loaded vesicle moves to a docking site before releasing its content into the extracellular space. Model 1 predicts that following exocytosis, the vesicle membrane does not collapse into the plasmalemma but releases its content via a transient fusion pore. If the synaptic vesicle membrane does not collapse (models 2 and 3) then the synaptic proteins may be retrieved via clathrin-coated pits and vesicles (model 2) or after fusion to, and resorting from, an early endosome (model 3). (b) Reproduced by permission from Geppert and Sudhof.[137]*

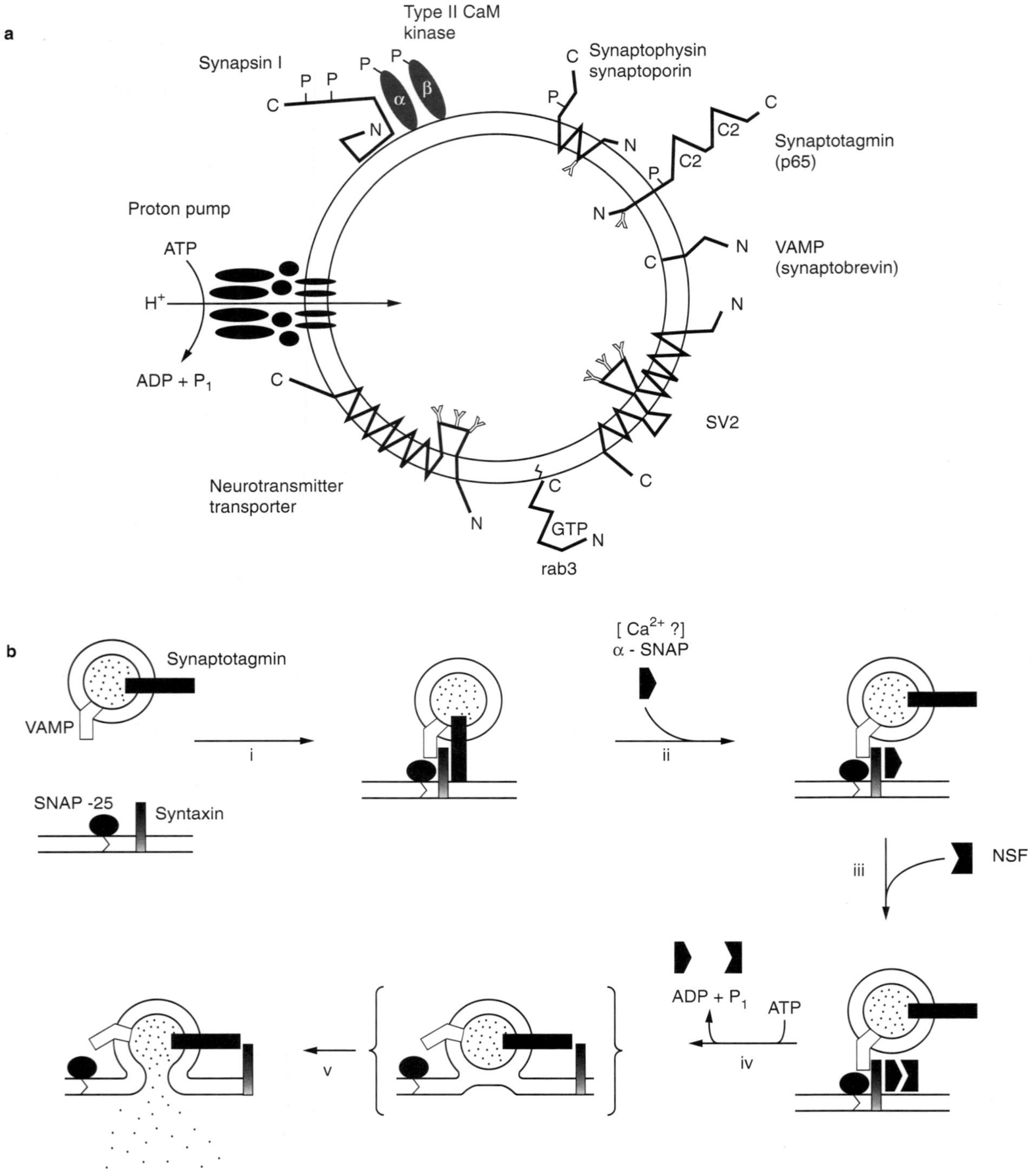

Figure 1.19 *Schematic representations depicting the membrane localization of proteins associated with the synaptic vesicles (a) and the sequence of events leading to docking and membrane fusion (b). The initial docking of the vesicle to the plasma membrane through interactions between VAMP, synaptotagmin, syntaxin and SNAP25 is depicted in step i. To initiate the assembly of the 20S particle, a-SNAP is bound and NSF is able to bind (step iii). The disassembly of the a-SNAP–NSF complex occurs in an ATP-hydrolysis dependent manner (step iv), presumably through the ATPase activity of NSF. A possible partly fused intermediate transition state may precede complete fusion of the membranes. Reproduced by permission from Wendland.[469]*

being amphiphilic or with post-translational modifications.[108,194,469] The integral membrane proteins remain associated with vesicles throughout their cycle, while the peripheral proteins may be associated with the vesicle only during part of it.

Integral membrane proteins

The main proteins included in the membrane of the vesicle involved in exocytosis are synaptotagmin, synaptobrevin and synaptophysin. The synaptotagmin (P65) variants I and II are present in all synaptic vesicles.[244] They are most likely to constitute the Ca^{2+} sensor triggering exocytosis.[136] The synaptobrevins, or vesicle-associated membrane proteins (VAMPs, also called synaptic t-SNARE) are the major substrate for tetanus and botulinum toxins.[361] They increase the catalytic rate, allowing the fusion process necessary for exocytosis.[466] Synaptophysin I and its isoform synaptoporin (synaptophysin II) are redundant and their functions are still not well understood, but their combined deficit in knockout (KO) mice produces impairments in synaptic plasticity (pair pulse facilitation, post-tetanic facilitation and LTP).[196]

Peripheral membrane proteins

Synapsins[178,179,451] exist in five isoforms, synapsin Ia and Ib, synapsin IIa and IIb and synapsin III, which are coded by three genes. According to the initially proposed mode of action, synapsins immobilize synaptic vesicles via a link to the actin-based cytomatrix.[451] Action potential propagation to the synaptic ending by elevating the cytosolic Ca^{2+} would allow a rapid shift from a resting to an active pool. It has recently been shown that Ca^{2+} differentially regulates the activity of synapsins which actually are high-affinity ATP-binding proteins that may have enzymic activity.[178,179] Analysis of KO mice first revealed that synapsins are unnecessary for synaptic vesicle exocytosis and secondly that short-term[350] but not long-term[407] plasticity is impaired in these animals. Another important component is a 25 kDa protein (SNAP-25; synaptosomal associated protein of 25 kDa) which is associated with the cytoplasmic face of the presynaptic plasma membrane.[469] A direct involvement of SNAP-25 in synaptic exocytosis is supported by the fact that it is specifically cleaved by the botulinum toxins A and E.[186] Synaptobrevin-2, syntaxin-1a and SNAP-25 assemble to form a ternary complex also named the core complex. This complex has been crystallized and its ternary structure clarified.[418] This core complex forms during the docking of the synaptic vesicle at the presynaptic plasma membrane, before vesicular opening.[193]

The ras-related small GTP binding (Rab) proteins are also involved in intracellular membrane traffic including exocytosis. Three isoforms of Rab3 are associated with synaptic vesicles. Rab3a is present at all synapses, while Rab3b and c are detected within a subset of terminal endings.[111,244] It has been shown that in synaptosomes Rab3 is associated with synaptic vesicles and separates from them upon stimulation.[111] Rab3a would regulate negatively the late steps of synaptic vesicle fusion with the presynaptic plasma membrane,[137] by activating the effector molecules rabphilin and RIM through GTP-dependent mechanisms.[411,463]

DOCKING AND FUSION OF SYNAPTIC VESICLES

A tempting sequence of molecular interactions and events for docking and liberation of vesicle content, which may well be modified by subsequent discoveries, is proposed in Fig. 1.19b.[386,469] In the case of synaptic vesicles, the vesicle-associated proteins (VAMPs/synaptobrevins) interact with the plasma membrane, with the associated syntaxin, or both.[386] These molecules, together with synaptotagmins, can form complexes, and synaptotagmin is displaced by the addition of cytosolic a-SNAP (soluble NSF attachment protein; NSF: NEM sensitive factor; NEM: N-ethyl-maleimide). The association of a-SNAP with syntaxin would be a calcium-dependent step. As illustrated in Fig. 1.19b, this initial event in the docking is compatible with the inhibitory action of synaptotagmin on exocytosis. These molecular interactions may correspond not only to docking but also to activation that would secondarily lead to exocytosis. Subsequently, NSF interact with a-SNAP, and it has been proposed that the roles of these two molecules would be catalytic, providing energy to promote the fusion process mediated by VAMPs (synaptobrevins) and syntaxins. Then, upon ATP hydrolysis, NSF and a-SNAP would dissociate, leading to fusion of the membrane with still unknown intermediates.[469]

PRESYNAPTIC CALCIUM CHANNELS

A transient rise in intracellular calcium concentration is the starter for the exocytotic event. The delay between entry of Ca^{2+} and transmitter release is very short (200 ms).[249] Since Ca^{2+} diffuses slowly, the localization of calcium channels is critical. A study using confocal microscopy and labelled ω-conotoxin, a molecule that binds specifically to calcium channels,[345] showed that calcium channels are exclusively located at the level of the presynaptic nerve terminal, forming rows perpendicular to the axis of the end-plate which correspond to those of the facing nicotinic receptors. This distribution is consistent with that of the 10-nm large particles seen with freeze fracture and present along the active zone.[323] At the level of the calyx-type presynaptic nerve terminal of the chick ciliary ganglion, using a patch clamp to monitor calcium-channel currents and a luminescent enzymic assay for ACh, it was shown that the opening of a single channel was sufficient to trigger quantal secretion.[412]

Synaptic receptors

Autoradiographic binding studies with agonist and antagonist molecules have provided data on the global distribution of different receptors (receptor mapping), but the spatial resolution of these techniques did not allow a precise subcellular localization, nor have they been sufficient for the identification of receptor subtypes. Since the mid-1980s, *in situ* hybridization and, when appropriate, antibodies have become available, and immunocytochemistry has greatly increased in accuracy.

TYPES OF RECEPTOR: IONOTROPIC VERSUS METABOTROPIC

Binding of a transmitter to its receptor results in a change of ionic conductances. Currently, two large families of receptors can be differentiated on the basis of their physiological modes of action (Fig. 1.20): the ionotropic and the metabotropic receptors.[293] In the first case, the receptor is part of the ion channel molecule and the binding of the ligand induces conformational changes leading to its opening. Physiological responses of these receptors to agonist are very rapid (1 ms or less). The second type involves a receptor molecule coupled to the channel through at least one protein. The gating of the channel is in this case slower (30 ms or more) and can be modulated. Ionotropic and metabotropic receptors often exist for the same neurotransmitter, e.g. glutamate, GABA, serotonin or ACh. Further, various isotypes of subunits exist for all receptors, contributing to their pharmacological properties.

Ionotropic receptors

These respond to molecules such as ACh, glutamate, GABA, glycine or serotonin and their excitatory or inhibitory action is determined by the ions which transit through the channel. The structure of ligand-gated ion channels is comparable (Fig. 1.21) and it has been proposed that these receptors belong to the same superfamily[31,283] of allosteric proteins.[128]

The nicotinic muscular acetylcholine receptor (nAChR) has served as a prototype for ionotropic proteins (Fig. 1.21a, b). AchR, GABA, glycine and serotonin receptors are formed by five homologous subunits. A quasi-symmetrical pentameric complex of transmembrane polypeptides around a central pore has been proposed as the basic quaternary structure for all members of the ion channel receptor superfamily. Each subunit is a topographically oriented glycoprotein with four transmembrane spanning elements (M1 to M4) with the C- and the N-terminus of the molecule being localized extracellularly (Fig. 1.21d). This group of receptors is referred to as the nicotinic receptor subfamily (Fig. 1.21c). The constitutive subunits of the receptor include the one which bears the ligand binding site and may exist in two or three copies, and others which contribute to the formation of the channel and may regulate pharmacological modulations of channel opening kinetics. The subunits and their isotypes have strong homologies, suggesting that they evolve from a common ancestor gene.[31] In the case of the glutamate

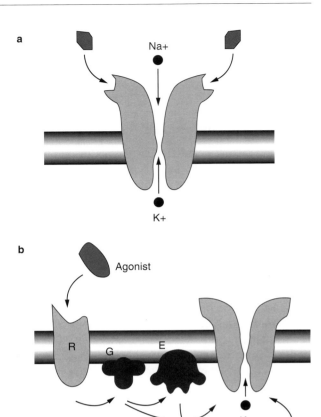

Figure 1.20 *Schematic example of direct (ionotropic) or second messenger-mediated (metabotropic) action of the neurotransmitter molecules. (a) A transmitter such as ACh can act directly on the channel protein, altering it to become permeable to Na⁺ and K⁺. (b) A molecule binds to a receptor (R) and activates a G-protein (G). The activated G-protein regulates the effector, which can be the channel or enzymes (E), which in turn control the intracellular second messengers. Modified by permission from Hall.[151]*

receptor subfamily, the transmembrane organization is not fully determined, but recent data support a model with the C-terminus being located intracellularly.[368] The transmembrane topology of the ionotropic glutamate receptors has three trans-membrane domains, TMD A, TMD B and TMD C, corresponding to the previously proposed M1, M3 and M4, respectively.[177] In this case the domain corresponding to M2 does not span the membrane but rather loops within it, so that its two extremities are intracellular. This domain between TMD A and TMD B therefore contributes to the formation of the channel.

Metabotropic receptors

The metabotropic receptors are a family of molecules coupled to receptors through GTP binding (G-) proteins (Fig. 1.20b).[367] They play a central role in signalling, and more than 100 G-coupled receptors have been cloned and

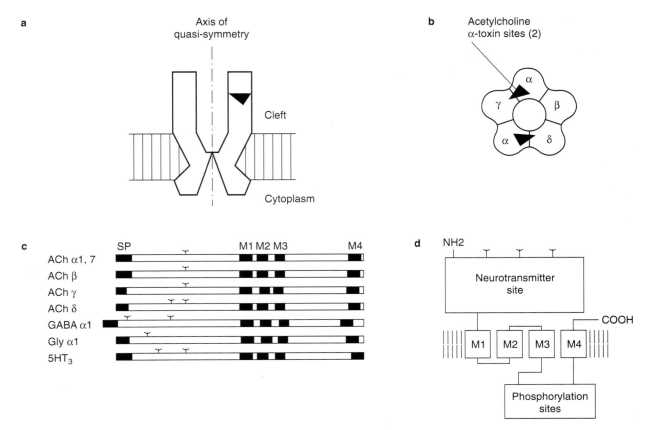

Figure 1.21 *Structural organization of the nicotinic receptor family. (a) Side view of the AChR. By electron image reconstructions the receptor molecule appears as a 11-nm long, 70-nm cylinder, projecting towards the synaptic cleft with a water-filled opening about 2 nm in diameter and 6 nm long, and exposing, towards the cytoplasm, a second 2-nm-diameter opening over about 2 nm. Across the lipid bilayer, it forms a more constricted region about 3 nm long. (b) Possible arrangement of the AChR subunits around the axis of quasi-symmetry delineating the ionic channel. In (a) and (b), the acetylcholine and α-toxin binding sites are located at the boundary between the α- and γ- or δ-subunits. (c) Diagrammatic representation of the primary structure of acetylcholine, glycine, GABA and serotoninergic (5-HT₃) receptor subunits. The sequences are aligned to bring homologous regions into phase; polypeptide lengths are normalized and glycosylation sites are indicated by branched bars. SP: signal peptide, M1–M4: hydrophobic stretches of 19–27 amino acids. (d) Model of transmembrane organization of nicotinic acetylcholine receptor subunits. The large hydrophilic amino-terminal domain of receptor subunits is exposed to the synaptic cleft and carries the neurotransmitter site and glycosylation sites (Y). Each subunit spans the membrane four times (transmembrane segments M1 and M4). The hydrophilic domain separating M3 from M4 faces the cytoplasm. It contains functional phosphorylation sites. Courtesy of Dr JL Galzi and JP Changeux.[128]*

sequenced. In the CNS, they contribute to signal transduction of classic neurotransmitters (e.g. glutamate, GABA, ACh, dopamine) or of neuropeptides (e.g. somatostatin, substance P and many peptidic hormones).

The receptors coupled to the G-proteins are composed of a single glycosylated molecule with seven transmembrane hydrophobic spanning domains and are members of a superfamily of genes.[176] These domains form helices which are linked together by hydrophilic domains. The glycosylated N-terminal domain is on the extracellular side of the membrane while the C-terminus is intracellularly localized.

The G-proteins are heterodimers with α-, β- and γ-subunits having independent and interactive func-

tions.[138] Schematically, the α-subunit binds the GTP and allows the coupling of receptor to the effector. The β- and the γ-subunits modulate the activity of the α-subunits, and contribute to the anchoring of the αβγ complex to the plasma membrane. In the resting states, α, β and γ form a stable complex. The binding of the agonist induces the binding of GTP to the α-subunit, and its subsequent dissociation from the β- and γ-subunits. The dissociated subunit α-GTP and less frequently the βγ-subunits modulate the effector system. The complex cascade of events that follows is reversible. Each molecule of receptor can activate many molecules of G-proteins through the hydrolysis of GTP to GDP. Thus, the intensity of signalling is determined by the relative amounts of receptor and G-proteins.

RECEPTOR SUBTYPES AND CELLULAR ORGANIZATION

Examples of the variability in the cellular distributions of receptors are given below for ACh, glutamate, GABA and glycine.

NICOTINIC ACETYLCHOLINE RECEPTORS

Molecular organization

The nAChR was initially purified from the electric organ of *Torpedo marmorata*. It is composed of four different subunits α, β, γ and δ, with an approximate molecular weight of 55 kDa. The receptor has a $\alpha_2\beta\gamma\delta$ stoichiometric ratio, and the molecular weight of the complex is around 275 kDa. Infrared spectroscopy indicates that the transmembrane portions of the subunits include α-helices and β-sheets. Image analysis and electron microscopy at 0.9 nm resolution[448] showed that the channel is formed by five transmembrane rods around the quasi-symmetrical axis, corresponding to the α-helices of the M2 segment of each subunit.

Cellular organization

The muscle postsynaptic membrane facing a motor neuron axon terminal is deeply enfolded with a thickening of the plasma membrane, a complex cytoskeletal apparatus and an overlaying basal lamina with many molecules specifically accumulated at this level.[152] The distribution of the nAChR was initially analysed with autoradiography using [^{125}I]α-bungarotoxin.[118,152] The quantitative analysis of autoradiograms revealed that receptors are concentrated in front of the presynaptic active zone at the level of the apex of the postsynaptic folds. In this zone the concentration reaches 8–10 000 receptors/μm^2, but it drops rapidly to 10/μm^2 a few micrometres away from the junction.[269] Sodium channels are also accumulated in these areas but, as shown with immunocytochemistry, they predominate in the depth of the postsynaptic folds.[113]

Neuronal acetylcholine receptors

There are two classes of neuronal AChR: ionotropic nicotinic and metabotropic muscarinic receptors. The physiological modulatory role of ACh transmission in the CNS is not fully understood, and it may be involved in some pathological conditions. For example, in Alzheimer's disease, the number of magnocellular neurons in the Meynert nucleus and in the nucleus of the diagonal band, which are the main source of the cortical ACh, is diminished (see Volume II, Chapter 4).[480]

Neuronal nicotinic receptors

The neuronal AChRs are encoded by a family of related genes, ten of which have been identified in rat and chicken neural tissues.[357] These are homologous to the muscle nAChR, and encode molecules with similar transmembrane organization. The similarity between the product of CNS and muscle genes is 40% and approaches 100% in the putative transmembrane domains of the subunits. Seven genes code for α- and three for β-isotypes. The α-subunit may contribute to the binding site. The functional nAChR is a pentamere formed by α- and β-subunits with a putative 2α and 3β stoichiometry,[9] and the combination of isotypes determines pharmacological specificities.[357] Thus, the mapping of the various isotypes of α- and β-subunits (Fig. 1.22) can provide a type of neuronal specificity that could be of great importance in the future development of new drugs.

In the CNS, ACh mediates fast excitation by opening cationic channels, therefore leading to membrane depolarization. Nicotinic responses can be elicited from many areas of the CNS, including the retina, spinal cord, hippocampus, thalamus and cerebral cortex.[284,357] However, synaptic events mediated by nicotinic receptors could only be demonstrated at the connection of motor neuron with Renshaw cells.[293] Various approaches suggest a chiefly presynaptic localization of central nAChR. For example, in the rat interpeduncular nucleus, nAChRs were found on axons from the medial habenula.[284] However, axo-axonal synapses have never been observed on nerve terminals bearing nAChR. This may imply that ACh acts through a paracrine interaction (see section below).

Immunostaining with an antiserum against the AChR β_2-subunit was predominantly on the neuronal perikaryon, dendrites (e.g. cortical pyramidal neurons and cerebellar Purkinje cells) or axons (e.g. in the striatum).[166] Ultrastructurally, the staining was associated with the intracellular and plasma membranes.

Muscarinic receptors

The muscarinic AChRs (mAChRs) are metabotropic and belong to a different gene superfamily. They are coupled to G-proteins, and so far five types, m1 to m5, of muscarinic receptor have been identified. However, their distribution and precise subcellular localization have not been unequivocally established.[454]

GLUTAMATE RECEPTORS

Glutamate is the main excitatory neurotransmitter in the CNS. The glutamate receptors display a high diversity, and three ionotropic families and one metabotropic family have been identified. The variability is increased by the existence of multiple subtypes for each family with different functions and patterns of expression. Activation of glutamate receptors forms the basis for most fast excitatory signalling and also plays a key role in neuronal plasticity and neurotoxicity.[176,288] Glutamate neurotransmission is directly involved in long-term potentiation in the hippocampus and long-term depression in the cerebellum. These changes are currently considered as being the synaptic mechanism underlying learning and memory.[36,266]

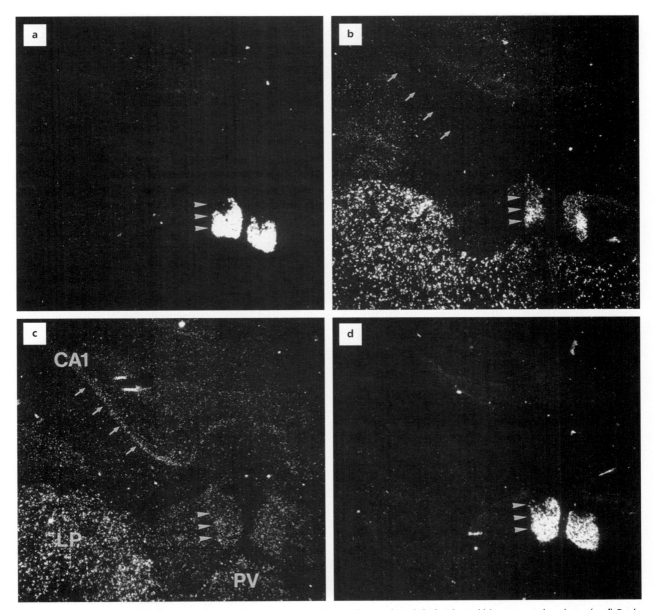

Figure 1.22 *Differential distribution of four different central AChR in the rat dorsal thalamic and hippocampal regions. (a–d) Dark-field emulsion autoradiograms showing the distribution of mRNA encoding for α_3, α_4, β_2 and β_4, respectively. Note that α_4- and β_2-subunit mRNAs are expressed in most areas shown here (with the exception of the CA1 field where only β_2 mRNA is at a detectable level), whereas α_3- and β_4-subunit mRNAs are selectively expressed in the inferior part of the medial habenula. Arrows and arrowheads indicate the pyramidal layer of CA1 hippocampal field and the medial habenula, respectively. CA1: CA1 field of the hippocampal formation; LP: lateral posterior thalamic nucleus; PV: paraventricular thalamic nucleus. Level of section: bregma –3.8 mm. Modified by permission from Hill et al.[166]*

Ionotropic glutamate receptors

Molecular organization

The amino acid glutamate binds to three pharmacologically defined ionotropic receptor subtypes. They are named for their selective agonists: AMPA (α-amino-3-hydroxy-5-methyl-4-isoxazole propionic acid), kainic acid and NMDA[133] (see Chapter 5, this Volume). Cloning and functional expression studies[288,368] revealed that each glutamate receptor subtype comprises multiple subunits.

More precisely, AMPA-sensitive receptors are formed by combinations of six subunits (GluR1 to 7); GluR5–7 actually belong to the kainate family. In addition, these subunits may occur with or without an alternatively spliced exonic sequence of 38 residues between the TMD B and TMD C segments. They are named 'flip' and 'flop', respectively. Moreover, the genomic sequence of GluR2 differs from the cDNA in the coding sequence between TMD A and TMD B. This nucleotide exchange results from RNA editing and produces an arginine (R) instead of a glutamine (Q). The locus of the modification is therefore named the Q/R site. GluR5 and 6 could also be edited, but with a lower efficiency. This single-residue modification within the channel has profound repercussions on the physiology of the receptor complex. The kainate receptors result from the expression of two protomers (GluR5–7) alone or combined with KA1 and KA2. The NMDA receptors are composed of the NR1 subunit combined with NR2A, B, C and D. Here again, alternative splicing generates eight isoforms with distinct physiological properties. One NR3A and two orphan δ_1 and δ_2 subunits have been identified. The latter two are not involved in the formation of functional channels, nor do they modify the function of other subunit combinations. At present, 17 glutamate ionotropic receptor cDNAs have been identified and sequenced. This variability results from six different gene families: a single one for AMPA receptors, two for kainate and three for NMDA. These genes are scattered over numerous chromosomes, and variability is increased by alternative splicing and mRNA editing. However, the subunit composition of synaptic AMPA, kainate and NMDA receptors has not yet been established at any synapse. This point is extremely important since their biophysical properties depend upon the combination of subunits present in the native multimeric protein.[368] Yet, recombinant expression of cDNA has allowed precise functional analysis of pure channel populations. Furthermore, the combination of patch-clamp and reverse transcription–polymerase chain reaction (RT-PCR) techniques showed significant differences in the mRNAs present in a single cell, which were correlated with differences in physiological properties.[40] All of these results, in addition to mapping analysis with *in situ* hybridization, clearly indicate that the physiological and pharmacological properties of native glutamate receptors are correlated with the subunit composition.

Moreover, although the distribution of glutamate ionotropic receptors parallels that of presynaptic glutamate innervation, each neuronal cell type seems to exhibit a proper pattern of subtype expression. This has been shown for neurons in the neostriatum[266] as well as in the cochlear nucleus.[185] Inherited diseases in man have not yet been associated with mutations in ionotropic glutamate receptor genes.

Subcellular distribution of ionotropic glutamate receptors

Ionotropic glutamate receptors are also expressed differentially on the neuronal membrane of single cells. For example, hippocampal pyramidal cells in the CA3 area of the hippocampus, enriched in GluR1–4 and NMDA-R1 subunits,[316] receive multiple excitatory afferent systems with precise dendritic locations. In CA3 pyramidal cells the NMDA-R1 subunits are postsynaptic in the medial segments of apical dendrites, on the receptive surface for commissural fibres, but are absent from proximal apical

dendrites which receive mossy fibre synapses.[381] Both the immunoperoxidase method and the more precise immunogold technique demonstrate that ionotropic AMPA receptors are located on the postsynaptic membrane and are concentrated in front of the presynaptic active zone.[299,316] Some neurological syndromes result from autoantibodies directed against defined types of glutamate receptors, including Rasmussen's encephalitis with autoantibodies against GluR3,[59,347] or against GluR2 in non-familial olivopontocerebellar degeneration,[125] and against various AMPA and kainate receptors in paraneoplastic neurodegenerative syndromes.[126,445] However, the relation between the immunological responses and the clinical symptoms has not yet been established.[163]

Metabotropic glutamate receptors

Molecular organization

The metabotropic glutamate receptors (mGluRs) are a unique and highly heterogeneous class of glutamate receptors coupled to multiple second messenger systems.[176] In addition to the first member (mGluR1),[180,267] there are variants with sequence homologies numbered mGluR2 to 8.[288,319] To add to this variability, spliced variants of mGluR1 named a, b and c also exist. Like other G-coupled proteins, they possess seven transmembrane segments, but they are considerably larger than other similar receptors and have no sequence homology with other G-coupled receptors.[367]

Pharmacological responses of this subfamily of glutamate receptor are plentiful, indicating that they are involved in a large number of neuronal operations. The cellular response to glutamate depends upon the subtypes of receptors.[288] According to their pharmacology, G-protein coupling and sequence relations, they have been divided into three groups. Group I (mGluR1 and mGluR5) activate phospholipase C, induce the formation of IP_3 and stimulate the mobilization of internal calcium, while group II (mGluR2 and mGluR3) and group III (mGluR4, mGluR6, mGluR7 and mGluR8) inhibit forskolin-stimulated cyclic adenosine monophosphate (cAMP) formation.[140,287,305,320,367]

Subcellular distribution of metabotropic glutamate receptors

Metabotropic glutamate receptors of group I are found at postsynaptic sites, while those of groups II and III can be presynaptic or postsynaptic.[47,289,320]

The metabotropic glutamate receptors of group I, mGluR1a[265] and mGluR5,[378] were initially found to be postsynaptic in Purkinje cells. As for the ionotropic glutamate receptors, autoantibodies against mGluR1 induce a specific cerebellar disease: paraneoplastic cerebellar ataxia.[382] Immunogold labelling indicates that mGluR1a and mGluR5 are accumulated at the periphery of the postsynaptic differentiation, and are also detected at a distance from all synaptic contacts.[19,257] Group I, metabotropic glutamate receptors, are stabilized by a PDZ domain molecule named homer (see section below).[49,444] The physiological importance of this perisynaptic organization is not established. However, mGluR is activated with high-frequency stimulation of the presynaptic fibres, but only produces a weak response at low frequency.[277] It has, therefore, been hypothesized that the low amount of released glutamate following low-frequency stimulation would be sufficient to activate synaptically located ionotropic receptors, but not perisynaptic G-coupled receptors.

Group II mGluR2 and mGluR3 subunits are present in the cerebellum, in some Golgi cells, and not only in the somato-dendritic compartment, but also in axon terminals. Metabotropic glutamate receptors of group III also exhibit a complex pattern of distribution. mGluR7 is a good example. It is mainly presynaptic and concentrated at the active zone and in the hippocampus and it was found to be apposed to mGluR1-positive interneurons.[47,377] In the olfactory bulb and locus coeruleus, mGluR7 has been detected at the postsynaptic level.[210,212]

RECEPTORS TO INHIBITORY AMINO ACIDS

In the mammalian CNS, GABA and glycine are the major inhibitory neurotransmitters.[25] Mature GABA and glycine receptors are distinct molecular entities with specific pharmacology, the action of the latter being selectively antagonized by the convulsant alkaloid strychnine. In the spinal cord, glycine mediates its inhibitory effects on the postsynaptic target cells through activation of a specific glycine-dependent chloride conductance.[42] In contrast, GABA has more complex actions. The presynaptic action is due to a weak depolarization of the nerve terminal membrane that blocks the propagation of action potentials.[484] The postsynaptic effect results from the opening of a chloride conductance that hyperpolarizes the target membrane.[42] The GABA$_B$ receptor acts to open K$^+$ or close Ca^{2+} channels via G-proteins and can regulate presynaptically the transmitter release.[46] In contrast, the GABA$_A$ receptor is a ligand-gated chloride ion channel, modulated by barbiturates, benzodiazepines, steroids and ethanol, which primarily generates inhibitory postsynaptic potentials.[306]

GABA$_A$ receptors

Molecular organization

Biochemical and molecular biological studies show that the GABA$_A$ receptor belongs to the superfamily of ligand-gated ion channels and thus probably displays a pentameric structure arising from the assembly of several different subunits.[31] Molecular cloning studies have identified seven types of subunit (α, β, γ, δ, ϵ, π and τ) with around 40% peptidic identity, including isoforms (α_1–α_6, β_1–β_3, γ_1–γ_3) with 70–80% identity.[471] The combination of subunits creates GABA$_A$ receptors with

different pharmacological and electrophysiological characteristics.[165] Strikingly, the γ_2-subunit, which is an integral component of the native GABA$_A$ receptor, is required for benzodiazepine sensitivity, although α-subunits primarily bear the benzodiazepine binding site.[165] Impairment of GABAergic neurotransmission involving GABA$_A$ receptors, thus reducing inhibition, has been described in cortical dysfunction in man or in mouse models of human pathologies, including temporal lobe epilepsy[117,256] and focal cortical malformations.[338]

The GABA$_C$ receptors are another class of ionotropic GABA receptors with distinct electrophysiological and pharmacological properties,[41,105] being formed of ρ-subunits.[41,321] They have specific pharmacological features since they are insensitive to benzodiazepines and barbiturates and are not blocked by the GABA$_A$ receptor antagonist bicuculline.[104] In contrast, they are specifically activated by the GABA analogue cis-aminocrotonic acid (CACA)[104] and blocked by the competitive inhibitor, TPMPA (1,2,5,6-tetrahydropyridine-4-methylphosphinic acid).[327] Although they were initially found in the retina,[74] their presence was later reported in the superior colliculus and hippocampus.[43]

Subtypes and cellular organization of GABA$_A$ receptors

On central neurons, the subcellular distribution of GABA$_A$ receptor subunits varies according to isotype,[20] thus contributing to the pharmacological heterogeneity of the neuronal membrane. However, postembedding immunogold studies have shown that the GABA$_A$ receptors are highly enriched in the postsynaptic membrane. Subunits α_1 and $\beta_{2/3}$ were detected postsynaptically at both synaptic differentiations and extrasynaptic membranes in the cerebellar cortex.[20,298,387,388] In contrast, the α_6-subunit was found only at synaptic sites on granule cells of the cerebellum.[20] The $\beta_{2/3}$-subunit was also detected on the presynaptic membrane at axodendritic and axo-somatic contacts in the rat substantia nigra and globus pallidus or in the dendate gyrus.[300,342] An interesting observation of differential distribution at a single cell level is to be found at hippocampal pyramidal cells, where the α_2-subunit is localized on the initial segment of axon and the α_1-subunit is found at synapses on the soma and on dendrites.[301]

Glycine receptors

Glycine, the smallest and simplest amino acid is, after GABA, one of the most abundant inhibitory neurotransmitters in the CNS.[25] In addition to its inhibitory role, glycine may facilitate excitatory transmission in the brain by potentiating the response to glutamate of the NMDA receptor.[200] As an inhibitory transmitter, glycine predominates in the spinal cord and brainstem,[482] and is mainly involved in the inhibition of motor neurons through their recurrent collateral network. In mice, mutations of various subunits of the glycine receptor (GlyR) are responsible for motor diseases characterized by exaggerated startle reflexes.[32] In man, the GlyR α_1-subunit gene (see below, Molecular organization of the GlyR) is mutated in the familial hyperekplexia or startle disease, hereditary neurological disorder.[11,376] These observations underline the role of the glycine receptor in the control of movements, since this disease is characterized by marked and sustained muscle hypertonia and by an exaggerated startle reflex which persists throughout life. Cases of hyperekplexia-like syndromes not involving the GlyR α_1-subunit gene have also been described,[456] involving other α- or β-subunit genes.[32]

Molecular organization of the GlyR

The GlyR is composed of two major polypeptides of 48 kDa (α) and 58 kDa (β), the binding site being associated with the α-subunit.[25,31] Sedimentation and cross-linking experiments suggest that the purified GlyR is composed of three α- and two β-subunits, ($\alpha_3\beta_2$), this stoichiometry with five subunits being comparable with that of the nAChR.[31] The subunit composition is determined by sequences in the first half of the N-terminal domain[232] and the sequence of assembly of GlyR as well as the post-translational modifications required for the transit from one intracellular compartment to another have been determined.[149]

A strong homology and a similar structural organization of the α- and β-subunits were revealed by cDNA sequencing.[25,32,455] Both proteins possess a putative cleavable signal sequence, a large hydrophilic extracellular domain, four hydrophobic membrane-spanning segments (M1 to M4), and an extended cytoplasmic domain between the third and fourth transmembrane regions. The M3–M4 intracellular loop of the GlyR β-subunit interacts with gephyrin, contributing to the stabilization of the GlyR at the postsynaptic domain (see below).

Glycine receptor a-subunit subtypes

Subtype heterogeneity of the glycine receptor was first detected during development of the rat spinal cord.[25,31] There, a neonatal α-isoform prevalent at birth differs from the adult isoform by a lower strychnine binding affinity. Within 2–3 weeks after birth, this form is progressively replaced in spinal cord by the adult form of receptor. This heterogeneity was confirmed by DNA sequencing data. A novel GlyR subunit, designated α_2 and isolated from human and rat cDNA libraries, displayed about 80% amino acid identity with the α_1-subunit. In addition, an α_3-isoform has been isolated from a rat brain cDNA library and a novel α_4-subunit from a mouse genomic library.[32] So far, no variants of the β-subunit have been detected. Additional diversity results from alternative splicing of α_1-, α_2- and β-subunits. Further, a rat α_2 variant (α_{2^*}) has been identified, and forms homomeric receptors

with low strychnine affinity corresponding to the neonatal isoform.[32]

Synaptic distribution and cellular organization of GlyR

Once the GlyR had been purified, monoclonal antibodies raised against the receptor revealed a patchy immunoreactivity at the neuronal surface in the ventral horn of the rat spinal cord and in the goldfish brainstem (Fig. 1.23).[25,369,440] A comparable punctate distribution was found in many regions of the CNS, including neurons in the spinal cord, cerebellum, cochlear nucleus or olfactory bulb of the rat or on the Mauthner (M-) cell of teleosts.[25] Ultrastructurally, immunoperoxidase and immunogold labelling has demonstrated that the receptors and the associated gephyrin (see section below) are concentrated on the postsynaptic membrane adjacent to the presynaptic release site (Fig. 1.24). Glycine-activated chloride channels have the same extension as the postsynaptic differentiation, and form functional microdomains at the surface of the target cell. These microdomains exhibit a somato-dendritic gradient comparable to that seen for the presynaptic active zones on the Mauthner cells,[417,442] on neurons of the goldfish brainstem (Fig. 1.23b) and on the motor neuron of the rat spinal cord.[122] This topological organization may be an important structural feature for neuronal integration, since larger patches of receptor may lead to an increased inhibition. *In vitro* experiments in which controlled inhibitory innervation was added to purified motor neurons have allowed the direct demonstration that the formation of the GlyR-enriched postsynaptic microdomains depends directly on the chemical nature of the presynaptic innervation.[242] The activity of the GlyR is needed to promote the GlyR microdomains, since treatment with the antagonist strychnine prevents their formation.[214,243]

RECEPTOR LOCALIZATIONS: CLUSTERED AND/OR DIFFUSE

A key question in synaptic signalling and the neuronal integration of afferent signals is whether postsynaptic receptors are clustered facing sites of transmitter release, or whether they are diffusely distributed on the membrane of the postsynaptic neuron. Local specialization of the postsynaptic somato-dendritic membrane is a central issue for two reasons: first, many active molecules are involved in neurotransmission, and secondly, receptors may exist as ionotropic and metabotropic with various isoforms having distinct physiological and pharmacological properties.

Some neurotransmitters, such as glycine or glutamate, are also intermediate cellular metabolites and are present at relatively low concentrations in the extracellular fluid. Therefore, receptors for these molecules have to be accumulated in front, or in the immediate vicinity of the presynaptic release sites in order to face the highest con-

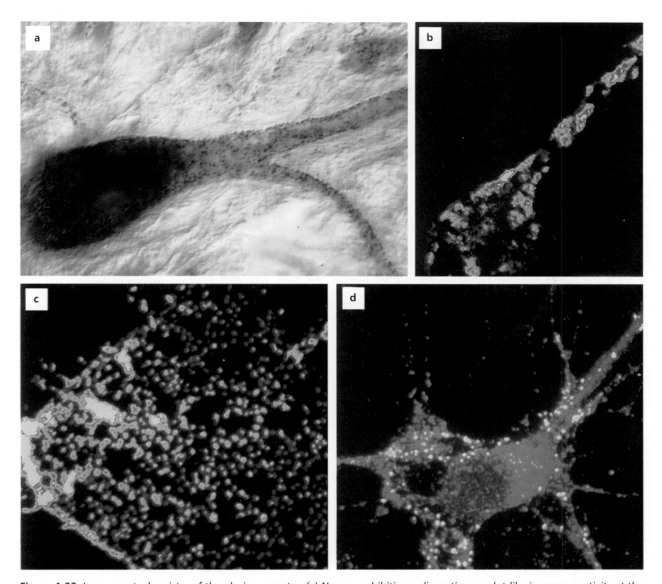

Figure 1.23 *Immunocytochemistry of the glycine receptor. (**a**) Neuron exhibiting a discontinuous dot-like immunoreactivity at the dendritic level. The immunoreactivity was enhanced with nickel and cobalt salt. (**b**) Colour-coded immunofluorescence illustrating larger patches of receptors on a dendritic process. (**c**) Clusters of receptors are disposed over the surface of the soma of this large neuron; (**a–c**) are from the brainstem reticulata of goldfish. (**d**) Example of spinal neuron kept in culture for 10 days and expressing clusters of receptors at its surface; (**b–d**) obtained with confocal microscopy.*

centration of agonist molecule during activation of the presynaptic ending. Alternatively, other molecules such as GABA are not involved in cellular metabolism, leaving open the question of their localization. Biological amines, such as ACh or serotonin, may be released at a distance from the target membrane. In this 'volume transmission', the receptors might be distributed in large patches or all along the membrane. Studies of serotonin receptors (5-HTR), using antibodies against the 5-HT$_{1A}$R, have provided evidence for this. In the dorsal raphe nucleus, the immunoperoxidase reaction product was not patchy but localized along the neuronal surface, outlining the contours of cell bodies and dendrites in an uneven, but continuous manner (Fig. 1.25). Double

labelling with anti-serotonin and 5-HT$_{1A}$R has shown that these receptors, in the dorsal raphe nucleus, are autoreceptors.[399] Another complex situation is the co-localization of neurotransmitters: in this case the postsynaptic receptors may form a mosaic, or may have differential distribution, one type being in the centre and the other at the periphery of the postsynaptic membrane facing the sites of release.

IMMOBILIZATION OF RECEPTORS

In the neuromuscular junction and in most of the central synapses, receptors are clustered in high concentrations on the postsynaptic membrane facing the sites of

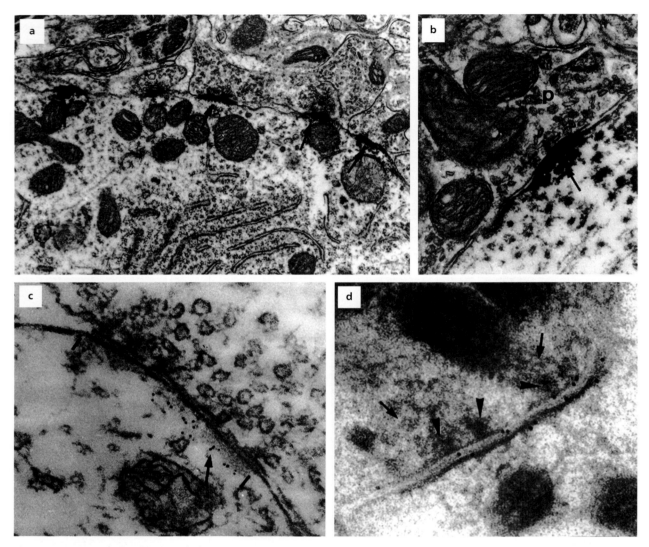

Figure 1.24 *Synaptic localization of glycine receptor in the ventral horn of the rat spinal cord. (a, b) Immunoperoxidase reaction showing accumulation of the glycine receptor-associated gephyrin (arrows) at postsynaptic differentiations in front of the boutons containing pleomorphic vesicles (p). High- and low-power magnifications, respectively. (c) Pre-embedding immunogold (5-nm particles) detection of the gephyrin (arrows) within the limit of the synaptic complex (between the bars). (d) Postembedding immunogold (10-nm particles) detection of an extracellular epitope on the transmembrane components of the receptor. The tissue was cryoembedded in a lowicryl resin. The presynaptic element can be identified by the presence of small vesicles (arrows) and of presynaptic dense projections (arrowheads). Modified from Triller et al.[440]*

presynaptic transmitter release. This is constantly the case for the GlyR, and also for some subtypes of glutamate and GABA receptors. This precise localization at defined loci of the plasmalemma of the target cell raises the problem of the biogenesis and maintenance of the postsynaptic membrane. This problem was initially studied at the neuromuscular junction and then applied to central synapses, first at the glycinergic and then at the GABA and glutamatergic connections.

Neuromuscular junction

At the neuromuscular junction, various factors contribute to the localization of nAChR. These include neurally derived molecules and elements of the postsynaptic cytoskeleton, including agrin and the 43 kDa nicotinic associated protein.

Agrin

The synaptic basal lamina differs from the rest of the basal lamina that surrounds the muscle fibres in that it contains agrin, which is able to induce nAChR clustering. Agrin is synthesized by motor neurons, secreted at the axon terminal and included in the basal lamina. Muscles also synthesize and secrete agrin, which is also integrated into the basal lamina. The agrin gene codes for multiple different proteins generated by alternative splicing. Functional

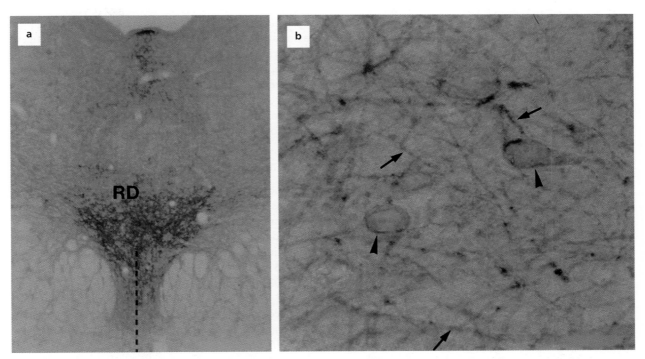

Figure 1.25 *Immunohistochemistry of 5-HT$_{1A}$ receptors. (a) Neurons in the raphe dorsalis exhibiting immunoreactivity (RD). The midline is indicated by a broken line. (b) High magnification showing a continuous but uneven labelling of the perikaryal (arrowhead) and dendritic (arrows) membrane.*

analysis has revealed that two sites underlie the activity of the molecule, the most important one being present in neuronal agrin splice variants.[151]

Analysis of the distribution of agrin splice variants with *in situ* hybridization and PCR indicates that neurons other than motor neurons also express active forms of agrins. Whether or not this molecule is involved in receptor aggregation at neuron–neuron synapses is still open to question.

Other presynaptic molecules may contribute to the appropriate localization of receptors at the end-plate. One of them, named ARIA (AchR inducing activity),[198] stimulates the synthesis of muscle nAChR, and also promotes the formation and the maintenance of postsynaptic components at appropriate sites.[99] Another example is CGRP (calcitonin gene-related peptide) which is synthesized by motor neurons and is involved, among other factors, in the compartmentalization of nAChR gene expression during end-plate development.[92]

The 43-kDa protein

An extrinsic membrane protein of 43 kDa, closely associated with the nAChR, was initially purified from the *Torpedo* electric organ, and it is strictly co-localized with the receptor.[92] The removal of the 43-kDa protein by alkaline treatment increased the rotational and lateral motility of the nAChR.[60] The 43-kDa protein, which is beneath the channel pore, interacts with the β-subunit of the receptor.[118] However, it must be stressed that the

nAChR–43-kDa complex is also stabilized by other interactions with the submembranous cytoskeleton, including actin and other molecules belonging to the spectrin/dystrophin family.[118] Whether or not the 43-kDa protein is involved in nAChR clustering during synaptogenesis still remains to be clarified, but it is likely to stabilize the receptor clusters once they have formed.[60]

Inhibitory glycinergic and GABAergic synapses

In the CNS, receptor clustering in front of the presynaptic active zone was initially documented for the glycine receptor. Immunocytochemistry has revealed that clusters of transmembrane α- and/or β-subunits appear progressively at the neuronal surface and that they are contemporaneous with the formation of synaptic contacts.[25]

In contrast to the α- and the β-subunits of the glycine receptor, the 93-kDa polypeptide is a non-glycosylated peripheral membrane protein.[217] This polypeptide, named gephyrin, binds with high affinity to polymerized tubulin[217] and has been localized by immunoelectron microscopy (Fig. 1.24b, c) at the cytoplasmic face of glycinergic postsynaptic membranes (Fig. 1.24a–c).[25] Within the CNS, these gephyrin transcripts are found in most regions of the brain, including those that do not express the glycine binding α-subunit.[216] This distribution, revealed by *in situ* hybridization, coincides with that of the β-subunit. These observations raise the possibility that gephyrin may have a function comparable with that of the 43-kDa peptide associated with the nAChR.[60]

The importance of gephyrin for the organization of the postsynaptic membrane was tested: inhibition of gephyrin synthesis by antisense depletion[218] or gene knockout in mice[107] led to the absence of GlyR clusters at the neuronal surface.

In either case, these results demonstrate unambiguously that gephyrin plays a central role in the formation of glycine-enriched microdomains at the neuronal surface. Gephyrin stabilizes the glycine receptors at synapses by binding to microtubules,[215] and acts as a dominant localization signal for the GlyR β-subunit.[220] However, the function of gephyrin is probably more complex owing to the high number of splice variants generated from the gephyrin gene[322] and which are highly heterogeneous in their binding to the GlyR β-subunit.[274] Other molecules were found, with yeast two-hybrid screen or GST pulldown assays, to bind to gephyrin. Collybistin, a GDP–GTP exchange factor, was identified, and co-transfection experiments have demonstrated that it promoted the transfer of gephyrin to the plasma membrane.[211] The actin monomere binding protein profilin was also identified as being a possible partner of gephyrin, and the gephyrin–profilin interaction could be involved in the regulation of GlyR cluster size.[262] The kinase RAFT1 (rapamycin and FKBP12 target protein) may act as a regulator of mRNA translation in dendrites.[353] High levels of GlyR α-subunit mRNAs were found in dendrites,[326] the translation of which could then be regulated specifically at glycinergic synapses.

Although a direct association of gephyrin to GABA receptor could not be demonstrated *in vivo*, a good demonstration of the role of gephyrin in the postsynaptic accumulation of GABA receptor was obtained from KO mice.[98,221] Analysis of the mutant in which the GABAR γ2-subunit gene was invalidated indicated that this subunit was responsible for the synaptic localization of the heteromeric GABAR through an interaction with gephyrin.[98] The GABAR γ2-subunit also binds to a microtubule-associated protein named GABARAP (GABA receptor-associated protein).[462] Similarly, in the retina, the GABAc receptor subunit ρ1 binds to MAP1-B.[154] Yet the interplay between glycine, GABA receptor, gephyrin and GABARAP is far from being understood. Experiments in which cholinergic, GABAergic, glycinergic or mixed glycine/GABAergic innervation were provided to cultured motor neurons indicated that given receptors accumulated only under the endings with matching neurotransmitters, despite the fact that gephyrin formed a subsynaptic matrix under any of these chemically defined synapses.[242] It is still not known how the gephyrin variants[274] are involved in the acquisition of this synaptic specificity. Impairment of gephyrin function may be responsible for a paraneoplastic stiff-man syndrome (SMS), which is characterized by chronic rigidity, spasms and autoimmunity against synaptic antigens. These paraneoplastic syndromes occur in association with cancer but do not result from the tumour or compression by metastasis.[79] Much evidence indicates that SMS are associated with autoimmunity to neural antigens impairing synaptic inhibition such as GAD[275] or amphiphysin.[80] Recently, a case was reported[56] in which SMS resulted from an autoimmunity to gephyrin. The motor symptoms observed in this case are in line with the function of gephyrin as a stabilizer of glycine and GABA receptors.

Glutamatergic synapses

The molecular analysis of excitatory postsynaptic densities has demonstrated the presence of a family of proteins containing PDZ domains and being involved in the assembly and regulation of the postsynaptic microdomains. The most important among these proteins are the SAP90/PSD95 family (SAP97/hDlg, SAP102 and Chapsyn110/PSD103), CASK, GRIP/ABP, S-SCAM, Mint1 and PICK1.[71,131,132] The PDZ domain is a common 90-amino-acid sequence present in PSD95/SAP90, DLG and ZO1. The structure of PDZ domains of SAP90/PSD95, SAP97/hDlg CASK has been unravelled by X-ray crystallography.[77,90] The PDZ domain binds to short specific sequences with a 10–100-μM affinity to short peptide sequences which are found almost always at the C-terminus of interacting proteins and the PDZ binding domain.[132,208] All of the SAP90/PSD95 family members have some structural features in common: they contain three N-terminal PDZ domains, a Src-homology 3 (SH3) domain and a C-terminal inactive guanylate kinase (GK) domain. In yeast, two hybrids, the cytoplasmic C-terminus of the K+ channel and of the NR2 subunit of the NMDA receptor, were found to interact with the second and first PDZ domains of SAP90/PSD95.[207,228] The kainate KA1 and KA2 subunits interact with the SH3 and GK domains of SAP90/PSD95.[129] In addition, SAP90/PSD95 interacts with neuroligin through the third PDZ domain, and with FAS2.[190,432] The postsynaptic receptor cluster formation is driven by the capacity of the SAP90/PSD95 family members to polymerize through their N-terminus domains and to anchor to the plasma membrane through the palmitoylation of N-terminal cystein residues.[181,436] The SAP90/PSD95 PDZ domains interact with the microtubule-associated protein CRIPT.[294] Further, the SAP90/PSD95 is indirectly bound via its GK domain to the subsynaptic actin cytoskeleton through indirect interactions involving GKAP/SAPAP, ProSAP/Shank and cortactin.[132] Therefore, SAP90/PSD95 can be considered as being a genuine scaffold protein involved in the anchoring of receptor to cytoskeleton but also in defining the locus of presynaptic–postsynaptic interaction (see below).

The AMPA GluR2 and GluR3 subunits bind to PDZ domains of GRIP1, GRIP2/ABP (AMPA-receptor binding protein),[87,410] which both contain seven PDZ domains, and PICK1,[477] which contains a single PDZ domain. Another AMPA-receptor interacting protein, SAP97, specifically binds to the AMPA-receptor GluR1 subunit.[355] The interaction of GRIP1, GRIP2/ABP and SAP97 with the underlying cytoskeleton is not as strong as the one of the NMDA receptor with SAP90/PSD95. This may reflect the mobility of AMPA receptor seen during plastic modifications of the postsynaptic membrane composition in processes such as long-term potentiation and depression (see below).

ADHESION, SYNAPSE FORMATION AND SYNAPTIC PLASTICITY

The adhesive processes probably play a key role in the correct matching between the presynaptic and postsynaptic elements. These types of interaction at synapses involve homophilic cadherin–cadherin and heterophilic neurexin–neuroligin interactions. Both neurexins[279] and cadherins[372,478] display a high variability that may account for the chemical complementarity between the presynaptic bouton and the apposed postsynaptic membrane, thus being involved in a 'synaptic adhesive code'.[372]

Cadherins

More than 80 members of the cadherin family have been identified so far. Most of them have a single transmembrane stretch and an extracellular domain with characteristic calcium-binding sequence motifs, which varies from one cadherin to another.[425] A structure–function analysis of cell adhesion by neural (N) cadherin has revealed that cadherins may exist in a stable monomeric or dimeric form and that their lateral dimerization increases their intercellular adhesivity.[426] As cadherins are involved in homophilic interactions, the variability of the cadherin structure and the regulation of adhesiveness by dimerization may provide a switchable 'key–lock' code for the stabilization of complex network. The intracellular domains that are conserved among cadherins interact with catenin P120 and β-catenin. The latter binds with α-catenin which itself associates with cytoskeletal compounds.[478] Classic cadherins and associated catenins are found at synaptic junctions bordering the active zones.[446] They are symmetrically distributed on the presynaptic and postsynaptic elements. The various classes of cadherins have specific patterns of distribution in the brain, delineating neural pathways.[419] Cadherin accumulation at neuro-neuronal contacts is one of the first steps in synapse formation, and it has been proposed that the differential distribution of cadherins and homophilic interaction would 'lock in' the newly formed synaptic contact.[100] During synaptogenesis in the hippocampus, N-cadherin and β-catenin are found in axons and dendrites. Subsequently, they are clustered at all synaptic sites. Later on, N-cadherin is detected only at excitatory synaptic contacts, while β-catenins are present at both excitatory and inhibitory synapses, which therefore may contain another type of cadherin.[29]

Regulation of the adhesion process at synapses is also involved in plastic modification of transfer of information between neurons in the hippocampus, as observed during LTP. Modifications of the homophilic cadherin–cadherin interactions with extracellularly applied antibodies or peptides lead to an impairment of LTP.[428]

Other cell-surface molecules of the cadherin family, referred to as protocadherins or cadherin-related neuronal receptors (CNR), have been identified. They have the same gross structure as classic cadherins, and their intracellular domains interact with Fyn tyrosine kinase. Unlike classic cadherins, CNR are localized at the active zone.[223] Mice lacking Fyn have deficits in their LTP at excitatory synapses, GABAergic synapses are abnormal and they have deficits in the neuronal migration.[478] Arcadlin, a member of the CNR, was initially identified as an immediate-early gene, the expression of which is induced by NMDA-dependent LTP. Antibodies against arcadlin reduced the excitatory response and blocked LTP induction.[479] It was therefore proposed that this protocadherin could also be involved in the activity-dependent structural reorganization of the synapse.

Neurexin–neuroligin

Neurexins which bind to neuroligins at synapses constitute a family of molecules which display a very high variability: more than 1000 variants can be generated from three different genes, alternative promoters and alternative splicing.[279] Both neurexins and neuroligins have a single transmembrane domain, and contain at their intracellular N-terminus a sequence which is able to interact with PDZ domains. On the presynaptic side, neurexins may interact with CASK, a scaffolding protein which contains kinase-like and PDZ domains.[158] CASK is present on both sides of the synapse and forms a complex with molecules such as Velis and Mint1, but on the presynaptic side indirect evidence indicates that this complex interacts with vesicular fusion machinery.[57] Neurexin may also bind directly to synaptotagmin, a synaptic vesicle protein.[159] Neuroligins, which are concentrated at the active zone of most glutamatergic, but not GABAergic synapses,[389] interact through their PDZ binding domain with the third PDZ domain of SAP90/PSD95.[190] PSD95/SAP90 is a postsynaptic scaffolding protein which contributes to the stabilization of the NMDA-type glutamate receptor at the synapse (see above). Neurexins bind to neuroligin (neurexin-1β and neuroligin-1) and may function as heterophilic adhesion molecules;[188,189,292] the specificity is most likely to depend on the structure of their extracellular domains.

It has been shown *in vitro* that the expression of neuroligin is sufficient to provoke the differentiation of the presynaptic element:[360] in these experiments, the expression of neuroligin-1 or -2 by fibroblasts determined the formation of functional presynaptic differentiation. This was mediated through an interaction with neurexin-1β. It is highly probable that this effect resulted from the recruitment by neurexin-1β of a presynaptic scaffold containing the CASK molecule. It was then postulated[335] that, in turn, the presynaptic neurexin-1β could, by interacting with neuroligin, induce the formation of a glutamate receptive membrane containing PSD95, thus leading to the accumulation of NMDA receptors.

These co-ordinated molecular interactions allowing the formation of a transcellular macromolecular complex and subsequent differentiation of the presynaptic and postsynaptic membrane are compatible with rapid synapse formation, a process which was demonstrated, at least for glutamatergic synapses, to last for less than 1–2 h.[115] This rapid formation of synapses is probably facilitated by the preassembled presynaptic components[2] and postsynaptic preassembled microdomains containing receptors and scaffolding molecules.[242,303,336]

Paracrine signalling: volume transmission

Neuronal networks in sensory and motor systems are organized in a very precise manner, and constitute the 'point-to-point' systems.[397] Their functions are based on the precision of the axonal wiring and the consequent synaptic specificity. In 'point-to-point' systems, the numerical relationship between a projecting neuron and its targets does not go beyond one to several hundreds, and the synaptic junction is considered to be the only valid site for chemical transmission. Conversely, neuronal networks in modulatory systems, termed 'global' or 'diffuse' systems,[397] are characterized by the ratio between a remarkably small number of projecting neurons and an extremely large number of target cells. Neurons in these systems can communicate in a widespread but still organized manner, where their modulatory action may be exerted through paracrine release of their neuroactive compounds into the extracellular space. These compounds diffuse locally for some distances to affect numerous target cells equipped with adequate receptors. In the wider concept of 'volume transmission', neuronal communication occurs not only through paracrine but also through endocrine signalling, the latter operating via the blood circulation.[121]

The synaptic communication in global or diffuse systems can be as fast as in point-to-point systems, although in general it is a much slower process. This slow rate also characterizes the neuronal systems using neuropeptides as neuroactive messengers. Both the onset of the response (from a few milliseconds in classical transmission to several hundreds) and its duration (it can last for seconds, or even hours) are much slower. By this criterion, neuropeptidergic systems, also of modulatory action, can be included in the global systems. Finally, another common point is that in monoaminergic and neuropeptidergic systems the postsynaptic receptor is not directly related to an ion channel but belongs to the category of G-protein-linked receptors.

NON-JUNCTIONAL VERSUS JUNCTIONAL AXON TERMINALS: MORPHOLOGICAL CORRELATES OF PARACRINE AND SYNAPTIC SIGNALLING, RESPECTIVELY

The ultrastructural studies of Descarries and Beaudet,[23,85] have shown that the monoaminergic innervation in the CNS can follow two different modalities depending on the territory of innervation. In some regions such as the cerebral cortex monoaminergic axons do not establish synaptic contacts or junctional complexes (non-junctional innervation),[85] whereas in other regions such as the subcommissural organ the terminals form junctional complexes.[22] The cerebellar cortex has a non-junctional modality of innervation. Neither tyrosine hydroxylase-immunoreactive axons, even in weaver mutant cerebellum with numerous free postsynaptic specializations (Fig. 1.26),[1] nor those able to up take tritiated 5-HT, establish synaptic junctions.[24] These ultrastructural features of noradrenergic and serotoninergic innervation of the cerebellum match with the modulatory role reported with electrophysiological methods. For instance, it is known that noradrenaline potentiates the inhibition of Purkinje cells elicited by the release of GABA, and provokes the increase in spontaneous inhibitory synaptic currents of basket and stellate cells.[246] Hence, the morphological bimodality observed in monoaminergic systems has been considered to represent the two different types of chemical neuronal signalling, the junctional modality being the correlate of synaptic interactions, and the non-junctional modality corresponding to paracrine signalling.

Coexistence of neuroactive substances in neurons

Dale et al.,[76] following their demonstration that ACh is released from motor nerves, suggested that neurons synthesize and release the same messenger molecules at all of their terminals (a notion later called 'Dale's principle'). Dale's ideas can be viewed as the metabolic correlate of the neuron theory: neurons not only are anatomically independent, but also represent metabolic units. Therefore, each neuron has its own cellular organization and its own biochemical properties, which underlie a common mechanism for chemical synaptic transmission at all of its axonal terminals. This metabolic unity of the neuron has since been interpreted and extended in several ways, the most commonly accepted view being that each neuron is able to synthesize and release only one transmitter; this idea was never stated by Dale but became almost axiomatic until the beginning of the 1980s.

ANATOMICAL EVIDENCE OF COEXISTENCE OF NEUROTRANSMITTERS

The number of neuroactive compounds presumably used by neurons in chemical communication has increased

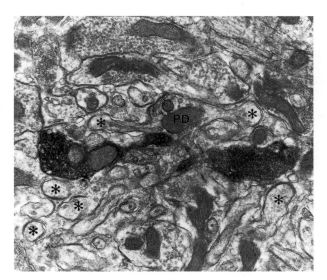

Figure 1.26 *Electron micrograph of the cerebellar cortex of the adult weaver mutant mouse. Catecholaminergic innervation visualized with tyrosine hydroxylase (TH) immunostaining. Two labelled varicosities in close vicinity to a Purkinje cell dendrite (PD) and a cluster of free spines (asterisks). Despite the large number of non-innervated postsynaptic specializations, note the absence of synaptic complexes between the labelled axon terminals and the surrounding dendritic elements. This micrograph illustrates the non-junctional modality of the catecholaminergic innervation in the cerebellar cortex. Reproduced by permission from Abbott and Sotelo.[1]*

tremendously. Double or triple immunolabelling has confirmed that two or more of these substances may coexist in a single neuron. At neuronal cell bodies, *in situ* hybridization with specific molecular probes to visualize mRNA coding for synthesizing enzymes and/or neuropeptides has been combined with immunohistochemistry of classic neurotransmitters. These studies[175] have shown that all possible combinations of neurotransmitter coexistence may occur in mammalian central neurons. According to their frequency, such combinations are: a classic transmitter and one or several peptides, up to seven peptides in a single neuron, and two or more classic transmitters.[174]

THE PROBLEM OF RELEASE IN NEURONS CONTAINING MULTIPLE TRANSMITTERS

Neurochemical and electrophysiological proof that neurons that synthesize and store multiple neuroactive compounds are also able to release them under physiological conditions has been obtained in several neuronal systems.[174] The main problem has been to determine whether these substances are released simultaneously or sequentially by a different process. The existence of two types of storage organelle in most nerve endings has largely facilitated the understanding of the releasing mechanisms. Moreover, high-frequency stimulation favours

neuropeptide release from large, dense-core vesicles. As concluded by Changeux,[63] the ability of the nerve endings to translate a frequency code into a chemical one provides the coexistence of neuronal messengers with a new and powerful mechanism of information transfer in the CNS.

Electrical synapses

In the most common case of electrical interactions, the current flow spreads electrotonically (passively) from the neuron in which it is generated into a neighbouring one. In contrast with chemical synapses, transmission occurs with or without some synaptic delay. In addition, the electrotonic spread of the depolarizing current is bidirectional (with the exception of the rectifying electrical junctions, still not found in the mammalian brain). These two properties, high speed and reciprocity, contribute to a shorter latency of postsynaptic excitation and to a synchronous discharge of groups of coupled neurons. These two properties, together with the absence of fatiguability (the current passage through the synapse is passive), underlie the main functional features of this mode of synaptic transmission: fast speed and synchronization.[224]

At sites where neurons are in direct apposition, they are still separated by their own plasma membranes and the intercalated extracellular space, 15–30 nm in width. The high electrical resistance of the membranes and the cleft is great enough to prevent significant electrotonic coupling between cells.[203] Electrical interactions between neurons must necessarily occur at specific sites on the neuronal membranes which could constitute low-resistance pathways. Indeed, combined electrophysiological and structural studies have shown that electrical transmission takes place through specific membrane junctions, termed gap junctions by Revel and Karnovsky.[340] These junctions, present in all mature cell types with the exceptions of skeletal muscle, erythrocytes and spermatozoa, are intercellular communicating channels capable of allowing an exchange of diffusible molecules between the linked cells.

MORPHOLOGY OF GAP JUNCTIONS

Gap junctions between mammalian neurons (electrical synapses) share all of their internal features with those extensively studied between other classes of cells, mainly liver, heart and lens. They appear as small plaques where the junctional membranes run straight and parallel. Under favourable conditions, gap junctions exhibit a heptalaminar configuration (Fig. 1.27b), resulting from the closeness of the junctional membranes, which narrows the extracellular space to a minute gap of 1–2 nm. A specific constituent of interneuronal gap junctions is the almost constant presence of a cytoplasmic semi-dense band undercoating the whole length of the inner membrane surface at the gap-junctional plaque.

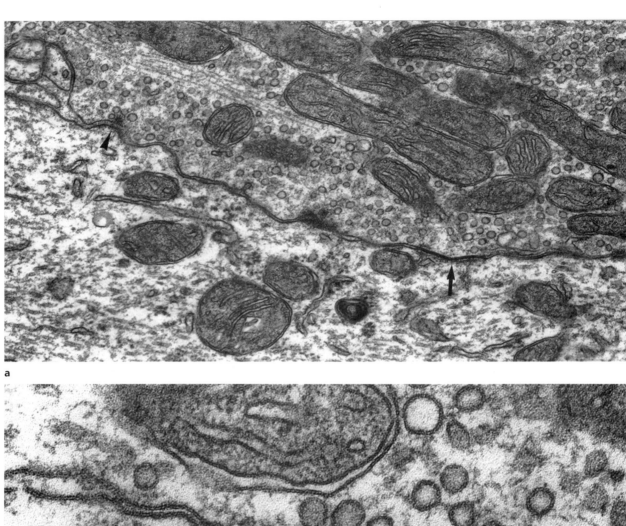

a

b

Figure 1.27 *Mixed synapse in the rat lateral vestibular nucleus. (a) Primary vestibular fibre synapsing on the cell body of a giant cell of Deiters' nucleus with synaptic complex (arrowhead) and gap junction (arrow). (b) Higher magnification, from a serial section of the gap junction in (a), showing its typical heptalaminar organization. Note the cytoplasmic dense material (arrows) undercoating the junctional membranes.*

Using the freeze-fracture technique, these junctions appear as polygonal lattices of particles protruding on the P-face of the junctional membranes, and a complementary lattice of pits on the E-face. These particles measure 8 nm in diameter and are arranged in a crystalline manner, forming hexagonal arrays, with a centre-to-centre spacing of about 9 nm. The disposition of the gap-junction particles is symmetrical in both junctional membranes, such as the particles on one P-face are in register with those on the other P-face. Each of the opposing particles, protruding in the extracellular narrow cleft, spans the gap separating the two junctional membranes.[401] Electron-microscopical image reconstruction of isolated junctions indicates that a gap-junction channel is a dodecamer, with six monomers in the membrane of each of the two coupled cells. In a proposed model, the walls of the hemichannels (gap-junction particles) contact each other at the centre of the inter-membrane cleft.[28,260]

PROTEIN COMPOSITION AND MOLECULAR BIOLOGY OF GAP JUNCTIONS

The intercellular channels in gap junctions are formed by structural proteins called connexins (Cx). After the cloning of the first Cx,[314] it became evident that these proteins are encoded by a multigene family. Differences in the predicted molecular weights of the encoded proteins differentiate the individual connexin (Cx26, Cx32, Cx36, Cx43, Cx45, the examples of those most abundantly present in the CNS). Today, 14 mouse Cx genes are known, and at least six others have been cloned in other vertebrate species. Hence, there are over 20 known Cx genes,[470] all of which encode membrane proteins with four trans-membrane domains. However, despite the great homology between Cx genes, their encoded proteins frequently exhibit regions of unique sequence, to adapt channel properties to specific tissue and/or cell requirements. Based on these structural differences, Cx genes can be classified into three large groups: α-(Cx26, Cx32) and β-(Cx43) connexins, which are the two classical subgroups, and γ-connexins (perch Cx34.7, skate Cx35 and rodent Cx36), which constitute a novel subgroup.[68,302]

Six connexins form a single-membrane channel (the hemichannel) which is called a connexon. Two connexons, spanning the two plasma membranes and aligning in the extracellular space, form the intercellular channel and, finally, the clustering of intercellular channels constitutes one gap junction. Each connexon can be formed by the same (homomeric) or different (heteromeric) types of connexins. In addition, intercellular channels can be homotypic, when the two apposed connexons are of identical molecular composition, or they can be heterotypic when they differ.[470] All these possible combinations explain the great molecular heterogeneity of gap junctions which, in turn, determines their unique molecular permeability.[233] Each intercellular channel has a minimum diameter of 1.2 nm, which constitutes an aqueous path. The size and the dynamic regulation of this path exclude the access of nuclei acids and proteins. However, they permit the passage of second messengers and small metabolites, in addition to ions. Hence, cells linked through gap junctions are not only electrotonically but also metabolically coupled.

Specific antibodies and nucleotide probes, together with RT-PCR analysis, have allowed the sites of Cx expression in the CNS to be identified. Until recently, the expressed Cxs were not tissue specific, and belonged to α- and β-subgroups. For instance, Cx26 and Cx32 from liver, and Cx43 from heart were also visualized in the brain and the spinal cord, Cx32 in oligodendrocytes and a few neurons, Cx26 and Cx43 in leptomeningeal and ependymal cells,

and Cx43 in astrocytes.[84] The cloning of the rodent Cx36 by the group of Cicirata[68] has changed our ideas about gap junctions in the neural system, since Cx36 is the first one to be almost exclusively expressed in nervous tissue and, more importantly, to be expressed almost solely in neurons (Fig. 1.28). Hence, the γ-subgroup of Cxs seems to contain the proteins structurally implicated in electrical synapses.

For years electrotonic transmission, discovered in invertebrates,[120] has been thought to be a kind of synaptic mediation almost exclusive to phylogenetically primitive forms. Some investigators even considered that the occurrence of electrical synapses in the mammalian CNS was not of functional importance but a phylogenetic remnant.[95] Now, advances in molecular biology have provided some evidence against this unreasonable conclusion. Indeed, invertebrates have also gap junctions that, although they differ in gap width, interchannel separation and channel diameter, share most of the morphological and pharmacological features with vertebrate gap junctions. However, the genes encoding for gap junctions in invertebrates, called innexins,[470] are not invertebrate orthologues of any connexin, although they also encode membrane proteins with four transmembrane domains. Hence, in contrast to the molecules implicated in chemical synaptic transmission, most of which have homologues in invertebrates and vertebrates, those involved in electrotonic coupling are different and exhibit later evolutionary development.

Finally, the cloning of connexins has also revealed that they can be molecular targets in neurological disease. Hence, connexin 32 is the molecular target of the X-linked forms of Charcot–Marie–Tooth disease, with mutations exclusively affecting Schwann cells (reviewed in Ref. 27).

CONFORMATIONAL CHANGES IN CONNEXON MORPHOLOGY ASSOCIATED WITH FUNCTIONAL STAGES OF GAP JUNCTIONS

Gap-junction permeability can be regulated by physiological and experimental conditions. The fast and reversible effects of some of these conditions on junctional conductance suggest that gap-junctional channels can undergo rapid conformational changes in parallel with functional changes. Zampighi et al.[483] examined the gap junctions of the crayfish electrical synapses in control conditions (coupled stage) and after experimentally increasing axonal acidification (uncoupled stage). In both instances, the lateral axons were fixed in the same aldehyde fixative before freeze-fracture of the membranes. In control experiments, when the junctional resistance is about 60–80 kΩ the two synaptic membranes are separated by a narrow gap (4–6 nm). In freeze-fracture replicas 90% of the junctional particles are arranged in characteristic gap-junctional plaques. Moreover, the correlation between the total number of junctional

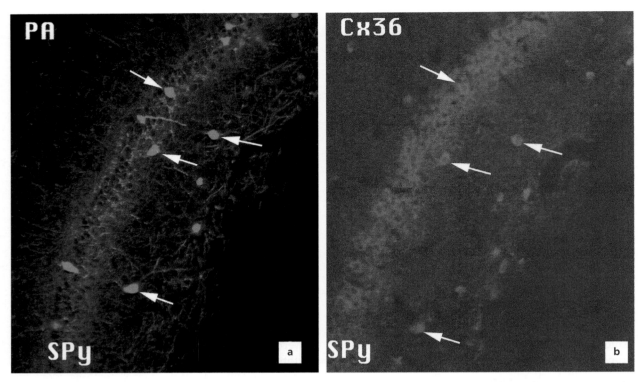

Figure 1.28 *Double immunohistochemistry of interneurons in CA3 of the adult rat hippocampus. (a) Parvalbumin immunostaining (PA); (b) connexin 36 immunostaining (Cx36). The interneurons marked by arrows are double labelled, showing that a majority of this class of cells expresses connexin 36. Thus, inhibitory interneurons are electrotonically coupled. From F Cicirata and C Sotelo (unpublished micrographs).*

particles and the junctional resistance indicates that all of those particles correspond to open channels. After axonal acidification, there is a large increase in junctional resistance (~300 kΩ) and axon potentials fail to propagate. Under these conditions, the extracellular cleft increases up to 10–20 nm and the total number of junctional particles participating in plaque formation substantially decreases. This decrease parallels the increase in the number of isolated junctional particles dispersed in the axolemmae. These observations suggest that dissembly of hemichannels in the junctional plaques is related to the closure of the channels. In a recent model it has been proposed that in low Ca^{2+} solution (coupled stage) the connexins in each cell membrane forming the channel have their subunits slightly tilted. In Ca^{2+}-containing solution (uncoupled stage), the channel closure may be achieved by the twisting of each subunit, which will progressively reduce the central core of the channel to total closure.[449]

ELECTRICAL SYNAPTIC TRANSMISSION IN THE MAMMALIAN BRAIN

Morphologically, the best evidence for electrotonic coupling is the ultrastructural detection of interneuronal gap junctions, although this method has obvious limitations. For this reason, since 1967[404] (the date of one of the first

discoveries of electrical synapses in the mammalian brain), the number of neuronal systems with reported interneuronal gap junctions, although highly increased (reviewed in Ref. 406), remains low. Electrophysiologically, the problem seems even more complicated. For direct evidence of electrotonic coupling, the two coupled neurons need to be simultaneously impaled, and the depolarization in one neuron needs to provoke a fast, smaller but clear depolarization in the adjacent neuron. Even with the advances of *in vitro* slices, the number of direct demonstrations of neuronal coupling is extremely low.[247] The indirect method appears to be easier, through recording of graded antidromic depolarizations, also termed 'short-latency depolarizations', under strictly controlled conditions.[225] However, even this method has not given a complete picture of the incidence of this mode of synaptic communication in the mammalian brain (reviewed in Refs. 247, 401 and 406).

The demonstration of gap-junctional coupling between neurons has been facilitated by the introduction of dye-coupling methods,[259] which has increased the number of known electrical synapses in the mammalian brain.[304] However, since the recent discovery of neuron-specific connexins,[68] riboprobes and antibodies have begun to be available, as well as the mapping of Cx36 expression.[26,66,313] Neuronal cell bodies expressing Cx36 have been identified in the neocortex and allocortex. They belong to GABAergic interneurons in layers V and II of the cerebral cortex and CA1, CA3 and the dentate gyrus of the hippocampus, particularly those expressing parvalbumin.[119] Hence, in these cortices, inhibitor interneurons are organized into complex networks of neurons with synchronized activity, which could impose a rhythmic and/or oscillatory activity to the principal projecting neurons. These kinds of activity have been proposed to play important roles in cognition and other higher neural functions,[346] and could result from gap junctions linking the dendritic network of the interneurons.[119] Neuronal cell bodies expressing Cx36 are also present in the ventrobasal and ventral nuclear complex of the thalamus, the cerebellar cortex (stellate and basket cells), the spinal cord and brainstem motor neurons, and inferior olivary neurons, among others. Hence, electrical transmission appears to be a major mechanism of neuronal interaction in the CNS of vertebrates, including mammals.[401]

CHEMICAL TRANSMISSION AND ELECTROTONIC COUPLING: MUTUAL INTERACTIONS

As stated previously, chemical and electrical transmission do not always exclude each other but, in precise morphological situations, both may operate between the same two neurons.

Mixed synapses: morphological substratum for a dual mode of synaptic transmission

In electrically transmitting synapses between a presynaptic axon and a postsynaptic neuron, the axon terminal often contains synaptic vesicles. Furthermore, at the synaptic interface of axon terminals linked through gap junctions to their postsynaptic partners, two other types of junctional zone are almost constantly present: (1) synaptic complexes or synaptic junctions, and (2) intermediary junctions similar to attachment plaques. The synaptic vesicles are associated not with the gap junction but with the presynaptic vesicular grid, forming active zones, the releasing sites of chemically transmitting synapses.

The association of electrical and chemical synapses was first demonstrated electrophysiologically in the avian ciliary ganglion.[264] The term 'mixed synapses' has been proposed by Sotelo and Palay,[405] who reported the first example of these electrical and chemical junction associations in the mammalian brain, between large axon terminals (presumably primary vestibular fibres) and giant cells of Deiters, in the lateral vestibular nucleus of the rat (Fig. 1.27). Mixed synapses have, thereafter, been described in many other regions of the rodent brain stem, where it is apparent that most of the axo-somatic and axo-dendritic electrical synapses are in fact mixed synapses.[401,406] A dual mode of synaptic transmission through mixed synapses has been proven only in a few instances, and always in non-mammalian vertebrates.[406] The presence of these junctional associations raises the question

of what possible functions they serve. They may represent a more subtle and refined type of neuronal communication than either electrotonic coupling or chemical transmission alone, since they offer the possibility of local interactions that could modulate synaptic efficiency. Because gap junctions are known to allow passage of second messenger molecules (Ca^{2+}, cAMP, IP_3), they may regulate synaptic efficiency by modulation of presynaptic neurotransmitter release for postsynaptic diffusion of second messengers.

Chemical synaptic modulation of electrotonic coupling

Besides the mixed synapses, other co-operative interactions between electrical and chemical modes of synaptic transmission have been reported. They concern a specific mechanism for increase and decrease in the electrotonic coupling of neurons. Theoretically, transmission across gap junctions can be modulated either by directly changing the junctional conductance or indirectly by changing the extrajunctional membrane resistance.[58,62,153,238,290,408]

One of the most exciting examples of co-operative interactions between the two modes of synaptic transmission occurs in the inferior olive of all mammalian species analysed. Studies carried out in two invertebrates, the molluscs *Navanax* and *Aplysia*,[58,408] have shown that a decrease in extrajunctional membrane resistance, as a result of the synaptic firing of inhibitory afferent fibres, diminishes the efficacy of the coupling by short-circuiting the membranes of the coupled neurons. Conversely, excitatory synaptic transmission increases the extrajunctional membrane resistance and, for the converse reason, facilitates the rate of electrotonic coupling. Therefore, in both situations the degree of coupling is under chemical synaptic control. In both situations the chemical synapses must be strategically placed near the gap junction. This is precisely what happens in the inferior olive of mammals (mouse, rat, cat and monkey),[13,400,402] where gap junctions appear to be restricted, for the most part, to specialized arrangements of the neuropil, the inferior olivary glomeruli. The glomerulus consists of a central core of dendritic elements, some of them linked by gap junctions (Fig. 1.29), surrounded by a peripheral ring of axon terminals. GABAergic axon terminals, originating from the deep cerebellar nuclei, synapse on the two coupled dendritic elements between those forming the peripheral ring (Fig. 1.29).[13] Thus, the coupling of these neurons is controlled by the olivo-cerebello-olivary feedback loop. Llinas and collaborators[237,248] recorded simultaneously from 30 to 96 Purkinje cells in the crus 1 and 2a of the rat cerebellum. Cross-correlation analysis of the recordings revealed the organization of Purkinje cells to be in sagittal stripes. Those Purkinje cells within one stripe are correlated, whereas the activity of these cells in the mediolateral direction is not correlated. This

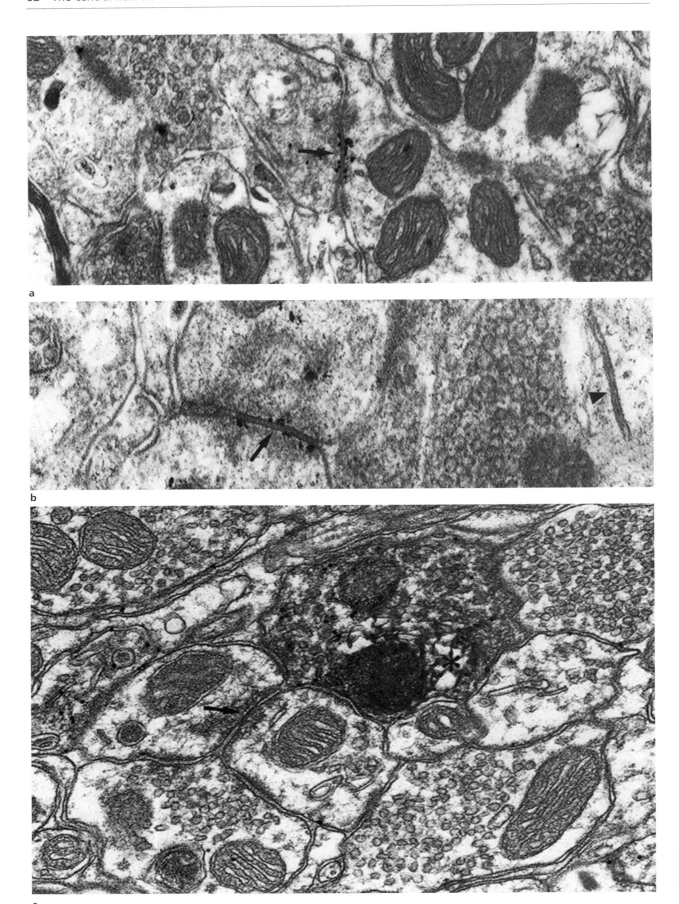

a

b

c

Figure 1.29 *Electrical interactions between neurons in the rat inferior olive. (a, b) Electron micrographs of dendro-dendritic gap junctions in the neuropil of the inferior olive. Immunocytochemical localization of connexin 36. The arrows point to dendro-dendritic gap junctions decorated with silver-intensified gold particles. In (a) the gap junction links a small and a medium-sized, extraglomerular, dendritic profile, while in (b) the gap junction is between two small dendritic profiles in a glomerulus. Note that the gap junction between two astrocytic processes (arrowhead) is not labelled. (c) Electron micrograph of an olivary glomerulus, showing that the GABAergic innervation of the dendritic profiles linked through a gap junction (arrow) originates in the lateral cerebellar nucleus. The axon terminal straddling the two linked dendrites is double labelled: anterogradely, with WGA-HRP injected in the cerebellar lateral nucleus (asterisk), and with GABA immunocytochemistry (colloidal gold postembedding). The strategic location of these dentato-olivary synapses suggests that they can modulate the electrotonic coupling rate between sets of inferior olivary neurons. (a, b) From F Cicirata and C Sotelo (unpublished micrographs), (c) reproduced by permission from Angaint and Sotelo.[13]*

basic pattern of activity disappears when the activity of the cerebellar inhibitory feedback to the inferior olive, via the deep cerebellar nuclei, is blocked by GABA receptor antagonists or when the deep nuclei are lesioned. Thus, for Llinas, the inferior olive organizes movement in time. In this way, the inferior olive, through the intrinsic properties of its neurons and the organization of its ensembles by co-operation between chemical and electrical synapses, become the key element in the co-ordination of movements.

Acknowledgements

The authors wish to thank Drs Serge Duckett, Louise Abbott and Richard Miles for critical reading of the manuscript, as well as Mr Denis Le Cren for photographic work and Anne-Marie Skévis and Claudine Nguyen for excellent and patient secretarial assistance.

REFERENCES

1 Abbott LC, Sotelo C. Ultrastructural analysis of catecholaminergic innervation in weaver and normal mouse cerebellar cortices. *J Comp Neurol* 2000; **426**: 316–29.

2 Ahmari SE, Buchanan J, Smith SJ. Assembly of presynaptic active zones from cytoplasmic transport packets. *Nat Neurosci* 2000; **3**: 445–51.

3 Ainger K, Avossa D, Diana AS et al. Transport and localization elements in myelin basic protein mRNA. *J Cell Biol* 1997; **138**: 1077–87.

4 Alcantara S, Ruiz M, D'Arcangelo G et al. Regional and cellular patterns of reelin mRNA expression in the forebrain of the developing and adult mouse. *J Neurosci* 1998; **18**: 7779–99.

5 Alcantara S, Ruiz M, De Castro F et al. Netrin 1 acts as an attractive or as a repulsive cue for distinct migrating neurons during the development of the cerebellar system. *Development* 2000; **127**: 1359–72.

6 Ales E, Tabares L, Poyato JM et al. High calcium concentrations shift the mode of exocytosis to the kiss-and-run mechanism. *Nat Cell Biol* 1999; **1**: 40–4.

7 Altman J, Bayer S. Embryonic development of the rat cerebellum. I. Delineation of the cerebellar primordium and early cell movements. *J Comp Neurol* 1985; **231**: 1–26.

8 Altman J, Das G. Autoradiographic and histological studies of postnatal neurogenesis. I. A longitudinal investigation of the kinetics, migration and transformation of cells incorporating tritiated thymidine in neonatal rats, with special reference to postnatal neurogenesis in some brain regions. *J Comp Neurol* 1966; **126**: 337–89.

9 Anand R, Conroy WG, Schoepfer R et al. Neuronal nicotinic acetylcholine receptors expressed in *Xenopus* oocytes have a pentameric quaternary structure. *J Biol Chem* 1991; **266**: 11192–8.

10 Anderson SA, Eisenstat DD, Shi L, Rubenstein JL. Interneuron migration from basal forebrain to neocortex: dependence on Dlx genes. *Science* 1997; **278**: 474–6.

11 Andrew M, Owen MJ. Hyperekplexia: abnormal startle response due to glycine receptor mutations. *Br J Psychiatry* 1997; **170**: 106–8.

12 Andrews SB, Leapman RD, Landis DM, Reese TS. Activity-dependent accumulation of calcium in Purkinje cell dendritic spines. *Proc Natl Acad Sci USA* 1988; **85**: 1682–5.

13 Angaut P, Sotelo C. Synaptology of the cerebello-olivary pathway. Double labelling with anterograde axonal tracing and GABA immunocytochemistry in the rat. *Brain Res* 1989; **479**: 361–5.

14 Baas PW. Microtubules and neuronal polarity: lessons from mitosis. *Neuron* 1999; **22**: 23–31.

15 Baas PW, Black MM, Banker GA. Changes in microtubule polarity orientation during the development of hippocampal neurons in culture. *J Cell Biol* 1989; **109**: 3085–94.

16 Baas PW, Deitch JS, Black MM, Banker GA. Polarity orientation of microtubules in hippocampal neurons: uniformity in the axon and nonuniformity in the dendrite. *Proc Natl Acad Sci USA* 1988; **85**: 8335–9.

17 Bamburg JR, Bernstein BW. Actin and actin-binding proteins in neurons. In: Burgoyne RD ed. *The neuronal cytoskeleton*. New York: Wiley-Liss, 1991: 121–60.

18 Barr M, Bertram L, Lindsay A. The morphology of the cell nucleus, according to sex. *Anat Rec* 1950; **107**: 283–97.

19 Baude A, Nusser Z, Roberts JD et al. The metabotropic glutamate receptor (mGluR1 alpha) is concentrated at perisynaptic membrane of neuronal subpopulations as detected by immunogold reaction. *Neuron* 1993; **11**: 771–87.

20 Baude A, Sequier JM, McKernan RM et al. Differential subcellular distribution of the alpha 6 subunit versus the alpha 1 and beta 2/3 subunits of the GABAA/benzodiazepine receptor complex in granule cells of the cerebellar cortex. *Neuroscience* 1992; **51**: 739–48.

21 Bayer S, Yackel J, Puri P. Neurons in the rat dentate gyrus granular layer substantially increase during juvenile and adult life. *Science* 1982; **216**: 890–2.

22 Beaudet A, Descarries L. The fine structure of central serotonin neurons. *J Physiol* 1981; **77**: 193–203.

23 Beaudet A, Descarries L. The monoamine innervation of rat cerebral cortex: synaptic and nonsynaptic axon terminals. *Neuroscience* 1978; **3**: 851–60.

24 Beaudet A, Sotelo C. Synaptic remodeling of serotonin axon terminals in rat agranular cerebellum. *Brain Res* 1981; **206**: 305–29.

25 Bechade C, Sur C, Triller A. The inhibitory neuronal glycine receptor. *Bioessays* 1994; **16**: 735–44.

26 Belluardo N, Mudo G, Trovato-Salinaro A *et al*. Expression of connexin36 in the adult and developing rat brain. *Brain Res* 2000; **865**: 121–38.

27 Bennett MV. Connexins in disease (News). *Nature* 1994; **368**: 18–9.

28 Bennett MV, Barrio LC, Bargiello TA *et al*. Gap junctions: new tools, new answers, new questions. *Neuron* 1991; **6**: 305–20.

29 Benson DL, Tanaka H. N-cadherin redistribution during synaptogenesis in hippocampal neurons. *J Neurosci* 1998; **18**: 6892–904.

30 Bertoni-Freddari C, Giuli C, Pieri C, Paci D. Quantitative investigation of the morphological plasticity of synaptic junctions in rat dentate gyrus during aging. *Brain Res* 1986; **366**: 187–92.

31 Betz H. Ligand-gated ion channels in the brain: the amino acid receptor superfamily. *Neuron* 1990; **5**: 383–92.

32 Betz H, Kuhse J, Schmieden V *et al*. Structure and functions of inhibitory and excitatory glycine receptors. *Ann NY Acad Sci* 1999; **868**: 667–76.

33 Betz WJ, Bewick GS. Optical analysis of synaptic vesicle recycling at the frog neuromuscular junction. *Science* 1992; **255**: 200–3.

34 Bilak SR, Morest DK. Differential expression of the metabotropic glutamate receptor mGluR1alpha by neurons and axons in the cochlear nucleus: *in situ* hybridization and immunohistochemistry. *Synapse* 1998; **28**: 251–70.

35 Blichenberg A, Schwanke B, Rehbein M *et al*. Identification of a *cis*-acting dendritic targeting element in MAP2 mRNAs. *J Neurosci* 1999; **19**: 8818–29.

36 Bliss TV, Collingridge GL. A synaptic model of memory: long-term potentiation in the hippocampus. *Nature* 1993; **361**: 31–9.

37 Blochl A, Thoenen H. Localization of cellular storage compartments and sites of constitutive and activity–dependent release of nerve growth factor (NGF) in primary cultures of hippocampal neurons. *Mol Cell Neurosci* 1996; **7**: 173–90.

38 Bloch-Gallego E, Ezan F, Tessier-Lavigne M, Sotelo C. Floor plate and netrin-1 are involved in the migration and survival of inferior olivary neurons. *J Neurosci* 1999; **19**: 4407–20.

39 Bloom FE, Aghajanian GK. Cytochemistry of synapses: selective staining for electron microscopy. *Science* 1966; **154**: 1575–7.

40 Bochet P, Audinat E, Lambolez B *et al*. Subunit composition at the single-cell level explains functional properties of a glutamate-gated channel. *Neuron* 1994; **12**: 383–8.

41 Bormann J. The 'ABC' of GABA receptors. *Trends Pharmacol Sci* 2000; **21**: 16–19.

42 Bormann J, Hamill OP, Sakmann B. Mechanism of anion permeation through channels gated by glycine and gamma-aminobutyric acid in mouse cultured spinal neurones. *J Physiol (Lond)* 1987; **385**: 243–86.

43 Boue-Grabot E, Roudbaraki M, Bascles L *et al*. Expression of GABA receptor rho subunits in rat brain. *J Neurochem* 1998; **70**: 899–907.

44 Bourrat F, Sotelo C. Early development of the rat precerebellar system: migratory routes, selective aggregation and neuritic differentiation of the inferior olive and lateral reticular nucleus neurons. An overview. *Arch Ital Biol* 1990; **128**: 151–70.

45 Bourrat F, Sotelo C. Migratory pathways and neuritic differentiation of inferior olivary neurons in the rat embryo. Axonal tracing study using the *in vitro* slab technique. *Brain Res* 1988; **467**: 19–37.

46 Bowery N. GABA$_B$ receptors and their significance in mammalian pharmacology. *Trends Pharmacol Sci* 1989; **10**: 401–7.

47 Bradley SR, Levey AI, Hersch SM, Conn PJ. Immunocytochemical localization of group III metabotropic glutamate receptors in the hippocampus with subtype-specific antibodies. *J Neurosci* 1996; **16**: 2044–56.

48 Brady ST. Molecular motors in the nervous system. *Neuron* 1991; **7**: 521–33.

49 Brakeman PR, Lanahan AA, O'Brien R *et al*. Homer: a protein that selectively binds metabotropic glutamate receptors. *Nature* 1997; **386**: 284–8.

50 Brose K, Tessier-Lavigne M. Slit proteins: key regulators of axon guidance, axonal branching, and cell migration. *Curr Opin Neurobiol* 2000; **10**: 95–102.

51 Bruckenstein DA, Lein PJ, Higgins D, Fremeau RT Jr. Distinct spatial localization of specific mRNAs in cultured sympathetic neurons. *Neuron* 1990; **5**: 809–19.

52 Brustle O, Spiro AC, Karram K *et al*. In vitro-generated neural precursors participate in mammalian brain development. *Proc Natl Acad Sci USA* 1997; **94**: 14809–14.

53 Burack MA, Silverman MA, Banker G. The role of selective transport in neuronal protein sorting. *Neuron* 2000; **26**: 465–72.

54 Burgess TL, Kelly RB. Constitutive and regulated secretion of proteins. *Annu Rev Cell Biol* 1987; **3**: 243–93.

55 Burgoyne R. *The neuronal cytoskeleton*. New York: Wiley-Liss, 1991.

56 Butler MH, Hayashi A, Ohkoshi N *et al*. Autoimmunity to gephyrin in Stiff-Man syndrome. *Neuron* 2000; **26**: 307–12.

57 Butz S, Okamoto M, Sudhof TC. A tripartite protein complex with the potential to couple synaptic vesicle exocytosis to cell adhesion in brain. *Cell* 1998; **94**: 773–82.

58 Carew TJ, Kandel ER. Two functional effects of decreased conductance EPSPs: synaptic augmentation and increased electrotonic coupling. *Science* 1976; **192**: 150–3.

59 Carlson NG, Gahring LC, Twyman RE, Rogers SW. Identification of amino acids in the glutamate receptor, GluR3, important for antibody-binding and receptor-specific activation. *J Biol Chem* 1997; **272**: 11295–301.

60 Cartaud J, Changeux JP. Post-transcriptional compartmentalization of acetylcholine receptor biosynthesis in the subneural domain of muscle and electrocyte junctions. *Eur J Neurosci* 1993; **5**: 191–202.

61 Cattaneo E, McKay R. Proliferation and differentiation of neuronal stem cells regulated by nerve growth factor. *Nature* 1990; **347**: 762–5.

62 Cepeda C, Walsh JP, Hull CD *et al*. Dye-coupling in the neostriatum of the rat: I. Modulation by dopamine-depleting lesions. *Synapse* 1989; **4**: 229–37.

63 Changeux JP. Coexistence of neuronal messengers and molecular selection. *Prog Brain Res* 1986; **68**: 373–403.

64 Chazal G, Durbec P, Jankovski A *et al*. Consequences of neural cell adhesion molecule deficiency on cell migration in the rostral migratory stream of the mouse. *J Neurosci* 2000; **20**: 1446–57.

65 Chuong CM, Crossin KL, Edelman GM. Sequential expression and differential function of multiple adhesion molecules during the formation of cerebellar cortical layers. *J Cell Biol* 1987; **104**: 331–42.

66 Cicirata F, Corte G, Wehrle R et al. Regional distribution and cellular characterization of the connexin 36 protein in the brain of adult mouse. Eur J Neurosci 2000; 12 (Suppl): 11–52.

67 Colonnier M. Synaptic patterns on different cell types in the different laminae of the cat visual cortex. An electron microscope study. Brain Res 1968; 9: 268–87.

68 Condorelli DF, Parenti R, Spinella F et al. Cloning of a new gap junction gene (Cx36) highly expressed in mammalian brain neurons. Eur J Neurosci 1998; 10: 1202–8.

69 Couteaux R, Pécot-Dechavassine M. Vésicules synaptiques et poches au niveau des zones actives de la jonction neuromusculaire. CR Acad Sci Ser D Paris 1970; 271: 2346–9.

70 Craig AM, Banker G. Neuronal polarity. Annu Rev Neurosci 1994; 17: 267–310.

71 Craven SE, Bredt DS. PDZ proteins organize synaptic signaling pathways. Cell 1998; 93: 495–8.

72 Cremer H, Lange R, Christoph A et al. Inactivation of the N-CAM gene in mice results in size reduction of the olfactory bulb and deficits in spatial learning. Nature 1994; 367: 455–9.

73 Cremona O, De Camilli P. Synaptic vesicle endocytosis. Curr Opin Neurobiol 1997; 7: 323–30.

74 Cutting GR, Lu L, O'Hara BF et al. Cloning of the gamma-aminobutyric acid (GABA) rho 1 cDNA: a GABA receptor subunit highly expressed in the retina. Proc Natl Acad Sci USA 1991; 88: 2673–7.

75 Dahmane N, Ruiz-i-Altaba A. Sonic hedgehog regulates the growth and patterning of the cerebellum. Development 1999; 126: 3089–100.

76 Dale HH, Feldberg H, Vogt M. Release of acetylcholine at voluntary motor nerve endings. J Physiol (Lond) 1936; 86: 353–80.

77 Daniels DL, Cohen AR, Anderson JM, Brunger AT. Crystal structure of the hCASK PDZ domain reveals the structural basis of class II PDZ domain target recognition. Nat Struct Biol 1998; 5: 317–25.

78 D'Arcangelo G, Miao GG, Chen SC et al. A protein related to extracellular matrix proteins deleted in the mouse mutant reeler. Nature 1995; 374: 719–23.

79 Darnell RB. The importance of defining the paraneoplastic neurologic disorders (Editorial; comment). N Engl J Med 1999; 340: 1831–3.

80 De Camilli P, Thomas A, Cofiell R et al. The synaptic vesicle-associated protein amphiphysin is the 128-kD autoantigen of Stiff-Man syndrome with breast cancer. J Exp Med 1993; 178: 2219–23.

81 de Carlos JA, Lopez-Mascaraque L, Valverde F. Dynamics of cell migration from the lateral ganglionic eminence in the rat. J Neurosci 1996; 16: 6146–56.

82 Decker CJ, Parker R. Diversity of cytoplasmic functions for the 3'-untranslated region of eukaryotic transcripts. Curr Opin Cell Biol 1995; 7: 386–92.

83 De Duve C. The lysosome concept. In: De Reuck AVS, Cameron, MP eds. Lysosomes. Boston, MA: Little Brown and Co., 1963: 1–31.

84 Dermietzel R, Spray DC. Gap junctions in the brain: where, what type, how many and why? Trends Neurosci 1993; 16: 186–92.

85 Descarries L, Watkins KC, Lapierre Y. Noradrenergic axon terminals in the cerebral cortex of rat. III. Topometric ultrastructural analysis. Brain Res 1977; 133: 197–222.

86 Doetsch F, Caille I, Lim DA et al. Subventricular zone astrocytes are neural stem cells in the adult mammalian brain. Cell 1999; 97: 703–16.

87 Dong H, O'Brien RJ, Fung ET et al. GRIP: a synaptic PDZ domain-containing protein that interacts with AMPA receptors. Nature 1997; 386: 279–84.

88 Dotti CG, Banker GA, Binder LI. The expression and distribution of the microtubule-associated proteins tau and microtubule-associated protein 2 in hippocampal neurons in the rat in situ and in cell culture. Neuroscience 1987; 23: 121–30.

89 Dotti CG, Simons K. Polarized sorting of viral glycoproteins to the axon and dendrites of hippocampal neurons in culture. Cell 1990; 62: 63–72.

90 Doyle DA, Lee A, Lewis J et al. Crystal structures of a complexed and peptide-free membrane protein-binding domain: molecular basis of peptide recognition by PDZ. Cell 1996; 85: 1067–76.

91 Droz B, Leblond CP. Axonal migration of proteins in the central nervous system and peripheral nerves as shown by radioautography. J Comp Neurol 1963; 121: 325–46.

92 Duclert A, Changeux JP. Acetylcholine receptor gene expression at the developing neuromuscular junction. Physiol Rev 1995; 75: 339–68.

93 Dunaevsky A, Tashiro A, Majewska A et al. Developmental regulation of spine motility in the mammalian central nervous system. Proc Natl Acad Sci USA 1999; 96: 13438–43.

94 Dunphy WG, Rothman JE. Compartmental organization of the Golgi stack. Cell 1985; 42: 13–21.

95 Eccles JC. The physiology of synapses. Berlin: Springer, 1964.

96 Engert F, Bonhoeffer T. Dendritic spine changes associated with hippocampal long-term synaptic plasticity. Nature 1999; 399: 66–70.

97 Eriksson P, Perfilieva E, Björk-Eriksson T et al. Neurogenesis in the adult human hippocampus. Nat Med 1998; 11: 1313–17.

98 Essrich C, Lorez M, Benson JA et al. Postsynaptic clustering of major GABA$_A$ receptor subtypes requires the gamma 2 subunit and gephyrin. Nat Neurosci 1998; 1: 563–71.

99 Falls DL, Rosen KM, Corfas G et al. ARIA, a protein that stimulates acetylcholine receptor synthesis, is a member of the neu ligand family. Cell 1993; 72: 801–15.

100 Fannon AM, Colman DR. A model for central synaptic junctional complex formation based on the differential adhesive specificities of the cadherins. Neuron 1996; 17: 423–34.

101 Faundez V, Horng JT, Kelly RB. A function for the AP3 coat complex in synaptic vesicle formation from endosomes. Cell 1998; 93: 423–32.

102 Fawcett DW. Cilia and flagella. In: Brachet J, Mirsky AE eds. The cell. New York: Academic Press, 1961: 217–97.

103 Feddersen RM, Ehlenfeldt R, Yunis WS et al. Disrupted cerebellar cortical development and progressive degeneration of Purkinje cells in SV40 T antigen transgenic mice. Neuron 1992; 9: 955–66.

104 Feigenspan A, Bormann J. Differential pharmacology of GABAA and GABAC receptors on rat retinal bipolar cells. Eur J Pharmacol 1994; 288: 97–104.

105 Feigenspan A, Wassle H, Bormann J. Pharmacology of GABA receptor Cl$^-$ channels in rat retinal bipolar cells. Nature 1993; 361: 159–62.

106 Feldman ML, Peters A. Intranuclear rods and sheets in rat cochlear nucleus. J Neurocytol 1972; 1: 109–27.

107 Feng G, Tintrup H, Kirsch J et al. Dual requirement for gephyrin in glycine receptor clustering and molybdoenzyme activity. Science 1998; 282: 1321–4.

108 Fernandez-Chacon R, Sudhof TC. Genetics of synaptic vesicle function: toward the complete functional anatomy of an organelle. Annu Rev Physiol 1999; 61: 753–76.

109 Ferro-Novick S, Jahn R. Vesicle fusion from yeast to man. *Nature* 1994; **370**: 191–3.

110 Fischer M, Kaech S, Knutti D, Matus A. Rapid actin-based plasticity in dendritic spines. *Neuron* 1998; **20**: 847–54.

111 Fischer von Mollard G, Stahl B, Khokhlatchev A *et al*. Rab3C is a synaptic vesicle protein that dissociates from synaptic vesicles after stimulation of exocytosis. *J Biol Chem* 1994; **269**: 10971–4.

112 Fischer von Mollard G, Stahl B, Li C *et al*. Rab proteins in regulated exocytosis. *Trends Biochem Sci* 1994; **19**:164–8.

113 Flucher BE, Daniels MP. Distribution of Na⁺ channels and ankyrin in neuromuscular junctions is complementary to that of acetylcholine receptors and the 43 kd protein. *Neuron* 1989; **3**: 163–75.

114 Foster GA, Johansson O. Ultrastructural morphometric analysis of somatostatin-like immunoreactive neurones in the rat central nervous system after labelling with colloidal gold. *Brain Res* 1985; **342**: 117–27.

115 Friedman HV, Bresler T, Garner CC, Ziv NE. Assembly of new individual excitatory synapses: time course and temporal order of synaptic molecule recruitment. *Neuron* 2000; **27**: 57–69.

116 Friend DS, Farquhar MG. Functions of coated vesicles during protein absorption in the rat vas deferens. *J Cell Biol* 1967; **35**: 357–76.

117 Fritschy JM, Kiener T, Bouilleret V, Loup F. GABAergic neurons and GABA(A)-receptors in temporal lobe epilepsy. *Neurochem Int* 1999; **34**: 435–45.

118 Froener SC. Regulation of ion channel distribution at synapses. *Annu Rev Neurosci* 1993; **16**: 347–68.

119 Fukuda T, Kosaka T. Gap junctions linking the dendritic network of GABAergic interneurons in the hippocampus. *J Neurosci* 2000; **20**: 1519–28.

120 Furshpan EJ, Potter DD. Transmission at the giant motor synapses of the crayfish. *J Physiol* 1959; **145**: 289–325.

121 Fuxe K, Agnati LF. Two principal modes of electrochemical communication in the brain: volume versus wiring transmission. In: Fuxe K, Agnati LF eds. *Volume transmission in the brain: novel mechanisms for neural transmission*. New York: Raven Press, 1991: 1–9.

122 Fyffe REW, Alvarez FJ, Harrington D. Differential distribution of glycine receptors on motoneurons in the cat spinal cord. *Soc Neurosci Abstr* 1993; **19**: 983.

123 Gad H, Low P, Zotova E *et al*. Dissociation between Ca²⁺-triggered synaptic vesicle exocytosis and clathrin-mediated endocytosis at a central synapse. *Neuron* 1998; **21**: 607–16.

124 Gage FH. Mammalian neural stem cells. *Science* 2000; **287**: 1433–8.

125 Gahring LC, Rogers SW, Twyman RE. Autoantibodies to glutamate receptor subunit GluR2 in nonfamilial olivopontocerebellar degeneration. *Neurology* 1997; **48**: 494–500.

126 Gahring LC, Twyman RE, Greenlee JE, Rogers SW. Autoantibodies to neuronal glutamate receptors in patients with paraneoplastic neurodegenerative syndrome enhance receptor activation. *Mol Med* 1995; **1**: 245–53.

127 Galileo DS, Majors J, Horwitz AF, Sanes JR. Retrovirally introduced antisense integrin RNA inhibits neuroblast migration *in vivo*. *Neuron* 1992; **9**: 1117–31.

128 Galzi JL, Changeux JP. Neurotransmitter-gated ion channels as unconventional allosteric proteins. *Curr Opin Struct Biol* 1994; **4**: 554–65.

129 Garcia EP, Mehta S, Blair LA *et al*. SAPGO binds and clusters kainate receptors causing incomplete desensitization. *Neuron* 1998; **21**: 727–39.

130 Gardiol A, Racca C, Triller A. Dendritic and postsynaptic protein synthetic machinery. *J Neurosci* 1999; **19**: 168–79.

131 Garner CC, Kindler S. Synaptic proteins and the assembly of synaptic junctions. *Trends Cell Biol* 1996; **6**: 429–33.

132 Garner CC, Nash J, Huganir RL. PDZ domains in synapse assembly and signalling. *Trends Cell Biol* 2000; **10**: 274–80.

133 Gasic GP, Hollmann M. Molecular neurobiology of glutamate receptors. *Annu Rev Physiol* 1992; **54**: 507–36.

134 Gazzaley AH, Benson DL, Huntley GW, Morrison JH. Differential subcellular regulation of NMDAR1 protein and mRNA in dendrites of dentate gyrus granule cells after perforant path transection. *J Neurosci* 1997; **17**: 2006–17.

135 Geppert M, Bolshakov VY, Siegelbaum SA *et al*. The role of Rab3A in neurotransmitter release. *Nature* 1994; **369**: 493–7.

136 Geppert M, Goda Y, Hammer RE *et al*. Synaptotagmin I: a major Ca²⁺ sensor for transmitter release at a central synapse. *Cell* 1994; **79**: 717–27.

137 Geppert M, Sudhof TC. RAB3 and synaptotagmin: the yin and yang of synaptic membrane fusion. *Annu Rev Neurosci* 1998; **21**: 75–95.

138 Gilman AG. G proteins: transducers of receptor-generated signals. *Annu Rev Biochem* 1987; **56**: 615–49.

139 Goldstein LS, Yang Z. Microtubule-based transport systems in neurons: the roles of kinesins and dyneins. *Annu Rev Neurosci* 2000; **23**: 39–71.

140 Gomeza J, Joly C, Kuhn R *et al*. The second intracellular loop of metabotropic glutamate receptor 1 cooperates with the other intracellular domains to control coupling to G-proteins. *J Biol Chem* 1996; **271**: 2199–205.

141 Gonzalez-Gaitan M, Jackle H. Role of Drosophila alpha-adaptin in presynaptic vesicle recycling. *Cell* 1997; **88**: 767–76.

142 Gordon N. Epilepsy and disorders of neuronal migration. II: Epilepsy as a symptom of neuronal migration defects. *Dev Med Child Neurol* 1996; **38**: 1131–4.

143 Goud B, McCaffrey M. Small GTP-binding proteins and their role in transport. *Curr Opin Cell Biol* 1991; **3**: 626–33.

144 Gray EG. A morphological basis for pre-synaptic inhibition. *Nature* 1962; **193**: 82–3.

145 Gray EG. Axo-somatic and axo-dendritic synapses of the cerebellar cortex: an electron microscope study. *J Anat* 1959; **93**: 420–33.

146 Gray E. Electron microscopy of presynaptic organelles of the spinal cord. *J Anat* 1963; **97**: 101–6.

147 Gray EG, Pease HL. On understanding the organisation of the retinal receptor synapses. *Brain Res* 1971; **35**: 1–15.

148 Graziadei PP, Graziadei GA. Neurogenesis and neuron regeneration in the olfactory system of mammals. I. Morphological aspects of differentiation and structural organization of the olfactory sensory neurons. *J Neurocytol* 1979; **8**: 1–18.

149 Griffon N, Buttner C, Nicke A *et al*. Molecular determinants of glycine receptor subunit assembly. *EMBO J* 1999; **18**: 4711–21.

150 Haass C, Koo EH, Capell A *et al*. Polarized sorting of beta-amyloid precursor protein and its proteolytic products in MDCK cells is regulated by two independent signals. *J Cell Biol* 1995; **128**: 537–47.

151 Hall ZW. *Molecular neurobiology*. Sunderland, MA: Sinauer, 1992.

152 Hall ZW, Sanes JR. Synaptic structure and development: the neuromuscular junction. *Cell* 1993; **72** (Suppl): 99–121.

153 Hampson EC, Vaney DI, Weiler R. Dopaminergic modulation of gap junction permeability between amacrine cells in mammalian retina. *J Neurosci* 1992; **12**: 4911–22.

154 Hanley JG, Koulen P, Bedford F *et al*. The protein MAP-1B links GABA(C) receptors to the cytoskeleton at retinal synapses. *Nature* 1999; **397**: 66–9.

155 Hannah MJ, Schmidt AA, Huttner WB. Synaptic vesicle bio-genesis. *Annu Rev Cell Dev Biol* 1999; **15**: 733–98.

156 Harada A, Oguchi K, Okabe S *et al*. Altered microtubule organization in small-calibre axons of mice lacking tau pro-tein. *Nature* 1994; **369**: 488–91.

157 Harris KM, Landis DM. Membrane structure at synaptic junctions in area CA1 of the rat hippocampus. *Neuro-science* 1986; **19**: 857–72.

158 Hata Y, Butz S, Sudhof TC. CASK: a novel dlg/PSD95 homolog with an N-terminal calmodulin-dependent pro-tein kinase domain identified by interaction with neurex-ins. *J Neurosci* 1996; **16**: 2488–94.

159 Hata Y, Davletov B, Petrenko AG *et al*. Interaction of synap-totagmin with the cytoplasmic domains of neurexins. *Neu-ron* 1993; **10**: 307–15.

160 Hatten ME. Central nervous system neuronal migration. *Annu Rev Neurosci* 1999; **22**: 511–39.

161 Hatten ME. Riding the glial monorail: a common mecha-nism for glial-guided neuronal migration in different regions of the developing mammalian brain. *Trends Neu-rosci* 1990; **13**: 179–84.

162 Hatten ME, Liem RK, Mason CA. Two forms of cerebellar glial cells interact differently with neurons *in vitro*. *J Cell Biol* 1984; **98**: 193–204.

163 He XP, Patel M, Whitney KD *et al*. Glutamate receptor GluR3 antibodies and death of cortical cells. *Neuron* 1998; **20**: 153–63.

164 Heuser JE, Reese TS. Structural changes after transmitter release at the frog neuromuscular junction. *J Cell Biol* 1981; **88**: 564–80.

165 Hevers W, Luddens H. The diversity of GABAA receptors. Pharmacological and electrophysiological properties of GABA_A channel subtypes. *Mol Neurobiol* 1998; **18**: 35–86.

166 Hill JA Jr, Zoli M, Bourgeois JP, Changeux JP. Immunocyto-chemical localization of a neuronal nicotinic receptor: the beta 2-subunit. *J Neurosci* 1993; **13**: 1551–68.

167 Hill MA, Schedlich L, Gunning P. Serum-induced signal transduction determines the peripheral location of beta-actin mRNA within the cell. *J Cell Biol* 1994; **126**: 1221–9.

168 Hirano A. Neurons, astrocytes and ependyma. In: Davis RL, Robertson DM eds. *Textbook of neuropathology*. Baltimore, MD: Williams and Wilkins, 1985: 1–91.

169 Hirokawa N. Kinesin and dynein superfamily proteins and the mechanism of organelle transport. *Science* 1998; **279**: 519–26.

170 Hirokawa N. Mechanism of axonal transport. Identification of new molecular motors and regulations of transports. *Neurosci Res* 1993; **18**: 1–9.

171 Hirokawa N. Molecular architecture and dynamics of the neuronal cytoskeleton. In: Burgoyne RD ed. *The neuronal cytoskeleton*. New York: Wiley-Liss, 1991: 5–74.

172 Hirokawa N. The arrangement of actin filaments in the postsynaptic cytoplasm of the cerebellar cortex revealed by quick-freeze deep-etch electron microscopy. *Neurosci Res* 1989; **6**: 269–75.

173 Hockfield S, McKay RD. Identification of major cell classes in the developing mammalian nervous system. *J Neurosci* 1985; **5**: 3310–28.

174 Hokfelt T. Neuronal communication through multiple coexisting messengers. In: Edelman G, Gall W, Cowan W eds. *Synaptic function*. New York: John Wiley, 1987: 179–211.

175 Hokfelt T, Lundberg J, Schultzberg M. Coexistence of peptides and putative transmitters in neurons. In: Costa E, Trabucchi M eds. *Neural peptides and neuronal commu-nication*. New York: Raven Press, 1980: 1–23.

176 Hollmann M, Heinemann S. Cloned glutamate receptors. *Annu Rev Neurosci* 1994; **17**: 31–108.

177 Hollmann M, Maron C, Heinemann S. *N*-Glycosylation site tagging suggests a three transmembrane domain topolo-gy for the glutamate receptor GluR1. *Neuron* 1994; **13**: 1331–43.

178 Hosaka M, Sudhof TC. Synapsin III, a novel synapsin with an unusual regulation by Ca^{2+}. *J Biol Chem* 1998; **273**: 13371–4.

179 Hosaka M, Sudhof TC. Synapsins I and II are ATP-binding proteins with differential Ca^{2+} regulation. *J Biol Chem* 1998; **273**: 1425–9.

180 Houamed KM, Kuijper JL, Gilbert TL *et al*. Cloning, expression, and gene structure of a G protein-coupled glutamate receptor from rat brain. *Science* 1991; **252**: 1318–21.

181 Hsueh YP, Kim E, Sheng M. Disulfide-linked head-to-head multimerization in the mechanism of ion channel cluster-ing by PSD-95. *Neuron* 1997; **18**: 803–14.

182 Hu H. Chemorepulsion of neuronal migration by Slit2 in the developing mammalian forebrain. *Neuron* 1999; **23**: 703–11.

183 Hu H, Rutishauser U. A septum-derived chemorepulsive fac-tor for migrating olfactory interneuron precursors. *Neuron* 1996; **16**: 933–40.

184 Hu H, Tomasiewicz H, Magnuson T, Rutishauser U. The role of polysialic acid in migration of olfactory bulb interneu-ron precursors in the subventricular zone. *Neuron* 1996; **16**: 735–43.

185 Hunter C, Petralia RS, Vu T, Wenthold RJ. Expression of AMPA-selective glutamate receptor subunits in morpho-logically defined neurons of the mammalian cochlear nucle-us. *J Neurosci* 1993; **13**: 1932–46.

186 Huttner WB. Cell biology. Snappy exocytoxins (News; Com-ment). *Nature* 1993; **365**: 104–5.

187 Ichimura T, Hashimoto PH. Structural components in the synaptic cleft captured by freeze-substitution and deep etching of directly frozen cerebellar cortex. *J Neurocytol* 1988; **17**: 3–12.

188 Ichtchenko K, Hata Y, Nguyen T *et al*. Neuroligin 1: a splice site-specific ligand for beta-neurexins. *Cell* 1995; **81**: 435–43.

189 Ichtchenko K, Nguyen T, Sudhof TC. Structures, alternative splicing, and neurexin binding of multiple neuroligins. *J Biol Chem* 1996; **271**: 2676–82.

190 Irie M, Hata Y, Takeuchi M *et al*. Binding of neuroligins to PSD-95. *Science* 1997; **277**: 1511–15.

191 Jacobson M. *Developmental neurobiology* 3rd edn. New York: Plenum Press, 1991.

192 Jacques TS, Relvas JB, Nishimura S *et al*. Neural precursor cell chain migration and division are regulated through different beta1 integrins. *Development* 1998; **125**: 3167–77.

193 Jahn R, Sudhof TC. Membrane fusion and exocytosis. *Annu Rev Biochem* 1999; **68**: 863–911.

194 Jahn R, Sudhof TC. Synaptic vesicles and exocytosis. *Annu Rev Neurosci* 1994; **17**: 219–46.

195 Jankovski A, Sotelo C. Subventricular zone–olfactory bulb migratory pathway in the adult mouse: cellular composi-tion and specificity as determined by heterochronic and heterotopic transplantation. *J Comp Neurol* 1996; **371**: 376–96.

196 Janz R, Sudhof TC, Hammer RE *et al*. Essential roles in synaptic plasticity for synaptogyrin I and synaptophysin I. *Neuron* 1999; **24**: 687–700.

197 Jareb M, Banker G. The polarized sorting of membrane pro-teins expressed in cultured hippocampal neurons using viral vectors. *Neuron* 1998; **20**: 855–67.

198 Jessell TM, Siegel RE, Fischbach GD. Induction of acetyl-choline receptors on cultured skeletal muscle by a factor

extracted from brain and spinal cord. *Proc Natl Acad Sci USA* 1979; **76**: 5397–401.

199 Johansson CB, Momma S, Clarke DL *et al*. Identification of a neural stem cell in the adult mammalian central nervous system. *Cell* 1999; **96**: 25–34.

200 Johnson JW, Ascher P. Glycine potentiates the NMDA response in cultured mouse brain neurons. *Nature* 1987; **325**: 529–31.

201 Kaech S, Fischer M, Doll T, Matus A. Isoform specificity in the relationship of actin to dendritic spines. *J Neurosci* 1997; **17**: 9565–72.

202 Kaiserman-Abramof IR, Palay SL. Fine structural studies of the cerebellar cortex in a mormyrid fish. In: Llinas R ed. *Neurobiology of cerebellar evolution and development*. Chicago, IL: American Medical Association, 1969: 171–205.

203 Katz B. *Nerve, muscle and synapse*. New York: McGraw-Hill, 1966.

204 Kelly RB, Grote E. Protein targeting in the neuron. *Annu Rev Neurosci* 1993; **16**: 95–127.

205 Kennedy MB. The postsynaptic density. *Curr Opin Neurobiol* 1993; **3**: 732–7.

206 Kiebler MA, DesGroseillers L. Molecular insights into mRNA transport and local translation in the mammalian nervous system. *Neuron* 2000; **25**: 19–28.

207 Kim E, Niethammer M, Rothschild A *et al*. Clustering of Shaker-type K$^+$ channels by interaction with a family of membrane-associated guanylate kinases. *Nature* 1995; **378**: 85–8.

208 Kim JH, Huganir RL. Organization and regulation of proteins at synapses (Published erratum appears in *Curr Opin Cell Biol* 1999; **11**: 407–8). *Curr Opin Cell Biol* 1999; **11**: 248–54.

209 Kim S, Masurowsky E, Benitez H, Murray M. Histochemical studies of the intranuclear rodlet in neurons of chicken sympathetic and sensory ganglia. *Histochemie* 1970; **24**: 33–40.

210 Kinoshita A, Shigemoto R, Ohishi H *et al*. Immunohistochemical localization of metabotropic glutamate receptors, mGluR7a and mGluR7b, in the central nervous system of the adult rat and mouse: a light and electron microscopic study. *J Comp Neurol* 1998; **393**: 332–52.

211 Kins S, Betz H, Kirsch J. Collybistin, a newly identified brain-specific GEF, induces submembrane clustering of gephyrin. *Nat Neurosci* 2000; **3**: 22–9.

212 Kinzie JM, Shinohara MM, van den Pol AN *et al*. Immunolocalization of metabotropic glutamate receptor 7 in the rat olfactory bulb. *J Comp Neurol* 1997; **385**: 372–84.

213 Kirchhausen T. Adaptors for clathrin-mediated traffic. *Annu Rev Cell Dev Biol* 1999; **15**: 705–32.

214 Kirsch J, Betz H. Glycine-receptor activation is required for receptor clustering in spinal neurons. *Nature* 1998; **392**: 717–20.

215 Kirsch J, Betz H. The postsynaptic localization of the glycine receptor-associated protein gephyrin is regulated by the cytoskeleton. *J Neurosci* 1995; **15**: 4148–56.

216 Kirsch J, Betz H. Widespread expression of gephyrin, a putative glycine receptor-tubulin linker protein, in rat brain. *Brain Res* 1993; **621**: 301–10.

217 Kirsch J, Langosch D, Prior P *et al*. The 93-kDa glycine receptor-associated protein binds to tubulin. *J Biol Chem* 1991; **266**: 22242–5.

218 Kirsch J, Wolters I, Triller A, Betz H. Gephyrin antisense oligonucleotides prevent glycine receptor clustering in spinal neurons. *Nature* 1993; **366**: 745–8.

219 Kleiman R, Banker G, Steward O. Development of subcellular mRNA compartmentation in hippocampal neurons in culture. *J Neurosci* 1994; **14**: 1130–40.

220 Kneussel M, Betz H. Receptors, gephyrin and gephyrin-associated proteins: novel insights into the assembly of inhibitory postsynaptic membrane specializations. *J Physiol (Lond)* 2000; **525** (Pt 1): 1–9.

221 Kneussel M, Brandstatter JH, Laube B *et al*. Loss of postsynaptic GABA(A) receptor clustering in gephyrin-deficient mice. *J Neurosci* 1999; **19**: 9289–97.

222 Koenig JH, Ikeda K. Synaptic vesicles have two distinct recycling pathways. *J Cell Biol* 1996; **135**: 797–808.

223 Kohmura N, Senzaki K, Hamada S *et al*. Diversity revealed by a novel family of cadherins expressed in neurons at a synaptic complex. *Neuron* 1998; **20**: 1137–51.

224 Korn H, Faber DS. Electrical interactions between vertebrate neurons: field effects and electrotonic coupling. In: Schmitt FO, Worden F eds. *The neurosciences 4th study program*. Cambridge, MA: MIT Press, 1979: 333–58.

225 Korn H, Sotelo C, Crepel F. Electronic coupling between neurons in the rat lateral vestibular nucleus. *Exp Brain Res* 1973; **16**: 255–75.

226 Korn H, Sur C, Charpier S *et al*. The one vesicle hypothesis and multivesicular release. In: Stjärne L, Greengard P, Grillner S *et al*. eds. *Molecular and cellular mechanisms of neurotransmitter release*. New York: Raven Press, 1993: 301–22.

227 Kornack DR, Rakic P. Continuation of neurogenesis in the hippocampus of the adult macaque monkey. *Proc Natl Acad Sci USA* 1999; **96**: 5768–73.

228 Kornau HC, Schenker LT, Kennedy MB, Seeburg PH. Domain interaction between NMDA receptor subunits and the postsynaptic density protein PSD-95. *Science* 1995; **269**: 1737–40.

229 Kreis TE. Regulation of vesicular and tubular membrane traffic of the Golgi complex by coat proteins. *Curr Opin Cell Biol* 1992; **4**: 609–15.

230 Kristensson K. Retrograde transport of macromolecules in axons. *Annu Rev Pharmacol Toxicol* 1978; **18**: 97–110.

231 Kuffler SW, Nicholls JG, Martin AR. *From neuron to brain. A cellular approach to the function of the nervous system*. Sunderland, MA: Sinauer, 1984.

232 Kuhse J, Betz H, Kirsch J. The inhibitory glycine receptor: architecture, synaptic localization and molecular pathology of a postsynaptic ion-channel complex. *Curr Opin Neurobiol* 1995; **5**: 318–23.

233 Kumar NM, Gilula NB. The gap junction communication channel. *Cell* 1996; **84**: 381–8.

234 Kuromi H, Kidokoro Y. Two distinct pools of synaptic vesicles in single presynaptic boutons in a temperature-sensitive *Drosophila* mutant, shibire. *Neuron* 1998; **20**: 917–25.

235 Landis DM, Hall AK, Weinstein LA, Reese TS. The organization of cytoplasm at the presynaptic active zone of a central nervous system synapse. *Neuron* 1988; **1**: 201–9.

236 Landis DM, Weinstein LA, Reese TS. Substructure in the postsynaptic density of Purkinje cell dendritic spines revealed by rapid freezing and etching. *Synapse* 1987; **1**: 552–8.

237 Lang EJ, Sugihara I, Llinas R. GABAergic modulation of complex spike activity by the cerebellar nucleoolivary pathway in rat. *J Neurophysiol* 1996; **76**: 255–75.

238 Lasater EM, Dowling JE. Dopamine decreases conductance of the electrical junctions between cultured retinal horizontal cells. *Proc Natl Acad Sci USA* 1985; **82**: 3025–9.

239 Lavdas AA, Grigoriou M, Pachnis V, Parnavelas JG. The medial ganglionic eminence gives rise to a population of early neurons in the developing cerebral cortex. *J Neurosci* 1999; **19**: 7881–8.

240 Leblond C. Classification of cell populations on the basis of their proliferative behavior. *Natl Cancer Inst Monogr* 1964; **14**: 119–50.

241 Legouis R, Hardelin JP, Levilliers J *et al*. The candidate gene for the X-linked Kallmann syndrome encodes a protein related to adhesion molecules. *Cell* 1991; **67**: 423–35.

242 Levi S, Chesnoy-Marchais D, Sieghart W, Triller A. Synaptic control of glycine and GABA(A) receptors and gephyrin expression in cultured motoneurons. *J Neurosci* 1999; **19**: 7434–49.

243 Levi S, Vannier C, Triller A. Strychnine-sensitive stabilization of postsynaptic glycine receptor clusters. *J Cell Sci* 1998; **111**: 335–45.

244 Li C, Ullrich B, Zhang JZ *et al*. Ca(2+)-dependent and -independent activities of neural and non-neural synaptotagmins. *Nature* 1995; **375**: 594–9.

245 Lindner J, Rathjen FG, Schachner M. L1 mono- and polyclonal antibodies modify cell migration in early postnatal mouse cerebellum. *Nature* 1983; **305**: 427–30.

246 Llano I, Gerschenfeld HM. Beta-adrenergic enhancement of inhibitory synaptic activity in rat cerebellar stellate and Purkinje cells. *J Physiol (Lond)* 1993; **468**: 201–24.

247 Llinas R. Electronic transmission in the mammalian central nervous system. In: Bennett MVL, Spray DC eds. *Gap junctions*. Cold Spring Harbor, NY: Cold Spring Harbor Laboratory Press, 1985: 337–53.

248 Llinas R, Sasaki K. The functional organization of the olivo-cerebellar system as examined by multiple Purkinje cell recordings. *Eur J Neurosci* 1989; **1**: 587–602.

249 Llinas R, Steinberg IZ, Walton K. Presynaptic calcium currents in squid giant synapse. *Biophys J* 1981; **33**: 289–321.

250 Llinas RR. The intrinsic electrophysiological properties of mammalian neurons: insights into central nervous system function. *Science* 1988; **242**: 1654–64.

251 Loewi O. Uber humorale ubertragbarkeit der herzn-erzvenwirkung. *Pflugers Archiv Gesamte Physiol Menschen Tiere* 1921; **189**: 239–42.

252 Lois C, Alvarez-Buylla A. Long-distance neuronal migration in the adult mammalian brain. *Science* 1994; **264**: 1145–8.

253 Lois C, Alvarez-Buylla A. Proliferating subventricular zone cells in the adult mammalian forebrain can differentiate into neurons and glia. *Proc Natl Acad Sci USA* 1993; **90**: 2074–7.

254 Lois C, Garcia-Verdugo JM, Alvarez-Buylla A. Chain migration of neuronal precursors. *Science* 1996; **271**: 978–81.

255 Lo Nigro C, Chong CS, Smith AC *et al*. Point mutations and an intragenic deletion in LIS1, the lissencephaly causative gene in isolated lissencephaly sequence and Miller–Dieker syndrome. *Hum Mol Genet* 1997; **6**: 157–64.

256 Loup F, Wieser HG, Yonekawa Y *et al*. Selective alterations in GABAA receptor subtypes in human temporal lobe epilepsy. *J Neurosci* 2000; **20**: 5401–19.

257 Lujan R, Nusser Z, Roberts JD *et al*. Perisynaptic location of metabotropic glutamate receptors mGluR1 and mGluR5 on dendrites and dendritic spines in the rat hippocampus. *Eur J Neurosci* 1996; **8**: 1488–500.

258 Luskin MB. Restricted proliferation and migration of postnatally generated neurons derived from the forebrain subventricular zone. *Neuron* 1993; **11**: 173–89.

259 MacVicar BA, Dudek FE. Electrotonic coupling between pyramidal cells: a direct demonstration in rat hippocampal slices. *Science* 1981; **213**: 782–5.

260 Makowski L, Caspar DL, Phillips WC, Goodenough DA. Gap junction structures. II. Analysis of the x-ray diffraction data. *J Cell Biol* 1977; **74**: 629–45.

261 Maletic-Savatic M, Malinow R. Calcium-evoked dendritic exocytosis in cultured hippocampal neurons. Part I: Trans-Golgi network-derived organelles undergo regulated exocytosis. *J Neurosci* 1998; **18**: 6803–13.

262 Mammoto A, Sasaki T, Asakura T *et al*. Interactions of drebrin and gephyrin with profilin. *Biochem Biophys Res Commun* 1998; **243**: 86–9.

263 Mariani J, Crepel F, Mikoshiba K *et al*. Anatomical, physiological and biochemical studies of the cerebellum from Reeler mutant mouse. *Phil Trans R Soc Lond B Biol Sci* 1977; **281**: 1–28.

264 Martin A, Pilar G. Dual mode of synaptic transmission in the avian ciliary ganglion. *J Physiol (Lond)* 1963; **168**: 93–115.

265 Martin LJ, Blackstone CD, Huganir RL, Price DL. Cellular localization of a metabotropic glutamate receptor in rat brain. *Neuron* 1992; **9**: 259–70.

266 Martin SJ, Grimwood PD, Morris RG. Synaptic plasticity and memory: an evaluation of the hypothesis. *Annu Rev Neurosci* 2000; **23**: 649–711.

267 Masu M, Tanabe Y, Tsuchida K *et al*. Sequence and expression of a metabotropic glutamate receptor. *Nature* 1991; **349**: 760–5.

268 Mathisen PM, Johnson JM, Kawczak JA, Tuohy VK. Visinin-like protein (VILIP) is a neuron-specific calcium-dependent double-stranded RNA-binding protein. *J Biol Chem* 1999; **274**: 31571–6.

269 Matthews-Bellinger J, Salpeter MM. Distribution of acetylcholine receptors at frog neuromuscular junctions with a discussion of some physiological implications. *J Physiol (Lond)* 1978; **279**: 197–213.

270 Matus A. Microtubule-associated proteins: their potential role in determining neuronal morphology. *Annu Rev Neurosci* 1988; **11**: 29–44.

271 Mayford M, Baranes D, Podsypanina K, Kandel ER. The 3′-untranslated region of CaMKII alpha is a *cis*-acting signal for the localization and translation of mRNA in dendrites. *Proc Natl Acad Sci USA* 1996; **93**: 13250–5.

272 McAllister AK, Katz LC, Lo DC. Neurotrophins and synaptic plasticity. *Annu Rev Neurosci* 1999; **22**: 295–318.

273 McPherson PS, De Camili P. Recycling and biogenesis of synaptic vesicles. *Semin Neurosci* 1994; **6**: 137–47.

274 Meier J, De Chaldee M, Triller A, Vannier C. Functional heterogeneity of gephyrins. *Mol Cell Neurosci* 2000; **16**: 566–77.

275 Meinck HM, Ricker K, Hulser PJ, Solimena M. Stiff man syndrome: neurophysiological findings in eight patients. *J Neurol* 1995; **242**: 134–42.

276 Miale I, Sidman R. An autoradiographic analysis of histogenesis in the mouse cerebellum. *Exp Neurol* 1961; **4**: 277–96.

277 Miles R, Poncer JC. Metabotropic glutamate receptors mediate a post-tetanic excitation of guinea-pig hippocampal inhibitory neurones. *J Physiol (Lond)* 1993; **463**: 461–73.

278 Miller TM, Heuser JE. Endocytosis of synaptic vesicle membrane at the frog neuromuscular junction. *J Cell Biol* 1984; **98**: 685–98.

279 Missler M, Sudhof TC. Neurexins: three genes and 1001 products. *Trends Genet* 1998; **14**: 20–6.

280 Miyashiro K, Dichter M, Eberwine J. On the nature and differential distribution of mRNAs in hippocampal neurites: implications for neuronal functioning. *Proc Natl Acad Sci USA* 1994; **91**: 10800–4.

281 Momma S, Johansson CB, Frisen J. Get to know your stem cells. *Curr Opin Neurobiol* 2000; **10**: 45–9.

282 Morris NR. Nuclear migration. From fungi to the mammalian brain. *J Cell Biol* 2000; **148**: 1097–101.

283 Morris SM, Albrecht U, Reiner O *et al*. The lissencephaly gene product Lis1, a protein involved in neuronal migra-

tion, interacts with a nuclear movement protein, NudC. *Curr Biol* 1998; **8**: 603–6.

284 Mulle C, Vidal C, Benoit P, Changeux JP. Existence of different subtypes of nicotinic acetylcholine receptors in the rat habenulo-interpeduncular system. *J Neurosci* 1991; **11**: 2588–97.

285 Mundigl O, Matteoli M, Daniell L *et al*. Synaptic vesicle proteins and early endosomes in cultured hippocampal neurons: differential effects of Brefeldin A in axon and dendrites. *J Cell Biol* 1993; **122**: 1207–21.

286 Nakajima Y. Fine structure of the synaptic endings on the Mauthner cell of the goldfish. *J Comp Neurol* 1974; **156**: 379–402.

287 Nakanishi S. Metabotropic glutamate receptors: synaptic transmission, modulation, and plasticity. *Neuron* 1994; **13**: 1031–7.

288 Nakanishi S. Molecular diversity of glutamate receptors and implications for brain function. *Science* 1992; **258**: 597–603.

289 Neki A, Ohishi H, Kaneko T *et al*. Pre- and postsynaptic localization of a metabotropic glutamate receptor, mGluR2, in the rat brain: an immunohistochemical study with a monoclonal antibody. *Neurosci Lett* 1996; **202**: 197–200.

290 Neyton J, Piccolino M, Gerschenfeld HM. Neurotransmitter-induced modulation of gap junction permeability in retinal horizontal cells. In: Bennett MVL, Spray DC eds. *Gap junctions*. Cold Spring Harbor, NY: Cold Spring Harbor Laboratory Press, 1985: 381–91.

291 Nguyen Ba-Charvet KT, Brose K, Marillat V *et al*. Slit2-Mediated chemorepulsion and collapse of developing forebrain axons. *Neuron* 1999; **22**: 463–73.

292 Nguyen T, Sudhof TC. Binding properties of neuroligin 1 and neurexin 1beta reveal function as heterophilic cell adhesion molecules. *J Biol Chem* 1997; **272**: 26032–9.

293 Nicoll RA, Malenka RC, Kauer JA. Functional comparison of neurotransmitter receptor subtypes in mammalian central nervous system. *Physiol Rev* 1990; **70**: 513–65.

294 Niethammer M, Valtschanoff JG, Kapoor TM *et al*. CRIPT, a novel postsynaptic protein that binds to the third PDZ domain of PSD-95/SAP90. *Neuron* 1998; **20**: 693–707.

295 Nixon RA. Dynamic behavior and organization of cytoskeletal proteins in neurons: reconciling old and new findings. *Bioessays* 1998; **20**: 798–807.

296 Nonet ML, Staunton JE, Kilgard MP *et al*. Caenorhabditis elegans rab-3 mutant synapses exhibit impaired function and are partially depleted of vesicles. *J Neurosci* 1997; **17**: 8061–73.

297 Nowakowski RS, Lewin SB, Miller MW. Bromodeoxyuridine immunohistochemical determination of the lengths of the cell cycle and the DNA-synthetic phase for an anatomically defined population. *J Neurocytol* 1989; **18**: 311–18.

298 Nusser Z, Lujan R, Laube G *et al*. Cell type and pathway dependence of synaptic AMPA receptor number and variability in the hippocampus. *Neuron* 1998; **21**: 545–59.

299 Nusser Z, Mulvihill E, Streit P, Somogyi P. Subsynaptic segregation of metabotropic and ionotropic glutamate receptors as revealed by immunogold localization. *Neuroscience* 1994; **61**: 421–7.

300 Nusser Z, Roberts JD, Baude A *et al*. Immunocytochemical localization of the alpha 1 and beta 2/3 subunits of the GABA$_A$ receptor in relation to specific GABAergic synapses in the dentate gyrus. *Eur J Neurosci* 1995; **7**: 630–46.

301 Nusser Z, Sieghart W, Benke D *et al*. Differential synaptic localization of two major gamma-aminobutyric acid type A receptor alpha subunits on hippocampal pyramidal cells. *Proc Natl Acad Sci USA* 1996; **93**: 11939–44.

302 O'Brien J, Bruzzone R, White TW *et al*. Cloning and expression of two related connexins from the perch retina define a distinct subgroup of the connexin family. *J Neurosci* 1998; **18**: 7625–37.

303 O'Brien RJ, Xu D, Petralia RS *et al*. Synaptic clustering of AMPA receptors by the extracellular immediate-early gene product Narp. *Neuron* 1999; **23**: 309–23.

304 O'Donnell P, Grace AA. Dopaminergic modulation of dye coupling between neurons in the core and shell regions of the nucleus accumbens. *J Neurosci* 1993; **13**: 3456–71.

305 Okamoto N, Hori S, Akazawa C *et al*. Molecular characterization of a new metabotropic glutamate receptor mGluR7 coupled to inhibitory cyclic AMP signal transduction. *J Biol Chem* 1994; **269**: 1231–6.

306 Olsen RW, Tobin AJ. Molecular biology of GABA$_A$ receptors. *FASEB J* 1990; **4**: 1469–80.

307 Ono K, Tomasiewicz H, Magnuson T, Rutishauser U. N-CAM mutation inhibits tangential neuronal migration and is phenocopied by enzymatic removal of polysialic acid. *Neuron* 1994; **13**: 595–609.

308 Palay S, Palade G. The fine structure of neurons. *J Biophys Biochem Cytol* 1955; **1**: 69–88.

309 Palay SL. The morphology of synapses in the central nervous system. *Exp Cell Res* 1958; **5** (Suppl): 275–93.

310 Palay SL, Chan-Palay V. *Cerebellar cortex. Cytology and organization*. Berlin: Springer, 1974.

311 Palay SL, Sotelo C, Peters A, Orkand PM. The axon hillock and the initial segment. *J Cell Biol* 1968; **38**: 193–201.

312 Pannese E. *Neurocytology. Fine structure of neurons, nerve processes, and neuroglial cells*. Stuttgart: G Thieme, 1994.

313 Parenti R, Gulisano M, Zappala A, Cicirata F. Expression of connexin36 mRNA in adult rodent brain. *NeuroReport* 2000; **11**: 1497–502.

314 Paul DL. Molecular cloning of cDNA for rat liver gap junction protein. *J Cell Biol* 1986; **103**: 123–34.

315 Peters A, Palay SL, Webster HdF. *The fine structure of the nervous system. Neurons and their supporting cells*. New York: Oxford University Press, 1991.

316 Petralia RS, Yokotani N, Wenthold RJ. Light and electron microscope distribution of the NMDA receptor subunit NMDAR1 in the rat nervous system using a selective anti-peptide antibody. *J Neurosci* 1994; **14**: 667–96.

317 Pfenninger K, Akert K, Moor H, Sandri C. The fine structure of freeze-fractured presynaptic membranes. *J Neurocytol* 1972; **1**: 129–49.

318 Pfenninger K, Sandri C, Akert K, Eugster CH. Contribution to the problem of structural organization of the presynaptic area. *Brain Res* 1969; **12**: 10–18.

319 Pin JP, Duvoisin R. The metabotropic glutamate receptors: structure and functions. *Neuropharmacology* 1995; **34**: 1–26.

320 Pin JP, Joly C, Heinemann SF, Bockaert J. Domains involved in the specificity of G protein activation in phospholipase C-coupled metabotropic glutamate receptors. *EMBO J* 1994; **13**: 342–8.

321 Polenzani L, Woodward RM, Miledi R. Expression of mammalian gamma-aminobutyric acid receptors with distinct pharmacology in *Xenopus* oocytes. *Proc Natl Acad Sci USA* 1991; **88**: 4318–22.

322 Prior P, Schmitt B, Grenningloh G *et al*. Primary structure and alternative splice variants of gephyrin, a putative glycine receptor-tubulin linker protein. *Neuron* 1992; **8**: 1161–70.

323 Pumplin DW, Reese TS, Llinas R. Are the presynaptic membrane particles the calcium channels? *Proc Natl Acad Sci USA* 1981; **78**: 7210–13.

324 Purves D, Lichtman JW. *Principles of neural development*. Sunderland, MA: Sinauer, 1985.

325 Quinlan EM, Philpot BD, Huganir RL, Bear MF. Rapid, experience-dependent expression of synaptic NMDA receptors in visual cortex *in vivo*. *Nat Neurosci* 1999; **2**: 352–7.

326 Racca C, Gardiol A, Triller A. Dendritic and postsynaptic localizations of glycine receptor alpha subunit mRNAs. *J Neurosci* 1997; **17**: 1691–700.

327 Ragozzino D, Woodward RM, Murata Y *et al*. Design and in vitro pharmacology of a selective gamma-aminobutyric acidC receptor antagonist. *Mol Pharmacol* 1996; **50**: 1024–30.

328 Rakic P. Contact regulation of neuronal migration. In: Edelman GE, Thiery JP ed. *The cell in contact*. New York: John Wiley, 1985: 67–90.

329 Rakic P. Defects of neuronal migration and the pathogenesis of cortical malformations. *Prog Brain Res* 1988; **73**: 15–37.

330 Rakic P. Neuron–glia relationship during granule cell migration in developing cerebellar cortex. A Golgi and electronmicroscopic study in Macacus Rhesus. *J Comp Neurol* 1971; **141**: 283–312.

331 Rakic P. Principles of neural cell migration. *Experientia* 1990; **46**: 882–91.

332 Rakic P, Cameron RS, Komuro H. Recognition, adhesion, transmembrane signaling and cell motility in guided neuronal migration. *Curr Opin Neurobiol* 1994; **4**: 63–9.

333 Rall W, Shepherd GM, Reese TS, Brightman MW. Dendrodendritic synaptic pathway for inhibition in the olfactory bulb. *Exp Neurol* 1966; **14**: 44–56.

334 Ramon y Cajal S. *Histologie du système nerveux de l'homme et des vertèbres* Vol. 2. Paris: Maloine ed., 1911.

335 Rao A, Harms KJ, Craig AM. Neuroligation: building synapses around the neurexin–neuroligin link (News). *Nat Neurosci* 2000; **3**: 747–9.

336 Rao A, Kim E, Sheng M, Craig AM. Heterogeneity in the molecular composition of excitatory postsynaptic sites during development of hippocampal neurons in culture. *J Neurosci* 1998; **18**: 1217–29.

337 Raviola E, Gilula NB. Intramembrane organization of specialized contacts in the outer plexiform layer of the retina. A freeze-fracture study in monkeys and rabbits. *J Cell Biol* 1975; **65**: 192–222.

338 Redecker C, Luhmann HJ, Hagemann G *et al*. Differential downregulation of GABAA receptor subunits in widespread brain regions in the freeze-lesion model of focal cortical malformations. *J Neurosci* 2000; **20**: 5045–53.

339 Regnier-Vigouroux A, Tooze SA, Huttner WB. Newly synthetised synaptophysin is transported to synaptic-like microvesicles via constitutive secretory vesicles and the plasmamembrane. *EMBO J* 1991; **10**: 3589–601.

340 Revel JP, Karnovsky MJ. Hexagonal array of subunits in intercellular junctions of the mouse heart and liver. *J Cell Biol* 1967; **33**: C7–12.

341 Reynolds BA, Weiss S. Generation of neurons and astrocytes from isolated cells of the adult mammalian central nervous system. *Science* 1992; **255**: 1707–10.

342 Richards JG, Schoch P, Haring P *et al*. Resolving GABAA/benzodiazepine receptors: cellular and subcellular localization in the CNS with monoclonal antibodies. *J Neurosci* 1987; **7**: 1866–86.

343 Ringstad N, Gad H, Low P *et al*. Endophilin/SH3p4 is required for the transition from early to late stages in clathrin-mediated synaptic vesicle endocytosis. *Neuron* 1999; **24**: 143–54.

344 Rio C, Rieff HI, Qi P, Khurana TS, Corfas G. Neuregulin and erbB receptors play a critical role in neuronal migration (Published erratum appears in *Neuron* 1997; **19**: 1349). *Neuron* 1997; **19**: 39–50.

345 Robitaille R, Adler EM, Charlton MP. Strategic location of calcium channels at transmitter release sites of frog neuromuscular synapses. *Neuron* 1990; **5**: 773–9.

346 Rodriguez E, George N, Lachaux JP *et al*. Perception's shadow: long-distance synchronization of human brain activity. *Nature* 1999; **397**: 430–3.

347 Rogers SW, Andrews PI, Gahring LC *et al*. Autoantibodies to glutamate receptor GluR3 in Rasmussen's encephalitis. *Science* 1994; **265**: 648–51.

348 Rohrer H. The role of growth factors in the control of neurogenesis. *Eur J Neurosci* 1990; **2**: 1005–15.

349 Roos J, Kelly RB. Preassembly and transport of nerve terminals: a new concept of axonal transport (News; Comment). *Nat Neurosci* 2000; **3**: 415–17.

350 Rosahl TW, Spillane D, Missler M *et al*. Essential functions of synapsins I and II in synaptic vesicle regulation. *Nature* 1995; **375**: 488–93.

351 Rothman JE, Orci L. Molecular dissection of the secretory pathway. *Nature* 1992; **355**: 409–15.

352 Ryan TA, Reuter H, Wendland B *et al*. The kinetics of synaptic vesicle recycling measured at single presynaptic boutons. *Neuron* 1993; **11**: 713–24.

353 Sabatini DM, Barrow RK, Blackshaw S *et al*. Interaction of RAFT1 with gephyrin required for rapamycin-sensitive signaling. *Science* 1999; **284**: 1161–4.

354 Saga Y, Yagi T, Ikawa Y *et al*. Mice develop normally without tenascin. *Genes Dev* 1992; **6**: 1821–31.

355 Sans N, Petralia RS, Wang YX *et al*. A developmental change in NMDA receptor-associated proteins at hippocampal synapses. *J Neurosci* 2000; **20**: 1260–71.

356 Sapir T, Elbaum M, Reiner O. Reduction of microtubule catastrophe events by LIS1, platelet-activating factor acetylhydrolase subunit. *EMBO J* 1997; **16**: 6977–84.

357 Sargent PB. The diversity of neuronal nicotinic acetylcholine receptors. *Annu Rev Neurosci* 1993; **16**: 403–43.

358 Sauer F. Mitosis in the neural tube. *J Comp Neurol* 1935; **62**: 377–405.

359 Scheetz AJ, Nairn AC, Constantine-Paton M. NMDA receptor-mediated control of protein synthesis at developing synapses. *Nat Neurosci* 2000; **3**: 211–16.

360 Scheiffele P, Fan J, Choih J, Fetter R, Serafini T. Neuroligin expressed in nonneuronal cells triggers presynaptic development in contacting axons. *Cell* 2000; **101**: 657–69.

361 Schiavo G, Benfenati F, Poulain B *et al*. Tetanus and botulinum-B neurotoxins block neurotransmitter release by proteolytic cleavage of synaptobrevin. *Nature* 1992; **359**: 832–5.

362 Schmid SL, McNiven MA, De Camilli P. Dynamin and its partners: a progress report. *Curr Opin Cell Biol* 1998; **10**: 504–12.

363 Schmidt A, Huttner WB. Biogenesis of synaptic-like microvesicles in perforated PC12 cells. *Methods* 1998; **16**: 160–9.

364 Schmidt A, Wolde M, Thiele C *et al*. Endophilin I mediates synaptic vesicle formation by transfer of arachidonate to lysophosphatidic acid. *Nature* 1999; **401**: 133–41.

365 Schmied R, Holtzman E. A phosphatase activity and a synaptic vesicle antigen in multivesicular bodies of frog retinal photoreceptor terminals. *J Neurocytol* 1987; **16**: 627–37.

366 Schmitt RO, Dev P, Smith BH. Electrotonic processing of information by brain cells. *Science* 1976; **193**: 114–20.

367 Schoepp DD, Conn PJ. Metabotropic glutamate receptors in brain function and pathology. *Trends Pharmacol Sci* 1993; **14**: 13–20.

368 Seeburg PH. The TINS/TiPS Lecture. The molecular biology of mammalian glutamate receptor channels. *Trends Neurosci* 1993; **16**: 359–65.

369 Seitanidou T, Triller A, Korn H. Distribution of glycine receptors on the membrane of a central neuron: an immunoelectron microscopy study. *J Neurosci* 1988; **8**: 4319–33.

370 Serafini T, Colamarino SA, Leonardo ED *et al*. Netrin-1 is required for commissural axon guidance in the developing vertebrate nervous system. *Cell* 1996; **87**: 1001–14.

371 Sever S, Muhlberg AB, Schmid SL. Impairment of dynamin's GAP domain stimulates receptor-mediated endocytosis. *Nature* 1999; **398**: 481–6.

372 Shapiro L, Colman DR. The diversity of cadherins and implications for a synaptic adhesive code in the CNS. *Neuron* 1999; **23**: 427–30.

373 Shepherd GM. *Neurobiology*. New York: Oxford University Press, 1983.

374 Shepherd GM. *Foundations of the neuron doctrine*. New York: Oxford University Press, 1991: 1–338.

375 Shi G, Faundez V, Roos J, Dell'Angelica EC, Kelly RB. Neuroendocrine synaptic vesicles are formed *in vitro* by both clathrin-dependent and clathrin-independent pathways. *J Cell Biol* 1998; **143**: 947–55.

376 Shiang R, Ryan SG, Zhu YZ *et al*. Mutations in the alpha 1 subunit of the inhibitory glycine receptor cause the dominant neurologic disorder, hyperekplexia. *Nat Genet* 1993; **5**: 351–8.

377 Shigemoto R, Kulik A, Roberts JD *et al*. Target-cell-specific concentration of a metabotropic glutamate receptor in the presynaptic active zone. *Nature* 1996; **381**: 523–5.

378 Shigemoto R, Nomura S, Ohishi H *et al*. Immunohistochemical localization of a metabotropic glutamate receptor, mGluR5, in the rat brain. *Neurosci Lett* 1993; **163**: 53–7.

379 Shupliakov O, Low P, Grabs D *et al*. Synaptic vesicle endocytosis impaired by disruption of dynamin–SH3 domain interactions. *Science* 1997; **276**: 259–63.

380 Sidman RL, Rakic P. Neuronal migration, with special reference to developing human brain: a review. *Brain Res* 1973; **62**: 1–35.

381 Siegel SJ, Brose N, Janssen WG *et al*. Regional, cellular, and ultrastructural distribution of *N*-methyl-d-aspartate receptor subunit 1 in monkey hippocampus. *Proc Natl Acad Sci USA* 1994; **91**: 564–8.

382 Sillevis Smitt P, Kinoshita A, De Leeuw B *et al*. Paraneoplastic cerebellar ataxia due to autoantibodies against a glutamate receptor. *N Engl J Med* 2000; **342**: 21–7.

383 Simons K, Zerial M. Rab proteins and the road maps for intracellular transport. *Neuron* 1993; **11**: 789–99.

384 Sinden JD, Rashid-Doubell F, Kershaw TR *et al*. Recovery of spatial learning by grafts of a conditionally immortalized hippocampal neuroepithelial cell line into the ischaemia-lesioned hippocampus. *Neuroscience* 1997; **81**: 599–608.

385 Smeyne RJ, Chu T, Lewin A *et al*. Local control of granule cell generation by cerebellar Purkinje cells. *Mol Cell Neurosci* 1995; **6**: 230–51.

386 Sollner T, Rothman JE. Neurotransmission: harnessing fusion machinery at the synapse. *Trends Neurosci* 1994; **17**: 344–8.

387 Somogyi P, Fritschy JM, Benke D *et al*. The gamma 2 subunit of the GABAA receptor is concentrated in synaptic junctions containing the alpha 1 and beta 2/3 subunits in hippocampus, cerebellum and globus pallidus. *Neuropharmacology* 1996; **35**: 1425–44.

388 Somogyi P, Takagi H, Richards JG, Mohler H. Subcellular localization of benzodiazepine/GABAA receptors in the cerebellum of rat, cat, and monkey using monoclonal antibodies. *J Neurosci* 1989; **9**: 2197–209.

389 Song JY, Ichtchenko K, Sudhof TC, Brose N. Neuroligin 1 is a postsynaptic cell-adhesion molecule of excitatory synapses. *Proc Natl Acad Sci USA* 1999; **96**: 1100–5.

390 Soriano E, Alvarado-Mallart RM, Dumesnil N *et al*. Cajal-Retzius cells regulate the radial glia phenotype in the adult and developing cerebellum and alter granule cell migration. *Neuron* 1997; **18**: 563–77.

391 Soriano E, Dumesnil N, Auladell C *et al*. Molecular heterogeneity of progenitors and radial migration in the developing cerebral cortex revealed by transgene expression. *Proc Natl Acad Sci USA* 1995; **92**: 11676–80.

392 Sotelo C. Cerebellar synaptogenesis: what we can learn from mutant mice. *J Exp Biol* 1990; **153**: 225–49.

393 Sotelo C. Formation of presynaptic dendrites in the rat cerebellum following neonatal X-irradiation. *Neurosciences* 1977; **2**: 275–283.

394 Sotelo C. General features of the synaptic organization in the central nervous system. In: Paoletti R, Davison AN eds. *Chemistry and brain development*. New York: Plenum Press, 1971: 239–80.

395 Sotelo C. Permanence and fate of paramembranous synaptic specializations in 'mutants' experimental animals. *Brain Res* 1973; **62**: 345–51.

396 Sotelo C. Permanence of postsynaptic specializations in the frog sympathetic ganglion cells after denervation. *Exp Brain Res* 1968; **6**: 294–305.

397 Sotelo C, Alvarado-Mallart RM. Reconstruction of the defective cerebellar circuitry in adult Purkinje cell degeneration mutant mice by Purkinje cell replacement through transplantation of solid embryonic implants. *Neuroscience* 1987; **20**: 1–22.

398 Sotelo C, Alvarado–Mallart RM, Frain M, Vernet M. Molecular plasticity of adult Bergmann fibers is associated with radial migration of grafted Purkinje cells. *J Neurosci* 1994; **14**: 124–33.

399 Sotelo C, Cholley B, El Mesikawi S. Direct immunohistochemical evidence of the existence of 5-HT1A autoreceptors on serotoninergic neurons in the midbrain raphenuclei. *Eur J Neurosci* 1990; **2**: 1144–54.

400 Sotelo C, Gotow T, Wassef M. Localization of glutamic-acid-decarboxylase-immunoreactive axon terminals in the inferior olive of the rat, with special emphasis on anatomical relations between GABAergic synapses and dendrodritic gap junctions. *J Comp Neurol* 1986; **252**: 32–50.

401 Sotelo C, Korn H. Morphological correlates of electrical and other interactions through low-resistance pathways between neurons of the vertebrate central nervous system. *Int Rev Cytol* 1978; **55**: 67–107.

402 Sotelo C, Llinas R, Baker R. Structural study of inferior olivary nucleus of the cat: morphological correlates of electrotonic coupling. *J Neurophysiol* 1974; **37**: 541–59.

403 Sotelo C, Palay S. The fine structure of the lateral vestibular nucleus in the rat. I. Neurons and neuroglial cells. *J Cell Biol* 1968; **36**: 151–179.

404 Sotelo C, Palay SL. Synapses avec des contacts étroits (tight junctions) dans le noyau vestibulaire latéral du rat. *J Microscopie* 1967; **6**: 83a.

405 Sotelo C, Palay SL. The fine structure of the later vestibular nucleus in the rat. II. Synaptic organization. *Brain Res* 1970; **18**: 93–115.

406 Sotelo C, Triller A. Morphological correlates of electrical, chemical and dual modes of transmission. In: Stjärne L, Hedquist P, Lagerzantz H, Wennmaln A eds. *Chemical neurotransmission 75 years*. London: Academic Press, 1981: 13–28.

407 Spillane DM, Rosahl TW, Sudhof TC, Malenka RC. Long-term potentiation in mice lacking synapsins. *Neuropharmacology* 1995; **34**: 1573–9.

408 Spira ME, Bennett MV. Synaptic control of electrotonic coupling between neurons. *Brain Res* 1972; **37**: 294–300.

409 Spruston N, Schiller Y, Stuart G, Sakmann B. Activity-dependent action potential invasion and calcium influx into hippocampal CA1 dendrites. *Science* 1995; **268**: 297–300.

410 Srivastava S, Osten P, Vilim FS *et al*. Novel anchorage of GluR2/3 to the postsynaptic density by the AMPA receptor-binding protein ABP. *Neuron* 1998; **21**: 581–91.

411 Stahl B, Chou JH, Li C *et al*. Rab3 reversibly recruits rabphilin to synaptic vesicles by a mechanism analogous to raf recruitment by ras. *Embo J* 1996; **15**: 1799–809.

412 Stanley EF. Single calcium channels and acetylcholine release at a presynaptic nerve terminal. *Neuron* 1993; **11**: 1007–11.

413 Steward O. mRNA localization in neurons: a multipurpose mechanism? *Neuron* 1997; **18**: 9–12.

414 Steward O, Levy WB. Preferential localization of polyribosomes under the base of dendritic spines in granule cells of the dentate gyrus. *J Neurosci* 1982; **2**: 284–91.

415 Stowell JN, Craig AM. Axon/dendrite targeting of metabotropic glutamate receptors by their cytoplasmic carboxy–terminal domains (published erratum appears in *Neuron* 1999 24: following 762). *Neuron* 1999; **22**: 525–36.

416 Sur C, Korn H, Triller A. Colocalization of somatostatin with GABA or glutamate in distinct afferent terminals presynaptic to the Mauthner cell. *J Neurosci* 1994; **14**: 576–89.

417 Sur C, Triller A, Korn H. Morphology of the release site of inhibitory synapses on the soma and dendrite of an identified neuron. *J Comp Neurol* 1995; **351**: 247–60.

418 Sutton RB, Fasshauer D, Jahn R, Brunger AT. Crystal structure of a SNARE complex involved in synaptic exocytosis at 2.4 A resolution. *Nature* 1998; **395**: 347–53.

419 Suzuki SC, Inoue T, Kimura Y *et al*. Neuronal circuits are subdivided by differential expression of type-II classic cadherins in postnatal mouse brains. *Mol Cell Neurosci* 1997; **9**: 433–47.

420 Svendsen CN, Smith AG. New prospects for human stem-cell therapy in the nervous system. *Trends Neurosci* 1999; **22**: 357–64.

421 Takahashi T, Nowakowski RS, Caviness VS Jr. Cell cycle parameters and patterns of nuclear movement in the neocortical proliferative zone of the fetal mouse. *J Neurosci* 1993; **13**: 820–33.

422 Takei K, Mignery GA, Mugnaini E *et al*. Inositol 1,4,5-trisphosphate receptor causes formation of ER cisternal stacks in transfected fibroblasts and in cerebellar Purkinje cells. *Neuron* 1994; **12**: 327–42.

423 Takei K, Mundigl O, Daniell L, De Camilli P. The synaptic vesicle cycle: a single vesicle budding step involving clathrin and dynamin. *J Cell Biol* 1996; **133**: 1237–50.

424 Takei K, Stukenbrok H, Metcalf A *et al*. Ca^{2+} stores in Purkinje neurons: endoplasmic reticulum subcompartments demonstrated by the heterogeneous distribution of the InsP3 receptor, Ca(2+)-ATPase, and calsequestrin. *J Neurosci* 1992; **12**: 489–505.

425 Takeichi M. Cadherins: a molecular family important in selective cell–cell adhesion. *Annu Rev Biochem* 1990; **59**: 237–52.

426 Tamura K, Shan WS, Hendrickson WA *et al*. Structure–function analysis of cell adhesion by neural (N-) cadherin. *Neuron* 1998; **20**: 1153–63.

427 Tan SS, Breen S. Radial mosaicism and tangential cell dispersion both contribute to mouse neocortical development. *Nature* 1993; **362**: 638–40.

428 Tang L, Hung CP, Schuman EM. A role for the cadherin family of cell adhesion molecules in hippocampal long-term potentiation. *Neuron* 1998; **20**: 1165–75.

429 Tatsuoka H, Reese TS. New structural features of synapses in the anteroventral cochlear nucleus prepared by direct freezing and freeze-substitution. *J Comp Neurol* 1989; **290**: 343–57.

430 Taxi J. Etude de l'ultrastructure des zones synaptiques dans les ganglions sympathiques de la grenouille. *CR Acad Sci Ser D, Paris* 1961; **252**: 174–6.

431 Terrazas R. Notas sobre la neuroglia del cerebelo y el crecimiento de los elementos nerviosos. *Rev Trim Microgr* 1897; **2**: 49–65.

432 Thomas U, Kim E, Kuhlendahl S *et al*. Synaptic clustering of the cell adhesion molecule fasciclin II by discs – large and its role in the regulation of presynaptic structure. *Neuron* 1997; **19**: 787–99.

433 Tienari PJ, De Strooper B, Ikonen E *et al*. The beta-amyloid domain is essential for axonal sorting of amyloid precursor protein. *Embo J* 1996; **15**: 5218–29.

434 Todd AJ, Spike RC, Price RF, Neilson M. Immunocytochemical evidence that neurotensin is present in glutamatergic neurons in the superficial dorsal horn of the rat. *J Neurosci* 1994; **14**: 774–84.

435 Tongiorgi E, Righi M, Cattaneo A. Activity-dependent dendritic targeting of BDNF and TrkB mRNAs in hippocampal neurons. *J Neurosci* 1997; **17**: 9492–505.

436 Topinka JR, Bredt DS. N-terminal palmitoylation of PSD-95 regulates association with cell membranes and interaction with K$^+$ channel Kv1.4. *Neuron* 1998; **20**: 125–34.

437 Torre ER, Steward O. Demonstration of local protein synthesis within dendrites using a new cell culture system that permits the isolation of living axons and dendrites from their cell bodies. *J Neurosci* 1992; **12**: 762–72.

438 Torre ER, Steward O. Protein synthesis within dendrites: glycosylation of newly synthesized proteins in dendrites of hippocampal neurons in culture. *J Neurosci* 1996; **16**: 5967–78.

439 Torri-Tarelli F, Haimann C, Ceccarelli B. Coated vesicles and pits during enhanced quantal release of acetylcholine at the neuromuscular junction. *J Neurocytol* 1987; **16**: 205–14.

440 Triller A, Cluzeaud F, Pfeiffer F *et al*. Distribution of glycine receptors at central synapses: an immunoelectron microscopy study. *J Cell Biol* 1985; **101**: 683–8.

441 Triller A, Korn H. Transmission at a central inhibitory synapse. III. Ultrastructure of physiologically identified and stained terminals. *J Neurophysiol* 1982; **48**: 708–36.

442 Triller A, Seitanidou T, Franksson O, Korn H. Size and shape of glycine receptor clusters in a central neuron exhibit a somato-dendritic gradient. *New Biol* 1990; **2**: 637–41.

443 Trommsdorff M, Gotthardt M, Hiesberger T *et al*. Reeler/Disabled-like disruption of neuronal migration in knockout mice lacking the VLDL receptor and ApoE receptor 2. *Cell* 1999; **97**: 689–701.

444 Tu JC, Xiao B, Yuan JP *et al*. Homer binds a novel proline-rich motif and links group 1 metabotropic glutamate receptors with IP3 receptors. *Neuron* 1998; **21**: 717–26.

445 Twyman RE, Rogers SW, Gahring LC *et al*. Antibodies to glutamate receptors: a role in excitatory dysregulation of the central nervous system? *Adv Neurol* 1999; **79**: 535–41.

446 Uchida N, Honjo Y, Johnson KR *et al*. The catenin/cadherin adhesion system is localized in synaptic junctions bordering transmitter release zones. *J Cell Biol* 1996; **135**: 767–79.

447 Uchizono K. Characteristics of excitatory and inhibitory synapses in the central nervous system of the cat. *Nature* 1965; **207**: 642–3.

448 Unwin N. Nicotinic acetylcholine receptor at 9 A resolution. *J Mol Biol* 1993; **229**: 1101–24.

449 Unwin N. The structure of ion channels in membranes of excitable cells. *Neuron* 1989; **3**: 665–76.

450 Valdivia O. Methods of fixation and the morphology of synaptic vesicles. *J Comp Neurol* 1971; **142**: 257–73.

451 Valtorta F, Benfenati F, Greengard P. Structure and function of the synapsins. *J Biol Chem* 1992; **267**: 7195–8.

452 Valverde F, De Carlos JA, Lopez-Mascaraque L. Time of origin and early fate of preplate cells in the cerebral cortex of the rat. *Cereb Cortex* 1995; **5**: 483–93.

453 Van Der Loos H. Fine structure of synapses in the cerebral cortex. *Zellforsch Mikrosk Anat* 1963; **60**: 815–25.

454 van Huizen F, Strosberg AD, Cynader MS. Cellular and subcellular localisation of muscarinic acetylcholine receptors during postnatal development of cat visual cortex using immunocytochemical procedures. *Brain Res Dev Brain Res* 1988; **44**: 296–301.

455 Vannier C, Triller A. Biology of the postsynaptic glycine receptor. *Int Rev Cytol* 1997; **176**: 201–44.

456 Vergouwe MN, Tijssen MA, Shiang R et al. Hyperekplexia-like syndromes without mutations in the GLRA1 gene. *Clin Neurol Neurosurg* 1997; **99**: 172–8.

457 Vrensen G, Cardozo JN, Muller L, van der Want J. The presynaptic grid: a new approach. *Brain Res* 1980; **184**: 23–40.

458 Wagner J, Akerud P, Castro DS et al. Induction of a midbrain dopaminergic phenotype in Nurr1-overexpressing neural stem cells by type 1 astrocytes . *Nat Biotechnol* 1999; **17**: 653–9.

459 Wallace CS, Lyford GL, Worley PF, Steward O. Differential intracellular sorting of immediate early gene mRNAs depends on signals in the mRNA sequence. *J Neurosci* 1998; **18**: 26–35.

460 Walsh C, Cepko CL. Widespread dispersion of neuronal clones across functional regions of the cerebral cortex. *Science* 1992; **255**: 434–40.

461 Walsh CA. Genetic malformations of the human cerebral cortex. *Neuron* 1999; **23**: 19–29.

462 Wang H, Bedford FK, Brandon NJ et al. GABA(A)-receptor-associated protein links GABA(A) receptors and the cytoskeleton. *Nature* 1999; **397**: 69–72.

463 Wang Y, Okamoto M, Schmitz F et al. Rim is a putative Rab3 effector in regulating synaptic-vesicle fusion. *Nature* 1997; **388**: 593–8.

464 Warnock DE, Schmid SL. Dynamin GTPase, a force-generating molecular switch. *Bioessays* 1996; **18**: 885–93.

465 Waxman SG. Molecular neurobiology of myelinated nerve fiber: ion-channel distributions and their implications for demyelinating diseases. In: Kandel ER ed. *Molecular neurobiology in neurology and psychiatry*. New York: Raven Press, 1987: 7–37.

466 Weber T, Zemelman BV, McNew JA et al. SNAREpins: minimal machinery for membrane fusion. *Cell* 1998; **92**: 759–72.

467 Wechsler-Reya RJ, Scott MP. Control of neuronal precursor proliferation in the cerebellum by Sonic Hedgehog. *Neuron* 1999; **22**: 103–14.

468 Weiss P, Hiscoe H. Experiments in the mechanism of nerve growth. *J Exp Zool* 1948; **107**: 315–95.

469 Wendland B. Molecular mechanisms of synaptic vesicle docking and membrane fusion. *Semin Neurosci* 1994; **6**: 167–76.

470 White TW, Paul DL. Genetic diseases and gene knockouts reveal diverse connexin functions. *Annu Rev Physiol* 1999; **61**: 283–310.

471 Whiting PJ, Bonnert TP, McKernan RM et al. Molecular and functional diversity of the expanding GABA-A receptor gene family. *Ann NY Acad Sci* 1999; **868**: 645–53.

472 Wichterle H, Garcia-Verdugo JM, Alvarez-Buylla A. Direct evidence for homotypic, glia–independent neuronal migration. *Neuron* 1997; **18**: 779–91.

473 Wilhelm JE, Vale RD. RNA on the move: the mRNA localization pathway (Published erratum appears in *J Cell Biol* 1993; **123**(6 Pt 1):1625). *J Cell Biol* 1993; **123**: 269–74.

474 Wilson DB. Proliferation in the neural tube of the splotch (Sp) mutant mouse. *J Comp Neurol* 1974; **154**: 249–55.

475 Wozniak M, Limbird LE. Trafficking itineraries of G protein-coupled receptors in epithelial cells do not predict receptor localization in neurons. *Brain Res* 1998; **780**: 311–22.

476 Wu W, Wong K, Chen J et al. Directional guidance of neuronal migration in the olfactory system by the protein Slit. *Nature* 1999; **400**: 331–6.

477 Xia J, Zhang X, Staudinger J, Huganir RL. Clustering of AMPA receptors by the synaptic PDZ domain-containing protein PICK1. *Neuron* 1999; **22**: 179–87.

478 Yagi T, Takeichi M. Cadherin superfamily genes: functions, genomic organization, and neurologic diversity. *Genes Dev* 2000; **14**: 1169–80.

479 Yamagata K, Andreasson KI, Sugiura H et al. Arcadlin is a neural activity-regulated cadherin involved in long term potentiation. *J Biol Chem* 1999; **274**: 19473–9.

480 Yankner BA, Mesulam MM. Seminars in Medicine of the Beth Israel Hospital, Boston. beta-Amyloid and the pathogenesis of Alzheimer's disease. *N Engl J Med* 1991; **325**: 1849–57.

481 Yee KT, Simon HH, Tessier-Lavigne M, and O'Leary DM. Extension of long leading processes and neuronal migration in the mammalian brain directed by the chemoattractant netrin-1. *Neuron* 1999; **24**: 607–22.

482 Young AB, MacDonald RL. Glycine as a spinal cord neurotransmitter. In: Davidoff RA ed. *Handbook of the spinal cord*. New York: Marcel Dekker, 1983: 1–43.

483 Zampighi G, Kreman M, Ramon F et al. Structural characteristics of gap junctions. I. Channel number in coupled and uncoupled conditions. *J Cell Biol* 1988; **106**: 1667–78.

484 Zhang SJ, Jackson MB. GABA-activated chloride channels in secretory nerve endings. *Science* 1993; **259**: 531–4.

485 Zhu PC, Thureson-Klein A, Klein RL. Exocytosis from large dense cored vesicles outside the active synaptic zones of terminals within the trigeminal subnucleus caudalis: a possible mechanism for neuropeptide release. *Neuroscience* 1986; **19**: 43–54.

486 Zhu Y, Li H, Zhou L, Wu JY, Rao Y. Cellular and molecular guidance of GABAergic neuronal migration from an extracortical origin to the neocortex. *Neuron* 1999; **23**: 473–85.

2

Structure and function of glia in the central nervous system

MARTIN BERRY, ARTHUR M. BUTT, GRAHAM WILKIN AND V. HUGH PERRY

INTRODUCTION

Glial cells in the central nervous system (CNS) are classified as macroglia (subclasses of which include oligodendrocytes, astrocytes, novel NG-2$^+$ glia, and ependymal cells and their derivatives) and microglia. Most of these glial types were recognized in the late nineteenth century by Ramony Cajal, Del Rio-Hortega and Golgi using specialized metallic impregnation techniques, many of which were specific for particular glia. Today, these morphological methods have been superseded by immunocytological and lectin stains, electron microscopy, *in situ* hybridization (ISH) and iontophoretic intracellular dye injection, augmented by physiological recording techniques, Ca^{2+} imaging and ion channel expression measurement. The former methods use phenotypic marker antibodies, which recognize cellular constituents (or epitopes) unique to, or characteristic of, the different types of glia. Some of the classical stains and electron microscopy remain useful techniques, not only for the identification of glial types according to morphological criteria, but also, as in the case of electron microscopy, for the clear definition of otherwise unresolvable cytoplasmic organelles, fine cytoplasmic processes and intercellular membrane interrelationships.

An early concept of their function envisaged that glia provided the structural and functional support for neurons, much like the connective tissues of organs in the periphery. It is now known that glia have a widespread range of physiological roles in the normal brain, and that most react in a protective capacity to all forms of pathology.

MACROGLIA

Oligodendrocytes

Oligodendrocytes produce the myelin sheaths that insulate CNS axons. The importance of myelin in axonal function is clearly illustrated by the demyelinating disease multiple sclerosis (MS) in man, in which loss of myelin causes the conduction block underlying the debilitating clinical episodes of the disease (see Chapter 8, Volume II). Mature myelin-producing oligodendrocytes are process-bearing cells and each terminal oligodendrocyte process ensheaths an axon to form one internodal myelin segment of variable thickness and length (Fig. 2.1).[74,75,322] Each oligodendrocyte and the internodal myelin segment that it forms are collectively called a unit (Figs 2.1–2.3). Myelinating oligodendrocytes are located within the CNS white matter tracts (Fig. 2.4), but many oligodendrocytes are also found in grey matter, where they are associated with neuronal perikarya,[228] although little is known about either the anatomy, or function of these 'satellite oligodendrocytes'.

STRUCTURE OF OLIGODENDROCYTES

In electron micrographs, the cell bodies of oligodendrocytes have a small profile. The nucleus is round with dense chromatin and the cytoplasm is usually scanty and opaque, rich in granular endoplasmic reticulum, ribosomes and mitochondria. Mori and Leblond[259] described three classes of oligodendrocyte on the basis of their fine structural appearances. Light oligodendrocytes are large

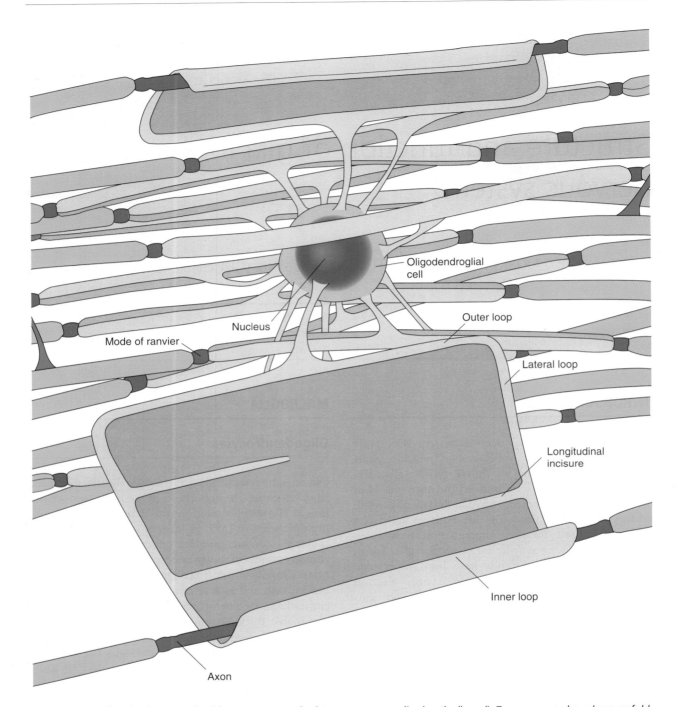

Figure 2.1 *An oligodendrocyte unit with processes attached to numerous myelin sheaths (in red). Two processes have been unfolded to different degrees to demonstrate their enormous surface area. Note also the displacement of the oligodendrocyte cytoplasm to narrow ridges, mainly at the margins of the flattened sheet of myelin; the outer cytoplasmic rim actually spirals around the myelin sheath and does not run longitudinally as depicted here (see Figs 2.3, 2.4, 2.11). Axons: mauve; adjacent intersegmental myelin sheaths: green. Modified by permission from Morell and Norton*[258] *by Raine.*[315]

with a pale nucleus; these cells show rapid mitotic activity. Medium-shade oligodendrocytes, in comparison with the light cells, are smaller with a denser nucleus, and have reduced mitotic activity. Dark oligodendrocytes are the smallest cells with the most dense nucleus and are mitotically inactive. The relative frequencies of each type are 9%, 35% and 56%, respectively. This classification may reflect a maturation sequence of oligodendrocytes in which light cells represent the adult oligodendrocyte progenitor cell pool for the production of a stable population of dark cells through an intermediate medium-shade type.

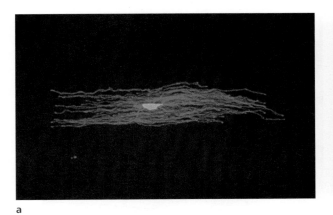
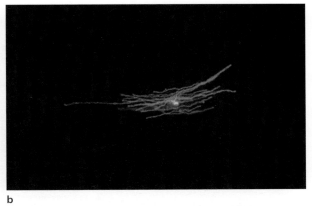

a   b

Figure 2.2 *Confocal epifluorescent microscopy of lysinated rhodamine dextran microinjected oligodendrocyte units from (**a**) adult rat and (**b**) mouse optic nerves. Axons run through the optic nerve in parallel and the inner and outer tongues of oligodendrocyte cytoplasm of each internodal myelin segment units are clearly seen as 10–20 longitudinal parallel processes of approximately the same length in each unit, connected by stems to the soma. The terminal swellings of each process probably represent the paranodal loops.*

Myelin is a fatty insulating layer of high electrical resistance and low capacitance facilitating the rapid saltatory conduction of axonal action potentials. A single myelin sheath is an extraordinarily large trapezoid sheet which is an extension of the oligodendrocyte plasma membrane with most of the cytoplasm extruded (except within isolated strands which form the Schmidt–Lantermann incisures), so that the two plasma membranes are directly apposed to form a single lamella of compacted myelin containing Schmidt–Lantermann cytoplasmic clefts, and surrounded by a ridge of cytoplasm which forms the inner and outer mesaxons and paranodal loops (Fig. 2.1). The myelin sheath spirals around the axon to form multiple concentric lamellae (Fig. 2.5a). The myelin lamellae are formed by the fusion of opposed inner leaflets of plasma membrane to form the major dense line; the juxtaposed outer leaflets form the minor dense line or intraperiod line, typically seen in cross-sections of myelin sheaths in electron micrographs.[158] The internodal myelin segments are separated by nodes of Ranvier, an area of naked axolemma specialized for action potential propagation, where the terminal paranodal loops of the sheath are opposed to the axolemma at a myelin attachment zone (Fig. 2.5b). The paranodal loops form a spiral linear junctional complex with the axolemma within this zone believed to be important in the differential distribution of sodium and potassium channels in the nodal and juxtaparanodal axolemma, respectively (Fig. 2.6).[411]

The number of lamellae (N) determines the insulating properties of the sheath, whereas internodal myelin sheath length (L) determines the speed of conduction. Both N and L are directly and positively correlated with axon diameter (D), so thick axons conduct more rapidly than slimmer ones.[70,155,156,264] Individual oligodendrocytes support 1–50 myelin sheaths and have L values ranging from 50 to 1000 μm^3, and each myelin sheath has dimensions of approximately $\pi\, D\, N\, L$.[70,156] This places a con-

siderable metabolic load on individual oligodendrocytes and, since myelin is not static but replaced by continuous turnover, it is perhaps not surprising that oligodendrocyte function is confined exclusively to the formation and maintenance of CNS myelin.

MYELIN COMPOSITION

CNS myelin contains galactolipids and myelin-related proteins. The main lipids are galactocerebroside (GalC) and its sulfated derivative sulfatide,[280] whereas the most abundant proteins are proteolipid protein (PLP), the myelin basic proteins (MBP), myelin-associated oligodendrocytic basic protein (MOBP), myelin-associated glycoprotein (MAG), myelin-associated oligodendrocyte glycoprotein (MOG), myelin-associated oligodendrocyte specific protein (MOSP), carbonic anhydrase II (CA-II) and 2′,3′-cyclic nucleotide 3′-phosphodiesterase (CNPase). All these proteins can be monitored immunohistochemically and by ISH using appropriate messenger RNA (mRNA) probes (Fig. 2.7).[56,68–73,143,386,400,401] Another useful marker for oligodendrocytes and myelin is the mouse monoclonal antibody Rip, which labels an unknown epitope specific to both, and thus has the unique property of labelling entire units (Fig. 2.3).[36,73,122] MBP and MOBP mRNA are of interest because they are translocated into oligodendrocyte processes, where both proteins are synthesized on free polysomes and inserted locally into the myelin sheaths, whereas mRNA encoding for the myelin proteins remains in the perinuclear cytoplasm and their products are transported distally for insertion in the myelin membrane.[78,401] The microtubule network plays a key role in translocating myelin components to their distal domains.[79,401] In general, the lipids provide the insulating properties of myelin, while the proteins function to stabilize the myelin lamellae and maintain membrane-to-membrane interactions, both within compacted myelin

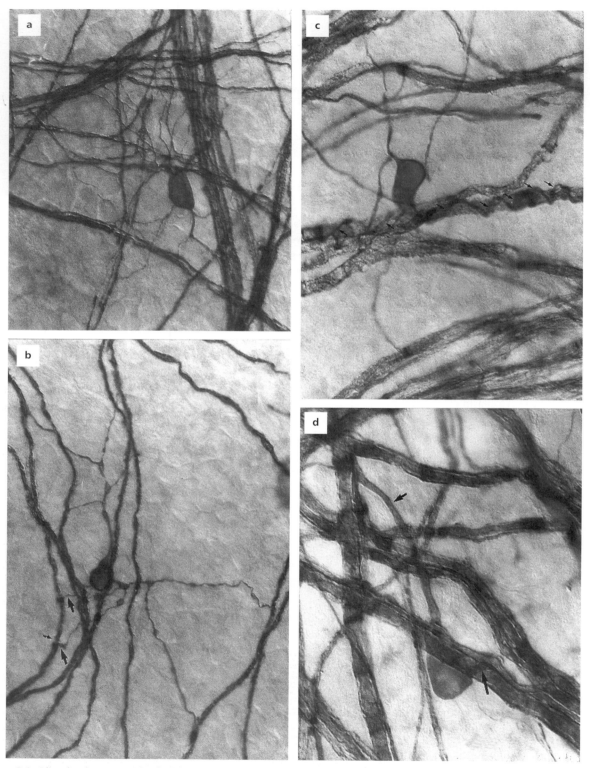

Figure 2.3 *Oligodendrocytes stained with Rip. A whole mount of the rat anterior medullary velum shows (**a**) type I, (**b**) type II, (**c**) type III and (**d**) type IV oligodendrocyte units. Note that the sizes of the oligodendrocyte cell bodies and the diameters of the axons myelinated are directly and positively correlated, but that the number of processes is inversely related to unit type. In these examples, the processes of a type I oligodendrocyte (**a**) engage multiple small-diameter fibres, while the two thick processes of the type IV (**d**) unit form the thick myelin sheaths of two large-diameter fibres (arrows). Type II and III units have intermediate axon/glial relationships. Note that the type III unit in (**c**) engages medium-sized axons and that the outer rim of oligodendrocyte cytoplasm of one myelin sheath forms a conspicuous Rip-positive reversed spiral on either side of a point of engagement of the axon (arrows) – PAP stained, DIC photomicrograph.*

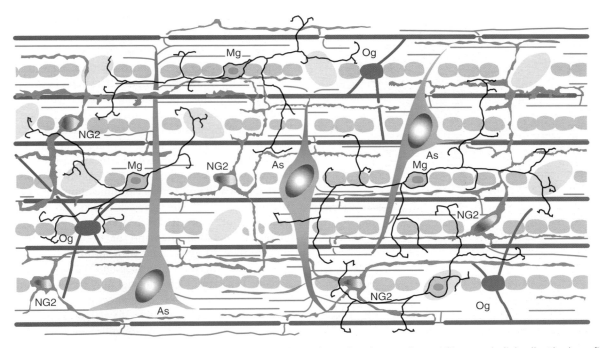

Figure 2.4 *Long fibre tract of the central nervous system with myelinated and unmyelinated fibres and glial cells. The long fibre tracts of the brain and the spinal cord consist of myelinated and unmyelinated nerve fibres running through a regular meshwork of four types of glial cell: astrocytes (As), oligodendrocytes (Og), NG-2 glia (see page 17), and microglia (Mg) The glia cell bodies lie in unicellular rows, which are of considerable length, and are aligned along the long axis of the tracts. Stretches of 5–10 contiguous oligodendrocytes are separated by solitary astrocytes. Microglia and NG-2 glia are also regularly spaced, with a lower frequency than astrocytes. All three glia give rise to both transverse and longitudinally orientated processes, which interweave among axon bundles to form a complex meshwork. For astrocytes, oligodendrocytes and NG-2 glia, the processes of individual cells penetrate into the territory of adjacent cells; the branching domains of microglia tend not to overlap (see Fig. 2.22). Both astrocytes and NG-2 glia have processes terminating on naked axolemma at nodes of Ranvier. Modified by permission from Suzuki and Raisman.[394]*

sheaths and between the axolemma and myelin sheath.[272] MBP fuses the two cytoplasmic membrane bilayers to form the major dense line, whereas PLP has a similar role in fusion of the extracellular membranes to form the intraperiod line (Fig. 2.5a). Studies on mutant mice have indicated key roles for MAG and the galactolipids in axon–glial interactions, and the latter may play an essential role in the formation of nodes of Ranvier.

OLIGODENDROCYTE PHENOTYPES

Classical studies defined four subtypes of oligodendrocyte,[60,99,290] on the basis of the number and size of myelin sheaths in the unit (Fig. 2.3). This hypothesis is supported by findings on the toad spinal cord,[384] and more recently in the mammalian spinal cord[39,122,156,329,330,414] and rodent anterior medullary velum.[36,70,72,73] Oligodendrocytes

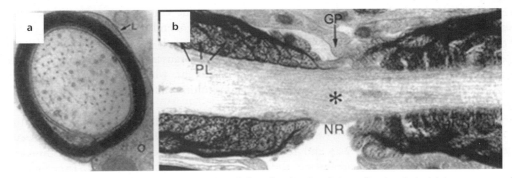

Figure 2.5 *Ultrastructure of myelin. Electron micrographs of the oligodendroglial myelin sheath in (a) transverse and (b) longitudinal section. (a) There is direct continuity between the oligodendrocyte process (O) and the outermost lamella (L) of the myelin sheath (from Hirano[158] with permission). (b) Myelin sheaths terminate as paranodal loops (PL) either side of bare regions of axon (asterisk), known as the node of Ranvier (NR). Perinodal glial processes (GP) from astrocytes and NG-2 glia (see Figs 2.6, 2.14, 2.20) give rise to delicate extensions which pass into the nodal gap.*

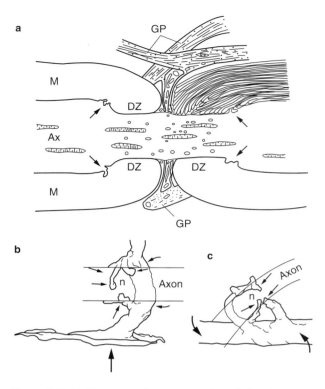

Figure 2.6 *(a) Diagrammatic representation of the ultrastructure of a nodal region in a large central nervous system axon of the cat. AX, axon; M, myelin; GP, glial processes from astrocytes and NG-2 glia (see also Figs 2.4, 2.5, 2.14, 2.20); arrows indicate abnodal axoglial interdigitations.[156] (b, c) Artist's reconstruction of perinodal astrocyte processes from serial electron micrographs of nodes. Larger processes (curved arrows) branch perinodally to give two or more finger-like projections (arrows), which loop around the axon and make discrete contacts with the axolemma at the node (n). The perinodal astrocyte processes stem in (b) from along the length of a collateral branch and, in (c), from a primary process, which also forms an end-foot at the pial surface (broad arrow). Representative sections through the node depicted in (b) are shown in Fig. 2.20. Putative perinodal astrocyte processes can be recognized at the level of the light microscope as (i) microscopic barbs and offshoots, ranging from submicrometre to 5–10 μm in length, and (ii) collateral branches which end freely in the nerve and form terminal contacts with nodes. However, individual nodal contacts cannot be resolved using the light microscope. The perinodal astrocyte processes contact the same node along with processes of NG2 glia (Figs 2.4 and 2.14) (see also Fig. 2.1). Reproduced by permission from (a) Hildebrand et al.[156] and (b, c) Butt et al.[66,67]*

are phenotypically heterogeneous (Fig. 2.7) and units exhibit direct relationships between fibre diameters and myelin biochemistry, the number of myelin sheaths per unit, and both the longitudinal (internodal lengths) and radial (number of lamellae) dimensions of the myelin sheaths.[39,70,72,73,155,329,330] Oligodendrocyte types I and II are morphologically similar,[384] in that they myelinate numer-

ous small-diameter axons, and myelin sheaths have few lamellae and short internodal lengths. Type III oligodendrocytes myelinate a small number of larger diameter axons, supporting myelin sheaths with numerous lamellae and long internodal lengths. The type IV oligodendrocyte unit phenotype is similar to type III, but has a cell body directly applied to an individual axon of large diameter which it myelinates. The distribution densities of oligodendrocyte phenotypes in the CNS are determined by the spatial dispersion of axons with a critical diameter of below or above approximately 2–4 μm.[63] Type II/IV units support at least a 50 times greater volume of myelin than type I/II units.[70,156,329,330] The large cell bodies and thick radial processes of type III/IV units probably reflect the increased metabolic demand of the greater mass of myelin they support, and their prominent Schmidt–Lantermann incisures may facilitate the distribution of myelin gene products throughout the large myelin sheaths. There are subtle differences in the myelin composition of small- relative to large-diameter CNS fibres,[5,151,156,249,420] and the oligodendrocytes of such units exhibit phenotypic differences in expression of CA-II and the L- and S-isoforms of MAG.[72,73] Two extreme variants are S-MAG$^-$/CA-II$^+$ type I/II units and S-MAG$^+$/CA-II$^-$ type III/IV units, which myelinate the smallest and largest diameter fibres, respectively (Fig. 2.8).[72] However, transplant studies indicate that oligodendrocytes are not inherently programmed to myelinate a specific size of axon.[114] Moreover, oligodendrocyte phenotype changes in pathology (e.g. levels of CA-II increase when the volume of myelin supported decreases)[35,283] and oligodendrocytes that remyelinate axons in the adult have shorter and thinner sheaths than normal.[35,44,136,316] It has been suggested that biochemical and metabolic differences between oligodendrocytes may determine their susceptibility to demyelination and capacity for remyelination.

DEVELOPMENT OF OLIGODENDROCYTES

Oligodendrocyte progenitors are derived from neuroepithelial precursors in the ventricular and subventricular layers of the embryonic brain and spinal cord neural tube. Oligodendrocyte progenitors express platelet-derived growth factor α-receptor (PDGF-αR) and *plp/dm*-20 transcripts,[338,380] and migrate to their final sites in the brain, where they begin to express the NG-2 chondroitin sulfate proteoglycan and the O4 sulfatide.[90,112,113,149,216,217,277,410] They undergo local proliferation before either differentiating into myelinating oligodendrocytes (Fig. 2.9) or dying by apoptosis. As they differentiate, oligodendrocyte progenitors lose PDGF-αR and NG-2, but not O4 expression. They first produce GalC as newly formed oligodendrocytes, and then as pre-myelinating oligodendrocytes begin to express the myelin-related proteins as they initiate axonal myelination.[69,71,76,112,150,217,374,401] A small but significant population of PDGF-αR$^+$/NG-2$^+$/O4$^+$ cells persists in the mature

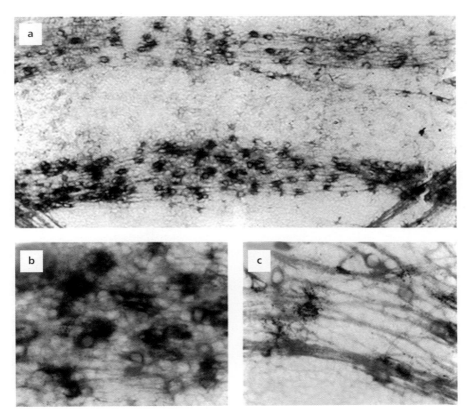

Figure 2.7 *Double* in situ *hybridization to demonstrate oligodendrocyte lineage in the anterior medullary velum of neonatal rats. (a) Platelet-derived growth factor-α receptor (PDGF-αR) mRNA expressing oligodendrocyte progenitors (blue) are localized to the tracts of myelinated axons, interpolated between (b) myelin basic protein (MBP) mRNA expressing oligodendrocytes (red). (c) Multipolar PDGF-αR mRNA expressing oligodendrocyte progenitors closely resemble MBP mRNA expressing myelinating oligodendrocytes. Reproduced by permission from Butt* et al.[68]

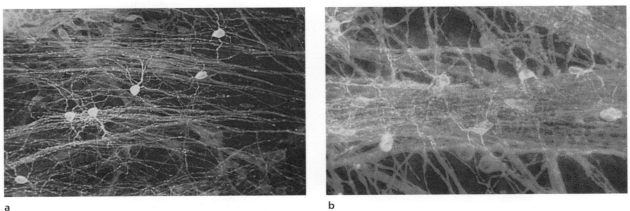

Figure 2.8 *Double immunofluorescence of oligodendrocytes with Rip and CAH. Confocal micrographs of oligodendrocytes in the rat anterior medullary velum, double immunofluorescence labelled with Rip (fluorescein conjugated) and carbonic anhydrase II (CA-II; rhodamine conjugated), showing two biochemical subtypes of oligodendrocyte which are either Rip$^+$/CA-II$^+$ (yellow cells, since both antibodies are co-localized), or Rip$^+$/CA-II$^-$ (green cells). In (a), Rip$^+$/CA-II$^+$ oligodendrocytes (yellow) are multipolar with small somata which myelinate numerous small-diameter axons (corresponding to type I and II units). In (b), Rip$^+$/CA-II$^-$ oligodendrocytes (green) have large somata with few thick radial processes which myelinate a small number of large-diameter fibres (corresponding to type III and IV units). This field also contains typical Rip$^+$/CA-II$^+$ oligodendrocytes (yellow). The Rip provided complete labelling of oligodendrocyte somata, radial processes and myelin sheaths. Reproduced by permission from Butt* et al.[73]

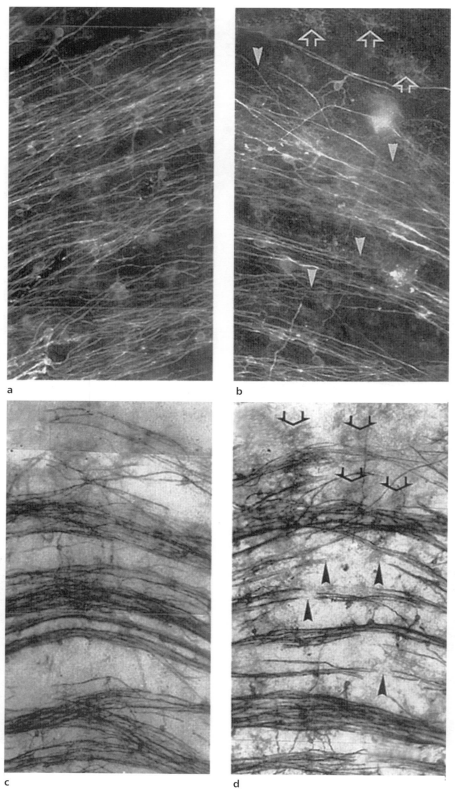

Figure 2.9 *Differentiation of oligodendrocytes. Oligodendrocytes and myelin stained with Rip in whole mounts of the rat anterior medullary velum, visualized by immunofluorescence (**a**, **b**) and immunoperoxidase (**c**, **d**), following intraventricular injection of saline (**a**, **c**), platelet-derived growth factor (PDGF)-AA (**b**), or basic fibroblast growth factor (FGF-2) (**d**). In controls, loops of myelinated axon bundles are present and the area is densely populated by myelinating oligodendrocytes (**a**, **c**). Following treatment with either PDGF-AA (**b**), or FGF-2 (**d**) myelination is retarded, unmyelinated gaps appear (arrowheads, **b**, **d**), and there is an increase in the frequency of premyelinating oligodendrocytes (open arrows, **b**, **d**). Reproduced by permission from Butt et al.,[68] Goddard et al.,[137] and Butt and Berry.[63]*

brain and these are considered to be adult oligodendrocyte progenitors,[67,69,118,216,277,331,421,422] but the cells of a part or all of this population appear differentiated and may have definitive functional roles in the mature CNS unrelated to myelination (see below). The definitive number of myelin producing oligodendrocytes is determined by the balance between cell division, survival and differentiation under the control of environmental cues, including trophic factors and cell contact-mediated signals.[26,138,148]

Most of the factors that control oligodendrocyte differentiation *in vitro* have been defined (reviewed by Goldman).[138] A key factor is the AA isoform of PDGF, which acts as a mitogen and survival signal for oligodendrocyte progenitors,[23] and prevents their premature development into oligodendrocytes.[279,337] Basic fibroblast growth factor (bFGF or FGF-2) is another potent mitogen for cells of the early oligodendrocyte lineage and conserves the expression of PDGF-αR on oligodendrocyte progenitors, blocking their differentiation into GalC+/O4+ oligodendrocytes.[46,131,133,234] Insulin-like growth factor-I (IGF-I) is a potent cell survival agent for both oligodendrocyte progenitors and GalC+ oligodendrocytes, promoting their differentiation into myelin-producing oligodendrocytes.[23,29,234,235,238] Other key factors *in vitro* include thyroid hormone, which affects the internal clock that controls the timing of oligodendrocyte differentiation, and neurotrophin-3 (NT-3), which controls oligodendrocyte numbers.[25,28] A few studies have begun to dissect the roles of these trophic factors *in vivo* in genetically altered mice.[76] Butt and colleagues have intraventricularly injected these agents and analysed their effects on oligodendrocyte development and differentiation in the rat anterior medullary velum, a tissue that roofs part of the IVth ventricle.[36,68,137] Using this technique PDGF-AA (Fig. 2.9a, b) and FGF-2 (Fig. 2.9c, d) retard oligodendrocyte differentiation and myelination, increasing the numbers of both oligodendrocyte progenitors and early oligodendrocytes. Conversely, IGF-I promotes myelination and increases the numbers of myelin-producing oligodendrocytes and the amount of myelin in the velum. These factors are abundant in astrocytes and neurons in both the developing and adult brain,[31,152,245,313,424] the latter providing a potential mechanism by which axons control the number of oligodendrocytes.[27,61] These factors may also be regulators of adult progenitor cells *in vitro*,[422] but their effects *in vivo* are unknown and the role of these cells in remyelination after demyelination *in vivo* is at present conjectural (see below).

Although the synthesis of myelin proteins may be intrinsic to oligodendrocytes *in vitro*,[301,427] it appears that *in vivo* myelination is driven by axon–oligodendrocyte interactions via contact-mediated signals, possibly involving interactions between neural cell adhesion molecules (NCAMs), FGF-R, MAG and PLP-DM20, among many molecules.[20,106,143,400,425]

In vivo, myelination proceeds through three sequential, interdependent maturation phases[63] (Fig. 2.10a–c).

Phase I: axon contact

Premyelinating oligodendrocytes (GalC+/O4+) extend profuse filipodia that form multiple contacts with numerous axons prior to ensheathment, and begin to express CNPase, MBP, PLP and Rip.[69,71,132,143,150,401] At the same time, axonal neurofilament protein is phosphorylated, axons thicken to a critical diameter of approximately 0.2 μm and presumptive nodes of Ranvier are induced.[71,157,341]

Phase II: axon ensheathment, establishment of both nodes and incipient internodal myelin segments.

As premyelinating oligodendrocytes engage axons, they immediately begin myelination.[71,150] Remahl and Hildebrand[329] showed that the initial lamellar ensheathments are uncompacted E-sheaths. After a remodelling phase, when non-ensheathing processes are lost, the definitive number of sheaths per unit and incipient internodal lengths are established,[71] and the number of axons per oligodendrocyte unit decreases throughout the transition from E- to M-compaction.[39,329] Correlated with the observation that the first axons to be myelinated generally grow into fibres with diameters larger than those ensheathed later, the type III/IV oligodendrocyte phenotype differentiates first to myelinate the prospective large axons, while type I/II differentiate last to myelinate the small-diameter axons.[39,71,246,329] At the time of ensheathment, all axons have a small diameter,[71] and axonal growth depends on oligodendrocyte contact, possibly mediated by the galactolipids.[305] Divergence of oligodendrocyte unit phenotype therefore occurs during ensheathment, when all axons have a small diameter. The remodelling that underlies phenotypic specification presumably occurs in response to unresolved contact-mediated recognition signals derived from axons within the unit, which could be qualitatively and/or quantitatively different for prospective large- and small-diameter axons.[63] Bjartmar *et al.*[39] suggested that the E-phase is a period during which units compete for axons by axolemmal engagement and disengagement. The rules of competition, whereby myelinated internodal segments become serially arranged along an axon, separated by nodes of Ranvier, and ultimately attain approximately equal lengths along a given axon, are unknown.[168]

Phase III: maturation

The maturational phase comprises myelin compaction, nodal and juxtaparanodal axolemmal ion channel aggregation,[179,325] radial growth of myelinated axons, redistribution of MBP and PLP within oligodendrocytes, and increased unit expression of MOG and S-MAG.[400] The clustering of ion channels at nodes of Ranvier occurs at the same time as incipient internodal segments and axon–glial contacts at paranodal junctions are established,

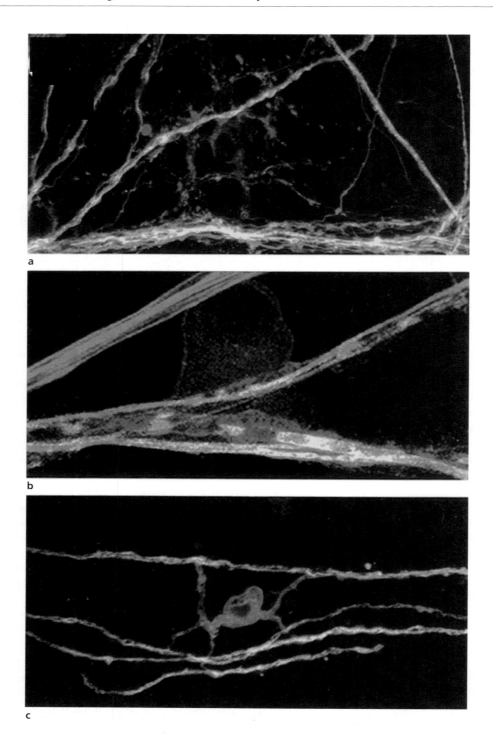

a

b

c

Figure 2.10 *Differentiation of oligodendrocytes. Confocal micrographs of developing oligodendrocytes in the rat anterior medullary velum, double immunofluorescence labelled with either Rip and NF-200 (a, b), or Rip and myelin basic protein (MBP) (c). The Rip is fluorescein conjugated and NF-200 (a, b) and the MBP (c) are rhodamine conjugated. Oligodendrocytes appear green and unmyelinated axons appear red (a, b). Premyelinating oligodendrocytes (green) extend profuse branching processes that form multiple filopodial associations with numerous axons (red) in the immediate vicinity; juxtapositions of oligodendrocyte processes on axons appear yellow (a). The definitive number of sheaths supported by oligodendrocyte units is established after a period of remodelling, when non-ensheathing processes are lost, but even at this stage there is incomplete circumferential axonal ensheathment (b). Myelinating oligodendrocytes establish incipient internodal myelin sheaths, and at this stage, while Rip continues to label the entire unit, MBP is redistributed from the entire unit to the myelin sheaths alone, so co-expression of Rip and MBP appears yellow (c). Reproduced by permission from Butt et al.[71] and Butt and Berry.[63]*

and is mediated by Caspr, ankyrin-3/G and the galacto-lipids.[305,325] Finally, there is interdependent maturation of axon–oligodendrocyte unit function and radial growth of the axon and its myelin sheath which, in the rat and cat, attain their adult dimensions late in development, many weeks after the start of myelination.[246,329,330] Myelin lamellae are probably formed by growth of the inner mesaxon around the axolemma. Thus, during myelination, the inner lamellae grow first towards the nodal area and the outer lamellae follow later, staggered at increasing distances behind the juxtaparanodal lamellae. Consequently, the outer tongue of oligodendrocyte cytoplasm of the internodal myelin segment forms a conspicuous abnodal ridge (Fig. 2.11).

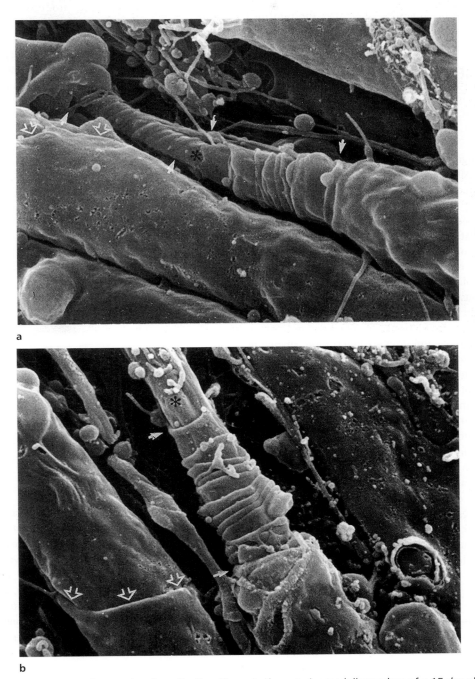

a

b

Figure 2.11 *Scanning electron micrographs of myelinating fibres. In the anterior medullary velum of a 15-day-old rat they show the paranodal loops (between arrows) spiralling towards naked axolemma (asterisks at presumptive nodes). In the upper micrograph, adjacent paranodal loops (between arrows) of consecutive myelin segments exhibit reverse spirals. Note the outer ridges (open arrows) on the surface of the myelin sheaths in both micrographs, which probably correspond to the outer cytoplasmic rims of oligodendrocyte cytoplasm. (Electron micrographs prepared by Dr U Mangold and Professor J Sievers at the Universities of Hamburg and Kiel, Germany, respectively.)*

In the adult, axons and oligodendrocytes continue to be interdependent. For example, loss of axonal function induces disruption of myelin-related gene products in oligodendrocytes whereas, after loss of oligodendrocytes and/or their myelin sheaths, axolemmal ion channels become dispersed and axonal conduction is impaired. It is not known whether the re-establishment of units is a function of mature oligodendrocytes or oligodendrocyte progenitors, but the functions of neither the reformed oligodendrocyte unit nor the axons associated with it completely recover.

FUNCTIONS OF OLIGODENDROCYTES

Oligodendrocytes function to provide myelin sheaths for CNS axons. The myelin sheaths impose saltatory conduction on axons, the speed of conduction being determined by the lengths of the internodal myelin segments. Oligodendrocytes interact with axons to determine the siting of nodes, aggregation of axolemmal ion channels and maintenance of the stability of myelin. Destruction of oligodendrocytes or myelin leads to disastrous consequences for CNS function. Remyelination after demyelination occurs to a limited degree and could be a function of either the surviving oligodendrocytes or newly differentiated cells formed from the adult progenitor pool.

Gap junctions between astrocytes and oligodendrocytes account for the spread of intracellularly injected dyes between the two populations. These oligodendrocyte–astrocyte junctional complexes are heterotypic, involving the juxtaposition of one hemichannel of the specific oligodendrocyte connexin-32 and the astrocytic connexin-43.[101] The functions of astrocytic–oligodendrocytic membrane couplings are unknown. Connexin-32 gap junctions are also expressed at the myelin–axon interface at paranodes and mediate axon–oligodendrocyte signalling of unknown function. At different stages of their development, oligodendrocytes also express a wide range of ion channels and pumps, as well as neurotransmitter receptors and transporters.[24] For example, oligodendrocyte progenitors transiently express receptors for glutamate and GABA, the major excitatory and inhibitory neurotransmitters in the CNS.[408] Glutamate- and/or GABA-induced changes in intracellular calcium (Fig. 2.12) may play a role in oligodendrocyte differentiation.

NG-2 GLIA

A population of glial cells which express the NG2 chondroitin sulfate proteoglycan has been identified in both the grey and the white matter.[67,214,216] These cells are phenotypically distinct from astrocytes, oligodendrocytes and microglia (Fig. 2.13), but have the antigenic phenotype of oligodendrocyte progenitors.[277,331] Butt and colleagues suggested that NG-2 glia may represent a novel population of glial cells in the CNS, although it remains a possibility

that they may give rise to oligodendrocytes in both the developing and adult CNS.[67]

RELATION OF NG-2 GLIA TO OLIGODENDROCYTE PROGENITORS

Oligodendrocyte progenitors are labelled in culture with the A2B5 monoclonal antibody and are defined as bipotential O-2A cells, capable of producing both GalC+ oligodendrocytes and a class of astrocyte called the type II astrocyte, expressing glial fibrillary acidic protein (GFAP).[312,314] Type II astrocytes were purportedly specialized to send perinodal processes exclusively to nodes of Ranvier.[117,118,255] However, it is now generally believed that, *in vivo*, O-2A cells are oligodendrocyte progenitors that

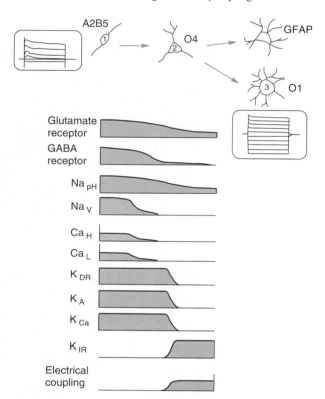

Figure 2.12 *Current and receptor expression by oligodendrocytes. Schematic representation of current and receptor expression by cells of the oligodendrocyte lineage in vitro. A2B5-positive oligodendrocyte progenitors (1) develop into O4 positive progenitors (2), which can give rise to either GFAP+ astrocytes or O1/GalC+ oligodendrocytes (3), depending on the culture conditions. Oligodendrocyte progenitors co-express O4, PDGF-αR and NG-2.[277,331] Insets on the left and right show currents in the progenitors and oligodendrocytes, respectively, activated by depolarizing and hyperpolarizing voltage steps. The densities of ion channels and gap junctions during oligodendrocyte differentiation are displayed below. Na_{pH}, pH-activated Na$^+$ current; Na_V, voltage-activated Na$^+$ current; Ca_H, high voltage-activated Ca^{2+} current; Ca_L, low voltage-activated Ca^{2+} current; K_{DR}, delayed rectifier K$^+$ current; K_A, A-type K$^+$ current; K_{Ca}, Ca-dependent K$^+$ current; K_{IR}, time-dependent inwardly rectifying K$^+$ current. Reproduced by permission from Kettenmann et al.[183]*

constitutively develop into oligodendrocytes, and do not give rise to type II astrocytes,[62,124] a conclusion corroborated by the *in vivo* morphological findings of Butt and colleagues.[64,65]

In an ultrastructural study, Butt *et al.*[67] observed that a significant population of adult NG-2 glia have a complex stellate morphology, with processes exclusively terminating on axolemma at nodes of Ranvier (Fig. 2.14) to form a nodal network to which the microprocesses of astrocytes also contribute (see below). Since NG-2 labels O-2A cells *in vitro* and NG-2 glia have an oligodendrocyte progenitor antigenic phenotype *in vivo*, in the developing and adult CNS,[277,331,382] it is reasonable to conclude that NG-2 glia and oligodendrocytes are derived from a common bipotential stem cell (reviewed by Nishiyama *et al.*[276]) and

so NG-2 glia may represent the *in vivo* counterpart of the type II astrocyte. However, NG-2 glia do not form end-feet at the glia limitans of the pia or cerebral blood vessels,[67] nor do they support myelin sheaths or express GFAP, Rip, MBP, CA-II, lectin, glutamine synthetase (GS) or S-100,[67,278,331] and so are phenotypically distinct from astrocytes, oligodendrocytes and microglia. Adult NG-2 glia apparently have the antigenic phenotype of oligodendrocyte progenitors, expressing PDGF-αR and O4, and have been referred to as adult oligodendrocyte progenitors.[277,331] It is possible that NG-2 glia may retain the capacity to give rise to oligodendrocytes in the adult,[216] which has implications for oligodendrocyte regeneration in MS,[362] particularly since NG-2 glia are found in MS lesions.[81] Significantly, NG-2 is upregulated in glial

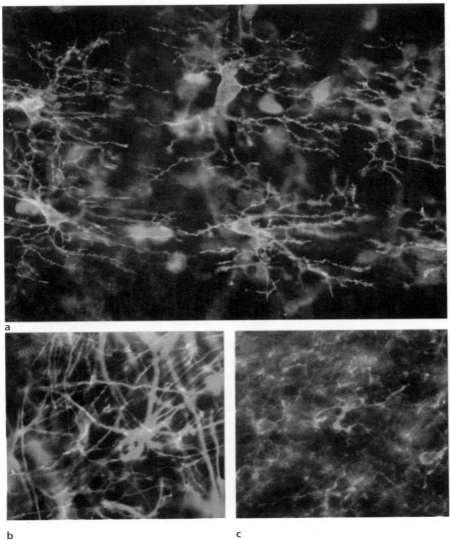

Figure 2.13 *NG-2 glia. Photomicrographs of NG-2 glia in the rat anterior medullary velum double immunofluorescence labelled with NG-2 and CA-II (**a**), GFAP (**b**), or lectin (**c**). NG-2 was fluorescein conjugated (green) and the other markers were rhodamine-conjugated (red). NG-2 glia are smaller than oligodendrocytes (**a**) and astrocytes (**b**), and are similar in size and morphology to microglia (**c**), but do not express markers for oligodendrocytes, astrocytes or microglia. Reproduced by permission from Butt* et al.[67]

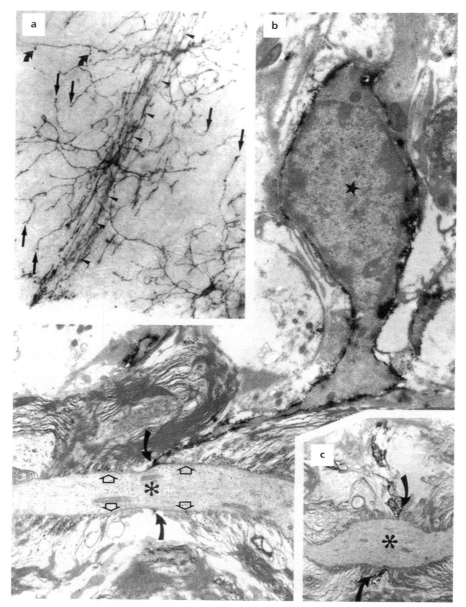

Figure 2.14 *NG-2 glia. Micrographs of NG-2 glia in the rat anterior medullary velum, visualized by immunoperoxidase staining in whole-mounted tissue (a) and by pre-embedding electron microscope immunocytochemistry (b, c). DIC optics superimpose the images of NG-2-positive dendritic cells and myelinated axons (a). Typically, NG-2-positive cells have small soma with multiple branched varicose primary processes, which ramify in the long axes of axon bundles (arrowheads, b) or terminate on individual axons (arrows, a). Processes bear spines along their lengths, which also terminate on axons (curved arrows, a). Electron micrographs show the surface labelling of the NG-2 glial cell membrane (star, b) that wraps processes (curved arrows, b, c) around the axolemma at nearby nodes of Ranvier (asterisks, b, c), defined by the juxtaposed paranodal loops of adjacent myelin sheaths (open arrows, b). Reproduced by permission from Butt et al.[67]*

neoplasms, including glioblastomas, oligodendrogliomas and astrocytomas,[83,370] suggesting that they may all be derived from NG-2 glia.

In adult CNS grey matter, in which myelin is largely absent, there is no apparent necessity for a pool of regenerative adult oligodendrocyte progenitors, but there is a significant population of multibranched NG-2 glia that send processes to form intimate associations with axodendritic synapses (Fig. 2.15).[34,284]

FUNCTIONS OF NG-2 GLIA

NG-2 glia are ideally suited to respond to changes in axonal function and, being a reactive phenotype, respond rapidly to CNS injury by upregulation of NG-2 expression, proliferation and outgrowth of processes.[188,213,215,278,328] Significantly, the NG-2 chondroitin sulfate proteoglycan, a component of the glial scar matrix, has been shown to inhibit CNS axon regeneration.[119] In addition, NG-2 glia express quisqualate-sensitive glutamate receptors which stimulate raised cytosolic calcium,[124] and so glutamate released synaptically or non-synaptically from axons could control the function of NG-2 glia[34] (Fig. 2.16). In addition, NG-2 glia may play a role in the establishment of nodes of Ranvier and the nodal aggregation of sodium channels.[63,67] The function of the nodal (Figs 2.4, 2.5, 2.14) and synaptic (Fig. 2.15) contacts is presently unknown.

In summary, it is likely that all or some NG-2 glia are a morphologically unique and a functionally specialized class of glia which exclusively form axonal contacts at both nodes of Ranvier in the white matter and synapses in the grey matter.[34,67,284] Thus, it may be germane to rename these unique differentiated mature glia 'synantocytes' (from the Greek *synant*, meaning contact), to distinguish them from oligodendrocyte progenitors, O-2A cells and type II astrocytes.

Astrocytes

The term astrocyte was first used by Santiago Ramon y Cajal in a description of this macroglial cell type in the early twentieth century.[320] Even at this early time, there was argument about what their function might be. In 1907, Lugaro[229] suggested that astrocytes played a role in maintaining an equable environment for neurons whereas, in 1909, Ramon y Cajal[321] thought they might be more important for the insulation of neurons and in forming scar tissue after CNS damage (see also Ref. 309). The functions of astrocytes remained a mystery for several decades, after the early pioneering studies, until an ever-growing armory of techniques became available to examine astrocyte function (for reviews see Refs 185, 263).

The techniques used to study astrocytes all have their limitations. Perhaps the most insidious is seen in culture,

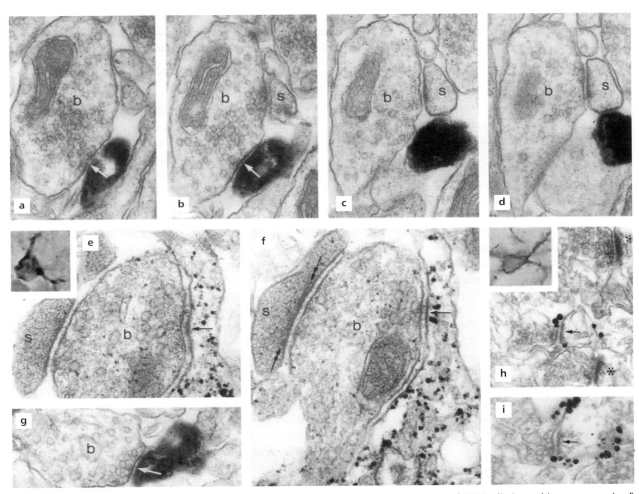

Figure 2.15 *NG-2 glia. Electron micrographs of the synaptic relationships of the processes of NG-2 glia in rat hippocampus. (a–d) Serial sections of a process (black, peroxidase reaction) from a physiologically identified, biocytin-labelled NG-2 glial cell receives a synapse (arrow) from a bouton (b) that also gives a synapse to a dendritic spine (s). (e, f) Silver-intensified gold reaction of an NG-2 glial (inset, light micrograph) process revealing the postsynaptic membrane specialization (arrows), compared with that (between double arrows) of a spine (s) innervated by the same bouton (b). (g) Another bouton (b) makes a synapse (arrow) only with an NG-2 glial cell process. (h, i) NG-2 glial cell (inset) in the stratum radiatum of the adult rat, showing the postsynaptic membrane specialization (arrows) and those of neighbouring synapses on dendritic spines (asterisks). Reproduced by permission from Bergles et al.*[34]

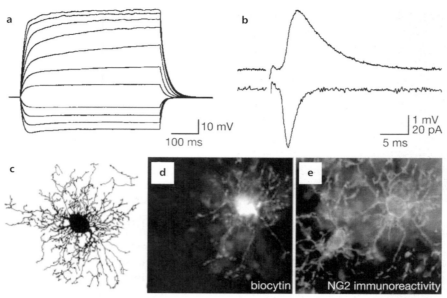

Figure 2.16 *NG-2 glia. Synaptic responses from identified NG-2 glia in rat hipocampal slices. (**a**) Current-clamp recording of membrane response to current injection. (**b**) Evoked response to Schaffer collateral/commissural fibre stimulation, recorded in voltage clamp and current clamp. (**c**) Reconstruction of a biocytin-filled (**d**) NG-2 glia (**e**). Reproduced by permission from Bergles et al.[34]*

where astrocytes express novel phenotypes not seen *in vivo*.[89,191,237] While cultured cells offer the advantages of purity and accessibility, experiments *in vivo* are required to confirm that *in vitro* data are representative of the developmental and phenotypic state of the cell under investigation. ISH is increasingly used, but there is often uncertainty about the identity of the cell expressing the mRNA unless further confirmation is sought. Unfortunately, the conditions for ISH do not often allow for concomitant immunocytochemistry, although GFAP filaments are usually stable. However, the presence of mRNA does not necessarily mean the expression of cognate protein. Immunocytochemistry, using antibodies specific for particular proteins, is very useful as long as cell identity is confirmed with an astrocyte-specific marker. Recently, electrophysiologists, using the technique originally described by Edwards *et al.*,[110] have patch clamped astrocytes in brain sections. After recording, the cells can be identified by filling with fluorescent dyes and/or immunocytochemical labelling (Fig. 2.17). Removal of cell contents through a microelectrode allows identification of the mRNA transcripts present with reverse transcription–polymerase chain reaction (RT-PCR).

STRUCTURE OF ASTROCYTES

Astrocytes are multipolar cells; their long processes radiate from the cell body and frequently branch dichotomously (Figs 2.4, 2.17, 2.18). The processes are both stem-like and velate, and have multiple functions. Junctional complexes at sites of contact between different astrocytic processes imply that astrocytes form an interconnected functional syncytium within the neuropil. Many processes terminate as end-feet which contact the basal laminae of both blood vessels and the pia mater. End-feet are bound together by tight junctions to form a contiguous coat, contributing to the glia limitans of the blood–brain barrier (BBB) (Fig. 2.19) and cerebrospinal fluid (CSF)–brain barrier (Fig. 2.20), respectively. Other fine processes are closely associated with nodal axolemma and, along with NG2 glia terminals, probably serve a specialized function unique to nodal activity (Figs 2.4, 2.20) (see below). Many dendritic and somatic neuronal membranes are ensheathed by astrocyte processes, except at sites of membrane apposition at synapses. In electron micrographs (Fig. 2.21), astrocyte profiles are larger and more translucent than those of oligodendrocytes. Their pale nuclei contain heterochromatin concentrated in a rim below the nuclear envelope. The relatively translucent cytoplasm has many lysosomes and glycogen granules, a prominent Golgi apparatus, and bundles of 10 nm GFAP intermediate filaments which fill the remaining cytoplasm and extend into all processes,[222] being particularly abundant in fibrous astrocytes. Antibodies to GFAP[38] are used immunohistochemically to identify astrocytes (Figs 2.18, 2.22, 2.23). Astrocytes also contain glutamate synthetase,[302] vimentin and S-100 protein. Some astrocytes are GFAP negative and their subclassification relies on the use of the latter markers and also upon electrophysiological observations.[366,383,409]

Two morphologically distinct astrocytic phenotypes,[298] called protoplasmic and fibrous types, predominate in the grey and the white matter (Fig. 2.21), but it is not known whether they are functionally distinct. Other astrocytic morphologies are regionally specific and

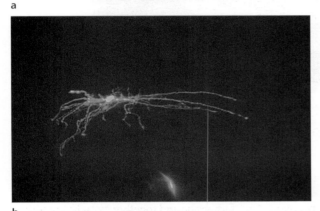

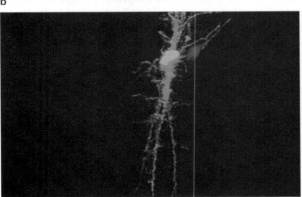

c

Figure 2.17 *Astrocytes. Lysinated rhodamine dextran-microinjected astrocytes from the adult rat anterior medullary velum (**a**) and adult mouse optic nerve (**b**). (**c**) A higher power view of (**b**) rotated through 90°. Astrocytes have a stellate morphology; most processes are stem-like but some near the cell body are vellate and some have bulbous swellings which are subpial end-feet. Most processes bear fine off-shoots and spines along their lengths. (Confocal micrographs.)*

tion are that the functional heterogeneity of astrocytes, reflected in local astrocyte expression of homologous receptors for neurotransmitters released by neighbouring neurons, is ignored.[418] Expression of neurotransmitter receptors enables astrocytes to respond to ligands released by neurons[306] (see below).

Astrocyte functions include roles in normal developing and adult CNS and after either damage or disease. The latter functions are discussed in Chapter 3, this Volume. Here, astrocyte functions in the normal developing and adult CNS are discussed.

DEVELOPMENT OF ASTROCYTES

Origins of astrocytes

Current opinion holds that neurons and the macroglia derive from neuroepithelial stem cells in periventricular areas of the developing CNS. Most rodent neurons are generated prenatally while the macroglia arise postnatally, suggesting separate precursors. Recent tissue culture experiments have revealed the multipotential nature of stem cells (for reviews see Refs 127, 413), with restricted differentiation potentials (for references see Ref. 413). In

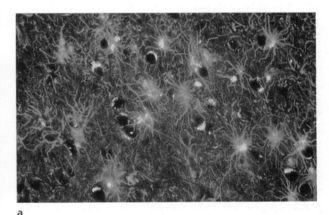

a

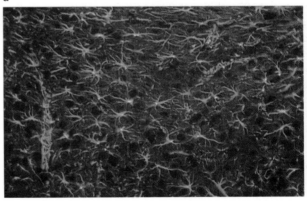

b

Figure 2.18 *GFAP+ astrocytes in the adult human (**a**) and rat (**b**) cerebral cortices. Note the end-feet of astrocytes enclosing a blood vessel in (**b**). Such perivascular end-feet are components of the blood–brain barrier. (Immunofluorescence micrographs.)*

include Bergmann glia in the cerebellar cortex (Fig. 2.23), Müller cells in the retina, radial glia in the walls of the neural tube (Fig. 2.24) and cerebral vesicle during development, and a variety of ependymal cells which line the ventricular system and spinal canal of the adult CNS (see below). The limitations of this morphological classifica-

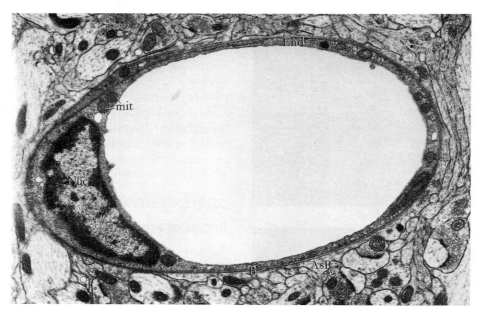

Figure 2.19 *Cerebral capillary. Transverse section through a capillary in the rat cerebral cortex. The nucleus (Nuc) of an endothelial cell (End) thickens the capillary wall, which is surrounded by a basal lamina (B) upon which abut astrocyte end-feet (AsP), forming a complete covering. Reproduced by permission from Peters* et al.[298]

culture, stem cells are nestin positive and respond to epidermal growth factor (EGF) by dividing and forming large, multicellular spheres, termed 'neurospheres' (Fig. 2.22) which also contain more differentiated progenitor cells.[413] Weiss and colleagues suggest that these latter cells have a limited capacity for further proliferation when stimulated by FGF. Two progenitor populations are of particular interest: one that gives rise only to neurons, and another that forms both neurons and astrocytes, i.e. is bipotential, requiring the addition of serum to the cultures (Fig. 2.25).

The question of which serum factors are necessary for the differentiation of a particular glial precursor was addressed by Raff and colleagues in their *in vitro* studies on the A2B5-positive O-2A progenitor cell (for review see Ref. 311). Initially isolated from the developing rat optic nerve, the O-2A progenitor cell differentiates into either an oligodendrocyte, in the absence of serum, or a process-bearing, GFAP-positive type II astrocyte, in the presence of serum. The fibroblast-like type I astrocyte (Fig. 2.25) is believed to derive from a different progenitor. Ciliary neurotrophic factor (CNTF) and an as yet undefined protein constituent of the extracellular matrix are essential for the differentiation of the O-2A cell into a type II astrocyte.[219] The type II astrocyte does not appear to have an *in vivo* counterpart[255] and, until such a cell is found *in vivo*, the possibility that this astrocyte is a peculiarity of culture will be debated. With respect to the more recent experiments on neurospheres (Fig. 2.22), Chiang *et al.*[84] report that retinol induces the differentiation of spindle-shaped, GFAP-positive astrocytes following removal of EGF. Other astrocyte differentiation agents are bone morphogenic protein-2 (BMP-2),[144] interferon[47] and leukaemia

inhibitory factor (LIF).[195,267,335] The LIF receptor is required not only for the expression of GFAP, but also for the astrocytic induction of neuronal differentiation and survival, by astrocyte-derived trophic factors.[195] These putative agents are absent from LIF receptor-negative precursor populations obtained from mice with a disrupted LIFR gene. Clearly, more work needs to be done to resolve this issue. In particular, how many astrocyte differentiation stages require induction agents and is local astrocyte heterogeneity determined by the actions of combinations of such factors within different CNS regions?

Radial glia (RG)

Many cells of the astrocyte lineage pass through a RG phenotypic stage before becoming fully differentiated astrocytes. RG are crucial elements in the guidance of developing neurons in CNS regions such as the cerebral cortex, cerebellum and spinal cord[318] (Fig. 2.24). RG are characterized by an extended bipolar shape and the expression of a number of markers including nestin, brain lipid-binding protein, intermediate filament-associated protein, and antigens bound by the monoclonal antibodies RC1 and RC2 and the D4 antiserum.[77,111,115,116,126,159,256,423] Recent work by Soriano and colleagues[378] suggests that the differentiation of RG is controlled, at least in part, by transitory Cajal–Retzius neurons through the release of soluble factors. The biochemical mechanisms involved in the migration of developing neurons along RG are by no means completely understood, but progress has been made in investigating the functions of astrotactin and glial growth factor (or neuregulin), respectively.[6,339,428] Both these molecules are expressed by migrating cerebellar

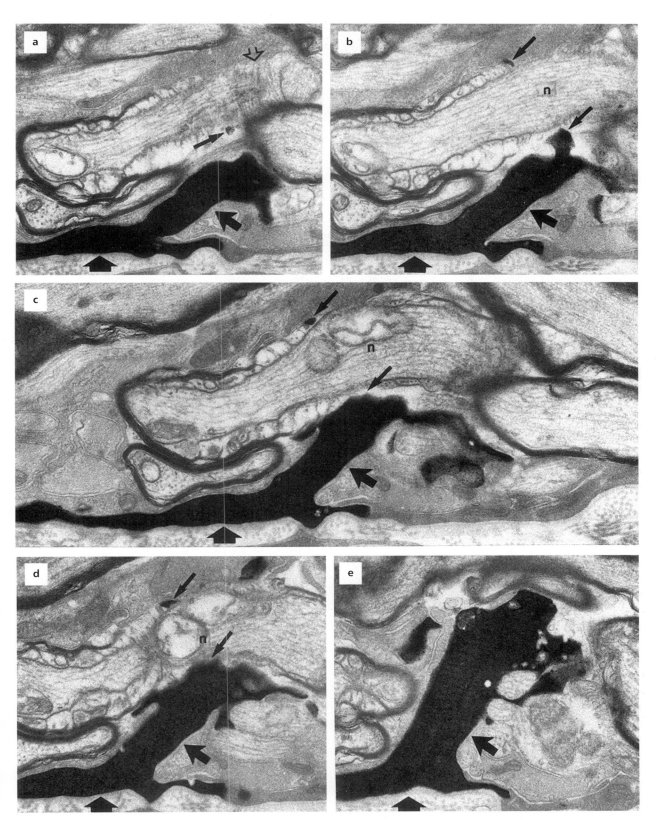

Figure 2.20 *Electron micrographs of the optic nerve. Serial longitudinal section show a process of a horseradish peroxidase (HRP)-filled astrocyte which forms both nodal contacts and an end-foot at the subpial glia limitans. The primary HRP-filled process (large arrows) contacts one side of the nodal axolemma; the rest of the node (n) is partially invested by small processes (small arrows in a–d) which branch from the main stem. The same primary HRP-filled process forms a typical end-foot (broad arrow) juxtaposed to the pial basal lamina to form a glia limitans externa (paranodal loops are indicated by an open arrow). A reconstruction of the node is illustrated in Figure 2.6. Reproduced by permission from Butt et al.[66]*

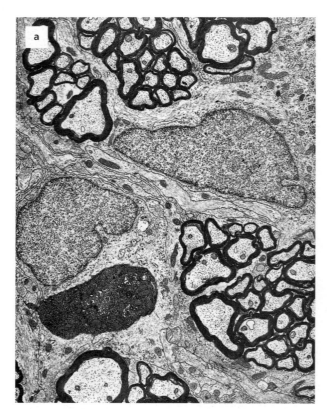
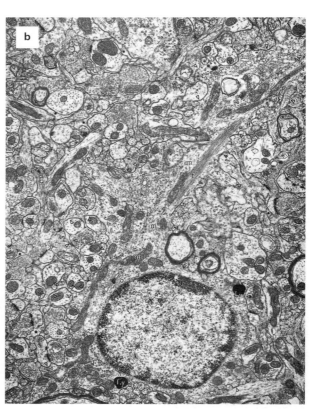

Figure 2.21 *Fibrous and protoplasmic astrocytes. (a) Electron micrographs of two fibrous astrocytes and part of a dark oligodendrocyte (O) in the optic nerve of the rat. The nuclei (Nuc) of the astrocytes are homogeneous in density and irregular in shape. Both astrocytes contain profiles of mitochondria, endoplasmic reticulum (ER) and Golgi apparatus (G). Fibrils are present and occupy much of the cytoplasm. (b) Electron micrograph of a protoplasmic astrocyte in the cerebral cortex of the adult rat containing a nucleus (Nuc). Within the cytoplasm (outlined by open arrows) are bundles of filaments (f), mitochondria (mit), microtubules (m), endoplasmic reticulum (ER), free ribosomes (r), lysosomes (Ly) and a Golgi apparatus (G). Reproduced by permission from Peters et al.[298]*

granule cells. A specific glial receptor for astrotactin has yet to be found; however, neuregulin is known to activate the ErbB receptor tyrosine kinase of the EGF receptor family present on glia.

Astrocytic control of neuronal shape

In addition to acting as guides for migrating developing neurons, astrocytes may participate in the growth of dendrites and axons. The results of tissue culture studies from a number of laboratories are generally consistent with a hypothesis that astrocytes derived from the local region of neurons (homotypic) support dendritic growth, while astrocytes from target regions preferentially support axonal growth. In early studies, Prochiantz and coworkers co-cultured either rat or mouse embryonic mesencephalic neurons with either mesencephalic or striatal astrocytes, and showed that homotypic astrocytes stimulate dendritic growth, whereas target-derived, striatal astrocytes preferentially stimulate mesencephalic neurons to elongate their axons.[17,80,100] Astrocyte-derived factors regulate neuronal polarity by modifying the adhesion of neurons to the culture substratum.[344] Other data, obtained using different combinations

of astrocytes and neurons from other regions, only partly support the hypothesis.[105,211,212,310] Nonetheless, all studies report astrocytic effects on either dendritic, or axonal growth.

ASTROCYTE-DERIVED GROWTH FACTORS IN THE DEVELOPING AND MATURE CNS

The large number of growth factors and their receptors precludes an attempt at a comprehensive coverage of this topic. Instead, the potential importance of astrocytic synthesis and release of growth factors in the developing CNS is indicated. In addition, rather than separating information on individual growth factors which relate to either the developing or mature CNS, local release and possible functions in the normal adult CNS are discussed here. Refer to Chapter 3 in this volume for the importance of astrocyte growth factors following CNS damage and disease.

Classical neurotrophins

During normal CNS development neurotrophins and other growth factors are required to support cell division and maturation. The classical neurotrophins comprise nerve growth factor (NGF), brain-derived neurotrophic factor (BDNF), NT-3 and NT-4/5, which bind to the Trk (tyrosine kinase) receptors. NGF binds preferentially to TrkA, BDNF and NT-4/5 (and with lesser affinity, NT-3) to TrkB, while NT-3 is the preferred ligand for TrkC. Studies on the Trk receptors are complicated by the discovery of seven different TrkB transcripts encoding both full-length and truncated receptors, and TrkC transcripts encoding at least three variants of this receptor (for review

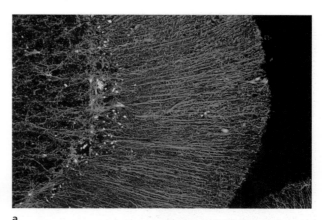

a

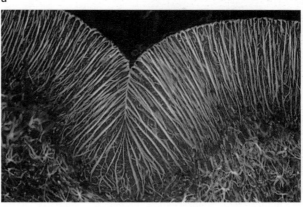

b

Figure 2.23 *Astrocytic fibres. Glial fibrillary acidic protein (GFAP)-positive Bergmann glial fibres in the cerebellar cortex of the human (**a**) and rat (**b**).*

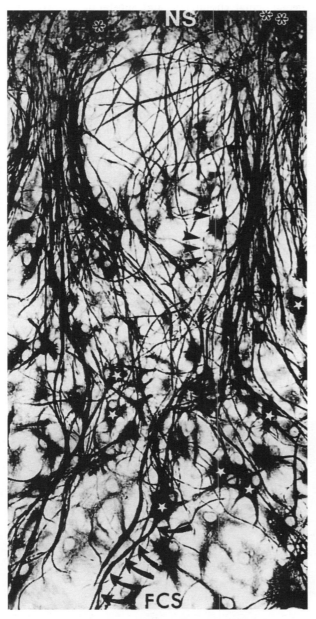

Figure 2.22 *Astrocytes in neurospheres. Glial fibrillary acidic protein (GFAP) immunostaining of 14-day-old subcultured rat cortical neurospheres (NS) maintained in 2% fetal calf serum-containing medium. Cell bodies of astrocytes within the neurosphere are marked with an asterisk. Cell bodies that have migrated away are marked with white stars. Reproduced by permission from Chiang et al.[84]*

see Ref. 231). The other receptor that binds all neurotrophins with the same low affinity is the p75 receptor, which co-operates with the Trk receptors to either increase or decrease neurotrophin binding and/or signalling efficiency, and may also act independently to activate mechanisms leading to apoptosis.[21] It has long been known that astrocytes can produce neurotrophins either in culture or after lesions *in vivo*.[202,345] However, only recently have specific antisera been developed allowing immunohistochemical protein localization in brain sections. The neurotrophins are mostly synthesized in neurons, with few observers noting neurotrophins in astrocytes in developing or adult CNS. Friedman *et al.*[123] reported immunoreactive NT-3 and NT-4/5 in GFAP-positive astrocytes in scattered cells in the rat brainstem, but these cells are not widespread through the rest of the CNS. It is not clear whether the neurotrophins are synthesized or taken up by the astrocytes, and what their functions may be. Astrocytes expressing internally truncated TrkB and TrkC receptors are widely distributed in the rat brain.[346] It has been suggested that binding to these truncated receptors might limit diffusion and thus control neurotrophin access to non-targeted neurons.

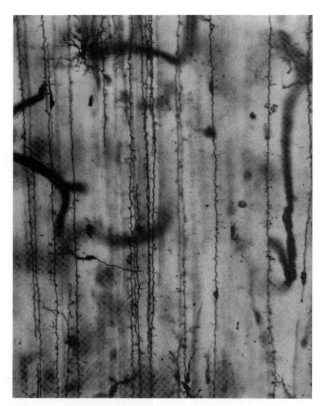

Figure 2.24 *Radial glial fibres. Section of Golgi-impregnated wall of a monkey fetal cerebral vesicle showing the elongated shafts of radial glial fibres. Reproduced by permission from Rakic.[318]*

Other growth factors

Although CNTF acts through a different type of receptor to that for the classical neurotrophins, it displays neurotrophic effects on a range of central neurons[11,171,349] and also has effects on oligodendrocytes and their O-2A progenitor in culture.[29,165,226] In normal, unlesioned adult CNS, CNTF is expressed at very low levels in most regions, with the exception of the optic nerve and olfactory bulb, where the levels of CNTF rise rapidly postnatally, the synthetic compartment being the astrocyte.[387] Thus, astrocytes could provide CNTF locally during development. Although CNTF lacks a normal signal sequence, it is released from both undamaged cultured astrocytes[178] and damaged astrocytes *in vivo*.[172] Possible CNTF targets following damage are neurons, e.g. motor, medial septal cholinergic and substantia nigra dopaminergic neurons, all of which are rescued from cell death by CNTF *in vivo*.[146,147,368] Astrocytic autocrine or paracrine upregulation of the CNTF receptor after CNS lesions[172,208,347] may induce components of their reactive response.[164,177,218]

The FGF family now comprises some 18 members.[282] Most is known about FGF-1 and FGF-2, although their distribution in the CNS is still uncertain,[18] at least FGF-2 is synthesized in astrocytes. Kuzis *et al*.[201] demonstrated the presence of FGF-2 in some astrocytes from postnatal day 7 onwards, and its level increases in hippocampal, neocortical and subcortical astrocytes up to adulthood. Like CNTF, FGF-2 has no signal sequence for directing the protein into the secretory pathway and this, together with its rather late appearance in development, has led to the suggestion that FGF-2 may be active after damage rather than during normal development.[201]

PDGF is a 30-kDa homodimeric or heterodimeric protein comprising disulfide-bonded A- and B-polypeptide chains. The isoform found in astrocytes is PDFG-AA. mRNA is located in type I rat astrocytes in culture and in glial cells in brain sections, albeit at lower levels than in neurons (for review see Ref. 403). A well-documented function of PDGF is that of mitogen for the O2A

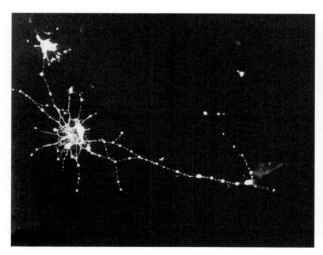
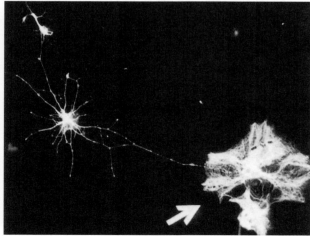

Figure 2.25 *Type I and II astrocytes. Immunofluorescence micrograph of type I and II astrocytes in cultures of newborn optic nerve cells after 2 weeks in culture. On the right both the single stellate type II and the group of type I astrocytes are stained for glial fibrillary acidic protein (GFAP). On the left the single type II astrocyte displays binding of the monoclonal antibody A2B5. Reproduced by permission from Lillien and Raff.[219]*

oligodendrocyte precursor.[308,311] Recently, Calver and colleagues[76] examined the effects of PDGF knockouts in mouse development. They found a marked reduction in the number of O-2A progenitors and oligodendrocytes in the spinal cords of mice lacking the PDGF-A but not in mice lacking the PBGF-B gene, implicating the PDGF-AA homodimer in the control of progenitor proliferation *in vivo*. However, it is uncertain whether the PDGF-AA, which acts on the O-2A cells, derives from astrocytes or from axons.

Astrocytic involvement in the development of the blood–brain barrier

The barrier arises when the tight junctions of vascular endothelial cells develop, inhibiting the movement of molecules between these cells. The abluminal membranes of capillary endothelial cells are covered with a thin basal lamina (30–40 nm thick) overlain by the end-feet of astrocytes (Figs 2.18, 2.19). Pericytes, totally enveloped in basal lamina, are often found between the endothelial cells and the astrocytic end-feet.[419] What is responsible for the induction of the endothelial cell tight junctions in CNS blood vessels? Are the endothelial cells able to construct these junctions on their own or are other cell types involved? Both *in vivo* and *in vitro* experimental approaches have been used in attempts to answer these questions. Janzer and Raff[176] demonstrated that cultured astrocytes transplanted on to the surface of the rat iris became vascularized and induced a permeability barrier for dyes in the capillary endothelia. However, Holash *et al.*[160] also undertook experiments of this type and claimed that they led to inconclusive results. Brain endothelial cells rapidly lose their blood–brain characteristics in culture, even though certain characteristics are regained by growing them with astrocytes. Thus, there is no optimal *in vitro* barrier model presently available (for review see Ref. 129). Although astrocytes almost certainly are involved in the induction and possibly the maintenance of the barrier, much remains to be done to determine the mechanisms involved.

THE MATURE CNS

Morphological relationships to neurons

The relationship between astrocytes and different populations of neurons is variable. In the cerebellum, for example, Purkinje cell perikarya and dendritic trees are encased by Bergmann glial processes (Fig. 2.23), except where the afferents of excitatory granule and inhibitory interneurons make synapses. In contrast, the perikarya of granule neurons are rarely covered (Fig. 2.26). The individual terminal elements of the complex cerebellar glomeruli are not associated with astrocytic processes, although neighbouring glomeruli are separated by such extensions.[289] In the neocortex, only 29% of synapses make contact with astrocytes and these are not fully covered.[379]

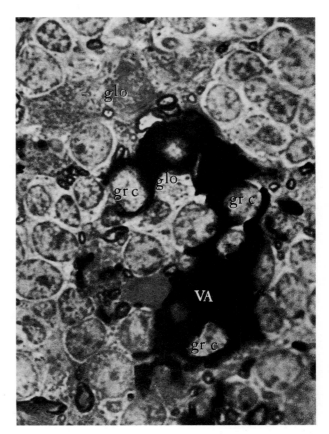

Figure 2.26 *Golgi-stained astrocyte in the internal granule layer of the adult rat cerebellum. Sheets of astroglial cytoplasm either completely or partially enwrap some granule cells (grc) and a complex synaptic terminal, the glomerulus (glo), whereas other granule cells are not covered. Reproduced by permission from Palay and Chan Palay.[289]*

A recent study of the stratum radiatum of the CA1 hippocampal area found that 57% of synapses have associated astrocytic processes. Ventura and Harris[406] suggest that this might mean that 'glutamate, released at approximately two-thirds of hippocampal synapses, might diffuse to other synapses, unless neuronal glutamate transporters are more effective than previously reported'. The amount of astrocyte covering of particular neuronal compartments is almost certainly related to the dependency of that compartment on astrocyte support. Such support may mean immediate or long-term dependency on astrocyte-released substances, such as metabolic substrates or growth factors, or simply insulation from the activity of other neurons by, for example, astrocyte neurotransmitter uptake.

White-matter tracts and fibrous astrocytes

In the white-matter, glia are arranged in long unicellular rows, which lie parallel with the axon bundles through which the primary glial processes course orthogonally.[64,65,394] In the adult rat fimbria, for example, solitary astrocytes are regularly spaced between a series of five to ten oligodendrocytes (Fig. 2.4); solitary microglia and NG-2 glia are also interposed regularly within the rows, but at a lower frequency than astrocytes. White-matter astrocytes are mainly of the fibrous phenotype, their processes terminating either as end-feet over the basal lamina of both the pia and vasculature to form a glia limitans, or as minute *en passant* collaterals which engage nodes of Ranvier[66] (Figs 2.4, 2.6, 2.20). A single node of Ranvier is contacted by the perinodal microprocesses of different astrocytes and also by those of NG-2 glia (Figs 2.4, 2.14).[67] Astrocyte perinodal processes secrete proteoglycans at CNS nodes[37,117] which could act either as a cationic exchange resin or as a maintenance factor of nodal cytoarchitecture.[156,204] Perinodal astrocytic processes also have high densities of sodium channels,[41,42] which may be activated by ephaptic (non-synaptic cell-to-cell membrane electrical) transmission at perinodal sites.[82] Astrocytes are functionally coupled with oligodendrocytes through heterotypic connexin-32/43 gap junctions between the membrane of the paranodal myelin loops and perinodal astrocyte processes, and also homotypically coupled via connexin-43 gap junctions.[101,244,412] Gap junctions offer a potential for intercellular signalling providing a basis for modulation of astrocyte function in response to neural/oligodendrocyte damage over a range of normal activities and also after injury. Calcium may act as an intercellular signal in many of these responses. For example, astrocytes interconnected via connexin-43 gap junctions propagate a Ca^{2+} wave through the network at a rate of 7–27 µm/s.[87,92,101] Wave propagation may be initiated in response to a variety of physiological and pathological stimuli, and Ca^{2+} may in turn act as an intracellular messenger regulating astrocyte functions including energy metabolism, vascular interactions, neurotransmitter uptake and metabolism, membrane transport, and the secretion of a multitude of substances including trophic factors, peptides and nitric oxide.[87,92]

Astrocytes and endothelia: orthogonal arrays

Astrocytic end-feet surround the capillary endothelial cells in the CNS. This morphological arrangement separates the endothelium from the neuronal perikarya and their processes. However, it is uncertain how much of a barrier the astrocytic processes present to molecules crossing from the blood to neurons and in the reverse direction. One membrane element pertinent to the movement of molecules at the astrocyte–endothelial cell interface is the 'orthogonal array' seen in freeze-fracture replicas of the astroglial end-foot (Fig. 2.27). These groupings of particles of individual size 6–7 nm in diameter were long believed to be transmembrane proteins. Recent observations seem to confirm this idea. Aquaporin-4, a member of the family of membrane water channels (for review see Ref. 193), has been shown to be present within astrocytic end-feet and within the orthogonal arrays.[266,275,326] These observations indicate that astrocytes possess specific

membrane domains for water transport facilitating movement between themselves and the intravascular space. Aquaporin-4 may not be the only molecule within the orthogonal arrays. Nagelhus *et al.*[265] also showed that the inwardly rectifying K^+ channel, Kir 4.1 (see Voltage-gated ion channels, below), is also located in Müller cell plasma membrane domains which abut blood vessels and form the glia limitans at the retina/vitreous body interface.

Voltage-gated ion channels

A major physiological difference between neurons and astrocytes is that the former generate an action potential, whereas the latter do not. Nonetheless, astrocytes possess a variety of voltage-gated ion channels. These include sodium, potassium, calcium and certain anion channels (for reviews see Refs 107, 375, 377). Here, by way of an introduction to a rapidly expanding research area, the channels for the cations Na^+, K^+ and Ca^{2+} are reviewed.

Sodium channels

Two types of Na^+ channel have been identified in cultured astrocytes, those that are neuron like, tetrododotoxin (TTX)-sensitive ones in stellate astrocytes and those that are TTX insensitive in non-process-bearing astrocytes (reviewed in Ref. 377). In culture, expression in stellate astrocytes is constitutive, whereas expression in non-process-bearing cells declines with time.[376] Neurons have a modulatory effect on channel expression in both types of astrocyte. In cultures of optic nerve non-process-bearing astrocytes, the presence of neurons maintains channel expression[24] whereas, in spinal cord cultures, neurons cause a downregulation in both astrocyte

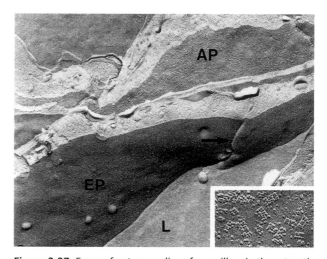

Figure 2.27 *Freeze-fracture replica of a capillary in the rat optic nerve. L, vessel lumen; EP, protoplasmic fracture face (P-face) of the luminal membrane of the endothelial cell; AP, P-face of an astrocytic end-foot with orthogonal arrays of particles (higher magnification in the insert); arrow, an endothelial cell tight junction (membrane plane not exposed). Reproduced by permission from Wolburg and Risau.*[419]

types.[399] The reasons for these differential effects are not clear. Oh *et al.*[281] undertook the combined technique of RT-PCR on mRNA from rat optic nerve. This tissue contains astrocytes, oligodendrocytes and axons, but not neurons. The Na$^+$ channel subtypes I, II and III are all detected. However, immunocytochemical examination with specific antibodies revealed no labelling of astrocytes within the optic nerve, although the type II channel is expressed by spinal cord astrocytes *in vivo*.[43] More recently, patch-clamp experiments on astrocytes in rodent hippocampal slices revealed the presence of Na$^+$ channels.[1,50,197] During mouse ontogeny, TTX-sensitive Na$^+$ currents decline to very low or undetecable levels in the stratum radiatum of the hippocampal CA1 subfield.[197] With respect to function, the low density of sodium channels on astrocytes rules out the possibility of action potential generation. However, raised extracellular K$^+$, possibly from local neuronal activity, may facilitate Na$^+$ channel opening and Na$^+$ entry. Subsequent activation of Na$^+$/K$^+$-ATPase results in a net uptake of K$^+$.[272,396]

Potassium channels

In astrocytes delayed rectifier, transient A-type and calcium-activated potassium channels have all been identified, but their functions await clarification (for reviews see Refs 107, 375). In contrast, the major K$^+$ channel type in astrocytes, the inward rectifier (Kir), is almost certainly involved in the uptake of excess extracellular K$^+$ resulting from local neuronal activity. One idea is that these K$^+$ are removed from regions of high concentration, into glia linked by gap junctions and from there to regions of low concentration, through a process known as 'spatial buffering'.[286] The distal regions of glial cells such as retinal Müller cells display more positive resting membrane potentials than the equilibrium potential for K$^+$, causing an efflux of K$^+$ into the extracellular fluid, dubbed 'siphoning' in retinal Müller cells.[273] Electrophysiologists have demonstrated that Kirs are present in glia *in vivo* and that their expression is strongly regulated during development and in response to brain damage and disease.[54,197,361] Several Kirs have been cloned and sequenced, and Kir 4.1 is expressed in certain populations of astrocytes in the rat cerebral cortex, hippocampus and cerebellum.[304] Not all astrocytes display the channel, however. For example, in the cerebellum, Bergmann glia are immunoreactive, whereas astrocytes in white-matter tracts are unreactive. Oligodendrocytes also express Kir 4.1 (Fig. 2.28). A question to be addressed is do astrocytes that do not express Kir 4.1 have other mechanisms for the removal of K$^+$, or does this function only reside in certain populations of astrocytes?

Calcium channels

Purified astrocytes in culture usually do not express Ca^{2+} channels, but they will do so in the presence of neurons when both L-type and T-type Ca^{2+} currents are present.[89] These currents are also detected in astrocytes acutely dis-

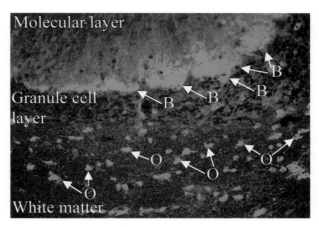

Figure 2.28 *Potassium channels in astrocytes. Fluorescence micrograph showing the expression of the K$^+$ inwardly rectifying channel, Kir 4.1, in the adult rat cerebellum. Arrows labelled 'B' indicate the position of the Bergmann glial cell bodies in the molecular layer from which their immunoreactive processes arise. Arrows labelled 'O' indicate oligodendrocyte somata in the white matter.*

sociated from excised optic nerve using a 'tissue-print' procedure.[24] The function of such channels is not clear, but if they are functional *in vivo*, the consequent influx of Ca^{2+} into the cell could precipitate a number of physiological processes such as cell proliferation, regulation of cell volume and cell death.[375] The discovery of intracellular Ca^{2+} waves in astrocytes and Müller cells after neurotransmitter exposure suggests a possible important role for intracellular Ca^{2+} in signalling in gap junction-connected glia.[88,274] However, it seems that the raised levels of Ca^{2+} within astrocytes probably derive from intracellular stores rather than from the extracellular source (for review see Ref. 12).

Uptake of neurotransmitters

Synaptic clearance of neurotransmitters is important for both limiting the duration of action and preventing concentration build-up. Astrocytes take up the amino acids, glutamate and γ-aminobutyric acid (GABA), and the monoamines dopamine, noradrenaline and serotonin. The rank order of uptake is glutamate > GABA > monoamines (reviewed in Ref. 192). Isolated preparations are used for most of the studies on monoamine uptake, in particular by cultured astrocytes. It has been more difficult to demonstrate uptake *in vivo*. Kimelberg[192] suggests that this may simply be attributable to a lack of microscopic resolution, coupled with a poor efficiency. It would seem then that neurons are capable of maintaining their own environment, with astrocytes possibly acting as a secondary clearance system.

Glutamate

In contrast to monoamines, astrocytes are exceptionally effective transporters of extracellular glutamate. As excessive extracellular concentrations of glutamate may lead to neuronal excitotoxicity, glutamate removal is crucial to the well-being of many neuronal populations in the CNS.[250] The uptake of either radiolabelled glutamate or non-metabolized D-aspartate (carried on the same transporters) into astrocytes in culture or in slices can be readily demonstrated.[416,417] Astrocytes contain the enzyme glutamine synthetase, responsible for the conversion of glutamate to glutamine, which is then released and returned to local neurons. Using specific antibodies for glutamate and glutamine, together with gold labelling immunohistochemistry, a differential distribution was seen by Ottersen and colleagues[287] in rat cerebellum. Glutamate was concentrated predominantly in neurons, and glutamine in astrocytes. As pointed out by Ottersen et al.,[287] this economic recycling of carbon units is advantageous, since glutamine can cross the extracellular space without causing activation of glutamate or other receptors. Over the past few years, great strides have been taken in understanding the membrane transporters responsible for the uptake of glutamate (for review see Ref. 372). Sodium-dependent transporters have the highest capacity for glutamate and aspartate and the most efficient extracellular removal of excitatory amino acids. The protein(s) that mediate Na^+-independent uptake are of low capacity and have not yet been cloned. Family members of the Na^+-dependent transporters in rodents include GLT-1, EAAC1, GLAST, EAAT4 and EAAT5. GLT-1 and GLAST (human homologues EAAT2 and EAAT1, respectively) are solely glial transporters. EAAC1 is found mainly in neurons but occasionally in astrocytes.[85] GLT-1 immunoreactive protein is most concentrated in forebrain astrocytes but it is also seen in astrocytes throughout the rest of the brain and spinal cord.[125,209,343] GLAST is primarily found in the cerebellum, where it is located in the Bergmann glia.[388] Estimations of the contribution of GLT-1 to forebrain glutamate uptake have been undertaken using gene deletion and antisense oligonucleotides. Each resulting deletion reduced forebrain or striatal transport by up to 90%.[342,397] Because neurons die after these procedures this estimate of uptake into astrocytes may be somewhat exaggerated, but does indicate a critical role for these cells in the prevention of glutamate-induced damage.

GABA

GABA transport, like glutamate transport, is Na^+ dependent. Three transporters, termed GAT-1, 2 and 3, have been cloned and sequenced from rat brain,[49,145] while a fourth is found in mouse and human brains.[48,225] Studies in rat brain using ISH reveal that GAT-1 mRNA is restricted to neurons and GAT-2 expressed only over leptomeninges, while GAT-3 mRNA is mainly located in glia, but also found in neurons of the retina and olfactory bulb.[108] Subsequent light- and electron-microscopic immunohistochemical studies of the rat cerebellum have

located GAT-1 mainly in presynaptic terminals and GAT-3 in glial processes.[174] In contrast to these studies, De Biasi et al.[95] found immunoreactive GAT-1 and 3 in astrocytes, but not in neurons in rat thalamus. The reasons for these regional differences in GABA transporter distribution are not known. However, although astrocytes possess GABA transporters and take up GABA, autoradiographical studies indicate that most glial cells exhibit little GABA uptake in vivo.[175,180] Their contribution to the uptake in any one area, however, is probably determined by the type of GABAergic neuron with which they associate. In the cerebellum, for example, Bergmann glia possess neither GAT-1 nor GAT-3, and GABA would appear to be taken up by the interneurons in the molecular layer which express GAT-1. In the synaptic glomeruli of the granule cell layer, the GABA-releasing Golgi terminals also possess GAT-1 and nearby astrocytes express GAT-3.[174] In the deep cerebellar nuclei, the GABA-releasing Purkinje cell terminals express neither transporter, while strong GAT-3 and weaker GAT-1 immunostaining is located in the surrounding astrocytes.[334]

Neurotransmitter receptors on astrocytes

Initial studies investigating neurotransmitter receptors on astrocytes relied on cultured cells as a model system. Cultured astrocytes can express phenotypic characteristics which may be associated with developmental, mature, reactive or possibly a unique pluripotential state only occurring in particular in vitro conditions. Thus, while astrocytes in culture express most of the receptors found on neurons in the CNS,[190,306] a continuing task has been to determine when and where they are expressed in vivo (for review see Ref. 306).

In vivo, astrocytes, like neurons, express receptors for the major excitatory and inhibitory amino acids, glutamate and GABA, respectively, as well as for noradenaline, serotonin, ATP, acetylcholine (muscarinic), and various peptides.[306] Evidence for the expression of glutamate and GABA receptors and the involvement of others in the breakdown of glycogen and the possible transfer of carbon units from astrocytes to neurons will now be reviewed.

Glutamate receptors

There are both ionotropic and metabotropic glutamate receptors; the ionotropic receptors comprise α-amino-3-hydroxy-5-methyl-4-isoxazolepropionic acid (AMPA), kainate and N-methyl-D-aspartate (NMDA) (for review see Ref. 288; also Chapter 1, this Volume).

AMPA

Although all mRNAs for all four AMPA subunits are located in subsets of GFAP-positive astrocytes in the cerebral cortex,[86] these data and immunocytochemical examination[243,300] indicate that the R4 subunit is the most prevalent. Its expression is characteristic of astrocytes throughout the brain, e.g. R4-positive cells have been detected in the olfactory bulb, the dentate gyrus, the amygdala[243] and the cerebral cortex.[243,300] Although not as prevalent as R4, the R1, R2 and R3 subunits are expressed by select populations of astrocytes.[94,247,381] Astrocytes in the mouse hippocampus exhibit an AMPA-induced depolarizing response with low Ca^{2+} permeability.[365,367]

Kainate

There is little evidence of kainate receptor subunits on astrocytes, an exception being cerebellar Bergmann glia which are immunohistochemically positive for GluR6/7.[299]

NMDA

Astroglial NMDA receptors are different from those of neurons in that they are not blocked by Mg^{2+}, enhanced by glycine or coupled to an influx of Ca^{2+}.[262] Immunohistochemical studies have revealed that astrocytes in the visual cortex, amygdala and locus coeruleus possess R1 subunits.[10,404]

Metabotropic glutamate receptors (mGluRs)

There is little evidence for mGluRs on astrocytes in vivo. Of the eight cloned subunits, the most likely to be present in vivo is GluR-5. Recent results examining acutely isolated hippocampal astrocytes indicate expression of mGluR-3 and mGluR-5 subunits.[360]

GABA receptors

Astrocytes can express the $GABA_A$ receptor, which possesses an intrinsic Cl^- channel. GABA activation of the receptor depolarizes astrocytes by an efflux of Cl^-, because the $Na^+/K^+/2Cl^-$ cotransporter and the Cl^-/HCO_3^- exchanger maintain an outward Cl^- gradient.[186] Although the $GABA_A$ subunits expressed by most astrocytes in vivo are not known, it has been shown that Bergmann glia express α_2-, α_3- and δ-subunits.[261]

Functions of amino acid receptors on astrocytes

The functional importance of these receptors remains unknown. Speculations, however, include $GABA_A$ receptor involvement in Cl^- homoeostasis, AMPA receptor-induced astrocyte swelling, possible control of synaptic activity and mGluR control of astrocyte proliferation (for reviews see Refs 12, 408).

Receptors for monoamines and peptides

The monoamines, noradrenaline, serotonin and histamine, and the peptide vasoactive intestinal peptide (VIP) have a common function in that they all promote glycogenolysis in mouse cerebrocortical slices (for review see Ref. 402). It is uncertain whether the glycosyl units, mobilized by glycogenolysis, are used by astrocytes themselves, or

metabolized further to lactate, to be released for use by local neurons. Such potential metabolic coupling between astrocytes and neurons is discussed below. There is substantial immunohistochemical evidence for the existence of β-adrenergic receptors on astrocytes.[7–9] The case for astrocytic serotonin receptors is, however, unclear, since although 5-HT$_{1A}$ receptor-like immunoreactivity in neurons and astrocytes throughout the CNS has been reported,[415] staining is probably restricted to neurons.[134,187] There is little evidence so far for the expression of astrocytic histaminic receptors. However, Bergmann glia in vivo respond to histamine with an increase in Ca^{2+} levels and are inhibited by the selective histamine antagonist chlorpheniramine.[194] As with many other receptors, VIP receptors have been demonstrated on cultured astrocytes.[13] However, the situation in vivo is still unclear. VIP receptor mRNA is expressed in neurons and possibly also in glia.[173]

Neuronal–astrocyte signalling and metabolic coupling

In the normal mammalian CNS, the principal energy source is glucose. To pass from blood to brain, glucose must cross the membranes of the capillary endothelial cells and the astrocytic end-feet. An important, but as yet unanswered question is: how much of this glucose passes directly to neurons and how much is distributed to neurons through local astrocytes? Although higher affinity antisera are needed to be sure of certain localizations, there is evidence that both astrocytes and neurons express glucose transporters (reviewed in Ref. 405). Whether all neurons in vivo are capable of transporting all the glucose necessary for normal self-sufficiency remains to be determined. However, if the hypothesis proposed by Magistretti and co-workers (see below) is true then, at least in some circumstances, certain populations of neurons may be dependent on their partner astrocytes for the supply of metabolic substrates.

Glycogen, the single largest energy reserve in the brain, is localized in astrocytes. Magistretti and Pellerin[239] suggest that glycogen should be viewed as providing a metabolic buffer during physiological activity. Glycogen turnover in the brain is rapid and co-ordinated with synaptic activity.[241] As reported above, various neurotransmitters have been shown to induce glycogenolysis in rodent brain slices. It seems that glucose itself is not released from astrocytes, but possibly lactate is. The release of lactate is intimately linked to the uptake of glutamate released from local glutamatergic synaptic terminals[240] (Fig. 2.29).

In summary, functional investigations during the 1980s and 1990s have shown that astrocytes and their precursors may participate in many events in the normal, developing and mature CNS to the benefit of neighbouring neurons. The two cell types are inexorably linked at many levels, and further technical developments will undoubtedly reveal greater and possibly surprising evidence of these linkages.

Ependymal cells

STRUCTURE OF EPENDYMAL CELLS

Most of the ventricular system is lined by either cuboidal, or columnar ependymal cells (Fig. 2.30). Their apical ventricular surfaces have cilia and microvilli, and adjacent cells are anchored to each other by desmosomes with prominent tonofibrils and connexin-26 gap junctions.[102] Ependymal cells have an indented heterochromatic nucleus and their cytoplasm contains many mitochondria, lysosomes, microfilaments and microtubules.[45,53] The ependyma covering white and grey matter differs in that the cells of the latter are more flattened, with highly folded interdigitating lateral margins, and many of the cells lack cilia. Ependymal cells express GFAP, vimentin, cytokeratins, glycoproteins and S-100β during development, but in adults they are largely GFAP/S-100 negative.[353]

The ependyma of the circumventricular organs of the third and fourth ventricles is specialized, and may represent the vestige of a phylogenetically ancient group of CSF-contacting protoneurons in the vertebrate brain.[407] Indeed, these organs are classified as either ependymal or para-ependymal:[199] ependymal circumventricular organs are the choroid plexi and the subcommissural organs; para-ependymal circumventricular organs include the subfornical organ, the neurohypophysis, the median eminence, the pineal gland and the area postrema (see review by McKinley and Oldfield[233]). Only the ependymal organs will be considered here. Choroid plexus secretory cells are cuboidal epithelial cells opposed to the basal lamina of the tela choroidea and vascular core of the plexus (Fig. 2.31). The ventricular surfaces of the choroid plexus cells have numerous long microvilli, but few cilia except during development. The nuclei are basally located and the cytoplasm has a large Golgi complex and many mitochondria. A blood–CSF barrier is maintained in the epithelium by tight junctions (zonula occludens) and desmosomes between the highly folded lateral margins of adjacent cells.[363] Secretion of CSF by the choroid plexus

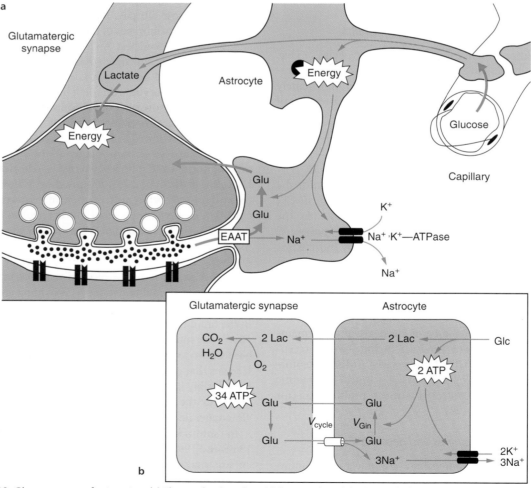

Figure 2.29 *Glucose usage of astrocytes. (a) The mechanisms by which synaptic activity is coupled to glucose usage. (b) Stoichiometry of glutamate-mediated synaptic transmission and glucose usage V_{cycle}, rate of tricarboxylic acid (TCA) cycle; V_{Gln} and rate of neurotransmitter cycle. EAAT, Excitatory Amino Acid Transporter; glc, glucose; lac, lactate. Reproduced by permission from Magistretti et al.[240]*

cells is dependent on the Na/K pump and the enzyme carbonic anhydrase C.[350] The microvilli of the epithelium are rich in Na/K-ATPase.[51]

The subcommissural organ is formed by columnar ependymal cells extending from the rostral to the ventral surface of the posterior commissure, at the anterior entrance to the midbrain aqueduct. In the human brain, it is prominent in the fetus but vestigial in the adult. The organ has unknown secretory functions; in some mammals, glycoproteins secreted by the gland aggregate as a strand of material called Reissner's fibre which extends the full length of the central spinal canal.[340,385]

Associated with circumventricular organs is a specialized ependymal cell called the tanycyte.[59,120] In the hypothalamic wall of the third ventricle, for example, tanycytes have long basal processes which ramify among parvocellular neurosecretory neurons in the paraventricular area. Tanycyte processes terminate in the arcuate nucleus as end-feet, bound by tight junctions, either on the portal blood vessels of the median eminence, or at the pial surface. These basal processes are rich in mitochondria, intermediate filaments and microtubules. The end-feet contain dense-core vesicles. The cell bodies line the ventricular lumen and are joined by tight junctions. Their apical surfaces are devoid of cilia, but abundant microvilli and pleomorphic blebs protrude into the ventricular lumen. Most tanycytes are GFAP⁻/S-100⁺.

DEVELOPMENT OF EPENDYMAL CELLS

In the rat brain, definitive ependymal cells first appear within the neuroependymal epithelium during the proliferative/migratory phase of neurogenesis.[3,4,58,93,319] Differentiation proceeds along a caudorostral axis starting in the fourth ventricle on about embryonic day (E) 14, the third ventricle on E15 and the lateral ventricles on E17. The ependymal lining may continue to be formed until postnatal day (P) 14. At around E17–19 GFAP-positive tanycytes in the hypothalamic wall of the third ventricle appear and most have differentiated by P7.[3,4,93,348] Matu-

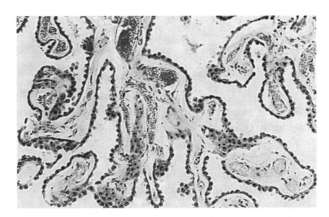

Figure 2.31 *Choroid plexus. Choroid plexus from the lateral recess of the fourth ventricle of a 52-year-old woman. (Toluidine blue.)*

ration is complete by P12. In mature ependyma, the frequency of mitotic activity is very low. A similar ontogenetic pattern probably occurs in man. The choroid plexus develops from proliferation of the ependyma at an early ontogenetic stage, and mitosis and differentiation could be induced by the vascular core of the invaginating tela choroidea.

During development ependymal cells synthesize cell adhesion molecules, proteoglycans, S-100 protein and neurotrophins supporting specialized roles for guiding migratory neuroblasts to their destinations (radial glial), and establishing commissural connections (floor and roof plate ependyma).[58,97,353,354] Specialized junctional complexes are present in the embryonic choroid plexi, including plate, strap and wafer junctions which allow the differential diffusion of proteins from the blood into the CSF.[356,357,364] Proteins in fetal CSF are excluded from the extracellular fluid of the immature brain by specific barriers at the CSF–brain interface not present in the adult.[109,355] CSF proteins are differentially taken up by neuroependymal cells, including radial glia and neuroblasts, and probably affect brain development as a whole.

FUNCTIONS OF MATURE EPENDYMA

The speculative activities of ependymal cells in the adult include secretion, absorption, transport, receptor functions and the provision of a barrier between the brain and CSF.[97,355] The strongest evidence for a role in transport is provided by tanycytes, which link the CSF with the hypophyseal portal blood vessels through the hypothalamic neuropil. Thus, when horseradish peroxidase (HRP) is injected into the third ventricle, the protein is excluded from regions of the hypothalamus lined by tanycytes, presumably because intercellular tight junctions render the tanycyte epithelium impermeable. However, HRP is found, within tanycytes and their basal processes, suggesting uptake from the CSF and intracellular transport to end-feet.

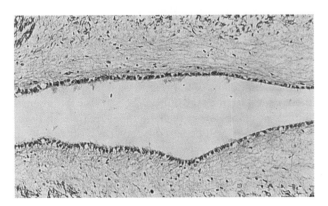

Figure 2.30 *Ependymal cells. Ependymal lining of the floor of the fourth ventricle of the brainstem of a 60-year-old man. (Toluidine blue.)*

Ependyma does not regenerate after injury at any age, probably because the epithelium is non-mitotic and is incapable of re-expressing fetal cytoskeletal and secretory proteins.[59,352] Thus, tearing of the ventricular linings leaves discontinuities of exposed and herniated neuropil, and nodules of reactive subventricular astrocytes[35] and ependymal rosettes form.[352] Ependymal rupture associated with subependymal heterotopia may be an aetiological factor in epilepsy.[327]

An important extension of the ependymal epithelium is the subependymal layer, a collection of primitive, mitotically active dark and light nucleated cells scattered along the margins of the ventricles and spinal canal immediately below the ependyma.[373] The layer contains astrocyte and oligodendrocyte progenitor cells,[230] which give rise to both types of macroglial phenotypes after birth and into adulthood. More recently, the subependymal region has gained importance as a potential source of adult neural stem cells[200,398] which, when implanted into the adult CNS could replace tissue lost after trauma and degenerative diseases. The layer may have clinical relevance because it has been implicated in the formation of periventricular glial tumours.[162,205] On the apical surfaces of ependymal cells scattered supraependymal epiplexus (Kolmer) cells are found.[221] They are mostly macrophages (see below), unidentified glial forms and probably also some neurons. Supraependymal cells are more frequent over the choroid plexus than elsewhere, where they have been called epiplexus cells.[2,236,393] They are probably macrophages which pinocytose cellular debris and proteins present in the ventricular lumen,[227] and also partake in immunological responses and iron regulation in the ventricular system.[221]

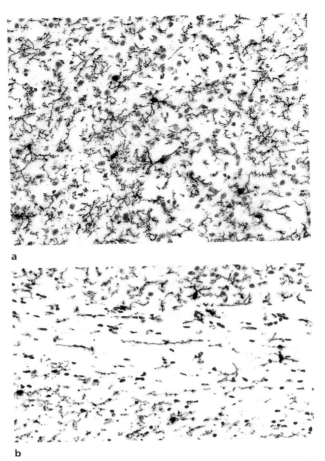

a

b

Figure 2.32 *Microglia in the mouse brain. (**a**) Regular distribution of microglia in the ventral striatum; (**b**) elongated microglia in the white matter. (HB1 immunohistochemistry.)*

MICROGLIA

In all tissues of the body there is a population of resident macrophages,[140] and the CNS and its associated tissues are no exception. Macrophages are present in the meninges, and brain vasculature and parenchyma. The term microglia is used to describe those cells with a distinct morphology and phenotype that lie within the parenchyma of the CNS (Figs 2.32, 2.33). These cells, first described and named by Del Rio-Hortega,[98] are the resident macrophages of the CNS parenchyma. There is an extensive literature debating whether microglia are derived from the mononuclear phagocyte lineage, the consensus of which supports the idea that microglia are indeed members of this lineage (for useful reviews on this historical debate see Refs 220, 223).

In addition to microglia, several other populations of macrophages are associated with the CNS which have different and contrasting functions compared with those of microglia. Perivascular macrophages[141] lie adjacent to the abluminal surface of endothelial cells, separated from the parenchyma by a basement membrane, and do not have the long, fine processes of microglia (Fig. 2.34). There are

macrophages with short, stout processes and a stellate morphology lying within the stroma of the choroid plexus, in addition to a small population of macrophages over the surface of the choroid plexus (epiplexus, or Kolmer cells).[248] There is also a substantial population of macrophages and dendritic cells associated with the leptomeninges.[52,236,296]

Now that the microglial lineage debate has been resolved, it is appropriate that attention becomes focused on the cell biology and functions of microglia and other macrophages in the brain. There is increasing evidence to show that microglia and their relatives of the mononuclear phagocyte lineage may contribute to CNS homoeostasis, and to the outcome of brain injury and disease. Many of these issues are more readily addressed in experimental models of pathology in the laboratory and, for this reason, this review will be based largely on observations in laboratory rodents.

STRUCTURE OF MICROGLIA

Microglia are small elongated cells with two or three branches stemming from each pole, which characteristically bifurcate into fine, curved, claw-like terminals (Fig.

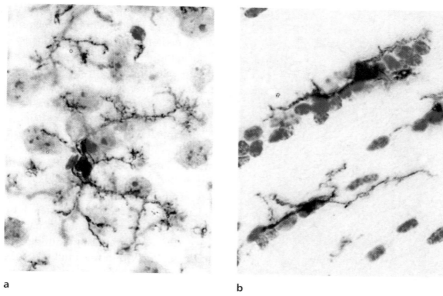

a   b

Figure 2.33 *Microglia. High-power fields of microglia in grey (**a**) and white (**b**) matter from Figure 2.32. Note the fine, bristle-like protrusions in the branches of the microglia. (HB1 immunohistochemistry.)*

2.35). Electron-micrographic profiles are small and flattened containing an elongated nucleus with dense peripheral chromatin, surrounded by a thin rim of pale cytoplasm which is more plentiful at each pole.[70,259] There is a small Golgi apparatus, scattered lysosomal granules and isolated rough endoplasmic reticulum.[223] Microglia are classically stained by the silver carbonate method developed by Del Rio-Hortega.[98] The fact that it took so long to establish that the microglia were the resident macrophages of the brain parenchyma gives an important indication of just how unusual these macrophages are compared with other tissue macrophages. It is now well recognized that the microenvironment in the normal adult brain dramatically downregulates or switches off these cells. The atypical phenotype of microglia, in both rodent and human CNS, is characterized not only by their morphology but also by the lack of expression of molecules usually associated with tissue macrophages. For example, the major histocompatibility complex (MHC) antigens class I and class II and CD45 (the leukocyte common antigen) are expressed at very low or undetectable levels[292,389] and the scavenger receptor[33] and the macrophage cytosolic protein EDI, a molecule expressed on the lysosomal compartment,[104,292] are also downregulated in normal adult rodent microglia. Resident microglia do, however, express F4/80, the complement type 3 receptor (CR3) and Fc receptors.[296] Other useful reagents which reveal resident microglia in rodents and human brain are the lectins, *Griffonia simplicifolia*,[390] *Ricinus communis* and several others,[426] but the antigens expressing particular sugar moieties are not known. Microglia also express the GD3 ganglioside and may thus be confused with the adult and perinatal macroglial progenitors in the nervous system (see Ref. 421 for discussion).

The molecular events involved in this downregulation are not well understood: they could involve either a lack of stimulation or active suppression induced by other cells in the microenvironment. The presence of the BBB and the exclusion of plasma proteins from the CNS has an influence on microglial phenotype.[293,295] In the circumventricular organs, sites in the brain where the BBB is lacking, or after damage to the BBB, microglia have a more upregulated phenotype. The substrate to which macrophages adhere can have a profound effect on their phenotype, and it has been suggested that the adhesion of microglia to a ligand in the CNS microenvironment may contribute to their unusual phenotype.[294] A novel protein which could underlie the molecular basis of macrophage adhesion to

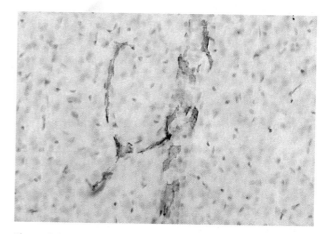

Figure 2.34 *Macrophages. Perivascular macrophages with a relatively simple morphology in the rat brain. Microglia in the brain parenchyma are not stained. (Immunohistochemistry with monoclonal antibody ED2.)*

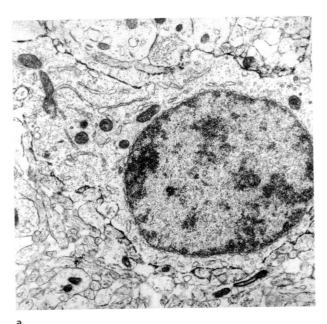

a

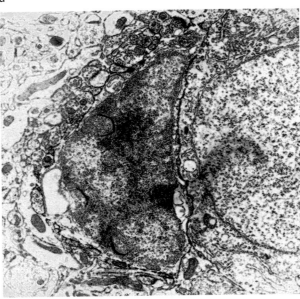

b

Figure 2.35 *Microglial cells. Electron micrographs illustrating immunohistochemically identified amoeboid, or immature, microglial cell in the developing mouse brain (**a**) and a microglia cell in the adult brain (**b**). The immature microglial cell has the typical appearance of a tissue macrophage, while the mature microglia is remarkable for the sparse cytoplasm and scant cytoplasmic organelles.*

brain tissue has been identified by an *in vitro* adhesion assay.[57] The adhesion of macrophages to brain tissue, using this assay, is blocked by *Griffonia simplicifolia* and *Ricinus communis*, suggesting that galactose residues on the microglia may bind a lectin-like molecule in brain tissue.

Another approach to define the factors involved in the generation of the microglial phenotype has been to try and reproduce the adult microglia phenotype in culture. These

studies have in part been hindered by the fact that microglia are largely defined by their morphology and lack of expression of a variety of antigens. Although it is possible to induce macrophages to grow long processes, simply by selecting the appropriate medium, this does not mean that these cells are now microglia. Convincing evidence for expression of the microglial phenotype in an *in vitro* system comes from Sievers *et al.*,[371] who showed that both contact with astrocytes and the products secreted by astrocytes play a part (see above). These studies demonstrated that macrophages derived from the blood and the spleen would adopt a microglia-like morphology and express the inwardly rectifying K channel associated with microglia. Neurotrophins secreted by neurons downregulate MHC expression by macrophages in culture, suggesting an important influence of neurons on microglia.[271] Within the adult CNS, there are yet further nuances of the neural microenvironmental influence on microglia. Microglia are ubiquitous, but their distribution is heterogeneous. Quantitative studies in the rodent demonstrate that the density of microglia varies between the grey and the white matter, and also from cytoarchitectural region to region, with as much as a six-fold difference between low-density regions (e.g. cerebellum) and high-density regions (e.g. ventral striatum).[207] It is not known what controls the variation in microglial density, but it is not related to variation in either neuronal or glial density, the distribution of a particular neurotransmitter or the frequency of developmental cell death in a particular locality. Along with the variation in cell density, there are subtle but consistent variations in the morphology of microglia, some of which are obviously related to the tissue structure, for example, the elongated microglia in white matter. Microglia in the circumventricular organs are exposed to plasma proteins and have a relatively simple morphology compared with those in the parenchyma protected by the BBB.

DEVELOPMENT OF MICROGLIA

In view of the long debate surrounding the origin of microglia, it is worth briefly summarizing the evidence that microglia are indeed mononuclear phagocytes. Radiation chimaeras are animals in which the host bone marrow has been destroyed by a lethal dose of radiation, and then reconstituted by bone marrow from another animal. By using different strain polymorphisms in the MHC locus, it is possible to arrange matters so that the donor and host haematopoietic cells carry different markers that can be detected immunocytochemically, but which do not give rise to graft-versus-host disease in the chimaeras. Hickey and colleagues,[153,154] using such chimaeras, have shown that bone marrow-derived cells can enter the CNS compartments and adopt the position and morphology of macrophages in the choroid plexus, the meninges and the perivascular space, and of microglia within the parenchyma. The number of donor cells that replace host cells over a given period will depend on the lifespan of the host macrophages in the different tissue compartments. The meningeal and perivascular macrophages turn over relatively rapidly and within a few months donor derived cells make up 30–50% of the total population.[154] In contrast, over the same period, microglia carrying the donor MHC marker are relatively rare. Studies using [³H]thymidine to study microglial kinetics also conclude that microglia turn over rather slowly compared with other tissue macrophages.[206] While these studies demonstrate conclusively that the CNS macrophages including microglia are of haematopoietic origin, the use of MHC polymorphisms is not without its problems, particularly in the assessment of the turnover of the different populations. MHC antigen expression is significantly downregulated on the resident quiescent microglia of adult rodents and it is necessary to activate microglia to reveal expression.[297,389]

The use of a donor cell marker that is not influenced by the CNS microenvironment would avoid this problem but, even in these chimaeras, there is no universal agreement about the validity of the data on the kinetics. De Groot et al.[96] reconstituted newborn and 3-month old mice with bone marrow from a transgenic mouse bearing multiple copies of a bacteriophage lambda gene, and found that up to 22 months later only 10% of the microglia in the white matter, and none in the grey matter, were of donor type. A study using donor cells carrying a human glucocerebroside gene, inserted with a retroviral vector, showed that the number of donor microglia may be as high as 20%, 3–4 months after reconstitution.[196] In another system, cells constitutively expressing β-galactosidase were used as the donor cells and it was the perivascular and meningeal macrophages that were predominantly of donor origin.[181] In summary, the results from the chimaera studies suggest that some variable proportion of the resident microglia is either very long lived or replenished by the division of cells which entered the CNS during embryogenesis.

There is now a significant number of studies in which immunocytochemical and histochemical techniques have provided evidence for a monocytic origin of microglia. When the details of the cellular morphology of mononuclear phagocytes are revealed, the sequence of development and differentiation of microglia provide a clear picture of the transition from monocytes.[296] This has also been shown by labelling the monocyte and immature microglia population with dyes which can then be detected later in life, when the cells have matured to fully differentiated microglia.[210] Earlier studies on microglia, and the other CNS-associated macrophages, suffered from limitations of the reagents and immunocytochemical detection systems. With improvements, a large number of cell-surface and cytoplasmic antigens restricted to leukocytes or other tissue macrophages are found to be expressed by microglia in the CNS and not by other cell types within the brain parenchyma such as astrocytes, oligodendrocytes or neurons.[291,294]

There is little doubt that microglia are derived from a haematopoietic precursor of the myeloid lineage, but there is still speculation about the possibility that microglia are a specialized branch of this lineage. There are two alternatives. In one, microglia are derived from monocytes which enter tissues, including the CNS, randomly, and there the distinct morphology and phenotype of microglia are induced in monocytes by the neural microenvironment. The other alternative envisages a distinct subset of myeloid cells, or monocytes, that are in some manner destined for the CNS parenchyma. This latter point of view received some support from the finding that immature microglia isolated from the neonatal CNS express an unusual pattern of ionic conductances.[184] Macrophages from the peritoneal cavity show predominantly outward K^+ currents, but cultured microglia express only an inward rectifying K^+ channel. This channel is expressed by immature microglia in fresh in vitro slices of neonatal CNS, demonstrating that this property is not simply an unusual feature of culture conditions.[55] Banati et al.[19] found that this inward rectifying K^+ channel is expressed on a subset of mononuclear phagocytes in the bone marrow, raising the possibility that bone marrow cells expressing this particular K^+ channel property are destined for the CNS. The importance of the CNS microenvironment per se has, however, been highlighted in studies by Sievers and colleagues,[359,371] who showed that macrophages derived from blood, or indeed the spleen, express both a microglial morphology and inwardly rectifying K^+ channels when cultured with astrocytes. The morphological phenotype is induced only by contact with the astrocytes and not by astrocyte conditioned medium, but the pattern of channel expression could be induced by astrocyte condition medium alone. At present, there is little reason to believe that microglia are derived from a distinct subset of monocytes.

MACROPHAGES AND MICROGLIA IN THE DEVELOPING CNS

Recruitment of monocytes into the developing CNS

The ontogeny of the haematopoietic system has been studied in considerable detail[252] and the sequence of development and migration of stem cells has been documented from the yolk sac to the liver, and from there to the bone marrow.[260] The growth factors that control the proliferation and differentiation of the macrophage lineage have been cloned and manipulated both in vitro and in vivo.[251] However, the ontogeny of the mononuclear phagocyte system in tissues has received relatively little attention. A major problem for the study of the distribution of mononuclear phagocytes in tissues, and for their study in development, is the unequivocal identification of these cells. The development of antibodies specific for mononuclear phagocytes has contributed significantly to our knowledge of the distribution of these cells,[166] and has served to highlight the regional expression of different antigens and the influence of the local microenvironment.[140] The macrophage is the only haematopoietic derived cell, apart from the mast cell, that takes up residence in tissues. These cells in the adult organism have a ubiquitous distribution, found in large numbers in almost all organs, particularly at potential portals of entry, where they act as the first line of defence against injury and infection.

Studies on the development of the mononuclear phagocyte populations in non-neuronal tissues are few, and little is known about the mechanisms by which monocytes enter tissues in development. There is a large body of evidence on the molecular events involved in leukocyte recruitment to an inflammatory site in the adult.[142] The monocyte is first tethered to the endothelium at the site of inflammation and then binding by integrins, on the surface of the monocyte to ligands on the endothelium, results in firmer attachment and subsequent diapedesis into the tissue. Chemoattractant cytokines, known as chemokines, which are synthesized by tissue macrophages and stromal cells, have a role to play in the specific recruitment and activation of leukocytes at inflammatory sites.[254] There is an increasing body of evidence to implicate chemokines in inflammatory processes in the brain.[323] On the endothelium of the developing embryo, the adhesion molecules that mediate recruitment of monocytes are not known, although observations in the developing rodent brain suggest that they are different from those involved in recruitment to an inflammatory stimulus. The signals that regulate the timing of recruitment during development and the number of cells that will enter a particular tissue are not known. It was suggested that programmed cell death in association with the development of many organs could play a part in driving the recruitment process.[67,296]

In the mouse embryo macrophages first appear in the yolk sac at about E10, rapidly followed by their appearance in the liver, then in the spleen and the differentiating mesenchymal tissues.[260] With the onset of haematopoiesis in the liver, the spleen and subsequently the bone marrow, there is a concomitant rapid increase in the number of macrophages. At E12, macrophages are seen in the connective tissue surrounding the neuroectoderm, and also within the developing nervous system.[260] Since some macrophages/microglia appear in the developing nervous system before haematopoiesis is initiated in the bone marrow, they cannot be bone marrow derived, although they are of the mononuclear phagocyte lineage and originate from the haematopoietic system. In the human embryo, microglia are present within the ventricular and subventricular zones by the ninth week of gestation and invade the cerebrum by the second trimester.[332,333] As in studies on the developing rodent, mononuclear phagocytes first appear in white matter and then migrate into grey matter.[332]

The early appearance of haematopoietic derived cells in the developing brain led to a search for a haematopoietic stem cell in the developing nervous system. The first report of a pluripotential stem cell within the CNS of adult mice[30] was later contested and attributed to blood contamination.[161] Observations that 'microglial progenitor cells' may arise in cultures of either neonatal brain tissue or astroglia again raised the question of the possible presence of a haematopoietic stem cell in the brain.[336] However, neural stem cells may have a differentiation potential that is far greater than previously suspected. This offers an explanation for these apparently contradictory results, since transplantation of genetically labelled neural stem cells into irradiated hosts gives rise not only to myeloid cells, but also to lymphoid and haematopoietic cells.[40] The plasticity of these stem cells is remarkable, but their functional significance within the adult CNS remains unclear.

Function of macrophages and microglia in the developing CNS

Since the first observations by Del Rio-Hortega,[98] it has been repeatedly documented that there are large numbers of macrophages, or amoeboid microglia, within the developing brain. The term amoeboid macrophage is used to describe the rounded macrophages seen in the developing brain prior to their differentiation to the more highly branched adult microglia (Fig. 2.35). It is now well established that, during the development of the CNS, there is a substantial loss of neurons, glia and their processes.[285] The overlap in the timing of this programmed cell death and the invasion of the CNS by cells of the mononuclear phagocyte lineage has aroused interest in the possible role of these phagocytes in CNS development.

The phenomenon of programmed cell death in developing embryos is well known; the cells die by a process called apoptosis.[182] Although programmed cell death has now been well documented in the development of many organs, the molecular mechanisms by which the dying cells are cleared from tissues has only recently been described. It has been shown, for example, that the apoptotic cells in the interdigital regions of the developing mouse footplate are cleared not by neighbouring mesenchymal cells, as was originally thought,[130] but by monocyte-derived macrophages.[163] Similarly, in the developing CNS, macrophages are involved in tissue remodelling. For example, Innocenti[169] showed in the developing forebrain that large numbers of cortical cells send axons across the corpus callosum, which do not survive into adulthood. The axon is eliminated during development without the loss of the parent cell body. At the time that these 'exuberant projections' are disappearing large numbers of macrophages are present in the cortical white matter.[170] Macrophages may be involved in the removal of these axons, although examples of axonal phagocytosis by macrophages are rare. The presence of macrophages in the developing corpus callosum had been documented before the work of Innocenti and colleagues, and the possible relationship of macrophages to sporadic degeneration alluded to,[220] but the significance and magnitude of the numbers of fibres, neurons and glia that degenerate in the developing CNS had not been appreciated, largely because apoptosis is detectable only over a very brief period and is not accompanied by an inflammatory response. It is only with detailed quantitative studies that the widespread loss of axons, neurons and glia from the developing nervous system has been recognized as a major developmental event.[285]

Macrophages and microglia in the clearance of apoptotic neurons and glia

Studies documenting the entry of monocytes into the developing CNS, at about the time of programmed cell death suggest that apoptosis may be a signal driving the recruitment of monocytes.[167,296] In the developing CNS, programmed cell death may drive the migration of an immature microglial population into the parenchyma, whereas rounded macrophages (amoeboid microglia) engulf apoptotic cells.[167] In the developing retina, programmed cell death passes in a wave roughly from the inner retinal layers to the outer layers, and the appearance of macrophages and microglia in the mouse retina apparently follows this gradient. However, macrophages are present in the ganglion cell layer of the retina prior to cell death.[16] Although it is an attractive hypothesis, there is no direct evidence that programmed cell death is the stimulus for the recruitment of macrophages into the developing brain. Indeed, one of the key features of apoptosis is the absence of an accompanying inflammatory response, since apoptotic cells degenerate without liberating their cytoplasmic contents, a possible means by which large numbers of cells could be removed without the potentially harmful effects of an inflammatory response.[358] The recruitment of macrophages at the time of programmed cell death would require the synthesis of a chemoattractant, for example, one of the chemokines released by the apoptotic cells. This appears to be unlikely since the distribution of apoptotic cells and the distribution of macrophages in the forebrain are only partially overlapping.[14] There are both apoptotic cells surrounded by processes of a macrophage, and apoptotic cells unaccompanied by macrophage processes. One approach to investigating the relationship between the mononuclear phagocyte population, their recruitment and distribution, and apoptosis of cells in the developing brain, is to examine the consequences of enhanced, or reduced, cell death on both monocyte recruitment and their differentiation to microglia.

In the developing retina, the invading monocytes follow the wave of cell death across the retina from the ganglion cell layer to the outer plexiform layer, but do not enter the outer nuclear layer, where cell death appears to be relatively rare, at least in rodents.[32] In the rd/rd mutant mouse, the photoreceptors begin to degenerate as the outer segments form,[351] and macrophages now invade the outer nuclear layer in large numbers and phagocytose the

dying cells. It would appear that, as in the developing footpad,[163] if large enough numbers of cells synchronously undergo apoptosis then macrophages are recruited. It is not known whether this is a primary event, due to the generation of chemoattractants by dying cells, or secondary to chemokines released by macrophages phagocytosing large numbers of apoptotic cells. A similar picture is seen in the brain following exposure of embryos to the cytotoxin methylazoxymethanol. Macrophages are recruited to the sites where large numbers of cells undergo apoptosis[15] but, after an initial large increase in macrophage number, the debris is cleared, cells mature into microglia and their density returns close to normal. The territorial arrangement of the microglia, so characteristic of the normal CNS, is maintained.

If macrophages are not recruited to the brain by a chemokine released from the apoptotic cells, how do macrophages recognize neurons and glia undergoing apoptosis? It seems likely that macrophages are opportunistic phagocytes that recognize changes on the surfaces of cells undergoing apoptosis. There are multiple cell surface molecules expressed on dying cells which macrophages recognize, including the vitronectin receptor, the scavenger receptor, CD14 and CD44, to name but a few,[303] but the mechanisms by which dying neurons and glia are recognized are not known.

To investigate whether macrophages play an essential part in tissue remodelling during CNS development, it would be useful to manipulate macrophage populations relatively specifically. This is not a simple matter, but has been done in several circumstances. In transgenic mice overexpressing the murine granulocyte–macrophage colony-stimulating factor (GM-CSF), the number of macrophages within the eye is increased.[91] In these mice, the photoreceptor layer of the retina degenerates coincident with the onset of transgene expression and is correlated with the appearance of large numbers of macrophages expressing the transgene. It is unclear why the animals do not show more widespread defects in other CNS structures, given that macrophages are virtually ubiquitous in the developing CNS. It is possible that the photoreceptors are extremely sensitive to various toxins or insults.

Another approach to manipulating the macrophage population has been to generate transgenic mice in which diphtheria toxin is expressed from a macrophage-specific gene, resulting in the destruction of the macrophage when the gene is activated.[203] In the eyes of these mice, the hyaloid artery and the pupillary membrane are abnormally persistent, suggesting that macrophages are necessary for the removal of these structures. In a further series of experiments, macrophages were eliminated from the anterior chamber of the eye by the injection of toxic liposomes.[103] The data show for the first time that macrophages not only remove the pupillary membrane but actually induce apoptotic cell death in the endothelial cells. Extension of these studies, demonstrating the active participation of the macrophage in inducing cell death during tissue remodelling, to other regions of the CNS, or indeed other tissues, would be of considerable interest.

Thus, it is clear that macrophages play a part in the removal of dying cells and debris from the developing CNS and, in specialized sites, they may actually initiate cell death. The mechanisms by which they recognize apoptotic cells of the CNS are not known. Studies on the eye show that the failure of macrophage recruitment or excessive recruitment in development may result in abnormalities of eye development. Whether the failure of macrophages to clear debris, or excessive phagocyte activity, could result in other abnormalities of CNS development with functional consequences is an interesting possibility. The generation of PU.1 null transgenic mice, which lack mononuclear phagocytes, but can survive into the postnatal period,[232] will allow further investigation of the role of macrophages in CNS development. Details of the organization of fibre tracts and commissural pathways, where macrophages are known to cluster during development, could shed light on the role of these cells in CNS tissue modelling.

Other functions of macrophages in the developing CNS

Not only are macrophages motile and phagocytic cells, but they also have a remarkably diverse secretory repetoire.[270,324] Molecules secreted by activated macrophages are involved in functions such as the killing of micro-organisms, tissue remodelling and wound repair. Thus, it is possible that macrophages are involved in aspects of CNS development other than the removal of apoptotic cells, but there is surprisingly little information on the secretory products of macrophages in the developing brain. *In vitro*, immature microglia secrete many different molecules, including interleukin-1 (IL-1),[135] NGF,[242] IL-3,[128] IL-6,[121] elastase,[268] and plasminogen activator.[269] However, culture conditions do not represent the microenvironment of the brain, and although demonstrating that the macrophages and immature microglia have the potential to secrete cytokines, they provide little information about the complex regulation of such macrophage-derived molecules in the developing CNS.

MICROGLIA IN ADULT CNS

Normal function of microglia

While there has been extensive analysis of the cell surface antigen expression of resting microglia, evidence that they secrete molecules that may influence neurons, astrocytes or the cerebral endothelium is lacking.

Given the downregulated phenotype of microglia within the adult CNS, it is hard to imagine what their function may be. Do they contribute to homoeostasis in the CNS, as macrophages do in other tissues? Are they waiting for something to happen: the first line of defence of the CNS? The only homoeostatic function so far described in the normal adult CNS is that of pruning the

terminal arbors of magnocellular axons in the neural lobe.[307] The evidence suggests that these cells phagocytose the endings of magnocellular neurons that have penetrated the capillary bed in the neural lobe. It is not clear whether microglia at other sites play a role in synaptic remodelling but, given the sparseness of their processes relative to synaptic density, it seems unlikely. In the aged nervous system, microglia have a more upregulated phenotype[297,369] and contain large amounts of debris, indicating maintenance of their phagocytic role.

MICROGLIA ACTIVATION IN PATHOLOGY

A remarkable feature of microglia is their very rapid and robust response to almost any type of disturbance of CNS homoeostasis or neuronal injury.[198,224,291] Their activation, revealed by the enhanced or *de novo* expression of particular antigens and altered morphology, is often the very first indicator that there is some form of deviation from normality in the CNS. The differential microglial response to different pathological states in the CNS has been extensively reviewed elsewhere,[198,291,294] but a number of important distinctions must be made. The activation of microglia is an important indicator that host defence mechanisms against tissue injury or infection have been awakened. In keeping with the tenets of Metchnikoff[253] that inflammation is the activation or delivery of phagocytes to the site of a tissue injury, it is valuable to consider the differential inflammatory responses of these different pathologies. In particular, it is important to distinguish between innate and acquired inflammatory responses, and responses that are acute and chronic.

Activation of microglia

The reaction of microglia to a particular brain injury is a graded rather than an all-or-nothing response. The more severe the injury, the greater the activation and de-differentiation of microglia from the resting state. The graded response of microglia has been studied in particular detail by Kreutzberg, using the facial nerve model.[198] Transection of the facial nerve results in a retrograde response in the neurons of the facial nucleus. In the absence of both neuronal degeneration and damage to the BBB, microglia become activated, proliferate, upregulate a number of cell surface antigens, including MHC antigens,[389] and synthesize several cytokines, including IL-6 and transforming growth factor-β (TGF-β).[392] If the neurons of the facial nerve are induced to undergo retrograde degeneration by the retrograde transport of *Ricinus communis*, then the microglia will undergo further de-differentiation, and become rounded phagocytic cells.[391] The experiments in this system suggest that, while the neuropil remains intact, aspects of the microglial morphology will be retained but, the more degenerated or disrupted the tissue, the more microglia are released from local microenvironmental influences, and the more they de-differentiate to become typical macrophages.

Although there are now numerous descriptions of microglial activation in this model and its variants, remarkably little is known about the signals that pass from the injured neuron to the microglia. The proliferation of microglia in this model appears to be driven largely by the cytokine macrophage colony-stimulating factor (M-CSF). In the op/op mouse, which lacks functional M-CSF protein, the proliferation of microglia in the facial nucleus does not take place after facial nerve axotomy.[317]

The retrograde response of the motor neurons of the facial nucleus is accompanied by loss of synaptic input onto the cell body and dendrites. This phenomenon is associated with microglial proliferation, leading to the suggestion that the microglia may be actively involved in the removal of the synapses, known as synaptic stripping.[198] This attractive idea would be consistent with microglia playing a protective role after nerve injury. However, recent evidence, in which microglial proliferation in the hypoglossal nucleus was blocked by intrathecal delivery of cytosine arabinoside, suggests that microglia are not essential for either synaptic stripping or the successful regeneration of the motor neuron axons.[395] The role of the microglia in this model remains enigmatic. The functions of activated microglia in CNS injury and disease are discussed in Chapter 3 of this volume.

In summary, microglia are the resident macrophages of the brain parenchyma. They are derived from mononuclear phagocyte precursors that enter the embryonic brain during the period of developmental cell death. Immature microglia phagocytose clear apoptotic cells before they mature to form a stable long-lived population of cells in the brain parenchyma. It is not known what determines the proportions of microglia in different regions of the brain, but developmental abnormalities are very unlikely to be reflected in activated or an atypical microglia distribution in later life.

In the adult brain, microglia are ubiquitous and are characterized by their highly differentiated morphology, regular distribution and downregulated phenotype. Changes in morphology and increases in expression of cell-surface or cytoplasmic antigens characterize the activated microglia. Microglial activation accompanies all forms of CNS injury and disease and is often the first evidence of a homoeostatic disturbance. Careful characterization of the phenotype of these cells in the developing and adult brain, and in different disease states, will further our understanding of the role of these cells in the normal and diseased CNS.

REFERENCES

1 Akopian G, Kuprijanova E, Kressin K, Steinhäuser C. Analysis of ion channel expression by astrocytes in red nucleus brain stem slices of the rat. *Glia* 1997; **19**: 234–46.

2 Allen DJ. Scanning EM of epiplexus macrophages (Kolmer cells) in the dog. *J Comp Neurol* 1975; **161**: 197–214.

3 Altman J, Bayer SA. Development of the diencephalon in the rat. I. Autoradiographic study of the time of origin and setting patterns of neurons of the hypothalamus. *J Comp Neurol* 1978; **182**: 945–72.

4 Altman J, Bayer SA. Development of the diencephalon in the rat. III. Ontogeny of the specialized ventricular linings of the hypothalamic third ventricle. *J Comp Neurol* 1978; **182**: 995–1016.

5 Amaducci L, Pazzaglia A, Pessina G. The relation of proteolipids and phosphatides to tissue elements in the bovine nervous system. *J Neurochem* 1962; **9**: 509–18.

6 Anton ES, Marchionni MA, Rakic P. Role of GGF/neuregulin signalling in interactions between migrating neurons and radial glia in the developing cerebral cortex. *Development* 1997; **124**: 3501–10.

7 Aoki C. Beta-adrenergic receptors: astrocytic localization in the adult visual cortex and their relation to catecholaminergic axon terminals as revealed by electron microscopic immunocytochemistry. *J Neurosci* 1992; **12**: 781–92.

8 Aoki C, Joh TH, Pickel VM. Ultrastructural localization of beta-adrenergic receptor-like immunoreactivity in the cortex and neostriatum of rat brain. *Brain Res* 1987; **437**: 264–82.

9 Aoki C, Lubin M, Fenstemaker S. Columnar activity regulated astrocytic beta-adrenergic receptor-like immunoreactivity in VI of adult monkeys. *Neuroscience* 1994; **11**: 179–87.

10 Aoki C, Venkatesan C, Go CG et al. Cellular and subcellular localization of NMDA-R1 subunit immunoreactivity in the visual cortex of adult and neonatal rats. *J Neurosci* 1994; **14**: 5202–22.

11 Arakawa Y, Sendtner M, Thoenen H. Survival effect of ciliary neurotrophic factor (CNTF) on chick embryonic motoneurons in culture: comparison with other neurotrophic factors and cytokines. *J Neurosci* 1990; **10**: 3507–15.

12 Araque A, Sanzgiri RP, Parpura V, Haydon PG. Astrocyte-induced modulation of synaptic transmission. *Can J Physiol Pharmacol* 1999; **77**: 699–706.

13 Ashur-Fabian O, Giladi E, Brenneman DE, Gozes I. Identification of VIP/PACAP receptors on rat astrocytes using antisense oligodeoxynucleotides. *J Molec Neurosci* 1998; **9**: 211–22.

14 Ashwell KWS. The distribution of microglia and cell death in the fetal rat forebrain. *Brain Res Dev Brain Res* 1991; **58**: 1–12.

15 Ashwell KWS. The effects of prenatal exposure to methylazoxymethanol acetate on microglia. *Neuropathol Appl Neurobiol* 1992; **18**: 610–18.

16 Ashwell KWS, Hollander H, Streit W, Stone J. The appearance and distribution of microglia in the developing retina of the rat. *Vis Neurosci* 1989; **2**: 437–48.

17 Autillo-Touati A, Chamak B, Araud D et al. Region-specific neuro-astroglial interactions: ultrastructural study of the *in vitro* expression of neuronal polarity. *J Neurosci* 1988; **19**: 326–42.

18 Baird A. Fibroblast growth factors: activities and significance of non-neurotrophin neurotrophic factors. *Curr Opin Neurobiol* 1994; **4**: 78–86.

19 Banati R, Hoppe D, Gottmann K et al. A subpopulation of bone marrow derived macrophages share a unique ion channel pattern with microglia. *J Neurosci Res* 1991; **30**: 593–600.

20 Bansal R, Kumar M, Murray K et al. Regulation of FGF receptors in the oligodendrocyte lineage. *Mol Cell Neurosci* 1996; **7**: 263–75.

21 Barker PA. p75[NTR]: a study in contrasts. *Cell Death Diff* 1998; **5**: 346–56.

22 Barres BA, Chun LLY, Corey DP. Ion channels in vertebrate glia. *Annu Rev Neurosci* 1990; **13**: 441–74.

23 Barres BA, Hart IK, Coles HSR et al. Cell death and control of cell survival in the oligodendrocyte lineage. Cell 1992; 70: 31–46.

24 Barres BA, Koroshetz WJ, Swartz KJ et al. Ion channel expression by white matter glia: the O2A glial progenitor cell. Neuron 1990; 4: 507–24.

25 Barres BA, Lazar MA, Raff MC. A novel role for thyroid hormone, glucocorticoids, and retinoic acid in timing oligodendrocyte development. Development 1994; 120: 1097–1108.

26 Barres BA, Raff MC. Control of oligodendrocyte number in the developing rat optic nerve. Neuron 1994; 12: 935–42.

27 Barres BA, Raff MC. Proliferation of oligodendrocyte precursor cells depends on electrical activity in axons. Nature 1993; 361: 258–60.

28 Barres BA, Raff MC, Gaese F et al. A crucial role for neurotrophin-3 in oligodendrocyte development. Nature 1994; 356: 371–5.

29 Barres BA, Schmidt R, Sendtner M, Raff MC. Multiple extracellular signals are required for long-term oligodendrocyte survival. Development 1993; 118: 283–95.

30 Bartlett PF. Pluripotential hemopoietic stem cells in adult mouse brain. Proc Natl Acad Sci USA 1982; 82: 2722–5.

31 Bartlett WP, Li XS, Williams M, Benkovic S. Localization of insulin-like growth factor-1 mRNA in murine central nervous system during postnatal development. Dev Biol 1991; 147: 239–50.

32 Beazley LD, Perry VH, Baker B, Darby J. An investigation into the role of ganglion cells in the regulation of division and death of other retinal cells. Brain Res Dev Brain Res 1987; 33: 169–84.

33 Bell MD, Lopez-Gonzalez R, Lawson L et al. Upregulation of the macrophage scavenger receptor in response to different forms of injury in the CNS. J Neurocytol 1994; 23: 605–13.

34 Bergles DE, Roberts JDB, Somogyl P, Jahr CE. Glutamatergic synapses on oligodendrocyte precursor cells in the hippocampus. Nature 2000; 405: 187–91.

35 Berry M, Hunter AS, Duncan A et al. Axon–glial relations during regeneration of axons in the adult rat anterior medullary velum. J Neurocytol 1998; 27: 915–37.

36 Berry M, Ibrahim M, Carlile J et al. Axon glial relations in the anterior medullary velum of the adult rat. J Neurocytol 1995; 24: 965–83.

37 Bertolotto A, Rocca G, Schiffer D. Chondoitin 4-sulphate proteoglycan forms an extracellular network in human and rat central nervous system. J Neurol Sci 1990; 100: 113–23.

38 Bignami A, Dahl D. The astroglial response to stabbing. Immunofluorescence studies with antibodies to astrocyte-specific protein (GFP) in mammalian and submammalian vertebrates. Neuropath Appl Neurobiol 1976; 2: 99–110.

39 Bjartmar C, Hildebrand C, Loinder K. Morphological heterogeneity of rat oligodendrocytes: electron microscopic studies on serial sections. Glia 1994; 11: 235–44.

40 Bjornson CRR, Rietze RL, Reynolds BA et al. Turning brain into blood: a hematopoietic fate adopted by adult neural stem cells in vivo. Science 1999; 283: 534–7.

41 Black JA, Firedman B, Waxman SG et al. Immuno-ultrastructural localisation of sodium channels at nodes of Ranvier and perinodal astrocyte processes in the rat optic nerve. Proc R Soc Lond Ser B 1989; 238: 39–51.

42 Black JA, Waxman SG, Friedman B et al. Sodium channels in astrocytes of rat optic nerve in situ: immunoelectron microscopic studies. Glia 1989; 2: 353–69.

43 Black JA, Westenbroek R, Ransom BR et al. Type II sodium channels in spinal cord astrocytes in situ: immunocytochemical observations. Glia 1994; 12: 219–27.

44 Blakemore WF, Murray JA. Quantitative examination of internodal length of myelinated fibres in the central nervous system. J Neurol Sci 1981; 49: 273–84.

45 Bleier R. Ultrastructure of supraependymal cells and ependyma of the hypothalamic third ventricle of mouse. J Comp Neurol 1977; 174: 359–76.

46 Bögler O, Wren D, Barnett SC et al. Cooperation between two growth factors promotes extended self-renewal and inhibits differentiation of oligodendrocyte-type-2 astrocyte (O-2A) progenitor cells. Proc Natl Acad Sci USA 1990; 87: 6368–72.

47 Bonni A, Sun Y, Nadal-Vicens M et al. Regulation of gliogenesis in the central nervous system by the JAK-STAT signalling pathway. Science 1995; 278: 477–82.

48 Borden LA, Smith KE, Gustafson EL et al. Cloning and expression of a betaine/GABA transporter from human brain. J Neurochem 1995; 64: 977–84.

49 Borden LA, Smith KE, Hartig PR et al. Molecular heterogeneity of the GABA transporter system: cloning of two novel high affinity transporters from rat brain. J Biol Chem 1992; 267: 21098–104.

50 Bordey A, Sontheimer H. Postnatal development of ionic currents in rat hippocampal astrocytes in situ. J Neurophysiol 1997; 78: 461–77.

51 Bradbury MWB. Anatomy and physiology of cerebrospinal fluid. In: Schur AH, Bokley CE eds. Hydrocephalus. Oxford: Oxford University Press, 1993: 19–47.

52 Braun JS, Kaisling B, Le Hir M. Cellular components of the immune barrier in the spinal meninges and dorsal root ganglia of the rat: immunohistochemical (MHC class II) and electron microscopic observations. Cell Tissue Res 1993; 273: 209–17.

53 Brightman MW, Palay SC. The fine structure of ependyma in the brain. J Cell Biol 1963; 19: 415–39.

54 Bringmann A, Francke M, Pannicke T et al. Role of glial K$^+$ channels in ontogeny and gliosis: a hypothesis based upon studies on Müller cells. Glia 2000; 29: 35–44.

55 Brockhaus J, Ilschner S, Banati RB, Kettenmann H. Membrane properties of amoeboid microglia cells in the corpus callosum from early postnatal mice. J Neurosci 1994; 13: 4412–21.

56 Brophy PJ, Boccaccio GL, Colman DR. The distribution of myelin basic protein mRNAs within myelinating oligodendrocytes. Trends Neurosci 1993; 16: 515–21.

57 Brown HC, Townsend MJ, Fearn S, Perry VH. An adhesion molecule for macrophages in the brain. J Neurocytol 1998; 27: 867–76.

58 Bruni JE. Ependymal development, proliferation, and functions: a review. Microsc Res Tech 1998; 41: 2–13.

59 Bruni JE, del Bigio MR, Chattenburg RE. Ependyma: normal and pathological. A review of the literature. Brain Res Rev 1985; 9: 1–19.

60 Bunge RP. Glial cells and the central myelin sheath. Physiol Rev 1968; 48: 197–251.

61 Burne JF, Staple JK, Raff MC. Glial cells are increased proportionally in transgenic optic nerves with increased numbers of axons. J Neurosci 1996; 7: 2469–72.

62 Butt AM. Macroglial cell types, lineage, and morphology in the CNS. Ann N Y Acad Sci 1991; 633: 90–5.

63 Butt AM, Berry M. Oligodendrocytes and the control of myelination in vivo: new insights from the rat anterior medullary velum. J Neurosci Res 2000; 59: 477–88.

64 Butt AM, Colquhoun K, Berry M. Confocal imaging of glial cells in the intact rat optic nerve. Glia 1994; 10: 315–22.

65 Butt AM, Colquhoun K, Tutton M, Berry M. Three dimensional morphology of astrocytes and oligodendrocytes in the intact mouse optic nerve. J Neurocytol 1994; 23: 469–85.

66 Butt AM, Duncan A, Berry M. Astrocyte associations with nodes of Ranvier: ultrastructural analysis of HRP–filled astrocytes in the mouse optic nerve. *J Neurocytol* 1994; **23**: 486–99.

67 Butt AM, Duncan A, Hornby MF *et al*. Cells expressing the NG2 antigen contact nodes of Ranvier in adult CNS white matter. *Glia* 1999; **26**: 84–91.

68 Butt AM, Hornby MF, Ibrahim M *et al*. PDGF-α receptor and myelin basic protein mRNAs are not coexpressed by oligodendrocytes *in vivo*: a double *in situ* hybridization study in the anterior medullary velum of the neonatal rat. *Mol Cell Neurosci* 1997; **8**: 311–22.

69 Butt AM, Hornby, MF, Kirvell S, Berry M. Platelet-derived growth factor delays oligodendrocyte differentiation and axonal myelination *in vivo* in the anterior medullary velum of the developing rat. *J Neurosci Res* 1997; **48**: 588–96.

70 Butt AM, Ibrahim M, Berry M. Axon–myelin sheath relations of oligodendrocyte unit phenotypes in the adult rat anterior medullary velum. *J Neurocytol* 1998; **27**: 259–69.

71 Butt AM, Ibrahim M, Berry M. The relationship between developing oligodendrocyte units and maturing axons during myelinogenesis in the anterior medullary velum of neonatal rats. *J Neurocytol* 1997; **26**: 327–38.

72 Butt AM, Ibrahim M, Gregson N, Berry M. Differential expression of the L- and S-isoforms of myelin associated glycoprotein (MAG) in oligodendrocyte unit phenotypes in the adult rat anterior medullary velum. *J Neurocytol* 1998; **27**: 271–80.

73 Butt AM, Ibrahim M, Ruge FM, Berry M. Biochemical subtypes of oligodendrocytes in the anterior medullary velum of the rat as revealed by the monoclonal antibody RIP. *Glia* 1995; **14**: 185–97.

74 Butt AM, Ransom BR. Morphology of astrocytes and oligodendrocytes during development in the intact rat optic nerve. *J Comp Neurol* 1993; **338**: 141–58.

75 Butt AM, Ransom BR. Visualization of oligodendrocytes and astrocytes in the intact rat optic nerve by intracellular injection of Lucifer Yellow and horse radish peroxidase. *Glia* 1989; **2**: 470–5.

76 Calver AR, Hall AC, Yu W-P *et al*. Oligodendrocyte population dynamics and the role of PDGF *in vivo*. *Neuron* 1998; **20**: 869–82.

77 Cameron RS, Rakic P. Identification of membrane proteins that comprise the plasmalemmal junction between migrating neurons and radial glial cells. *J Neurosci* 1994; **14**: 3139–55.

78 Campagnoni AT. Molecular biology of myelination. In: Kettenmann H, Ransom BR eds. *Neuroglial cells*. Oxford: Oxford University Press, 1995: 555–70.

79 Carson JH, Worboys K, Ainger K, Barbarese E. Translocation of myelin basic protein mRNA in oligodendrocytes requires microtubules and kinesin. *Cell Motil Cytoskeleton* 1997; **38**: 318–28.

80 Chamak B, Fellous A, Glowinski J, Prochiantz A. MAP2 expression and neuritic outgrowth and branching are co-regulated through region-specific neuro-astroglial interactions. *J Neurosci* 1987; **7**: 3163–70.

81 Chang A, Nishiyama A, Peterson J *et al*. NG2-positive oligodendrocyte progenitor cells in adult human brain and multiple sclerosis lesions. *J Neurosci* 2000; **20**: 6404–12.

82 Chao TI, Skachkov SN, Eberhardt W, Reichenbach, A. Na⁺ channels of Müller (glial) cells isolated from retinae of various mammalian species including man. *Glia* 1994; **10**: 173–85.

83 Chekenya M, Rooprai HK, Davies D *et al*. The NG2 chondroitin sulfate proteoglycan: role in malignant progression of human brain tumours. *Int J Dev Neurosci* 1999; **17**: 421–35.

84 Chiang YH, Silani V, Zhou FC. Morphological differentiation of astroglial progenitor cells from EGF-responsive neurospheres in response to fetal calf serum, basic fibroblast growth factor, and retinol. *Cell Transplant* 1996; **5**: 179–89.

85 Conti F, Debiasi S, Minelli A *et al*. EAACl, a high-affinity glutamate transporter, is localised to astrocytes and GABAergic neurons besides pyramidal cells in the rat cerebral cortex. *Cereb Cortex* 1998; **8**: 108–16.

86 Conti F, Minelli A, Brecha NC. Cellular localization and laminar distribution of AMPA glutamate receptor subunits mRNAs and proteins in the rat cerebral cortex. *J Comp Neurol* 1994; **350**: 241–59.

87 Cornell-Bell AH, Finkheimer SM. Ca²⁺ waves in astrocytes. *Cell Calcium* 1991; **12**: 185–204.

88 Cornell-Bell AH, Finkbeiner SM, Cooper MS, Smith SJ. Glutamate induces calcium waves in cultured astrocytes: long–range glial signalling. *Science* 1990; **247**: 470–3.

89 Corvalan V, Cole R, deVellis J, Hagawara S. Neuronal modulation of calcium channel activity in cultured rat astrocytes. *Proc Natl Acad Sci USA* 1990; **87**: 4345–8.

90 Curtis R, Cohen J, Fok–Seang J *et al*. Development of macroglial cells in rat cerebellum. I. Use of antibodies to follow early *in vivo* development and migration of oligodendrocytes. *J Neurocytol* 1988; **17**: 43–54.

91 Cuthbertson RA, Lang RA. Developmental ocular disease in GM–CSF transgenic mice is mediated by autostimulated macrophage. *Dev Biol* 1989; **134**: 119–29.

92 Dani JW, Cherujavsky A, Smith SJ. Neuronal activity triggers calcium waves in hippocampal astrocyte networks. *Neuron* 1992; **8**: 429–40.

93 Das GD. Gliogenesis and ependymogenesis during embryonic development of the rat. *J Neurol Sci* 1979; **43**: 193–204.

94 Day NC, Williams TL, Ince PG *et al*. Distribution of AMPA-selective glutamate receptor subtypes in the human hippocampus and cerebellum. *Brain Res Molec Brain Res* 1995; **31**: 17–32.

95 De Biasi S, Vitellaro-Zuccarello L, Brecha NC. Immunoreactivity for the GABA transporter-1 and GABA transporter-3 is restricted to astrocytes in the rat thalamus. A light and electron-microscopic immunolocalization. *Neuroscience* 1998; **83**: 815–28.

96 De Groot CJ, Huppes W, Sminia T *et al*. Determination of the origin and nature of brain macrophages and microglia cells in mouse central nervous system, using non-radioactive *in situ* hybridisation and immunoperoxidase techniques. *Glia* 1992; **6**: 301–9.

97 Del Bigio MR. The ependyma: a protective barrier between brain and cerebrospinal fluid. *Glia* 1995; **14**: 1–13.

98 Del Rio-Hortega P. Microglia. In: Penfield W ed. *Cytology and cellular pathology of the nervous system*. New York: Hoeber PB, 1932: 482–534.

99 Del Rio-Hortega P. Tercera apotación al conocimiento morfologica e interpretacion funcional de la oligodendroglia. *Mem Real Soc Soc Española Hist Nat Madrid* 1928; **14**: 5–122.

100 Denis-Donini S, Glowinski J, Prochiantz A. Glial heterogeneity may define the three-dimensional shape of mouse mesencephalic dopaminergic neurones. *Nature* 1984; **307**: 641–3.

101 Dermietzel R, Spray DC. Gap junctions in the brain: where, what type, how many and why? *Trends Neurosci* 1993; **16**: 186–92.

102 Dermietzel R, Traub O, Hwang TK *et al*. Differential expression of three gap junction proteins in developing and mature brain tissue. *Proc Natl Acad Sci USA* 1989; **86**: 10148–52.

103 Diez-Roux G, Lang RA. Macrophages induce apoptosis in normal cells *in vivo*. *Development* 1997; **124**: 3633–8.

104 Dijkstra CD, Dopp EA, Joling P, Krall G. The heterogeneity of mononuclear phagocytes in the lymphoid organs: distinct macrophage subpopulations in the rat recognized by monoclonal antibodies ED1, ED2 and ED3. *Immunology* 1985; **54**: 589–99.

105 Dijkstra S, Bär PR, Gispen WH, Joosten EAJ. Selective stimulation of dendritic outgrowth from identified cortical neurons by homotopic astrocytes. *Neuroscience* 1999; **92**: 1331–42.

106 Doherty P, Walsh FS. CAM-FGF receptor interactions: a model for axonal growth. *Mol Cell Neurosci* 1996; **8**: 99–111.

107 Duffy S, Fraser DD, MacVicar BA. Potassium channels. In: Kettenmann H, Ransom BE eds. *Neuroglia*. Oxford: Oxford University Press, 1995: 185–201.

108 Durkin MM, Smith KE, Borden LA *et al*. Localization of messenger RNAs encoding three GABA transporters in rat brain: an *in situ* hybridization study. *Brain Res Mol Brain Res* 1995; **33**: 7–21.

109 Dziegielewska KM, Knott GW, Saunders NR. The nature and composition of the internal environment of the developing brain. *Cell Mol Neurobiol* 2000; **20**: 41–56.

110 Edwards FA, Konnerth A, Sakmann B, Takahishi T. A thin slice preparation for patch-clamp recordings from neurones of the mammalian central nervous system. *Pflügers Arch* 1989; **414**: 600–12.

111 Edwards MA, Yamamoto M, Caviness VS. Organization of radial glial and related cells in the developing murine CNS: an analysis based upon a new monoclonal antibody marker. *Neuroscience* 1990; **36**: 121–44.

112 Ellison J, de Vellis J. Platelet derived growth factor receptor is expressed by cells in the early oligodendrocyte lineage. *J Neurosci Res* 1994; **37**: 116–28.

113 Ellison JA, de Vellis J. Amoeboid microglia expressing GD3 ganglioside are concentrated in regions of oligodendrogenesis during development of the rat corpus callosum. *Glia* 1995; **14**: 123–32.

114 Fanarraga ML, Griffiths IR, Zhao M, Duncan ID. Oligodendrocytes are not inherently programmed to myelinate a specific size of axon. *J Comp Neurol* 1998; **399**: 94–100.

115 Feng L, Hatten ME, Heintz N. Brain lipid-binding protein (BLBP): a novel signalling system in the developing mammalian CNS. *Neuron* 1994; **12**: 895–908.

116 Feng L, Heintz N. Differentiating neurons activate transcription of the brain lipid-binding protein gene in radial glial through a novel regulatory element. *Development* 1995; **121**: 1719–30.

117 ffrench-Constant C, Miller, RH, Hruse J *et al*. Molecular specialisation of astrocyte processes at nodes of Ranvier in the rat optic nerve. *J Cell Biol* 1986; **102**: 844–52.

118 ffrench-Constant C, Raff MC. The oligodendrocyte-type-2 astrocyte cell lineage is specialized for myelination. *Nature* 1986; **323**: 335–8.

119 Fidler PS, Schutte K, Asher RA *et al*. Comparing astrocytic cell lines that are inhibitory or permissive for cell growth: the major axon-inhibitory proteoglycan is NG2. *J Neurosci* 1999; **19**: 8778–88.

120 Flament-Durand J, Brion JP. Tanycytes: morphology and functions. A review. *Int Rev Cytol* 1985; **96**: 121–55.

121 Frei K, Malipiero UV, Leist TP *et al*. On the cellular source and function of interleukin 6 produced in the central nervous system in viral diseases. *Eur J Immunol* 1989; **19**: 689–94.

122 Friedman B, Hockfield S, Black JA *et al*. *In situ* demonstration of mature oligodendrocytes and their processes: an immunocytochemical study with a new monoclonal antibody, Rip. *Glia* 1989; **2**: 380–90.

123 Friedman WJ, Black IB, Kaplan DR. Distribution of the neurotrophins brain-derived neurotrophic factor, neurotrophin-3, and neurotrophin-4/5 in the postnatal brain: an immunocytochemical study. *Neuroscience* 1998; **84**: 101–14.

124 Fulton BP, Burne JF, Raff MC. Visualization of O-2A progenitor cells in developing and adult rat optic nerve by quisqualate-stimulated cobalt uptake. *J Neurosci* 1992; **12**: 4816–33.

125 Furuta A, Rothstein JD, Martin LJ. Glutamate transporter protein subtypes are expressed differentially during rat central nervous system development. *J Neurosci* 1997; **17**: 8363–75.

126 Gadisseux JF, Evard PH, Misson JP, Caviness VS. Dynamic changes in the density of radial glial fibers of the developing murine cerebral wall: a quantitative immunohistological analysis. *J Comp Neurol* 1992; **322**: 246–54.

127 Gage FH, Ray J, Fisher LJ. Isolation, characterization and use of stem cells from the CNS. *Neuroscience* 1995; **18**: 159–62.

128 Ganter S, Northoff H, Mannel D, Gebicke-Haerter PJ. Growth control of cultured microglia. *J Neurosci Res* 1992; **33**: 218–30.

129 Garberg P. *In vitro* models of the blood–brain barrier. *ATLA* 1998; **26**: 821–47.

130 Garcia-Martinez V, Macias D, Ganan Y *et al*. Internucleosomal DNA fragmentation and programmed cell death (apoptosis) in the interdigital tissue of the embryonic chick leg bud. *J Cell Sci* 1993; **106**: 201–8.

131 Gard AL, Pfeiffer SE. Glial cell mitogens bFGF and PDGF differentially regulate development of O4+Galc− oligodendrocyte progenitors. *Dev Biol* 1993; **159**: 618–30.

132 Gard AL, Pfeiffer SE. Oligodendrocyte progenitors isolated directly from developing telencephalon at a specific phenotypic stage: myelinogenic potential in a defined environment. *Development* 1989; **106**: 119–32.

133 Gard AL, Pfeiffer SE. Two proliferative stages of oligodendrocyte lineage (A2B5+O4− and O4+GalC−) under different mitogenic control. *Neuron* 1990; **5**: 615–25.

134 Gerard C, Langlois J, Gingrich J *et al*. Production and characterization of polyclonal antibodies recognizing the intracytoplasmic loop of the 5-hydroxytryptamine (1A) receptor. *Neuroscience* 1994; **62**: 721–39.

135 Giulian D, Young DG, Woodward J *et al*. Interleukin-1 is an astroglial growth factor in the developing brain. *J Neurosci* 1988; **8**: 709–14.

136 Gledhill RF, McDonald WI. Morphological characteristics of central demyelination and remyelination, a single fibre study. *Ann Neurol* 1977; **1**: 552–6.

137 Goddard DR, Berry M, Butt AM. *In vivo* actions of fibroblast growth factor-2 and insulin like growth factor-I on oligodendrocyte development and myelination in the central nervous system. *J Neurosci Res* 1999; **57**: 74–85.

138 Goldman JE. Regulation of oligodendrocyte differentiation. *Trends Neurosci* 1992; **15**: 359–62.

139 Gonzalez AM, Berry M, Maher PA *et al*. A comprehensive analysis of the distribution of FGF-2 and FGFR1 in the rat brain. *Brain Res* 1995; **701**: 201–26.

140 Gordon S, Lawson L, Rabinowitz S *et al*. Antigen markers of macrophage differentiation in murine tissues. *Curr Top Microbiol Immunol* 1992; **181**: 1–37.

141 Graeber MB, Streit WJ, Kreutzberg GW. Identity of ED2-positive perivascular cells in rat brain. *J Neurosci Res* 1989; **2**: 103–6.

142 Granger DN, Kubes P. The microcirculation and inflammation: modulation of leucocyte–endothelial cell adhesion. *J Leukoc Biol* 1994; **55**: 662–75.

143 Griffiths IR, Klugman M, Anderson TJ et al. Current concepts of PLP and its role in the nervous system. Microsc Res Tech 1998; 41: 344–58.

144 Gross RE, Mehler MF, Mabie PC et al. Bone morphogenic proteins promote astroglial lineage commitment by mammalian subventricular zone progenitor cells. Neuron 1996; 17: 595–606.

145 Guastella J, Nelson N, Nelson H et al. Cloning and expression of a rat brain GABA transporter. Science 1990; 249: 1303–6.

146 Hagg T, Quon D, Higaki J, Varon S. Ciliary neurotrophic factor prevents neuronal degeneration and promotes low affinity NGF receptor expression in the adult rat CNS. Neuron 1992; 8: 145–58.

147 Hagg T, Varon S. Ciliary neurotrophic factor prevents degeneration of adult rat substantia nigra dopaminergic neurons in vivo. Proc Natl Acad Sci USA 1993; 90: 6315–19.

148 Hardy R, Reynolds R. Neuron–oligodendroglial interactions during central nervous system development. J Neurosci Res 1993; 36: 121–6.

149 Hardy R, Reynolds R. Proliferation and differentiation potential of rat forebrain oligodendroglial progenitors both in vitro and in vivo. Development 1991; 111: 1061–80.

150 Hardy RJ, Friedrich VL. Progressive remodelling of the oligodendrocyte process arbor during myelinogenesis. Dev Neurosci 1996; 18: 243–54.

151 Hartman BK, Agrawal CH, Agrawal D, Kalmbach S. Development and maturation of central nervous system myelin: comparison of immunohistochemical localisation of proteolipid protein and basic protein in myelin and oligodendrocytes. Proc Natl Acad Sci USA 1982; 79: 4217–20.

152 Hatten ME, Lynch M, Rydel RE et al. In vitro neurite extension by granule neurons is dependent upon astroglial derived fibroblast growth factor. Dev Biol 1988; 125: 280–9.

153 Hickey WF, Kimura H. Perivascular microglia are bone marrow derived and present antigen in vivo. Science 1988; 239: 290–2.

154 Hickey WF, Vass K, Lassmann H. Bone marrow derived elements in the central nervous system: an immunohistochemical and ultrastructural analysis of rat chimera. J Neuropathol Exp Neurol 1992; 51: 246–56.

155 Hildebrand C, Hahn R. Relation between myelin sheath thickness and axon size in spinal cord white matter of some vertebrate species. J Neurol Sci 1978; 38: 421–34.

156 Hildebrand C, Remahl S, Persson H, Bjartmar C. Myelinated nerve fibres in the CNS. Prog Neurobiol 1993; 40: 319–84.

157 Hildebrand C, Waxman SG. Postnatal differentiation of rat optic nerve fibres: electron microscopic observations on the development of nodes of Ranvier and axoglial relations. J Comp Neurol 1984; 224: 25–37.

158 Hirano A. A confirmation of oligodendroglial origin of myelin in the adult rat. J Cell Biol 1968; 38: 637–40.

159 Hockfield S, McKay RDG. Identification of major classes in the developing brain. J Neurosci 1985; 5: 3310–28.

160 Holash JA, Noden DM, Stewart PA. Re-evaluating the role of astrocytes in blood–brain barrier induction. Dev Dyn 1993; 197: 14–25.

161 Hoogerbrugge PM, Wagemaker G, van Bekkum DW. Failure to demonstrate pluripotential hemopoietic stem cells in mouse brains. Proc Natl Acad Sci USA 1985; 82: 4268–9.

162 Hopewell JW. The subependymal plate and the genesis of gliomas. J Pathol 1975; 117: 101–3.

163 Hopkinson-Woolley J, Hughes D, Gordon S, Martin P. Macrophage recruitment during limb development and wound healing in the embryonic and foetal mouse. J Cell Sci 1994; 107: 1159–67.

164 Hudgins SN, Levison SW. Ciliary neurotrophic factor stimulates astroglial hypertrophy in vivo and in vitro. Exp Neurol 1998; 150: 171–82.

165 Hughes SM, Lillien LE, Raff MC et al. Ciliary neurotrophic factor induces type-2 astrocyte differentiation in culture. Nature 1988; 335: 70–3.

166 Hume DA, Gordon S. The mononuclear phagocyte system of the mouse defined by the immunohistochemical localization of antigen F4/80. In: Van Furth R ed. Mononuclear phagocytes: characteristics, physiology and function. Dordrecht: Martinus Nijhoff, 1985: 9–17.

167 Hume DA, Perry VH, Gordon S. Immunohistochemical localization of macrophage-specific antigen in developing mouse retina: phagocytosis of dying neurons and differentiation of microglia cells to form a regular array in the plexiform layers. J Cell Biol 1983; 97: 253–7.

168 Ibrahim M, Butt AM, Berry M. The relationship between myelin sheath diameter and internodal length in the anterior medullary velum of the rat. J Neurol Sci 1995; 133: 119–27.

169 Innocenti GM. Growth and reshaping of axons in the establishment of visual callosal connections. Science 1981; 212: 824–7.

170 Innocenti GM, Koppel H, Clarke S. Transitory macrophages in the white matter of the developing visual cortex. I. Light and electron microscopic characteristics and distribution. Brain Res Dev Brain Res 1983; 11: 39–53.

171 Ip NY, Li Y, van der Stadt I et al. Ciliary neurotrophic factor enhances neuronal survival in embryonic rat hippocampal cultures. J Neurosci 1991; 11: 3124–34.

172 Ip NY, Wiegand SJ, Morse J, Rudge JS. Injury-induced regulation of ciliary neurotrophic factor mRNA in the adult rat brain. Eur J Neurosci 1993; 5: 25–33.

173 Ishihara T, Shigemoto R, Mori K et al. Functional expression and tissue distribution of a novel receptor for vasoactive intestinal polypeptide. Neuron 1992; 8: 811–19.

174 Itouji A, Sakai N, Tanaka C, Saito N. Neuronal and glial localization of two GABA transporters (GAT1 and GAT3) in the rat cerebellum. Brain Res Mol Brain Res 1996; 37: 309–16.

175 Iversen LL, Schon FE. The use of autoradiographic techniques for the identification and mapping of transmitter-specific neurones in the CNS. In: Mandell A ed. New concepts in neurotransmitter regulation. Plenum, New York, 1973: 153–93.

176 Janzer RC, Raff MC. Astrocytes induce blood–brain barrier properties in endothelial cells. Nature 1987; 325: 253–7.

177 Kahn MA, Ellison JA, Speight GJ, de Vellis J. CNTF regulation of astrogliosis and the activation of microglia in the developing rat central nervous system. Brain Res 1995; 685: 55–67.

178 Kamiguchi H, Yoshida K, Sagoh M et al. Release of ciliary neurotrophic factor from cultured astrocytes and its modulation by cytokines. Neurochem Res 1995; 20: 1187–93.

179 Kaplan MR, Meyer-Franke A, Lambert S et al. Induction of sodium channel clustering by oligodendrocytes. Nature 1997; 386: 724–8.

180 Kelly JS, Fabienne D. Differential labelling of glial cells and GABA-inhibitory interneurones and nerve terminals following the microinjection of [β-³H]alanine, [³H]DABA and [³H]GABA into single folia of the cerebellum. Cold Spring Harb Symp Quant Biol 1976; 40: 93–106.

181 Kennedy DW, Abkowitz JL. Kinetics of central nervous system microglial and macrophage engraftment: analysis using a transgenic bone marrow transplantation model. Blood 1997; 1997; 90: 986–93.

182 Kerr JFR, Harmon BV. Definition and incidence of apoptosis: an historical perspective. In: Tomei LD, Cope FO eds. *Apoptosis: the molecular basis of cell death*. Cold Spring Harbor, NY: Cold Spring Harbor Laboratory, 1991: 5–29.

183 Kettenmann H, Blankenfeld GV, Trotter J. Physiological properties of oligodendrocytes during development. *Ann N Y Acad Sci* 1991; **633**: 64–77.

184 Kettenmann H, Hoppe D, Gottmann K. Cultured microglial cells have a distinct pattern of membrane channels different from peritoneal macrophages. *J Neurosci Res* 1990; **26**: 278–87.

185 Kettenmann H, Ransom BE. *Neuroglia*. Oxford: Oxford University Press, 1995.

186 Kettenmann H, Schachner M. Pharmacological properties of GABA, glutamate and aspartate induced depolarizations in cultured astrocytes. *J Neurosci* 1985; **5**: 3295–301.

187 Kia HK, Miquel MC, Brisorgueil MJ *et al*. Immunocytochemical localization of serotonin$_{1A}$ receptors in the rat central nervous system. *J Comp Neurol* 1996; **365**: 289–305.

188 Keirstead HS, Levine JM, Blakemore WF. Response of the oligodendrocyte progenitor cell population (defined by NG2 labelling) to demyelination of the adult spinal cord. *Glia* 1998; **22**: 161–70.

189 Kimelberg HK. Current methods and approaches to studying astrocytes: a forum position paper. *Neurotoxicology* 1999; **20**: 703–12.

190 Kimelberg HK. *Glial cell receptors*. New York: Raven Press, 1988.

191 Kimelberg HK. Methodological concerns: commentary on forum position paper. *Neurotoxicology* 1998; **19**: 27–34.

192 Kimelberg HK, Jalonen T, Walz W. Regulation of the brain microenvironment: transmitters and ions. In: Murphy S ed. *Astrocytes: pharmacology and function*. San Diego, CA: Academic Press, 1993: 193–228.

193 King LS, Agre P. Pathophysiology of the aquaporin water channels. *Annu Rev Physiol* 1996; **58**: 619–48.

194 Kirischuk S, Tuschick S, Verkhratsky A, Kettenmann H. Calcium signalling in mouse Bergmann glial cells mediated by α_1-adrenoceptors and H_1 histamine receptors. *Eur J Neurosci* 1996; **8**: 1198–208.

195 Koblar SA, Turnley AM, Classon BJ *et al*. Neural precursor differentiation into astrocytes requires signaling through the leukemia inhibitory factor receptor. *Proc Natl Acad Sci USA* 1998; **95**: 3178–81.

196 Krall WJ, Challita PM, Perlmutter LS *et al*. Cells expressing glucocerebroside from a retroviral vector repopulate macrophages and central nervous system microglia after murine bone marrow transplantation. *Blood* 1994; **83**: 2737–48.

197 Kressin K, Kuprijanova E, Jabs R *et al*. Developmental regulation of Na and K conductances in glial cells of mouse hippocampal brain slices. *Glia* 1995; **15**: 173–87.

198 Kreutzberg GW. Microglia: a sensor for pathological events in the CNS. *Trends Neurosci* 1996; **19**: 312–18.

199 Kuhlenbeck H. *The central nervous system of vertebrates* Vol. 3, Part 1. Basel: Karger, 1970: 299–367.

200 Kuhn HG, Svendsen CN. Origins, functions, and potential of adult neural stem cells. *Bioessays* 1999; **21**: 625–30.

201 Kuzis K, Reed S, Cherry NJ *et al*. Developmental time course of acidic and basic fibroblast growth factors' expression in distinct cellular populations of the rat central nervous system. *J Comp Neurol* 1995; **358**: 142–53.

202 LaBourdette G, Sensenbrenner M. Growth factors and their receptors in the central nervous system. In: Kettenmann H, Ransom BE eds. *Neuroglia*. Oxford: Oxford University Press, 1995: 441–59.

203 Lang RA, Bishop JM. Macrophages are required for cell death and tissue remodelling in the developing mouse eye. *Cell* 1993; **74**: 453–62.

204 Langley OK. Ion exchange at the node of Ranvier. *Histochem J* 1990; **100**: 113–23.

205 Lantos PL. The fine structure of perivascular pleomorphic gliomas induced transplacentally by *N*-ethyl-*N*-nitrosourea in BD-IX rats. With a note on their origin. *J Neurol Sci* 1972; **17**: 443–60.

206 Lawson LJ, Perry VH, Gordon S. Turnover of resident microglia in the normal adult mouse brain. *Neuroscience* 1992; **48**: 405–15.

207 Lawson LJ, Perry VH, Dri P, Gordon S. Heterogeneity in the distribution and morphology of microglia in the normal adult mouse brain. *Neuroscience* 1990; **39**: 151–70.

208 Lee M-Y, Kim C-J, Shin S-L *et al*. Increased ciliary neurotrophic factor expression in reactive astrocytes following spinal cord injury in the rat. *Neurosci Lett* 1998; **255**: 79–82.

209 Lehre KP, Levy LM, Ottersen OP *et al*. Differential expression of two glial glutamate transporters in the rat brain: quantitative and immunocytochemical observations. *J Neurosci* 1995; **15**: 1835–53.

210 Leong SK, Ling EA. Amoeboid and ramified microglia: their interrelationship and response to brain injury. *Glia* 1992; **7**: 39–47.

211 Le Roux IPD, Reh TA. Independent regulation of primary dendritic and axonal growth by maturing astrocytes *in vitro*. *Neurosci Lett* 1995; **198**: 5–8.

212 Le Roux IPD, Reh TA. Regional differences in glial-derived factors that promote dendritic outgrowth from mouse cortical neurons *in vitro*. *J Neurosci* 1994; **14**: 4639–55.

213 Levine JM. Increased expression of the NG2 chondroitin-sulfate proteoglycan after brain injury. *J Neurosci* 1994; **14**: 4716–30.

214 Levine JM, Card JP. Light and electron microscopic localization of a cell surface antigen (NG2) in the rat cerebellum: association with smooth protoplasmic astrocytes. *J Neurosci* 1987; **7**: 2711–20.

215 Levine JM, Reynolds R. Activation and proliferation of endogenous oligodendrocyte precursor cells during ethidium bromide-induced demyelination. *Exp Neurol* 1999; **160**: 333–47.

216 Levine JM, Stincone F, Lee Y-S. Development and differentiation of glial precursor cells in the rat cerebellum. *Glia* 1993; **7**: 307–21.

217 LeVine SM, Goldman JE. Spatial and temporal patterns of oligodendrocyte differentiation in rat cerebrum and cerebellum. *J Comp Neurol* 1988; **227**: 441–5.

218 Levison SW, Ducceschi MH, Young GM, Wood TL. Acute exposure to CNTF *in vivo* induces multiple components of reactive gliosis. *Exp Neurol* 1996; **141**: 256–68.

219 Lillien LE, Raff MC. Analysis of the cell–cell interactions that control type-2 astrocyte development *in vitro*. *Neuron* 1990; **4**: 525–34.

220 Ling EA. The origin and nature of microglia. *Adv Cell Neurobiol* 1981; **2**: 33–82.

221 Ling EA, Kaur C, Lu J. Origin, nature, and some functional considerations of intraventricular macrophages, with special reference to epiplexus cells. *Microsc Res Tech* 1998; **41**: 43–56.

222 Ling EA, Paterson JA, Privat A *et al*. Investigation of glial cells in semithin sections I. Identification of glial cells in the brain of young rats. *J Comp Neurol* 1973; **149**: 43–72.

223 Ling EA, Wong WC. The origin and nature of ramified and amoeboid microglia: a historical review and current concepts. *Glia* 1993; **7**: 9–18.

224 Lipton SA. Similarity of neuronal cell injury and death in AIDS dementia and focal cerebral ischemia: potential treatment with NMDA open-channel blockers and nitric oxide-related species. *Brain Pathol* 1996; **6**: 507–17.

225 Liu Q-R, Lopez-Corcuera B, Mandiyan S et al. Molecular characterization of four pharmacologically distinct γ-aminobutyric acid transporters in mouse brain. *J Biol Chem* 1993; **268**: 2106–12.

226 Louis J-C, Magal E, Takayama S, Varon S. CNTF protection of oligodendrocytes against natural and tumor necrosis factor-induced death. *Science* 1992; **259**: 689–92.

227 Lu J, Kaur C, Ling EA. Uptake of tracer by epiplexus cells via the choroid plexus epithelium following an intravenous or intraperitoneal injection of horseradish peroxidase in rats. *J Anat* 1993; **183**: 609–18.

228 Ludwin SK. The perineuronal satellite oligodendrocyte. A role in remyelination. *Acta Neuropathol* 1979; **47**: 49–53.

229 Lugaro E. Sulle funzioni della nevroglia. *Riv Patol Nerv Ment* 1907; **12**: 225–33.

230 Luskin MB, McDermott K. Divergent lineages for oligodendrocytes and astrocytes originating in the neonatal forebrain subventricular zone. *Glia* 1994; **11**: 211–26.

231 McAllister KA, Katz LC, Lo DC. Neurotrophins and synaptic plasticity. *Annu Rev Neurosci* 1999; **22**: 295–318.

232 McKercher SR, Torbett BE, Anderson KL et al. Targeted disruption of the Pu.1 gene results in multiple hematopoietic abnormalities. *EMBO J* 1996; **15**: 5647–58.

233 McKinley MJ, Oldfield BJ. Circumventricular organs. In: Paxinos G ed. *The human nervous system*. San Diego, CA: Academic Press, 1990: 415–38.

234 McKinnon RD, Matsui T, Dubois-Dalcq M, Aaronson SA. FGF modulates the PDGF-driven pathway of oligodendrocyte development. *Neuron* 1990; **5**: 603–14.

235 McKinnon RD, Smith C, Behar T et al. Distinct effects of bFGF and PDGF on oligodendrocyte progenitor cells. *Glia* 1993; **7**: 245–54.

236 McMenamin PG. Distribution and phenotype of dendritic cells and resident tissue macrophages in the dura mater, leptomeninges, and choroid plexus of the rat brain as demonstrated in wholemount preparations. *J Comp Neurol* 1999; **405**: 553–62.

237 McMillan MK, Thai L, Hong J-S et al. Brain injury in a dish: a model for reactive gliosis. *Trends Neurosci* 1994; **17**: 138–42.

238 McMorris FA, Dubois-Dalcq M. Insulin-like growth factor I promotes cell proliferation and oligodendroglial commitment in rat glial progenitor cells developing *in vitro*. *J Neurosci Res* 1988; 21: 199–209.

239 Magistretti PJ, Pellerin L. Cellular bases of brain energy metabolism and their relevance to functional brain imaging: evidence for a functional role of astrocytes. *Cereb Cortex* 1996; **6**: 50–61.

240 Magistretti PJ, Pellerin L, Rothman D, Shulman RG. Energy on demand. *Science* 1999; **283**: 496–7.

241 Magistretti PJ, Sorg O, Martin JL. Regulation of glycogen metabolism in astrocytes: physiological, pharmacological and pathological aspects. In: Murphy S ed. *Astrocytes: pharmacology and function*. San Diego, CA: Academic Press, 1993: 243–65.

242 Mallat M, Houlgatte R, Brachet P, Prochiantz A. Lipopolysaccharide-stimulated rat brain macrophages release NGF *in vitro*. *Dev Biol* 1989; **133**: 309–11.

243 Martin LJ, Blackstone CD, Levy AI et al. AMPA glutamate receptor subunits are differentially distributed in rat brain. *Neuroscience* 1993; **53**: 327–58.

244 Massa PT, Mugnaimi E. Cell junctions and intramembrane particles of strocytes and oligodendrocytes. *Neuroscience* 1982; **7**: 523–38.

245 Matsuyama A, Iwata H, Okumura N et al. Localization of basic fibroblast growth factor-like immunoreactivity in the rat brain. *Brain Res* 1992; **587**: 49–65.

246 Matthews MA, Duncan D. A quantitative study of morphological changes accompanying the initiation and progress of myelin production in the dorsal funiculus of the rat spinal cord. *J Comp Neurol* 1971; **142**: 1–22.

247 Matute C, Gutierrez-Igarza K, Rio C, Miledi R. Glutamate receptors in astrocytic end-feet. *NeuroReport* 1994; **5**: 1205–8.

248 Matyszak MK, Lawson LJ, Perry VH, Gordon S. Stromal macrophages of the choroid plexus situated at an interface between the brain and the peripheral immune system constitutively express MHC class II antigens. *J Neuroimmunol* 1992; **40**: 173–82.

249 Mehl E, Wolfgang F. Myelin types with different protein components in the same species. *J Neurochem* 1969; **16**: 1510–14.

250 Meldrum B, Garthwaite J. EAA pharmacology: excitatory amino acid neurotoxicity and neurodegenerative disease. *Trends Pharmacol* 1990; **11**: 379–87.

251 Metcalf D. The molecular control of normal and leukaemic granulocytes and macrophages. *Proc R Soc Lond B Biol Sci* 1987; **230**: 389–423.

252 Metcalf D, Moore MAS. Embryonic aspects of haemopoiesis. In: *Haemopoietic cells. Frontiers of biology* 1971; **24**: 172–271.

253 Metchnikoff E. *Lectures on the comparative pathology of inflammation* Starling FA, Starling EH trans. London: Kegan, Paul, Trench and Trubner, 1891.

254 Miller M, Krangel M. Biology and biochemistry of the chemokines: a family of chemotactic and inflammatory cytokines. *Crit Rev Immunol* 1992; **12**: 17–46.

255 Miller RH, Ffrench-Constant C, Raff MC. The macroglial cells of the rat optic nerve. *Annu Rev Neurosci* 1989; **12**: 5417–34.

256 Misson JP, Edwards ME, Yamamoto M, Caviness VS. Identification of radial glial cells within the developing murine central nervous system: studies based upon a new histochemical marker. *Dev Brain Res* 1988; **44**: 95–108.

257 Misson JP, Takahashi T, Caviness VS. Ontogeny of radial and other astroglial cells in the murine cerebral cortex. *Glia* 1991; **4**: 138–48.

258 Morel P, Norton WT. Myelin. *Sci Am* 1980; **242**: 88–118.

259 Mori S, Leblond CP. Electron microscopic identification of three classes of oligodendrocytes and a preliminary study of their proliferatice activity in the corpus callosum of young rats. *J Comp Neurol* 1970; **139**: 1–30.

260 Morris L, Graham CF, Gordon S. Macrophages in haemopoietic and other tissues of the developing mouse detected by the monoclonal antibody F4/80. *Development* 1991; **112**: 517–26.

261 Muller T, Fritschy JM, Grosche J et al. Developmental regulation of voltage-gated K+ channel and GABA_A receptor expression in Bergmann glial cells. *J Neurosci* 1994; **14**: 2503–14.

262 Muller T, Grosche J, Ohlemeyer C, Kettenmann H. NMDA-activated currents in Bergmann glial cells. *NeuroReport* 1993; **4**: 671–4.

263 Murphy S. *Astrocytes: pharmacology and function*. San Diego, CA: Academic Press, 1993.

264 Murray JA, Blakemore WF. The relationship between internodal length and fibre diameter in the spinal cord of the cat. *J Neurol Sci* 1980; **45**: 29–41.

265 Nagelhus EA, Inanobe A, Fujita A et al. Immunogold evidence suggests that coupling of K^+ siphoning and water transport in rat retinal Müller cells is mediated by a coenrichment of Kir4.1 and AQP4 in specific membrane domains. Glia 1999; 26: 47–54.

266 Nagelhus EA, Veruki ML, Torp R et al. Aquaporin-4 water channel protein in the rat retina and optic nerve: polarized expression in Müller cells and fibrous astrocytes. J Neurosci 1988; 18: 2506–19.

267 Nakagaito Y, Yoshida T, Motonobu S, Takeuchi M. Effects of leukemia inhibitory factor on the differentiation of astrocyte progenitor cells from embryonic mouse cerebral hemispheres. Brain Res Dev Brain Res 1995; 87: 220–3.

268 Nakajima K, Shimojo M, Hamanoue M et al. Identification of elastase as a secretory protease from cultured rat microglia. J Neurochem 1992; 58: 1401–8.

269 Nakajima K, Tuzaki N, Nagata K et al. Production and secretion of plasminogen in cultured rat brain microglia. FEBS Lett 1992; 308: 179–82.

270 Nathan CF. Secretory products of macrophages. J Clin Invest 1987; 79: 319–26.

271 Neumann H, Misgeld T, Matsumuro K, Wekerle H. Neurotrophins inhibit major histocompatibility class II inducibility of microglia: involvement of the p75 neurotrophin receptor. Proc Natl Acad Sci USA 1998; 95: 5779–84.

272 Newman EA. Glial cell regulation of extracellular potassium. In: Kettenmann H, Ransom BE eds. Neuroglia. Oxford: Oxford University Press, 1995: 717–31.

273 Newman EA, Frambach DA, Odette LL. Control of extracellular potassium levels by retinal glial cell K^+ siphoning. Science 1984; 225: 1174–5.

274 Newman EA, Zahs KR. Calcium waves in retinal glial cells. Science 1997; 275: 844–7.

275 Nielson S, Nagelhus EA, Amiry-Moghaddam M et al. Specialized membrane domains for water transport in glial cells: high-resolution immunogold cytochemistry of aquaporin-4 in rat brain. J Neurosci 1997; 19: 171–80.

276 Nishiyama A, Chang A, Trapp BD. $NG2^+$ glial cells: a novel glial cell population in the adult brain. J Neuropathol Exp Neurol 1999; 58: 1113–24.

277 Nishiyama A, Lin X-L, Giese N et al. Co-localization of NG2 proteoglycan and PDGF α-receptor on O2A progenitor cells in the developing rat brain. J Neurosci Res 1996; 43: 299–314.

278 Nishiyama A, Yiu M, Drazba JA, Tuohy VK. Normal and reactive NG2 +ve flial cells are distinct from resting and activated microglia. J Neurosci Res 1997; 48: 299–312.

279 Noble M, Murray K, Stroobant P et al. Platelet-derived growth factor promotes division and motility and inhibits premature differentiation of the oligodendrocyte/type-2 astrocyte progenitor cell. Nature 1988; 333: 560–3.

280 Norton WT, Cammer W. Isolation and characterization of myelin. In: Morell P ed. Myelin. New York: Plenum, 1984: 147–95.

281 Oh Y, Black JA, Waxman SG. The expression of rat brain voltage-sensitive Na^+ channel mRNAs in astrocytes. Brain Res Mol Brain Res 1994; 23: 57–65.

282 Ohbayashi N, Hoshikawa M, Kimura S et al. Structure and expression of the mRNA encoding a novel fibroblast growth factor, FGF-18. J Biol Chem 1998; 273: 18161–4.

283 O'Leary MT, Blakemore WF. Use of a rat Y chromosome probe to determine the long-term survival of glial cells transplanted into areas of CNS demyelination. J Neurocytol 1997; 26: 191–206.

284 Ong WY, Levine JM. A light and electron microscopic study of NG2 chondroitin sulfate proteoglycan-positive oligodendrocyte precursor cells in the normal and kainate-lesioned rat hippocampus. Neuroscience 1999; 92: 83–95.

285 Oppenheim RW. Cell death during development of the nervous system. Annu Rev Neurosci 1991; 14: 453–501.

286 Orkand RK, Nicholls JG, Kuffler SW. Effect of nerve impulses on the membrane potential of glial cells in the central nervous system of amphibia. J Neurophysiol 1966; 29: 788–806.

287 Ottersen OP, Chaudhry FA, Danbolt NC et al. Molecular organization of cerebellar glutamate synapses. Prog Brain Res 1997; 114: 97–107.

288 Ozawa S, Kamiya H, Tsuzuki K. Glutamate receptors in the mammalian central nervous system. Prog Neurobiol 1998; 54: 581–618.

289 Palay SL, Chan-Palay Y. Cerebellar cortex: cytology and organization. New York: Springer, 1974.

290 Penfield W. Neuroglia and microglia. The interstitial tissue of the central nervous system. In: Cowdry EV ed. Special cytology Section XXXI, Vol III. New York: Hoeber, 1932: 1445–82.

291 Perry VH. Macrophages and the nervous system. Austin, TX: RG Landes Co., 1994.

292 Perry VH, Anderson PB, Gordon S. Macrophages and inflammation in the nervous system. Trends Neurosci 1993; 16: 268–73.

293 Perry VH, Crocker PR, Gordon S. The blood–brain barrier regulates the expression of a macrophage scialic acid-binding receptor on microglia. J Cell Sci 1992; 101: 201–7.

294 Perry VH, Gordon S. Macrophages and the nervous system. Int Rev Cytol 1991; 125: 203–44.

295 Perry VH, Gordon S. Modulation of CD4 antigen on macrophages and microglia in rat brain. J Exp Med 1987; 166: 1138–43.

296 Perry VH, Hume DA, Gordon S. Immunohistochemical localization of macrophages and microglia in the adult and developing mouse brain. Neuroscience 1985; 15: 313–26.

297 Perry VH, Matyszak MK, Fearn S. Altered antigen expression of microglia in the aged rodent CNS. Glia 1993; 7: 60–7.

298 Peters A, Palay SL, Webster H. The fine structure of the nervous system: the neurons and supporting cells. Philadelphia, PA: WB Saunders, 1991.

299 Petralia RS, Wang YX, Wenthold RJ. Histological and ultrastructural localization of the kainate receptor subunits, KA2 and GluR6/7 in the rat nervous system using selective antipeptide antibodies. J Comp Neurol 1994; 349: 85–110.

300 Petralia RS, Wenthold RJ. Light and electron immunocytochemical localization of AMPA-selective glutamate receptors in the rat brain. J Comp Neurol 1992; 318: 329–54.

301 Pfeiffer S, Barbarese E, Bhat S. Noncoordinate regulation of myelinogenic parameters in primary cultures of dissociated fetal rat brain. J Neurosci Res 1981; 6: 369–80.

302 Pilkington GL, Lantos PL. Biological markers for tumors of the brain. Adv Tech Stand Neurosurg 1994; 21: 3–41.

303 Platt N, da Silva RP, Gordon S. Recognizing death: the phagocytosis of apoptotic cells. Trends Cell Biol 1998; 8: 365–72.

304 Poopalasundaram S, Knott C, Shamotienko OG et al. Glial heterogeneity in the expression of the inwardly-rectifying K^+ channel, Kir4.1 in adult rat CNS. Glia 2000; 30: 362–72.

305 Popko B. Myelin galactolipids: mediators of axon–glial interactions? Glia 2000; 29: 149–53.

306 Porter JT, McCarthy JD. Astrocytic neurotransmitter receptors in situ and in vivo. Prog Neurobiol 1997; 51: 439–55.

307 Pow DV, Perry VH, Morris JF, Gordon S. Microglia in the neurohypophysis associate with and endocytose terminal portions of neurosecretory neurons. *Neuroscience* 1989; **33**: 567–78.

308 Pringle NP, Mudhar HS, Collarini EJ, Richardson WD. PDGF receptors in the rat CNS: during late neurogenesis, PDGF alpha-receptor expression appears to be restricted to glial cells of the oligodendrocyte lineage. *Development* 1992; **115**: 535–51.

309 Privat A, Gimenez-Ribotta M, Ridet J-L. Morphology of astrocytes. In: Kettenmann H, Ransom BE eds. *Neuroglia*. Oxford: Oxford University Press, 1995: 3–22.

310 Qian J, Bull MS, Levitt P. Target-derived astroglia regulate axonal outgrowth in a region-specific manner. *Dev Biol* 1992; **149**: 278–94.

311 Raff MC. Glial cell diversification in the rat optic nerve. *Science* 1989; **243**: 1450–5.

312 Raff MC, Abney ER. Miller RH. Two glial cell lineages diverge prenatally in rat optic nerve. *Dev Biol* 1984; **106**: 53–60.

313 Raff MC, Lillien LE, Richardson WD *et al*. Platelet-derived growth factor from astrocytes drives the clock that times oligodendrocyte development in culture. *Nature* 1988; **333**: 562–5.

314 Raff MC, Miller RH, Noble MA. A glial precursor cell that develops *in vitro* into an astrocyte or an oligodendrocyte depending on culture medium. *Nature* 1983; **303**: 390–6.

315 Raine CS. Morphology of myelin and myelination. In: Morell P ed. *Myelin*. New York: Plenum Press, 1984: 1–50.

316 Raine CS, Dolich M. The anterior medullary velum and its involvement during autoimmunodemyelination. *J Neurocytol* 1986; **15**: 261–72.

317 Raivich G, Moreno-Flores MT, Moller JC, Kreutzberg GW. Inhibition of post-traumatic microglial proliferation in a genetic model of macrophage colony-stimulating factor deficiency in the mouse. *Eur J Neurosci* 1994; **6**: 1615–18.

318 Rakic P. Radial glial cells: scaffolding for brain construction. In: Kettenmann H, Ransom BE eds. *Neuroglia*. Oxford: Oxford University Press, 1995: 746–62.

319 Rakic P, Sidman RL. Subcommissural organ and adjacent ependyma: autoradiographic study of their origin in the mouse brain. *Am J Anat* 1968; **122**: 317–36.

320 Ramony Cajal S. Contributión al conocimiento de la neuroglía del cerebro humano. *Trab Lab Invest Biol Univ Madrid* 1913; **18**: 225–315.

321 Ramony Cajal S. *Histologie du système nerveux de l'homme et des vertébrés*. Paris: A Maloine, 1909.

322 Ransom BR, Butt AM, Black J. Ultrastructural identification of HRP-injected oligodendrocytes in the intact rat optic nerve. *Glia* 1991; **4**: 37–45.

323 Ransohoff RM, Tani M. Do chemokines mediate leukocyte recruitment in post-traumatic CNS inflammation? *Trends Neurosci* 1998; **21**: 154–9.

324 Rappolee DA, Werb Z. Macrophage-derived growth factors. *Curr Top Microbiol Immunol* 1992; **181**: 87–140.

325 Rasband MN, Peles E, Trimmer JS *et al*. Dependence of nodal sodium channel clustering on paranodal axoglial contact in developing CNS. *J Neurosci* 1999; **19**: 7516–28.

326 Rash JE, Yasumura T, Hudson CS *et al*. Direct immunogold labeling of aquaporin-4 in square arrays of astrocyte and ependymocyte plasma membranes in rat brain and spinal cord. *Proc Natl Acad Sci USA* 1998; **95**: 11981–6.

327 Raymond AA, Fish DR, Stevens JM *et al*. Subependymal heterotopia: a distinct neural migration disorder associated with epilepsy. *J Neurol Neurosurg Psychiatry* 1994; **57**: 1195–202.

328 Redwine JM, Armstrong RC. *In vivo* proliferation of oligodendrocyte progenitors expressing PDGFaR during early remyelination. *J Neurobiol* 1998; **34**: 413–28.

329 Remahl S, Hildebrand C. Relation between axons and oligodendroglial cells during initial myelination. I. The glial unit. *J Neurocytol* 1990; **19**: 313–28.

330 Remahl S, Hildebrand C. Relation between axons and oligodendroglial cells during initial myelination. II. The individual axon. *J Neurocytol* 1990; **19**: 883–98.

331 Reynolds R, Hardy R. Oligodendroglial progenitors labeled with the O4 antibody persist in the adult rat cerebral cortex *in vivo*. *J Neurosci Res* 1997; **47**: 455–70.

332 Rezaie P, Cairns NJ, Male DK. Expression of adhesion molecules on human fetal cerebral vessels: relationship to microglial colonisation during development. *Brain Res Dev Brain Res* 1997; **104**: 175–89.

333 Rezaie P, Patel K, Male DK. Microglia in the human fetal spinal cord – patterns of distribution, morphology and phenotype. *Brain Res Dev Brain Res* 1999; **115**: 71–81.

334 Ribak CE, Tong WMY, Brecha NC. Astrocytic processes compensate for the apparent lack of GABA transporters in the axon terminals of cerebellar Purkinje cells. *Anat Embryol* 1996; **194**: 379–90.

335 Richards LJ, Kilpatrick TJ, Dutton R *et al*. Leukaemia inhibitory factor or related factors promote the differentiation of neuronal and astrocytic precursors within the developing murine spinal cord. *Eur J Neurosci* 1996; **8**: 291–9.

336 Richardson A, Hao C, Federoff S. Microglia progenitor cells: a subpopulation in cultures of mouse neopallial astroglia. *Glia* 1993; **7**: 25–33.

337 Richardson WD, Pringle N, Mosley MJ *et al*. A role for platelet-derived growth factor in normal gliogenesis in the central nervous system. *Cell* 1988; **53**: 309–19.

338 Richardson WD, Smith HK, Sun T *et al*. Oligodendrocyte lineage and the motor neuron connection. *Glia* 2000; **29**: 136–42.

339 Rio C, Rieff HI, Qi P, Corfas G. Neuregulin and rebB receptors play a critical role in neuronal migration. *Neuron* 1997; **19**: 39–50.

340 Rodriguez EM, Rodriguez S, Hein S. The subcommissural organ. *Microsc Res Tech* 1998; **41**: 98–123.

341 Rosenbluth J. Role of glial cells in the differentiation and function of myelinated axons. *Int J Dev Neurosci* 1988; **6**: 3–24.

342 Rothstein JD, Dykes-Hoberg M, Pardo CA *et al*. Knockout of glutamate transporters reveals a major role for astroglial transport in excitotoxicity and clearance of glutamate. *Neuron* 1996; **16**: 675–86.

343 Rothstein JD, Martin L, Levy AI *et al*. Localization of neuronal and glial glutamate transporters. *Neuron* 1994; **13**: 713–25.

344 Rousselet A, Autillo-Touati A, Araud D, Prochiantz A. *In vitro* regulation of neuronal morphogenesis and polarity by astrocyte-derived factors. *Dev Biol* 1990; **137**: 33–45.

345 Rudge JS. Astrocyte-derived neurotrophic factors. In: Murphy S ed. *Astrocytes: pharmacology and function*. San Diego, CA: Academic Press, 1993: 267–305.

346 Rudge JS, Li Y, Pasnikowski EM *et al*. Neurotrophic factor receptors and their signal transduction capabilities in rat astrocytes. *Eur J Neurosci* 1994; **6**: 693–705.

347 Rudge JS, Pasnikowski EM, Holst P, Lindsay RM. Changes in neurotrophic factor expression and receptor activation following exposure of hippocampal neuron/astrocyte cocultures to kainic acid. *J Neurosci* 1995; **15**: 6856–67.

348 Rutzel H, Schiebel TH. Prenatal and early post natal development of glial cells in the median eminence of the rat. *Cell Tissue Res* 1980; **211**: 117–37.

349 Saadat S, Sendtner M, Rohrer H. Ciliary neurotrophic factor induces cholinergic differentiation of rat sympathetic neurons in culture. *J Cell Biol* 1989; **108**: 1807–16.

350 Saito Y, Wright EM. Regulation of bicarbonate transport across the brush border membrane of the bull-frog choroid plexus. *J Physiol Lond* 1984; **350**: 327–42.

351 Sanyal S, Bal AK. Comparative light and electron microscopic study of retinal histogenesis in normal and rd mutant mice. *Z Anat Entwickl Gesch* 1973; **142**: 219–38.

352 Sarnat HB. Ependymal reactions to injury: a review. *J Neuropathol Exp Neurol* 1995; **54**: 1–15.

353 Sarnat HB. Histochemistry and immunocytochemistry of the developing ependyma and choroid plexus. *Microsc Res Tech* 1998; **41**: 14–28.

354 Sarnat HB. Role of fetal ependyma. *Pediatr Neurol* 1992; **8**: 163–78.

355 Saunders NR, Habgood MD, Dziegielewska KM. Barrier mechanisms in the brain, I. Adult brain. *Clin Exp Pharmacol Physiol* 1999; **26**: 11–19.

356 Saunders NR, Habgood MD, Dziegielewska KM. Barrier mechanisms in the brain, II. Immature brain. *Clin Exp Pharmacol Physiol* 1999; **26**: 85–91.

357 Saunders NR, Habgood MD, Dziegielewska KM. Barriers in the immature brain. *Cell Mol Neurobiol* 2000; **20**: 29–40.

358 Savill JS, Fadok V, Henson PM. Phagocyte recognition of cells undergoing apoptosis. *Immunol Today* 1993; **14**: 131–6.

359 Schmidtmayer J, Jacobsen C, Miksch G, Sievers J. Blood monocytes and spleen macrophages differentiate into microglia-like cells on monolayers of astrocytes: membrane currents. *Glia* 1994; **12**: 259–67.

360 Schools GP, Kimmelberg HK. mGluR3 and mGluR5 are the predominant metabotropic glutamate receptor mRNAs expressed in hippocampal astrocytes acutely isolated from young rats. *J Neurosci Res* 1999; **58**: 533–43.

361 Schroder W, Hager G, Kouprijanova E et al. Lesion-induced changes of electrophysiological properties in astrocytes of the rat dentate gyrus. *Glia* 1999; **28**: 166–74.

362 Scolding N, Franklin R, Stevens S et al. Oligodendrocyte progenitors are present in the normal adult human CNS and in lesions of multiple sclerosis. *Brain* 1998; **121**: 2221–8.

363 Scott DE, Van Dyke DH, Paul WK et al. Ultrastructural analysis of human cerebral ventricular system 3. The choroid plexus. *Cell Tissue Res* 1974; **150**: 389–97.

364 Segal MB. The choroid plexuses and the barriers between the blood and the cerebrospinal fluid. *Cell Mol Neurobiol* 2000; **20**: 183–96.

365 Seifert G, Rehn L, Weber M, Steinhäuser C. AMPA receptor subunits expressed by single astrocytes in the juvenile mouse hippocampus. *Brain Res Mol Brain Res* 1997; **47**: 286–94.

366 Seifert G, Steinhäuser C. Glial cells in the mouse hippocampus express AMPA receptors with an intermediate Ca^{2+} permeability. *Eur J Neurosci* 1997; **7**: 1872–81.

367 Seifert G, Zhou M, Steinhäuser C. Analysis of AMPA receptor properties during postnatal development of mouse hippocampal astrocytes. *J Neurophysiol* 1997; **78**: 2916–23.

368 Sendtner M, Kreutzberg GW, Thoenen H. Ciliary neurotrophic factor prevents the degeneration of motor neurons after axotomy. *Nature* 1990; **345**: 440–1.

369 Sheffield LG, Berman NE. Microglial expression of MHC class II increases in normal aging of nonhuman primates. *Neurobiol Aging* 1998; **19**: 47–55.

370 Shoshan Y, Nishiyama A, Chang A et al. Expression of oligodendrocyte progenitor cell antigens by gliomas: implications for the histogenesis of brain tumors. *Proc Natl Acad Sci USA* 1999; **96**: 10361–6.

371 Sievers J, Parwaresch R, Wottge HU. Blood monocytes and spleen macrophages differentiate into microglia-like cells on monolayers of astrocytes: morphology. *Glia* 1994; **12**: 245–58.

372 Sims KD, Robinson MB. Expression patterns and regulation of glutamate transporters in the developing and adult nervous system. *Crit Rev Neurobiol* 1999; **13**: 169–97.

373 Smart I. The ependymal layer of the mouse brain and its cell production by radio-autography after thymidine-H^3 injection. *J Comp Neurol* 1961; **116**: 325–47.

374 Sommer I, Schachner M. Monoclonal antibody (O1 to O4) to oligodendrocyte cell surface: an immunocytological study in the central nervous system. *Dev Biol* 1981; **83**: 311–27.

375 Sontheimer H. Voltage-dependent ion channels in glial cells. *Glia* 1994; **11**: 156–72.

376 Sontheimer H, Minturn JE, Black JA et al. Two types of Na^+ currents in cultured rat optic nerve astrocytes: changes with time in culture and with age of culture derivation. *J Neurosci Res* 1991; **30**: 275–87.

377 Sontheimer H, Ritchie JM. Voltage-gated sodium and calcium channels. In: Kettenmann H, Ransom BE eds. *Neuroglia*. Oxford: Oxford University Press, 1995: 202–20.

378 Soriano E, Alvarado-Mallart RM, Dumesnil N et al. Cajal-Retzius cells regulate the radial glia phenotype in the adult and developing cerebrum and alter granule cell migration. *Neuron* 1997; **18**: 563–77.

379 Spacek J. Three-dimensional analysis of dendritic spines. III. Glial sheath. *Anat Embryol (Berl)* 1985; **171**: 245–52.

380 Spassky N, Olivier C, Perez-Villegas E et al. Single or multiple oligodendroglial lineages: a controversy. *Glia* 2000; **29**: 143–8.

381 Spreafico R, Frassoni C, Arcelli P et al. Distribution of AMPA selective glutamate receptors in the thalamus of adult rats and during postnatal development. *Brain Res Dev Brain Res* 1994; **82**: 231–44.

382 Stallcup WB, Beasley L. Bipotential glial precursor cells of the optic nerve express the NG2 proteoglycan. *J Neurosci* 1987; **7**: 2737–44.

383 Steinhäuser C, Kressin K, Kuprijanova E et al. Properties of voltage–activated Na^+ and K^+ currents in mouse hippocampal glial cells *in situ* and after acute isolation from tissue slices. *Pflügers Arch* 1994; **428**: 610–20.

384 Stensaas LJ, Stensaas SS. Astrocytic neuroglial cells, oligodendrocytes and microgliacytes in the spinal cord of the toad. I. Light microscopy. *Z Zellforsch* 1968; **84**: 473–89.

385 Sterba G, Clein I, Naumann W, Petter H. Immunocytochemical investigation of the subcommissural organ in the rat. *Cell Tissue Res* 1981; **218**: 659–62.

386 Sternberger NH, Quarles RH, Itoyama T, Webster H de F. Myelin-associated glycoprotein demonstrated immunocytochemically in myelin and myelin-forming cells of developing rat. *Proc Natl Acad Sci USA* 1979; **76**: 1510–14.

387 Stöckli KA, Lillien LE, Näher-Noé M. et al. Regional distribution, developmental changes, and cellular localization of CNTF-mRNA and protein in the rat brain. *J Cell Biol* 1991; **115**: 447–59.

388 Storck T, Schulte S, Hofmann K, Stoffel W. Structure, expression and functional analysis of a Na^+-dependent glutamate/aspartate transporter from rat brain. *Proc Natl Acad Sci USA* 1992; **89**: 10955–9.

389 Streit WJ, Graeber MB, Kreutzberg GW. Expression of Ia antigen on perivascular and microglial cells after sublethal and lethal motor neuron injury. *Exp Neurol* 1989; **105**: 115–26.

390 Streit WJ, Kreutzberg GW. Lectin binding by resting and reactive microglia. *J Neurocytol* 1987; **16**: 249–60.

391 Streit WJ, Kreutzberg GW. Response of endogenous glial cells to motor neuron degeneration induced by toxic ricin. *J Comp Neurol* 1988; **268**: 248–63.

392 Streit WJ, Semple-Rowland SL, Hurley SD *et al*. Cytokine mRNA profiles in contused spinal cord and axotomized facial nucleus suggest a beneficial role for inflammation and gliosis. *Exp Neurol* 1998; **152**: 74–87.

393 Sturrock RR. A developmental study of epiplexus cells and subependymal cells and their possible relationship to microglia. *Neuropathol Appl Neurobiol* 1978; **4**: 307–22.

394 Suzuki M, Raisman G. The glial framework of central white matter tracts: segmental rows of contiguous interfascicular oligodendrocytes and solitary astrocytes give rise to a continuous meshwork of transverse and longitudinal processes in the adult rat fimbria. *Glia* 1992; **6**: 222–35.

395 Svensson M, Aldskogius H. Synaptic density of axotomized hypoglossal motorneurons following pharmacological blockade of the microglial cell proliferation. *Exp Neurol* 1993; **120**: 123–31.

396 Sweadner KJ. Na, K-ATPase and its isoforms. In: Kettenmann H, Ransom BE eds. *Neuroglia*. Oxford: Oxford University Press, 1995: 259–72.

397 Tanaka K, Watase K, Manabe T *et al*. Epilepsy and exacerbation of brain injury in mice lacking the glutamate transporter GLT-1. *Science* 1997; **276**: 1699–702.

398 Temple S. CNS development: the obscure origins of adult stem cells. *Curr Biol* 1999; **9**: 397–9.

399 Thio CL, Waxman SG, Sontheimer H. Ion channels in spinal cord astrocytes *in vitro*: III. Modulation of channel expression by co-culture with neurons and neuron-conditioned medium. *J Neurophysiol* 1993; **69**: 819–31.

400 Trapp BD. Myelin-associated glycoprotein: location and potential functions. *Ann N Y Acad Sci* 1990; **605**: 29–43.

401 Trapp BD, Moench T, Pullety M *et al*. Spatial segregation of mRNA encoding myelin-specific proteins. *Proc Natl Acad Sci USA* 1987; **84**: 7773–7.

402 Tsacopoulos M, Magistretti PJ. Metabolic coupling between glia and neurons. *J Neurosci* 1996; **16**: 877–85.

403 Valenzuela CF, Kazlauskas A, Weiner JL. Roles of platelet-derived growth factor in the developing and mature nervous system. *Brain Res Rev* 1997; **24**: 77–89.

404 Van Bockstaele EJ, Colago EEO. Selective distribution of the NMAD-R1 glutamate receptor in astrocytes and presynaptic axon terminals in the nucleus locus coeruleus of the rat brain: an immunoelectron microscopic study. *J Comp Neurol* 1996; **369**: 483–96.

405 Vannucci SJ, Maher F, Simpson IA. Glucose transporter proteins in brain: delivery of glucose to neurons and glia. *Glia* 1997; **21**: 2–21.

406 Ventura R, Harris KM. Three-dimensional relationships between hippocampal synapses and astrocytes. *J Neurosci* 1999; **19**: 6897–906.

407 Vigh B, Vigh-Teichmann I. Actual problems of the cerebrospinal fluid-contacting neurons. *Microsc Res Tech* 1998; **41**: 57–83.

408 Von Blankenfeld G, Enkvist K, Kettenmann H. Gamma-aminobutyric acid and glutamate receptors. In: Kettenmann H, Ransom BE eds. *Neuroglia*. Oxford: Oxford University Press, 1995: 335–45.

409 Walz W, Lang MK. Immunocytochemical evidence for a distinct GFAP-negative subpopulation of astrocytes in the adult rat hippocampus. *Neurosci Lett* 1998; **257**: 127–30.

410 Warrington AE, Pfeiffer SE. Proliferation and differentiation of O4$^+$ oligodendrocytes in postnatal rat cerebellum: analysis in unfixed tissue slices using anti-glycolipid antibodies. *J Neurosci Res* 1992; **33**: 338–53.

411 Waxman SG, Ritchie JM. Molecular dissection of the myelinated axon. *Ann Neurol* 1993; **33**: 121–36.

412 Waxman SG, Black JA. Freeze fracture ultrastructure of the perinodal astrocyte and associated glial junctions. *Brain Res* 1946; **308**: 77–88.

413 Weiss S, Reynolds BA, Vescovi AL *et al*. Is there a neural stem cell in the mammalian forebrain? *Trends Neurosci* 1996; **19**: 387–93.

414 Weruaga-Prieto E, Eggli P, Celio MR. Topographic variations in rat brain oligodendrocyte morphology elucidated by injection of lucifer yellow in fixed tissue slices. *J Neurocytol* 1996; **25**: 19–31.

415 Whitaker Azmitia PM, Clarke C, Azmitia EC. Localization of 5-HT$_{1A}$ receptors to astroglial cells in adult rats: implications for neuronal–glial interactions and psychoactive drug mechanism of action. *Synapse* 1993; **14**: 201–5.

416 Wilkin GP, Garthwaite J, Balazs R. Putative acidic amino acid transmitters in the cerebellum. 2. Electron microscopic localisation of transport sites. *Brain Res* 1982; **244**: 69–80.

417 Wilkin GP, Levy G, Johnstone SR, Riddle SR. Cerebellar astroglial cells in primary culture: expression of different morphological appearances and different ability to take up ^{3}H-aspartate and ^{3}H-GABA. *Brain Res Dev Brain Res* 1983; **10**: 265–77.

418 Wilkin GP, Marriott DR, Cholewinkski AJ. Astrocyte heterogeneity. *Trends Neurosci* 1990; **13**: 43–6.

419 Wolburg H, Risau W. Formation of the blood–brain barrier. In: Kettenmann H, Ransom BE eds. *Neuroglia*. Oxford: Oxford University Press, 1995: 763–76.

420 Wolfgram F, Kotorii K. The composition of myelin proteins of the central nervous system. *J Neurochem* 1968; **15**: 1281–90.

421 Wolswijk G. GD3 cells in the adult rat optic nerve are ramified microglia rather than 0-2A adult progenitor cells. *Glia* 1994; **10**: 244–9.

422 Wolswijk G, Noble M. *In vitro* studies in the development and maintenance of the oligodendrocyte type-2 astrocyte (O-2A) lineage in the adult central nervous system. In: Kettenmann H, Ransom BR eds. *Neuroglial cells*. Oxford: Oxford University Press, 1994: 149–61.

423 Yang H-Y, Lieska N, Shao D *et al*. Immunotyping of radial glia and their glial derivatives during development of the rat spinal cord. *J Neurocytol* 1993; **22**: 558–71.

424 Yeh H-J, Ruit KG, Wang Y-X *et al*. PDGF A-chain gene is expressed by mammalian neurons during development and in maturity. *Cell* 1991; **64**: 209–16.

425 Yin X, Crawford TO, Griffin JW *et al*. Myelin-associated glycoprotein is a myelin signal that modulates the caliber of myelinated axons. *J Neurosci* 1998; **18**: 1953–62.

426 Zambenedett P, Giordano R, Zatta P. Histochemical localization of glycoconjugates on microglial cells in Alzheimer's disease brain samples by using Abrus precatorius, Maackia amurensis, Momordica charantia, and Sambucus nigra lectins. *Exp Neurol* 1998; **153**: 167–71.

427 Zeller NK, Behar TN, Dubois-Dalcq ME, Lazzarini RA. The timely expression of myelin basic protein gene in cultured rat brain oligodendrocytes is independent of continuous neuronal influences. *J Neurosci* 1985; **5**: 2955–62.

428 Zheng C, Heintz N, Hatten ME. CNS gene encoding astrotactin, which supports neuronal migration along glial fibers. *Science* 1996; **272**: 417–19.

3

Cellular pathology of the central nervous system

MANUEL B. GRAEBER, WILLIAM F. BLAKEMORE AND GEORG W. KREUTZBERG

THE NEURON

The great variety of neuronal morphology demonstrates that in reality there is no prototypical nerve cell. Considering all the different shapes and sizes of sensory or autonomic ganglion cells, motor neurons, Purkinje cells, granule cells, cortical interneurons or pyramidal cells, it is astonishing that they are all built for the same purpose: to receive, process and transmit information by means of bioelectrical signals. Neurons share all the features of basic metabolism, cytoarchitecture, organelles and functional cell biology with other somatic cells. The usually spherical nucleus shows relatively little heterochromatin and contains one or even two nucleoli. There are mitochondria, lysosomes, Golgi complexes and a rough endoplasmic reticulum (RER) organized in Nissl bodies. Neurons possess an especially elaborate cytoskeleton with microtubules, intermediate filaments and microfilaments used as scaffolds or motors to manage the enormous task of cytoplasmic transport in the axons and the dendrites. This reflects the need to support the unique morphology of neurons which are asymmetrical and polarized to an extent not seen in any other cell. A sophisticated transport system is needed to supply the axon, which does not have any protein synthesis of its own, and the dendrites (see Chapter 1, this volume). The enormous variety of molecules needed to sustain information processing at the synapse and along the neuronal membranes may be the reason for another outstanding feature of the nerve cell: the great variety of genes transcribed in neurons. Up to 50% of all genes may be expressed only in the nervous system to a significant extent.[88,603]

It is important to realize that neurons change under pathological conditions. This has been investigated most extensively in the motor neurons of the spinal cord and the brainstem after axotomy.[226,321] Much knowledge on the plasticity of regulatory mechanisms in injured neurons has been gained through studies of the nerve cell body's response to axonal lesions (see below).

Neuronal cell death

During fetal development neurons are mitotically active in the walls of both the neural tube and the ventricular cavities (Fig. 3.1). In the developing central nervous system (CNS), proliferating and migrating neurons are abundant. Excess neuronal cell populations, however, are usually eliminated by programmed cell death at the critical late stages of development when proliferation, migration, neurite outgrowth and initial synaptogenesis occur. After birth, production of neurotrophins is rapidly downregulated in the CNS and neuronal proliferation subsides. Adult mammalian neurons, with the exception of the olfactory epithelium,[230] are postmitotic and cannot be replaced. Thus, neuronal loss without replacement by proliferation is a characteristic feature of CNS injury. Although the natural capacity for neuronal regeneration is extremely limited in the adult mammalian brain, the

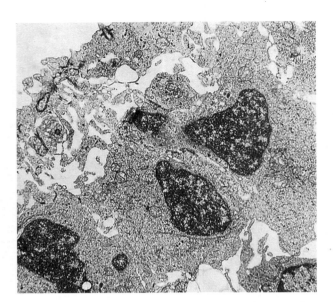

Figure 3.1 *Dividing neuroblast in the periventricular zone of rat embryo at embryonic day 14. Electron micrograph.*

factors which are involved are now beginning to be elucidated. It is only very recently that convincing evidence has been obtained in support of the existence of stem cells in the adult CNS that may contribute to neuronal renewal.[98,132,197,328]

Nerve cell death in the CNS may take different forms representing a spectrum of morphologies and mechanisms ranging from classical apoptosis during development to necrosis in ischaemia and infectious diseases.[133,299] Examples in ageing, common neurodegenerative diseases such as Alzheimer's, Parkinson's and amyotrophic lateral sclerosis (ALS), ischaemia and neuronal cell death after infectious and toxic insults are given in Chapters 5 and 13, this Volume, and Chapters 1–6, Volume II.

APOPTOSIS AND 'PROGRAMMED' CELL DEATH

Cell death as a sporadic event was first recognized more than a century ago. In 1885 Flemming[154] observed cell death characterized by conspicuous chromatin condensation in the ovarian follicle of the rabbit. This description of physiologically occurring cell death was confirmed by Nissen in the lactating mammary glands.[426] The term apoptosis (in Greek *apo* means 'from' and *ptosis* means 'a fall'; i.e. the term literally suggests the image of leaves dropping off here and there from a tree as a natural process) refers to cell death which occurs as a normal event during development in many growing tissues.[106,260,296,365,545,668] Since this type of cell death is primarily controlled by an internal programme, i.e. activation of 'cell death genes', rather than external factors,[538] it represents a form of 'programmed' cell death.

Classical apoptosis has a distinct nuclear morphology studied in detail by Kerr *et al.*[296] At an early stage of apop-

tosis the outer nuclear membrane emits several pseudopodia, a process aptly described as budding and also referred to as zeiosis (in Greek *zio* means 'I boil'). The process of budding is not yet completely understood but it appears to involve disconnection between the cell membrane and the underlying cytoskeleton. Upon DNA fragmentation the chromatin condenses into various shapes:[365,503,668] occasionally, two half-moons or variations of curved profiles of fragmented DNA are observed in apoptotic cells. At its final stage the nuclear DNA often disintegrates into several apoptotic bodies which may be rapidly removed by neighbouring cells and/or invading mononuclear phagocytes. An apoptotic cell, however, may also shrink into one dense mass and form a single apoptotic body. A detailed description of the morphological characteristics of apoptosis can be found in Wyllie *et al.*[668]

Apoptosis can run its course in minutes to hours. It may thus be relatively unobtrusive in tissue sections.[545,668] Apoptotic cells can be recognized by their characteristic morphology of nuclear break-up (karyorrhexis). Morphological evaluation is greatly facilitated in semithin sections. Since forms of apoptosis can vary morphologically, identification of apoptotic cells in tissue sections has been improved by molecular biological techniques.[173,195] These techniques, also referred to as TUNEL (terminal transferase-mediated nick-end labelling) or ISEL (*in situ* end labelling), take advantage of the fact that internucleosomal DNA cleavage exposes endings of DNA strands which can be labelled enzymically by adding tails of either biotinylated or digoxigenin-labelled nucleotides. Yet, TUNEL or ISEL labelling per se does not prove the occurrence of apoptotic cell death.[93,228,273,658] Importantly, TUNEL-negative neuronal cell death also occurs (see below).[119] The biochemical hallmark of apoptosis is internucleosomal DNA fragmentation into relatively small fragments of approximately 180–200 base pairs which is achieved by activation of a Ca^{2+}/Mg^{2+}-dependent endonuclease.[24] This DNA fragmentation gives rise to a characteristic DNA laddering if DNA extracted from apoptotic cells is separated by gel electrophoresis. In contrast to necrosis, apoptotic cells rarely occur in clusters but are usually single cells throughout a given tissue.[296,365]

Programmed cell death requires *de novo* gene expression.[539] It is initiated by the activation of specific genes, the expression of which can be triggered by external agents such as hormones, cytokines, physical or chemical agents and viruses.[371] Over the past few years, numerous genes have been identified which regulate cell proliferation and cell death by either promoting or inhibiting the entry of a cell into a cell death pathway.[387] Genetic control of cell survival has been intensively studied in a nematode (*Caenorhabditis elegans*).[142] The adult worm possesses 959 cells which remain after death of another 131 cells during development. Apoptosis in *C. elegans* requires three genes: *ced-3*, *ced-4* and *egl-1*. If *ced-3*, *ced-4* or *egl-1* is eliminated, apoptosis does not take place and the 131 extra cells

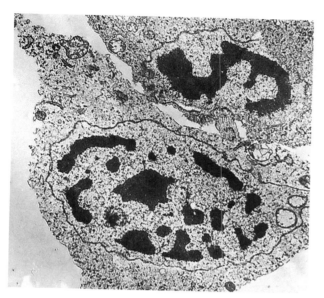

Figure 3.2 *Apoptotic neuron. Electron micrograph of an apoptotic neuron exhibiting DNA fragmentation in the dorsal root ganglion of a rat embryo at embryonic day 16.*

survive. In mammals, one important protein inhibiting apoptosis is the 25 kDa protein bcl-2, first identified in non-Hodgkin's lymphoma. bcl-2 shows sequence homology to *ced-9*, which also prevents cell death in the nematode *C. elegans*.[251,261] *ced-3* resembles the human caspases which act as proteases, whereas *ced-4* is similar to a human gene called *Apaf-1*.[674]

Another important development in recent years is the realization that mitochondria play a crucial role in the control of cell death mechanisms. They can be regarded as the 'cellular centres of death control'.[326,345,588]

Apoptosis plays its most prominent role in the developing nervous system. Many neurons undergo apoptosis at defined stages of development. One of the best examples of apoptosis as a mechanism to eliminate excessive neurons by growth factor deprivation is the dorsal root ganglion (DRG) (Fig. 3.2). Between embryonic day (E) 14 and E16 in the rat, almost half of the DRG neurons undergo apoptosis.[101] This phenomenon is most probably related to the downregulation of nerve growth factor (NGF) synthesis. NGF is produced and released by the peripheral targets of sympathetic and sensory neurons and thus determines, after synaptic uptake and retrograde axonal transport, neuronal maintenance or death.[120] Other neurotrophins (see below) and ciliary neurotrophic factor (CNTF) may also be important for motor neuron survival.[548] Growth factor deprivation is a common mechanism by which apoptosis of sensory and motor neurons is induced in the developing nervous system. Among glial cells, oligodendrocytes appear to be particularly vulnerable to programmed cell death. Apoptosis of oligodendrocytes predominates in multiple system atrophy,[337,474] which may well represent a primary gliodegenerative disorder (see Chapter 6, Volume II). Glial cells are more

sensitive than neurons to the action of a number of toxins.[167,236,591] In human immunodeficiency virus-1 (HIV-1) encephalitis, single-stranded DNA breaks are detected in neurons, in reactive astrocytes and rarely in multinucleated giant cells (see Chapter 1, Volume II).[465] In multiple sclerosis (MS), DNA fragmentation is predominantly found in T lymphocytes and in oligodendrocytes at the edges of actively demyelinating lesions (see Chapter 7, Volume II).[447] This observation is in line with the finding that autoreactive, encephalitogenic T-lymphocytes undergo DNA fragmentation within 72–96 h after CNS infiltration in experimental autoimmune encephalomyelitis (EAE).[455,525] Thus, elimination of autoreactive T-lymphocytes is achieved mainly by induction of programmed cell death in the brain.

INJURY-INDUCED OR ACCIDENTAL CELL DEATH: NECROSIS

Necrosis is the term used for non-apoptotic, accidental cell death, occurring in response to external stimuli such as mild heat or toxic agents. A common form of necrosis occurs after ischaemia. Light microscopical changes are preceded by ultrastructural changes such as disintegration of ribosomes and cytoskeleton, and by biochemical alterations such as disturbed protein synthesis. By light microscopy, necrosis is signalled by nuclear alterations (karyolysis, pyknosis and karyorrhexis) and by cytoplasmic changes (intensive cytoplasmic eosinophilia, loss of structure and fragmentation; see below). These changes are not specific for necrosis, but may also be seen in apoptosis. Unlike apoptotic cells, however, which tend to die singly, necrotic cells usually die in large clusters giving rise to large lesions, e.g. ischaemic infarcts.

In necrosis, morphological changes in mitochondria and an increased influx of calcium across cell membranes are the pathological hallmarks, whereas nuclear changes are less obvious, particularly in the early stages. Increased calcium passage through neuronal membranes can occur via two main cytoplasmic membrane channels: voltage-dependent and receptor-activated. Excitotoxic amino acids bind to *N*-methyl-D-aspartate (NMDA) channels which open receptor-associated sodium channels. The resulting membrane depolarization opens voltage-dependent calcium channels, thus causing an influx of calcium into the cell. Nerve cells which are highly vulnerable to ischaemia express NMDA receptors on their surface, and cell death of such neurons can be prevented by administration of NMDA receptor antagonists such as dizocilpine maleate (MK-801). Other types of non-NMDA receptors involved in excitotoxic cell death are AMPA (α-amino-3-hydroxy-5-methyl-4-isoxazole propionic acid) receptors, which can be antagonized, for example, by NBQX [2,3-dihydroxy-6-nitro-7-sulphamoylbenzo(F)-quinoxaline].

After ischaemia, vulnerable neurons undergo a sequence of characteristic morphological changes.[75]

Within the first 6 h after ischaemia neurons are slightly shrunken and the perikaryon shows microvacuolation, corresponding chiefly to swollen mitochondria. After more prolonged survival ischaemic cell death develops as a gradual transition from the stage of microvacuolation to one in which the neuron is shrunken and stains darkly with cresyl violet. The cytoplasm becomes markedly eosinophilic in haemotoxylin and eosin (H&E)-stained sections and contains fine, granular, dispersed Nissl substance. The nucleus is also shrunken, often triangular and darkly stained. A later stage is homogenizing cell change: the cytoplasm is uniformly structureless and eosinophilic. The nucleus shows advanced degeneration with disintegration of the nuclear membrane. The end-stage of hypoxic cell damage is a shrunken and fragmented nucleus without distinguishable cytoplasm.

Neuronophagia is an acute process that follows fatal injuries to nerve cells. It is seen most prominently in infectious and toxic lesions (see Fig. 3.61). In ischaemic lesions its frequency decreases with the severity of the damage. By light microscopy, groups of activated microglial cells accumulate around dying neurons. Mitotic figures and transformation of microglia into brain macrophages are common. Nerve cell bodies and dendrites are the main targets of phagocytosis. Pyramidal cells of the cerebral cortex, fatally damaged by inflammatory or toxic events, can be invaded by activated microglial cells. In this case the former contour of the large neurons can be preserved and the cluster of microglia often assumes the shape of the dying cell. Thus, neuronophagia is a process of active phagocytosis in which microglia act as scavengers. In Fig. 3.60, this process is documented in a remote CNS lesion caused by retrograde axonal transport of toxic ricin via the facial nerve.[582] This leads to death of the affected motor neurons and phagocytosis of the neuronal soma and dendrites by resident microglia-derived brain macrophages.

TYPES OF CELL DEATH

Apoptosis has become an important research field. However, while the classical definition of apoptosis is a morphological one,[668] the term is now being used in a much broader sense.[382] This causes some problems. For instance, whereas the role of apoptosis during CNS development is unquestioned, its contribution to neurodegeneration is controversial.[20,35,249,313,369,401,403,573,595,597,667] The matter is complicated further by the fact that the 'death phenotype' of cells depends on their energy status,[344] with apoptosis and necrosis possibly representing stages of a metabolic and morphological spectrum.[471] In addition, there is increasing evidence that other forms of cell death exist in the CNS[21,105,123,126,168,210,293,396,448,621] which are likely to be influenced by genetic factors.[616] Aposklesis[210] (withering) has been proposed as a term to denote the slow fading away of nerve cells after axotomy in the adult and in the parkinsonian nigra where TUNEL

staining is detectable in the absence of apoptotic and necrotic morphology. Furthermore, non-apoptotic 'dark' degenerating neurons can be observed in a mouse model of experimental Huntington's disease.[119,616] The dying nerve cells in the latter are even TUNEL negative. Both aposklesis and dark degeneration take a much slower course than apoptosis. Furthermore, the following types of dark neuron must be distinguished from the above: (1) the dark cells of Cammermeyer which represent a preparation artefact;[74] (2) reversible (early stages of hypoglycaemic neuronal injury, epilepsy, ischaemia, spreading depression); (3) irreversible dark cell changes in ischaemic neurons[305] (for a detailed discussion see Chapter 5, this Volume). Importantly, intravital, non-artefactual neuronal damage shows a time course and often conforms to a pattern of selective vulnerability ('pathoclisis'). Thus, the term apoptosis should be used with caution, especially in the context of the adult nervous system. Often it is difficult for the neuropathologist to know with certainty which of the above processes has taken place. However, the correct interpretation of the observed phenomena may be of importance in medicolegal cases.

Regenerative response of motor neurons

The capacity for regeneration and repair after injury of CNS neurons is very limited although extrinsic neurons, i.e. nerve cells whose axons leave the CNS environment, generally do better (see below). By the use of peripheral nerve grafts, Aguayo and his colleagues were able to stimulate axotomized retinal ganglion cells and other CNS neurons to grow new axons out of the proximal stump (Fig. 3.3) and elongate over several millimetres into the graft and the brainstem.[5,47] It has also been demonstrated that various types of CNS graft transplanted into the brain can survive and form connections in the host organ.

A pivotal observation that has been used to explain the limited capacity of axonal elongation in the injured CNS came from studying the interactions of oligodendroglial

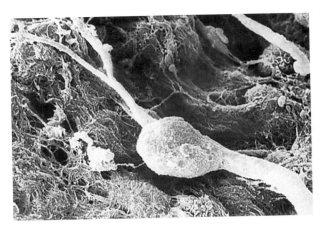

Figure 3.3 *Axonal growth cone. Scanning electron micrograph of an axonal growth cone in a regenerating peripheral nerve.*

cells and neurons in cell cultures.[536] Oligodendroglia produce molecules inhibitory to axonal elongation and if these inhibitory molecules are blocked, considerable axonal growth can be observed in the lesioned spinal cord.[528,534] This growth process is significantly enhanced if growth factors, called neurotrophins, are simultaneously applied.[87,527] Extrinsic neurons such as the motor neurons located in the spinal cord, the medulla oblongata and the midbrain as well as the ganglion cells of the peripheral nervous system (PNS), e.g. the dorsal root ganglia, are constitutively capable of growing new axons and thus anatomically reconnect to the lost peripheral target.

REACTION OF THE NEURONAL CELL BODY TO AXON DAMAGE

Axonal injury can occur after trauma, compression, inflammation or other types of lesion. Interrupting the continuity of axons leads to a characteristic retrograde reaction in the neurons of origin accompanied by marked alterations in the satellite glial cells. The terms 'axon reaction' and 'retrograde' or 'axonal response' are all used synonymously. The term 'chromatolysis' can be misleading and should be defined strictly as a decrease or loss of compact basophilia in the perinuclear region of the neuron[614] (Fig. 3.4).

The light microscopical changes occurring after axotomy can be best studied in Nissl-stained sections. Within the first week after lesioning, the axotomized neurons

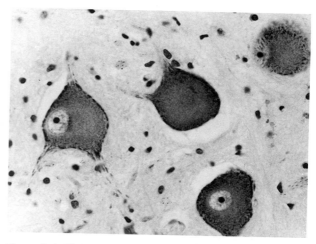

Figure 3.4 *Chromatolysis. Chromatolysis in anterior horn cells of the lumbar cord in a case with long-standing peripheral neuropathy. Note the rounded shape of the neurons, eccentric nuclei, the loss of Nissl bodies from the central part of the cell and their persistence at its periphery. (Cresyl violet.) Reproduced by permission from Ref. 134.*

display swelling of the cell body, dispersal of the Nissl substance (Fig. 3.5) and peripheral displacement and deformation of the nucleus.[427] However, the use of basic dyes shows increased staining of the perikaryon, reflecting the increase in ribosomal RNA lacking the usual organization of structured Nissl bodies. In brief, these neurons are

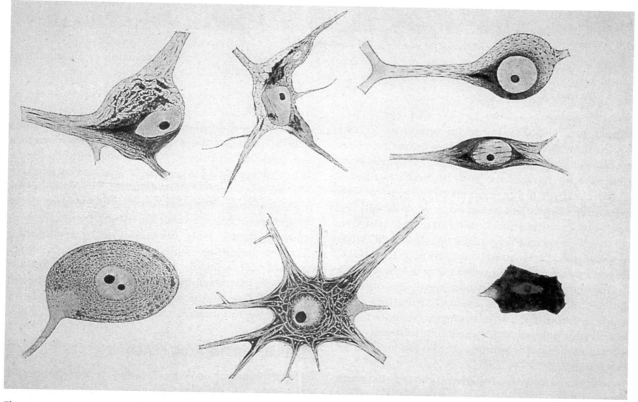

Figure 3.5 *Neurons drawn by Franz Nissl (reproduced from his original drawing).*

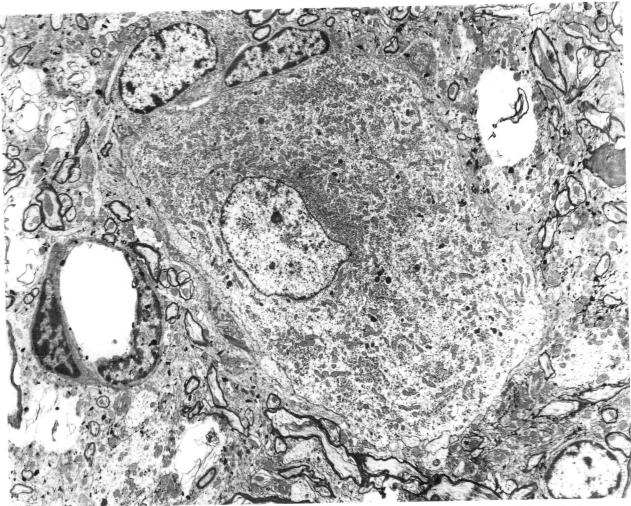

Figure 3.6 *Axonal reaction. Injured rat facial motor neuron exhibiting fine structural changes characteristic of the cell body response: peripheral displaced nucleus, dense nuclear cap consisting of granular endoplasmic reticulum, disappearance of organized Nissl bodies, increased free ribosomes/polysomes, and undulating plasmalemma covered by glial cell processes with loss of synaptic terminals. Electron micrograph.*

hypertrophic and will stay so for several weeks, even beyond the time when reinnervation of the peripheral target has been achieved.[237] In adult rat primary sensory neurons, axotomy-induced apoptosis has been described.[235]

The ultrastructure of axotomized neurons has been extensively studied and described in great detail[44] (Fig. 3.6). Comparative studies in central and peripheral nerve cells serving different functional modalities have revealed differences as well as common alterations.[42] Important factors which modify the neuronal responses to axotomy include: species and age of the organism, nature of the axonal injury (axotomy, neurotmesis, avulsion), contact with the distal stump (to enable or prevent regeneration), proximity of the lesion to the nerve cell soma, and the type of neuron according to function and localization.[137,425,585,677]

Axotomized neurons display conspicuous ultrastructural changes. The nucleus is peripherally displaced (eccentric) and loses its spherical shape by developing indentations and scalloping of the nuclear envelope facing the centre of the cell. A large Nissl body with an extremely high density of ribosomes can often be seen as a 'nuclear cap'. Of all the organelles that have increased in the cell body, the free ribosomes and polysomes are the most prominent. The cisternae of the RER become shorter and are no longer arranged in parallel arrays. The contour of the cell body, normally smooth and concave between the parting primary dendrites, becomes convex and wavy, reflecting the hypertrophy of the cell and the instability of the cell membrane. The surface of the cell body and also the stem dendrites are covered by glial profiles having lost most, if not all, presynaptic terminals.[68]

SIGNAL FOR THE AXON REACTION

Hypertrophy, organelle increase and nuclear changes are structural correlates of an enhanced or changed gene expression in the neuron after axotomy. The identity of the

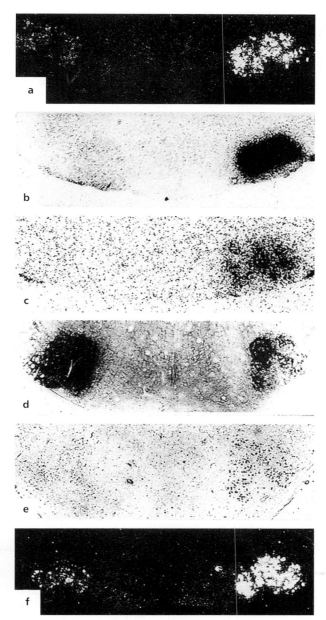

Figure 3.7 *Molecular changes in the regenerating facial nucleus of experimental animals. (a) Induction of c-jun mRNA 8 h after axotomy. In situ hybridization, dark-field exposure. (b) Increase in glucose uptake by deoxyglucose accumulation 7 days after axotomy. (c) Induction of transforming growth factor (TGF)β₁ mRNA 7 days after axotomy. In situ hybridization, bright-field exposure. (d) Decrease in acetylcholinesterase (AChE) activity 18 days after axotomy. (e) Induction of NADPH enzyme activity, an isoenzyme of the neuronal nitric oxide synthase (NOS), 4 days after axotomy. Enzyme histochemistry. (f) Induction of calcitonin gene-related peptide (CGRP) mRNA, a neurotransmitter of cholinergic neurons, 1 day after axotomy. In situ hybridization, dark-field exposure.*

signal for the response of the nerve cell body to axotomy is still unknown. It could be bioelectrical, structural (e.g. interruption of cytoskeleton) or molecular (e.g. the lack of a trophic factor coming from the periphery, the action of a factor derived from the lesion site or a premature return of previously anterogradely transported substances).[115,225] The most favoured view is the interruption of the supply of a trophic factor, e.g. neurotrophins or neurocytokines, conveyed to the cell body by retrograde axonal transport. There is experimental evidence that blocking retrograde transport by colchicine delays axotomy-induced retrograde changes.[561] In otherwise intact hypoglossal nerves, blockade of anterograde and retrograde axonal transport leads to retrograde neuronal and glial reactions similar to those seen after axotomy.[11]

THE NEURONAL REGENERATION PROGRAMME

There is abundant evidence for a significant change in gene expression of neurons after axotomy. Increases in cytoskeletal and other housekeeping proteins can be observed. Neurotransmitter-related enzymes and receptors are down-regulated and satellite glial cells become activated. After axotomy in sympathetic and motor neurons, a fast upregulation of the immediate-early genes (IEGs) and transcription factors occurs.[238,252,283] Some IEGs (such as *c-fos*, *c-jun* or *junB*) encode transcription factors that bind to DNA at sites known to regulate gene expression and therefore could contribute to long-term changes in motor neurons. Hours after injury, Northern blot analysis has revealed that injured motor neurons show a unique pattern of IEG induction: high levels of *c-jun* and *junB* messenger RNAs (mRNAs) are maintained up to 8 days after axotomy. However, *c-fos*, which is known to act in concert with *c-jun* in other systems, is not expressed, nor is it induced by axotomy in regenerating neurons. The mRNA of the transcription factor *TIS-11* increases in a fashion similar to *c-jun* and *junB* with an early rise at 10 h that lasts for many days (Fig. 3.7). In addition, there are complex and co-ordinated changes in the glial cell population (see below; see also Fig. 3.58).

In situ hybridization histochemistry has demonstrated that *c-jun* mRNA is localized in motor neurons, indicating that *c-jun* induction occurs in the course of the retrograde reaction that accompanies the response in the axotomized neurons, but not in satellite glial cells. In the injured facial nucleus *junB* and *TIS-11* mRNAs are localized in neurons.

CYTOSKELETAL PROTEINS

Proteins forming the cytoskeleton of the axon are known to be delivered by slow axonal transport[265] (see Chapter 1, this Volume). The main components are the neurofilament triplet and the tubulins moving with the 'slow component a' (SCa) and actin transported with the 'slow component b' (SCb).[224] These proteins exhibit profound changes in the amounts transported in axons after lesioning and during regeneration: neurofilament proteins decrease, while tubulins and actin increase.[264,562] Corresponding changes in the cell bodies of axotomized neurons have been demonstrated. In a wide variety of sensory sympathetic and motor neurons in lower vertebrates, birds and mammals, axotomy induces an increase in the synthesis of tubulins and actin and a decrease in synthesis of the neurofilament triplet proteins.[250,263,433,600]

Neurofilaments may serve as spacers in the axoplasm that contribute to the stability and the rigidity of the axon. The decrease in these intermediate filaments thus could lead to an increase in the fluidity of axoplasm; this could facilitate and enhance axonal bulk transport. It has been shown that SCb carrying, for example, actin, is accelerated by 20% in axons conditioned by a lesion.[279] In the goldfish optic nerve, protein transport is also enhanced during regeneration.[227] The changes in neurofilament protein expression were correlated with changes in the calibre of the axons.[472]

Microtubules are composed of α- and β-tubulins. Synthesis of tubulins is increased in neurons during regeneration.[422,562,600] Therefore, they are prominent organelles in the axon and are the carriers to the molecular motor kinesin that drives axonal transport.[623]

A detailed analysis of the molecular forms of tubulin in axotomized neurons has yielded insights into a highly specific gene induction.[175,262,375,402] There are six different α-tubulin genes in mammals.[633] The embryonic α-tubulin, $T\alpha_1$, is highly expressed in the developing nervous system.[402] It is also strongly upregulated in axotomized facial and spinal motor neurons, in sympathetic neurons and in hippocampal pyramidal cells after an entorhinal lesion. Thus, it seems that, during axonal regeneration, gene expression is switched to a growth-associated programme reverting to the developmental state.

NERVE GROWTH FACTORS AND THEIR RECEPTORS

A gene family of growth factors has been designated as neurotrophins. They include NGF, brain-derived neurotrophic factor (BDNF), neurotrophin-3 (NT-3) and neurotrophin-4/5.[439,440,606] These factors are all target derived, i.e. they are produced by the innervated cells or tissue to reach the neurons via retrograde axonal transport. In nerve cells, the efficacy and specificity of the neurotrophins depend on the presence and number of receptors. They are synthesized by the neurons and are highly regulated after axotomy.[118,285,489] Injury to the sciatic nerve leads to a rapid disappearance of NGF receptors in the severed axons but they are strongly induced in the Schwann cells of the denervated distal stump.[487,488] In dorsal root ganglia, β-NGF receptors quickly vanish from the sensory neurons. This coincides with the disappearance of the receptors from the axons in the proximal stump. The production of NGF receptors is resumed in the perikarya after successful nerve regeneration.[486,632] Two types of NGF receptor have been characterized: the high-affinity trkA glycoprotein and the low-affinity p75 NGF

receptor, which also binds BDNF and NT-3.[138] In sensory neurons, axotomy leads to downregulation of mRNA of both receptors, eventually causing a temporary deprivation of NGF in the perikarya because of the lack of receptors. In addition, the rapid induction of NGF receptors in Schwann cells at the lesion site leads to an advantage of these non-neuronal cells over axons when competing for NGF released at the stump regions.[489] Regeneration of adult sensory nerves does not depend on exogenous NGF. Application of antibodies against NGF has no influence on the speed of nerve regeneration and restoration of sensory function.[127]

Neurotrophins are maintenance factors for a variety of neurons, not only during development, but also after axonal damage. In the neonatal period, BDNF and NT-4/5 are able to save spinal or facial motor neurons.[310,548,670] NGF is effective in protecting DRG cells, sympathetic neurons, and retinal ganglion cells *in vivo* from post-traumatic degeneration.[89,500–502] An action of NGF on lesioned motor neurons also seems possible because axotomy induces the new expression of NGF receptors in spinal motor neurons,[148,310,661] in contrast to the sensory neurons, which downregulate both NGF receptors.

In addition to the known retrograde transport of neurotrophins, there is evidence to suggest that endogenous BDNF is transported anterogradely in peripheral and central neurons. Increased anterograde transport of BDNF has been suggested to play a role in the early neuronal response to peripheral nerve injury at sites distal to the cell body.[14,610]

The function of other neurotrophic agents that are not necessarily target derived is also of interest. CNTF has a strong protective action on lesioned motor neurons and suppresses even the chromatolysis of axotomized neurons.[547,548] Glial cell-line derived neurotrophic factor (GDNF) was initially identified as a trophic factor for dopaminergic neurons of the substantia nigra.[348] In testing its potential in the facial nucleus, GDNF was demonstrated to have a profound neurotrophic effect on lesioned motor neurons *in vivo*.[420,441,671]

Basic fibroblast growth factor (bFGF) has a similar, although much weaker, action on immature motor and on sensory neurons.[234,445] FGF also supports the survival of mammalian retinal ganglion cells after optic nerve section.[558] Its efficacy depends on the post-injury interval.[267] Insulin-like growth factor-I (IGF-I) promotes sciatic nerve regeneration.[291] Transforming growth factor-β (TGF-β) has also been suggested to play a functional role in the regeneration of motor neurons.[108]

Growth-associated proteins (GAPs)

GAP-43/B50 is a membrane phosphoprotein that is associated with neuronal development and plasticity, especially with axonal sprouting and elongation.[15,187,652] Although its precise function is not yet known, GAP-43/B50 seems to be a substrate for protein kinase C13 and thus could be modulated by extracellular signals instrumental in establishing axonal connectivities.[395] GAP-43/B50 is synthesized in neurons and its mRNA is upregulated quickly in central and peripheral neurons after axotomy.[117,599,666] The protein is transported rapidly down the axons and is present in the axonal sprouts as soon as they are formed.[267,626,666]

Transferrin is a plasma protein that functions as a transporter for iron into the cell. Iron is an essential element in the biotransport of oxygen and in electron transfer. Tissue cultures of normal and malignant cells require this factor for maintenance and particularly for cell proliferation.[400] The key molecule for iron delivery to the tissue is the transferrin receptor, which is expressed constitutively at brain capillaries.[372] Transection of the facial nerve leads to a dramatic upregulation of transferrin receptors in the motor neurons with subsequent transport to the growing axon. This is another example of neuronal capacity to change from stability to a growth process to provide the necessary means for formation of a new axon.[215,485]

OXIDATIVE METABOLISM IN THE REGENERATION PROCESS

Among the many changes which occur in a neuron that responds to axonal lesioning, there are interesting alterations in the intermediate metabolism of carbohydrates (Fig. 3.7). One day after facial or hypoglossal nerve transection, the corresponding motor nuclei in the brainstem show a significant increase in glucose uptake that remains elevated for 4–6 weeks.[323,559,560] It seems possible that the increase in glucose uptake is needed to supply the hexose monophosphate shunt, which can produce riboses for the enhanced synthesis of RNA. The key enzymes of this shunt, glucose-6-dehydrogenase and 6-phosphogluconate dehydrogenase, both display an increase in activity after axotomy.[245,317,602]

Quantitative measurements in the regenerating hypoglossal nucleus have revealed an increase of 84% in glucose utilization over control values.[567] It is not clear for what processes such a large additional amount of energy is required. Enzymes of the glycolytic pathway and the Krebs cycle do not show any changes in their activity. A substantial increase in the level of glycogen phosphorylase in axotomized sciatic motor neurons indicates a switch to active glycogen production, which also could account for the large increase in glucose uptake.[665] Nitric oxide synthase (NOS) expression in motor neurons after nerve injury appears to be regulated by signals derived from peripheral reinnervation targets.[677]

NEUROTRANSMISSION-RELATED CHANGES FOLLOWING AXOTOMY

Most of the changes discussed previously reflect increased cellular activity, the metabolic counterpart of neuronal hypertrophy. Several changes, however, point in another direction, namely that of reduced functional activity. This applies especially to neurotransmitter-related proteins, such as receptors or enzymes involved in the biosynthesis or degradation of transmitters, e.g. muscarinic receptors, dopamine-β-hydroxylase, tyrosine hydroxylase and choline acetyltransferase (AChE).

AChE is probably the best investigated representative of this group (Fig. 3.7). It decreases to about 60% of normal activity in the rat facial nucleus and stays at this value for about 4 weeks before slowly recovering. Light and electron microscopic histochemistry shows enzyme activity to disappear quickly from the dendrites, while staining of perikarya is still visible. In the facial nucleus of the guinea-pig, AChE is secreted from the dendrites to the extracellular space, leading to enzyme accumulation in the basal laminae of the local capillaries.[324] Moreover, a downregulation of other cholinergic proteins (e.g. choline acetyltransferase, the muscarinic and the nicotinic cholinergic receptors) has been reported in axotomized neurons of various types.[26,546]

Glycine receptors, demonstrated in the form of binding sites, decreased by about 50% for 25 days in the hypoglossal nucleus in response to nerve transection.[509] Similarly, the expression of γ-aminobutyric acid-A (GABA$_A$) receptors seems to decrease in axotomized DRGs. As a consequence, GABA sensitivity of the dorsal roots decreases.[304] This injury-induced decline in the GABA response is modulated by the type of surgery employed, suggesting a regulatory influence of neurotrophic factors from the periphery.[49] In central and peripheral catecholaminergic neurons, decreases to various degrees of norepinephrine, tyrosine hydroxylase, dopamine-β-hydroxylase and monoamine oxidase have been reported.[94,508]

NEUROPEPTIDES

Neuropeptides are abundant in the sensory neurons but relatively rare in motor neurons. Their role in regeneration and repair is not fully understood, although they are also differentially regulated after axotomy in the affected nerve cell bodies. The best studied is calcitonin gene-related peptide (CGRP) (Fig. 3.7) which, although present in sensory neurons, is most prominent in motor neurons. It shows a marked increase in both mRNA and peptide in motor neurons after peripheral section of the facial, hypoglossal and sciatic nerves.[28,239,280,406,469,577] An initial increase in peptide immunoreactivity is seen as early as 15 h after axotomy, with a first peak at 3 days and a second peak 3 weeks after surgery. In the facial nucleus, CGRP mRNA is present in 50% of the motor neurons. Specific probes used for in situ hybridization have shown that this increase is due only to upregulation of α-CGRP,[430] which differs from β-CGRP by only one amino acid. In contrast to the motor neurons, the primary sensory neurons of the spinal ganglia respond to axotomy with a decrease in CGRP.[135,136] Again, in contrast to the motor neurons, α-CGRP and β-CGRP mRNA decreases, returning to normal values when regeneration is allowed to take place.[430,513]

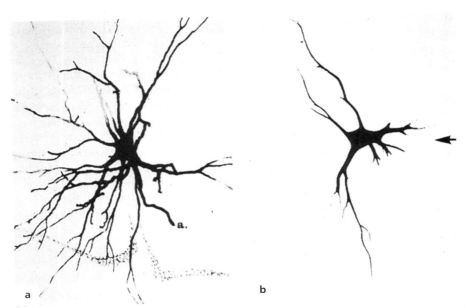

a　　　　　　　　　　　　　　b

Figure 3.8 *Dendritic tree of motor neurons. Reconstruction of the labelled dendritic tree of two motor neurons intracellularly injected with [³H]glycine. (a) Control neuron. All the dendrites and their individual branches can be followed throughout their length, many beyond the level of reconstruction (1000 μm). (b) Colchicine-treated neuron. Dendrites are devastated and radioactivity is transported no further than 100–200 μm from the soma, indicating disruption of dendritic transport by colchicine. Reproduced by permission from Ref. 532.*

The expression of various neuropeptides and their mRNAs has been extensively studied in the rat spinal cord after sciatic nerve transection.[29] Sensitive *in situ* hybridization methods have revealed the plasticity of peptide expression. Surprisingly, it was found that only subpopulations and occasionally only a few neurons upregulated mRNA for peptides: this occurred for galanin, vasoactive intestinal peptide (VIP) and substance P, for periods of 2–3 weeks after injury.[550,683] Tyrosine and somatostatin seem to be upregulated for a slightly longer time in both motor and sensory neurons.[638] A downregulation was seen for enkephalin mRNA in spinal neurons.[683] In summary, peptide expression is altered strongly after axon lesioning. In addition, the upregulation or downregulation of metabolic parameters and their time course may considerably vary. The relationship between these responses and the capacity of the individual neuron to regenerate remains to be determined.

Importantly, downregulation of μ-opioid receptors has been observed after peripheral axotomy of DRG neurons in rats and non-human primates. and in the spinal interneurons of the dorsal horn. This may represent one factor underlying the well-known insensitivity of neuropathic pain to opioid analgesics.[682]

Pathology of dendrites

The general features of dendritic morphology and ultrastructure are described in Chapter 1 of this Volume. Damage to the dendrites sooner or later extends also to the presynaptic or axonal compartment. Unlike axons, dendrites have a machinery to synthesize proteins. Like axons, however, they are also supplied by components produced and transported from the neuronal cell body. Dendritic transport has a speed of at least 3 mm/h.[531] This means that large neurons, e.g. motor neurons, neurons of the reticular formation, Purkinje cells or pyramidal cells with a dendritic field extending 1000 μm into the neuropil, can reach their periphery with newly synthesized proteins within 20 min. The transport can be blocked by

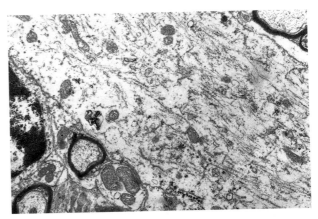

Figure 3.9 *Dendritic damage. Local application of colchicine to the spinal cord of an experimental animal causes severe disease in the stem dendrite of a motor neuron. The most conspicuous organelles of normal dendrites, the microtubules with their bridges of microtubulin-associated proteins (MAPs), have disintegrated. Electron micrograph.*

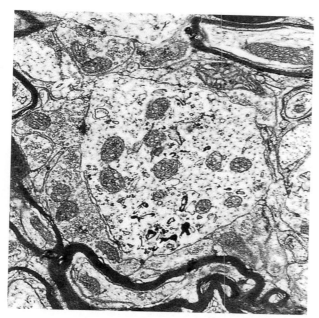

Figure 3.10 *Dendritic changes in a 'knockout' mouse. Electron micrograph of dendritic changes in a CNTF 'knockout' mouse. Courtesy of Dr M Sendtner, University of Würzburg, Germany.*

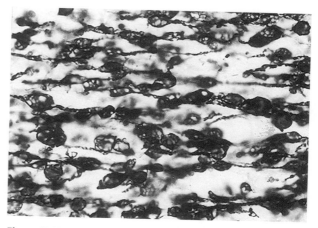

Figure 3.12 *Wallerian degeneration. Degenerating myelinated fibres in the superior cerebellar peduncle 10 days after infarction of the dentate nucleus. Myelin sheaths are broken up into ovoids. (Luxol fast blue–cresyl violet.) Reproduced by permission from Ref. 134.*

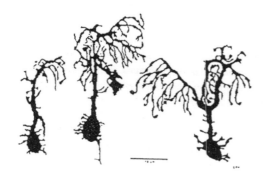

Figure 3.11 *Purkinje cells in Menkes' disease. Dendritic pathology of Purkinje cells in Menkes' kinky hair disease. The main dendritic system is atrophic and devoid of tertiary branchlets. Camera lucida drawing of a silver impregnation. Adapted by permission from Ref. 476.*

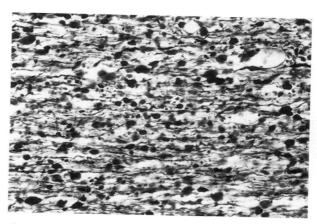

Figure 3.13 *Degenerating nerve fibre. Degenerating nerve fibres in the white matter near an infarct of 10 days' duration. Silver impregnation shows the axons broken up into argyrophilic fragments. (Glees silver impregnation.) Reproduced by permission from Ref. 134.*

colchicine, indicating that it depends on intact microtubules,[532] since colchicine severely affects the dendritic cytoskeleton (Figs 3.8, 3.9). After axotomy dendrites of motor neurons become retracted and lose some presynaptic terminals.[68,586] A certain degree of plasticity in dendritic spines has also been observed in neurons under the influence of gonadal steroids:[203] hypothalamic neurons are subjected to periodic changes in dendritic physiology and synaptic morphology according to their functional state controlled by various hormones.[27,477,604] Dendritic atrophy has been reported in sympathetic ganglion cells in aged rats. Treatment with exogenous NGF can reverse the age-related dendritic and axonal changes.[18]

In man, abnormalities in dendritic spines have been reported in cases of developmental retardation. The shape, length and number of spines seem to be reduced in Down's syndrome, and in Patau's syndrome (trisomy 13) and in handicapped children without an obvious karyotype.[369,584] Dendritic spine dysgenesis seems to be related to age and the severity of mental retardation.[475]

Biopsy material from patients undergoing surgery for temporal lobe epilepsy revealed dendritic pathology in the pyramidal cells and dentate granule cells of the hippocampus. Loss of spines, irregular beading, and both swelling and shrinkage of the shaft segment have been observed and interpreted as a progressive degeneration leading to neuronal cell death[521] (see also Chapter 15, this Volume).

Several hereditary diseases of the CNS in man and mice show remarkable alterations to the dendritic

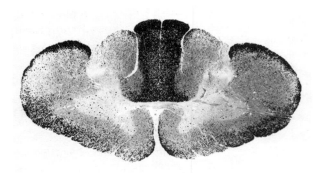

Figure 3.14 *Myelin damage in the spinal cord. Frozen section of cervical (C8) spinal cord after destruction of the lower thoracic cord by metastatic carcinoma. (Products of myelin degeneration in ascending tracts are stained black by the Marchi method.) Reproduced by permission from Ref. 134.*

morphology (Fig. 3.10). Menkes' kinky-hair disease is a sex-linked disorder with developmental retardation based on a defective copper binding protein. The neuropathology shows focal cerebral and cerebellar degeneration, the latter being particularly severe in Purkinje cells: their dendrites are smaller, show irregular and fewer branches and have an anomalous orientation. The Purkinje cell bodies that normally have a smooth surface covered by astrocytic processes show numerous pseudodendritic sprouts that give the neurons the spiny appearance of a cactus[476] (Fig. 3.11).

Pathology of axons

In the middle of the nineteenth century Augustus Waller[639] made the seminal observation that in a severed peripheral nerve the nerve fibres of the distal stump degenerate while those of the proximal stump survive: nerve fibres need to be connected to the cell body as their nutritive centre. This process, called wallerian degeneration, occurs in the distal stump and has four main events: axolysis as a decay of axonal processes, myelinolysis leading to a dissolution of the myelin sheath, phagocytosis of the debris by resident and invading macrophages, and finally the proliferation of Schwann cells (Figs 3.12–3.14). They form the Büngner bands, i.e. rows of Schwann cell nuclei orientated in the longitudinal axis of the nerve. They are covered by continuous basal laminae used as guides for regeneration by ingrowing axons. In the CNS axolysis and myelinolysis are similar to those occurring in the periphery. However, axonal regeneration does not take place spontaneously after fibre tract interruption in the CNS.

The complex, multifunctional axonal transport system is the target of many different noxious insults (Figs 3.15, 3.16). Substances such as colchicine that disrupt microtubules interfere with axonal transport.[139] Lack of oxygen in ischaemia leads to a decrease in adenosine triphosphate

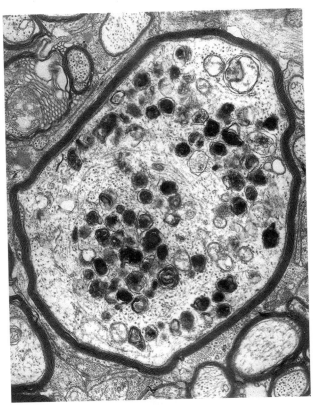

Figure 3.15 *Degenerating nerve fibre. An early stage of nerve fibre degeneration in the CNS. This electron micrograph shows the accumulation of dense bodies, filaments and tubules in the degenerating axon while the myelin sheath is still intact. Preparation by Dr Jean M Jacobs, Institute of Neurology, London, UK. Reproduced by permission from Ref. 134.*

(ATP) necessary to drive the molecular motors. Mechanical irritation of axons, as in spinal injury or brain trauma, influences the phosphorylation state of the neurofilament proteins and thus changes the viscosity of axoplasm, leading to traumatic axonal injury (see Chapter 14 in this Volume).

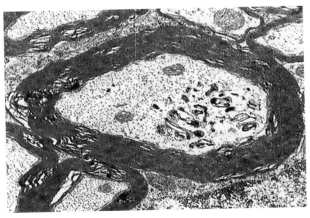

Figure 3.16 *Axonal damage. Axonal pathology in a CNTF 'knockout' mouse. Electron micrograph. Courtesy of Dr M Sendtner, University of Würzburg, Germany.*

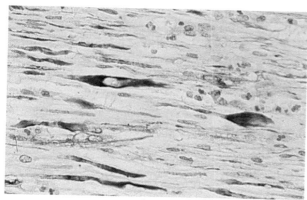

Figure 3.17 *Retraction balls. 'Retraction balls' indicating the presence of swollen, injured axons in white matter in diffuse axonal injury. (Immunostaining for the 68-kDa neurofilament protein.)*

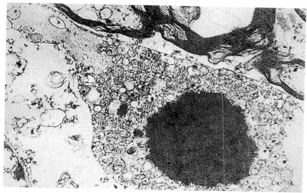

Figure 3.18 *Neuroaxonal spheroids. Large, electron-dense neuroaxonal spheroids in a case of infantile neuroaxonal dystrophy. Electron micrograph. Reproduced by permission from Ref. 134.*

Traumatically induced axonal damage involves a cascade of changes that culminates in the interruption of axons. This 'delayed or secondary axotomy' has been studied successfully in detail by Povlishock.[472] A relatively mild injury may cause a misalignment of neurofilaments such that they lose their typical longitudinal and parallel orientation within 30 min. Neurofilaments lose their phosphorylated sidearms, leading to their close packing and a diminution of microtubules. Impaired axonal transport, with a damming back of organelles, vesiculotubular structures and swelling, can lead to axonal disruption. This delayed axotomy is part of the post-traumatic secondary damage occurring within the first 24 h of injury. It appears to be the most common axonal pathology in traumatic brain injury. For human neuropathology the use of antibodies against the 68 kDa neurofilament protein, the low molecular weight component of the neurofilament triplet, has been proposed as a helpful marker for diffuse axonal injury[205] (Fig. 3.17). However, β-amyloid precursor protein (β-APP) appears to be even more sensitive.[174]

Neuroaxonal dystrophy was first recognized by Seitelberger[541,542] as a pathognomonic substrate for several neurological diseases. Hallervorden-Spatz disease, infantile neuroaxonal dystrophy or Seitelberger's disease, late

infantile and juvenile neuroaxonal dystrophy and the neuroaxonal leukodystrophy are considered primary neuroaxonal dystrophies (Fig. 3.18) (see Chapters 8 and 9, this Volume, and Chapter 6, Volume II).

Secondary or symptomatic forms of neuroaxonal dystrophy occur in the brain with ageing[524] and under various conditions, e.g. chronic alcoholic encephalopathies, mucoviscidosis, and Parkinson's and Wilson's diseases. The morphology of the diseased axons is characterized by the appearance of axonal swellings, the larger of which, measure up to 120 μm in diameter, are designated axonal spheroids. They contain densely packed axoplasmic organelles, including tubulovesicular structures, residual and dense bodies, disintegrated mitochondria and other abnormal profiles. The changes are first seen in the most distal parts of the axon and their terminals. They progress in a retrograde direction leading to demyelination, axonal disconnection and reactive astrocytosis.[541]

Neuronal vacuolation

Neuronal vacuolation is often associated with prominent astrocytosis. Diffuse vacuolation in the grey or white matter is a characteristic change seen in cytotoxic oedema, probably reflecting enlargement of the extracellular space[307] (see Chapter 4, this Volume). In addition, it is seen in some diseases involving the white matter such as subacute degeneration of the spinal cord and spongy degeneration of the white matter in children (Canavan's disease). Neuronal vacuolation also occurs as a degenerative change after fibre tract degeneration or after axotomy. Vacuolation, neuronal loss and disproportionally prominent astrocytosis with massive glial fibrillary acidic protein (GFAP) expression (see below) are typical of transmissible spongiform encephalopathies or prion diseases such as Creutzfeldt–Jakob disease (CJD)[374] (Figs 3.19, 3.20). Ultrastructurally, the spongiform changes in CJD consist of intraneuronal, clear vacuoles often with membranous

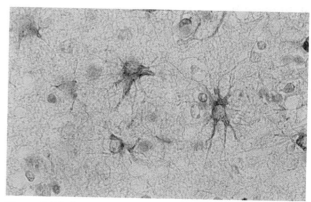

Figure 3.19 *Astrocytoses. Hypertrophic, cortical astrocytes in Creutzfeldt–Jakob disease. [Immunostaining for the astrocytic marker glial fibrillary acidic protein (GFAP) with haematoxylin counterstain.]*

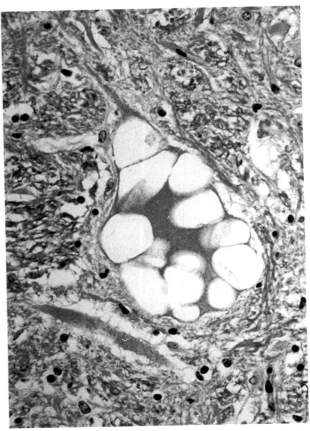

Figure 3.20 *Spongiform change in BSE. Vacuolated neuron from the midbrain in bovine spongiform encephalopathy. The perikaryon is nearly filled with vacuoles which have thin walls, vary in size and appear to be coalescing. (H&E.) Courtesy of Dr GAH Wells. Reproduced by permission from Ref. 134.*

septa, and sometimes containing granular debris (Fig. 3.21). Occasionally, membrane-bound vacuoles may also be seen in axons (see Chapter 5, Volume II).

Physiological changes in neurons associated with ageing

LIPOFUSCIN

Accumulation of lipofuscin granules is a common feature in ageing (see Chapter 4, Volume II). In H&E-stained sections, they retain their typical yellow–brown colour. Lipofuscin granules are abundant in the inferior olive, in the dentate nucleus of the cerebellum and in motor neurons in the anterior horn of the spinal cord. Histochemically, lipofuscin is heterogeneous and consists of lipids, proteins and carbohydrates. Ultrastructurally, it is composed of membrane-bound particles which contain mainly electron-dense, homogeneous material with a granular appearance (Fig. 3.22). These granules are generally considered to be residual bodies derived from lysosomes. In lipofuscinosis, there is a widespread increase in

the number of lipofuscin granules. In addition, lipid inclusions, linked to metabolic diseases such as gangliosidosis, exist, but are morphologically and biochemically distinct from lipofuscin accumulation.

NEUROMELANIN

Neuromelanin, being a byproduct of catecholamine synthesis, is structurally and biochemically distinct from melanin which is confined to melanophores found only in the leptomeninges. It is particularly abundant in the substantia nigra (Fig. 3.23), the locus coeruleus and the dorsal motor nucleus of the vagus nerve. In children, the substantia nigra appears macroscopically pale, although histochemical techniques demonstrate low levels of neuromelanin. Compared with lipofuscin, neuromelanin is much darker in H&E-stained sections and is strongly argentophilic. Ultrastructurally, neuromelanin granules are 1–2.5 μm in diameter and appear as inhomogeneous bodies with irregularly shaped surfaces. They contain coarse dense complexes and light globules in a granular matrix. In Parkinson's disease, there is a typical loss of neuromelanin-containing, dopaminergic neurons in the pars compacta of the substantia nigra.

Additional neuronal changes are discussed in the following chapters: granulovacuolar degeneration (Chapter 4, Volume II), neurofibrillary change (Chapter 4, Volume II), senile plaques (Chapter 4, Volume II), argentophilic inclusions (Pick bodies; Chapter 4, Volume II), Hirano bodies (Chapter 4, Volume II), Lafora bodies (Chapter 15, this Volume), Lewy bodies (Chapter 6, Volume II), Bunina bodies (Chapter 6, Volume II) and viral inclusions (Chapter 1, Volume II).

Molecular genetic basis of neuronal and glial pathology

During the past few years, a large number of neurological 'disease genes', malfunction of which underlies neurogenetic disorders, have been cloned (for detailed information see http://www.ncbi.nlm.nih.gov/Omim/searchomim.html). Two types of neurogenetic disorder can be distinguished. Type 1 neurogenetic diseases are caused by the malfunction of a gene or genes expressed in the neuroectoderm. This results in various classical inherited neurological diseases, including neuromuscular and movement disorders and neurodevelopmental defects. Type 2 neurogenetic diseases comprise disorders in which the neurological disease arises indirectly by the malfunction of a gene not expressed in the nervous system. Various metabolic diseases belong to this category.[413]

While the sequencing of the human genome nears completion, it is becoming evident that neuropathology will be of increasing importance for bridging the gap between the clinical symptomatology and functional biology of CNS diseases.[314,336,470] Microarray analyses,[76] in particular, will play an important role in the development of

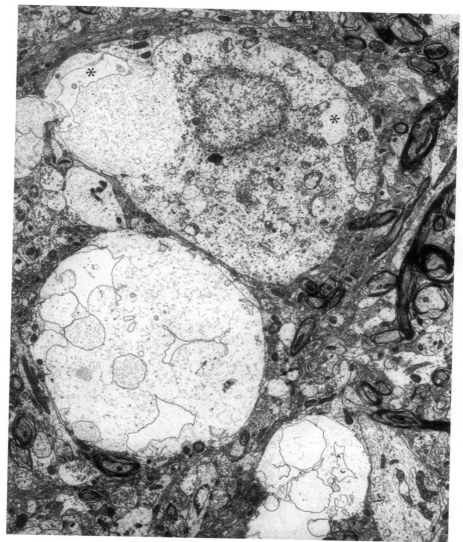

Figure 3.21 *Neuronal vacuolation in experimental prion disease. Neuronal vacuolation in spongiform encephalopathy transmitted experimentally to a marmoset. This electron micrograph shows several membrane-bound vacuoles in the perikaryon of a thalamic neuron as well as large vacuoles lying, probably, in neuronal processes. Reproduced by permission from Ref. 134.*

cell type-, brain region- and disease-specific neurogenetic expression databases. Neuropathologists, equipped with new tools such as laser capture microdissection,[143,533] could take a leading role in this development. The correlation between expression profiles of diseased tissues and classical morphological findings may include the analysis of experimental systems such as transgenic and knockout mice, zebra fish, *C. elegans* and *Drosophila*.[150]

REACTION AND RESPONSES OF OLIGODENDROCYTES TO INJURY

Morphological changes associated with oligodendrocyte and myelin pathology

The majority of oligodendrocytes are present within the white matter tracts of the brain and spinal cord (Fig. 3.24).

Degenerative changes affecting the oligodendrocyte–myelin sheath complex elicit, or are accompanied by, an astrocytic and/or macrophage response except in some forms of hypomyelination, mild forms of spongiform myelinopathies and the early stages of primary demyelination. The increased cellularity associated with this response can often be detected in routine H&E-stained preparations or can be visualized using staining methods which demonstrate astrocytes and microglia/macrophages.

WALLERIAN DEGENERATION OR DEMYELINATION SECONDARY TO AXON DEGENERATION

When axons degenerate myelin sheaths break down into a series of myelin ovoids (Fig. 3.25) which are separated from their supporting oligodendrocytes. The ovoids rapidly become isolated by astrocyte processes and these cells hypertrophy with a marked increase in GFAP

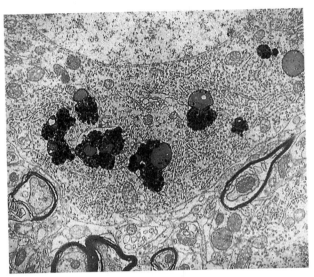

Figure 3.22 *Lipofuscin granules. Electron-dense lipofuscin granules are abundant in ageing neurons in the CA3 area of the hippocampus. Electron micrograph.*

filaments and accumulations of primary and secondary lysosomes.[52] Areas of wallerian degeneration therefore show an increase in GFAP staining which persists long after the myelin debris has been removed. At the same time as astrocytes respond, microglia become activated and begin to phagocytose the myelin ovoids[61] (Figs 3.26, 3.27). Although both astrocytes and microglia increase in numbers in response to axon degeneration (Fig. 3.27), this is minimal compared with the increase in cellularity seen in primary demyelination (Fig. 3.28). The combined activity of astrocytes and macrophages results in the slow degradation of the myelin ovoids over a period of weeks or months in lesions where there is not a breakdown of the blood–brain barrier (BBB).[182, 333] However, where the breakdown of the BBB occurs, such as in trauma and infarction, the clearance of myelin debris is rapid, and macrophages which are largely derived from monocytes become filled with neutral fat and accumulate in the damaged area. The oligodendrocytes that supported the myelin

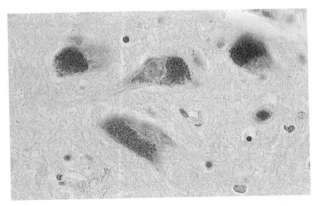

Figure 3.23 *Neuromelanin in the substantia nigra. Normal, neuromelanin-containing neurons in the human substantia nigra. (H&E.)*

sheaths around the degenerate axons atrophy, and most survive within the area of astrocytosis which eventually replaces the lost tissue.[359,394] In some instances these cells surround themselves with a thin layer of myelin[52] (Fig. 3.27). Recently, the view has been expressed that some oligodendrocytes undergo apoptosis as a consequence of the axon degeneration that follows spinal cord trauma.[557]

A feature of the early stages of wallerian degeneration is the presence of degenerate macrophages within myelin ovoids (Fig. 3.25). These cells, termed myelophages, are most readily appreciated when myelin tracts are cut longitudinally. They are formed because microglial cells enter the periaxonal space by penetrating beneath the paranodal loops at nodes of Ranvier just prior to the transformation of the myelin sheath into myelin ovoids.[9] Once isolated in the myelin ovoid, the cells undergo apoptosis. Since they are the only cells present within the ovoid, they are not phagocytosed and remain for long periods, acting as a hallmark of the process which generated them.

PRIMARY DEMYELINATION, REMYELINATION AND HYPOMYELINATION

The detection of these primary pathologies of the myelin–oligodendrocyte complex can sometimes pose problems in routine neuropathological examinations. However, the use of resin-embedded tissue or an appropriate selection of special stains on well-fixed tissue can usually identify the nature of the pathology.

The detection of active primary demyelination poses few problems since the pathology is often focal and the removal of myelin sheaths is accomplished by a florid infiltration of macrophages which quickly accumulate myelin debris and become transformed into typical fat-filled macrophages or gitter cells[447,473] (Fig. 3.28). Areas of primary demyelination can be aged by identifying the chemical nature of the myelin degradation products in macrophage phagosomes.[78] The macrophage infiltration is usually accompanied by a marked astrocytic hypertrophy and hyperplasia. Since this glial reaction is similar to that seen in areas of malacia, it is important that the presence of demyelinated axons is demonstrated by the use of axon stains, and when the axons are followed into the adjacent white matter there should be an absence of the pathological changes associated with wallerian degeneration. Areas of chronic demyelination, such as those which characterize MS, appear as areas of astrocytosis devoid of myelin in which demyelinated axons can be shown to be in continuity with normally myelinated axons in the surrounding white matter (see Chapter 8, Volume II).

The identification of remyelination, partial demyelination and hypomyelination can prove difficult in routine histological preparations. All of these changes appear as axons enveloped by myelin sheaths which are too thin for the axons that they surround.[58] Thinly myelinated axons, present in a focal area of astrocytosis in the

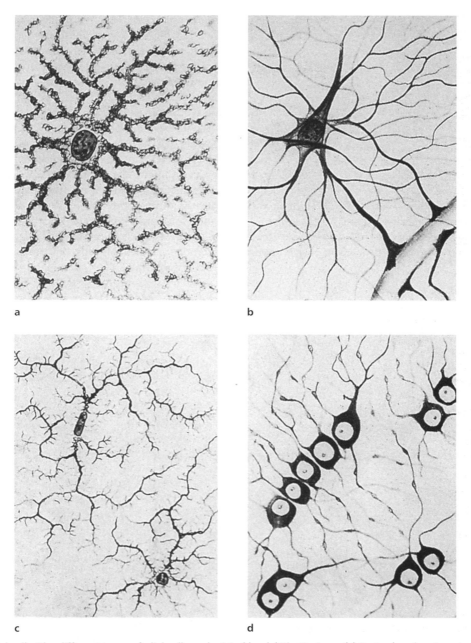

Figure 3.24 *Glial cells. The different types of glial cells as depicted by del Rio-Hortega. (a) Protoplasmic astrocyte in the grey mat-ter. (b) Fibrillary astrocyte in the white matter. (c) Resting, ramified microglia. (d) Oligodendrocytes aligned in rows in the white matter. Reproduced by permission from Ref. 571.*

...ite matter, such as is the case in the shadow ... can readily be identified as remyelination. ... circumstances the identification of ... separation from partial demyeli-... ion, can be difficult since these ... he absence of any other glial ... n initial examination may ... aining or a slight increase ... atter. The separation and ... ypes of change can only be ... on of well-fixed, plastic-... xons are cut in both longitu-

dinal and transverse planes. With a few exceptions in nor-mal tissue, myelin sheath thickness, internodal length and width of nodes of Ranvier show a constant relationship to axonal diameter.[256] These relationships result from the effect of growth on relationships established during myeli-nation.[256] Thus, if myelination is retarded relative to axon-al development, or takes place in a mature nervous system, the result will be a myelin sheath which appears too thin, and an internode too short, for the diameter of the asso-ciated axon (Fig. 3.29). Therefore, myelin sheaths which appear too thin and/or internodes which are too short indicate hypomyelination if present throughout the

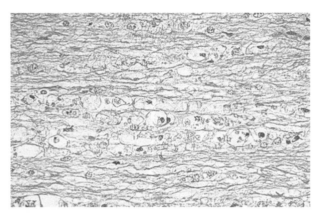

Figure 3.25 *Wallerian degeneration. Areas of wallerian degeneration contain a moderate increase in cell density. Pyknotic cells (myelophages) can be found within some myelin ovoids. (H&E.)*

white matter, and remyelination if found in otherwise normal white matter of an adult. Because of the relationship of myelin sheaths to axon size, such abnormalities are most easily appreciated in association with large-diameter axons. In contrast to hypomyelination and remyelination, in partial demyelination the dimensions of myelin sheaths are irregularly reduced (Figs 3.30, 3.31); thus, internodes can be of normal length but too thin for the diameter of the axons they enclose, or short, thinly myelinated internodes are interposed between internodes with normal dimensions.[154,192] Accumulations of displaced myelin are often associated with the thinned myelin internodes of partial demyelination and nodes of Ranvier may be widened. Astrocytosis may be a feature of partial demyelination but macrophages filled with myelin debris or neutral fat are generally absent.

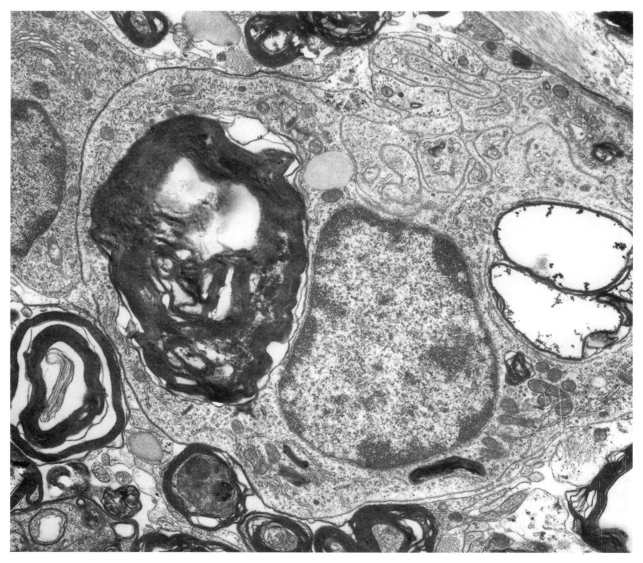

Figure 3.26 *Macrophage with myelin debris. Electron micrograph of phagocytosed myelin debris within a macrophage in an area of wallerian degeneration.*

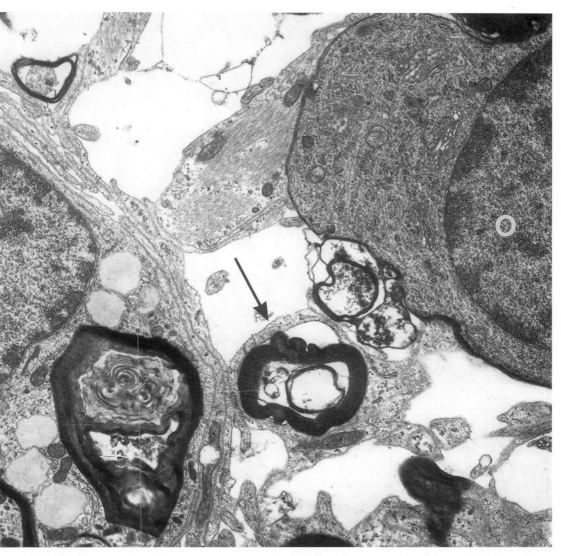

...xonal breakdown and myelin clearance. Following axonal breakdown and myelin clearance, oligodendrocytes (O) ...ay be covered by myelin membrane. The other cell is a macrophage which contains droplets of neutral fat and myelin ...te processes enclose a further myelin ovoid (arrow). Electron micrograph.

...rocyte pathology

...mmunocytochemistry and electron micro-
...ealed a number of changes that can be pre-
...godendrocyte cytoplasm. These include the
...vacuoles[59] (see section on myelin sheath
... below), increased numbers of micro-
...otein crystalline arrays,[258,437] dense bodies,[57]
...ribosomes, accumulations of autophago-
...otein accumulations within the endoplasmic
...Oligodendrocytes become tau positive after
...nd stroke[272] and tau-positive inclusions are
... a number of chronic neurodegenerative
...see Chapters 4 and 6, Volume II). In
...ental systems changes are seen in the cyto-
...s of myelin sheaths prior to demyelination,
...on which suggests, by analogy to the

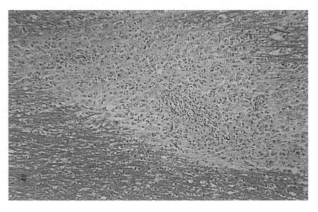

Figure 3.28 *'Foamy' macrophages in demyelination. Areas of active primary demyelination are characterized by accumulation of foamy macrophages which contain droplets of neutral fat and partially degraded myelin. (Luxol fast blue.)*

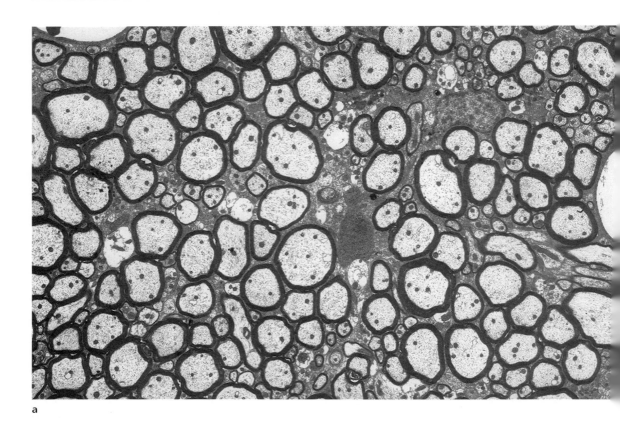

a

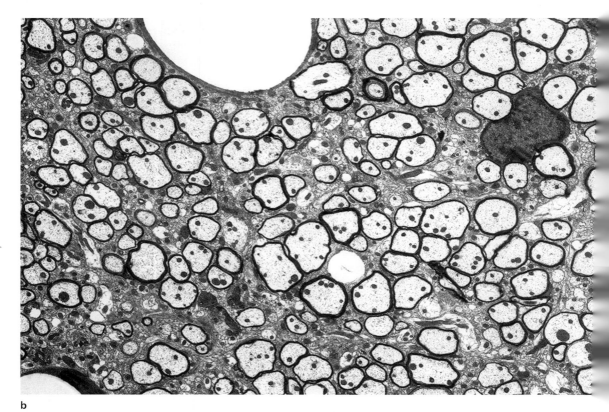

b

Figure 3.29 *Normal myelinated and remyelinated axons. In normal white matter there is a constant relationship betwee. ness of the myelin and the diameter of the axon that it encloses. This relationship changes after remyelination so that my appear thinner than normal. Myelinated axons in the superior cerebellar peduncle of mice of similar age: (a) normal; nated following cuprizone-induced demyelination. Electron micrographs.*

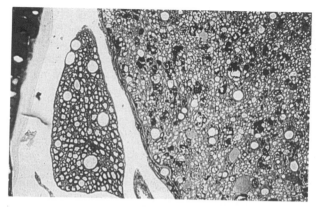

Figure 3.30 *Partial demyelination. Partial demyelination due to chronic compression arising from a misligned vertebra in the spinal cord of a dog. (Toluidine blue.)*

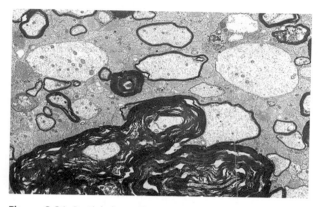

Figure 3.31 *Partial demyelination. Partial demyelination due to chronic compression arising from a malaligned vertebra in the spinal cord of a dog. Some axons have no myelin sheath, while others are surrounded by a thin myelin sheath or irregular accumulations of myelin. Electron micrograph of an area corresponding to the area shown by light microscopy in Figure 3.30.*

axonopathies, that metabolically compromised oligodendrocytes are 'dying back'.[59,363,505] Although often difficult to evaluate, there is increasing evidence that oligodendrocytes in areas of damage may undergo hypertrophy and perhaps even division.[360,410]

Common myelin artefacts

MYELINOID BODIES

Myelinoid bodies are myelin-like lamellar bodies found in association with paranodes of large axons, over 5 μm in diameter. The Marchi-positive bodies range in size from 1 μm to 8–25 μm in diameter and resemble myelin fragments seen in early wallerian degeneration. Myelinoid bodies were thought to be related to myelin metabolism and recent studies support the view that these bodies represent paranodal budding off of 'old'

myelin for local breakdown and reutilization.[256] Since these structures are not seen in association with nerve fibres under 5 μm, it is suggested that they represent a form of myelin turnover, balanced by the production of new myelin by the oligodendrocyte, specific for large-diameter fibres. An alternative explanation may be that these bodies represent the physiological manifestation of partial demyelination seen under pathological circumstances.

BUSCAINO BODIES OR MUCOCYTES

Metachromatic deposits of mucin-like material can sometimes be found in the white matter in association with a variety of neurological conditions and in normal individuals. This material, which appears in the form of multiple or single round bodies of varying size or as multiple multilobulated grape-like areas, has been variously termed mucocytes, metachromatic bodies or Buscaino bodies[569] (Fig. 3.32). Although originally considered to be associated with some form of degenerative change in oligodendrocytes, the change represents an artefact arising from post-mortem degeneration of myelin sheaths. The cause of this change is unknown but it is frequently seen when well-fixed tissue has been retained for several weeks in formol saline. The absence of nuclei within the stained area provides a means of distinguishing this change from cellular accumulation of material and its presence in the white matter avoids confusion with corpora amylacea, which share many of the staining characteristics of this material.

PRESSURE-INDUCED DEMYELINATION AND MYELIN SHEATH ARTEFACTS

A series of artefacts can complicate the examination of resin-embedded white matter by light and electron microscopy.[259] Large myelin sheaths are particularly susceptible to artefactual separation of myelin lamellae and in certain instances the whole or part of the myelin sheath can become separated from axons, giving the impression of primary demyelination. Handling of unfixed or

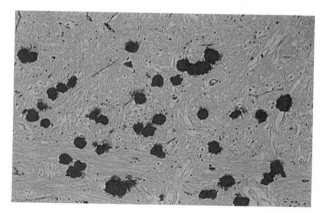

Figure 3.32 *Buscaino bodies or mucocytes in the normal white matter. (Periodic acid-Schiff.)*

partially fixed white matter predisposes to this change. These changes can be separated from true demyelination by the absence of any astrocytic or macrophage response. A further change which can be mistaken as demyelination is when osmium tetroxide fails to penetrate the full thickness of the tissue. This results in lack of staining of the myelinated areas which on superficial examination can appear as myelin loss. Again, the expected glial responses to myelin sheath breakdown are absent.

MYELIN VACUOLATION

Myelin sheath-related vacuoles can be found in the normal brain. The vacuoles tend to occur as single round holes in the otherwise adequately fixed white matter; their distribution may be symmetrical. Their presence may be associated with prolonged immersion in 70% alcohol.[648]

The genesis of myelin pathology

In order to appreciate the genesis of myelin pathology it is necessary to understand aspects of the oligodendrocyte–myelin sheath complex and the processes of myelination.

MYELINATION

The interaction between axons and oligodendrocytes which results in the formation of a myelin sheath is termed myelination (see also Chapter 2, this Volume). The process may be considered in terms of the response of one cell (an oligodendrocyte precursor) to signals from another cell (the neuron) which results in cell division, migration, differentiation and then association of the committed oligodendrocyte with the axon. In the appropriate cellular environment and in the absence of inhibitory factors this association results in the formation of a myelin sheath, the volume of which is appropriate for the area of axon covered.[58] In the young animal myelination proceeds in an orderly manner throughout the neuraxis, different tracts being myelinated at different times.[379] Thus in man, some of the axons of the ventral spinal cord are myelinated between 26 and 36 weeks of fetal life, while those of the corpus callosum are not myelinated until the second month of extrauterine life. Within a tract system, axons are not myelinated simultaneously.[379] In the optic system, although the precursors migrate into the optic nerve from the chiasm,[566] the nerve myelinates first at its ocular end. In the spinal cord myelination shows a craniocaudal progression with different tracts myelinating at different times during development.[158] Prior to myelination precursor cells migrate into and/or proliferate in the area to be myelinated, a process termed myelination gliosis. Although myelination of the CNS takes place over a prolonged period, only the phases of cell recruitment and the initial phase of myelin-sheath formation represent vulnerable periods

and these occur at different times in different parts of the nervous system. Once the myelin sheath is established axons are no longer susceptible to agents which were capable of producing damage during the earlier vulnerable period. Thus, doses of X-irradiation which will inhibit myelination[65,185] have no effect on the established myelin sheath[66] and drugs such as AY9944 which inhibit cholesterol biosynthesis and cause demyelination in myelinating animals do not have a similar effect in the myelinated animal.[589]

Immediately before, during and after myelination, axons increase in diameter and the myelin sheath is quickly formed. The myelination process therefore demands a rapid synthesis and delivery of myelin proteins and lipids.[467] Although the mechanisms which control the synthesis of the various myelin components are not yet fully understood, it is clear that the synthesis of the various myelin sheath components is normally well coordinated. For example, when one myelin protein cannot be synthesized, the other components of the myelin sheath are not overproduced.[554] Thus, in the shiverer mouse, where myelin basic protein (MBP) cannot be synthesized because of a deletion within the MBP gene, the myelin that is produced has, with the exception of MBP, a reduced but correct ratio of myelin constituents. The myelin sheaths that are produced are thin and have an uncompacted period line, but otherwise both the oligodendrocyte cell body and the pockets of cytoplasm associated with the myelin sheath have a normal appearance. Thus, myelination can be likened to a production line in which there is feedback control from the region of insertion into the membrane which controls the production of individual components. Whether the control occurs at transcription or translation is unclear; however, in certain situations this regulation fails and the result is abnormal myelin or death of myelinating oligodendrocytes.[649] This is particularly seen when there is overproduction of a normal protein or formation of an abnormal protein that has to pass through the endoplasmic reticulum. Point mutations of the PLP gene, such as occur in the jimpy mouse, the shaking pup, the myelin-deficient rat and in Pelizaeus–Merzbacher disease, lead to a toxic gain of function and there is severe hypomyelination associated with death of oligodendrocytes when they start to myelinate.[277] In the degenerating cells, the cisterns of the RER and the Golgi complex are dilated by protein as a result of the misfolded protein not being recognized by the transporter required for its export from this organelle.[204] The introduction of additional PLP genes[289] or the JC virus T antigen[240,565] leads to severe hypomyelination. When the copy number is low additional PLP genes result in demyelination,[289] or axon degeneration,[17] when the transgenic animals are several months old. Deletion of the PLP genes has little effect on myelin sheath formation but leads to widespread late-onset axon degeneration, particularly of smaller diameter myelinated axons.[232] Axon degeneration is also a feature of transgenic animals in which the myelin-associated glycoprotein (MAG) gene is deleted.[673] These transgenic studies in which myelin sheaths appear unstable are revealing the importance of a normal myelin sheath for the long-term integrity of axons. The signalling pathways involved have not been resolved; however, it is recognized that phosphorylation of neurofilaments and thus axon calibre is influenced by the ensheathment process.[107,514]

Although genetic disease is one of the most common causes of hypomyelination,[419] the myelination process in animals can be disrupted by virus infections in the first trimester of pregnancy (which lead to persistent infection),[404] by chemical intoxication,[278] or by exposure to X-irradiation at the time of myelination.

THE OLIGODENDROCYTE–MYELIN SHEATH COMPLEX

The myelin sheaths that surround axons in the CNS are made and then maintained by oligodendrocytes for the life of the individual. There is no evidence of turnover of oligodendrocytes since this could not occur without leaving evidence for its occurrence by the presence of axons surrounded by thin myelin sheaths. In the CNS the majority of axons over 0.6 μm in diameter are surrounded by a myelin sheath. In normal individuals myelin sheath thickness is directly related to axonal diameter in all but the largest diameter axons.[256] Internodal length also increases with fibre diameter.[414] Exceptions to these generalizations may be found, notably in those parts of the nervous system where there is a change in the myelination status of an axon, for example at the initial myelin segment, the PNS–CNS transition zone where unmyelinated PNS axons become myelinated by oligodendrocytes and Schwann cell myelin changes to oligodendrocyte myelin, and at the retina–optic nerve junction. At such sites, nodes of Ranvier are wider than normal, with aberrant axon–glial contacts, and myelin internodes are short, with myelin sheaths thinner than would be expected for the axon's diameter.[256]

Unlike Schwann cells which myelinate axons in the PNS on a one cell to one internode basis, an oligodendrocyte can form variable numbers of internodes. These internodes are generally considered to be on different axons which may or may not be in the same tract system.[575] When located within the same tract system, the internodes supported by an individual cell are myelinated at the same time and are often of similar length, which results in a clustering of the nodes of Ranvier. An individual oligodendrocyte may support from one to 60 internodes. Silver impregnations, immunocytochemical studies and recently visualization of individual oligodendrocyte by intracellular injection of dyes[85] show that there is an inverse relationship between axonal diameter and oligodendrocyte size and the number of internodes supported by individual oligodendrocytes.[82,83] Thus, large oligodendrocytes are associated with a single or few internodes on large-diameter axons, while small oligodendrocytes support many internodes on small-diameter

axons. Since the volume of myelin present in internodes associated with large-diameter axons greatly exceeds that present in internodes associated with small-diameter axons, the cells supporting myelin sheaths on large-diameter axons are supporting a far greater volume of myelin than the cells associated with a much greater number of internodes on small-diameter axons.[58] That large oligodendrocytes are the most metabolically active cells is reflected in their ultrastructural appearance,[54] the heterogeneity of their immunocytochemical staining,[16,84] and the different signal intensity seen following in situ hybridization for myelin-related mRNA.[394]

PARTIAL DEMYELINATION

Partial demyelination differs from primary demyelination in that only a portion of the myelin sheath is lost and occurs as a consequence of oligodendrocytes failing to maintain their normal myelin load.[58] Although the various molecules of myelin are turned over slowly, the oligodendrocytic metabolism must keep pace with such turnover if internodes are to be sustained at their established dimensions. In addition, it appears that myelin sheaths on large-diameter axons are inherently unstable, as reflected by their susceptibility to artefactual demyelination. Thus, in situations when large-diameter axons with their thick myelin sheaths are exposed to focal pressure, a portion of the internodal myelin becomes rearranged to form a myelin figure. Such accumulations of myelin remain in contact with the remaining myelin sheath, which appears thinner because of the rearranged myelin. With time, the myelin figures disappear and although the internodes have a normal morphology and length, the myelin sheath is thinner than it should be for the axon that it surrounds. At the nodes of Ranvier one paranode may be of normal dimensions, while the other has a myelin sheath which is thinner. Occasionally, paranodes become completely detached from the axon and nodes of Ranvier are wider than normal. If such nodal widening is sufficient to stimulate remyelination then a short, thinly myelinated internode is formed, intercalated between internodes which have normal myelin sheaths.

Although partial demyelination can effect internodes on both large and small diameter axons, it is most obvious on large-diameter axons, particularly following acute pressure lesions. It can only be appreciated on small-diameter axons by plotting myelin sheath thickness against axon diameter.

WHOLE INTERNODE DEMYELINATION AND REMYELINATION

Although it is possible that myelin sheaths can be destroyed, leaving the oligodendrocytes intact in most instances, selective loss of whole internodes of myelin results from the death of oligodendrocytes. This can arise for many reasons, but the most common causes are: lytic virus infection, the result of allergy to normal cell components, allergy to antigens expressed as a result of virus infection, specific chemical intoxication, or as a result of 'bystander damage' in inflammatory reactions.[384,438] Oligodendrocytes have functional AMPA/kainate glutamate receptors and are thus vulnerable to AMPA/kainate receptor-mediated excitotoxicity.[388] *In vitro* studies have also incriminated a number of other mediators of cell death, such as oxidative stress, tumour necrosis factor (TNF)/NGF receptor interactions and complement;[398] however, the extent to which these operate *in vivo* has yet to be established.

Although the events after the death of oligodendrocytes appear to follow a stereotyped pattern in natural disease states, in experimental models the speed of these responses can be very different and has a marked effect on the efficiency of the remyelinating process. In most instances of whole internode demyelination, the myelin sheath undergoes changes before it is shed from the axon; these changes include honeycombing, vesiculation and fragmentation[58] (Fig. 3.33). In other instances the myelin sheath appears to peel off the axon unchanged to form myelin ovoids similar to those seen in wallerian degeneration.[55] When demyelination is occurring in areas where there has not been concurrent loss of astrocytes, clearance of myelin debris rapidly progresses.[55] However, when astrocytes are absent, large arrays of honeycombed myelin surround the demyelinated axons and these can persist for many weeks or months. In these cases, remyelination is poor or delayed.[205] There may be a delay

between an insult which will lead to degeneration of oligodendrocytes and initiation of demyelination. Thus, after injection of the intercalating agent ethidium bromide, demyelination may not occur for 7 days, during which time oligodendrocytes show nuclear and cytoplasmic changes related to the effects of disruption of nucleic acid metabolism.[56] In cuprizone intoxication abnormal oligodendrocytes can be found in white matter tracts for several weeks prior to the onset of myelin sheath breakdown.[59] Areas of demyelination are invaded by many macrophages, and in the case of immune-mediated demyelination lymphocytes are also present. When demyelination is progressing rapidly, macrophages often insinuate their processes into the myelin sheath and clathrin-coated vesicles can be seen adjacent to fragments of partly ingested myelin sheath (micropinocytosis vermiformis).[480] In the past, much has been made of macrophage stripping off myelin sheaths as an indication of immune-mediated demyelination; although a feature of experimental allergic encephalomyelitis, this form of myelin sheath degradation is not restricted to this condition and can be observed in most rapidly demyelinating diseases (Fig. 3.33). As removal of the myelin sheath progresses, macrophages become replete with droplets of neutral fat and, when present, astrocytes hypertrophy, with their processes separating individual demyelinated axons. When demyelination occurs in areas devoid of astrocytes the demyelinated axons clump together owing to the presence of adhesion molecules, such as L1, N-CAM and Ng-CAM.

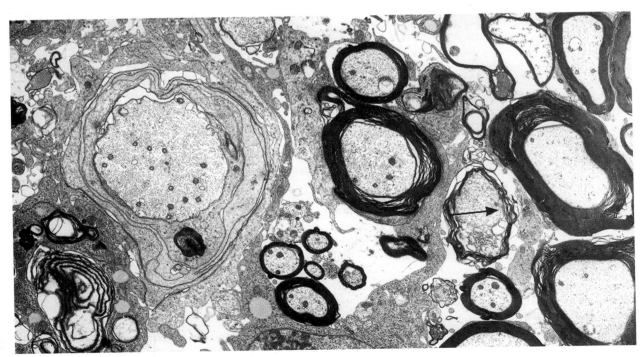

Figure 3.33 *Active primary demyelination. An electron micrograph of active primary demyelination: macrophage processes can be seen stripping a myelin sheath from an axon while a further myelin sheath shows evidence of fragmentation (arrow). The macrophage cell body (bottom left) contains myelin debris and droplets of neutral lipid.*

REMYELINATION

Since its first description in the 1960s using the model cerebrospinal fluid barbotage,[81] remyelination has been recorded in a number of experimental models of demyelination (see Chapter 8, Volume II). It has also been documented in naturally occurring demyelinating disease, including MS where it is thought to occur in most acute plaques.[473,482] Remyelination can be a very efficient process (Fig. 3.34), and in experimental models, especially those involving the use of gliotoxins, entire areas of demyelination may undergo repair. However, a number of factors can impair the efficiency of remyelination, including the age of the individual in which demyelination is induced[552] and the mode of induction.[663] There is some evidence to suggest that remyelination becomes progressively less efficient if the same area of white matter is subjected to repeated episodes of demyelination followed by remyelination[284,341] or after prolonged demyelination.[358] This phenomenon may in part account for the poor or absent remyelination associated with chronic plaques in MS.

The precise mechanisms and cellular events that occur during CNS remyelination have not yet been fully elucidated. However, a widely accepted model of the events that occur in demyelinating lesions arising from the death of oligodendrocytes involves the generation of new remyelinating cells from surrounding intact tissue and their migration into the lesioned area, where they proceed to remyelinate the demyelinated axons. There is now good evidence from both ultrastructural and immunocytochemical studies that the newly generated and recruited cell is an immature oligodendrocyte[90,194,498] similar to oligodendrocyte progenitors that occur during development.[479] Tissue culture and developmental studies indicate that such cells possess degrees of motility and responsiveness to mitogens which distinguish them from more mature oligodendrocytes and therefore they possess those properties that are required for remyelination.[429]

What are the factors that govern the division, migration and differentiation of remyelinating cells? The identity of many of these factors remains obscure but, again, clues are provided by tissue culture and developmental studies. Various growth factors and cytokines have been shown to have relevant effects on oligodendrocyte progenitors.[664] For example, platelet-derived growth factor (PDGF), bFGF, IGF, NT-3 and interleukin-2 (IL-2) have all been shown to be mitogens for rodent oligodendrocyte progenitors. The effects of other growth factors on these cells include chemotaxis (PDGF), promotion of myelinogenesis (PDGF and IGF) and protection against

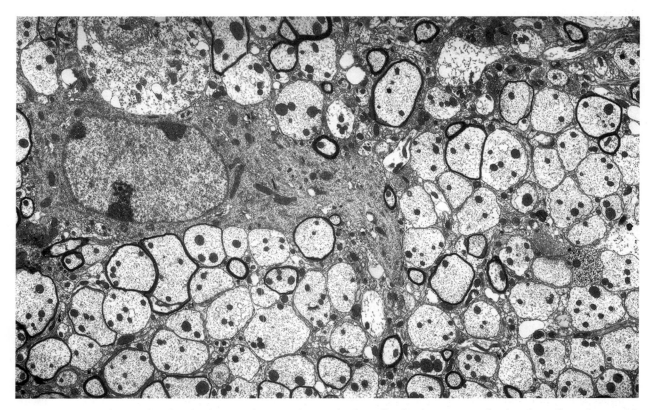

Figure 3.34 *Remyelination by oligodendrocyte. Electron micrograph of an oligodendrocyte remyelinating demyelinated axons following cuprizone intoxication in the mouse. The cell has a large nucleolus and cytoplasm rich in ribosomes. The various stages of axon ensheathment can be seen. Initially axons are engulfed by oligodendrocyte processes and as the processes commence the first spiral of the sheath, their inner surface comes together to form the period line.*

apoptosis (PDGF, IGF and NT-3). The potential importance of a protective effect is illustrated by the ability of CNTF to protect oligodendrocyte progenitors from TNF-induced injury,[357] indicating that the presence of protective factors may be required for remyelination to occur in the otherwise hostile environment of a demyelinating lesion. Direct evidence that growth factors are involved in CNS remyelination is scarce, although IGF, FGF and PDGF[391] have all been implicated in the remyelination of gliotoxin-induced demyelination using a range of molecular, immunocytochemical and pharmacological approaches.[257] Activated microglia/macrophages and reactive astrocytes are known to be potent sources of growth factors and cytokines, and there is some evidence that the presence and status of these cell types are critical for the efficacy of the remyelinating process.[163,284]

While it is clear that the cells responsible for remyelination are generated by mitosis and are of an immature phenotype, the origin of these cells is still a matter of controversy with two schools of thought. The first, the adult progenitor theory, proposes that remyelinating cells are derived from a small pool of oligodendrocyte progenitors to be found within the differentiated adult CNS. Persuasive evidence that such a cell exists comes from tissue culture studies where it has been possible to isolate a progenitor cell which resembles, but is distinct from, the oligodendrocyte progenitor that occurs during development.[152] This cell can be induced to become more motile and divide more rapidly by exposure to combinations of growth factors such as might occur in association with demyelinating lesions but not in undamaged tissue.[429] Several studies offer proof for a progenitor origin of remyelinating cells.[91,181,295] The alternative view, the de-differentiation theory, argues that new remyelinating cells are derived from mature oligodendrocytes that divide to give rise to a progeny of a less mature phenotype.[660] There is some evidence from ultrastructural autoradiography studies that a small number of mature myelin-forming oligodendrocytes may be capable of division.[362] Moreover, exposure of mature oligodendrocytes in tissue culture to appropriate growth factors causes them to revert to a less mature phenotype.[233]

An alternative form of remyelination has been suggested for situations where oligodendrocytes survive the loss of their myelin sheaths. Recent analysis of acute, repairing MS lesions has identified cells within the lesions that express myelin oligodendrocyte glycoprotein (MOG), a glycoprotein associated with myelin-forming oligodendrocytes, which are thought to have survived the demyelinating events and be able to regenerate new myelin sheaths.[77,447] The evidence for this form of remyelination is limited since it is by no means clear whether an oligodendrocyte that has already established one complement of internodes can do so for a second time, and studies involving transplantation and X-irradiation question this suggestion.[63,596]

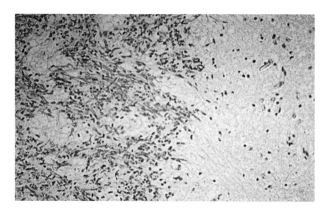

Figure 3.35 *Remyelination by Schwann cells. Schwann cells myelinating demyelinated axons in an area of demyelination in the CNS. (Immunostaining for the peripheral myelin sheath protein P₀.)*

Schwann cell myelination of CNS axons

Although Schwann cells can occasionally be associated with axons in the normal CNS they are not a normal cellular component of the undamaged CNS. They may remyelinate CNS axons, often in large numbers, in several lesions (Fig. 3.35). From experimental studies it is now clear that for this to happen two conditions must prevail: first, there must be disturbance of the integrity of the glia limitans, and secondly, axons which should or have been myelinated by oligodendrocytes must be present.[162] However, with the demonstration that CNS-derived glial precursors can give rise to both oligodendrocytes and Schwann cells the assumption that Schwann cells observed remyelinating CNS axons are always of PNS origin can be questioned.[294,412]

MYELIN SHEATH VACUOLATION

Myelin sheath vacuolation forms the basis of a light-microscopic change known as status spongiosus. It is a common form of myelin abnormality which may develop alone or may accompany or precede primary demyelination. In myelin vacuolation, fluid accumulates in the form of vacuoles in certain portions of the myelin sheath (Fig. 3.36). The most common location, and the only one where the change is brought about by amphipathic compounds such as triethyltin[642] and hexochlorophene,[615] is within the myelin sheath proper where the accumulation of fluid is focal and results from separation of the intraperiod line (Figs 3.37, 3.38). However, the change can also involve the periaxonal space, occurring between the inner and outer tongues of oligodendrocyte cytoplasm, or appear as vacuoles within oligodendrocyte cytoplasm. Vacuolation associated with the myelin sheath–oligodendrocyte complex may resolve completely without leaving residual pathology, as is the case in hexochlorophene and triethyltin intoxication, or may be followed or accompanied by primary demyelina-

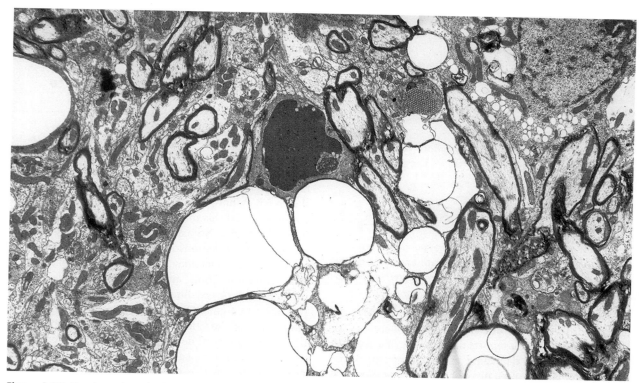

Figure 3.36 *Cuprizone intoxication. Electron micrograph of an oligodendrocyte with marked clumping of nuclear chromatin surrounded by myelin sheath-associated vacuoles following cuprizone intoxication in the mouse. This area will undergo primary demyelination which will be remyelinated.*

tion. The latter situation occurs in intoxications such as cuprizone intoxication in mice,[59] isoniazide intoxication in dogs,[64] certain genetic diseases[242] and in virus and autoimmune disorders.[67] Because of its frequent association with demyelinating conditions, myelin-associated vacuolation can be used as a sensitive indicator of the well-being of the myelin sheath–oligodendrocyte complex. However, this change can arise artefactually. In most instances where vacuolation represents a significant pathological change it is accompanied by disturbances in astrocytes and/or microglia.

Normal maintenance of myelin sheaths in the CNS is dependent on viable oligodendrocytes. Experimental intoxications of oligodendrocytes indicates that when oligodendrocyte function is impaired, fluid invariably accumulates in myelin sheaths, while a more generalized myelin sheath vacuolation arises as a consequence of incorporation of certain lipophilic chemicals into myelin sheaths. It is suggested that myelin sheath vacuolation restricted to certain white-matter tracts is a sign of primary oligodendrocyte injury, while myelin sheath vacuolation that is diffusely distributed throughout the CNS is a sign of exposure to a primary myelinotoxic agent.

The experimental spongy myelinopathies with restricted distribution within the CNS show astrocytic lesions in addition to the changes in myelin sheaths. A consequence of myelin sheath vacuolation may be that intramyelinic vacuoles rupture and release their contents into the extra-cellular space.[59] As astrocytes are known to respond by hypertrophy to an abnormal environment, the astrocytic hypertrophy may be a secondary phenomenon due to a reaction to the extracellular fluid accumulation and/or myelin degeneration. However, primary astrocytic changes also frequently occur since many of the agents damaging oligodendrocytes also injure the astrocytes. Thus, both local injection of ethidium bromide into the white matter[56] and systemic administration of 6-aminonicotinamide[442] cause not only demyelination and

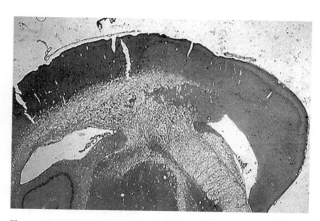

Figure 3.37 *Hexochlorophene intoxication in the rat. This change, although dramatic, is reversible when the drug administration is discontinued. (H&E.)*

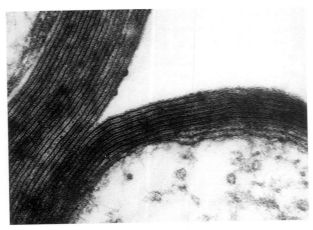

Figure 3.38 *Isoniazide intoxication. In the spongiform myelino-pathies most vacuoles in the myelin sheath appear to be the result of fluid accumulation within the space created by the separation of the intraperiod line. Electron micrograph.*

oligodendrocyte death but also necrosis of astrocytes. Unfortunately, in most reports the response of astrocytes to oligodendrocyte damaging agents is poorly documented, so that it is often not clear whether or not these

compounds are generally gliotoxic and, if so, whether there is variation in the relative susceptibility of oligodendrocytes and astrocytes.

The relationship of oligodendrocytes to other cells

Although the main function of oligodendrocytes is to make and maintain the myelin sheaths around CNS axons, they have a number of relationships of pathological significance. There are proteins associated with the myelin sheath which have an inhibitory effect on axonal regeneration[95,535] and this may be one of the reasons for poor regeneration of CNS axons in white-matter tracts. Gap junctions can be demonstrated between oligodendrocytes and astrocytes which may have implications for intercellular communication and spread of viruses.[492] The perineuronal or satellite oligodendrocyte (Fig. 3.39) remains an enigma. Oligodendrocytes seem to have an affinity for this location, since not only do they cluster there during normal development, but it also represents a site where infiltrating glioma cells and transplanted glial progenitor cells aggregate.[41] Satellite oligodendrocytes do

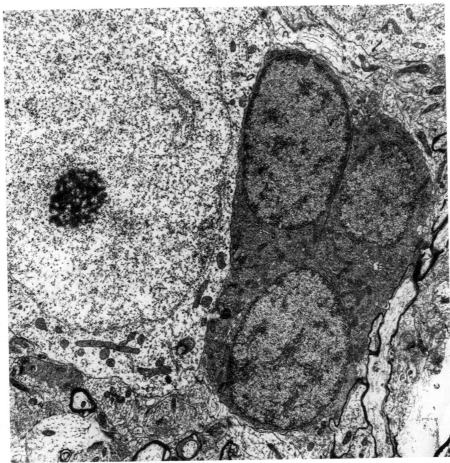

Figure 3.39 *Satellite oligodendrocytes. Cluster of three satellite oligodendroglial cells in the normal superior colliculus showing both intimate contact with the nerve cell body (left of cluster) and also myelin formation (right of cluster). Electron micrograph.*

not increase in number during chromatolysis. They are myelinating cells and can be immunostained for MBP and MAG.[361] The relationship between astrocytes and cells of the oligodendrocyte lineage during remyelination has already been considered in the section on remyelination.

ASTROCYTES

Basic cell biological parameters of reactive astrocytes

Astrocytes have been traditionally classified as protoplasmic or fibrous based on morphological criteria (Fig. 3.24), the former being typically found in the normal grey matter and the latter occurring in normal white matter. This morphological classification has significance for pathology, since the presence of increased amounts of glial fibres in reactive astrocytes which assume a more fibrous phenotype may be of diagnostic use. The main biochemical constituent of glial filaments is GFAP (Figs 3.40, 3.41), a type III intermediate filament protein.[7,52,146,271] Several alternative transcripts exist.[111] Not all astrocytes express detectable levels of GFAP in their normal state. However, GFAP is an excellent marker for labelling most, if not all, reactive astrocytes.[139,144] GFAP may be detected immunocytochemically in both surgical biopsy tissue and postmortem material. It is also widely used as a marker for astrocytes in experimental neuropathology. In the rat, the GFAP gene has been shown to possess tissue-specific methylation domains.[598] However, cell type and tissue specificity of GFAP expression are not absolute.[392] Furthermore, if longstanding fibrillary gliosis is to be detected, the classical Holzer stain may be a better choice than GFAP immunocytochemistry.

The question of astrocyte development has attracted much attention. It is now clear that astrocytes comprise a functionally diverse cell population with many specialized subtypes which have complex interactions with their local microenvironment.[268,325,643,651,659] This heterogeneity seems important with respect to the establishment of regionally specific synaptic patterning.[405] Thus, the classification of type 1 and type 2 astrocytes[478] should be confined to in vitro models and not be applied to reactive astrocytes. It was first thought that type 1 and type 2 astrocytes would correspond to protoplasmic and fibrous astrocytes, but this does not seem to be the case.

There are striking discrepancies between in vitro and in vivo properties of astrocytes regarding development,[564] electrophysiological parameters[643] and the capacity of astrocytes to participate in immune reactions.[125] Striking species differences also exist. Therefore, when considering astrocyte functions in the living organism, it should be kept in mind that much of our current knowledge on astrocytes is based on in vitro findings.[30,139] The phenotye of astrocytes is especially dependent on neighbouring neurons.[338,611,643] This is in line with the enormous sophistication of the receptive machinery of astrocyte membranes (see Chapter 2, this Volume). Considering the extremely large surface area of the 'sheet-like' astrocyte periphery[258] and their intercellular communication via a 'functional syncytium',[411] astrocytes are likely to monitor continuously the state of neighbouring neurons and adjust closely to their functional activity.

Pathophysiology of astrocytes

Support of the structure and metabolism of the CNS is a function traditionally ascribed to astrocytes.[34,288] The physiological interaction between astrocytes and neurons begins early during development and is important for neuronal migration, neurite outgrowth and axonal pathfinding. Processes of radial glial cells guide migrating neurons to their permanent positions in the cerebral and cerebellar cortex[346] and it is known from work on mutant mice that aberrant astrocyte development leads to developmental disturbances.[678] The production of extracellular matrix and adhesion molecules as well as of neurotrophic and neurite-promoting factors by astrocytes seems crucial for normal CNS development, maintenance and repair.[139,170] Astrocytes play an important role in cerebral energy metabolism and in the synthesis of complex lipids. Glycogen synthesis, storage and catabolism are glial functions which are unique to astrocytes.[160,512] Glycogen found in reactive astrocytes can, through generation of lactate and pyruvate,[243,491] serve as an important source of energy.

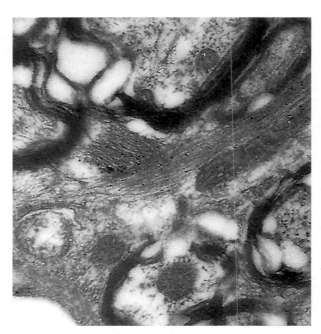

Figure 3.40 *GFAP in a Bergmann astrocyte. Immunogold labelling for GFAP of glial filaments in a Bergmann astrocyte. Reproduced by permission from Ref. 214.*

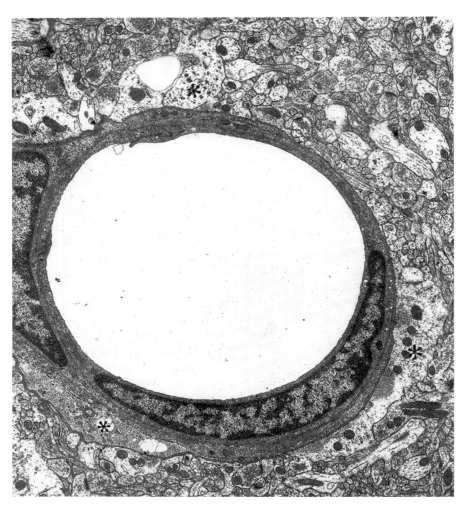

Figure 3.41 *Astrocytic foot processes. Electron micrograph showing attachment of astrocytes to the basal lamina around a cerebral capillary. Astrocytic processes (*) contain glial filaments or granules of glycogen. Reproduced by permission from Ref. 134.*

Another widely accepted function of astrocytes which is of great relevance to pathophysiology is to secure homoeostasis through uptake of neuroactive substances such as neurotransmitters and regulation of pH, ion concentrations and osmolarity. This fits well with the important role attributed to astrocytes in various disease states such as disturbances of the BBB causing vasogenic oedema or metabolic dysregulation resulting in cytotoxic oedema (see below). Thus, astrocytes, which are the most numerous cell type in the CNS, appear to act as 'controllers' of the extracellular milieu. Astrocytic 'spatial buffering' of potassium which is released from neurons is thought to limit the spread of excitation,[576] and astrocyte processes adjoining nodes of Ranvier may act as boundaries of the nodal microenvironment and could be involved in ion channel replacement.[643]

Knowledge on the involvement of astrocytes in the metabolism of certain neurotransmitters is of relevance when attempting to appreciate the role of astrocytes in the protection against excitotoxins. Astrocytes play an important role in the metabolism of glutamate, the most plentiful amino acid and the major excitatory neurotransmitter in the adult CNS.[32,253,676,679] Nerve cells are metabolically 'handicapped' with respect to glutamate synthesis because they depend for its production on a supply of several compounds from astrocytes.[530] Much of this supply is provided through glutamine, a non-neuroactive compound which can be shuttled safely between astrocytes and neurons and which is hydrolysed to glutamate via a phosphate-dependent glutaminase within neurons.[679] Astrocytes rapidly remove glutamate from the synaptic cleft via a high-affinity uptake system.[32,679] This is important as extracellular concentrations of glutamate must be kept low in order to maximize the signal-to-noise ratio following its release from presynaptic terminals and to avoid potentially neurotoxic effects.[679] Astrocytic conversion of glutamate into glutamine occurs in the presence of ammonia.[32,432] Thus, astrocytes protect neurons not only from excitatory amino acid (EAA)-induced neurotoxicity, but also from negative effects of high extracellular concentrations of ammonia.[248,378] These crucial metabolic pathways have been collectively termed the 'glutamate–glutamine cycle'.[530,679] However, it should be borne in mind that astrocytes can also act as the site for bioactivation of neurotoxins.[131]

Table 3.1 *Molecules expressed by human astrocytes* in situ

Function[a]	Designation	FFPE[b]	Reference(s)
Actin-binding protein	Ezrin	+	180
Adhesion molecule	CD44	+	185
Adhesion molecule	HNK-1	+	193
Calcium-binding protein	S-100	+	231
Cytokine	IL-1	+	231
Cytokine/growth factor	TGF-β_1	+	637
Cytokine	TNF	–	266, 543, 617
Cytolytic protein	Perforin	–	172
Cytoskeletal constituent	GFAP	+	53, 146, 332
Cytoskeletal constituent	Vimentin	+	193, 332
ECM molecule	Laminin	+	193
Glycolytic pathway	NSE	+	634
Growth factor	FGFa, b	F	199, 612
Growth factor receptor	EGF-R	+	55
Intracellular protein	J1-31	F	366
Lens protein	αB-crystallin	+	276
Lysosomal protease	Cathepsins B, D	+	130, 418
Neurotransmitter metabolism	MAO-B (HC)	–	417
Neurotransmitter metabolism	Peptide receptors	–	124
Serine protease inhibitor	α_1-ACT (ISH)	–	451
Signal transduction	PKC	–	103, 495
Transport of iron	Transferrin	+	112, 193
Transport of lipids	Apolipoprotein E	+	72, 130

[a]Some molecules may have additional functions.

[b]FFPE, formalin-fixed and paraffin-embedded tissue: +, may be detected in FFPE; F, formalin fixation (paraformaldehyde fixation) without subsequent paraffin embedding; –, frozen tissue only, not detectable in FFPE.

α_1-ACT, α_1-Antichymotrypsin; ECM, extracellular matrix; EGF-R, epidermal growth factor receptor; FGF, fibroblast growth factor (a, acidic; b, basic); GFAP, glial fibrillary acidic protein; IL-1, interleukin-1; MAO-B, monoamine oxidase B; NSE, neuron-specific enolase; PKC, protein kinase C; TGF-β_1, transforming growth factor beta-1; TNF, tumour necrosis factor; HC, histochemical detection; ISH, *in situ* hybridization.

Among the many cellular functions ascribed to astrocytes in CNS pathology, none has caused more controversy than their role as antigen-presenting cells (APCs). In general, T-cells do not respond to free, intact protein antigen but require presentation of processed peptide fragments in the molecular context of major histocompatibility complex (MHC) molecules which are expressed on the surface of APCs. It is generally believed that MHC restriction of T-cell recognition of encephalitogenic antigens is a function of MHC class II molecules. It has been established that non-neoplastic human astrocytes are incapable of expressing MHC class II molecules *in vivo*.[71,125,208] In addition, the important costimulatory molecule B7, a ligand of the T-cell-specific activational proteins CD28/CTLA-4, is not inducible on human astrocytes but is present on microglia and perivascular cells.[125] There is an inhibitory influence of cortical neurons on the induction of MHC class II molecules in astrocytes.[423,611] Thus, astrocytes are unlikely to play a prominent role as antigen presenters to Th$_1$-cells but may stimulate Th$_2$ responses[12] and modulate the activity of microglia and infiltrating peripheral immune cells by the production of cytokines (Table 3.1).[139,625] The relative incapacity of astrocytes to present antigen is paralleled by their expression of Fas ligand (FasL)[100] and their ability to prime T-cells for apoptotic cell death.[196]

Phagocytosis by astrocytes is an uncommon phenomenon and can be mainly observed during development.[6,506,507] Support for the view that protection of neurons[31,466,654,672] is an important function of astrocytes comes from the observation that astrocytes serve as a 'sink' for toxic substances such as lead (Pb) in the brain.[349]

ASTROCYTE SWELLING

Astrocytes respond rapidly to various types of CNS injury. It appears that protoplasmic and fibrous astrocytes are similar in this capacity. Swelling is one of the earliest responses of astrocytes to CNS injury. Astrocyte swelling occurs in hypoxia, hypoglycaemia, hepatic encephalopathy, status epilepticus, exposure to certain neurotoxins and trauma.[32,355,431] If associated with an overall increase in brain water content, swelling may lead to increased intracranial pressure and mass effects[431] (see Chapter 4, this Volume). Swollen astrocytes are less capable of maintaining their homoeostatic functions, such as uptake of ions and neurotransmitters. In addition, astrocyte swelling is associated with a release of intracellular EAAs including glutamate, aspartate and taurine,[32] which may further damage injured neurons. One of the mechanisms likely to be involved in glial swelling is the inhibition of membrane Na^+/K^+-ATPase activity and the subsequent accumulation of cytoplasmic Na^+ and loss of K^+.[32,355]

Astrocyte swelling is of particular importance in the context of cytotoxic brain oedema (see Chapter 4, this Volume). The most commonly encountered cytotoxic oedema is observed in cerebral ischaemia, where an interruption of energy supply leads to failure of the ion pump and osmoregulation, resulting in an intracellular increase in sodium and water.[306] Neurotoxic effects of excitatory amino acids such as glutamate may play an important role in postischaemic injury. Glutamate toxicity is considered to lead to astrocytic swelling through stimulation of K^+ influx.[46] The underlying mechanisms are complex and involve the activation of different K^+ channels, pertussis toxin-sensitive G-proteins, the glutamate carrier, at least one cotransporter and an increase in intracellular Ca^{2+}.[244] Arachidonic acid, which is released and accumulates in the brain in cerebral ischaemia and trauma, may also play an important role in cell swelling and irreversible cell injury.[574] In a rat model of *Haemophilus influenzae* type b meningitis, bacterially mediated cytokine release, free radical production in the meninges by neutrophils and the release of neurotoxic factors by microglia have been suggested to contribute to astrocytic swelling.[386]

It has been speculated that changes in astroglial volume with secondary effects on the extracellular space could modulate neuronal excitability.[244] Astrocyte swelling could also serve to limit the diffusion of toxic substances, such as glutamate, from sites of injury.[385]

Nuclear 'swelling' constitutes a characteristic of Alzheimer type 2 astrocytes, which are commonly found in chronic hepatic encephalopathy and in Wilson's disease (see Chapter 10, this Volume).

HYPERTROPHY AND HYPERPLASIA OF ASTROCYTES

One of the most prominent features of reactive astrocytes is their increase in GFAP. Thus, a rise in the number of GFAP-positive cells can be observed in most CNS pathologies.[50,147,159,211,405,464,522] The *de novo* appearance of GFAP-immunoreactive astrocytes in brain areas with normally low levels of GFAP expression has led to the suggestion that reactive astrocytosis is typically associated with astrocytic hyperplasia,[342] and that it may also involve migration of astrocytes.[583] However, studies using immunocytochemistry for GFAP in combination with tritiated thymidine autoradiography or bromodeoxyuridine labelling have demonstrated that, at least in acute CNS lesioning models, mitotic cell division and migration of astrocytes are unlikely to account for the

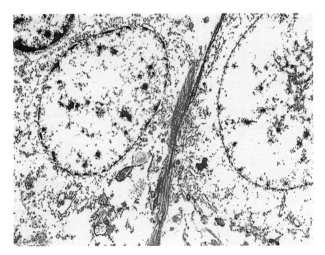

Figure 3.42 *Neuron and astrocyte in Creutzfeldt–Jakob disease (CJD). Electron micrograph of a cortical neuron with spongiform change and neighbouring astrocyte in CJD.*

majority of GFAP-positive cells.[139,223,415] Yet, regional specialization of astrocytes may influence their mitotic potential. Proliferation of Bergmann astrocytes represents a common finding after hypoxic damage to Purkinje cells, and hyperplasia of cortical astrocytes characteristically occurs in CJD (Figs 3.19, 3.42) and subacute sclerosing panencephalitis (SSPE). In these conditions, nuclei of astrocytes may be seen arranged in pairs or small groups (Fig. 3.43), indicating nerve cell death. In contrast, proliferation of brainstem astrocytes is less commonly observed.

Marked hypertrophy of astrocytes is seen in acute as well as in chronic, slowly progressive disease. In oedematous white matter, in the vicinity of brain tumours and of metastases or around abscesses, reactive astrocytes become enlarged, exhibit a homogeneous, eosinophilic cytoplasm and stain strongly for GFAP. Their nuclei are often enlarged and eccentric, lying close to the cytoplasmic membrane. Such cells are known as gemistocytic (or

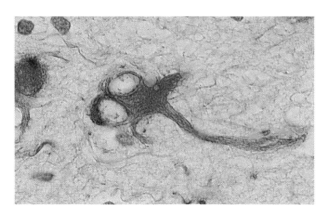

Figure 3.43 *GFAP immunostaining of a binucleated astrocyte. Binucleated astrocyte in the neocortex in a case of CJD indicating astrocytic proliferation. (Immunostaining for GFAP counterstained with haematoxylin.)*

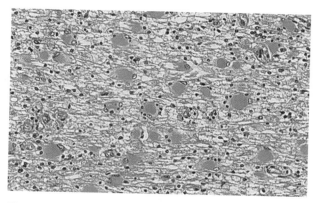

Figure 3.44 *Reactive astrocytes. Reactive, hypertrophic ('gemistocytic') astrocytes in an actively demyelinating corpus callosum lesion in multiple sclerosis. (H&E.)*

swollen-bodied) astrocytes (Figs 3.44, 3.45). Resolution of acute lesions and of white matter oedema is usually followed by an extensive formation of astrocytic glial filaments, leaving a firm 'gliotic scar'. Such tissue areas are readily visualized using the classical Holzer stain. Hypertrophy of astrocytes can also be seen in leukodystrophies where astrocytes in the white matter may become markedly enlarged. Gliotic tissue is firmer than normal tissue and tends to appear grey upon macroscopic examination. The finding of fibrillary gliosis indicates abnormality in the CNS, although visualization of microglial activation through staining for MHC class II antigens may prove to be an even more subtle indicator of tissue pathology. Increased GFAP immunoreactivity often extends beyond the actual lesion site, probably as a result of the electrotonic coupling of astrocytes via gap junctions.[183,497] Another molecule which is significantly upregulated in reactive astrocytes is *N*-cadherin,[493,631] which may be of relevance to the adhesive properties of CNS scar tissue. A role for endothelin B receptor signal transduction in reactive astrocytes has been proposed.[70]

SIGNIFICANCE OF REACTIVE GFAP EXPRESSION AND GLIAL FIBRE FORMATION

Although reactive GFAP expression is a hallmark of astrocytic involvement in tissue pathology, the finding of increased tissue levels of GFAP is not specific for any disease. Reactive upregulation of GFAP expression has been observed in numerous human diseases and experimental conditions, indicating that astrocytes can respond to diverse alterations in neurons such as retrograde and transganglionic changes, wallerian degeneration and direct neuronal injury.[50,147,159,211,415,464] Expression of vimentin in adult reactive astrocytes[522,669] may help to identify tissue areas where structural brain damage has occurred and persists for prolonged periods.[219,464] In some astrocytes vimentin appears necessary to stabilize GFAP filaments.[171] The biological significance of reactive astrocytes in glial scar formation is of great interest as their cell processes may form a barrier to growing axons and thus impede CNS regeneration.[281,353,537] However, astrocytes may also support CNS regeneration[170,494] and these cells should therefore not be viewed as purely adverse elements in the damaged CNS.[355,494]

In view of the obvious complexity of the astrocytic response to injury, it has been suggested that the therapeutic challenge for the future may not be so much to inhibit or exaggerate this response as to modify the promoting and inhibitory phenomena associated with it.[431]

The mechanisms underlying regulation of expression of the GFAP gene and the function of reactive GFAP expression have attracted considerable attention. Since the induction of GFAP expression may be considered the main indicator of astroglial activation,[139] it is interesting to note that in EAE a reactive increase in GFAP immunoreactivity may be observed in the absence of a detectable elevation of cellular GFAP content.[147] Increased GFAP immunostaining has, however, been associated with elevated GFAP synthesis in reactive astrocytes challenged by axotomy of motor neurons.[601] Changes in GFAP expression can occur at both transcriptional and translational levels and may be modulated by steroids, cytokines and growth factors.[338] Microglia-derived IL-1[453] may be especially important as this cytokine has been shown to stimulate astrocytosis and neovascularization.[191] Astrocyte heterogeneity is of great significance in this context as GFAP expression shows brain region-specific responses to sex steroids and astrocytic–neuronal interactions.[338] From a functional point of view, GFAP seems to be required for the formation of stable astrocytic processes and their interaction with neurons *in vitro*.[373,645] However, the relevance of these findings has been questioned in the light of *in vivo* experiments demonstrating that transgenic mice lacking GFAP develop and reproduce normally.[454]

The above findings are in line with the *in vivo* observation that both the extent and time course of reactive GFAP expression may be related to specific astrocytic activation states. For instance, astrocytes responding to postaxotomy changes in rat facial motor neurons undergo hypertrophy

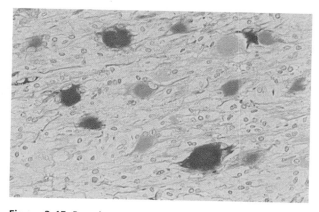

Figure 3.45 *Reactive astrocytes. Reactive, hypertrophic astrocytes similar to those shown in Fig. 3.44. (Immunostained for GFAP.)*

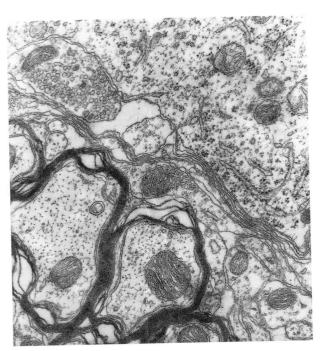

Figure 3.46 *Astrocytic processes in repair. Electron micrograph of astrocytic lamellar cell processes surrounding a regenerating facial motor neuron in the rat, 30 days following nerve transection. Reproduced by permission from Ref. 213.*

and newly synthesize GFAP but they do not proliferate.[211,223] The amount of GFAP synthesized depends on the success of neuronal regeneration, i.e. the rate of GFAP synthesis is higher after peripheral nerve cut and when peripheral reinnervation of the musculature is prevented than after simple nerve crush.[601] After axotomy, the juxtaneuronal reactive astrocytes reshape their processes and form thin cytoplasmic lamellae which become interposed between neuronal surface membranes and afferent synaptic terminals (Fig. 3.46). This astrocytic lamellar reaction leads to an increased compartmentalization of the deafferented motor nucleus and seems strongly dependent upon a well-controlled reorganization of the astrocytic cytoskeleton. After lethal motor neuron injury, reactive astrocytes undergo hypertrophy without subtle reshaping of cell processes. The increase in GFAP expression is massive and a typical glial scar develops.[582]

JUXTASYNAPTIC ASTROCYTE PROCESSES CO-OPERATE AND COMPETE WITH SYNAPTIC TERMINALS

Almost a century ago (1909) Cajal suggested that neuroglial cells have an insulating function within the CNS. He proposed that neuroglial cells are always distributed in such a way as to prevent the flow of impulses from neurons in a haphazard manner.[462] Indirect evidence in support of this concept comes from electron-microscopic studies indicating an insulating morphology of astrocytes under both physiological and reactive conditions. In the anterior horns

and the substantia gelatinosa of the spinal cord there is a close contact between astrocyte processes and synaptic terminals. Afferent axons synapsing on the surfaces of anterior horn cells are segregated either individually or in small groups,[462] so that they appear to lie in astrocytic compartments. Glial ensheathment can also be seen on Purkinje cells. During development, Purkinje cells receive axosomatic climbing fibre input but lose those afferents during postnatal maturation. Later, Bergmann astrocytes wrap the vacated synaptic sites.[463] Astrocytic ensheathment of neuronal surfaces is also seen in sensory ganglia of the spinal and cranial nerves, including the mesencephalic primary sensory nucleus of the trigeminal nerve which has neurons closely covered by astrocytes.[113] From a functional point of view, it would seem useful to improve the signal-to-noise ratio in those neurons which process basic information from the outside world by covering input sites which could attract additional axon terminals. In contrast, in brain regions where a more generalized multiple input is the rule, as in the cerebral cortex, glial wrapping is rare.[463] Importantly, synaptic transmission between neurons can be modulated by astrocytes.[22,23,551]

Several other types of mammalian neuron are insulated by glial cell processes. Wrapping of neuronal and dendritic surfaces by astrocytic lamellar cell extensions is especially prominent in the hypothalamus, e.g. the arcuate nucleus, the ventromedial nucleus, the preoptic area, the supraoptic nucleus, the nucleus circularis, and in the neurophypophysis.[320,604] A high degree of neuronal plasticity can be observed in these brain areas where the density of synapses is regulated by hormones. Depending on physiological stimuli such as dehydration/rehydration, oestrus, parturition, lactation and suckling, synaptic densities change and vacated synaptic sites in these nuclei become occupied by astrocytic processes.

There can be little doubt that astrocytes play a role in synaptic transmission. In fact, it has been suggested that a functional synapse consists not only of the presynaptic terminal and the postsynaptic membrane but also of its glial ensheathment.[298] The latter is usually provided by astrocytes. Therefore, the involvement of juxtasynaptic astrocytic processes in the regulation of the density of synaptic connections under pathological conditions, e.g. after CNS injury, has attracted considerable attention. In the rat phrenic nucleus, the dendrites of motor neurons are normally separated from each other by thin, intervening astrocytic processes.[201] Within hours after hemisection of the spinal cord, the territories of dendro-dendritic appositions and the number of synapses increase at the expense of astrocytic coverings. An active retraction of astrocytic processes appears to occur and seems to enable synaptic contacts to become functional.[201] In the facial nucleus of the rat, detachment and displacement of afferent axon terminals from the surface membrane of motor neurons,[68] known as 'synaptic stripping', occurs during regeneration. Microglial cells seem to play an important role in this process. As described previously, astrocytes stimulated by axotomy of motor neurons increase their expression of GFAP and reshape their cell processes. Beginning 2–3 weeks after axotomy, stacks of astrocytic lamellar cell extensions (Fig. 3.46) closely surround the cell bodies and stem dendrites of the regenerating motor neurons.[212] The resulting synaptic insulation of the regenerating motor neurons is a long-lasting phenomenon and may even be permanent.[212] Reactive astrocytes thus maintain the state of synaptic deafferentation that is initially associated with the microglial response. As synaptic stripping has been shown to occur in the human CNS,[209] prolonged and incomplete functional recovery after peripheral nerve injury may in part be explained by central glial reactions. Reactive astrocytes have the capacity to limit increases in extracellular K^+ that are produced by hyperactive surviving neurons.[641] Considering the high sophistication of central neuronal circuitry, it may be better for some systems to have no input than the wrong input.

ROSENTHAL FIBRES

Rosenthal fibres are intracytoplasmic, filamentous inclusions of astrocytes that are found in several neurological disorders. In H&E-stained sections, they appear as homogeneous hyaline, eosinophilic, bright red structures which may be rounded, oval or elongated and greatly variable in size (Fig. 3.47). They are remarkably stable and cannot be removed from sections by vigorous treatment with fat solvents such as ether or chloroform. Mallory's phosphotungstic acid haematoxylin (PTAH) stain renders them a red to purple colour, while periodic acid–Schiff (PAS) staining is negative. Immunocytochemically, Rosenthal fibres stain positively with GFAP,[568] ubiquitin and the lens protein αB-crystallin. The function of the latter lies in the reorganization of intermediate filament aggregates into a filamentous network in normal astrocytes.[315] However, an excess of GFAP may be detrimental to normal astrocyte function.[145] Immunoultrastructural studies have suggested that Rosenthal fibres are huge aggregation products of αB-cystallin, GFAP and ubiquitin.[609] In addition, the 27-kDa heat shock protein (HSP27) has been detected in Rosenthal fibres.[275]

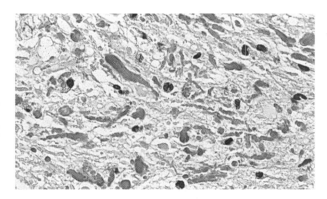

Figure 3.47 *Rosenthal fibres. Abundant Rosenthal fibres around the third ventricle in a case of congenital hydrocephalus. (H&E.)*

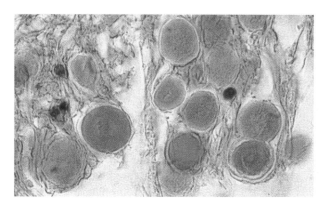

Figure 3.48 *Corpora amylacea. (H&E.)*

Rosenthal fibres are usually found in association with long-lasting, intense fibrillary gliosis, e.g. around syringomyelic cavities and in pilocytic astrocytomas of the cerebellum and optic nerve. They have also been described in some cases of Alzheimer's disease.[644] Rosenthal fibres accumulate massively in the brain of patients suffering from Alexander's disease.[275,609]

CORPORA AMYLACEA

Corpora amylacea are spherical, laminated hyaline bodies composed of polyglucosans.[92] They are most abundant at surfaces: close to pia (Fig. 3.48), around blood vessels and beneath the ependymal lining.[519] Their accumulation in the CNS is associated with ageing and they can be formed in response to neuronal loss.[627] Corpora amylacea contain an amorphous basophilic material, sometimes with a more deeply staining central core. They stain positively with iodine, methyl violet and PAS. An origin of corpora amylacea in the CNS from both neurons and glia has been suggested.[92,520] Antigens detected in corpora amylacea include ubiquitin, tau-2 and heat shock proteins.[102,354] About 4% of the total weight of corpora amylacea is consistently composed of protein.[102] It should be noted that many antibodies as well as nucleic acid hybridization probes tend to bind unspecifically to corpora amylacea. A method for the experimental induction of corpora amylacea has been devised.[523]

OTHER INCLUSIONS

Astrocytic hyaline inclusions containing advanced glycation endproducts have been observed in familial amyotrophic lateral sclerosis with a superoxide dismutase 1 gene mutation.[292] Tau-positive glial inclusions occur in several 'tauopathies'.[25,311] Coarse, paranuclear, eosinophilic inclusions in astrocytes have been described in Aicardi syndrome.[80] (For a review see Ref. 99.)

EPENDYMA

The ependyma reacts to injury with a few stereotypical responses and, if at all, has a very limited capacity for regeneration.[79] Thus, once the ependymal surface is broken, e.g. by stretching during ventricular dilatation or inflammation, it is probably not repaired. Typical ependymal reactions to injury include atrophy, reactive cell loss with the formation of ependymal discontinuities and subventricular gliosis.[515] Beneath the ependyma there is a layer of subependymal glial cells, most of which are astrocytes that have retained their capacity for proliferation and expression of GFAP and S-100. These cells give rise to 'subventricular glial nodules'[515] which are rich in glial fibres (Fig. 3.49). The macroscopic appearance of these nodules is that of tiny clear granules looking like droplets of water. They are best seen in the floor of the fourth ventricle but may occur throughout the ventricular system. These granules may or may not be covered by a layer of ependyma and may have a row, small nests or acini of ependymal cells deeper in the granules. The formation of subventricular glial nodules is especially pronounced in neurosyphilis. However, subventricular glial nodules may develop after any irritative process and thus lack disease specificity, as do most glial reactions. In hydrocephalus, subependymal astrocytes form stacks of processes which may 'seal' and protect the subependymal neuropil against increased cerebrospinal fluid pressure (Fig. 3.50). It should be noted that the subependymal zone as well as the ependymal lining represent sources of adult neural stem cells.[98,132,197,328]

MICROGLIA

The resting microglial cell

Microglia, the resident macrophages of the nervous system, are ubiquitously distributed in non-overlapping territories throughout the CNS (Fig. 3.24). These resident cells comprise up to 20% of the total glial cell population.[343] The role of microglia in various pathological conditions was clearly recognized by del Rio-Hortega, who also coined the term.[121,503] Their nature and identity have long been debated but it is now generally accepted that they are ontogenetically related to cells of the mononuclear phagocyte lineage, unlike all other cell types in the CNS.[43,116,216,351,459,460,578,580] In functional terms, microglia form a network of immune accessory cells throughout the brain and spinal cord and they respond even to the slightest alterations in their microenvironment, functioning as an intrinsic 'sensor' to threats[318] (see also Chapter 2, this Volume). This is of practical diagnostic use[434] (Figs 3.51–3.53).

Microglial turnover

The question of microglial origin is closely linked to the problem of microglial turnover *in vivo*. Bone marrow chimaera experiments have proved to be a particularly valuable tool for analysing microglial turnover. In these experiments, the presence or absence of bone marrow-derived cells has been examined in the brains of rat chimaeras.[255] These studies show that resident microglia have an extremely low turnover with bone marrow precursor cells (less than 1%) while the percentage of replaced cells is high for macrophages in the leptomeninges (60%) and for perivascular cells (30%).[255] These results confirm that the resident microglia form a relatively stable cell population with little turnover with extrinsic bone marrow-derived cells. Similar results have been obtained in the brains of sex-mismatched humans with bone marrow transplantation.[622] Analysis of bone marrow turnover in the PNS demonstrates that a high percentage of satellite

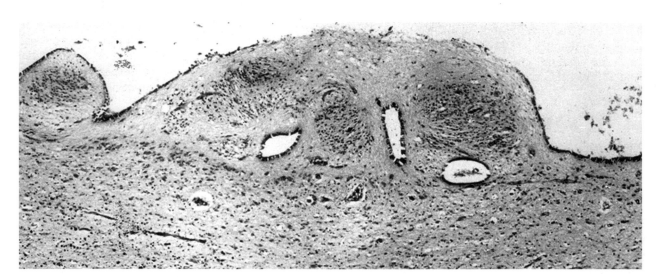

Figure 3.49 *Subventricular glial nodules. Subventricular glial nodules (formerly called 'granular ependymitis') in the lateral ventricle. The ependyma, partially deficient, is elevated over aggregations of astrocytes. Small nests of ependymal cells are seen beneath the glial cells. (H&E.) Reproduced by permission from Ref. 134.*

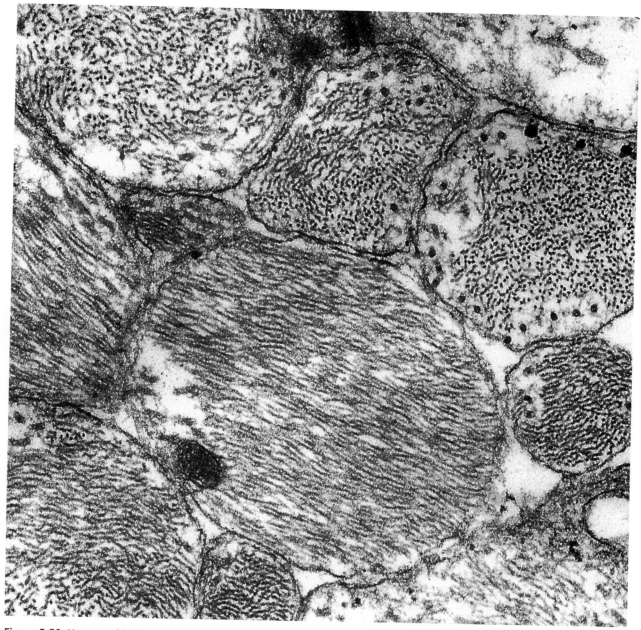

Figure 3.50 *Hypertrophied astrocytic processes. Stacks of hypertrophic astrocytic processes in the periventricular zone of a child suffering from hydrocephalus. Electron micrograph. Courtesy of Professor RO Weller, University of Southampton, UK.*

cells in dorsal root ganglia (80%) and of resident macrophages in the peripheral nerve (60%) undergoes replacement by bone marrow cells.[628] The functional implications of these bone marrow chimaera studies have particular importance for the trafficking of foreign agents into the CNS. In HIV encephalitis, for example, HIV-infected bone marrow cells may reach the CNS perivascular compartment or the endoneurial PNS compartment, respectively, via such a homing mechanism. These results lend support to the Trojan horse hypothesis, whereby HIV-infected macrophages carry the virus into the brain and eventually spread it within the brain to resident microglia.[129,169]

The general activation concept

FROM RESTING MICROGLIA TO BRAIN MACROPHAGE

Resting microglia show a downregulated immuno-phenotype and are in a functionally quiescent state.[460,580] However, observations in neuropathology indicate that microglia can most rapidly respond to injury in the CNS.[318] Activated microglia were first described by Franz Nissl in the form of 'rod cells'[428] (Figs 3.54, 3.55). To define better the stages of microglial activation, animal models which leave the BBB unimpaired and thus allow the study

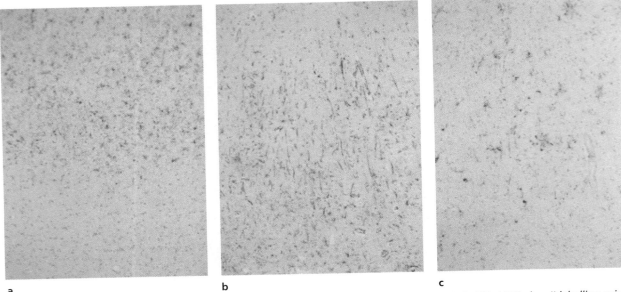

a   b   c

Figure 3.51 *Microglia in various diseases. Microglia, comparative cortical pathology (CJD, SSPE, AD), MHC class II labelling using the CR3/43 monoclonal antibody. The microglial pattern of reactiveness is essentially diagnostic of the respective disease. Modified from Ref. 207.*

of the activation of microglia in the absence of infiltrating haematogenous macrophages have proved invaluable. In this context, the model of facial nerve axotomy has been particularly useful.[580] After facial nerve transection, microglia but not astrocytes rapidly proliferate[223,316,563] (Fig. 3.56), become hypertrophic and express several marker molecules on their surface. These marker molecules comprise not only macrophage-related antigens such as CR3,[218] but also MHC class I and II antigens,[579,581] as well as CD4 and cell adhesion molecules which are otherwise only found on cells of the immune system.[308,483,580] In addition, APP is newly expressed by activated, perineuronal microglia.[36] After facial nerve axotomy, the intermediate filament protein, vimentin, has been found to constitute the main cytoskeletal protein of activated, motile microglia.[221] In other pathologies, e.g. cerebral ischaemia, however, vimentin is expressed by reactive astrocytes but not by activated microglia. In response to facial nerve transection, microglia, particularly in a perineuronal position (Figs 3.56–3.59), proliferate and start to ensheath the injured motor neuron, interposing processes between afferent synaptic terminals and the neuronal surface.[322] This phenomenon, originally described by Blinzinger and Kreutzberg,[69] is now generally referred to as 'synaptic stripping'. Detachment of synaptic terminals from the motor neuron surface may have an impact on the synaptic reorganization of injured motor neurons. Under the condition of facial nerve axotomy, microglia become activated but not phagocytic (Fig. 3.59). However, if motor neuron death is induced by injection of toxic ricin into the facial nerve, microglia rapidly transform into phagocytic cells.[582] Clusters of microglia-derived brain macrophages gradually remove the neuronal

cell debris (Fig. 3.60). These microglia-derived brain macrophages also express *de novo* the ED1 epitope which is otherwise typical of peripheral macrophages.

In summary, the microglial response to injury occurs gradually.[318,580] First, microglia become activated, but do not become phagocytic. Secondly, following neuronal and/or axonal terminal degeneration, microglia transform into intrinsic brain phagocytes. Thus, the transformation of microglia into a potentially cytotoxic effector cell is under strict control *in vivo* and only takes place if cell death occurs. A mechanism of cellular communication between neurons and microglia, involving fractalkine and CX3CR1, has been proposed[246] and questioned.[287]

In view of their morphological and functional characteristics, at least four different phenotypes of microglia can be distinguished:

- the amoeboid microglia found perinatally;
- the ramified, resting microglia in the mature CNS;
- the activated, but non-phagocytic microglia in response to sublethal CNS injury; and
- the phagocytic microglia ('brain macrophages') found in areas of trauma, inflammation and neuronal necrosis where they participate in neuronophagy (Fig. 3.61).

In animal models, microglial activation occurs in response to several pathological stimuli including brain trauma,[179] T-cell-mediated inflammation,[177] global and focal ischaemia,[176,409] transplants into the brain, experimental gliomas,[408] and viral and bacterial infections.[200] Microglial activation may even occur rapidly in response to remote and relatively mild injuries suggesting that fast

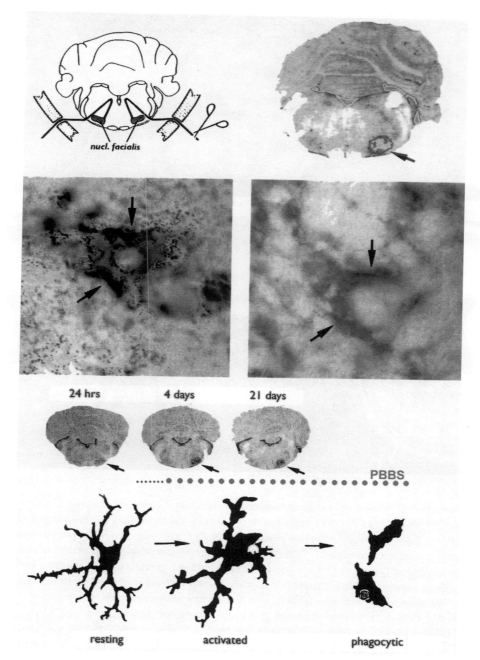

Figure 3.52 *Activated microglia. Microautoradiographic detection of [³H]PK11195 binding to activated microglia. The arrows on the cross-sections of the brainstem point to the facial nuclei and the arrows arould the nerve cell point to perineuronal microglia, respectively. Modified from Ref. 39.*

activation pathways are operating. There is hardly any disease of the nervous system without microglial activation. Under all of these conditions microglia upregulate an almost stereotypic pattern of activation markers including the CR3 complement receptor, cell adhesion molecules, leukocyte common antigen (CD45), MHC class I and class II antigens, CD4 and APP. Moreover, they secrete cytokines, for example TGF-β₁.

The factors other than neuronal cell death that induce microglial activation are just beginning to be elucidated.

Cortical spreading depression and changes in extracellular ATP levels[178,297] as well as intrathecal application of inflammatory cytokines[629] are sufficient to induce a microglial activation in the absence of obvious pathological tissue damage. Moreover, colony-stimulating factors such as macrophage colony-stimulating factor (M-CSF) and granulocyte–macrophage colony-stimulating factor (GM-CSF) are involved in microglial proliferation and activation.[483] These factors are strong mitogens for microglia and influence their differentiation *in*

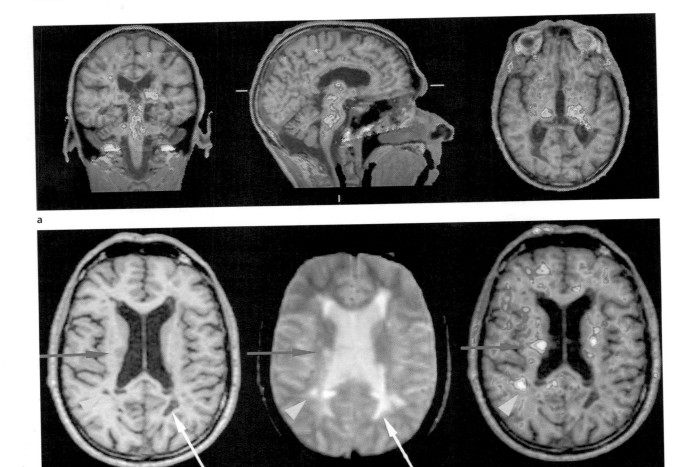

Figure 3.53 *Activated microglia. [^{11}C](R)-PK11195 positron emission tomography imaging of activated microglia in vivo in multiple sclerosis. MRI and [^{11}C](R)-PK11195 RET. All images follow the radiological convention, i.e. the left side of the image corresponds to the subject's right side. (a) Three orthogonal views of [^{11}C](R)-PK11195 images co-registered and overlaid on the MRI of a atient showing spinothalamic tract-associated [^{11}C](R)-PK11195 signals extending through the brainstem and pons into the thalamus. (b–d) T$_1$-weighted (b) and T$_2$-weighted (c) MRI and [^{11}C](R)-PK11195 PET (overlaid onto T$_1$-weighted MRI) (d) of this patient show lesions in all different spin-echo MRI seqences that partially overlap with areas of significantly increased [^{11}C](R)-PK11195 binding (red arrow). The white arrow ponts to a 'black hole' in an area that appears strongly hypointense in the T$_1$-weighted MRJ and has little binding of [^{11}C](R)-PK11195. Note, however, that a similar black hole (yellow arrowhead) adjacent to the right occipital horn of the lateral ventricle shows significant [^{11}C](R)-PK11195 binding. Courtesy of Dr Richard Banati, MRC Cyclotron Unit and Imperial College School of Medicine, London, UK; reproduced by permission from Ref. 40.*

vitro.[188,590] *In vivo*, the expression of M-CSF and GM-CSF receptors is increased on the surface of activated microglia already in the premitotic stage.[484] Moreover, in the osteopetrotic (op) mouse mutant, which is deficient in M-CSF, microglial proliferation is reduced by about 90% if these mice are challenged by facial nerve axotomy.[490] In pathological conditions which give extrinsic, haematogenous cells access to the lesion site in the brain following breakdown of the BBB, it is not possible to distinguish intrinsic, microglia macrophages derived from extrinsic, infiltrating ones.

Experimental autoimmune encephalomyelitis is an inflammatory CNS disease which is induced by auto-reactive T-lymphocytes recognizing CNS autoantigens[646] (see also Chapter 8, Volume II). BBB function is impaired at an early stage of the disease. Microglia/macrophages proliferate strongly in the vicinity of perivascular T-cell infiltrates and upregulate the expression of MHC class II antigens and cell adhesion molecules.[86,376,377,630] During the clinical recovery stage, these inflammatory foci consisting of microglia/macrophages are surrounded by hypertrophic astrocytes so that the activated microglia exist somewhat separated from the inflammatory lesion. Macrophage depletion experiments using silica or liposomes purport to show a crucial role of extrinsic macrophages in the development of

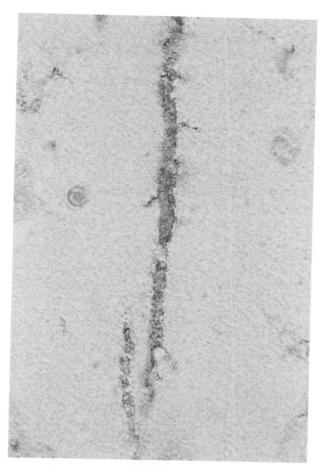

Figure 3.54 *Microglial rod cell. Microglial rod cell in a case of subacute sclerosing panencephalitis. (HLA-DR immunostaining counterstained with haematoxylin.) Reproduced by permission from Ref. 208.*

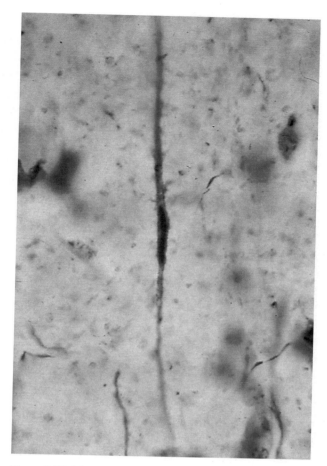

Figure 3.55 *Microglial rod cell in general paralysis of the insane. (Penfield's silver impregnation.)*

lesions.[270] If EAE is induced in bone marrow chimaeric rats, the turnover of meningeal macrophages and perivascular cells (see below) is accelerated but the resident microglia remain a relatively stable cell population with limited replacement by donor-derived macrophages.[340] Donor-derived macrophages are accordingly detected in the CNS parenchyma at the peak but not at the recovery stage of EAE. Therefore, resident microglia may proliferate and become activated in the absence of considerable turnover of haematogenous macrophages.

CYTOTOXICITY

A characteristic property of microglia *in vivo* is their swift activation after CNS injury and their capacity for site-directed phagocytosis. There are two principal ways by which microglia can act as cytotoxic cells. First, they may act as brain phagocytes removing tissue debris.[582] Microglia express Fc and complement receptors on their surface. In particular, during antibody-mediated demyelination activated microglia can lyse antibody-coated target cells via interaction of Fc and complement receptors

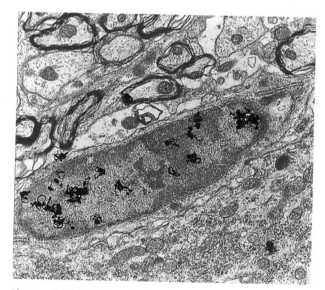

Figure 3.56 *Mitotic microglial cell. Mitotic, perineuronal microglia in the regenerating rat facial nucleus 2 days after facial nerve axotomy. [³H]Thymidine autoradiography at ultrastructural level.*

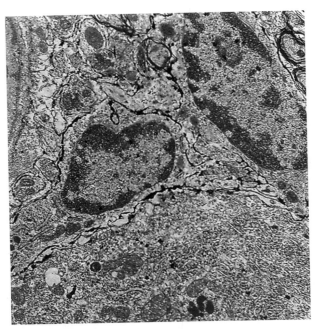

Figure 3.57 *Activated microglial cell. Activated, perineuronal microglial cell exhibiting prominent deposits of the ectoenzyme 5'-nucleotidase on its surface. Regenerating rat facial nucleus 7 days after facial nerve axotomy.*

on their surface with immune complexes and complement-opsonized antigens.[680] Secondly, activated microglia are capable of releasing several potentially cytotoxic substances such as free oxygen intermediates, nitric oxide, proteinases, arachidonic acid derivates, excitatory amino acids, quinolinic acid and cytokines.[36,110,309,397,468,592] Microglia-produced TNF-α can cause bystander damage during demyelination.[544] Free oxygen radicals released by microglia have a neurotoxic effect in cocultures of neurons and microglia.[605] HIV-infected mononuclear cells have also been shown to produce low molecular weight neurotoxins, possibly causing neuronal damage in an NMDA receptor-mediated fashion.[190] However, much of the information on the cytotoxic properties of activated microglia pertains to *in vitro* observations and remains to be confirmed *in vivo*. Furthermore, the cytotoxic properties of microglia are subject to considerable species variation.[110] The cytotoxic properties of microglia can be modulated by cytokines and neurotransmitters.

While cytokines such as interferon-γ (IFN-γ) prime microglia to become activated, other cytokines such as TGF-β₁ or IL-4 downregulate microglial cytotoxicity.[37] Both the phagocytic and the cytotoxic activation of microglia can be ameliorated by TGF-β₁, suggesting that autocrine regulation of microglial activation may also occur during tissue damage.[399] Neuronal activity may furthermore control microglial activation. Noradrenaline has been shown to reduce IL-1 and free radical production in macrophages, and β-adrenergic agonists such as isoproterenol may reduce IL-1 and TNF-α production of microglia. Furthermore, neurotrophins inhibit major

histocompatibility class II inducibility of microglia *in vivo*.[424] In turn, pharmacological intervention with macrophage/microglial activation has been shown to reduce the extent of tissue damage in animal models of cerebral ischaemia.[189] Strategies to rescue neuronal function after suppressing microglial activation, however, must be viewed with caution. Function will not be recovered from necrotic or irreversibly damaged neurons. Any therapeutic strategy must therefore aim at interfering with microglial cytotoxicity in the early, still reversible, stage of neuronal damage.

Phagocytosis by microglia includes apoptotic[331] cells which, however, have to display phosphatidylserine.[3] It is noteworthy that microglia-derived phagocytes eliminate certain CNS constitutents such as myelin degradation products rather slowly, presumably because they fail to release molecules which facilitate phagocytosis.[10] Adhesive properties between microglia and peripheral macrophages also differ.[608]

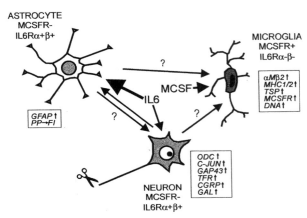

Figure 3.58 *Microglial activation. A schematic summary of the changes occurring at the level of the injured neuronal cell body after axotomy. In the axotomized neuron, there is a rapid increase in nucleic acid metabolism-associated enzymes (ornithine decarboxylase, ODC), immediate-early gene proteins (IEG), growth-associated proteins (GAP43) and neuropeptides (NP) such as CGRP and galanin. Adjacent astrocytes produce growth factors and cytokines (GF/CK), show an increase in GFAP content and change shape from a protoplasmic to a fibrillary-like type. The third cell type, the microglia, shows enhanced expression of cell adhesion molecules (α_M β_2-integrin, thrombospondin/TSP), major histocompatibility complex antigens (MHCI,II) and receptors for microglial mitogens (MCSFR). These activated microglia move into direct apposition to the neuronal cell body, where they begin to proliferate (DNA). Absence of MCSF leads to a strong reduction in the activation of MCSF receptor-positive microglia (MCSFR+) but does not affect the receptor-negative neurons and astrocytes (MCSFR–). Absence of interleukin-6 (IL–6) affects IL-6 receptor-postive astrocytes and neurons (IL–6Rα+β+), but also the receptor-negative microglia (IL–6Rα–β–), indicating an indirect effect. Molecular factors, symbolized by question marks, mediating this neuroglial cross-talk are still to be identified. Modified from Ref. 483.*

Microglial and astroglial activation often occurs in concert during CNS injury (Fig. 3.58). Since microglial activation frequently precedes astrocytic reactions, it is reasonable to assume that activated microglia may release at an early stage mediators such as IL-1 which induce astro-cytic activation.[149] Reactive astrocytes may, in turn, contribute to CNS regeneration by secreting neurotrophic factors.

Although activated microglia are generally regarded as cytotoxic effector cells, they also play a tissue-protective

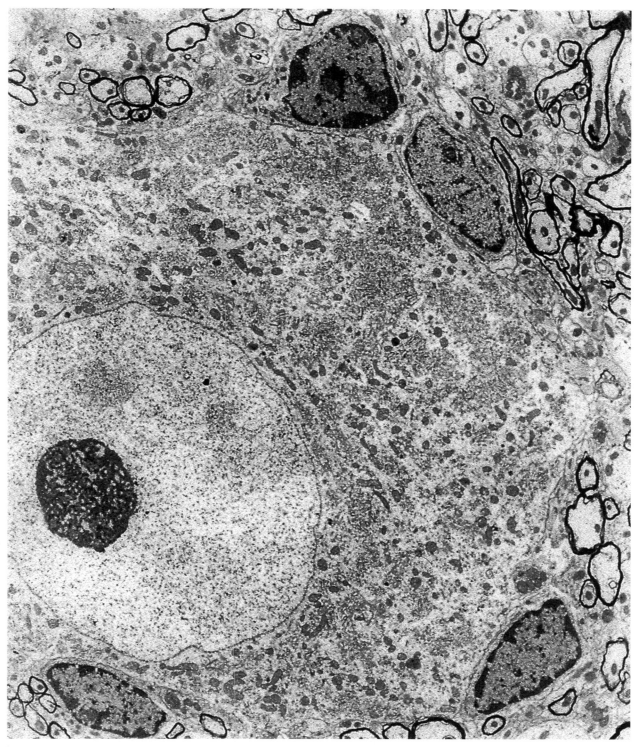

Figure 3.59 *Microglial activation. Sublethal motor neuron injury, i.e. facial nerve axotomy, leads to microglial activation. Microglia proliferate around injured motor neurons but they do not become phagocytic. Regenerating rat facial nucleus 7 days after facial nerve axotomy. Electron micrograph.*

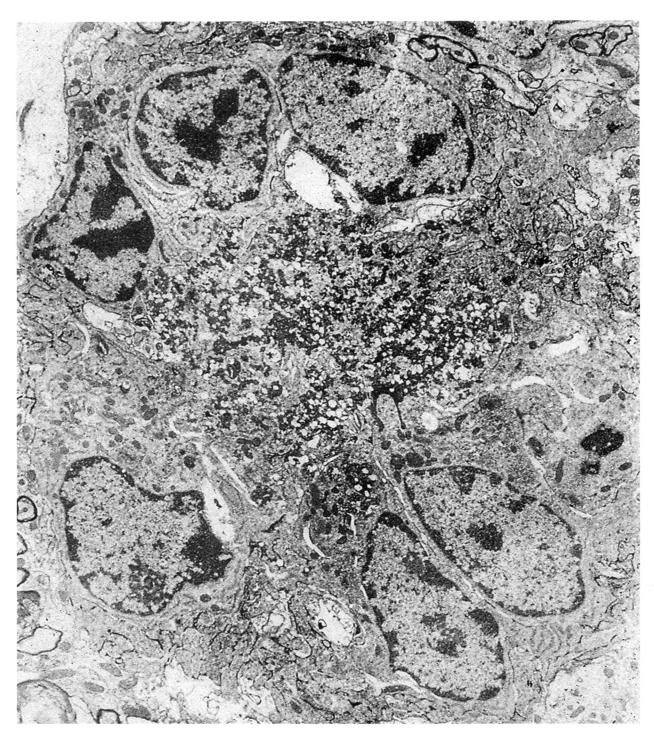

Figure 3.60 *Neuronophagy. Lethal motor neuron injury induced by toxic ricin injection into the facial nerve leads to the transformation of microglia into macrophages and neuronophagia. Clusters of these microglia-derived brain macrophages phagocytose the debris of necrotic facial motor neurons 7 days after the lesion. Electron micrograph. Reproduced by permission from Ref. 582.*

role. The TGF-β_1 produced by activated microglia, for example after direct cortical trauma or after global cerebral ischaemia, may promote tissue repair either directly or indirectly by reducing astrocytic scar formation.[350,650] Microglia-secreted plasminogen promotes neurite outgrowth and may be involved in extracellular matrix

proteolysis, thereby regulating cell migration and synaptogenesis.[416] Tissue remodelling by intervening, activated microglia is well exemplified in the regenerating optic nerve of fish or amphibia which, unlike mammals, have a high capacity for CNS regeneration. Regeneration of the optic nerve is preceded by a pronounced

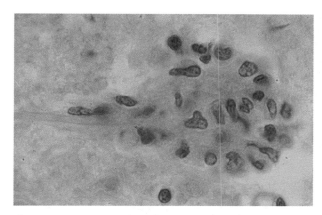

Figure 3.61 *Neuronophagy in a case of acute poliomyelitis. Clusters of activated microglia with prominent, elongated nuclei have invaded an anterior horn motor neuron in the spinal cord. (H&E.)*

macrophage/microglial response which supports regeneration. Thus, microglial activation has two faces: under conditions of cell death microglia act as scavengers removing tissue debris, whereas in more subtle injury they exert a surveillance function to play a protective role.[38]

IMMUNE FUNCTIONS: MHC EXPRESSION AND ANTIGEN PRESENTATION

The low level of MHC antigen expression in the brain has contributed to the traditional view of the brain as an immunologically privileged site.[646] In rodent and human brain, MHC class I antigen expression is low in the intact nervous system and normally confined to blood vessels. MHC class II antigens are expressed together with the processed antigen and additional costimulatory molecules such as B7 on the surface of an APC. They are required for antigen presentation leading to stimulation of antigen-specific T-lymphocytes. In the brain of Lewis rats, MHC class II antigen expression is low and mainly found in macrophages in the leptomeninges and in the choroid plexus, as well as in the perivascular cells. In addition, a subpopulation of resident microglia appears to express MHC class II immunoreactivity constitutively, particularly in the white matter of the cerebellum and in the white matter of the lumbar spinal cord. *In vivo*, a hierarchy of MHC class II antigen expression exists. MHC class II antigens can be rapidly upregulated in the entire population of resident microglia by intrathecal administration of inflammatory cytokines such as TNF-α and IFN-γ.[629] In contrast, MHC class II antigens can only be induced at extremely low levels by high doses of cytokines in endothelial cells and cells of neuroectodermal origin including astrocytes. Accordingly, MHC class II antigen expression has not been convincingly demonstrated in reactive astrocytes *in vivo*. However, MHC class II expression in microglia is subject to considerable species variation. In the

black Norway rat, which is resistant to the induction of T-cell-mediated autoimmune inflammation, almost all resident microglia constitutively express MHC class II antigens.[540]

Following both inflammatory and remote non-inflammatory lesions, MHC class II molecules are rapidly upregulated in activated microglia but not in reactive astrocytes. During inflammatory reactions this MHC class II induction is widespread. In contrast, MHC class II induction in microglia after more subtle and non-inflammatory lesions such as peripheral nerve axotomy is restricted to the primary projection areas.[579] Under these non-inflammatory conditions, microglial MHC class II expression does not necessarily imply antigen-presenting function. This high degree of immune alertness, however, may facilitate delayed-type hypersensitivity reactions. In fact, increased MHC class II antigen expression induced by peripheral nerve injury targets T-cell-mediated inflammation at specific sites within the CNS such as the deafferented superior colliculus or the axotomized facial nucleus.[157,364] These results strongly suggest a crucial role of MHC class II-positive, activated microglia in T-cell recruitment and point to a possible link between brain trauma and inflammation. In turn, massive class II expression by microglia in various neurodegenerative diseases[389] occurring in the absence of co-stimulatory molecules (glial inflammation) could protect the CNS against immune-mediated injury like a 'firewall'.[38,125,458]

In the human brain, analysis of MHC class II expression is strongly influenced by technical factors including post-mortem survival times, tissue collection and embedding procedures.[381] In fresh-frozen human brains, MHC class II expression is typically found in perivascular cells and in some, mainly white matter microglia.[247] Although these brains may be classified as histologically normal, it is almost impossible to exclude that a subtle brain injury might have contributed to the MHC class II expression observed in resident microglia. Genetic variation is another possibility. In formalin-fixed, routinely processed and paraffin wax-embedded material, MHC class II expression appears to be restricted to activated microglia.[208] The extent of constitutive MHC class II expression by human microglia remains debatable. A possible role of human microglia in local stimulation of T-cell proliferation and antigen presentation is further supported by the presence of costimulatory molecules such as B7 on the surface of activated microglia, e.g. in acute MS.[125]

Microglial involvement in CNS diseases

Classical examples of microglial activation in CNS diseases are the appearance of rod-shaped microglia in cortical degeneration during neurosyphilis (general paralysis of the insane) or SSPE and the formation of nodules of neuronophagic microglia around anterior horn motor neurons in poliomyelitis.[128,208,389,390] Activated microglia, however, are found in almost any CNS pathology and thus serve as an early and sensitive marker of tissue damage (Fig. 3.62).[318] Human microglia can be identified by RCA-1 lectin histochemistry[368] and by immunocytochemical detection with several antibodies such as anti-CD45, anti-CD68, anti-MHC class II (e.g. CR3/43), HAM56, anti-ferritin and Iba1.[2,208,274,675] For routine application on formalin-fixed, paraffin-embedded tissue the following staining techniques are particularly useful. RCA-1 lectin histochemistry is easy to perform and sensitive but has the disadvantage of cross-reacting with the endothelium of blood vessels. Anti-CD68 (KP1) typically associates with lysosomal structures and is an excellent marker for macrophages but does not label all activated microglia. In contrast, the anti-MHC class II antibody CR3/43 stains activated microglia in paraffin sections reliably, and HAM56 preferentially labels phagocytic foamy macrophages in ischaemic brain lesions or in acute MS lesions.[2] Another good marker is Ki-M1P,[452] although this antibody is less sensitive than CR3/43 and shows a somewhat granular labelling pattern. Iba-1[274] is reactive across several species and works well in paraffin-embedded human material; the antibody is ideal for double-labelling microglia as it is polyclonal. All of these stains are specific for human microglia in the sense that they do not recognize other glial cell types or neurons but cross-react with macrophages and related cells.

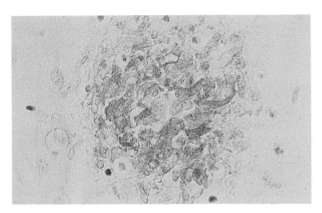

Figure 3.63 *Microglial nodule in HIV encephalitis. (HLA-DR immunostaining counterstained with haematoxylin.) Reproduced by permission from Ref. 208.*

HIV ENCEPHALITIS

In addition to CD4-positive T-lymphocytes, cells of the monocyte/macrophage lineage are a primary target of HIV-1. Microglia express the chemokine receptors CCR5 and CCR3 together with CD4 and also express CXCR4, but their infection by HIV-1 viruses that use only CXCR4 as a coreceptor is relatively inefficient.[169] CCR5 is the principal coreceptor for HIV-1 dementia isolates.[8]

The pathological hallmark of HIV-1 encephalitis is the multinucleated giant cell (MGC).[549] These cells express macrophage/microglial markers and HIV-1 coat proteins such as gp25 and gp41, and contain high copy numbers of HIV-1 nucleic acids.[329] It is likely that MGCs arise from fusion of HIV-1-infected microglia, possibly as a result of the cytopathic, fusion-inducing properties of HIV-1. In addition, activated microglia are present in the form of microglial nodules (Fig. 3.63). It is rare in HIV-1 encephalitis to have infection of cell types other than microglia/macrophages. Thus, microglia are now established as the CNS target of HIV-1.[169] Bone marrow chimaera experiments[255] lend support to the Trojan horse hypothesis according to which HIV-1-infected bone marrow cells initially target the perivascular space, a site close to the BBB, and traverse it to enter the brain parenchyma. HIV-1 would then spread to parenchymal cells. Thus, HIV-1-infected glia and MGC harbour a persisting virus reservoir in the brain which is difficult to reach by pharmacological approaches.

In HIV-1 encephalitis, about 25% of the macrophage/microglial population contain high copy numbers of HIV-1 DNA and RNA.[202] An even greater percentage of macrophages/microglia contain HIV-1-specific proteins, e.g. gp41.[330] Studies on the distribution of proviral and viral HIV sequences show that infected macrophages/microglia are concentrated in areas of potentially HIV-1-induced tissue damage. Thus, the pattern of HIV-1-induced CNS lesions is largely correlated with the extent of regional HIV-1 replication in microglia. In cortical areas, activated microglia frequently enwrap cortical neu-

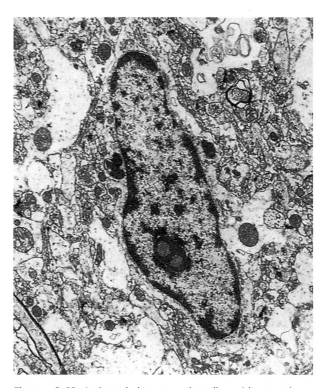

Figure 3.62 *Activated human microglia with prominent nuclear heterochromatin. Electron micrograph.*

rons. In addition, activated microglia may be abundant in deep grey matter nuclei.[129] Neuronal cell death does not correlate with dementia in HIV infection but is related to microglial activation and axonal damage.[4]

Examination of brains of asymptomatic HIV-1-positive individuals who died accidentally and of rare cases with acute fatal encephalopathy revealing HIV infection, and comparison with experimental simian immunodeficiency virus and feline immunodeficiency virus infections, suggest that invasion of the CNS by HIV-1 occurs at the time of primary infection and induces an immunological process.[229] This includes an increase in the number of microglial cells, upregulation of MHC class II antigens and local production of cytokines.

Transgenic mice overexpressing gp120 show neuropathological changes such as dendritic and synaptic loss, astrocytosis and microglial proliferation in the form of a 'nodular' encephalitis.[607] In vitro, gp120-induced neurotoxicity depends on the presence of macrophages/microglia, suggesting that these cells process gp120 and possibly shed a smaller, neurotoxic fragment of gp120. In addition to processing viral proteins, microglia may release several cytotoxic substances, particularly reactive oxygen intermediates, proteases, quinolinic acid and excitatory amino acids. HIV-1-infected microglia synthesize high levels of TNF mRNA. In the spinal cord, activated microglia may play a crucial role in mediating tissue damage in vacuolar myelopathy. In addition to causing tissue damage, activated microglia may help to restrict opportunistic infections occurring in the acquired immunodeficiency syndrome (AIDS), particularly toxoplasmosis and fungal infections caused by *Cryptococcus neoformans*, *Nocardia* or *Candida* (see Chapter 1, Volume II).

ALZHEIMER'S DISEASE AND OTHER NEURODEGENERATIVE DISORDERS

In the aged brain, there is an increased number of microglial cells. In aged non-human primates compared with young ones the number of microglia is increased by about 40%. Moreover, microglia of aged rodents show morphological changes, MHC class II upregulation and an altered cellular distribution of iron-binding proteins.[461]

In Alzheimer's disease MHC class II-positive microglia are prominent in the core of senile plaques.[241,389] These activated microglial cells in the core as well as activated microglia at the outer border of the senile plaque express several immune-related antigens such as β_2-integrins, complement receptors, vitronectin receptor, α_2-macroglobulin, IL-1, IL-6, TNF-α and human leukocyte antigen (HLA)-DR[390] (Fig. 3.64). Microglia are associated not only with senile plaque amyloid (Fig. 3.51) but also with extracellular neurofibrillary tangles.[115] The relationship between microglial activation in Alzheimer's disease and amyloid formation is under intense scrutiny. It has been suggested that the interaction of microglial scavenger receptors with fibrillar β-amyloid

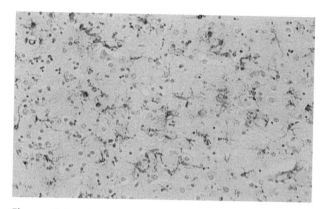

Figure 3.64 *Microglial activation in Alzheimer's disease. Microglial activation in the cerebral cortex of an apolipoprotein E ε_4 homozygote Alzheimer case. (HLA-DR immunostaining.)[140]*

may stimulate microglia to secrete apolipoprotein E (ApoE) and complement proteins which may contribute to neurotoxicity and neuronal degeneration.[141] Importantly, the allele status at the ApoE locus has an influence on microglial activation in Alzheimer's disease.[140,446] CD40–CD40L interaction may be necessary for Aβ-induced microglial activation.[593]

Wisniewski *et al.*[656] have ultrastructurally described amyloid fibrils within the endoplasmic reticulum of activated microglia in the immediate vicinity of amyloid deposition, suggesting that activated microglia may not only process but also synthesize amyloid. In addition, amyloid fibrils have been described in perivascular cells, suggesting that they may form a source of vascular amyloid.[657] However, other authors maintain the view that microglia are not associated with initial plaque formation but rather phagocytose and possibly process the amyloid.[161,553] It is not yet clear whether microglial activation around senile plaques in Alzheimer's disease is a primary event actively supporting amyloidogenesis or a secondary phenomenon (see Chapter 4, Volume II).

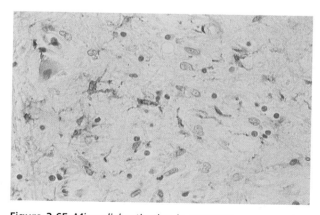

Figure 3.65 *Microglial activation in progressive supranuclear palsy. Microglial activation in the dentate nucleus in a case of progressive supranuclear palsy. (HLA-DR immunostaining.) Reproduced by permission from Ref. 208.*

Activated, MHC class II-positive microglia have also been demonstrated in a number of neurodegenerative disorders such as Parkinson's disease, multiple system atrophy and progressive supranuclear palsy[35,313,389,390] (Fig. 3.65). In amyotrophic lateral sclerosis activated microglia are abundant in areas of degenerating motor neurons in the ventral horn of the spinal cord as well as in the central motor cortex. In addition to phagocytosing necrotic neurons, these activated microglial cells surround degenerating motor neurons with their hypertrophic processes (see Chapter 6, Volume II). Activated microglia are also abundant in transmissible spongiform encephalopathies (prion diseases), including CJD[184,516,635] (see Chapter 5, Volume II).

MULTIPLE SCLEROSIS

In MS demyelination occurs in the proximity of phagocytic macrophages/microglia. Macrophages outnumber T-lymphocytes by far in acute and chronic MS lesions. In acute lesions with rapid myelin breakdown activated macrophages/microglia are abundant and appear morphologically as lipid-laden cells throughout the lesion, but they are most conspicuous at the border between the demyelinating plaque and the still intact, but reactive surrounding tissue.[347] The presence of oil-red-O-positive, lipid-laden foamy macrophages is thought, in combination with T-lymphocyte infiltration, to indicate active lesions (Fig. 3.66). Early demyelinating activity may be recognized on the basis of Luxol fast blue (LFB)-positive blue granules in macrophages.[339]

Although difficult to assess only by morphological criteria, reactive, ramified microglia appear to be concentrated at the edge of acute lesions and express high levels of MHC class II molecules[69] (Fig. 3.67). In contrast, MHC class II expression by astrocytes in MS has not been confirmed. Moreover, activated microglia express high levels of CD45, intercellular adhesion molecule-1 (ICAM-1), Fc receptors, CR1, CR3 and CR4 complement receptors,[620]

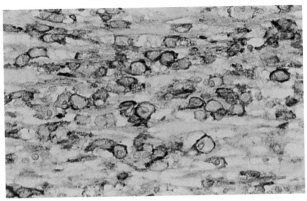

Figure 3.67 *Macrophages in multiple sclerosis. Foamy macrophages in an actively demyelinating white matter lesion in acute 'Marburg type' of multiple sclerosis. (HLA-DR immunostaining.)*

low-density lipoprotein receptor[347] as well as costimulatory molecules required for 'positive' antigen presentation to T-lymphocytes[125] (for review see Refs 48 and 481). Microglia are considered to play a key role in MS pathogenesis.[572,594] Importantly, they induce MBP-specific T-cell anergy or T-cell activation, according to their state of activation.[383] Activated microglia can damage antibody-coated targets, i.e. mainly oligodendrocytes and the myelin sheath via interaction of Fc and complement receptors and complement-opsonized antigens on the myelin sheath. Such cross-linking will further stimulate the microglial oxidative burst response and the release of inflammatory cytokines such as IL-1, IL-6 and TNF-α which have been shown to be expressed by microglia in MS lesions (see Chapter 8, Volume II). It should be noted, however, that many macrophages in EAE lesions, the rodent model of MS, have been shown to be recently derived from the blood.

HEAD INJURY

In animal models, direct or indirect cortical trauma induces an immediate local microglial reaction at the site of primary lesion as well as a delayed microglial reaction at more distant projection areas.[613] At the lesion site activated microglia have been shown by microdialysis measurements and by *in situ* hybridization to release high levels of IL-1, IL-6 and TGF-β_1 within 24–48 h of the lesion occurring.[662] Microglia-derived IL-1 may induce astrogliosis and neovascularization around the lesion,[191] while microglia-derived IL-6 and TGF-β_1 may directly support tissue repair.[350] Clusters of activated microglia are frequently observed in diffuse axonal lesions of the cerebrum, cerebellum and brainstem in man following head injury.[104,434] After penetrating brain lesions including intracerebral stereotactic biopsies, activated microglia may persist for years. Thus, microglial reactions may serve as a sensitive indicator for even relatively subtle or long-pending local brain damage (see Chapter 14, this Volume).

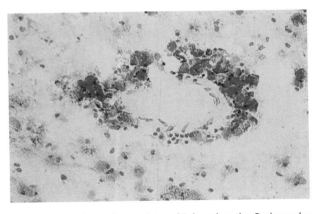

Figure 3.66 *Macrophages in multiple sclerosis. Perivascular accumulation of oil-red-O-positive macrophages in acute multiple sclerosis indicating rapidly progressive myelin degradation and uptake of neutral lipids by macrophages/microglia.*

ISCHAEMIA

In both global and focal cerebral ischaemia in rats, microglia become rapidly activated not only in selectively vulnerable brain regions such as the hippocampal CA1 area or in the penumbra of a focal infarct, but also at remote projection sites. At the primary site of ischaemic damage microglial proliferation and activation occur within the first 24 h after ischaemia.[73,153,176,409] In addition to upregulating the expression of several immune-related antigens such as MHC class II antigens on their surface, microglia transform into brain phagocytes and synthesize cytokines such as TGF-β_1.[650]

In cerebral infarcts in man, numerous activated MHC class II-positive microglia occur at the edge of the lesion as well as in the surrounding tissue. Activated microglia occasionally start to isolate morphologically still intact cortical neurons as if to protect them from cytotoxic damage. Within the infarct, mononuclear phagocytes are abundant within a few days after the ischaemic injury and persist for several months. These cells assume the classical morphology of foamy macrophages: round cells measuring 20–30 μm in diameter, with a granular, lipid-laden cytoplasm and a small, dark, eccentric nucleus (Fig. 3.68). In the case of intraparenchymal bleeding, these cells as well as activated microglia with a more ramified morphology rapidly transform into typical haemosiderophages. In the absence of any marker positively distinguishing extrinsic macrophages from intrinsic microglia, however, the precise contribution of these two cell populations to the overall pool of mononuclear phagocytes remains to be established in ischaemia (see Chapter 5, this Volume).

The functional consequences of microglial activation in ischaemia are not yet understood. Activated microglia may contribute to tissue damage by their pronounced cytotoxicity.[189] In line with this assumption, pharmacological interference with the reaction of mononuclear phagocytes has been shown to attenuate the extent of tissue damage in animal models. However, activated microglia may also be neuroprotective.[684]

BRAIN TUMOURS

Gliomas and secondary brain tumours are infiltrated extensively by macrophages/microglia.[456] These cells are found throughout the tumour with an increased density at the periphery; many have become phagocytic.[408] In human gliomas, however, the histological grading is not correlated with the degree of microglial activation.[393] Although microglia show pronounced tumour cell cytotoxicity *in vitro*,[166] the macrophage/microglial response does not appear to mount an effective tumour defence *in vivo*. This weak cytotoxic action may at least in part be due to active suppression of microglial cytotoxicity. Microglia may even increase proliferation and migratory activity in human glioma cell lines,[636] and only weakly present glioma antigen.[156] Tumour cells secrete cytokines such as TGF-β_1 which downregulate microglial cytotoxicity.[301,356,526] Thus, blockade of TGF-β production by brain tumours may enhance microglial anti-tumour cytotoxicity (see Chapter 11, Volume II).

PERIVASCULAR CELLS AND OTHER BRAIN MACROPHAGES

The term brain macrophage refers to at least five anatomically and probably also functionally distinct cell types of which only one, the microglia cell, is actually resident in the CNS parenchyma. All the other types, however, are located within the bony confinements of the CNS; these include the meningeal macrophages, supraependymal macrophages, epiplexus macrophages (Kolmer cells) and perivascular macrophages, a subpopulation of which has been termed 'perivascular cells'.[19,165,220,380]

Perivascular cells are located outside the CNS parenchyma proper, from which they are separated by the parenchymal basement membrane and the glial lamina limitans (Figs 3.69, 3.70). They are relatively large, spindle-shaped cells of the perivascular space lacking

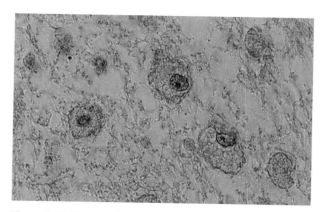

Figure 3.68 *Phagocytic microglia/macrophages ('gitter cells') in ischaemic necrosis. (H&E.)*

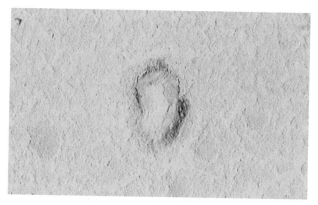

Figure 3.69 *Perivascular cell. HLA-DR-positive perivascular cell in a histologically normal human brain. Reproduced by permission from Ref. 222.*

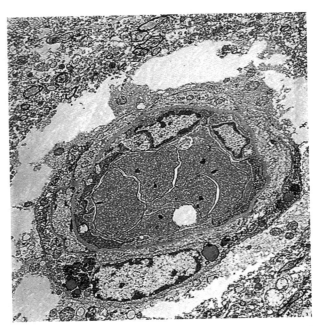

Figure 3.70 *Perivascular cell. HLA-DR-positive perivascular cell from histologically normal human cerebral cortex. Immuno-electron microscopy for HLA-DR molecules. Reproduced by permission from Ref. 217.*

direct contact with neural cellular elements. Perivascular cells constitutively express several myelomonocytic antigens which are commonly absent from resting microglia.[164] This immunophenotype, their location in the perivascular space and their morphology distinguish perivascular cells from microglia and from resident cells of the outer blood vessel wall, i.e. pericytes, smooth-muscle cells and fibroblasts (Figs 3.69, 3.70). Perivascular cells are also distinct from mast cells as they lack the histochemical and morphological characteristics of the latter. In the adult, perivascular cells are continuously renewed from peripheral bone marrow precursors.[254,255,622]

For a long time, there was confusion in the literature regarding the terminology of perivascular cells because they bear little resemblance to full-blown macrophages in their resting state. 'Perivascular clasmatocyte',[327] 'granular pericyte', 'neurolipomastocyte', 'fluorescent granular perithelial cell', 'granular perithelial cell', 'perivascular macrophage' and 'adventitial cell' have all been used to describe these cells. The distinction between perivascular cells and perivascular microglia[216] was first made by del Rio-Hortega,[503] who referred to the former as 'perivascular histiocytes'. In recent years, the term perivascular cell has been widely accepted as it is both non-committal and anatomically correct.[19,125,300,517,622,655]

The question of identity of perivascular cells is an important one as this cell type may represent the Trojan horse of HIV-1 and other CNS infections.[220] Furthermore, there is evidence to suggest that perivascular cells play a role in vascular β-amyloid deposition and plaque forma-

tion in Alzheimer's disease.[655] Perivascular cells of the human brain may constitutively express MHC class II antigens[217] and are capable of synthesizing T-cell costimulatory molecules such as B-7.[125,312,619,653] The cells are therefore likely to be involved in CNS immune reactions.[647] Considering their unique position at the BBB, perivascular cells may represent the very first line of CNS defence.

EFFECTS OF IRRADIATION ON THE NERVOUS SYSTEM

Unlike tissues with a high rate of cell division such as the intestinal epithelium, the mature nervous system with a rather low rate of cell turnover and renewal is relatively resistant to X-irradiation. The developing nervous system, however, is highly sensitive.[303,587] If the developing human nervous system is exposed to X-irradiation, severe malformations may occur such as microgyria or agyria-pachygyria. Germinal cells, dividing neuroblasts, endothelial cells, vascular smooth-muscle cells, choroid plexus cells, astrocytes in the white matter, Bergmann glia, oligodendrocytes as well as oligodendrocyte and astrocyte precursor cells are among the most radiosensitive cell populations.[290,352,499,555,624] Irradiation blocks mitosis and kills sensitive cells mainly in the late G_1- and S-phases of the cell cycle, probably via induction of apoptosis through a protein synthesis-mediated process.[151] In addition, X-irradiation inactivates DNA repair enzymes and generates the production of free hydroxyl groups and protons. As a consequence, an irradiated cell may lose its capacity to repair cellular damage and will eventually die. X-irradiation of the developing rat optic nerve at birth, for example, prevents oligodendrocyte development and hence myelination. As oligodendrocytes express neurite growth inhibitory molecules, optic nerve fibre outgrowth is increased in these myelin-free X-irradiated nerves.[518] In the mature mammalian nervous system oligodendrocytes also remain more sensitive to X-irradiation than, for example, astrocytes and neurons. Thus, X-irradiated white matter is more susceptible to partial demyelination than normal white matter[59] and the loss of endothelial integrity has its most profound effect on white matter.[63] The threshold dose for delayed necrosis of white matter in most species is 20–25 Gy.

In the nervous system X-irradiation causes damage in an almost dose-dependent manner. A whole-body X-ray dose of 100 Gy leads to death within a few hours. Local X-irradiation with doses above 70 Gy leads to acute necrosis of both exposed white and grey matter, while doses between 50 and 70 Gy usually give rise only to partial tissue necrosis. The spinal cord is generally more vulnerable to X-irradiation than the supratentorial brain regions.[529,681]

Radiation effects on the nervous system are often delayed and can be divided into three catagories. Acute reactions are related to impaired BBB function and lead to oedema formation.[510] They are usually mild and sensitive to treatment with corticosteroids, and are thus transient. Increases in leukocyte–endothelial cell interactions have been seen 24 h and 3 weeks after single high doses of radiation.[1] Early delayed reactions occur several weeks after radiotherapy and are almost always non-lethal. In these cases damage is mainly to the white matter, affecting both myelin and axons. In addition, mild focal vascular hyalinization, but without fibrinoid necrosis, is observed.[282,286,334] The late delayed reactions are the most common postirradiation changes seen in autopsy material. They consist of coagulative tissue necrosis with some glial reaction and characteristic vascular changes. The vascular abnormalities include fibrinoid or hyaline changes of blood vessel walls with abnormal endothelial cells and perivascular fibrosis.[367,457] In experimental studies, astrocytosis and fibrillary gliosis have been shown to increase with radiation dose. Astrocytes become hypertrophic and increase their expression of GFAP, whereas microglia proliferate and express immunomolecules or cytokines such as TNF.[97] TNF-α has been suggested to be involved in late brain responses to irradiation and to contribute to clinical symptoms.[96]

In tumour therapy, X-irradiation of intracranial neoplasms often exposes the non-tumorous surrounding tissue to therapeutic doses of irradiation. In particular, the radiation effects on the cerebellar cortex can be striking.[511] Following irradiation of primary extracranial head and neck tumours as well as of meningiomas located at the skull base, optic neuropathy may occur.[198] In addition, irradiation of the spinal cord may occur during radiation therapy of adjacent non-neuronal neoplasms such as those located in the neck region, in the oropharynx or nasopharynx and at paravertebral sites. Brain tumours may develop in survivors of childhood acute lymphoblastic leukaemia after cranial radiotherapy.[496] Meningiomas and to a lesser degree sarcomas have been reported to occur after skull X-irradiation, in particular if the X-ray exposure took place during early childhood.[45,640] In one study[570] a higher incidence of atypical and malignant meningiomas was found in patients after X-irradiation of the skull than in age-matched controls. In addition, neoplasms such as astrocytic and other neuroectodermal tumours have been reported to occur more frequently in patients following X-irradiation than in patients who have not been treated.[504] A high incidence of meningiomas and abnormalities in neuronal migration leading to mental retardation has been observed among Japanese survivors of the atomic bombs (see Chapter 11, Volume II).[443,556]

Studying the effects of heavy-ion irradiation on the spinal cord of the rat, it has been found that the effective dose that induces a 50% incidence of hindlimb paralysis and destructive cavity formation ($_{ED50}$) was 18.5 and 19.5 Gy, respectively, and that the latent period was shorter than that for X-irradiation.[436]

Other types of radiation, e.g. laser and ultraviolet irradiation, can also cause tissue necrosis in the nervous system. These changes are not specific but usually involve coagulation necrosis and local oedema induced by hyperthermia and absorption of high-energy waves. Laser irradiation of the skull may cause circumscribed coagulation necrosis surrounded by a zone of oedema in the brain.[302,335] In glioma therapy, stereotactic laser surgery has been introduced particularly for targeted therapy of deep-seated intracerebral tumours.[444]

Other physical injuries include electrical trauma (including injury by lightning) and damage produced by focused ultrasound waves. After electrical trauma, both thermic and functional changes, on the basis of ion disturbances and hence disturbed nerve conduction, may occur. Thermic damage causes local tissue coagulation necrosis which may extend to widespread and/or complete necrosis and burning. Other morphological changes seen after lightning or electric current damage are venous hyperaemia, haemorrhages around the third ventricle and in the floor of the fourth ventricle, as well as severe brain oedema. As a delayed consequence of electrical trauma, atrophy of the dorsal and/or lateral columns can occur in the spinal cord several weeks to months after the injury.[449]

Focused ultrasound waves may produce a circumscribed lesion in the target area with relatively little haemorrhage while the tissue in the path of the beam remains relatively unimpaired.[33,421]

Following stressful conditions such as hyperthermia, injured neural and non-neural cells respond by exhibiting a changing pattern of gene expression and elevated protein synthesis. All cells share this molecular response to stress which is characterized by the increased production of HSPs.[407,618] Thus, HSP expression and induction appear to be universal features of environmental stress that ensure cellular survival by participating in the mechanisms of synthesis, transport and folding of new proteins. However, HSPs are also expressed constitutively at normal growth temperatures and have basic and indispensable functions in the life cycle of proteins as molecular chaperones, as well as playing a role in protecting cells.[435]

ARTEFACTS

Artefacts occur too readily at various stages of neuropathological tissue preparation and may confuse interpretation. A main obstacle to good tissue fixation and adequate histological tissue preservation is autolytic changes which occur after brain death in intensive-care patients with artificially supported respiration and ventilation or undue delay between death and autopsy. After more than 24–36 h on a respirator, brains fail to become adequately fixed and allow the proliferation of anaerobic organisms which may render histological analysis difficult. Macroscopically, these respirator brains show 'Swiss cheese'-like changes with large bullous cavities visible to the naked eye. If inadequately fixed, brain tissue appears pinkish and soft to the touch, particularly in the white matter.

Other artefactual changes include the formation of metachromatic bodies in the white matter, selective granule cell necrosis in the cerebellum, and shrinkage artefacts giving rise to an extreme widening of perivascular spaces and perineuronal halos. These artefactual changes are often due to insufficient dehydration and inadequate impregnation with paraffin wax upon embedding. Microscopically, a common neuronal artefact is the presence of dark, shrunken neurons (Fig. 3.71). They are irregular in outline, the apical dendrite has a twisted, corkscrew-like appearance, the nucleus and cytoplasm stain darkly and the Nissl substance cannot be identified.[74] The precise causes of these changes may be multiple, but dark shrunken neurons probably arise as an artefactual tissue change by applying extensive pressure on tissue and/or too rapid fixation. Glial cell artefacts often involve myelin-forming oligodendrocytes and include myelinoid bodies, mucocytes and miscellaneous myelin sheath artefacts previously discussed in the section on oligodendrocyte pathology.

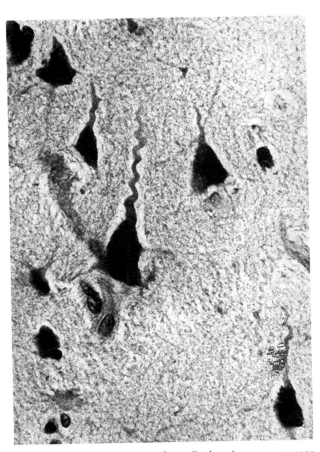

Figure 3.71 *Dark neuron. Artefactually shrunken neurons near the cut edge of a cortical biopsy. These cells are darkly stained and the apical dendrite has a twisted corkscrew-like appearance. (Haematoxylin and van Gieson.) Reproduced by permission from Ref. 134.*

Acknowledgements

We thank K. Brückner for help with the artwork, Dr J. Chalcroft for concordance analysis of the text file and K. Chalcroft for secretarial assistance.

REFERENCES

1 Acker JC, Marks LB, Spencer DP *et al.* Serial *in vivo* observations of cerebral vasculature after treatment with a large single fraction of radiation. *Radiat Res* 1998; **149**: 350–9.

2 Adams CW, Poston RN. Macrophage histology in paraffin-embedded multiple sclerosis plaques is demonstrated by the monoclonal pan macrophage marker HAM-56: correlation with chronicity of the lesion. *Acta Neuropathol (Berl)* 1990; **8**: 208–11.

3 Adayev T, Estephan R, Meserole S *et al.* Externalization of phosphatidylserine may not be an early signal of apoptosis in neuronal cells, but only the phosphatidylserine-displaying apoptotic cells are phagocytosed by microglia. *J Neurochem* 1998; **71**: 1854–64.

4 Adle-Biassette H, Chretien F, Wingertsmann L *et al.* Neuronal apoptosis does not correlate with dementia in HIV infection but is related to microglial activation and axonal damage. *Neuropathol Appl Neurobiol* 1999; **25**: 123–33.

5 Aguayo AD, David S, Bray GM. Influences of the glial environment on the elongation of axons after injury: transplantation studies in adult rodents. *J Exp Biol* 1981; **95**: 231–40.

6 Al-Ali SY, Al-Hussain SM. An ultrastructural study of the phagocytic activity of astrocytes in adult rat brain. *J Anat* 1996; **188**: 257–62.

7 Albers K, Fuchs E. The molecular biology of intermediate filament proteins. *Int Rev Cytol* 1992; **134**: 243–79.

8 Albright AV, Shieh JTC, Itoh T *et al.* Microglia express CCR5, CXCR4, and CCR3, but of these, CCR5 is the principal coreceptor for human immunodeficiency virus type 1 dementia isolates. *J Virol* 1999; **73**: 205–13.

9 Aldskogius H. Indirect and direct Wallerian degeneration in the intramedullaray root fibres of the hypoglossal nerve. *Adv Anat Embryo Cell Biol* 1974; **50**: 1–78.

10 Aldskogius H, Kozlova EN. Central neuron–glial and glial–glial interactions following axon injury. *Prog Neurobiol* 1998; **55**: 1–26.

11 Aldskogius H, Svensson M. Effect on the rat hypoglossal nucleus of vinblastine and colchicine applied to the intact or transected hypoglossal nerve. *Exp Neurol* 1988; **99**: 461–73.

12 Aloisi F, Ria F, Penna G, Adorini L. Microglia are more efficient than astrocytes in antigen processing and in Th1 but not Th2 cell activation. *J Immunol* 1998; **160**: 4671–80.

13 Aloyo VJ, Zwiers H, Gispen WH. Phosphorylation of B-50 protein by calcium-activated, phospholipid-dependent protein kinase and B-50 protein kinase. *J Neurochem* 1983; **41**: 649–53.

14 Altar CA, DiStefano PS. Neurotrophin trafficking by anterograde transport. *Trends Neurosci* 1998; **21**: 433–7.

15 Andersen LB, Schreyer DJ. Constitutive expression of GAP-43 correlates with rapid, but not slow regrowth of injured dorsal root axons in the adult rat. *Exp Neurol* 1999; **155**: 157–64.

16 Anderson ES, Bjartmar C, Westermark G, Hildebrand C. Molecular heterogeneity of oligodendrocytes in chicken white matter. *Glia* 1999; **27**: 15–21.

17 Anderson TJ, Schneider A, Barrie JA *et al*. Late-onset neurodegeneration in mice with increased dosage of the proteolipid protein gene. *J Comp Neurol* 1998; **394**: 506–19.

18 Andrews TJ, Cowen T. Nerve growth factor enhances the dendritic arborization of sympathetic ganglion cells undergoing atrophy in aged rats. *J Neurocytol* 1994; **23**: 234–41.

19 Angelov DN, Walther M, Streppel M *et al*. The cerebral perivascular cells. *Adv Anat Embryol Cell Biol* 1998; **147**: 1–87.

20 Anglade P, Vyas S, Javoy-Agid F *et al*. Apoptosis and autophagy in nigral neurons of patients with Parkinson's disease. *Histol Histopathol* 1997; **12**: 25–31.

21 Aoki MP, Maldonado CA, Aoki A. Apoptotic and non-apoptotic cell death in hormone-dependent glands. *Cell Tissue Res* 1998; **291**: 571–4.

22 Araque A, Sanzgiri RP, Parpura V, Haydon PG. Astrocyte-induced modulation of synaptic transmission. *Can J Physiol Pharmacol* 1999; **77**: 699–706.

23 Araque A, Sanzgiri RP, Parpura V, Haydon PG. Calcium elevation in astrocytes causes an NMDA receptor-dependent increase in the frequency of miniature synaptic currents in cultured hippocampal neurons. *J Neurosci* 1998; **18**: 6822–9.

24 Arends MJ, Morris RG, Wyllie AH. Apoptosis. The role of the endonuclease. *Am J Pathol* 1990; **136**: 593–608.

25 Arima K, Izumiyama Y, Nakamura M *et al*. Argyrophilic tau-positive twisted and non-twisted tubules in astrocytic processes in brains of Alzheimer-type dementia: an electron microscopical study. *Acta Neuropathol* 1998; **95**: 28–39.

26 Armstrong DM, Brady R, Hersh LB *et al*. Expression of choline acetyltransferase and nerve growth factor receptor within hypoglossal motor neurons following nerve injury. *J Comp Neurol* 1991; **304**: 596–607.

27 Arnold AP. Gonadal steroid-induced organization and reorganization of neural circuits involved in bird song. In: Cotman CW ed. *Synaptic plasticity*. New York: Guilford Press, 1985: 263–85.

28 Arvidsson U, Johnson H, Piehl F *et al*. Peripheral nerve section induces increased levels of calcitonin gene-related peptide (CGRP)-like immunoreactivity in axotomized motor neurons. *Exp Brain Res* 1990; **79**: 212–16.

29 Arvidsson U, Piehl F, Johnson H *et al*. The peptidergic motor neuron. *NeuroReport* 1993; **4**: 849–56.

30 Aschner M. Astrocytic functions and physiological reactions to injury: the potential to induce and/or exacerbate neuronal dysfunction – a forum position paper. *Neurotoxicology* 1998; **19**: 7–17.

31 Aschner M. Astrocyte metallothioneins (MTs) and their neuroprotective role. *Ann N Y Acad Sci* 1997; **825**: 334–47.

32 Aschner M, LoPachin RMJ. Astrocytes: targets and mediators of chemical-induced CNS injury. *J Toxicol Environ Hlth* 1993; **38**: 329–42.

33 Astrom KE, Bell E, Ballantine HT, Heidensleben E. An experimental neuropathological study of the effect of high frequency focused ultrasound on the brain of the cat. *J Neuropathol Exp Neurol* 1961; **20**: 484–520.

34 Baba A. Role of endothelin B receptor signals in reactive astrocytes. *Life Sci* 1998; **62**: 1711–15.

35 Bacci A, Verderio C, Pravettoni E, Matteoli M. The role of glial cells in synaptic function. *Phil Trans R Soc Lond Ser B Biol Sci* 1999; **354**: 403–9.

36 Banati RB, Daniel SE, Blunt SB. Glial pathology but absence of apoptotic nigral neurons in long-standing Parkinson's disease. *Mov Disord* 1998; **13**: 221–7.

37 Banati RB, Gehrmann J, Czech C *et al*. Early and rapid de novo-synthesis of Alzheimer betaA4-amyloid precursor protein (APP) in activated microglia. *Glia* 1993; **9**: 199–210.

38 Banati RB, Gehrmann J, Schubert P, Kreutzberg GW. Cytotoxicity of microglia. *Glia* 1993; **7**: 111–18.

49 Banati RB, Graeber MB. Surveillance, intervention and cytotoxicity: is there a protective role of microglia? *Dev Neurosci* 1994; **16**: 114–27.

40 Banati RB, Myers R, Kreutzberg GW. PK ('peripheral benzodiazepine')-binding sites in the CNS indicate early and discrete brain lesions: microautoradiographic detection of [³H]PK11195 binding to activated microglia. *J Neurocytol* 1997; **26**: 77–82.

41 Banati RB, Newcombe J, Gunn RN *et al*. The peripheral benzodiazepine binding site in the brain in multiple sclerosis: quantitative *in vivo* imaging of microglia as a measure of disease activity. *Brain* 2000; **123**: 2321–37.

42 Barnett SC, Franklin RJM, Blakemore WF. *In vitro* and *in vivo* analysis of a rat bipotential O-2A progenitor cell line containing the temperature sensitive mutant gene of the SV 40 large T antigen. *Eur J Neurosci* 1993; **5**: 1247–60.

43 Barron KD. Comparative observations on the cytologic reactions of central and peripheral nerve cells to axotomy. In: Kao CC, Bunge RP, Reier JP eds. *Spinal cord reconstruction*. New York: Raven Press, 1983: 7–40.

44 Barron KD. The microglial cell. A historical review. *J Neurol Sci* 1995; **134** (Suppl): 57–68.

45 Barron KD, Chiang TY, Daniels AC, Doolin PF. Subcellular accompaniments of axon reaction in cervical motor neurons of the cat. In: Zimmerman HM ed. *Progress in neuropathology* Vol. 1. New York: Grune and Stratton, 1971: 255–80.

46 Beller AJ, Feinsod M, Sahar A. The possible relationship between small dose irradiation to the scalp and intracranial meningeomas. *Neurochirurg Stuttgart* 1972; **15**: 135–43.

47 Bender AS, Norenberg MD. The role of K⁺ influx on glutamate induced astrocyte swelling: effect of temperature. *Acta Neurochirurg* 1994; **60** (Suppl): 28–30.

48 Benfey M, Aguayo AJ. Extensive elongation of axons from rat brain into peripheral nerve grafts. *Nature* 1982; **296**: 150–2.

49 Benveniste EN. Role of macrophages/microglia in multiple sclerosis and experimental allergic encephalomyelitis. *J Mol Med* 1997; **75**: 165–73.

50 Bhisitkul RB, Kocsis JD, Gordon TR, Waxman SG. Trophic influence of the distal nerve segment on GABAA receptor expression in axotomized adult sensory neurons. *Exp Neurol* 1990; **109**: 273–8.

51 Bignami A, Dahl D. The astroglial response to stabbing. Immunofluorescence studies with antibodies to astrocyte-specific protein (GFA) in mammalian and submammalian vertebrates. *Neuropathol Appl Neurobiol* 1976; **2**: 99–110.

52 Bignami A, Eng LF, Dahl D, Uyeda CT. Localization of the glial fibrillary acidic protein in astrocytes by immunofluorescence. *Brain Res* 1972; **43**: 429–35.

53 Bignami A, Ralston HJ. The cellular reaction to Wallerian degeneration in the central nervous system of the cat. *Brain Res* 1969; **13**: 444–61.

54 Birecree E, Whetsell WO, Stoscheck C *et al*. Immunoreactive epidermal growth factor receptors in neuritic plaques from patients with Alzheimer's disease. *J Neuropathol Exp Neurol* 1988; **47**: 549–60.

55 Bjartmar C, Hildebrand C, Loinder K. Morphological heterogeneity of rat oligodendrocytes: electron microscopic studies on serial sections. *Glia* 1994; **11**: 235–44.

56 Blakemore WF. Demyelination of the superior cerebellar peduncle in the mouse induced by cuprizone. *J Neurol Sci* 1973; **20**: 63–72.

57 Blakemore WF. Ethidium bromide induced demyelination in the spinal cord of the cat. *Neuropathol Appl Neurobiol* 1982; **8**: 365–75.

58 Blakemore WF. Invasion of Schwann cells into the spinal cord of the rat following local injections of lysolecithin. *Neuropathol Appl Neurobiol* 1976; **2**: 21–39.

59 Blakemore WF. Myelination, demyelination and remyelination in the CNS. In: Thomas Smith W, Cavanagh JB eds. *Recent advances in neuropathology*. Edinburgh: Churchill Livingstone, 1982: 53–82.

60 Blakemore WF. Observations on oligodendrocyte degeneration, the resolution of status spongiosus and remyelination in cuprizone intoxication in mice. *J Neurocytol* 1972; **1**: 413–26.

61 Blakemore WF. Partial demyelination of cat spinal cord after X-irradiation and surgical interference. *Neuropathol Appl Neurobiol* 1978; **4**: 381–92.

62 Blakemore WF, Cavanagh JB. 'Neuroaxonal dystrophy–occurring in an experimental 'dying back– process in the rat. *Brain* 1969; **92**: 789–804.

63 Blakemore WF, Keirstead HS. The origin of remyelinating cells in the CNS. *J Neuroimmunol* 1999; **98**: 69–76.

64 Blakemore WF, Palmer AC. Delayed infarction of spinal cord white matter following X-irradiation. *J Pathol* 1982; **137**: 273–80.

65 Blakemore WF, Palmer AC, Noel PRB. Ultrastructural changes in isoniazid-induced brain oedema in the dog. *J Neurocytol* 1972; **1**: 263–78.

66 Blakemore WF, Patterson RC. Observations on the interaction of Schwann cells and astrocytes following X-irradiation of neonatal rat spinal cord. *J Neurocytol* 1975; **4**: 573–85.

67 Blakemore WF, Patterson RC. Suppression of remyelination in the CNS by X-irradiation. *Acta Neuropathol (Berl)* 1978; **42**: 105–13.

68 Blakemore WF, Welsh CJR, Tonks P, Nash AA. Observations on demyelinating lesions induced by Theiler's virus in CBA mice. *Acta Neuropathol (Berl)* 1988; **76**: 581–9.

69 Blinzinger K, Kreutzberg G. Displacement of synaptic terminals from regenerating motor neurons by microglial cells. *Z Zellforsch Mikrosk Anat* 1968; **85**: 145–57.

70 Bo L, Mrk S, Kong PA *et al.* Detection of MHC class II antigens on macrophages and microglia, but not on astrocytes and endothelia in active multiple sclerosis lesions. *J Neuroimmunol* 1994; **51**: 135–46.

71 Boyle EA, McGeer PL. Cellular immune response in multiple sclerosis plaques. *Am J Pathol* 1990; **137**: 575–84.

72 Boyles JK, Pitas RE, Wilson E *et al.* Apolipoprotein E associated with astrocytic glia of the central nervous system and with nonmyelinating glia of the peripheral nervous system. *J Clin Invest* 1985; **76**: 1501–13.

73 Brierley JB, Brown AW. The origin of lipid phagocytes in the central nervous system: I. the intrinsic microglia. *J Comp Neurol* 1982; **211**: 397–406.

74 Brown AW. Structural abnormalities in neurones. *J Clin Pathol Suppl (R Coll Pathol)* 1977; **11**: 155–69.

75 Brown AW, Brierley JB. Evidence for early anoxic–ischaemic cell damage in the rat brain. *Experientia* 1966; **22**: 546–7.

76 Brown PO, Botstein D. Exploring the new world of the genome with DNA microarrays. *Nature Genet* 1999; **21**: 33–7.

77 Brück W, Schmied M, Suchanek G *et al.* Oligodendrocytes in the early course of multiple sclerosis. *Ann Neurol* 1994; **35**: 65–73.

78 Brück W, Sommermeier N, Bergmann M *et al.* Macrophages in multiple sclerosis. *Immunobiology* 1996; **195**: 588–600.

79 Bruni JE. Ependymal development, proliferation, and functions: a review. *Microsc Res Technique* 1998; **41**: 2–13.

80 Buchino JJ, Nicol KK, Parker JCJ. Aicardi syndrome: a morphologic description with particular reference to intracytoplasmic inclusions in cortical astrocytes. *Pediatr Pathol Lab Med* 1996; **16**: 285–91.

81 Bunge MB, Bunge RP, Ris H. Ultrastructural study of remyelination in an experimental lesion in the adult cat spinal cord. *J Biophys Biochem Cytol* 1961; **10**: 67–94.

82 Bunge RP. Glial cells and the central myelin sheath. *Physiol Rev* 1968; **48**: 197–251.

83 Butt AM, Ibrahim M, Berry M. Axon–myelin sheath relations of oligodendrocyte unit phenotypes in the adult rat anterior medullary velum. *J Neurocytol* 1998; **27**: 259–69.

84 Butt AM, Ibrahim M, Ruge FM, Berry M. Biochemical subtypes of oligodendrocyte in the anterior medullary velum of the rat as revealed by the monoclonal antibody Rip. *Glia* 1995; **14**: 185–97.

85 Butt AM, Ransom BR. Morphology of astrocytes and oligodendrocytes during development in the rat optic nerve. *J Comp Neurol* 1993; **338**: 141–58.

86 Butter C, O'Neil JK, Baker D *et al.* An immunoelectron microscopical study of class II major histocompatibility complex during chronic relapsing experimental allergic encephalomyelitis in Biozzi AB/H mice. *J Neuroimmunol* 1991; **33**: 37–42.

87 Cai DM, Shen YJ, De Bellard M *et al.* Prior exposure to neurotrophins blocks inhibition of axonal regeneration by MAG and myelin via a cAMP-dependent mechanism. *Neuron* 1999; **22**: 89–101.

88 Cantor CR, Smith CL. Consequences of mapping and sequencing the human genome for neurologic diseases. In: Rosenberg RN, Prusiner SB, DiMauro S *et al.* eds. *The molecular and genetic basis of neurological disease*. Boston, MA: Butterworth-Heinemann, 1993: 977–87.

89 Carmignoto G, Maffei L, Candeo P *et al.* Effect of NGF on the survival of rat retinal ganglion cells following optic nerve section. *J Neurosci* 1989; **9**: 1263–72.

90 Carroll WM, Jennings AR. Early recruitment of oligodendrocyte precursors in CNS demyelination. *Brain* 1994; **117**: 563–78.

91 Carroll WM, Jennings AR, Ironside LJ. Indentification of the adult resting progenitor cell by autoradiographic tracking of oligodendrocyte precursors in experimental CNS demyelination. *Brain* 1998; **121**: 293–302.

92 Cavanagh JB. Corpora-amylacea and the family of polyglucosan diseases. *Brain Res Rev* 1999; **29**: 265–95.

93 Charriaut-Marlangue C, Ben-Ari Y. A cautionary note on the use of the TUNEL stain to determine apoptosis. *NeuroReport* 1995; **7**: 61–4.

94 Cheah TB, Geffen LB. Effects of axonal injury on norepinephrine, tyrosine hydroxylase and monoamine oxidase levels in sympathetic ganglia. *J Neurobiol* 1973; **4**: 44 3–52.

95 Chen MS, Huber AB, Van der Haar ME *et al.* Nogo-A is a myelin-associated neurite outgrowth inhibitor and an antigen for monoclonal antibody IN-1. *Nature* 2000; **403**: 434–9.

96 Chiang CS, Hong JH, Stalder A *et al.* Delayed molecular responses to brain irradiation. *Int J Radiat Biol* 1997; **72**: 45–53.

97 Chiang CS, McBride WH, Withers HR. Radiation-induced astrocytic and microglial responses in mouse brain. *Radiother Oncol* 1993; **29**: 60–8.

98 Chiasson BJ, Tropepe V, Morshead CM, van der Kooy D.

Adult mammalian forebrain ependymal and subependymal cells demonstrate proliferative potential, but only subependymal cells have neural stem cell characteristics. *J Neurosci* 1999; **19**: 4462–71.

99 Chin SS, Goldman JE. Glial inclusions in CNS degenerative diseases. *J Neuropathol Exp Neurol* 1996; **55**: 499–508.

100 Choi C, Park JY, Lee J et al. Fas ligand and Fas are expressed constitutively in human astrocytes and the expression increases with IL-1, IL-6, TNF-alpha, or IFN-gamma. *J Immunol* 1999; **162**: 1889–95.

101 Chu Wang IW, Oppenheim RW. Cell death of motor neurons in the chick embryo spinal cord. I. A light and electron microscopic study of naturally occurring and induced cell loss during development. *J Comp Neurol* 1978; **177**: 33–58.

102 Cisse S, Perry G, Lacoste-Royal G et al. Immunochemical identification of ubiquitin and heat-shock proteins in corpora amylacea from normal aged and Alzheimer's disease brains. *Acta Neuropathol (Berl)* 1993; **85**: 233–40.

103 Clark EA, Leach KL, Trojanowski JQ, Lee VM. Characterization and differential distribution of the three major human protein kinase C isozymes (PKC alpha, PKC beta, and PKC gamma) of the central nervous system in normal and Alzheimer's disease brains. *Lab Invest* 1991; **64**: 35–44.

104 Clark JM. Distribution of microglial clusters in the brain after head injury. *J Neurol Neurosurg Psychiat* 1974; **37**: 463–74.

105 Clarke PGH. Developmental cell death: morphological diversity and multiple mechanisms. *Anat Embryol Berlin* 1990; **181**: 195–213.

106 Cohen JJ. Programmed cell death in the immune system. *Adv Immunol* 1991; **50**: 55–85.

107 Cole JS, Messing A, Trojanowski JQ, Lee VMY. Modulation of axon diameter and neurofilaments by hypomyelinating Schwann cells in transgenic mice. *J Neurosci* 1994; **14**: 6956–66.

108 Colosetti P, Olsson T, Miyazono K, Funa K. Axotomy of rat facial nerve induces TGF-beta and latent TGF-beta binding protein. *Brain Res Bull* 1995; **37**: 561–7.

109 Colton AC, Gilbert DL. Production of superoxide by a CNS macrophage, the microglia. *FEBS Lett* 1987; **223**: 284–8.

110 Colton C, Wilt S, Gilbert D et al. Species differences in the generation of reactive oxygen species by microglia. *Mol Chem Neuropathol* 1996; **28**: 15–20.

111 Condorelli DF, Nicoletti VG, Barresi V et al. Structural features of the rat GFAP gene and identification of a novel alternative transcript. *J Neurosci Res* 1999; **56**: 219–28.

112 Connor JR, Menzies SL, St Martin SM, Mufson EJ. A histochemical study of iron, transferrin, and ferritin in Alzheimer's disease brains. *J Neurosci Res* 1992; **31**: 75–83.

113 Copray JCVM, Liem RSB, van Willigen JD. Morphological arrangement between astrocytes and trigeminal mesencephalic primary afferent neurons in the rat. *Exp Brain Res* 1990; **83**: 215–18.

114 Cragg BG. What is the signal for chromatolysis? *Brain Res* 1970; **23**: 1–21.

115 Cras P, Kawai M, Siedlak S, Perry G. Microglia are associated with the extracellular neurofibrillary tangles of Alzheimer disease. *Brain Res* 1991; **558**: 312–14.

116 Cuadros MA, Navascues J. The origin and differentiation of microglial cells during development. *Prog Neurobiol* 1998; **56**: 173–89.

117 Curtis R, Green D, Lindsay RM, Wilkin GP. Up-regulation of GAP-43 and growth of axons in rat spinal cord after compression injury. *J Neurocytol* 1993; **22**: 51–64.

118 Curtis R, Tonra JR, Stark JL et al. Neuronal injury increases

119 Davies SW, Turmaine M, Cozens BA et al. From neuronal inclusions to neurodegeneration: neuropathological investigation of a transgenic mouse model of Huntington's disease. *Phil Trans R Soc Lond B* 1999; **354**: 971–9.

120 Deckwerth TL, Johnson EM. Neurotrophic factor deprivation-induced death. *Ann NY Acad Sci* 1993; **679**: 121–31.

121 del Rio-Hortega P. El tercer elemento de los centro nerviosos. *Boll Soc Espanol Biol* 1919; **9**: 68–120.

122 del Rio-Hortega P. Microglia. In: Penfield W ed. *Cytology and cellular pathology of the nervous system*. New York: Paul B Hoeber, 1932: 483–534.

123 Depraetere V, Golstein P. Dismantling in cell death: molecular mechanisms and relationship to caspase activation. *Scand J Immunol* 1998; **47**: 523–31.

124 Deschepper CF. Peptide receptors on astrocytes. *Front Neuroendocrinol* 1998; **19**: 20–46.

125 De Simone R, Giampaolo A, Giometto B et al. The costimulatory molecule B7 is expressed on human microglia in culture and in multiple sclerosis acute lesions. *J Neuropathol Exp Neurol* 1995; **54**: 175–87.

126 de Torres C, Munell F, Ferrer I et al. Identification of necrotic cell death by the TUNEL assay in the hypoxic–ischemic neonatal rat brain. *Neurosci Lett* 1997; **230**: 1–4.

127 Diamond J, Foester A, Holmes M, Coughlin M. Sensory nerves in adult rats regenerate and restore sensory function to the skin independently of exogenous NGF. *J Neurosci* 1992; **12**: 1467–76.

128 Dickson DW, Lee SC, Mattiace LA et al. Microglia and cytokines in neurological disease, with special reference to AIDS and Alzheimer's disease. *Glia* 1993; **7**: 75–83.

129 Dickson DW, Mattiace LA, Kure K et al. Microglia in human disease, with an emphasis on the aquired immune deficiency syndrome. *Lab Invest* 1991; **64**: 135–56.

130 Diedrich JF, Minnigan H, Carp RI et al. Neuropathological changes in scrapie and Alzheimer's disease are associated with increased expression of apolipoprotein E and cathepsin D in astrocytes. *J Virol* 1991; **65**: 4759–68.

131 DiMonte DA, Royland JE, Irwin I, Langston JW. Astrocytes as the site for bioactivation of neurotoxins. *Neurotoxicology* 1996; **17**: 697–703.

132 Doetsch F, Caille I, Lim DA et al. Subventricular zone astrocytes are neural stem cells in the adult mammalian brain. *Cell* 1999; **97**: 703–16.

133 Dorandeu A, Wingertsmann L, Chretien F et al. Neuronal apoptosis in fatal familial insomnia. *Brain Pathol* 1998; **8**: 531–7.

134 Duchen LW. General pathology of neurons and neuroglia. In: Hume Adams J, Duchen LW eds. *Greenfield's neuropathology* 5th edn. London: Edward Arnold, 1992: 1–68.

135 Dumoulin FL, Raivich G, Haas CA et al. Calcitonin gene-related peptide and peripheral nerve regeneration. *Ann N Y Acad Sci* 1992; **657**: 351–60.

136 Dumoulin FL, Raivich G, Streit WJ, Kreutzberg GW. Differential regulation of calcitonin gene-related peptide (CGRP) in regenerating rat facial nucleus and dorsal root ganglion. *Eur J Neurosci* 1991; **3**: 338–42.

137 Dusart I, Airaksinen MS, Sotelo C. Purkinje cell survival and axonal regeneration are age dependent: an *in vitro* study. *J Neurosci* 1997; **17**: 3710–26.

138 Ebendal T. Function and evolution in the NGF family and its receptors. *J Neurosci Res* 1992; **32**: 461–70.

139 Eddleston M, Mucke L. Molecular profile of reactive astrocytes – implications for their role in neurologic disease.

Neuroscience 1993; **54**: 15–36.

140 Egensperger R, Kösel S, Von Eitzen U, Graeber MB. Microglial activation in Alzheimer disease: Association with APOE Genotype. *Brain Pathol.* 1998; **8**: 439–47.

141 El Khoury J, Hickman SE, Thomas CA *et al.* Microglia, scavenger receptors, and the pathogenesis of Alzheimer's disease. *Neurobiol Aging* 1998; **19**: S81–4

142 Ellis H, Horvitz HR. Genetic control of programmed cell death in the nematode *C. elegans. Cell* 1986; **44**: 817–29.

143 Emmert-Buck MR, Bonner RF, Smith PD *et al.* Laser Capture Microdissection. *Science* 1996; **274**: 998–1001.

144 Eng LF, Ghirnikar RS. GFAP and astrogliosis. *Brain Pathol* 1994; **4**: 229–37.

145 Eng LF, Lee YL, Kwan H *et al.* Astrocytes cultured from transgenic mice carrying the added human glial fibrillary acidic protein gene contain Rosenthal fibers. *J Neurosci Res* 1998; **53**: 353–60.

146 Eng LF, Vanderhaeghen JJ, Bignami A, Gerstl B. An acidic protein isolated from fibrous astrocytes. *Brain Res* 1971; **28**: 351–4.

147 Eng LF, Yu AC, Lee YL. Astrocytic response to injury. *Prog Brain Res* 1992; **94**: 353–65.

148 Ernfors P, Henschen A, Olson L, Persson H. Expression of nerve growth factor receptor mRNA is developmentally regulated and increased after axotomy in rat spinal cord motor neurons. *Neuron* 1989; **2**: 1605–13.

149 Fagan AM, Gage FH. Cholinergic sprouting in the hippocampus: a proposed role for IL-1. *Exp Neurol* 1990; **110**: 105–20.

150 Feany MB, Bender WW. A *Drosophila* model of Parkinson's disease. *Nature* 2000; **404**: 394–8.

151 Ferrer I, Serrano T, Rivera R *et al.* Radiosensitive populations and recovery in X-ray-induced apoptosis in the developing cerebellum. *Acta Neuropathol (Berl)* 1993; **86**: 491–500.

152 ffrench-Constant C, Raff MC. Proliferating bipotential glial progenitor cells in adult optic nerve. *Nature* 1986; **319**: 499–502.

153 Finsen BR, Jorgensen MB, Diemer NH, Zimmer J. Microglial MHC antigen expression after ischemic and kainic acid lesions of the adult rat hippopcampus. *Glia* 1993; **7**: 41–9.

154 Fish CJ, Blakemore WF. A model of chronic spinal cord compression in the cat. *Neuropathol Appl Neurobiol* 1983; **9**: 109–20.

155 Flemming W. Ueber die Bildung von Richtungsfiguren in Saeugetiereiern beim Untergang Graaf'scher Follikel. *Arch Anat Entwicklungsgeschichte* 1885; **18**: 221–44.

156 Flügel A, Labeur MS, Grasbon-Frodl EM *et al.* Microglia only weakly present glioma antigen to cytotoxic T cells. *Int J Dev Neurosci* 1999; **171**: 547–56.

157 Flügel A, Schwaiger FW, Neumann H *et al.* Neuronal FasL induces cell death of encephalitogenic T lymphocytes. *Brain Pathol* 2000; **10**: 353–64.

158 Foran DR, Peterson AC. Myelin aquisition in the central nervous system of the mouse revealed by an MBP-LacZ transgene. *J Neurosci* 1992; **12**: 4890–7.

159 Forno LS, DeLanney LE, Irwin I *et al.* Astrocytes and Parkinson's disease. *Prog Brain Res* 1992; **94**: 429–36.

160 Forsyth RJ. Astrocytes and the delivery of glucose from plasma to neurons. *Neurochem Int* 1996; **28**: 231–41.

161 Frackowiak J, Wisniewski HM, Wegiel J *et al.* Ultrastructure of the microglia that phagocytose amyloid and the microglia that produce beta-amyloid fibrils. *Acta Neuropathol (Berl)* 1992; **84**: 225–33.

162 Franklin RJM, Blakemore WF. Requirements for Schwann cell migration within CNS environments: a viewpoint. *Int J Dev Neurosci* 1993; **11**: 641–9.

163 Franklin RJM, Crang AJ, Blakemore WF. The role of astro-

cytes in the remyelination of glial-free areas of demyelination. In: Seil FJ ed. *Neural regeneration.* New York: Raven Press, 1993: 125–33.

164 Franklin WA, Mason DY, Pulford K *et al.* Immunohistological analysis of human mononuclear phagocytes and dendritic cells by using monoclonal antibodies. *Lab Invest* 1986; **54**: 322–35.

165 Franson P, Ronnevi LO. Myelin breakdown and elimination in the posterior funiculus of the adult cat after dorsal rhizotomy: a light and electron microscopic qualitative and quantitative study. *J Comp Neurol* 1984; **223**: 138–51.

166 Frei K, Siepl C, Groscurth P *et al.* Antigen presentation and tumor cytotoxicity by interferon-γ-treated microglial cells. *Eur J Immunol* 1987; **12**: 237–43.

167 Fukuda A, Deshpande SB, Shimano Y, Nishino H. Astrocytes are more vulnerable than neurons to cellular Ca^{2+} overload induced by a mitochondrial toxin, 3-nitropropionic acid. *Neuroscience* 1998; **87**: 497–507.

168 Fukuda T, Wang H, Nakanishi H *et al.* Novel non-apoptotic morphological changes in neurons of the mouse hippocampus following transient hypoxic-ischemia. *Neurosci Res* 1999; **33**: 49–55.

169 Gabuzda D, He J, Ohagen A, Vallat AV. Chemokine receptors in HIV-1 infection of the central nervous system. *Semin Immunol* 1998; **10**: 203–13.

170 Gage FH, Olejniczak P, Armstrong DM. Astrocytes are important for sprouting in the septohippocampal circuit. *Exp Neurol* 1988; **102**: 2–13.

171 Galou M, Colucci-Guyon E, Ensergueix D *et al.* Disrupted glial fibrillary acidic protein network in astrocytes from vimentin knockout mice. *J Cell Biol* 1996; **133**: 853–63.

172 Gasque P, Jones J, Singhrao SK, Morgan B. Identification of an astrocyte cell population from human brain that expresses perforin, a cytotoxic protein implicated in immune defense. *J Exp Med* 1998; **187**: 451–60.

173 Gavrieli Y, Sherman Y, Ben-Sasson SA. Identification of programmed cell death *in situ* via specific labeling of nuclear DNA fragmentation. *J Cell Biol* 1992; **119**: 493–501.

174 Geddes JF, Whitwell HL, Graham DI. Traumatic axonal injury: practical issues for diagnosis in medicolegal cases. *Neuropathol Appl Neurobiol* 2000; **26**: 105–16.

175 Geddes JW, Cotman CW, Miller FD. *In situ* hybridisation of tubulin α-1 mRNA as a marker of neurons participating in reactive synaptogenesis. *Soc Neurosci Abstr* 1988; **14**: 823.

176 Gehrmann J, Bonnekoh P, Miyazawa T *et al.* Immunocytochemical study of an early microglial activation in ischemia. *J Cereb Blood Flow Metab* 1992; **12**: 257–69.

177 Gehrmann J, Gold R, Linington C *et al.* Spinal cord microglia in experimental allergic neuritis: evidence for fast and remote activation. *Lab Invest* 1992; **67**: 100–13.

178 Gehrmann J, Mies G, Bonnekoh P *et al.* Microglial reaction in the rat cerebral cortex induced by cortical spreading depression. *Brain Pathol* 1993; **3**: 11–18.

179 Gehrmann J, Schoen SW, Kreutzberg GW. Lesion of the rat entorhinal cortex leads to a rapid microglial reaction in the dentate gyrus. A light and electron microscopical study. *Acta Neuro pathol (Berl)* 1991; **82**: 442–55.

180 Geiger KD, Stoldt P, Schlote W, Derouiche A. Ezrin immunoreactivity with increasing malignancy of astrocytic tumors but is absent in oligodendrogliomas. *Am J Pathol* 2000; **157**: 1785–93.

181 Gensert JM, Goldman JE. Endogenous progenitors remyelinate demyelinated axons in the adult CNS. *Neuron* 1997; **19**: 197–203.

182 George R, Griffin JW. Delayed macrophage responses and

myelin clearance during Wallerian degeneration in the central nervous system: the dorsal radiculotomy model. *Exp Neurol* 1994; **129**: 225–36.

183 Giaume C, Venance L. Intercellular calcium signaling and gap junctional communication in astrocytes. *Glia* 1998; **24**: 50–64.

184 Giese A, Brown DR, Groschup MH *et al*. Role of microglia in neuronal cell death in prion disease. *Brain Pathol* 1998; **8**: 449–57.

185 Gilmore SA. The effects of X-irradiation on the spinal cords of neonatal rats. II. Histological observation. *J Neuropathol Exp Neurol* 1963; **22**: 294–301.

186 Girgrah N, Letarte M, Becker LE *et al*. Localization of the CD44 glycoprotein to fibrous astrocytes in normal white matter and to reactive astrocytes in active lesions in multiple sclerosis. *J Neuropathol Exp Neurol* 1991; **50**: 779–92.

187 Gispen WH, Nielander HB, De Graan PNE *et al*. Role of the growth-associated protein B-50/GAP-43 in neuronal plasticity. *Mol Neurobiol* 1992; **5**: 61–85.

188 Giulian D, Ingeman JE. Colony-stimulating factors as promoters of ameboid microglia. *J Neurosci* 1988; **8**: 4707–17.

189 Giulian D, Robertson C. Inhibition of mononuclear phagocytes reduces ischemic injury in the spinal cord. *Ann Neurol* 1990; **27**: 33–42.

190 Giulian D, Vaca K, Noonan C. Secretion of neurotoxins by mononuclear phagocytes infected with HIV-1. *Science* 1990; **250**: 1593–6.

191 Giulian D, Woodward J, Young DG *et al*. Interleukin-1 injected into mammalian brain stimulates astrogliosis and neovascularisation. *J Neurosci* 1988; **8**: 2485–90.

192 Gledhill RE, Harrison BM, McDonald WI. Demyelination and remyelination after acute spinal cord compression. *Exp Neurol* 1973; **35**: 239–53.

193 Gocht A, Löhler J. Changes in glial cell markers in recent and old demyelinated lesions in central pontine myelinolysis. *Acta Neuropathol (Berl)* 1990; **80**: 46–58.

194 Godfraind C, Friedrich VL, Holmes KV, Dubois-Dalcq M. *In vivo* analysis of glial cell phenotypes during a viral demyelinating disease in mice. *J Cell Biol* 1989; **109**: 2405–16.

195 Gold R, Schmied M, Rothe G *et al*. Detection of DNA fragmentation in apoptosis: application of *in situ* nick translation to cell culture systems and tissue sections. *J Histochem Cytochem* 1993; **41**: 1023–30.

196 Gold R, Schmied M, Tontsch U *et al*. Antigen presentation by astrocytes primes rat T lymphocytes for apoptotic cell death. A model for T-cell apoptosis *in vivo*. *Brain* 1996; **119**: 651–9.

197 Goldman SA, Kirschenbaum B, Harrison-Restelli C, Thaler HT. Neuronal precursors of the adult rat subependymal zone persist into senescence, with no decline in spatial extent or response to BDNF. *J Neurobiol* 1997; **32**: 554–66.

198 Goldsmith BJ, Rosenthal SA, Wara WM, Larson DA. Optic neuropathy after irradiation of meningeoma. *Radiology* 1992; **185**: 71–6.

199 Gomez-Pinilla F, Cummings BJ, Cotman CW. Induction of basic fibroblast growth factor in Alzheimer's disease pathology. *NeuroReport* 1990; **1**: 211–14.

200 Gonzalez-Scarano F, Baltuch G. Microglia as mediators of inflammatory and degenerative diseases. *Ann Rev Neurosci* 1999; **22**: 219–40.

201 Goshgarian HG. Possible morphological and physiological correlates to the unmasking of a latent motor pathway after spinal cord injury. In: Seil FJ ed. *Advances in neural regeneration research*. New York: Wiley-Liss, 1990: 341–53.

202 Gosztonyi G, Artigas J, Lamperth L, Webster deFH. Human immunodeficiency virus (HIV) distribution in HIV encephalitis: study of 19 cases with combined use of *in situ* hybridisation and immunocytochemistry. *J Neuropathol Exp Neurol* 1994; **53**: 521–34.

203 Gould E, Woolley CS, Frankfurt M, McEwen BS. Gonadal steroids regulate dendritic spine density in hippocampal pyramidal cells in adulthood. *J Neurosci* 1990; **10**: 1286–91.

204 Gow A, Friedrich VL Jr, Lazzarini RA. Many naturally occurring mutations of myelin proteolipid protein impair its intracellular transport. *J Neurosci Res* 1994; **37**: 574–83.

205 Graca DL, Blakemore WF. Delayed remyelination in rat spinal cord following ethidium bromide injection. *Neuropathol Appl Neurobiol* 1986; **12**: 593–605.

206 Grady MS, McLaughlin MR, Christman CW *et al*. The use of antibodies targeted against the neurofilament subunits for the detection of diffuse axonal injury in humans. *J Neuropathol Exp Neurol* 1993; **52**: 143–52.

207 Graeber MB. The microglial 'sensor' of pathology. In: Ling EA, Tan CK, Tan CBC eds. *Topical issues in microglia research*. Singapore: Singapore Neuroscience Association, 1996: 237–53.

208 Graeber MB, Bise K, Mehraein P. CR3/43, a marker for activated human microglia: application to diagnostic neuropathology. *Neuropathol Appl Neurobiol* 1994; **20**: 406–8.

209 Graeber MB, Bise K, Mehraein P. Synaptic stripping in the human facial nucleus. *Acta Neuropathol (Berl)* 1993; **86**: 179–81.

210 Graeber MB, Grasbon-Frodl E, Abell-Aleff P, Kosel S. Nigral neurons are likely to die of a mechanism other than classical apoptosis in Parkinson's disease. *Parkinsonism Relat Disord* 1999; **5**: 187–92.

211 Graeber MB, Kreutzberg GW. Astrocytes increase in glial fibrillary acidic protein during retrograde changes of facial motor neurons. *J Neurocytol* 1986; **15**: 363–73.

212 Graeber MB, Kreutzberg GW. Astrocytic reactions accompanying motor neuron regeneration. In: Seil FJ ed. *Advances in neural regeneration research*. New York: Wiley-Liss, 1990: 215–24.

213 Graeber MB, Kreutzberg GW. Delayed astrocyte reaction following facial nerve axotomy. *J Neurocytol* 1988; **17**: 209–20.

214 Graeber MB, Kreutzberg GW. Immuno gold staining (IGS) for electron microscopical demonstration of glial fibrillary acidic (GFA) protein in LR White embedded tissue. *Histochemistry* 1985; **83**: 497–500.

215 Graeber MB, Raivich G, Kreutzberg GW. Increase of transferrin receptors and iron uptake in regenerating motor neurons. *J Neurosci Res* 1989; **23**: 342–5.

216 Graeber MB, Streit WJ. Perivascular microglia defined. *Trends Neurosci* 1990; **13**: 366.

217 Graeber MB, Streit WJ, Büringer D *et al*. Ultrastructural location of major histocompatibility complex (MHC) class II positive perivascular cells in histologically normal human brain. *J Neuropathol Exp Neurol* 1992; **51**: 303–11.

218 Graeber MB, Streit WJ, Kreutzberg GW. Axotomy of the rat facial nerve leads to increased CR3 complement receptor expression by activated microglial cells. *J Neurosci Res* 1988; **21**: 18–24.

219 Graeber MB, Streit WJ, Kreutzberg GW. Formation of microglia-derived brain macrophages is blocked by adriamycin. *Acta Neuropathol (Berl)* 1989; **78**: 348–58.

220 Graeber MB, Streit WJ, Kreutzberg GW. Identity of ED2-positive perivascular cells in rat brain. *J Neurosci Res* 1989; **22**: 103–6.

221 Graeber MB, Streit WJ, Kreutzberg GW. The microglial

cytoskeleton: vimentin is localized within activated cells in situ. *J Neurocytol* 1988; **17**: 573–80.

222 Graeber MB, Streit WJ, Kreutzberg GW. Toward an immunological definition of the blood–brain barrier: significance of MHC class II positive perivascular cells. In: Yonezawa T ed. *Proceedings of the XIth International Congress of Neuropathology: Satellite symposium on demyelination, mechanisms and background. Neuropathology* Suppl 4. Kyoto: Japanese Society for Neuropathology, 1991: 74–9.

223 Graeber MB, Tetzlaff W, Streit WJ, Kreutzberg GW. Microglial cells but not astrocytes undergo mitosis following rat facial nerve axotomy. *Neurosci Lett* 1988; **85**: 317–21.

224 Grafstein B. Axonal transport: function and mechanisms. In: Waxman SG, Kocsis JD, Stys PK eds. *The axon, structure, function and pathophysiology*. Oxford: Oxford University Press, 1995: 185–99.

225 Grafstein B. Chromatolysis reconsidered: a new view of the nerve cell body in axonal regeneration. In: Seil FJ ed. *Nerve, organ and tissue regeneration: research perspectives*. New York: Academic Press, 1983: 37–50.

226 Grafstein B, McQuarrie IG. Role of the nerve cell body in axonal regeneration. In: Cotman CW ed. *Neuronal plasticity*. New York: Raven Press, 1978: 155–95.

227 Grafstein B, Murray M. Transport of protein in goldfish optic nerve during regeneration. *Exp Neurol* 1969; **25**: 494–508.

228 Grasl-Kraupp B, Ruttkaynedecky B, Koudelka H et al. *In situ* detection of fragmented DNA (TUNEL assay) fails to discriminate among apoptosis, necrosis, and autolytic cell death: a cautionary note. *Hepatology* 1995; **21**: 1465–8.

229 Gray F, Scaravilli F, Everall I et al. Neuropathology of early HIV-1 infection. *Brain Pathol* 1996; **6**: 1–15.

230 Graziadei PPC, Monti-Graziadei GA. Neurogenesis and neuron regeneration in the rat olfactory system of mammals. I. Morphological aspects of differentiation and structural organization of the olfactory sensory neurons. *J Neurol* 1979; **8**: 1–18.

231 Griffin WS, Stanley LC, Ling C et al. Brain interleukin 1 and S-100 immunoreactivity are elevated in Down syndrome and Alzheimer disease. *Proc Natl Acad Sci USA* 1989; **86**: 7611–15.

232 Griffiths I, Klugmann M, Anderson T et al. Axonal swellings and degeneration in mice lacking the major proteolipid of myelin. *Science* 1998; **280**: 1610–13.

233 Grinspan JB, Stern JL, Franceschini B, Pleasure D. Trophic effects of basic fibroblast growth factor (bFGF) on differentiated oligodendroglia: a mechanism for regeneration of the oligodendroglial lineage. *J Neurosci Res* 1993; **36**: 672–80.

234 Grothe C, Unsicker K. Basic fibroblast growth factor in the hypoglossal system: specific retrograde transport, trophic, and lesion-related responses. *J Neurosci Res* 1992; **32**: 317–28.

235 Groves MJ, Christopherson T, Giometto B, Scaravilli F. Axotomy-induced apoptosis in adult rat primary sensory neurons. *J Neurocytol* 1997; **26**: 615–24.

236 Guerri C, Renau-Piqueras J. Alcohol, astroglia, and brain development. *Mol Neurobiol* 1997; **15**: 65–81.

237 Guntinas-Lichius O, Schulte E, Stennert E, Neiss WF. The use of texture analysis to study the time course of chromatolysis. *J Neurosci Meth* 1997; **78**: 1–6.

238 Haas CA, Donath C, Kreutzberg GW. Differential expression of immediate early genes after transection of the facial nerve. *Neuroscience* 1993; **53**: 91–9.

239 Haas CA, Streit WJ, Kreutzberg GW. Rat facial motor neu-rons express increased levels of calcitonin gene-related peptide mRNA in response to axotomy. *J Neurosci Res* 1990; **27**: 270–5.

240 Haas S, Haque NS, Beggs AH et al. Expression of the myelin basic protein gene in transgenic mice expressing human neurotropic virus, JCV, early protein. *Virology* 1994; **202**: 89–96.

241 Haga S, Akai K, Ishii T. Demonstration of microglial cells in and around senile (neuritic) plaques in the Alzheimer brain – an immunohistochemical study using a novel monoclonal antibody. *Acta Neuropathol (Berl)* 1989; **77**: 569–75.

242 Hagen G, Blakemore WF, Bjerkas I. Ultrastructural findings in spongy degeneration of white matter in silver foxes (*Vulpes vulpes*). *Acta Neuropathol (Berl)* 1990; **80**: 590–6.

243 Hamprecht B, Dringen R, Pfeiffer B, Kurz G. The possible roles of astrocytes in energy metabolism of the brain. In: Fedoroff S, Juurlink, BHJ, Doucette R eds. *Biology and pathology of astrocyte–neuron interactions*. New York: Plenum Press, 1993: 83–91.

244 Hansson E, Johansson BB, Westergren I, Rönnbäck L. Mechanisms of glutamate induced swelling in astroglial cells. *Acta Neurochirurg* 1994; **60** (Suppl): 12–14.

245 Härkönen MHA, Kauffman FC. Metabolic alterations in the axotomized superior cervical ganglion of the rat. II. The pentose phosphate pathway. *Brain Res* 1974; **65**: 141–57.

246 Harrison JK, Jiang Y, Chen S et al. Role for neuronally derived fractalkine in mediating interactions between neurons and CX3CR1-expressing microglia. *Proc Natl Acad Sci USA* 1998; **95**: 10896–901.

247 Hayes GM, Woodroofe MN, Cuzner ML. Microglia are the major cell type expressing MHC class II in human white matter. *J Neurol Sci* 1987; **80**: 25–37.

248 Hazell AS, Butterworth RF. Hepatic encephalopathy: an update of pathophysiologic mechanisms. *Proc Soc Exp Biol Med* 1999; **222**: 99–112.

249 He BP, Strong MJ. Motor neuronal death in sporadic amyotrophic lateral sclerosis (ALS) is not apoptotic. A comparative study of ALS and chronic aluminium chloride neurotoxicity in New Zealand white rabbits. *Neuropathol Appl Neurobiol* 2000; **26**: 150–60.

250 Heacock AM, Agranoff BW. Enhanced labeling of a retinal protein during regeneration of optic nerve in goldfish. *Proc Natl Acad Sci USA* 1976; **73**: 828–32.

251 Hengartner MO, Ellis RE, Horvitz HR. *Caenorhabditis elegans* gene ced-9 protects cell from programmed cell death. *Nature* 1992; **356**: 494–9.

252 Herdegen T, Kummer W, Fiallos CE et al. Expression of c-JUN, JUNB and JUN D proteins in rat nervous system following transection of vagus nerve and cervical sympathetic trunk. *Neuroscience* 1991; **45**: 413–22.

253 Hertz L, Dringen R, Schousboe A, Robinson SR. Astrocytes: glutamate producers for neurons (Review). *J Neurosci Res* 1999; **57**: 417–28.

254 Hickey WF, Kimura H. Perivascular microglial cells of the CNS are bone marrow-derived and present antigen *in vivo*. *Science* 1988; **239**: 290–2.

255 Hickey WF, Vass K, Lassmann H. Bone marrow-derived elements in the central nervous system: an immunohistochemical and ultrastructural survey of rat chimeras. *J Neuropathol Exp Neurol* 1992; **51**: 246–56.

256 Hildebrand C, Remahl S, Persson H, Bjartmar C. Myelinated nerve fibres in the CNS. *Prog Neurobiol* 1993; **40**: 319–84.

257 Hinks GL, Franklin RJM. Distinctive patterns of PDGF-A, FGF-2, IGF-1, and TGF-beta1 gene expression during remyelination of experimentally-induced spinal cord demyelination. *Mol Cell Neurosci* 1999; **14**: 153–68.

258 Hirano A. Neuronal and glial processes in neuropathology. *J Neuropathol Exp Neurol* 1978; **37**: 365–74.

259 Hirano A. Some postmortem structural changes in peripheral myelinated fibers. In: Adachi M, Hirano A, Aronson SM eds. *The pathology of the myelinated axon.* New York: Igaku-Shoin, 1985: 30–48.

260 Hockenbery D. Defining apoptosis. *Am J Pathol* 1995; **146**: 16–18.

261 Hockenbery D, Nunez C, Milliman RD *et al.* Bcl-2 is an inner mitochondrial membrane protein that blocks programmed cell death. *Nature* 1990; **348**: 334–6.

262 Hoffman PN, Cleveland DW. Neurofilament and tubulin expression recapitulates the developmental pattern during axonal regeneration: induction of a specific β-tubulin isotype. *Proc Natl Acad Sci USA* 1988; **85**: 4530–3.

263 Hoffman PN, Cleveland DW, Griffin JW *et al.* Neurofilament gene expression: a major determinant of axonal caliber. *Proc Natl Acad Sci USA* 1987; **84**: 3472–6.

264 Hoffman PN, Lasek RJ. Axonal transport of the cytoskeleton in regenerating motor neurons: constancy and change. *Brain Res* 1980; **202**: 317–33.

265 Hoffman PN, Lasek RJ. The slow component of axonal transport. Identification of major structural polypeptides of the axon and their generality among mammalian neurons. *J Cell Biol* 1975; **66**: 351–66.

266 Hofman FM, Hinton DR, Johnson K, Merrill JE. Tumor necrosis factor identified in multiple sclerosis brain. *J Exp Med* 1989; **170**: 607–12.

267 Holtmaat AJ, Oestreicher AB, Gispen WH, Verhaagen J. Manipulation of gene expression in the mammalian nervous system: application in the study of neurite outgrowth and neuroregeneration-related proteins. *Brain Res Rev* 1998; **26**: 43–71.

268 Hösli E, Hösli L. Receptors for neurotransmitters on astrocytes in the mammalian central nervous system. *Prog Neurobiol* 1993; **40**: 477–506.

269 Houle JD, Ye JH. Changes occur in the ability to promote axonal regeneration as the post-injury period increases. *NeuroReport* 1997; **8**: 751–5.

270 Huitinga I, Van Rooijen N, DeGroot CJA *et al.* Suppression of experimental allergic encephalo myelitis in Lewis rats after elimination of macrophages. *J Exp Med* 1990; **172**: 1025–33.

271 Inagaki M, Nakamura Y, Takeda M *et al.* Glial fibrillary acidic protein: Dynamic property and regulation by phosphorylation. *Brain Pathol* 1994; **4**: 239–43.

272 Irving EA, Nicholl J, Graham DI, Dewar D. Increased tau immunoreactivity in oligodendrocytes following human stroke and head injury. *Neurosci Lett* 1996; **213**: 189–92.

273 Ishimaru MJ, Ikonomidou C, Tenkova TI *et al.* Distinguishing excitotoxic from apoptotic neurodegeneration in the developing rat brain. *J Comp Neurol* 1999; **408**: 461–76.

274 Ito D, Imai Y, Ohsawa K *et al.* Microglia-specific localization of a novel calcium-binding protein, iba1. *Mol Brain Res* 1998; **57**: 1–9.

275 Iwaki T, Iwaki A, Tateishi J *et al.* Alpha B-crystallin and 27-kD heat shock protein are regulated by stress conditions in the central nervous system and accumulate in Rosenthal fibers. *Am J Pathol* 1993; **143**: 487–95.

276 Iwaki T, Wisniewski T, Iwaki A *et al.* Accumulation of alpha B-crystallin in central nervous system glia and neurons in pathologic conditions. *Am J Pathol* 1992; **140**: 345–56.

277 Jackson KF, Duncan ID. Cell kinetics and cell death in the optic nerve of the myelin deficent rat. *J Neurocytol* 1988; **17**: 657–70.

278 Jackson KF, Hammang JP, Worth SF, Duncan ID. Hypomyelination in the neonatal rat central nervous system following tellurium intoxication. *Acta Neuropathol (Berl)* 1989; **78**: 301–9.

279 Jacob JM, McQuarrie IG. Axotomy accelerates slow component b of axonal transport. *J Neurobiol* 1991; **22**: 570–82.

280 Jacobsson G, Piehl F, Meister B. VAMP-1 and VAMP-2 gene expression in rat spinal motoneurones: differential regulation after neuronal injury. *Eur J Neurosci* 1998; **10**: 301–16.

281 Jakeman LB, Reier PJ. Axonal projections between fetal spinal cord transplants and the adult rat spinal cord: a neuronanatomical tracing study of local interactions. *J Comp Neurol* 1991; **307**: 311–34.

282 Jellinger K, Sturm KW. Delayed radiation myelopathy in man. Report of twelve necropsy cases. *J Neurol Sci* 1971; **14**: 389–408.

283 Jenkins R, Hunt SP. Long-term increase in the levels of c-jun RNA and Jun protein-like immunoreactivity in motor and sensory neurons following axon damage. *Neurosci Lett* 1991; **129**: 107–10.

284 Johnson ES, Ludwin SK. The demonstration of recurrent demyelination and remyelination of axons in the central nervous system. *Acta Neuropathol (Berl)* 1981; **53**: 93–8.

285 Johnson H, Hökfelt T, Ulfhake B. Expression of p75(NTR), trkB and trkC in nonmanipulated and axotomized motoneurons of aged rats. *Mol Brain Res* 1999; **69**: 21–34.

286 Jones A. Transient radiation myelopathy. *Br J Radiol* 1964; **37**: 727–44.

287 Jung S, Aliberti J, Graemmel P *et al.* Analysis of fractalkine receptor CX(3)CR1 function by targeted deletion and green fluorescent protein reporter gene insertion. *Mol Cell Biol* 2000; **20**: 4106–14.

288 Kacem K, Lacombe P, Seylaz J, Bonvento G. Structural organization of the perivascular astrocyte endfeet and their relationship with the endothelial glucose transporter: a confocal microscopy study. *Glia* 1998; **23**: 1–10.

289 Kagawa T, Ikenaka K, Inoue Y *et al.* Glial cell degeneration and hypomyelination caused by overexpression of myelin proteolipid protein gene. *Neuron* 1994; **13**: 427–42.

290 Kamiryo T, Kassell NF, Thai QA *et al.* Histological changes in the normal rat brain after gamma irradiation. *Acta Neurochir* 1996; **138**: 451–9.

291 Kanje M, Skottner A, Sjberg J, Lundborg G. Insulin-like growth factor I (IGF-I) stimulates regeneration of the rat sciatic nerve. *Brain Res* 1989; **486**: 396–8.

292 Kato S, Horiuchi S, Nakashima K *et al.* Astrocytic hyaline inclusions contain advanced glycation endproducts in familial amyotrophic lateral sclerosis with superoxide dismutase 1 gene mutation: immunohistochemical and immunoelectron microscopical analyses. *Acta Neuropathol* 1999; **97**: 260–6.

293 Kazzaz JA, Horowitz S, Li Y, Mantell LL. Hyperoxia in cell culture. A non-apoptotic programmed cell death. *Ann N Y Acad Sci* 1999; **887**: 164–70.

294 Keirstead HS, Ben-Hur T, Rogister B *et al.* PSA-NCAM positive CNS precursors generate both oligodendrocytes and Schwann cells to remyelinate the CNS following transplantation. *J Neurosci* 1999; **19**: 7529–36.

295 Keirstead HS, Levine JM, Blakemore WF. Response of the oligodendrocyte progenitor cell population (defined by NG2 labelling) to demyelination in the adult spinal cord. *Glia* 1998; **22**: 161–70.

296 Kerr JFR, Wyllie AH, Currie AR. Apoptosis: a basic biological phenomenon with wide ranging implications in tissue kinetics. *Br J Cancer* 1972; **26**: 239–57.

297 Kettenmann H, Banati R, Walz W. Electrophysiological

behavior of microglia. *Glia* 1993; **7**: 93–101.

298 Kettenmann H, Faissner A, Trotter J. Neuron–glia interactions in homeostasis and degeneration. In: Greger R, Koepchen HP, Mommaerts W, Windhorst U eds. *Human physiology*. Heidelberg: Springer, 1996: 533–43.

299 Ketzler S, Weis S, Haug H, Budka H. Loss of neurons in the frontal cortex in AIDS brains. *Acta Neuropathol (Berl)* 1990; **80**: 92–4.

300 Kida S, Steart PV, Zhang ET, Weller RO. Perivascular cells act as scavengers in the cerebral perivascular spaces and remain distinct from pericytes, microglia and macrophages. *Acta Neuropathol (Berl)* 1993; **85**: 646–52.

301 Kiefer R, Supler ML, Toyka KV, Streit WJ. *In situ* detection of transforming growth factor-beta mRNA in experimental rat glioma and reactive glial cells. *Neurosci Lett* 1994; **166**: 161–4.

302 Kiessling M, Herchenhan E, Eggert HR. Cerebrovascular and metabolic effects on the rat brain of focal Nd:YAG laser irradiation. *J Neurosurg* 1990; **73**: 909–17.

303 Kimler BF. Prenatal irradiation: a major concern for the developing brain. *Int J Radiat Biol* 1998; **73**: 423–34.

304 Kingery WS, Fields RD, Kocsis JD. Diminished dorsal root GABA sensitivity following chronic peripheral nerve injury. *Exp Neurol* 1988; **100**: 478–90.

305 Kirino T. Delayed neuronal death. *Neuropathology* 2000; **20** (Suppl): S95–7.

306 Klatzo I. Evolution of brain edema concepts. *Acta Neurochirurg* 1994; **60** (Suppl): 3–6.

307 Klatzo I. Neuropathological aspects of brain edema. *J Neuropathol Exp Neurol* 1967; **26**: 1–14.

308 Kloss CUA, Werner A, Klein MA *et al.* Integrin family of cell adhesion molecules in the injured brain: Regulation and cellular localization in the normal and regenerating mouse facial motor nucleus. *J Comp Neurol* 1999; **411**: 162–78

309 Koennecke LA, Zito MA, Proescholdt MG *et al.* Depletion of systemic macrophages by liposome-encapsulated clodronate attenuates increases in brain quinolinic acid during CNS-localized and systemic immune activation. *J Neurochem* 1999; **73**: 770–9.

310 Koliatsos VE, Crawford TO, Price DL. Axotomy induces nerve growth factor receptor immunoreactivity in spinal motor neurons. *Brain Res* 1991; **549**: 297–304.

311 Komori T. Tau-positive glial inclusions in progressive supranuclear palsy, corticobasal degeneration and Pick's disease. *Brain Pathol* 1999; **9**: 663–79.

312 Kösel S, Egensperger R, Bise K *et al.* Long-lasting perivascular accumulation of major histocompatibility complex class II-positive lipophages in the spinal cord of stroke patients: possible relevance for the immune privilege of the brain. *Acta Neuropathol* 1997; **94**: 532–8.

313 Kösel S, Egensperger R, von Eitzen U *et al.* On the question of apoptosis in the parkinsonian substantia nigra. *Acta Neuropathol* 1997; **93**: 105–8.

314 Kösel S, Graeber MB. Use of neuropathological tissue for molecular genetic studies: parameters affecting DNA extraction and polymerase chain reaction. *Acta Neuropathol (Berl)* 1994; **88**: 19–25.

315 Koyama Y, Goldman JE. Formation of GFAP cytoplasmic inclusions in astrocytes and their disaggregation by alpha B-crystallin. *Am J Pathol* 1999; **154**: 1563–72.

316 Kreutzberg GW. Autoradiographische Untersuchung über die Beteiligung von Gliazellen an der axonalen Reaktion im Fazialiskern der Ratte. *Acta Neuropathol (Berl)* 1966; **7**: 149–61.

317 Kreutzberg GW. Changes of coenzyme (TPN) diaphorase and TPN-linked dehydrogenase during axonal reaction of the nerve cell. *Nature* 1963; **199**: 393–4.

318 Kreutzberg GW. Microglia: a sensor for pathological events

in the CNS. *Trends Neurosci* 1996; **19**: 312–18.

319 Kreutzberg GW. Neuronal dynamics and axonal flow. IV. Blockage of intra-axonal enzyme transport by colchicine. *Proc Natl Acad Sci USA* 1969; **62**: 722–8.

320 Kreutzberg GW. Perineuronal glial reactions in regeneration of motor neurons. In: Fedoroff S, Juurlink BHJ, Doucette R eds. *Biology and pathology of astrocyte–neuron interactions*. New York: Plenum Press, 1993: 283–90.

321 Kreutzberg GW. Reaction of the neuronal cell body to axonal damage. In: Waxman SG, Kocsis JD, Stys PK eds. *The axon, structure, function and pathophysiology*. Oxford: Oxford University Press, 1995: 355–74.

322 Kreutzberg GW, Barron KD. 5'-nucleotidase of microglial cells in the facial nucleus during axonal reaction. *J Neurocytol* 1978; **7**: 601–10.

323 Kreutzberg GW, Emmert H. Glucose utilization of motor nuclei during regeneration: a 14C-2-deoxyglucose study. *Exp Neurol* 1980; **70**: 712–16.

324 Kreutzberg GW, Toth L, Kaiya H. Acetylcholinesterase as a marker for dendritic transport and dendritic secretion. *Adv Neurol* 1975; **12**: 269–81.

325 Krisch B, Mentlein R. Neuropeptide receptors and astrocytes. *Int Rev Cytol* 1994; **148**: 119–69.

326 Kroemer G, Dallaporta B, Rescherigon M. The mitochondrial death/life regulator in apoptosis and necrosis. *Annu Rev Physiol* 1998; **60**: 619–42.

327 Kubie LS. A study of the perivascular tissues of the central nervous system, with the supravital technique. *J Exp Med* 1927; **46**: 615–26.

328 Kuhn HG, Svendsen CN. Origins, functions, and potential of adult neural stem cells. *Bioessays* 1999; **21**: 625–30.

329 Kure K, Lyman W, Weidenheim K, Dickson DW. Cellular localization of an HIV-1 antigen in subacute AIDS encephalitis using an improved double-labeling immunohistochemical method. *Am J Pathol* 1992; **136**: 1085–92.

330 Kure K, Weidenheim KM, Lyman WD, Dickson DW. Morphology and distribution of HIV-1 gp41-positive microglia in subacute aids encephalitis: pattern of involvement resembling a multisystem degeneration. *Acta Neuropathol (Berl)* 1990; **80**: 393–400.

331 Lafarga M, Andres MA, Calle E, Berciano MT. Reactive gliosis of immature Bergmann glia and microglial cell activation in response to cell death of granule cell precursors induced by methylazoxymethanol treatment in developing rat cerebellum. *Anat Embryol* 1998; **198**: 111–22.

332 Lafarga M, Berciano MT, Suarez I *et al.* Cytology and organization of reactive astroglia in human cerebellar cortex with severe loss of granule cells: A study on the ataxic form of Creutzfeldt–Jakob disease. *Neuroscience* 1991; **40**: 337–52.

333 Lampert PW, Cressman MR. Fine-structural changes of myelin sheaths after axonal degeneration in the spinal cord of rats. *Am J Pathol* 1966; **49**: 1139–55.

334 Lampert PW, Davies RL. Delayed effects of radiation on the human central nervous system. *Neurology* 1964; **14**: 912–17.

335 Lampert PW, Fox JL, Earle KM. Cerebral edema after laser irradiation. An electron microscopic study. *J Neuropathol Exp Neurol* 1966; **25**: 531–41.

336 Landwehrmeyer GB, McNeil SM, Dure LS *et al.* Huntington's disease gene: regional and cellular expression in brain of normal and affected individuals. *Ann Neurol* 1995; **37**: 218–30.

337 Lantos PL, Papp MI. Cellular pathology of multiple system atrophy: a review. *J Neurol Neurosurg Psychiatr* 1994; **57**: 129–33.

338 Laping NJ, Teter B, Nichols NR *et al.* Glial fibrillary acidic

protein: Regulation by hormones, cytokines, and growth factors. *Brain Pathol* 1994; **4**: 259–75.

339 Lassmann H, Raine CS, Antel J, Prineas JW. Immunopathology of multiple sclerosis: report on an international meeting held at the Institute of Neurology of the University of Vienna. *J Neuroimmunol* 1998; **86**: 213–17.

340 Lassmann H, Schmied M, Vass K, Hickey WF. Bone marrow derived elements and resident microglia in brain inflammation. *Glia* 1993; **7**: 19–24.

341 Lassmann H, Suchanek G, Schmied M. Mechanisms of de- and remyelination in an autoimmune encephalomyelitis and mutiple sclerosis. In: Salvati S ed. *A multidisciplinary approach to myelin diseases* Vol. II. New York: Plenum Press, 1994: 137–42.

342 Latov N, Nilaver G, Zimmerman EA *et al*. Fibrillary astrocytes proliferate in response to brain injury. A study combining immunoperoxidase technique for glial fibrillary acidic protein and radioautography of tritiated thymidine. *Dev Biol* 1979; **72**: 381–4.

343 Lawson LJ, Perry VH, Dri P, Gordon S. Heterogeneity in the distribution and morphology of microglia in the normal, adult mouse brain. *Neuroscience* 1991; **39**: 151–70.

344 Leist M, Single B, Castoldi AF *et al*. Intracellular adenosine triphosphate (ATP) concentration: a switch in the decision between apoptosis and necrosis. *J Exp Med* 1997; **185**: 1481–6.

345 Lemasters JJ, Nieminen AL, Qian T *et al*. The mitochondrial permeability transition in cell death: a common mechanism in necrosis, apoptosis and autophagy. *Biochim Biophys Acta – Bioenergetics* 1998; **1366**: 177–96.

346 Levitt P, Rakic P. Immunoperoxidase localization of glial fibrillary acidic protein in radial glial cells and astrocytes of the developing Rhesus monkey brain. *J Comp Neurol* 1980; **193**: 815–40.

347 Li H, Newcombe J, Groome NP, Cuzner ML. Characterization and distribution of phagocytic macrophages in multiple sclerosis plaques. *Neuropathol Appl Neurobiol* 1993; **19**: 214–23.

348 Lin LFH, Doherty DH, Lile JD *et al*. GDNF -- a glial cell line derived neurotrophic factor for midbrain dopaminergic neurons. *Science* 1993; **260**: 1130–2.

349 Lindahl LS, Bird L, Legare ME *et al*. Differential ability of astroglia and neuronal cells to accumulate lead: dependence on cell type and on degree of differentiation. *Toxicol Sci* 1999; **50**: 236–43.

350 Lindholm D, Castren E, Kiefer R *et al*. Transforming growth factor-beta 1 in the rat brain: increase after injury and inhibition of astrocyte proliferation. *J Cell Biol* 1992; **117**: 395–400.

351 Ling EA, Wong WC. The origin and nature of ramified and amoeboid microglia: a historical review and current concepts. *Glia* 1993; **7**: 9–18.

352 Little JB. Cellular effects of ionizing radiation. *N Engl J Med* 1968; **278**: 308–15.

353 Liuzzi FJ, Lasek RJ. Astrocytes block axonal regeneration in mammals by activating the physiological stop pathway. *Science* 1987; **237**: 642–5.

354 Loeffler KU, Edward DP, Tso MOM. Tau-2 immunoreactivity of corpora amylacea in the human retina and optic nerve. *Invest Ophthalmol Vis Sci* 1993; **34**: 2600–3.

355 LoPachin RMJ, Aschner M. Glial-neuronal interactions: relevance to neurotoxic mechanisms. *Toxicol Appl Pharmacol* 1993; **118**: 141–58.

356 Lorusso L, Rossi ML. The phagocyte in human gliomas. *Ann N Y Acad Sci* 1997; **832**: 405–25.

357 Louis J-C, Magal E, Takayama S, Varon S. CNTF protection of oligodendrocytes against natural and tumor necrosis

factor-induced death. *Science* 1993; **259**: 689–92.

358 Ludwin SK. Chronic demyelination inhibits remyelination in the central nervous system. *Lab Invest* 1980; **43**: 382–7.

359 Ludwin SK. Oligodendrocytes from optic nerves subjected to long-term Wallerian degeneration retain the capacity to myelinate. *Acta Neuropathol (Berl)* 1992; **84**: 530–7.

360 Ludwin SK. Proliferation of mature oligodendrocytes after trauma to the central nervous system. *Nature* 1984; **308**: 274–5.

361 Ludwin SK. The function of perineuronal satellite oligodendrocytes: an immunohistochemical study. *Neuropathol Appl Neurobiol* 1984; **10**: 143–9.

362 Ludwin SK, Bakker DA. Can oligodendrocytes attached to myelin proliferate? *J Neurosci* 1988; **8**: 1239–44.

363 Ludwin SK, Johnson ES. Evidence for a 'dying-back–gliopathy in demyelinating disease. *Ann Neurol* 1981; **9**: 301–5.

364 Maehlen J, Olsson T, Zachau A *et al*. Local enhancement of major histocompatibility complex (MHC) class I and II expression and cell infiltration in experimental allergic encephalomyelitis around axotomized motor neurons. *J Neuroimmunol* 1989; **23**: 125–32.

365 Majno G, Joris I. Apoptosis, oncosis, and necrosis. *Am J Pathol* 1995; **146**: 3–15.

366 Malhotra SK, Predy R, Johnson ES *et al*. Novel astrocytic protein in multiple-sclerosis plaques. *J Neurosci Res* 1989; **22**: 36–49.

367 Mandybur TI, Gore I. Amyloid in late post-irradiation necrosis of brain. *Neurology* 1969; **19**: 983–92.

368 Mannoji H, Yeger H, Becker LE. A specific histochemical marker (lectin Ricinus communis agglutinin-1) for normal human microglia, and application to routine histopathology. *Acta Neuropathol (Berl)* 1986; **71**: 341–4.

369 Marin-Padilla M. Structural abnormalities of the cerebral cortex in human chromosomal aberrations: a Golgi study. *Brain Res* 1972; **44**: 625–9.

370 Martin LJ. Neuronal death in amyotrophic lateral sclerosis is apoptosis: possible contribution of a programmed cell death mechanism. *J Neuropathol Exp Neurol* 1999; **58**: 459–71.

371 Martin SJ, Green DR, Cotter TG. Dicing with death: dissecting the components of the apoptosis machinery. *Trends Biochem Sci* 1994; **19**: 26–30.

372 Mash DC, Pablo J, Flynn DD *et al*. Characterization and distribution of transferrin receptors in the rat brain. *J Neurochem* 1990; **55**: 1972–9.

373 Mason CA, Edmondson JC, Hatten ME. The extending astroglial process: Development of glial cell shape, the growing tip, and interactions with neurons. *J Neurosci* 1988; **8**: 3124–34.

374 Masters CL, Richardson EP Jr. Subacute spongiform encephalopathy (Creutzfeldt–Jakob disease): the nature and progression of spongiform change. *Brain* 1978; **101**: 333–44.

375 Mathew TC, Jackson P, Murphy R *et al*. The neuronal growth-associated α-tubulin mRNA, Tα1, is induced during regeneration and collateral sprouting of sympathetic neurons. *J Cell Biol* 1988; **107**: 727a.

376 Matsumoto Y, Hara N, Tanaka R, Fujiwara M. Immunohistochemical analysis of the rat central nervous system during experimental allergic encephalomyelitis, with special reference to Ia-positive cells with dendritic morphology. *J Immunol* 1986; **136**: 3668–76.

377 Matsumoto Y, Ohmori K, Fujiwara M. Microglial and astroglial reactions to inflammatory lesions of experimental autoimmune encephalomyelitis in the rat central nervous system. *J Neuroimmunol* 1992; **37**: 23–33.

378 Matsushita M, Yamamoto T, Gemba H. The role of astrocytes in the development of hepatic encephalopathy. *Neurosci Res* 1999; **34**: 271–80.

379 Matthews MA, Duncan D. A quantitative study of morphological changes accompanying the initiation and progress of myelin production in the dorsal funiculus of the rat spinal cord. *J Comp Neurol* 1971; **142**: 1–22.

380 Matthews MA, Kruger L. Electron microscopy of non-neuronal cellular changes accompanying neural degeneration in thalamic nuclei of the rabbit. I. Reactive hematogenous and perivascular elements within the basal lamina. *J Comp Neurol* 1973; **148**: 285–312.

381 Mattiace LA, Davies P, Dickson DW. Detection of HLA-DR on microglia in the human brain is a function of both clinical and technical factors. *Am J Pathol* 1990; **136**: 1101–14.

382 Mattson MP, Keller JN, Begley JG. Evidence for synaptic apoptosis. *Exp Neurol* 1998; **153**: 35–48.

383 Matyszak MK, Denis-Donini S, Citterio S et al. Microglia induce myelin basic protein-specific T cell anergy or T cell activation, according to their state of activation. *Eur J Immunol* 1999; **29**: 3063–76.

384 Matyszak MK, Townsend MJ, Perry VH. Ultrastructural studies of an immune-mediated inflammatory response in the CNS parenchyma directed against a non-CNS antigen. *Neuroscience* 1997; **78**: 549–60.

385 Maxwell WL, Bullock R, Landholt H, Fujisawa H. Massive astrocytic swelling in response to extracellular glutamate – a possible mechanism for post-traumatic brain swelling? *Acta Neurochirurg* 1994; **60** (Suppl): 465–7.

386 Maxwell WL, Bullock R, Scott A et al. Diffuse astrocytic swelling and increased second messenger activity following acute *Haemophilus influenzae* meningitis – evidence from a rat model. *Acta Neurochirurg* 1994; **60** (Suppl): 45–7.

387 McConkey DJ, Orrenius S, Jondal M. Cellular signaling in programmed cell death (apoptosis). *Immunol Today* 1990; **11**: 120–1.

388 McDonald JW, Althomsons SP, Hyrc KL et al. Oligodendrocytes from forebrain are highly vulnerable to AMPA/ kainate receptor-mediated excitotoxicity. *Nature Med* 1998; **4**: 291–7.

389 McGeer PL, Itagaki S, Boyes BE, McGeer EG. Reactive microglia are positive for HLA-DR in the substantia nigra of Parkinson's and Alzheimer's disease brains. *Neurology* 1988; **38**: 1285–91.

390 McGeer PL, Kawamata T, Walker DG et al. Microglia in degenerative neurological disease. *Glia* 1993; **7**: 84–92.

391 McKay JS, Blakemore WF, Franklin RJM. Trapidil-mediated growth factor-inhibition during CNS remyelination results in reduced numbers of oligodendrocytes. *Neuropath Appl Neurobiol* 1998; **24**: 498–506.

392 McLendon RE, Bigner DD. Immunohistochemistry of the glial fibrillary acidic protein: basic and applied considerations. *Brain Pathol* 1994; **4**: 221–8.

393 McMorris CS, Esiri M. Immunocytochemical study of macrophages and microglial cells and extracellular matrix components in human CNS disease. 1. Gliomas. *J Neurol Sci* 1991; **101**: 47–58.

394 Mcphilemy K, Griffiths IR, Mitchell LS, Kennedy PGE. Loss of axonal contact causes down-regulation of the PLPgene in oligodendrocytes – evidence from partial lesions of the optic nerve. *Neuropathol Appl Neurobiol* 1991; **17**: 275–87.

395 Meiri KF, Willard M, Johnson MI. Distribution and phosphorylation of the growth-associated protein GAP-43 in regenerating sympathetic neurons in culture. *J Neurosci* 1988; **8**: 2571–81.

396 Mengubas K, Riordan FA, Bravery CA et al. Ceramide-induced killing of normal and malignant human lymphocytes is by a non-apoptotic mechanism. *Oncogene* 1999; **18**: 2499–506.

397 Merrill JE, Ignarro LJ, Sherman MP et al. Microglial cell cytotoxicity of oligodendrocytes is mediated through nitric oxide. *J Immunol* 1993; **151**: 2132–41.

398 Merrill JE, Scolding NJ. Mechanisms of damage to myelin and oligodendrocytes and their relevance to disease. *Neuropath Appl Neurobiol* 1999; **25**: 435–58.

399 Merrill JE, Zimmermann RP. Natural and induced cytotoxicity of oligodendrocytes by microglia is inhibitable by TGF-β1. *Glia* 1991; **4**: 327–31.

400 Mescher AL. Trophic activity of regenerating peripheral nerves. *Comments Dev Neurobiol* 1992; **1**: 373–90.

401 Migheli A, Atzori C, Piva R et al. Lack of apoptosis in mice with ALS. *Nat Med* 1999; **5**: 966–7.

402 Miller FD, Naus CCG, Durand M et al. Isotypes of α-tubulin are differentially regulated during neuronal maturations. *J Cell Biol* 1987; **105**: 3065–73.

403 Mochizuki H, Goto K, Mori H, Mizuno Y. Histochemical detection of apoptosis in Parkinson's disease. *J Neurol Sci* 1996; **137**: 120–3.

404 Möller JR, McLenigan M, Potts BJ, Quarles RH. Effects of congenital infection of sheep with border disease virus on myelin proteins. *J Neurochem* 1993; **61**: 1808–12.

405 Mong JA, McCarthy MM. Steroid-induced developmental plasticity in hypothalamic astrocytes: Implications for synaptic patterning. *J Neurobiol* 1999; **40**: 602–19.

406 Moore RY. Cranial motor neurons contain either galanin or calcitonin gene-related peptide like immunoreactivity. *J Comp Neurol* 1989; **282**: 512–22.

407 Morimoto RI. Cells in stress: transcriptional activation of heat shock genes. *Science* 1993; **259**: 1409–10.

408 Morioka T, Baba T, Black KL, Streit WJ. The response of microglial cells to experimental rat glioma. *Glia* 1992; **6**: 75–9.

409 Morioka T, Kalehua AN, Streit WJ. Characterization of microglial reaction after middle cerebral artery occlusion in rat brain. *J Comp Neurol* 1993; **327**: 123–32.

410 Morris CS, Esiri MM, Sprinkle TJ, Gregson N. Oligodendrocyte reactions and cell proliferation markers in human demyelinating diseases. *Neuropathol Appl Neurobiol* 1994; **20**: 272–81.

411 Mugnaini E. Cell junctions of astrocytes, ependyma, and related cells in the mammalian central nervous system, with emphasis on the hypothesis of a generalized functional syncytium of supporting cells. In: Fedoroff S, Vernadakis A eds. *Astrocytes*. New York: Academic Press, 1986: 329–71.

412 Mujtaba T, Mayer-Proschel M, Rao MS. A common neural progenitor for the CNS and PNS. *Dev Biol* 1998; **200**: 1–15.

413 Müller U, Graeber MB. Neurogenetic diseases: molecular diagnosis and therapeutic approaches. *J Mol Med* 1996; **74**: 71–84.

414 Murray JA, Blakemore WF. The relationship between internodal length and fibre diameter in the spinal cord of the cat. *J Neurol Sci* 1980; **45**: 29–41.

415 Murray M, Wang SD, Goldberger ME, Levitt P. Modification of astrocytes in the spinal cord following dorsal root or peripheral nerve lesions. *Exp Neurol* 1990; **110**: 248–57.

416 Nagata K, Takei N, Nakajima K et al. Microglial conditioned medium promotes survival and development of cultured mesencephalic dopaminergic neurons from embryonic rat brain. *J Neurosci Res* 1993; **34**: 357–63.

417 Nakamura S, Kawamata T, Akiguchi I et al. Expression of monoamine oxidase B activity in astrocytes of senile plaques. *Acta Neuropathol (Berl)* 1990; **80**: 419–25.

418 Nakamura Y, Takeda M, Suzuki H et al. Abnormal distrib-

ution of cathepsins in the brain of patients with Alzheimer's disease. *Neurosci Lett* 1991; **130**: 195–8.

419 Nave K-A. Neurological mouse mutants and the genes of myelin. *J Neurosci Res* 1994; **38**: 607–12.

420 Naveilhan P, ElShamy WM, Ernfors P. Differential regulation of mRNAs for GDNF and its receptors Ret and GDNFR alpha after sciatic nerve lesion in the mouse. *Eur J Neurosci* 1997; **9**: 1450–60.

421 Nelson E, Linstrom PL, Haymaker W. Pathological effects of ultrasound on the human brain. A study of 25 cases in which ultrasonic irradiation was used as a lobotomy procedure. *J Neuropathol Exp Neurol* 1959; **18**: 489–508.

422 Neumann D, Scherson T, Ginzburg I et al. Regulation of mRNA levels for microtubule proteins during nerve regeneration. *FEBS Lett* 1983; **162**: 270–6.

423 Neumann H, Boucraut J, Hahnel C et al. Neuronal control of MHC class II inducibility in rat astrocytes and microglia. *Eur J Neurosci* 1996; **8**: 2582–90.

424 Neumann H, Misgeld T, Matsumuro K, Wekerle H. Neurotrophins inhibit major histocompatibility class II inducibility of microglia: involvement of the p75 neurotrophin receptor. *Proc Nat Acad Sci USA* 1998; **95**: 5779–84.

425 Nicholls JG, Adams WB, Eugenin J et al. Why does the central nervous system not regenerate after injury? *Surv Ophthalmol* 1999; **43**: S136–41.

426 Nissen F. Ueber das Verhalten der Kerne in den Milchdruesenzellen bei der Absonderung. *Arch Mikrosk Anat* 1885; **26**: 337–42.

427 Nissl F. Ueber die Veraenderungen der Ganglienzellen am Facialiskern des Kaninchens nach Ausreissung des Nerven. *Allg Z Psychiat* 1892; **48**: 197–8.

428 Nissl F. Ueber einige Beziehungen zwischen Nervenzellenerkrankungen und glioesen Erscheinungen bei verschiedenen Psychosen. *Arch Psychiat* 1899; **32**: 1–21.

429 Noble M, Fokseang J, Wolswijk G, Wren D. Development and regeneration in the central nervous system. *Phil Trans R Soc B* 1990; **327**: 127–43.

430 Noguchi K, Senba E, Morita Y et al. Alpha-CGRP and beta-CGRP mRNAs are differentially regulated in the rat spinal cord and dorsal root ganglion. *Mol Brain Res* 1990; **7**: 299–304.

431 Norenberg MD. Astrocyte responses to CNS injury. *J Neuropathol Exp Neurol* 1994; **53**: 213–220.

432 Norenberg MD. The distribution of glutamine synthetase in the rat central nervous system. *J Histochem Cytochem* 1979; **27**: 756–62.

433 Oblinger MM, Szumlas RA, Wong J, Liuzzi FJ. Changes in cytoskeletal gene expression affect the composition of regenerating axonal sprouts elaborated by dorsal root ganglion neurons *in vivo*. *J Neurosci* 1989; **9**: 2645–53.

434 Oehmichen M, Theuerkauf I, Meissner C. Is traumatic axonal injury (AI) associated with an early microglial activation? Application of a double-labeling technique for simultaneous detection of microglia and AI. *Acta Neuropathol* 1999; **97**: 491–4.

435 Ohtsuka K, Hata M. Molecular chaperone function of mammalian Hsp70 and Hsp40: a review. *Int J Hyperthermia* 2000; **16**: 231–45

436 Okada S, Okeda R, Matsushita S, Kawano A. Histopathological and morphometric study of the late effects of heavy-ion irradiation on the spinal cord of the rat. *Radiat Res* 1998; **150**: 304–15.

437 Okamoto K, Hirai S, Hirano A. Hirano bodies in myelinated fibers of hepatic encephalopathy. *Acta Neuropathol (Berl)* 1982; **58**: 307–10.

438 O'Leary MT, Bujdoso R, Blakemore WF. Rejection of wild type and genetically engineered major histocompatibility complex-deficient glial cell xenografts in the central nervous system results in bystander demyelination and Wallerian degeneration. *Neuroscience* 1998; **85**: 269–80.

439 Oppenheim RW. Cell death during development of the nervous system. *Annu Rev Neurosci* 1991; **14**: 453–501.

440 Oppenheim RW. The neurotrophic theory and naturally occurring motor neuron death. *Trends Neurosci* 1989; **12**: 252–5.

441 Oppenheim RW, Houenou LJ, Johnson JE et al. Developing motor neurons rescued from programmed and axotomy-induced cell death by GDNF. *Nature* 1995; **373**: 344–6.

442 O'Sullivan BM, Blakemore WF. Acute nicotinamide deficency in the pig induced by 6-aminonicotinamide. *Vet Pathol* 1980; **17**: 748–58.

443 Otake M, Schull WJ. Radiation-related brain damage and growth retardation among the prenatally exposed atomic bomb survivors. *Int J Radiat Biol* 1998; **74**: 159–71.

444 Otsuki T, Yoshimoto T, Jokura H, Katakura R. Stereotactic laser surgery for deep-seated brain tumours by open-system endoscopy. *Stereotactic Funct Neurosurg* 1990; **54**: 404–8.

445 Otto D, Unsicker K, Grothe C. Pharmacological effects of nerve growth factor and fibroblast growth factor applied to the transectioned sciatic nerve on neuron death in adult rat dorsal root ganglia. *Neurosci Lett* 1987; **83**: 156–60.

446 Overmyer M, Helisalmi S, Soininen H et al. Reactive microglia in aging and dementia: an immunohistochemical study of postmortem human brain tissue. *Acta Neuropathol* 1999; **97**: 383–92.

447 Ozawa K, Suchanek G, Breitschopf H et al. Patterns of oligodendroglial pathology in multiple sclerosis. *Brain* 1994; **117**: 1311–22.

448 Palyi I, Kremmer T, Kalnay A et al. Effects of methylacetylenic putrescine, an ornithine decarboxylase inhibitor and potential novel anticancer agent, on human and mouse cancer cell lines. *Anticancer Drugs* 1999; **10**: 103–11.

449 Panse F. Electrical trauma. In: Braakman W ed. *Handbook of clinical neurology*. Amsterdam: North Holland, 1975: 683–729.

450 Papp MI, Lantos PL. Accumulation of tubular structures in oligodendroglial and neuronal cells as the basic alteration in multiple system atrophy. *J Neurol Sci* 1992; **107**: 172–82.

451 Pasternack JM, Abraham CR, Van Dyke BJ et al. Astrocytes in Alzheimer's disease gray matter express alpha1-antichymotrypsin mRNA. *Am J Pathol* 1989; **135**: 827–33.

452 Paulus W, Roggendorf W, Kirchner T. Ki-M1P as a marker for microglia and brain macrophages in routinely processed human tissues. *Acta Neuropathol (Berl)* 1992; **84**: 538–44.

453 Pearson VL, Rothwell NJ, Toulmond S. Excitotoxic brain damage in the rat induces interleukin-1beta protein in microglia and astrocytes: correlation with the progression of cell death. *Glia* 1999; **25**: 311–23.

454 Pekny M, Leveen P, Pekna M et al. Mice lacking glial fibrillary acidic protein display astrocytes devoid of intermediate filaments but develop and reproduce normally. *EMBO J* 1995; **14**: 1590–8.

455 Pender MP, Nguyen KB, McCombe PA, Kerr JFR. Apoptosis in the nervous system in experimental allergic encephalomyelitis. *J Neurol Sci* 1991; **104**: 81–7.

456 Penfield W. Microglia and the process of phagocytosis in gliomas. *Am J Pathol* 1925; **1**: 77–97.

457 Pennybaker J, Russell DS. Necrosis of the brain due to radiation therapy: Clinical and pathological observations. *J*

Neurol Neurosurg Psychiat 1948; **11**: 183–98.

458 Perry VH. A revised view of the central nervous system microenvironment and major histocompatibility complex class II antigen presentation. *J Neuroimmunol* 1998; **90**: 113–21.

459 Perry VH, Andersson P-B, Gordon S. Macrophages and inflammation in the central nervous system. *Trends Neurosci* 1993; **16**: 268–73.

460 Perry VH, Gordon S. Macrophages and microglia in the nervous system. *Trends Neurosci* 1988; **11**: 273–7.

461 Perry VH, Matyszak MK, Fearn S. Altered antigen expression of microglia in the aged rodent CNS. *Glia* 1993; **7**: 60–7.

462 Peters A, Palay SL, Webster HdeF. *The fine structure of the nervous system. Neurons and their supporting cells.* Oxford: Oxford University Press, 1991.

463 Peters A, Palay SL, Webster HdeF. *The fine structure of the nervous system: The cells and their processes.* New York: Harper & Row, 1970.

464 Petito CK, Morgello S, Felix JC, Lesser ML. The two patterns of reactive astrocytosis in postischemic rat brain. *J Cereb Blood Flow Metab* 1990; **10**: 850–9.

465 Petito CK, Roberts B. Evidence for apoptotic cell death in HIV encephalitis. *Am J Pathol* 1995; **146**: 1121–30.

466 Peuchen S, Bolanos JP, Heales SJ *et al.* Interrelationships between astrocyte function, oxidative stress and antioxidant status within the central nervous system. *Prog Neurobiol* 1997; **52**: 261–81.

467 Pfeiffer SE, Warrington AE, Bansal R. The oligodendrocyte and its many processes. *Trends Cell Biol* 1993; **3**: 191–7.

468 Piani D, Frei K, Do KQ *et al.* Murine brain macrophages induce NMDA receptor mediated neurotoxicicty by secreting glutamate. *Neurosci Lett* 1991; **133**: 159–62.

469 Piehl F, Arvidsson U, Johnson H *et al.* Calcitonin gene-related peptide (CGRP)-like immunoreactivity and CGRP mRNA in rat spinal cord motor neurons after different types of lesions. *Eur J Neurosci* 1991; **3**: 737–57.

470 Plomin R, Owen MJ, McGuffin P. The genetic basis of complex human behaviors. *Science* 1994; **264**: 1733–9.

471 Portera-Cailliau C, Price DL, Martin LJ. Excitotoxic neuronal death in the immature brain is an apoptosis–necrosis morphological continuum. *J Comp Neurol* 1997; **378**: 70–87.

472 Povlishock JT. Traumatically induced axonal injury: Pathogenesis and pathobiological implications. *Brain Pathol* 1992; **2**: 1–12.

473 Prineas JW, Barnard RO, Kwon EE *et al.* Multiple sclerosis: remyelination of nascent lesions. *Ann Neurol* 1993; **33**: 137–51.

474 Probst-Cousin S, Rickert CH, Schmid KW, Gullotta F. Cell death mechanisms in multiple system atrophy. *J Neuropathol Exp Neurol* 1998; **57**: 814–21.

475 Purpura DP. Dendritic spine 'dysgenesis– and mental retardation. *Science* 1974; **186**: 1126–8.

476 Purpura DP, Hirano A, French JH. Polydendritic Purkinje cells in X-chromosome linked copper malabsorption: a Golgi study. *Brain Res* 1976; **117**: 125–9.

477 Purves D ed. *Neural activity and the growth of the brain.* Cambridge: Cambridge University Press, 1994: 1–108.

478 Raff MC. Glial cell diversification in the rat optic nerve. *Science* 1989; **243**: 1450–5.

479 Raff MC, Miller RH, Noble M. A glial progenitor cell that develops *in vitro* into an astrocyte or an oligodendrocyte depending on culture medium. *Nature* 1983; **303**: 390–6.

480 Raine CS. Biology of disease: analysis of autoimmune demyelination: its impact on multiple sclerosis. *Lab Invest* 1984; **50**: 608–35.

481 Raine CS. Multiple sclerosis: immune system molecule expression in the central nervous system. *J Neuropathol Exp Neurol* 1994; **53**: 328–37.

482 Raine CS, Traugott U. Remyelination in chronic relapsing experimental allergic encephalomyelitis and multiple sclerosis. In: Adachi A, Hirano A, Aronson SM eds. *The pathology of the myelinated axon.* New York: Igaku-Shoin, 1985: 229–75.

483 Raivich G, Bluethmann H, Kreutzberg GW. Signaling molecules and neuroglial activation in the injured central nervous system. *Keio J Med* 1996; **45**: 239–47.

484 Raivich G, Gehrmann J, Kreutzberg GW. Increase of colony-stimulating factor and granulocyte-macrophage colony-stimulating factor receptors in the regenerating rat facial nucleus. *J Neurosci Res* 1991; **30**: 682–6.

485 Raivich G, Graeber MB, Gehrmann J, Kreutzberg GW. Transferrin receptor expression and iron uptake in the injured and regenerating rat sciatic nerve. *Eur J Neurosci* 1991; **3**: 919–27.

486 Raivich G, Hellweg R, Graeber MB, Kreutzberg GW. The expression of growth factor receptors during nerve regeneration. *Rest Neurol Neurosci* 1990; **1**: 217–23.

487 Raivich G, Hellweg R, Kreutzberg GW. NGF receptor-mediated reduction in axonal NGF uptake and retrograde transport following sciatic nerve injury and during regeneration. *Neuron* 1991; **7**: 151–64.

488 Raivich G, Kreutzberg GW. Expression of growth factor receptors in injured nerve tissue. I. Axotomy leads to a shift in the cellular distribution of specific b-nerve growth factor binding in the injured and regenerating PNS. *J Neurocytol* 1987; **16**: 687–700.

489 Raivich G, Kreutzberg GW. Peripheral nerve regeneration: role of growth factors and their receptors. *Int J Dev Neurosci* 1993; **11**: 311–24.

490 Raivich G, Moreno-Flores MT, Moeller JC, Kreutzberg GW. Inhibition of microglial proliferation in a genetic model of macrophage colony stimulating factor deficiency. *Eur J Neurosci* 1994; **6**: 1615–18.

491 Ransom BR, Fern R. Does astrocytic glycogen benefit axon function and survival in CNS white matter during glucose deprivation? *Glia* 1997; **21**: 134–41.

492 Ransom BR, Kettenmann H. Electrical coupling, without dye coupling, between mammalian astrocytes and oligodendrocytes in cell culture. *Glia* 1990; **3**: 258–66.

493 Redies C. Cadherins in the central nervous system. *Prog Neurobiol* 2000; **61**: 611–48.

494 Reier PJ, Eng LF, Jakeman L. Reactive astrocyte and axonal outgrowth in the injured CNS: is gliosis really an impediment to regeneration? In: Seil FJ ed. *Neural regeneration and transplantation.* New York: Alan R Liss, 1989: 183–209.

495 Reifenberger G, Deckert M, Wechsler W. Immunohistochemical determination of protein kinase C expression and proliferative activity in human brain tumors. *Acta Neuropathol (Berl)* 1989; **78**: 166–75.

496 Relling MV, Rubnitz JE, Rivera GK *et al.* High incidence of secondary brain tumours after radiotherapy and antimetabolites. *Lancet* 1999; **354**: 34–9.

497 Reuss B, Unsicker K. Regulation of gap junction communication by growth factors from non-neural cells to astroglia: a brief review. *Glia* 1998; **24**: 32–8.

498 Reynolds R, Wilkin GP. Cellular reaction to an acute demyelinating/remyelinating lesion of the rat brain stem: localisation of GD3 ganglioside immunoreactivity. *J Neurosci Res* 1993; **36**: 405–22.

499 Rezvani M, Hopewell JW, Robbins ME. Initiation of nonneoplastic late effects: the role of endothelium and connective tissue. *Stem Cells* 1995; **13** (Suppl 1): 248–56.

500 Rich KM, Disch SP, Eichler ME. The influence of regenera-

tion and nerve growth factor on the neuronal cell body reaction to injury. *J Neurocytol* 1989; **18**: 569–76.

501 Rich KM, Luszczynski JR, Osborne PA, Johnson EJ. Nerve growth factor protects adult sensory neurons from cell death and atrophy caused by nerve injury. *J Neurocytol* 1987; **16**: 261–8.

502 Rich KM, Yip HK, Osborne PA *et al*. Role of nerve growth factor in the adult dorsal root ganglia neuron and its response to injury. *J Comp Neurol* 1984; **230**: 110–18.

503 Rich T, Watson CJ, Wyllie A. Apoptosis: the germs of death. *Nature* Cell Biology 1999; **1**: E69–71.

504 Robinson RG. A second brain tumour and irradiation. *J Neurol Neurosurg Psychiat* 1978; **41**: 1005–12.

505 Rodriguez M, Scheithauer BW, Forbes G, Kelly PJ. Oligodendrocyte injury is an early event in lesions of multiple sclerosis. *Mayo Clin Proc* 1993; **68**: 627–36.

506 Ronnevi LO. Origin of the glial processes responsible for the spontaneous postnatal phagocytosis of boutons on cat spinal motor neurons. *Cell Tissue Res* 1978; **189**: 203–17.

507 Ronnevi LO. Spontaneous phagocytosis of boutons on spinal motor neurons during early postnatal development. An electron microscopical study in the cat. *J Neurocytol* 1977; **6**: 487–504.

508 Ross RA, Joh TH, Reis DJ. Reversible changes in the accumulation and activities of tyrosine hydroxylase and dopamine-β-hydroxylase in neurons of nucleus locus coeruleus during the retrograde reaction. *Brain Res* 1975; **92**: 57–72.

509 Rotter A, Schultz CM, Frostholm A. Regulation of glycine receptor binding in the mouse hypoglossal nucleus in response to axotomy. *Brain Res Bull* 1984; **13**: 487–92.

510 Rubin P, Gash DM, Hansen JT *et al*. Disruption of the blood–brain barrier as the primary effect of CNS irradiation. *Radiother Oncol* 1994; **31**: 51–60.

511 Russel DS, Rubinstein LJ. *Pathology of tumours of the nervous system*. 5 edn. Edward Arnold, London, 1989.

512 Rust RS. Energy metabolism of developing brain. *Curr Opin Neurol* 1994; **7**: 160–5.

513 Saika T, Senba E, Noguchi K *et al*. Changes in expression of peptides in rat facial motor neurons after facial nerve crushing and resection. *Mol Brain Res* 1991; **11**: 187–96.

514 Sanchez I, Hassinger L, Paskevich PA *et al*. Oligodendroglia regulate the regional expansion of axon caliber and local accumulation of neurofilaments during development independently of myelin formation. *J Neurosci* 1996; **16**: 5095–105.

515 Sarnat HB. Ependymal reactions to injury. A review. *J Neuropathol Exp Neurol* 1995; **54**: 1–15.

516 Sasaki A, Hirato J, Nakazato Y. Immunohistochemical study of microglia in the Creutzfeldt–Jakob diseased brain. *Acta Neuropathol (Berl)* 1993; **86**: 337–44.

517 Sasaki A, Nakazato Y. The identity of cells expressing MHC class II antigens in normal and pathological human brain. *Neuropathol Appl Neurobiol* 1992; **18**: 13–26.

518 Savio T, Schwab M. Lesioned corticospinal tract axons regenerate in myelin-free rat spinal cord. *Proc Natl Acad Sci USA* 1990; **87**: 4130–3.

519 Sbarbati A, Carner M, Colletti V, Osculati F. Extrusion of corpora amylacea from the marginal gila at the vestibular root entry zone. *J Neuropathol Exp Neurol* 1996; **55**: 196–201.

520 Sbarbati A, Carner M, Colletti V, Osculati F. Myelin-containing corpora amylacea in vestibular root entry zone. *Ultrastruct Pathol* 1996; **20**: 437–42.

521 Scheibel ME, Crandall PH, Scheibel AB. The hippocampal–dentate complex in temporal lobe epilepsy. *Epilepsia* 1974; **15**: 55–80.

522 Schiffer D, Giordana MT, Migheli A *et al*. Glial fibrillary

acidic protein and vimentin in the experimental glial reaction of the rat brain. *Brain Res* 1986; **374**: 110–18.

523 Schipper HM. Experimental induction of corpora amylacea in adult rat brain. *Microsc Res Technique* 1998; **43**: 43–8.

524 Schmidt RE. Neuroaxonal dystrophy in aging rodent and human sympathetic autonomic ganglia: synaptic pathology as a common theme in neuropathology. *Adv Pathol Lab Med* 1993; **6**: 505–22.

525 Schmied M, Breitschopf H, Gold R *et al*. Apoptosis of T lymphocytes in experimental autoimmune encephalomyelitis. Evidence for programmed cell death as a mechanism to control inflammation in the brain. *Am J Pathol* 1993; **143**: 446–52.

526 Schneider J, Hofman FM, Apuzzo ML, Hinton DR. Cytokines and immunoregulatory molecules in malignant glial neoplasms. *J Neurosurg* 1992; **77**: 265–73.

527 Schnell L, Schneider R, Kolbeck R *et al*. Neurotrophin-3 enhances sprouting of corticospinal tract during development and after adult spinal cord lesion. *Nature* 1994; **367**: 170–3.

528 Schnell L, Schwab ME. Axonal regeneration in the rat spinal cord produced by an antibody against myelin-associated neurite growth inhibitors. *Nature* 1990; **343**: 269–72.

529 Scholz W, Hs YK. Late damage from Roentgen irradiation of the human brain. *Arch Neurol Psychiat* 1938; **40**: 928–37.

530 Schousboe A, Westergaard N, Hertz L. Neuronal–astrocytic interactions in glutamate metabolism. *Biochem Soc Trans* 1993; **21**: 49–53.

531 Schubert P, Kreutzberg GW. Parameters of dendritic transport. *Adv Neurol* 1975; **12**: 255–68.

532 Schubert P, Kreutzberg GW, Lux HD. Neuroplasmic transport in dendrites: effect of colchicine on morphology and physiology of motor neurons in the cat. *Brain Res* 1972; **47**: 331–43.

533 Schütze, K, Clement-Sengewald A. Catch and move-cut or fuse. *Nature* 1994; **368**: 667–70.

534 Schwab ME. Experimental aspects of spinal cord regeneration. *Curr Opin Neurol Neurosurg* 1993; **6**: 549–53.

535 Schwab ME, Bartholdi D. Degeneration and regeneration of axons in the lesioned spinal cord. *Physiol Rev* 1996; **76**: 319–70.

536 Schwab ME, Caroni P. Oligodendrocytes and CNS myelin are nonpermissive substrates for neurite growth and fibroblast spreading *in vitro*. *J Neurosci* 1988; **8**: 2381–93.

537 Schwab ME, Kapfhammer JP, Brandtlow CE. Inhibitors of neurite growth. *Annu Rev Neurosci* 1993; **16**: 565–95.

538 Schwartz LM, Kosz L, Kay BK. Gene activation is required for developmentally programmed cell death. *Proc Natl Acad Sci USA* 1990; **87**: 6594–8.

539 Schwartz LM, Osborne BA. Programmed cell death, apoptosis and killer genes. *Immunol Today* 1993; **14**: 582–90.

540 Sedgwick JD, Schwender J, Gregersen R *et al*. Resident macrophages (ramified microglia) of the adult brown Norway rat central nervous system are constitutively major histocompatibility complex II positive. *J Exp Med* 1990; **177**: 1145–52.

541 Seitelberger F. Neuroaxonal dystrophy: its relation to aging and neurological diseases. In: Vinken PJ, Bruyn GW, Klawans HL eds. *Handbook of clinical neurology* Vol. 5 *Extrapyramidal disorders*. Amsterdam: Elsevier, 1986: 391–415.

542 Seitelberger F, Weingarten K. On the participation of the optic nerve in some degenerative brain processes. *J Gen Hum* 1966; **15**: 284–301.

543 Selmaj K, Raine CS, Cannella B, Brosnan CF. Identification

of lymphotoxin and tumor necrosis factor in multiple sclerosis lesions. *J Clin Invest* 1991; **87**: 949–54.

544 Selmaj KW, Raine CS. Tumor necrosis factor mediates myelin and oligodendrocyte damage *in vitro*. *Ann Neurol* 1988; **23**: 339–46.

545 Sen S. Programmed cell death: concept, mechanism and control. *Biol Rev* 1992; **67**: 287–319.

546 Senba E, Simmons DM, Wada E *et al*. RNA levels of neuronal nicotinic acetylcholine receptor subunits are differentially regulated in axotomized facial motor neurons: an *in situ* hybridisation study. *Mol Brain Res* 1990; **8**: 349–53.

547 Sendtner M, Kreutzberg GW, Thoenen H. Ciliary neurotrophic factor prevents the degeneration of motor neurons after axotomy. *Nature* 1990; **345**: 440–1.

548 Sendtner M, Schmalbruck H, Stckli KA *et al*. Ciliary neurotrophic factor prevents degeneration of motor neurons in mouse mutant progressive motor neuronopathy. *Nature* 1992; **358**: 502–4.

549 Sharer L, Cho E-S, Epstein L. Multinucleated giant cells and HTLV-III in AIDS encephalopathy. *Hum Pathol* 1985; **16**: 760.

550 Shehab SA, Atkinson ME. Vasoactive intestinal polypeptide (VIP) increases in the spinal cord after peripheral axotomy of the sciatic nerve originate from primary afferent neurons. *Brain Res* 1986; **372**: 37–44.

551 Shelton MK, Mccarthy KD. Mature hippocampal astrocytes exhibit functional metabotropic and ionotropic glutamate receptors in situ. *Glia* 1999; **26**: 1–11.

552 Shields SA, Gilson JM, Blakemore WF, Franklin RJM. Remyelination occurs as extensively but more slowly in old rats compared to young rats following gliotoxin-induced CNS demyelination. *Glia* 1999; **28**: 77–83.

553 Shigematsu K, McGeer PL Walker DG *et al*. Reactive microglia/macrophages phagocytose amyloid precursor protein produced by neurons following neural damage. *J Neurosci Res* 1992; **31**: 443–53.

554 Shine HD, Readhead C, Popko B *et al*. Morphometric analysis of normal, mutant, and transgenic CNS: correlation of myelin basic protein expression and myelinogenesis. *J Neurochem* 1992; **58**: 342–9.

555 Shinohara C, Gobbel GT, Lamborn KR *et al*. Apoptosis in the subependyma of young adult rats after single and fractionated doses of X-rays. *Cancer Res* 1997; **57**: 2694–702.

556 Shintani T, Hayakawa N, Hoshi M *et al*. High incidence of meningioma among Hiroshima atomic bomb survivors. *J Radiat Res* 1999; **40**: 49–57.

557 Shuman SL, Bresnahan JC, Beattie MS. Apoptosis of microglia and oligodendrocytes after spinal cord contusion in rats. *J Neurosci Res* 1997; **50**: 798–808.

558 Sievers J, Hausmann B, Unsicker K, Berry M. Fibroblast growth factors promote the survival of adult rat retinal ganglion cells after transection of the optic nerve. *Neurosci Lett* 1987; **76**: 157–62.

559 Singer P, Mehler S. Glucose, leucine uptake in the hypoglossal nucleus after hypoglossal nerve transection with and without prevented regeneration in the Sprague–Dawley rat. *Neurosci Lett* 1986; **67**: 73–7.

560 Singer PA, Mehler S. 2-Deoxy [^{14}C]glucose uptake in rat hypoglossal nucleus after nerve transection. *Exp Neurol* 1980; **69**: 617–26.

561 Singer PA, Mehler S, Fernandez HL. Blockade of retrograde axonal transport delays the onset of metabolic and morphologic changes induced by axotomy. *J Neurosci* 1982; **2**: 1299–306.

562 Sinicropi DV, McIlwain DL. Changes in the amounts of cytoskeletal proteins within the perikarya and axons of regenerating frog motor neurons. *J Cell Biol* 1983; **96**: 240–7.

563 Sjöstrand J. Proliferative changes in glial cells during nerve regeneration. *Z Zellforsch Mikrosk Anat* 1965; **68**: 481–93.

564 Skoff RP, Knapp PE. Division of astroblasts and oligodendroblasts in postnatal rodent brain: evidence for separate astrocyte and oligodendrocyte lineages. *Glia* 1991; **4**: 165–74.

565 Small JA, Scangos GA, Cork L *et al*. The early region of human papovarirus JC induces dysmyelination in transgenic mice. *Cell* 1986; **46**: 13–18.

566 Small RK, Riddle P, Noble M. Evidence for migration of oligodendrocyte-type-2 astrocyte progenitor cell into the rat optic nerve. *Nature* 1987; **328**: 155–7.

567 Smith CB, Crane AM, Kadekaro M *et al*. Stimulation of protein synthesis and glucose utilization in the hypoglossal nucleus induced by axotomy. *J Neurosci* 1984; **4**: 2489–96.

568 Smith DA, Lantos PL. Immunocytochemistry of cerebellar astrocytomas: with a special note on Rosenthal fibres. *Acta Neuropathol (Berl)* 1985; **66**: 155–9.

569 Smith MC. Metachromatic bodies in the brain. *J Neurol Neurosur Psychiat* 1949; **12**: 100–10.

570 Soffer D, Pittalugua S, Feiner M, Beller AJ. Intracranial meningeomas following low dose irradiation to the head. *J Neurosurg* 1983; **59**: 1048–53.

571 Somjen GG. Nervenkitt. Notes on the history of the concept of neuroglia. *Glia* 1988; **1**: 2–9.

572 Sriram S, Rodriguez M. Indictment of the microglia as the villain in multiple sclerosis. *Neurology* 1997; **48**: 464–70.

573 Stadelmann C, Deckwerth TL, Srinivasan A *et al*. Activation of caspase-3 in single neurons and autophagic granules of granulovacuolar degeneration in Alzheimer's disease: evidence for apoptotic cell death. *Am J Pathol* 1999; **155**: 1459–66.

574 Staub F, Winkler A, Peters J *et al*. Swelling, acidosis, and irreversible damage of glial cells from exposure to arachidonic acid *in vitro*. *J Cereb Blood Flow Metab* 1994; **14**: 1030–9.

575 Sternberger NH, Itoyama Y, Kies MW, Webster H de F. Immunocytochemical method to identify basic protein in myelin-forming oligodendrocytes of newborn rat CNS. *J Neurocytol* 1978; **7**: 251–63.

576 Steward O, Torre ER, Tomasulo R, Lothman E. Seizures and the regulation of astroglial gene expression. *Epilepsy Res Suppl* 1992; **7**: 197–209.

577 Streit WJ, Dumoulin FL, Raivich G, Kreutzberg GW. Calcitonin gene-related peptide increases in rat facial motor neurons after peripheral nerve transection. *Neurosci Lett* 1989; **101**: 143–8.

578 Streit WJ, Graeber MB. Microglia: a pictorial. *Prog Histochem Cytochem* 1996; **31**: 1–89.

579 Streit WJ, Graeber MB, Kreutzberg GW. Expression of Ia antigen on perivascular and microglial cells after sublethal and lethal motor neuron injury. *Exp Neurol* 1989; **105**: 115–26.

580 Streit WJ, Graeber MB, Kreutzberg GW. Functional plasticity of microglia: a review. *Glia* 1988; **1**: 301–7.

581 Streit WJ, Graeber MB, Kreutzberg GW. Peripheral nerve lesion produces increased levels of MHC antigens in the CNS. *J Neuroimmunol* 1989; **21**: 117–23.

582 Streit WJ, Kreutzberg GW. Response of endogenous glial cells to motor neuron degeneration induced by toxic ricin. *J Comp Neurol* 1988; **268**: 248–63.

583 Strömberg I, Björklund H, Dahl D *et al*. Astrocyte responses to dopaminergic denervations by 6-hydroxydopamine and 1-methyl-4-phenyl-1,2,3,6-tetrahydropyridine as evidenced by glial fibrillary acidic protein immunohistochemistry. *Brain Res Bull* 1986; **17**: 225–36.

584 Suetsugu M, Mehraein P. Spine distribution along the apical dendrites of the pyramidal neurons in Down's syn-

drome. A quantitative Golgi study. *Acta Neuropathol (Berl)* 1980; **50**: 207–10.

585 Sugimoto T, Xiao C, Ichikawa H. Neonatal primary neuronal death induced by capsaicin and axotomy involves an apoptotic mechanism. *Brain Res* 1998; **807**: 147–54.

586 Sumner BEH, Watson WE. Retraction and expansion of the dendritic tree of motor neurones of adult rats induced *in vivo. Nature* 1971; **233**: 273–5.

587 Sundaresan N, Guiterrez FA, Larsen MB. Radiation myelopathy in children. *Ann Neurol* 1978; **4**: 47–50.

588 Susin SA, Zamzami N, Kroemer G. Mitochondria as regulators of apoptosis: doubt no more. *Biochim Biophys Acta – Bioenergetics* 1998; **1366**: 151–65.

589 Suzuki K, Zagoren JC. Degeneration of oligodendroglia in the central nervous system of rats treated with A79944 or triparanol. *Lab Invest* 1974; **31**: 503–15.

590 Suzumura A, Sawada M, Yanamoto H, Maranouchi T. Effects of colony stimulating factors on isolated microglia *in vitro. J Neuroimmunol* 1990; **30**: 111–20.

591 Tacconi MT. Neuronal death: is there a role for astrocytes? *Neurochem Res* 1998; **23**: 759–65.

592 Takeuchi A, Isobe KI, Miyaishi O *et al.* Microglial NO induces delayed neuronal death following acute injury in the striatum. *Eur J Neurosci* 1998; **10**: 1613–20.

593 Tan J, Town T, Paris D *et al.* Microglial activation resulting from CD40-CD40L interaction after beta-amyloid stimulation. *Science* 1999; **286**: 2352–5.

594 Tan J, Town T, Paris D *et al.* Activation of microglial cells by the CD40 pathway: relevance to multiple sclerosis. *J Neuroimmunol* 1998; **97**: 77–85.

595 Tan S, Wood M, Maher P. Oxidative stress induces a form of programmed cell death with characteristics of both apoptosis and necrosis in neuronal cells. *J Neurochem* 1998; **71**: 95–105.

596 Targett MP, Sussman J, O'Leary MT *et al.* Failure to achieve remyelination of demyelinated rat axons following transplantation of glial cells obtained from the adult human brain. *Neuropath Appl Neurobiol* 1996; **22**: 199–206.

597 Tatton WG, Olanow CW. Apoptosis in neurodegenerative diseases: the role of mitochondria. *Biochim Biophys Acta – Bioenergetics* 1999; **1410**: 195–213.

598 Teter B, Osterburg HH, Anderson CP, Finch CE. Methylation of the rat glial fibrillary acidic protein gene shows tissue-specific domains. *J Neurosci Res* 1994; **39**: 680–93.

599 Tetzlaff W, Alexander SW, Miller FD, Bisby MA. Response of facial and rubrospinal neurons to axotomy: changes in mRNA expression for cytoskeletal proteins and GAP-43. *J Neurosci* 1991; **11**: 2528–44.

600 Tetzlaff W, Bisby MA, Kreutzberg GW. Changes in cytoskeletal proteins in the rat facial nucleus following axotomy. *J Neurosci* 1988; **8**: 3181–9.

601 Tetzlaff W, Graeber MB, Bisby MA, Kreutzberg GW. Increased glial fibrillary acidic protein synthesis in astrocytes during retrograde reaction of the rat facial nucleus. *Glia* 1988; **1**: 90–5.

602 Tetzlaff W, Kreutzberg GW. Enzyme changes in the rat facial nucleus following a conditioning lesion. *Exp Neurol* 1984; **85**: 547–64.

603 The Genome Directory. *Nature* 1995; **377** (Suppl).

604 Theodosis DT, Poulain DA. Activity-dependent neuronal-glial and synaptic plasticity in the adult mammalian hypothalamus. *Neuroscience* 1993; **57**: 501–35.

605 Thery C, Chamak B, Mallat M. Free radical killing of neurons. *Eur J Neurosci* 1991; **3**: 1155–64.

606 Thoenen H. The changing scene of neurotrophic factors. *Trends Neurosci* 1991; **14**: 165–170.

607 Toggas S, Masliah E, Rockenstein E *et al.* Central nervous system damage produced by expression of HIV-1 coat protein gp120 in transgenic mice. *Nature* 1994; **367**: 188–93.

608 Toku K, Tanaka J, Fujikata S *et al.* Distinctions between microglial cells and peripheral macrophages with regard to adhesive activities and morphology. *J Neurosci Res* 1999; **57**: 855–65.

609 Tomokane N, Iwaki T, Tateishi J *et al.* Rosenthal fibers share epitopes with alpha B-crystallin, glial fibrillary acidic protein, and ubiquitin, but not with vimentin. Immunoelectron microscopy with colloidal gold. *Am J Pathol* 1991; **138**: 875–85.

610 Tonra JR, Curtis R, Wong V *et al.* Axotomy upregulates the anterograde transport and expression of brain-derived neurotrophic factor by sensory neurons. *J Neurosci* 1998; **18**: 4374–83.

611 Tontsch U, Rott O. Cortical neurons selectively inhibit MHC class II induction in astrocytes but not in microglial cells. *Int Immunol* 1993; **5**: 249–54.

612 Tooyama I, Akiyama H, McGeer PL *et al.* Acidic fibroblast growth factor-like immunoreactivity in brain of Alzheimer patients. *Neurosci Lett* 1991; **121**: 155–8.

613 Töpper R, Gehrmann J, Schwarz M *et al.* Remote microglial activation in the quinolinic acid model of Huntington's disease. *Exp Neurol* 1993; **123**: 271–83.

614 Torvik A. Central chromatolysis and the axon reaction: a re-appraisal. *Neuropathol Appl Neurobiol* 1976; **2**: 423–32.

615 Towfighi J. Hexachlorophene. In: Spencer PS, Schaumburg HH eds. *Experimental and clinical neurotoxicology*. Baltimore, MD: Williams and Wilkins, 1980: 440–55.

616 Turmaine M, Raza A, Mahal A *et al.* Nonapoptotic neurodegeneration in a transgenic mouse model of Huntington's disease. *Proc Natl Acad Sci USA* 2000; **97**: 8093–97.

617 Tyor WR, Glass JD, Griffin JW *et al.* Cytokine expression in the brain during the acquired immunodeficiency syndrome. *Ann Neurol* 1992; **31**: 349–60.

618 Tytell M, Barbe MF, Brown IR. Stress (heat shock) protein accumulation in the central nervous system. *Adv Neurol* 1993; **59**: 293–303.

619 Ulvestad E, Williams K, Bo L *et al.* HLA class II molecules (HLA-DR, -DP, -DQ) on cells in the human CNS studied *in situ* and *in vitro. Immunology* 1994; **82**: 535–41.

620 Ulvestad E, Williams K, Vedeler C *et al.* Reactive microglia in multiple sclerosis lesions have an increased expression of receptors for the Fc part of IgG. *J Neurol Sci* 1994; **121**: 125–31.

621 Unchern S, Saito H, Nishiyama N. Death of cerebellar granule neurons induced by piperine is distinct from that induced by low potassium medium. *Neurochem Res* 1998; **23**: 97–102.

622 Unger ER, Sung JH, Manivel JC *et al.* Male donor-derived cells in the brains of female sex- mismatched bone marrow transplant recipients: a Y-chromosome specific *in situ* hybridisation study. *J Neuropathol Exp Neurol* 1993; **52**: 460–70.

623 Vale RD, Reese TS, Sheetz MP. Identification of a novel force-generating protein, kinesin, involved in microtubule-based motility. *Cell* 1985; **42**: 39–50.

624 Van der Maazen RW, Verhagen I, Kleiboer BJ, Van der Kogel AJ. Radiosensitivity of glial progenitor cells of the perinatal and adult rat optic nerve studied by *in vitro* clonogenic assay. *Radiother Oncol* 1991; **20**: 258–64.

625 Van der Voorn P, Tekstra J, Beelen RH *et al.* Expression of MCP-1 by reactive astrocytes in demyelinating multiple sclerosis lesions. *Am J Pathol* 1999; **154**: 45–51.

626 Van der Zee CEEM, Nielander HB, Vos JP *et al.* Expression of growth-associated protein B-50 (GAP43) in dorsal root ganglia and sciatic nerve during regenerative sprouting. *J Neurosci* 1989; **9**: 3505–12.

627 Van Paesschen W, Revesz T, Duncan JS. Corpora amylacea in hippocampal sclerosis. *J Neurol Neurosurg Psychiatry* 1997; **63**: 513–5.

628 Vass K, Hickey WF, Schmidt RE, Lassmann H. Bone marrow-derived elements in the peripheral nervous system. An immunohistochemical and ultrastructural investigation in chimeric rats. *Lab Invest* 1993; **69**: 275–82.

629 Vass K, Lassmann H. Intrathecal application of interferon-γ: progressive appearance of MHC antigens within the nervous system. *Am J Pathol* 1990; **137**: 789–800.

630 Vass K, Lassmann H, Wekerle H, Wisniewski HM. The distribution of Ia antigen in the lesions of rat acute experimental allergic encephalomyelitis. *Acta Neuropathol (Berl)* 1986; **70**: 149–60.

631 Vazquez-Chona F, Geisert EE. N-Cadherin at the glial scar in the rat. *Brain Res* 1999; **838**: 45–50.

632 Verge VMK, Merlio J-P, Grondin J *et al*. Colocalization of NGF binding sites, trk mRNA, and low-affinity NGF receptor mRNA in primary sensory neurons: Responses to injury and infusion of NGF. *J Neurosci* 1992; **12**: 4011–22.

633 Villasante A, Wang D, Dobner P *et al*. Six mouse α-tubulin mRNAs encode five distinct isotypes: testis-specific expression of two sister genes. *Mol Cell Biol* 1986; **6**: 2409–19.

634 Vinores SA, Rubinstein LJ. Simultaneous expression of glial fibrillary acidic (GFA) protein and neuron-specific enolase (NSE) by the same reactive or neoplastic astrocytes. *Neuropathol Appl Neurobiol* 1985; **11**: 349–59.

635 Von Eitzen U, Egensperger R, Kösel S *et al*. Microglia and the development of spongiform change in Creutzfeldt–Jakob disease. *J Neuropathol Exp Neurol* 1998; **57**: 246–56.

636 Wagner S, Czub S, Greif M *et al*. Microglial macrophage expression of interleukin 10 in human glioblastomas. *Int J Cancer* 1999; **82**: 12–6.

637 Wahl SM, Allen JB, McCartney-Francis N *et al*. Macrophage-derived and astrocyte-derived transforming growth factor-beta as a mediator of central nervous system dysfunction in acquired immune deficiency syndrome. *J Exp Med* 1991; **173**: 981–91.

638 Wakisaka S, Kajander KC, Bennett GJ. Increased neuropeptide Y(NPY)-like immunoreactivity in rat sensory neurons following peripheral axotomy. *Neurosci Lett* 1991; **124**: 200–3.

639 Waller AV. Experiments on the section of the glossopharyngeal and hypoglossal nerves of the frog, and observations of the alterations produced thereby in the structure of their primitive fibres. *Phil Trans R Soc Lond* 1850; **140**: 423–69.

640 Waltz TA, Brownell B. Sarcoma: a possible late result of effective radiation therapy for pituitary adenoma. Report of two cases. *J Neurosurg* 1966; **24**: 901–7.

641 Walz W, Wuttke WA. Independent mechanisms of potassium clearance by astrocytes in gliotic tissue. *J Neurosci Res* 1999; **56**: 595–603.

642 Watanabe I. Organotins (Triethyltin). In: Spencer PS, Schaumburg HH eds. *Experimental and clinical neurotoxicology*. Baltimore, MD: Williams and Wilkins, 1980: 545–57.

643 Waxman SG, Sontheimer H, Black JA, Minturn JE, Ransom BR. Dynamic aspects of sodium channel expression in astrocytes. *Adv Neurol* 1993; **59**: 135–55.

644 Wegiel J, Wisniewski HM. Rosenthal fibers, eosinophilic inclusions, and anchorage densities with desmosome-like structures in astrocytes in Alzheimer's disease. *Acta Neuropathol (Berl)* 1994; **87**: 355–61.

645 Weinstein DE, Shelanski ML, Liem RKH. Suppression by antisense mRNA demonstrates a requirement for the glial fibrillary acidic protein in the formation of stable astrocytic processes in response to neurons. *J Cell Biol* 1991; **112**: 1205–13.

646 Wekerle H, Linington C, Lassmann H, Meyermann R. Cellular immune reactivity within the CNS. *Trends Neurosci* 1986; **9**: 271–7.

647 Weller RO, Engelhardt B, Phillips MJ. Lymphocyte targeting of the central nervous system: a review of afferent and efferent CNS-immune pathways. *Brain Pathol* 1996; **6**: 275–88.

648 Wells GAH, Wells M. Neuropil vacuolation in brain: a reproducible histological processing artefact. *J Comp Pathol* 1989; **101**: 355–62.

649 Werner H, Jung M, Klugmann M *et al*. Mouse models of myelin diseases. *Brain Pathol* 1998; **8**: 771–93.

650 Wiessner C, Gehrmann J, Lindholm D *et al*. Expression of transforming growth factor-β1 and interleukin-1b mRNA in rat brain following transient forebrain ischemia. *Acta Neuropathol (Berl)* 1993; **86**: 439–47.

651 Wilkin GP, Marriott DR, Cholewinski AJ. Astrocyte heterogeneity. *Trends Neurosci* 1990; **13**: 43–6.

652 Willard M, Meiri KF, Johnson MI. The role of GAP-43 in axon growth. In: Smith RS, Bishop MA eds. *Axonal transport*. New York: Alan R Liss, 1987: 407–20.

653 Williams K, Ulvestad E, Antel JP. B7/BB-1 antigen expression on adult human microglia studied *in vitro* and *in situ*. *Eur J Immunol* 1994; **24**: 3031–7.

654 Wilson JX. Antioxidant defense of the brain: a role for astrocytes. *Can J Physiol Pharmacol* 1997; **75**: 1149–63.

655 Wisniewski HM, Wegiel J. Migration of perivascular cells into the neuropil and their involvement in b-amyloid plaque formation. *Acta Neuropathol (Berl)* 1993; **85**: 586–95.

656 Wisniewski HM, Wegiel J, Wang KC *et al*. Ultrastructural studies of the cells forming amyloid fibers in classical plaques. *Can J Neurol Sci* 1989; **16**: 535–42.

657 Wisniewski HM, Wegiel J, Wang KC, Lach B. Ultrastructural studies of the cells forming amyloid in the cortical vessel wall in Alzheimer's disease. *Acta Neuropathol (Berl)* 1992; **84**: 117–27.

658 Wolvekamp MCJ, Darby IA, Fuller PJ. Cautionary note on the use of end-labeling DNA fragments for detection of apoptosis. *Pathology* 1998; **30**: 267–71.

659 Wong SS, Li RHY, Stadlin A. Oxidative stress induced by MPTP and MPP+: selective vulnerability of cultured mouse astrocytes. *Brain Res* 1999; **836**: 237–44.

660 Wood PM, Mora J. Source of remyelinating oligodendrocytes. *Adv Neurol* 1993; **59**: 113–23.

661 Wood SJ, Pritchard J, Sofroniew MW. Reexpression of nerve growth factor receptor after axonal injury recapitulates a developmental event in motor neurons: differential regulation when regeneration is allowed or prevented. *Eur J Neurosci* 1990; **2**: 650–7.

662 Woodroofe MN, Sarna GS, Wadhwa M *et al*. Detection of interleukin-1 and interleukin-6 in adult rat brain, following mechanical injury, by *in vitro* microdialysis: evidence of a role of microglia in cytokine production. *J Neuroimmunol* 1991; **33**: 227–36.

663 Woodruff RH, Franklin RJM. Demyelination and remyelination of the caudal cerebellar peduncle of adult rats following stereotaxic injection of lysolecithin, ethidium bromide and complement/anti-galactocerebroside – a comparative study. *Glia* 1999; **25**: 216–28.

664 Woodruff RH, Franklin RJM. Growth factors and remyelination in the CNS. *Histol Histopathol* 1997; **12**: 459–66.

665 Woolf CJ Chong MS, Ainsworth A. Axotomy increases glycogen phosphorylase activity in motor neurons. *Neuroscience* 1984; **12**: 1261–9.

666 Woolf CJ, Reynolds ML, Molander C *et al*. The growth-associated protein GAP-43 appears in dorsal root ganglion cells and in the dorsal horn of the rat spinal cord following peripheral nerve injury. *Neuroscience* 1990; **34**: 465–78.

667 Wüllner U, Kornhuber J, Weller M *et al.* Cell death and apoptosis regulating proteins in Parkinson's disease: a cautionary note. *Acta Neuropathol* 1999; **97**: 408–12.

668 Wyllie AH, Kerr JFR, Currie AE. Cell death: the significance of apoptosis. *Int Rev Cytol* 1980; **68**: 251–306.

669 Yamada T, Kawamata T, Walker DG, McGeer PL. Vimentin immunoreactivity in normal and pathological human brain tissue. *Acta Neuropathol (Berl)* 1992; **84**: 157–62.

670 Yan Q, Elliott J, Snider WD. Brain-derived neurotrophic factor rescues spinal motor neurons from axotomy-induced cell death. *Nature* 1992; **360**: 753–5.

671 Yan Q, Matheson C, Lopez OT. *in vivo* neurotrophic effects of GDNF on neonatal and adult facial motor neurons. *Nature* 1995; **373**: 341–4.

672 Ye ZC, Sontheimer H. Astrocytes protect neurons from neurotoxic injury by serum glutamate. *Glia* 1998; **22**: 237–48.

673 Yin XH, Crawford TO, Griffin JW *et al.* Myelin-associated glycoprotein is a myelin signal that modulates the caliber of myelinated axons. *J Neurosci* 1998; **18**: 1953–62.

674 Yoshida H, Kong YY, Yoshida R *et al.* Apaf1 is required for mitochondrial pathways of apoptosis and brain development. *Cell* 1998; **94**: 739–50.

675 Yoshioka M, Shapshak P, Sun NCJ *et al.* Simultaneous detection of ferritin and HIV-1 in reactive microglia. *Acta Neuropathol (Berl)* 1992; **84**: 297–306.

676 Yu AC, Lee YL, Eng LF. Glutamate as an energy substrate for neuronal–astrocytic interactions. *Prog Brain Res* 1992; **94**: 251–9.

677 Yu WH. Regulation of nitric oxide synthase expression in motoneurons following nerve injury. *Dev Neurosci* 1997; **19**: 247–54.

678 Yuasa S, Kitoh J, Oda S, Kawamura K. Obstructed migration of Purkinje cells in the developing cerebellum of the reeler mutant mouse. *Anat Embryol* 1993; **188**: 317–29.

679 Yudkoff M, Nissim I, Hertz L, Pleasure D, Erecinska M. Nitrogen metabolism: neuronal–astroglial relationships. *Prog Brain Res* 1992; **94**: 213–24.

680 Zajicek JP, Wing M, Scolding NJ, Compston A. Interactions between oligodendrocytes and microglia: a major role for complement and tumor necrosis factor in oligodendrocyte adherence and killing. *Brain* 1992; **115**: 1611–31.

681 Zeman W. Veränderungen durch ionisierende Strahlen. In: Scholz W ed. *Handbuch der speziellen pathologischen Anatomie und Histologie* Vol. XIII/3. Berlin: Springer, 1955.

682 Zhang X, Bao L, Shi TJ *et al.* Down-regulation of mu-opioid receptors in rat and monkey dorsal root ganglion neurons and spinal cord after peripheral axotomy. *Neuroscience* 1998; **82**: 223–40.

683 Zhang X, Verge VMK, Wiesenfeld-Hallin Z *et al.* Expression of neuropeptides and neuropeptide mRNAs in spinal cord after axotomy in the rat, with special reference to motor neurons and galanin. *Exp Brain Res* 1993; **93**: 4 50–61.

684 Zietlow R, Dunnett SB, Fawcett JW. The effect of microglia on embryonic dopaminergic neuronal survival *in vitro*: diffusible signals from neurons and glia change microglia from neurotoxic to neuroprotective. *Eur J Neurosci* 1999; **11**: 1657–67.

4

Raised intracranial pressure, oedema and hydrocephalus

JAMES W. IRONSIDE AND JOHN D. PICKARD

INTRODUCTION

Many of the early concepts of raised intracranial pressure (ICP) were based on the Monro–Kellie doctrine,[100,145] which stated that once the fontanelles and sutures of the skull have closed, the intracranial contents consist of incompressible brain and blood contained within a rigid unyielding bony structure. These concepts were subsequently modified by Burrows[23] to account for the presence of cerebrospinal fluid (CSF). Further important modifications were developed by Duret,[46] von Bergmann[10] and Kocher[112] in promoting the important concept of spatial compensation within the skull, and in defining four clinical stages of cerebral compression. As an intracranial mass lesion increases in size, compensatory reduction of other intracranial contents can temporarily prevent or modify an increase in ICP. Once this compensatory capacity has become exhausted, ICP will rise slowly at first, and then rapidly to levels approaching that of arterial blood pressure. Other modifying factors in the inter-relationship of intracranial CSF, blood volume and ICP (such as spinal dural sac elasticity and the spinal epidural venous plexus) were introduced by Weed and McKibben,[225] Weed,[224] and Flexner et al.[62] and in several papers from the Evans–Ryder group in Cincinnati, USA.[53,187–189]

In experimental non-human primate studies, Langfitt and his group[114–116,277] defined stages of brain compression similar to those previously described clinically by Duret[46] and Kocher.[112] This experimental model also established the importance of cerebral vasomotor paralysis as the end-stage consequence of intracranial expanding lesions. Intrinsic vasomotor tone is lost in the arteries and the arterioles, capillaries and veins become distended, ICP becomes equal to systemic arterial pressure and the cerebral blood flow (CBF) ceases, resulting in brain death.

Many intracranial pathologies, including tumour, abscess, haematoma, recent infarction, oedema, infection or metabolic encephalopathy, eventually produce a life-threatening increase in ICP. Brain swelling in association with these pathological processes is an additional important factor which contributes to the effect of size of many intracranial expanding lesions. Most of these lesions are localized to a single site within the brain or its surrounding structures, and produce distortion and eventual herniation of the brain, leading to pressure gradients between the supratentorial and infratentorial compartments of the skull (by occluding the subarachnoid space at the tentorial incisure), or between the intracranial compartment and the spinal subarachnoid space (by obliterating the subarachnoid space at the foramen magnum). It was not until the existence of these pressure gradients was recognized[19,20,117,118,199] that it was appreciated that CSF pressure obtained from lumbar puncture could be normal in a patient with raised intracranial CSF pressure, and this procedure may therefore precipitate brain herniation by increasing the pressure gradient between the intracranial compartment and spinal subarachnoid space.

Although the pathological processes involved in raised ICP and distortion of the brain can be defined and discussed separately, they act in concert in individual cases, each process contributing to the dynamic sum of the pathophysiological changes experienced by the patient. In general, the more slowly a focal mass expands, the more likely it is to produce displacement of the brain without an early increase in ICP, since intrinsic compensatory mechanisms, particularly reduced CSF volume, can operate at their maximum efficiency. It is in such cases that distortion and herniation of the brain are most pronounced. In contrast, if focal lesions expand rapidly it is more likely that distortion of the brain will be accompanied by a high ICP, and in such cases brain death usually supervenes before considerable brain distortion or intracranial herniation can occur. These factors may be further modified by the age of the patient; in the elderly, if there is pre-existing cerebral atrophy with a corresponding increase in the volume of intracranial CSF, the compensatory capacity is potentially greater than in a younger individual in whom the brain is not atrophic. In infants, the unfused skull may expand as ICP increases, long before brain distortion and intracranial herniation occur. Even when ICP has been normal in the presence of a slowly expanding mass lesion, a further small increase in the volume of any of the intracranial contents (e.g. the vasodilatation that occurs during sleep) is likely to result in an increase in ICP because of the nature of the intracranial volume–pressure relationship.

This chapter describes the mechanisms by which ICP can be increased and the pathological consequences to the brain, its blood supply and rest of the body. Various patterns of distortion and herniation of the brain will be reviewed and the interactions between them and ICP defined in physiological and pathological terms. Recent advances in imaging techniques have allowed an unparalleled opportunity to use dynamic and functional imaging studies as part of the multimodality monitoring in patients with raised ICP; the results of these investigations will be discussed not only in terms of our understanding of the pathophysiological mechanisms operating under such conditions, but also in relation to the clinical investigation and management of raised ICP.

Table 4.1 *Comparison of the major types of cerebral oedema in man*

	Vasogenic	Cytotoxic	Hydrostatic	Hypo-osmolar	Interstitial
Pathogenesis	Blood–brain barrier breakdown	Impairment of cellular Na/K membrane pump	High vascular transmural pressure	Low plasma osmotic pressure; intact blood–brain barrier	High CSF pressure
Ultrastructure	Enlarged extracellular spaces in white matter with swelling of perivascular astrocyte foot process	No enlargement of extracellular spaces Cytoplasmic hydropic swelling in neurons or glia	Varies as underlying condition evolves	Glial swelling in cerebral cortex Extracellular oedema in white matter	Periventricular white-matter extracellular oedema
Site of accumulation	Local: around tumours or traumatic lesions Diffuse: in cerebral white matter	Intracellular swelling, mostly in grey matter	Extracellular	Intracellular and extracellular	Periventricular white-matter extracellular space
Fluid composition	Plasma filtrate (with plasma proteins)	Plasma ultrafiltrate (mostly water and sodium)	Water (Na^+) Perivascular protein extravasation in hypertensive encephalopathy	Water (Na^+)	Presumed to be CSF or interstitial fluid in composition
Clinical significance	Major component of most clinically significant examples of cerebral oedema, particularly focal lesions	Hypoxia and ischaemia are the most common causes; most cases are eventually accompanied by vasogenic oedema	Systemic hypertension; loss of autoregulation; post-brain decompression	Hyponatraemia: dilutional or due to SIADH CSF formation may be increased	Acute hydrocephalus

SIADH, inappropriate secretion of antidiuretic hormone.

RAISED INTRACRANIAL PRESSURE

The brain is an expansile structure that expands and contracts with each heartbeat. As there are not any valves within the venous drainage from the brain, any changes in intrathoracic pressure are transmitted to ICP. To illustrate the concept of ICP, such phenomena can readily be seen and palpated simply by examining the fontanelle of a baby.

The 'four-lump' concept describes most simply the causes of raised ICP: the mass, CSF accumulation, vascular congestion and cerebral oedema (Table 4.1). Of course, brain, blood and CSF per se are incompressible within the confines of a rigid box once the fontanelles and sutures have closed (the Monro–Kellie doctrine as modified by Burrows;[23,100,145] see above) but, given time, there are intracranial compensatory mechanisms that can prevent or ameliorate an increase in ICP. To understand these compensatory mechanisms, it is necessary to understand the dependence of normal ICP both on the CSF circulation and on the cerebral circulation.

ICP in the steady state

Resting ICP in the steady state is the equilibrium pressure at which CSF production and absorption are in balance and is associated with an equivalent equilibrium volume of CSF (see below). Eighty per cent of CSF is the product of active secretion by the choroid plexus at about 0.35 ml/min, a process which slows down with age. The remainder of the CSF is contributed by movement of interstitial fluid into the ventricles and the subarachnoid space. CSF production remains relatively constant provided cerebral perfusion pressure (CPP) is adequate.[43] The normal range of ICP is 0–0.13 kPa (0–10 mmHg). The upper limit in patients undergoing continuous ICP monitoring is usually 2 kPa (15 mmHg) in adults; upper limits in children are considerably lower.

CSF absorption is a passive process through the arachnoid granulations into both the superior sagittal sinus and the venous drainage of the spinal root sleeves and increases with rising CSF pressure (Davson's equation):[43,132]

$$CSF\ drainage = (CSF\ pressure - sagittal\ sinus\ pressure)/outflow\ resistance$$

or:

$$P_{csf}\ (= ICP) = I_{csf} \times R_{out} + P_{sss}$$

where I_{csf} is the CSF production rate, R_{out} is the CSF outflow resistance and P_{sss} is the superior sagittal sinus pressure. Note the similarity of this equation to Ohm's law (voltage = current × resistance).

CSF outflow resistance, CSF production rate and brain compliance may be determined in patients by the infusion of artificial CSF into the ventricles or lumbar sac while measuring the change in CSF pressure.[41] Such tests also reveal the interplay between the CSF and cerebrovascular circulations (Fig. 4.1). These measurements are of considerable clinical utility when assessing

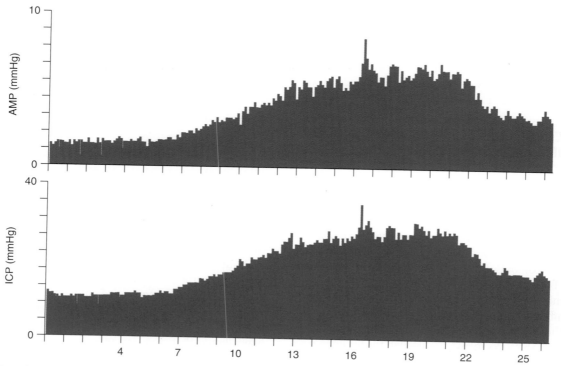

Figure 4.1 *Time course of mean ICP (bottom) and its pulse amplitude (AMP – top) in response to constant rate infusion of saline into CSF spaces. Infusion at a rate of 1.5 ml/min was started in the seventh minute (x-axis – time from start of recording) and finished after 22 min. From Czosnyka et al. (1996).[41]*

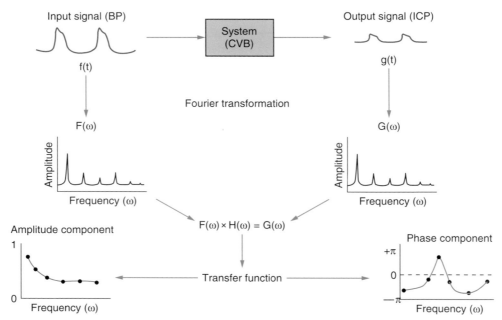

Figure 4.2 *Raised ICP: pressure waveform analysis. A systems analysis methodology applying pressure waveform analysis techniques to study the pressure transmission characteristics of the cerebrovascular bed (CVB). The input blood pressure [f(t)] and output intracranial [g(t)] wave forms recorded from locations across the CVB can be described by spectral analysis in terms of their harmonic components [F(ω) and G(ω)]. Spectral analysis of the blood pressure and ICP signals resolved each waveform as a series of sine waves consisting of a fundamental component and five harmonics of the fundamental. The transfer function [H(ω)] defines how the input signal is transformed into the output signal and consists of amplitude and phase components. The amplitude curve describes how much pressure is transmitted through the CVB at each harmonic frequency. The phase curve describes how much each pressure sine wave is shifted in its cycle as it is transmitted through the CVB. Courtesy of Dr I Piper, University of Glasgow, UK.*

patients with possible CSF disturbances, including all forms of hydrocephalus, benign intracranial hypertension, cerebral atrophy and shunt malfunction. Continuous ICP monitoring often shows that both the amplitude of the CSF pulsewave and its shape become altered during elevation of ICP. Spectral analysis allows the complex ICP waveform to be resolved into a single fundamental wave and a series of harmonics (Fig. 4.2).

EFFECTS OF CHANGES IN CEREBRAL BLOOD VOLUME AND CSF PRESSURE

The normal ICP waveform consists of both cardiac and respiratory components superimposed on baseline ICP. Any change in cerebral blood volume on the arterial side of the cerebral circulation must be compensated for either by a reduction in cerebral venous volume or by phasic movement of CSF out of the skull through the foramen magnum. Both pneumoencephalography and, more recently, dynamic MRI have revealed that the cerebral mantle expands and compresses the lateral ventricles during systole thereby propelling CSF through the aqueduct of Sylvius. CSF moves to and fro through the foramen magnum during the cardiac cycle. Inevitably there is a lag phase between the systolic increase in cerebral blood volume and the effect of the compensatory mechanisms so that CSF pressure increases to reflect in part the systolic waveform.

However, the CSF pressure waveform is not an exact replica of the arterial waveform as it has been 'filtered' and loses certain frequency components through the combined effects of the compliance of the wall of the cerebral arteries, cerebrovascular resistance and intracranial compliance (brain + venous drainage + CSF drainage) (Fig. 4.3).

Hence, an additional term, 'ICP vasogenic', is required to complete Davson's formula:[38,131]

$$ICP = ICP_{CSF\ circulation} + ICP_{vasogenic}$$
$$= R_{out} \times I_{csf} + P_{SSS} + ICP_{vasogenic}$$

Cerebrovascular smooth muscle (and hence CBF/volume) responds to changes in arterial carbon dioxide, arterial oxygen tension and CPP. Both hypercapnia and hypoxia cause cerebral vasodilatation resulting in a rise in ICP.

Over the physiological range of arterial blood pressure (from the lower limit of about 50 mmHg to an upper limit of about 140 mmHg), cerebral arterioles relax with falling blood pressure and constrict with increasing blood pressure, a phenomenon called autoregulation that takes some 5–15 s to develop.[163] For example, brief carotid compression for 5–10 s is followed by a transient reactive hyperaemia that can be detected with transcranial Doppler.

These changes in cerebral arterial diameter in the healthy brain are reflected in alterations in cerebral blood volume and hence ICP: arterial hypotension increases ICP

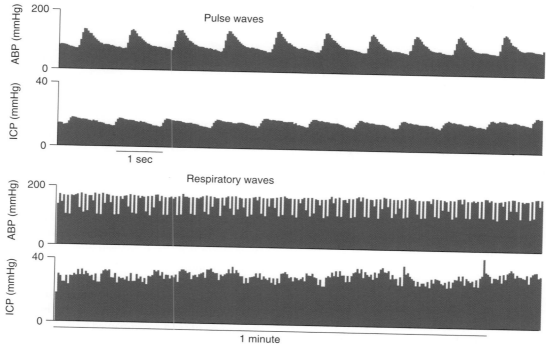

Figure 4.3 *ICP and arterial waveforms. When autoregulation is intact, the ICP waveform is not an exact replica of the arterial blood pressure (ABP) waveform as it loses frequency components by the effects of cerebrovascular compliance and resistance, and intracranial compliance. Top: pulse component. Bottom: respiratory component (in a mechanically ventilated patient). Courtesy of Dr M Czosnyka, University of Cambridge, UK.*

and arterial hypertension decreases ICP within the physiological range. Slow fluctuations in arterial blood pressure, lasting for 30 s to a few minutes, are almost always present in ventilated patients and their effect on ICP can be used to assess the state of autoregulation.[39] Where autoregulation is defective, cerebral arterioles respond passively to changes in arterial blood pressure so that ICP increases with increasing mean arterial blood pressure. There is an interaction between arterial blood gases and autoregulation, and surprisingly small degrees of hypercapnia impair autoregulation.

If mean arterial blood pressure increases acutely beyond about 140 mmHg, there is 'break-through' of autoregulation, with microfractures of the arteriolar and capillary endothelium, focal breakdown of the blood–brain barrier

(BBB) and extravasation of protein and water into the brain.[129] This process is the basis of hypertensive encephalopathy. With arterial hypotension, below about 50 mmHg, CBF falls and the brain becomes ischaemic.

INTRACRANIAL PRESSURE–VOLUME RELATIONSHIPS

As a mass increases in size within the skull, ICP does not rise initially because of a reduction in CSF volume and cerebral blood volume but, once such mechanisms are exhausted, ICP rises and its pulse pressure increases. Spontaneous waves of pressure (plateau and B-waves) begin to appear[70,127] (Fig. 4.4). There is an exponential

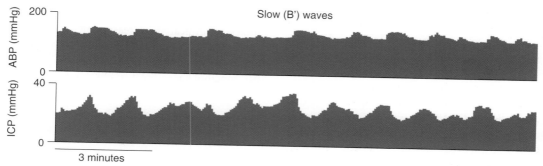

Figure 4.4 *Intracranial pressure–volume relationships. Spontaneous waves of raised ICP (B-waves) occur when compensatory mechanisms of accommodating an expanding intracranial mass have failed; these B-waves bear no relationship to the arterial blood pressure (ABP). Courtesy of Dr M Czosnyka, University of Cambridge, UK.*

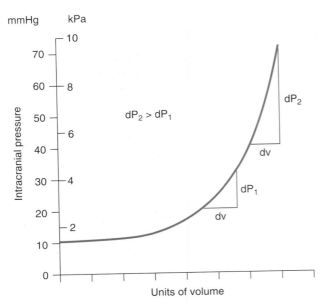

Figure 4.5 *Theoretical intracranial pressure–volume curve. As volume increases and ICP rises, uniform increments of volume (dv) produce progressively larger increases in ICP (dP$_1$ and dP$_2$). Increases or decreases in volume cause correspondingly greater changes in ICP on the steep part of the curve.*

relationship between increase in volume and intracranial mass and increase in ICP, at least within the clinically important range (Fig. 4.5). On the left side of the curve, changes in volume provoke little change in ICP and the brain is said to be compliant. However, on the right side, quite small changes in volume of the order of 1 ml provoke large increases in ICP. The brain is now stiffer or less compliant.[114,143]

Cerebral perfusion pressure

Mean ICP closely approximates to mean cerebral venous pressure and hence CPP is defined as:[141]

$$CPP = MABP - mean\ ICP$$

The response of CBF to changing CPP largely reflects alterations in mean arterial blood pressure. As CPP falls with increasing ICP, intracranial pulse pressure increases. First, the brain is stiffer and a given systolic injection of cerebral blood volume provokes a larger ICP response. Secondly, cerebral arterioles dilate to maintain cerebral perfusion through the autoregulatory mechanism and hence the pulsatile component of CBF increases with falling CPP. If autoregulation is defective, ICP pulse pressure amplitude starts to decrease as ICP increases.[8]

When ICP equals arterial blood pressure, angiographic pseudo-occlusion occurs[127] and reverberation, systolic spikes or no flow may be seen on transcranial Doppler sonography.[106]

The 'split brain'

There is a paradox between the lower limit of CPP compatible with autoregulation and the level of CPP below which outcome after acute brain injury deteriorates. In the healthy brain, autoregulation continues down to a CPP of 40 mmHg, whereas the patient's CPP must be maintained above 60–65 mmHg if outcome is not to be jeopardized. Conventionally, any elevation of ICP requires treatment if the cerebral perfusion pressure is below 60 mmHg in adults for over 5 min. This paradox may partly reflect the 'split-brain' problem: autoregulation of CBF to changes in CPP or cerebrovascular tone in response to changes in arterial carbon dioxide tension may be impaired focally, leaving reactivity intact in other areas of the brain. If vasospasm is present, an even higher perfusion pressure may be required to provide adequate levels of CBF. Total CBF may be increased or decreased in areas with absent reactivity. Hyperaemia is non-nutritional 'luxury perfusion', where CBF is in excess of the brain's metabolic requirements and accompanied by early filling of veins on angiography and the appearance of 'red veins' at operation. Cerebral vasodilators such as carbon dioxide will dilate normal arterioles, thereby increasing ICP with the risk of reducing flow in damaged areas of brain 'intracerebral steal'. Inverse 'steal' is a theoretical treatment for raised ICP by the use of hyperventilation: an acute reduction of arterial carbon dioxide tension vasoconstricts the normal cerebral arterioles, thereby directing blood to focally abnormal areas. In practice, however, prolonged hyperventilation may provoke cerebral ischaemia.[149] Positron emission tomography (PET) can identify focal areas of abnormal cerebral blood flow and oxygen utilization in patients without evidence of ischaemia on conventional monitoring (Fig. 4.6).

Status epilepticus leads to gross cerebral vasodilatation and intracranial hypertension[45] as the result of greatly increased cerebral metabolism, respiratory dysfunction with hypoxia and hypercapnia and local release of endogenous vasodilatatory agents within the brain. Depression of cerebral oxidative metabolism by anaesthesia and hypothermia may reduce CBF and ICP where there is a large area of brain with reasonable electrical activity and where normal flow–metabolism coupling mechanisms are intact, as indicated by reasonable CBF carbon dioxide reactivity.[151] Functional imaging techniques can also demonstrate abnormalities of cerebral glucose and oxygen metabolism in focal cerebral ischaemia (Fig. 4.7).

Waves of ICP

In addition to the physiological cardiac and respiratory waves, spontaneous waves of ICP may develop and are associated with cerebrovascular dilation. These are conventionally described as B-waves (1/min) or plateau waves

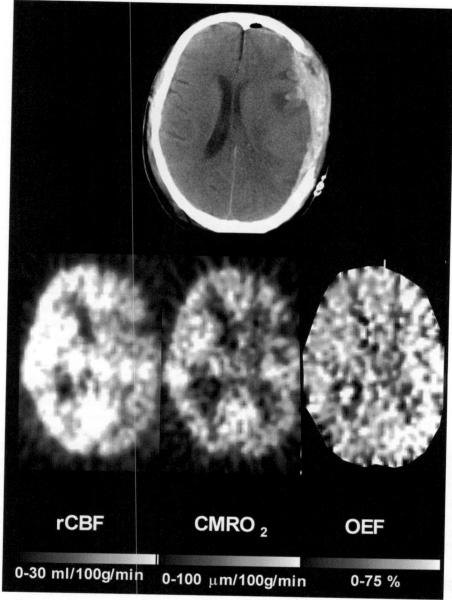

rCBF   CMRO$_2$ OEF

0-30 ml/100g/min   0-100 μm/100g/min   0-75 %

Figure 4.6 *Functional imaging: focal cerebral ischaemia. CT and PET scans obtained 16 h following head injury, after evacuation of an acute left subdural haematoma. Note the area of critically low cerebral blood flow (CBF) and high oxygen extraction fraction (OEF > 75%) underlying the remains of the evacuated haematoma. The perfusion defect is severe enough to compromise cerebral metabolism of oxygen (CRMO$_2$). These perfusion deficits are present despite an acceptably low ICP (18 mmHg), acceptable cerebral perfusion pressure (90 mmHg), relative normocapnia (P$_a$CO$_2$ 4.9 kPa) and no evidence of ischaemia on global bedside monitors of cerebrovascular adequacy. Courtesy of Professor D Menon, University of Cambridge, UK.*

(ICP exceeding 50 mmHg for more than 5 min[70,127]) (Fig. 4.4). Cerebral blood volume increases during plateau waves and may be the result in some cases of inappropriate autoregulatory vasodilatation (described by Rosner as a vasodilatatory cascade).[183] Increase in cerebral blood volume causes an increase in ICP, a decrease in CPP, vasodilatation, further increase in ICP, etc., until the system reaches a state of maximum vasodilatation. Plateau waves are observed in patients with preserved cerebral autoregulation with reduced pressure–volume compensatory reserves or compliance. Two other types of wave may be confused with the classical plateau waves. First, in autoregulating patients when CPP decreases and ICP increases this type of increase in ICP lasts only as long as CPP remains reduced, and a self-sustaining vasodilatory cascade is never initiated. Secondly, in non-autoregulating patients, ICP waves may be seen with a sharply rising edge relating to a sudden increase in CPP and a characteristic passive transmission of pressure changes from the arterial to the intracranial compartment. Finally, impressive vasogenic ICP waves may be seen during episodes of spontaneous hyperaemia.[40]

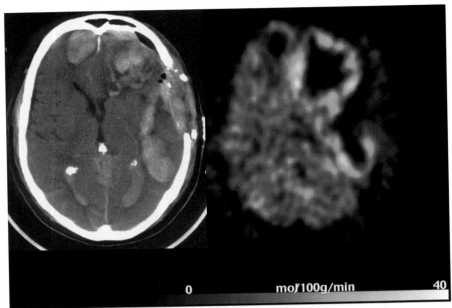

Figure 4.7 *Functional imaging: glucose and oxygen metabolism in focal cerebral ischaemia. CT and* [18]*fluorodeoxyglucose PET scan 48 h after head injury. Note the pericontusional increases in glucose uptake. These may be accompanied by commensurate increases in oxygen metabolism and represent hyperglycolysis, which may be due to anaerobic glucose metabolism in ischaemia. Courtesy of Professor D Menon, University of Cambridge, UK.*

ICP may rise uncontrollably, an event which is termed refractory intracranial hypertension. Mean ICP may increase to well above 80 mmHg, probably owing to rapid brain swelling over a period of a few hours compounded by herniation and brainstem compression (see below). Pulse amplitude of ICP is commonly secondly reduced with activation of a Cushing response and a gradual rise in mean arterial pressure.[35] The moment of brainstem herniation is commonly marked by a rapid decrease in mean arterial pressure, a rise in heart rate and a terminal decrease in CPP to negative values.[114]

Intracranial gradients of pressure

Much mystique surrounds this subject. In the steady state, pressure should be equal between any points within a freely communicating system. However, transient pressure gradients are essential to normal brain function:

- the pressure gradient from the arterial side of the circulation to the venous side;
- the pressure gradients created by systolic expansion of the cerebral mantle and choroid plexus with transient gradients across the aqueduct of Sylvius, foramina of Magendie and Luschka and foramen magnum;
- subtle interplay of pressures between cerebral bridging veins, CSF pressure and sagittal sinus pressure:[95]

$$P_v > P_{csf} > P_{sss}$$

- the intraparenchymal pressure gradient that causes interstitial fluid flow from the brain through the ependyma into the ventricle.[33]

Pathologically, as a mass increases in size, at first it causes local effects through local distortion and compression and irritation and is compounded by local cerebral oedema. Vasogenic oedema may develop, which involves bulk flow of the fluid through the disrupted BBB of the affected blood vessel through the white matter and into the ventricles (see below).[178,182] As the mass increases further in size, brain shift occurs that may cause compression of the ventricular system and hence contralateral hydrocephalus. Such brain shift is a result of compression and there must be some pressure gradient to create it, however difficult it may be to measure it using simplistic pressure transducers. The concept of tissue pressure has recently been advanced through the application of continuum mechanics to include the concepts of fluid flow through a porous medium and hence the concepts of compression, shear and fluid pressures. Finally, herniation occurs: subfalcine, transtentorial or via the foramen magnum (see below). When herniation occurs, there is no longer free communication between two adjacent compartments and ICP rises abruptly and brainstem ischaemia supervenes.

THE BLOOD–BRAIN BARRIER

The neural and glial cells of the brain are isolated from the bloodstream and their interior environment is tightly regulated. The BBB consists of both structural and functional components located within the complex formed by the cerebrovascular endothelial cells, pericytes and astroglial end-feet.[174] The concept of the BBB started in

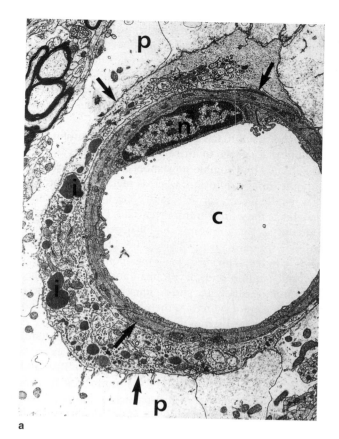

the late nineteenth century with Ehrlich's observation of the failure of vital dye injected into the bloodstream to enter the brain when all other organ systems of the body were stained by the dye. Subsequently, Goldmann demonstrated that dyes introduced into the CSF space entered the brain freely, indicating that there was not a CSF–brain barrier. The location of the BBB is the capillary endothelium which has three structural features not found generally elsewhere in the body: tight junctions without fenestrations, a paucity of pinocytotic intracellular vesicles and abundant mitochondria.[156] The tight junctions seal the endothelial cells together and prohibit intercellular passage of substances.[174] The small number of pinocytotic intracellular vesicles suggests a minor role for vesicular transendothelial transport under normal conditions. However, a marked increase in the number of endothelial vesicles has been observed in experimental head injury and in the vicinity of brain tumours following seizure activity, so that the statement about the paucity of vesicular transport may not always hold true under pathological conditions[165,169,173] (Fig. 4.8).

The endothelial cells contain numerous enzyme systems, many of which are involved in BBB functions. Some of these (e.g. the hydrolases) exhibit differential activity on the luminal and abluminal endothelial surfaces.[84] The continuous layer of endothelium is in turn surrounded by

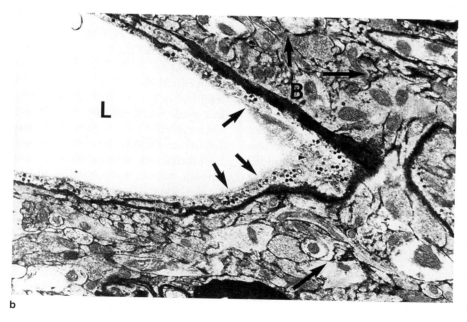

Figure 4.8 *Blood–brain barrier: normal and adjacent to tumour.* **(a)** *Electron microscopy of a normal cerebral capillary (c) showing the relationship between the endothelial cell (n), pericyte (i) and astrocyte foot processes (p). Basement membrane around the endothelial cells and pericyte is indicated by arrowheads.* **(b)** *Electron microscopy of perivascular area of brain adjacent to a tumour fixed by perfusion 15 min after intraventricular injection of horseradish peroxidase. The narrow extracellular space (arrows) and basement membrane (B) are densely stained with horseradish peroxidase reaction product. Lumen (L). Courtesy of* **(a)** *Professor G Pilkington, and* **(b)** *Professor PL Lantos, Institute of Psychiatry, London, UK;* **(b)** *reproduced by permission from Elsevier, Amsterdam.*

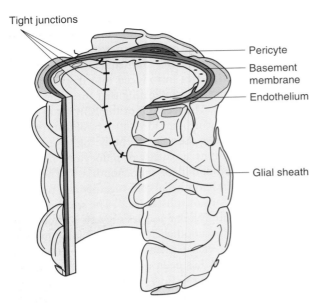

Figure 4.9 *Diagrammatic representation of the blood–brain barrier. This shows the relationships between capillary endothelium, basement membrane, pericytes and astrocytic foot processes. Capillary endothelial cells are attached to each other by tight junctions.*

a basement membrane which is 40–50 nm thick and contains proteoglycans, heparin sulfate, laminin, entactin and type IV collagen.[133] Astrocytic foot processes have direct contact with the basement membrane of the cerebral capillaries, extending around the blood vessels to form a complete envelope (Fig. 4.9). The functional BBB must include the astrocytic end-feet applied to the abluminal surface of the endothelium because of the considerable evidence for interaction between astrocytes and endothelial cells in respect of barrier function.[66,196] There is good evidence both *in vitro* and *in vivo* that the permeability properties of endothelial cells can be induced by the astrocytic end-feet.[89] Pericyte processes are also present around cerebral capillaries and are surrounded completely by a duplication of the endothelial basement membrane, with which they have direct contact. Pericytes are not thought to influence functional aspects of the BBB, but they may represent at least part of the population of perivascular cells which react to barrier breakdown.[102]

Brain oedema is directly related to the passage of free water from the vascular compartment to either an intracellular location or the extracellular or interstitial fluid space.[161] Fluxes of water are not caused by a change in the BBB, since free water can diffuse almost without hindrance across the capillary membrane according to hydrostatic and more powerful osmotic gradients.[65] Water, therefore, will passively follow movements in sodium and other ions and other molecules of various sizes. However, the significance of the recently discovered water channels (aquaporins) in the BBB requires additional considera-

tion.[218] The ability of mannitol to shrink the brain depends in part on the integrity of the BBB; normally, it crosses the barrier very poorly and thereby creates an osmotic gradient with water moving from brain to blood. However, mannitol has other effects, including viscosity-induced changes in autoregulation and direct effects on cerebrovascular smooth muscle.[148]

The normal BBB has a number of mechanisms for controlling the passage of these substances across the cell wall.[16,43,172] Lipid-soluble substances can move across the endothelium by diffusion, whereas metabolic substrates may require specific carrier systems, one of the most abundant being the glucose transporter (GLUT-1)[126] consistent with the fact that the brain is highly dependent upon glucose as a source of energy. There is free passage for amino acids required as precursors and metabolic intermediates, (neutral L-amino acids, tryptophan and phenylalumine; basic amino acids, lysine and arginine), particularly where the brain cannot synthesize them.[162] The entry of amino acids which are used as neurotransmitters [glycine, γ-aminobutyric acid (GABA), glutamate and aspartate] occurs very slowly, since specific carriers do not exist.

The rate at which substances can cross the BBB and enter the brain is determined by the product of the permeability of the barrier to that particular substance and the total surface area of capillary endothelium to which it is exposed. If the permeability is very high, the quantity of substance entering the brain is related mainly to its delivery to the brain, that is the CBF. For less freely diffusible compounds the permeability is the limiting factor and this may be influenced not only by the size of the molecule and whether it is bound to a protein, but also by the ionic charge and polarity.

The Na^+/K^+-ATPase on the abluminal surface of the brain endothelial cells is used to maintain the potassium level within the extracellular space of only 3 mM. With increased neural activity the extracellular potassium concentration rises, which is buffered by concerted action between astroglial cells, the abluminal surface of the endothelial cells and vasodilatation of cerebrovascular smooth muscle. Mitochondria provide the energy to service ionic channels and activate pumps in the endothelial cell wall. There are many components of the enzymatic BBB which both protect the brain from circulating vascular toxins and also assist with breakdown of neurotransmitters (monoamine oxidase, cholinesterase and GABA transaminase).[97] Advantage can be taken of properties of the BBB when designing drugs (e.g. the barrier-permeable L-dopa in combination with barrier-impermeable dopa-decarboxylase inhibitor in the treatment of Parkinson's disease). Endothelial cells produce substances such as nitric oxide and various derivatives of arachidonic acid that modulate the effects of other neighbouring cells.[27,47] There are certain structures within the brain that do not have an intact BBB, including the circumventricular organs, the area postrema and pituitary gland.[16,43,172] Specialized neurons at these sites may act as sensors for circulating levels of hormones in the blood-stream and thereby act as part of the feedback loops through the hypothalamus that control the blood pressure, for example.

Endogenous systems exist that modulate BBB function under physiological conditions, but the details are scanty: an ascending noradrenergic control of barrier permeability from the locus coeruleus; the effects of endogenous hormones including atrial natriuretic peptide, aldosterone and adrenocorticotropic hormone (ACTH); endogenously derived histamine, serotonin (5-hydroxytryptamine), bradykinin, nitric oxide and derivatives of arachidonic acid.[47,134]

Three possible mechanisms may operate in opening the BBB:

- separation of the interendothelial tight junctions;
- increased vesicular transport and the formation of transendothelial channels;
- biochemical and structural alteration of the endothelial membrane, resulting in an increase in its permeability.

Opening of tight interendothelial junctions has not been observed in experimental simulations of conditions associated with failure of the BBB.[172] Transient opening of this part of the barrier system has been observed following administration of substances of very high osmolality. Recent studies have identified a series of proteins which are integral to the structure and maintenance of the tight endothelial junctions, including occludin ZO-1 and claudin.[213] Loss of the tight endothelial junctions in glioma blood vessels may occur as a consequence of vascular endothelial growth factor secretion by tumour cells; the abnormal proliferating vessels are deficient in these essential structural proteins.[160,223]

While increased pinocytotic activity has been observed after a number of pathological stimuli (Fig. 4.8), the changes are usually transient and formation of open channels across the capillary endothelium has not been observed. Other work has suggested that after brain damage there may be perturbation of the endothelial plasmalemma. Stimulation of the arachidonic acid cascade with increased synthesis of prostaglandins and leukotrienes and stimulation of nitric oxide synthesis are mechanisms whereby free oxygen radicals may be produced in brain tissue.[26,168] This process is considered to take place in the endothelial cells, and the highly reactive oxygen species result in lipid peroxidation and damage to membrane structure, thereby disrupting the selectivity of components of the BBB. Other mechanisms may include the rapid production of cytokines, such as tumour necrosis factor-α (TNF-α) and interleukin-1B (IL-1B) in response to injury and inflammation.[193,201] Among other effects, intercellular adhesion molecule-1 (ICAM-1) may be induced, thereby attracting and facilitating the migration of leukocytes into the brain and activation of microglia.[1]

BRAIN SWELLING AND OEDEMA

An increase in the volume of all, or part, of the brain is a potential complication of head injury, ischaemia, haemorrhage, tumours, infection and metabolic disturbances. If the process is generalized, the subarachnoid space is obliterated and the ventricles are decreased in size (Fig. 4.10). If localized there is a mass effect that may considerably augment the size of the causative lesion itself; for example, a meningioma or a cerebral metastasis (Fig. 4.11). While such processes will eventually cause raised

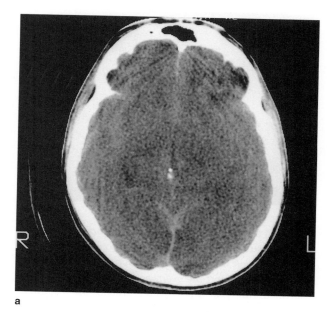

a

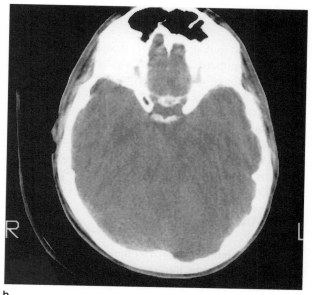

b

Figure 4.10 *Diffuse brain swelling. Non-contrast-enhanced cranial CT scan of a patient with post-traumatic diffuse brain swelling, showing obliteration of the basal cisterns and compression of the third ventricle to a slit-like structure. Courtesy of Dr R Gibson, Western General Hospital, Edinburgh, UK.*

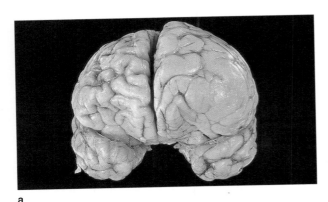

a

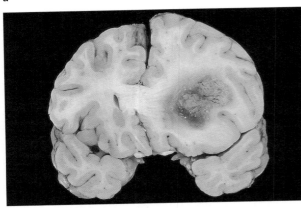

b

Figure 4.11 *Localized brain swelling. Cerebral oedema and brain swelling around a metastatic small cell anaplastic lung carcinoma in the left frontal lobe. (a) The surfaces of the gyri have been flattened against the overlying dura and the sulci partly obliterated. (b) The white matter around the metastatic deposit is oedematous, resulting in displacement of midline structures to the right, with a left subfalcine hernia.*

ICP, computed tomographic (CT) studies in patients with early post-traumatic brain swelling have shown that a reduction in the volume of the ventricular system does not necessarily indicate that ICP is elevated at that time, but it does increase the likelihood that it will become elevated at a later stage. Expansion of brain tissue may be due to an increase in the intravascular blood volume in that area of the brain, known as congestive brain swelling, or it may be due to an increase in the water content of the brain tissue, termed cerebral oedema.

Congestive brain swelling

There is considerable debate over the contribution of cerebral blood volume to intracranial hypertension, mainly because of the difficulty in measuring cerebral blood volume in critically ill patients. Hypoxia, hypercapnia and halothane all cause cerebral vasodilatation and raised ICP. Raised ICP is an adverse prognostic factor in most patients; failure of autoregulation of CBF and hence of cerebral blood volume are major contributors to this process. Refractory intracranial hypertension is accompanied by

failure of autoregulation, and cerebral blood volume increases during a plateau wave of elevated ICP. ICP waveform analysis and jugular venous oxygen saturation measurements may suggest the presence of hyperaemia (CBF in excess of metabolic requirement) even in the absence of epileptic seizures; raised venous pressure is also a potent cause of raised ICP. Unfortunately, the technology to measure cerebral blood volume, unlike that for cerebral oedema, is poorly developed. Only patients who are stable can be transported for research scans, be they CT, magnetic resonance imaging (MRI) or PET scans. Cerebral blood volume images are noisy and difficult to quantify, cannot distinguish arteriolar from venous components and cannot reveal dynamic changes, only steady state. Hence, although CBV may not increase at all or only moderately in the steady state after acute brain injury, this does not mean that cerebrovascular dysautoregulation and congestive brain swelling are not very important.

Congestive brain swelling may occur with startling rapidity in patients, especially children, who have sustained a head injury, in patients with traumatic acute subdural haematoma and in patients in whom aneurysms rupture intraoperatively or whose brain swells after removal of a large arteriovenous malformation. The increase in cerebral blood volume is claimed to be mainly in the capillary and postcapillary part of the cerebrovascular beds, but it is not yet possible to determine this in man. In spite of its frequency, the pathophysiology of the process is not entirely clear. There has to be relaxation of arterioles to permit flooding of the vascular bed at high intravascular pressure and/or a relative constriction of the venous outflow into the more protected and rigid dural sinuses. Some (but not all) cranial window studies of subarachnoid bridging veins during intracranial hypertension suggest that there is indeed an element of segmental vasoconstriction. The congested brain expands particularly rapidly when arterial pressure is high.[120] There is a reduction in the subarachnoid and intraventricular CSF volume and when ICP does rise the increase is often in the form of pressure waves. While cerebrovascular dilatation may result from clearly identifiable causes such as hypoxaemia, hypercapnia or severe elevations of arterial pressure, other instances are less easily explained and are usually attributed to an ill-defined central neurogenic mechanism. Lesions or stimuli in the hypothalamus and in the medulla oblongata have been shown not only to interfere with the reactivity of the cerebral circulation to physiological stimuli, but also, on occasions, to produce a marked primary cerebral vasodilatation with elevation of ICP.[85,195] When such vasodilatation is combined with arterial hypertension and loss of the capacity of cerebral arterioles to constrict, as occurs in vasomotor paralysis, the rapidity and severity of brain swelling can be devastating. ICP soon attains the level of systemic arterial pressure, perfusion of the brain ceases and brain death supervenes. Should the skull and dura be opened at this stage, massive external brain herniation will rapidly occur.[116]

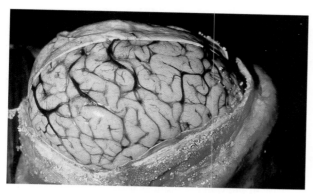

Figure 4.12 *Diffuse brain swelling. This was found at autopsy due to vasogenic oedema following closed head injury. The gyri are flattened, the sulci are compressed and the swollen brain is closely applied to the tightened dura mater.*

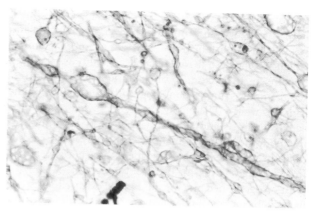

Figure 4.13 *Chronic cerebral oedema. The myelin sheaths within the white matter become widely separated, and exhibit numerous irregular areas of swelling and blebbing. (Solochrome cyanin.)*

The neuropathologist infrequently encounters congestive brain swelling, since it may subside as a result of the ante-mortem fall in blood pressure, leaving only the less specific evidence of a previous episode of high ICP such as pressure necrosis in one or both parahippocampal gyri. When there has been prolonged congestive brain swelling, however, vasogenic cerebral oedema supervenes, water accumulates in the extracellular space and in that event the brain will remain swollen after death (Fig. 4.12). The interrelationship between arterial blood pressure and the severity of congestive brain swelling has been exploited in one approach to the management of post-traumatic intracranial hypertension, in which β-blocking agents are used to produce a modest reduction in arterial pressure with the aim of reducing the severity of the swelling. The risk with such a strategy is, however, that the fall in arterial pressure, even if accompanied by a modest reduction in ICP, may still reduce CPP (the driving intravascular pressure) and result in brain ischaemia.[140]

Cerebral oedema

Cerebral oedema is defined as an increase in brain tissue volume that is due to an increased tissue water content.[58,65] This definition distinguishes oedema from hydrocephalus, cerebral atrophy and congestive brain swelling, but does not differentiate between intracellular and extracellular location of the water. In the past, German authors distinguished between Hirnschwellung, in which the water was intracellular, and Hirnödem, in which the water was located in the extracellular space.[175] Nowadays, the term 'brain swelling' is widely accepted as being synonymous with an increase in cerebral blood volume and therefore best prefaced by the term 'congestive'. The term 'brain oedema' is often used loosely by clinicians to denote a condition in which it is suspected that ICP is elevated. As with 'vasospasm' this imprecise use of terminology is to be deprecated.

The normal water content of grey matter is 80% of the wet weight (800 mg/g) while that of the white matter is considerably lower, at 68% of wet weight (680 mg/g), with the exception of the subcortical arcuate fibres of white matter in which the water content approaches that of grey matter.[2] In cerebral oedema typical water content values would be 81–82% in grey matter and 76–79% in white matter. The greater accumulation of water therefore occurs in white matter owing to the greater freedom with which water can move through the parallel fibre bundles (Fig. 4.13). This propensity of oedema fluid to accumulate in white matter is usually apparent on brain slices and on CT or MRI, both of which clearly show expansion of the centrum semiovale.

The causes of cerebral oedema are an increase in intravascular pressure, damage with increased permeability of the cerebral capillary wall and/or a decrease in plasma colloid osmotic pressure. Any of these, alone or in combination, may upset the Starling equilibrium to favour a greater net outflow of water, ionic solutes and even larger molecules into brain tissue or into the extracellular space, or to accumulate within brain cells, principally astrocytes.

In laboratory studies, six principal varieties of cerebral oedema have been distinguished.[138] These may also be encountered in clinical practice either singly or, more frequently, in combination.[68,107] A comparison between the major clinical forms of cerebral oedema is given in Table 4.1.

Vasogenic oedema

The type of cerebral oedema encountered most frequently in clinical practice is vasogenic oedema, in which an incompetent BBB permits extravasation of plasma-like fluid into the extracellular space. This type of oedema can be produced experimentally by application of intense cold to the surface of the brain;[28,107] in clinical practice it occurs in the vicinity of brain tumours,[204] intracerebral haematomas, cerebral abscesses and contusions. The formation rate of oedema is increased by systemic hypertension (if local autoregulation is impaired), fever, hypercapnia and vasodilatory substances.[29,220] The actual mechanism by which the increase in vascular permeability is produced remains far from clear. In brain tumours, the blood vessels themselves may be abnormal with fenestrations in the capillary wall.[203] There may also be increased pinocytotic activity in the endothelium. Cleaving, or separation of interendothelial tight junctions has been proposed, but only observed clearly in cases where there have been dramatic changes in plasma osmolality.

In vasogenic oedema the fluid in the extracellular space has a high content of plasma protein and the fluid spreads by bulk flow rather than diffusion, the rate of spread being proportional to the capillary hydrostatic pressure.[178,179] The oedema fluid tends to collect in the white matter by extension from the grey matter along adjacent white-matter tracts. Vasogenic oedema is often, thereby, a major factor contributing to the effective mass of an intracranial expanding lesion such as a glioma, meningioma or metastatic carcinoma (Fig. 4.11). The region of disruption of the BBB is essential to development of vasogenic oedema: surgical removal of a 'cold lesion' reduces such oedema. The oedema occurs mainly in the white matter and if present for some time, produces a pale-green discoloration on macroscopic examination. On histological examination there is pallor of myelin staining, the myelin sheaths often appearing abnormally swollen, vacuolated and beaded, and less closely packed than in normal white matter (Fig. 4.13). This is accompanied by astrocytic hypertrophy and hyperplasia. These cells take up and digest extravasated serum proteins; perivascular macrophage-like cells in the white matter may also perform these functions.[102] The oligodendrocytes within the affected white matter usually do not show any structural abnormalities, but if the vasogenic oedema has persisted for some time, the myelin sheaths undergo fragmentation and their lipid breakdown products are phagocytosed by macrophages and perivascular cells. This irreparable damage may result in the formation of small cystic spaces in the affected white matter.

Cytotoxic or cellular oedema

One of the earliest responses of brain tissue to injury is swelling of astrocytes. Klatzo[107] defined cytotoxic oedema as cellular swelling associated with a reduced extracellular space, but an intact BBB (at least to macromolecules in the initial stages). This can occur because energy failure disables the Na^+/K^+ membrane pump systems, allowing large amounts of sodium accompanied by chloride to enter the cell. Coupling of sodium influx with hydrogen ion efflux and chloride influx with bicarbonate efflux via ion-exchanger (antiporter) mechanisms may aggravate the process. Energy failure cannot be the only explanation of interference with these mechanisms, all of which will cause the cell to become swollen owing to influx of osmotically drawn water. These

membrane transporters can be induced or inhibited by a range of neurotransmitters and other agents.

In the case of energy failure, not only is the Na^+/K^+-ATPase pump system impaired, but the voltage and lig-and-gated mechanisms for regulating calcium entry into the cell are also disturbed. The destructive sequence of calcium-mediated events that begins with cerebral ischaemia and ends with cerebral infarction is dealt with in greater detail in Chapter 6 of this Volume. In the context of the present discussion, the important issue is the range of mechanisms that may, in the end, result in an increase in the water content of astrocytes and other cellular elements in the brain, resulting in cellular swelling.

Ischaemic oedema formation depends not only on the degree of reduction in CBF, but also on the duration of the ischaemia.[9] Cellular oedema after cerebral contusion observed by Bullock and his associates[22] may also be related to ischaemia. Because the metabolically active cellular constituents of brain tissue are located more in the grey matter than in the white matter, cytotoxic or cellular oedema is more prominent in grey matter,[154] but can involve adjacent white matter (Fig. 4.14). In the initial stages of ischaemic oedema, cytotoxic intracellular accumulation of water is related to acute tissue deprivation of oxygen and glucose, resulting in failure of the ATPase-dependent Na^+/K^+ exchange pump. Experimental studies of ischaemic oedema (reviewed by Klatzo)[107] have shown that after permanent occlusion of a major blood vessel the initial cytotoxic oedema is followed by irreversible ischaemic cell damage, resulting in a secondary vasogenic component when endothelial cells are damaged. In temporary ischaemia, when occlusion of a major cerebral artery is followed by reperfusion of the affected territory, there is a biphasic opening of the BBB (relating initially to reactive hyperaemia, and then to ischaemic cell damage to the endothelium) which also results in a vasogenic component to the cerebral oedema. Similar mechanisms are thought to operate in ischaemic brain injury in man.[68]

Hydrostatic oedema

Even if vascular endothelium remains intact, a sudden increase in intravascular pressure or transmural pressure can overcome the cerebrovascular resistance, producing high-pressure flooding of the capillary bed, and a hydrostatic pressure gradient sufficient to drive water across the capillary wall into the extracellular space. This can occur when arterial pressure suddenly becomes high during craniotomy, or when an intracranial mass lesion that has been causing severe intracranial hypertension is abruptly decompressed. The initial response of congestive brain swelling is followed after some minutes by extravasation of protein-poor fluid into and through the extracellular space of the brain.[197] An experimental preparation of this form of oedema was developed by Ishii et al.[86] who inflated an intracranial balloon in experimental animals

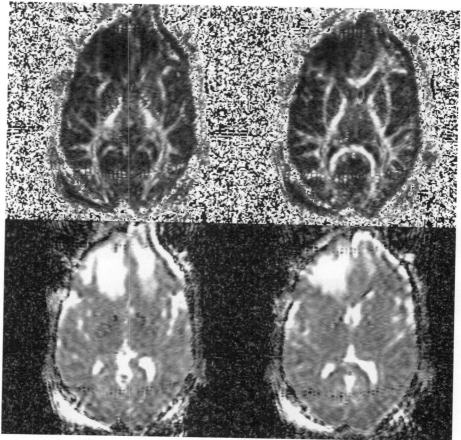

Figure 4.14 *Cytotoxic oedema. Relative anisotropy image from a diffusion-weighted MRI imaging data set, showing disruption of white-matter tracts in the region of a right frontal contusion. The lower images show the extent of the diffusion-weighted hyperintensity, which is thought to represent cytotoxic oedema. Courtesy of Professor D Menon, University of Cambridge, UK.*

to the point of incipient tentorial herniation. After the balloon was inflated for several hours, it was abruptly deflated and this was followed by severe brain swelling, close examination of which revealed an increase in extracellular water content typical of cerebral oedema. This model has clinical parallels in patients suffering from space-occupying lesions in whom surgical decompression has been undertaken.

A particularly severe example of this form of oedema may be seen in patients with a very high ICP in whom a bony decompression has been carried out, leading to rapid external herniation of the brain. The marked decrease in radiodensity of the extruded brain, typical of oedematous tissue is best shown by CT scans. Repeat PET studies have revealed that the CBF to such herniating brain is often adequate to maintain viability. Such brain should not be excised but a wider defect created to allow swelling and to avoid venous infarction at the edges of the defect.

Interstitial oedema

In patients with acute obstructive high-pressure hydrocephalus (see below) there is an increase in water content in the periventricular white matter. CT or MRI shows the process to be most pronounced around the frontal and occipital horns of the lateral ventricles (Fig. 4.15). In these cases, it appears that fluid under high pressure is forced through the ependyma into periventricular white matter. Fishman[58] termed this process interstitial cerebral oedema. Initially, the radiological appearance of interstitial oedema was held to indicate that intraventricular pressure would be high when measured, but experience shows that this is not invariably so. Damage to the stretched ependyma has been invoked to explain the periventricular oedema under circumstances of normal ICP. In the elderly, periventricular changes on CT or MRI more often reflect gliosis, demyelination and infarction rather than interstitial oedema.

Hypo-osmotic oedema

Stern and Coxon[202] infused distilled water into the peritoneal cavity of experimental subjects to produce a marked reduction of serum osmolality, and demonstrated associated diffuse brain swelling. Others have demonstrated that any reduction in serum osmolality to less than

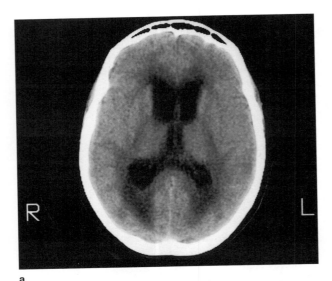

a

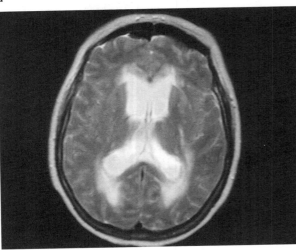

b

Figure 4.15 *Interstitial oedema. Chronic hydrocephalus with interstitial oedema in the periventricular white matter. (a) Non-contrast-enhanced cranial CT scan showing symmetrical lucency in the white matter. (b) T2-weighted cranial MRI scan (post-gadolinium) showing areas of increased signal in the periventricular white matter in a similar distribution to the lucent areas in the CT scan. Courtesy of Dr R Gibson, Western General Hospital, Edinburgh, UK.*

120 mmol/1 achieved by either intraperitoneal water infusion or intravenous administration of hypo-osmolar solutions will produce diffuse expansion of the brain associated with raised ICP, increased tissue water content and reduced CBF.[135] Comparable reductions in serum osmolality occur not infrequently in head-injured patients and after other severe cerebral insults, but have also been associated with episodes of raised ICP. Such reductions in osmolality may be the result of the excessive replacement of fluid loss by intravenous dextrose and water solutions, or may be due to the development of syndromes of appropriate or inappropriate secretion of antidiuretic hormone. The neurological sequelae of hyponatraemia can include

epilepsy, coma and respiratory arrest. Arieff[7] showed these to be more pronounced and to occur at a higher level of serum sodium in premenopausal women than in post-menopausal women or in men.

Spread and resolution of cerebral oedema

Klatzo,[108] Clasen *et al.*,[29] Hochwald *et al.*,[78] and Reulen *et al.*,[179] have investigated the factors that regulate the rate and extent of the spread of oedema fluid through the brain from a focal point by labelling with dyes or radioisotopes. Factors responsible for cerebral arterial or arteriolar vasodilatation (hypercapnia, hypoxaemia, severe arterial hypertension, hyperthermia and certain drugs) accelerate the rate of formation of oedema and the rate of passage of labelled elements of oedema fluid across the brain. Conversely, any factor that causes cerebral vasoconstriction tends to impede this process. Diffuse elevation of ICP also impedes the progress of oedema fluid across the brain. For several years it was considered that all oedema fluid passed eventually into the ventricles to be absorbed with CSF. While this may be true for the most part, uptake of labelled protein molecules has been observed in glial cells in periventricular regions, within blood vessels in the same area, and in regional lymph nodes draining the tissues of the head and neck, indicating that several different routes of absorption of the components of oedema fluid exist.[104,111] Double-labelling techniques also suggest that different components of the oedema fluid migrate at different rates through the extracellular space in the white matter.[71,155] In earlier studies of vasogenic oedema the concept of an oedema front was proposed, referring to the advancing wave of fluid emerging from a damaged area of the brain. The discovery that protein, water and other components pass through the extracellular space at different rates, depending on molecular weight and ionic charge, has modified this concept of the dynamics of brain oedema. While it is accepted that the factors which increase intracapillary pressure and reduce plasma osmotic pressure both favour the formation and spread of the vasogenic oedema, the exact mechanisms by which this occurs are incompletely understood.

Effects of cerebral oedema on neuronal function

There is no firm evidence that an increase in brain water, whether local or generalised, can directly interfere with neuronal activity or the patient's neurological state. In contrast, patients with perifocal brain oedema frequently manifest corresponding focal neurological deficit that improves after treatment with corticosteroids, a therapy aimed at ameliorating the oedema. Penn[164] convincingly demonstrated a lack of correlation between areas of cerebral oedema demonstrated by CT and signs of focal neurological dysfunction; patients showing improvement with corticosteroid therapy may still show oedema on CT scanning. Two possibilities exist for the inconstant relationship between focal brain oedema and corresponding neurological dysfunction. First, oedema causes brain dysfunction only when it is sufficiently severe to cause cerebral ischaemia or distortion and herniation of the brain. Secondly, in some circumstances the oedema fluid carries within it agents that may themselves be responsible for localised brain dysfunction.[220]

Whittle and his associates[242] have shown, using an infusion model of brain oedema with instillation of a number of putative oedema-inducing agents including arachidonic acid, bradykinin, plasma and glioma cyst fluid, that vascular reactivity in the oedematous brain region is impaired even if electroencephalographic activity and resting blood flow have not been reduced.[238–241] It has also been proposed that brain tissue pressure within the oedematous area may be elevated well above the prevailing ICP.[154] Convincing evidence for persistence of such major pressure gradients has not, however, been forthcoming.

When regional CBF is measured within areas of cerebral oedema, the flow levels are often low, indicating that when ICP is sufficiently elevated by the mass effect of the oedema, CPP becomes reduced. If CBF reactivity has been impaired, particularly autoregulatory activity, then even a relatively small reduction in CPP may be sufficient to induce a reduction in blood flow. It has also been proposed that because local CBF is measured in ml/min per 100 g tissue perfused, an apparent fall in blood flow in areas of brain oedema may, in fact, represent an unchanged volume of blood perfusing a greater weight of tissue. Such arguments overlook the increased diffusion distances involved from capillary to neuron.

Papilloedema

Papilloedema has long been regarded as a reliable index of raised ICP, with the implication that when it is absent ICP is not elevated. This is simply not true and has led to mindless dilatation of pupils to obtain a better view with an ophthalmoscope. It is indefensible to lose the pupillary light reflex in this way in patients with an impaired level of consciousness. It has proved possible to induce papilloedema experimentally by the slow expansion of an intracranial mass lesion. Bordley and Cushing[11] injected wax into the subdural space. Hayreh[76] expanded an intracranial balloon slowly with continuous measurement of ICP, and confirmed Cushing's result that the slow expansion of the mass lesion produced raised ICP and papilloedema. Hayreh also showed that development of the papilloedema depended on extension of the subarachnoid space around the optic nerve into the orbit so that the nerve could be exposed to the CSF pressure. Incision of the optic sheath in this space prevented papilloedema, even when ICP was elevated.[212,246]

The swelling of the optic nerve head that characterizes papilloedema is not due to increased water content, but represents an accumulation of axoplasm in the optic papilla consequent to a blockage of axoplasmic flow from the ganglion cells along the optic nerve. The relative lack of myelin around these axons may facilitate papillary swelling when sustained intracranial hypertension compresses the optic nerve and blocks centripetal axoplasmic flow. Changes in fast axonal transport occur only after the development of disc swelling, implying that changes in slow transport may be the primary abnormality.

In patients with benign intracranial hypertension in its initial episodes, chronic subdural haematoma and brain tumour, there is a close relationship between elevation of ICP and papilloedema. Even so, the older the patient, the less likely is papilloedema to develop. Papilloedema does not occur in an eye in which antecedent optic atrophy has destroyed most or all of the nerve fibres. In acute severe head injury the position is different, since papilloedema (of low grade only) is found in less than 5% of cases within a week of injury, although the ICP is high in more than 50% of cases. It is possible that the intracranial hypertension does not persist for a time sufficient for papilloedema to develop. Persistent elevation of ICP for 2 or more weeks is, however, well recognized in head injury, so that it remains unclear why papilloedema should be so uncommon in this circumstance. It must, however, be concluded that while papilloedema is a valuable indicator of the presence of chronically elevated ICP, its absence in acute conditions cannot be taken to mean that ICP is normal.

THE PATHOLOGY OF INTRACRANIAL EXPANDING LESIONS

An expanding mass lesion within a rigid cranial cavity will trigger a number of closely interrelated events, the first of which is distortion of the adjacent brain.[222] Schettini and Walsh[192] showed that when a pressure-sensitive transducer is driven downwards to indent the surface of the brain, the pressure recorded on the face of the transducer diminishes over time as the brain accommodates the distortion. While this might suggest that local properties of brain tissue can contribute to the prevention of an increase in ICP, the major factor responsible for spatial compensation is a reduction in the volume of intracranial CSF. This is achieved by a reduction in the volume of the cerebral ventricles, subarachnoid space and extracerebral CSF cisterns. Compression of the major intracranial venous sinuses may also contribute to spatial compensation within the cranial cavity.

The basic sequence of events can therefore be summarized as local deformity, reduced volume of CSF, shift and distortion of the brain and eventually (in the intact skull) the appearance of internal herniae, i.e. displacement of brain tissue from one intracranial component into another, or into the spinal canal (Fig. 4.16). These displacements result from the development of pressure gradients between intracranial compartments and lead to secondary vascular complications such as haemorrhage and ischaemia.[146,226] When the skull surrounding an expanding intracranial mass is not rigid, e.g. the unfused skull in infants or a displaced flap of bone resulting from skull fracture or surgery, displacement of the brain may occur through the bony defect as an external cerebral hernia.

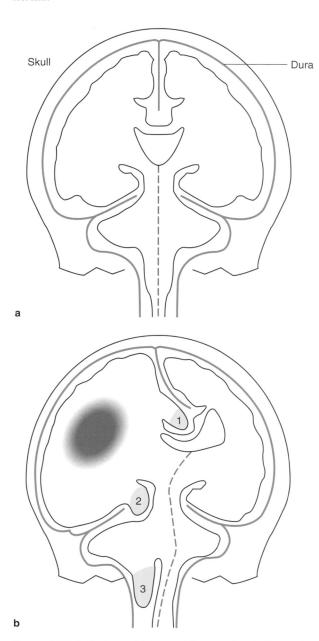

a

b

Figure 4.16 *Pathology of intracranial expanding lesions. Diagrammatic representation of (a) normal intracranial compartments and (b) the effects of an expanding lesion within a cerebral hemisphere, showing anatomical distortion and shift of the midline structures. The sites of (1) subfalcine, (2) transtentorial, and (3) foramen magnum herniae are indicated.*

Supratentorial expanding lesions

Expansion of an intrinsic lesion within a cerebral hemisphere results in compression of adjacent brain structures and overall expansion of the hemisphere. Sulci on the surface of the brain become narrowed and overlying gyri are flattened against the dura mater, obliterating the subarachnoid space. At autopsy the dura mater may be so tense that it is difficult to incise it without damaging the underlying cerebral cortex. Lindenberg[123] suggested that these circumstances may be sufficient to produce compression of the terminal branches of the cerebral arteries, resulting in ischaemic cortical neurons within the depth of sulci. However, it appears more likely that reduced CPP in a patient with a high ICP is the major factor contributing to these perisulcal infarcts.[88]

As the mass continues to expand, the lateral ventricles on the side of the lesion and the third ventricle become reduced in size and there is contralateral displacement of the midline structures: the pericallosal arteries, interventricular septum, thalamus, hypothalamus, third ventricle and midbrain (Fig. 4.17). Recent clinical and neuroradiological studies have suggested that acute lateral displacement of the midbrain and hypothalamus may be fatal in the absence of established cerebral herniation.[142,180] Obliteration of the contralateral foramen of Monro may lead to enlargement of the contralateral lateral ventricle and a further increase in ICP. The sylvian fissure becomes narrowed and the lesser wing of the sphenoid bone may produce a groove on the inferior surface of the frontal lobe. The floor of the third ventricle is displaced towards the basal cisterns and the mamillary bodies become wedged into a narrowed interpeduncular fossa.

While this sequence of events may occur with any expanding lesion within a cerebral hemisphere, certain dis-

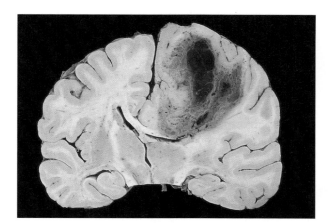

Figure 4.17 *Supratentorial expanding lesions. A haemorrhagic right parietal glioblastoma has resulted in lateral shift of cerebral structures with a large right subfalcine hernia, obliteration of the right lateral ventricle and third ventricle and distortion of the thalamus.*

placements are selectively affected by the site of the lesion. An expanding lesion in the frontal lobe will produce displacement of the free margin of the anterior part of the falx cerebri; the posterior part of the falx is rarely displaced laterally because it is firmly tethered at this level. A lesion in the temporal lobe will produce disproportionately severe shift of the third ventricle and will displace upwards the sylvian fissure and the adjacent branches of the middle cerebral artery.

As the lesion continues to expand, the next stage is the development of internal cranial herniae. The major sites of intracranial herniation were described early in the twentieth century at the falx cerebri, tentorium cerebelli and foramen magnum.[36,119,136,191]

Supracallosal subfalcine (or cingulate) hernia

Expansion of a mass in the frontal or parietal lobe will eventually result in herniation of the ipsilateral cingulate gyrus under the free edge of the falx to produce selective displacement of the pericallosal arteries away from this lesion and from the midline (Fig. 4.17). This may compromise circulation through the pericallosal arteries and result in infarction of the parietal parasagittal cortex, manifesting clinically as a weakness or sensory loss in one or both legs. The posterior end of the falx is tethered, so a posterior supracallosal hernia can occur only after there has been downward displacement of the roof of the ipsilateral ventricle. A wedge of pressure necrosis may occur along the groove where the cingulate gyrus makes contact with the falx[184] (Fig. 4.18). If the brain returns to its normal shape as a result of treatment, this wedge of necrosis can be taken as a reliable marker of previous herniation at this site.

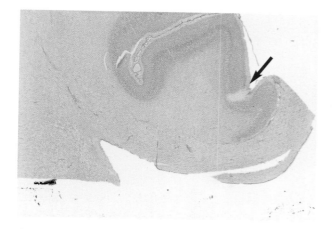

Figure 4.18 *Supracallosal subfalcine hernia: pressure necrosis. Pressure necrosis in the cingulate gyrus. Recent rarefaction necrosis (arrow) in relation to a subfalcine hernia. Cresyl violet stain. Courtesy of Professor DI Graham, University of Glasgow, UK.*

Tentorial (uncal or lateral transtentorial) hernia

Any supratentorial expanding hemispheric mass may produce herniation of the ipsilateral uncus and medial part of the parahippocampal gyrus medially and downward through the tentorial incisura; this occurs most frequently when the mass is located in the temporal lobe. The width of this hernia is influenced by variations in the capacity of the tentorial incisura[32] as well as the size and location of the mass lesion. As the parahippocampal gyrus herniates, the midbrain is narrowed in its transverse axis and the cerebral aqueduct becomes compressed. The contralateral cerebral peduncle is pushed against the opposite free tentorial edge,[56] and the ipsilateral oculomotor nerve becomes compressed between the petroclinoid ligament or the free edge of the tentorium and the posterior cerebral artery (Fig. 4.19). The oculomotor nerve is at first only flattened where it is compressed

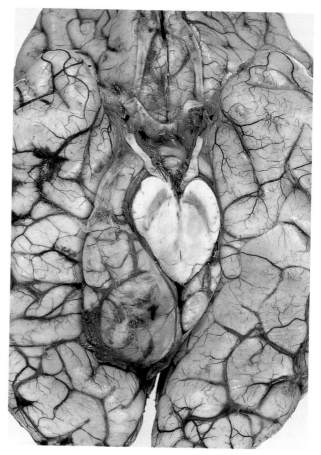

Figure 4.19 *Transtentorial hernia: compression of upper brainstem. An extensive transtentorial hernia on the right has resulted in compression of the midbrain and cerebral aqueduct, with flattening of the right IIIrd nerve against the parahippocampal gyrus. The hernia is demarcated by a prominent groove, and shows early haemorrhagic necrosis in its posterior aspect.*

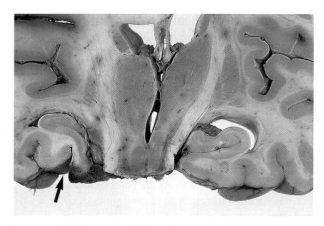

Figure 4.20 *Transtentorial hernia: pressure necrosis. Unilateral haemorrhagic necrosis (arrow) in the left parahippocampal gyrus following a transtentorial hernia in a patient with a left parietal glioblastoma.*

and angulated over the posterior cerebral artery, but later there is often haemorrhage into the nerve. The resulting paralysis of oculomotor nerve produces ptosis and dilatation of the pupil ipsilateral to the lesion, with loss of the direct response to light shone in the affected eye and of the consensual response to light shone in the opposite eye. There is loss of upward and medial movement of the eye and in its resting position it deviates laterally, due to unopposed action of the VIth cranial nerve. Dilatation of the pupil is the earliest consistent sign of tentorial herniation and may occur before there is any impairment of consciousness.[57,90,91,136,177,205,219]

As the tentorial hernia enlarges, a wedge of haemorrhagic necrosis appears along the lines of the groove in the parahippocampal gyrus (Fig. 4.20). Compression of the contralateral cerebral peduncle against the free edge of the tentorium may lead to infarction with or without haemorrhage in the dorsal part of the peduncle and adjacent tegmentum.[101] This lesion may produce weakness followed by extensor rigidity in the limbs ipsilateral to the expanding lesion. This phenomenon has been studied by MRI, and is seen most often in older patients with brain atrophy and a pronounced degree of midbrain shift as a complication of chronic subdural haematoma.[30] It is much more common for tentorial herniation to be associated with a contralateral limb weakness and eventual extensor rigidity, owing to compression of the cerebral peduncle on the side of the mass lesion by direct pressure from the herniating brain.

Because some degree of shift and herniation of the brain can occur during the period of spatial compensation without a significant increase in ICP, it may be difficult to establish after death whether ICP has been high during life. Adams and Graham[3] suggested that the pathognomonic feature of high ICP due to a supratentorial expanding lesion is the presence of a wedge of pressure necrosis in one or both parahippocampal gyri, best seen in coronal sections of the brain. Haemorrhagic pres-

sure necrosis can be identified macroscopically (Fig. 4.20), but if haemorrhage is absent, necrosis may only be identifiable microscopically (Fig. 4.21). This form of pressure necrosis can be distinguished from a herniation contusion by its more lateral situation. Pressure necrosis of this type was found in every patient known to have had an ICP of more than 5.4 kPa (40 mmHg) during life, and in most of the patients with ICP levels between 2.7 and 5.3 kPa (20–40 mmHg), but in none of the patients with ICP levels of less than 2.7 kPa (20 mmHg).[3]

Any change in the ICP which results in accentuation of the pressure gradient across the tentorial incisura may worsen the degree of tentorial herniation. This mechanism was modelled in experiments by Fitch and McDowall,[60] Miller[139] and Takizawa et al.,[207] in which an intracranial balloon is gradually inflated to the point where the pressure gradient has just begun to develop between the lateral ventricle and the cisterna magna. At this point, the pupil ipsilateral to the balloon begins to dilate. If inflation of the balloon is now stopped so that the size of the mass lesion remains the same, and an agent that causes cerebral vasodilatation (e.g. carbon dioxide or halothane) is administered, there is an increase in supratentorial pressure without an equivalent increase in infratentorial pressure, and the dilatation of the pupil now becomes complete. Transient rises in ICP recorded supratentorially in response to small volume changes are not transmitted to the infratentorial compartment. Studies in patients with head injury and with intracranial tumours[99] have shown that transtentorial pressure gradients are not uncommon and, when present, are frequently accompanied by clinical signs of tentorial herniation.

Any increase in the pressure gradient is commonly associated with abrupt worsening of the patient's neurological status, such as onset of decerebrate rigidity and loss of consciousness. Expansion of a supratentorial mass lesion may therefore be responsible for initiating tentorial

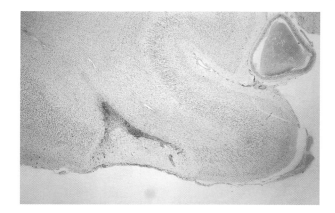

Figure 4.21 *Transtentorial hernia: pressure necrosis. A wedge of longstanding pressure necrosis is present in the parahippocampal gyrus, indicative of previous transtentorial herniation. (The patient survived in a vegetative state for 6 weeks after evacuation of an intracerebral haematoma.) (Cresyl violet.) Courtesy of Professor DI Graham, University of Glasgow, UK.*

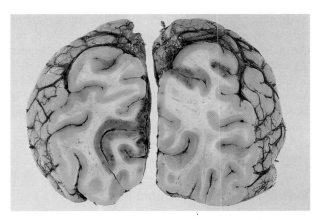

Figure 4.22 *Transtentorial hernia: medial occipital infarction. Recent asymmetrical haemorrhagic infarction of the medial occipital lobes following transtentorial herniation and posterior cerebral artery compression as a consequence of a left temporal glioblastoma. The left occipital cortex is more extensively damaged than the right.*

herniation and establishing the beginnings of a transtentorial pressure gradient. Subsequently, any process that would normally induce a diffuse increase in ICP will increase the transtentorial pressure gradient and accentuate the process of herniation; major degrees of lateral midline shift may cause blockage of the foramen of Monro and narrowing of the cerebral aqueduct, resulting in hydrocephalus.

Other sequelae of raised ICP and tentorial herniation include the compression of arteries; occlusion of the anterior choroidal artery may lead to infarction in the medial part of the globus pallidus, in the internal capsule and in the optic tract. Compression of a posterior cerebral artery, the blood vessel most commonly affected, may lead to infarction in the thalamus, in the temporal lobe including the hippocampus, and of the medial and inferior surfaces of the cortex of the occipital lobe (Fig. 4.22). Compression of a superior cerebellar artery may lead to cerebellar infarction. Infarction of the occipital cortex and cerebellum under these circumstances is often intensely haemorrhagic. These vascular effects usually occur on the same side as the tentorial hernia, but they may also be bilateral and very occasionally contralateral.[208] Clinical and neuroradiological studies of survivors of transtentorial herniation have revealed a spectrum of complications which range from a transient 'locked-in' syndrome[244] to more profound neurological deficits, the severity of which is generally related to the degree of herniation as assessed neuroradiologically.[215]

Central transtentorial herniation

This form of herniation occurs particularly in response to frontal and parietal lesions or to bilateral expanding lesions such as chronic subdural haematomas. It results from caudal displacement of the diencephalon and the

rostral brainstem and may be preceded by a lateral transtentorial hernia. If ICP increases rapidly in association with lesions of this type, both parahippocampal gyri may herniate through the tentorial incisure, leading to the formation of a circular or ring hernia which is most evident posteriorly and may compress the tectal plate. The clinical manifestations are bilateral ptosis and failure of upward gaze, followed by loss of the pupillary light reflex.

Although major degrees of 'diencephalic downthrust'[52] are readily identifiable on neuropathological examination, minor degrees of caudal displacement of the brainstem are less easy to identify, even in a properly fixed brain. The evidence for downward axial displacement of the brainstem in the herniation process has emerged from both experimental[209] and human post-mortem studies.[74] More recently, Ropper[181] has obtained MRI of a patient showing the clinical manifestations of central transtentorial herniation and failed to establish downward axial displacement of the brainstem. Autopsy studies in patients in whom central herniation has been clinically established show backwards and downwards displacement of the mamillary bodies, compression of the pituitary stalk and caudal displacement of the posterior part of the floor of the third ventricle, which comes to lie below the level of the tentorial incisure. Focal infarction may occur in the mamillary bodies and in the anterior lobe of the pituitary gland owing to impaired blood flow through the long hypothalamohypophysial portal vessels. The thalamus becomes distorted with elongation of individual neurons, and the occulomotor nerves become elongated and angulated. Infarction in territories supplied by the anterior choroidal, posterior cerebral and superior cerebellar arteries is also a frequent occurrence.

The clinical correlates of this state are loss of consciousness, decerebrate rigidity and bilateral dilatation of the pupils with loss of light response. The systemic blood pressure becomes elevated as a result of increased sympathetic activity and the heart rate slows. Important areas in the brainstem associated with arterial hypertension appears to be the floor of the fourth ventricle and the nucleus of the tractus solitarius, especially on the left side.[54,80] Alterations in respiration are also common.[81,209]

Haemorrhage and infarction of the midbrain and pons

This is a common and often terminal event in patients with supratentorial expanding lesions, high ICP and tentorial herniation. Emphasis is usually placed on the occurrence of haemorrhage because this is obvious macroscopically, but microscopic examination shows infarction to be at least as frequent as haemorrhage. Both types of lesion occur adjacent to the midline in the tegmentum of the midbrain (Fig. 4.23) and in the tegmental and basal parts of the pons. First described by Duret, there has always been considerable debate about the pathogenesis of the haemorrhage and

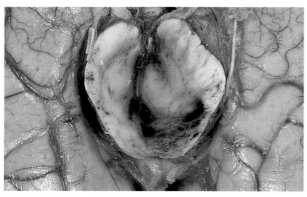

Figure 4.23 *Transtentorial hernia: brainstem haemorrhage. A large centrally located haemorrhage is present in the midbrain as a consequence of transtentorial herniation. The cerebral peduncle on the right is compressed and distorted.*

ischaemia. The most important factors are likely to be caudal displacement and anterior–posterior elongation of the rostral brainstem caused by side-to-side compression by

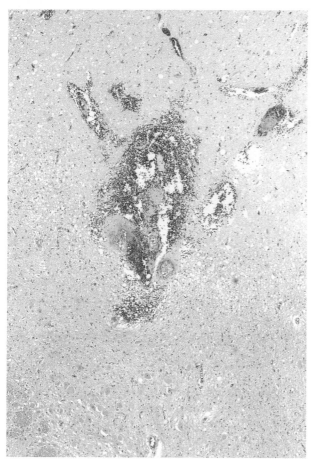

Figure 4.24 *Transtentorial hernia: brainstem haemorrhage. Histological examination of the midbrain from the case illustrated in Fig. 4.23 shows distortion of the white matter and multiple perivascular haemorrhages extending into the parenchyma as a consequence of transtentorial herniation. (H&E.)*

the tentorial hernia, coupled with relative immobility of the basilar artery. With progressive displacement, the central perforating branches of the basilar artery that supply the rostral brainstem become stretched and narrowed,[74] leading to spasm, infarction or haemorrhage[92] (Fig. 4.24). According to Klintworth,[109,110] brainstem haemorrhage is more likely when high ICP and axial brainstem shift have suddenly been reduced by surgical decompression, resulting in an increase in blood flow in the previously ischaemic brainstem.

Tonsillar hernia (foraminal impaction, cerebellar cone)

Downward displacement of the cerebellar tonsil through the foramen magnum occurs as an early complication of expanding masses in the posterior cranial fossa (Fig. 4.25), but it may also occur in association with supratentorial space-occupying lesions.[99] The pathognomonic indication of this form of brain herniation is haemorrhagic necrosis at the tips of the cerebellar tonsils (Fig. 4.26) and a groove on the ventral surface of the medulla, where it is compressed against the anterior border of the foramen magnum. The accompanying distortion of the spinal medullary junction results in apnoea, which may occur at a stage when consciousness is still preserved. However, tonsillar herniation is usually the last in a sequence of intracranial events, at least one of which will already have been responsible for loss of consciousness. Most patients at this stage will also exhibit other abnormal neurological signs, such as decerebrate rigidity and impairment of brainstem reflexes. This latter situation is the more likely and the source of raised ICP is a supratentorial expanding lesion; isolated apnoea is usually a sequel to an expanding lesion within the posterior cranial fossa.

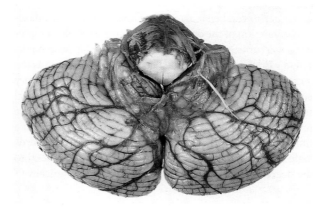

Figure 4.25 *Tonsillar hernia: pressure necrosis. Herniation of the cerebellar tonsils into the foramen magnum has resulted in haemorrhagic necrosis on the inferior surface of the tonsils, which are surrounded by a well-defined groove on the lateral aspect. On the medial aspect the tonsils are closely applied to the medulla, which is correspondingly flattened.*

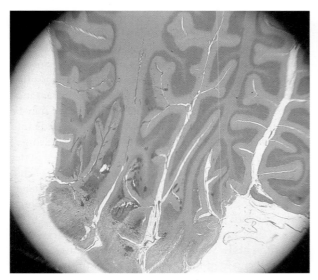

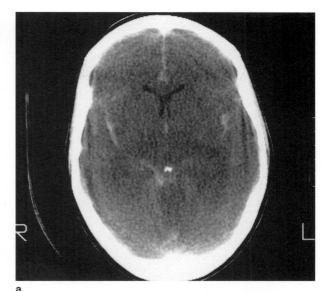

Figure 4.26 *Tonsillar hernia: pressure necrosis. Histological examination of the cerebellum from the case illustrated in Fig. 4.25 showing haemorrhagic necrosis at the tip of the impacted tonsil. (H&E.) Courtesy of Professor JE Bell, University of Edinburgh, UK.*

Diffuse brain swelling

When ICP has become elevated as a result of diffuse brain swelling, the ventricles become small but remain symmetrical and there is no lateral shift of midline structures[6] (Fig. 4.27). Nevertheless, bilateral tentorial herniae may occur, their size depending on the rate and severity of brain swelling and the dimensions of the tentorial incisura. Caudal displacement of the diencephalon and brainstem, and central transtentorial herniation are the major contributors to the neurological dysfunction and vegetative disturbance that may result in a fatal outcome in such patients.

Infratentorial expanding lesions

Hydrocephalus, with enlargement of both lateral ventricles and the third ventricle, is the most common abnormality associated with expanding lesions in the posterior cranial fossa, whether they be in the fourth ventricle, within or outside the cerebellum (Fig. 4.28). When the lesion is not in the midline, the aqueduct and fourth ventricle are both compressed and displaced contralaterally. Tonsillar herniation occurs most rapidly with a supratentorial expanding lesion. Occasionally, the posterior inferior cerebellar arteries may be compressed, resulting in infarction in the inferior part of one or both cerebellar hemispheres. Herniation of the superior surface of the cerebellum may occur in an upward direction through the tentorial incisure, and is termed reversed tentorial hernia. If the posterior cranial fossa lesion has been expanding very slowly, upward herniation of the superior vermis of the cerebellum can produce considerable distortion of the temporal lobes.

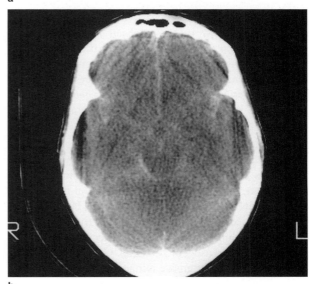

a

b

Figure 4.27 *Diffuse brain swelling. Non-contrast-enhanced cranial CT scan showing diffuse brain swelling in a patient with subarachnoid haemorrhage. The lateral and third ventricles are compressed, with obliteration of the perimesencephalic cisterns, but no displacement of the midline structures. Courtesy of Dr R Gibson, Western General Hospital, Edinburgh, UK.*

The clinical manifestations of upward tentorial herniation are sudden appearance of bilateral extensor rigidity and loss of the pupillary light reflex. This is most likely to occur when sudden decompression by CSF drainage of enlarged lateral ventricles is carried out in the presence of an undecompressed expanding lesion in the posterior fossa.

External cerebral herniae

These occur as rare complications of rapidly expanding supratentorial masses when there is a displaceable defect

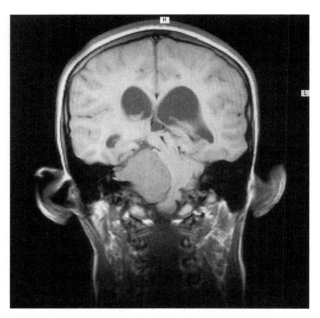

Figure 4.28 *Asymmetrical hydrocephalus. T1-weighted cranial MRI scan showing asymmetrical hydrocephalus resulting from a severe compression and distortion of the cerebral aqueduct and fourth ventricle by a large right acoustic schwannoma, which is displacing the cerebellum and brainstem. Courtesy of Dr R Gibson, Western General Hospital, Edinburgh, UK.*

in the skull, usually surgical or traumatic. This may amount to small protrusions of cortex through cranial burr holes, but if a larger cerebral decompression has been undertaken, major portions of the cerebral hemisphere may herniate through the calvarial defects. Haemorrhagic pressure necrosis occurs at the edge of the hernia, with swelling of brain tissue within the defect due to venous obstruction and vasogenic oedema. Continuing herniation will result in extensive ischaemic or haemorrhagic necrosis of the involved cortex and white matter. A recent study of acute intraoperative brain herniation during elective surgery found that most cases were due to extraaxial haemorrhage (subarachnoid or intraventricular), rather than the intraparenchymal haemorrhages and acute brain oedema occurring in patients with severe head injury who undergo emergency neurosurgery.[243] Accordingly, the outcome for such elective surgical patients is better than for those with severe head injury.

OTHER CRANIAL EFFECTS OF RAISED ICP

Bony changes

Bony changes usually occur only if ICP has been elevated for a considerable period. In adults, the dorsum sellae is the first structure to be affected. At first, there is loss of detail of the cortex (lamina dura) anteriorly at the lower part of the dorsum. With the passage of time, the bony changes in the dorsum may become more extensive and the floor of the pituitary fossa may also become involved. These changes are often visible on lateral skull X-rays and may be attributed to downward pressure on the diaphragma sellae. A deeply cupped diaphragma is often seen in patients with slowly expanding intracranial lesions. Pressure effects on the floor of the sellae may be accentuated where the subarachnoid space extends into the pituitary fossa, the so-called 'empty sella syndrome'; cerebral cortex may also extrude through the dura mater to produce small pits in the bone of the base of the skull, particularly in the middle cranial fossa, and ultimately there may be erosion of the orbital plates and lesser wings of the sphenoid bone. In infants and children up to 10 years of age, an early sign of raised ICP is separation of the sutures at the vault of the skull. In such cases, there is also enlargement of the skull, thinning of the bone of the vault and prominence of the convolutional impressions.

Clinical symptoms and signs of raised ICP and herniation

The initial effects of a developing mass will reflect loss of local brain function and, if cortical, possibly focal seizures. If the mass is very slowly growing, there may be remarkably few, if any, clinical symptoms or signs. As the mass enlarges and is surrounded by swollen brain, the local signs expand in type and severity; for example, a tumour in the sylvian fissure on the dominant side may present with focal seizures or wild expressive dysphasia, and progress to severe dysphasia and hemiparesis worse in the arm than the leg. As ICP starts to rise, the symptoms may be of novel headaches, nausea and visual disturbances. The previously unencountered nature of the headache is the most important feature, and helps to distinguish it from a patient's other, more longstanding, headaches (migraine, tension, period, cervical spondylosis, etc.). Classically, the headaches are worse upon waking because of both venous congestion on lying flat (there are no valves between the head and the right atrium) and mild carbon dioxide retention while asleep. Both phenomena reverse on waking and standing. The headache is probably related to stretching and distortion of the dura and major intracranial blood vessels, all of which are pain sensitive. The vomiting is related to distortion or pressure on the floor of the fourth ventricle where the vomiting centre is located.

Visual disturbance due to raised ICP may reflect the lateral diplopia of a VIth nerve palsy or the blurring of vision, an enlarged blind spot or obscurations of vision (usually on standing) associated with papilloedema. A IIIrd nerve palsy is a late sign and reflects tentorial herniation and midbrain compression: the patient seldom complains as unconsciousness has supervened. Three signs are the hallmark of midbrain compression in the following order: deterioration in the level of consciousness through compression and ischaemia of the reticular activating system, hemiparesis ipsilateral to the hemispheric lesion (the cerebral peduncle at risk of Kernohan's notch is contralateral to the lesion and contains the corticospinal tract from the other hemisphere) and finally a IIIrd nerve palsy, usually starting on the side of the lesion. The crucial process is shift and distortion of the brainstem as much as the hernia itself.

Systemic sequelae of raised ICP

Changes in blood pressure and heart rate are associated with axial brainstem shift and raised ICP. The usual pattern of response is of one or more surges of arterial hypertension, when systolic blood pressure may rise to 40 kPa (300 mmHg) or more, followed by a steadily falling blood pressure that soon becomes unresponsive to central vasopressor drugs. At this stage, brainstem death supervenes and circulatory arrest will eventually follow. The rise in arterial pressure is due to increased sympathetic activity and can be blocked by surgery or drug-induced interruption of the pathway.[61,79]

Signs of myocardial damage may also be present in patients with raised ICP and distortion of the brain. These consist of electrocardiographic changes, elevation of the ST segment and T-wave inversion, suggestive of myocardial ischaemia, and pathological changes consisting of subendocardial haemorrhage and widespread focal myocardial cell necrosis.[31] These changes can also be prevented by autonomic blockade, both sympathetic and parasympathetic.[75,121] Respiratory disturbances are frequent before the occurrence of apnoea. Plum and Posner[167] propose that various disorders of respiratory pattern could be associated with dysfunction in particular areas of the brain: periodic respiration with the forebrain, central neurogenic hyperventilation with the midbrain, and ataxic respiration and apnoea with the lower pons and medulla. North and Jennett[152,153] failed to confirm this hierarchy of respiratory disorder in an extensive study of patterns of respiration in patients with various forms of brain damage. They observed different respiratory patterns in the same patient at different times and concluded only that the lower the brain damage or dysfunction extended down the brainstem, the more likely it was that some form of respiratory abnormality would be present.

A further problem in patients with raised ICP and brain distortion is related to pulmonary dysfunction. This may be observed in its most dramatic form in the neurogenic pulmonary oedema that may complicate the course of patients with severe subarachnoid haemorrhage which is associated with severely elevated ICP. Ducker[44] proposed that sympathetic overactivity was responsible for alterations in pulmonary capillary blood flow, with a consequent alteration of the ventilation/perfusion ratio. This is, however, a difficult area to investigate since patients with severe acute brain dysfunction related to head injury, brain tumour or intracranial haemorrhage may also have areas of pulmonary atelectasis related to aspiration of gastric contents consequent upon loss of protective reflexes and the changes in the respiratory pattern with periods of apnoea.[64]

The mucosa of the digestive and urogenital tracts can become haemorrhagic, eroded and ulcerated in patients with raised ICP and brain distortion, the most frequent sites being the gastric mucosa, the distal duodenum, proximal jejunum and urinary bladder. Cushing[34] drew attention to the problem of acute gastroduodenal ulceration and suggested that it was due to sympathetic overactivity and increased gastric acid production.

Endoscopic studies have confirmed that gastric erosions are common in comatose patients with raised ICP. Although gastric acidity is increased under these circumstances, the levels are not higher than those seen in individuals with chronic peptic ulceration.[69] The administration of histamine receptor antagonists reduces gastric acidity in these patients and diminishes the incidence and severity of gastric bleeding, but does not appear to affect the frequency of gastric erosion.[73] This suggests that mucosal ischaemia is the most likely explanation for gastroduodenal mucosal ulceration, but that high gastric acidity increases the likelihood of haemorrhage.

HYDROCEPHALUS

Definitions

The term hydrocephalus refers to an accumulation of CSF within the head as a result of a disturbance of its secretion, circulation or absorption. This definition distinguishes hydrocephalus from cerebral atrophy. The term is commonly used as synonymous with enlargement of at least the lateral ventricles, but there are circumstances when that supposition will mislead. Patients with a blocked shunt inserted previously to treat their hydrocephalus may not always enlarge their ventricles ('unresponsive ventricles'), leading the unwary to presume that the shunt is patent. Labels can be dangerous: a wide range of terms is used to describe various forms of hydrocephalus.

Obstructive or non-communicating hydrocephalus occurs when a lesion or stricture impedes free passage of the CSF from the lateral ventricles to the subarachnoid space, causing dilatation of the portion of the CSF pathway that lies proximal to the obstruction. This is virtually always located at an isthmus in the internal CSF pathway. Thus, obstructive hydrocephalus may be caused by lesions located at the foramen of Munro, within the third ventricle at its anterior or posterior portion, in the aqueduct of Sylvius, within the fourth ventricle or at the outlet foramina of Magendie and Luschka.

Communicating hydrocephalus refers to the abnormality in which there is free passage of CSF from within the ventricular system into the subarachnoid space but there is still failure of CSF absorption with dilatation of the lateral ventricles and the third and fourth ventricles. The reabsorptive problem lies within the subarachnoid space, impeding the passage of CSF around the cerebellum through the cisterna ambiens, or at the arachnoid villi, impeding the reabsorption of CSF into the cerebral venous system at the superior sagittal sinus. The distinction between obstructive and communicating hydrocephalus is important, not least because lumbar puncture may be lethal in the former but safe in the latter.

In active or progressive hydrocephalus, sequential imaging shows the ventricles becoming progressively enlarged. This is contrasted with arrested hydrocephalus in which ventricular enlargement has occurred in the past but continued observation over a period of time shows no further enlargement of the lateral ventricles. Arrested hydrocephalus is a treacherous and unstable condition. ICP monitoring has revealed that there are often episodes of raised ICP with enhanced B-wave activity, particularly when asleep. There is an incidence of rapid deterioration and death in teenagers with 'arrested' hydrocephalus.

In hydrocephalus *ex vacuo*, or cerebral atrophy, there is loss of white matter and enlargement of the ventricular system as a consequence of brain atrophy (see also Chapter 4, Volume II). This condition may commonly be found in patients who have suffered severe head injury, vascular disease with multi-infarct dementia or other forms of progressive degenerative brain disorder. However, there is growing awareness of patients who have a combination of hydrocephalus with cerebral atrophy: the clinical problem is to define which patients have a remediable hydrocephalic component and to give a realistic prognosis as each separate process progresses (see below).

The terms high-pressure, normal-pressure and low-pressure hydrocephalus are self-explanatory, although it is widely recognized that a number of patients with so-called normal-pressure hydrocephalus will manifest repeated brief episodes of raised ICP if ventricular pressure is monitored continuously and especially if an overnight period of recording is included. This form of normal-pressure hydrocephalus is sometimes referred to as intermittent pressure or occult hydrocephalus. For the most part the causes of ventricular enlargement are obstructive, malreabsorptive or postatrophic. In theory, the ventricles can also enlarge if there is an overproduction of CSF beyond the capacity of the system to absorb it. Thus, some authors refer to hypersecretory hydrocephalus in the specific case of papillomas of the choroid plexus, rare examples of which have been shown to be associated with an excess of secretion of CSF.[48] Referral to Davson's equation (see above) demonstrates that even a five-fold increase in CSF production rate will only increase ICP by about 12 mmHg. However, such lesions not infrequently shed debris into the CSF, which may impede CSF absorption at the arachnoid villi and granulations or block off either the occipital horn of the

ipsilateral ventricle or, through midline shift, the contralateral ventricle. There may, therefore, also be an obstructive and a malreabsorptive element even in this form of hydrocephalus.

In the past, otitic hydrocephalus was used to refer to the development of raised ICP associated with middle ear infection that was complicated by sigmoid sinus thrombosis. This mechanism was considered to be but one of a number of possible causes of the condition of benign intracranial hypertension (see below).

Finally, external hydrocephalus has sometimes been used to describe a phenomenon of excessive CSF within the head, not in the ventricular system but over the surface of the brain. This condition predominantly occurs in young children and may be associated with asymptomatic macrocephaly. There is debate as to whether the excess fluid is in the subarachnoid or the subdural space. Treatment is only indicated if the head circumference continues to increase across percentiles or the child fails to progress through the developmental milestones. External hydrocephalus should not be confused with the widened cortical sulci associated with cerebral atrophy.

Functional anatomy and physiology of the CSF pathway

For an understanding of the pathophysiology of hydrocephalus it is necessary to review briefly the anatomy and histology of the meninges and the normal dynamics of the CSF system (see above). For more extensive information, the reviews of Davson *et al.*,[43] Russell,[186] Fishman,[59] McComb,[128] Williams *et al.*,[245] McKinnon.,[130] Weller *et al.*[231–233] and Ekstedt[50] may be consulted.

The meninges

The brain and spinal cord are enclosed by three layers of connective tissue known as the meninges, which are derived from a variety of embryonic structures. These include the neural crest for the telencephalic meninges, the cephalic mesoderm for the brainstem meninges, and the somatic mesoderm for the spinal meninges.[25,158] The outermost layer (pachymeninges) or dura mater is closely attached to the periosteum of the inner skull. In contrast, the spinal dura mater and vertebral periosteum are distinct structures separated by the spinal epidural space which contains the inner vertebral venous (Batson's) plexuses. At the base of the skull, a connective tissue bridge has recently been described between the dura mater and the rectus capitis posterior minor muscle, which extends from the first cervical vertebra to the occipital bone.[210] The dura mater is composed of dense fibres of collagen and elastic fibres arranged in laminae, and contains numerous small blood vessels. Within the skull, the dura mater is reflected to fold inwards as four septi which divide the cranial cavity into communicating spaces within which the main subdivisions of the brain are lodged: the falx cerebri, the tentorium cerebelli, the falx cerebelli and the diaphragma sellae. The first two of these are of major importance in relation to brain swelling and herniation (see above). These dural folds separate to form the cerebral venous sinuses, which are lined by endothelium and are involved in the drainage of blood from the cerebral, meningeal and diploic veins, and in the reabsorption of CSF (see below). The dura mater contains pressure and stretch receptors, and is innervated by sensory and postganglionic sympathetic nerves, the latter being involved in vasomotor regulation.[245] The inner aspect of the dura mater is closely attached to the outer layer of the arachnoid mater, previously known as the subdural mesothelium,[5] from which it can be separated to form a subdural space.

The inner layers, or leptomeninges, comprise the arachnoid and pia mater. The arachnoid mater consists of a subdural mesothelial layer and a compact central layer.[5] The cells of the central region of the arachnoid mater are polygonal with round nuclei and pale cytoplasm. These tightly packed cells possess desmosomes and intercellular tight junctions which form a barrier to the diffusion of substances into the subdural space.[5] The inner layer of the arachnoid is also composed of mesothelial cells and is vis-

ible as a translucent film over the surface of the brain and spinal cord. The cerebral part of the arachnoid mater covers the brain loosely and does not enter the sulci. The subarachnoid space, between the inner arachnoid and pia mater, is traversed by fine arachnoidal trabeculae, which are reflected over extracerebral and spinal blood vessels. This leptomeningeal coat over the blood vessels is then reflected on the surface of the cerebrum and spinal cord as the pia mater.[82] The relationship between these structures is illustrated in Fig. 4.29. The space is enlarged in several areas where the course of the arachnoid mater does not closely follow the surface of the underlying brain. These enlarged spaces are known as the subarachnoid cisterns, the largest of which (the cisterna magna) is continuous below with the subarachnoid space of the spinal cord.

The cells of the arachnoid mater form small aggregates known as the arachnoid granulations, which occur in clusters near the intracranial venous sinuses (particularly the superior sagittal sinus) and within the walls of veins associated with spinal nerve roots.[105] These granulations protrude into the sinuses and increase in size and number with age. In extreme old age, they may cause pressure atrophy of the skull, producing small pits on the internal aspect of the cranium. At the base of the granulations, narrow necks of arachnoid mater project into the venous sinus by

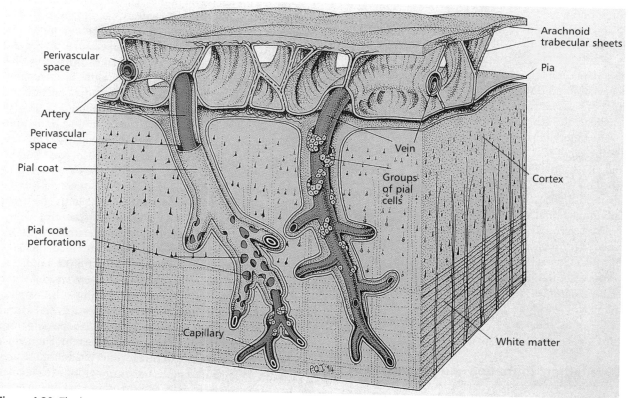

Figure 4.29 *The leptomeninges. Diagrammatic representation of the interrelationships between the leptomeninges and blood vessels entering and leaving the cerebral cortex. The subarachnoid space is divided by trabeculae and a layer of pia mater accompanies each artery as it enters the cortex. As the arterial diameter decreases, the pial coating becomes perforated and finally disappears at the capillary level. The perivascular space between the artery and the pia mater inside the brain is continuous with the perivascular space around the meningeal vessels. Veins do not have a similar coating of pia mater. Reproduced by permission from Weller.[230]*

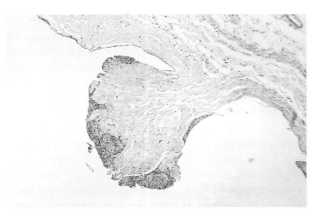

Figure 4.30 *Arachnoid villus. This consists of a core of collagenous tissue containing numerous fine channels, overlaid by the arachnoidal cap through which CSF is absorbed into the venous system. (H&E.)*

apertures in their dural lining. These expand to form the arachnoid villi, which comprise a core of collagenous tissue with a complex network of channels lined by compacted collagen and occasional macrophages (Fig. 4.30). These cores are overlaid by arachnoid caps, each around 150 μm thick, and composed of mesothelial cells which are attached to the endothelium lining the sinus.[105,215] The CSF is absorbed into the venous sinuses through various apertures, one-way valves within the arachnoid villi; the rate of absorption is directly proportional to the pressure difference between the CSF and the dural venous sinuses.[37,42,124,228,229] The cells of the arachnoid cap contain more abundant cytoplasm than other arachnoidal cells and form syncytial sheets which may contain small psammoma bodies.[214] These features are recapitulated in meningiomas, which are thought to originate from these cells.

The inner lining of the meninges, the pia mater, is also composed of loose connective tissue containing collagen and elastic fibres surrounding a thin intact sheet of flattened mesothelial cells which possess desmosomes and gap junctions.[82] The cerebral pia mater covers the whole surface of the brain, including the complex infoldings of the cerebral gyri and cerebellar foliae, and becomes invaginated to form the tela choroidea of the cerebral ventricles. The pia mater is reflected over the surface of small blood vessels entering and leaving the surface of the brain; a subpial space has been defined ultrastructurally which communicates with the perivascular space around blood vessels of the cerebrum.[105] The pia mater around the spinal cord has a similar structure.[150]

Distribution, formation and absorption of CSF

The normal CSF volume in an adult is approximately 140 ml, of which 20 ml is located in the lateral ventricles, 5 ml in the third, aqueduct and fourth ventricles, and the remainder in the subarachnoid space, the majority lying in the spinal canal. The rates of formation and absorp-

tion of CSF remain in balance under normal conditions. Whereas the rate of formation remains constant under most physiological conditions, the rate of absorption varies according to the level of ICP, which can therefore adjust to keep the system in overall balance (see above). CSF is produced at the rate of approximately 0.35 ml/min; this rate is reduced when the cerebral metabolic rate falls, and can be affected by a number of drugs and by the level of blood flow through the blood vessels of the choroid plexus.[43]

More than 75% of the daily CSF production is from the choroid plexus which lies within the lateral, third and fourth ventricles. This is formed by invagination of the ependyma into the ventricular system by the blood vessels of the pia mater. Choroid plexus epithelium is a single row of cuboidal cells folded into villi with a brush border of microvilli on the ventricular surface. The formation of CSF by the choroid plexus involves two distinct processes, filtration through the fenestrated capillaries of the choroid plexus into its interstitial spaces, and active secretion by the endothelium. Active transport of sodium over the choroidal epithelial wall depends on Na^+/K^+ATPase-pumps, which are energy dependent and may be blocked by ouabain. The passage of water from blood to the CSF is osmotically tied to sodium transport. Carbonic anhydrase is also presumed to play a role in this process because CSF secretion is markedly reduced by carbonic anhydrase inhibitors, e.g. the drug Acetazolamide.[185] Formation rates of CSF may also be inhibited by diuretic drugs, reduction of temperature and brain metabolism, changes in CSF osmolality and CPP below the autoregulatory threshold, which results in a reduction in CBF.[190] There is also an extrachoroidal contribution to CSF formation, which may simply represent seepage of fluid from the interstitial space of the brain into the ventricular system across into the ependyma. This contribution can, however, be considerably increased under certain conditions. For example, high levels of CSF production can follow ablation of large portions of the choroid plexus, a procedure carried out in the past that was generally unsuccessful in attempts to control hydrocephalus.[137] CSF production remains relatively constant provided that cerebral perfusion pressure is adequate.

CSF circulates as the result of a force from behind, created by active secretion, together with expansion of the cerebral mantle during systole and the impact of respiratory and postural changes in venous pressure. CSF circulates slowly through the ventricular system, passing from the lateral and third ventricles via the cerebral aqueduct into the fourth ventricle. The aqueduct in adults measures around 15 mm in length and varies from a triangular shape in its rostral aspect to an oval region with a centre 2 mm in diameter, ending with a T-shaped outline adjacent to the fourth ventricle.[245] The CSF leaves the ventricular system by the exit foramina in the fourth ventricle, the midline foramen of Magendie and the lateral foramina of Luschka that open into the subarachnoid space in the cerebellopontine angle. The CSF flows from there over the surface of the brain and spinal cord within the subarachnoid space to be absorbed into the venous system by the arachnoid villi (see above).

CSF absorption is a passive process through the arachnoid granulations into the superior sagittal sinus and the venous drainage of the spinal root sleeves, and increases with rising CSF pressure according to Davson's equation (see above). Since the pressure within the posterior parts of the cerebrovenous sinuses does not increase substantially during intracranial hypertension in the adult, a considerable pressure gradient can develop between CSF and venous blood in these areas. Tripathi[211] and Levine et al.[122] showed that the pathway for absorption of CSF consists of pressure-sensitive microvesicles that enlarge and link to form open channels as the pressure gradient increases. Thus, absorption of CSF by bulk flow can increase rapidly in patients with lesions associated with raised ICP, to make a major contribution to spatial compensation. One of the striking features in patients who die of major space-occupying lesions is an obliteration of the subarachnoid space and reduction in size of the ventricles. In addition to CSF reabsorption into venous sinuses, there is increasing evidence for lymphatic drainage of CSF both in experimental models and in man.[103,232] CSF can be transported through the cribriform plate into the nasal submucosa, where it is absorbed by cervical lymphatics.[14,198] Experimental blockage of this pathway reduces CSF clearance, and it has been suggested recently that this pathway may represent the major route of CSF absorption at low or normal ICP.[144] This view challenges the traditional concepts of CSF absorption via arachnoid villi and further studies are required to assess its functional significance in man.[15]

When there is an obstruction to CSF outflow, it is possible for CSF to be absorbed transependymally. In cases of high-pressure hydrocephalus, the periventricular lucency observed on CT scans and termed interstitial brain oedema is considered to be an example of this process (Fig. 4.15). However, in the elderly, such periventricular lucency is more likely to represent gliosis, infarction or demyelination (see below on normal-pressure hydrocephalus).

Pathogenesis of ventricular enlargement and cortical atrophy

Although the rate of CSF absorption varies with changes in ICP, while the rate of CSF production remains constant over a wide range of values of ICP, an equilibrium is established in the normal subject which corresponds to that point where CSF formation and absorption rates are equal: the ventricular system is of normal volume at the normal level of ICP. When the system is perturbed, new equilibrium levels may be set at which CSF formation and absorption are once again in balance, but in which the ventricular system may be larger or smaller and the ICP may be normal or elevated. It seems clear that as long as CSF is produced at 20 ml/h, an imbalance between the formation and absorption cannot be sustained for long, and elevated CSF pressure is found only in the more florid examples of obstructive or acute malresorptive hydrocephalus.

Experimental hydrocephalus has been produced by injection of silicon oils or kaolin into the cisterna magna.[235,236] This produces progressive ventricular enlargement associated with disruption of the ependyma, interstitial oedema and destruction of nerve fibres in the periventricular white matter. The ventricular enlargement occurs over a period of weeks, but after 10 weeks the ventricular enlargement becomes constant, a state of arrested hydrocephalus has occurred and there is re-establishment of a continuous (although attenuated) ependymal lining. Periventricular oedema reduces, but there is a persisting decrease in the number of axons and a corresponding increase in glial tissue in the periventricular brain. Similar features have been found in man.[234] If ventricular drainage is established even at this late stage, reduction in ventricular size occurs with restoration of all or part of the thickness of the cerebral mantle.

Cerebral cortical atrophy in chronic hydrocephalus was usually thought to be due to a combination of factors, including direct pressure effects and oedema. However, the contribution of cerebral ischaemia has been increasingly recognized, and recent magnetic resonance spectroscopic studies have shown changes in high-energy phosphate metabolism, intracellular pH and lactate production which reflect cerebral ischaemia.[17] Further information on the mechanisms of neuronal damage has come from

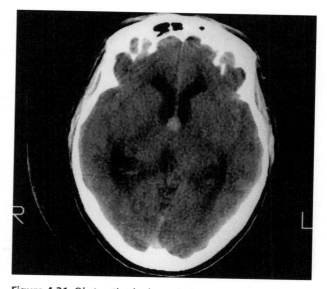

Figure 4.31 *Obstructive hydrocephalus: at the third ventricle. Cranial CT scan showing hydrocephalus with dilated lateral ventricles due to obstruction of the third ventricle by a colloid cyst, which appears as a hyperdense round lesion (centre). Courtesy of Dr R Gibson, Western General Hospital, Edinburgh, UK.*

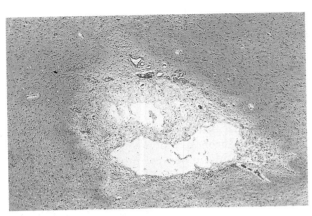

Figure 4.32 *Obstructive hydrocephalus: at the aqueduct of Sylvius. Post-inflammatory aqueduct stenosis resulting from cytomegalovirus infection in infancy is characterized by partial obstruction of the aqueduct by an irregular accumulation of glial tissue, surrounded by numerous ependymal proliferations forming small canalicular structures. (H&E.)*

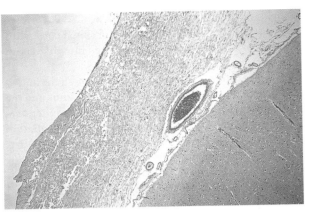

Figure 4.34 *Obstructive hydrocephalus: in the subarachnoid space. Fibrous obliteration of the subarachnoid space following partially treated pneumococcal meningitis, which resulted in hydrocephalus due to impaired CSF resorption. (H&E.)*

studies of soluble Fas (CD95/Apo-1) in the CSF in hydrocephalus, with increased levels suggesting that an apoptotic mechanism may be responsible for neuronal loss.[55]

Causes of hydrocephalus in man

Obstructive hydrocephalus affecting the lateral ventricles only may be the result of a colloid cyst of the third ventricle (Fig. 4.31), intraventricular haemorrhage or progressive enlargement of suprasellar tumours to invaginate the anterior part of the third ventricle. These include pituitary adenoma, craniopharyngioma, meningioma and astrocytoma.

Obstruction of the posterior end of the third ventricle and aqueduct may be due to aqueduct stenosis (Fig. 4.32), or to tumours or other lesions in the pineal region or

affecting the tectal plate. Lesions within the fourth ventricle which may affect CSF flow include choroid plexus papilloma, medulloblastoma and ependymoma (Fig. 4.33). Cerebellar tumours such as astrocytomas and haemangioblastomas, as well as infective lesions such as cerebellar abscess, may produce sufficient distortion and compression of the fourth ventricle to result in proximal hydrocephalus.

Obstruction of the outlet of the fourth ventricle may result from acute inflammatory exudate related to meningitis, chronic inflammation (as in sarcoidosis) or aggregation of neoplastic cells in cases of carcinomatous meningitis. Organization and fibrosis around the outlet of the fourth ventricle are also common complications after subarachnoid haemorrhage. Under these circumstances, the production of fibroblasts and extracellular matrix problems may be stimulated by the release of transforming growth factor-β_1 into the CSF. This has been observed recently in a recent study of neonatal hydrocephalus after intraventricular haemorrhage, where it may explain the failure of conventional fibrinolytic therapy.[237]

Obstruction to the flow of CSF across the tentorial hiatus may be caused by large tumours in the cerebellopontine angle, such as acoustic Schwannoma (Fig. 4.28), while obstruction to CSF reabsorption may also be a sequel to severe subarachnoid haemorrhage or meningitis,[51] as organization of haemorrhage or inflammatory exudate proceeds within the arachnoid granulations (Fig. 4.34).

More unusual causes of hydrocephalus include vascular lesions, such as ectasia of the basilar artery or aneurysmal dilatation of the great vein of Galen. Communicating hydrocephalus has many causes (see Table 4.2).

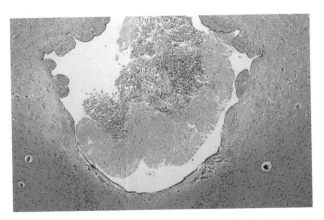

Figure 4.33 *Obstructive hydrocephalus: at the fourth ventricle. Autopsy specimen from a patient who died following a severe posterior fossa head injury. Necrotic cerebellar tissue occludes the fourth ventricle and had resulted in obstructive hydrocephalus. (H&E.)*

Normal-pressure hydrocephalus

This term is commonly used for a syndrome in elderly individuals, classically characterized by disturbance of gait,

Table 4.2 *Types of communicating hydrocephalus*

(a) Defects of flow in the subarachnoid space
  Leptomeningeal inflammation
    infections
    pyogenic
    tuberculosis
    haemorrhage
  Subarachnoid haemorrhage secondary to aneurysm or
  arteriovenous malformation
  Head injury
  Craniotomy
  Meningitis carcinomatosis
  Foreign matter
  Cockayne's syndrome[21]
  Tonsillar elongation/prolapse basilar impression (Paget's)
  Masses (neoplastic and non-neoplastic)

(b) Defects of absorption of CSF at the arachnoid
granulations
  Congenital deficiency of arachnoid granulation
  Raised cerebral venous sinus pressure
  GM2 gangliosidosis[157]

(c) Abnormalities of the CSF
  Excessive production or abnormally high intraventricular
  CSF pulse pressure
  Choroid plexus papilloma
  Increased CSF viscosity secondary to high protein content
  (e.g. spinal neurofibromas, Guillain–Barré)

(d) Idiopathic

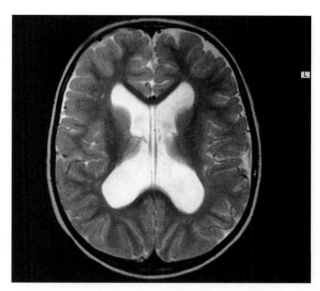

Figure 4.35 *Normal pressure hydrocephalus. T2-weighted cranial MRI scan in a 44-year-old female with normal-pressure hydrocephalus, showing symmetrical ventricular dilatation with no other structural abnormality. Courtesy of Dr R Gibson, Western General Hospital, Edinburgh, UK.*

progressive dementia associated with slowing of cognitive processes and urinary incontinence (through a combination of urgency, inability to reach the toilet in time and lack of concern).[4] Cases have been described in childhood and adolescence,[18] while in many patients (regardless of age) the principal symptom is gait impairment, with subtle and occasionally unrecognized cognitive deterioration[166,216] (see also Chapter 4, Volume II). Normal-pressure hydrocephalus (NPH) is seldom the cause of severe dementia alone in adults. Overall, cognitive function but not frontal executive function may improve after CSF diversion in over 70% of patients with normal-pressure hydrocephalus secondary to a known cause, but in only 30–50% of idiopathic cases[72,83] (Fig. 4.35). Although the lateral ventricles are widely enlarged (Fig. 4.8), the mean CSF pressure at lumbar puncture is not elevated. In patients who respond to shunting, however, continuous monitoring of ICP can demonstrate episodes of moderate intracranial hypertension, often in the form of B-waves, particularly during sleep.[166] In some patients there is a known possible antecedent cause such as head injury, subarachnoid haemorrhage, ischaemic vascular encephalopathy or meningitis,[72,166] but in some cases no cause can be found even after post-mortem examination.

The CSF dynamics of this state have been widely studied by a number of investigators who have proposed that the causative mechanism in normal-pressure hydro-

cephalus is an increase in CSF outflow resistance.[12,13,49,125] This leads to a resetting of the equilibrium with the re-establishment of a normal CSF production and absorption after a period of increased ICP which then returns to normal, but with ventricular enlargement persisting.[147] It has also been claimed that regional CBF in this condition is altered as a consequence of the altered CSF hydrodynamic state, particularly in the subcortical white matter and the frontotemporal cortex.[113] However, it is very difficult to measure white-matter blood flow in patients with very dilated ventricles, so such observation requires corroboration with modern imaging techniques.[159]

The clinical importance of this syndrome is that in a proportion of cases a dramatic improvement in the patient's clinical status may follow an operation to shunt CSF from the lateral ventricles or the lumbar subarachnoid space into the peritoneal cavity. Cognition but not frontal executive function may return to normal, the gait improves and urinary continence is restored.[67,83,170,216] The higher the CSF outflow resistance, the greater the probability that the patient will respond to a shunt. The absence of deep white-matter lesions on MRI is also a good prognostic sign. There is a large amount of literature which is difficult to interpret because of a failure to characterize the patients in a uniform way and to ensure that the CSF shunt is patent post-operatively.[24,67,170,217] Finally, there are patients with continued dementia who have a remediable hydrocephalic component to their condition, combined with cerebrovascular disease, Alzheimer's disease, etc. Pre-existing hypertensive cerebrovascular disease may predispose to the development of normal-pressure hydrocephalus through changes in the physical properties of the cerebral mantle. Any benefit from shunting in patients with combined

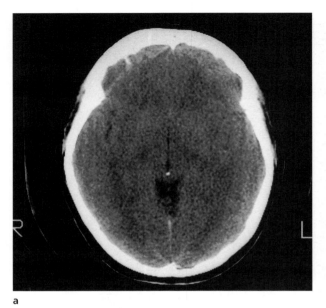 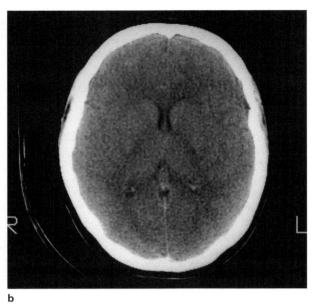

a

b

Figure 4.36 *Benign intracranial hypertension. Contrast-enhanced cranial CT scan in a case of benign intracranial hypertension, showing a symmetrical reduction in size of the lateral ventricles, with narrowing of the third ventricle and basal cisterns. Courtesy of Dr R Gibson, Western General Hospital, Edinburgh, UK.*

normal-pressure hydrocephalus will be undermined by the natural history of progression of the other components. Great care has to be taken when managing patients with normal-pressure hydrocephalus, as they are often fragile. The advent of programmable valves has helped to reduce the risk of subdural haematomas.

Benign intracranial hypertension (idiopathic, intracranial hypertension; pseudotumour cerebri)

This term is used for a small group of patients (1:100 000 population) in whom symptoms and signs of raised ICP occur without a demonstrable cause. Papilloedema and headache occur commonly, sometimes accompanied by palsy of the VIth cranial nerve.[171] Many cases present as a chronic progressive disorder, but acute and subacute presentations have been recognized, sometimes in the absence of detectable papilloedema.[96] Most cases occur in adult females, often associated with obesity,[96,221] but presentations in childhood have been reported in the absence of obesity, but with other associated conditions.[194] A wide range of associated disorders has been reported in adults and children, including obesity, coagulopathy, endocrine diseases, hypervitaminosis A and tetracycline use, but the majority of cases appear to be idiopathic.[171] Neurological studies reveal a normal ventricular system or sometimes ventricles that are smaller than normal (Fig. 4.36). Since the comprehensive reviews by Foley[63] and Johnston and Paterson[94] the important relationship between raised ICP and papilloedema has been confirmed and it has been recognized that consciousness may be pre-

served in patients with benign intracranial hypertension, despite pressures in excess of 60 mmHg. Because ICP is evenly distributed throughout the craniospinal axis in this condition, there are no ICP gradients, nor is there any shift or herniation of the brain.

Benign intracranial hypertension does not represent a single clinical entity but it is the endpoint of several different pathological processes, all of which cause raised ICP and none of which causes brain shift or herniation except after surgical intervention. Four mechanisms have been proposed to explain benign intracranial hypertension:[87,93,176,200,206] diffuse cerebral oedema, increased cerebral blood volume, hypersecretion of CSF and impaired CSF absorption. There is little evidence for diffuse cerebral oedema or CSF hypersecretion. In extensive, angiographic investigations of a group of patients with benign intracranial hypertension, Janny and his colleagues[87] found that in half of their cases there was evidence of occlusion of at least one of the major dural venous sinuses, and high CSF outflow resistance has also been implicated as a causative factor.[93] With the recent availability of magnetic resonance angiography and imaging sequences that allow the specific delineation of venous flow patterns, it has become well established that a number of cases of benign intracranial hypertension, but not all, are indeed associated with segmental occlusions within the major dural venous sinuses (Fig. 4.37).[98]

There is evidence for impaired CSF absorption, but not in all patients. Impaired CSF absorption may be a more important mechanism in patients with normal venous sinuses. For the present, however, the causes of intracranial hypertension in patients in whom venous occlusion is not identified remain a mystery. Treatment

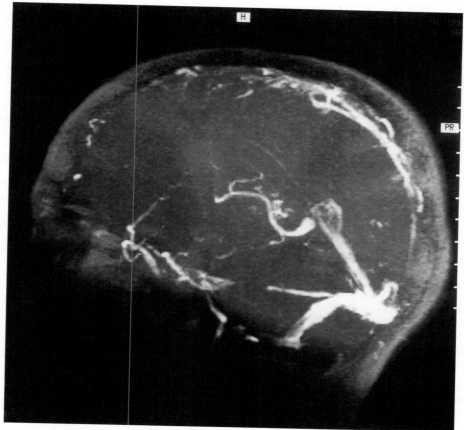

Figure 4.37 *Benign intracranial hypertension. Cranial MRI venogram in a patient with benign intracranial hypertension showing absence of flow in the anterior portion of the superior sagittal sinus and adjacent cortical veins as a consequence of venous thrombosis. Courtesy of Dr R Gibson, Western General Hospital, Edinburgh, UK.*

includes weight reduction for the obese, diuretics including Acetazolamide, ventriculoperitoneal or lumboperitoneal shunting (with the risk in the latter of secondary Chiari malformation), optic nerve sheath fenestration, bitemporal decompression and, most recently, venous stenting for patients with transverse sinus stenosis.[77]

Acknowledgement

This chapter is an update of that written by the late and much missed Professor J Douglas Miller, and Professor James Ironside for the previous edition.

REFERENCES

1 Abbott NJ. Inflammatory mediators and modulation of blood–brain barrier permeability. *Cell Mol Neurobiol* 2000; **20**: 131–47.

2 Adachi M, Feigin I. Cerebral oedema and the water content of normal white matter. *J Neurol Neurosurg Psychiatry* 1966; **29**: 446–50.

3 Adams JH, Graham DI. The relationship between ventricular fluid pressure and the neuropathology of raised intracranial pressure. *Neuropathol Appl Neurobiol* 1976; **2**: 323–32.

4 Adams RD, Fisher CM, Hakim S et al. Symptomatic occult hydrocephalus with 'normal' cerebrospinal fluid pressure. *N Engl J Med* 1965; **273**: 117–26.

5 Alcolado R, Weller RO, Parrish E, Garrod D. The cranial arachnoid and pia mater in man: anatomical and ultra-structural observations. *Neuropathol Appl Neurobiol* 1988; **14**: 1–18.

6 Aldrich EF, Eisenberg HM, Saydjari C et al. Diffuse brain swelling in severely head inured children. A report from the NIH Traumatic Coma Data Bank. *J Neurosurg* 1992; **76**: 450–4.

7 Arieff AI. Hyponatremia, convulsions, respiratory arrest and permanent brain damage after elective surgery in healthy women. *N Engl J Med* 1986; **314**: 1529–35.

8 Avezaat CJJ, Eindhoven JHM van, Wyper DJ. Cerebrospinal fluid pulse pressure and intracranial volume–pressure relationships. *J Neurol Neurosurg Psychiatry* 1979; **42**: 687–700.

9 Bell BA, Symon L, Branston NM. CBF and time thresholds for the formation of ischemia, cerebral edema and effect of reperfusion in baboons. *J Neurosurg* 1985; **62**: 31–41.

10 Bergmann E von. Über den Hirndruck. *Arch Klin Chir* 1885; **32**: 705–32.

11 Bordley J, Cushing H. Observations on chocked disc with special reference to decompressive cranial operations. *JAMA* 1909; **52**: 353–64.

12 Borgesen SE, Gjerris F. Relationship between intracranial pressure, ventricular size and resistance to CSF outflow. *J Neurosurg* 1987; **67**: 535–9.

13 Borgesen SE, Gjerris F. The predictive value of conductance to outflow of CSF in normal pressure hydrocephalus. *Brain* 1982; **105**: 65–86.

14 Boulton M, Armstrong D, Flessner M *et al*. Raised intracranial pressure increases CSF drainage through arachnoid villi and extracranial lymphatics. *Am J Physiol* 1998; **275**: 889–96.

15 Boulton M, Flessner M, Armstrong D *et al*. Contribution of extracranial lymphatics and arachnoid villi to the clearance of a CSF tracer in the rat. *Am J Physiol* 1999; **276**: 818–23.

16 Bradbury M. *The concept of a blood–brain barrier*. Chichester: John Wiley, 1979.

17 Braun KP, Vandertop WP, Goodkens RH *et al*. NMR spectroscopic evaluation of cerebral metabolism in hydrocephalus: a review. *Neurol Res* 2000; **22**: 51–64.

18 Bret P, Chazal J. Chronic ('normal pressure') hydrocephalus in childhood and adolescence. A review of 16 cases and reappraisal of the syndrome. *Childs Nerv Syst* 1995; **11**: 687–91.

19 Browder J, Meyers R. Behaviour of systemic blood pressure, pulse rate and spinal fluid pressure associated with acute changes in intracranial pressure artificially produced. *Arch Surg* 1938; **35**: 1–19.

20 Browder J, Meyers R. Observations on the behaviour of the systemic blood pressure, pulse and spinal fluid pressure following craniocerebral injury. *Am J Surg* 1936; **31**: 403–27.

21 Brumback RA, Yoder FW, Andrews AD *et al*. Normal pressure hydrocephalus. Recognition and relationship to neurological abnormalities in Cockayne's syndrome. *Arch Neurol* 1978; **35**: 337–45.

22 Bullock R, Maxwell WL, Graham DI *et al*. Glial swelling following human cerebral contusion: an ultrastructural study. *J Neurol Neurosurg Psychiatry* 1991; **54**: 427–34.

23 Burrows G. *On disorders of the cerebral circulation and on the connection between affections of the brain and diseases of the heart*. London: Longman, Brown, Green & Longman, 1846: 55–6.

24 Caruso R, Cervoni L, Vitale AM, Salvati M. Idiopathic normal-pressure hydrocephalus in adults: result of shunting correlated with clinical findings in 18 patients with a review of the literature. *Neurosurg Rev* 1997; **20**: 104–7.

25 Catala M. Embryonic and fetal development of structures associated with the cerebrospinal fluid in man and other species. Part I: The ventricular system, meninges and choroid plexuses. *Arch Anat Cytol Pathol* 1998; **46**: 153–69.

26 Cazaubon SM, Couraud PO. Nitric oxide and endothelin at the blood–brain barrier. In: Partridge WM ed. *Introduction to the blood–brain barrier*. Cambridge: Cambridge University Press, 1998: 338–44.

27 Chen Y, McCarron RM, Ohara Y *et al*. Human brain capillary endothelium: 2-arachidonoglycerol (endocannabinoid) interacts with endothelin-1. *Circ Res* 2000; **87**: 323–7.

28 Clasen RA, Cooke PM, Pandolfi S, Boyd D, Raimondi AJ. Experimental cerebral edema produced by focal freezing. *J Neuropathol Exp Neurol* 1962; **21**: 579–96.

29 Clasen RA, Pandolfi S, Laing I, Casey D. Experimental study of relation of fever to cerebral edema. *J Neurosurg* 1974; **41**: 576–81.

30 Cohen AR, Wilson J. Magnetic resonance imaging of Kernohan's notch. *Neurosurgery* 1990; **27**: 205–7.

31 Connor RCR. Heart damage associated with intracranial lesions. *BMJ* 1968; **iii**: 29–31.

32 Corsellis JAN. Individual variation in the size of the tentorial opening. *J Neurol Neurosurg Psychiatry* 1958; **21**: 279–83.

33 Cserr HF, Depasquale M, Patlak CS. Convection of cerebral interstitial fluid and its role in brain volume regulation. *Ann N Y Acad Sci* 1989; **481**: 123–34.

34 Cushing H. Peptic ulcers and the interbrain. *Surg Gynecol Obstet* 1932; **55**: 1–34.

35 Cushing H. Some experimental and clinical observations concerning rates of increased intracranial tension. *Am J Med Sci* 1902; **124**: 375–400.

36 Cushing H. Some principles of cerebral surgery. *JAMA* 1909; **52**: 184–95.

37 Cutler RWP, Page LK, Galicich J, Watters GV. Formation and absorption of cerebrospinal fluid in man. *Brain* 1968; **91**: 707–20.

38 Czosynka M, Richards HK, Czosnyka Z *et al*. Vascular components of cerebrospinal fluid compensation. *J Neurosurg* 1999; **90**: 732–9.

39 Czosnyka M, Smielewski P, Kirkpatrick PJ *et al*. Continuous assessment of the cerebral vasomotor reactivity in head injuries. *Neurosurgery* 1997; **41**: 11–19.

40 Czosnyka M, Smielewski P, Piechnik S. Hemodynamic characterisation of intracranial pressure plateau waves in head injured patients. *J Neurosurg* 1999; **91**: 11–19.

41 Czosnyka M, Whitehouse H, Smielewski P *et al*. Testing of cerebrospinal compensatory reserve in shunted and non-shunted patients: a guide to interpretation based on an observational study. *J Neurol Neurosurg Psychiatry* 1996; **60**: 549–58.

42 Davson H, Hollingsworth G, Segal MB. The mechanism of drainage of the cerebrospinal fluid. *Brain* 1970; **93**: 665–78.

43 Davson H, Welch K, Segal M. *Physiology and pathology of cerebrospinal fluid*. Edinburgh: Churchill Livingstone, 1987.

44 Ducker TB. Control of brain endothelial permeability. *Cerebrovasc Brain Metab Rev* 1968; **3**: 39–72.

45 Duffy TE, Howse DC, Plum F. Cerebral energy metabolism during experimental status epilepticus. *J Neurochem* 1975; **24**: 925–33.

46 Duret H. *Études expérimentales et cliniques sur les traumatismes cérébraux*. Paris: Delahaye, 1878.

47 Easton AS, Fraser PA. Arachidonic acid increases cerebral microvascular permeability by free radicals in single pial microvessels of the anaesthetized rat. *J Physiol* 1998; **507**: 541–7.

48 Eisenberg HM, McComb JG, Lorenzo AV. Cerebrospinal fluid overproduction and hydrocephalus associated with choroid plexus papilloma. *J Neurosurg* 1974; **40**: 381–5.

49 Ekstedt J. CSF hydrodynamic studies in man. *J Neurol Neurosurg Psychiatry* 1978; **41**: 345–53.

50 Ekstedt J. CSF hydrodynamic studies in man. 2. Normal hydrodynamic variables related to CSF pressure and flow. *J Neurol Neurosurg Psychiatry* 1978; **41**: 345–53.

51 Ellington E, Margolis G. Block of arachnoid villus by subarachnoid haemorrhage. *J Neurosurg* 1969; **30**: 651–7.

52 Esiri MM. *Oppenheimer's diagnostic neuropathology* 2nd edn. Oxford: Blackwell Science, 1996: 26–7.

53 Evans JP. Increased intracranial pressure: its physiology and management. *Surg Clin North Am* 1956; **36**: 233–42.

54 Fein JM. Hypertension and the central nervous system. *Clin Neurosurg* 1982; **29**: 666–721.

55 Felderhoff-Mueser U, Herold R, Hochhaus F *et al*. Increased cerebrospinal fluid concentrations of soluble Fas (CD95.Apo-1) in hydrocephalus. *Arch Dis Child* 2001; **84**: 369–72.

56 Feldman E, Gandy SE, Becker R *et al*. MRI demonstrates descending transtentorial herniation. *Neurology* 1988; **39**: 622–7.

57 Finney LA, Walker AE. *Transtentorial herniation*. Springfield, IL: Thomas, 1962.

58 Fishman RA. Brain edema. *N Engl J Med* 1975; **293**: 706–11.

59 Fishman RA. *Cerebrospinal fluid in diseases of the nervous system*. Philadelphia, PA: WB Saunders, 1980.

60 Fitch W, McDowall DG. Effect of halothane on intracranial pressure gradients in the presence of intracranial space-occupying lesions. *Br J Anaesth* 1971; **43**: 904–12.

61 Fitch W, McDowall DG. System vascular responses to increased intracranial pressure. *J Neurol Neurosurg Psychiatry* 1977; **40**: 833–42.

62 Flexner LB, Clark JH, Weed LH. The elasticity of the dural sac and its contents. *Am J Physiol* 1932; **101**: 292–303.

63 Foley J. Benign forms of intracranial hypertension – 'toxic' and otitic hydrocephalus. *Brain* 1955; **78**: 1–41.

64 Frost EAM. Respiratory problems associated with head trauma. *Neurosurgery* 1977; **1**: 300–6.

65 Go KG. The normal and pathological physiology of brain water. *Adv Techn Stand Neurosurg* 1997; **23**: 47–142.

66 Goldstein GW. Endothelial cell–astrocyte interactions. A cellular model of the blood–brain barrier. *Ann NY Acad Sci* 1988; **529**: 31–9.

67 Graff-Radford NR, Godersky JC, Jones MP. Variables predicting surgical outcome in symptomatic hydrocephalus in the elderly. *Neurology* 1989; **39**: 1601–4.

68 Greenwood J. Mechanisms of blood–brain barrier breakdown. *Neuroradiology* 1991; **33**: 95–100.

69 Gudeman SK, Wheeler CB, Miller JD et al. Gastric secretory and mucosal injury response to severe head trauma. *Neurosurgery* 1983; **12**: 175–9.

70 Guillaume J, Janny P. Manometric intracrannienne contuivé: interest de la methods et premiers resultants. *Rev Neurol* 1951; **84**: 131–42.

71 Hahm H, Ferzt R, Muller J, Cervos-Navarro J. Topography of diffuse brain edema. In: Cervos-Navarro J, Ferzt R eds. *Brain edema – pathology, diagnosis and therapy*. New York: Raven Press, 1980: 299–316.

72 Hakim S, Adams RD. The special clinical problems of symptomatic hydrocephalus with normal cerebrospinal pressure. *J Neurol Sci* 1965; **2**: 307–27.

73 Halloran LG, Zfass AM, Gayle WE et al. The prevention of acute gastrointestinal complications after severe head injury. *Am J Surg* 1980; **139**: 44–8.

74 Hassler O. Arterial pattern of human brain stem. Normal appearance and deformation in expanding supratentorial conditions. *Neurology* 1967; **17**: 368–75.

75 Hawkins WE, Clower BR. Myocardial damage after head trauma in simulated intracranial haemorrhage in mice: the role of the autonomic nervous system. *Cardiovasc Res* 1971; **5**: 524–9.

76 Hayreh SS. Pathogenesis of oedema of the optic disc (papilloedema). *Br J Ophthalmol* 1964; **48**: 522–43.

77 Higgins JNP, Owler BK, Cousins C, Pickard JD. Venous sinus stenting for refractory benign intracranial hypertension. *Lancet* 2001; **259**: 228–30.

78 Hochwald GM, Marlin AE, Wald A, Malhan C. Movement of water between blood, brain and CSF in cerebral edema. In: Pappius HM, Feindel W eds. *Dynamics of brain edema*. Berlin: Springer, 1976: 29–31.

79 Hoff JT, Mitchell RA. The effect of hypoxia on the Cushing response. In: Brock M, Dietz H eds. *Intracranial pressure*. Berlin: Springer, 1972: 205–9.

80 Hoff JT, Reis DJ. Localization of regions mediating the Cushing response in the central nervous system of the cat. *Arch Neurol* 1970; **22**: 228–40.

81 Howell DA. Upper brain stem compression and foraminal impaction with intracranial space-occupying lesions and brain swelling. *Brain* 1959; **82**: 525–50.

82 Hutchings M, Weller RO. Anatomical relationships of the pia mater to the cerebral blood vessels in man. *J Neurosurg* 1986; **65**: 316–25.

83 Iddon JL, Pickard JD, Cross JJL et al. Specific patterns of cognitive impairment in patients with idiopathic normal pressure hydrocephalus and Alzheimer's disease: a pilot study. *J Neurol Neurosurg Psychiatry* 1999; **67**: 723–31.

84 Inomata M, Yoshioka T, Nasu F, Mayahara H. Ultracytochemical studies of capillary endothelial cells in the rat central nervous system. *Acta Anat* 1984; **118**: 243–8.

85 Ishii S. Brain swelling. In: Caveness WE, Walker AE eds. *Head injury*. Philadelphia, PA: Lippincott, 1966: 276–99.

86 Ishii S, Hayner R, Kelly WA, Evans JP. Studies of cerebral swelling. II. Experimental cerebral swelling produced by supratentorial extradural compression. *J Neurosurg* 1959; **16**: 152–66.

87 Janny P, Chazel J, Colnet G. Benign intracranial hypertension and disorders of the CSF absorption. *Surg Neurol* 1981; **15**: 168–74.

88 Janzer RC, Friede RL. Perisulcal infarcts: lesions caused by hypotension during increased intracranial pressure. *Ann Neurol* 1979; **6**: 339–404.

89 Janzer RC, Raff MC. Astrocytes induce blood–brain barrier properties in endothelial cells. *Nature* 1987; **325**: 2513–17.

90 Jefferson G. The tentorial pressure cone. *Arch Neurol Psychiatry* 1938; **40**: 857–76.

91 Jennett WB, Stern WE. Tentorial herniation, the mid-brain and pupil. Experimental studies in brain compression. *J Neurosurg* 1960; **17**: 598–608.

92 Johnson RT, Yates PO. Brain stem haemorrhages in expanding supratentorial conditions. *Acta Radiol (Stockh)* 1956; **46**: 250–6.

93 Johnston I. The reduced CSF absorption syndrome: a reappraisal of benign intracranial hypertension and related conditions. *Lancet* 1973; **iii**: 418–20.

94 Johnston I, Paterson A. Benign intracranial hypertension II. CSF pressure and circulation. *Brain* 1974; **97**: 301–12.

95 Johnston IH, Rowan JO. Raised intracranial pressure and cerebral blood flow. 4. Intracranial pressure gradients and regional cerebral blood flow. *J Neurol Neurosurg Psychiatry* 1974; **37**: 585–92.

96 Jones JS, Nevai J, Freeman MP, McNinch DE. Emergency department presentation of idiopathic intracranial hypertension. *Am J Emerg Med* 1999; **17**: 517–21.

97 Kalaria RN, Harik SI. Blood–brain barrier monoamine oxidase: enzyme characterization in cerebral microvessels and other tissues from six mammalian species, including human. *J Neurochem* 1987; **49**: 856–64.

98 Karahalios DG, Rekate HL, Khayata MH. Elevated intracranial venous pressure as a universal mechanisms in pseudotumour cerebri of varying etiologies. *Neurology* 1996; **46**: 198–202.

99 Kaufmann GE, Clark K. Continuous simultaneous monitoring of intraventricular and cervical subarachnoid cerebrospinal fluid pressure to investigate the development of cerebral or tonsillar herniation. *J Neurosurg* 1970; **33**: 145–50.

100 Kellie G. An account of the appearances observed in the dissection of two of three individuals presumed to have perished in the storm of the 3rd and whose bodies were discovered in the vicinity of Leith on the morning of 4th November 1821, with some reflections on the pathology of the brain. *Trans Med Chir Soc Edin* 1824; **1**: 84–169.

101 Kernohan JW, Woltman HW. Incisura of the crus due to contralateral brain tumour. *Arch Neurol Psychiatry* 1929; **21**: 274–87.

102 Kida S, Ellison DW, Steart V, Weller RO. Characterisation of perivascular cells in astrocytic tumours and peritumoural oedematous brain. *Neuropathol Appl Neurobiol* 1995; **21**: 121–9.

103 Kida S, Pantazis A, Weller RO. CSF drains directly from the subarachnoid space into nasal lymphatics in the rat. Anatomy, histology and immunological significance. *Neuropathol Appl Neurobiol* 1993; **19**: 480–8.

104 Kida S, Weller RO, Zhang E-T et al. Anatomical pathways for lymphatic drainage of the brain and their pathological significance. Neuropathol Appl Neurobiol 1995; 21: 181–4.

105 Kida S, Yamashima T, Kubota T et al. A light and electron microscopic and immunohistochemical study of human arachnoid villi. J Neurosurg 1988; 69: 429–35.

106 Kirkham FJ, Levin SD, Padaychee J. Transcranial pulsed Doppler ultrasound findings in brainstem death. J Neurol Neurosurg Psychiatry 1987; 50: 1504–13.

107 Klatzo I. Neuropathological aspects of brain edema. J Neuropathol Exp Neurol 1967; 26: 1–14.

108 Klatzo I. Pathophysiological aspects of brain edema. In: Reulen HJ, Schurmann K eds. Steroids and brain edema. Berlin: Springer, 1972: 1–8.

109 Klintworth GK. Secondary brain stem haemorrhage. J Neurol Neurosurg Psychiatry 1966; 29: 423–5.

110 Klintworth GK. The pathogenesis of secondary brain stem hemorrhage as studied with an experimental model. Am J Pathol 1965; 47: 525–36.

111 Knopf PM, Cserr SC, Nolan T et al. Physiology and immunology of lymphatic drainage of interstitial and cerebrospinal fluid from the brain. Neuropathol Neurobiol 1995; 21: 175–80.

112 Kocher T. Hirnerschütterung, Hirndruck und chirurgische Eingriffe bein Hirnerkrankungen. In: Nothnagel: Specialle Pathologie und Therapie Vol. I9, Part 3. Vienna: Holder, 1885: 92–134.

113 Kristensen B, Malm J, Fagerland M et al. Regional cerebral blood flow, white matter abnormalities, and cerebrospinal fluid hydrodynamics in patients with idiopathic adult hydrocephalus syndrome. J Neurol Neurosurg Psychiatry 1996; 60: 282–8.

114 Langfitt TW. Increased intracranial pressure. Clin Neurosurg 1969; 16: 436–71.

115 Langfitt TW, Kassell NF, Weinstein JD. Cerebral blood flow with intracranial hypertension. Neurology 1965; 15: 761–73.

116 Langfitt TW, Weinstein JD, Kassell NF. Cerebral vasomotor paralysis produced by intracranial hypertension. Neurology 1965; 15: 632–41.

117 Langfitt TW, Weinstein JD, Kassell NF, Galiardi W. Transmission of increased intracranial pressure II. Within the supratentorial space. J Neurosurg 1964; 21: 998–1005.

118 Langfitt TW, Weinstein JD, Kassell NF, Simeone FA. Transmission of increased intracranial pressure I. Within the craniospinal axis. J Neurosurg 1964; 21: 989–97.

119 Le Beau J. L'oedème du Cerveau. Paris: Recht, 1938.

120 Leech PJ, Miller JD. Intracranial volume/pressure relationships during experimental brain compression in primates. II Effect of induced changes in arterial pressure. J Neurol Neurosurg Psychiatry 1974; 37: 1099–104.

121 Levett JM, Johns LM, Replogie RL, Mullan S. Cardiovascular effects of experimental cerebral missile injury in primates. Surg Neurol 1980; 13: 59–64.

122 Levine JE, Povlishock JT, Becker DP. The morphological correlates of primate cerebrospinal fluid absorption. Brain Res 1982; 241: 31–41.

123 Lindenberg R. Compression of brain arteries as a pathogenic factor for tissue necrosis and their areas of predilection. J Neuropathol Exp Neurol 1955; 14: 233–43.

124 Lorenzo AV, Page LK, Watters GV. Relationship between cerebrospinal fluid formation, absorption and pressure in human hydrocephalus. Brain 1970; 93: 679–92.

125 Lorenzo AW, Bresnan MJ, Barlow CF. Cerebrospinal fluid absorption defect in normal pressure hydrocephalus. Arch Neurol 1974; 30: 387–93.

126 Lund-Anderson H. Transport of glucose from blood to brain. Physiol Rev 1991; 59: 305–53.

127 Lundberg N. Continuous recording and control of ventricular fluid pressure in neurosurgical practice. Acta Psychiatr Neurol Scand 1960; 36: 1–193.

128 McComb JG. Recent research into the nature of the cerebrospinal fluid formation and absorption (Review article). J Neurosurg 1983; 59: 369–83.

129 MacKenzie ET, Stragaard S, Graham DI et al. Effects of induced hypertension in cats on pial arteriolar calibre, local cerebral blood flow and the blood brain barrier. Circ Res 1976; 39: 33–41.

130 McKinnon SG. Anatomy of the cerebral veins, dural sinuses, sella, meninges, and CSF spaces. Neuroimag Clin North Am 1998; 8: 101–17.

131 Marmarou A, Maset AL, Ward JD. Contribution of CSF and vascular factors to elevation of ICP in severely head injured patients. J Neurosurg 1987; 66: 883–90.

132 Marmarou A, Shulman K, Rosende RM. A non-linear analysis of the CSF system and intracranial pressure dynamics. J Neurosurg 1978; 48: 332–44.

133 Martinez-Hernendez A, Amenta PS. The basement membrane in pathology. Lab Invest 1983; 48: 656–77.

134 Mayhan WG. Nitric oxide donor-induced increase in permeability of the brain barrier. Brain Res 2000; 866: 101–8.

135 Meinig G, Reulen HJ, Magavly C. Regional cerebral blood flow and cerebral perfusion pressure in global brain edema induced by water intoxication. Acta Neurochir 1973; 29: 1–13.

136 Meyer A. Herniation of the brain. Arch Neurol Psychiatry 1920; 4: 387–400.

137 Milhorat TH. Failure of choroid plexectomy as treatment for hydrocephalus. Surg Gynecol Obstet 1974; 139: 505–8.

138 Miller JD. Clinical management of cerebral oedema. Br J Hosp Med 1979; 20: 152–66.

139 Miller JD. Effects of hypercapnia on pupillary size, intracranial pressure and cerebral venous PO_2 during experimental brain compression. In: Lundberg N, Ponten U, Brock M eds. Intracranial pressure II. Berlin: Springer, 1975: 444–6.

140 Miller JD. Vasoconstriction as head injury treatment – right or wrong? Intens Care Med 1994; 20: 249–50.

141 Miller JD, Stanek A, Langfitt TW. Concepts of cerebral perfusion pressure and vascular compression during intracranial hypertension. Prog Brain Res 1972; 35: 411–32.

142 Miller Fisher C. Brain herniation: a revision of classical concepts. Can J Neurol Sci 1995; 22: 83–91.

143 Miver JD, Garibi J, Pickard JD. Induced changes of cerebrospinal fluid volume. Effects during continuous monitoring of ventricular fluid pressure. Arch Neurol 1973; 28: 265–9.

144 Mollanji R, Bozanovic-Sosic R, Silver I et al. Intracranial pressure accommodation is impaired by blocking pathways leading to extracranial lymphatics. Am J Physiol Regul Integr Comp Physiol 2001; 5: 1573–81.

145 Monro A. Observations on the structure and function of the nervous system. Edinburgh: Creech & Johnston, 1783.

146 Moore MT, Stern K. Vascular lesions of the brain stem and occipital lobe occurring in association with brain tumours. Brain 1938; 61: 70–81.

147 Mori K, Mima T. To what extent has the pathophysiology of normal-pressure hydrocephalus been clarified? Crit Rev Neurosurg 1998; 20: 232–43.

148 Muizelaar JP, Lutz HA, Becker DP. Effect of mannitol on intracranial pressure and cerebral blood flow and correlation with pressure autoregulation in severely head-injured patients. J Neurosurg 1984; 61: 700–6.

149 Muizelaar JP, Marmarou A, Ward JD *et al*. Adverse effects of prolonged hyperventilation in patients with severe head injury: a randomised controlled trial. *J Neurosurg* 1991; **75**: 731–9.

150 Nicholas DS, Weller RO. The fine anatomy of the human spinal meninges. A light and scanning electron microscopic study. *J Neurosurg* 1988; **69**: 276–82.

151 Nordstrom CH, Messeter K, Sundberg G. Cerebral blood flow, vasoreactivity and oxygen consumption during barbiturate therapy in severe traumatic brain lesions. *J Neurosurg* 1988; **68**: 424–31.

152 North JB, Jennett S. Abnormal breathing patterns associated with acute brain damage. *Arch Neurol* 1974; **31**: 338–44.

153 North JB, Jennett S. Response of ventilation and of intracranial pressure during rebreathing of carbon dioxide in patients with acute brain damage. *Brain* 1976; **99**: 169–82.

154 O'Brien MD, Waltz AG. Intracranial pressure gradients caused by experimental cerebral ischaemia and edema. *Stroke* 1973; **4**: 694–8.

155 Ohata K, Marmarou A. Clearance of brain edema and macromolecules through the cortical extracellular space. *J Neurosurg* 1992; **77**: 387–96.

156 Oldendorf WH, Canford WE, Brown WJ. The age apparent work capability of the blood–brain barrier: a study of the mitochondrial content of the capillary endothelial cells in brain and other tissues of the rat. *Ann Neurol* 1977; **1**: 409–17.

157 O'Neill B, Butler AB, Young E *et al*. Adult-onset GM2 gangliosidosis. Seizures, dementia, and normal pressure hydrocephalus associated with glycolipid storage in the brain and arachnoid granulation. *Neurology* 1978; **28**: 1117–23.

158 O'Rahilly R, Muller F. The meninges in human development. *J Neuropathol Exp Neurol* 1986; **45**: 588–608.

159 Owler B, Pickard JD. Normal pressure hydrocephalus and cerebral blood flow: a review. *Acta Neurol Scand* 2001; **104**: 325–42.

160 Papadopoulos MC, Sasdoun S, Davies DC, Bell BA. Emerging molecular mechanisms of brain tumour oedema. *Br J Neurosurg* 2001; **15**: 101–8.

161 Pappius HM. Fundamental aspects of brain oedema. In: Vinken PJ, Bryn GW eds. *Handbook of clinical neurology. Part I, Tumours of the brain and skull*. New York: Elsevier, 1974: 167–85.

162 Pardridge WM. Brain metabolism: a perspective from the blood–brain barrier. *Physiol Rev* 1983; **63**: 1481–535.

163 Paulson OB, Strangaard J, Edvinsson L. Cerebral autoregulation. *Cerebrovasc Brain Metab Rev* 1990; **2**: 161–92.

164 Penn RD. Cerebral edema and neurological function: CT, evoked responses and clinical examination. In: Cervos-Navarro J, Ferzt R eds. *Brain edema – pathology, diagnosis and therapy*. New York: Raven Press, 1980: 383–94.

165 Petito CK, Schaefer JA, Plum F. The blood brain barrier in experimental seizures. In: Pappius HM, Feindel W eds. *Dynamics of brain edema*. Berlin: Springer, 1976: 38–42.

166 Pickard JD. Adult communicating hydrocephalus. *Br J Hosp Med* 1982; **27**: 35–44.

167 Plum F, Posner JB. *The diagnosis of stupor and coma* 3rd edn. Philadelphia, PA: Davis, 1980.

168 Povlishock JT. The pathophysiology of blood–brain barrier dysfunction due to traumatic brain injury. In: Partridge WM ed. *Introduction to the blood–brain barrier*. Cambridge: Cambridge University Press, 1998: 441–53.

169 Povlishock JT, Becker DP, Sullivan HG, Miller JD. Vascular permeability alterations to horseradish peroxidase in experimental brain injury. *Brain Res* 1978; **153**: 223–39.

170 Raftopoulos C, Deleval J, Chaskis C *et al*. Cognitive recovery in idiopathic normal pressure hydrocephalus: a prospective study. *Neurosurgery* 1994; **35**: 397–405.

171 Ramadan NM. Headache caused by raised intracranial pressure and intracranial hypotension. *Curr Opin Neurol* 1996; **9**: 214–18.

172 Rapoport SI. *Blood brain barrier in physiology and medicine*. New York: Raven Press, 1976.

173 Rapoport SI, Robinson PJ. Tight junctional modification as the basis of osmotic opening of the blood brain barrier. *Ann N Y Acad Sci* 1986; **481**: 250–66.

174 Reese TS, Kamovsky MJ. Five structural localisations of the blood–brain barrier to exogenous peroxidase. *J Cell Biol* 1967; **34**: 207–17.

175 Reichardt M. Über Hirnschwellung. *Z Gesamte Neurol Psychiatrie* 1911; **3**: 1–43.

176 Reid AC, Matheson MS, Teasdale G. Volume of the ventricles in benign intracranial hypertension. *Lancet* 1980; **ii**: 7–8.

177 Reid WL, Cone WV. The mechanism of fixed dilation of the pupil resulting from ipsilateral cerebral compression. *JAMA* 1939; **112**: 2030–4.

178 Reulen HJ, Graham R, Spatz M and Klatzo I. Role of pressure gradients and bulk flow in dynamics of vasogenic brain edema. *J Neurosurg* 1977; **46**: 24–35.

179 Reulen HJ, Tsuyumu M, Tack A *et al*. Clearance of edema fluid in cerebrospinal fluid. *J Neurosurg* 1978; **48**: 754–64.

180 Ropper AH. Lateral displacement of the brain and level of consciousness in patients with an acute hemispheral mass. *N Engl J Med* 1986; **314**: 953–8.

181 Ropper AH. Syndrome of transtentorial herniation: is vertical displacement necessary? *J Neurol Neurosurg Psychiatry* 1993; **56**: 932–5.

182 Rosenberg GA, Estrada E, Wesley M, Kyner WT. Autoradiographic patterns of brain interstitial fluid flow after collagenase-induced haemorrhage in rat. *Acta Neurochir Suppl* 1990; **51**: 280–2.

183 Rosner MJ, Becker DP. Origins and evolutions of plateau waves. Experimental observations and theoretical model. *J Neurosurg* 1984; **60**: 312–24.

184 Rothfus WE, Goldberg AL, Tabas JH, Deeb ZL. Callosomarginal infarction secondary to transfalial herniation. *Am J Neuroradiol* 1987; **8**: 1073–6.

185 Rubin RC, Henderson ES, Ommaya AK *et al*. The production of cerebrospinal fluid in man and its modification by acetazolamide. *J Neurosurg* 1966; **25**: 430–6.

186 Russell DS. Observations on the pathology of hydrocephalus. *Special Report Series of the Medical Research Council* 1949; **265**.

187 Ryder HW, Espey FF, Kimball FD *et al*. Effect of changes in systemic venous pressure on the cerebrospinal fluid pressure. *Arch Neurol Psychiatry* 1952; **68**: 175–9.

188 Ryder HW, Espey FF, Kimball FD *et al*. Influence of changes in cerebral blood flow on the cerebrospinal fluid pressure. *Arch Neurol Psychiatry* 1952; **68**: 165–9.

189 Ryder HW, Espey FF, Kimball FD *et al*. Mechanism of the change in cerebrospinal fluid pressure following an induced change in the volume of the fluid space. *J Lab Clin Med* 1953; **41**: 428–35.

190 Sahar A, Hochwald GM, Ransohoff J. Experimental hydrocephalus: cerebrospinal fluid formation and ventricular size as a function of intraventricular pressure. *J Neurol Sci* 1970; **11**: 81–91.

191 Scheinker IM. Transtentorial herniation of the brain stem; a characteristic clinicopathologic syndrome: pathogenesis of hemorrhages in the brain stem. *Arch Neurol Psychiatry* 1945; **53**: 289–98.

192 Schettini A, Walsh EK. Pressure relaxation of the intracranial system *in vivo*. *Am J Physiol* 1973; **225**: 513–17.

193 Schilling L, Wahl M. Mediators of cerebral edema. *Adv Exp Med Biol* 1999; **474**: 123–41.

194 Scott IU, Siatkowski RM, Eneyni M *et al*. Idiopathic intracranial hypertension in children and adolescents. *Am J Ophthalmol* 1997; **124**: 253–5.

195 Shalit MN, Reinmuth OM, Shimoyo S, Scheinberg P. Carbon dioxide and cerebral circulatory control III. The effects of brain stem lesions. *Arch Neurol* 1967; **17**: 342–53.

196 Shivers RR, Arthur FE, Bowman PD. Induction of gap junctions and brain enthothelium-like tight junctions in cultured bovine endothelial cells: local control of cell specialization. *J Submicrosc Cytol* 1988; **20**: 1–14.

197 Shutta HS, Lassell NF, Langfitt TW. Brain swelling produced by injury and aggravated by arterial hypertension – a light and electron microscopic study. *Brain* 1968; **9**: 281–94.

198 Silver I, Li B, Szalai J, Johnston M. Relationship between intracranial pressure and cervical lymphatic pressure and flow rates in sheep. *Am J Physiol* 1999; **277**: 1712–17.

199 Smyth GE, Henderson WR. Observations on the cerebrospinal fluid pressure on simultaneous ventricular and lumbar punctures. *J Neurol Psychiatry* 1938; **1**: 226–37.

200 Sorensen PS, Thomsen C, Gjerris F *et al*. Increased brain water content in pseudotumour cerebri measured by magnetic resonance imaging of the brain water self diffusion. *Neurol Res* 1989; **11**: 160–4.

201 Stanimirovic D, Satoh K. Inflammatory mediators of cerebral endothelium: a role in brain inflammation. *Brain Pathol* 2000; **10**: 113–26.

202 Stern WE, Coxon RV. Osmolality of brain tissue and its relation to brain bulk. *Am J Physiol* 1964; **206**: 1–7.

203 Stewart PA, Hayakawa K, Farrell CL. Quantitation of blood–brain barrier ultrastructure. *Microsc Res Techn* 1994; **27**: 516–27.

204 Stewart PA, Hayakawa K, Farrell CL, Del Maestro RF. Quantitative study of microvessel ultrastructure in human peritumoral brain tissue. *J Neurosurg* 1987; **67**: 697–705.

205 Sunderland S. The tentorial notch and complications produced by herniation through that aperture. *Br J Surg* 1958; **45**: 422–38.

206 Sussman J, Sarkies NJ, Pickard JD. Benign intracranial hypertension. *Adv Techn Stand Neurosurg* 1998; **24**: 261–305.

207 Takizawa H, Gabra-Sanders T, Miller JD. Analysis of changes in intracranial pressure and pressure volume index at different locations in the craniospinal axis during supratentorial epidural balloon inflation. *Neurosurgery* 1986; **19**: 1–8.

208 Teasdale E, Cardos E, Galbraith S, Teasdale G. CT scan in severe diffuse head injury: physiological and clinical correlations. *J Neurol Neurosurg Psychiatry* 1984; **47**: 600–3.

209 Thompson RK, Malina S. Dynamic axial brain stem distortion as a mechanism explaining the cardiorespiratory changes in increased intracranial pressure. *J Neurosurg* 1959; **16**: 664–75.

210 Thompson VP. Anatomical research lives! *Nat Med* 1995; **i**: 297–8.

211 Tripathi R. Tracing the bulk outflow route of cerebrospinal fluid by transmission and scanning electron microscopy. *Brain Res* 1974; **80**: 503–11.

212 Tso MOM, Hayreh SS. Optic disc edema in raised intracranial pressure III. A pathologic study of experimental apapilledema. *Arch Ophthalmol* 1977; **95**: 1148–57.

213 Tsukita S, Furuse M, Itoh M. Molecular dissection of tight junctions: occludin and ZO-1. In: Partridge WM ed. *Introduction to the blood–brain barrier*. Cambridge: Cambridge University Press, 1998: 322–9.

214 Upton ML, Weller RO. The morphology of cerebrospinal fluid drainage pathways in human arachnoid granulations. *J Neurosurg* 1985; **63**: 867–75.

215 Uzan M, Yentur E, Hanci M *et al*. Is it possible to recover from uncal herniation? Analysis of 71 head injured cases. *J Neurosurg Sci* 1998; **42**: 89–94.

216 Vanneste JAL. Diagnosis and management of normal-pressure hydrocephalus. *J Neurol* 2000; **247**: 5–14.

217 Vanneste JAL. Three decades of normal pressure hydrocephalus: are we wiser now? *J Neurol Neurosurg Psychiatry* 1994; **57**: 1021–5.

218 Venero JL, Vizute ML, Machado A, Cano J. Aquaporins in the central nervous system. *Prog Neurobiol* 2001; **63**: 321–36.

219 Vincent C, David M, Thiebault F. Le cône de pression temporal dans les tumeurs des hémisphères cérébraux. Sa symptomatologie: sa gravité: les traitments qu'il convient de lui opposer. *Rev Neurol* 1936; **65**: 536–45.

220 Wahl M, Unterberg A, Baethmann A, Schilling L. Mediators of blood–brain barrier dysfunction and formation of vasogenic brain oedema. *J Cereb Blood Flow Metab* 1988; **8**: 621–34.

221 Wall M. Idiopathic intracranial hypertension: mechanisms of visual loss and disease management. *Semin Neurol* 2000; **20**: 89–95.

222 Walsh EK, Schettini A. Elastic behaviour of brain tissue *in vivo*. *Am J Physiol* 1976; **230**: 1058–62.

223 Wang W, Dentler WL, Borchardt RT. VEGF increases BMEC monolayer permeability by affecting occluding expression and tight junction assembly. *Am J Physiol Heart Circ Physiol* 2001; **280**: 434–40.

224 Weed LH. Some limitations of the Monro–Kellie hypothesis. *Arch Surg* 1929; **18**: 1049–68.

225 Weed LH, McKibben PS. Pressure changes in cerebrospinal fluid following intravenous injection of solutions of various concentrations. *Am J Physiol* 1919; **48**: 512–30.

226 Weinstein JD, Langfitt TW, Bruno L *et al*. Experimental study of patterns of brain distortion and ischaemia produced by an intracranial mass. *J Neurosurg* 1968; **28**: 513–21.

227 Weinstein JD, Langfitt TW, Kassell JF. Vasopressor response to increased intracranial pressure. *Neurology* 1964; **14**: 1118–31.

228 Welch K, Friedman V. The cerebrospinal fluid valves. *Brain* 1960; **83**: 454–69.

229 Welch K, Pollay M. Perfusion of particles through arachnoid villi of the monkey. *Am J Physiol* 1961; **201**: 651–4.

230 Weller RO. Fluid compartments and fluid balance in the central nervous system. In: Williams PL ed. *Gray's anatomy* 38th edn. Edinburgh: Churchill Livingstone, 1995: 1202–23.

231 Weller RO. Pathology of cerebrospinal fluid and interstitial fluid of the CNS: significance for Alzheimer disease, prion disorders and multiple sclerosis. *J Neuropathol Exp Neurol* 1998; **57**: 885–94.

232 Weller RO, Kida S, Zhang E-T. Pathways of fluid drainage from the brain – morphological aspects and immunological significance in rat and man. *Brain Pathol* 1992; **2**: 277–84.

233 Weller RO, Massey A, Kuo YM, Roher AE. Cerebral amyloid angiopathy: accumulation of A beta in interstitial fluid drainage pathways in Alzheimer's disease. *Ann N Y Acad Sci* 2000; **903**: 110–17.

234 Weller RO, Shulman K. Infantile hydrocephalus: clinical, histological and ultrastructural study of brain damage. *J Neurosurg* 1972; **36**: 255–65.

235 Weller RO, Wisniewski H. Histological and ultrastructural changes with experimental hydrocephalus in adult rabbits. *Brain* 1969; **92**: 819–28.

236 Weller RO, Wisniewski H, Shulman K, Terry RD. Experimental hydrocephalus in young dogs: histological and ultrastructural study of the brain tissue damage. *J Neuropathol Exp Neurol* 1971; **30**: 613–24.

237 Whitelaw A, Christie S, Pople I. Transforming growth factor-beta1: a possible signal molecule for posthemorrhagic hydrocephalus? *Pediatr Res* 1999; **46**: 576–80.

238 Whittle IR. Origins and management of peritumoural brain dysfunction. *Neurosurg Q* 1992; **2**: 174–98.

239 Whittle IR, Clark M, Gregori A *et al*. Interstitial white matter brain edema does not alter the electroencephalogram. *Br J Neurosurg* 1992; **6**: 433–7.

240 Whittle IR, Piper IR, Ironside J, Miller JD. Neuropathological and neurophysiological effects of interstitial white matter autologous and non-autologous protein-containing solutions. Further evidence for a glioma-derived permeability factor. *Acta Neurochir* 1993; **120**: 164–74.

241 Whittle IR, Piper IR, Miller JD. The contribution of arachidonic acid to the etiology and pathophysiology of vasogenic brain edema. Studies using an infusion edema model. *Acta Neurochir* 1991; **113**: 57–68.

242 Whittle IR, Piper IR, Miller JD. The role of bradykinin in the etiology of vasogenic brain edema and perilesional brain dysfunction. *Acta Neurochir* 1992; **115**: 53–9.

243 Whittle IR, Viswanathan R. Acute intraoperative brain herniation during elective neurosurgery: pathophysiology and management considerations. *J Neurol Neurosurg Psychiatry* 1996; **61**: 584–90.

244 Wijdicks EF, Miller GM. Transient locked-in syndrome after uncal herniation. *Neurology* 1999; **12**: 1296–7.

245 Williams PL, Warwick R, Dyson M, Bannister LH. *Gray's anatomy – neurology*. Edinburgh: Churchill-Livingstone, 1989.

246 Wittschafter JD, Rizzo FJ, Smiley BC. Optic nerve axoplasm and papilledema. *Surv Ophthalmol* 1975; **20**: 157–89.

5

Hypoxia and related conditions

ROLAND N. AUER AND GARNETTE R. SUTHERLAND

INTRODUCTION

When considering the pathogenesis of brain damage, hypoxia is often equated with ischaemia, although they are biochemically and pathologically quite different. The hallmark, defining feature of ischaemia is impairment of the blood supply, while hypoxia can be defined most generally as a reduction in either oxygen supply or oxygen use, to a level that does not sustain normal cellular metabolism. Even cursory reflection suggests that hypoxia is different, in that it might not significantly impair cerebral blood flow (CBF). In most forms of hypoxia, CBF is in fact increased. Therefore, the pathophysiology of hypoxia and ischaemia must be considered separately. This chapter will review ventilation, circulation, respiration and cerebral energy metabolism, all components of the delivery of oxygen to intracellular loci where it chemically reacts to sustain biological processes. Neuronal mechanisms of injury will be discussed, in an attempt to explain the pathogenesis of selective neuronal necrosis, while sparing glia and blood vessels. A classification of hypoxia will be given, emphasizing which forms of hypoxia cause cerebral necrosis, as well as the non-necrotizing adaptations to chronic hypoxia.

Some definitions and comments on terminology are in order at the outset. The word 'hypoxia' has a number of possible meanings, each of which carries more precision than the unqualified term. Hypoxia can be classified based on the normal pathway of delivery and utilization of the molecule. Hypoxic, anaemic and histotoxic thus describe hypoxic states in which, respectively, oxygen supply, blood oxygen transport or tissue utilization of oxygen are impaired. Precision of terminology is helpful here (Table 5.1). Hypoxaemia denotes low blood oxygen content, and anoxaemia (an impossibility) zero blood oxygen content. Anoxia is a term often used, but no oxygen whatsoever is also impossible in aerobic, living biological systems. What could be correctly described by anoxia is zero ambient oxygen, as in human inhalation of pure nitrogen.[286]

Hypoxia is often combined with the term ischaemia, although hypoxaemia usually does not accompany ischaemia. These authors decry the use of the term 'hypoxia/ischaemia' or 'hypoxia–ischaemia' for several reasons. First, hypoxia and focal ischaemia rarely occur together clinically. Secondly, these terms mix two separate pathophysiological entities and cloud thinking about brain events that transpire in each insult. Lastly, pure hypoxaemia to the brain can result in coma from which recovery is eminently possible, whereas prolonged coma after global ischaemia carries a grave prognosis. Since pure hypoxia tends to occur in younger patients, recognition of a pure hypoxic insult, without accompanying ischaemia, is important in determining a clinical prognosis. Clinically and pathophysiologically, hypoxia needs to be distinguished from ischaemia.

Attempts are often made to define precise thresholds below which damage consistently takes place. In stagnant hypoxia (global ischaemia), there is not an absolute threshold below which damage regularly occurs at all ages, in all brain locations. Instead, damage depends on the presence or absence of crucial biochemical events that may transpire at different thresholds of age, temperature, blood glucose level, ischaemic duration and depth, all interacting. Magnetic resonance imaging (MRI) and MR spectroscopy illustrate the effect of hypoxia and ischaemia on brain chemistry, structure and function, and can help to define thresholds of tissue damage. This chapter also

Table 5.1 *Hypoxia: definitions and terms*

Term	Meaning	Necrosis in brain tissue	Comment
Hypoxia	Low oxygen, not further specified (tissue, blood, atmosphere)	See specific entities	Unqualified, not a useful term
Hypoxia/ischaemia or hypoxia–ischaemia	Combination of hypoxia and ischaemia	If hypoxia is superadded to ischaemia, necrosis is exacerbated	Widely used, non-specific term combining hypoxia and ischaemia. Cardiac arrest encephalopathy or global ischaemia is a better term, if that is what is meant
Hypoxaemia	Low oxygen in blood	Reversible synaptic alterations, but without neuronal cell body necrosis	Seen in respiratory tract disease (larynx, trachea, bronchi, bronchioles), not in pure cardiovascular disease. Tends to occur in younger patients
Hypobaric hypoxia	Hypoxaemia accompanying ↓ ambient P_{O_2}	Reversible synaptic alterations (at very high altitudes), but without neuronal cell body necrosis	Temporary synaptic alterations produce 'high altitude stupid' (HAS) syndrome, with impaired thinking and decision making, which reverses on descent to lower altitudes
Anoxia	No oxygen	Not a specific or useful term by itself	Carries no specific meaning in the intact organism
Anoxaemia	No oxygen in blood	Impossible to assess in intact animal	An impossibility, without cardiac bypass and removal of all blood O_2
Anaemic hypoxia	Low blood haemoglobin	No brain-damaging potential	Actually protective for stroke owing to favourable rheology[284,320,345,597]
Histotoxic hypoxia	Tissue utilization of oxygen impaired	No brain-damaging potential without accompanying hypotension	Examples: poisoning by cyanide, sulfide, azide
Carbon monoxide poisoning	CO in blood, displacing O_2 from haemoglobin binding sites	Necrosis in pallidoreticularis, plus typical ischaemic distribution	Complex triad effected: (1) anaemia (occupation of haemoglobin binding sites by CO), (2) histotoxic hypoxia (by binding to Fe-rich globus pallidus), and (3) stagnant hypoxia due to heart failure
Stagnant hypoxia	Low tissue P_{O_2} due to global ischaemia	Necrosis (both pan-necrosis and selective neuronal necrosis) in well-defined distributions	Not often used term, conceptually focusing on ↓ tissue P_{O_2} in global ischaemia

discusses selective vulnerability, a fascinating principle that holds in most of neuropathology, whereby exposure of the entire brain to an insult nevertheless gives rise to damage in remarkably restricted and unique places that are characteristic for each type of brain insult.

OXYGEN DELIVERY AND METABOLISM

The entire process of delivery of oxygen to the brain can be envisaged as a cascade, the partial pressure of oxygen (P_{O_2}) decreasing in steps from the ambient air, through the lungs, blood and finally to the brain itself (Fig. 5.1). Each step in this cascade allows oxygen molecules to 'flow down' a portion of the gradient, allowing further delivery of oxygen to the tissue. At sea level, these steps give rise to an overall drop in P_{O_2} from 158 mmHg in ambient air (21% × 760 mmHg), to approximately 28–30 mmHg as the normal value for tissue P_{O_2} in non-ischaemic brain. Values for focal oxygen in mitochondria are even lower.

Ventilation

Vertebrates can absorb oxygen directly from their body surfaces only a very short distance into the skin. This mechanism would suffice for minute organisms, but the utilization of a capillary system in the tissue allows delivery and diffusion of oxygen to loci deep within a larger body. Ventilation and circulation deliver oxygen from outside the body to where oxygen is needed in the tissue,

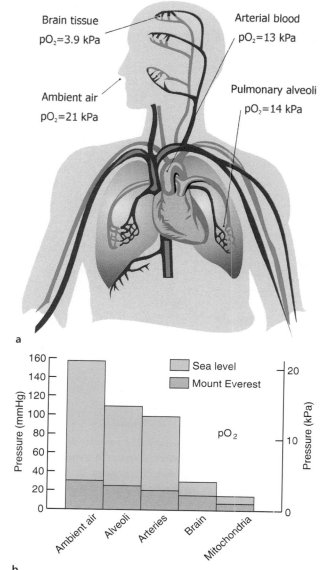

Figure 5.1 *Oxygen cascade. (a) Brain tissue receives oxygen from ambient air only after it passes from outside the body through ventilatory and circulatory systems, each delivering the molecule at successively reduced partial pressures, finally to reach brain tissue, where P_{O_2} is lowest. (b) There is a progressive 'oxygen cascade' with oxygen running down a gradient to brain mitochondria, where oxygen is utilized. In the cascade, the lowest oxygen tensions are in the brain mitochondria. Note that on Mount Everest, ambient P_{O_2} equals the brain tissue P_{O_2} at sea level, and the steps in the oxygen cascade are considerably flattened. The lowest recorded arterial P_{O_2} in a living human was 1 kPa (7.5 mmHg) and the corresponding venous P_{O_2} was 0.27 kPa (2 mmHg),[232] and the cascade under such conditions would involve only very small steps.*

allowing the existence of vertebrate organisms of any size from mouse to whale.

Skeletal muscles draw air into the chest by changing its shape, effectively expanding thoracic volume on inspiration. The chest then collapses because of its natural elas-ticity, during expiration. The two muscle sets that cause inspiration are the external intercostals and the dia-phragm, although forced expiration is also possible, via the internal intercostal muscles. All the intercostals are innervated by the thoracic spinal cord, but the diaphragm is innervated from a higher source via the phrenic nerve, arising from the cervical spinal cord levels C2–C4. Sever-ance of the spinal cord at thoracic and low cervical levels thus allows spontaneous breathing, but ventilation is instantly stopped when the cord is severed above C4, since both the diaphragm and the intercostal muscles are paralysed.

ONDINE'S CURSE

Control of ventilation is normally automatic, not voli-tional; but some conscious breathing is possible via the corticospinal tracts, as in 'taking a deep breath' at will. The automatic control descends in pathways separate from the corticospinal tracts. Anterolateral fibres in the spinal cord originate in the medulla oblongata. Failure of this para-llel automatic ventilatory system results in total depen-dence on the corticospinal pathways for continuous breathing. It seems that conscious attention to breathing during day and night is all but impossible. The consequent failure to ventilate during sleep is lethal.[51,174]

The term Ondine's curse for such failure of automatic ventilation comes from Ondine, the water nymph in a story from Greek mythology involving a curse that required conscious breathing to avoid death. It is heuris-tic for the study of hypoxic brain damage that when death occurs due to Ondine's curse, there is no evidence of neu-ronal necrosis in the cerebral cortex or hippocampus,[52] structures often stated to be 'brain structures selectively vulnerable to hypoxia'. Instead, autopsy usually reveals only the cause of the chronic hypoventilation and even-tual fatal ventilatory failure, an anatomical cause inevitably located in the medulla.[52,222] Lesions need not even be bilateral to cause hypoxic ventilatory failure and death, as autopsy has shown unilateral medullary lesions in death due to Ondine's curse.[73,428] Chronic hypoxia due to longstanding ventilatory failure gives rise to eventual death of the organism, but without brain damage (see page 240).

THE OXYGEN CASCADE: FROM AIR TO BLOOD

Once breathing is initiated at birth, ventilation continues uninterrupted throughout life, delivering inspired oxygen from ambient air to pulmonary alveoli. At sea level, inspired air, which consists of just under 21% oxygen, has a pressure of 101 kPa (760 mmHg), with a P_{O_2} of 21.2 kPa (158 mmHg). The ambient P_{O_2} decreases at altitudes above sea level, dropping to 4 kPa (30 mmHg) at the summit of Mount Everest.

When air is inhaled, along the course of the respirato-ry passages, gaseous water and carbon dioxide are added, and their respective partial pressures must be subtracted from the total air pressure to reduce further the partial pressure of oxygen in the inspired air. When the alveoli are reached, there is a small difference between the alveolar and the arterial P_{O_2}, due to diffusion of oxygen across the alveolar wall. Pulmonary vascular shunts causing admixture of venous blood reduce the partial pressure of oxygen still further, resulting in an arterial P_{O_2} near 13.3 kPa (100 mmHg) in the lower altitudes on the planet. Once the process of ventilation has delivered oxygen to the pulmonary alveoli, and oxygen crosses into the pulmonary blood vessels, it becomes the function of the circulatory system to deliver oxygen to the brain.

Circulation

Disease of the blood vessels is covered in Chapter 6, this Volume. Here, different aspects of the cerebral circulation are emphasized, including the phylogenetic and ontogenetic variations, especially those which may explain differential brain effects of hypoxic and ischaemic states.

THE OXYGEN CASCADE: FROM BLOOD TO BRAIN

Although the usual focus is brain oxygen delivery and use, removal of metabolic wastes, such as lactate,[589] is equally important when considering cerebral function and cerebral damage. For example, there is good evidence that accumulation of H^+ plays a role in producing cerebral necrosis.[351,352,453,455]

As the cerebral blood vessels penetrate the brain parenchyma, they branch repeatedly, reducing in size until they end in capillaries which only allow red blood cells (RBCs) to pass single file through the circulation. These capillaries vary in density throughout the brain, being richer in areas with high metabolic rates. Capillaries have long been known to be denser in grey (Fig. 5.2) than in the white matter,[153] and the rate of 50 ml/100 g per minute for human cerebral blood flow is an integrated average of grey matter, where flow rates are >80 ml/100 g per minute, and white matter, where rates can be as low as 20–25 ml/100 g per minute. Even within either grey or white matter, this principle appears to hold: capillary density is richer where metabolic, and consequently oxygen delivery rates, are highest. Within white matter, for example, capillary density was found to be twice as high in the pyramidal tract as in the fasciculus cuneatus.[153] Within the grey matter of the inferior colliculus, capillary density closely correlates with both the cerebral metabolic rate for glucose and the CBF, suggesting that capillary density could even be estimated from the local metabolic rate.[239]

The cerebral metabolic rate for glucose and for oxygen, per gram of brain tissue, is higher in species with small brains[608] and in infants.[62] The increased rate of metabolism in small brains is due to a greater density of neurons, not glia, which have remained constant in density during phylogenesis.[204,257,556]

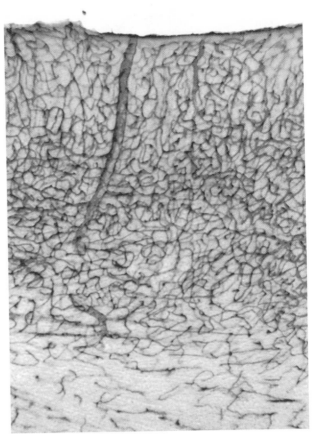

Figure 5.2 *Cerebral blood vessels. The vascular density in the white matter, seen at the bottom, is sparse in comparison with the grey matter. Capillary density increases in response to chronic hypoxia, as in adaptation to high altitude (see text). (Factor VIII immunocytochemistry.)*

The metabolic correlate of this is that the glycolytic rate, largely carried out by glia (Fig. 5.3), remains constant across species[609] whereas the rate of aerobic metabolism (oxidative phosphorylation) increases in smaller brains[608,609] owing to increased neuronal density. Figure 5.4 shows the metabolism of glucose to lactate and transport of this lactate to neurons for tricarboxylic acid (TCA) metabolism. The decreased density of neurons as one progresses from the brain of the mouse (~142 500 neurons mm^{-3}) to rat (~105 000 neurons mm^{-3}), cat (~30 800 neurons mm^{-3}), man (~10 500 neurons mm^{-3}) and whale (~6800 neurons mm^{-3})[606,607] is immediately apparent on inspection of brain sections, and is well known to those regularly examining central nervous system (CNS) tissue from different species.

Cerebral blood flow is dictated by cerebral metabolism, and like the metabolic rate, is thus also higher per gram of tissue in smaller brains of, say, rat or gerbil compared with man. This is reflected anatomically in a higher capillary density (and reduced diffusion distance for oxygen) in species with small brains, and in the immature brain. A similar increase in capillary density occurs on adaptation to high altitude (see page 240).

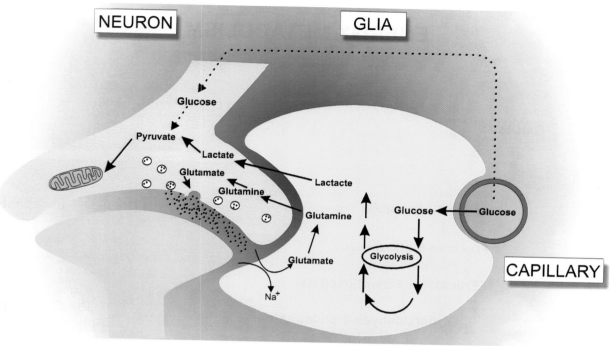

Figure 5.3 *Neuron–glia relationships. Carrier-mediated transport of glucose from the capillary delivers glucose across the endothelium into the glia. Astrocytic glycolysis then yields lactate, which is passed on to the neuron. Glutamine is also passed from astrocyte to neuron, where glutaminase regenerates glutamate. Glutamate molecules must be removed efficiently from synapses, and this is done by high-affinity axonal reuptake and by uptake into glia. Some glucose can be metabolized directly by neurons (dotted pathway), but their chief substrate under normal conditions is lactate.*

CBF ischaemic thresholds (see Chapter 6, this Volume) also vary in line with these differences in metabolism. CBF ischaemic thresholds for infarction are higher in species with small brains, being roughly 12 ml/100 g per minute in the larger non-human primate brain,[30,313,435,588] but 45 ml/100 g per minute in the small rodent brain.[300] However, the ratio of the normal blood flow to the threshold for infarction remains roughly constant across species at 3:1. It may be envisaged that animals with small brains have higher rates of basal blood flow to satisfy higher rates of metabolism, and therefore have higher absolute CBF thresholds for infarction. The neuronal density, which decreases as brains become larger, primarily determines not only metabolic rates but also CBF and blood flow thresholds for ischaemic damage.[300]

CEREBRAL AUTOREGULATION

CBF is thus a largely dependent variable in the schema of brain circulation and metabolism. Mechanisms controlling CBF have been intensively investigated, and are local rather than global: hypoxic increases in brain blood flow occur independent of sensorineural input from peripheral hypoxia sensors.[429,611] Rather, local brain activity determines not only oxygen and glucose consumption, but also blood flow in any particular brain region. In the intact brain, all three are normally coupled, rising and falling in synchrony. This is termed local autoregulation, and per 100 g of human brain, every minute roughly 50 ml of

blood is delivered, from which 25 µmol of glucose is extracted, requiring the simultaneous extraction of 150 µmol (3 ml) of O_2 for its oxidization.

The normal coupling mechanism matching CBF to cerebral metabolism is unknown. Candidates include pH (H^+),[362,537] adenosine[287,346,436,505,640] and nitric oxide (NO).[349,369,403,542] Whatever the mechanism, coupling normally occurs between increases or decreases in brain glucose metabolism, oxygen utilization and blood flow. Hypoxaemia seems to impair neither this CBF–metabolism coupling nor cerebral circulatory responses in general,[178,346,401] whereas most of the other pathophysiological states discussed in this chapter do.

Respiration

Respiration refers to the cellular combination of oxygen with substrates containing carbon and hydrogen, producing carbon dioxide and water. Respiration is to be distinguished from ventilation, which refers to the act of breathing and the passage of oxygen from the surrounding air to the pulmonary alveoli.

Because of the stoichiometric relationship of glucose consumption to oxygen utilization, with six molecules of oxygen required to burn one molecule of glucose, oxygen consumption should parallel glucose utilization if the brain does not burn fuel other than glucose. This is in fact

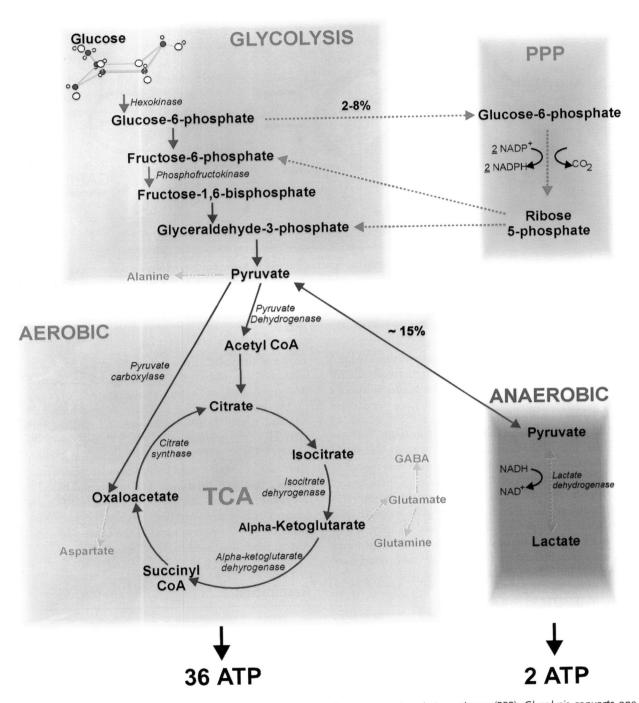

Figure 5.4 *Schema of glycolysis, oxidative phosphorylation and the pentose phosphate pathway (PPP). Glycolysis converts one molecule of glucose to two molecules of pyruvate, which in turn is interconvertible with lactate via the enzyme lactate dehydrogenase (LDH). This process yields two molecules of ATP per lactate, or four per glucose molecule. Oxidative phosphorylation yields 36 molecules of ATP, but can only proceed in the presence of oxygen as an electron acceptor. Reducing the flux of glycolysis, as in hypoglycaemia, causes a shortage of acetate moieties for oxaloacetate to condense with, to turn the Krebs cycle. Oxaloacetate thus builds up, causing a secondary build-up of aspartate in hypoglycaemia.*

true,[223] and only under special circumstances is the brain able to burn substrates other than glucose, such as lactate, ketone bodies, endogenous fats or proteins. This will be discussed in the section on hypoglycaemia.

CEREBRAL ENERGY METABOLISM

Unlike other organs of the body, the adult brain burns only glucose as a fuel. Respiration in the brain oxidizes glucose to carbon dioxide and water in two metabolic sequences, first, glycolysis and then the TCA cycle (Fig. 5.4). After glucose is taken up from the bloodstream and into glia by specific transporters, it is metabolized via glycolysis to 2 equivalents of pyruvate, producing 2 equivalents of adenosine triphosphate (ATP) overall. The rate of glycolysis is controlled by the enzymes hexokinase and phosphofructokinase, both of which are strongly affected by the level of ATP. Lactate, interconvertible with pyruvate via the action of lactate dehydrogenase (LDH), is preferentially metabolized by glia and is then transported to neurons from glia. This lactate is converted to pyruvate through LDH and is then able to enter the mitochondrion to be introduced into the TCA cycle.

Once phosphorylated by hexokinase, glucose may be diverted into one of two, parallel pathways: Embden–Meyerhof glycolysis or the pentose shunt, the latter also termed the pentose phosphate pathway (PPP). The PPP itself consists of two parts: an oxidative and a non-oxidative branch. The oxidative branch serves to produce equivalents of NADPH (the reduced form of nicotinamide-adenine dinucleotide phosphate), hence coupling the PPP to glutathione metabolism, one of the primary free-radical scavenging mechanisms. It is the $NADP^+$/NADPH ratio that controls the rate-limiting enzyme of the oxidative branch, glucose-6-phosphate dehydrogenase. The non-oxidative branch produces ribose-5-phosphate for nucleic acid synthesis. Under physiological conditions some 2–8% of glucose is metabolized through the PPP, but under oxidative stress this value is able to rise to nearly 40%, indicating a large reserve capacity of the pathway. Hypothermia (see below) increases the proportion of glucose diverted into the PPP.

Glia differ from neurons in that there is a second entry point of pyruvate into the TCA cycle. In both glia and neurons, conversion of pyruvate to acetyl coenzyme A (CoA) through pyruvate dehydrogenase is active, while the conversion of pyruvate into oxaloacetate by the action of pyruvate carboxylase occurs only in glia. Pyruvate carboxylase, a biotin-dependent CO_2-fixing enzyme, is important in the replenishment of amino acid pools and it is estimated that some 10% of glucose enters the TCA cycle in this manner.

The TCA cycle is a source of substrate for the synthesis of several amino acids, such as glutamate, glutamine and γ-aminobutyric acid (GABA) (from α-ketoglutarate) and aspartate (from oxaloacetate), and produces NADH and $FADH_2$ (the reduced forms of nicotinamide-

adenine dinucleotide and flavin adenine dinucleotide) used in oxidative phosphorylation. There are three main points of control for the TCA cycle rate: the conversion of oxaloacetate to citrate (citrate synthase), the production of α-ketoglutarate from isocitrate (isocitrate dehydrogenase), and the synthesis of succinyl CoA from α-ketoglutarate (α-ketoglutarate dehydrogenase). Through these rate-limiting enzymes the level of ATP controls the rate of the TCA cycle.

NADH and $FADH_2$ produced in the TCA cycle can then be used in oxidative phosphorylation. These energy-rich compounds have a pair of electrons with a high transfer potential, and when these electrons are donated to O_2 a large amount of energy is freed which can be used in the production of ATP. While the TCA cycle enzymes occupy the mitochondrial matrix, oxidative phosphorylation takes place on the inner membrane of the mitochondrion where 34 of the 36 ATP molecules per molecule of glucose are produced. The electrons from NADH and $FADH_2$ are transferred by proteins containing haem moieties, and it is here that poisons of the cyctochrome oxidase system and carbon monoxide (CO) act to inhibit respiration.

The energy freed by respiration would be simply released as heat if it were not stored in high-energy chemical bonds. The short-term intracellular currency of energy is the ATP molecule. Longer term intracellular energy-storing molecules include phosphocreatine and, for very long-term storage, glycogen. The brain contains only small amounts of glycogen, mostly localized in astrocytes.

When the third high-energy phosphate bond of ATP is broken, energy is passed to other subcellular processes utilizing energy in the form of a phosphate group. A molecule of adenosine diphosphate (ADP) results. Two molecules of ADP can be converted to one molecule of ATP and one molecule of adenosine monophosphate (AMP), the former capable of transferring another high-energy phosphate to other molecules. The concept of the energy charge of the tissue[31] expressed as a fraction, places the high-energy molecules in the numerator and the total adenosine nucleotide pool in the denominator. The energy charge is typically 0.93, and falls from this value in all conditions impairing cellular respiration.

$$\text{Energy charge} = \frac{[ATP] + {}^1/_2[ADP]}{\Sigma[ATP] + [ADP] + [AMP]}$$

CLASSIFICATION OF HYPOXIA

Hypoxia, as used by physiologists, is a generic term. It is apparent from the previous description of the oxygen cascade that difficulties may arise at several points along the pathway of oxygen delivery and utilization sequence. This naturally gives rise to a classification of hypoxia.

Hypoxaemia

Hypoxaemia (Table 5.1) refers to low blood levels of oxygen, from whatever cause. This may be due to either restrictive or obstructive pulmonary parenchymal disease, upper airway obstruction, or a low inspired oxygen concentration such as during high-altitude mountain climbing. The haemoglobin molecule has four sites that bind oxygen. At normal P_{O_2} values, over 98% of the oxygen carrying sites on the haemoglobin molecule are occupied by oxygen in arterial blood. In the superior sagittal sinus venous blood returned from the brain, roughly 70% of the oxygen-carrying sites on haemoglobin molecules are occupied, i.e. three sites on most haemoglobin molecules and two sites on most of the remaining molecules of haemoglobin. The oxygen extraction fraction is thus said to be 28%, implying that 28% of the oxygen carried into the brain on haemoglobin molecules was extracted by the brain. This oxygen extraction fraction can increase in states of hypoxia, as part of the brain adjustments allowing adaptation to hypoxia.

BRAIN COMPENSATION IN HYPOXAEMIA

The brain compensates for hypoxaemia in several ways. First, the dissociation of oxygen from haemoglobin increases at lower P_{O_2} values, but not in a linear fashion. The curve relating arterial oxygen saturation (S_aO_2) to arterial P_{O_2} is sigmoid shaped. This curve can be shifted by factors such as acidosis, which causes haemoglobin to give up oxygen more easily in the tissue (Bohr effect). Secondly, even mild hypoxia[517] causes more oxygen to be extracted from the blood, and a lower oxygen content of venous blood results.[505] Thirdly, CBF increases with hypoxia,[1,64,136,184,224,308,402,505] compensating for the decreased oxygen content of arterial blood by increasing flow through the tissue microcirculation.[350] Chronic hypoxia increases the haemoglobin, further adding to oxygen delivery.[358]

These mechanisms supplement the hyperventilation that accompanies hypoxaemia,[555] acting to uphold cerebral oxygenation and the cerebral metabolic rate of oxygen consumption ($CMRO_2$).[110] Cerebral energy levels are maintained in the tissue. Most experiments show that there can be a slight decline in phosphocreatine and ATP, and an increase in tissue lactate which occurs early in hypoxia, followed by achievement of a new, hypoxic steady state.[41,182,183,241,256,307,398,399,564] After these metabolic adjustments, brain pH and tissue P_{CO_2} remain stable during hypoxaemia,[276] indicating that tissue washout and removal of wastes is unimpaired in hypoxia.

TISSUE P_{O_2} MEASUREMENT IN HYPOXIA

It has become possible to measure brain tissue P_{O_2} directly in man for a period of days.[173] The oxygen cascade above described a progressive step-wise reduction in the partial pressure of oxygen from air to lung, to blood, to brain,

where normal tissue P_{O_2} values are 3.7–4.0 kPa (28–30 mmHg). As expected, hypoxaemia leads to a further decrease in the tissue P_{O_2} from the normal, and a flattening of the steps in the oxygen delivery cascade (see Fig. 5.1). Tissue P_{O_2} levels can fall from 2.7–5.4 kPa (20–40 mmHg) to ≤1 kPa (5 mmHg) during severe hypoxaemia[350] and can reach ≤0.25 kPa (0–2 mmHg) when breathing only 2–3.5% O_2.[549]

Brain tissue P_{O_2} monitoring appears to offer prognostic value in head injury, correlating with CBF better than either brain P_{CO_2} or pH.[179] Poor outcome in head injury was found to correlate with tissue P_{O_2} of ≤2.5 kPa (19 mmHg).[180] In the non-injured brain subjected to iatrogenic ischaemia, as in neurosurgical aneurysm clipping, a tissue P_{O_2} of 1.3 kPa (10 mmHg) can be tolerated before tissue hypoxia becomes critical and tissue pH rises.[187,274]

High-altitude hypoxia and brain damage

Whether high-altitude hypoxia causes loss of neurons has been a vexatious question. The issue is important not only to climbers who frequent the Himalayas, but also to the science of brain damage. The compensatory mechanisms, already alluded to earlier in this chapter, that account for the lack of brain damage after exposure to high altitude, are reviewed.

When arterial oxygen levels acutely drop to 4 kPa (30 mmHg) or less, consciousness is dulled and memory is impaired, unless considerable time elapses for adaptation and inspired oxygen is lowered gradually. This can be demonstrated experimentally.[24,185] Although neuronal necrosis is not produced,[430] synapses are affected by hypoxia.[571]

Synaptic dysfunction causes a syndrome that has been termed 'high-altitude stupid' (HAS) in mountaineering circles, due to errors of judgement and poor decisions made by experienced climbers at high altitudes. This reverses on return to low altitudes, and permanent deficits are not detectable on neuropsychological testing.[303] High-altitude mountaineers experience very low arterial oxygen pressures, and ambient P_{O_2} is < 4 kPa (30 mmHg) at the summit of Mount Everest. Such low oxygen pressures, when acutely experienced in other settings without time for compensation, produce reversible coma but not neuronal necrosis.[232,540] Thus, hypoxia causes synaptic abnormalities, without causing neuronal necrosis, explaining why hypoxia causes behavioural abnormality with normal neuropathology, free of neuronal necrosis.

Detailed neuropsychological testing 2–7 weeks after return from base camp after an Everest expedition shows no permanent neuropsychological impairment, in spite of the fact that one summitteer tested descended without oxygen.[303] Another group tested 22 mountaineers 16–221 days after Himalayan climbing, and did not find any neurological or psychological impairment.[132] These studies indicate that chronic, severe hypobaric, high-altitude hypoxia is unaccompanied by brain damage.

Adaptation occurs after several days at high altitude, a fact exploited by experienced climbers and guides in the Himalayas.[354] Brain blood flow increases with chronic hypoxia, reaching an asymptote after roughly 6 days.[185,555] Exposure to hypobaric hypoxia is accompanied by remodelling of the brain vasculature (see Fig. 5.2).[72,113,255,358,425] Leakage of the new capillaries formed at elevation may explain the phenomenon of high-altitude cerebral (o)edema (HACE). This unpredictable form of potentially lethal cerebral oedema can only be cured by return to lower altitude, and is probably due to a state of high CBF through a neovascular, leaky microcirculation. It is not known whether high-altitude pulmonary (o)edema (HAPE) is due to such neocapillaries, or a hyperdynamic pulmonary circulation. In summary, high-altitude hypoxia is accompanied by several distinct complications (HAS, HACE, HAPE), but causes more change in tissue capillaries and brain synapses than neuronal cell bodies. High-altitude mountaineers are at risk for losing appendages as a result of freezing, but not their brain cells.

Severe hypoxia other than at altitude

If the chronic hypoxia of mountaineering seems not to harm the brain permanently, what of acute hypoxia, where adaptation periods are absent? Very low arterial P_{O_2} levels of ~3 kPa (20 mmHg) are widely held to be incompatible with survival. Nevertheless, survivors of such extreme hypoxia do not have any permanent physiological impairment when followed for many months.[232] A decerebrate state after hypoxia is also compatible with long-term recovery, free of neurological signs or symptoms.[232,540] One 2-year-old boy with obstructive bronchitis remained in a coma for over 2 weeks, without neurological residua after profound hypoxia without heart stoppage.[540] Such cases illustrate that acute, severe, hypoxic hypoxia occurring without cardiac failure is unaccompanied by brain damage. In contrast, cases where acute hypoxia is accompanied by cardiac arrest, such as near drowning or pure nitrogen inhalation,[286] there is severe brain damage, identical to that seen after cardiac arrest.[81,142]

The question of whether uncomplicated acute hypoxic hypoxia can give rise to brain damage can be tested in controlled laboratory experiments. The well-known Levine model consists of unilateral carotid occlusion and immersion in nitrogen, causing damage ipsilateral to the occlusion.[366] Experiments where 7.7% O_2 was administered for 2 h to neonatal rat pups with unilateral carotid artery ligation did not show brain damage in the hemisphere exposed only to hypoxia, opposite the occluded artery.[6] The neonatal brain, however, differs considerably from the adult brain in its response to global ischaemia (see Chapter 9, this Volume). For example, glutamate is not released in newborn animals.[119]

In adult, spontaneously breathing animals, hypoxia causes a precipitous fall in blood pressure, the animals sustaining damage in arterial boundary zones.[88] Animal data

indicate that profound hypoxic hypoxia itself does not produce cerebral necrosis in the intact animal, and[150] concomitant hypotension, either spontaneous (i.e. due to the hypoxia) or induced, is necessary to produce cerebral necrosis.[150,430]

Although there is no evidence that necrosis of cells or tissue results from uncomplicated hypoxic hypoxia, synaptic alterations occur. Electron microscopy has shown abnormalities in presynaptic terminals after exposure to hypoxia, consisting of expansion of presynaptic terminals containing multilamellar bodies, aggregated or clumped synaptic vesicles, and various tubular arrays and profiles. Some of these changes, which are of uncertain significance, were also seen in other elements of the brain, including neuronal perikarya, glia, and vascular components.[654,655] Hamster brains exposed to hypoxia showed swelling of mitochondria in neuronal perikarya,[243] a reversible finding.

Another study which exposed infant non-human primates to hypoxia of 4% O_2 (3 kPa, 20–22 mmHg) found selective synaptic degeneration of GABAergic terminals using electron microscopy but neuronal cell body necrosis was not seen by light or electron microscopy.[571] Hypoxia of 3 h duration caused selective GABAergic loss in cultures of neurons from cerebral cortex.[526] The lateral reticular nucleus of the thalamus, a solely GABAergic nucleus, also showed neuronal necrosis.[533,575] These findings may explain posthypoxic seizures, by removal of inhibitory GABAergic mechanisms.[577] The time course of clinical recovery from pure hypoxic insults, consisting of days to weeks,[232,540] also fits with synaptic degeneration and regeneration. Although ganglioside breakdown has been found in human infant brains that have been hypoxic,[513] adult brains did not show change in free fatty acids, and only small changes in prostaglandins and eicosanoids.[504]

Anaemia

Anaemia is low blood haemoglobin from whatever cause, one consequence of which is decreased oxygen carrying capacity of the blood. As in hypoxic hypoxia, compensatory mechanisms intervene to preserve brain oxygenation. When haemoglobin levels drop, there is an increase in CBF, which actually shows an inverse relationship with the haemoglobin level.[75,593,596] Conversely, polycythaemia lowers CBF[284,592] and increases the risk for ischaemic stroke.[320,345,496,597] Patients with leukaemia can have very low haemoglobin levels, but these are not accompanied by signs of inadequate cerebral oxygenation, unless leukostasis and very high white blood cell (WBC) counts (>300 000) supervene, when cerebral haemorrhage (not 'anaemic hypoxia') can result.[201] There is thus no evidence that uncomplicated anaemia can cause brain damage, whereas there is considerable evidence that polycythaemia and high haemoglobin levels lower CBF, as well as predispose to intravascular thrombosis.

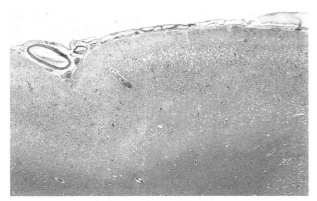

Figure 5.5 *Cardiac arrest. This 64-year-old male survived for 5 weeks. Cystic laminar necrosis is seen in cortical layers II and III, with vascular proliferation in layers IV and V.*

Stagnant hypoxia (cardiac arrest encephalopathy; transient global ischaemia)

When the blood supply to the brain is impaired, tissue P_{O_2} levels fall. Hence the name stagnant hypoxia can be applied, but it will be noted that this is tantamount to ischaemia. The impairment of blood flow can affect the entire brain, termed global ischaemia, or only a portion thereof, termed focal ischaemia. Focal ischaemia and the underlying vascular diseases are covered in Chapter 6, this Volume.

The potential structural consequences of global ischaemia comprise selective neuronal necrosis if ischaemia is less severe, and infarction if ischaemia is more profound and/or prolonged (Fig. 5.5). These two degrees of tissue damage can occur anywhere in the brain.

Global ischaemia, like focal ischaemia, can be either transient or permanent. The difference lies in whether blood flow to the intracranial contents is or is not restored. A critical parameter here is the duration of interruption of the cerebral circulation. If flow is immediately restored through the cerebral vasculature, as in successfully resuscitated cardiac arrest, then some degree of global ischaemic damage, or cardiac arrest encephalopathy, may result. If flow is not restored in time, then an increase in the intrinsic resistance of the cerebrovascular bed occurs, precluding reperfusion, and non-perfused brain, or permanent global ischaemia, inevitably results.

The consequences of transient global ischaemia can roughly be predicted from a number of factors. The basic importance of the duration of global ischaemia is obvious from clinical experience. A second factor is the completeness of the ischaemic insult. Some degree of residual perfusion (and resuscitative cardiac massage) gives a better outcome than total cardiac standstill and no blood pressure whatsoever during the insult.

Thirdly, brain temperature during the period of stagnant hypoxia or transient global ischaemia is clearly critical in determining the degree of resulting brain dam-

age.[100] Clinical cases of stagnant hypoxia with hypothermia clearly illustrate this. One well-documented case is that of a 14-year-old girl who fell through the ice into freezing water and suffered total hypoxia for 40 minutes. In spite of this prolonged submersion, there were ultimately no long-term neurological deficits.[559] The powerful neuroprotective effect of hypothermia has given rise to a resurgent interest in using controlled hypothermia as a neuroprotective tool against ischaemia (see Ischaemic neuroprotection, below). Conversely, mild hyperthermia of 1–2°C augments ischaemic brain necrosis,[100,171,226] acidosis[129,254] and glutamate release.[427] Hypothermia has been shown to reduce H^+ proton production in total circulatory arrest in man.[277] Fever should be scrupulously avoided in clinical states of brain hypoperfusion.

It is probable that enhanced tissue acidosis also accounts for the aggravating effect of the fourth major factor in determining the outcome after transient global ischaemia, the blood glucose level. The major role of blood glucose in determining outcome in ischaemic states was first suggested by studies in which rabbits fed a diet of carrot had markedly better survival after ischaemia, than animals given a regular diet.[108,155,456] Metabolic studies have shown that restricting substrate supply improves recovery of energy metabolism, and reduces accumulation of lactate.[217] The ketotic or starved state improves tolerance to ischaemia[189,342,386] and reduces neuronal death.[408] High glucose is detrimental.[160,512,576] Inhibition of glycolysis with 2-deoxyglucose appears to protect[145,424] and blocking glycolysis also inhibits post-mortem tissue changes.[206] Together, these experimental results suggest that glycolysis can damage tissue, probably by producing acid equivalents.

In man, the pioneering studies of cardiac arrest by Longstreth showed that high blood glucose levels worsened the outcome of out-of-hospital cardiac arrest.[379–382] The same was found in near-drowning.[28] In focal ischaemia, the poorer outcome with high blood glucose levels has been shown to occur with or without diabetes.[511]

Transient global ischaemia: density and distribution of damage

The four major factors determining the amount of brain damage seen after cardiac arrest are thus the duration of ischaemia, the degree of ischaemia, the temperature during the period of circulatory stagnation and the blood glucose levels. When damage is severe, owing to any combination of these factors, it is clinically accompanied by epileptic activity.[112,355,569,638,652] Such epileptic activity is associated with augmented necrosis, both being treatable with insulin and diazepam.[625] Although global ischaemia occurs most commonly with cardiac arrest, it also accompanies the onset of heat stroke (cerebral hyperthermia).[375]

Global ischaemia, in animals and in man, damages specific neuroanatomical locations: the cerebral cortex, the striatum, the hippocampus and the cerebellar Purkinje cells.[85,142,635] In the cortex, damage usually affects the middle cortical laminae (Fig. 5.5), and is accentuated over the boundary zones of the cerebral hemisphere,[82] i.e. territories between the areas irrigated by the anterior, middle and posterior cerebral arteries. The parasagittal convexity is the junction between the anterior and middle cerebral artery, and can be unilaterally affected in global ischaemia due to asymmetry in the circle of Willis (Fig. 5.6). Occlusion of a carotid artery, since it reduces flow to both anterior and middle cerebral arteries, also gives this boundary zone pattern.[230] If hypotension is mild or less prolonged, stagnant hypoxia only occurs in the triple watershed zone, located more posteriorly than often realized (Fig. 5.7). If hypotension is severe and prolonged, then the entire cerebral cortex becomes involved along with the rest of the brain (Fig. 5.8).

Hippocampal damage may be unilateral, and its degree may relate not only to the factors listed above, but also to the survival period: more damage may be seen after longer survival times after the cardiac arrest[279,501] (see section below on Delayed neuronal death). Sometimes, the hippocampus is relatively spared, in spite of necrosis in the cerebral cortex, the thalamus and the cerebellum.[84] Within the hippocampus, the cells first affected by the mildest ischaemic insults comprise the CA1 area of Lorente de Nó[383] also termed, in man, the H_1 cells of Rose (Fig. 5.9).[529] As in the cerebral cortex, however, the selectivity of lesions is lost with severe insults, in which necrosis of CA3 (H_2) and even dentate gyrus can be seen.

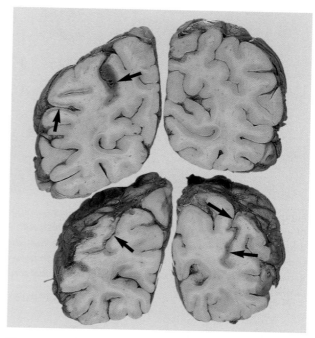

Figure 5.7 *Boundary zone infarction. This 67-year-old man had surgical hypotension, from cross-clamping of the aorta for 44 min. The cortex is discoloured yellow or brown in necrotic areas (arrows). The lesions are in the triple watershed between the three territories of the anterior, middle and posterior cerebral arteries, and are located quite posteriorly, especially on the right. They did not extend anteriorly into the double watershed zones, seen here by the normal section of brain in the upper right, nor was the hippocampus affected.*

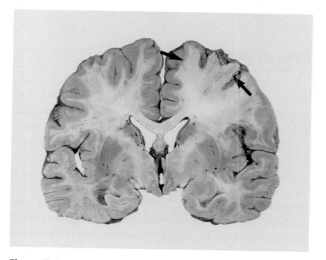

Figure 5.6 *Boundary zone infarction. Double watershed lesion on the right side, in a 57-year-old man with cardiac arrest 4 days prior to death. Liver disease and jaundice accompanied heart disease. Leakage of bile pigments into the watershed infarct causes yellow discoloration in the centrum semiovale on the right. There is no breach of the blood–brain barrier on the left, however, owing to asymmetry in the circle of Willis and sparing of the left side from ischaemic necrosis.*

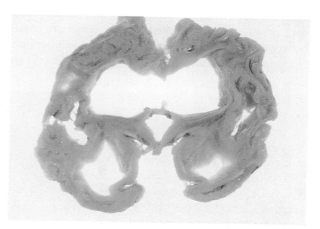

Figure 5.8 *Cardiac arrest. This occurred during hip surgery in a 79-year-old woman who survived for 9 years in a decerebrate state. Her brain shows severe necrosis everywhere, weighing only 600 g. Loss of any selectivity of damage is due to the severity of the insult. Necrosis in the telencephalon and diencephalon results in hydrocephalus ex vacuo of the third and lateral ventricles.*

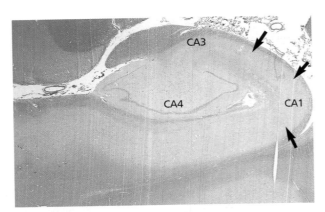

Figure 5.9 *Cardiac arrest: the hippocampus. The hippocampus of a man, aged 49 years, who suffered a cardiac arrest, with 7 weeks of survival. The lateral geniculate body is seen at the upper left corner. Neuronal fallout is visible under high power in the hilus (CA4) and in the neurons of the CA1 pyramidal zone (arrows).*

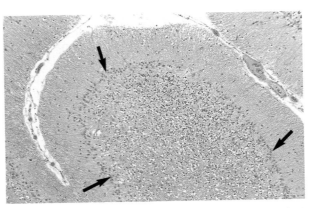

Figure 5.11 *Cardiac arrest: Purkinje cells. Female, aged 79 years, with cardiac arrest 2 years prior to death. Purkinje neurons have now been replaced by a row of astrocytes (arrows) termed Bergmann glia. Damage is relatively severe and there is thinning of the granule cell layer as well (cf. Fig. 5.10).*

Global ischaemia may also selectively affect the basal ganglia, either the corpus striatum or specifically the globus pallidus.[214] Necrosis in the brainstem can also occur, with a clinical picture of irreversible coma and absent brainstem reflexes,[302,520] clinically simulating non-perfused brain (see page 247). Alternatively, the forebrain structures may be necrotic, with relative sparing of the brainstem.[644] Necrosis of the pars reticularis of substantia nigra may occur.[81,84] This is noteworthy in view of necrosis in the identical midbrain region seen in experimental status epilepticus[459] (see Chapter 15, this Volume) and the tendency for epileptiform activity to appear in the postischaemic brain.[112,355,569,638,652]

The cerebellum, like the cerebrum, is supplied by three major arteries, and in global ischaemia can show widespread necrosis in severe cardiac arrest[142] or in shorter cardiac arrest, necrosis limited to the boundary zones between the superior, posterior inferior and anterior inferior cerebellar arteries. Microscopically, Purkinje cells are affected first, and will show acidophilic necrosis after short survival (Fig. 5.10). Longer survival will allow development of a characteristic form of fibrillary gliosis in the cerebellar cortex,[142] Bergmann gliosis (Fig. 5.11), signifying previous loss of Purkinje neurons.

Unusually, the spinal cord may be selectively affected in some cases of global ischaemia due to cardiac arrest.[304] As in CO poisoning (see page 250), global ischaemia may sometimes selectively affect the white matter, especially when hypotension complicates intensive care.[98]

Neuroimaging allows unprecedented definition of the brain during life. Computed tomographic (CT) and especially MR scanning allow anatomical structures to be identified with considerable precision (Fig. 5.12).

Hypoxia and ischaemia compared

When the cerebral circulation is interrupted, two processes fail: lack of delivery and lack of removal. Glucose and oxygen are not delivered, and metabolic waste products are not removed in ischaemia. Hypoxia is quite different from ischaemia. In hypoxaemia, only delivery is impaired, not removal. Any shortage involves delivery of only one molecule, O_2. Since CBF is maintained or increased in hypoxia,[1,64,136,184,224,308,402,505] other molecules continue to be delivered to the brain in hypoxia. Waste products such as CO_2 and H^+ also continue to be removed unabatedly during hypoxia, accounting for normal tissue P_{CO_2} and pH in pure hypoxaemia.[275] Hypoxia is thus a much simpler and a priori a less dire primary insult to the brain than ischaemia.

The consequence is that uncomplicated hypoxia, in the intact organism, does not by itself give rise to brain necrosis. With added ischaemia, however, necrosis appears, and hypoxia then modulates the degree of damage.[430] This is easily seen in the original Levine model[366] of experimen-

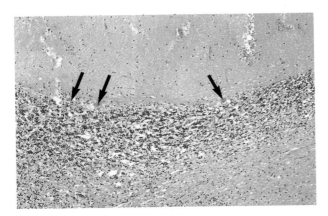

Figure 5.10 *Cardiac arrest: ischaemic neurons. Male, 38 years old, with cardiac arrest 1 week prior to death. Acidophilic Purkinje cells are seen (arrows) in the necrotic cerebellar cortex.*

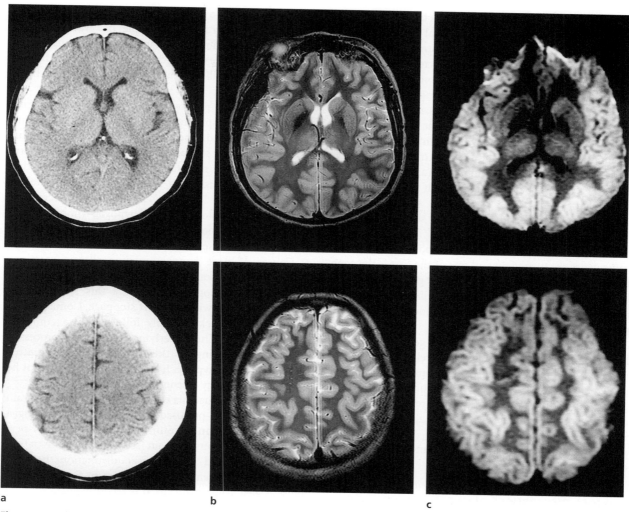

Figure 5.12 *(a) CT scans, (b) T2-weighted MRI, and (c) diffusion-weighted MRI scans obtained post cardiac arrest. The top row is taken through the basale ganglia and thalamus, and the bottom row more superiorly, over the convexity. CT and T2-weighted MR studies show subtle changes while the diffusion study is markedly abnormal with extensive cortical hyperintensity consistent with cytotoxic oedema.*

tal ischaemia, where necrosis occurs only ipsilateral to carotid ligation during hypoxia.

NEUROTRANSMISSION FAILURE AND ENERGY FAILURE

In the hypoxic brain, neurotransmission and electrical failures precede energy failure.[17,30,402] Thus, for example, there is no evidence for cellular energy failure in the medulla at an appropriately early time that would account for hypoxic apnoea.[183] Lactate accumulation occurs without energy failure,[544] and so energy failure cannot be invoked to explain hypoxic lactate accumulation. Lactate already begins to increase when the oxygen content of inspired air drops to 12%, corresponding to an $S_{a_{O_2}}$ of 50%.[241] When inspired oxygen is 7%, corresponding to an $S_{a_{O_2}}$ of 23–35%, there is some hydrolysis of phosphocreatine, but ATP levels are maintained.[241] Still lower inspired oxygen concentrations of 2–3% cause electroencephalographic (EEG) changes and the phosphocreatine/creatine ratio decreases.[549]

Events in hypoxia do not progress beyond this reversible pathophysiological state of electrical failure and early energy failure. A steady state is reached,[241] unlike in ischaemia. The glutamate release in ischaemia[59] is absent in pure hypoxaemia.[495] The consequence of all this is that the stage of tissue necrosis is never reached in the brain in hypoxaemia.

Younger mammals are more resistant to hypoxia (and, as will be seen below, to hypoglycaemia) than adults. Infants have lower basal metabolic rates,[62] an adaptation also to high altitude[272,273] and hibernation.[202,337]

GENE ACTIVATION IN HYPOXIA AND ISCHAEMIA

Analysis of gene activation in hypoxia and ischaemia is heuristic for understanding the fundamental differences between these two kinds of insult. A new steady state is achieved in hypoxia, with mainly regulatory genes turned on. Ischaemia involves a mass activation of genes, in association with large-scale tissue destruction.

Many classes of genes can be activated by brain insults, such as genes for transcriptional regulators (*c-fos*, *c-jun*, *junB*, *TIS8* = *zif-268*, *krox-20*), stress proteins (e.g. heat-shock proteins), glucose transporters, haem oxygenase, growth factors, interleukin converting enzyme (ICE)-like proteases; bcl family (e.g. ICE, Nedd2, Yama/CPP32; bcl-2, bcl-x) and caspases, involved in apoptosis. Some genes have adaptive value when stimulated,[118,164,332,650] while others may be harmful.[27,157,191]

Thresholds for the activation of gene transcription vary. Even physiological stimuli and neurotransmitter (acetylcholine) release can activate genes such as transcriptional regulator *c-fos*.[235,285,523,536] Stronger stimuli turn on heat-shock proteins, and still stronger stimuli, the genes for apoptosis.

Although pure hypoxaemia is not a potent brain insult, some genes are turned on and one of the first is the gene for erythropoietin production.[413] Other genes activated by hypoxia, such as HIF (hypoxia-inducible factor), affect angiogenesis and glycolysis.[590] Some genes stimulated are pro-apoptotic, such as *BNIP-3*.[91]

Ischaemia activates many more genes than does hypoxaemia, owing to an augmented cellular stress compared with hypoxaemia. The genes coding for heat-shock proteins such as hsp72[127,169,338,466] and tumour suppressor genes,[128] in addition to transcriptional regulators, such as *c-fos*, *c-jun*, *junA* or *junB*,[143,485] are all stimulated by ischaemia.

Differences between hypoxaemia and ischaemia are outlined in Table 5.2.

CLINICAL DIFFERENCES BETWEEN HYPOXIA AND ISCHAEMIA

The difference between hypoxia and ischaemia has been emphasized in the clinical literature.[430,568] A major reason to distinguish sharply these insults clinically is to be able to predict the ultimate outcome of global insults that result in coma. Hypoxic coma, although rare, is reversible, and tends to occur in young people. If a grave prognosis is spuriously ascribed to a coma accompanying a pure hypoxic insult, treatment could be withdrawn from a patient who actually has not suffered widespread brain necrosis.

In medicolegal review, it is important to determine whether cardiorespiratory arrest or merely respiratory arrest has occurred. The clinical prognosis is vastly different if the heart stoppage has not occurred and blood pressure has been maintained. Cerebral ischaemia, that most potent of insults, is then unlikely. Total cerebral ischaemia of only 2 min can cause neuronal necrosis.[575] However, even profound arterial hypoxia, without cardiac arrest or hypotension (i.e. without cerebral ischaemia) is inadequate to cause brain necrosis.[232,522,540]

Causes of pure hypoxia include allergic reactions and infectious disease of the tracheobronchial tree, and mostly young people demonstrate this syndrome of respiratory arrest without heart stoppage. Coma persists for around 2 weeks, usually followed by a complete recovery.[232,522,540] The underlying brain repair process is synaptic, accounting for this time course and eventual recovery. If only hypoxia has occurred, there will not be any neuropathology on conventional examination,[232,522,540] whereas global ischaemia will show either extensive brain necrosis[142] or non-perfused brain. The neuropathologist is often called upon to confirm a diagnosis of non-perfused brain or respirator brain (see page 247). This pathophysiological and pathological distinction between hypoxia and ischaemia is thus important for the pathologist as well as the clinician. It is recommended that the imprecise term hypoxia/ischaemia be abandoned in favour of more precise definitions. Thus, hypoxia or hypoxaemia should be used to describe low oxygen due to altitude or pulmonary disease, for example. Global ischaemia should be used when hypotension or cardiac arrest has occurred.

Table 5.2 *Differences between hypoxaemia and ischaemia*

	Global ischaemia	Hypoxaemia
Electrical failure	+	+
↓ ATP	+++	+
↓ Phosphocreatine	+++	+
↑ Lactate	+++	+
Fatty acid catabolism	+++	0
Protein catabolism	+++	0
Steady state attained	No	Yes
Gene activation	HIF	All genes studied affected
Tissue pathology	Selective neuronal necrosis and infarction	Synaptic alterations
Clinical context	Cardiac arrhythmia or arrest, profound hypotension (older age group)	Anaphylaxis, asthma, bronchitis, bronchiolitis, epiglottitis, short anaesthetic accidents (younger age group)
Clinical decerebration	+++	+
Clinical recovery	±	+++

+++ = severe, + = present, ± = possible.

Non-perfused brain (respirator brain; permanent global ischaemia)

If perfusion never returns to the intracranial contents after transient global ischaemia,[196] there is brain death, or non-perfused brain.[68] Blood flow stops at the level of the foramen lacerum in the carotid arteries. This was formerly termed respirator brain, owing to the association with a clinical history of the patient being on a 'respirator' (ventilator).[605]

Brain perfusion depends on the mean arterial blood pressure exceeding the intracranial pressure (ICP), in order to drive the blood through the resistance of the cerebral vasculature. The cerebral perfusion pressure (CPP) equals the mean arterial blood pressure minus the (ICP). When the CPP drops below a critical value, around 6 kPa (45 mmHg), non-perfused brain can occur if flow is not restored immediately. Clearly, non-perfused brain can be due to either an increase in ICP (see Chapter 4, this Volume) or a decrease in arterial blood pressure. Relevant causes include ischaemic brain oedema (e.g. the oedema associated with recent infarction), sudden hypotension (e.g. during anaesthesia or due to cardiac arrhythmia) or traumatic brain injury, with its associated drop in CBF and rise in ICP.[409] Whatever the cause of the increased ICP, perfusion stops and blood stagnates in the microcirculation throughout the brain.

Initially, series of cases were described[4,20,240] with patients on a respirator for prolonged periods, and the neuropathological effects were thought to be related somehow to the respirator. It is now clear, however, that the medulla oblongata can in some cases be perfused in respirator brain, and such patients need not be on a respirator to develop the classical neuropathological changes of respirator brain, as they are breathing spontaneously. Thus, the term non-perfused brain is more descriptive and pathophysiologically accurate. Non-perfused brain is the extreme, irreversible form of stagnant hypoxia, in which blood flow to the intracranial contents is never restored. It is the neuropathological correlate of clinical brain death, and marks the end of useful life, since brain circulation and function can never be restored again.

Grossly, cases of non-perfused brain show a different appearance from cardiac arrest encephalopathy (Fig. 5.13). The non-perfused brain shows dusky brown discoloration of the cerebral cortex, blurring of the junction of the cortex and the white matter, and general friability of the brain. With longer survival, there is increasing brown discoloration of the entire brain, which becomes harder to fix in formalin owing to protein alterations, resulting in symmetrical patches of pink, unfixed white matter in the portions of the centrum semiovale farthest away from the ventricles.

Microscopically, the histology is far better preserved than expected from the gross appearance (Fig. 5.14). Although acidophilic neurons may be seen, this is not the

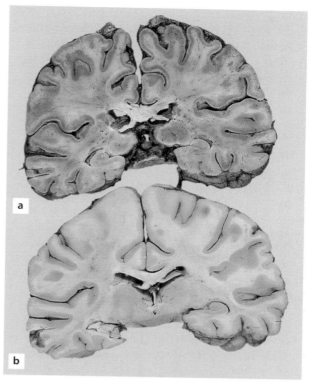

Figure 5.13 *Cardiac arrest. Gross appearance of (**a**) non-perfused brain or respirator brain, and (**b**) recent cardiac arrest encephalopathy. The non-perfused brain is from a 59-year-old man who survived for 8 days after cardiac arrest. Note the dusky brown discoloration of the cortex and the red colour in the white matter, indicative of the poor fixation characteristic of non-perfused brain. (**b**) Brain is from a 44-year-old woman who lived for 2 days after cardiac arrest, and is pale by comparison. The junction between the cortex and white matter is blurred.*

rule, and neuronal cell membranes are preserved. There is a general pallor of the tissue, including stagnant red blood corpuscles in the circulation, appearing pale owing to lysed haemoglobin. Because of the lack of perfusion, there is no tissue reaction except possibly at the border of perfused and non-perfused tissue, usually at the level of the high cervical spinal cord or medulla oblongata. The pathological changes of non-perfused brain take about 12 h to develop,[68] although they become more obvious in 24 h, an important point if the neuropathologist is called upon to confirm brain death.

The spinal cord, the venous sinuses and the pituitary gland should be also examined. The cord is usually well preserved pathologically, and clinically may show autonomous neurophysiological activity (Lazarus sign).[270] Fragments of autolysed cerebellum[475] can be found around the spinal cord. The dural venous sinuses are thrombosed.[490] The pituitary gland invariably undergoes infarction (Fig. 5.15), owing to the vulnerability to increased ICP, of its portal venous blood supply from the hypothalamus.

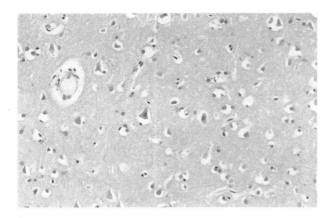

a

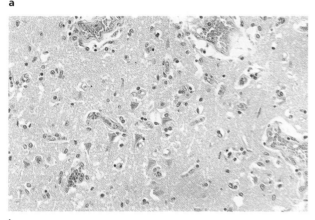

b

Figure 5.14 *Non-perfused brain. (a) Non-perfused brain compared with (b) transient global ischaemia. The cortex of the non-perfused brain shows pallor of the neuropil, and no tissue reaction, although there are acidophilic neurons in this field. Blood vessels appear empty, as RBCs have been stagnant, and have lysed haemoglobin. The cortex from transient ischaemia, in contrast, shows tissue reaction as vascular proliferation, as well as numerous acidophilic neurons.*

Usually, respiratory support is discontinued if non-perfused brain, accompanied by the clinical criteria for brain death, is diagnosed. Non-perfused brain is generally followed after a variable period by somatic death, even if ventilatory support is continued. This is due to the cardiac consequences of increased ICP[558] and poorly understood brain–body relationships. Subsequent deterioration can occur in haemodynamic stability[524] and cardiac arrest after many hours to a few days, but cases with long somatic survival (74 days) have been reported.[490] Such cases show a leukocytic tissue reaction superficially in the brain, with WBCs infiltrating the brain parenchyma from the perfused skull and meninges.[490,551] Since the entire brain produces lactic acid through anaerobic metabolism, cerebrospinal fluid (CSF) lactate levels are higher in brain death than in other neurological states.[493] Furthermore, the normal cisternal-to-lumbar gradient of acidity is reversed until resuscitation occurs.[318]

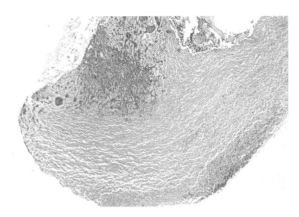

Figure 5.15 *Pituitary gland. Pale necrosis of most of the adenohypophysis is seen. There is only an island of preserved tissue, and a thin rim of tissue at the lower right, supplied by meningohypophyseal arteries. The gland is vulnerable to infarction in the non-perfused brain because of its dependence on portal blood from the hypothalamus. This supply is interrupted in the non-perfused brain. The pituitary should always be examined in cases of brain death.*

Histotoxic hypoxia

If oxygen delivery to the tissues is intact, oxygen utilization may still be impaired at the tissue level as a result of poisoning of the cellular machinery for oxidation of glucose to carbon dioxide and water. This can occur through poisoning of proteins in the electron transport chain of oxidative metabolism.

Of such agents inducing histotoxic hypoxia, cyanide and sulfide are two of the most common clinically encountered. Both inhibit cytochrome enzymes in the mitochondria, sulfide actually being the more potent agent of the two in inhibiting respiration.[574] Human exposures to cyanide have suggested that brain damage might result from exposure.[188,263,359,550] Similarly, cases where workers are exposed to hydrogen sulfide in sewers and especially in the oil and gas industry[99] have suggested that sulfide might cause brain damage.[5] Inhalation of hydrogen sulfide causes immediate 'knock down' due to apnoea. However, the question of whether cardiac hypotension or cardiac standstill accounts for the cerebral damage in resuscitated survivors cannot be answered in physiologically uncontrolled human observations. Cardiac function and blood pressure remain unknown at the time of the exposure, and global ischaemia to the brain can thus never be ruled out in man exposed to these agents in the field.

Animal experiments have shed light on the problem, since physiological parameters such as blood oxygenation, carbon dioxide, pH, haemoglobin and blood pressure could be controlled. Such experiments have uniformly demonstrated that exposure to even very high concentrations of these agents is incapable of producing cerebral necrosis unless hypotension supervenes. They have also shown that cyanide and sulfide are themselves potent and immediate depressors of blood pressure.[46,87] Experiments with cyanide encephalopathy have shown that although cyanide causes severe perturbations in cerebral energy metabolism including reduction in cytochrome oxidase activity, depletion of ATP and production of lactate, brain necrosis is not seen.[400] The situation is similar with sulfide exposure, where, like cyanide encephalopathy, several hours of EEG isoelectricity (flat EEG) are produced by the agent. In a recent series, only in one ventilated animal receiving a very high dose of sulfide (exceeding the lethal dose in the unventilated animal), was cerebral necrosis seen.[46] Persistent hypotension to ≤35 mmHg for more than 30 min accompanied the cerebral necrosis. Rare animals that do show necrosis in studies of both cyanide and sulfide encephalopathy do so in the hippocampus and/or the cerebral cortex, i.e. in a distribution resembling that seen after global ischaemia.[46,400]

Another agent which poisons oxidative metabolism, although with a lower potency than either sulfide or cyanide, is sodium azide (NaN_3).[574] Again, it has been shown experimentally that this cytochrome poison also causes profound hypotension, the effects of which cannot be separated from any presumed direct cytotoxic effect.[418] It is concluded from these animal studies that agents that produce histotoxic hypoxia all produce profound hypotension, and that, like hypoxic hypoxia and anaemic hypoxia, histotoxic hypoxia does not, by itself, damage the brain.[46,87,400]

CARBON MONOXIDE POISONING

CO is a well-known lethal poison, produced by incomplete combustion of carbon. Accidental exposure is common and due to cooking or heating indoors, or in tents. Intentional exposure occurs with suicidal or homicidal intent using automobile exhaust. Fires potentially expose building occupants to CO. The mechanisms of brain damage after CO poisoning are more complex than in the other hypoxic states in this chapter, because CO poisoning involves an interesting interplay of several parallel mechanisms, and because white matter can be prominently affected.

Mechanisms of brain damage in CO poisoning

CO BINDING TO HAEMOGLOBIN

Anaemic hypoxia due to displacement by the CO molecule of oxygen from its binding site on the haemoglobin was a phenomenon understood in 1856 by Claude Bernard.[63] The displacement of O_2 molecules reduces the effective oxygen-carrying haemoglobin concentration and thus is pathophysiologically equivalent to anaemic hypoxia.

The affinity of the CO molecule for haemoglobin is almost 200 times that of oxygen. In survivors of CO poisoning, the reduced effective haemoglobin level is thus permanent until new RBCs (which have a lifespan of

roughly 120 days) are produced. However, there is no evidence for anaemic hypoxia playing a role in the pathogenesis of cerebral necrosis (see above). Whether the anaemic hypoxia caused by CO poisoning contributes to the other mechanisms is doubtful. Compared with arterial hypoxaemia, CO hypoxia decreases cerebrovascular resistance even more,[612] but then, CO has more effects than simply hypoxia.

CO BINDING TO BRAIN

By analogy to blood binding of CO to haemoglobin, the second effect of CO is a direct binding to brain regions rich in iron. The globus pallidus and the pars reticularis of the substantia nigra (together termed the pallidoreticularis) are the brain regions with the highest iron content. CO binds directly to haem iron in these two brain regions. This direct histotoxicity explains the selective vulnerability of the pallidoreticularis to CO poisoning (Fig. 5.16). The identical localization can now be visualized during life using modern neuroimaging techniques (Fig. 5.17).

CARDIAC EFFECTS OF CO

Although it is tempting to base explanations of the distribution of cerebral necrosis in CO poisoning on the binding of CO to brain regions rich in iron, this explains

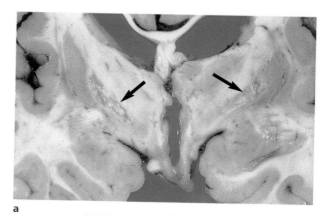

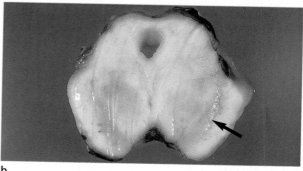

Figure 5.16 *Carbon monoxide poisoning: necrosis of globus pallidus. Brain changes in a 5-year-old girl who was asphyxiated in a house fire. Death occurred 9 weeks later. (a) Characteristic necrosis of the globus pallidus (arrows); (b) necrosis of the pars reticulata of the substantia nigra (arrow).*

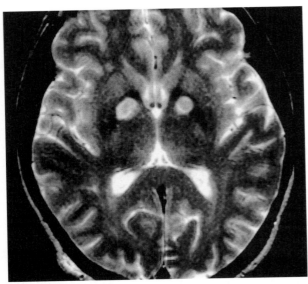

Figure 5.17 *Carbon monoxide poisoning. This was a result of a suicide attempt using an automobile exhaust. The increased water content of the necrotic globus pallidus causes it to be bright in this T2-weighted MRI scan.*

only the necrosis in the globus pallidus and the pars reticularis of the substantia nigra. Other brain regions regularly affected in CO poisoning are not especially iron rich.

Experimental evidence derived from laboratory animals[478] indicates that CO cardiotoxicity and hypotension are pathogenic factors in CO encephalopathy. It is instructive to compare CO with uncomplicated hypoxaemia: while the onset of hypoxaemia causes hypertension, CO causes hypotension.[612] In human CO poisoning, cardiac failure develops, with actual myocardial necrosis.[458] Anaemia causes high output failure, and effective anaemia is produced by CO in blood (binding to haemoglobin, see above).

The distribution of brain damage in the cerebral cortex, the hippocampus and the cerebellar Purkinje cells in human cases of CO poisoning[420,509,518] gives further support for a prominent role for hypotension in the pathogenesis of the damage,[478] in common with other forms of histotoxic hypoxia.

Not only may clinical CO poisoning resemble global ischaemia pathologically, but conversely, global ischaemia may surprisingly mimic some features of the pathology of CO poisoning. Cardiac arrest can give rise to metabolic and structural lesions focally in the globus pallidus or the substantia nigra.[168,214,423,506] The pallidoreticular pattern of damage has been seen in experimental epilepsy.[459] It is not known whether the postischaemic epileptiform activity seen after human global ischaemia correlates with this pattern of vulnerability in the globus pallidus or pars reticularis of the substantia nigra.

A prominent role for hypotension in the pathogenesis of brain damage in general, is further suggested by cyanide poisoning, another form of histotoxic hypoxia marked by cardiac failure, where it can produce selective lesions of the globus pallidus.[419] Indeed, the pallidum may be normal in CO intoxication.[360] These considerations indicate that the pallidoreticular pattern of brain damage, although associated with CO poisoning, is neither 100% sensitive nor specific for CO, and that any condition leading to cardiac failure may give rise to lesions of the globus pallidus and the pars reticularis of the substantia nigra.

Like global ischaemia, CO poisoning is exacerbated by high blood glucose levels.[499] In common with other forms of hypoxia is the paucity of permanent brain damage in survivors of CO poisoning, considering the total number of cases exposed to the gas.[219] It is unknown whether cases of documented CO poisoning without brain damage had less hypotension.

White-matter damage in CO poisoning

In addition to grey-matter disease, CO poisoning can lead to demyelination and destruction of cerebral white matter, sometimes termed Grinker's myelinopathy.[238,458] The destruction of the white matter can be delayed after exposure to CO[301] and be accompanied by delayed neurological deterioration as occasionally seen in global ischaemia.[506,627] It is important to note, however, that white-matter lesions can also be produced under controlled laboratory conditions by cyanide.[87] Thus, as in the other features of CO poisoning, white-matter lesions and delayed neurological deterioration are not specific for CO. The occurrence of white-matter lesions in hypoxic states may be favoured by less severe insults.[367]

Brain appearance in CO poisoning

Examination of the brain in CO poisoning reveals features dependent upon the length of survival. Acutely, the brain is pink owing to the appearance of the bright red carboxyhaemoglobin. Oedema may be seen, as in global ischaemia, up to several days after the insult. Later, sharply demarcated necrosis appears in the globus pallidus. A granular appearance of the white matter may suggest Grinker's myelinopathy, if survival has been long enough. Atrophy of the cerebral cortex and the hippocampus is seen. Over time, this may become extreme, depending upon the severity of the initial insult. Lesions may be seen in the substantia nigra on close gross examination. Microscopically, the lesions in CO poisoning follow the typical course of necrosis in the CNS.

AIR EMBOLISM AND DECOMPRESSION SICKNESS

Air consists of 78% nitrogen, just under 21% oxygen and almost 1% argon. All other gases, including CO_2, comprise the tiny remaining fraction. Nitrogen is the least soluble gas contained in air. When decompression occurs after there has been equilibrium at a higher pressure, as in divers who are surfacing after spending some time at considerable depth, previously dissolved nitrogen will leave the liquid phase of blood and spontaneously form intravascular bubbles. These bubbles vary in size, determining where they lodge in the circulation. This has been termed 'the bends' and is a hazard in professional and amateur divers.

Target organs in decompression sickness include the spinal cord, where microinfarcts are seen,[103,262,487] as well as the skin, bone, retina[507] and ear.[486] Bubbles can be demonstrated in the blood vessels of the spinal cord 20 min after return to atmospheric pressure in experimental decompression sickness.[486] Examination of the spinal cord of amateur and professional divers regularly reveals spinal cord microinfarcts, even in asymptomatic individuals.[487] Thus, the clinical neurological spectrum of spinal cord lesions due to air embolism extends from patients who are frankly paraplegic[103] to divers who were asymptomatic during life and totally unaware of their subclinical spinal cord neuropathology.

Air embolism also plays a role in the neurological damage seen after cardiac bypass surgery,[472] in the vernacular called 'pump head' because of the neurological symptoms associated with the patient having been on the bypass pump. Air introduced into the cardiac chambers during open-heart surgery can embolize to the brain.[348] One study found, in addition to hippocampal necrosis suggestive of global ischaemia, microinfarcts in the white matter and in the cerebral cortex, but no crystalline emboli, a combination suggesting microbubble air embolism.[614] Since air requires a considerable time to dissolve in the blood, similar to that required for a thromboembolus, air embolism can be considered a form of transient ischaemia, where the duration of vascular obstruction is long enough to cause infarction (see Chapter 6, this Volume). Permanent neurological damage may result by this ischaemic mechanism.[95,348]

SELECTIVE NEURONAL NECROSIS

Classified by the degree of tissue damage, lesions in any brain region generally fall into two types, depending upon whether neurons only, or neurons plus the other elements of neural tissue are damaged. If neurons only are affected, the degree of tissue damage is termed selective neuronal necrosis (Fig. 5.18). If all tissue elements die, i.e. glia and blood vessels as well as neurons, the lesion is termed pan-necrosis, or infarction in the case of ischaemia. Selective neuronal necrosis and pan-necrosis can each occur in virtually any brain region.

The distinction between the two degrees of tissue damage is not to be confused with the concept of selective vulnerability, which refers to the phenomenon whereby global brain insults give rise to focal lesions in certain

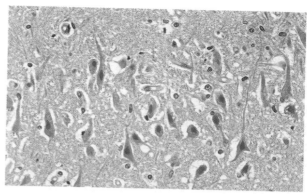

Figure 5.18 *Selective neuronal necrosis. There is sparing of glial elements in the neuropil, in contrast to infarction (pan-necrosis). The hallmark change of neuronal acidophilia is evident. Such neurons do not have a chance of recovery, and are removed from the tissue over time. The electron-microscopic appearance of such neurons is shown in Fig. 5.20. (Hippocampus, CA1 zone; cardiac arrest with 7-day survival.)*

brain regions. In other words, selective vulnerability within the brain gives rise to local brain lesions in specific locations according to the disease process, and these lesions can be either pan-necrosis or selective neuronal necrosis.

The very existence of selective neuronal necrosis as a phenomenon is likely to be due in some way to the neuronal possession of receptors for the excitatory neurotransmitter glutamate.[534] Infarction, in contrast, probably occurs when all cell types are overwhelmed by a drop in tissue pH,[562,599] damaging neurons and glia.[229,352,453,455,465] Lactic acid is more toxic than HCl, since it can permeate the cell interior.[229] The drop in pH is not, however, simply due to equimolar H^+ and lactate production, but results from protons released by the hydrolysis of ATP under anaerobic conditions,[492] and from the Krebs cycle, which lacks oxygen as a hydrogen acceptor.

Conditions altering lactate production can leave pH_i unaltered,[441] and low tissue pH does not always accompany high lactate levels.[283,492] Intracellular buffering and compartmentation of lactate in the glia[351] further account for dissociation between lactate levels and acidosis.[353] The dissociation of acid from lactate production has led to a call for the terms lactosis and acidosis to describe accumulation of lactate and protons, respectively.[492] Acidosis of only a mild degree can be protective against neuronal death mediated by hyperexcitation.[600] Pan-necrosis in ischaemia[563] and its relationship to lactic acidosis will be dealt with in Chapter 6, this Volume. Here, mechanisms involved in selective neuronal necrosis will be discussed, beginning with a comparison of the cellular properties of neurons and glia.

Neurons and glia compared

It was first thought that neurons are selectively vulnerable because they are generally larger than glia or other cell types. It could be envisaged, for example, that the diffusion distance for oxygen is greater for a larger cell, or that other nutrients traverse a greater distance reaching neurons and their cellular interior. The problem with this thesis is that selective neuronal necrosis occurs in both large and small neurons, and there is not a correlation between neuronal size and the capacity to undergo neuronal necrosis. Large neurons such as Betz cells, second in size only to the human ovum, are spared in global brain ischaemia.[439] A better correlate than size with neuronal resistance is neuronal NADPH activity,[163] probably due to protection against oxidative stress.

Neurons were once thought to be vulnerable because of their unique metabolic activity. Glycolysis and oxidative phosphorylation under hypoxic conditions differ in glia and neurons.[248] The surrounding glia and other cell types in the nervous system by implication have been held to be relatively inactive metabolically. It is true that neurons have considerable energy demands. However, neurons divide their energy expenditure roughly equally among axoplasmic transport, ion pumping and refurbishing the cell structurally. Axoplasmic transport is lacking in glia, but not the other two basic processes, ion pumping and protein synthesis. Astrocytes have been shown to have ionic currents and cell-surface receptors for glutamate, and also for the inhibitory neurotransmitter GABA.[250,305,404,581] Astrocytes regulate the extracellular space, and are not merely passive sinks. The sum total of astrocytic activity modulates both extracellular[452] and intracellular ionic concentrations[491] of $[Ca^{2+}]$ in CNS tissue.

In addition to their demonstrated receptors and ionic fluxes, glia have very active metabolism,[516] and are the cells in which most of CNS anaerobic glycolysis takes place.[609] Oligodendrocytes are active in the formation and maintenance of myelin, and astrocytes in the maintenance of the extracellular milieu of the CNS. Glia may be more vulnerable to apoptosis (see page 257) in certain pathological conditions,[502] possibly explaining selective white-matter lesions such as CO leukoencephalopathy (see above). The idea that uniquely demanding metabolic levels of the neuron account for selective neuronal necrosis in any brain region thus seems simplistic and untenable. Neuronal perikarya, after all, are repositories of genetic information and sites of protein synthesis, most of the remaining metabolic action in the nervous system taking place far from the cell body, i.e. in the neuropil, where axons, dendrites, synapses and glia are located.

Furthermore, metabolic rates vary widely among the different brain regions, and show little correlation with the distribution of selective neuronal necrosis. It seems unlikely that the occurrence of selective neuronal necrosis can be explained by any unique metabolic rate.

Excitotoxicity

If simplistic ideas of neuronal size or rates of metabolism cannot explain selective neuronal necrosis, there must be additional factors. One potential Achilles' heel of neurons, but not other cell types, is their capability of demonstrating long-term changes in synaptic efficiency which may persist for hours to days or even longer, and are likely to be involved in memory mechanisms. This lasting synaptic facilitation is termed long-term potentiation (LTP)[69] and is due to postsynaptic alterations in dendrites and spines.[387] This probably accounts for the characteristic 'axon-sparing, dendritic lesion' of excitotoxicity (Fig. 5.19). LTP can allow potentially damaging calcium influx into the neuron, activating protein kinase C[21] and proteases,[390] for example. Calcium appears essential for the production of LTP[356,389] and LTP can be induced by calcium.[616]

The synaptic facilitation of LTP is probably involved in forming memory traces in the brain.[259,387,388,566,567] It is likely that an exaggeration of this normal, physiological mechanism makes neurons vulnerable to long-term deterioration in their ion gradients, especially calcium, and long-term changes in excitability.

The fundamental idea that neurons can be damaged by overstimulation, rather than by merely depriving them of oxygen or glucose, was pioneered by John Olney with his observations on glutamate toxicity.[479–481,484] Not only glutamate but also other amino acids were toxic. The neuroexcitatory potential of acidic amino acids was found to coincide with their neurotoxic potential.[480] This correspondence of the ability to excite with the ability to destroy led Olney to formulate the concept of excitotoxicity.

For years, it was not appreciated that the early neuronal lesion in selective neuronal necrosis lies neither in the axon nor in the perikaryon,[86,89,90,391] but in neuronal dendrites. This holds in ischaemia,[310,646,647] hypoglycaemia[38] and epilepsy.[295] Selective dendritic lesions, sparing axons (Fig. 5.19), are characteristic of neuronal death due to hyperexcitation.[482,483] The dendrites appear to swell

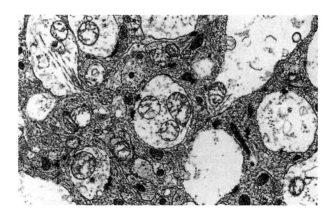

Figure 5.19 *Excitotoxicity. Characteristic of the dendritic lesion is axon sparing. Dendrites and their contained mitochondria show clear swelling. The surrounding neuropil shows normal electron density of cell processes and normal, dark mitochondria. The selective swelling of dendrites is due to the dendritic location of receptors for excitatory amino acids. (Dentate gyrus, hypoglycaemia, 10 min of flat EEG.)*

because of loss of ion and water homoeostasis, other tissue elements in the neuropil, such as astrocytes, neuronal perikarya or axons, escaping this process because of fewer receptors or absence of receptors. Long-lasting redistribution of calcium also occurs in dendrites,[146] although it is still unclear whether there are morphological changes.[15]

Since ischaemia releases large quantities of glutamate into the restricted extracellular space of the brain,[59,242] and axon-sparing, selective dendritic lesions are seen in the cells later destined to die in ischaemia,[310,646,647] it seems that a component of ischaemic neuronal death is excitotoxic, glutamate being the chief excitant. In hypoglycaemia (see page 260) the excitotoxin is chiefly aspartate.

Glutamate is a ubiquitous neurotransmitter in the brain,[197,631] but does not act at only one single receptor. The four receptors activated can be classified[443] as follows: (1) N-methyl-D-aspartate (NMDA) receptors, (2) kainate receptors, a favoured agonist (although domoic acid appears to have even higher affinity), (3) α-amino-3-hydroxy-5-methyl-4-isoxazole propionic acid (AMPA) receptors, and (4) metabotropic receptors, so named because they lead to activation of intracellular regulatory transduction events without necessarily generating transmembrane ion fluxes (see Chapter 1, this Volume).

Activation of one or more subtypes of glutamate receptor may lead to overstimulation of intracellular mechanisms normally involved in homoeostatic cell regulation. Such sequences may in many cases be thought of as exaggerated responses of normal cell regulatory mechanisms, and can pass all the way through the cytoplasm to activate the genome. One good example is the ischaemia-induced production of cellular proteins which can be classed as molecular chaperones. Since global ischaemia prominently induces the cellular production of chaperone proteins, and since they may be involved in cellular protection, the concept of molecular chaperone proteins will be briefly reviewed.

Molecular chaperone and heat-shock proteins

It was once thought that the one-dimensional, linear information in the peptide sequence of proteins was sufficient to lead to a correct three-dimensional configuration of the final protein. This is the principle of protein self-assembly. However, it is now clear that when protein translation is complete, incorrect interactions, if not prevented, may take place among portions of the newly synthesized linear peptide chain. It is the function of chaperone proteins to prevent such incorrect interactions that would cause assembly to proceed along pathways leading to non-functional proteins.[190]

Although chaperone proteins do not contain steric information regarding the final protein structure, they function by inhibiting interaction of exposed surfaces (hence their name) of the protein, which might incorrectly interact with other molecules. They thus function to stabilize proteins during assembly. Since specific steric information regarding the final assembled protein product is not contained in the chaperone, a single chaperone molecule can assist the assembly of many different protein molecules.

In addition to their role in protein synthesis, chaperone proteins can obviate the breakdown of existing completely assembled protein molecules occurring under conditions of cellular stress. A good example is the response of cells to heat. Thermal energy transmitted to protein molecules causes increased molecular motion and exposure of protein surfaces which might interact in an undesirable way with other proteins (termed denaturation if permanent) or with reactive moieties within the cell. The neuronal response to heat thus consists of a stepped-up production of proteins with molecular weights of 60 and 70 kDa, termed heat-shock proteins. These proteins confer cellular protection by preventing denaturation of existing perfectly functional cellular proteins under certain conditions of cellular stress. Proteins which do break down are removed by an extralysosomal degradative system, via conjugation with ubiquitin, a protein that earmarks damaged cellular molecules for non-lysosomal destruction in proteaosomes. Such breakdown occurs during ischaemia.[261]

Global ischaemia (and hyperthermia) both result in expression of heat-shock proteins,[468] a more sensitive indicator of cell stress than ubiquitin.[468,469] Infarction causes heat-shock proteins to be activated in astrocytes as well as neurons.[557] Hyperthermia alone also induces expression of genes for heat-shock proteins in astrocytes as well as endothelial cells.[372]

The heat-shock response is a useful indicator of the localization of cells undergoing stress in the nervous system,[470] but the response is more than a marker: it is also a survival factor for the cell, since blocking heat-shock gene expression reduces the cell's ability to withstand heat stress.[312] Prior exposure to a potentially injurious stress such as ischaemia, heat shock, arsenic or a calcium ionophore promotes neuronal survival against subsequent glutamate toxicity, and the protective effect is blocked by inhibiting protein synthesis.[384,528] Hypothermia reduces heat-shock protein expression caused by ischaemia,[126] either by mitigating the stress of ischaemia or via a direct effect of reduced temperature on the temperature-sensitive process of heat-shock protein expression.[372] The heat-shock protein response may explain not only the neuronal neuroprotective effect of hyperthermic treatment prior to ischaemia,[125,344] but also the neuroprotective ischaemic preconditioning effect.

Ischaemic preconditioning

If ischaemia is preceded by a small ischaemic insult that would not, by itself, cause necrosis ('conditioning lesion'), damage is reduced.[341,343,377] The mechanism of protection probably involves the activation of genes by the small, preconditioning stress, with induction of protein synthesis[442] and production of heat-shock proteins.[378,447,462] Indeed, protein synthesis itself is better preserved after ischaemia if preceded by ischaemic preconditioning.[329] Molecular chaperone proteins could conceivably make the cell more robust toward subsequent insults by stabilizing pre-existing intracellular proteins against incorrect molecular surface interactions of cellular proteins.[190]

Clearly, the time necessary for an immediate-early gene response must be allowed to elapse between the conditioning lesion and the second ischaemic insult, otherwise proteins will not have been produced, and protection not expected. For example, hsp70 synthesis begins to be stimulated at 2 h, increases at 8 h and is stimulated throughout the first week after ischaemia,[378,462,467] synthesis appearing maximal at 3 days.[378] This corresponds to the time course of the ischaemic preconditioning effect,[331] suggesting that if not hsp70, some similar chaperone proteins may be induced and account for the neuroprotective effect. The entire process of gene turn-on and subsequent protection may be initiated by ischaemia-induced activation of the NMDA subtype of glutamate receptor.[325,330]

If there is insufficient time for gene turn-on and protein synthesis, i.e. if the time elapsed between the first ischaemic insult and the second is short, the situation of two ischaemic insults can be considered as repetitive ischaemia, the first insult being detrimental rather than beneficial. Periods of shorter ischaemia are better survived than uninterrupted ischaemia of the same duration.[25,325,326,328] For example, CA1 neurons tolerate a 3-min ischaemic insult better when it is broken up into three 1-min periods with interspersed periods of reperfusion.[25] These observations concur with other investigations indicating that the impact of a period of brain ischaemia is lessened if it is broken up by intermittent reperfusion.[228,417]

The cumulative detrimental effect of repetitive ischaemia[601] is not due to exaggerated release of glutamate after each successive ischaemic insult,[446,449] and the protective effect of a preconditioning lesion is not due to reduced extracellular release of glutamate.[448] Accumulation of lactate is a feature of repetitive ischaemia[269] and may exacerbate damage, since even a single bout of ischaemia leaves lactate elevated for up to a week.[497] In the hippocampus, selective loss of CA4 neurons secreting somatostatin onto GABAergic neurons in the dentate hilus may play a role in protecting CA1 from subsequent damage by virtue of dampening their excitatory input.[412] Whatever the mechanism, the resultant accumulated cell damage in repetitive ischaemia, as in a single bout of ischaemia,[525] correlates with the behavioural deficit.[648]

Immediately after ischaemia, within 6 h, the brain is more vulnerable to a global ischaemic insult than the normal brain,[331,601] whereas after 1 day to 1 week, the previous ischaemia confers increased resistance.[331] Tolerance or susceptibility to ischaemia thereafter returns to control levels. The term 'conditioning' lesion is apt, since the time course corresponds to the beneficial effect of physical conditioning in exercise.

Nitric oxide

NO is a vasodilator, free radical and messenger molecule in the brain[78–80,163] and is a retrograde messenger across synapses. Its synthesizing enzyme, nitric oxide synthase (NOS), comes in three isoforms, a neuronal NOS (nNOS) that is localized to neurons, an inducible isoform that is induced in astroglia, microglia and endothelial cells (iNOS, NOS2) and a constitutive form that is localized in the endothelium (eNOS, NOS3).[474,633]

NO produced by nNOS and iNOS has been implicated in ischaemic brain injury secondary to free radicals, while NO produced by eNOS is known to be neuroprotective owing to its vasodilatory effects. NO thus appears to have two opposing effects on cell death,[161] explaining the opposite effects seen with experimental NOS inhibition.[96,97,162,365,434,494,519,628] There is further complication by the occurrence of the endothelial form of NOS in neurons, neuronal NO possibly representing the long-sought diffusible retrograde messenger[552] which crosses the synaptic cleft in long-term potentiation to cause presynaptic changes.[172,246,633]

NO produced by iNOS in non-neuronal cells may contribute to ischaemic brain injury, peaking at 24–48 h after ischaemia, localizing to infiltrating neutrophils and endothelial cells.[288,290] NO is involved in regulating platelets and, thereby, haemostasis and thrombosis.[407] Being a free radical, neuronal NO is a potent cytotoxin,[406] as is macrophage NO.[74,114] NO acts by forming peroxynitrite radicals[161,515] that may damage DNA.[656] It is possible to inhibit NO production and reduce ischaemic brain damage.[289,471]

NADPH diaphorase activity is co-localized with messenger RNA (mRNA) and protein of NOS,[78] but not with haem oxygenase,[619] which has the same relationship to CO that NOS has to NO.[659] NADPH diaphorase activity confers resistance to NMDA,[347] but not to non-NMDA excitation.[194] Diaphorase activity is absent in cortical neurons of knockout mice lacking the neuronal form of NOS,[281] and such mice demonstrate reduced vulnerability to ischaemic neuronal necrosis.[282] This suggests that neuronal NO seems to operate in exacerbating ischaemic neuronal death, overshadowing any beneficial effects of vasodilatation due to NO.

Morphology of selective neuronal necrosis and infarction

Whatever the pathophysiology of selective neuronal necrosis, a common appearance results. Acidophilic neurons are seen after hours to days (Fig. 5.18). These

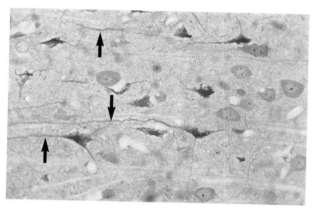

Figure 5.20 *Dark neurons. These need to be distinguished from acidophilic neurons (cf. Fig. 5.18), and show condensation, and affinity for basic as well as acid dyes, giving a purple appearance. The cell membranes of dark neurons are intact by electron microscopy (see Fig. 5.22), allowing dendritic cytoplasm to take on a corkscrew appearance during shrinkage. Such corkscrew dendrites (arrows) allow distinction of dark (i.e. reversibly damaged) from acidophilic (i.e. irreversibly damaged) neurons, in addition to the colour changes in double-stained (i.e. stained with an acid–base stain pair) sections. (Cortex, layer III, hypoglycaemia, 30 min of flat EEG, no recovery; in the rat.)*

represent dead neurons.[36] Dark and light neurons (Fig. 5.20), in contrast, represent early, reversible alterations.[36,37,578] Dark neurons and their profiles are also occasionally seen in normal tissue.[135] Early microvacuolation seen by light microscopy corresponds to swollen mitochondria by electron microscopy[86] and is also reversible.[237]

The necrotic nature of acidophilic neurons can be established first by the fact that they are removed from the tissue over time, either with or without accompanying macrophages.[36,37] Secondly, the corresponding electron micrograph of the acidophilic neuron[37,38] reveals the ultrastructural features of cellular necrosis, including mitochondrial flocculent densities and large, confluent breaks in the nuclear and cell membrane (Fig. 5.21). Dark neurons, in contrast, show only marked condensation ultrastructurally (Fig. 5.22). Volumetric recovery can be demonstrated through serial study over time, with reversal of the appearance of cytoplasmic condensation.[36]

In pan-necrosis (termed infarction if the cause is ischaemia), the intervening neuropil is removed as well as the neurons. In contrast to selective neuronal necrosis, this degree of tissue damage is always accompanied by the infiltration of macrophages. After days to weeks, astrocytic division occurs (hyperplasia). The astrocytes become hypertrophic by virtue of accumulation of eosinophilic cytoplasm (reactive astrocytes or gemistocytes), and accumulations of intermediate filaments of glial fibrillary acidic protein (GFAP). These cytoplasmic fibrils can be visualized with glial stains such as the Holzer stain or phosphotungstic acid–haematoxylin (PTAH), or by immunocytochemistry. Many months later, pan-necrosis appears as a fluid-filled cyst surrounded by neuropil containing fibre-forming astrocytes.

Dark neurons

Dark neurons (Fig. 5.20) are commonly seen in clinical and experimental neuropathology, and have plagued the

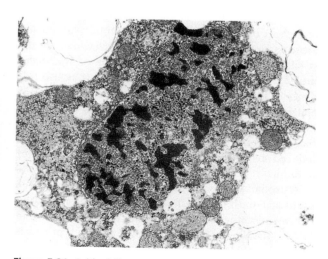

Figure 5.21 *Acidophilic neuron. Ultrastructurally, it shows large, confluent breaks in the nuclear membrane, and a coarse stippling of nuclear chromatin. The cytoplasm is amorphous and the mitochondria show flocculent densities. The cell membrane, like the nuclear membrane, is not intact. (Hypoglycaemia, 60 min of flat EEG with 18-h recovery, cerebral cortex, lamina III; in the rat.)*

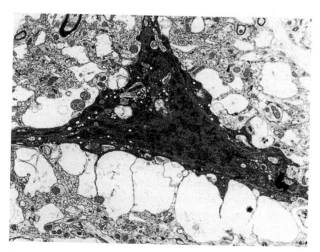

Figure 5.22 *Dark neurons. In spite of their appearance light microscopy (LM) (Fig. 5.20), ultrastructurally the cell is intact, as are the organelle and nuclear membranes (cf. Fig. 5.21). Recovery appears over time (see text), signifying this appearance as a neuron 'at risk', not a dead neuron. (Hypoglycaemia, 60 min of flat EEG with 5-min recovery, cerebral cortex, lamina III; in the rat.)*

interpretation of tissue sections since their early observation.[106] Although very dark, they have visibly intact cell membranes (Fig. 5.22) and internal organelles.[36] They do not, in spite of their appearance, signify neuronal death. Dark neurons occur in the early, reversible stages of neuronal injury due to ischaemia,[158] hypoglycaemia[36] and epilepsy.[579] They can be shown to recover longitudinally over time, in many brain insults, including hypoglycaemia[36] and epilepsy.[578]

Mechanically stimulating the cortex causes a wave of depolarization termed spreading depression[364] and such mechanical handling of living neural tissue easily produces dark neurons.[105] However, spreading depression produces no permanent neuronal damage.[454] Together with the intact organelles and cell membranes, and reversibility in controlled, sequentially examined experimental material,[36,578] the data establish the reversibility of dark neurons.

Other causes for dark neurons also involve mild cellular perturbation of the neuron. Trans-synaptic stimulation and release of glutamate,[144,213,573,618] or simply inhibition of the Na^+/K^+-ATPase pump, induces dark neurons in the tissue.[148,610] Mechanical touch and spreading depression can also cause dark neurons.[105,333,514] The sheer variety of conditions that can perturb the neuron into undergoing dark transformation has been recognized.[212]

In human neurosurgically excised material, in addition to spreading depression caused by mechanical excision, the tissue has been exposed to complete glucose deprivation en route from the operating theatre. The common cause of dark neurons in neurosurgical material thus can only be attributed to an undefined combination of at least two potential causes for dark neurons: spreading depression and hypoglycaemia. In this context, dark neurons are termed 'biopsy artefact' (see also Chapter 3, this Volume).

In experimental material, delayed fixation after death causes the tissue to be deprived of glucose, and dark neurons then appear with delayed fixation.[105] A short postmortem interval in man will give similar results to an experiment in the laboratory with delayed fixation: dark neurons will appear. Dark neurons do not occur in autopsy material unless the post-mortem interval is short. They seem to represent a contraction process of a perturbed neuron at the time of fixation. Neurons seem very sensitive to the perturbation that causes the cellular contraction at the time of fixation: dark neurons are occasionally seen in normal, aldehyde-fixed neural tissue.[135]

It is concluded that dark neurons represent reversibly perturbed neurons in aldehyde-fixed tissue. They must be distinguished from slow forms of neuronal degeneration where the cytoplasm undergoes progressive darkening accompanied by systematic organelle changes.[615]

Delayed neuronal death

The term delayed neuronal death, or maturation phenomenon, was first applied to observations in the hippocampus of rodents subjected to global ischaemia,[297,339,340] although there is evidence that a similar biological phenomenon occurs after brief, focal ischaemia.[444] The fundamental observation is that neurons do not die immediately after the 5–10 min period of global ischaemia, but rather die in the hours to days afterwards. Delayed neuronal death, as the term is commonly used, refers to the slow neuronal degeneration occurring days after an episode of complete ischaemia of short duration, not that following chronic, partial incomplete ischaemia.[461,603] In man, there is evidence for delayed neuronal death.[279,501]

Hypothermia delays the process of neuronal necrosis still further.[170] If the hypothermia is prolonged, permanent protection against neuronal necrosis may occur.[138–140] Certainly, however, the bulk of neuronal necrosis in the hippocampus after normothermic cardiac arrest is completed within the first week after global brain ischaemia. Clinical criteria cannot be used to gauge ongoing neuronal death: it is characteristic of global ischaemic encephalopathy that while neurons continue to die,[279,501] the clinical status improves[582] owing to the variety of recovery mechanisms available to the brain.

Delayed neuronal death is due to deleterious secondary processes in the recovery period, after the primary ischaemic insult has ended. The nature of these secondary deleterious processes is incompletely understood. Factors which have been studied are neuronal hyperactivity in the postischaemic period,[23,587] possibly due to enhanced sensitivity of postischaemic neurons to afferent stimuli,[22] mitochondrial perturbations,[2] as well as postischaemic alterations in calcium[22] and glutamate[23] homoeostasis. In the hippocampus, this may be due to early loss of neurons using somatostatin in the hilus,[412] rather than loss of GABAergic interneurons per se.[309] However, in the remainder of the brain it is the GABAergic neurons that are destroyed selectively by global ischaemia, in the striatum,[198] the lateral reticular nucleus of the thalamus[532,575,577] and the cerebral cortex.[571] There is also evidence in man that electrical hyperactivity or even status epilepticus occurs after cardiac arrest and that this is associated with a negative outcome.[112,355,569,652] Some animal studies have confirmed this electrical hyperactivity induced by ischaemia,[22,264,587] while others have not found it.[102,208,291,306,426]

Neuronal protein synthesis is inhibited during the postischaemic interval before cell death,[591] but inhibition of protein synthesis is not unique to neurons destined to die.[71,335] Rather, the failure to recover protein synthesis is unique, but this may be an epiphenomenon in dying neurons. Fasting actually prevents, not exacerbates, delayed neuronal necrosis.[408] Delayed death can be demonstrated to be calcium dependent in neuronal cultures exposed to glutamate.[120,122,535] Ischaemia leads to a marked increase in glutamate within the extracellular space of the brain,[59,242] which comprises only 15–20% of brain volume. Structurally, delayed neuronal death is accompanied early by selective dendritic lesions, sparing axons.[310,646,647] This suggests an excitotoxic component[479–481] to ischaemic cell death, since dendrites are predominantly where excitatory receptors are located.

Structural findings have suggested that delayed neuronal death is not due to a nuclear, or programmed cell death (apoptosis, see below). Death of neurons in brain regions other than the hippocampus, such as the neocortex,[444,510] the striatum[444,510] or the cerebellar Purkinje cells,[279] is less delayed than in the hippocampus. The importance of delayed neuronal death lies in the implication that neurons are not destroyed simply and directly at the end of the period of ischaemia. It is now accepted that delayed neuronal death is not due to a normal appearance of dead neurons in sections, neurons which merely take time to alter their appearance and undergo cytolysis at later time points. Rather, delayed neuronal death is a true biological phenomenon in which the cells have a normal appearance early after ischaemia because they are still viable, and are not yet irreversibly committed to die. The important clinical implication is that therapeutic intervention during this postischaemic period before the neurons have died, i.e. in the 'therapeutic window', is theoretically possible and may be fruitful.[139]

Ischaemic apoptosis, caspases and neuronal cell suicide

Although apoptosis is usually a counterforce to mitosis in biology (as in tumours[643] or in neural development), it has become fashionable to consider death of neurons, essentially postmitotic cells, as apoptosis in the context of ischaemia.[123] Apoptosis arises in the regulation of the cell cycle,[595] but neurons do not have a cell cycle. Exceptions include the olfactory bulb and the subgranular zone of the dentate gyrus, where neurogenesis occurs in association with blood vessels.[488] This burgeoning field of the study of neuronal death as potentially apoptotic is extremely controversial, not only in ischaemia, but also in other degenerative diseases such as Alzheimer's disease.[500]

Apoptosis basically constitutes an active, gene-directed dismantling and shrinking of a functioning cell by an intracellular programme for cell suicide.[334] The process takes place by an orderly process resulting in the sequential activation of enzymes.[396] These are unlike digestive enzymes, however, and have very restricted specificity for sites on the protein chain. The appellation caspase derives from 'cysteine protease cleaving after an aspartate residue'. Since caspases are more akin to molecular scissors than other, less discriminating enzymic destroyers of protein, cells appear remarkably preserved in outline during the process of dismantling. Cell membranes are intact, for example, and the mitochondrial flocculent densities seen in necrosis only appear very late in apoptosis.

The numerous experimental morphological studies of apoptosis in ischaemia almost always rely solely on light microscopy and terminal deoxytransferase-mediated dUTP nick end labelling (TUNEL). This cannot resolve cell membranes and makes it impossible to determine whether mitochondrial flocculent densities are present. TUNEL is non-specifically activated in necrosis.[231,604]

Activation of genes favouring programmed neuronal death has been documented by numerous groups[27,56,57,66,278,464,477] and transgenic mice overexpressing bcl-2 are resistant to ischaemia.[410] Endonucleases have been shown to be activated after ischaemia.[115,602] DNA fragmentation has been seen,[117,192,252,268,298,336,370,371,393,394,397,554] but was found to occur too late, i.e. after cell death in one experiment.[503] Studies using electron microscopy to look specifically for features of apoptosis have not found them,[166,207] even under experimental conditions theoretically favouring apoptosis, such as borderline insults to CA1 neurons of the hippocampus.[141] Some electron-microscopic studies have not focused on the presence or absence of the important, hallmark features distinguishing necrosis from apoptosis: absence of cell membrane integrity and mitochondrial flocculent densities.[373,463]

In focal ischaemic infarction, apoptosis would require a simultaneous suicide of neurons, astrocytes and oligodendrocytes. In some ischaemic situations, glia have curiously been found to be more vulnerable to apoptosis than neurons.[502]

Apoptosis is characterized by lack of a cellular inflammatory reaction, yet ischaemic necrosis shows a prominent mixed (neutrophilic–histiocytic) inflammatory component,[215,216,539] the magnitude of which is dependent on the severity of the insult.[411] Strategies combating the inflammatory component of the ischaemic cascade have been successful, against both neutrophils and histiocytes.[53,77,116,130,133,134,137,186,227,247,541,629] The presence of prominent inflammation in the ischaemic cascade also argues against apoptosis as the mechanism of cell death.

Necrosis occurs in conditions of energy failure, while apoptosis is a programme executing a cell with intact energy stores. Ischaemia is a well-documented cause of energy failure[560] causing cell death in rough proportion to the degree of energy failure.[415]

Another problem to be resolved out in this field is the activation of PARP (poly-ADPribose polymerase), which kills cells by NAD depletion, energy failure and necrosis. PARP has been shown to be activated in focal ischaemia,[192] a finding more compatible with necrosis than apoptosis. Some workers have proposed both mechanisms, apoptosis and necrosis,[327,376] or a different kind of apoptosis.[395,450,583] Caspase-3, the final executioner in the apoptotic cascade, is expressed in neurons.[450] Why important, postmitotic cells in the brain would be executed seems unclear, although some kinds of programmed cell death distinct from apoptosis or necrosis[583] might occur in slow neuronal degeneration.[159] Although initial reports with caspase inhibitors in some models seem promising,[368] the results in this controversial field will require confirmation, in different models, and in clinical trials.

Relationship of selective neuronal necrosis to infarction

Pathologically, the hypoxic states seem to give rise to only two degrees of damage: selective neuronal necrosis and pan-necrosis. In the former, only neurons are destroyed, but in the latter, all cell types are damaged, save perhaps endothelial cells.[104,271] Other contexts for pan-necrosis include the mitochondrial encephalopathy with lactic acidois and stroke (MELAS) syndrome, where necrosis is in a non-vascular distribution, unaccompanied by ischaemia. Pan-necrosis in MELAS and other mitochondrial disease probably relates to local tissue acidosis (see below).

There is no pathological evidence for the concept of incomplete infarction. The fact that the neuropil is either preserved or necrotic, in selective neuronal necrosis and infarction, respectively, without any intermediate state, argues against this concept. In selective neuronal necrosis, recovery is abetted by the surviving neuropil. Although small infarcts can close the gap caused by a tissue defect and present histologically as a glial scar, larger areas of infarction leave only a fluid-filled cyst.

Excitatory amino acids lead to selective neuronal necrosis,[19,121] and acidosis leads to pan-necrosis, the latter by damaging both neurons and glia.[50,352,453] However, the pathogenic relationships may not always be straightforward.

In neuropathological conditions characterized by pan-necrosis and acidosis, axon-sparing dendritic lesions may be seen. This is the case in Wernicke's encephalopathy, where there is dendritic swelling[630] and tissue acidosis,[245] and in ischaemic or epileptic pan-necrosis of the substantia nigra, where dendritic swelling[292,293] also accompanies a profound tissue acidosis.[294] Clearly, characteristic excitotoxic pathology occurs in acidotic CNS tissue.

Conversely, neuropathological conditions characterized by a primary action of excitatory amino acids can give rise to pan-necrosis, as seen in tissue acidosis below a certain threshold.[296] In excitotoxicity, the original descriptions by Olney of hypothalamic damage due to the excitotoxin glutamate clearly show pan-necrosis, not merely selective neuronal necrosis.[479,480,482]

In conclusion, the neuropathology in acidotic tissue states, and in excitotoxicity, may have some overlap. Some interaction between the two mechanisms is thus implied. It is likely that the metabolic stimulation due to glutamate and its analogues, if severe, causes metabolic activation enough to engender a severe, necrotizing tissue acidosis.

ISCHAEMIC NEUROPROTECTION

Excitatory amino acid antagonism

Since glutamate is released into the extracellular space with cerebral ischaemia,[59] obvious targets for neurotherapeutic intervention are the receptors for excitatory amino acids,[124,416] both NMDA[18,93] and non-NMDA receptors such as ionotropic AMPA receptors[225] and metabotropic receptors. As depolarization follows cell excitation via these receptors, and depolarization leads to activation of voltage-sensitive calcium channels (VSCCs), blockade of VSCCs has also been attempted.[32] Another strategy uses an endogenous neuroprotectant system within the brain, stimulated normally by adenosine, to confer ischaemic neuroprotection.[538] Success has been variable in these experiments and, in general, results are more favourable in focal than in global ischaemia.

A major concern has been raised regarding the purity of the alleged pharmacological mechanism of action in many of these experiments, since the drugs involved often induce hypothermia which, if abolished, also abolishes neuroprotection.[92,147,253] Although such an action via hypothermia may still be useful clinically, the mechanism of action of numerous pharmacological agents may have to be reconsidered if benefit is merely due to a drug-induced hypothermia.

Hypothermia

The protective effect of hypothermia in global hypoxic states has long been known, including effectiveness if hypothermia was begun before[67,508] or even after the insult.[58,639,642,660] A temperature of 20°C has been used to allow repair of intrathoracic fistulae with 19 min of complete circulatory arrest, without neurological sequelae.[76] Profound hypothermia of <20°C is used in surgical practice to protect the brain against iatrogenic global ischaemia.[149,236,617] The protective effect of hypothermia extends to the immature brain in infant asphyxia,[422] as can be demonstrated in the laboratory[438,586,645,653] and clinically.[236,422]

The effect of lowered temperature is so powerful that overlooked hypothermia may explain many of the experimental neuroprotective effects of pharmacological agents in global ischaemia.[92,147,253]

Despite the evidence that hypothermia is very effective, its mechanism of neuroprotective action is relatively poorly understood.[226] The cerebral utilization of oxygen is reduced[110] but improvement in brain tissue P_{O_2} does not seem to play a role.[42] The cerebral metabolic rate is lowered by hypothermia, such that oxygen consumption is only 25% of normal at 22°C.[244] Cerebral blood flow undergoes a similar hypothermic reduction,[3,244] in line with the coupling of CBF to metabolism (see above), but flow is still above the metabolic requirements at hypothermic temperatures.[156] Hypothermia reduces ischaemic brain oedema (Fig. 5.23).[165]

Metabolic benefits include slowed depletion of high-energy phosphates and increased diversion of glucose into the potentially neuroprotective pentose phosphate pathway (Fig. 5.4).[315] Hypothermia decreases free radical production,[322] and derangement of intracellular regulatory

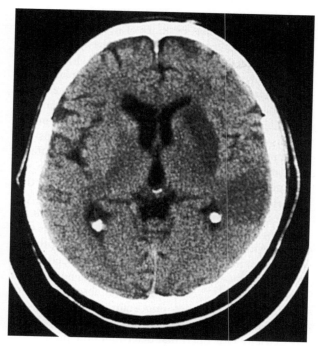

Figure 5.23 *Ischaemic oedema. This 71-year-old male had ischaemia due to thromboembolism 2 days prior to this CT scan. There is dark lucency in the right internal capsule and basal ganglia, signifying increased brain water. As a result of oedema, there is slightly greater indentation of the lateral ventricle on the right, owing to the mass effect of the focally increased brain water.*

enzymes such as calcium-calmodulin dependent protein kinase II[26,131] and protein kinase C,[109,175] and improved resynthesis of ubiquitin.[405,649] Peripheral blood lactate levels increase in hypothermia.[3] CO_2 further contributes to a peripheral acidosis, which may serve to maintain ventilation in hypothermia.[154] Cardiac function and blood pressure are also well maintained in hypothermia until near death.[251] The preservation of ventilatory and cardiac functions, together with hypothermic neuroprotection of the brain, explain the miraculous appearance of survival after hypothermia.[354,632]

In contrast to blood lactate, cerebral lactate levels are reduced, even if temperature is lowered by only 1°C.[65] Brain acidosis may or may not be reduced by hypothermia.[361,374,451]

Although intraischaemic hypothermia may operate by mitigating the intraischaemic rise in the excitatory compounds glutamate, glycine and dopamine,[44,45,101,427,445] the effectiveness of postischaemic hypothermia,[58,639] which acts when extracellular glutamate levels have returned to normal in the extracellular space,[473] cannot be explained by this mechanism.

Postischaemic temperature reduction may hold promise as a treatment for global cerebral ischaemia.[47,138–140] Focal ischaemia is also protected by intraischaemic[530] and postischaemic[321,531] hypothermia, and may be a treatment for focal ischaemic stroke in man.[319]

Insulin

Preischaemic or postischaemic insulin offers neuroprotection against global ischaemia.[626] High blood glucose levels are known to be damaging[217,440] and insulin lowers glucose, but also has a direct action on brain tissue.[624,658] Lowering high blood glucose levels with insulin may also be useful in focal ischaemia,[249] although optimum blood glucose levels that minimize brain damage remain to be determined.[151]

Hyperoxia

Before considering neuroprotection with oxygen, hyperoxic brain damage must be considered. By itself, hyperoxia at normobaric pressures does not seem to damage the adult brain, but at hyperbaric pressures, such as those encountered during diving,[55,176,177] 100% oxygen is toxic and causes brain necrosis.[48] Early changes are seen in cell processes and especially in mitochondria.[49] In the neonate, the situation is different, in that even normobaric hyperoxia can cause widespread neuronal necrosis.[16]

The combination of hyperoxia and carotid ligation gives a novel result. In hyperoxia, the hemisphere contralateral to the ligation undergoes necrosis, but in the ipsilateral one there is none,[48] exactly opposite to the results after hypoxia/carotid ligation. Thus, the reduced flow protects the ligated ipsilateral hemisphere from hyperoxic damage.

High arterial P_{O_2} levels of > 27 kPa (200 mmHg) have been shown to protect against ischaemic brain damage.[430] It may thus be possible to capitalize on this interactive effect of hyperoxia and ischaemia in therapy of acute cerebral ischaemia. Another effect of hyperoxaemia, one relevant to neuroimaging, is increased tissue contrast due to offloading of dissolved plasma oxygen at P_{aO_2} > 47 kPa (350 mmHg).[61]

Other measures protecting against ischaemia

A change in blood pressure of even 20 mmHg profoundly affects infarct size in animals[657] and also in man with ischaemic stroke.[314] There is experimental evidence that increasing the blood pressure reduces ischaemic damage,[260] and iatrogenic hypertension reduces brain damage in vasospasm accompanied by ischaemia.[323]

Magnesium is an NMDA receptor glutamate antagonist with a long, demonstrated history of safety in human pregnancy. Increasing the serum magnesium reduces focal ischaemic damage, especially if insulin is used to counteract the hyperglycaemia due to the Mg^{2+}.[299] In addition to glutamate antagonism, blood flow is improved, and clinical trials with Mg^{2+} have begun.[437]

HYPOGLYCAEMIC BRAIN DAMAGE

History of hypoglycaemic brain damage

Severe hypoglycaemia became much more common since the 1921 discovery of insulin, which was immediately put to use to treat diabetes. Thereafter, suspected brain damage due to hypoglycaemia associated with the use of insulin to treat diabetes became of increasing clinical concern. This led to numerous investigations into the fatal cases.[43,70,193,317,547,548,641]

An entirely new use for insulin, in the form of insulin shock as a 'therapy', was devised in the 1930s by a psychiatrist in Vienna, Dr Manfred Sakel. Insulin was thus used to treat schizophrenia.[543] One of the complications of therapy, aiming to produce 30 min of hypoglycaemic coma, was that the period of coma continued to be followed by death. Thus, cases of insulin therapy and insulin coma resulting in death were closely examined neuropathologically. Insulin shock therapy received support from some experimental results proclaiming no brain damage,[220] but other reports demonstrated permanent brain damage in the form of neuronal loss and gliosis with long-term survival.[107,181,324,363,392] The neuropathological autopsy thus contributed to the eventual abandonment of insulin therapy for schizophrenia, which fell into disuse by the 1950s.[414]

Neuropathologists still see hypoglycaemic brain damage in several settings. One is accidental or intentional (i.e. homicidal or suicidal) insulin overdose,[317] which may require the neuropathologist to demonstrate the presence of hypoglycaemic, as opposed to ischaemic, brain damage in medicolegal cases. A second is medication error, with insulin or another hypoglycaemic agent being inadvertently substituted for another drug, or given in an erroneously high dose.[317] The most common setting, however, is in the treatment of diabetes mellitus,[111] and it has been estimated that 5–8% of children with type I diabetes mellitus suffer bouts of severe hypoglycaemia (defined as accompanied by stupor or coma).[60] Recent clinical trials have shown a benefit of tight blood sugar control on the complications of diabetes mellitus, but possibly an increase in the incidence of hypoglycaemic brain damage.[167,266]

Although the early work focused on demonstrating the presence or absence of hypoglycaemic brain damage and its distribution over time, attention turned to the mechanism. Insulin itself was suspected to be neurotoxic at one time,[585] but laboratory experiments and human autopsy studies established hypoglycaemia as the mediator of neuronal damage. Morphological studies of cellular lesions focused on early microvacuolation, shown ultrastructurally to be due to swollen mitochondria,[8,10,11,316] and the term 'ischaemic cell change' was used because of the identical appearance of necrotic neurons to that seen in ischaemia, without emphasizing the important cardinal alteration of increased tinctorial affinity for acid dyes.[83,86]

The hallmark of neuronal death in both ischaemia and hypoglycaemia is the appearance of neuronal acidophilia,[40] which occurs concomitantly with the appearance of mitochondrial flocculent densities (Fig. 5.21), as demonstrated in hypoglycaemic brain damage,[36,37] and probably relates to irreversible protein alterations in the cell causing increased affinity for acid dyes. Mitochondrial flocculent densities have been shown to be proteinaceous, as they disappear when the tissue is injected with trypsin or proteinase.[613] Since necrotic neurons develop an affinity for acid dyes whatever the cause of neuronal death, the term neuronal acidophilia would seem more descriptive, accurate and inclusive.

The cause of the hypoglycaemia is immaterial to the resulting brain damage. Oral hypoglycaemic agents such as sulfonylureas release endogenous insulin and produce hypoglycaemia which has identical pathogenic effects on the brain as does hypoglycaemia due to exogenous insulin administration.[317,620] Surprisingly, the absolute level of blood sugar is also not important once it drops to < 1.5 mM; it is the presence or absence of cerebral EEG isoelectricity (flat EEG) that determines the presence or absence of brain damage. The flat EEG is preceded by the appearance of large, high-amplitude delta-waves in the frequency range of 1–4 Hz (the clinical counterpart of which is stupor).[421] Without EEG silence (the clinical counterpart of which is coma), brain damage in the form of neuronal necrosis is absent.

The brain uses principally glucose as a fuel, with few exceptions. The infant brain is capable of oxidizing lactate,[265,267,594] bestowing some protection against hypoglycaemia. This capability disappears with the progressive inability of lactate to enter the brain with maturation,[594] although some lactate can probably be burned during hypoglycaemia even by the adult brain.[218,457,553] Starvation is accompanied by brain utilization of ketone bodies, which circulate at elevated levels,[258] and the profoundly hypoglycaemic brain also burns ketones.[218,221,258,553] Lastly, hypoglycaemia, if profound enough to cause a flat EEG, can cause the breakdown of endogenous brain substrates, which can be used as fuel.[7,221] Thus, the energy of the brain is derived from the oxidative metabolism of glucose. Glycolysis yields four molecules of ATP and oxidative metabolism a further 38, for a total of 42 molecules of ATP per molecule of glucose that totally combines with oxygen to form carbon dioxide and water.

Hypoglycaemia was long thought to injure the brain simply by starving the neurons of glucose. Such a theory suggests that depriving neurons of either oxygen or glucose should have identical patterns of damage. As in global ischaemia, large neurons should be most vulnerable to necrosis according to such a theory, but hypoglycaemia, like global ischaemia,[439] does not preferentially affect large neurons in the brain.

Other flaws in the glucose starvation hypothesis of hypoglycaemic brain injury appeared after work demonstrating that the pathogenesis of selective neuronal necrosis in many cases involves the release of excitatory and toxic (excitotoxic) compounds in the brain. Work had already suggested that excitatory receptors play a role in ischaemic brain damage, since blockade of NMDA excitatory receptors reduced ischaemic damage.[570] Hypoglycaemic neuronal death could be blocked by pharmacological antagonists of NMDA excitatory receptors, reducing neuronal necrosis in spite of exposure to identical levels of hypoglycaemia in untreated animals.[637] These findings were accompanied by morphological demonstration of selective abnormalities in the dendritic tree of hippocampal neurons, where excitatory receptors are located, sparing axons of passage.[38] Such morphological lesions had been described earlier when the excitotoxins were discovered by Olney,[482,483] and are due to the dendritic location of excitatory receptors. Thus, it became clear that, although internal cellular mechanisms may initiate hypoglycaemic neuronal necrosis, at least part of the pathogenic mechanisms which subsequently give rise to hypoglycaemic neuronal death involve binding of an excitatory compound to external neuronal receptors. The pathogenic chain leading from a low blood sugar to neuronal death is thus somewhat longer and more indirect than might initially be suspected.

Biochemical basis of hypoglycaemic brain damage

Profound hypoglycaemia is accompanied by complex biochemical alterations.[33,561] Salient biochemical features include energy failure, reflected by a reduction in the energy charge (see above) to about 25–35% of normal. Protein and lipid catabolism occurs. Flux through the glycolytic pathway is reduced, with a consequent reduction in tissue levels of lactate and pyruvate. Proton production in the Krebs cycle, which turns more slowly, is reduced. The shortage of protons and organic acids together leads to a tissue alkalosis,[498] in contrast to ischaemia, in which these events do not take place.

Decarboxylation of pyruvate to yield carbon dioxide and acetate is reduced. The resulting shortage of acetyl CoA, with which oxaloacetate condenses (Fig. 5.4), leads to the tissue build-up of oxaloacetate. Oxaloacetate is the α-keto-acid in a transamination reaction with glutamate, yielding aspartic acid and α-ketoglutarate:

$$\text{Oxaloacetate} + \text{Glutamate} \rightleftarrows \text{Aspartate} + \alpha\text{-Ketoglutarate}$$

The excess oxaloacetate resulting from reduced glycolytic flux drives this reaction to the left by the chemical law of mass action (le Chetalier's principle). The result is an actual depletion of tissue levels of glutamate, with a marked increase in aspartate.[9,10,54] However, as a result of general failure of the cellular ability to maintain chemical compartmentation in profound hypoglycaemia, both aspartate and, to a lesser degree, glutamate increase in the extracellular space of the brain.[545]

The origin of the aspartate that is released in hypoglycaemia is metabolic, resulting from a shift in the aspartate–glutamate transaminase reaction towards aspartate. This occurs during hypoglycaemia due to a primary decrease in glycolytic flux, causing a shortage of moieties with which oxaloacetate can condense in the citric acid cycle. Inhibiting glycolytic flux, even without peripheral hypoglycaemia, causes an identical increase in aspartate.[546] The extracellular aspartate then damages neurons by an excitotoxic mechanism. The aspartate in the interstitial fluid of the brain drains into the CSF, explaining a unique aspect of the localization of hypoglycaemic brain damage to the dentate gyrus (see page 262).

Pharmacology of hypoglycaemic brain damage

The aspartate released into the extracellular space by the brain rendered isoelectric (flat EEG) due to profound hypoglycaemia is present in the interstitial space of the brain and in the CSF. Glutamate is also released, but to a lesser extent than aspartate. The ratio of aspartate to glutamate increases is the reverse of that in ischaemia, with glutamate predominating in ischaemia and aspartate in hypoglycaemia. Glutamate, being the naturally occurring endogenous neurotransmitter, is a broad-spectrum agonist at multiple receptors (see section on excitotoxicity). Since aspartate is more selective for NMDA receptors than glutamate, pharmacological blockade of NMDA receptors may be more effective in hypoglycaemia than in ischaemia. This indeed has been the case.[489,636,637] Although AMPA antagonists have not been studied in hypoglycaemic brain damage, voltage-sensitive calcium channel blockade has been found to be ineffective[476] or detrimental,[34] again in contrast with ischaemia, where a protective effect of calcium antagonists is generally seen.[32] Another difference is that the selective destruction of GABAergic neurons seen in hypoxia or ischaemia (see above) does not take place in hypoglycaemia.[527] Hypothermia has only a slight effect on hypoglycaemic brain damage,[14] compared with its universal and powerful protective effect in ischaemia (see above).

Morphology of hypoglycaemic brain damage

Hypoglycaemic brain damage, like ischaemic brain damage, affects the hippocampus and cerebral cortex, causing selective neuronal necrosis. Thus, in human neuropathological material, it is often impossible to distinguish hypoglycaemic from ischaemic brain damage,[460,521] and these two insults have long been considered identical.[86,152] However, controlled animal experiments delivering insults of hypoglycaemia and ischaemia to the brain, under close physiological monitoring, demonstrated differences between the morphological picture of hypoglycaemic and ischaemic brain damage.[39]

Lactate and pyruvate production is reduced in hypoglycaemia owing to reduced glycolytic flux, whereas in ischaemia anaerobic glycolysis is stimulated. Proton production by the Krebs cycle is reduced in hypoglycaemia, but increased in ischaemia. This, in conjunction with ammonia production from deamination of amino acids in hypoglycaemia, contributes to a tissue alkalosis. The pH change is opposite in ischaemia, where an acidosis develops. This lack of acidosis in hypoglycaemia probably accounts for the impossibility of producing hypoglycaemic pan-necrosis, whereas pan-necrosis is commonly seen in more severe tissue ischaemia, since acidosis seems a critical link in the pathogenesis of cerebral infarction. The lack of infarction in hypoglycaemic brain damage thus probably has a simple biochemical explanation. Hypoglycaemic brain damage, in its pure form, no matter how severe, is limited to selective neuronal necrosis. Infarction is not a feature.

Neuronal necrosis in hypoglycaemia usually involves the cerebral cortex, the hippocampus[35,70,107,181,317,324] and the caudate nucleus.[70,107,317,324] Changes were rarely reported in the spinal cord,[431,565,598] but never in the cerebellum.[392]

In rats,[38] rabbits[634] and sometimes in human material,[35,392] necrosis of the dentate gyrus is seen. The granule cells of the dentate gyrus are usually conspicuously normal in ischaemic brain damage, being the last neuronal type within the hippocampus to be recruited in ischaemia. In hypoglycaemia, however, perhaps due to the extracellular overflow of large quantities of aspartate,[545] necrosis of dentate granule cells, which contain excitatory receptors on the superficial molecular layer close to the ventricular fluid, is seen.

A second potentially distinguishing neuropathological feature is the presence of Purkinje cell necrosis in ischaemia, but absent in hypoglycaemia. This probably relates to the glucose transporter of the cerebellum, which is more efficient than elsewhere in the brain.[357] Reversible changes, such as mitochondrial swelling seen by electron microscopy in experimental material, do occur in the cerebellum in profound hypoglycaemia.[13]

Thirdly, the distribution of neuronal necrosis in the cerebral cortex, and its degree, may give a clue distinguishing hypoglycaemia from ischaemia. A superficial distribution of neuronal necrosis has been described in hypoglycaemic brain damage in man[107,324,363,548] and animals.[195,233] This contrasts with an intracortical distribution of neuronal necrosis to the middle cortical laminae in global ischaemic insults. Hypoglycaemic brain damage also gives a paucity of intracortical necrosis, with a widespread, even distribution of necrotic neurons over the hemisphere,[35,317] accounting for the high CBF in the presence of persistent coma.[12] The hemispheric distribution of neuronal necrosis does not show the predilection for arterial boundary zones as seen in ischaemic brain damage. Contrasting features between the neuropathology of global ischaemia, and that of hypoglycaemia, are given in Table 5.3.

Ultrastructurally, axon-sparing lesions imply that excitatory compounds are present in the extracellular space, binding selectively to dendrites and causing selective dendritic swelling due to receptor activation, followed by ion and water fluxes across the dendritic membrane. A salient feature of hypoglycaemic neuronal death by electron microscopy is just such dendritic swelling (Fig. 5.19). However, in contrast to ischaemia, where glutamate is released in large quantities,[59] hypoglycaemia releases more aspartate[545] than glutamate (see above).

SELECTIVE VULNERABILITY

All diseases in neuropathology show selective vulnerability. That is to say, an insult is delivered to the entire brain, yet only restricted brain regions show damage. This adds an extra dimension of complexity to the pathology of the brain compared with other organs, and partially accounts for separate study of CNS diseases in neuropathology. Homogeneous uniform damage affecting all parts of the brain equally is non-existent: the brain is the most inhomogeneous organ of the body.

Knowledge of selective vulnerability may give a clue to the origin or nature of the disease process, but elucidating why certain brain regions are vulnerable is doubly important, for it may also give rise to improved understanding of the mechanism(s) of damage, and may thence lead to treatment for neurological disease.

Table 5.3 *Differences between the neuropathology of global ischaemia and hypoglycaemia*

	Stagnant hypoxia (global ischaemia)	Hypoglycaemia
Cerebral cortex: gross distribution	Watershed	Uniform
Cerebral cortex: layers involved	Middle laminae	Superficial laminae
Hippocampus	CA1 > CA3 (dentate only if severe)	CA1 dentate
Cerebellum	Watershed	Absent
Brainstem	Can be involved	Absent

Theories attempting to explain selective vulnerability

Cogent explanations for selective vulnerability are lacking in most disease states. Significant progress has been made, however, in a few instances of selective vulnerability, as seen in stagnant hypoxia or global ischaemia. A seminal finding was the demonstration by Benveniste and Diemer that transient global ischaemia releases glutamate into the extracellular fluid of the brain.[59] Glutamate is now known to be the ubiquitous neurotransmitter of the brain and has the capability of causing neuronal necrosis by hyperexcitation, often termed excitotoxic neuronal death. In the hippocampus, a structure exquisitely vulnerable to global cerebral ischaemia, excitatory receptors are abundant. One subtype of glutamate receptor, named the NMDA receptor after its most favoured agonist, N-methyl-D-aspartate, is nowhere more abundant in the brain than in the dendritic fields of the vulnerable neurons[234,432,433] in CA1.[383,580] This is the best current explanation available for the dramatic difference in damage in two adjacent zones of the hippocampus in global ischaemia (Fig. 5.24), both of which are subjected to an identical primary insult, the reduction in blood flow. Modern receptor studies have thus shed light on the old problem of selective vulnerability in neuropathology. The argument of the Vogts of a neuronal difference or 'pathoklisis'[621–623] versus the vascular argument of Spielmeyer[584] accounting for why the CA1[529] field of cells die in ischaemia has been decidedly tipped in favour of the Vogts' argument of neuronal differences.

Other pathogenic mechanisms may operate to explain selective vulnerability, and treatment with NMDA antagonists has not always been shown to be of benefit in the hippocampus after global ischaemia. For example, other excitatory receptors such as AMPA receptors may play a prominent role in neuronal death after transient global ischaemia.[94,199,225] Neurotoxicity may be enhanced by zinc, known to be present in synaptic vesicles and co-released with transmitter.[200,572] Zinc released into the synaptic cleft has been estimated to reach potentially neurotoxic concentrations.[29,280] However, zinc in the hippocampus is present primarily in *en passant* axonal dilatations of mossy fibres ending on CA3,[209–211] which is relatively resistant. There are numerous enzymic differences shown histochemically between the vulnerable CA1 zone and the resistant CA3 zone.[205]

Dentate granule cells are rich in NMDA receptors, yet are not vulnerable. However, in hypoglycaemic brain damage, where massive quantities of aspartate and glutamate are released into the brain extracellular fluid,[545] the dentate gyrus is clearly vulnerable, in a pattern showing a relationship to CSF spaces, in rat,[38] rabbit[634] and man.[35] It thus seems that access of an excitatory compound to vulnerable neurons and their receptive fields must be considered, in addition to the intrinsic properties of the neuron, to give the most comprehensive explanation of selective vulnerability.

Satisfying explanations of selective vulnerability in other brain regions have been even more elusive than in the hippocampus. It seems clear that in most brain regions, stagnant hypoxia (global ischaemia) causes selective loss of GABAergic neurons. In the cerebral cortex,[571] the thalamus (lateral reticular nucleus)[203,532,575] and the striatum,[198] selective loss of GABAergic neurons has been shown. However, in the hippocampus, the CA1 zone shows actual preservation of GABAergic interneurons,[309] in spite of the stronger excitatory input that CA1 GABAergic neurons receive.[651] The hilus of the hippocampus shows loss of somatostatinergic innervation of GABAergic neurons, rather than loss of GABAergic neurons themselves.[311] Selective GABAergic neuron loss is one plausible explanation for epilepsy after hypoxic states.[571,577] The fundamental cause of selective destruction of neurons containing GABA is far from clear, but may be related to activation of excitatory receptors other than those of the NMDA subtype.[532] Clearly, our understanding of selective vulnerability of neuronal populations to ischaemia is still incomplete.

Other instances can be given where neuropathological observations of selective vulnerability lack a cogent explanation. Cerebellar Purkinje cells are vulnerable to transient global ischaemia. This was initially difficult to reconcile with the calcium hypothesis of neuronal cell death, since calcium was thought to enter neurons mainly by NMDA-gated channels, or by voltage-sensitive Ca^{2+} channels activated by depolarization. However, the recent use of cerebellar cultures enriched in Purkinje cells has allowed the discovery of an AMPA subtype of glutamate receptor with direct Ca^{2+} permeability,[385] perhaps

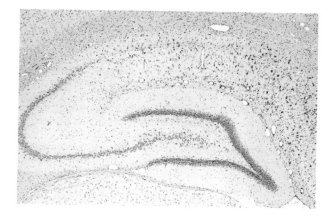

Figure 5.24 *Selective vulnerability. The hippocampus of the rat after global ischaemia is shown. The stain shows cell bodies in blue and glial fibrillary acidic protein in brown. There is striking limitation of both cell loss (seen as absence of the blue band of cells) and gliosis (seen as brown astrocytes) to the selectively vulnerable CA1 zone. This is probably related to glutamate receptor subtype distributions (see text). (Cresyl violet/GFAP immunocytochemistry.)*

explaining the long-known vulnerability of cerebellar Purkinje cells to degeneration in excitotoxic situations such as global ischaemia.

Sometimes, selective vulnerability of a particular brain region is striking, and easily correlated with a known pathogenic factor. An example is the long-known vulnerability of the globus pallidus and pars reticularis of the substantia nigra, the two brain regions richest in iron content, to necrosis in CO poisoning (see above). The extreme affinity of the CO molecule for the cytochrome haem iron in these regions, far exceeding the affinity of oxygen itself, is a true example of histotoxic hypoxia. However, explanations such as large neuronal size attempting to account for selective vulnerability do not hold up on close scrutiny: the largest neurons in the brain, the Betz cells of the motor cortex, are resistant to transient global ischaemic insult.[439] The explanation for selective vulnerability in most cases will depend on gaining a deeper understanding of the molecular constituents of the various brain regions which are unique to that region, and the interaction of such critical molecular characteristics with the environmental alterations impinging on the neuron. The resulting neuronal perturbations may be common to several disease processes, and partly unique to the disease process in question, giving rise to selective vulnerability of different brain regions.

REFERENCES

1 Abdul-Rahman A, Dahlgren N, Ingvar M et al. Local versus regional cerebral blood flow in the rat at high (hypoxia) and low (phenobarbital anesthesia) flow rates. Acta Physiol Scand 1979; 106: 53–60.

2 Abe K, Aoki M, Kawagoe J et al. Ischemic delayed neuronal death. A mitochondrial hypothesis. Stroke 1995; 26: 1478–89.

3 Adams JE, Elliot H, Sutherland VC et al. Cerebral metabolic studies of hypothermia in the human. Surg Forum 1956; 7: 535–9.

4 Adams RD, Jéquier M. The brain death syndrome: hypoxemic panencephalopathy. Schweiz Med Wochenschr 1969; 99: 65–73.

5 Adelson L, Sunshine I. Fatal hydrogen sulfide intoxication. Arch Pathol 1966; 81: 375–80.

6 Ådén U, Bona E, Hagberg H, Fredholm B. Changes in c-fos mRNA in the neonatal rat brain following hypoxic ischemia. Neurosci Lett 1994; 180: 91–5.

7 Agardh C-D, Chapman AG, Nilsson B, Siesjö BK. Endogenous substrates utilized by rat brain in severe insulin-induced hypoglycemia. J Neurochem 1981; 36: 490–500.

8 Agardh CD, Chapman AG, Pelligrino D, Siesjö BK. Influence of severe hypoglycemia on mitochondrial and plasma membrane function in rat brain. J Neurochem 1982; 38: 662–8.

9 Agardh C-D, Folbergrová J, Siesjö BK. Cerebral metabolic changes in profound insulin-induced hypoglycemia, and in the recovery period following glucose administration. J Neurochem 1978; 31: 1135–42.

10 Agardh C-D, Kalimo H, Olsson Y, Siesjö BK. Hypoglycemic brain injury. I. Metabolic and light microscopic findings in rat cerebral cortex during profound insulin-induced hypoglycemia and in the recovery period following glucose administration. Acta Neuropathol (Berl) 1980; 50: 31–41.

11 Agardh C-D, Kalimo H, Olsson Y, Siesjö BK. Hypoglycemic brain injury: Metabolic and structural findings in rat cerebellar cortex during profound insulin-induced hypoglycemia and in the recovery period following glucose administration. J Cereb Blood Flow Metab 1981; 1: 71–84.

12 Agardh C-D, Rosén I, Ryding E. Persistent vegetative state with high cerebral blood flow following profound hypoglycemia. Ann Neurol 1983; 14: 482–6.

13 Agardh C-D, Siesjö BK. Hypoglycemic brain injury: phospholipids, free fatty acids, and cyclic nucleotides in the cerebellum of the rat after 30 and 60 minutes of severe insulin-induced hypoglycemia. J Cereb Blood Flow Metab 1981; 1: 267–75.

14 Agardh CD, Smith M-L, Siesjö BK. The influence of hypothermia on hypoglycemia-induced brain damage in the rat. Acta Neuropathol (Berl) 1992; 83: 379–85.

15 Agnihotri N, Lopez-Garcia JC, Hawkins RD, Arancio O. Morphological changes associated with long-term potentiation. Histol Histopathol 1998; 13: 1155–62.

16 Ahdab-Barmada M, Moossy J, Nemoto EM, Lin MR. Hyperoxia produces neuronal necrosis in the rat. J Neuropathol Exp Neurol 1986; 45: 233–46.

17 Albaum HG, Noell WK, Chinn HI. Chemical changes in the rabbit brain during anoxia. Am J Physiol 1953; 174: 408–12.

18 Albers GW, Goldberg MP, Choi DW. Do NMDA antagonists prevent neuronal injury? Yes. Arch Neurol 1992; 49: 418–20.

19 Albin RL, Greenamyre JT. Alternative excitotoxic hypotheses. Neurology 1992; 42: 733–8.

20 Alderete JF, Jeri FR, Richardson EP Jr et al. Irreversible coma: a clinical, electroencephalographic and neuropathological study. Trans Am Neurol Assoc 1968; 93: 16–20.

21 Alkon DL, Rasmussen H. A spatial–temporal model of cell activation. Science 1988; 239: 998–1005.

22 Andiné P, Jacobson I, Hagberg H. Calcium uptake evoked by electrical stimulation is enhanced postischemically and precedes delayed neuronal death in CA1 of rat hippocampus: involvement of NMDA receptors. J Cereb Blood Flow Metab 1988; 8: 799–807.

23 Andiné P, Orwar O, Jacobson I et al. Changes in extracellular amino acids and spontaneous neuronal activity during ischemia and extended reflow in the CA1 of the rat hippocampus. J Neurochem 1991; 57: 222–9.

24 Ando S, Kametani H, Osada H et al. Delayed memory dysfunction by transient hypoxia, and its prevention with forskolin. Brain Res 1987; 405: 371–4.

25 Araki T, Kato H, Kogure K. Neuronal damage and calcium accumulation following repeated brief cerebral ischemia in the gerbil. Brain Res 1990; 528: 114–22.

26 Aronowski J, Grotta JC, Waxham MN. Ischemia-induced translocation of Ca^{2+}/calmodulin-dependent protein kinase II: potential role in neuronal damage. J Neurochem 1992; 58: 1743–53.

27 Asahi M, Hoshimaru M, Uemura Y et al. Expression of interleukin-1β converting enzyme gene family and bcl-2 gene family in the rat brain following permanent occlusion of the middle cerebral artery. J Cereb Blood Flow Metab 1997; 17: 11–18.

28 Ashwal S, Schneider S, Tomasi L, Thompson J. Prognostic implications of hyperglycemia and reduced cerebral blood flow in childhood near-drowning. Neurology 1990; 40: 820–3.

29 Assaf SY, Chung SH. Release of endogenous Zn^{2+} from brain tissue during activity. Nature 1984; 308: 734–6.

30 Astrup J, Siesjö BK, Symon L. Thresholds in cerebral ischemia – the ischemic penumbra. *Stroke* 1981; **12**: 723–5.

31 Atkinson DE. The energy charge of the adenylate pool as a regulatory parameter. Interaction with biofeedback modifiers. *Biochemistry* 1968; **7**: 4030–4.

32 Auer RN. Calcium channel antagonists in cerebral ischemia: a review. *Drug Dev* 1993; **2**: 307–17.

33 Auer RN. Hypoglycemic brain damage. *Stroke* 1986; **17**: 488–96.

34 Auer RN, Anderson LG. Hypoglycemic brain damage: effect of a dihydropyridine calcium antagonist. *Diabetologia* 1996; **39**: 129–34.

35 Auer RN, Hugh J, Cosgrove E, Curry B. Neuropathologic findings in three cases of profound hypoglycemia. *Clin Neuropathol* 1989; **8**: 63–8.

36 Auer RN, Kalimo H, Olsson Y, Siesjö BK. The temporal evolution of hypoglycemic brain damage. I. Light and electron microscopic findings in the rat cerebral cortex. *Acta Neuropathol (Berl)* 1985; **67**: 13–24.

37 Auer RN, Kalimo H, Olsson Y, Siesjö BK. The temporal evolution of hypoglycemic brain damage. II. Light and electron microscopic findings in the rat hippocampus. *Acta Neuropathol (Berl)* 1985; **67**: 25–36.

38 Auer RN, Kalimo H, Olsson Y, Wieloch T. The dentate gyrus in hypoglycemia. Pathology implicating excitotoxin-mediated neuronal necrosis. *Acta Neuropathol (Berl)* 1985; **67**: 279–88.

39 Auer RN, Siesjö BK. Biological differences between ischemia, hypoglycemia, and epilepsy. *Ann Neurol* 1988; **24**: 699–707.

40 Auer RN, Wieloch T, Olsson Y, Siesjö BK. The distribution of hypoglycemic brain damage. *Acta Neuropathol (Berl)* 1984; **64**: 177–91.

41 Bachelard HS, Lewis LD, Pontén U, Siesjö BK. Mechanisms activating glycolysis in the brain in arterial hypoxia. *J Neurochem* 1974; **22**: 395–401.

42 Bacher A, Kwon JY, Zornow MH. Effects of temperature on cerebral tissue oxygen tension, carbon dioxide tension, and pH during transient global ischemia in rabbits. *Anesthesiology* 1998; **88**: 403–9.

43 Baker AB. Cerebral lesions in hypoglycemia. II. Some possibilities of irrevocable damage from insulin shock. *Arch Pathol* 1938; **26**: 765–76.

44 Baker AJ, Zornow MH, Grafe MR et al. Hypothermia prevents ischemia-induced increases in hippocampal glycine concentrations in rabbits. *Stroke* 1991; **22**: 666–73.

45 Baker CJ, Fiore AJ, Frazzini VI et al. Intraischemic hypothermia decreases the release of glutamate in the cores of permanent focal cerebral infarcts. *Neurosurgery* 1995; **36**: 994–1001.

46 Baldelli RJ, Green FHY, Auer RN. Sulfide toxicity: the role of mechanical ventilation and hypotension in determining survival rate and brain necrosis. *J Appl Physiol* 1993; **75**: 1348–53.

47 Baldwin WA, Kirsch JR, Hurn PD et al. Hypothermic cerebral reperfusion and recovery from ischemia. *J Physiol (Lond)* 1991; **261**: H774–81.

48 Balentine JD. Pathogenesis of central nervous system lesions induced by exposure to hyperbaric oxygen. *Am J Pathol* 1968; **53**: 1097–109.

49 Balentine JD. Ultrastructural pathology of hyperbaric oxygenation in the central nervous system, observations in the anterior horn gray matter. *Lab Invest* 1974; **31**: 580–92.

50 Balentine JD, Greene WB. Myelopathy induced by lactic acid. *Acta Neuropathol (Berl)* 1987; **73**: 233–9.

51 Beal F, Richardson EP Jr. Localized brainstem ischemic damage and Ondine's curse after near drowning. *Neurology* 1983; **33**: 717–21.

52 Beal MF, Richardson EP Jr, Brandstetter R et al. Localized brainstem ischemic damage and Ondine's curse after near-drowning. *Neurology* 1983; **33**: 717–21.

53 Bednar MM, Raymond S, McAuliffe T et al. The role of neutrophils and platelets in a rabbit model of thromboembolic stroke. *Stroke* 1991; **22**: 44–50.

54 Behar KL, Hollander JA den, Petroff OAC et al. Effect of hypoglycemic encephalopathy upon amino acids, high-energy phosphates, and pH$_i$ in the rat brain *in vivo*: detection by sequential ^{1}H and ^{31}P NMR spectroscopy. *J Neurochem* 1985; **44**: 1045–55.

55 Behnke AR, Johnson FS, Poppen JR, Motley EP. The effects of oxygen on man at pressures from one to four atmospheres. *Am J Physiol* 1935; **110**: 565–72.

56 Beilharz EJ, Williams CE, Dragunow M et al. Mechanisms of delayed cell death following hypoxic–ischemic injury in the immature rat: evidence for apoptosis during selective neuronal loss. *Mol Brain Res* 1995; **29**: 1–14.

57 Bennett SAL, Tenniswood M, Chen J-H et al. Chronic cerebral hypoperfusion elicits neuronal apoptosis and behavioral impairment. *Neuroreport* 1998; **9**: 161–6.

58 Benson DW, Williams GR, Spencer FC, Yates AJ. The use of hypothermia after cardiac arrest. *Anesth Analg* 1959; **38**: 423–8.

59 Benveniste H, Drejer J, Schousboe A, Diemer NH. Elevation of the extracellular concentrations of glutamate and aspartate in rat hippocampus during transient cerebral ischemia monitored by intracerebral microdialysis. *J Neurochem* 1984; **43**: 1369–74.

60 Bergada I, Suissa S, Dufresne J, Schiffrin A. Severe hypoglycemia in IDDM children. *Diabetes Care* 1989; **12**: 239–44.

61 Berkowitz BA. Role of dissolved plasma oxygen in hyperoxia-induced contrast. *Magn Reson Imaging* 1997; **15**: 123–6.

62 Berlet HH. Hypoxic survival of normoglycaemic young adult and adult mice in relation to cerebral metabolic rates. *J Neurochem* 1976; **26**: 1267–74.

63 Bernard C. In: Greene HG ed. trans. *An introduction to the study of experimental medicine*. New York: MacMillan, 1927.

64 Berntman L, Carlsson C, Siesjö BK. Cerebral oxygen consumption and blood flow in hypoxia: influence of sympathoadrenal activation. *Stroke* 1979; **10**: 20–5.

65 Berntman L, Welsh FA, Harp JR. Cerebral protective effect of low grade hypothermia. *Anesthesiology* 1981; **55**: 495–8.

66 Bhat RV, DiRocco R, Marcy VR et al. Increased expression of IL-1β converting enzyme in hippocampus after ischemia: selective localization in microglia. *J Neurosci* 1996; **16**: 4146–54.

67 Bigelow WG, Callaghan JC, Hopps JA. General hypothermia for experimental intracardiac surgery. *Ann Surg* 1950; **132**: 531–7.

68 Black PMcL. Brain death. *N Engl J Med* 1978; **299**: 338–44, 393–401.

69 Bliss TVP, Lømo T. Long-lasting potentiation of synaptic transmission in the dentate area of the anaesthetized rabbit following stimulation of the perforant path. *J Physiol (Lond)* 1973; **232**: 331–56.

70 Bodechtel G. Der Hypoglykämische Shock und seine Wirkung auf das Zentralnervensystem. *Dtsch Arch Klin Med* 1933; **175**: 188–201.

71 Bodsch W, Barbier A, Oehmichen M et al. Recovery of monkey brain after prolonged ischemia. II. Protein synthesis and morphological alterations. *J Cereb Blood Flow Metab* 1986; **6**: 22–33.

72 Boero JA, Ascher J, Arregui A et al. Increased brain capillaries in chronic hypoxia. *J Appl Physiol* 1999; **86**: 1211–19.

73 Bogousslavsky J, Khurana R, Deruaz JP et al. Respiratory failure and unilateral caudal brainstem infarction. Ann Neurol 1990; 28: 668–773.

74 Boje KM, Arora PK. Microglial-produced nitric oxide and reactive nitrogen oxides mediate neuronal cell death. Brain Res 1992; 587: 250–6.

75 Borgström L, Jóhannsson H, Siesjö BK. The influence of acute normovolemic anemia on cerebral blood flow and oxygen consumption of anesthetized rats. Acta Physiol Scand 1975; 93: 505–14.

76 Borst HG, Schaudig A, Rudolph W. Arteriovenous fistula of the aortic arch: repair during deep hypothermia and circulatory arrest. J Thorac Cardiovasc Surg 1964; 48: 443–7.

77 Bowes MP, Zivin JA, Rothlein R. Monoclonal antibody to the ICAM-1 adhesion site reduces neurological damage in a rabbit cerebral embolism stroke model. Exp Neurol 1993; 119: 215–19.

78 Bredt DS, Glatt CE, Hwang PM et al. Nitric oxide synthase protein and mRNA are discretely localized in neuronal populations of the mammalian CNS together with NADPH diaphorase. Neuron 1991; 7: 615–24.

79 Bredt DS, Hwang PM, Snyder SH. Localization of nitric oxide synthase indicating a neural role for nitric oxide. Nature 1990; 347: 768–70.

80 Bredt DS, Snyder SH. Nitric oxide, a novel neuronal messenger. Neuron 1992; 8: 3–11.

81 Brierley JB, Adams JH, Graham DI, Simpson JA. Neocortical death after cardiac arrest. A clinical, neurophysiological, and neuropathological report of two cases. Lancet 1971; ii: 560–5.

82 Brierley JB, Brown AW, Excell BJ, Meldrum BS. Brain damage in the rhesus monkey resulting from profound arterial hypotension. 1. Its nature, distribution and general physiological correlates. Brain Res 1969; 13: 68–100.

83 Brierley JB, Brown AW, Meldrum BS. The nature and time course of the neuronal alterations resulting from oligaemia and hypoglycemia in the brain of Macaca mulatta. Brain Res 1971; 25: 483–99.

84 Brierley JB, Cooper JE. Cerebral complications of hypotensive anaesthesia in a healthy adult. J Neurol Neurosurg Psychiatry 1962; 25: 24–30.

85 Brierley JB, Excell BJ. The effects of profound systemic hypotension upon the brain of M. rhesus: physiological and pathological observations. Brain 1966; 89: 269–98.

86 Brierley JB, Meldrum BS, Brown AW. The threshold and neuropathology of cerebral 'anoxic–ischemic' cell change. Arch Neurol 1973; 29: 367–74.

87 Brierley JB, Prior PF, Calverley J, Brown AW. Cyanide intoxication in Macaca mulatta. J Neurol Sci 1977; 31: 133–57.

88 Brierley JB, Prior PF, Calverley J, Brown AW. Profound hypoxia in Papio anubis and Macaca mulatta – physiological and neuropathological effects. I. Abrupt exposure following normoxia. II. Abrupt exposure following moderate hypoxia. J Neurol Sci 1978; 37: 1–29.

89 Brown AW, Brierley JB. Anoxic–ischemic cell change in rat brain. Light microscopic and fine-structural observations. J Neurol Sci 1972; 16: 59–84.

90 Brown AW, Brierley JB. The earliest alterations in rat neurones and astrocytes after anoxia–ischaemia. Acta Neuropathol (Berl) 1973; 23: 9–22.

91 Bruick RK. Expression of the gene encoding the proapoptotic Nip3 protein is induced by hypoxia. Proc Natl Acad Sci USA 2000; 97: 9082–7.

92 Buchan A, Pulsinelli WA. Hypothermia but not the N-methyl-d-aspartate antagonist, MK-801, attenuates neuronal damage in gerbils subjected to transient global ischemia. J Neurosci 1990; 10: 311–16.

93 Buchan AM. Do NMDA antagonists prevent neuronal injury? No. Arch Neurol 1992; 49: 420–1.

94 Buchan AM, Li H, Cho S, Pulsinelli WA. Blockade of the AMPA receptor prevents CA1 hippocampal injury following severe but transient forebrain ischemia in adult rats. Neurosci Lett 1991; 132: 255–8.

95 Budabin M. Neurologic complications of open heart surgery. Mt Sinai J Med 1982; 49: 311–13.

96 Buisson A, Margaill I, Callebert J et al. Mechanisms involved in the neuroprotective activity of a nitric oxide synthase inhibitor during focal cerebral ischemia. J Neurochem 1993; 61: 690–6.

97 Buisson A, Plotkine M, Boulu RG. The neuroprotective effect of a nitric oxide inhibitor in a rat model of focal cerebral ischaemia. Br J Pharmacol 1992; 106: 766–7.

98 Burger PC, Vogel FS. Hemorrhagic white matter infarction in three critically ill patients. Hum Pathol 1977; 8: 121–32.

99 Burnett WW, King EG, Grace M, Hall WF. Hydrogen sulfide poisoning: a review of 5 years' experience. Can Med Assoc J 1977; 117: 1277–81.

100 Busto R, Dietrich WD, Globus MY-T, Ginsberg MD. The importance of brain temperature in cerebral ischemic injury. Stroke 1989; 20: 1113–14.

101 Busto R, Globus MY-T, Dietrich WD et al. Effect of mild hypothermia on ischemia-induced release of neurotransmitters and free fatty acids in rat brain. Stroke 1989; 20: 904–10.

102 Buzsáki G, Freund TF, Bayardo F, Somogyi P. Ischemia-induced changes in the electrical activity of the hippocampus. Exp Brain Res 1989; 78: 268–78.

103 Calder IM, Palmer AC, Hughes JT et al. Spinal cord degeneration associated with type II decompression sickness: case report. Paraplegia 1989; 27: 51–7.

104 Calhoun CL, Mottaz JH. Capillary bed of the rat cerebral cortex. The fine structure in experimental cerebral infarction. Arch Neurol 1966; 15: 320–8.

105 Cammermeyer J. Is the solitary dark neuron a manifestation of postmortem trauma to the brain inadequately fixed by perfusion? Histochemistry 1978; 56: 97–115.

106 Cammermeyer J. The importance of avoiding 'dark' neurons in experimental neuropathology. Acta Neuropathol (Berl) 1961; 1: 245–70.

107 Cammermeyer J. Über Gehirnveränderungen, entstanden unter Sakelscher Insulintherapie bei einem Schizophrenen. Z Ges Neurol Psychiatrie 1938; 163: 617–33.

108 Campbell JA. Diet and resistance to oxygen want. Q J Exp Physiol 1939; 29: 259–75.

109 Cardell M, Boris-Möller F, Wieloch T. Hypothermia prevents the ischemia-induced translocation and inhibition of protein kinase C in the rat striatum. J Neurochem 1991; 57: 1814–17.

110 Carlsson C, Hägerdal M, Siesjö BK. Protective effect of hypothermia in cerebral oxygen deficiency caused by arterial hypoxia. Anesthesiology 1976; 44: 27–35.

111 Casparie AF, Elving LD. Severe hypoglycemia in diabetic patients: frequency, causes, prevention. Diabetes Care 1985; 8: 141–5.

112 Celesia GG, Grigg MM, Ross E. Generalized status myoclonicus in acute anoxic and toxic–metabolic encephalopathies. Arch Neurol 1988; 45: 781–4.

113 Cervos-Navarro J, Sampaolo S, Hamdorf G. Brain changes in experimental chronic hypoxia. Exp Pathol 1991; 42: 205–12.

114 Chao CC, Hu S, Molitor TW et al. Activated microglia mediate neuronal cell injury via a nitric oxide mechanism. J Immunol 1992; 149: 2736–41.

115 Charriaut-Marlangue C, Margaill I, Plotkine M, Ben-Ari Y. Early endonuclease activation following reversible focal

ischemia in the rat brain. *J Cereb Blood Flow Metab* 1995; **15**: 385–8.

116 Chen H, Chopp M, Bodzin G. Neutropenia reduces the volume of cerebral infarct after transient middle cerebral artery occlusion in the rat. *Neurosci Res Commun* 1992; **11**: 93–9.

117 Chen J, Jin K, Chen M *et al.* Early detection of DNA strand breaks in the brain after transient focal ischemia: implications for the role of DNA damage in apoptosis and neuronal cell death. *J Neurochem* 1997; **69**: 232–45.

118 Chen J, Uchimura K, Stetler RA *et al.* Transient global ischemia triggers expression of the DNA damage-inducible gene GADD45 in the rat brain. *J Cereb Blood Flow Metab* 1998; **18**: 646–57.

119 Cherici G, Alesiani M, Pellegrini-Giampietro DE, Moroni F. Ischemia does not induce the release of excitotoxic amino acids from the hippocampus of newborn rats. *Dev Brain Res* 1991; **60**: 235–40.

120 Choi DW. Calcium-mediated neurotoxicity: relationship to specific channel types and role in ischemic damage. *Trends Neurosci* 1988; **11**: 465–9.

121 Choi DW. Glutamate neurotoxicity and diseases of the nervous system. *Neuron* 1988; **1**: 623–34.

122 Choi DW. Ionic dependence of glutamate neurotoxicity. *J Neurosci* 1987; **7**: 369–79.

123 Choi DW. Ischemia-induced neuronal apoptosis. *Curr Opin Neurobiol* 1996; **6**: 667–72.

124 Choi DW. Methods for antagonizing glutamate neurotoxicity. *Cerebrovasc Brain Metab Rev* 1990; **2**: 105–47.

125 Chopp M, Chen H, Ho K-L *et al.* Transient hyperthermia protects against subsequent forebrain ischemic cell damage in the rat. *Neurology* 1989; **39**: 1396–8.

126 Chopp M, Li Y, Dereski MO *et al.* Hypothermia reduces 72-kDa heat-shock protein induction in rat brain after transient forebrain ischemia. *Stroke* 1992; **23**: 104–7.

127 Chopp M, Li Y, Dereski MO *et al.* Neuronal injury and expression of 72-kDa heat-shock protein after forebrain ischemia in the rat. *Acta Neuropathol (Berl)* 1991; **83**: 66–71.

128 Chopp M, Li Y, Zhang ZG, Freytag SO. p53 expression in brain after middle cerebral artery occlusion in the rat. *Biochem Biophys Res Commun* 1992; **182**: 1201–7.

129 Chopp M, Welch KMA, Tidwell CD, Helpern JA. Global cerebral ischemia and intracellular pH during hyperglycemia and hypoglycemia in cats. *Stroke* 1988; **19**: 1383–7.

130 Chopp M, Zhang RL, Chen H *et al.* Postischemic administration of an anti-mac-1 antibody reduces ischemic cell damage after transient middle cerebral artery occlusion in rats. *Stroke* 1994; **25**: 869–76.

131 Churn SB, Taft WC, Billingsley MS *et al.* Temperature modulation of ischemic neuronal death and inhibition of calcium/calmodulin-dependent protein kinase II in gerbils. *Stroke* 1990; **21**: 1715–21.

132 Clark CF, Heaton RK, Wiens AN. Neuropsychological functioning after prolonged high altitude mountaineering. *Aviat Space Environ Med* 1983; **54**: 202–7.

133 Clark WM, Madden KP, Rothlein R, Zivin JA. Reduction of central nervous system ischemic injury by monoclonal antibody to intercellular adhesion molecule. *J Neurosurg* 1991; **75**: 623–7.

134 Clark WM, Madden KP, Rothlein R, Zivin JA. Reduction of central nervous system ischemic injury in rabbits using leukocyte adhesion antibody treatment. *Stroke* 1991; **22**: 877–83.

135 Cohen EB, Pappas GD. Dark profiles in the apparently normal central nervous system: a problem in the electron microscopic identification of early anterograde axonal degeneration. *J Comp Neurol* 1969; **136**: 375–96.

136 Cohen PJ, Alexander SC, Smith TC *et al.* Effects of hypoxia and normocarbia on cerebral blood flow and metabolism in conscious man. *J Appl Physiol* 1967; **23**: 183–9.

137 Coimbra C, Drake M, Boris-Möller F, Wieloch T. Long-lasting neuroprotective effect of postischemic hypothermia and treatment with an anti-inflammatory/antipyretic drug. Evidence for chronic encephalopathic processes following ischemia. *Stroke* 1996; **27**: 1578–85.

138 Colbourne F, Auer RN, Sutherland GR. Characterization of postischemic behavioral deficits in gerbils with and without hypothermic neuroprotection. *Brain Res* 1998; **803**: 69–78.

139 Colbourne F, Corbett D. Delayed and prolonged postischemic hypothermia is neuroprotective in the gerbil. *Brain Res* 1994; **654**: 265–72.

140 Colbourne F, Corbett D. Delayed postischemic hypothermia: a six month survival study using behavioral and histologic assessments of neuroprotection. *J Neurosci* 1995; **15**: 7250–60.

141 Colbourne F, Sutherland GR, Auer RN. Electron microscopic evidence against apoptosis as the mechanism of neuronal death in global ischemia. *J Neurosci* 1999; **19**: 4200–10.

142 Cole G, Cowie VA. Long survival after cardiac arrest: case report and neuropathological findings. *Clin Neuropathol* 1987; **6**: 104–9.

143 Collaco-Moraes Y, Aspey BS, Belleroche JS de, Harrison MJ. Focal ischemia causes an extensive induction of immediate early genes that are sensitive to MK-801. *Stroke* 1994; **25**: 1855–60.

144 Collins RC, Olney JW. Focal cortical seizures cause distant thalamic lesions. *Science* 1982; **218**: 177–9.

145 Combs DJ, Reuland DS, Martin DB *et al.* Glycolytic inhibition by 2-deoxyglucose reduces hyperglycemia-associated mortality and morbidity in the ischemic rat. *Stroke* 1986; **17**: 989–94.

146 Connor JA, Wadman WJ, Hockberger PE, Wong RKS. Sustained dendritic gradients of Ca^{2+} induced by excitatory amino acids in CA1 hippocampal neurons. *Science* 1988; **240**: 649–53.

147 Corbett D, Evans S, Thomas C *et al.* MK-801 reduces cerebral ischemic injury by inducing hypothermia. *Brain Res* 1990; **514**: 300–4.

148 Cornog JL Jr, Gonatas NK, Feierman JR. Effects of intracerebral injection of ouabain on the fine structure of rat cerebral cortex. *Am J Pathol* 1967; **51**: 573–90.

149 Coselli JS, Crawford ES, Beall AC *et al.* Determination of brain temperatures for safe circulatory arrest during cardiovascular operation. *Ann Thorac Surg* 1988; **45**: 638–42.

150 Courten-Myers GM de, Fogelson HM, Kleinholz M, Myers RE. Hypoxic brain and heart injury thresholds in piglets. *Biomed Biochim Acta* 1989; **48**: S143–8.

151 Courten-Myers GM de, Kleinholz M, Wagner KR, Myers RE. Normoglycemia (not hypoglycemia) optimizes outcome from middle cerebral artery occlusion. *J Cereb Blood Flow Metab* 1994; **14**: 227–36.

152 Courville CB. Late cerebral changes incident to severe hypoglycemia (insulin shock). Their relation to cerebral anoxia. *Arch Neurol Psychiatry (Chic)* 1957; **78**: 1–14.

153 Craigie EH. On the relative vascularity of various parts of the central nervous system of the albino rat. *J Comp Neurol* 1920; **31**: 429–64.

154 Cranston WI, Pepper MC, Ross DN. Carbon dioxide and control of respiration during hypothermia. *J Physiol (Lond)* 1955; **127**: 380–9.

155 Craven C, Chinn H, MacVicar R. Effect of carrot diet and restricted feeding on the resistance of the rat to hypoxia. *J Aviat Med* 1950; **21**: 256–8.

156 Croughwell N, Smith LR, Quill T. The effect of temperature on cerebral metabolism and blood flow in adults during cardiopulmonary bypass. *J Thorac Cardiovasc Surg* 1992; **103**: 549–54.

157 Crumrine RC, Thomas AL, Morgan PF. Attenuation of p53 expression protects against focal ischemic damage in transgenic mice. *J Cereb Blood Flow Metab* 1994; **14**: 887–91.

158 Czurko A, Nishino H. 'Collapsed' (argyrophilic, dark) neurons in rat model of transient focal cerebral ischemia. *Neurosci Lett* 1993; **162**: 71–4.

159 Dal Canto MC, Gurney ME. Development of central nervous system pathology in a murine transgenic model of human amyotrophic lateral sclerosis. *Am J Pathol* 1994; **145**: 1271–9.

160 D'Alecy L, Lundy EF, Barton KJ, Zelenock GB. Dextrose containing intravenous fluid impairs outcome and increases death after eight minutes of cardiac arrest and resuscitation in dogs. *Surgery* 1986; **100**: 505–11.

161 Dalkara T, Yoshida T, Irikura K, Moskowitz MA. Dual role of nitric oxide in focal cerebral ischemia. *Neuropharmacology* 1994; **33**: 1447–52.

162 Dawson DA, Kusumoto K, Graham DI et al. Inhibition of nitric oxide synthesis does not reduce infarct volume in a rat model of focal cerebral ischaemia. *Neurosci Lett* 1992; **142**: 151–4.

163 Dawson TM, Dawson VL, Snyder SH. A novel neuronal messenger molecule in brain: the free radical, nitric oxide. *Ann Neurol* 1992; **32**: 297–311.

164 De Bilbao F, Guarin E, Nef P et al. Cell death is prevented in thalamic fields but not in injured neocortical areas after permanent focal ischaemia in mice overexpressing the anti-apoptotic protein Bcl-2. *Eur J Neurosci* 2000; **12**: 921–34.

165 Dempsey RJ, Combs DJ, Edwards Maley M et al. Moderate hypothermia reduces postischemic edema development and leukotriene production. *Neurosurgery* 1987; **21**: 177–81.

166 Deshpande J, Bergstedt K, Lindén T et al. Ultrastructural changes in the hippocampal CA1 region following transient cerebral ischemia: evidence against programmed cell death. *Exp Brain Res* 1992; **88**: 91–105.

167 Diabetes Control and Complications Trial Research Group. The effect of intensive treatment of diabetes on the development and progression of long-term complications in insulin-dependent diabetes mellitus. *N Engl J Med* 1993; **329**: 977–86.

168 Diemer NH, Siemkowicz E. Increased 2-deoxyglucose uptake in hippocampus, globus pallidus and substantia nigra after cerebral ischemia. *Acta Neurol Scand* 1980; **61**: 56–63.

169 Dienel GA, Kiessling M, Jacewicz M, Pulsinelli WA. Synthesis of heat shock proteins in rat brain cortex after transient ischemia. *J Cereb Blood Flow Metab* 1986; **6**: 505–10.

170 Dietrich WD, Busto R, Alonso O et al. Intraischemic but not postischemic brain hypothermia protects chronically following global forebrain ischemia in rats. *J Cereb Blood Flow Metab* 1993; **13**: 541–9.

171 Dietrich WD, Busto R, Valdes I, Loor Y. Effects of normothermic versus mild hyperthermic forebrain ischemia in rats. *Stroke* 1990; **21**: 1318–25.

172 Dinerman JL, Dawson TM, Schell MJ et al. Endothelial nitric oxide synthase localized to hippocampal pyramidal cells: implications for synaptic plasticity. *Proc Natl Acad Sci USA* 1994; **91**: 4214–18.

173 Dings J, Meixensberger J, Jager A, Roosen K. Clinical experience with 118 brain tissue oxygen partial pressure catheter probes. *Neurosurgery* 1998; **43**: 1082–95.

174 Doling EC, Richardson EP Jr. Ophthalmoplegia and Ondine's curse. *Arch Ophthalmol* 1977; **95**: 1790–3.

175 Domanska-Janik K, Zablocka B. Protein kinase C as an early and sensitive marker of ischemia-induced progressive neuronal damage in gerbil hippocampus. *Mol Chem Neuropathol* 1993; **20**: 111–23.

176 Donald KW. Oxygen poisoning in man. Part I. *BMJ* 1947; **i**: 667–72.

177 Donald KW. Oxygen poisoning in man. Part II. *BMJ* 1947; **i**: 712–17.

178 Donegan JH, Traystman RJ, Koehler RC et al. Cerebrovascular hypoxic and autoregulatory responses during reduced brain metabolism. *Am J Physiol* 1985; **249**: H421–9.

179 Doppenberg EM, Zauner A, Bullock R et al. Correlations between brain tissue oxygen tension, carbon dioxide tension, pH, and cerebral blood flow – a better way of monitoring the severely injured brain? *Surg Neurol* 1998; **49**: 650–4.

180 Doppenberg EM, Zauner A, Watson JC, Bullock R. Determination of the ischemic threshold for brain oxygen tension. *Acta Neurochir Suppl (Wien)* 1998; **71**: 166–9.

181 Döring G. Zur Histopathologie und Pathogenese des tödlichen Insulinshocks. *Dtsch Ztschr Nervenheilkunde* 1938; **147**: 217–27.

182 Duffy TE, Cavazzuti M, Cruz NF, Sokoloff L. Local cerebral glucose metabolism in newborn dogs: effects of hypoxia and halothane anesthesia. *Ann Neurol* 1982; **11**: 233–46.

183 Duffy TE, Nelson SR, Lowry OH. Cerebral carbohydrate metabolism during acute hypoxia and recovery. *J Neurochem* 1972; **19**: 959–77.

184 Dumke PR, Schmidt CF. Quantitative measurements of cerebral blood flow in the macaque monkey. *Am J Physiol* 1943; **138**: 421–31.

185 Dunn JF, Grinberg O, Roche M et al. Noninvasive assessment of cerebral oxygenation during acclimation to hypobaric hypoxia. *J Cereb Blood Flow Metab* 2000; **20**: 1632–5.

186 Dutka AJ, Kochanek PM, Hallenbeck JM. Influence of granulocytopenia on canine cerebral ischemia induced by air embolism. *Stroke* 1989; **20**: 390–5.

187 Edelman GJ, Hoffman WE, Charbel FT. Cerebral hypoxia after etomidate administration and temporary cerebral artery occlusion. *Anesth Analg* 1997; **85**: 821–5.

188 Edelmann F. Ein Beitrag zur Vergiftung mit gasförmiger Blausäure insbesondere zu den dabei auftretenden Gehirnveränderungen. *Deutsche Ztschr Nervenheilkunde* 1921; **72**: 259–87.

189 Eiger SM, Kirsch JR, D'Alecy LG. Hypoxic tolerance enhanced by β-hydroxybutyrate-glucagon in the mouse. *Stroke* 1980; **11**: 513–17.

190 Ellis RJ, Vies SM van der. Molecular chaperones. *Annu Rev Biochem* 1991; **60**: 321–47.

191 Endres M, Namura S, Shimizu-Sasamata M et al. Attenuation of delayed neuronal death after mild focal ischemia in mice by inhibition of the caspase family. *J Cereb Blood Flow Metab* 1998; **18**: 238–47.

192 Endres M, Wang ZQ, Namura S et al. Ischemic brain injury is mediated by the activation of poly(ADP-ribose)polymerase. *J Cereb Blood Flow Metab* 1997; **17**: 1143–51.

193 Fazekas JF, Alman RW, Parrish AE. Irreversible posthypoglycemic coma. *Am J Med Sci* 1951; **222**: 640–1.

194 Ferriero DM, Simon RP. Neonatal striatal NADPH-diaphorase neurons are vulnerable to quisqualate and its analogue α-amino-3-hydroxy-5-methyl-4-isoxazole propionate (AMPA). *Neurosci Lett* 1991; **126**: 52–6.

195 Finley KH, Brenner C. Histologic evidence of damage to the brain in monkeys treated with Metrazol and insulin. *Arch Neurol Psychiatry (Chic)* 1941; **45**: 403–38.

196 Fischer EG. Impaired perfusion following cerebrovascular stasis. A review. *Arch Neurol* 1973; **29**: 361–6.

197 Fonnum F, Storm-Mathisen J, Divac I. Biochemical evidence for glutamate as neurotransmitter in corticostriatal and corticothalamic fibres in rat brain. *Neuroscience* 1981; **6**: 863–73.

198 Francis A, Pulsinelli W. The response of GABAergic and cholinergic neurons to transient cerebral ischemia. *Brain Res* 1982; **243**: 271–8.

199 Frank L, Bruhn T, Diemer NH. The effect of an AMPA antagonist (NBQX) on postischemic neuron loss and protein synthesis in the rat brain. *Exp Brain Res* 1993; **95**: 70–6.

200 Frederickson CJ, Hernandez MD, McGinty JF. Translocation of zinc may contribute to seizure-induced death of neurons. *Brain Res* 1989; **480**: 317–21.

201 Freireich EJ, Thomas LB, Frei E III *et al.* A distinctive type of intracerebral hemorrhage associated with 'blastic crisis' in patients with leukemia. *Cancer* 1960; **13**: 146–54.

202 Frerichs KU, Kennedy C, Sokoloff L, Hallenbeck JM. Local cerebral blood flow during hibernation, a model of natural tolerance to 'cerebral ischemia'. *J Cereb Blood Flow Metab* 1994; **14**: 193–205.

203 Freund TF, Buzsáki G, Leon A, Baimbridge KG, Somogyi P. Relationship of neuronal vulnerability and calcium binding protein immunoreactivity in ischemia. *Exp Brain Res* 1990; **83**: 55–66.

204 Friede R. Der quantitative Anteil der Glia an der Cortexentwicklung. *Acta Anat* 1954; **20**: 290–6.

205 Friede RL. The histochemical architecture of Ammon's horn as related to selective vulnerability. *Acta Neuropathol (Berl)* 1966; **6**: 1–13.

206 Friede RL, Houten WH van. Relations between post-mortem alterations and glycolytic metabolism in the brain. *Exp Neurol* 1961; **4**: 197–204.

207 Fukuda T, Wang H, Nakanishi H *et al.* Novel non-apoptotic morphological changes in neurons of the mouse hippocampus following transient hypoxic–ischemia. *Neurosci Res* 1999; **33**: 49–55.

208 Furukawa K, Yamana K, Kogure K. Postischemic alterations of spontaneous activities in rat hippocampal CA1 neurons. *Brain Res* 1990; **530**: 257–60.

209 Gaarskjaer FB. Organization of the mossy fiber system of the rat studied in extended hippocampi. I. Terminal area related to number of granule and pyramidal cells. *J Comp Neurol* 1978; **178**: 49–72.

210 Gaarskjaer FB. Organization of the mossy fiber system of the rat studied in extended hippocampi. II. Experimental analysis of fiber distribution with silver impregnation methods. *J Comp Neurol* 1978; **178**: 73–88.

211 Gaarskjaer FB. The hippocampal mossy fiber system of the rat studied with retrograde tracing techniques. Correlation between topographic organization and neurogenetic gradients. *J Comp Neurol* 1982; **203**: 717–35.

212 Gallyas F, Zoltay G, Dames W. Formation of 'dark' (argyrophilic) neurons of various origin proceeds with a common mechanism of biophysical nature (a novel hypothesis). *Acta Neuropathol (Berl)* 1992; **83**: 504–9.

213 Gallyas F, Zoltay G, Horvath Z *et al.* An immediate morphopathologic response of neurons to electroshock; a reliable model for producing 'dark' neurons in experimental neuropathology. *Neurobiology (Bp)* 1993; **1**: 133–46.

214 Garcia JH. Morphology of global cerebral ischemia. *Crit Care Med* 1989; **16**: 979–87.

215 Garcia JH, Cox JV, Hudgins WR. Ultrastructure of the microvasculature in experimental cerebral infarction. *Acta Neuropathol (Berl)* 1971; **18**: 273–85.

216 Garcia JH, Liu KF, Yoshida Y *et al.* Influx of leukocytes and platelets in an evolving brain infarct (Wistar rat). *Am J Pathol* 1994; **144**: 188–99.

217 Gardiner M, Smith M-L, Kägström E *et al.* Influence of blood glucose concentration on brain lactate accumulation during severe hypoxia and subsequent recovery of brain energy metabolism. *J Cereb Blood Flow Metab* 1982; **2**: 429–38.

218 Gardiner RM. The effects of hypoglycaemia on cerebral blood flow and metabolism in the new-born calf. *J Physiol (Lond)* 1980; **298**: 37–51.

219 Garland H, Pearce J. Neurological complications of carbon monoxide poisoning. *Q J Med* 1967; **36**: 445–55.

220 Gellhorn E. Effects of hypoglycemia and anoxia on the central nervous system. *Arch Neurol Psychiatry (Chic)* 1938; **40**: 125–46.

221 Ghajar JBG, Plum F, Duffy TE. Cerebral oxidative metabolism and blood flow during acute hypoglycemia and recovery in unanaesthetised rats. *J Neurochem* 1982; **38**: 397–409.

222 Giangaspero F, Schiavina M, Sturani C *et al.* Failure of automatic control of ventilation (Ondine's curse) associated with viral encephalitis of the brainstem: a clinicopathologic study of one case. *Clin Neuropathol* 1988; **7**: 234–7.

223 Gibbs EL, Lennox WG, Nims LF, Gibbs FA. Arterial and cerebral venous blood: arterial–venous differences in man. *J Biol Chem* 1942; **144**: 325–32.

224 Gibbs FA, Gibbs EL, Lennox WG. Changes in human cerebral blood flow consequent to alterations in blood gases. *Am J Physiol* 1935; **111**: 557–63.

225 Gill R. The pharmacology of α-amino-3-hydroxy-5-methyl-4-isoxazole propionate (AMPA)/kainate antagonists and their role in cerebral ischaemia. *Cerebrovasc Brain Metab Rev* 1994; **6**: 225–56.

226 Ginsberg MD, Sternau LL, Globus MY-T *et al.* Therapeutic modulation of brain temperature: relevance to ischemic brain injury. *Cerebrovasc Brain Metab Rev* 1992; **4**: 189–225.

227 Giulian D, Robertson C. Inhibition of mononuclear phagocytes reduces ischemic injury in the spinal cord. *Ann Neurol* 1990; **27**: 33–42.

228 Goldman MS, Anderson RE, Meyer FB. Effects of intermittent reperfusion during temporary focal ischemia. *J Neurosurg* 1992; **77**: 911–16.

229 Goldman SA, Pulsinelli WA, Clarke WY *et al.* The effects of extracellular acidosis on neurons and glia *in vitro*. *J Cereb Blood Flow Metab* 1989; **9**: 471–7.

230 Graham DI, Mendelow AD, Tuor U, Fitch W. Neuropathologic consequences of internal carotid artery occlusion and hemorrhagic hypotension in baboons. *Stroke* 1990; **21**: 428–34.

231 Grasl-Kraupp B, Ruttkay-Nedecky B, Koudelka H *et al.* In situ detection of fragmented DNA (TUNEL assay) fails to discriminate among apoptosis, necrosis, and autolytic cell death: a cautionary note. *Hepatology* 1995; **21**: 1465–8.

232 Gray FD Jr, Horner GJ. Survival following extreme hypoxemia. *JAMA* 1970; **211**: 1815–17.

233 Grayzel DM. Changes in the central nervous system due to convulsions due to hyperinsulinism. *Arch Intern Med* 1934; **54**: 694–701.

234 Greenamyre JT, Olson JMM, Penney JB Jr, Young AB. Autoradiographic characterization of N-methyl-d-aspartate-, quisqualate- and kainate-sensitive glutamate binding sites. *J Pharmacol Exp Ther* 1985; **233**: 254–63.

235 Greenberg ME, Ziff EB, Greene LA. Stimulation of neuronal acetylcholine receptors induces rapid gene transcription. *Science* 1986; **234**: 80–3.

236 Greene KA, Marciano FF, Hamilton MG *et al.* Cardiopulmonary bypass, hypothermic circulatory arrest and barbiturate cerebral protection for the treatment of giant vertebrobasilar aneurysms in children. *Pediatr Neurosurg* 1994; **21**: 124–33.

237 Griffiths T, Evans MC, Meldrum BS. Status epilepticus: the reversibility of calcium loading and acute neuronal pathological changes in the rat hippocampus. *Neuroscience* 1984; **12**: 557–67.

238 Grinker RR. Über einen Fall von Leuchtgasvergiftung mit doppelseitiger Pallidumerweichung und schwerer Degeneration des tieferen Grosshirn Marklagers. *Z Ges Neurol Psychiatrie* 1925; **98**: 433–56.

239 Gross PM, Sposito NM, Pettersen SE et al. Topography of capillary density, glucose metabolism, and microvascular function within the rat inferior colliculus. *J Cereb Blood Flow Metab* 1987; **7**: 154–60.

240 Grunnet ML, Paulson G. Pathological changes in irreversible brain death. *Dis Nerv Syst* 1971; **32**: 690–4.

241 Gurdjian ES, Stone WE, Webster JE. Cerebral metabolism in hypoxia. *Arch Neurol Psychiatry (Chic)* 1944; **5**: 472–7.

242 Hagberg H, Lehmann A, Sandberg M et al. Ischemia-induced shift of inhibitory and excitatory amino acids from intra- to extracellular compartments. *J Cereb Blood Flow Metab* 1985; **5**: 413–19.

243 Hager H, Hirschberger W, Scholz W. Electron microscopic changes in the brain tissue of Syrian hamsters following acute hypoxia. *Aerospace Med* 1960; **31**: 379–87.

244 Hägerdal M, Harp J, Nilsson L, Siesjö BK. The effect of induced hypothermia upon oxygen consumption in the rat brain. *J Neurochem* 1975; **24**: 311–16.

245 Hakim AM. The induction and reversibility of cerebral acidosis in thiamine deficiency. *Ann Neurol* 1984; **16**: 673–9.

246 Haley JE, Malen PL, Chapman PF. Nitric oxide synthase inhibitors block long-term potentiation induced by weak but not strong tetanic stimulation at physiological brain temperatures in rat hippocampal slices. *Neurosci Lett* 1993; **160**: 85–8.

247 Hallenbeck JM, Dutka AJ, Tanishima T et al. Polymorphonuclear leukocyte accumulation in brain regions with low blood flow during the early postischemic period. *Stroke* 1986; **17**: 246–53.

248 Hamberger A, Hydén H. Inverse enzyme changes in neurons and glia during increased function and hypoxia. *J Cell Biol* 1963; **16**: 521–5.

249 Hamilton MG, Tranmer BI, Auer RN. Insulin reduction of cerebral infarction due to transient focal ischemia. *J Neurosurg* 1995; **82**: 262–8.

250 Hansen AJ. Effect of anoxia on ion distribution in the brain. *Physiol Rev* 1985; **65**: 101–48.

251 Hansen DB. Arterial blood pressure in unanesthetized hypothermic rats. *J Appl Physiol* 1954; **6**: 645–9.

252 Hara A, Yoshimi N, Mori H et al. Hypothermic prevention of nuclear DNA fragmentation in gerbil hippocampus following transient forebrain ischemia. *Neurol Res* 1995; **17**: 461–4.

253 Hara H, Onodera H, Kogure K. Effects of hyperthermia on the effectiveness of MK-801 treatment in the gerbil hippocampus following transient forebrain ischemia. *Brain Res Bull* 1992; **29**: 659–65.

254 Haraldseth O, Nygård Ø, Grønås T et al. Hyperglycemia in global cerebral ischemia and reperfusion: a 31-phosphorous NMR spectroscopy study in rats. *Acta Anaesthesiol Scand* 1992; **36**: 25–30.

255 Harik SI, Hritz MA, LaManna JC. Hypoxia-induced brain angiogenesis in the adult rat. *J Physiol* 1995; **485**: 525–30.

256 Harik SI, Lust WD, Jones SC et al. Brain glucose metabolism in hypobaric hypoxia. *J Appl Physiol* 1995; **79**: 136–40.

257 Hawkins A, Olszewski J. Glia/nerve cell index for cortex of the whale. *Science* 1957; **126**: 76–7.

258 Hawkins RA, Williamson DH, Krebs HA. Ketone-body utilization by adult and suckling rat brain *in vivo*. *Biochem J* 1971; **122**: 13–18.

259 Hawkins RD, Son H, Arancio O. Nitric oxide as a retrograde messenger during long-term potentiation in hippocampus. *Prog Brain Res* 1998; **118**: 155–72.

260 Hayashi S, Nehls DG, Kieck CF et al. Beneficial effects of induced hypertension on experimental stroke in awake monkeys. *J Neurosurg* 1984; **60**: 151–7.

261 Hayashi T, Takada K, Matsuda M. Changes in ubiquitin and ubiquitin–protein conjugates in the CA1 neurons after transient sublethal ischemia. *Mol Chem Neuropathol* 1991; **15**: 75–82.

262 Haymaker W, Davison C. Fatalities resulting from exposure to simulated high altitudes in decompression chambers. *J Neuropathol Exp Neurol* 1950; **9**: 29–59.

263 Haymaker W, Ginzler AM, Ferguson RL. Residual neuropathological effects of cyanide poisoning. A study of the central nervous system of 23 dogs exposed to cyanide compounds. *Military Surgeon* 1952; **iii**: 231–46.

264 Heiss WD, Hayakawa T, Waltz AG. Cortical neuronal function during ischemia. Effects of occlusion of one middle cerebral artery on single-unit activity in cats. *Arch Neurol* 1976; **33**: 813–20.

265 Hellmann J, Vannucci RC, Nardis EE. Blood–brain barrier permeability to lactic acid in the newborn dog: lactate as a cerebral metabolic fuel. *Pediatr Res* 1982; **16**: 40–4.

266 Henry RR, Gumbiner B, Ditzler T et al. Intensive conventional insulin therapy for type II diabetes. Metabolic effects during a 6-mo outpatient trial. *Diabetes Care* 1993; **16**: 21–31.

267 Hernández MJ, Vannucci RC, Salcedo A, Brennan RW. Cerebral blood flow and metabolism during hypoglycemia in newborn dogs. *J Neurochem* 1980; **35**: 622–8.

268 Heron A, Pollard H, Dessi F et al. Regional variability in DNA fragmentation after global ischemia evidenced by combined histological and gel electrophoresis observations in the rat brain. *J Neurochem* 1993; **61**: 1973–6.

269 Hetherington HP, Tan MJ, Luo KL et al. Evaluation of lactate production and clearance kinetics by ^{1}H NMR in a model of brief repetitive cerebral ischemia. *J Cereb Blood Flow Metab* 1994; **14**: 591–6.

270 Heytens L, Verlooy J, Gheuens J, Bossaert L. Lazarus sign and extensor posturing in a brain-dead patient. Case report. *J Neurosurg* 1989; **71**: 449–51.

271 Hills CP. Ultrastructural changes in the capillary bed of the rat cerebral cortex in anoxic–ischemic brain lesions. *Am J Pathol* 1964; **44**: 531–43.

272 Hochachka PW. Patterns of O_2-dependence of metabolism. *Adv Exp Med Biol* 1988; **222**: 143–51.

273 Hochachka PW, Clark CM, Brown WD et al. The brain at high altitude: hypometabolism as a defense against chronic hypoxia? *J Cereb Blood Flow Metab* 1994; **14**: 671–9.

274 Hoffman WE, Charbel FT, Edelman G. Brain tissue oxygen, carbon dioxide, and pH in neurosurgical patients at risk for ischemia. *Anesth Analg* 1996; **82**: 582–6.

275 Hoffman WE, Charbel FT, Edelman G, Ausman JI. Brain tissue oxygen pressure, carbon dioxide pressure, and pH during hypothermic circulatory arrest. *Surg Neurol* 1996; **46**: 75–9.

276 Hoffman WE, Charbel FT, Edelman G et al. Brain tissue oxygen pressure, carbon dioxide pressure and pH during ischemia. *Neurol Res* 1996; **18**: 54–6.

277 Hoffman WE, Charbel FT, Munoz L, Ausman JI. Comparison of brain tissue metabolic changes during ischemia at 35- and 18°C. *Surg Neurol* 1998; **49**: 85–8.

278 Honkaniemi J, Massa SM, Breckinridge M, Sharp FR. Global ischemia induces apoptosis-associated genes in hippocampus. *Mol Brain Res* 1996; **42**: 79–88.

279 Horn M, Schlote W. Delayed neuronal death and delayed neuronal recovery in the human brain following global ischemia. *Acta Neuropathol (Berl)* 1992; **85**: 79–87.

280 Howell GA, Welch MG, Frederickson CJ. Stimulation-induced uptake and release of zinc in hippocampal slices. *Nature* 1984; **308**: 736–8.

281 Huang PL, Dawson TM, Bredt DS *et al*. Targeted disruption of the neuronal nitric oxide synthase gene. *Cell* 1993; **75**: 1273–86.

282 Huang Z, Huang PL, Panahian N *et al*. Effects of cerebral ischemia in mice deficient in neuronal nitric oxide synthase. *Science* 1994; **265**: 1883–5.

283 Hugg JW, Duijn JH, Matson GB *et al*. Elevated lactate and alkalosis in chronic human brain infarction observed by ^{1}H and ^{31}P MR spectroscopic imaging. *J Cereb Blood Flow Metab* 1992; **12**: 734–44.

284 Humphrey PR, Du Boulay GH, Marshall J *et al*. Cerebral blood flow and viscosity in relative polycythaemia. *Lancet* 1979; **ii**: 873–7.

285 Hunt SP, Pini A, Evan G. Induction of c-fos-like protein in spinal cord neurons following sensory stimulation. *Nature* 1987; **328**: 632–4.

286 Hunter S, Ballinger WE, Greer M. Nitrogen inhalation in the human. *Acta Neuropathol (Berl)* 1985; **68**: 115–21.

287 Hylland P, Nilsson GE, Lutz PL. Time course of anoxia-induced increase in cerebral blood flow rate in turtles: evidence for a role of adenosine. *J Cereb Blood Flow Metab* 1994; **14**: 877–81.

288 Iadecola C, Xu X, Zhang F *et al*. Marked induction of calcium-independent nitric oxide synthase activity after focal cerebral ischemia. *J Cereb Blood Flow Metab* 1995; **15**: 52–9.

289 Iadecola C, Zhang F, Xu X. Inhibition of nitric oxide synthase ameliorates cerebral ischemic damage. *Am J Physiol* 1995; **268**: R286–92.

290 Iadecola C, Zhang F, Xu S *et al*. Inducible nitric oxide synthase gene expression in brain following cerebral ischemia. *J Cereb Blood Flow Metab* 1995; **15**: 378–84.

291 Imon H, Mitani A, Andou Y *et al*. Delayed neuronal death is induced without postischemic hyperexcitability: continuous multiple-unit recording from ischemic CA1 neurons. *J Cereb Blood Flow Metab* 1991; **11**: 819–23.

292 Inamura K, Olsson Y, Siesjö BK. Substantia nigra damage induced by ischemia in hyperglycemic rats. A light and electron microscopic study. *Acta Neuropathol (Berl)* 1987; **75**: 131–9.

293 Inamura K, Smith M-L, Olsson Y, Siesjö BK. Pathogenesis of substantia nigra lesions following hyperglycemic ischemia: changes in energy metabolites, cerebral blood flow, and morphology of pars reticulata in a rat model of ischemia. *J Cereb Blood Flow Metab* 1988; **8**: 375–84.

294 Ingvar M, Folbergrová J, Siesjö BK. Metabolic alterations underlying the development of hypermetabolic necrosis in the substantia nigra in status epilepticus. *J Cereb Blood Flow Metab* 1987; **7**: 103–8.

295 Ingvar M, Morgan PF, Auer RN. The nature and timing of excitotoxic neuronal necrosis in the cerebral cortex, hippocampus and thalamus due to flurothyl-induced status epilepticus. *Acta Neuropathol (Berl)* 1988; **75**: 362–9.

296 Ingvar M, Schmidt-Kastner R, Meller D. Immunohistochemical markers for neurons and astrocytes show pannecrosis following infusion of high-dose NMDA into rat cortex. *Exp Neurol* 1994; **128**: 249–59.

297 Ito U, Spatz M, Walker JT Jr, Klatzo I. Experimental cerebral ischemia in Mongolian gerbils. I. Light microscopic observations. *Acta Neuropathol (Berl)* 1975; **32**: 209–23.

298 Iwai T, Hara A, Niwa M *et al*. Temporal profile of nuclear DNA fragmentation *in situ* in gerbil hippocampus following transient forebrain ischemia. *Brain Res* 1995; **671**: 305–8.

299 Izumi Y, Roussel S, Pinard E, Seylaz J. Reduction of infarct volume by magnesium after middle cerebral artery occlusion in rats. *J Cereb Blood Flow Metab* 1991; **11**: 1025–30.

300 Jacewicz M, Tanabe J, Pulsinelli WA. The CBF threshold and dynamics for focal cerebral infarction in spontaneously hypertensive rats. *J Cereb Blood Flow Metab* 1992; **12**: 359–70.

301 Jacob H. Über die diffuse Hemisphärenmarkerkrankung nach Kohlenoxydvergiftung bei Fallen mit Klinisch intervallere Verlaufsform. *Z Ges Neurol Psychiatrie* 1939; **167**: 161–79.

302 Janzer RC, Friede RL. Hypotensive brain stem necrosis of cardiac arrest encephalopathy. *Acta Neuropathol (Berl)* 1980; **50**: 53–6.

303 Jason GW, Pajurkova EM, Lee RG. High-altitude mountaineering and brain function: neuropsychological testing of members of a Mount Everest expedition. *Aviat Space Environ Med* 1989; **60**: 170–3.

304 Jennings GH, Newton MA. Persistent paraplegia after repeated cardiac arrests. *BMJ* 1969; **3**: 572–3.

305 Jensen AM, Chiu SY. Fluorescence measurement of changes in intracellular calcium induced by excitatory amino acids in cultured cortical astrocytes. *J Neurosci* 1990; **10**: 1165–75.

306 Jensen MS, Lambert JD, Johansen FF. Electrophysiological recordings from rat hippocampus slices following *in vivo* brain ischemia. *Brain Res* 1991; **554**: 166–75.

307 Johannsson H, Siesjö BK. Blood flow and oxygen consumption of the rat brain in profound hypoxia. *Acta Physiol Scand* 1974; **90**: 281–2.

308 Jöhannsson H, Siesjö BK. Cerebral blood flow and oxygen consumption in the rat in hypoxic hypoxia. *Acta Physiol Scand* 1975; **93**: 269–76.

309 Johansen FF, Jørgensen MB, Diemer NH. Resistance of hippocampal CA-1 interneurons to 20 min of transient cerebral ischemia in the rat. *Acta Neuropathol (Berl)* 1983; **61**: 135–40.

310 Johansen FF, Jørgensen MB, Lubitz DKJE von, Diemer NH. Selective dendrite damage in hippocampal CA1 stratum radiatum with unchanged axon ultrastructure and glutamate uptake after transient cerebral ischemia in the rat. *Brain Res* 1984; **291**: 373–7.

311 Johansen FF, Zimmer J, Diemer NH. Early loss of somatostatin neurons in dentate hilus after cerebral ischemia in the rat precedes CA-1 pyramidal cell loss. *Acta Neuropathol (Berl)* 1987; **73**: 110–14.

312 Johnston RN, Kucey BL. Competitive inhibition of hsp70 gene expression causes thermosensitivity. *Science* 1988; **242**: 1551–4.

313 Jones TH, Morawetz RB, Crowell RM *et al*. Thresholds of focal cerebral ischemia in awake monkeys. *J Neurosurg* 1981; **54**: 773–82.

314 Jørgensen HS, Nakayama H, Raaschou HO, Olsen TS. Effect of blood pressure and diabetes on stroke in progression. *Lancet* 1994; **344**: 156–9.

315 Kaibara T, Sutherland GR, Colbourne F, Tyson RL. Hypothermia: depression of tricarboxylic acid cycle flux and evidence for pentose phosphate shunt upregulation. *J Neurosurg* 1999; **90**: 339–47.

316 Kalimo H, Agardh C-D, Olsson Y, Siesjö BK. Hypoglycemic brain injury. II. Electron microscopic findings in rat cerebral neurons during profound insulin-induced hypoglycemia and in the recovery period following glucose administration. *Acta Neuropathol (Berl)* 1980; **50**: 43–52.

317 Kalimo H, Olsson Y. Effect of severe hypoglycemia on the human brain. *Acta Neurol Scand* 1980; **62**: 345–56.

318 Kalin EM, Tweed WA, Lee J, MacKeen WL. Cerebrospinal-fluid acid–base and electrolyte changes resulting from cerebral anoxia in man. *N Engl J Med* 1975; **293**: 1013–16.

319 Kammersgaard LP, Rasmussen BH, Jorgensen HS *et al*. Feasibility and safety of inducing modest hypothermia in awake patients with acute stroke through surface cooling: a case–control study. The Copenhagen Stroke Study. *Stroke* 2000; **31**: 2251–6.

320 Kannel WB, Gordon T, Wolf PA, McNamara P. Hemoglobin and the risk of cerebral infarction: the Framingham study. *Stroke* 1972; **3**: 409–20.

321 Karibe H, Chen J, Zarow GJ *et al*. Delayed induction of mild hypothermia to reduce infarct volume after temporary middle cerebral artery occlusion in rats. *J Neurosurg* 1994; **80**: 112–19.

322 Karibe H, Chen SF, Zarow GJ *et al*. Mild intraischemic hypothermia suppresses consumption of endogenous antioxidants after temporary focal ischemia in rats. *Brain Res* 1994; **649**: 12–18.

323 Kassell NF, Peerless SJ, Durward QJ *et al*. Treatment of ischemic deficits from vasospasm with intravascular volume expansion and induced arterial hypertension. *Neurosurgery* 1982; **11**: 337–43.

324 Kastein GW. Insulinvergiftung. II. Neurologische und anatomisch–histologische Beschreibung. *Z Ges Neurol Psychiatrie* 1938; **163**: 342–61.

325 Kato H, Araki T, Kogure K. Role of the excitotoxic mechanism in the development of neuronal damage following repeated brief cerebral ischemia in the gerbil: protective effects of MK-801 and pentobarbital. *Brain Res* 1990; **516**: 175–9.

326 Kato H, Araki T, Murase K, Kogure K. Alterations in [³H]MK-801, [³H]muscimol, [³H]cyclic AMP, and [³H]rolipram binding in the gerbil hippocampus following repeated ischemic insults. *Neuroscience* 1993; **52**: 245–53.

327 Kato H, Kanellopoulos GK, Matsuo S *et al*. Neuronal apoptosis and necrosis following spinal cord ischemia in the rat. *Exp Neurol* 1997; **148**: 464–74.

328 Kato H, Kogure K. Neuronal damage following non-lethal but repeated cerebral ischemia in the gerbil. *Acta Neuropathol (Berl)* 1990; **79**: 494–500.

329 Kato H, Kogure K, Nakata N *et al*. Facilitated recovery from postischemic suppression of protein synthesis in the gerbil brain with ischemic tolerance. *Brain Res Bull* 1995; **36**: 205–8.

330 Kato H, Liu Y, Araki T, Kogure K. MK-801, but not anisomycin, inhibits the induction of tolerance to ischemia in the gerbil hippocampus. *Neurosci Lett* 1992; **139**: 118–21.

331 Kato H, Liu Y, Araki T, Kogure K. Temporal profile of the effects of pretreatment with brief cerebral ischemia on the neuronal damage following secondary ischemic insult in the gerbil: cumulative damage and protective effects. *Brain Res* 1991; **553**: 238–42.

332 Kawahara N, Mishima K, Higashiyama S *et al*. The gene for heparin-binding epidermal growth factor-like growth factor is stress-inducible: its role in cerebral ischemia. *J Cereb Blood Flow Metab* 1999; **19**: 307–20.

333 Kepes JJ, Malone DG, Griffin W *et al*. Surgical 'touch artifacts' of the cerebral cortex. An experimental study with light and electron microscopic analysis. *Clin Neuropathol* 1995; **14**: 86–92.

334 Kerr JFR. Shrinkage necrosis: a distinct mode of cellular death. *J Pathol* 1971; **105**: 13–20.

335 Kiessling M, Dienel GA, Jacewicz M, Pulsinelli WA. Protein synthesis in postischemic rat brain: a two-dimensional electrophoretic analysis. *J Cereb Blood Flow Metab* 1986; **6**: 642–9.

336 Kihara S, Shiraishi T, Nakagawa S *et al*. Visualization of DNA double strand breaks in the gerbil hippocampal CA1 following transient ischemia. *Neurosci Lett* 1994; **175**: 133–6.

337 Kilduff TS, Miller JD, Radeke CM *et al*. ¹⁴C-2-deoxyglucose uptake in the ground squirrel brain during entrance to and arousal from hibernation. *J Neurosci* 1990; **10**: 2463–75.

338 Kinouchi H, Sharp FR, Hill MP *et al*. Induction of 70-kDa heat shock protein and hsp70 mRNA following transient focal cerebral ischemia in the rat. *J Cereb Blood Flow Metab* 1993; **13**: 105–15.

339 Kirino T. Delayed neuronal death in the gerbil hippocampus following ischemia. *Brain Res* 1982; **239**: 57–69.

340 Kirino T, Tamura A, Sano K. Delayed neuronal death in the rat hippocampus following transient forebrain ischemia. *Acta Neuropathol (Berl)* 1984; **64**: 139–47.

341 Kirino T, Tsujita Y, Tamura A. Induced tolerance to ischemia in gerbil hippocampal neurons. *J Cereb Blood Flow Metab* 1991; **11**: 299–307.

342 Kirsch JR, D'Alecy LG, Mongroo PB. Butanediol induced ketosis increases tolerance to hypoxia in the mouse. *Stroke* 1980; **11**: 506–13.

343 Kitagawa K, Matsumoto M, Tagaya M *et al*. 'Ischemic tolerance' phenomenon found in the brain. *Brain Res* 1990; **528**: 21–4.

344 Kitagawa K, Matsumoto M, Tagaya M *et al*. Hyperthermia-induced neuronal protection against ischemic injury in gerbils. *J Cereb Blood Flow Metab* 1991; **11**: 449–52.

345 Kiyohara Y, Ueda K, Hasuo Y *et al*. Hematocrit as a risk factor of cerebral infarction: long-term prospective population survey in a Japanese rural community. *Stroke* 1986; **17**: 687–92.

346 Ko KR, Ngai AC, Winn HR. Role of adenosine in regulation of regional cerebral blood flow in sensory cortex. *Am J Physiol* 1990; **259**: H1703–8.

347 Koh J-Y, Choi DW. Vulnerability of cultured cortical neurons to damage by excitotoxins: differential susceptibility of neurons containing NADPH-diaphorase. *J Neurosci* 1988; **8**: 2153–63.

348 Kol S, Ammar R, Weisz G, Melamed Y. Hyperbaric oxygenation for arterial air embolism during cardiopulmonary bypass. *Ann Thorac Surg* 1993; **55**: 401–3.

349 Kozniewska E, Oseka M, Stys T. Effects of endothelium-derived nitric oxide on cerebral circulation during normoxia and hypoxia in the rat. *J Cereb Blood Flow Metab* 1992; **12**: 311–17.

350 Kozniewska E, Weller L, Höper J *et al*. Cerebrocortical microcirculation in different stages of hypoxic hypoxia. *J Cereb Blood Flow Metab* 1987; **7**: 464–70.

351 Kraig RP, Chesler M. Astrocytic acidosis in hyperglycemic and complete ischemia. *J Cereb Blood Flow Metab* 1990; **10**: 104–14.

352 Kraig RP, Petito CK, Plum F, Pulsinelli WA. Hydrogen ions kill brain at concentrations reached in ischemia. *J Cereb Blood Flow Metab* 1987; **7**: 379–86.

353 Kraig RP, Pulsinelli WA, Plum F. Carbonic acid buffer changes during complete brain ischemia. *Am J Physiol* 1986; **250**: R348–57.

354 Krakauer J. *Into thin air: a personal account of the Mount Everest disaster*. New York: Random House, 1997.

355 Krumholz A, Stern BJ, Weiss HD. Outcome from coma after cardiopulmonary resuscitation: relation to seizures and myoclonus. *Neurology* 1988; **38**: 401–5.

356 Kullmann DM, Perkel DJ, Manabe T, Nicoll RA. Ca²⁺ entry via postsynaptic voltage-sensitive Ca²⁺ channels can transiently potentiate excitatory synaptic transmission in the hippocampus. *Neuron* 1992; **9**: 1175–83.

357 LaManna JC, Harik SI. Regional comparisons of brain glucose influx. *Brain Res* 1985; **326**: 299–305.

358 LaManna JC, Vendel LM, Farrell RM. Brain adaptation to chronic hypobaric hypoxia in rats. *J Appl Physiol* 1992; **72**: 2238–43.

359 Lambert SW. Poisoning by hydrocyanic acid gas with special reference to its effects upon the brain. *Neurol Bull* 1919; **2**: 93–105.

360 Lapresle J, Fardeau M. The central nervous system and carbon monoxide poisoning. II. Anatomical study of brain lesions following intoxication with carbon monoxide (22 cases). *Prog Brain Res* 1967; **24**: 31–74.

361 Laptook AR, Corbett RJT, Burns D, Sterett R. Neonatal ischemic neuroprotection by modest hypothermia is associated with attenuated brain acidosis. *Stroke* 1995; **26**: 1240–6.

362 Lassen NA. Brain extracellular pH; The main factor controlling cerebral blood flow. *Scand J Clin Lab Invest* 1968; **22**: 247–51.

363 Lawrence RD, Meyer R, Nevin S. The pathological changes in the brain in fatal hypoglycemia. *Q J Med* 1942; **11**: 181–201.

364 Leão AAP. Spreading depression of activity in the cerebral cortex. *J Neurophysiol* 1944; **7**: 359–90.

365 Lerner-Natoli M, Rondouin G, Bock F de, Bockaert J. Chronic NO synthase inhibition fails to protect hippocampal neurones against NMDA toxicity. *Neuroreport* 1992; **3**: 1109–12.

366 Levine S. Anoxic-ischemic encephalopathy in rats. *Am J Pathol* 1960; **36**: 1–17.

367 Levine S, Stypulkowski W. Experimental cyanide encephalopathy. *Arch Pathol* 1959; **67**: 306–23.

368 Li H, Colbourne F, Sun P *et al.* Caspase inhibitors reduce neuronal injury after focal but not global cerebral ischemia in rats. *Stroke* 2000; **31**: 176–82.

369 Li J, Iadecola C. Nitric oxide and adenosine mediate vasodilation during functional activation in cerebellar cortex. *Neuropharmacology* 1994; **33**: 1453–61.

370 Li Y, Chopp M, Jiang N *et al.* Temporal profile of *in situ* DNA fragmentation after transient middle cerebral artery occlusion in the rat. *J Cereb Blood Flow Metab* 1995; **15**: 389–97.

371 Li Y, Chopp M, Jiang N *et al.* Induction of DNA fragmentation after 10 to 120 minutes of focal cerebral ischemia in rats. *Stroke* 1995; **26**: 1252–8.

372 Li Y, Chopp M, Yoshida Y, Levine SR. Distribution of 72-kDa heat-shock protein in rat brain after hyperthermia. *Acta Neuropathol (Berl)* 1992; **84**: 94–9.

373 Li Y, Sharov VG, Jiang N *et al.* Ultrastructural and light microscopic evidence of apoptosis after middle cerebral artery occlusion in the rat. *Am J Pathol* 1995; **146**: 1045–51.

374 Lin B, Busto R, Globus MY-T *et al.* Brain temperature modulations during global ischemia fail to influence extracellular lactate levels in rats. *Stroke* 1995; **26**: 1634–8.

375 Lin MT, Lin SZ. Cerebral ischemia is the main cause for the onset of heat stroke syndrome in rabbits. *Experientia* 1992; **48**: 225–7.

376 Lipton P. Ischemic cell death in brain neurons. *Physiol Rev* 1999; **79**: 1431–568.

377 Liu Y, Kato H, Nakata N, Kogure K. Protection of rat hippocampus against ischemic neuronal damage by pretreatment with sublethal ischemia. *Brain Res* 1992; **586**: 121–4.

378 Liu Y, Kato H, Nakata N, Kogure K. Temporal profile of heat shock protein 70 synthesis in ischemic tolerance induced by preconditioning ischemia in rat hippocampus. *Neuroscience* 1993; **56**: 921–7.

379 Longstreth WT Jr, Diehr P, Cobb LA *et al.* Neurologic outcome and blood glucose levels during out-of-hospital cardiopulmonary resuscitation. *Neurology* 1986; **36**: 1186–91.

380 Longstreth WT Jr, Diehr P, Inui TS. Prediction of awakening after out-of-hospital cardiac arrest. *N Engl J Med* 1983; **308**: 1378–82.

381 Longstreth WT Jr, Inui TS. High blood glucose level on hospital admission and poor neurological recovery after cardiac arrest. *Ann Neurol* 1984; **15**: 59–63.

382 Longstreth WT Jr, Inui TS, Cobb LA, Copass MK. Neurologic recovery after out-of-hospital cardiac arrest. *Ann Intern Med* 1983; **98**: 588–92.

383 Lorente de Nó R. Studies on the striation of the cerebral cortex. II. Continuation of the study of the Ammonic system. *J Psychol Neurol* 1934; **46**: 113–77.

384 Lowenstein DH, Chan PH, Miles MF. The stress protein response in cultured neurons: characterization and evidence for a protective role in excitotoxicity. *Neuron* 1991; **7**: 1053–60.

385 Lu YM, Yin H-Z, Weiss JH. Ca^{2+} permeable AMPA/kainate channels permit rapid injurious Ca^{2+} entry. *Neuroreport* 1995; **6**: 1089–92.

386 Lundy EF, Klima LD, Huber TS *et al.* Elevated blood ketone and glucagon levels cannot account for 1,3-butanediol induced cerebral protection in the Levine rat. *Stroke* 1987; **18**: 217–22.

387 Luscher C, Nicoll RA, Malenka RC, Muller D. Synaptic plasticity and dynamic modulation of the postsynaptic membrane. *Nat Neurosci* 2000; **3**: 545–50.

388 Lynch G, Baudry M. The biochemistry of memory: a new and specific hypothesis. *Science* 1984; **224**: 1057–63.

389 Lynch G, Larson J, Kelso S *et al.* Intracellular injections of EGTA block induction of hippocampal long-term potentiation. *Nature* 1983; **305**: 719–21.

390 Lynch G, Seubert P. Links between long-term potentiation and neuropathology. An hypothesis involving calcium-activated proteases. *Ann N Y Acad Sci* 1989; **568**: 171–80.

391 McGee-Russell SM, Brown AW, Brierley JB. A combined light and electron microscope study of early anoxic–ischaemic cell change in the rat brain. *Brain Res* 1970; **20**: 193–200.

392 MacKeith SA, Meyer A. A death during insulin treatment of schizophrenia; with pathological report. *J Ment Sci* 1939; **85**: 96–105.

393 Mackey ME, Wu Y, Hu R *et al.* Cell death suggestive of apoptosis after spinal cord ischemia in rabbits. *Stroke* 1997; **28**: 2012–17.

394 MacManus JP, Buchan AM, Hill IE *et al.* Global ischemia can cause DNA fragmentation indicative of apoptosis in rat brain. *Neurosci Lett* 1993; **164**: 89–92.

395 MacManus JP, Fliss H, Preston E *et al.* Cerebral ischemia produces laddered DNA fragments distinct from cardiac ischemia and archetypal apoptosis. *J Cereb Blood Flow Metab* 1999; **18**: 502–10.

396 MacManus JP, Linnik MD. Gene expression induced by cerebral ischemia: an apoptotic perspective. *J Cereb Blood Flow Metab* 1997; **17**: 815–32.

397 MacManus JP, Rasquinha I, Tuor U, Preston E. Detection of higher-order 50- and 10-kbp DNA fragments before apoptotic internucleosomal cleavage after transient cerebral ischemia. *J Cereb Blood Flow Metab* 1997; **17**: 376–87.

398 MacMillan V, Siesjö BK. Brain energy metabolism in hypoxemia. *Scand J Clin Lab Invest* 1972; **30**: 127–36.

399 MacMillan V, Siesjö BK. The effect of hypercapnia upon the energy metabolism of the brain during arterial hypoxemia. *Scand J Clin Lab Invest* 1972; **30**: 237–44.

400 MacMillan VH. Cerebral energy metabolism in cyanide encephalopathy. *J Cereb Blood Flow Metab* 1989; **9**: 156–62.

401 McPherson RW, Eimerl D, Traystman RJ. Interaction of hypoxia and hypercapnia on cerebral hemodynamics and brain electrical activity in dogs. *Am J Physiol* 1987; **253**: H890–7.

402 McPherson RW, Zeger S, Traystman RJ. Relationship of somatosensory evoked potentials and cerebral oxygen consumption during hypoxic hypoxia in dogs. *Stroke* 1986; **17**: 30–6.

403 Macrae IM, Dawson DA, Norrie JD, McCulloch J. Inhibition of nitric oxide synthesis: effects on cerebral blood flow and glucose utilisation in the rat. *J Cereb Blood Flow Metab* 1993; **13**: 985–92.

404 MacVicar BA, Tse FW, Crichton SA, Kettenmann H. GABA-activated Cl⁻ channels in astrocytes of hippocampal slices. *J Neurosci* 1989; **9**: 3577–83.

405 Magnusson K, Wieloch T. Impairment of protein ubiquitination may cause delayed neuronal death. *Neurosci Lett* 1989; **96**: 264–70.

406 Maiese K, Boniece I, DeMeo D, Wagner JA. Peptide growth factors protect against ischemia in culture by preventing nitric oxide toxicity. *J Neurosci* 1993; **13**: 3034–40.

407 Marcus AJ, Safier LB. Thromboregulation: multicellular modulation of platelet reactivity in hemostasis and thrombosis. *FASEB J* 1993; **7**: 516–22.

408 Marie C, Bralet AM, Gueldry S, Bralet J. Fasting prior to transient cerebral ischemia reduces delayed neuronal necrosis. *Metab Brain Dis* 1990; **5**: 65–75.

409 Marion DW, Darby J, Yonas H. Acute regional cerebral blood flow changes caused by severe head injuries. *J Neurosurg* 1991; **74**: 407–14.

410 Martinou JC, Dubois-Dauphin M, Staple JK *et al*. Overexpression of BCL-2 in transgenic mice protects neurons from naturally occurring cell death and experimental ischemia. *Neuron* 1994; **13**: 1017–30.

411 Matsuo Y, Onodera H, Shiga Y *et al*. Correlation between myeloperoxidase-quantified neutrophil accumulation and ischemic brain injury in the rat. Effects of neutrophil depletion. *Stroke* 1994; **25**: 1469–75.

412 Matsuyama T, Tsuchiyama M, Nakamura H *et al*. Hilar somatostatin neurons are more vulnerable to an ischemic insult than CA1 pyramidal neurons. *J Cereb Blood Flow Metab* 1993; **13**: 229–34.

413 Maxwell PH, Pugh CW, Ratcliffe PJ. Inducible operation of the erythropoietin 3′ enhancer in multiple cell lines: evidence for a widespread oxygen-sensing mechanism. *Proc Natl Acad Sci USA* 1993; **90**: 2423–7.

414 Mayer-Gross W. Insulin coma therapy of schizophrenia: some critical remarks on Dr. Sakel's report. *J Ment Sci* 1951; **97**: 132–5.

415 Mehmet H, Yue X, Squier MV *et al*. Increased apoptosis in the cingulate sulcus of newborn piglets following transient hypoxia–ischaemia is related to the degree of high energy phosphate depletion during the insult. *Neurosci Lett* 1994; **181**: 121–5.

416 Meldrum B. Protection against ischaemic neuronal damage by drugs acting on excitatory neurotransmission. *Cerebrovasc Brain Metab Rev* 1990; **2**: 27–57.

417 Memezawa H, Smith M-L, Siesjö BK. Penumbral tissues salvaged by reperfusion following middle cerebral artery occlusion in rats. *Stroke* 1992; **23**: 552–9.

418 Mettler FA, Sax DS. Cerebellar cortical degeneration due to acute azide poisoning. *Brain* 1972; **95**: 505–16.

419 Meyer A. Intoxications. *Greenfield's neuropathology* 2nd edn. London: Edward Arnold, 1963: 235–87.

420 Meyer A. Über die Wirkung der Kohlenoxydvergiftung auf das Zentralnervensystem. *Z Ges Neurol Psychiatric* 1926; **100**: 201–47.

421 Meyer JS, Portnoy HD. Localized cerebral hypoglycemia simulating stroke. *Neurology* 1958; **8**: 601–14.

422 Miller JA Jr. New approaches to preventing brain damage during asphyxia. *Am J Obstet Gynecol* 1971; **110**: 1125–33.

423 Miller JR, Myers RE. Neuropathology of systemic circulatory arrest in adult monkeys. *Neurology* 1972; **22**: 888–904.

424 Miller LP, Villeneuve JB, Braun LD, Oldendorf WH. Effect of pharmacological doses of 3-*O*-methyl-d-glucose and 2-deoxy-d-glucose on rat brain glucose and lactate. *Stroke* 1986; **17**: 957–61.

425 Mironov V, Hritz MA, LaManna JC *et al*. Architectural alterations in rat cerebral microvessels after hypobaric hypoxia. *Brain Res* 1994; **660**: 73–80.

426 Mitani A, Imon H, Iga K *et al*. Gerbil hippocampal extracellular glutamate and neuronal activity after transient ischemia. *Brain Res Bull* 1990; **25**: 319–24.

427 Mitani A, Kataoka K. Critical levels of extracellular glutamate mediating gerbil hippocampal delayed neuronal death during hypothermia: brain microdialysis study. *Neuroscience* 1991; **42**: 661–70.

428 Mito T, Becker LE, Takashima S. Neuropathology of central respiratory dysfunction in infancy. *Pediatr Neurosurg* 1991; **17**: 80–7.

429 Miyabe M, Jones MD Jr, Koehler RC, Traystman RJ. Chemodenervation does not alter cerebrovascular response to hypoxic hypoxia. *Am J Physiol* 1989; **257**: H1413–18.

430 Miyamoto O, Auer RN. Hypoxia, hyperoxia, ischemia and brain necrosis. *Neurology* 2000; **54**: 362–71.

431 Moersch FP, Kernohan JW. Hypoglycemia. Neurologic and neuropathologic studies. *Arch Neurol Psychiatry (Chic)* 1938; **39**: 242–57.

432 Monaghan DT, Cotman CW. Distribution of *N*-methyl-d-aspartate-sensitive l-[³H]glutamate-binding sites in rat brain. *J Neurosci* 1985; **5**: 2909–19.

433 Monaghan DT, Holets VR, Toy DW, Cotman CW. Anatomical distributions of four pharmacologically distinct ³H-l-glutamate binding sites. *Nature* 1983; **306**: 176–9.

434 Moncada C, Lekieffre D, Arvin B, Meldrum B. Effect of NO synthase inhibition on NMDA- and ischaemia-induced hippocampal lesions. *Neuroreport* 1992; **3**: 530–2.

435 Morawetz RB, Crowell RH, DeGirolami U *et al*. Regional cerebral blood flow thresholds during cerebral ischemia. *Fed Proc* 1979; **38**: 2493–4.

436 Morii S, Ngai AC, Ko KR, Winn HR. Role of adenosine in regulation of cerebral blood flow: effects of theophylline during normoxia and hypoxia. *Am J Physiol* 1987; **253**: H165–75.

437 Muir KW. New experimental and clinical data on the efficacy of pharmacological magnesium infusions in cerebral infarcts. *Magnes Res* 1998; **11**: 43–56.

438 Mujsce DJ, Towfighi J, Yager JY, Vannucci RC. Neuropathologic aspects of hypothermic circulatory arrest in newborn dogs. *Acta Neuropathol (Berl)* 1993; **85**: 190–8.

439 Murayama S, Bouldin TW, Suzuki K. Selective sparing of Betz cells in primary motor area in hypoxic-ischemic encephalopathy. *Acta Neuropathol (Berl)* 1990; **80**: 560–2.

440 Myers RE, Yamaguchi S. Nervous system effects of cardiac arrest in monkeys. *Arch Neurol* 1977; **34**: 65–74.

441 Nagai Y, Naruse S, Weiner MW. Effect of hypoglycemia on changes of brain lactic acid and intracellular pH produced by ischemia. *NMR Biomed* 1993; **6**: 1–6.

442 Nakagomi T, Kirino T, Kanemitsu H *et al*. Early recovery of protein synthesis following ischemia in hippocampal neurons with induced tolerance in the gerbil. *Acta Neuropathol (Berl)* 1993; **86**: 10–15.

443 Nakanishi S. Molecular diversity of glutamate receptors and implications for brain function. *Science* 1992; **258**: 597–603.

444 Nakano S, Kogure K, Fujikura H. Ischemia-induced slowly progressive neuronal damage in the rat brain. *Neuroscience* 1990; **38**: 115–24.

445 Nakashima K, Todd MM. Effects of hypothermia on the rate of excitatory amino acid release after ischemic depolarization. *Stroke* 1996; **27**: 913–18.

446 Nakata N, Kato H, Kogure K. Effects of repeated cerebral ischemia on extracellular amino acid concentrations measured with intracerebral microdialysis in the gerbil hippocampus. *Stroke* 1993; **24**: 458–64.

447 Nakata N, Kato H, Kogure K. Inhibition of ischaemic tolerance in the gerbil hippocampus by quercetin and anti-heat shock protein-70 antibody. *Neuroreport* 1993; **4**: 695–8.

448 Nakata N, Kato H, Kogure K. Ischemic tolerance and extracellular amino acid concentrations in gerbil hippocampus measured by intracerebral microdialysis. *Brain Res Bull* 1994; **35**: 247–51.

449 Nakata N, Kato H, Liu Y, Kogure K. Effects of pretreatment with sublethal ischemia on the extracellular glutamate concentrations during secondary ischemia in the gerbil hippocampus evaluated with intracerebral microdialysis. *Neurosci Lett* 1992; **138**: 86–8.

450 Namura S, Zhu J, Fink K et al. Activation and cleavage of caspase-3 in apoptosis induced by experimental cerebral ischemia. *J Neurosci* 1998; **18**: 3659–68.

451 Natale JA, D'Alecy LG. Protection from cerebral ischemia by brain cooling without reduced lactate accumulation in dogs. *Stroke* 1989; **20**: 770–7.

452 Nedergaard M. Direct signalling from astrocytes to neurons in cultures of mammalian brain cells. *Science* 1994; **263**: 1768–71.

453 Nedergaard M, Goldman SA, Desai S, Pulsinelli WA. Acid-induced death in neurons and glia. *J Neurosci* 1991; **11**: 2489–97.

454 Nedergaard M, Hansen AJ. Spreading depression is not associated with neuronal injury in the normal brain. *Brain Res* 1988; **449**: 395–8.

455 Nedergaard M, Kraig RP, Tanabe J, Pulsinelli WA. Dynamics of interstitial and intracellular pH in evolving brain infarct. *Am J Physiol* 1991; **260**: R581–8.

456 Nelson D, Goetzl S, Robins S, Ivy AC. Carrot diet and susceptibility to acute 'anoxia'. *Proc Soc Exp Biol Med* 1943; **52**: 1–2.

457 Nemoto EM, Hoff JT. Lactate uptake and metabolism by brain during hyperlactatemia and hypoglycemia. *Stroke* 1974; **5**: 48–53.

458 Neubuerger KT, Clarke ER. Subacute carbon monoxide poisoning with cerebral myelinopathy and multiple myocardial necroses. *Rocky Mountain Med J* 1945; **42**: 29–34.

459 Nevander G, Ingvar M, Auer RN, Siesjö BK. Status epilepticus in well oxygenated rats causes neuronal necrosis. *Ann Neurol* 1985; **18**: 281–90.

460 Ng T, Graham DI, Adams JH, Ford I. Changes in the hippocampus and the cerebellum resulting from hypoxic insults: frequency and distribution. *Acta Neuropathol (Berl)* 1989; **78**: 438–43.

461 Ni JW, Matsumoto K, Li HB et al. Neuronal damage and decrease of central acetylcholine level following permanent occlusion of bilateral common carotid arteries in rat. *Brain Res* 1995; **673**: 290–6.

462 Nishi S, Taki W, Uemura Y et al. Ischemic tolerance due to the induction of HSP70 in a rat ischemic recirculation model. *Brain Res* 1993; **615**: 281–8.

463 Nitatori T, Sato N, Waguri S et al. Delayed neuronal death in the CA1 pyramidal cell layer of the gerbil hippocampus following transient ischemia is apoptosis. *J Neurosci* 1995; **15**: 1001–11.

464 Niwa M, Hara A, Iwai T et al. Expression of Bax and Bcl-2 protein in the gerbil hippocampus following transient forebrain ischemia and its modification by phencyclidine. *Neurol Res* 1997; **19**: 629–33.

465 Norenberg MD, Mozes LW, Gregorios JB, Norenberg L-OB. Effects of lactic acid on astrocytes in primary culture. *J Neuropathol Exp Neurol* 1987; **46**: 154–66.

466 Nowak TS Jr. Localization of 70 kDa stress protein mRNA induction in gerbil brain after ischemia. *J Cereb Blood Flow Metab* 1991; **11**: 432–9.

467 Nowak TS Jr. Synthesis of a stress protein following transient ischemia in the gerbil. *J Neurochem* 1985; **45**: 1635–41.

468 Nowak TS Jr, Bond U, Schlesinger MJ. Heat shock RNA levels in brain and other tissues after hyperthermia and transient ischemia. *J Neurochem* 1990; **54**: 451–8.

469 Nowak TS Jr, Jacewicz M. The heat shock/stress response in focal cerebral ischemia. *Brain Pathol* 1994; **4**: 67–76.

470 Nowak TS Jr, Osborne OC, Suga S. Stress protein and proto-oncogene expression as indicators of neuronal pathophysiology after ischemia. *Prog Brain Res* 1993; **96**: 195–208.

471 Nowicki JP, Duval D, Poignet H, Scatton B. Nitric oxide mediates neuronal death after focal cerebral ischemia in the mouse. *Eur J Pharmacol* 1991; **204**: 339–40.

472 Nussmeier NA, Arlund C, Slogoff S. Neuropsychiatric complications after cardiopulmonary bypass: cerebral protection by a barbiturate. *Anesthesiology* 1986; **64**: 165–70.

473 Obrenovitch TP, Richards DA. Extracellular neurotransmitter changes in cerebral ischaemia. *Cerebrovasc Brain Metab Rev* 1995; **7**: 1–54.

474 O'Dell TJ, Huang PL, Dawson TM et al. Endothelial NOS and the blockade of LTP by NOS inhibitors in mice lacking neuronal NOS. *Science* 1994; **265**: 542–6.

475 Ogata J, Yutani C, Imakita M et al. Autolysis of the granular layer of the cerebellar cortex in brain death. *Acta Neuropathol (Berl)* 1986; **70**: 75–8.

476 Ohta S, Smith M-L, Siesjö BK. The effect of a dihydropyridine calcium antagonist (isradipine) on selective neuronal necrosis. *J Neurol Sci* 1991; **103**: 109–15.

477 Okamoto M, Matsumoto M, Ohtsuki T et al. Internucleosomal DNA cleavage involved in ischemia-induced neuronal death. *Biochem Biophys Res Commun* 1993; **196**: 1356–62.

478 Okeda R, Funata N, Song S-J et al. Comparative study on pathogenesis of selective cerebral lesions in carbon monoxide poisoning and nitrogen hypoxia in cats. *Acta Neuropathol (Berl)* 1982; **56**: 265–72.

479 Olney JW. Brain lesions, obesity, and other disturbances in mice treated with monosodium glutamate. *Science* 1969; **164**: 719–21.

480 Olney JW. Glutamate-induced neuronal necrosis in the infant mouse hypothalamus. *J Neuropathol Exp Neurol* 1971; **30**: 75–90.

481 Olney JW. Glutamate-induced retinal degeneration in neonatal mice. Electron microscopy of the acutely evolving lesions. *J Neuropathol Exp Neurol* 1969; **28**: 455–74.

482 Olney JW, Ho OL, Rhee V. Cytotoxic effects of acidic and sulphur containing amino acids on the infant mouse central nervous system. *Exp Brain Res* 1971; **14**: 61–76.

483 Olney JW, Rhee V, Ho OL. Kainic acid: a powerful neurotoxic analogue of glutamate. *Brain Res* 1974; **77**: 507–12.

484 Olney JW, Sharpe LG, Feigin R. Glutamate-induced brain damage in infant primates. *J Neuropathol Exp Neurol* 1972; **31**: 464–88.

485 Oorschot DE, Black MJ, Rangi F, Scarr E. Is Fos protein expressed by dying striatal neurons after immature hypoxic–ischemic brain injury? *Exp Neurol* 2000; **161**: 227–33.

486 Palmer AC. Target organs in decompression sickness. *Prog Underwater Sci* 1990; **15**: 15–23.

487 Palmer AC, Calder IM, Hughes JT. Spinal cord degeneration in divers. *Lancet* 1987; **ii**: 1365–6.

488 Palmer TD, Willhoite AR, Gage FH. Vascular niche for adult hippocampal neurogenesis. *J Comp Neurol* 2000; **425**: 479–94.

489 Papagapiou MP, Auer RN. Regional neuroprotective effects of the NMDA receptor antagonist MK-801 (dizocilpine) in hypoglycemic brain damage. *J Cereb Blood Flow Metab* 1990; **10**: 270–6.

490 Parisi JE, Kim RC, Collins GH, Hilfinger MF. Brain death with prolonged somatic survival. *N Engl J Med* 1982; **306**: 14–16.

491 Parpura V, Basarsky TA, Liu F et al. Glutamate-mediated astrocyte–neuron signalling. *Nature* 1994; **369**: 744–7.

492 Paschen W, Djuricic B, Mies G et al. Lactate and pH in the brain: association and dissociation in different pathophysiological states. *J Neurochem* 1987; **48**: 154–9.

493 Paulson GW, Wise G, Conkle R. Cerebrospinal fluid lactic acid in death and in brain death. *Neurology* 1972; **22**: 505–9.

494 Pauwels PJ, Leysen JE. Blockade of nitric oxide formation does not prevent glutamate-induced neurotoxicity in neuronal cultures from rat hippocampus. *Neurosci Lett* 1992; **143**: 27–30.

495 Pearigen P, Gwinn R, Simon RP. The effects of *in vivo* hypoxia on brain injury. *Brain Res* 1996; **725**: 184–91.

496 Pearson TC, Wetherley-Mein G. Vascular occlusive episodes and venous hematocrit in primary proliferative polycythemia. *Lancet* 1978; **ii**: 1219–22.

497 Peeling J, Wong D, Sutherland GR. Nuclear magnetic resonance study of regional metabolism after forebrain ischemia in rats. *Stroke* 1989; **20**: 633–40.

498 Pelligrino D, Almquist L-O, Siesjö BK. Effects of insulin-induced hypoglycemia on intracellular pH and impedance in the cerebral cortex of the rat. *Brain Res* 1981; **221**: 129–47.

499 Penney DG, Helfman CC, Dunbar JC Jr, McCoy LE. Acute severe carbon monoxide exposure in the rat: effects of hyperglycemia and hypoglycemia on mortality, recovery, and neurologic deficit. *J Physiol (Lond)* 1991; **69**: 1168–77.

500 Perry G, Zhu X, Smith MA. Do neurons have a choice in death? *Am J Pathol* 2001; **158**: 1–2.

501 Petito CK, Feldmann E, Pulsinelli WA, Plum F. Delayed hippocampal damage in humans following cardiorespiratory arrest. *Neurology* 1987; **37**: 1281–6.

502 Petito CK, Olarte JP, Roberts B et al. Selective glial vulnerability following transient global ischemia in rat brain. *J Neuropathol Exp Neurol* 1998; **57**: 231–8.

503 Petito CK, Torres-Munoz J, Roberts B et al. DNA fragmentation follows delayed neuronal death in CA1 neurons exposed to transient global ischemia in the rat. *J Cereb Blood Flow Metab* 1997; **17**: 967–76.

504 Petroni A, Borghi A, Blasevich M et al. Effects of hypoxia and recovery on brain eicosanoids and carbohydrate metabolites in rat brain cortex. *Brain Res* 1987; **415**: 226–32.

505 Phillis JW, DeLong RE, Towner JK. Adenosine deaminase inhibitors enhance cerebral anoxic hyperemia in the rat. *J Cereb Blood Flow Metab* 1985; **5**: 295–9.

506 Plum F, Posner JB, Hain RF. Delayed neurological deterioration after anoxia. *Arch Intern Med* 1962; **110**: 56–63.

507 Polkinghorne PJ, Sehmi K, Cross MR et al. Ocular fundus lesions in divers. *Lancet* 1988; **ii**: 1381–3.

508 Pontius RG, Bloodwell RD, Cooley DA, De Bakey ME. The use of hypothermia in the prevention of brain damage following temporary arrest of cerebral circulation: experimental observations. *Surg Forum* 1954; **5**: 224–8.

509 Poursines Y, Alliez J, Toga M. Étude des lésions corticales d'un cas d'intoxication oxycarbonée. *Rev Neurol (Paris)* 1956; **94**: 731–5.

510 Pulsinelli WA, Brierley JB, Plum F. Temporal profile of neuronal damage in a model of transient forebrain ischemia. *Ann Neurol* 1982; **11**: 491–8.

511 Pulsinelli WA, Levy DE, Sigsbee B et al. Increased damage after ischemic stroke in patients with hyperglycemia with or without diabetes mellitus. *Am J Med* 1983; **74**: 540–4.

512 Pulsinelli WA, Waldman S, Rawlinson D, Plum F. Moderate hyperglycemia augments ischemic brain damage: a neuropathologic study in the rat. *Neurology* 1982; **32**: 1239–46.

513 Qi Y, Xue QM. Ganglioside levels in hypoxic brains from neonatal and premature infants. *Mol Chem Neuropathol* 1991; **14**: 87–97.

514 Queiroz L de Sousa, Eduardo RMP. Occurrence of dark neurons in living mechanically injured rat neocortex. *Acta Neuropathol (Berl)* 1977; **38**: 45–8.

515 Radi R, Beckman JS, Bush KM, Freeman BA. Peroxynitrite oxidation of sulfhydryls. The cytotoxic potential of superoxide and nitric oxide. *J Biol Chem* 1991; **266**: 4244–50.

516 Raley-Susman KM, Miller KR, Owicki JC, Sapolsky RM. Effects of excitotoxin exposure on metabolic rate of primary hippocampal cultures: application of silicon microphysiometry to neurobiology. *J Neurosci* 1992; **12**: 773–80.

517 Rapoport SI, Lust WD, Fredericks WR. Effects of hypoxia on rat brain metabolism: unilateral *in vivo* carotid infusion. *Exp Neurol* 1986; **91**: 319–30.

518 Raskin N, Mullaney OC. The mental and neurological sequelae of carbon monoxide asphyxia in a case observed for 15 years. *J Nerv Ment Dis* 1940; **92**: 640–59.

519 Reif DW. Delayed production of nitric oxide contributes to NMDA-mediated neuronal damage. *Neuroreport* 1993; **4**: 566–8.

520 Révész T, Geddes JF. Symmetrical columnar necrosis of the basal ganglia and brain stem in an adult following cardiac arrest. *Clin Neuropathol* 1988; **7**: 294–8.

521 Richardson JC, Chambers RA, Heywood PM. Encephalopathies of anoxia and hypoglycemia. *Arch Neurol* 1959; **1**: 178–90.

522 Rie MA, Bernad PG. Prolonged hypoxia in man without circulatory compromise fails to demonstrate cerebral pathology. *Neurology* 1980; **30**: 443.

523 Robertson GS, Pfaus JG, Atkinson LJ et al. Sexual behavior increases c-fos expression in the forebrain of the male rat. *Brain Res* 1991; **564**: 352–7.

524 Robertson KM, Hramiak IM, Gelb AW. Endocrine changes and haemodynamic stability after brain death. *Transplant Proc* 1989; **21**: 1197–8.

525 Rod MR, Whishaw IQ, Auer RN. The relationship of structural ischemic brain damage to neurobehavioural deficit: the effect of postischemic MK-801. *Can J Psychol* 1990; **44**: 196–209.

526 Romijn HJ. Preferential loss of GABAergic neurons in hypoxia-exposed neocortex slab cultures is attenuated by the NMDA receptor blocker d-2-amino-7-phosphonoheptanoate. *Brain Res* 1989; **501**: 100–4.

527 Romijn HJ, Jong BM de. Unlike hypoxia, hypoglycemia does not preferentially destroy GABAergic neurons in developing rat neocortex explants in culture. *Brain Res* 1989; **480**: 58–64.

528 Rordorf G, Koroshetz WJ, Bonventre JV. Heat shock protects cultured neurons from glutamate toxicity. *Neuron* 1991; **7**: 1043–51.

529 Rose M. Die sogenannte Riechrinde beim Menschen und beim Affen. *J Psychol Neurol* 1926; **34**: 261–401.

530 Rosomoff HL. Hypothermia and cerebral vascular lesions. I. Experimental interruption of the middle cerebral artery during hypothermia. *J Neurosurg* 1956; **13**: 244–55.

531 Rosomoff HL. Hypothermia and cerebral vascular lesions. II. Experimental middle cerebral artery interruption followed by induction of hypothermia. *Arch Neurol Psychiatry (Chic)* 1957; **78**: 454–64.

532 Ross DT, Duhaime AC. Degeneration of neurons in the thalamic reticular nucleus following transient ischemia due to raised intracranial pressure: excitotoxic degeneration mediated via non-NMDA receptors? *Brain Res* 1989; **501**: 129–43.

533 Ross DT, Graham DI. Selective loss and selective sparing of neurons in the thalamic reticular nucleus following human cardiac arrest. *J Cereb Blood Flow Metab* 1993; **13**: 558–67.

534 Rothman SM, Olney JW. Glutamate and the pathophysiology of hypoxic/ischemic brain damage. *Ann Neurol* 1986; **19**: 105–11.

535 Rothman SM, Thurston JH, Hauhart RE. Delayed neurotoxicity of excitatory amino acids *in vitro*. *Neuroscience* 1987; **22**: 471–80.

536 Rouiller EM, Wan XS, Moret V, Liang F. Mapping of c-fos expression elicited by pure tones stimulation in the auditory pathways of the rat, with emphasis on the cochlear nucleus. *Neurosci Lett* 1992; **144**: 19–24.

537 Roy CS, Sherrington CS. The regulation of the blood supply of the brain. *J Physiol (Lond)* 1890; **11**: 85.

538 Rudolphi KA, Schubert P, Parkinson FE, Fredholm BB. Adenosine and brain ischemia. *Cerebrovasc Brain Metab Rev* 1992; **4**: 346–69.

539 Rupalla K, Allegrini PR, Sauer D, Wiessner C. Time course of microglia activation and apoptosis in various brain regions after permanent focal cerebral ischemia in mice. *Acta Neuropathol (Berl)* 1998; **96**: 172–8.

540 Sadove MS, Yon MK, Hollinger PH *et al*. Severe prolonged cerebral hypoxic episode with complete recovery. *JAMA* 1961; **175**: 1102–4.

541 Saito K, Levine L, Moskowitz MA. Blood components contribute to rise in gerbil brain levels of leukotriene-like immunoreactivity after ischemia and reperfusion. *Stroke* 1988; **19**: 1395–8.

542 Saito S, Wilson DA, Hanley DF, Traystman RJ. Nitric oxide synthase does not contribute to cerebral autoregulatory phenomenon in anesthetised dogs. *J Auton Nerv Syst* 1994; **49**: 73–6.

543 Sakel M. The methodical use of hypoglycemia in the treatment of psychoses. *Am J Psychiatry* 1937; **94**: 111–29.

544 Salford LG, Siesjö BK. The influence of arterial hypoxia and unilateral carotid artery occlusion upon regional blood flow and metabolism in the rat brain. *Acta Physiol Scand* 1974; **92**: 130–41.

545 Sandberg M, Butcher SP, Hagberg H. Extracellular overflow of neuroactive amino acids during severe insulin-induced hypoglycemia: *in vivo* dialysis of the rat hippocampus. *J Neurochem* 1986; **47**: 178–84.

546 Sandberg M, Nyström B, Hamberger A. Metabolically derived aspartate – elevated extracellular levels *in vivo* in iodoacetate poisoning. *J Neurosci Res* 1985; **13**: 489–95.

547 Schereschewsky NA, Mogilnitzky N, Gorjaewa AW. Zur Pathologie und pathologischen Anatomie der Insulinvergiftung. *Endokrinologie* 1929; **5**: 204.

548 Schleussing H, Schumacher H. Grosshirnschädigung im Verlauf eines Diabetes mellitus. *Dtsch Arch Klin Med* 1933; **176**: 45–51.

549 Schmahl FW, Betz E, Dettinger E, Hohorst HJ. Energiestoffwechsel der Großhirnrinde und Elektroencephalogramm bei Sauerstoffmangel. *Pflugers Arch Ges Physiol* 1966; **292**: 46–59.

550 Schmorl. Demonstration. 3. Gehirn bei Blausäurevergiftung. *Münch Med Wochenschr* 1920; **67**: 913.

551 Schröder R. Later changes in brain death. Signs of partial recirculation. *Acta Neuropathol (Berl)* 1983; **62**: 15–23.

552 Schuman EM, Madison DV. Locally distributed synaptic potentiation in the hippocampus. *Science* 1994; **263**: 532–6.

553 Schurr A, West CA, Rigor BM. Lactate-supported synaptic function in the rat hippocampal slice preparation. *Science* 1988; **240**: 1326–8.

554 Sei Y, Von Lubitz KJ, Basile AS *et al*. Internucleosomal DNA fragmentation in gerbil hippocampus following forebrain ischemia. *Neurosci Lett* 1994; **171**: 179–82.

555 Severinghaus JW, Chiodi H, Eger EI II *et al*. Cerebral blood flow in man at high altitude. Role of cerebrospinal fluid pH in normalization of flow in chronic hypocapnia. *Circ Res* 1966; **19**: 274–82.

556 Shariff GA. Cell counts in the primate cerebral cortex. *J Comp Neurol* 1953; **98**: 381–400.

557 Sharp FR, Lowenstein D, Simon R, Hisanaga K. Heat shock protein hsp72 induction in cortical and striatal astrocytes and neurons following infarction. *J Cereb Blood Flow Metab* 1991; **11**: 621–7.

558 Shivalkar B, Van Loon J, Wieland W *et al*. Variable effects of explosive or gradual increase of intracranial pressure on myocardial structure and function. *Circulation* 1993; **87**: 230–9.

559 Siebke H, Breivik H, Rod T, Lind B. Survival after 40 minutes' submersion without cerebral sequelae. *Lancet* 1975; **i**: 1275–7.

560 Siesjö BK. Cell damage in the brain: a speculative synthesis. *J Cereb Blood Flow Metab* 1981; **1**: 155–85.

561 Siesjö BK. Hypoglycemia, brain metabolism, and brain damage. *Diabetes/Metab Rev* 1988; **4**: 113–41.

562 Siesjö BK. Pathophysiology and treatment of focal cerebral ischemia. Part II: Mechanisms of damage and treatment. *J Neurosurg* 1992; **77**: 337–54.

563 Siesjö BK, Ekholm A, Katsura K, Theander S. Acid–base changes during complete brain ischemia. *Stroke* 1990; **21** (Suppl III): 194–9.

564 Siesjö BK, Nilsson L. The influence of arterial hypoxemia upon labile phosphates and upon extracellular and intracellular lactate and pyruvate concentrations in the rat brain. *Scand J Clin Lab Invest* 1971; **27**: 83–96.

565 Silfverskiöld BP. 'Polyneuritis hypoglycemia'. Late peripheral paresis after hypoglycemic attacks in two insulinoma patients. *Acta Med Scand* 1946; **125**: 502–4.

566 Silva AJ, Paylor R, Wehner JM, Tonegawa S. Impaired spatial learning in α-calcium-calmodulin kinase II mutant mice. *Science* 1992; **257**: 206–11.

567 Silva AJ, Stevens CF, Tonegawa S, Wang Y. Deficient hippocampal long-term potentiation in α-calcium-calmodulin kinase II mutant mice. *Science* 1992; **257**: 201–6.

568 Simon RP. Hypoxia versus ischemia. *Neurology* 1999; **52**: 7–8.

569 Simon RP, Aminoff MJ. Electrographic status epilepticus in fatal anoxic coma. *Ann Neurol* 1986; **20**: 351–5.

570 Simon RP, Swan JH, Griffiths T, Meldrum BS. Blockade of N-methyl-d-aspartate receptors may protect against ischemic damage in the brain. *Science* 1984; **226**: 850–2.

571 Sloper JJ, Johnson P, Powell TPS. Selective degeneration of interneurons in the motor cortex of infant monkeys following controlled hypoxia: a possible cause of epilepsy. *Brain Res* 1980; **198**: 204–9.

572 Sloviter RS. A selective loss of hippocampal mossy fiber Timm stain accompanies granule cell seizure activity induced by perforant path stimulation. *Brain Res* 1985; **330**: 150–3.

573 Sloviter RS, Dempster DW. 'Epileptic' brain damage is replicated qualitatively in the rat hippocampus by central injection of glutamate or aspartate but not by GABA or acetylcholine. *Brain Res Bull* 1985; **15**: 39–60.

574 Smith L, Kruszyna H, Smith RP. The effect of methemoglobin on the inhibition of cytochrome c oxidase by cyanide, sulfide or azide. *Biochem Pharmacol* 1977; **26**: 2247–50.

575 Smith M-L, Auer RN, Siesjö BK. The density and distribution of ischemic brain injury in the rat after 2–10 minutes of forebrain ischemia. *Acta Neuropathol (Berl)* 1984; **64**: 319–32.

576 Smith M-L, Hanwehr R von, Siesjö BK. Changes in extra- and intracellular pH in the brain during and following ischemia in hyperglycemic and in moderately hypoglycemic rats. *J Cereb Blood Flow Metab* 1986; **6**: 574–83.

577 Smith M-L, Kalimo H, Warner DS, Siesjö BK. Morphological lesions in the brain preceding the development of postischemic seizures. *Acta Neuropathol (Berl)* 1988; **76**: 253–64.

578 Söderfeldt B, Kalimo H, Olsson Y, Siesjö BK. Bicuculline-induced epileptic brain injury. Transient and persistent cell changes in rat cerebral cortex in the early recovery period. *Acta Neuropathol (Berl)* 1983; **62**: 87–95.

579 Söderfeldt B, Kalimo H, Olsson Y, Siesjö BK. Pathogenesis of brain lesions caused by experimental epilepsy. Light and electron microscopic changes in the rat cerebral cortex following bicuculline-induced status epilepticus. *Acta Neuropathol (Berl)* 1981; **54**: 219–31.

580 Sommer W. Erkrankung des Ammonshorns als aetiologisches Moment der Epilepsie. *Arch Psychiatrie* 1880; **10**: 631–75.

581 Sontheimer H, Kettenmann H, Backus KH, Schachner M. Glutamate opens Na$^+$/K$^+$ channels in cultured astrocytes. *Glia* 1988; **1**: 328–36.

582 Sowden GR, Robins DW, Baskett PJF. Factors associated with survival and eventual cerebral status following cardiac arrest. *Anaesthesia* 1984; **39**: 39–43.

583 Sperandio S, Belle I de, Bredesen DE. An alternative, non-apoptotic form of programmed cell death. *Proc Natl Acad Sci USA* 2000; **97**: 14376–81.

584 Spielmeyer W. Pathogenese örtlich elektiver Gehirnveränderungen. *Z Ges Neurol Psychiatrie* 1925; **99**: 756–76.

585 Stief A, Tokay L. Weitere experimentelle Untersuchungen über die cerebrale Wirkung des Insulins. *Z Ges Neurol Psychiatrie* 1935; **153**: 561–72.

586 Sutton LN, Clark BJ, Norwood CR et al. Global cerebral ischemia in piglets under conditions of mild and deep hypothermia. *Stroke* 1991; **22**: 1567–73.

587 Suzuki R, Yamaguchi T, Li C-L, Klatzo I. The effects of 5-minute ischemia in Mongolian gerbils: II. Changes of spontaneous neuronal activity in the cerebral cortex and CA1 sector of the hippocampus. *Acta Neuropathol (Berl)* 1983; **60**: 217–22.

588 Symon L, Crockard HA, Dorsch NW et al. Local cerebral blood flow and vascular reactivity in a chronic stable stroke in baboons. *Stroke* 1975; **6**: 482–92.

589 Symon L, Dorsch NWC, Ganz JC. Lactic acid efflux from ischaemic brain. An experimental study. *J Neurol Sci* 1972; **17**: 411–18.

590 Talks KL, Turley H, Gatter KC et al. The expression and distribution of the hypoxia-inducible factors HIF-1a and HIF-2a in normal human tissues, cancers, and tumor-associated macrophages. *Am J Pathol* 2000; **157**: 411–21.

591 Thilmann R, Xie Y, Kleihues P, Kiessling M. Persistent inhibition of protein synthesis precedes delayed neuronal death in postischemic gerbil hippocampus. *Acta Neuropathol (Berl)* 1986; **71**: 88–93.

592 Thomas DJ, DuBoulay GH, Marshall J et al. Cerebral blood flow in polycythemia. *Lancet* 1977; **ii**: 161–3.

593 Thomas DJ, DuBoulay GH, Marshall J et al. Effect of haematocrit on cerebral blood flow in man. *Lancet* 1977; **ii**: 941–3.

594 Thurston JH, Hauhart RE, Schiro J. Lactate reverses insulin-induced hypoglycemic stupor in suckling-weanling mice: biochemical correlates in blood, liver, and brain. *J Cereb Blood Flow Metab* 1983; **3**: 498–506.

595 Timsit S, Rivera S, Ouaghi P et al. Increased cyclin D1 in vulnerable neurons in the hippocampus after ischaemia and epilepsy: a modulator of *in vivo* programmed cell death? *Eur J Neurosci* 1999; **11**: 263–78.

596 Todd MM, Weeks JB, Warner DS. Cerebral blood flow, blood volume, and brain tissue hematocrit during isovolemic hemodilution with hetastarch in rats. *Am J Physiol* 1992; **263**: H75–82.

597 Tohgi H, Yamanouchi H, Murakami M, Kameyama M. Importance of the hematocrit as a risk factor in cerebral infarction. *Stroke* 1978; **9**: 369–74.

598 Tom MI, Richardson JC. Hypoglycemia from islet cell tumor of pancreas with amyotrophy and cerebrospinal nerve cell changes. *J Neuropathol Exp Neurol* 1951; **10**: 57–66.

599 Tombaugh GC, Sapolsky RM. Mechanistic distinctions between excitotoxic and acidotic hippocampal damage in an *in vitro* model of ischemia. *J Cereb Blood Flow Metab* 1990; **10**: 527–35.

600 Tombaugh GC, Sapolsky RM. Mild acidosis protects hippocampal neurons from injury induced by oxygen and glucose deprivation. *Brain Res* 1990; **506**: 343–5.

601 Tomida S, Nowak TS Jr, Vass K et al. Experimental model for repetitive ischemic attacks in the gerbil: the cumulative effect of repeated ischemic insults. *J Cereb Blood Flow Metab* 1987; **7**: 773–82.

602 Tominaga T, Kure S, Narisawa K, Yoshimoto T. Endonuclease activation following focal ischemic injury in the rat brain. *Brain Res* 1993; **608**: 21–6.

603 Torre JC de la, Fortin T. Partial or global rat brain ischemia: the SCOT model. *Brain Res Bull* 1991; **26**: 365–72.

604 Torres C de, Munell F, Ferrer I et al. Identification of necrotic cell death by the TUNEL assay in the hypoxic–ischemic neonatal rat brain. *Neurosci Lett* 1997; **230**: 1–4.

605 Towbin A. The respirator brain death syndrome. *Hum Pathol* 1973; **4**: 583–94.

606 Tower DB. Structural and functional organization of mammalian cerebral cortex: the correlation of neurone density with brain size. Cortical neurone density in the fin whale (*Balaenoptera physalus* L.) with a note on cortical neurone density in the Indian elephant. *J Comp Neurol* 1954; **101**: 19–52.

607 Tower DB, Elliott KAC. Activity of acetylcholine system in cerebral cortex of various unanesthetized mammals. *Am J Physiol* 1952; **168**: 747–59.

608 Tower DB, Young OM. Interspecies correlations of cerebral cortical oxygen consumption, acetylcholinesterase activity and chloride content: studies on the brains of the fin whale (*Balaenoptera physalus*) and the sperm whale (*Physeter catadon*). *J Neurochem* 1973; **20**: 253–67.

609 Tower DB, Young OM. The activities of butyrylcholinesterase and carbonic anhydrase, the rate of anaerobic glycolysis, and the question of a constant density of glial cells in cerebral cortices of various mammalian species from mouse to whale. *J Neurochem* 1973; **20**: 269–78.

610 Towfighi J, Gonatas NK. Effect of intracerebral injection of ouabain in adult and developing rats. An ultrastructural and autoradiographic study. *Lab Invest* 1973; **28**: 170–80.

611 Traystman RJ, Fitzgerald RS. Cerebrovascular response to hypoxia in baroreceptor- and chemoreceptor-denervated dogs. *Am J Physiol* 1981; **241**: H724–31.

612 Traystman RJ, Fitzgerald RS, Loscutoff SC. Cerebral circulatory responses to arterial hypoxia in normal and chemodenervated dogs. *Circ Res* 1978; **42**: 649–57.

613 Trump BF, McDowell EM, Arstila AU. Cellular reaction to injury. In: Hill RB, LaVia MF eds. *Principles of pathobiology* 3rd edn. New York: Oxford University Press, 1980: 20–111.

614 Tufo HM, Ostfeld AM, Shekelle R. Central nervous system dysfunction following open-heart surgery. *JAMA* 1970; **212**: 1333–40.

615 Turmaine M, Raza A, Mahal A et al. Nonapoptotic neurodegeneration in a transgenic mouse model of Huntington's disease. *Proc Natl Acad Sci USA* 2000; **97**: 8093–7.

616 Turner RW, Baimbridge KG, Miller JJ. Calcium-induced long-term potentiation in the hippocampus. *Neuroscience* 1982; **7**: 1411–16.

617 Ueda Y, Miki S, Kusuhara K et al. Deep hypothermic systemic circulatory arrest and continuous retrograde cerebral perfusion for surgery of aortic arch aneurysm. *Eur J Cardiothorac Surg* 1992; **6**: 36–41.

618 Van Harreveld A, Fifková E. Light- and electron-microscopic changes in central nervous tissue after electrophoretic injection of glutamate. *Exp Mol Pathol* 1971; **15**: 61–81.

619 Vincent SR, Das S, Maines MD. Brain heme oxygenase isoenzymes and nitric oxide synthase are co-localized in select neurons. *Neuroscience* 1994; **63**: 223–31.

620 Vital Cl, Picard J, Arné L, Aubertin J, Fenelon J, Mouton L. Pathological study of three cases of hypoglycemic encephalopathy (one of which occurred after sulfamidotherapy). *Le Diabète* 1967; **15**: 291–6.

621 Vogt C, Vogt O. Erkrankungen der Grosshirnrinde im Lichte der Topistik, Pathoklise, und Pathoarchitectonik. *J Psychol Neurol* 1922; **28**: 1–171.

622 Vogt C, Vogt O. Sitz und Wesen der Krankheiten im Lichte der topistischen Hirnforschung und des Varierens der Tiere. *J Psychol Neurol* 1937; **47**: 237–457.

623 Vogt O. Der Begriff der Pathoklise. *J Psychol Neurol* 1925; **33**: 245–55.

624 Voll CL, Auer RN. Insulin attenuates ischemic brain damage independent of its hypoglycemic effect. *J Cereb Blood Flow Metab* 1991; **11**: 1006–14.

625 Voll CL, Auer RN. Postischemic seizures and necrotizing ischemic brain damage: neuroprotective effect of postischemic diazepam and insulin. *Neurology* 1991; **41**: 423–8.

626 Voll CL, Auer RN. The effect of post-ischemic blood glucose levels on the density and distribution of ischemic brain damage in the rat. *Ann Neurol* 1988; **24**: 638–46.

627 Wagner KR, Kleinholz M, Myers RE. Delayed neurologic deterioration following anoxia: brain mitochondrial and metabolic correlates. *J Neurochem* 1989; **52**: 1407–17.

628 Wallis RA, Panizzon K, Wasterlain CG. Inhibition of nitric oxide synthase protects against hypoxic neuronal injury. *Neuroreport* 1992; **3**: 645–8.

629 Wang PY, Kao CH, Mui MY, Wang SJ. Leukocyte infiltration in acute hemispheric ischemic stroke. *Stroke* 1993; **24**: 236–40.

630 Watanabe I, Tomita T, Hung K-S, Iwasaki Y. Edematous necrosis in thiamine-deficient encephalopathy of the mouse. *J Neuropathol Exp Neurol* 1981; **40**: 454–71.

631 Watkins JC, Evans RH. Excitatory amino acid transmitters. *Annu Rev Pharmacol Toxicol* 1981; **21**: 165–204.

632 Weathers B. *Left for dead*. New York: Villard Books, a division of Random House, 2000.

633 Wei G, Dawson VL, Zweier JL. Role of neuronal and endothelial nitric oxide synthase in nitric oxide generation in the brain following cerebral ischemia. *Biochim Biophys Acta* 1999; **1455**: 23–34.

634 Weil A, Liebert E, Heilbrunn G. Histopathologic changes in the brain in experimental hyperinsulinism. *Arch Neurol Psychiatry (Chic)* 1938; **39**: 467–81.

635 Weinberger LM, Gibbon MH, Gibbon JH. Temporary arrest of the circulation to the central nervous system. II. Pathologic effects. *Arch Neurol Psychiatry (Chic)* 1940; **43**: 961–86.

636 Westerberg E, Kehr J, Ungerstedt U, Wieloch T. The NMDA-antagonist MK-801 reduces extracellular amino acid levels during hypoglycemia and prevents striatal damage. *Neurosci Res Commun* 1988; **3**: 151–8.

637 Wieloch T. Hypoglycemia-induced neuronal damage prevented by an N-methyl-d-aspartate antagonist. *Science* 1985; **230**: 681–3.

638 Wijdicks EF, Parisi JE, Sharbrough FW. Prognostic value of myoclonus status in comatose survivors of cardiac arrest. *Ann Neurol* 1994; **35**: 239–43.

639 Williams GR, Spencer FC. The clinical use of hypothermia following cardiac arrest. *Ann Surg* 1958; **148**: 462–6.

640 Winn HR, Rubio GR, Berne RM. The role of adenosine in the regulation of cerebral blood flow. *J Cereb Blood Flow Metab* 1981; **1**: 239–44.

641 Wohlwill F. Über Hirnbefunde bei Insulin Überdosierung. *Klin Wochenschr* 1928; **7**: 344–6.

642 Wolfe KB. Effect of hypothermia on cerebral damage resulting from cardiac arrest. *Am J Cardiol* 1960; **6**: 809–12.

643 Wyllie AH, Bellamy CO, Bubb VJ et al. Apoptosis and carcinogenesis. *Br J Cancer* 1999; **80** (Suppl 1): 34–7.

644 Wytrzes LM, Chatrian GE, Shaw CM, Wirch AL. Acute failure of forebrain with sparing of brain-stem function. Electroencephalographic, multimodality evoked potential, and pathologic findings. *Arch Neurol* 1989; **46**: 93–7.

645 Yager JY, Asselin J. Effect of mild hypothermia on cerebral energy metabolism during the evolution of hypoxic–ischemic brain damage in the immature rat. *Stroke* 1996; **27**: 919–26.

646 Yamamoto K, Hayakawa T, Mogami H et al. Ultrastructural investigation of the CA1 region of the hippocampus after transient cerebral ischemia in gerbils. *Acta Neuropathol (Berl)* 1990; **80**: 487–92.

647 Yamamoto K, Morimoto K, Yanagihara T. Cerebral ischemia in the gerbil: transmission electron microscopic and immunoelectron microscopic investigation. *Brain Res* 1986; **384**: 1–10.

648 Yamamoto M, Takahashi K, Ohyama M et al. Behavioral and histological changes after repeated brief cerebral ischemia by carotid artery occlusion in gerbils. *Brain Res* 1993; **608**: 16–20.

649 Yamashita K, Eguchi Y, Kajiwara K, Ito H. Mild hypothermia ameliorates ubiquitin synthesis and prevents delayed neuronal death in the gerbil hippocampus. *Stroke* 1991; **22**: 1574–81.

650 Yan C, Chen J, Chen D et al. Overexpression of the cell death suppressor Bcl-w in ischemic brain: implications for a neuroprotective role via the mitochondrial pathway. J Cereb Blood Flow Metab 2000; 20: 620–30.

651 Yao ZB, Li X, Xu ZC. GABAergic and asymmetrical synapses on somata of GABAergic neurons in CA1 and CA3 regions of rat hippocampus. A quantitative electron microscopic analysis. Stroke 1996; 27: 1411–16.

652 Young GB, Gilbert JJ, Zochodne DW. The significance of myoclonic status epilepticus in postanoxic coma. Neurology 1990; 40: 1843–8.

653 Young RSK, Olenginski TP, Yagel SK, Towfighi J. The effect of graded hypothermia on hypoxic–ischemic brain damage: a neuropathologic study in the neonatal rat. Stroke 1983; 14: 929–34.

654 Yu MC, Bakay L, Lee JC. Ultrastructure of the central nervous system after prolonged hypoxia. I. Neuronal alterations. Acta Neuropathol (Berl) 1972; 22: 222–34.

655 Yu MC, Bakay L, Lee JC. Ultrastructure of the central nervous system after prolonged hypoxia. II. Neuroglia and blood vessels. Acta Neuropathol (Berl) 1972; 22: 235–44.

656 Zhang J, Dawson VL, Dawson TM, Snyder SH. Nitric oxide activation of poly(ADP-ribose) synthetase in neurotoxicity. Science 1994; 263: 687–9.

657 Zhu CZ, Auer RN. Graded hypotension and MCA occlusion duration: effect in transient focal ischemia. J Cereb Blood Flow Metab 1995; 15: 980–8.

658 Zhu CZ, Auer RN. Intraventricular administration of insulin and IGF-1 in transient forebrain ischemia. J Cereb Blood Flow Metab 1994; 14: 237–42.

659 Zhuo M, Small SA, Kandel ER, Hawkins RD. Nitric oxide and carbon monoxide produce activity-dependent long-term synaptic enhancement in hippocampus. Science 1993; 260: 1946–50.

660 Zimmerman JM, Spencer FC. The influence of hypothermia on cerebral injury resulting from circulatory occlusion. Surg Forum 1959; 9: 216–18.

6

Vascular diseases

HANNU KALIMO, MARKKU KASTE AND MATTI HALTIA

INTRODUCTION

The central nervous system (CNS) requires a continuous supply of glucose and oxygen to sustain its high expenditure of energy. The transportation of these fuel molecules requires sufficient blood flow through a cerebral vasculature with adequate capacity. This chapter deals with diseases that affect the cerebral blood vessels and consequently cause disturbances of the cerebral blood flow (CBF), which in turn lead to tissue damage. It has been divided in five parts: (1) a short summary of the normal angiogenesis and anatomy of the cerebral vasculature; (2) a general account of the epidemiology of stroke; (3) a description of the diseases that afflict the blood-vessel walls; (4) a discussion of the equilibrium between the procoagulant and anticoagulant factors and how disturbances of this balance lead to pathological coagulation of the blood; and (5) the consequences of these pathological changes, i.e. with ischaemic damage and haemorrhage.

DEVELOPMENT AND ANATOMY

Development of cerebral vasculature

The formation of the cerebral vascular system is a tightly regulated developmental process, which requires an intricate interplay between the mesodermally derived vascular cells and neuroectodermally derived CNS. This process is controlled by signalling systems which include a large number of specific receptor molecules and their ligands, in addition to other necessary molecules involved for example in mitogenic, chemotactic, proteo-

lytic and adhesive activities. These signalling systems are subject to intensive research, because in adult brain the same molecules participate in the regulation of hypoxia- and tumour-induced angiogenesis, both of which are of great therapeutic importance.[403,421]

The development of the vascular system is initiated around the third week of gestation, when mesodermal precursor cells in paraxial mesoderm differentiate into haemangioblasts. This occurs under the influence of mesoderm inducing factors of the fibroblast growth factor family, which interact with vascular endothelial growth factor receptor-2 (VEGFR-2) on mesodermal precursor cells. Haemangioblasts in turn differentiate into vessel-forming angioblasts and into haematopoetic stem cells. Angioblasts cluster and acquire lumen forming interconnecting tubes, which comprise the primitive vascular plexus, a process called vasculogenesis. During this process vascular endothelial growth factor (VEGF), the essential ligand for VEGFR-2 and VEGFR-1 on angioblasts, is produced by surrounding cells and it is needed to maintain angioblast differentiation. VEGFR-1 is expressed later than VEGFR-2 and appears to be necessary for the assembly of angioblasts into functional blood vessels. Angioblasts also migrate into the head region to form a perineural vascular plexus around the developing brain (extracerebral vascularization).

After the primitive vascular plexus has been constructed, new blood vessels are formed by sprouting from the pre-existing vessels, a process termed angiogenesis, by which new blood vessels are also formed in adult organs. During sprouting the extracellular matrix is degraded by proteolysis, enabling migration of the proliferating endothelial cells, which are attracted by chemotactic factors, and of these VEGF appears to be the most important. Cerebral blood vessels are formed by capillary sprouts which originate from the perineural plexus and penetrate into the developing brain (intracerebral vascularization). VEGF produced by cells in the periventricular matrix zone appears to be the main chemotactic stimulus to the endothelial cells actively expressing VEGFR-2.[50] However, sprouting in angiogenesis requires additional ligand/ receptor sets, angiopoetin-1 and angiopoetin-2/tie-1 and tie-2, which may regulate the interaction between the endothelial and perivascular cells.[403] The penetrating blood vessels begin to form intracerebral branches of various sizes creating the vascular tree, by a remodelling process known as pruning. Finally, the blood vessels mature, which includes recruitment of pericytes and in larger blood vessels also of smooth-muscle cells and fibroblasts, and the formation of contacts with astrocytic processes.

The active phase of vascular proliferation ceases soon after birth, after which the cerebral vasculature is expanded only to meet the needs of the growing brain mainly by elongation of the pre-existing blood vessels. This occurs at the same time as downregulation of the receptor/ligand systems. In the normal adult brain angiogenesis is minimal, but it may be reactivated in some pathological conditions, e.g. in hypoxia/ischaemia, trauma or the presence of brain tumours. This newly activated angiogenesis is mainly regulated by the same signalling molecules as during development. VEGF has been demonstrated to be hypoxia inducible in many cell types, and accordingly VEGF expression is upregulated in glial cells at the periphery of infarcts. Similarly, it has been shown that VEGF expression in glioblastomas is enhanced up to 50-fold and it is accompanied by a parallel increase in VEGFRs on the endothelium of the neoplastic blood vessels. Analogous upregulations have been reported in the angiopoetin/tie systems.[403]

Arterial blood supply

The metabolism of the brain is almost solely aerobic (see Chapter 5, this Volume) and without any significant energy reserves. Therefore, the brain requires a constant, ample supply of well-oxygenated blood. The exceptionally high demand for circulating blood and oxygen is reflected in the disproportionately high rate of CBF compared with flow to other parts of the body, comprising 20% of the cardiac output and 15% of oxygen consumption in a resting adult person, even though the brain makes up only 2% of the body weight. This ample blood flow to the brain is supplied by two pairs of large arteries. The main, anterior flow (approx. 70% of the CBF) enters the intracranial cavity through the internal carotid arteries, and the posterior flow (approx. 30% of the CBF) is furnished by the vertebral arteries. These two systems anastomose via the anterior and posterior communicating arteries at the base of the brain to form the circle of Willis (Fig. 6.1).[27,136,196] There is considerable variation in the relative

size of the vertebral and communicating arteries. This does not have functional significance under normal conditions, but may become important if an obstruction develops in any of the main trunks. Another important anastomotic pathway is between the external and internal carotid arteries via the ophthalmic arteries. If this anastomotic network is normal, even the occlusion of one of the four main arteries may not necessarily lead to insufficient regional CBF. For example, in the case of a fusiform aneurysm arising from the distal segment of an internal carotid artery, this blood vessel may be slowly clamped surgically without causing infarction, and the slow obliteration of an arterial lumen by atherosclerosis also allows sufficient time for the collateral circulation to adjust.[196] Patients with only one patent vertebral artery have been cited as good examples of an efficient collateral circulation.

The leptomeningeal anastomoses are organized in the subarachnoid space over the surface of the brain, where the territories of the distal branches of the anterior, middle and posterior cerebral arteries overlap in the border or watershed zones (Fig. 6.1a–c). Corresponding border zones are also formed between the superior and inferior cerebellar arteries (Fig. 6.1d). These leptomeningeal anastomoses are located at the periphery of the arterial tree and therefore an adequate blood pressure is needed to maintain flow in these areas. By the same token, these zones are the first to be deprived of sufficient blood flow in the event of arterial hypotension.

The branches of the arteries running in the subarachoid space penetrate the brain parenchyma. These branches include both deep and superficial perforating arteries. The deep perforators leave the main cerebral arteries at the base of the brain and consist of: (1) the lenticulostriate arteries, which emerge from the first segments of the anterior and middle cerebral artery to supply the basal ganglia, and (2) perforant branches, which leave the posterior cerebral and posterior communicating arteries and nourish the thalamic nuclei. The superficial perforators originate from the pial branches of the anterior, middle and posterior cerebral arteries over the surface of the brain, and are of variable length: short ones supply the cortex and longer ones, the medullary arteries, nourish the deep white matter. Short penetrators also exist in the brainstem as paramedian branches of the basilar artery. The perforators are end arteries, i.e. they have very limited collateral connections with neighbouring blood vessels until they divide into capillaries. The capillaries do interconnect, but their collateral flow is so local and small that the occlusion of a perforator usually results in a small area of ischaemic damage, commonly described as lacunar infarcts (see below). The deep and superficial perforators do not anastomose deep in the brain, but meet in a junctional zone, where subcortical infarction can occur.[41] Interest in these perforators has increased considerably in parallel with improved resolution of the imaging methods which allows identification of small lacunar lesions in life (see Fig. 6.41a, b). The distribution territo-

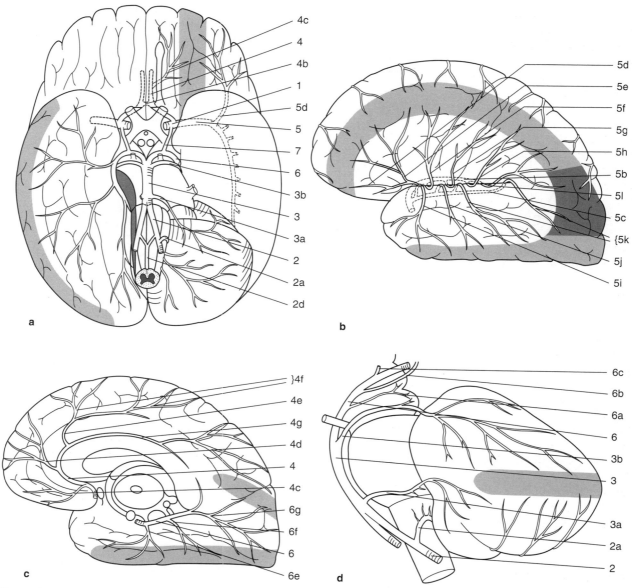

Figure 6.1 *Supply territories of the cerebral and cerebellar arteries. The border zones (watershed areas) between the territories are indicated by hatching. 1, Internal carotid artery; 1a, anterior choroidal artery; 2, vertebral artery; 2a, posterior interior cerebellar artery; 2b, paramedian branch; 2c, lateral bulbar branch; 2d, anterior spinal artery; 3, basilar artery; 3a, anterior inferior cerebellar artery; 3b, superior cerebellar artery; 3c, paramedian branch; 3d, short circumferential branch; 4, anterior cerebral artery; 4a, recurrent artery of Heubner; 4b, anterior communicating artery; 4c, medial orbitofrontal artery; 4d, frontopolar artery; 4e, callosomarginal artery; 4f, internal frontal branches; 4g, pericallosal artery; 5, middle cerebral artery; 5a, lenticulostriate artery; 5b, upper division; 5c, lower division; 5d, lateral orbitofrontal artery; 5e, ascending frontal (candelabra) branch; 5f, central (Rolandic) artery; 5g, anterior parietal artery; 5h, posterior parietal artery; 5i, temporal polar artery; 5j, anterior temporal artery; 5k, posterior temporal branches; 5l, angular artery; 6, posterior cerebral artery; 6a, quadrigeminal artery; 6b, posterior choroidal artery; 6c, thalamogeniculate artery; 6d, thalamoperforating artery; 6e, anterior temporal artery; 6f, posterior temporal artery; 6g, calcarine artery; 6h, paramedian branch; 6i, short circumferential branch; 6j, long circumferential branch; 7, posterior communicating artery; 7a, hypothalamic artery. Adapted from Ref. 423.*

ries of the main arteries in the brain and brainstem are depicted in the coronal and tomographic planes in Figs 6.2 and 6.3.

The microscopic structure of the extracranial parts of the carotid and vertebral arteries is similar to that of all other large arteries, whereas intracranial cerebral blood vessels have many structural features tailor-made for the specific requirements of the CNS. First, the endothelial cells of the intracranial blood vessels are joined by tight junctions, they have no fenestrations and their

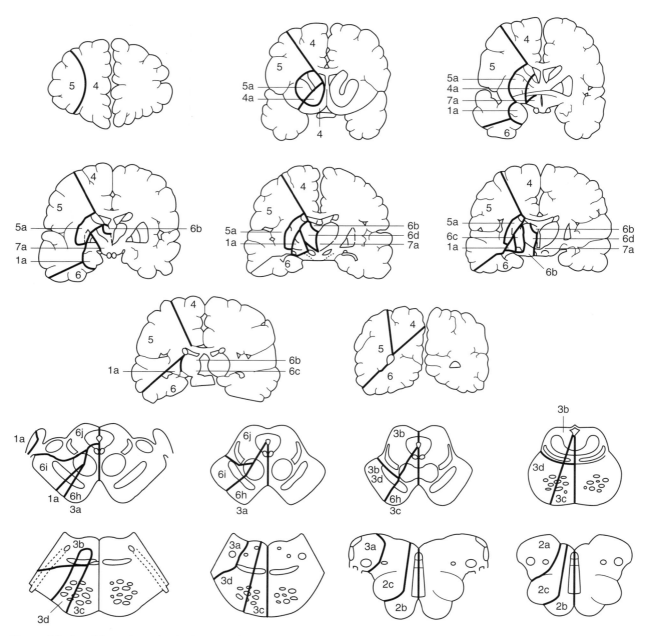

Figure 6.2 *Arterial supply territories in coronal planes of the cerebrum and brainstem. Explanations for the numbers are given in the legend to Fig. 6.1. Adapted from Ref. 423.*

metabolism has specific features related to their barrier and transcellular transport functions [for details of the blood–brain barrier (BBB) see Chapter 4, this Volume]. Further, the muscle coat of intracranial arteries is thinner than in the extracranial arteries of the corresponding size, the external elastic lamina is lacking and the adventitia is very thin.

Venous drainage

The venous circulation of the CNS (Fig. 6.4) is exceptional, differing from the common antiparallel (i.e. running in

parallel to opposite directions) orientation of arteries and veins in many other organs. In addition, the cerebral venous drainage employs unique dural sinuses as the final intracranial collecting blood vessels.[8,423] The blood from most of the white matter and cortex of the cerebral hemispheres is drained by veins of various lengths, which are still conventionally orientated antiparallel to the pial penetrating arteries. In general, the number of veins is less than the number of perforating arteries, and the long veins also drain cerebral cortex while passing through it.

When the veins of the superficial or cortical network exit the parenchyma and enter the subarachnoid space they turn towards the dural sinuses. In the suprasylvian and

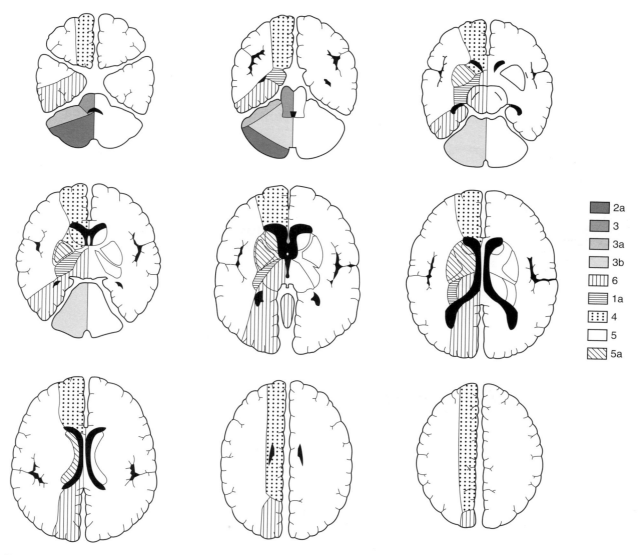

Figure 6.3 *Arterial supply territories in the tomographic planes. The numbering of the arteries is the same as in Figs 6.1 and 6.2. Adapted from Ref. 437, where it was originally modified from Ref. 448.*

paramedian regions the frontal, parietal and occipital superior cerebral veins run upwards to drain into the superior sagittal sinus. In the parasylvian region the middle cerebral veins drain via the superficial sylvian vein to the cavernous sinus. On the posterior lateral and inferior surfaces of the temporal lobe and on the lateral and inferior surface of the occipital lobe the veins drain into the lateral sinuses. In addition, the middle cerebral veins are connected upwards with the superior sagittal sinus by the vein of Trolard and downwards with the lateral sinus by the vein of Labbé. The number and location of the cortical veins vary considerably, which makes angiographic verification of their patency very difficult. The superficial veins have thin walls, no tunica muscularis and no valves, thus permitting dilatation and flow of venous blood in various directions. These features, together with numerous anastamoses, guarantee efficient collateral flow in the case of venous thrombosis.

Within the parenchyma of the hemispheres the veins of the superficial system anastomose extensively with the internal cerebral and basal veins of the deep network. The deep veins collect blood from the deep grey matter at the base of the brain and the choroid plexus of the lateral ventricles, and drain into the centrally located great cerebral vein of Galen. The latter joins the venous sinus system at the straight sinus at the apex of the cerebellar tentorium, into which the inferior sagittal sinus, running in the lower edge of falx, also empties. The straight sinus then merges with the superior sagittal and occipital sinuses at the confluence of sinuses (torcula Herophili). The bulk of the venous blood flows via the bilateral transverse and sigmoid sinuses (which together form the lateral sinus) and through the jugular foramen into the jugular veins. The right lateral sinus is commonly larger than the left, and in 14% of cases the transverse portion of the left sinus is not visualized in angiography, an anomaly which may be

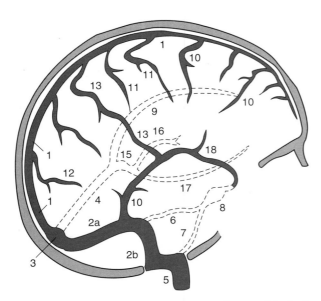

Figure 6.4 *Anatomy of venous drainage pathways of the brain. In the case of paired blood vessels only the right is depicted. The veins in black are located on the surface of the brain, those drawn with dashed lines are within the parenchyma. 1, Superior sagittal sinus; 2a, transverse portion of lateral sinus; 2b, sigmoid portion of lateral sinus; 3, confluence of sinuses; 4, straight sinus; 5, internal jugular vein; 6, superior petrosal vein; 7, inferior petrosal vein; 8, cavernous sinus; 9, inferior sagittal sinus; 10, frontal veins; 11, parietal vein; 12, occipital vein; 13, vein of Trolard; 14, vein of Labbé; 15, great vein of Galen; 16, internal cerebral vein; 17, basal vein; 18, superficial sylvian vein. Adapted from Ref. 8.*

Table 6.1 *Annual risk of stroke (all subtypes combined)*

Age group (years)	Approximate population risk
0–14	1 in 100 000
15–24	1 in 20 000
25–34	1 in 10 000
35–44	1 in 5000
45–54	1 in 1000
55–64	1 in 300
65–74	1 in 100
75–85	1 in 50
> 85	1 in 33

significant when searching for venous thrombosis. Dural sinuses also receive blood from the diploë of the skull bones, and they are connected with the extracranial veins via the emissary veins, which traverse the cranium.

The posterior fossa veins drain the cerebellum and brainstem. Having emerged on the surface the veins form a subarachnoid plexus, from where blood drains in three directions. Venous blood from the superior parts drains into the great cerebral vein of Galen, from the anterior parts into the petrosal sinuses and from the posterior and lateral parts into the adjacent straight, occipital and lateral sinuses.

The blood supply and vascular pathology of the spinal cord are described in Chapter 18, this Volume.

Physiology of the cerebral circulation

The physiology and regulation of the CBF and the exchange of metabolites between blood and parenchyma are described in detail in Chapter 5, this Volume.

DEFINITIONS AND EPIDEMIOLOGY OF VASCULAR DISORDERS OF THE CENTRAL NERVOUS SYSTEM

Stroke in general

Continuous sufficient blood flow through an intact cerebral vasculature is a prerequisite for undisturbed brain function. Stroke is defined as an 'abrupt onset of focal or global neurological symptoms caused by ischaemia or haemorrhage'.[439] By convention, these symptoms must continue for more than 24 h to qualify for the diagnosis of stroke, which is usually associated with permanent damage to brain. If the symptoms resolve within 24 h the episode is called a transient ischaemic attack (TIA). In TIA the tissue changes may also be transient, although with modern brain imaging it has been demonstrated that the attack may nevertheless have resulted in minor permanent yet symptomless lesions. Stroke is a common life-threatening neurological disease (Table 6.1) and the third leading cause of death. It is an important cause of hospital admissions and long-term disability in most industrialized populations,[439,542] and requires a major share of the economic resources of health-care systems.[493]

Although the clinical diagnosis of stroke is reasonably accurate, the diagnosis by pathological type, i.e. determination of the exact cause of the stroke, is considerably less accurate. According to the criteria of the MONICA project (Multinational MONItoring of trends and determinants in CArdiovacular disease) of the World Health Organization,[19] the pathological type of stroke should be determined by early brain imaging or by autopsy in fatal cases. Subarachnoid haemorrhage may be diagnosed by lumbar puncture. These criteria, greatly helped by the increasing sophistication of imaging methods and acceptance of a category of unspecified strokes, have definitely made the determination of the type of stroke more accurate. There are significant geographical, racial and ethnic variations in the frequency of the different pathological types of stroke (Table 6.2). In Western countries cerebral infarction accounts for approximately 60–80% of first-time strokes. In Far Eastern countries the figure is

Table 6.2 *Age-adjusted incidences and relative distributions of first-time stroke by pathological type in prospective studies of different populations (all age groups)*

Study	Year	Incidence per 100 000	CI (%)	ICH (%)	SAH (%)	US (%)
Oxfordshire, UK[24]	1981–1986	170	81	10	5	5
Jyväskylä, Finland[140,422]	1993	145 (227[a])	81	12	7	5
Umbria, Italy[414]	1986–1989	155	76	10	7	<1
Rochester, USA[61]	1985–1989	145	84[b]	11[b]	4	10
Taiwan[221]	1986–1990	330	71	22	5[b]	n.r.
Akita, Japan[481]	1983–1985	n.r.	56	30	1	6
Riyadh, Saudi Arabia[7]	1986–1990	n.r.	76	21	14	n.r.
			76	21	3	n.r.

CI, cerebral infarction; ICH, intracerebral haemorrhage; SAH, subarachnoid haemorrhage; US, unspecified type of stroke; n.r., not reported in the article.

The incidences are not fully comparable, because they are age-adjusted for different populations.

[a]When age-adjusted for European standard population aged >25 years; [b]for years 1980–1989.

about 50–60%, because the rate of intracerebral haemorrhage is as high as 16–44%, compared with equivalent Western figures of 5–11%. Subarachnoid haemorrhage has a smaller geographical variation, accounting for between 5 and 10% of cases. The frequency of unspecified strokes varies within a wide range from 3 to 25%, which is certainly influenced by the differential diagnostic policy adopted and resources available. The trend of change in the relative frequencies of different types of stroke has been similar in most countries, although quantitative differences exist. Since the 1970s the proportion of intracerebral haemorrhage has decreased, most significantly in Japan, whereas that of subarachnoid haemorrhage has remained fairly constant.[492] Details of these frequencies are given below.

Stroke incidence rates

The annual risk of stroke is highly age dependent. While the risk for a child under 15 years of age is 1 in 100 000, it is 1 in 33 for persons aged 85 years and over (Table 6.1). Because of this age dependence the incidence of stroke greatly varies according to the age structure of the population under study. It is higher in Western countries and Japan because of the higher proportion of elderly people compared with developing countries. When data from different countries are compared, the population to which the incidence rates have been age-adjusted must be known.[492] The age-adjusted annual incidence rates of all first-time strokes in different countries of the world vary between about 90 and 350 per 100 000. In Western countries the rates are often below 200, while in Oriental nations rates exceeding 300 have been reported (Table 6.2). For people aged 45–84 years European incidence rates are between 350 and 450, France having the lowest rate of 238, while in Russia the rate is 627.[438,531] The stroke incidence during the past 50 years has been declining in Western Europe and in Japan but increasing in Eastern

Europe.[531] This decline has occurred in all age groups, although it has been greatest in the elderly and it concerns both intracerebral haemorrhage and cerebral infarction, whereas the incidence of subarachnoid haemorrhage has remained constant. By contrast, the decreasing trend continued in Rochester, Minnesota, USA until the 1970s, but during the 1980s it began to rise again from the incidence rate (age adjusted to the 1970 US white population) of 205 in 1955–1959 to a low of 128 in 1975–1979 followed by a rise to 145 in 1985–1989. The explanation for this increase is not known.[61]

Racial, ethnic and social backgrounds have a definite impact on stroke incidence. In general, Caucasians have lower rates than non-Whites. In the USA several studies have verified significantly higher incidence rates for Blacks than for Whites.[440] In New Zealand the incidence was 44% higher among the original Maori population than the white population of predominantly British origin.[46] In Israel, the stroke incidence was 46–97% higher in Jewish women born in North Africa or Asia than among those born in Israel.[492] Differences may exist even within the same race: among Japanese males the incidence of stroke was three times higher in Japan than in Hawaii.[486]

Stroke mortality rates

The mortality rates for stroke in the USA have decreased steadily since 1915: the decline averaged 1% per year until the mid-1960s, after which it has accelerated to 5% per year.[543] Similar real decline has occurred in most Western industrialized nations, although stroke death rates vary more than 8-fold between different countries, from over 200 in 100 000 in some Eastern European countries to only 30 in Switzerland. The most striking decrease of over 7% per year in stroke mortality has occurred in Japan, whereas until the end of 1980s most Eastern European countries had experienced either an increase or no change. The stroke mortality rate rises with the patients' age: each

5 years doubles the age-specific death rates.[348] The overall rates for women and men run in parallel, but for men they are 25–50% higher than for women in all countries.

The key element in the decline in stroke mortality is thought to be a reduced incidence,[140] but the case fatality rates from stroke have also decreased due to either lesser severity or improved stroke management.[45] The most marked difference has been with intracerebral haemorrhage: for example, in Rochester, Minnesota, the 30-day case-fatality rate fell from 91% during 1945–1949 to 48% during 1980–1984.[45] Thus, ample evidence supports the contention that both declining incidence and falling case fatality rates contribute to the decline in stroke mortality in Western countries.

Risk factors for stroke

In addition to age, sex and race-related differences there are many potentially modifiable social habits and diseases that markedly increase the individual's risk for stroke. Among the former, cigarette smoking has been shown to be an independent determinant of stroke in a dose-dependent manner. Smokers have an approximately 3-fold increase of risk for subarachnoid haemorrhage, and a 2-fold increased risk for infarction, whereas the risk for intracerebral haemorrhage is not increased in comparison with non-smoking controls.[209,460] As with myocardial disease, there seems to be a J-shaped relationship between alcohol and stroke. Alcohol in small amounts appears to decrease slightly the risk of stroke, whereas heavy drinking increases the risk by up to 2.5-fold.[164]

Among the predisposing diseases,[531] hypertension is the most significant, increasing the risk by up to 4–5 times in a dose-dependent manner, and further accentuated by its high prevalence. The greatest numerical risk (5.6–17.6-fold) has been ascribed to atrial fibrillation, followed by many other cardiac diseases (2–4-fold risk), e.g. previous myocardial infarction, valvular heart disease and congestive heart disease, which all share a propensity for embolization. Carotid artery stenosis increases the risk of a completed stroke, especially if it is associated with previous TIAs. Hyperlipidaemia (up to 2-fold risk) and diabetes mellitus (1.5–3-fold risk) are the most common metabolic disorders associated with stroke. Certain medical treatments, such as open heart and coronary bypass surgery, increase the risk, as do the older oral contraceptives with a high oestrogen content.

The number of genetic risk factors of both ischaemic stroke and haemorrhages has increased in recent years as mutations in molecules regulating haemostasis have been identified. These strokes occur especially in the younger age group, as do also strokes induced by antiphospholipid autoantibodies, which cause an acquired immune-mediated thrombophilia and which have recently emerged as significant risk factors (see section on Haematological disorders).[275,374,487]

Migraine has also been reported as a risk factor (about 3.5-fold) in young women (below 45 years of age) for ischaemic but not haemorrhagic stroke.[86,507] Further, even a family history of migraine irrespective of personal history was found to increase the risk,[86] and the coexistence of other risk factors had more than any accumulative effect on odds ratios.[86,507] Besides, migraine is a common early symptom in cerebral autosomal dominant arteriopathy with subcortical infarcts and leukoencephalopathy (CADASIL; see below). In addition, there is a multitude of other incriminating factors, the effects of which are still controversial.[543]

DISEASES AFFECTING THE BLOOD VESSELS

Adequate flow of blood to the brain is normally delivered by a cerebral vasculature of sufficient calibre lined by intact endothelial cells on normal intima supported by structurally and functionally intact tunica muscularis and adventitia. Many disease processes may thicken the arterial wall and narrow the lumen, or may weaken the wall making it more susceptible to dilatation and rupture. Furthermore, these disorders frequently damage the endothelium or produce factors that may activate platelets and the clotting cascade and cause thrombosis.

Atherosclerosis

GENERAL ASPECTS

The most common vascular disease is atherosclerosis. It is a slowly developing disease, which often begins in childhood, although a small minority may have escaped it even by their ninth or tenth decade.[171] Atherosclerosis has many risk factors in common with stroke in general: dyslipidaemia, hypertension, diabetes mellitus and cigarette smoking. Atherosclerosis is a generalized disease of the whole arterial network, although marked regional variation exists. In the carotid arteries the rate of atheroma formation is about the same as in the aorta and coronary arteries. In these blood vessels the first structural alterations of atherosclerosis, called fatty streaks, may have appeared as early as by the first or second decade, whereas in the vertebral and intracranial cerebral arteries they develop a decade later.[171,356,411] The atherosclerotic lesions do not qualitatively differ between gender or various ethnic groups, although there is some anatomical variation: in the Caucasian population atherosclerosis is usually more severe in extracranial arteries and is less frequently localized to intracranial blood vessels than in African–Caribbean populations.[356] Quantitative differences between different ethnic groups are marked, which in part depends on the fact that many of the risk factors are associated with social and economic circumstances, although the real causes for the observed differences between ethnic groups are not known. Some generalizations about the risk factors have been made: high serum lipids and blood pressure are associated with a high incidence of atherosclerosis in both the extracranial and intracranial arteries, whereas low or normal lipids and high blood-pressure levels are mainly associated with intracranial and intracerebral arterial disease.[291]

PATHOGENESIS OF ATHEROSCLEROSIS

The hypotheses proposed to explain the development of atherosclerotic lesions in the arterial walls have become increasingly complex and elaborate. A key feature is accumulation of lipids in the arterial intima, which is initiated by dysfunction of endothelium. This leads to a series of interdependent cellular and molecular processes, including modification of the lipids, migration and proliferation of reactive smooth muscle and inflammatory cells, production of proinflammatory mediators, and possibly also invasion by infectious micro-organisms.[281,431,478]

Lipid metabolism

There is strong epidemiological and experimental evidence that increased dietary lipids, particularly cholesterol and saturated fats, correlate with the development of atherosclerotic lesions in the walls of large and medium-sized cerebral arteries (similarly in coronary arteries).[281,491] The normal metabolism (Fig. 6.5) of dietary cholesterol begins by its transport in serum chylomicrons together with triglycerides. The latter are removed by endothelial lipoprotein lipase in adipose tissue and skeletal muscle, and the remnants are taken up by hepatocytes for their own endogenous synthesis of cholesterol which is adjusted according to the amount of exogenous cholesterol. Cholesterol, phospholipids and triglycerides are delivered from the liver into the body tissues associated with apolipoproteins to guarantee solubility in serum. At first, these very low-density lipoprotein (VLDL) particles are rich in triglycerides, most of which are released in adipose tissue and muscle. Thus, VLDL particles are transformed into low-density lipoprotein (LDL) particles with diameter of about 20 nm. The physiological role of the LDL particles is to provide extrahepatic cells, including those of the CNS, with cholesterol.[60] To reach the extrahepatic cells LDL particles traverse the walls of capillaries and enter the extracellular fluid compartment of a given tissue. In tissue, LDL particles bind to LDL receptors on the surface of cells, in arterial intima on smooth-muscle cells, and are then taken up by receptor-mediated endocytosis to be used in ordinary metabolic pathways. Cells which have acquired sufficient cholesterol cease to produce LDL receptors and, consequently, to endocytose LDL particles. Excess LDL particles not taken up by the non-liver cells enter lymphatic capillaries and return into the circulation. The efflux of excess cholesterol is aided by high-density lipoprotein (HDL) particles, which enter the tissue from the blood, collect excess cholesterol from the cells and return to the circulation. In the blood, the HDL-

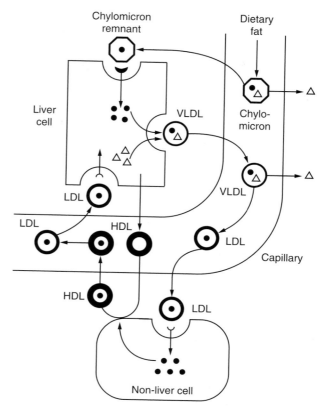

Figure 6.5 *Schematic figure of normal lipid metabolism. For details see the text. VLDL, very low-density lipoprotein; LDL, low-density lipoprotein; HDL, high density lipoprotein; ●, cholesterol; △, triglycerides; ⊤ , chylomicron remnant receptor; Y , LDL receptor.*

borne enzyme lecithin:cholesterol acyltransferase esterifies cholesterol and the product is transferred to LDL. LDL-cholesterol returned to the circulation is ultimately transported back to the liver for excretion in the bile. This phenomenon, called 'reverse cholesterol transport', normally keeps an equilibrium between the influx and efflux of cholesterol to and from the extrahepatic tissues, including the arterial intima.

Atherosclerotic lesions

Initial lesions

The lipid hypothesis implies that atherosclerosis begins to develop when a high plasma level of LDL is associated with excessive amounts of LDL-cholesterol in the arterial intima. LDL particles are retained much longer in the arterial intima than in other tissues, since in the intima there are no lymphatic capillaries, the nearest being located in the media. Furthermore, the proteoglycan matrix slows down the movement of LDL particles across the intima, which is separated from the media by poorly permeable internal elastic lamina. Because of the retarded passage, the concentration of LDL in the intima is at least 10 times higher than in the extracellular fluid of other extrahepatic tissues. Intimal cells do not express LDL receptors as do cells in the other extrahepatic tissues, which results in blockade of LDL uptake and further increase in the concentration LDL in the intima.[281]

According to the response to injury/inflammatory hypothesis, a further prerequisite for the initiation of the atherogenic process is disruption of the endothelial barrier function by an injury to the endothelial cells, which at the early stage is functional rather than structural.[431] The suggested causes of the injury include hypertension, hyperlipidaemia, free radicals and toxic substances such as cigarette smoke. The endothelial injury allows excessive egress of lipids and their deposition in the intima. Furthermore, it appears to be well established that chemical modification of LDL particles is essential for the initiation of the cascade which leads to pathological accumulation of lipids in the intima. Modified LDL particles are a potent chemoattractant for circulating monocytes[407] and, in addition, they impede the migration of macrophages from intima to the circulation. In the intima the attracted monocytes and, to a lesser extent, resident smooth-muscle cells take up and deposit modified LDL-cholesterol much more effectively than native LDL by exploiting specific 'scavenger receptors'.[169] These cells are transformed into intimal foam cells, clusters of which form the initial lesion visible to the naked eye as yellowish fatty streaks. Both the foam cells and extracellular lipids are strongly positive using common fat stains.

Most commonly, the modification of LDL is thought to mean oxidation by free radicals, which are produced by cells associated with the developing atherosclerotic plaque, i.e. endothelial cells, macrophages or smooth-muscle cells.[478,551] The process thus becomes self-perpetuating. The cholesterol derived from the modified LDL particles and stored in macrophages can be returned to the circulation by HDL, but commonly there is a simultaneous impairment of this initial stage of the 'reverse cholesterol transport' owing to low HDL levels in atherosclerotic patients. According to this view, atherogenesis depends on a close interplay between circulatory and cellular factors.

Fatty streaks may appear in the carotid arteries during the first decade, but their appearance does not always lead to more severe atherosclerosis,[468] nor do they cause any significant circulatory disturbances. Hence fatty streaks should not necessarily be regarded as pathological changes.[282]

Development of atherosclerotic plaques

Very slowly, and usually over decades, the fatty streaks develop into more advanced, elevated lesions atherosclerotic plaques (atheroma), which are called fibrous plaques, if the fibrous connective tissue predominates over lipids (Fig. 6.6a–c). These are usually located in specific sites, such as on the outer aspects of the bifurcations of arteries, where the intima is already developmentally thickened and the laminar blood flow is disturbed. Inflam-

matory cells enter the plaques from the circulation through interactions between various adhesion molecules and their ligands on the surface of the endothelial cells and leukocytes (Fig. 6.7). Inflammatory and endothelial cells secrete many different growth factors (e.g. platelet derived, epidermal, fibroblast and transforming growth factors) and cytokines [e.g. interleukins (ILs), tumour necrosis factor (TNF) and leukotrienes (LTs)], which most probably recruit additional cells, including smooth-muscle cells from the media into these lesions. They also induce the transformation of smooth-muscle cells from contractile cells into cells which actively synthesize proteins. These synthesizing smooth-muscle cells are alone responsible for the production of extracellular matrix components (mainly type I and III collagen) of the fibrous cap underneath the still intact endothelial cell layer. Beneath this cap, there are clusters of smooth-muscle cells, foam cells and lymphocytes, together with a central core of necrotic cell debris and extracellular lipids, frequently in the form of cholesterol crystals. As long as the fibrous cap remains whole the plaque is stable.

Fibrous plaques require as long as 20–30 years to form. Although they may already be advanced and stenose the lumen of the affected artery to a considerable extent, they usually do not reduce the blood flow sufficiently to cause neurological symptoms. In fact, as little as 5% of the cross-sectional area of the lumen is usually sufficient to maintain the blood flow at the level needed for normal brain function. However, the turbulences caused by the plaques contribute to progression of the disease.

Development of complicated plaques

Serious consequences occur when the atherosclerotic plaque is converted into an unstable complicated plaque, in which the size of the lipid core has increased and the fibrous cap has become thinner. The latter alteration is very important for the plaque becoming unstable, and according to the prevailing view it is modulated by inflammatory cells, which have been reported to be always present at the sites of ulceration or rupture of an atheromatous plaque.[74,281] Macrophages, T-lymphocytes and mast cells accumulated in the intima secrete cytokines which affect the rate of synthesis and lysis of the matrix proteins. In particular, γ-interferon (γ-IFN) secreted by T-lymphocytes decreases the number of smooth-muscle cells by inhibiting their proliferation and, together with other cytokines, e.g. TNF-α and IL-1β, also induces apoptotic death of smooth-muscle cells. Furthermore, γ-IFN inhibits collagen synthesis in smooth-muscle cells. By contrast, both vascular and inflammatory cells can produce matrix metalloproteinases which, if not sufficiently counteracted by specific tissue inhibitors, leads to degradation of the existing matrix and weakening of the fibrous cap.

A critical event is the damage to the endothelium: in detailed analyses of fatal cases with carotid artery occlusion the endothelial lining was always disrupted over com-

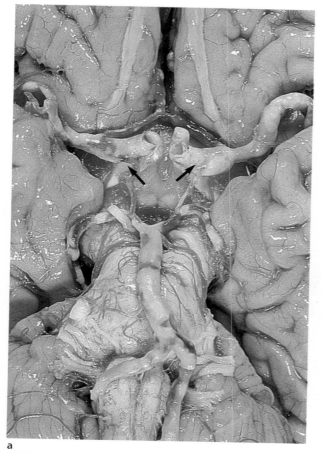

a

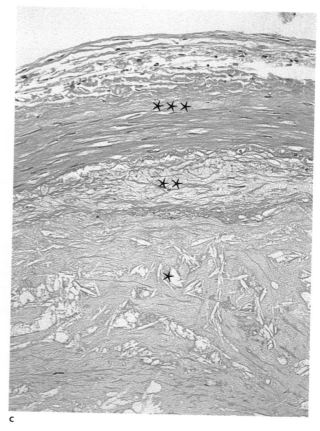

c

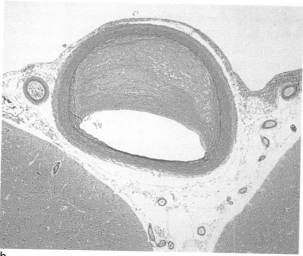

b

Figure 6.6 *Atherosclerosis. (a) Severe atherosclerosis has transformed the arteries of the circle of Willis into stiffened, tortuous, yellowish and non-transparent tubes, which in spite of the marked structural changes in the arterial walls had not caused overt cerebrovascular symptoms. Note also the incipient dilatation (dolichoectasia) of the internal carotid arteries (arrows). (b) The presence of a fibrous atherosclerotic plaque in a small leptomeningeal branch of the middle cerebral artery of only 1.8 mm in diameter demonstrates the aggravating effects of hypertension and diabetes mellitus, which make the atherosclerotic changes extend into more distant arterial branches. The plaque impinges on the lumen, but decreases of this magnitude should still allow adequate flow. (H&E.) (c) A higher magnification of the fibrous plaque shows the necrotic core with cholesterol crystals (*), foam cells (**) and fibrosis of the media with loss of smooth-muscle cells (***). (H&E.)*

plicated plaques.[377] Such disruption exposes tissue factors to activate coagulation (see below), and thrombus is formed over the plaque with increased risk of forming emboli and/or obstruction of the lumen. The high frequency of embolic strokes demonstrates that the formation of thromboemboli is obviously the most dangerous complication, because an embolus leads to an immediate occlusion of a blood vessel lumen, whereas a local thrombotic process is usually slow and there may be time for collateral channels to develop. Endothelial injury also occurs if the size of the plaque is abruptly increased by intramural bleeding from new blood vessels formed in the fibrous cap and at the margins of the plaque, although the blood may more frequently arise from the circulation through a rupture on the plaque surface.[71,135] With time, haemosiderin may accumulate within the lesion, and when calcium salts are precipitated in the necrotic core, the plaque acquires a characteristic hard consistency.

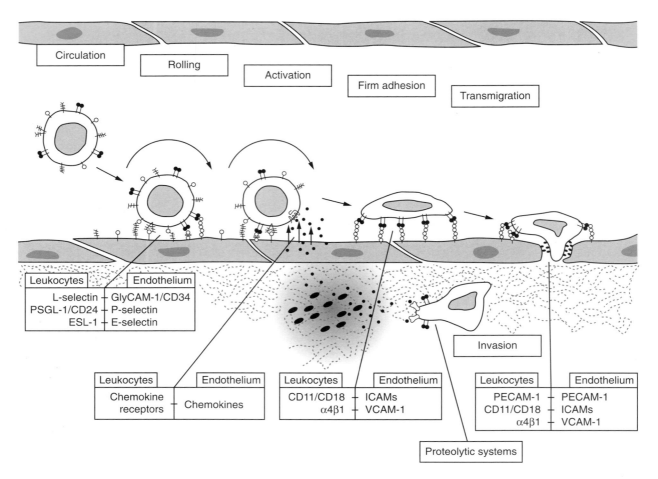

Figure 6.7 *Extravasation of inflammatory cells. Initially the circulating lymphocytes adhere to the endothelium only transiently and roll on it. This phase involves interaction between selectins and their ligands. During rolling lymphocytes are activated by cytokines and/or chemokines, which leads to activation of their integrin receptors CD11/CD18 and $\alpha_4\beta_1$. Shear stress and/or inflammatory mediators regulate endothelial cell expression of corresponding ligands, intercellular adhesion molecules (ICAMs) and vascular cell adhesion molecule-1 and (VCAM-1). These interactions result in firm adhesion and extravasation of inflammatory cells. The molecules involved are indicated in the boxes. Courtesy of Dr Leena Valmu, University of Helsinki.*

SMALL-ARTERY DISEASE

The pathogenesis and structural details of small-artery disease are less well established. It may have a different pathogenesis from that of atherosclerosis of larger arteries and therefore the non-specific term small-artery disease is most commonly used, although the term arteriolosclerosis and even the designation of small-artery atheriosclerosis are used.[106] Since this disease is often associated with hypertension, it will be described in the next section.

Hypertensive angiopathy

GENERAL ASPECTS

Experimental studies[31] have proved that chronic hypertension alters the autoregulation curve to the right towards higher pressure values (Fig. 6.8). This is a pro-tective reaction to delay the breakthrough of autoregulation and to maintain a constant level of CBF even at increased arterial pressure, thereby preventing the ill effects of the excessive systemic pressure on delicate capillaries. Clinical experience has shown that the same holds true for the human cerebral circulation.[175,299] The upper limit of autoregulation may be raised by up to 30 mmHg (Fig. 6.8), and as a consequence this shift to the right at the same time raises the lower limit of autoregulation at which adequate CBF can still be maintained. Symptoms of cerebral hypoperfusion develop when the mean arterial blood pressure is reduced to about 40% of the baseline levels. Consequently, in hypertensive patients such a reduction is reached at a correspondingly higher level of arterial pressure than in normotensives. Indeed, one-third of asymptomatic hypertensive patients have been found to have focal or diffuse cerebral hypoperfusion,[371] which may easily be reduced further to ischaemic levels; for example, by overefficient antihypertensive medication.

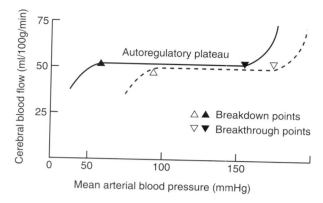

Figure 6.8 *Autoregulation. This maintains the cerebral blood flow (CBF) at a constant level between the mean arterial blood pressures of approximately 50 and 150 mmHg. Below and above these values the CBF varies with the arterial blood pressure. In hypertensive subjects the curve shifts to the right (dashed line).*

Such ischaemia may even become severe enough to cause brain damage, especially along the arterial border-zones.[175,299] By analogy, in a hypertensive patient with stroke, decrease in the blood pressure to levels tolerated by a normotensive may worsen the ischaemia.

CLINICAL PICTURE OF HYPERTENSIVE BRAIN DISEASE

The symptoms caused by arterial hypertension depend on the acuteness of the rise of the arterial pressure, as do the resulting vascular changes (below) and the brain damage. Sudden and severe 'malignant' hypertension, precipitated for example by renal disease, release of catecholamines from a phaeochromocytoma, disseminated vasculitis (e.g. polyarteritis nodosa) and eclampsia, or as a rebound effect after discontinuation of antihypertensives, may lead to hypertensive encephalopathy, an acute cerebral syndrome.[88,112,113,384] This syndrome is characterized by rapidly progressive signs of diffuse cerebral dysfunction, severe headache, altered state of consciousness, nausea and vomiting, i.e. symptoms of increased intracranial pressure. Brain oedema appears to be the cause of the increased intracranial pressure, since the patients usually have blurred discs and brain imaging discloses findings compatible with multifocal leakage of the blood–brain barrier (BBB).[198,410] These signs may be followed by additional neurological symptoms, both focal such as visual disturbances, and generalized such as convulsions and progressively decreased level of consciousness from drowsiness to deep coma. Focal ischaemic symptoms may also develop, and intracerebral haemorrhage is a potentially fatal complication.[415] In chronic arterial hypertension, the clinical symptoms are usually mild, e.g. minor headaches or tinnitus, and the patient may suddenly develop an unexpected intracerebral haemorrhage.

PATHOGENESIS AND PATHOLOGY OF HYPERTENSIVE ANGIOPATHY

Acute hypertension

Two different pathogenetic mechanisms have been proposed to be responsible for acute hypertensive brain injury. At present, the prevailing hypothesis states that the forced dilatation of the resistance vessels by the high arterial pressure, i.e. breakthrough of the autoregulation (Fig. 6.8), is crucial in the development of the encephalopathy, because this exposes distal smaller blood vessels to excessive pressure load and hyperperfusion.[295,321] In this situation, the blood flow increases passively after the rise in the blood pressure. At the same time, the high arterial pressure causes disruption of the BBB and, as a consequence, the transendothelial transport of plasma constituents either in pinocytotic vesicles or through specific channels increases, leading to vasogenic oedema (Fig. 6.9, see also Chapter 4, this Volume).[467,536] If the hypertension does not last too long, the BBB is rapidly closed again upon lowering of the blood pressure, which indicates that major structural injury has not occurred. However, with time plasma proteins, including fibrin, are deposited in the walls of small arteries, a process that leads to destruction of smooth-muscle cells (fibrinoid necrosis; see Fig. 6.10c).[147,415,429] Furthermore, acute hypertension may secondarily lead to ischaemia as a consequence of injury to endothelium and activation of platelets, the coagulation cascade and other procoagulative mechanisms.

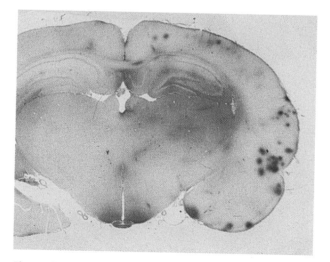

Figure 6.9 *Experimental acute hypertension. This has caused multifocal disruption of the blood–brain barrier and consequent vasogenic brain oedema. The acute rise in the arterial blood pressure was induced by clamping the abdominal aorta in rat for 10 min followed by survival for 2 h. These leakages are visible as small perivascular accumulations of albumin in the cortex. Diffuse spread of the oedema fluid to the surrounding parenchyma has already occurred in the deep grey matter, hippocampus and hypothalamus. (Antialbumin and haematoxylin counterstain.)*

According to the vasospasm hypothesis,[500] autoregulation of the cerebral circulation attempts to protect the brain by an exaggerated arteriolar vasoconstriction, which may focally be severe enough to result in ischaemia. In favour of this hypothesis, such a phenomenon may be visually observed in the retinal arteries,[156] and the pattern of CBF is heterogeneous, with wide variations in regional blood flow.[114]

Chronic hypertension

Chronic hypertension in man has two main consequences. First, it clearly aggravates atherosclerotic changes in both extracranial and intracranial larger arteries. Yet, a critical level of circulating lipoproteins is a prerequisite for this aggravating effect.[91] This has been also verified experimentally, since a special lipid-rich diet is needed to induce atherosclerosis in spontaneously hypertensive rats.[218] The atherosclerotic changes are qualitatively similar to those described above. In addition, hypertension makes atherosclerosis extend more distally into the intracranial compartment to affect blood vessels smaller than 2 mm in diameter (see Fig. 6.6b). The leptomeningeal arteries over the convexities are usually spared in normotensive atherosclerotic subjects, whereas in hypertensive patients they stand out as hardened non-collapsed yellowish blood vessels. Lesions similar to those seen in large blood vessel atherosclerosis are present in the walls of small arterioles down to 100 μm in diameter, and are called microatheroma.

Small-artery disease

The second sequel, often called small-artery disease, is considered to be more or less specific for hypertension. The arterial lesions in spontaneously hypertensive and stroke-prone rats seem to be in many respects a good model of hypertensive small-artery disease in man.[146,147] At the early stages of the development of such lesions, endothelial and smooth muscle cells show increased numbers of micropinocytotic vesicles, similar to that which has been demonstrated in acute hypertension.[536] However, the augmented transendothelial transport from blood to brain does not yet exceed the drainage and resolution capacity of the blood vessels, since major leakage of plasma constituents into the surrounding tissue is not detectable.[147] Instead, increased numbers of phagocytosed inclusions are observed in pericytes, which appear to take up and degrade the extravasated proteins.

At a later stage the persistent high blood pressure leads to focal disruptions of the BBB (Fig. 6.10a–c).[146,147] At these sites the basal lamina under the damaged or regenerated endothelial cells becomes thickened and reduplicated. The brightly eosinophilic 'fibrinoid' material in the thickened

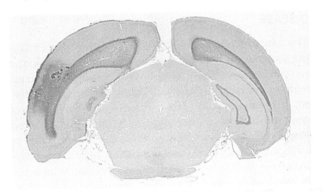

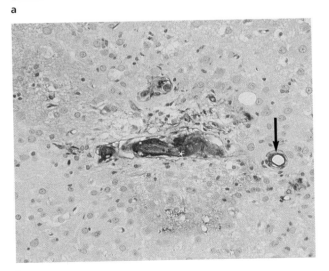

Figure 6.10 *Chronic hypertension. (a) Long-standing hypertension in a stroke-prone spontaneously hypertensive rat has caused multifocal disruption of the blood–brain barrier (BBB) with extravasation of plasma proteins. Evans-blue–albumin. (b) In a coronal section the site of disruption in the cortex is surrounded by leaked plasma constituents, which spread only focally in the cortex but diffusely in the underlying white matter. Note that the long-standing hypertension does not cause generalized leakage of the BBB and the cortical disruption has not resulted in a major haemorrhage. (c) A higher magnification of the BBB disruption in (b). The wall of the small artery (arrow) is thickened by the deposited plasma proteins ('fibrinoid necrosis'). The lumen of another artery (asterisk) is filled by a thrombus and there is leakage of plasma proteins into the surrounding cortical parenchyma. (b, c: antifibrinogen and haematoxylin counterstain.) (a) Courtesy of Dr K Fredriksson and Professor BB Johansson. (b, c) Reproduced by permission from Ref. 146.*

blood vessel walls is immunoreactive with antisera to different plasma proteins (Fig. 6.10c), and electron microscopy reveals extracellular deposits of proteinaceous material. Smooth-muscle cells in the tunica media gradually degenerate and are replaced by phagocytes and fibroblasts, and the latter produce increased amounts of collagen deposited in the blood vessel walls. This results in an increased ratio between the thickness of the media and the luminal radius in both the extracranial and intracranial arteries, leading to narrowing of the lumen.[147]

This change must be of haemodynamic importance[372,373] and, in association with decreased distensibility of the arterial walls, it contributes to the increased risk of ischaemia when blood pressure is lowered. In hypertensive rats focal dilatations of the diseased blood vessel walls seem to appear at sites of severe fibrinoid change. These are considered to indicate yielding of the weakened vessel wall.[147] These dilatations correspond to the controversial Charcot–Bouchard microaneurysms, which have been considered a characteristic feature of hypertension (see below).

The above sequence of events is also found in human cerebral blood vessels.[133,428,429] In general, the small intraparenchymal arteries and arterioles in hypertensive subjects have thickened walls, most characteristically in the basal ganglia. As an early change, which most likely precedes the more destructive alterations, this thickening may result from proliferation of smooth-muscle cells in response to the increased intraluminal pressure (Fig. 6.11). In longstanding hypertension the thickened eosinophilic walls become more homogeneous and less structured. The most commonly used term for this degenerative change in the arterial walls is lipohyalinosis.[133] Despite its common use it is poorly defined, and it is often incorrectly used.[429] The homogeneous eosinophilia in haematoxylin and eosin (H&E)-stained sections may result from either fibrinoid change (necrosis) or collagenous fibrosis (hyalinosis).[124] These two, most probably consecutive changes are readily distinguishable from each other by special stains, but are deceptively similar in H&E-stained sections.[429] The fibrinoid material in the blood vessel wall appears to be composed mainly of plasma proteins, with abundant fibrin, formed by the leakage of the BBB (see above, Fig. 6.10c) and of remnants of smooth-muscle cells. The latter have been claimed to undergo necrosis although others rather regard the process as degenerative. Lipids are usually only a minor component in these lesions. With time the fibrinoid material is replaced by fibrosis, i.e. collagen produced by fibroblasts, and when the fibroblasts disappear fibrosis is referred to as hyalinosis. For these reasons, the term lipohyalinosis perhaps should be abandoned and be replaced by correct terms, based on appropriate stains: fibrinoid change if histological or immunocytochemical stains verify the presence of fibrinoid/fibrin and fibrosis if collagen is the main constituent of the thickened arterial walls. Amyloid angio-

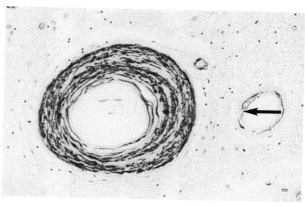

Figure 6.11 *The wall of an artery in the basal ganglia of a patient with chronic hypertension is markedly thickened due to smooth muscle hyperplasia, whereas the wall of the other artery (arrow) is fibrotic. (Antismooth-muscle actin and haematoxylin counterstain.)*

pathy and CADASIL (see below) need to be considered as differential diagnostic alternatives for thickened arterial walls.

Microaneurysms

Although there is a fairly good unanimity about the development of degenerative changes in the walls of small arteries, the traditional view of the formation of Charcot–Bouchard microaneurysms (or miliary aneurysms) as a result of the weakening of the blood vessel walls has been seriously questioned in recent years. According to the traditional view, microaneurysms arise as millimetre-thick outpouchings from parent arteries, the diameter of which vary between 25 and 250 µm.[131,526,527] When the microaneurysms rupture they appear as globular haemorrhages[131] and if 'healed' by thrombosis and fibrosis they are transformed into fibrous balls.[428] Evidence supporting this view has been gathered from studies using intravascular injections of contrast or casting media and serial microscopic sections,[97,131,428] but views opposing the significance of microaneurysms have also been presented; for example, in one study[485] only two aneurysms were found among 61 hypertensive patients with intracerebral haemorrhage. This long-lived controversy about the role of microaneurysms is still unsettled and the question was in the 1990s again addressed by two research groups who came to opposite conclusions. Wakai *et al.* identified microaneurysms in patients who had lobar haemorrhages and negative angiography, both under the operating microscope and in serial paraffin sections[526] (Fig. 6.12a, b). Interestingly, half of those patients whose haemorrhage was caused by a ruptured microaneurysm did not have a history of hypertension. By contrast, using elaborate enzyme histochemistry and high-resolution microradiography, Challa *et al.*[82] presented good evidence for a great majority of 'microaneurysms' actually being complex tortuosities, which may assume six basic patterns.[471] These

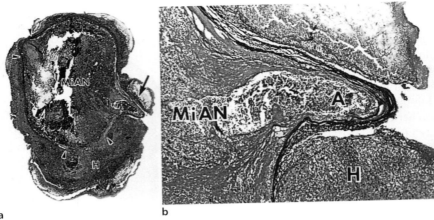

a   b

Figure 6.12 *Microaneurysm. (a) A surgical specimen from a 72-year-old hypertensive woman. The parent artery (arrow) with diameter of about 140 µm dilates into a microaneurysm (MiAN) of about 1700 µm in diameter. The collagenous wall of the microaneurysm has ruptured at two sites (between arrowheads), giving rise to a haematoma (H). (b) A higher magnification shows how the internal elastica of the artery (A) becomes frayed at the orifice of the microaneurysm (MiAN). (Elastica–van Gieson stain.) Reproduced by permission from Ref. 526.*

were most common in the interface between the grey and white matter and their number increased with ageing, yet hypertension had no effect on their frequency (Fig. 6.13a, b). True microaneurysms in their surgical intracerebral haemorrhage (ICH) material were virtually non-existent, nor did they find them in connection with lacunar infarcts.[80] The reason for this discrepancy might not be only methodical. It may well be that the degenerative changes in the arterial walls in the Japanese population with high frequency of ICH are truly different from those in Caucasian populations, e.g. resulting from genetic, dietary or environmental differences. The definite identification of microaneurysms in routine diagnostic paraffin sections is virtually impossible.

Inflammatory diseases

GENERAL ASPECTS

Inflammatory diseases of the CNS blood vessels are a heterogeneous group with multiple aetiologies including infections and immunological processes, and according to the present view, even atherosclerosis is regarded as an inflammatory disease (see above).[431] The vascular wall is invaded by blood-borne inflammatory cells (Fig. 6.7). Vasculitides present a real challenge to the clinician, because of the highly variable clinical symptomatology, difficulties in establishing the correct diagnosis, the need for specific therapy, and poor outcome. The American College

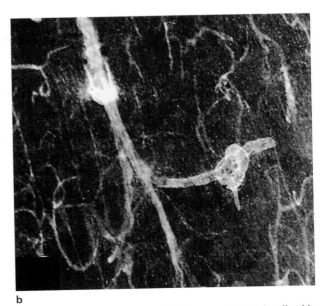

a   b

Figure 6.13 *(a) A complex vascular coil taken from a hypertensive patient who died of an intracellular haemorrhage visualized in 1000 µm celloidin sections reacted for alkaline phosphatase. (b) High-resolution microradiographs of similarly reacted sections of 500-µm thickness show an arteriolar knot-like structure. Reproduced by permission from (a) Ref. 82 and (b) Ref. 471.*

of Rheumatology has published clinical diagnostic criteria for several vasculitides with an immunological pathogenesis.[126] For the pathologist they are also perplexing, since their aetiology and pathogenesis are controversial and their histopathological features are quite variable and non-specific. No generally accepted classification of vasculitides is available.

Inflammatory CNS vascular diseases may be classified thus:

Non-infectious vasculitides:
- Primary cranial and/or cerebral inflammations
  - Takayasu's arteritis (TA)
  - giant cell or temporal arteritis (GCA)
  - primary angiitis of the central nervous system (PACNS)
  - Kawasaki disease
- Manifestations of systemic diseases:
  - systemic lupus erythematosus (SLE)
  - polyarteritis nodosa (PAN)
  - Wegener's granulomatosis
  - Churg–Strauss syndrome
  - Sjögren's syndrome
  - Behçet's syndrome
  - malignancy related
  - various
- Drug-induced vasculitis.

Infectious vasculitides:
- Bacterial
  - spirochaetal (e.g. lues, borreliosis)
  - purulent (e.g. streptococcus)
  - granulomatous (tuberculosis)
- Viral (e.g. herpes zoster, Epstein–Barr virus)
- Other microbial (fungal, protozoal, mycoplasmal, rickettsial).

The following classification of vasculitides (adapted from Ref. 238) is based on proposed pathogenetic mechanisms:

Immunological injury:
- Cell-mediated inflammation
  - Takayasu's arteritis (TA)
  - giant cell or temporal arteritis (GCA)
  - primary angiitis of the central nervous system (PACNS)
  - Kawasaki's disease
- Immune complex-mediated inflammation
  - systemic lupus erythematosus (SLE)
  - polyarteritis nodosa (PAN)
  - Behçet's syndrome
  - infection-induced (e.g. group A streptococcus or hepatitis B and C virus)
  - some malignancy-related vasculitides
  - some drug-induced vasculitides
- Antineutrophil cytoplasmic antibody (ANCA) mediated
  - Wegener's granulomatosis
  - Churg–Strauss syndrome
  - some drug-induced vasculitides
- Mixed immunological disorders
  - Sjögren's syndrome.

Direct infection of blood vessels:
- Bacterial (e.g. cocci, mycobacteria, spirochaetes)
- Viral (e.g. herpes zoster, Epstein–Barr virus)
- Other microbial (fungal, protozoal, mycoplasmal, rickettsial).

NON-INFECTIOUS VASCULITIDES

Primary cranial and/or cerebral vasculitides

In this group there are three main types, Takayasu's arteritis, giant cell arteritis (GCA) and primary angiitis of the central nervous system (PACNS), which share the histopathological features of granulomatous angiitis. Since the specific aetiologies of these diseases are still unknown, one view maintains that they could represent a topographic spectrum of the same disease, but so far the opposite view has been favoured.[308,463]

Takayasu's arteritis

In Takayasu's arteritis the aortic arch with its main arterial trunks and the descending aorta are the main sites of inflammation.[126,307,308] The involvement of the carotid and subclavian arteries is of special neuropathological interest. Patients are often relatively young (15–45 years) and Oriental females are the most frequently affected.[308] Takayasu's arteritis in about 20% of the cases is monophasic and self-limited, but the 10-year survival is only 90%.[126] The lymphoplasmacytic inflammation affects primarily the tunica media causing destruction of the elastic lamellae, inducing the formation of foreign body giant cells – a common finding wherever elastic tissue is excessively destroyed. Secondary fibrosis of all layers causes thickening and loss of compliance of the blood vessel walls, resulting in a characteristic loss of carotid pulsations. The involved arteries are finally transformed into rigid, thick-walled tubes with severe narrowing or occlusion by superimposed thrombosis. The obstruction to blood flow may result in cerebral ischaemia, which is usually due to embolism, although rarely affection of both carotids may cause severe haemodynamic changes. Revascularization of the obstructed carotid arteries may lead to a marked transient hyperperfusion syndrome.

The histopathology of recent lesions[308] is intimal proliferation and granulomatous inflammation with foreign body and Langhans'-type giant cells in the media. There is multifocal destruction of elastic lamellae in the aorta and of smooth-muscle cells in the carotids. The vertebral arteries are seldom affected. In the chronic phase fibrosis and thickening of the walls of the affected vessels prevail, although occasionally the arteries become dilated and rarely aortic dissection may ensue.

Giant cell arteritis

Giant cell or temporal arteritis (GCA) is the most common of the three granulomatous vasculitides, with an incidence of about 20 in 100 000 in individuals over 50 years of age.[76,126,307,308] The patients are usually over the age of 55 years. In rare fatal cases it has been possible to analyse the topography of the inflammation in detail. The primary target of GCA is the extracranial arteries of the head and neck, and it most often spares the intracranial blood vessels (see section on Primary angiitis of the central nervous system, below), although reports of involvement of the cerebral arteries exist. It may also affect more proximal vessels, i.e. the aorta and its branches and even the coronary arteries.[76,391] Involvement of the superficial temporal and ophthalmic arteries is well known, but the carotid and vertebral arteries may also be affected. The inflammation seems to fade as the affected arteries perforate the dura, at which point the amount of elastic component in the arterial wall also becomes markedly diminished.[541] The key symptom is headache and the serious sequel is blindness, either transient amaurosis fugax in about 10–12% or rarely permanent blindness in about 8% of patients.[77] The blindness is usually due to extension of the disease into the ocular, most commonly ophthalmic arteries and/or their branches, but it may also be caused by occipital ischaemic infarcts, most likely due to emboli from thrombosed vertebral arteries.[541] Stroke and TIA are, however, relatively rare manifestations (about 7%). GCA is commonly associated with polymyalgia rheumatica and a good diagnostic test is the very high erythrocyte sedimentation rate (ESR), as well as the prompt response to therapy with corticosteroids in most cases. The aetiology of GCA has remained obscure, but the histopathological features indicate a cell-mediated immunological reaction to an unknown antigen.

The affected blood vessel, especially the temporal artery, becomes tortuous, thickened and tender with diminished pulsations. The microscopical features of GCA vary to a considerable extent (Fig. 6.14). The inflammatory changes may extend along the length of the artery, but are most often focal. Therefore, a biopsy of 3–5 cm is recommended and a negative biopsy cannot completely rule out the possibility of GCA. The inflammation induces proliferation of the intima, which is infiltrated by a varying number of lymphocytes and plasma cells. The characteristic feature of multinucleated giant cells of either foreign body or Langhans'-type is most frequently seen in the inner media next to the irregularly frayed internal elastic lamina, where histiocytic cells of epithelioid appearance also accumulate. This type of infiltrate is often seen also in the adventitia. At later stages, both the media and adventitia may become fibrotic and thickened with blurring of their boundaries. The wall of the artery may rarely become weakened to such an extent that an aneurysm is formed. The local injury may also induce local thrombosis and if located in an anatomically critical blood vessel this may serve as a source of small emboli to the intracerebral arteries and be a rare cause of an infarct.[346]

Primary angiitis of the central nervous system

The rare, somewhat elusive entity of PACNS was originally delineated by Cravioto and Feigin in 1959.[100] It has previously been called granulomatous angiitis of the central nervous system and isolated angiitis,[463] and most recently the designation of primary angiitis has been given.[67,306] The clinical picture of PACNS is vague and non-specific: recurring headaches, multifocal neurological deficits, and diffuse encephalopathy with confusion and memory impairment.[68,355,463] The patients are usually adults (30–50 years old), but a paediatric case has also been reported.[330] Demonstration of multiple narrowed segments in cerebral arteries by angiography has been considered an essential finding for the diagnosis, but the

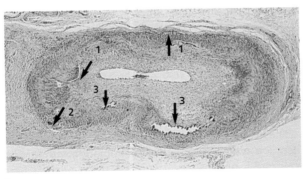

a

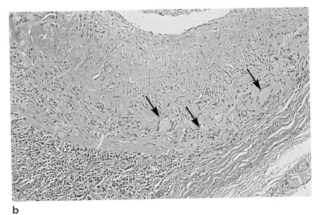

b

Figure 6.14 *Giant cell arteritis. (a) There are only fragments of internal elastic lamina remaining (arrows 1). The intima is markedly proliferated, causing severe narrowing of the lumen. In the adventitia and to a lesser extent in the media there are lymphocytes. In the media there are also histiocytes including one large multinucleated giant cell of Langhans' type (arrow 2). In addition, there are calcifications of Mönckeberg's sclerosis in the media (arrows 3). (Elastica–van Gieson.) (b) A higher magnification shows several multinucleated giant cells (arrows) and mild lymphocytic infiltration in the adventitia. (Van Gieson.)*

angiographic findings are not specific. There are several conditions that mimic PACNS, and one of them with a more benign clinical course has been suggested to be an entity of benign angiopathy of the CNS.[69] In contrast to GCA, the ESR in PACNS is usually mildly elevated at most[355] and the CSF often has a chronic meningitic pattern.[69] Histopathological verification of inflamed (blood vessels in a leptomeningeal or parenchymal biopsy has been considered pivotal in the confirmation of the diagnosis, although it may have limited diagnostic value (see below).[119] The prognosis of PACNS has been sinister: it used to be considered invariably fatal within a short time, but modern aggressive immunosuppressive therapy has proved effective.[355]

A biopsy from the tip of the non-dominant temporal lobe, which includes leptomeninges and a wedge of cortex, has been recommended, since this often provides a sufficient number of representative small arteries (200–500 µm in diameter).[306,355,463] Arteries are much more frequently affected than veins. PACNS may present in both granulomatous and non-granulomatous forms, either separately or coexisting in different parts of the brain of the same patient. The non-granulomatous form may appear as polyarteritis-type necrotizing inflammation or as simple lymphocytic vasculitis, which can create problems in differential diagnosis. The inflammatory infiltrate (Fig. 6.15) is composed mainly of lymphocytes accompanied by histiocytes and plasma cells. Giant cells of either Langhans' or foreign body type are scattered in varying numbers and, therefore, multiple sections may be needed to find them. They may be present in all layers, although the intima and the media appear to be the most common locations. A negative biopsy does not necessarily exclude the possibility of this focal disease[119,306] because in an experienced laboratory vasculitis was identified in only four of seven PACNS patients.[119] The interpretation of the findings may be hampered by the thinness of the intracerebral blood vessel walls. Immunofluorescence studies have been non-contributory.[355] Consequences in the surrounding parenchyma have been rarely described, but the lesions include focal infarction and rarely small haemorrhages.

Manifestations of systemic diseases

Systemic lupus erythematosus (SLE)

Involvement of the nervous system is very common in SLE: between 50 and 75% of patients develop neurological signs and symptoms such as epileptic seizures, hemiparesis/stroke and neuropathies, or psychiatric problems such as organic brain syndrome, psychosis and depression.[191,514] The complications of SLE, e.g. uraemia, hypertension and infections, as well as administration of steroid therapy, may be the cause of, or at least contribute to the neuropsychiatric problems.[514] Intracranial pathology has been considered to be the main cause of death in up to 19% of cases.[434]

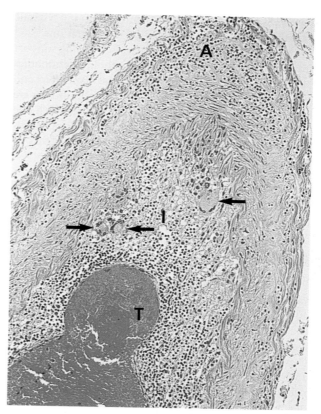

Figure 6.15 *Primary angiitis of the CNS. The thickened intima (I) and adventitia (A) are infiltrated by lymphocytes. Three multinucleated giant cells (arrows) are present just inside the frayed internal elastic lamina. The lumen of the parietal leptomeningeal artery is filled by a thrombus (T). (H&E.) Courtesy of Professor JT Lie, University of California, Davis Medical Center, Sacramento, USA.*

Cerebral perfusion deficits have been detected by imaging methods *in vivo*[482] and the most common change in the brain parenchyma is multiple foci of infarction.[110,191,222] Two different pathogenetic mechanisms have been proposed. Primary small vessel inflammatory vasculopathy has been considered the main cause of infarction by some,[191] whereas others emphasize thrombotic and thromboembolic mechanisms and ascribe minor significance to vasculitis.[110] Accordingly, the former have demonstrated histologically similar findings to those described in renal arteries and capillaries, i.e. fibrinoid necrosis, mononuclear inflammatory infiltrates and fibrotic thickening of the vessel walls, whereas the latter have not described marked vascular pathology. In support of the vasculitic view, deposition of immunoglobulins and complement in the blood vessel walls has been verified in biopsies from extracranial, more easily available tissues, but studies on intracranial blood vessels are very scarce.[191] Thus, immunocomplex-mediated vasculitis may well be one of the pathogenetic mechanisms, but in recent years thrombosis and thromboembolism appear to have become the more important alternative, and in some reviews SLE has not even been mentioned among systemic vasculitides that cause neurological manifestations.[110]

The thrombotic hypothesis has gained strong support from studies on circulating antiphospholipid antibodies (aPL), which have a well-known procoagulant effect and induce recurrent thromboses.[52,433,502] These antibodies are common in SLE patients,[315,502] on the basis of which one of the methods to detect their presence has been designated as a lupus anticoagulant assay. The prevalence of aPLs in SLE ranges from 7 to 85%.[315,502] However, they also occur in a wide variety of other diseases or as an independent syndrome,[38,52] and even in healthy subjects.[490] Details of aPLs are described below in the section on Haematological disorders.

Polyarteritis nodosa

Polyarteritis or panarteritis nodosa (PAN) is a generalized vasculitis. PAN may start at any age with the mean around 40–50 years and with a male to female ratio of about 2:1. It is a chronic disease with a fluctuating course and requires aggressive immunosuppressive therapy, which has improved its 5-year survival rate to 75–80% from less than 15% in untreated patients.[96,126,183,307] PAN causes necrotizing lesions in medium-sized and small arteries with frequent distal spread into arterioles. Veins and capillaries are usually spared. Its aetiology and pathogenesis have not been definitely established, but the mechanism most commonly implicated is an immune complex-mediated vasculitis. It is likely that there are various, often unknown, inciting antigens. Suspected antigens include microorganisms, autoantigens and drugs. For example, many PAN patients are seropositive for hepatitis B or C virus (about 10–50% or 20%, respectively), but the exact pathogenetic relationship between PAN and these viruses is still debatable.[75] The diagnosis of PAN is based on clinical, histopathological and angiographical findings after excluding other recognized causes of vasculitis.[96]

At present, two different forms of idiopathic PAN are recognized.[96] In the systemic PAN, the visceral organs (heart, kidneys and gastrointestinal tract) are mainly affected. In the limited form of PAN neurological manifestations frequently occur: skeletal muscle is affected in 40–80% of patients (see Chapter 10, Volume II) and peripheral nerves are involved almost as frequently, in 50–75% (see Chapter 9, Volume II). The reported frequencies of CNS involvement are highly variable, ranging from 4 to 53% of cases, but most seem to agree that it usually occurs at a later stage of the disease.[96,463] These discrepant figures most likely reflect the difficulties in diagnosing brain involvement with certainty in what is a fairly uncommon generalized vasculitis. CNS disease is the second most common cause of death among patients with PAN.[505]

The necrotizing lesions are always very patchy with a predilection for the branching points of the affected blood vessels. Most lesions are not more than 1 mm in length and vasculitis does not necessarily affect the whole circumference of the artery. Active lesions characteristically show fibrinoid necrosis, often with complete destruction of the blood vessel wall, and polymorphonuclear (PMN) leukocytes predominate in the inflammatory infiltrate. The necrotic wall may yield and lead to aneurysmal dilatation. In healed vessels all layers of the artery show fibrous scarring and the residual inflammation is represented by lymphocytes.[307]

Kawasaki's disease

Kawasaki's disease is an uncommon acute illness of childhood with unknown aetiology, which is clinically characterized by fever, mucosal inflammation with ulcerations, non-suppurative lymphadenopathy, oedema of hands and feet, polymorphous skin rash and ischaemic cardiac symptoms. Kawasaki's disease is a necrotizing arteritis with a similar distribution of vasculitic changes seen in PAN. It may also spread into cerebral arteries, as evidenced by the demonstration of cerebral hypoperfusion in positron emission tomography (PET)[226] and the occurrence of stroke or diffuse encephalopathy in children affected by this disease.[126]

Wegener's granulomatosis

Wegener's granulomatosis is characterized by necrotizing lesions in the respiratory tract frequently accompanied by a systemic vasculitis, which may also involve cranial and/or cerebral blood vessels. It is a chronic disease that may have its onset at any age, but the majority of patients are in their forties and fifties. The diagnosis is based on the clinical picture and demonstration of classic antineutrophil cytoplasmic autoantibodies (ANCA) directed against proteinase-3.[96,307] Neurological manifestations due to either vasculitis or granulomatous inflammation in the parenchyma are seen in about 30% of patients. The latter manifestation usually represents extension of the primary disease in the airway sinuses, orbit or auditory canal. CNS is usually involved at a late stage of the disease and with modern immunosuppressive therapy the disease only rarely spreads into the brain.[96,215]

Churg–Strauss syndrome

The neurological abnormalities in this disease are considered to be fairly similar to those in PAN.[184,354] However, the systemic symptoms, i.e. the presence of an allergic component manifesting itself as severe asthma and eosinophilia, and pulmonary involvement allow distinction of the Churg–Strauss syndrome – also called allergic angitis and granulomatosis (AAG) – from PAN. Besides, the pathogenetic mechanisms are considered to be different. PAN is recognized as an immune complex vasculitis, whereas in Churg–Strauss syndrome toxic proteins released from eosinophils have been implicated, although an association with p-ANCA antibodies against neutrophil-derived myeloperoxidase has been described. Histopathologically, there is a necrotizing vasculitis of medium and small sized arteries, sometimes also of capillaries and venules, with abundance of eosinophils among the inflammatory cells as well as the formation of extravascular granulomas.[354]

Sjögren's syndrome

Sjögren's syndrome is an autoimmune disorder characterized by multiple abnormalities of cellular and humoral immunity.[5,360] An important diagnostic feature is the involvement of exocrine glands, including salivary and lacrimal glands, which gives rise to the sicca syndrome due to decreased secretory activity of the affected glands. Sjögren's syndrome appears either as a primary (the only disease, pSS) or secondary (in association of other connective tissue disorder) disease. Peripheral nervous system affection in pSS is well documented, but the involvement of the CNS is a controversial issue. Involvement of the CNS may be a frequent systemic manifestation of pSS, with 20–25% in a highly selected group of pSS patients suffering from either focal (hemiparesis, focal epilepsy, loss of vision, transverse myelitis or a multiple sclerosis-like syndrome) or diffuse (aseptic meningoencephalitis, progressive encephalopathy or dementia) CNS disease.[5] Considerably lower figures have been reported by others; the discrepancies being ascribed mainly to a lack of generally accepted diagnostic criteria and the bias of patient referral.[360] Vasculitis has been reported to occur in about 10–15% of pSS patients.[307] CNS pathology has also been described as vasculitis or vasculopathy, which predominantly affects small venous vessels in the white matter. The inflammatory cells are mainly lymphocytes, plasma cells and macrophages, and they are usually found also in the meninges.[5] Vasculitis of medium-sized blood vessels resembling polyarteritis nodosa has also been described.[307]

Behçet's syndrome

This rare vasculitic multiorgan disorder is characterized by recurrent ulcers of oral and genital mucous membranes, uveitis and arthritis. In 30–40% of these patients the CNS is also affected, most commonly in the form of meningoencephalitis, which is often accentuated in the brainstem region (rhombencephalitis). The specific diagnosis is largely based on the associated systemic findings. The pathogenesis is unknown, but both viral and immunological mechanisms have been advocated. Histopathologically, there is a vasculitis of small blood vessels, mainly of venules.[354]

Drug-induced vasculitis

Vasculitis has been suggested to be one of the pathogenetic mechanisms that lead to an increased incidence of stroke among drug abusers. There are, however, very few neuropathological studies to verify this suspicion, but in some cocaine abusers definite vasculitis has been report-

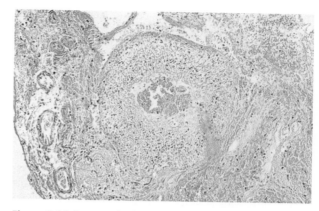

Figure 6.16 *Intracerebral haematoma caused by drug-induced vasculitis. A necrotic blood vessel is seen next to an intracerebral lobar haematoma of clinically undetermined origin from a 27-year-old abuser of multiple hard drugs. (Van Gieson.)*

ed.[145,286] The vasculitis seems to be non-infectious and possibly allergic. The inflammatory infiltrate is mainly lymphocytic and some patients respond to immunosuppressive therapy. There is a high frequency of intracerebral haemorrhage in users of cocaine, phenylpropanolamine and amphetamine,[168,464] suggesting that necrotizing vasculitis might be more common than presently thought (Fig. 6.16). The association between the possibly immune complex-mediated polyarteritis nodosa and hepatitis B and C viruses may be one explanation for necrotizing vasculitis in drug abusers.[75]

INFECTIOUS VASCULITIDES

Many infective agents are capable of invading the blood vessel walls and of inducing inflammation. For some agents blood vessel walls are even sites of predilection and neurological disease is their common manifestation. Since infectious diseases are covered in Chapters 1–3, Volume II, only certain specific features of the vascular involvement in infections are presented here.

Bacterial vasculitides

Spirochaetal vasculitis

A classical example of infectious vasculitis is the invasion of arterial walls by *Treponema pallidum* spirochaetes in syphilis.[162] This occurs most commonly in extracranial large arteries, but they also reach the arteries of the CNS. The vasculitis in the meningovascular neurosyphilis is called Heubner's arteritis. The intima and adventitia become thickened at the expense of thinned media. The inflammatory cell infiltrate consists of lymphocytes and plasma cells, but because of the small size of CNS blood vessels involvement of vasa vasorum is hardly detected beyond the carotid arteries. It is unusual to demonstrate treponema in the blood vessel wall. The end result of healed syphilitic vasculitis may be indistinguishable from an atherosclerotic fibrous plaque. Neurosyphilis has become increasingly prevalent as a complication of human immunodeficiency virus (HIV) infection[54] (see Chapter 1, Volume II).

Another spirochaete which has become increasingly important is *Borrelia burgdorferi*, the causative agent of Lyme neuroborreliosis. There is evidence that *B. burgdorferi* is able to penetrate the BBB and enter the brain parenchyma at a fairly early stage of the disease.[154] *Borrelia burgdorferi* seems to be able to bind also to connective tissue molecules in the blood vessel wall and induce a vasculitis.[339] As a consequence, the BBB is disrupted and multifocal enhancing lesions with mild oedematous tissue changes may develop (Fig. 6.17a, b). By this binding *B. burgdorferi* may escape eradication by antibiotics and give rise to recurrent disorders in the CNS.

Details on neurosyphilis and neuroborreliosis are presented in Chapter 3, Volume II.

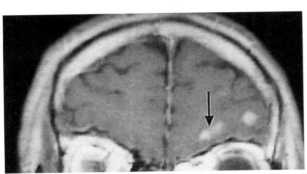

a

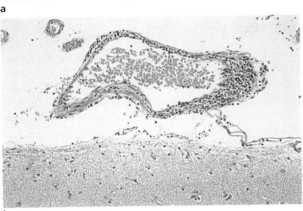

b

Figure 6.17 *Bacterial vasculitis. (a) Gadolinium-enhanced T1-weighted magnetic resonance (MR) image of the brain of a 40-year-old, previously healthy man, who had two episodes of epileptic seizures. There are two focal enhancing lesions, which disappeared with antibiotic therapy, but recurrences similarly amenable to antibiotics occurred three times in different locations. (b) Histopathology of the surgically removed lesion (arrow in a) discloses infiltration of the wall of a small leptomeningeal blood vessel by lymphocytes. The underlying parenchyma was slightly oedematous with minimal astrocytic reaction. Polymerase chain reaction analysis for presence of* B. burgdorferi *DNA was positive in three separate tissue samples. (H&E.) Courtesy of Dr J Oksi, University of Turku, Finland.*

Viral vasculitis

True cerebral vasculitis of the lymphocytic, necrotizing or granulomatous types may occur in viral infection,[469] particularly in immunosuppressed patients. Inflammatory alterations in the cerebral blood vessel walls have been reported, particularly in patients infected with the herpes viruses, notably herpes zoster-varicella virus[40,214,322] but direct evidence of viral presence in the vascular lesions remains scarce.[148] In some patients with polyarteritis nodosa not only have antibodies to hepatitis C virus been demonstrated (see above), but also viral nucleic acids by polymerase chain reaction. However, it is still unknown whether this virus can actually cause an arterial infection.[75]

In recent years, a spectrum of various types of vasculitis has been reported in association with HIV infection.[64–66,160,177] These include primary granulomatous angiitis of the CNS, polyarteritis nodosa-like conditions, hypersensitivity vasculitis and lymphomatoid granulomatosis. Cerebral vasculitis with transmural infiltration by mononuclear cells without necrosis, granulomas or leukocytoclasis was frequently found in early HIV infection.[177] The exact relationship between HIV infection and these various forms of inflammatory vascular disorders remains unclear.[65] Vascular inflammation in HIV infection appears to be multifactorial and may result from HIV-induced immunological abnormalities and exposure to a variety of xenoantigens, such as HIV, other infectious agents or drugs.[160]

Fungal vasculitis

In parallel with the increasing number of immunocompromised patients the frequency of opportunistic infections has also increased. Fungi with low pathogenicity are among the most common infectious agents. Fungal emboli may lodge in the intracranial arteries, penetrate the wall and induce vasculitis (Fig. 6.18), which may weaken the wall to such an extent that haemorrhage ensues. Among the most common fungi associated with cerebral vasculitides are *Aspergillus*, *Candida*, *Coccidioides* and *Mucor*[469] (see Chapter 2, Volume II).

Aneurysms

The term aneurysm is used to designate various forms of focal arterial dilatation. The principal forms of aneurysm related to the CNS include saccular, atherosclerotic, miliary (described above) and infectious aneurysms. By tradition, dissections of the arterial wall and arteriovenous fistulae are also considered.

SACCULAR ANEURYSMS

Saccular (berry) aneurysms are common lesions, which can be visualized by angiography and magnetic resonance

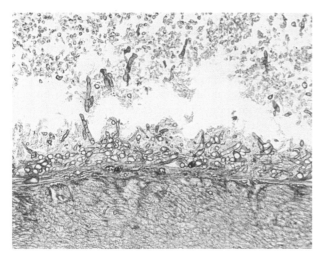

Figure 6.18 *Fungal vasculitis. Fungal hyphae of phycomycosis (mucormycosis) are seen attached to and partly invading the wall of an intracerebral artery of a 52-year-old male patient, who developed cerebro-rhino-ocular phycomycosis (CROP) in the context of keto-acidotic diabetes mellitus. (Silver methenamine stain.)*

imaging (MRI). They are of great clinical significance because of their propensity to spontaneous rupture. Ruptured saccular aneurysms are by far the most important cause of primary (non-traumatic) subarachnoid haemorrhage.

Epidemiology

The prevalence of intracranial saccular aneurysms in the general population, based on various autopsy series, is about 2–5% (range 0.2–9%), depending on whether the aneurysms were searched for or merely noted as incidental findings.[233,417,532] Aneurysms are rare in children and their prevalence increases with age. Less than 5% of aneurysms are encountered under the age of 20 years, about 60% being diagnosed in patients 40–60 years of age.[532] The overall prevalence of aneurysms is higher in women than in men (ratio 3:2), but this female preponderance does not become manifest until after the fifth decade, while in the younger age groups males predominate. About 12–15% cases of saccular aneurysms are familial, most often with an autosomal-dominant pattern of inheritance,[4] and these cases tend to be of younger age (by about 5 years) than non-familial cases.[426] About 40–70% of the aneurysms noted in various autopsy studies had ruptured before death.[250,532]

Aetiology, pathogenesis and risk factors

There is growing evidence that genetic factors are important in causing some early-onset familial saccular aneurysms/subarachnoid haemorrhage.[4] The age-adjusted prevalence of saccular aneurysms among first-degree relatives of affected families was reported to be four times

higher than in the general population.[425] Familial aneurysms were more often multiple and likely to rupture at a smaller size.[426] The causative molecular genetic mechanisms are still unestablished.[4] A few reports of type III collagen deficiency in the arteries of patients with saccular aneurysms have been published, but extensive sequencing of the *COL3A1* gene has not identified pathogenic mutations.[290]

Almost all saccular aneurysms arise at or very close to bifurcations of the main intracranial arteries and they rarely occur outside the cerebral circulation (Figs 6.19, 6.20). Intracranial arteries differ from their extracranial counterparts by the thinness of their walls, absence of an external elastic lamina and lack of perivascular support. Histological studies of major cerebral arteries of normal individuals have demonstrated frequent gaps in the muscular tunica media at the V-shaped distal divisions of bifurcations. In the area of the gap the arterial wall often consists only of the intima, the internal elastic lamina, which may be fenestrated, and some adventitial connective tissue.[532]

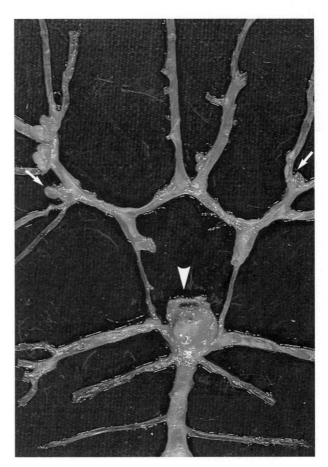

Figure 6.19 *Saccular aneurysm. The dissected circle of Willis from a patient who died of a subarachnoid haemorrhage from a ruptured saccular aneurysm at the tip of the basilar artery (large arrowhead). In addition, the patient had several unruptured small aneurysms in both middle cerebral arteries (two marked with small arrows).*

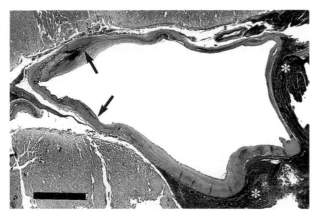

Figure 6.20 *Saccular aneurysm. A saccular aneurysm from the trifurcation of right middle cerebral artery. The aneurysm had ruptured and caused both an intracerebral haemorrhage into right temporal lobe and a subarchnoidal haemorrhage. The elastic lamina (black) stops at the arrows and the wall of the dilated aneurysm is composed of connective tissue with some atherosclerotic intimal thickening. The wall thins out towards the apex of the aneurysm on the right, but the actual rupture is not visible. The apex is covered by the blood (asterisks) in the subarachnoid space. (Elastica–van Gieson stain.)*

The majority of aneurysms do not appear until adulthood (see above), and new saccular aneurysms have been detected during angiographic follow-up monitoring of patients with a previously diagnosed aneurysm.[250] These observations and experimental work support the hypothesis that most saccular aneurysms are acquired degenerative lesions made worse by haemodynamic stress.[458,474] With increasing age, fibrous intimal pads are formed, particularly at the bifurcations of cerebral arteries, rendering their walls less elastic (Fig. 6.21). The configuration of the intimal arteriosclerotic thickening may alter the haemodynamic stress at sites of arterial bifurcation. In the presence of a gap in the muscular layer and fenestrated internal elastic lamina this stress may result in the outbulging of the thin arterial wall.[458] Alternatively, the elastic and muscular layers degenerate – without a pre-existing local defect – as the consequence of constant overstretching by haemodynamic stress at the apical angle of branching sites of major cerebral arteries.[474]

The haemodynamic hypothesis is compatible with the well-documented association of saccular aneurysms with arteriovenous malformations, which are characterized by increased regional blood flow. About 3–9% of patients with intracranial arteriovenous malformations have saccular aneurysms, especially in arteries haemodynamically related to the arteriovenous malformation.[32] An increased incidence of saccular aneurysms has also been noted in coarctation of the aorta and in patients with an asymmetrical circle of Willis, particularly of the proximal segments of the anterior cerebral arteries. Occlusion of one or more of the cerebral feeding blood vessels may enhance aneurysm formation, owing to augmented haemodynamic stress on the arteries involved in the collateral flow.[474]

The haemodynamic hypothesis is also supported by the observation that experimental manipulation of haemodynamic factors can produce arterial mural atrophy leading to aneurysmal dilatation.[474] In rats and non-human primates with induced hypertension and with unilateral carotid artery ligation, aneurysms arise on the anterior communicating artery, ipsilateral anterior cerebral artery and proximal segment of the posterior cerebral artery, whereas bilateral carotid ligation induces aneurysms in the posterior part of the circle of Willis, i.e. they develop in the segments of enhanced collateral blood flow. Under these experimental conditions, aneurysm formation was associated with apoptosis of medial smooth-muscle cells.[277]

Loss of tensile strength of the arterial wall may be a contributory factor, because aneurysms are associated with certain connective tissue disorders including Marfan's syndrome and Ehlers–Danlos syndrome type IV.[474] However, aneurysms associated with these conditions as well as with pseudoxanthoma elasticum tend to be of the fusiform variety[4] and occur in relatively young patients. An increased incidence of saccular aneurysms has also been reported in fibromuscular dysplasia[94] and moyamoya disease.[474,532]

In addition, many other factors have been implicated in the pathogenesis of saccular aneurysms, such as hypertension (e.g. renal hypertension associated with autosomal dominant polycystic kidney disease),[417] smoking, intake of alcohol, use of the contraceptive pill,

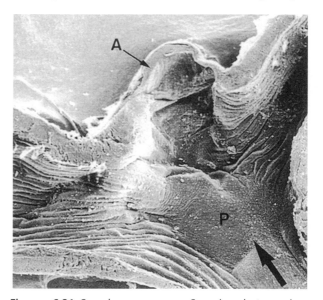

Figure 6.21 *Saccular aneurysm. Scanning-electron-microscopic picture of a small thin-walled aneurysm (A) at the bifurcation of a middle cerebral artery. A pad of vessel wall thickening (P) is seen proximal to the bifurcation and the rugose pattern of the normal vessel wall is disturbed. The direction of blood flow is indicated by the arrow. Reproduced by permission from Ref. 458.*

bacterial or viral infections, pituitary tumours and certain histocompatibility factors.[245,383,386,474,538] Although hypertension has been considered to be an important risk factor for the development of saccular aneurysms, its role has not been clearly established and the results are controversial. Hypertension has been shown to be associated with multiplicity of aneurysms.[12,387] However, no definite evidence of increased prevalence of hypertension over age- and sex-matched controls has been reported in patients with aneurysms, except for females aged 18–54 years.[12] Thus, saccular aneurysms can both arise and rupture in the absence of arterial hypertension.

Both cigarette smoking and alcohol consumption have been demonstrated to be independent modifiable risk factors for subarachnoid haemorrhage.[245] Current cigarette smokers have an approximately 3-fold relative risk, and smoking seems to increase the risk in a dose-dependent manner.[139,245] Proneness to subarachnoid haemorrhage among young men might be partly attributed to their heavier smoking and alcohol intake. The mechanisms of action of both smoking and alcohol intake have remained unknown, but it has been suggested that they might be mediated by frequent periods of augmented blood flow in cerebral arteries.[245] The effect of increased proteolytic activity in the sera of smokers on the aneurysmal wall has also been incriminated.[139]

Location

About 85–90% of saccular aneurysms occur on the terminal part of the internal carotid artery or on the major branches of the anterior portion of the circle of Willis.[532] The most frequent site is the internal carotid artery (approximately 40%), followed by the region of the anterior communicating artery (30%) and the proximal divisions of the middle cerebral artery (20%). Only about 5–10% are associated with the posterior cerebral or vertebrobasilar arteries, and less than 5% with other arteries, e.g. superior cerebellar artery. In children, in contrast to adults, 40–45% of aneurysms occur in the posterior cerebral circulation. Internal carotid artery aneurysms are twice as frequent in women as in men, this predominance being greatest proximally. In contrast, the anterior communicating artery predominates in men by a ratio of 3:2, and about 40% of the ruptured aneurysms in males are at that site.[532] The reported frequencies of multiple aneurysms in patients with subarachnoid haemorrhage vary from 8.6 to 31%, and their most frequent location is the middle cerebral artery.[420]

Macroscopic appearance

Saccular aneurysms vary widely in size and shape (Fig. 6.19). Their diameter at autopsy, is usually between 1 and 25 mm; those over 25 mm are called giant aneurysms.[532] A large proportion (30–45%) of saccular aneurysms of children are of giant size. In a detailed study the median greatest diameter of 181 unruptured aneurysms was 4 mm (range 2–26 mm), and that of 131 ruptured aneurysms (in patients with multiple aneurysms) was 10 mm (range 4–28 mm).[250] At the basilar bifurcation the average size was found to be twice that in other locations.[392] It should be kept in mind that aneurysms tend to shrink postmortem and that their angiographically registered diameters *in vivo* are at least 30–60% greater than values obtained at autopsy before fixation.[318]

Saccular aneurysms are also called berry aneurysms because of their shape. However, many are elongated and/or buckled and may show a somewhat narrow neck by which they communicate with the blood vessel lumen. The walls of some aneurysms are thin and translucent and tend to collapse at autopsy. Other aneurysms show opaque walls due to fibrous thickening or atherosclerosis, and protrude as rigid sacs from their site of origin. The walls may be calcified, particularly in large specimens. Large aneurysms also often contain a lamellated thrombus which may seed thromboemboli into distal arteries. Some aneurysms are completely fibrosed with obliteration of the lumen. Others are buried in adjoining brain tissue (see Fig. 6.47a, b) instead of protruding free into the subarachnoid space.

It may be difficult to recognize a ruptured aneurysm at autopsy, because small thin-walled aneurysms may be almost destroyed as they bleed and, even in the case of larger aneurysms, only their torn edges may remain. Ruptured aneurysms are often obscured by large amounts of surrounding subarachnoid and/or intracerebral blood clot. If the location of the aneurysm has not been established previously by angiography or brain imaging, it is advisable to remove first the blood clot with saline and then carry out a thorough search for the aneurysm before fixation, since dissection of fixed blood is tedious and the aneurysm may be difficult to identify in the clot. The distribution of the subarachnoid blood may indicate the site of the aneurysm (see below, Subarachnoid haemorrhage). In the absence of recent bleeding, orange–brown discoloration of the leptomeninges and the brain surface may reveal the site of previous haemorrhage. A more elaborate method for post-mortem visualization of ruptured aneurysms or malpositioned clips has been developed especially in forensic cases. Radio-opaque polymerizable rubber solution is perfused into the vasculature and the bleeding aneurysm, the patency of arteries or sometimes even associated arterial spasm can be detected by X-ray, and later also in brain sections, because the rubber cast can be cut. This method seems to be especially useful in forensic neuropathology (Fig. 6.22).[256]

Microscopic appearance

The relationship of saccular aneurysms to arterial branching is particularly well seen in small aneurysms. The pads of intimal thickening can be seen by scanning electron microscopy proximal either to normal divisions

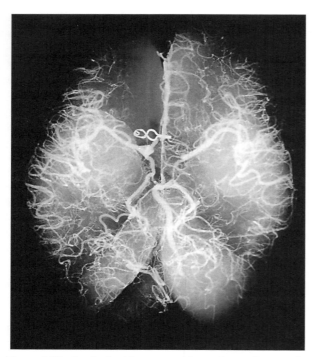

Figure 6.22 *Cerebral rubber cast angiography. A silicone rubber angiographic X-ray of a brain after an accidental kinking of the right anterior cerebral artery against the clip after ligating an aneurysm of the anterior communicating artery. As a consequence the territory of the right anterior cerebral artery has remained unfilled by the contrast medium. Reproduced by permission from Ref. 256.*

or to aneurysms (Fig. 6.21). The pads appear as flattened areas that have lost the rugose pattern of the blood vessel wall. The most characteristic histological feature of the aneurysm wall is the absence of both the muscular tunica media and the internal elastic lamina, both of which end abruptly at the neck of the aneurysm (Fig. 6.20). Apart from the endothelium, the wall of the aneurysmal pouch consists only of fibrous connective tissue of varying thickness. Even the endothelium may be incomplete, and a blood clot may line the luminal surface of the aneurysm. The wall of aneurysms frequently shows atherosclerotic changes, the severity of which appears to parallel their size.[280] After recent rupture the frayed remnants of the wall show necrosis and infiltration by inflammatory cells.[280]

Natural history of saccular aneurysms

The natural history of unruptured aneurysms is little known (for a discussion of their increase in size with time and rupture, see below).[250,532,538] Small saccular aneurysms of the basal cerebral arteries usually do not cause neurological symptoms. However, in a minority of cases, various well-recognized focal clinical syndromes may occur. An aneurysm may, for example, compress the optic tract or the IIIrd, IVth, Vth (ophthalmic division) or VIth cranial nerves. Epileptic fits may be associated with large aneurysms, particularly when buried within the temporal lobe.

The most common and serious complication of saccular aneurysms is its rupture, with consequent subarachnoid haemorrhage, possible arterial vasospasm and infarction and/or intracerebral haemorrhage (see below).[250,538] Rarely, a giant aneurysm may expand to such an extent that the patient dies from raised intracranial pressure.

DOLICHOECTASIA AND FUSIFORM ANEURYSMS

Dolichoectasia is characterized by elongation, widening and tortuosity of a cerebral artery.[532] The basilar artery[473] and the supraclinoid segment of the internal carotid artery[310] are the two most common sites involved (Figs 6.6a, 6.23), but the process may extend to the adjoining portions of the vertebral and middle cerebral arteries. The dolichoectatic basilar artery is often S-shaped with a luminal diameter exceeding 4.5 mm, the defined limit size of ectasia. The dilated portion of the artery may form a fusiform aneurysm (Fig. 6.23).

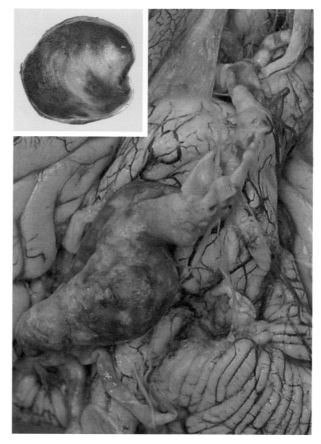

Figure 6.23 *Fusiform aneurysm. This patient had a tendency to develop dolichoectasia and fusiform aneurysms in her atherosclerotic cerebral arteries. The basilar artery is dilated and tortuous, to such an extent that the lesion constitutes a fusiform aneurysm, which also compresses and distorts the brainstem. Thrombosis of the basilar artery (inset) led to brainstem ischaemia and the patient's death. Courtesy of Dr L Paljärvi, Kuopio University Hospital, Finland.*

Dolichoectasia and fusiform aneurysms are commonly seen in patients with advanced cerebral atherosclerosis (Fig. 6.23) and have been associated with risk factors for atherosclerosis, such as hypertension, diabetes mellitus, hypercholesterolaemia and cigarette smoking. Dolichoectasia and/or fusiform aneurysms of the basal artery have been occasionally reported in children and young non-atheromatous patients, sometimes associated with conditions such as Ehler–Danlos syndrome type IV, Marfan's syndrome, pseudoxanthoma elasticum, α_1-antitrypsin deficiency[4,450,452] or various forms of arteritis. An increased risk of dolichoectasia has also been reported for patients with autosomal dominant polycystic kidney disease.[453] Apart from the intimal atherosclerotic lesions, the affected arterial segments may show a thin internal elastic lamina and an atrophic and fibrotic tunica media. These lesions have been interpreted by some authors to represent a unique form of arteriopathy.[310] Interestingly, in a recent review of 120 surgically treated giant fusiform aneurysms 111 had neither atherosclerosis nor other known arteriopathy.[118]

Progressive enlargement of the dolichoectatic arteries has been documented by serial computed tomography, and rapid *de novo* development of giant fusiform aneurysms has been angiographically documented in children.[240] Dolichoectasia and fusiform aneurysms may, by mechanical compression, cause cranial nerve palsies or hydrocephalus. Transient ischaemic attacks may ensue possibly due to emboli derived from thrombi or fragments of plaques in the walls of the enlarged arterial segment.[473] Brainstem and cerebellar infarction may occur as a result of intraluminal thrombosis (Fig. 6.23) or be due to atheromatous occlusion or distortion of the branches of the dilated basilar artery.[397] Spontaneous haemorrhage seems to be relatively rare.[310,547]

INFECTIOUS (SEPTIC) ANEURYSMS

Bacterial aneurysms arise from microbe-carrying emboli usually derived from an infected heart valve or pulmonary vein. About 3% of all patients with infective endocarditis have been claimed to develop such aneurysms.[144] However, it is possible that a great majority (up to 80–90%) of these patients only have a pyogenic infection of the arterial wall instead of a true infectious aneurysm, which may be difficult to identify with certainty.[195] The infected foci may rupture and lead to intracerebral haemorrhage, the risk of which has been estimated at 3–7% for patients with endocarditis.[195] The rupture tends to occur within the first 5 weeks of the endocarditis and the haemorrhage has a mortality rate in the order of 80%.[43] Most frequently, infectious aneurysms occur on the distal branches of the cerebral arteries, with particular predilection in the middle cerebral artery, and they are multiple in about 20% of cases.[43] The most common causative organisms include *Staphylococcus aureus* and *Streptococcus viridans*. Histologically, in the acute stage, an infected embolus may be seen adherent to an oedematous and necrotic arterial wall infiltrated by polymorphonuclear and other inflammatory cells. Experimental studies indicate that organisms spreading from the embolus may lead to weakening of the wall and aneurysmal dilatation within 24 h.[353]

Fungal ('mycotic' in the proper sense) aneurysms are caused by infected emboli from the heart or fungal meningitis, the primary focus of which usually resides in the lungs or paranasal sinuses.[219] A species of the genus *Aspergillus* is most commonly responsible. The angiophilic hyphae may be seen spreading along the intima or through the wall of the affected artery, accompanied by necrosis and a variable inflammatory response (see Fig. 6.18).

MILIARY ANEURYSMS

The miliary aneurysms or microaneurysms of Charcot–Bouchard are controversial. Because they have been considered to be caused by hypertension, they are discussed above in this context.

MISCELLANEOUS ANEURYSMAL LESIONS

Arterial dissections and dissecting aneurysms of intracranial arteries

Arterial dissection is characterized by extravasation of blood into the arterial wall, usually between the intima and media or less frequently between media and adventitia. The intramural haematoma may extend between the planes of the artery and re-enter the original lumen, creating a parallel false lumen. A dissection does not necessarily result in actual arterial dilatation, but if it does, the lesion is called a dissecting aneurysm. It should be noted that, apart from cases with severe atherosclerosis and large aneurysms, the intracranial blood vessels have only sparse vasa vasorum mainly supplying the adventitia[21] and thus the blood of the intramural haemorrhage must leak from the lumen of the artery through an intimal tear.

Dissections are most frequent in young and middle-aged adults, but also occur in children.[363] The vertebral, basilar, middle cerebral and internal carotid (above the clinoid processes), middle cerebral, vertebral and basilar arteries are particularly susceptible, and the lesions may be bilateral.[37,104] Many dissections are associated with blunt trauma to the head or neck or hyperextension injury, which stretches the arteries at the base of the brain sufficiently to rupture their intima. The trauma may apparently be trivial. Spontaneous dissection of intracranial arteries is less common than its extracranial counterpart, but has been increasingly diagnosed *intra vitam* in recent years by advanced imaging methods.[13] It has been reported in association with many conditions, such as arteritis, atherosclerosis, hypertension, the use of oral contraceptives, cystic medial necrosis and mucoid degeneration, fibromuscular dysplasia and segmental mediolytic 'arteritis'.[121,396] α_1-Antitrypsin deficiency and inherited connective tissue disorders seem to be common among patients with dissections.[49,449,454] Abnormalities of the internal elastic lamina are frequently encountered, and include focal absence, splitting, fraying and reduplication.[104] However, in approximately one-third of the pathologically documented cases no underlying vasculopathy has been noted.[121,375] Most intracranial dissections present with an ischaemic stroke due to stenosis or occlusion of the original lumen of the affected artery by the intramural haematoma.[446] Angiographic studies indicate that a benign course may be more frequent than suggested in the earlier literature.[274,405] Recurrent dissections seem to be rare. A persistent fusiform aneurysmal dilatation has been described as a sequel to dissection of the vertebral artery.[274,441]

Caroticocavernous sinus fistulae and dural arteriovenous fistulae

Within the base of the skull, the internal carotid artery passes along the wall of the cavernous sinus, with arterial and venous blood being separated only by the arterial wall and a thin venous endothelium. Most fistulae between the carotid artery and the venous cavernous sinus occur in adult males and are the immediate or sometimes delayed consequence of head injury.[292] Spontaneous fistulae are more frequent in women and they may develop secondary to rupture of saccular aneurysms on the internal carotid artery projecting into the cavernous sinus,[210] and to fibromuscular dysplasia or to connective tissue disorders such as Ehlers–Danlos syndrome type IV.[451] In some cases, a predisposing lesion cannot be found. Only occasional cases have been reported in infancy and childhood.[173,278] A caroticocavernous sinus fistula usually results in a distinctive clinical picture, characterized by ipsilateral pulsating exophthalmos with proptosis and a continuous bruit over the orbit. Large fistulae can divert sufficient blood from the brain to cause signs of cerebral ischaemia. Caroticocavernous sinus fistulae are usually treated by interventional neuroradiological techniques,[210] although spontaneous cure by thrombosis, particularly in the indirect (dural) type of fistula, may occasionally occur.

Dural arteriovenous fistula is an acquired arteriovenous shunt, which is located within the dura. It has a variable natural history and symptomatology, including venous hypertensive encephalopathy with progressive cognitive decline, and it may be a potentially reversible cause of vascular dementia.[225]

Vascular malformations

Vascular malformations have been classified on the basis of the calibre and configuration of the constituent vascular channels, their continuity with the normal cerebral vasculature, and the quantitative relation between blood vessels and the intervening parenchyma. Such classifications include discrete arteriovenous, venous, cavernous, capillary and mixed types (Table 6.3).[22,83] These malformations have been generally regarded as congenital lesions, which

Table 6.3 *Classification of vascular malformations of the intracranial cavity* [a]

I.   Congenital malformations in the brain parenchyma
Arteriovenous malformation
Variant: vein of Galen malformation (or 'aneurysm')
Cavernous haemangioma
Venous angioma and varicose vein
Capillary teleangiectasia
Mixed (or combined): cavernous and venous
cavernous and capillary
Other: haemangioma calcificans
II. Congenital malformations in the meninges
Arteriovenous malformation
Venous angioma and varicose vein (leptomeninges)
Cavernous haemangioma (dura)
III. Vascular malformations as a part of CNS or generalized syndromes
Phakomatoses (e.g. Sturge–Weber syndrome)
Hereditary haemorrhagic teleangiectasia (Rendu–Osler–Weber syndrome)
Other: e.g. Wyburn–Mason syndrome and cerebro-hepato-renal cavernous angiomas
IV. Acquired vascular lesions simulating vascular malformations
Radiation-induced lesions of the white matter
Lesions secondary to venous sinus obstruction

[a] The malformations of the spinal cord are presented in Chapter 18, this Volume.
Adapted from Ref. 83.

arise as a result of disordered mesodermal differentiation between the third and eighth weeks of gestation. However, recent studies indicate that radiation to the brain and dural sinus obstruction can cause acquired vascular lesions, which are radiologically and pathologically identical to vascular malformations. In addition, vascular malformations may occur as part of various syndromes, either generalized or limited to the CNS (Table 6.3).[83]

ARTERIOVENOUS MALFORMATIONS

Arteriovenous malformations, also called arteriovenous aneurysms or angiomas, are congenital abnormalities which consist of tangled masses of tortuous arteries, veins and abnormal connecting channels, and which apparently result from lack of development of the local capillary bed.[83,476,477] Familial occurrence is rare.[10] Because of their propensity to bleed, arteriovenous malformations clinically constitute the most significant group of vascular malformations and the most frequent type in surgical specimens.

Arteriovenous malformations can become symptomatic at any age, but they most commonly present in the second to fourth decade with recurrent subarachnoid or intracerebral bleeding.[174] Other common symptoms include seizures, headaches and various focal neurological deficits.[83] Some arteriovenous malformations are discovered as incidental findings at autopsy. Hormonal influences such as puberty or pregnancy may contribute to bleeding.[142]

Arteriovenous malformations range in size from grossly invisible (called cryptic vascular malformation) to those which involve a large part of an entire hemisphere. The great majority of arteriovenous malformations are supratentorial, occurring on the surface of the cerebral hemispheres (Fig. 6.24a) or deep in the basal ganglia or thalamus. Occasionally they may be confined to the dura or leptomeninges.[83] The superficial cerebral examples are frequently wedge-shaped, with the apex extending inwards into the centrum semiovale and approaching the ventricular surface. The overlying leptomeninges are often thickened and brownish, owing to previous haemorrhage, and the surrounding brain parenchyma is atrophic and

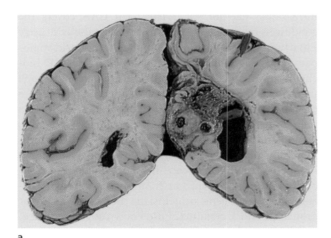

a

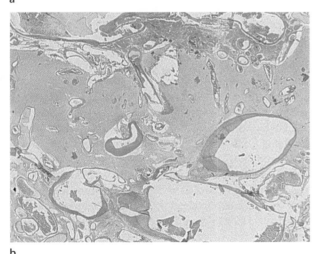

b

Figure 6.24 *Arteriovenous malformation. (a) An arteriovenous malformation on the medial surface of the right hemisphere in the parieto-occipital region. (b) Microscopically the arteriovenous malformation is composed of irregularly spaced blood vessels of variable sizes within, and separated by, the brain parenchyma. There are arteries, veins and 'arterialized' veins with walls of uneven thickness. (Van Gieson.)*

discoloured. Microscopically, the constituent blood vessels correspond to arteries with muscular and elastic laminae and veins dilated by the pressure to which they are exposed because of the shunting. The veins have usually thickened collagenous walls and appear 'arterialized', yet the increased cellularity in their walls depends on proliferation of fibroblasts, not of smooth-muscle cells (Fig. 6.24b). Segmental saccular dilatations are common. The pathological blood vessels are separated by brain parenchyma that often shows gliosis, haemosiderin pigmentation and foci of calcification.[83] The histological and immunocytochemical changes induced by preoperative embolization or laser treatment have recently been analysed.[457,556] The incidence of postoperative neurological complications correlates to a grading scheme, essentially based on size and location of the malformation.[190]

The arteriovenous malformations may enlarge over time by recruitment of contiguous blood vessels and usually cause shunting of blood from the arterial to the venous circulation. Large malformations may short-circuit ('steal') so much blood that the total cerebral blood flow is increased. Despite a drastically increased cerebral blood flow, however, tissue perfusion may be markedly reduced, resulting in chronic ischaemia.[311] In infants and children, excessive arteriovenous shunting may even lead to cardiac decompensation, particularly in arteriovenous malformations draining to and dilating the great vein of Galen ('vein of Galen aneurysms'). These lesions may also obstruct the aqueduct of Sylvius and result in hydrocephalus.[83,483] Occasionally, intracranial arteriovenous malformations communicate with extracranial arteries, usually branches of the external carotid, forming cirsoid aneurysms. Arteriovenous malformations are not infrequently associated with saccular aneurysms (see above).

VENOUS MALFORMATIONS

Venous malformations or venous angiomas are composed of conglomerates of varicose veins, separated from each other by more or less normal brain tissue. They may be the most common incidental vascular malformation found in imaging examinations. Most commonly these malformations are silent, but they may rarely present with epileptic seizures or haemorrhage.[157,362] Angiography discloses a cluster of small veins converging into a 'medusa head', from where blood is drained via a large central vein either peripherally into the leptomeninges or centrally into the galenic system. Histologically, only foci of dilated veins are usually detected, the three-dimensional structure of a 'medusa head' being difficult to appreciate in tissue sections.[83]

CAVERNOUS MALFORMATIONS

Cavernous malformations, usually called cavernous haemangiomas, are compact, occasionally multiple lesions up to several centimetres in diameter which may occur anywhere in the brain or the leptomeninges. They may present with seizures, headache and focal neurological

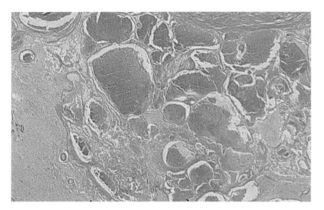

Figure 6.25 *Cavernous haemangioma. The 3-cm lesion in the frontal lobe of a 22-year-old female is composed of closely apposed dilated vascular channels with fibrotic walls and with little intervening brain parenchyma. (Van Gieson.)*

deficits and, less commonly, with haemorrhage, and may sometimes occur in a familial setting.[416] Many remain asymptomatic. Some autosomal-dominant cerebral cavernous malformations are caused by mutations of the *KRIT1* gene on chromosome 7q, encoding a protein that interacts with the *krev-1/rap1a* tumour suppressor gene.[442] Distinctive hyperkeratotic cutaneous venous malformations may co-occur in these patients.[293] Other familial cases are linked to loci at 7p and 3q.[99]

Cavernous haemangiomas may be macroscopically mistaken for fresh, sharply demarcated brain haemorrhages. Histologically, they are composed, of closely apposed dilated vascular channels with little or no intervening brain parenchyma (Fig. 6.25). The blood vessel walls are usually thin and consist of endothelium and a collageneous adventitia, but may show areas of calcification and even ossification.[83] A peripheral rim of haemosiderin deposits in the surrounding brain tissue is a characteristic feature, contributing to the almost diagnostic appearance of these lesions on MRI.[123,416] The vascular channels are often occluded, and the lesions may not fill on angiography, but enhance on computed tomographic (CT) scans. Histological studies have demonstrated the occurrence of small, 'cryptic', angiographically undetected cavernous or venous vascular malformations in a number of patients with brain haemorrhages but without evidence of hypertension, saccular aneurysms or arteriovenous malformations.[33,95] Cavernous haemangiomas may occasionally be associated with similar lesions in other organs, such as the kidney, liver, lung or skin.

CAPILLARY TELEANGIECTASIAS

Capillary teleangiectasia is composed of dilated (ectatic) capillary-type blood vessels, separated by relatively normal brain parenchyma. Haemorrhage from these lesions is very uncommon, and they are usually found incidentally at autopsy as small areas of haemorrhagic blush, most frequently in the pons.[83]

MIXED VASCULAR MALFORMATIONS

Some vascular malformations show features of more than one of the pathologically discrete categories mentioned above. For example, 14 out of 280 cases were found to represent such mixed vascular malformations.[22] Six were mixed cavernous and venous malformations, five were cases of predominantly cavernous malformations with features of arteriovenous malformation or capillary teleangiectasia in the same lesion, while three were examples of mixed venous and arteriovenous malformations.

Cerebral amyloid angiopathy

Cerebral amyloid angiopathy (CAA)[521] is characterized by the extracellular deposition of fibrillar proteins (amyloid) in the walls of blood vessels of the brain and meninges, and it may cause circulatory disturbances, including intracranial haemorrhage. The term CAA covers the conditions referred to by the earlier designations 'drüsige Entartung der Arterien und Kapillären', dyshoric angiopathy and congophilic angiopathy. To date, at least 17 biochemically distinct forms of amyloid are known. Despite their biochemical heterogeneity, all amyloid fibrils share certain unique physicochemical properties, such as a predominantly β-pleated sheet secondary structure, demonstrated by X-ray diffraction analyses.[167] Furthermore, amyloid fibrils bind stains, such as Congo red, showing apple-green birefringence in polarized light (Fig. 6.26) or fluorescent thioflavin S or T. Among the different varieties of amyloidogenic proteins, the β-amyloid precursor protein (β-APP), cystatin C (also known as gamma trace) and BRI protein are of particular interest in the genesis of CAA.

β-AMYLOID ANGIOPATHIES

The most common varieties of CAA are associated with the deposition of the β-amyloid peptide (Aβ), a cleavage product of β-APP encoded on chromosome 21 and expressed in endothelial, pericytic, smooth-muscle and adventitial cells of CNS blood vessels[365] (for further details on the molecular biology of β-APP see Chapter 4, Volume II). Deposition of Aβ in the walls of cerebral blood vessels is seen in sporadic CAA, in the CAA associated with Alzheimer's disease and Down's syndrome, as well as in the syndrome of hereditary cerebral haemorrhages with amyloid angiopathy of the Dutch and Flemish type (HCHWA-D and HCHWA-F; see below). Cerebrovascular Aβ accumulation has also been reported in patients with dementia pugilistica[498] and both cerebral and spinal vascular malformations.[194] Furthermore, some degree of Aβ-CAA has been found in 36% of consecutive autopsied patients aged ≥ 65 years of a general hospital, irrespective of the clinical diagnosis,[522] and the percentage of affected individuals increases with advancing age.[499,522] It has been suggested that the presence of the apolipoprotein Eε4 (ApoE ε4) allele is a risk factor for Aβ-

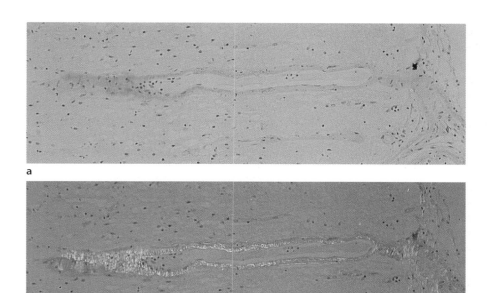

a

b

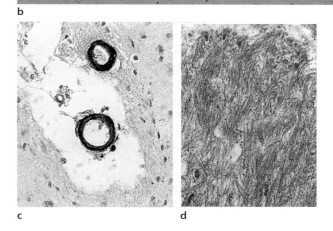

c   d

Figure 6.26 *Cerebral amyloid angiopathy. A penetrating artery from a non-demented patient who died of an intracerebral haematoma (see Fig. 6.47). The arterial walls are thickened by amorphous substance, which is coloured red with alkaline Congo stain (**a**) and gives typical apple-green birefringence (**b**). (**c**) The walls of intracerebral arteries from a patient with familial British dementia are strongly immunopositive with an antibody to amyloid BRI. (**d**) Electron micrograph of about 10 nm thick amyloid filaments in the wall of a cerebral artery from a patient with Aβ-CAA. Courtesy of Dr T Révész, Institute of Neurology, London, UK.*

CAA and Aβ-CAA-associated haemorrhage, independent of its association with Alzheimer's disease. The odds ratios increased approximately 3-fold for ε4 heterozygotes and 14-fold for ε4 homozygotes, relative to individuals without the ε4 allele.[179]

Sporadic Aβ-CAA most often has a patchy distribution and is usually most severe in the occipital and parietal cortex and meninges.[522] The hippocampus is usually spared and the white matter and basal ganglia are only rarely involved. Aβ-CAA-related haemorrhages tend to occur in the frontal or frontoparietal regions, so that factors other than the severity of angiopathy alone probably play a part in causing the haemorrhages.[522] Medium-sized and small arteries and arterioles are preferentially affected. Their walls are thickened by the deposition of amorphous, intensely eosinophilic, alkaline Congo red-positive and birefringent [also periodic acid-Schiff (PAS) positive] amyloid in the tunica media and adventitia, as a result of which the blood vessels become more rigid and fragile and assume characteristic round contours. A double barrel lumen is often seen. The presence of abnormally round, thick-walled blood vessels, particularly within the cortical parenchyma, should always raise the suspicion of CAA. It has been hypothesized that Aβ is deposited in the putative interstitial fluid drainage pathways of the brain.[535] The constituent protein of the amyloid deposits can be demonstrated immunocytochemically after formic acid pretreatment with antibodies against the Aβ peptide. The affected blood vessels may also show simultaneous but weaker immunoreactivity for cystatin C,[523,553] an associated feature that may be a significant cofactor in the pathogenesis of bleeding in Aβ-CAA. By electron microscopy, the extracellular deposits consist of randomly orientated straight, unbranched filaments of indefinite length with a diameter of approximately 6–9 nm. Most patients have variable numbers of senile plaques and neurofibrillary tangles[163] (for differential diagnostic criteria towards Alzheimer's disease see Chapter 4, Volume II). Several cases associated with granulomatous angiitis or a luxuriant giant cell reaction have been reported.[11]

The affected blood vessels in Aβ-CAA frequently show segmental dilatations or microaneurysms and fibrinoid necrosis.[326,382] The following sequential steps in the pathogenetic chain leading to blood vessel rupture and haemorrhage have been suggested on the basis of serial sections and computer-assisted three-dimensional image analysis:[323] (1) accumulation of amyloid in the arterial wall leading to (2) destruction of smooth muscle cells with (3) consequent dilatation (formation of microaneurysms) of the artery and (4) breakdown of the BBB with (5) deposition of plasma proteins in the vessel wall (fibrinoid necrosis), and finally (6) rupture and haemorrhage. Fibrinoid change was more marked than deposition of amyloid at the site of dilatation and rupture.

Sporadic Aβ-CAA is responsible for about 5–12% of primary non-traumatic intracerebral haemorrhages, being the most common cause of its lobar variant and giving also rise to petechial haemorrhages[163] (for details see below). Aβ-CAA may also lead to a rapidly progressive profound dementia with patchy loss of myelin in the white matter, petechial cortical haemorrhages and/or infarction. Many patients show both neuroradiological and neuropathological evidence of a Binswanger-like leukoencephalopathy, thought to be due to hypoperfusion of deep white matter[176,314] (for details see Chapter 4 , Volume II). A rare case of Aβ-CAA may present as a mass lesion.[53]

Aβ-CAA has also been observed in ageing dogs,[508] often associated with cerebral haemorrhage, in rhesus monkeys (*Macaca mulatta*[512]) and in squirrel monkeys (*Saimiri sciureus*[528]). Ageing squirrel monkeys showed a preferential deposition of Aβ in their meningeal blood vessels rather than in the brain parenchyma, in contrast to rhesus monkeys.[528]

The rare autosomal dominant disorder HCHWA-D was originally observed in two coastal villages of The Netherlands. It is clinically characterized by early death from recurrent brain haemorrhages in middle-aged normotensive individuals.[317] Many patients also show dementia, which may progress even without strokes, and a generalized radiological abnormality of the white matter, thought to be due to generalized hypoperfusion.[185] The vascular amyloid deposits contain variant Aβ-protein, but co-localization of immunoreactivity for cystatin C has been reported.[239] The affected individuals show an amino acid substitution (glutamine for glutamic acid) at position 22 of Aβ, caused by a point mutation (Dutch mutation) in the corresponding codon 693 of the β-APP gene.[303] A related disorder, due to a mutation (Flemish mutation) in the neighbouring codon 692 producing an alanine to glycine substitution, has been described in a Flemish Belgian family.[206] Mutations of Aβ which cause haemorrhages are located within the Aβ sequence, whereas those causing familial Alzheimer's disease are most often located in β-APP next to but outside Aβ.

OTHER CEREBRAL AMYLOID ANGIOPATHIES

Hereditary cerebral haemorrhages with amyloid angiopathy of the Icelandic type (HCHWA-I, hereditary cystatin C amyloid angiopathy) is another rare autosomal dominant disease associated with fatal brain haemorrhages in young or middle-aged normotensive adults.[182,239] In addition to the cerebral and meningeal arteries, the Icelandic patients show amyloid deposition in extracerebral tissues, including the skin.[35] The principal component of the amyloid is a variant of a cysteine proteinase inhibitor cystatin C.[161] The affected individuals show a T to A transversion at codon 68 in exon 2 of the cystatin C gene with consequent leucine to glutamine substitution.[304,389] Abnormal processing of cystatin C and a low extracellular concentration of this inhibitor of cysteine proteinases could contribute to destruction of the amyloidotic blood vessels.[495]

Several reports from the UK have described an autosomal dominant cerebral amyloid angiopathy with non-neuritic plaque formation.[334,402,546] This disorder, recently retermed familial British dementia (FBD), is clinically characterized by dementia, spastic paraparesis and ataxia with onset at around the fifth decade. Although the amyloid angiopathy is severe (Fig. 6.26c) it hardly ever causes haemorrhage. FBD is caused by single base substitution in the stop codon of a novel gene *BRI* (for British) located on chromosome 13 and encoding a putative type II single-spanning transmembrane precursor protein of 266 amino acids and relative molecular weight of 30 329 Da. The mutation results in a larger, 277-residue precursor and release of its 34 C-terminal amino acids generates the highly insoluble ABri amyloid subunit with relative molecular weight of about 4 kDa.[519] Another *BRI* mutation, a decamer duplication insertion before the normal stop codon 267, causes familial Danish dementia, associated with deposition of another 34-residue amyloid ADan in cerebral vessel walls.[520] For details see Chapter 4, Volume II.

Leptomeningeal microvascular amyloid has also been observed in another rare hereditary condition with widespread vascular amyloid in multiple organs and severe meningeal and vitreous amyloid deposits.[172,378,381] Furthermore, amyloid deposits in the walls of cerebral and/or meningeal blood vessels are found in various forms of systemic amyloidosis, e.g. transthyretin-related amyloid in familial amyloid polyneuropathy type I[513] and senile systemic amyloidosis,[231] or gelsolin-related amyloid in familial amyloidosis, Finnish.[188,276]

CADASIL

An autosomal-dominant inherited non-amyloid arteriopathy leading to multiple infarcts and dementia in patients without hypertension was described in 1977 by Sourander and Wålinder.[470] Interest in this entity and the number of patients diagnosed progressively increased in the 1990s, when the linkage to chromosome 19 was established in 1993, and the disease was at the same time given its present acronym: cerebral autosomal dominant arteriopathy with subcortical infarcts and leukoencephalopathy (CADASIL).[504] This was rapidly followed by the identification of the defective gene and protein in

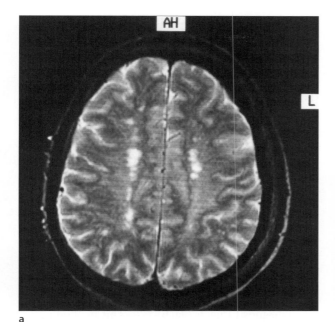
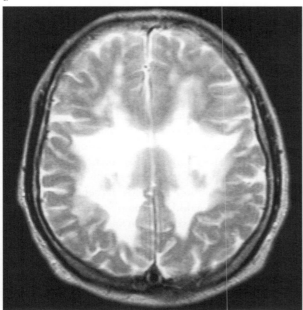

Figure 6.27 *CADASIL. (a) T2-weighted magnetic resonance (MR) image from a 38-year-old male with presymptomatic CADASIL. There are nodular hyperintensities in the periventricular white matter. (b) In a moderately demented homozygous CADASIL patient with a history of several strokes the MRI shows extensive confluent hyperintensities. Courtesy of Timo Kurki, Turku University Hospital, Finland.*

1996.[243] At present over 300 families world-wide with different ethnic backgrounds have been identified.

The cardinal symptoms of CADASIL are: (1) migraine with aura, often exceptionally severe causing sometimes even hemiparesis, (2) ischaemic strokes, (3) psychiatric symptoms, and (4) cognitive decline with eventual dementia. CADASIL patients may have their first stroke

before the age of 30, but the peak is around 40–50 years of age. Characteristic white matter changes (Fig. 6.27a, b) are detectable in T2-weighted MR images well before clinical symptoms (Fig. 6.27a) and decreased cerebral circulation can be demonstrated with PET.[506] Multiple infarcts cause cognitive decline between 40 and 70 years of age, primarily in executive frontal lobe functions, followed later by impairment of memory and other

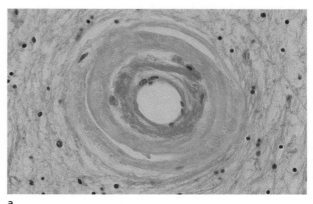
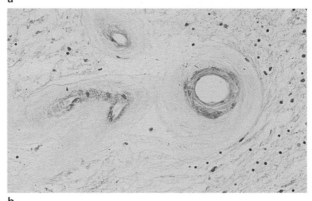
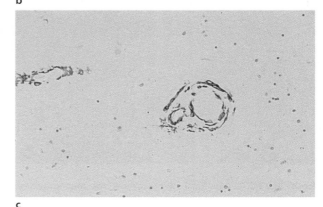

Figure 6.28 *CADASIL. Both the media and the adventitia of a penetrating artery from the parietal white matter of the patient in Fig. 6.27 are markedly thickened with accumulation of basophilic (a), PAS-positive (b) granular non-amyloid material in the media and fibrosis of the adventitia. Immunostaining for smooth-muscle actin (c) shows the irregular degeneration of the smooth-muscle cells. (a) H&E, (b) PAS, (c) antismooth-muscle actin and haematoxylin counterstain.*

cognitive functions, finally leading to the subcortical type of dementia. About 80% of CADASIL patients aged over 65 years are demented.[111] Death usually ensues within 15–25 years of the first strokes.

The characteristic neuropathological feature is non-arteriosclerotic and non-amyloid arteriopathy,[253,435,470]

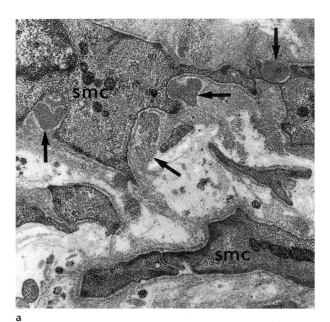

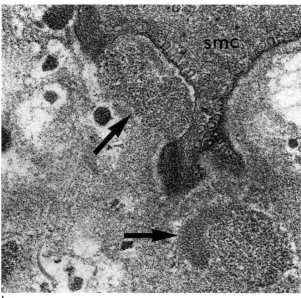

Figure 6.29 *CADASIL. (a) Low-power electron micrograph of a small dermal artery in a skin biopsy. There are numerous deposits of granular osmiophilic material (GOM; arrows) in indentations of and free between degenerative smooth-muscle cells with irregularly thickened basal lamina. (b) Higher magnification of a biopsy from a 19-year-old carrier of the defective gene demonstrates the typical granular appearance of GOM (arrows) and the common presence of pinocytotic vacuoles in the smooth-muscle cell cytoplasm beneath the upper GOM deposit. Smc, smooth-muscle cell.*

which mainly affects penetrating small and medium-sized arteries of the white matter, but it is also present in leptomeningeal blood vessels. There is marked concentric fibrous and/or hyaline thickening of the arterial walls with basophilic and PAS-positive granules in the tunica media (Figs 6.28a, b), and the muscle coat of the media is degenerated (Fig. 6.28c). Electron microscopy (EM) shows destruction of smooth-muscle cells and deposition of granular osmiophilic material (GOM; Fig. 6.29a, b). Extracellular domains of Notch3 accumulate at the plasma membrane of vascular smooth-muscle cells very close to but not within GOM, leaving the definite identity of GOM unknown.[242]

Although the symptoms are almost exclusively neurological, the arteriopathy is generalized and it also affects blood vessels outside the CNS, e.g. in skin, skeletal muscle and peripheral nerves.[435] GOM deposits appear to be specific for CADASIL, and EM analysis of small arteries in deep dermis or subcutis offers a reliable means for *intra vitam* diagnosis (Fig. 6.29a, b).[253,435] This method is recommended in new families with only suspected disease, because molecular genetic search for an unknown mutation may be very cumbersome. Furthermore, GOM is detectable already at the asymptomatic stage of the disease, even before the age of 20 years.

The defective gene in CADASIL is *Notch3*, located at chromosome 19p13. In man it has 33 exons and encodes a single transmembrane receptor protein Notch3 of 2321 amino acids. The structure of the *Notch3* gene and protein are depicted in Fig. 6.30. The function of Notch3 is pivotal during development in regulation of tissue differentiation. Genes of the *Notch* family are highly conserved during evolution, homologous genes having been identified from nematodes to man.[18] In adult human tissues, Notch3 is expressed only in vascular smooth-muscle cells.[242] Upon binding Notch3 is cleaved at two sites and the released intracellular fragment enters the nucleus to regulate transcription. The intramembranous cleavage of both Notch3 and β-amyloid precursor protein of Alzheimer's disease appears be performed by the same γ-secretase, which may be presenilin-1.[109] However, the ligands and the functional response to the Notch signalling in adult human tissues are still unknown.

The great majority of CADASIL cases are due to missense point mutations, but three small deletions have also been described (Fig. 6.30).[244] About 40 different point mutations have so far been identified. All these mutations seem to result in either a substitution of a wild-type cysteine with another amino acid or vice versa. The small deletions cause loss of one cysteine residue.[242] Thus, instead of the normal six cysteine molecules the mutated EGF repeat contains five or seven cysteines. Two *de novo* mutations of CADASIL have been diagnosed.[244]

The pathogenesis of CADASIL is still uncertain. The altered number of cysteine residues may affect the formation of sulfur bridges and therefore change the three-dimensional structure of the Notch3 receptor and

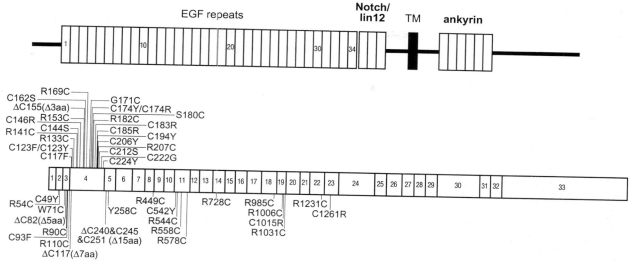

Figure 6.30 *Schematic representations of the Notch3 transmembrane receptor protein (upper scheme) and Notch3 gene (lower scheme). The positions of the point mutations causing a substitution of amino acid using the single-letter code are marked in the lower scheme. For the three small deletions the ordinal of the cysteine residue lost and the total number of amino acids (aa) deleted have been indicated. A great majority of the mutations is located within exons 3 and 4, which encode for the first five EGF repeats. EGF, epidermal growth factor; Notch/lin12, a specific motif of Notch receptors; TM, transmembrane; Δ, deletion.*

consequently its functions.[242,244] Since CADASIL is autosomally dominantly inherited, the mutations result either in toxic gain of function or in haploinsufficiency, i.e. one wild-type allele is not sufficient to maintain normal cellular function. Eventually, over the years smooth-muscle cells are destroyed, which leads to fibrous thickening of the arterial walls, narrowing of the lumen, impaired circulation and finally to thromboses, which cause focal ischaemic infarcts (Fig. 6.31).

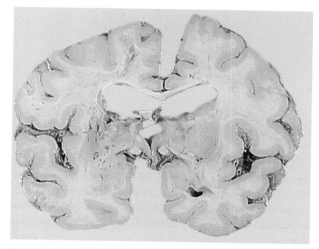

Figure 6.31 *CADASIL. The brain of a 63-year-old female patient, who had presented with adult-onset migraneous headache with visual aura, and who had her first stroke at the age of 52 years. Thereafter, strokes recurred several times per year and she became demented with other stroke-related deficits. There are multiple subcortical infarcts, predominantly in the deep grey matter and in the centrum semi-ovale on the upper left.*

Miscellaneous diseases of blood vessels

MOYAMOYA SYNDROME

The moyamoya syndrome is defined angiographically by spontaneous occlusion of the circle of Willis and the presence of abnormal collateral vascular networks at the base and on the convexity of the brain.[289,370] The angiographic appearance of these networks has given rise to the Japanese term *moyamoya*, meaning 'something hazy', like a puff of cigarette smoke drifting in the air (Fig. 6.32).[480] The term moyamoya syndrome covers both cases of primary moyamoya disease and cases of the angiographic moyamoya phenomenon, associated with various underlying disorders.[151] The moyamoya syndrome was first described in Japan[289,370,480] and was thought to be limited to the Japanese. However, an increasing number of cases have since been published from other countries, including all major racial and ethnic groups.[63,90] Two peaks of incidence have been found, one in the first decade and another in the fourth decade. About 50% of the reported patients are children under 15 years of age.[479] There is a slight preponderance of females. The most common clinical manifestation of moyamoya in children is alternating hemiparesis due to cerebral ischaemia, while in adults intracranial haemorrhage from the thin-walled collateral vessels predominates.[15]

The principal pathological alterations[189,548] include bilateral stenosis or occlusion of the distal portions of the internal carotid arteries and the proximal parts of the anterior and middle cerebral arteries, combined with numerous dilated, thin-walled collateral arteries branching from the posterior parts of the circle of Willis. These collateral blood vessels form an irregular network of pial anastomoses that also penetrate the brain. The outer diameter of the stenosed or occluded arteries is often severely reduced, and their walls may be whitish and nodular. Histologically, their intima shows massive fibrous thickening, usually without atheromatous features (Fig. 6.32b). The internal elastic lamina is usually preserved but extremely wavy and often duplicated or triplicated, whereas the media becomes atrophic (Fig. 6.32c). There is usually no inflammatory infiltration, but thrombosis, recanalization and aneurysm formation may occur. Electron microscopy shows that the intimal thickening is associated with proliferation of smooth-muscle-like cells and accumulation of collagen fibrils together with elastic material.[189]

Although the aetiology and pathogenesis of moyamoya disease remain unknown, most authors regard the abnormal vascular networks as evidence of collateral circulation secondary to occlusion of the anterior circle of Willis. Experimental mechanical, chemical or immunological damage to the endothelium, with subsequent platelet aggregation and release of platelet-derived growth factor (PDGF), may induce intimal thickening due to smooth-muscle-like cells and accumulation of collagen and elastic fibres. Local or systemic infections not infrequently precede the clinical manifestations of the moyamoya syndrome, and an inflammation-related humoral factor may thus induce repeated endothelial damage and intimal thickening.[189] Association of the moyamoya syndrome with a host of other acquired conditions, such as irradiation of the head and neck, suggests a multifactorial aetiology. However, there may be a genetic factor that predisposes to an exaggerated reaction of the immature vascular wall to noxious stimuli. Familial occurrence has been observed in about 7% of Japanese patients, mostly in pairs of siblings, including monozygotic twins.[273] Assuming an unknown mode of inheritance, a linkage was recently found between familial moyamoya disease and markers at 3p24.2-p26.[228] The moyamoya phenomenon has also been reported in patients with a number of unrelated inherited conditions such as neurofibromatosis-1, tuberous sclerosis, Marfan's syndrome, Alpert's syndrome, sickle-cell anaemia, Fanconi's anaemia and Schimke's immuno-osseous dysplasia.

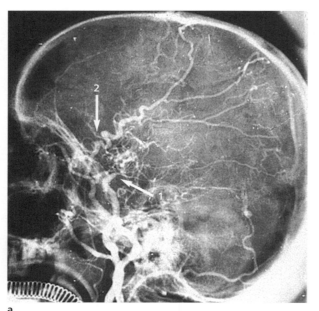

a

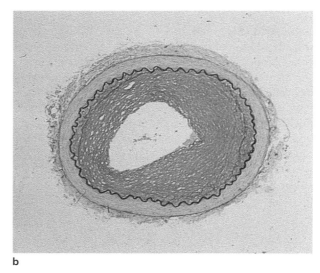

b

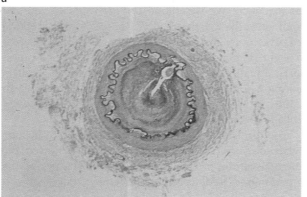

c

Figure 6.32 *Moyamoya disease. (a) Angiography of a patient discloses occlusion of the left internal carotid artery (arrow 1). Typical collateral circulation via the enlarged and meandering left middle menigeal artery (arrow 2) has developed, creating a network of collateral blood vessels between these two arteries. (b) Micrograph of the basilar artery from another moyamoya patient shows marked thickening of the intima and narrowing of the lumen. (c) The right posterior communicating artery of the same patient, with severe folding of the internal elastic lamina and probable thrombosis and recanalization of the lumen. (b, c: Elastica–van Gieson stain.) Reproduced by permission from Ref. 189.*

FIBROMUSCULAR DYSPLASIA

Fibromuscular dysplasia is a non-inflammatory segmental disease of the arterial wall, first described in the renal arteries[296] and later in the cervico-cephalic arterial tree.[98,316] Among patients undergoing carotid angiography fibromuscular dysplasia has been diagnosed in approximately 0.25–1%.[316] The disease occurs at all ages, but is unusual before adulthood and shows a clear predilection for females. Angiography shows luminal narrowing alternating with aneurysmal dilatations, giving a characteristic 'string of beads' appearance, while the two other patterns, 'tubular stenosis' and 'semicircumferential lesions', are much less common.[385] In the vast majority of cases, cervicocephalic fibromuscular dysplasia involves the midportion of the cervical internal carotid artery and has been thought to be the second most common stenosing lesion of the internal carotid artery after atheroma. The involvement is mostly bilateral. The extradural portion of the vertebral arteries is less frequently affected, while involvement of the intracranial arteries is rare. Any layer of the arterial wall can be affected, but most often the media bears the brunt of the lesion with hyperplasia of fibrous tissue and smooth muscle resulting in stenosis. These narrowed segments alternate with dilated portions, where the blood vessel wall is thinned and fibrosed with deficient media and disruption of the elastic laminae.[316,472] The aetiology of fibromuscular dysplasia has not been established. Occasional familial cases suggest genetic predisposition,[79] but local trauma, hormonal influences supported by female predominance, ischaemia of the blood vessel wall and viral infections have also been proposed as causative factors.[316]

Neurological symptoms of fibromuscular dysplasia are often trivial, such as headache, mental distress, tinnitus or audible bruits. Serious complications have been reported in about one-third[316] of patients. These arise since fibromuscular dysplasia is frequently associated with intracranial, often multiple aneurysms, which may cause subarachnoid haemorrhage, and with cervicocephalic arterial dissections. In addition, TIA or infarction may occur, probably caused by thromboembolism.

HAEMATOLOGICAL DISORDERS

Oxygen and all necessary substrates for cerebral metabolism are transported to the CNS by the cerebral circulation. Most often the disorders that compromise this carrier function impair the flow of blood itself, but there are also conditions in which the capacity of the blood to carry the essential ingredients of cerebral metabolism is limited to a critical extent. The majority of the diseases of the blood vessel walls do not usually cause sufficient narrowing of the vascular lumen to alone decrease the blood flow to ischaemic levels. It is commonly the associated thrombus formation induced by the vascular injury that finally obstructs the lumen. Alternatively, emboli detach from the thrombus to obstruct the flow in arteries. In the latter case the arteries are frequently otherwise healthy, as they are also in various thrombophilic conditions.

Haematological disorders are uncommon primary causes of acute cerebrovascular disorders, comprising only about 1% of all strokes, while the frequency in young adults is somewhat higher.[17] More than a dozen primary haematological disorders have been associated with ischaemic stroke[490] and another dozen may cause haemorrhage.

Thrombosis and antithrombosis

Under normal conditions when haemostasis is needed it is produced by promotion of two interdependent phenomena: aggregation of platelets and activation of the coagulation cascade. Endothelial damage induces aggregation of platelets and these release factors, for example thromboxane A_2 and adenosine diphosphate, which further recruit new platelets to adhere to the platelet thrombus. Platelets also release factors that activate

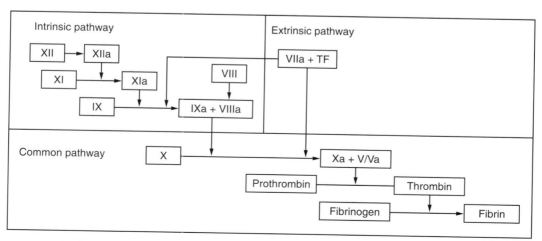

Figure 6.33 *The clotting cascade. a, Activated; TF, tissue factor.*

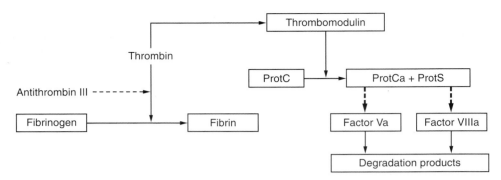

Figure 6.34 *Physiological antithrombotic mechanisms. Inhibitory effects are marked with dashed lines. The thick dashed line indicates that activated protein C and protein S inhibit the function of factors Va and VIIIa (which regulate formation of thrombin; see Fig. 6.33) by degrading these factors. a, Activated.*

the intrinsic pathway of coagulation. Tissue factor (factor VII receptor) capable of activating the extrinsic pathway becomes expressed on the surface of injured endothelium, exposed intima or accumulated inflammatory cells. Most commonly all these adverse events occur in complicated atherosclerotic plaques. The intrinsic and extrinsic pathways converge into the common pathway, as a result of which thrombin cleaves fibrinogen into fibrin (Fig. 6.33). If the flow conditions allow, a fibrin thrombus is formed on the platelet matrix.

Under normal conditions vascular patency and unhindered blood flow are guaranteed by an intact endothelium and the presence of antithrombotic molecules – many secreted by endothelial cells themselves – which prevent the aggregation of platelets and activation of the coagulation cascade (Fig. 6.34). Antithrombin III prevents the action of thrombin, and this inhibitory effect is amplified by heparin. Thrombin bound to thrombomodulin on endothelial surfaces participates in the counteraction of its own procoagulant effect by activating endothelium-derived protein C, which together with its circulating cofactor protein S forms a proteolytic complex that destroys activated factors V and VIII of the coagulation cascade. Finally, the fibrin thrombi are degraded by fibrinolysis (Fig. 6.35). Drug-induced fibrinolysis, which is an established therapy for acute myocardial infarction has been reintroduced in the 1990s for the treatment of ischaemic strokes.[341,529]

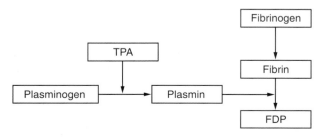

Figure 6.35 *Fibrinolysis. TPA, Tissue plasminogen activator (natural or iatrogenic such as recombinant TPA or streptokinase or urokinase); FDP, fibrin degradation products.*

Thrombophilia

Defects in the antithrombotic mechanisms (see Fig. 6.34), such as deficiency of antithrombin III, protein C or protein S, resistance of activated factor V to proteolysis by activated protein C (APC resistance with underlying mutation G1691A in factor V gene) and G20210A genotype of prothrombin can lead to a hypercoagulable state and thrombotic occlusion.[102,178,223,412,432] The first three deficiencies may be either inherited or acquired, while the latter two are hereditary. In these disorders thrombi are most often formed in the systemic venous circulation, and they appear to be risk factors of cerebral venous thrombosis,[101,412,447,489] whereas their role as the cause of arterial occlusions has not been fully analysed. Recent studies have demonstrated that many of them are also risk factors of ischaemic strokes in children or young adults,[374] but not necessarily in older adults.[412] These conditions are apparently more common than appreciated if special coagulation studies are performed among patients with atypical strokes.[432]

The increased incidence of cerebral infarction in certain generalized conditions such as malignancies, infections, use of oral contraceptives, pregnancy or chemotherapy may depend on acquired hypercoagulability due to deficient function of the antithrombotic molecules.[432]

In addition to the above factors increasing the formation of thrombin, high plasma levels of fibrinogen[515] and defective lysis of the incipient fibrin thrombi, e.g. due to deficiency of plasminogen (Fig. 6.35) can lead to full-blown thrombotic episodes. Homocysteinaemia has been recently shown to lead to impaired fibrinolysis, thereby increasing the risk of cardiovascular disease including ischaemic stroke.[287,534] In middle-aged populations the results have been contradictory: an elevated serum fasting level of homocysteine has been reported to have both an increased and unchanged risk of stroke. In a well-controlled study of young stroke patients, those with elevated serum homocysteine levels after methionine loading had a 4.8-fold increased risk, even though fasting levels of homocysteine did not differ between stroke patients and controls.[287] People with the C677T mutation in thermolabile 5,10-methylenetetrahydrofolate reductase, an enzyme associated with homocysteine metabolism, often have hyperhomocysteinaemia and in particular homozygosity for this mutation has been advocated as a risk factor of stroke. However, this genotype seems to carry either no or at most moderately increased risk.[192,287]

Antiphospholipid antibodies

Antiphospholipid antibodies (aPLs) are a heterogeneous family of autoantibodies which are associated with a spectrum of clinical manifestations collectively called antiphospholipid syndrome, the diagnosis of which requires the presence of a thrombotic or vasculopathic event and reliably identified presence of aPLs. Originally, aPLs were detected in patients with SLE (see above), but with improved testing methods and awareness of the multifaceted clinical picture of the antiphospholipid syndrome, aPLs have been found to occur in association with many other diseases, including malignancies, HIV infection, drug ingestion and various autoimmune disorders, such as rheumatoid arthritis, immune thrombocytopenic purpura as well as Sjögren's and Behcet's syndromes. These conditions have been classified as secondary aPL syndrome, as opposed to the more common primary one with no underlying medical condition.[38] However, population studies suggest that aPLs are present even in 2–5% of healthy people.[490]

The major clinical manifestations of the aPL syndrome are arterial and/or venous circulatory disturbances, recurrent miscarriages and thrombocytopenia. Its main neurological manifestation is ischaemic stroke, and aPLs have been verified to be an independent risk factor for first-time ischaemic stroke.[16,502] These strokes often occur at an exceptionally young age with no other apparent causes, which indicates a true causal relationship.[51,487,502] The prevalence of aPLs among young stroke patients has been estimated at 18–46%, but aPLs are also detected in 10–18% of older stroke patients.[368]

The thrombotic occlusions in patients with aPLs are most often venous, and thus the risk of paradoxical embolic strokes is increased. When thromboses occur in the arterial circulation, the brain is the most common site.[51,514] It is quite likely that the procoagulant state induced by the aPLs promotes full thrombosis in patients with other risk factors of stroke such as atherosclerosis, hypertension or diabetes. Furthermore, stroke patients with aPLs have an 8-fold risk of recurrence.[300] Smaller arteries may also become occluded with no associated vasculitis; for example, involvement of retinal arteries may give rise to different manifestations of ocular ischaemia. Fibrin thrombi, obstruction by intimal proliferation and recanalization with persistent fibrous webs across arteri-al lumina have been described as typical features, which at the same time suggest recurrent episodes of intravascular thrombosis and associated infarction.[222]

The two conventional assays for the presence of aPLs are: (1) demonstration of lupus anticoagulant (LA) phenomenon, the name of which derives from the fact that it was first detected in patients with SLE as a paradoxical prolongation of the in vitro coagulation time, even though an in vivo positive LA test indicates a thrombophilic state and a risk of ischaemic insults;[487] and (2) detection of anti-cardiolipin antibodies in patient's serum, presently using enzyme-linked immunosorbent assays (ELISAs).[487] Knowledge of the antigenic specificities and pathogenetic mechanisms of aPLs changed radically during the 1990s. It was demonstrated that the target of aPLs is not always only the phospholipid, but a 50-kDa protein in the patient's plasma, β_2-glycoprotein I (β_2-GPI, also called apolipoprotein H), is needed as a necessary cofactor for the binding of aPLs to the lipid antigens. Possibly, the combined β_2-GPI and phospholipid form neoepitopes to which the aPLs bind.[433] At present there are discrepant views as to whether β_2-GPI is the primary antigen or a necessary cofactor, or is not needed at all, and this probably also reflects variation in individual patients' aPL spectrum. Furthermore, it has been demonstrated that in addition to β_2-GPI, aPLs recognize other phospholipid binding plasma proteins, including prothrombin, protein C, protein S, thrombomodulin, annexin V and kininogens.[487]

Among non-cardiolipin phospholipids against which aPLs have been formed, both negatively charged (phosphatidylserine, -inositol, -glycerol and phosphatidic acid), and neutral (phosphatidylethanolamine and choline) ones have been identified. It has been shown that among 77 young non-SLE patients with stroke as many as 34 (44%) had aPLs against one or more of the phospholipids mentioned above. Among them, only 53% had antibodies to cardiolipin, the remainder having other phospholipid specificities, with phosphatidylinositol being the most common (65%). Remarkably, one single patient may have a variety of antibodies, i.e. to several different phospholipid antigens and of different immunoglobulin classes.[503]

The exact thrombogenic mechanisms of the aPLs have not been definitely established, although the following have been suggested: aPLs bind to phospholipids in the platelet membrane and cause their increased adhesion and aggregation. The expression or the amount of phospholipids needed in the anticoagulant system is altered. aPLs bind to endothelial phospholipids in combination with β_2-GPI, which induces endothelial damage with activation of different thrombosis-promoting processes. Conversely, β_2-GPI has also been proposed to be protective, like a 'Band-aid' which binds to phospholipids in damaged endothelial plasma membrane and thereby prevents the exposure of procoagulant factors in the endothelium to the circulation. This anticoagulant function could be lost, if β_2-GPI is excessively consumed by aPLs.[432,433]

Polycythaemia and hyperviscosity

In polycythaemia the number of red blood cells is increased with a high haemoglobin concentration (> 200 g/l) and haematocrit (> 60%). Patients with polycythaemia vera have been reported to have an up to five times greater risk of stroke than the age- and sex-matched controls.[89] Stroke has been reported to occur in as many as 20% of patients with polycythaemia vera, but is clearly less frequent in secondary polycythaemia.[195a,348] Even an abnormally high haematocrit without high red blood cell count carries an increased risk of stroke, since high haematocrit does not necessarily indicate true polycythaemia, but may be just secondary to dehydration.[369] In the Framingham study[255] if the haematocrit was over 45% in men and 42% in women, the risk of stroke was twice as high as among those with lower levels. In another study, the risk of cerebral infarction was not significantly affected by the haematocrit values when below 45%, but increased steeply above that value, especially in patients with severe atherosclerosis.[497]

The mechanism of stroke is considered to be the hyperviscosity of the hypercellular blood, which decreases CBF to levels at which multifocal small infarction results.[127] Whether the sluggish flow allows formation of thrombi or the stagnation of the blood is sufficient to cause ischaemia has not been definitely established.

An increased number of white blood cells can also cause a focal infarct, most probably due to stasis. Excessive concentrations of plasma proteins, e.g. in connection with different plasma cell dyscrasias, can also lead to hyperviscosity. Because of the high molecular weight of immunoglobulin M (IgM) molecules, the hyperviscosity syndrome is most likely to occur in Waldenström's macroglobulinaemia, but other paraproteinaemias may also give rise to this complication.[388]

Anaemias

Compensatory mechanisms during anaemia usually guarantee adequate oxygen transport to the brain. Thus, low haemoglobin as such is not a risk factor of stroke,[255] but additional factors interfering with the flow of blood are required.

SICKLE CELL DISEASE

This is a group of haemoglobinopathies in which under conditions of reduced oxygen supply the abnormal β-chains of the sickle haemoglobin S aggregate and polymerize to form rigid filamentous structures, 'tactoids', which in turn deform erythrocytes into sickle cells.[47] Although rheological properties of sickled erythrocytes suggest microvascular occlusion, the major pathology is extensive intracranial arterial disease with occlusions and stenosis in the internal carotid, and anterior, middle and posterior cerebral arteries. Massive intracranial haemorrhage and fat embolism may also occur.[436]

Of all the anaemias, sickle cell disease is the most commonly associated with stroke, which in turn most often occurs in children under the age of 15 years. About 15% of children with sickle cell disease experience cerebrovascular disorders. Cerebral infarction occurs in about 75% and intracerebral haemorrhages in some 20%, and these changes are commonly bilateral.[348]

β-THALASSAEMIA MAJOR

Thalassaemias are another group of hereditary anaemias associated with strokes.[47,343,544] In these either the α- or β-chain of the normal haemoglobin A carries a genetic defect. In the clinically most important β-thalassaemia major the patients have homozygous β-chain mutations, which at the molecular level encompass over 50 different mutations. The main clinical feature of β-thalassaemia major is hypochromic, microcytic anaemia due to impaired production and haemolysis of erythrocytes. The disease usually becomes manifest soon after birth. These patients have an increased risk of thrombotic stroke, to which the postsplenectomy thrombocytosis contributes. Haemorrhage after blood transfusions has also been reported.

Platelet abnormalities

Both thrombocytosis and thrombocytopenia have been associated with ischaemic stroke and TIA as well as with intracerebral haemorrhage. Thrombocytosis is believed to cause micro-occlusion, if the platelet count is above 400 000 or if the platelets are abnormally adhesive.

Among these disorders neurological complications are most common in thrombotic thrombocytopenic purpura (TTP), which is also called thrombotic microangiopathy or Moschowitz' disease.[388] It is a rare disorder, which primarily affects young and middle-aged women (20–50 years of age). In TTP platelets form thrombi, which occlude mainly cerebral and renal microvessels, and at the same time platelets are consumed to such an extent that thrombocytopenia and petechial haemorrhages (purpura) supervene.[393] The cause of TTP has been recently suggested to be overactivity of von Willebrand factor (vWF). In the familial form it is caused by constitutional deficiency of vWF-cleaving enzyme and in non-familial forms by inhibition of this enzyme by an IgG antibody.[150]

Neurological symptoms occur in nearly all patients with TTP,[488] and they are often very dramatic, including stupor, coma, seizures and stroke. The morphological changes, both in brain imaging[267] and by histopathological examination may be nil or only minimal even in lethal cases.[2] The lumina of microvessels, predominantly in the grey matter, are occluded by hyaline, eosinophilic platelet thrombi which, in addition, contain fibrin and factor VIII, among other substances. Endothelial hyperplasia is a characteristic feature, and sometimes the blood vessel wall is necrotic, whereas the surrounding parenchyma often discloses surprisingly few changes. In severe cases, however, multiple small cerebral infarcts corresponding to the territory of the occluded microvessel are present, and rarely, even large-vessel occlusion may occur.

$\alpha_2\beta_1$ integrin (glycoprotein Ia–IIa) is one of the major collagen receptors on platelets via which platelets adhere to collagen exposed in damaged blood vessel wall and become activated. The density of this receptor molecule is regulated by two linked silent polymorphisms (C807T and G873A) in the α_2 gene coding sequence. Platelets from individuals homozygous or heterozygous for T807 allele show higher expression of $\alpha_2\beta_1$ integrin and enhanced adhesion to collagen I compared with platelets from individuals homozygous for C807, which in practice means more active thrombus formation. Concordantly, it was demonstrated that the genotype T807 is an independent risk factor for stroke in young patients (≤50 years of age, odds ratio 3.02), in whom the conventional risk factors (hypertension, diabetes mellitus and smoking) had no effect on the risk.[73]

CONSEQUENCES OF CEREBROVASCULAR DISORDERS

The sequelae of diseases affecting the cerebral blood vessels can be broadly divided into two basic types: (1) obstruction of the blood vessels, which leads to ischaemia, and (2) rupture of the vessel wall, which leads to haemorrhage.

Cerebral ischaemia

GENERAL ASPECTS AND DEFINITIONS

Cerebral ischaemia defines a condition in which there is insufficient blood flow to the brain to maintain normal cellular functions. Since neurons have the highest demand for oxygen, neuronal function is affected first, followed in declining order of vulnerability by oligodendrocytes, astrocytes and vascular cells. Cerebral ischaemic insults to the human brain are of two basic types. By far the most important in clinical work is focal cerebral ischaemia (FCI). In FCI, narrowing or occlusion of the lumen of an artery reduces CBF in a defined territory in which the function of neurons becomes impaired or ultimately neurons are destroyed and a clinical 'stroke' ensues. In global cerebral ischaemia (GCI) the systemic circulation fails and consequently the blood flow of the whole brain becomes insufficient. The pathophysiology of GCI together with the basic cellular mechanisms involved in hypoxic and/or ischaemic nerve cell injury are detailed in Chapter 5, this Volume.

Although experimental models of ischaemia have been criticized as being poor replicants of human stroke[537] they are the only way to obtain detailed information about the various factors operative during the evolution of the ischaemic injury, on the basis of which rational therapeutic approaches are possible. In experimental studies FCI is most commonly induced by occlusion of the middle cerebral artery (MCA) with or without recirculation. This model of FCI differs from experimental GCI, commonly induced by forebrain ischaemia, in a number of important respects.[461] These differences are also applicable to man. For example, FCI is usually less severe and an irreversible injury develops more slowly than in GCI. The tissue damage in FCI consists of a central core of densely ischaemic tissue surrounded by a perifocal zone of less dense ischaemia perfused by critically reduced blood flow from the surrounding collaterals (penumbra zone, see below), whereas in GCI similar gradients do not usually exist. The cells in the central core of FCI rapidly become irreversibly injured, while cells in the latter zone are less severely injured, and may either become recruited into the core of the infarct, or be rescued by appropriate measures: there is a 'therapeutic window' during which the at-risk tissue may be salvaged.

ISCHAEMIC THRESHOLDS

The critical threshold values of CBF needed for the maintenance of functional and structural integrity of the brain were determined in a series of experimental studies in baboons and cats,[20,201,204] and in man approximately similar values were obtained in clinical studies using PET in stroke patients (Fig. 6.36). These studies showed that blood flow above about 40% of the normal value (i.e. approx. 20 ml/100 g per minute) ensures unimpaired spontaneous and evoked electrical activity of nerve cells. From about 40% to 30% increasing numbers of neurons are unable to produce sufficient energy to maintain the functions needed for the transmission of nerve impulses, and at about 30% of normal blood flow transmission

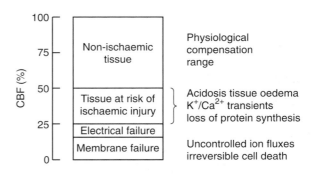

Figure 6.36 *Ischaemic thresholds of neuronal function. Courtesy of Dr P Lindsberg, Helsinki University Central Hospital, Finland.*

ceases completely, i.e. the threshold of transmission or electrical failure has been reached. The energy production in these spontaneously electrically silent neurons can still maintain basic household functions to keep the cells alive, e.g. the ion pumps of the plasma membrane. Thus, these neurons may resume transmission if adequate CBF is restored. If regional CBF further diminishes below about 15% of normal (10–12 ml/100 g per minute), a sudden rise in extracellular K^+ indicates that the threshold of membrane failure has been reached. At that stage, the energy produced can no longer maintain transmembrane ion gradients and the efflux of K^+ is accompanied by influx of Na^+, Ca^{2+} and Cl^- ions together with osmotically obligated water.[461] Membrane failure results in an irreversible nerve cell injury unless sufficient blood flow and energy production are restored. The absolute flow values of these thresholds depend on the species examined, being higher in smaller animals, and they are also influenced by physiological variables such as brain temperature. However, by and large, these levels seem to be proportional to the baseline blood flow rates in each animal and, thus, the relative values given seem to apply even to man.[28,201,461]

The fatal membrane failure is preceded at higher threshold levels of CBF by other disturbances of cellular metabolism. For example, brain oedema may begin to appear at a CBF level of 25% of normal,[241] intracellular and extracellular acidosis begins at a CBF level of around 40%,[193,340] and the synthesis of most proteins ceases in neurons at around 50–60% of normal blood flow (for details see Chapter 5, this Volume).[344]

The development of an irreversible injury depends not only on the severity of the ischaemic insult, i.e. the level of CBF, but also on its duration.[153,204] After MCA occlusion in cats, neurons appear to tolerate flow rates of near zero, 10 or 15 ml/100 g per minute for 25, 40 or 80 min, respectively, and at flow rates above 17–18 ml/100 g per minute most neurons are likely to recover. The noticeable variation in ischaemic tolerance of individual neurons indicates selective vulnerability.[204] Similar results have been obtained in macaque monkeys[105] and selective vulnerability is also a characteristic feature of global cerebral ischaemia (Chapter 5, this Volume).

The density and duration of ischaemia are, however, not always the only decisive factors, since under certain conditions nerve cell death may occur even after short ischaemic episodes followed by seemingly adequate reperfusion and often long after recovery of many neuronal functions. The pathophysiology of this delayed neuronal death and apoptotic neuronal death is described in Chapter 5, this Volume. Thus, the duration of the ischaemic insult after which nerve cells can still recover must be assessed after a sufficiently long recirculation period up to several days to guarantee that the recovery is permanent and not just due to the temporary restoration of some specific cellular functions (e.g. energy production or electrical activity). Therefore, quantitative histopathological analysis is the most reliable method for assessment of final outcome.

Information on the tolerance of human brain to focal ischaemia has emerged from temporary iatrogenic occlusion of an intracranial artery during saccular aneurysm surgery. Among normotensive and normothermic patients under normal neurosurgical anaesthesia no one subjected to ischaemia of less than 14 minutes' duration developed an infarct; 95% of them tolerated 19 minutes ischaemia, whereas all patients with occlusion for over 31 minutes had both clinical and radiological evidence of infarction.[444] The thresholds in man may be lowered by the longstanding effects of known cerebrovascular risk factors, such as hypertension and diabetes.

PRECONDITIONING (INDUCTION OF TOLERANCE)

Short-lived single or repetitive sublethal ischaemic episodes may stimulate brain cells to acquire tolerance to subsequent otherwise lethal ischaemia. In experimental studies it has been demonstrated that the ischaemic stress activates immediate-early genes (e.g. *c-fos*, *c-jun*, *jun B*). These then either turn on new genes or downregulate active genes, i.e. an 'after-stress' homoeostatic correction occurs; for example, production of antioxidants, neurotrophic factors, cytokines and heat-shock proteins is induced and alternative metabolic pathways as well as DNA repair mechanisms are activated.[87,107] Moreover, ischaemic tolerance in rodents is produced by repetitive nerve cell depolarizations (spreading depression) induced by glutamate, the excitatory amino acid transmitter which is also a mediator of ischaemic excitotoxic nerve cell injury.[87] Thus, it appears that depending on the intensity of the effect the same agents may be either cytoprotective or injurious.[107] If similar tolerance could be achieved by safe interventions in man, ischaemic preconditioning could be used before operations which harbour a substantial risk of ischaemic brain damage, such as extracranial or intracranial vascular surgery and open-heart surgery.

PENUMBRA

General aspects

The 'natural' evolution of a focal brain infarct has been analysed in detail using the model of permanent occlusion of MCA (Figs 6.37, 6.38). Astrup *et al.*[20] proposed that in FCI the central core, which has undergone membrane failure and becomes an infarct unless rapidly reperfused, is surrounded by a zone of tissue, which has passed only the upper threshold of electrical silence and, thus, has the capacity to recover if perfusion is restored. This zone was designated as penumbra (which means partly lighted area surrounding complete shadow, as around the moon in full eclipse). At the time of its definition the width, stability and duration of the penumbra could only be guessed.[20]

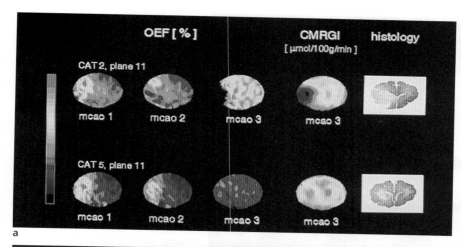

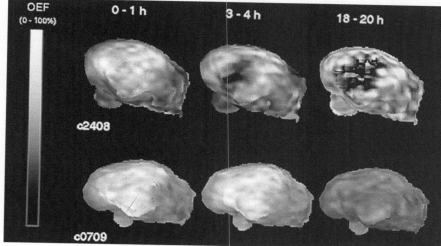

Figure 6.37 *Focal experimental ischaemic stroke. (a) Sequential multitracer PET scanning of the brains of two cats after middle cerebral artery occlusion for approx. 1 h (mcao 1), 2–3 h (mcao 2) or 18–24 h (mcao 3). In both cats, in the core of ischaemia the oxygen extraction fraction (OEF) has increased (misery perfusion) in the early phase (mcao 1) because of low blood flow. It has already markedly decreased by 2–3 h (mcao 2) in cat 2, in which the evolved infarct (after sacrifice verified by histology) finally stands out as an area with complete lack of oxygen and glucose utilization (mcao 3). In contrast, in cat 5 the early misery perfusion reverses, as verified by normalization of OEF and CMRO$_{GI}$ and preservation of tissue integrity. (b) The same phenomenon is demonstrated on the lateral aspect of the brain. Upper panel cat 2 with an evolving infarct; lower panel: cat 5 with reversal of the ischaemia. (a) Reproduced by permission from Ref. 16. (b) courtesy of Prof. W-D Heiss, Max-Planck Institut für Neurologische Forschung, Cologne, Germany.*

Because tissue in penumbra is considered potentially salvageable with appropriate therapy, attempts have been made to determine its exact pathogenesis and behaviour at different time intervals after the ischaemic insult. In the original penumbra study, electrodes inserted into the brain were used to measure the CBF and ion concentrations.[20] The only technique which allows non-invasive quantitative *in situ* analysis of the main physiological parameters of brain energy metabolism [i.e. regional CBF (rCBF), blood volume, oxygen extraction fraction (OEF) and cerebral metabolic rates of oxygen and glucose (CMRO$_2$ and CMRO$_{glc}$)] is PET.[28] PET was designed to be applied in human studies, although its technical complexity, practical difficulties, safety considerations and availability limit its use, especially for serial studies in practical clinical work. Thus, PET study in human stroke is described as only 'a snapshot of the complex dynamic events' and it has to be complemented by subsequent analyses using other imaging methods such as CT and different modalities of MRI.[28] Although PET could be performed only once on an individual stroke patient, the possible PET equivalent of penumbra, defined as zone of misery perfusion, was introduced in the early 1980s (see

below).[29] It is characterized by reduced CBF with relatively preserved or even normal CMRO$_2$. A hallmark of 'misery perfusion' is increased OEF, i.e. when the flow of oxygenated blood decreases more oxygen is extracted from the remaining flow to prevent a critical reduction in CMRO$_2$. Thus, as the definition of penumbra implies, the reduced blood flow can keep neurons alive, although only with difficulty.

The results of PET studies[30,203,328] may be summarized as follows. rCBF remained above 55% of normal in patients with TIA, i.e. when there was no tissue destruction. Cortical tissue became necrotic in areas, where rCBF was less than 30% (about 12 ml/100 g per minute) and/or CMRO$_2$ less than 40% of normal. In the peri-infarct zone with rCBF 30–45% of normal (or about 12–18 ml/100 g per minute) during the first 2 days, metabolic functions were unstable and infarction occurred if low flow values persisted. Tissue recovery occurred only in such peri-infarct zones, where misery perfusion was associated with CMRO$_2$ above a critical threshold level, i.e. such a peri-infarct zone represents penumbral tissue. Heiss *et al.*[205] compared early CBF values (measured with PET within 3 h after the onset of the stroke) with the final

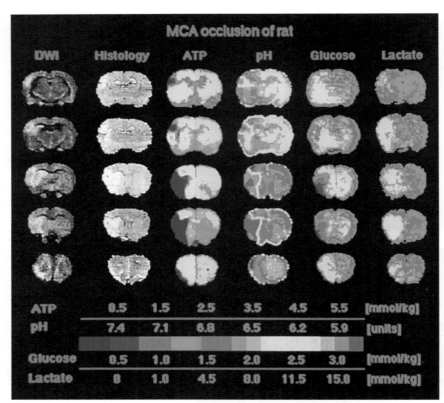

MCA occlusion of rat						
ATP	0.5	1.5	2.5	3.5	4.5	5.5	[mmol/kg]
pH	7.4	7.1	6.8	6.5	6.2	5.9	[units]
Glucose	0.5	1.0	1.5	2.0	2.5	3.0	[mmol/kg]
Lactate	0	1.0	4.5	8.0	11.5	15.0	[mmol/kg]

Figure 6.38 *Focal experimental ischaemic stroke. Colour-coded presentation of an early evolving infarct 7 h after middle cerebral artery occlusion in a rat. Diffusion-weighted magnetic resonance image (DWI) reveals the infarct in vivo as a pale area. Metabolic analysis of frozen sections of the same brain demonstrates a decrease in ATP and glucose concentration and lowering of pH parallel to the increase in lactate concentration in the infarct. Reproduced by permission from Ref. 23.*

infarct outlined on MRI. These revealed that initial penumbral tissue accounted for about 18% and initially sufficiently perfused tissue for about 12% of the final infarct volume, which could be interpreted as later enlargement and deterioration of the penumbra.

The development of high-resolution PET[202,539] made possible sequential analysis of the various physiological parameters of brain energy metabolism during the entire ischaemic episode in smaller experimental animals such as the cat (Fig. 6.37). Using such sequential multitracer PET scanning, Heiss *et al.*[202] demonstrated in the cat the interdependence of haemodynamic and metabolic events in the penumbra. They repeatedly measured rCBF, blood volume, OEF, $CMRO_2$ and $CMRO_{glc}$, and finally determined the infarct size on serial histological sections (Fig. 6.37). CBF in the core area was reduced to critical levels immediately after occlusion of the MCA. Around the core, in areas with reduced rCBF, $CMRO_2$ and $CMRO_{glc}$ remained relatively preserved and OEF was increased, i.e. this state corresponded to the misery perfusion described above. When the core of infarction expanded, defined as the area where the low rCBF became associated with low $CMRO_2$ and secondarily decreased OEF, the penumbral areas of increased OEF moved from the centre towards the periphery of the ischaemic territory as a sign of their dynamic nature. In contrast, in one animal with only transient misery perfusion indicated by later normalization of OEF, $CMRO_2$ and $CMRO_{glc}$, the infarct was of minimal size, demonstrating the viability of the penumbral tissue (Fig. 6.37). These findings verified that the sequence of events,

which had been deduced from single examinations in man at different poststroke time intervals, was correct.[28] These results also validated the present definition of penumbra as a dynamic zone around the core of an infarct. In penumbra, neurons are still viable but at risk of becoming recruited into the irreversibly injured core, which is continuously changing as the infarct evolves.[202]

Multiple pathogenetic processes occur in the penumbral zone when it becomes recruited into the evolving infarct.[461] These have been considered to cause 'molecular' injury as opposed to 'haemodynamic' injury in the infarct core.[270] The ischaemic core may evoke the spreading of repeated nerve cell depolarizations caused by excessive release of K^+ and excitatory amino acids (glutamate and aspartate)[213] from ischaemically injured neurons in the infarct core. The repeated depolarizations exhaust the already marginal energy supplies and thereby lead to transformation of hitherto non-lethal injury into an irreversible one, i.e. the infarct core serves as the centre for propagation of excitotoxic nerve cell injury[220] (for details see Chapter 5, this Volume). This interpretation is supported by therapeutic trials using either agents which decrease presynaptic release of excitatory amino acids or antagonists to glutamate receptors [both *N*-methyl-D-aspartate (NMDA) and α-amino-3-hydroxy-5-methyl-4-isoxazolepropionic acid (AMPA) type]: the frequency of perifocal depolarizations, the cortical volume with adenosine triphosphate (ATP) depletion or the infarct size were significantly reduced.[227,345,466] These agents seem to have real neuroprotective effects on penumbral neurons, since blood flow to the ischaemic region did not increase.[320,390] The microcirculation in the penumbral zone may also become progressively impaired. Since the penumbra lies next to irreversibly injured tissue, reactive inflammatory changes can occur in the subnormally perfused penumbral microvessels, which become secondarily shut down by a no-reflow process. This includes direct occlusion of capillaries by leukocytes or platelet aggregates adhering to endothelium, which is stimulated by ischaemia to express adhesion molecules and additional proinflammatory factors.[107,288] Finally, nitrous oxide (NO) rapidly increases in ischaemic cortex after MCA occlusion.[325] The cytotoxic effect of NO has been proposed to be due to inhibition of various enzymes of cellular respiration, oxidation of sulfydryl groups in proteins, nitration of DNA or formation of NO-based free radicals.[34,103]

The penumbral neurons at risk also activate their own defence mechanisms. Protein synthesis is suppressed at a relatively high threshold level of CBF, but the suppression appears to be selective and the proteins produced during ischaemia in the penumbral zone, e.g. protein products of immediate-early genes and heat shock/stress proteins, are considered to have an important, protective role (for details see Chapter 5, this Volume). The protective effect of NO molecules is brought about by their vasodilatory effect, which increases the blood flow in the penumbral area and decreases the volume of the infarct.[555] The opposite effects of NO reported in the literature have been explained by the site of action: in the vascular compartment NO has positive and in the parenchyma negative effects on FCI.

Utilization of PET in human stroke has several limitations. Therefore, simpler and more rapid methods were needed to detect penumbra and define relevant targets for therapy. The new modality of diffusion-weighted MRI (DWI) has made possible the detection of early (within a few minutes) ischaemic changes in vivo[23,137,165] and, when combined with perfusion MRI (PI), the presence of penumbral tissue at risk can be inferred and predictions made about the progression of the infarct (see below).[28] DWI offers a non-invasive method to detect ischaemic membrane failure, because it is considered to measure diffusion of protons of water molecules within different tissue compartments, including influx of water into the intracellular space, i.e. development of cytotoxic oedema as it occurs in ischaemia.[36] DWI changes also closely correlated with irreversibility of the ischaemic insult, both metabolically and histopathologically, validating DWI as a relevant indicator of acute infarction (Fig. 6.38).[23] However, recent human data have suggested that DWI lesion can also be reversed if reperfusion is achieved by thrombolysis very early after the onset of ischaemia. This indicates that a DWI lesion develops very rapidly and may partially represent salvageable ischaemic penumbra.[269]

Another MRI modality, PI makes use of the signal loss during the first pass of an intravenously administered paramagnetic contrast agent, on the basis of which relative CBF and blood volume can be calculated. Parallel assessment of DWI and PI has made possible concomitant identification of an infarct and perfusion in the ischaemic region. If the region of impaired perfusion at the moment of imaging is greater than the volume of infarct, the penumbral tissue around the infarct will be recruited to the infarct core unless CBF is restored. Thus, DWI and PI together provide rapid MRI techniques for determination of the potentially salvageble penumbral tissue in human stroke.[28]

REPERFUSION IN FOCAL CEREBRAL ISCHAEMIA

The best protective measure against tissue damage in FCI is natural reperfusion and restoration of normal aerobic energy production. For example, the Ca^{2+} antagonist nimodipine decreases the infarct volume by increasing rCBF.[351] Incomplete restoration of blood flow after prolonged ischaemic episodes of GCI is a well-known no-reflow phenomenon.[9] Its role in experimental FCI has been addressed more recently. Presumed causes of 'no-reflow' in GCI, such as endothelial swelling, perivascular oedema and increased blood viscosity may also occur in FCI. However, the main interest has been directed to the role of the intravascular inflammatory and clotting factors, which may significantly impede blood flow. Polymorphonuclear (PMN) leukocytes have been found to occlude the lumen of microvessels in perfusion-fixed animals, and analysis of the patency of microvessels by infusion of indian ink has revealed filling defects compatible with actual blockade of the lumen and flow hindrance.[108] It has been further demonstrated that the PMN leukocytes exploit their surface adhesion molecules to bind to endothelium, since antibody to CD18, the β-chain of the principal PMN leukocyte adhesion molecule CD11b/CD18 of the integrin superfamily, was able to inhibit the adherence and improve reperfusion, most significantly in non-capillary microvessels.[357] The ischaemic injury also stimulates endothelial expression of the ligands for leukocyte binding, e.g. intercellular adhesion molecule-1 (ICAM-1, the ligand of the CD11b/CD18), and P-selectin, an adhesion glycoprotein from the selectin superfamily.[380] P-selectin is also involved in clot formation, being expressed on platelets and promoting deposition of fibrin. Finally, the extrinsic coagulation system also seems to be involved, since infusion of an antibody against a key molecule in the extrinsic pathway of the coagulation cascade, tissue factor (see Fig. 6.33) increased reflow after 3 h of MCA occlusion in baboons.[494] Activation of the coagulation cascade may be even more likely in human stroke, where the artery is usually obstructed by a thrombotic mass instead of a suture or clip and the endothelium is often primarily injured, e.g. by atherosclerosis. The significance of these results in the pathogenesis and therapy of human stroke is still unknown.

Even successful reperfusion after FCI carries risks, especially if there is an increase in oxygen in excess of consumption, which may result in the formation of highly reactive oxygen free radicals, lipid peroxidation, protein oxidation and damage of DNA.[84] The production of such toxic free radicals has been considered to be possible even during the ischaemic period with low tissue oxygen, e.g. in the penumbra with misery perfusion.[462] These latter free radicals are possibly not oxygen related, as suggested by experiments using MCA occlusion in transgenic mice, which overexpress an enzyme that scavenges oxygen radicals, human CuZn-superoxide dismutase (CuZn-SOD).[84] In permanent FCI the overexpression of CuZn-SOD did not decrease the size of infarction,[85] whereas in FCI followed by reperfusion the extent of tissue damage was significantly reduced.[549]

FINAL OUTCOME OF FOCAL CEREBRAL ISCHAEMIA

After MCA occlusion in rats measurements of CBF showed that the transition from poorly to adequately perfused tissue is relatively abrupt. Similarly, the transition from infarct to surviving tissue in histopathological sections is surprisingly sharp. Around the core of infarction after MCA occlusion, there is only a narrow zone in which the transition from complete loss of neurons into tissue with a normal number of neurons occurs.[366] Similarly, the zone with selective neuronal necrosis and preservation of glial cells is also narrower than would be expected on the basis of the difference between neuronal and glial vulnerability to ischaemia.[501]

FOCAL CEREBRAL ISCHAEMIA AND INFARCTION IN CLINICAL PRACTICE

Transient ischaemic attack

In focal cerebral ischaemia the blood flow through an artery is compromised to such an extent that the tissue in its supply territory becomes ischaemic. In its mildest form the impaired regional CBF causes a TIA. This has an abrupt onset but is a rapidly diminishing neurological deficit of vascular origin which lasts for less than 24 h. The cause of

TIA in most cases is small emboli from extracranial sources, either cardiac or from atherosclerotic plaques in the carotid or vertebrobasilar arteries. Occasionally TIA has a haemodynamic cause, e.g. a regional flow deficit beyond a stenosed artery during transient hypotension.

Stroke and infarction

When the ischaemia is severe enough and lasts for long enough, permanent nerve cell damage ensues and if it results in a clinically detectable functional deficit it is called a 'stroke'. It has been recently re-emphasized that the ischaemia of moderate severity and/or of short duration can cause only selective necrosis of neurons, i.e. an incomplete infarction, instead of pan-necrosis of all tissue components, i.e. a full-blown infarction. The preservation of non-neuronal tissue components may make detection of incomplete infarction impossible or at least difficult, even with best imaging methods.[153]

The National Institute of Neurological Disease and Stroke (NINDS) Stroke Data Bank[437] has established the relative incidences of different causes of ischaemic insults leading to infarction exploiting all the new technologies available in highly specialized centres, e.g. magnetic resonance angiography in addition to conventional angiography, echocardiography and duplex Doppler sonography. With stringent criteria the causes of infarction have been classified as follows: (1) atherothrombotic group with two subgroups, (1A) large artery thrombosis and (1B) artery-to-artery embolism both of which have an atherosclerotic background; (2) cardioembolic group; (3) lacunar infarcts. The limitations of even the most advanced techniques have been acknowledged by creating the additional category of (4) infarcts of undetermined cause. The relative frequencies of the subtypes of infarcts are given in Table 6.4.

This classification demonstrates that the pathogenesis of vascular occlusions of large and medium-sized arteries differs from that of small arteries. In infarcts of known

Table 6.4 Relative frequencies of symptomatic stroke and infarcts[a] and incidence rates[b] according to subtypes of stroke

Subtype	'Strokes' (%)	Infarcts (%)	Infarction[b]
Infarction	68.6		
Atherothrombotic, large artery thrombosis	6.1	8.9	All 27, F 12, M 47
Atherothrombotic, artery-to-artery embolism	3.8	5.4	
Cardioembolic	13.2	19.3	All 40, F 37, M 42
Lacunar	18.1	26.6	All 25, F 22, M 29
Undetermined cause	27.4	39.9	All 52, F 50, M 51
Total (infarcts)		100.0	All 147, F 124, M 173
Haemorrhage	28.6		
Intracerebral	13.1		
Subarachnoid	13.5		
Other	2.8		
Total (all strokes)	100.0		

[a]In Stroke Data Bank of National Institute of Neurological Disorders and Stroke (adapted from Ref. 437).
[b]Age- and sex-adjusted incidence rates per 100 000 from Ref. 400. F, female; M, male.

cause, the lumen of intracranial large to medium-sized arteries is most commonly occluded by an embolus. Using the strict criteria of the Stroke Data Bank the frequency of locally formed thrombi in these arteries has proven to be much lower than previously estimated. In contrast, the small intraparenchymal penetrating arteries are most often occluded by a local process: thrombosis of a diseased small artery, microatheroma or occlusion of the origin of a penetrator by an atherosclerotic plaque. Furthermore, the presence of microemboli in retinal arteries has been presented as an indirect proof that they may also enter intracerebral penetrating arteries of corresponding small calibre.[347] The improved resolution of imaging methods has made the identification of small lacunar infarcts possible, so their relative frequency in the more recent statistics has increased markedly. Lacunar infarcts are now clearly the most common category of infarcts, and even though many are asymptomatic they are also the most commonly identified cause of stroke (Table 6.4).

Atherothrombotic, large artery thrombosis

Atherosclerosis is usually most severe in the extracranial carotid arteries, but it can involve the intracranial large and, in severe cases, also the medium-sized arteries, particularly when the aggravating effect of hypertension is superimposed (Fig. 6.6b). The atherosclerotic plaques serve as sites of thrombosis, when the endothelium has become ulcerated and/or stenosis has reduced the blood flow to such an extent that a thrombus can develop. Stenosis of greater than 90–95% severity may as such, under circumstances of decreased cerebral perfusion pressure, be sufficient to cause infarction on the basis of haemodynamic failure, a situation that is very difficult to verify *in vivo* and virtually impossible post-mortem.

Thromboembolic and related strokes

The Stroke Data Bank has separated embolic strokes into two categories: (1) strokes due to artery-to-artery embolism, and (2) cardioembolic strokes. Even though the emboli to the intracerebral arteries from the extracranial arteries or heart most often have identical pathological consequences, the clinical distinction is important, since the therapeutic strategies are different.[72]

Artery-to-artery embolism. Emboli breaking loose from thrombi formed on atherosclerotic often ulcerated lesions in the extracranial arteries may contain, in addition to coagulated blood and platelets, cholesterol and calcified particles from the underlying atheromatous plaque. The thrombus formed in severely stenosed arteries with reduced flow is usually of the fibrin-dependent red variety, whereas in arteries with brisker flow white platelet–fibrin thrombi are deposited on rough, sclerotic, often ulcerated surfaces. The artery-to-artery emboli into the anterior cerebral circulation most commonly arise from the vicinity of the bifurcation of the common carotid artery, and the emboli showering into the

posterior circulation originate in the vertebral arteries, either in the neck or within the cranial cavity.

Cardioembolic strokes. The causes and nature of emboli arising from the heart are manifold. Among the most common are fragments of thrombi formed because of atrial fibrillation or myocardial infarction (about 45% or 15% of cardioembolic strokes, respectively), in which cases the emboli are usually 'red clots'. Other common causes are emboli detaching from thrombi formed on damaged or prosthetic valves (10%) or cardiomyopathy and ventricular aneurysm (7.5%), and the less common ones include emboli from marantic vegetations of non-bacterial thrombotic endocarditis and paradoxical emboli via patent foramen ovale.[545] The emboli formed on valves are often of the white platelet and fibrin variety, and fragments of emboli from calcified valves frequently contain calcium precipitates.

Paradoxical emboli enter the arterial side of the heart from the venous circulation through a patent foramen ovale in the cardiac septum, usually during a temporary rise in the right cardiac chamber pressure (Valsalva manoeuvre) in association with conditions that favour venous thrombosis, e.g. phlebitis and recent surgery or delivery. With modern ultrasound methods, most effectively by using microbubbles in intravenously injected agitated saline as the contrast medium, a patent foramen ovale and paradoxical embolism have been shown to be more common than previously thought. However, the high prevalence of 25–30% in the general population indicates that patent foramen ovale in a stroke patient is not necessarily causative.[545] The frequency of a patent foramen was found to be higher in patients with stroke than in controls (40% vs 10%)[298] and in a French study paradoxical emboli comprised no less than 12.8% of all embolic strokes,[158] although a considerably lower figure (3.7%) was reported in an earlier American study.[39] Thus, the possibility of paradoxical emboli should be seriously considered in patients with embolic stroke without an apparent cause.

The distribution of cardiogenic thromboemboli fairly closely corresponds to the amount of blood that each major intracerebral artery receives from the heart. Therefore, the greatest numbers of these emboli lodge in the middle cerebral arteries. The carotid artery, even its common segment, may also be obstructed by a large embolus and approximately one-fifth of internal carotid artery occlusions are embolic.[72] Cardiogenic thrombi may also find their way to the posterior circulation, for example, they have accounted for 28.5% or 55% of infarcts in the territory of a posterior cerebral artery or superior cerebellar artery, respectively.[260,398]

Other embolic strokes

Tumour emboli. Emboli may also be composed of tumour cells, which either detach from a neoplasm located within the cardiovascular system or proliferate free in the circulating blood. The best known of these is cardiac myxoma, which is most often located in the left atrium. This tumour has a marked propensity to embolize, and embolic complications including neurological deficits are the presenting symptoms in about one-third of the patients. Cardiac myxoma occurs in two settings: sporadic tumour is most common among middle-aged female patients, whereas familial tumours occur most often in younger patients.[197] Intravascular malignant lymphomatosis (IML) is another 'embolizing' neoplasm, in which clusters of malignant lymphoid cells proliferating in the circulating blood may cause severe obstruction of CNS blood vessels and result in small focal infarcts both in the brain (Fig. 6.39a, b) and the spinal cord.

Fat embolism. Destruction of fat-containing tissues, e.g. in fractures of bones (bone marrow), pancreatitis, burns, and trauma to viscera or subcutaneous tissue, may lead to the formation of fat emboli, not uncommonly detectable in the lungs of such patients. For example, symptomatic fat embolism ensues in up to 2.2% of patients with fractures of long bones. After trauma, fat from the marrow of the fractured bone or from other traumatized adipose tissue enters the venous circulation, facilitated by an increased tissue pressure at the site of trauma.[361] In non-traumatic fat embolism factors that destabilize plasma lipids have been incriminated. Such factors, e.g. stress-induced neurohumoral substances or C-reactive protein, which agglutinates chylomicrons,[224] promote coalescence of fat into larger globules. If the number of blood-borne fat globules becomes so great that the trapping capacity of the pulmonary capillaries is exceeded, or if they bypass the lungs via a patent foramen ovale or pulmonary arteriovenous shunts,[122] the fat particles can enter the systemic circulation, including the cerebral arteries. The blockade of microvessels in the brain causes global cerebral ischaemia, which is aggravated by hypoxaemia due to pulmonary dysfunction. The BBB is disrupted and the vascular damage is often so extensive that petechial haemorrhages supervene.

The neurological symptoms include confusion, delirious restlessness, seizures, impairment of cognitive function and decreased levels of consciousness including coma, which usually appear 12–72 h after the injury.[361] CT scans may show diffuse brain oedema and focal low-density areas, but they may also be normal. MRI is considered to be more sensitive than CT, revealing scattered spotty areas of low and/or high intensity on T1-weighted images, and of high intensity on T2-weighted images. Definite proof of the cerebral hypoperfusion may be achieved by SPECT imaging.[120] Remarkable, even complete recovery is possible, but the reported mortality rates are high, varying from 13 to 87%. However, the underlying life-threatening disease makes it difficult to estimate the prognosis of fat embolism *per se*.[361]

The neuropathology of cerebral fat embolism has been reviewed by Kamenar and Burger.[254] Macroscopically, the brains of patients who died acutely after the onset of fat embolism may appear unremarkable, but usually oedema appears fairly rapidly. Multifocal petechial perivascular

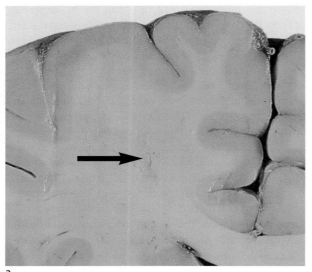

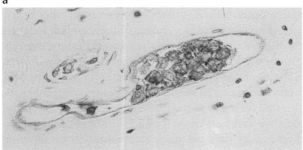

b

Figure 6.39 *(a) A small infarct (arrow) is seen in the white matter of a woman with intravascular malignant lymphomatosis, which had caused diffuse symptoms of encephalopathy. (b) Microscopically, the cause of the infarct was found to be an accumulation of malignant lymphoid cells within the lumen of a small artery. ((b) Antileukocyte common antigen and haematoxylin counterstain.)*

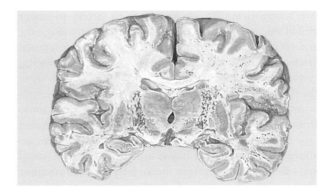

Figure 6.40 *Brain of a patient with acute pancreatitis, who subsequently developed generalized convulsions and became unconscious followed by cardiovascular collapse. He died within a couple of hours after the onset of the neurological symptoms. In the brain there are numerous small petachial haemorrhages, predominantly in the white matter. Courtesy of Dr H Aho, Turku University Central Hospital, Finland.*

haemorrhages predominate in the white matter (Fig. 6.40), a characteristic finding in patients surviving for several days, yet a similar picture may occur in some other conditions, e.g. hypoxic–ischaemic encephalopathy, acute haemorrhagic leukoencephalitis, malaria, air embolism and carbon monoxide intoxication. The diagnosis should be confirmed microscopically in frozen sections by demonstrating globules of neutral fat within microvessels surrounded by extravasated blood. Fat emboli may also cause perivascular anaemic microinfarcts, which are best seen with myelin stains. In long-term survivors there may be gross white matter atrophy. The grey matter is usually spared, even though its microvessels are also plugged by fat globules. They are more common in the blood vessels of the grey matter than in the white matter. The greater anastomotic potential of the grey matter vasculature has been offered as the most likely explanation for this discrepancy.[254]

Air embolism. The pathogenesis and consequences of air embolism and decompression sickness are described in Chapter 5, this Volume.

Lacunae and lacunar infarcts

Lacune was defined in 1901 by Pierre Marie as 'a cavity as a result of a healed infarct resulting from obstruction or rupture of a small perforating artery, most commonly in the lenticular nucleus'. Lacunar infarcts became a thoroughly analysed entity through the extensive studies of CM Fisher.[132,352] These studies gave rise to the concept that small lacunar infarcts (Fig. 6.41a, b) are responsible for specific types of stroke with focal neurological symptoms such as pure motor or sensory stroke, the dysarthria–clumsy hand syndrome and ataxia–hemiparesis. The underlying pathological substrates of these syndromes were lacunes, small trabeculated cavities, remnants of small infarcts ranging in diameter from 0.5 to 15 mm. These were suggested to be caused by occlusion of small arteries, diseased by lipohyalinosis, the main cause of which was considered to be hypertension.[132,199,352]

With the present high resolution of modern imaging methods, it has become possible to detect these small cavities by CT and MRI scans. They are defined as sharply defined areas with diameter of less than 15 mm corresponding to the territory of a single perforating artery (Fig. 6.41a).[338] Although they are often called lacunar infarcts, their aetiology cannot be conclusively determined *intra vitam*, although the clinical and radiological data most often agree with the eventual neuropathological findings (Fig. 6.41a, b). However, lacunar lesions may, in addition to infarction, have a variety of other aetiologies, including haemorrhage, infection and neoplasm.[81,271,347] Therefore, it would be preferable to use the general term lacune to describe all such lesions. Only if the clinical picture or the pathological findings allow determination of the cause of a lacune should the designation be more specific, e.g. lacunar infarct or lacunar haemorrhage. A

classification into lacunes into three types (type I, lacunar infarcts; type II, lacunar haemorrhages; type III, dilated perivascular spaces) has been suggested,[404] but the numerical designations are not in general use. In fact the verbal terms are suitably descriptive. Recently, an additional entity of incomplete lacunar infarction (type Ib) was suggested to exist and to be added to this classification.[294] It is the small counterpart of 'full-size' incomplete infarction, in which selective neuronal necrosis instead of pan-necrosis of all tissue components takes place.[153]

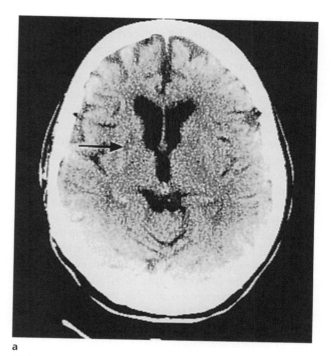

a

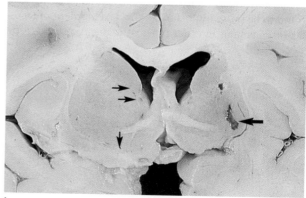

b

Figure 6.41 *Lacunar infarct. (a) CT scan of an 82-year-old female with longstanding arterial hypertension, who has a small lacune in the right basal ganglia (arrow), which had been symptomless. The patient died acutely of a large fresh atherothrombotic infarct in the territory of the left middle cerebral artery, which appears hypodense in this scan. (b) The lacunar change seen on the CT scan was verified as a lacunar infarct (thick arrow) elongated in the direction of the lenticulostriate perforating arteries. There are also perivascular cavities (thin arrows), best visible in the left caudate nucleus.*

Small perivascular cavities up to a couple of millimetres in diameter are a very common finding in the basal ganglia and deep white matter of elderly subjects (Fig. 6.41b). When these cavities are numerous the condition is called état lacunaire in the grey matter and état criblé in the deep white matter.[199] It is impossible to completely exclude the possibility that a cavity surrounding a central thickened blood vessel could be the remnant of a tiny complete or even incomplete lacunar infarct. However, since these perivascular cavities lack the definitive structural features of an infarct the alternative explanation[97] may be more likely, i.e. they are 'the result of spiralled elongation of small intracerebral arteries' in hypertensives (Figs 6.41b, 6.42). In these patients the small-artery alterations (e.g. due to hypertension) may lead to BBB leakage with chronic local vasogenic oedema, which by 'softening' the perivascular parenchyme would contribute to the cavitation. To avoid confusion, these perivascular empty spaces should perhaps be called (in accordance with the original interpretation of Durand-Fardel)[199] simply perivascular cavities instead of lacunes, and the condition with multiple alterations cavitary state (or état cavitaire).

Lacunar strokes and infarcts identified in vivo by high-resolution imaging[132,352] have been at the centre of active research and debate.[41,132,338,347,352] There seems to be good agreement that small infarcts with a diameter up to 15 mm are caused by occlusion of the perforating arteries with diameters between 100 and 200 μm. Originally, Fisher[132,199] claimed that the principal cause of 97% of lacunes was longstanding hypertension and that they were not related to carotid artery disease, cerebral embolism or diabetes mellitus. Several studies have, however, demonstrated that lacunar infarcts are associated with hypertension in only 24–75% of cases.[347] Furthermore, hypertension was not found to be more important in the development of lacunar infarcts than in other types of ischaemic stroke pre-

sumed to be due to atherosclerotic thromboembolism.[312] On the contrary, in a very large patient population from Japan lacunar infarcts were about three times more frequent in hypertensive than in normotensive patients. The likely cause of lacunar infarcts, also called 'infarcts limited to the territory of deep perforator',[41] was found to be small-artery disease alone in only 44% of the cases.[42] The proposal that lacunar infarcts have two different underlying pathophysiologies offers one explanation for this discrepancy. Single symptomatic lacunar infarcts, to which the usual risk factors apply, are presumably due to microemboli or microatheromatosis, whereas multiple, usually asymptomatic lacunar infarcts are due to arteriolosclerosis (lipohyalinosis) caused by hypertension and hyperinsulinism.[44,338]

The ultimate mechanism by which the lumen of the perforating small arteries is occluded has remained elusive, because lacunar stroke is usually non-lethal and, thus, direct proof at the critical time and site cannot be obtained. In addition, the laborious task of detailed post-mortem histopathological analyses has not been very attractive. Embolic occlusion is likely to be one of the mechanisms,[347] and the extracranial arteries and heart have been considered potential sources of emboli in 17–23% and 11–13% of lacunar infarcts, respectively.[42] Stenosis of the intracranial parent artery of the perforator supplying the infarct has been verified angiographically.[42] Microatheroma of the perforators has been considered the most common cause by some authors,[352] but the rapid onset of the 'stroke' makes either a superimposed thrombus or an intramural haemorrhage a likely adjuvant,[347] which would probably also be required when the lumen is slowly narrowed by arteriolosclerosis (lipohyalinosis).

Since the perforators are end arteries all the tissue of their cylinder-shaped territory is usually damaged (Fig. 6.41b). The ischaemic parenchyma undergoes the same sequence of changes as in larger infarcts, but the end-stage of a cystic remnant is much more rapidly achieved.

Arterial spasm

Focal ischaemia may develop in the territories of healthy intracerebral arteries, when a spastic contraction of the smooth-muscle cells reduces the arterial lumen to such a degree that the blood flow becomes insufficient. Since this is a common complication of subarachnoid haemorrhage, it is described in detail below.

CELLULAR CHANGES IN CEREBRAL ISCHAEMIA

Recanalization

The knowledge of what happens to the thrombus or thromboembolus that obstructs an artery in stroke patients is poor, the evidence being largely incidental rather than based on systematic follow-up. Approximately 20% of embolic (cardiac or artery-to-artery) MCA occlusions may recanalize spontaneously within 24 h, and

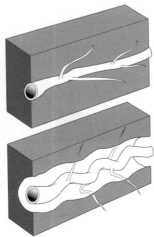

Figure 6.42 *Perivascular cavities. Diagram illustrating the changes in intracerebral arteries that bring about the condition of perivascular cavities; elongation, dilatation and spiralling of the artery with distortion of branches and separation from brain tissue.*

up to 80% may do so within 1 week.[128,530,554] The former figure does not include TIAs, but the disappearance of the symptoms within 24 h makes it necessary that rapid recanalization is achieved in the majority of those TIAs caused by small thromboemboli.

Evolution of infarcts

The transient nature of the neurological deficit in TIAs indicates that the neurons in the affected territory have not been permanently damaged but rather have reached the threshold of transmission failure. However, patients with TIA may have small infarcts on CT and MRI examinations if symptoms last for more than 4–5 h. Detailed clinicopathological correlative studies have not yet been performed, and the non-specific nature of the imaging findings leaves uncertainty.

The natural history of evolving brain infarcts follows a fairly constant time course:

Sequence of microscopical changes in brain infarcts

1 h:	microvacuoles within neurons (swollen mitochondria) followed by perineuronal vacuolation (swollen astrocytic processes);
4–12 h:	neuronal cytoplasm becomes increasingly eosinophilic, Nissl bodies disappear, nucleus becomes pyknotic and nucleoli are no more visible. BBB begins to leak;
15–24 h:	neutrophil leukocyte infiltration begins;
2 days:	macrophages (foam cells) appear. In larger infarcts these cells may be present for months;
5 days:	neutrophil leukocyte infiltration ceases;
Around 1 week:	proliferation of astrocytes around the core infarct begins.

The earliest way to visualize ischaemic necrosis appears to be DWI, which can detect apparent differences between normal and ischaemic tissue within minutes, whereas standard MRI can identify the increased water content, cytotoxic oedema, in the injured tissue within 6–12 h.[137] In post-mortem examination, infarction cannot be detected with the naked eye until about 12 h have elapsed from its onset. In unfixed brain it may take 24 h to become evident, but when the brain is properly fixed the infarct can be best delineated by palpation, because the necrotic tissue does not become fixed and gives a 'velvety' touch, which contrasts with the firmer consistency of non-necrotic fixed tissue. Visually, the smudging of the boundary between the grey and white matter is one of the earliest signs. Microscopically, the earliest and most characteristic hallmark is the eosinophilic neurons with pyknotic nuclei, 'red neurons' (Fig. 6.43a), visible after about 4 h. They are detectable by the traditional H&E staining, but with acid fuchsin these neurons stand out more prominently. The inflammatory reaction begins with

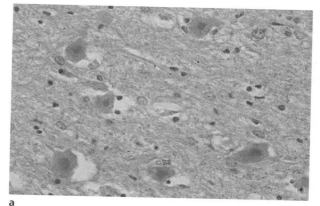

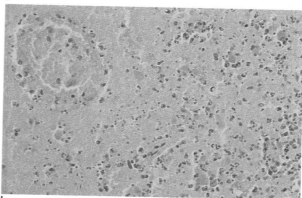

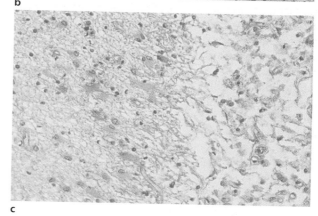

Figure 6.43 *Ischaemic infarct. (a) In acute ischaemic nerve cell injury the cytoplasm of the injured thalamic neurons stains bright red and their nuclei are pyknotic and have lost their characteristic nucleoli. (b) On the second day after the insult neutrophil leukocytes have invaded the infarct, where necrotic neurons appear as eosinophilic ghosts. (c) After 2 months the necrotic tissue has been removed by macrophages and transformed into a cyst, in which some lipid-containing macrophages are still present (on the right). The cystic cavity is bounded by reactive gemistocytic astrocytes. (H&E.)*

invasion of neutrophils, the earliest of which arrive by 15 h and in more significant numbers by 24 h (Fig. 6.43b); these are followed by entry of blood-derived phagocytes at 3 days. Reactive astrocytes begin to surround the necrotic tissue after 1 week, by which time the increased density of capillaries also becomes apparent. Phagocytosis of the tissue debris, visible as pools of foam or 'gitter' cells, may be apparent for months to years in large infarcts (Fig. 6.43c). The end result is a cavity lined by astrocytes and filled with clear fluid (see Fig. 6.29).

Ultrastructurally, ischaemic nerve cell injury was established in the classic studies of Brown and Brierley,[59] who used a model of global ischaemia combined with hypoxia in rats. The earliest morphological change in the sequence of 'ischaemic cell change' is the swelling of mitochondria, which renders the neurons microvacuolated. At the same time the cytoplasm of these neurons begins to condense to become electron dense, the nucleus becomes pyknotic with coarse chromatin, and the nucleoli disappear. These neurons correspond to the light-microscopic 'red neurons'. Swelling of astrocytes results in perineuronal and perivascular vacuolation.[59,152] An early sign of ischaemia in astrocytes is the clumping of the normally finely stippled chromatin due to the lowered pH. The difference between the structural changes in incomplete and/or temporary ischaemia (a condition that always prevails in focal ischaemia) as opposed to complete and/or permanent ischaemia was delineated in the late 1970s:[152,237,252] the classic dark ischaemically injured neurons with microvacuolation appeared only when the injured neurons were irrigated either during or after the ischaemic period by a trickle of blood flow, complete permanent ischaemia giving rise to pale, swollen neurons. In focal ischaemia the neurons in the central core undergo damage that is more akin to that in complete permanent ischaemia, possibly because the remaining blood flow is too low to allow the dark type of change to occur. The pathogenic mechanism of the dark injury has remained uncertain. It may be, for example, that the dark type of ischaemic nerve cell change reflects apoptosis, recently reported at the periphery of the infarct.[305] Alternatively, collapse of the cytoskeleton may possibly occur in ischaemically injured neurons, allowing condensation of the damaged neurons. For example, an early and marked degradation of a cytoskeletal protein, spectrin, by proteolytic enzymes has been reported after MCA occlusion,[550] the degradation of which can be markedly attenuated by administration of inhibitors of cytoplasmic calpain, a class of calcium-dependent cysteine proteases.[216]

Haemorrhagic infarction

On the basis of autopsy studies the frequency of haemorrhagic infarcts varies from 18 to 48%.[56,134] In a recent *in vivo* study of patients with first-time infarct haemorrhagic transformation was found in 14.9% of the patients by imaging (CT or MRI) within 7–10 days.[359] The majority of haemorrhagic infarcts are embolic arterial strokes: 51–71% of these become haemorrhagic compared with only 2–21% of non-embolic strokes.[313,395]

Two generally accepted mechanisms by which an infarct becomes haemorrhagic are (1) reperfusion of necrotic, leaking blood vessels, and (2) occlusion of venous drainage (see below). Reperfusion occurs when the embolus has been broken down by fibrinolytic enzymes, either naturally or by modern thrombolytic therapy.[529,530] Haemorrhagic infarction has been considered to carry a higher risk of clinical deterioration, but the small punctate (type I) haemorrhages do not result in an increased neurological deficit.[395] Clinicians know that non-anticoagulated 'stroke' patients with CT-verified haemorrhagic transformation of their infarct are either stable or clinically improving in a large majority of cases. Larger intraparenchymal (type II) haemorrhages, which are associated with clinical worsening of the patient's neurological status, occur less frequently. Their incidence is about 8% of all embolic infarcts[395] and 6.5% of all ischaemic hemispheric infarcts.[187a]

LEUKOARAIOSIS, BINSWANGER'S DISEASE AND MULTI-INFARCT DEMENTIA

Leukoaraiosis was introduced as a descriptive term for rarefaction of the white matter in radiological imaging (Fig. 6.27a, b),[186] but its use has been confused by associating specific pathogenic connotations with this term. It has multiple pathological counterparts, such as *état criblé*, white matter infarcts, foci of demyelination and vascular malformations. Leukoaraiosis should be used only to describe imaging finding as originally defined and not as a diagnosis for white matter ischaemia.[41]

Patients who suffer from multiple infarcts, commonly in deep parts of the brain and/or white matter, frequently develop a dementing disease, the name of which has evolved from atherosclerotic dementia through multi-infarct dementia to vascular dementia.[187,258] The causes of the infarcts are repeated thrombotic events and/or multiple emboli, which in turn may have various aetiologies such as atherosclerosis, vasculitides, coagulation disturbances, hypertensive angiopathy or certain sporadic or hereditary arteriopathies, e.g. 'classic' Binswanger's disease or CADASIL, both of which have similar pathological changes with patchy infarcts and small, deep-seated lacunar cavities in the white matter and basal ganglia together with thickening of the walls of the penetrant arteries. CADASIL is a genetic disorder with the defect in *Notch3* gene (see above). Binswanger's disease has a controversial causal relationship with hypertension. The symptoms, signs and structural alterations have been considered to be sufficiently specific to justify this disease as a separate clinicopathological entity.[41] Further details of multi-infarct dementias, including Binswanger's disease, are described in association with other dementing diseases in Chapter 4, Volume II.

VENOUS THROMBOSIS AND INFARCTION

Clinical picture and incidence

Cerebral venous thrombosis (CVT): (for anatomy of the venous drainage system, see above) as a cause of serious neurological symptoms and fatal outcome was described in the early nineteenth century.[413] For over a century CVT has been considered to be a rare disease with a fairly characteristic clinical picture of headache, seizures, focal signs, increased intracranial pressure, papilloedema and coma. The prognosis of CVT was considered to be grim, most often fatal, and the diagnosis was usually not established until post-mortem. With the introduction of angiography the concept of CVT began to change.[284] Today, using three-dimensional MR flow imaging[117] it has been shown that CVT is clearly more common and less serious than has been thought previously. The fairly non-specific symptoms, headache and the clinical picture of benign intracranial hypertension should initiate the appropriate imaging examinations (Fig. 6.44).[401] The true incidence of CVT is unknown, because adequate epidemiological studies are lacking.[8] The risk of CVT is considered to be approximately equal for both genders. CVT may occur in all age groups from neonates to old age, but among women there seems to be a peak in younger age groups, which most likely reflects the association of CVT with pregnancy and the use of oral contraceptives.[8,70,116] The fact that milder forms of CVT can now be recognized and a great majority of them recover with recanalization of the thrombosed blood vessel has certainly contributed to the decrease in mortality to 5.5–33%.[8,70,496] Thus, fatal CVT cases are infrequent in neuropathological practice.

Aetiology of venous thromboses

CVT can be caused by a multitude of different conditions. In the past, infections were by far the most common cause of CVT[283] whereas in the most recent large series of 110 cases only 8.2% had an infectious aetiology, the decrease being due to effective antimicrobial and anticoagulant therapy, and improved diagnostics of non-infectious CVTs.[8] The most common site of septic CVT is the cavernous sinus, where *Staphylococcus aureus* spreads from an infection in the middle third of the face, sphenoid or ethmoid air sinus, or a dental abscess. Otitis media and mastoiditis may induce septic thrombosis in the lateral sinus, and infections of the scalp may extend via the diploëic and emissary veins through the skull bone to the sagittal sinus. In immunosuppressed or chronically debilitated persons various opportunistic micro-organisms, including fungi and cytomegalovirus, have been found to be the cause of venous thrombosis.[115,342]

The altered hormonal status in young women during pregnancy, the puerperium or the intake of oral contraceptives is one of the most important non-infectious aetiologies of CVT[8,70,116] e.g. oral contraceptives were recorded as the sole cause in as many patients as infection

(8.2%).[8] Similarly, an altered state of coagulability associated with any surgery or conditions affecting the patient's general health, such as malignancies and malnutrition, predisposes to CVT. Thrombosis may be promoted simply by stagnation of blood flow, e.g. in congenital or congestive heart disease or dehydration. Certain haematological disorders, including thrombocythaemia and sickle cell disease, increase the risk of CVT. Disorders leading to thrombophilia, for example deficiencies of antithrombin III, protein C, protein S or plasminogen,[101,447,455,489] or the presence of acquired factors inducing hypercoagulability, e.g. antiphospholipid antibodies,[302,406] are fairly rare causes but should be considered, particularly when no other obvious cause is found, or in the former group if hereditary factors are suspected. A comprehensive account of the causes has been presented in a recent review.[8]

Pathogenesis and pathology

The cerebral venous network is extensive and there are well-developed collaterals (see above). Therefore, thrombosis must usually be fairly extensive, i.e. occlusion of a sinus or a major part of such, before the outflow channels are restricted to such an extent that the blood flow becomes greatly reduced and hypoxia/ischaemia ensues. Vasogenic oedema forms and it is severely aggravated by the engorgement of blood vessels proximal to the occlusion by the pressure within patent arteries; with more extensive ischaemic injury a haemorrhagic infarction occurs. Thrombolytic therapy in CVT does not carry the same risk of expansion of haemorrhage as in arterial thrombosis, since recanalization leads to lowered pressure in the region of haemorrhagic infarction.

The most common sites of CVT[8] are the superior sagittal sinus (72%; Figs 6.44, 6.45), lateral sinuses (70%

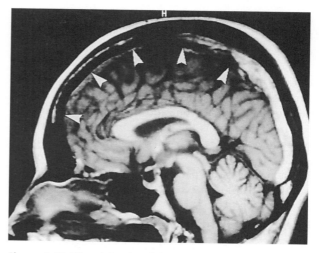

Figure 6.44 *T1-weighted gadolinium-enhanced magnetic resonance (MR) image of a patient with thrombosis of the anterior part of the sagittal sinus (arrowheads). Courtesy of Dr O Salonen, Helsinki University Central Hospital, Finland.*

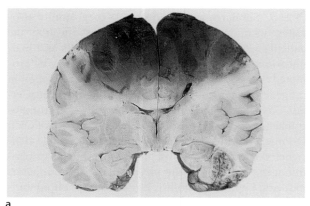

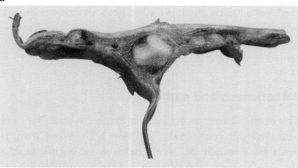

Figure 6.45 *(a) Thrombosis of the superior sagittal sinus has caused haemorrhagic necrosis and intraparenchymal haemorrhage in the parasagittal brain parenchyma. (b) The occluding thrombus is seen within the sinus.*

combined) and straight sinus (13%), but thrombosis commonly extends to several sinuses and/or veins. The anatomical variation of the left lateral sinus may be of importance: its thrombosis may cause infarction of the ipsilateral basal ganglia, if the sinus lacks connection with the confluence of sinuses, and its transverse portion may be hypoplastic, misleading the radiologist to suspect CVT. Localized thrombosis of cerebral veins, especially cortical ones, rarely results in tissue damage, but CVT of the deep internal veins and the great vein of Galen may cause severe damage to the basal ganglia and brainstem.[409]

The best-known pathological findings in CVT are those caused by superior sagittal sinus thrombosis, i.e. parasagittal haemorrhages extending to the white matter, haemorrhagic infarction and marked oedema (Fig. 6.45). Microscopy is the same as in any haemorrhagic infarct (see above) and haemorrhage (see below), but a specific feature appears to be more profuse leukocytic invasion, because the patent arteries allow ready inflow of reactive inflammatory cells.

Intracranial haemorrhages

GENERAL ASPECTS

Intracranial haemorrhage may occur as a result of head injury or asphyxia at birth, or it may be 'spontaneous', i.e.

the underlying cause can only be recognized by appropriate clinical investigations or, in fatal cases, at autopsy. The two main categories of spontaneous intracranial haemorrhage are intracerebral and subarachnoid. Extradural and subdural haemorrhages are virtually always due to trauma, whereas occasionally intracerebral haemorrhage and rarely massive subarachnoid haemorrhage are due to a head injury (see Chapter 14, this Volume). The subependymal and intraventricular haemorrhages in premature infants associated with perinatal hypoxia are described in Chapter 9, this Volume, and haemorrhage within the spinal cord in Chapter 18, this Volume.

INTRACEREBRAL HAEMORRHAGES (ICH)

Epidemiology and topography of ICH

The relative frequencies of ICH among first-time strokes in different populations are shown in Table 6.2. The annual incidence rates in studies based on Caucasian populations usually vary between 11 and 20 (crude) or 16 and 32 (age adjusted) per 100 000.[141] The incidence rate in a mixed population was higher for blacks than for whites, e.g. in Alabama, USA, 12 versus 32 (crude) per 100 000.[181] In Oriental populations ICH is still considerably more common than in African-Americans, the incidence rate being over 60 (crude) per 100 000.[221] In all populations a declining trend was recorded between 1945 and 1975.[149,509] Modern imaging methods have significantly improved *intra vitam* identification of ICHs. It has been claimed that the new imaging methods have revealed small encapsulated haematomas to such an extent that although the number of fatal cases has decreased, the incidence of ICH has remained at about the same level.[57b,500]

The frequency of the six major well-defined causes of ICH is presented in Table 6.5. Hypertension has remained the most important risk factor (for details see below). The relative frequencies of ICH in different anatomical locations are given in Table 6.6.[125] These data apply to the more common larger, and usually single, ICHs, which are also causes of small, petechial haemorrhages (see below).

Table 6.5 *Causes of non-traumatic intracerebral haemorrhage*

Cause	%
Hypertension	50
Cerebral amyloid angiopathy	12
Anticoagulants	10
Tumours	8
Illicit and licit drugs	6
Arteriovenous malformations and aneurysms	5
Miscellaneous	9

Adapted from Ref. 125.

Table 6.6 *Sites of non-traumatic intracerebral haemorrhage*

Haemorrhage	n	%	%	%
Lobar	65	31		
One lobe			46	
Frontal				17
Parietal				11
Temporal				9
Occipital				9
Two lobes			42	
Three lobes			12	
Deep supratentorial	107	51		
Putamen			48	
Thalamus			43	
Caudate			9	
Deep infratentorial	37	18		
Cerebellum			70	
Pons			30	
Total	209	100		

Adapted from Ref. 329.

Supratentorial haemorrhage

The larger ICHs within the hemispheres are commonly divided into lobar haemorrhages, as opposed to deep ones in the basal ganglia and thalamus.[57b,258] The ratio of lobar to deep haemorrhages has been reported to vary between 1:2 and 3:4.[141,155,329] Differences between the lobar and deep ICH were analysed and emphasized in a large patient group of the Stroke Data Bank.[329,437] Lobar and deep haemorrhages differ from each other not only in their location, but also in relative frequency of different causes and clinical picture. Hypertension is most common among patients with deep haemorrhages, occurring in up to 80% compared with 31–55% of patients with lobar haemorrhages. In the latter type CAA, arteriovenous malformations (often of very small size) and leukaemia are more common causes than hypertension.[200,258,329] On average, patients with lobar haemorrhages are 4–9 years older than those with deep haemorrhages (65–68 vs 59–61.5 years),[155,329] and the former are more common in men. Since the hemispheres are more voluminous than the deep nuclei, lobar haemorrhages on average are of larger size than the deep ones. Among the patients in the Stroke Data Bank the majority of the lobar haematomas exceeded 50 ml, whereas most deep ones were smaller than 15 ml.[329] The proximity of the ventricular system to the deep haemorrhages is the likely reason for their relatively greater frequency to extend into the ventricular system.[155,329]

Infratentorial haemorrhage

Cerebellar and brainstem haemorrhages constitute approximately 15–18% of all primary ICHs in Western populations.[141,155,333] However, in Oriental countries their relative frequency appears to vary considerably, e.g. in the

Chinese population of Hong Kong, with all ICHs amounting up to 27.1% of strokes, about 11% of the ICHs were infratentorial,[268] whereas in Korea pontine haemorrhages alone comprised 7.9% of all ICHs.[92] The ratio of cerebellar and brainstem haemorrhages is usually approximately 7:3–8:2. Most cerebellar haemorrhages are hemispheric in location and a great majority of brainstem haemorrhages are restricted to the pons, whereas the medulla oblongata is a rare primary site.[26] Pontine haemorrhages usually destroy large parts of the basal and/or tegmental pons. CT scanning has also allowed *intra vitam* detection of small, non-fatal, infratentorial haemorrhages. In the cerebellum these small ICHs are usually located in the vicinity of the fourth ventricle and in the pons unilaterally in the tegmentum.[92,271] Primary pontine haemorrhages have been classified on the basis of their size and anatomical location (up to four different types),[92,258,259] but it appears that only the unilateral tegmental lesion has special clinical relevance (see below).

Clinical picture of ICH

In general, the clinical picture of the larger supratentorial ICHs is usually related to its mass effect. This is further aggravated by oedema developing around the haematoma, which often causes deterioration of patients 24–76 h after the primary bleed. Among the clinical symptoms, severe headache and seizures[78,258] are more common in lobar haemorrhages, whereas visual deficits prevail in deep haemorrhages.[329] Motor deficit is common in both types, but it is more common in deep haemorrhages.

Decreased levels of consciousness (55–60%) or coma (20%) are observed approximately equally frequently in lobar and deep ICH. The mechanism for the decreased level of consciousness has been suggested to involve distortion and lateral displacement of the deep parts of the brain.[329,427] The raised intracranial pressure and the risk from transtentorial herniation rise with increasing size of the haematoma and its associated oedema surrounding the haematoma. Small pontine ICHs may cause different focal sensory or motor impairments,[258,259] whereas larger ones frequently lead to coma and fatal compression of the vital centres. Cerebellar haemorrhages are characteristically associated with vertigo and nausea, and they may fairly rapidly obstruct the circulation of cerebrospinal fluid, with consequent acute life-threatening hydrocephalus.[258,259]

In clinical practice the best way of diagnosing an ICH is by CT scan, which shows a hyperdense area for a couple of weeks, after which it is transformed into a hypodense lesion and occasionally becomes calcified.[143,285,533] Surprisingly, many smaller haemorrhages (2–20 ml in volume) leave no residual CT lesions, although ventricular enlargement may occur.[143,285] MRI reveals old haemorrhages more easily than CT on the basis of haemosiderin in T2-weighted images.

The prognosis of ICH is dependent on the size and location of the haemorrhage, whether there is intraventricular extension and the patient's age. For all supratentorial ICHs the 30-day case fatality percentages vary in population-based studies between 25 and 72% with a weighted mean of 48%, and in hospital-based reports between 27 and 54% with a weighted mean of 35%.[141] The deep ICHs have a 4–5% greater fatality rate, most probably reflecting the higher frequency of intraventricular extension, since the latter as a primary event increased the fatality rate to 78%.[141,329] The increase in the size of the haematoma from below 20 ml to over 80 ml raised the fatality rate from 16 to 82%.[141] The percentages for cerebellar haemorrhages are similar or somewhat greater than in the supratentorial ICHs. Over 80% of patients with larger pontine haemorrhages succumb, whereas only about 5% of unilateral tegmental haemorrhages are fatal.[92]

Pathology and pathogenesis of ICH

Most often pathologists do not diagnose ICH until at autopsy, since surgical removal of the haematoma is recommended only in selected patients.[200,266] However, if an operation is performed, careful sampling of the haematoma cavity and detailed histopathological analysis have been shown to reveal the definite cause of the ICH in a surprisingly high proportion of patients (Figs 6.12, 6.16, 6.18).[526] In post-mortem examinations it is usually not a problem to identify an ICH, as even small old lesions can be recognized by their orange tinge from haemosiderin. Determination of the definite cause of the bleeding may be difficult and even a thorough search of multiple sections may be inconclusive. The site, size and multiplicity of the ICHs and the structural changes in the blood vessels are helpful in this task. The size of the bleeding vessel is commonly correlated with the cause of the rupture: large blood vessels bleed in association with saccular aneurysms and arteriovenous malformations, whereas rupture of a small blood vessel, most commonly a lenticulostriate or pial perforating artery, occurs in association with hypertension, cerebral amyloid angiopathy, anticoagulation and neoplasia.[533]

Regardless of their causes, haematomas have a similar appearance. The time course of haematoma resorption and the response of the surrounding parenchyma have been analysed systematically in experimental animals and the findings have been extrapolated to man with similar results.[236,484] Fresh haematoma is a sharply demarcated collection of blood, from which erythrocytes spread a short distance to the adjacent parenchyma. A rim of surrounding neurons and glia undergoes necrosis during the first day and the amount of oedema increases. The inflammatory reaction in the surrounding tissue is similar to that in infarcts, although with the slightly later appearance of PMN leukocytes by 48 h, possibly because perifocal blood flow is impeded by compression. Macrophages assume the appearance of siderophages instead of foam cells, and blood-derived pigment may also be seen within astrocytes. The time course for the formation of haemosiderin in the CNS is the same as elsewhere in the body, and it may be detectable by the Prussian blue stain 1 day after initiation of phagocytosis. Haemosiderin may still be present several years later at the site of the haematoma within the astrocytes and macrophages in the walls of the residual cavity. It has been estimated that the clot is resorbed at 0.7 mm/day. Astrocyte proliferation to form an accessory glia limitans begins within 1 week with simultaneous neovascularization, which gives a characteristic ring enhancement around the haematoma on CT.[484]

The pathogenesis of the tissue damage in ICH has been of less interest to researchers than that in cerebral ischaemia. Mechanisms responsible for primary injury at or around the site of the haemorrhage include direct distortion and rupture of neuronal pathways. Bearing in mind the considerable size of the haematoma, the extent of this type of injury appears to be surprisingly small, as evidenced by the remarkable abatement or even complete disappearance of ICH on CT scans.[143] This has been attributed to the splitting rather than the destruction of nerve tracts. The role of ischaemia, both perifocal and global, in the development of permanent damage in ICH has been studied in a series of detailed experimental studies.[236,272,336,364,367] By comparing the effects of injected autologous blood and inflated balloon of the same volume in the caudate nucleus, in the rat it was demonstrated that the intracerebral mass alone causes a reduction in local blood flow below ischaemic threshold values, although ischaemia is further aggravated by substances derived from the blood clot. This occurred without a significant rise in the intracranial pressure providing support for the 'intracerebral squeeze' concept of brain damage in ICH.[350] However, uncontained (i.e. with intraventricular extension) haemorrhage raised the intracranial pressure to such an extent that cerebral perfusion pressure decreased. Furthermore, the ischaemic insult progressed even when the balloon was quickly deflated, indicating the existence of a penumbral zone around the mass. Only if the deflation took place within 10 min was the ischaemic penumbra reduced in size, i.e. the extent of the lesion at 24 h was smaller than with longer inflation times. Calcium-channel blockers and immunosuppression resulted in amelioration of the ischaemic injury, suggesting that there is a therapeutic window for ICH, although the permissible period seems to be very short.[336]

Hypertensive haemorrhage

The major decline in the incidence of haemorrhagic stroke in most Western countries over the past 40–50 years has been mainly due to the decline in intraparenchymal haemorrhages as a result of the greatly improved diagnosis and treatment of hypertension;[57a,335] simultaneously, the proportion of hypertension as the cause of ICH has declined: hypertension was the cause of almost 90% of all ICH in the 1940s, 70–80% in the 1970s[149] and only 45–56% in the

1980s[58,456] (Table 6.5). The relative frequency of ICH among 'stroke' patients of Far Eastern populations provides further evidence: in the People's Republic of China, Hong Kong and Korea, where the prevalence of hypertension is remarkably high (about 5–8% of adults), about 30% of the 'strokes' are ICHs,[268,279,459] whereas in Western countries their proportion is only about 10–15%. Hypertensive haemorrhages are usually a one-off event, with recurrent bleeding being rare, as opposed to rebleedings due to saccular aneurysms, vascular malformations or amyloid angiopathy.[258,259]

The most common sites of hypertensive ICH are the putamen and the thalamus (deep cerebral, about 60%), the hemispheres (lobar, 20%), the cerebellum (13%) and the pons (7%). The diameter of the arteries at these bleeding sites range from 50 to 200 μm, and many still regard Charcot–Bouchard microaneurysms as the likely cause of bleeding. Evidence supporting this view has been provided from studies using intravascular injections of contrast or casting media and serial microscopical sections,[82] but the role of microaneurysms is still unclear. Wakai and co-workers[526] identified microaneurysms in patients who had lobar haemorrhages and negative angiography and, remarkably, half of these patients did not even have a history of hypertension. In contrast, a study using elaborate enzyme histochemistry and high-resolution microradiography[82] presented strong evidence for microaneurysms being complex coils and twists of small arterioles (Fig. 6.13). Rupture of non-aneurysmal arteriolar wall damaged by hypertension was regarded as the likely cause of hypertensive haemorrhages. In clinical practice, this degenerative change is considerably easier to demonstrate than the tiny equivocal microaneurysm, which could well have been completely destroyed by the haemorrhage.

The bleeding arteries are fairly small considering the considerable size reached by some of the clots. The high arterial pressure provides additional power to enlarge the haematoma, simultaneously increasing the risk of intraventricular haemorrhage. The actual period of bleeding has been considered to be most often monophasic and short lasting, being completed in less than 2 h,[207] however, enlargement of the haematoma for up to 12 h has also been reported.[57] Thus, neurological deterioration may be due not only to the secondary oedema and ischaemia, but also to continuing bleeding.

Cerebral amyloid angiopathy

Sporadic CAA is responsible for up to 12% of primary non-traumatic intracerebral haemorrhages. It appears to be the most common (about 30%) cause of lobar, i.e. peripherally located intracerebral haemorrhage, particularly in elderly normotensive patients (Figs 6.26, 6.46). CAA carries a considerable risk of bleeding, as up to 20% of patients with CAA had experienced haemorrhage.[524] CAA haemorrhages may be multiple in site and time, and because of their common superficial location they are not

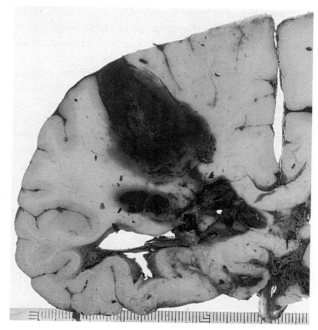

Figure 6.46 *A large lobar intracerebral haemorrhage in the same patient with congophilic amyloid angiopathy as in Fig. 6.26, a 68-year-old female without a history of dementia or arterial hypertension. The history of three previous haemorrhages in the same region and extension of the last one into the subarachnoid space are common features of haemorrhages related to cerebral amyloid angiopathy.*

infrequently associated with secondary subarachnoid haemorrhage (Fig. 6.46). The rigid and fragile arterial walls may make haemostasis very difficult to achieve after neurosurgical evacuation of the haematoma.[180,526] In addition to major lobar haemorrhage patients may show recurrent transient neurological symptoms suggestive of petechial haemorrhages. CAA may also be a precipitating factor behind those intraparenchymal haematomas which complicate fibrinolytic treatment of acute myocardial infarction.[394]

Haemorrhage caused by anticoagulants and antithrombolytics

Nearly 1% of patients treated with anticoagulants have been reported to suffer from an intracerebral haemorrhage during the therapy, the estimated risk being about three times higher than in controls.[3] About 10% of ICH are induced by anticoagulants. Understandably, the risk for ICH increases if the blood vessels are primarily damaged, i.e. when conventional anticoagulants are used in the treatment of ischaemic stroke, then not only may the infarct undergo haemorrhagic transformation (see above), but a frank haematoma may develop. Anticoagulation prolongs the time for which the breached vessels can bleed, making haematomas larger and their prognosis worse: the mortality of ICH patients with anticoagulation is about twice the overall mortality.[408]

Thrombolytic therapy may similarly cause an ICH. In several recent studies the incidence of ICH after this type of therapy for acute myocardial infarction has been about 0.3–0.8%.[232,324,511] Since this therapy clearly reduces the mortality of myocardial infarction, the increased risk of ICH is considered acceptable, despite the fact that these haemorrhages are often multiple with a high mortality rate.[48] The risk of ICH is considerably higher when the thrombolytic treatment is given for acute cerebral ischaemia. In a recent review of 17 trials the incidence of ICH was 3.5 times higher among patients treated with thrombolysis (5216 patients) than in placebo-treated patients and ICH was also frequently fatal. In spite of this, the thrombolytic therapy was considered beneficial, since there was a significant net reduction in the proportion of patients who died or became dependent in daily activities.[529] The frequency of haemorrhagic events increases with delay of treatment beyond 4–6 h, since then recanalization restores blood flow into more severely damaged and more easily leaking blood vessels.[510] The use of thrombolytic substances is especially dangerous in patients with extended early infarct signs because of the increase in fatal major ICH.[529]

Tumour haemorrhage

Both primary and metastatic intracranial tumours can cause major ICH, which in about half of the cases may be the first manifestation.[309,327] An excessive number of abnormal blood vessels in the tumours is thought to be the cause of the haemorrhage. This rich vascularity helps in differential diagnosis, since ring enhancement in CT is common in tumour haemorrhage, but unlikely to occur in fresh non-neoplastic ICH. Among primary tumours glioblastomas predominate, but their number is roughly proportional to their frequency. Considering the characteristic profusion of abnormal blood vessels with a disrupted BBB in malignant astrocytic tumours, more frequent major bleeds could have been anticipated. Despite their abundant 'chicken-wire' vasculature, oligodendrogliomas may not be as prone to bleeding as previously thought. Bronchogenic carcinoma, chorion-carcinoma. melanoma and renal cell carcinoma have been reported to be metastatic tumours most often responsible for an ICH.[259]

Drugs and intraparenchymal haemorrhage

The risk of ICHs among drug abusers is markedly increased, especially among those using cocaine, heroin, and sympathomimetics such as phenylpropanolamine, phencyclidine and amphetamines.[301,464] The age distribution corresponds to that of the abusers, i.e. young people are overrepresented compared with the general population.[251] In drug abusers the haematomas are commonly lobar, in the subcortical white matter, and the bleeding usually develops within minutes to a few hours after the use of the drug. Two main pathogenetic mechanisms have been proposed: either an acute rise in the blood pressure or arteritis, which histopathologically is similar to poly-arteritis nodosa.[301] Ethanol also increases the risk at the high end of the J-shaped relationship between haemorrhage and consumption: the risk for ICH was considered to be 2.4 if more than 400 g/week was consumed.[164] In alcoholics the haemorrhages also tend to be lobar.

Arteriovenous malformations and aneurysms

The common location of arteriovenous malformations at the interface of the parenchyma and the subarachnoid or intraventricular space makes possible haemorrhages in any or all of these three compartments, although subarachnoid haemorrhages are considerably less common than intraventricular and intracerebral bleeds.[14] The surgical specimen of an arteriovenous malformation rarely causes diagnostic difficulties. However, some small arteriovenous malformations may be difficult to detect within an ICH, but an otherwise unexplainable location of a small haematoma may give a hint. Sampling of all suspected areas for microscopic analysis in the wall of the haematoma cavity is recommended.[526]

Saccular aneurysm may cause an ICH, when its fundus is embedded in the parenchyma. Such aneurysms are

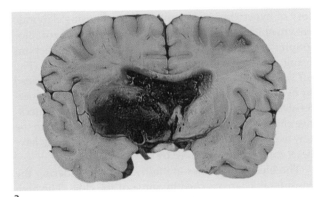

a

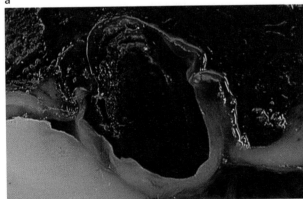

b

Figure 6.47 *Intraparenchymal and intraventricular haemorrhage caused by ruptured saccular aneurysm. (a) The tip of the ruptured aneurysm in the intracranial part of the left internal carotid artery is embedded in the overlying parenchyma. The massive haemorrhage has extended through the basal ganglia into the lateral ventricle. (b) A close-up shows the thinning of the wall of the aneurysm, which has eventually ruptured at its tip.*

located on the middle cerebral, anterior communicating or internal carotid artery, in descending order of incidence. Since the parent artery of these aneurysms resides in the subarachnoid space the haematoma originates close to the brain's basal surface and extends to a variable depth into the parenchyma, sometimes even all the way into the ventricle (Fig. 6.47). Bacterial emboli causing an infective aneurysm are commonly lodged within small intraparenchymal arteries, and therefore the ICH caused by these aneurysms may be indistinguishable from hypertensive haemorrhages. Because the infective aneurysms are small in size and fragile in structure, they are commonly destroyed by the haemorrhage and impossible to identify post-mortem. In these cases the clinical history and associated findings suggestive of infection, especially in the cardiac valves, may help in determining the cause of the bleed.

Subarachnoid haemorrhages caused by aneurysms or arteriovenous malformations are described below.

Subarachnoid haemorrhage

GENERAL

In subarachnoid haemorrhage the bleed takes place in the subarachnoid space alone or in connection with bleeding elsewhere in the CNS. In most populations primary non-traumatic subarachnoid haemorrhage represents about 5–9% of all strokes (Table 6.2). The annual incidence of subarachnoid haemorrhage from verified intracranial aneurysms is about 10–11 (range 6–17) per 100 000 in most Western countries, with somewhat higher figures reported, for example, from Japan, the USA and Finland, and lower figures from New Zealand, some parts of the USA and Scandinavia (excluding Finland).[46,229,337,445,532] The annual incidence of aneurysmal subarachnoid haemorrhage also increases almost linearly with age, from less than 1 per 100 000 before the age of 20 years to about 40 per 100 000 after the age of 65 years.[532] Deaths caused by ruptured aneurysms constitute 16–24% of all patients dying from cerebrovascular diseases.[138]

Modern neuroimaging techniques allow the demonstration of the cause of subarachnoid haemorrhage in the great majority of patients. Rupture of a saccular aneurysm is by far the most important cause of non-traumatic subarachnoid haemorrhage and accounts for about 80% (range 57–94%) of cases, while arteriovenous malformations are responsible for about 5–10% (range 0.6–16%). In 10–15% (range 5–28%) the cause cannot be identified by neuroimaging.[62,138,246,424] Secondary subarachnoid haemorrhage may occur in connection with ICH, blood being forced though the cortex into the subarachnoid space (Fig. 6.46) or with intraventricular haemorrhage, when the blood follows the pathway of the cerebrospinal fluid into the basal cisterns. Traumatic subarachnoid haemorrhage is described in Chapter 14, this Volume.

RUPTURE OF SACCULAR ANEURYSMS AND ANEURYSMAL SUBARACHNOID HAEMORRHAGE

The rate of rupture of saccular aneurysms has been estimated at approximately 1–2% per year. Aneurysms seem to increase in size with time, and their size appears to be the only independent predictive variable that indicates imminent rupture, the critical diameter being 10 mm.[538] In patients with multiple aneurysms, of which only the ruptured one had been clipped, the size of the other aneurysms that ruptured later increased significantly during the follow-up period, in contrast to those that did not rupture.[250] Although the initiation of saccular aneurysms seems to be associated with blood flow-related shear stress, further growth of the aneurysm fundus may occur by passive yield to blood pressure with simultaneous reactive formation of granulation tissue.[475] It has been proposed that atherosclerosis contributes to the growth, and the associated inflammation to the rupture of aneurysms, the latter being supported by the absence of inflammation in unruptured aneurysms.[265,280]

About 40–60% of major aneurysmal ruptures are preceded by warning symptoms, usually within 1–3 weeks, due either to local effects of aneurysmal expansion (e.g. localized head pain, cranial nerve palsies or visual defects) or to supposed 'warning leaks' (e.g. generalized headache lasting for hours or days, nausea, neck pain).[246,297] The rupture of a critically weakened aneurysm wall, most commonly at its fundus (Figs 6.20, 6.47b), is frequently associated with an acute rise in blood pressure during physical stress. It occurs significantly more often during the waking hours, particularly in the morning, than at night because of diurnal variations in blood pressure with much higher transient pressure peaks during waking hours.[465] The variations in blood pressure are accentuated in the elderly and in hypertensive subjects, owing to diminished compliance of their vascular walls.

The rupture most often causes a subarachnoid haemorrhage, which may, furthermore, be associated with vasospasm and ischaemic infarction (see below).[1,211] Less frequently the rupture results in an intracerebral haemorrhage (see above and Fig. 6.47).[1,517] The annual incidence of aneurysmal subarachnoid haemorrhage increases almost linearly with age, from less than 1 per 100 000 before the age of 20 years to about 23 (range 12–45) per 100 000 after the age of 60 years.[532] The median age of onset of the first subarachnoid haemorrhage is 50–60 years.

A ruptured aneurysm can usually be identified *in vivo* by angiography, CT or MRI (Fig. 6.48). The distribution of the resulting blood clot may indicate the position of the source of bleeding. Rupture of an aneurysm in the circle of Willis usually gives rise to blood in the basal cisterns. Bleeding from an aneurysm of the anterior communicating artery or an anterior cerebral

Table 6.7 *Cumulative mortality rates after aneurysmal subarachnoid haemorrhage*

Time after bleeding	Cumulative mortality (%)
Before medical care	15
Day 1	25–30
Week 1	40
Month 1	55
Month 6	60
Year 1	63
Year 5	65

Adapted from Refs 57b and 138.

artery often results in a haematoma between the frontal lobes which may extend backwards above the corpus callosum. Haemorrhages due to rupture of an aneurysm on a middle cerebral artery tend to have an asymmetrical distribution, with the bulk of the blood in and around the affected sylvian fissure. When the aneurysm (particularly those on the middle and anterior cerebral and anterior communicating arteries) is embedded in the surrounding brain parenchyma, the blood bursting from the ruptured aneurysm may penetrate into brain tissue, resulting in an intracerebral haemorrhage, which may even extend into the ventricular system (Fig. 6.47a, b). Intraventricular blood may spread throughout the ventricular system and into the subarachnoid space via the foramina of the fourth ventricle.[1,211,517] Occasionally, subarachnoid blood may even spontaneously penetrate into the subdural space.

Histologically, the blood in the subarachnoid space is contained by the arachnoid membrane and the pia mater surrounding the blood vessels. The pia mater on the surface of the brain appears to be continuous with the leptomeningeal coatings of the blood vessels in the subarachnoid space and seems to prevent direct passage of red blood cells from the subarachnoid space to the perivascular spaces within the brain.[225a]

Aneurysmal subarachnoid haemorrhage has a high mortality. It accounts for about 16–24% of all deaths due to cerebrovascular diseases.[445,532] Cumulative mortality rates after subarachnoid haemorrhage are presented in Table 6.7.[138] About 40% of all the patients die from the initial haemorrhage, 30% within the first 24 h. Without surgical intervention, one-third of the patients who survive the initial haemorrhage die of recurrent bleeding within 6 months after the initial episode, after which the surviving patients have a 3% per year risk of experiencing another haemorrhage.[235,247,262,430] Factors influencing survival include age, history of hypertension, and particularly the amount of subarachnoid blood seen by early brain imaging.[1,212,379] About 70% of patients who are still alive 6 months after the haemorrhage are able to

return to their normal life, while 20% are partially and 10% totally disabled.[138]

Rebleeding

There is a high risk of further bleeding, particularly during the first 24 h and at 1 week after the initial haemorrhage.[230,235,247,262,430] The cumulative risk of rebleeding after primary subarachnoid haemorrhage is approximately 15% at 7 days, 25% at 14 days and 50% at 6 months. After 6 months, the increase in the rate of rebleeding is about 3% per year, but after 10 years the risk approaches that of an unruptured aneurysm. Roughly two-thirds of the rebleedings are fatal, the mortality increasing with successive recurrences.

Platelets are responsible for primary haemostasis after the rupture of an aneurysm, and coagulation factors and collagen then secure the scar. The reduced ability of platelets to aggregate after primary subarachnoid haemorrhage has been invoked to explain the early rebleeds.[248,249,518] Later rebleedings have been attributed to lysis of the plugging clot by increased fibrinolytic activity in the CSF and plasma. Antifibrinolytic therapy has been reported to decrease the risk of rebleeding by about 50%, but the resulting reduction in mortality from rebleeding has been offset by deaths from delayed cerebral ischaemia.[263,516]

NON-ANEURYSMAL SUBARACHNOID HAEMORRHAGES

In 10–15% (range 5–28%) of patients with definite subarachnoid haemorrhage no aneurysm or arteriovenous malformation can be detected in angiography.[418] In the great majority of these patients the centre of bleeding was identified to be anterior to the midbrain and pons, i.e. perimesencephalic, the leaking blood vessels being veins or capillaries around the midbrain.[234,418] Other suggested sites of leakage have been lenticulostriate or thalamoperforating vessels,[6] microaneurysms or microangiomas obliterated by the haemorrhage, saccular aneurysms undergoing spontaneous thrombosis after rupture, or segmental defects or necrosis of the tunica media of small arteries.[6,93,170,234,418] These haemorrhages, especially the perimesencephalic ones, have a better prognosis than aneurysmal haemorrhages even without any specific treatment, and rebleeding or delayed cerebral ischaemia occurs very rarely.[376,419]

Arteriovenous malformations are the second most common (5–10%) identifiable cause of subarachnoid haemorrhage[62] but considerably lower and higher figures have been presented.[14,424] In general, intraventricular and intracerebral haemorrhages appear to be more common complications of arteriovenous malformations. The annual risk of rupture of previously unruptured arteriovenous malformations has been estimated at about 2–3%, and this risk persists over years.[174] Enlarging malformations and those with a single draining vein seem to carry a higher risk of bleeding.[349,525]

COMPLICATIONS OF SUBARACHNOID HAEMORRHAGE

Arterial vasospasm and delayed cerebral ischaemia

Vasospasm of the cerebral arteries and the associated delayed cerebral ischaemia and infarction are currently the most important cause of morbidity and mortality among patients with subarachnoid haemorrhage, although their frequency appears to be considerably diminished by improved therapy.[129,166,379] Vasospasm occurs with neurological deficits in about 15–35% of the patients with subarachnoid haemorrhage.[261] The clinical manifestations of delayed cerebral ischaemia do not usually begin before the fourth day after the initial subarachnoid haemorrhage and they reach their maximum around the seventh day after the haemorrhage. It is a serious complication: about 30% of the patients with delayed cerebral ischaemia die and another 30% become permanently disabled as a result of brain infarction, only 40% of the deficits being reversible.

Arterial vasospasm is usually demonstrable in patients by angiography (Fig. 6.48),[540] but it may persist

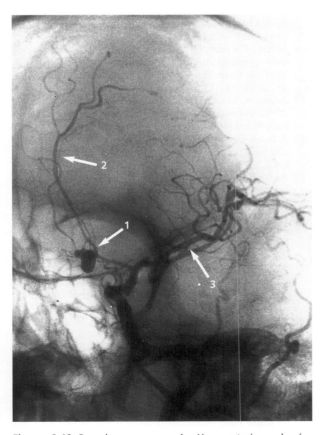

Figure 6.48 *Saccular aneurysm. An X-ray arteriography (an oblique projection) of a patient with subarachnoid haemorrhage discloses the ruptured saccular aneurysm to be localized in the anterior communicating artery (arrow 1). The secondary vasospasm in the pericallosal artery (arrow 2) has rendered it markedly narrower than the middle cerebral artery (arrow 3). Courtesy of Dr M Porras, Helsinki University Central Hospital, Finland.*

even after death and also be demonstrated by postmortem angiography.[257] Severe diffuse vasospasm with more than 50% reduction in blood vessel calibre is usually associated with reduced global and regional CBF. In fact, the latter correlates more closely with ischaemic symptoms than the severity of angiographic vasospasm.[159,540] In spite of severe vasospasm, CBF may remain sufficient by various compensatory mechanisms, e.g. adjustments of blood pressure and collateral circulation. However, CBF may be reduced below the critical level even in the absence of angiographic vasospasm, under the influence of such factors as intracerebral haematoma, oedema or hydrocephalus. Minimum global and regional CBFs of 30–33 and 15–20 ml/l00 g per minute, respectively, appear to be needed to guard against fixed neurological deficits or infarcts.[331,552]

The amount of subarachnoid blood in the basal cisterns and fissures seen by brain imaging within 3 days after the initial bleeding is highly predictive of the risk of delayed cerebral ischaemia and brain infarction, but the site of these complicating lesions need not be related to the location of the maximum subarachnoid blood clot.[1,212,379] The amount of intraventricular blood may also be an independent predictor of ischaemia.[212] Another strong predictor for the occurrence of delayed cerebral ischaemia is the duration of the initial unconsciousness.[217]

While the presence of blood in the cerebrospinal fluid seems to be the crucial initiating event, the definite pathogenesis of arterial vasospasm still remains poorly understood. For example, specific vasoconstrictive agents released from the subarachnoid blood clot have not been identified, although a host of such compounds has been proposed. The substances affecting arterial smooth muscle cells may also come from the circulation, because several morphological abnormalities that may result in increased transendothelial permeability have been described in the endothelial cells after subarachnoid haemorrhage both in man and in animal models.[129,261,540] These include increased endothelial pinocytosis and channel formation, opening of interendothelial tight junctions, and endothelial detachment and destruction, as well as intraluminal platelet adhesion and aggregation onto the damaged endothelium within a few hours after subarachnoid haemorrhage.[130,261] Contrast enhancement in the basal cisterns indicates increased arterial permeability in patients with subarachnoid haemorrhage.[261,540] Protracted contraction of the smooth-muscle cells may result from either the effect of vasoconstrictive agents (e.g. oxyhaemoglobin, endothelin-1, thromboxane A_2, catecholamines, serotonin), impairment of vasodilator activity (prostacyclin, endothelium-derived relaxing factor or NO) or an imbalance between the two (prostacyclin/thromboxane A_2, NO/endothelin).[129,261,319,540]

Alternative hypotheses invoked to explain arterial narrowing include immunological and/or inflammatory processes in the arterial wall initiated by the surrounding clot and a proliferative arteriopathy.[129,261,264,399]

Increased intracranial pressure and hydrocephalus

During the first few days after subarachnoid haemorrhage, the majority of patients show increased intracranial pressure which does not necessarily correlate with the amount of subarachnoid or intraventricular bleeding.[212] Instead, it seems to be largely caused by impaired reabsorption of the cerebrospinal fluid owing to blood in the subarachnoid space.[55] Increased intracranial pressure after subarachnoid haemorrhage may also be caused by the mass effect of a space-occupying haematoma or brain oedema.

Ventricular dilatation occurs in about 20% of the patients during the acute phase, and is related to the amount of intraventricular rather than subarachnoid haemorrhage.[208] About 10% of patients develop delayed communicating hydrocephalus, often with symptoms typical of 'normal-pressure hydrocephalus', which is usually alleviated by shunting.[208] This posthaemorrhagic hydrocephalus may be due to meningeal fibrosis.[443]

Other complications

Hypothalamic lesions (perivascular haemorrhages, microinfarcts) have been described in patients dying soon after subarachnoid haemorrhage, and may be associated with fluid and electrolyte imbalance.[532] Electrocardiographic abnormalities and elevations of serum creatine kinase activity frequently occur after subarachnoid haemorrhage and may be associated with a reduction in cardiac output, which increases the risk of cerebral ischaemia if vasospasm ensues.[332] Repeated subarachnoid haemorrhages may give rise to persistent leptomeningeal siderosis.

REFERENCES

1 Adams HP Jr, Kassell NF, Torner JC, Haley EC Jr. Predicting cerebral ischemia after aneurysmal subarachnoid hemorrhage: influences of clinical condition, CT results, and antifibronolytic therapy. A report of the Cooperative Aneurysm Study. *Neurology* 1987; **37**: 1586–91.

2 Adams RD, Cammermeyer J, Fitzgerald PJ. Neuropathological aspects of thrombocytic acro-angiothrombosis; clinico-anatomical study of generalized platelet thrombosis. *J Neurol Neurosurg Psychiatry* 1948; **11**: 27–43.

3 Albers GW, Sherman DG, Gress DR. Stroke prevention in nonvalvular atrial fibrillation: a review of prospective randomized trials. *Ann Neurol* 1991; **30**: 511–18.

4 Alberts MJ. Subarachnoid hemorrhage and intracranial aneurysms. In: Alberts MJ ed. *Genetics of cerebrovascular disease*. New York: Futura, 1999: 237–59.

5 Alexander EL. Neurologic disease in Sjögren's syndrome: mononuclear inflammatory vasculopathy affecting central/peripheral nervous system and muscle. A clinical review and update of immunopathogenesis. *Rheum Dis Clin North Am* 1993; **19**: 869–908.

6 Alexander MS, Dias PS, Uttley D. Spontaneous subarachnoid hemorrhage and negative cerebral panangiography. Review of 140 cases. *J Neurosurg* 1986; **64**: 537–42.

7 Al Rajeh S, Awada A, Niazi G, Larbi E. Stroke in a Saudi Arabian National Guard community. Analysis of 500 consecutive cases from a population-based hospital. *Stroke* 1993; **24**: 1635–9.

8 Ameri A, Bousser M-G. Cerebral venous thrombosis. *Neurol Clin* 1992; **10**: 87–111.

9 Ames A, Wright LW, Kowada M et al. Cerebral ischemia: II. The no-reflow phenomenon. *Am J Pathol* 1968; **52**: 437–53.

10 Amin-Hanjani S, Robertson R, Arginteanu MS, Scott RM. Familial intracranial arteriovenous malformations. Case report and review of the literature. *Pediatr Neurosurg* 1998; **29**: 208–13.

11 Anders KH, Wang ZZ, Kornfeld M et al. Giant cell arteritis in association with cerebral amyloid angiopathy: immunohistochemical and molecular studies. *Hum Pathol* 1997; **28**: 1237–46.

12 Andrews RJ, Spiegel PK. Intracranial aneurysms. Age, sex, blood pressure, and multiplicity in an unselected series of patients. *J Neurosurg* 1979; **51**: 27–32.

13 Anson J, Crowell RM. Cervicocranial arterial dissection. *Neurosurgery* 1991; **29**: 89–96.

14 Aoki N. Do intracranial arteriovenous malformations cause subarachnoid haemorrhage? Review of computed tomography features of ruptured arteriovenous malformations in the acute stage. *Acta Neurochir* 1991; **112**: 92–5.

15 Aoki N, Mizutani H. Does moyamoya disease cause subarachnoid hemorrhage? Review of 54 cases with intracranial hemorrhage confirmed by computerized tomography. *J Neurosurg* 1984; **60**: 348–53.

16 APASS. The antiphospholipid antibodies in stroke study (APASS) group. Anticardiolipin antibodies are an independent risk factor for first ischemic stroke. *Neurology* 1993; **43**: 2069–73.

17 Arboix A, Besses C. Cerebrovascular disease as the initial clinical presentation of haematological disorders. *Eur Neurol* 1997; **37**: 207–11.

18 Artavanis-Tsakonas S, Rand MD, Lake RJ. Notch signaling: Cell fate control and signal integration in development. *Science* 1999; **284**: 770–6.

19 Asplund K, Tuomilehto J, Stegmyr B et al. Diagnostic criteria and quality control of the registration of stroke events in the MONICA project. *Acta Med Scand* 1988; Suppl 728: 26–39.

20 Astrup J, Siesjö BK, Symon L. Thresholds in cerebral ischemia – the ischemic penumbra. *Stroke* 1981; **12**: 723–5.

21 Atkinson JL, Okazaki H, Sundt TM et al. Intracranial cerebrovascular vasa vasorum associated with atherosclerosis and large thick-walled aneurysms. *Surg Neurol* 1991; **36**: 365–9.

22 Awad IA, Robinson JRJ, Mohanty S, Estes ML. Mixed vascular malformations of the brain: clinical and pathogenetic considerations. *Neurosurgery* 1993; **33**: 179–88.

23 Back T, Hoehn-Berlage M, Kohno K, Hossmann K-A. Diffusion nuclear magnetic resonance imaging in experimental stroke. Correlation with cerebral metabolites. *Stroke* 1994; **25**: 494–500.

24 Bamford J, Sandercock P, Dennis M. A prospective study of acute cerebrovascular disease in the community: the Oxfordshire Community Stroke Project – 1981–86. *J Neurol Neurosurg Psychiatr* 1990; **53**: 16–22.

25 Barber PA, Darby DG, Desmond PM et al. Prediction of stroke outcome with echoplanar perfusion- and diffusion-weighted MRI. *Neurology* 1998; **51**: 418–26.

26 Barinagarrementeria F, Cantu C. Primary medullary hemorrhage. Report of four cases and review of the literature. *Stroke* 1994; **25**: 1684–7.

27 Barnett HJM, Mohr JP, Stein BM, Yatsu FM eds. *Stroke. Pathophysiology, diagnosis and management* 2nd edn. New York: Churchill Livingstone, 1992.

28 Baron JC. Mapping the ischaemic penumbra with PET: implications for acute stroke treatment. *Cerebrovasc Dis* 1999; **9**: 193–201.

29 Baron JC, Bousser MG, Rey A *et al*. Reversal of focal 'misery-perfusion syndrome' – by extra-intracranial arterial bypass in hemodynamic cerebral ischemia. A case study with ^{15}O positron emission tomography. *Stroke* 1981; **12**: 454–9.

30 Baron JC, Frackowiak RS, Herholz K *et al*. Use of PET methods for measurement of cerebral energy metabolism and hemodynamics in cerebrovascular disease. *J Cereb Blood Flow Metab* 1989; **9**: 723–42.

31 Barry DI, Strandgaard S, Graham DI *et al*. Cerebral blood flow in rats with renal and spontaneous hypertension: resetting of lower limit of autoregulation. *J Cereb Blood Flow Metab* 1982; **2**: 347–53.

32 Batjer H, Suss RA, Samson D. Intracranial arteriovenous malformations associated with aneurysms. *Neurosurgery* 1986; **18**: 29–35.

33 Becker D, Townsend JJ, Kramer RA, Newton TH. Occult cerebrovascular malformations: a series of 18 histologically verified cases with negative angiography. *Brain* 1979; **102**: 249–87.

34 Beckman JS. The double-edged role of nitric oxide in the brain function and superoxide-mediated injury. *J Dev Physiol* 1991; **15**: 53–9.

35 Benedikz E, Blöndal H, Guðmundsson G. Skin deposits in hereditary cystatin C amyloidosis. *Virchows Arch A Pathol Anat Histopathol* 1990; **417**: 325–31.

36 Benveniste H, Hedlund LW, Johnson GA. Mechanism of detection of acute cerebral ischemia in rats by diffusion-weighted magnetic resonance microscopy. *Stroke* 1992; **23**: 746–54.

37 Berkovic SF, Spokes RL, Anderson RM, Bladin PF. Basilar artery dissection. *J Neurol Neurosurg Psychiatry* 1983; **46**: 126–9.

38 Bick RL, Arun B, Frenkel EP. Antiphospholipid–thrombosis syndromes. *Haemostasis* 1999; **29**: 100–10.

39 Biller J, Adams HJ, Johnson MR *et al*. Paradoxical cerebral embolism: eight cases. *Neurology* 1986; **36**: 1356–60.

40 Blue MC, Rosenblum WI. Granulomatous angiitis of the brain with herpes zoster and varicella encephalitis. *Arch Pathol Lab Med* 1983; **107**: 126–8.

41 Bogousslavsky J. Subcortical infarcts. In: Fisher M, Bogousslavsky J eds. *Current review of cerebrovascular disease* 1st edn. Philadelphia, PA: Current Medicine, 1993: 31–40.

42 Bogousslavsky J, Regli F, Maeder P. Intracranial large artery disease and 'lacunar' infarction. *Cerebrovasc Dis* 1991; **1**: 154–9.

43 Bohmfalk GL, Story JL, Wissinger JP, Brown WE. Bacterial intracranial aneurysm. *J Neurosurg* 1978; **48**: 369–82.

44 Boiten J, Lodder J, Kessels F. Two clinically distinct lacunar infarct entities? A hypothesis. *Stroke* 1993; **24**: 652–6.

45 Bonita R, Beaglehole R. Stroke mortality. In: Whisnant JP ed. *Stroke: populations, cohorts, and clinical trials*. Oxford: Butterworth Heinemann, 1993: 59–79.

46 Bonita R, Beaglehole R, North JDK. Event incidence and case fatality rates of cerebrovascular disease in Auckland, New Zealand. *Am J Epidemiol* 1984; **120**: 236–43.

47 Bonner H, Erslev AJ. The blood and the lymphoid organs. In: Rubin E, Farber JL eds. *Pathology* 2nd edn. Philadelphia, PA: JB. Lippincott Co., 1994: 994–1096.

48 Boysen G. Primary intracerebral hemorrhage. In: Fisher M, Bogousslavsky J eds. *Current review of cerebrovascular disease* 1st edn. Philadelphia, PA: Current Medicine, 1993: 78–88.

49 Brandt T, Hausser I, Orberk E *et al*. Ultrastructural connective tissue abnormalities in patients with spontaneous cervicocerebral artery dissections. *Ann Neurol* 1998; **44**: 281–5.

50 Breier G, Risau W. The role of VEGF in blood vessel formation. *Trends Cell Biol* 1996; **6**: 454–6.

51 Brey RL, Escalante A. Neurological manifestations of antiphospholipid antibody syndrome. *Lupus* 1998; **7** (Suppl 2): S67–74.

52 Brey RL, Gharavi AE, Lockshin MD. Neurologic complications of antiphospholipid antibodies. *Rheum Dis Clin North Am* 1993; **19**: 833–50.

53 Briceno CE, Resch L, Bernstein M. Cerebral amyloid angiopathy presenting as a mass lesion. *Stroke* 1987; **18**: 234–9.

54 Brightbill TC, Ihmeidan IH, Post MJ *et al*. Neurosyphilis in HIV-positive and HIV-negative patients: neuroimaging findings. *Am J Neuroradiol* 1995; **16**: 703–11.

55 Brinker TS, Seifert V, Stolke D. Acute changes in the dynamics of the cerebrospinal fluid system during experimental subarachnoid hemorrhage. *Neurosurgery* 1990; **27**: 369–72.

56 Britton M, Gustafsson C. Non-rheumatic atrial fibrillation as a risk factor for stroke. *Stroke* 1985; **16**: 182–8.

57 Broderick JP, Brott TG, Tomsick T *et al*. Ultraearly evaluation of intracerebral hemorrhage. *J Neurosurg* 1990; **72**: 195–9.

57a Broderick JP, Phillips SJ, Whisnant JP *et al*. Incidence rates of stroke in the eighties: the end of the decline in stroke? *Stroke* 1989; **20**: 577–82.

57b Broderick JP, Brott TG, Tomsick T *et al*. Intracerebral hemorrhage more than twice as common as subarachnoid hemorrhage. *J Neurosurg* 1993; **78**: 188–91.

58 Brott T, Thalinger K, Hertzberg V. Hypertension as a risk factor for spontaneous intracerebral hemorrhage. *Stroke* 1986; **17**: 1078–83.

59 Brown AW, Brierley JB. The earliest alterations in rat neurones and astrocytes after anoxia-ischaemia. *Acta Neuropathol* 1973; **23**: 9–22.

60 Brown MS, Goldstein JL. A receptor-mediated pathway for cholesterol homeostasis. *Science* 1986; **232**: 34–47.

61 Brown RD, Whisnant JP, Sicks JD *et al*. Stroke incidence, prevalence, and survival: secular trends in Rochester, Minnesota, through 1989. *Stroke* 1996; **27**: 373–80.

62 Brown RD, Wiebers DO. Subarachnoid hemorrhage. In: Fisher M, Bogousslavsky J eds. *Current review of cerebrovascular disease*. Philadelphia, PA: Current Medicine, 1993: 89–99.

63 Bruno A, Adams JP Jr, Biller J *et al*. Cerebral infarction due to moyamoya disease in young adults. *Stroke* 1988; **19**: 826–33.

64 Budka H. Neuropathology of human immunodeficiency virus infection. *Brain Pathol* 1991; **1**: 163–75.

65 Budka H, Gray F. HIV-induced central nervous system pathology. In: Gray F ed. *Atlas of the neuropathology of HIV infection*. Oxford: Oxford University Press, 1993: 1–36.

66 Calabrese LH. Vasculitis and infection with the human immunodeficiency virus. *Rheum Dis Clin North Am* 1991; **17**: 131–47.

67 Calabrese LH, Duna GF. Evaluation and treatment of central nervous system vasculitis. *Curr Opin Rheumatol* 1995; **7**: 37–44.

68 Calabrese LH, Furlan AJ, Gragg LA, Ropos TJ. Primary angiitis of the central nervous system: diagnostic criteria and clinical approach. *Cleve Clin J Med* 1992; **59**: 293–306.

69 Calabrese LH, Gragg LA, Furlan AJ. Benign angiopathy: a distinct subset of angiographically defined primary angiitis of the central nervous system. *J Rheumatol* 1993; **20**: 2046–50.

70 Cantu C, Barinagarrementeria F. Cerebral venous thrombosis associated with pregnancy and puerperium. Review of 67 cases. *Stroke* 1993; **24**: 1880–4.

71 Caplan LR, Pessin MS. Symptomatic carotid artery disease and carotid endarterectomy. *Annu Rev Med* 1988; **39**: 273–99.

72 Caplan RC. Brain embolism, revisited. *Neurology* 1993; **43**: 1281–7.

73 Carlsson LE, Santoso S, Spitzer C et al. The alpha2 gene coding sequence T807/A873 of the platelet collagen receptor integrin alpha2beta1 might be a genetic risk factor for the development of stroke in younger patients. *Blood* 1999; **93**: 3583–6.

74 Carr SC, Farb A, Pearce WH et al. Activated inflammatory cells are associated with plaque rupture in carotid artery stenosis. *Surgery* 1997; **122**: 757–63.

75 Carson CW, Conn DL, Czaja AJ et al. Frequency and significance of antibodies to hepatitis C virus in polyarteritis nodosa. *J Rheumatol* 1993; **20**: 304–9.

76 Caselli RJ, Hunder GG. Neurologic aspects of giant cell (temporal) arteritis. *Rheum Dis Clin North Am* 1993; **19**: 941–53.

77 Caselli RJ, Hunder GG, Whisnant JP. Neurologic disease in biopsy-proven giant cell (temporal) arteritis. *Neurology* 1988; **38**: 352–9.

78 Cervoni L, Artico M, Salvati M et al. Epileptic seizures in intracerebral hemorrhage: a clinical and prognostic study of 55 cases. *Neurosurg Rev* 1994; **17**: 185–8.

79 Chabriat H, Tournier-Lasserve E, Bousser M-G. Vasculopathies. In: Alberts MJ ed. *Genetics of cerebrovascular disease*. New York: Futura, 1999: 195–208.

80 Challa VR, Bell MA, Moody DM. A combined hematoxylin–eosin, alkaline phosphatase and high-resolution microradiographic study of lacunes. *Clin Neuropathol* 1990; **9**: 196–204.

81 Challa VR, Moody DM. The value of magnetic resonance imaging in the detection of type II hemorrhagic lacunes. *Stroke* 1989; **20**: 822–5.

82 Challa VR, Moody DM, Bell MA. The Charcot–Bouchard aneurysm controversy: impact of a new histologic technique. *J Neuropathol Exp Neurol* 1992; **51**: 264–71.

83 Challa VR, Moody DM, Brown WR. Vascular malformations of the central nervous system. *J Neuropathol Exp Neurol* 1995; **54**: 609–21.

84 Chan PH. Oxygen radicals in focal cerebral ischemia. *Brain Pathol* 1994; **4**: 59–65.

85 Chan PH, Kamii H, Yang G et al. Brain infarction is not reduced in SOD-1 transgenic mice after a permanent focal cerebral ischemia. *NeuroReport* 1993; **5**: 293–6.

86 Chang CL, Donaghy M, Poulter N. Migraine and stroke in young women: case–control study. The World Health Organisation Collaborative Study of Cardiovascular Disease and Steroid Hormone Contraception. *BMJ* 1999; **318**: 13–18.

87 Chen J, Simon R. Ischemic tolerance in the brain. *Neurology* 1997; **48**: 306–11.

88 Chester EM, Agamanolis DP, Banker BW, Victor M. Hypertensive encephalopathy: a clinicopathologic study of 20 cases. *Neurology* 1978; **28**: 928–39.

89 Chievitz E, Thiede T. Complications and causes of death in polycythaemia vera. *Acta Med Scand* 1962; **172**: 513–23.

90 Chiu D, Shedden P, Bratina P, Grotta JC. Clinical features of moyamoya disease in the United States. *Stroke* 1998; **29**: 1347–51.

91 Chobanian AV, Prescott MF, Haudenschild CC. Recent advances in molecular pathology. The effects of hypertension on the arterial wall. *Exp Mol Pathol* 1984; **41**: 153–69.

92 Chung C-S, Park C-H. Primary pontine hemorrhage: a new CT classification. *Neurology* 1992; **42**: 830–4.

93 Cioffi F, Pasqualin A, Cavazzani P, Da PR. Subarachnoid haemorrhage of unknown origin: clinical and tomographical aspects. *Acta Neurochir* 1989; **97**: 31–9.

94 Cloft HJ, Kallmes DF, Kalmes MH et al. Prevalence of cerebral aneurysms in patients with fibromuscular dysplasia: a reassessment. *J Neurosurg* 1998; **88**: 436–40.

95 Cohen HCM, Tucker WS, Humphreys RP, Perrin RJ. Angiographically cryptic histologically verified cerebrovascular malformations. *Neurosurgery* 1982; **10**: 704–14.

96 Cohen Tervaert CJW, Kallenberg C. Neurologic manifestations of systemic vasculitides. *Rheum Dis Clin North Am* 1993; **19**: 913–40.

97 Cole FM, Yates PO. Comparative incidence of cerebrovascular lesions in normotensive and hypertensive patients. *Neurology* 1968; **18**: 255–9.

98 Connett MC, Lausche JM. Fibromuscular hyperplasia of the internal carotid artery. Report of a case. *Ann Surg* 1965; **162**: 59–62.

99 Craig HD, Gunel M, Cepeda O et al. Multilocus linkage identifies two new loci for a mendelian form of stroke, cerebral cavernous malformation, at 7p15–13 and 3q25.2–27. *Hum Mol Genet* 1998; **7**: 1851–8.

100 Cravioto H, Feigin I. Noninfectious granulomatous angiitis involving the central nervous system. *Neurology* 1959; **9**: 599–609.

101 Cros D, Comp PC, Beltran G, Gum G. Superior sagittal sinus thrombosis in a patient with protein S deficiency. *Stroke* 1990; **21**: 633–6.

102 Dahlbäck B, Hildebrand B. Inherited resistance to activated protein C is corrected by anticoagulant factory activity found to be a property of factor V. *Proc Natl Acad Sci USA* 1994; **91**: 1396–400.

103 Dalkara T, Moskowitz MA. The complex role of nitric oxide in the pathophysiology of focal cerebral ischemia. *Brain Pathol* 1994; **4**: 49–57.

104 Deck JHN. Pathology of spontaneous dissection of intracranial arteries. *Can J Neurol Sci* 1987; **14**: 88–91.

105 DeGirolami U, Crowell RM, Marcouz FW. Selective necrosis and total necrosis in focal cerebral ischemia. Neuropathologic observations on experimental middle cerebral artery occlusion in the macaque monkey. *J Neuropathol Exp Neurol* 1984; **43**: 57–71.

106 DeGraba TJ, Fisher M, Yatsu FM. Atherogenesis and strokes. In: Barnett HM ed. *Stroke: pathophysiology, diagnosis, and management*. New York: Churchill Livingstone, 1993: 29–48.

107 del Zoppo G, Ginis I, Hallenbeck JM et al. Inflammation and stroke: putative role for cytokines, adhesion molecules and iNOS in brain response to ischemia. *Brain Pathol* 2000; **10**: 95–112.

108 del Zoppo GJ, Schmid-Schönbein GW, Mori E et al. Polymorphonuclear leukocytes occlude capillaries following middle cerebral artery occlusion and reperfusion in baboons. *Stroke* 1991; **22**: 1276–83.

109 De Strooper B, Annaert W, Cupers P et al. A presenilin-1-dependent gamma-secretase-like protease mediates release of Notch intracellular domain. *Nature* 1999; **398**: 518–22.

110 Devinsky O, Petito CK, Alonso DR. Clinical and neuropathological findings in systemic lupus erythematosus: the role of vasculitis, heart emboli, and thrombotic thrombocytopenic purpura. *Ann Neurol* 1988; **23**: 380–4.

111 Dichgans M, Mayer M, Uttner I *et al.* The phenotypic spectrum of CADASIL: clinical findings in 102 cases. *Ann Neurol* 1998; **44**: 731–9.

112 Dinsdale HB. Hypertensive encephalopathy. In: Barnett HJM, Mohr JP, Stein BM, Yatsu FM eds. *Stroke* 2nd edn. New York: Churchill Livingstone, 1993: 787–92.

113 Dinsdale HB. Hypertensive encephalopathy. *Stroke* 1982; **13**: 717–19.

114 Dinsdale HB, Robertson DM, Haas RA. Cerebral blood flow in acute hypertension. *Arch Neurol* 1974; **31**: 80–7.

115 Dinubile MJ. Septic thrombosis of the cavernous sinuses. Neurological review. *Arch Neurol* 1988; **45**: 567–74.

116 Donaldson JO, Lee NS. Arterial and venous stroke associated with pregnancy. *Neurol Clin* 1994; **12**: 583–99.

117 Dormont D, Anxionnat R, Evrard S *et al.* MRI in cerebral venous thrombosis. *J Neuroradiol* 1994; **21**: 81–99.

118 Drake CG, Peerless SJ. Giant fusiform intracranial aneurysms: a review of 120 patients treated surgically from 1965 to 1992. *J Neurosurg* 1997; **87**: 141–62.

119 Duna GF, Calabrese LH. Limitations of invasive modalities in the diagnosis of primary angiitis of the central nervous system. *J Rheumatol* 1995; **22**: 662–7.

120 Erdem E, Namer IJ, Saribas O *et al.* Cerebral fat embolism studied with MRI and SPECT. *Neuroradiology* 1993; **35**: 199–201.

121 Eskenasy-Cottier AC, Leu HJ, Bassetti C *et al.* A case of dissection of intracranial cerebral arteries with segmental mediolytic 'arteries'. *Clin Neuropathol* 1994; **13**: 329–37.

122 Etchells EE, Wong DT, Davidson G, Houston PL. Fatal cerebral fat embolism associated with a patent foramen ovale. *Chest* 1993; **104**: 962–3.

123 Farmer JP, Cosgrove GR, Villemure JG *et al.* Intracerebral cavernous angiomas. *Neurology* 1988; **38**: 1699–704.

124 Feigin I, Prose P. Hypertensive fibrinoid arteritis of the brain and gross cerebral hemorrhage. A form of 'hyalinosis'. *Arch Neurol* 1959; **1**: 98–110.

125 Feldman E. Intracerebral hemorrhage. In: Fisher M ed. *Clinical atlas of cerebrovascular disorders*. Chicago, IL: Wolfe, 1994; **11**: 11–17.

126 Ferro JM. Vasculitis of the central nervous system. *J Neurol* 1998; **245**: 766–76.

127 Fiermonte G, Aloe-Spiriti MA, Latagliata R *et al.* Polycythaemia vera and cerebral blood flow: a preliminary study with transcranial Doppler. *J Intern Med* 1993; **234**: 599–602.

128 Fieschi C, Argentino C, Lenzi GL *et al.* Clinical and instrumental evaluation of patients with ischemic stroke within the first six hours. *J Neurol Sci* 1989; **91**: 311–22.

129 Findlay JM, Macdonald RL, Weir BKA. Current concepts of pathophysiology and management of cerebral vasospasm following aneurysmal subarachnoid hemorrhage. *Cerebrovasc Brain Metab Rev* 1991; **3**: 336–61.

130 Findlay JM, Weir BKA, Kanamaru K, Espinosa F. Arterial wall changes in cerebral vasospasm. *Neurosurgery* 1989; **25**: 736–46.

131 Fisher CM. Cerebral miliary aneurysms in hypertension. *Am J Pathol* 1972; **66**: 313–30.

132 Fisher CM. Lacunar infarcts: a review. *Cerebrovasc Dis* 1991; **1**: 311–20.

133 Fisher CM. Pathological observations in hypertensive cerebral hemorrhage. *J Neuropathol Exp Neurol* 1971; **30**: 536–50.

134 Fisher CM, Adams RD. Observations on brain embolism with special reference to the mechanism of hemorrhagic infarction. *J Neuropathol Exp Neurol* 1951; **10**: 92–4.

135 Fisher CM, Ojemann RG. A clinico-pathologic study of carotid endarterectomy plaques. *Rev Neurol (Paris)* 1986; **142**: 573–89.

136 Fisher M ed. *Clinical atlas of cerebrovascular disorders*. London: 1994.

137 Fisher M, Sotak CH, Minematsu K, Li L. New magnetic resonance techniques for evaluating cerebrovascular disease. *Ann Neurol* 1992; **32**: 115–22.

138 Fogelholm R, Hernesniemi J, Vapalahti M. Impact of early surgery on outcome after aneurysmal subarachnoid hemorrhage. A population-based study. *Stroke* 1993; **24**: 1649–54.

139 Fogelholm R, Murros K. Cigarette smoking and subarachnoid haemorrhage: a population-based case–control study. *J Neurol Neurosurg Psychiatry* 1987; **50**: 78–80.

140 Fogelholm R, Murros K, Rissanen A, Ilmavirta M. Decreasing incidence of stroke in central Finland, 1985–1993. *Acta Neurol Scand* 1997; **95**: 38–43.

141 Fogelholm R, Nuutila M, Vuorela A-L. Primary intracerebral haemorrhage in the Jyväskylä region, Central Finland, 1985–89: incidence, case fatality rate, and functional outcome. *J Neurol Neurosurg Psychiatry* 1992; **55**: 546–52.

142 Forster DM, Kunkler IH, Hartland P. Risk of cerebral bleeding from arteriovenous malformations in pregnancy: the Sheffield experience. *Stereotact Funct Neurosurg* 1993; **61** (Suppl): 20–2.

143 Franke CL, van Swieten JC, van Gijn J. Residual lesions on computed tomography after intracerebral hemorrhage. *Stroke* 1991; **22**: 1530–3.

144 Frazee JG, Cahan LD, Winter J. Bacterial intracranial aneurysm. *J Neurosurg* 1980; **53**: 633–41.

145 Fredericks RK, Lefkowitz DS, Challa VR. Cerebral vasculitis associated with cocaine abuse. *Stroke* 1991; **22**: 1437–9.

146 Fredriksson K, Auer RN, Kalimo H *et al.* Cerebrovascular lesions in stroke-prone spontaneously hypertensive rats. *Acta Neuropathol* 1985; **68**: 284–94.

147 Fredriksson K, Nordborg C, Kalimo H *et al.* Cerebral microangiopathy in stroke-prone spontaneously hypertensive rats. An immunohistochemical and ultrastructural study. *Acta Neuropathol* 1988; **75**: 241–52.

148 Fukumoto S, Kinjo M, Hokamura K, Tanaka K. Subarachnoid hemorrhage and granulomatous angiitis of the basilar artery: demonstration of the varicella-zoster virus in the basilar artery lesions. *Stroke* 1986; **17**: 1024–8.

149 Furlan AJ, Whisnant JP, Elveback LR. The decreasing incidence of primary intracerebral hemorrhage: a population study. *Ann Neurol* 1979; **5**: 367–73.

150 Furlan M, Robles R, Galbusera M *et al.* von Willebrand factor-cleaving protease in thrombotic thrombocytopenic purpura and the hemolytic–uremic syndrome. *N Engl J Med* 1998; **339**: 1578–84.

151 Gadoth N, Hirsch M. Primary and acquired forms of moyamoya syndrome. *Israel J Med Sci* 1980; **16**: 370–7.

152 Garcia JH, Kalimo H, Kamijyo Y, Trump BF. Cellular events during partial cerebral ischemia. I. Electron microscopy of feline cerebral cortex after middle-cerebral artery occlusion. *Virchows Arch Cell Pathol* 1977; **25**: 191–206.

153 Garcia JH, Lassen NA, Weiller C *et al.* Ischemic stroke and incomplete infarction. *Stroke* 1996; **27**: 761–5.

154 Garcia-Monco JC, Fernandez Villar B, Calvo Alen J, Benach JL. *Borrelia burgdorferi* in the central nervous system: experimental and clinical evidence for early invasion. *J Infect Dis* 1990; **161**: 1187–93.

155 Gårde A, Böhmer G, Seldén B, Neiman J. 100 cases of spontaneous intracerebral haematoma. *Eur Neurol* 1983; **22**: 161–72.

156 Garner A, Ashton N, Tripathi R *et al.* Pathogenesis of hypertensive retinopathy: an experimental study in the monkey. *Br J Ophthalmol* 1975; **59**: 3–44.

157 Garner TB, Del Gurling OJ, Kelly DLJ, Laster DW. The natural history of intracranial venous angiomas. *J Neurosurg* 1991; **75**: 715–22.

158 Gautier JC, Durr A, Koussa S *et al.* Paradoxical cerebral embolism with a patent foramen ovale. *Cerebrovasc Dis* 1991; **1**: 192–202.

159 Géraud G, Tremoulet M, Guell A, Bes A. The prognostic value of noninvasive CBF measurement in subarachnoid hemorrhage. *Stroke* 1984; **15**: 301–5.

160 Gherardi R, Belec L, Mhiri C *et al.* The spectrum of vasculitis in human immunodeficiency virus-infected patients. A clinicopathologic evaluation. *Arthritis Rheum* 1993; **36**: 1164–74.

161 Ghiso J, Jensson O, Frangione B. Amyloid fibrils in hereditary cerebral hemorrhage with amyloidosis of Icelandic type is a variant of γ-trace protein (cystatin C). *Proc Natl Acad Sci USA* 1986; **83**: 2974–78.

162 Giang DW. Central nervous system vasculitis secondary to infections, toxins, and neoplasms. *Semin Neurol* 1994; **14**: 313–19.

163 Gilbert JJ, Vinters HV. Cerebral amyloid angiopathy: incidence and complications in the aging brain. I. Cerebral hemorrhage. *Stroke* 1983; **14**: 915–23.

164 Gill JS, Shipley MJ, Tsementzis SA. Alcohol consumption: a risk factor for hemorrhagic and non-hemorrhagic stroke. *Am J Med* 1991; **90**: 489–97.

165 Gill R, Sibson NR, Hatfield RH *et al.* A comparison of the early development of ischaemic damage following permanent middle cerebral artery occlusion in rats as assessed using magnetic resonance imaging and histology. *J Cereb Blood Flow Metab* 1995; **15**: 1–11.

166 Gilsbach JM, Reulen HJ, Ljunggren B *et al.* Early aneurysm surgery and preventive therapy with intravenously administered nimodipine: a multicenter, double-blind, dose-comparison study. *Neurosurgery* 1990; **26**: 458–64.

167 Glenner GG. Amyloid deposits and amyloidosis. The β-fibrillosis. *N Engl J Med* 1980; **302**: 1283–92.

168 Glick R, Hoying J, Cerullo L, Perlman S. Phenylpropanolamine: an over-the-counter drug causing central nervous system vasculitis and intracerebral hemorrhage. Case report and review. *Neurosurgery* 1987; **20**: 969–74.

169 Goldstein JL, Ho YK, Basu SK, Brown MS. Binding site on macrophages that mediates uptake and degradation of acetylated low-density lipoprotein, producing massive cholesterol deposition. *Proc Natl Acad Sci USA* 1979; **76**: 333–7.

170 Gomez PA, Lobato RD, Rivas JJ *et al.* Subarachnoid haemorrhage of unknown aetiology. *Acta Neurochir* 1989; **101**: 35–41.

171 Gorelick PB. Distribution of atherosclerotic cerebrovascular lesions. Effects of age, race, and sex. *Stroke* 1993; **24** (Suppl I): I-16–19.

172 Goren H, Steinberg MC, Farboody GH. Familial oculoleptomeningeal amyloidosis. *Brain* 1980; **103**: 473–95.

173 Gossman MD, Berlin AJ, Weinstein MA *et al.* Spontaneous direct carotid-cavernous fistula in childhood. *Ophthal Plast Reconstr Surg* 1993; **9**: 62–5.

174 Graf CJ, Perret GE, Torner JC. Bleeding from cerebral anteriovenous malformations as part of their natural history. *J Neurosurg* 1983; **58**: 331–7.

175 Graham DI. Ischemic brain damage of cerebral perfusion failure type after treatment of severe hypertension. *BMJ* 1975; **iv**: 739.

176 Gray F, Dubas F, Roullet E, Escourolle R. Leukoencephalopathy in diffuse hemorrhagic cerebral amyloid angiopathy. *Ann Neurol* 1985; **18**: 54–9.

177 Gray F, Lescs MC, Keohane C *et al.* Early brain changes in HIV infection: neuropathological study of 11 HIV seropositive, non-AIDS cases. *J Neuropathol Exp Neurol* 1992; **51**: 177–85.

178 Green D, Otoya J, Oriba H, Rovner R. Protein S deficiency in middle-aged women with stroke. *Neurology* 1992; **42**: 1029–33.

179 Greenberg SM, Rebeck GW, Vonsattel JPG *et al.* Apolipoprotein E ε4 and cerebral hemorrhage associated with amyloid angiopathy. *Ann Neurol* 1995; **38**: 254–9.

180 Greene GM, Godersky JC, Biller J *et al.* Surgical experience with cerebral amyloid angiopathy. *Stroke* 1990; **21**: 1545–9.

181 Gross CR, Kase CS, Mohr JP *et al.* Stroke in south Alabama: incidence and diagnostic features – a population based study. *Stroke* 1984; **15**: 249–55.

182 Gudmundsson G, Hallgrimsson J, Jonasson TA, Bjarnason O. Hereditary cerebral haemorrhage with amyloidosis. *Brain* 1972; **95**: 387–404.

183 Guillevin L, Huong Du LT, Godeau P. Clinical findings and prognosis of polyarteritis nodosa and Churg–Strauss angiitis: a study in 165 patients. *Br J Rheumatol* 1988; **27**: 258–64.

184 Guillevin L, Lhote F, Jarrousse B, Fain O. Treatment of polyarteritis nodosa and Churg–Strauss syndrome. A meta-analysis of 3 prospective controlled trials including 182 patients over 12 years. *Ann Med Intern Paris* 1992; **143**: 405–16.

185 Haan J, Algra PR, Roos RA. Hereditary cerebral hemorrhage with amyloidosis, Dutch type. Clinical and computed tomographic analysis of 24 cases. *Arch Neurol* 1990; **47**: 649–53.

186 Hachinski VC. Leukoaraiosis. *Arch Neurol* 1987; **44**: 21–3.

187 Hachinski VC, Lasten NA, Marshall J. Multi-infarct dementia. A cause of mental deterioration in the elderly. *Lancet* 1974; **ii**: 207–10.

187a Hacke W, Kashe M, Fieschi C *et al.* Intravenous thrombolysis with recombinant tissue plasminogen activator. European Cooperative Acute Stroke Study (ECASS). *J Am Med Assoc* 1995; **274**: 1015–27.

188 Haltia M, Ghiso J, Prelli F *et al.* Amyloid in familial amyloidosis, Finnish type, is antigenically and structurally related to gelsolin. *Am J Pathol* 1990; **136**: 1223–8.

189 Haltia M, Iivanainen M, Majuri H, Puranen M. Spontaneous occlusion of the circle of Willis (moyamoya syndrome). *Clin Neuropathol* 1982; **1**: 11–22.

190 Hamilton MG, Spetzler RF. The prospective application of a grading system for arteriovenous malformations. *Neurosurgery* 1994; **34**: 2–6.

191 Hanly JG, Walsh NMG, Sangalang V. Brain pathology in systemic lupus erythematosus. *J Rheumatol* 1992; **19**: 732–41.

192 Harmon DL, Doyle RM, Meleady R *et al.* Genetic analysis of the thermolabile variant of 5,10-methylenetetrahydrofolate reductase as a risk factor for ischemic stroke. *Arterioscler Thromb Vasc Biol* 1999; **19**: 208–11.

193 Harris RJ, Symon L. Extracellular pH, potassium, and calcium activities in progressive ischaemia of rat cortex. *J Cereb Blood Flow Metab* 1984; **4**: 178–86.

194 Hart MN, Merz P, Bennett-Gray J *et al.* β-Amyloid protein in Alzheimer's disease is found in cerebral and spinal cord vascular malformations. *Am J Pathol* 1988; **132**: 167–72.

195 Hart RG, Kagan-Hallet K, Joerns SE. Mechanisms of intracranial hemorrhage in infective endocarditis. *Stroke* 1987; **18**: 1048–56.

195a Hart RG, Kanter MC. Hematologic disorders and ischemic stroke. A selective review. *Stroke* 1990; **21**: 1111–21.

196 Hartkamp MJ, van Der Grond J, van Everdingen KJ *et al.* Circle of Willis collateral flow investigated by magnetic resonance angiography. *Stroke* 1999; **30**: 2671–8.

197 Haught WH, Alexander JA, Conti CR. Familial recurring cardiac myxoma. *Clin Cardiol* 1991; **14**: 692–5.

198 Hauser RA, Lacey M, Knight MR. Hypertensive encephalopathy: magnetic resonance imaging demonstration of reversible cortical and white matter lesions. *Arch Neurol* 1988; **45**: 1078–83.

199 Hauw JJ. The history of lacunes. In: Donnan GA, Norrving B, Bamford J, Bogousslavsky J eds. *Lacunar and other subcortical infarctions*. New York: Oxford University Press, 1995: 3–15.

200 Heiskanen O. Treatment of spontaneous intracerebral and intracerebellar hemorrhages. *Stroke* 1993; **24** (Suppl I): I-94–5.

201 Heiss W-D. Experimental evidence of ischemic thresholds and functional recovery. *Stroke* 1992; **23**: 1668–72.

202 Heiss W-D, Graf R, Wienhard K et al. Dynamic penumbra demonstrated by sequential multitracer PET after middle cerebral artery occlusion in cats. *J Cereb Blood Flow Metab* 1994; **14**: 892–902.

203 Heiss W-D, Huber M, Fink G et al. Progressive derangement of peri-infarct viable tissue in ischemic stroke. *J Cereb Blood Flow Metab* 1992; **12**: 193–203.

204 Heiss WD, Rosner G. Functional recovery of cortical neurons as related to degree and duration of ischemia. *Ann Neurol* 1983; **14**: 294–301.

205 Heiss WD, Thiel A, Grond M, Graf R. Which targets are relevant for therapy of acute ischemic stroke? *Stroke* 1999; **30**: 1486–9.

206 Hendriks L, van Duijn DC, Cras P et al. Presenile dementia and cerebral haemorrhage linked to a mutation at codon 692 of the beta-amyloid precursor protein gene. *Nat Genet* 1992; **1**: 218–21.

207 Herbstein DJ, Schaumberg HH. Hypertensive intracerebral hematoma: an investigation of the initial hemorrhage and rebleeding using chromium Cr 51-labeled erythrocytes. *Arch Neurol* 1974; **30**: 412–14.

208 Heros RC. Acute hydrocephalus after subarachnoid hemorrhage. *Stroke* 1989; **20**: 715–17.

209 Higa M, Davanipour Z. Smoking and stroke. *Neuroepidemiology* 1991; **10**: 211–22.

210 Higashida RT, Halbach VV, Dowd C et al. Endovascular detachable balloon embolization therapy of cavernous carotid artery aneurysms: results of 87 cases. *J Neurosurg* 1990; **72**: 857–63.

211 Hijdra A, Brouwers PJAM, Vermeulen M, van Gijn J. Grading the amount of blood on computed tomograms after subarachnoid hemorrhage. *Stroke* 1990; **21**: 1156–61.

212 Hijdra A, van Gijn J, Nagelkerke NJD et al. Prediction of delayed cerebral ischemia, rebleeding, and outcome after aneurysmal subarachnoid hemorrhage. *Stroke* 1988; **19**: 1250–6.

213 Hillered L, Hallström A, Segersvard S et al. Dynamics of extracellular metabolites in the striatum after middle cerebral artery occlusion in the rat, monitored by intracerebral microdialysis. *J Cereb Blood Flow Metab* 1989; **9**: 607–16.

214 Hilt DC, Buchholz D, Krumhoiz A et al. Herpes zoster ophthalmicus and delayed contralateral hemiparesis caused by cerebral angiitis: diagnosis and management approaches. *Ann Neurol* 1983; **14**: 543–4.

215 Hoffman GS, Kerr GS, Leavitt RY. Wegener granulomatosis: an analysis of 158 patients. *Ann Intern Med* 1992; **116**: 488–98.

216 Hong SC, Goto Y, Lanzino G et al. Neuroprotection with a calpain inhibitor in a model of focal cerebral ischemia. *Stroke* 1994; **25**: 663–9.

217 Hop JW, Rinkel GJ, Algra A, van Gijn J. Initial loss of consciousness and risk of delayed cerebral ischemia after aneurysmal subarachnoid hemorrhage. *Stroke* 1999; **30**: 2268–71.

218 Horie R. Studies on stroke in relation to cerebrovascular atherogenesis in stroke-prone spontaneously hypertensive rats (SHRSP). *Arch Jpn Chir* 1977; **46**: 191–213.

219 Horten BC, Abbott GF, Porro RS. Fungal aneurysms of intracranial vessels. *Arch Neurol* 1976; **33**: 577–9.

220 Hossmann K-A. Glutamate-mediated injury in focal cerebral ischemia: the excitotoxin hypothesis revised. *Brain Pathol* 1994; **4**: 23–36.

221 Hu HH, Sheng WY, Chu FL et al. Incidence of stroke in Taiwan. *Stroke* 1992; **23**: 1237–1241.

222 Hughson MD, McCarty GA, Sholer CM, Brumback RA. Thrombotic cerebral arteriopathy in patients with the antiphospholipid syndrome. *Mod Pathol* 1993; **6**: 644–53.

223 Huisman MV, Rosendaal F. Thrombophilia. *Curr Opin Hematol* 1999; **6**: 291–7.

224 Hulman G. Pathogenesis of non-traumatic fat embolism. *Lancet* 1988; **338**: 1366–7.

225 Hurst RW, Bagley LJ, Galetta S et al. Dementia resulting from dural arteriovenous fistulae: the pathologic findings of venous hypertensive encephalopathy. *Am J Neuroradiol* 1998; **19**: 1267–73.

225a Hutchings M, Weller RO. Anatomical relationships of the pia mater to cerebral blood vessels in man. *J Neurosurg* 1986; **65**: 316–25.

226 Ichiyama T, Nishikawa M, Hayashi T et al. Cerebral hypoperfusion during acute Kawasaki disease. *Stroke* 1998; **29**: 1320-1.

227 Iijima T, Mies G, Hossmann K-A. Repeated negative DC deflections in rat cortex following middle cerebral artery occlusion are abolished by MK-801: effect on volume of ischemic injury. *J Cereb Blood Flow Metab* 1992; **12**: 727–33.

228 Ikeda H, Sasaki T, Yoshimoto T et al. Mapping of a familial moyamoya disease gene to chromosome 3p24.2–p26. *Am J Hum Genet* 1999; **64**: 533–7.

229 Inagawa T, Ishikawa S, Aoki H et al. Aneurysmal subarachnoid hemorrhage in Izumo City and Shimane Prefecture of Japan. Incidence. *Stroke* 1988; **19**: 170–5.

230 Inagawa T, Kamiya K, Ogasawara H, Yano T. Rebleeding of ruptured intracranial aneurysms in the acute stage. *Surg Neurol* 1987; **28**: 93–9.

231 Ishihara T, Nagasawa T, Yokota T et al. Amyloid protein of vessels in leptomeninges, cortices, choroid plexuses, and pituitary glands from patients with systemic amyloidosis. *Hum Pathol* 1989; **20**: 891–5.

232 ISIS-3, Group TISoISc. A randomised comparison of streptokinase vs tissue plasminogen activator vs anistreplase and of aspirin plus heparin vs aspirin alone among 41,299 cases of suspected acute myocardial infarction. *Lancet* 1992; **339**: 753–70.

233 Iwamoto H, Kiyohara Y, Fujishima M et al. Prevalence of intracranial saacular aneurysms in a Japanese community based on a consecutive autopsy series during a 30-year observation period. The Hisayama study. *Stroke* 1999; **30**: 1390–5.

234 Iwanaga H, Wakai S, Ochiai C et al. Ruptured cerebral aneurysms missed by initial angiographic study. *Neurosurgery* 1990; **27**: 45–51.

235 Jane JA, Winn HR, Richardson AE. The natural history of intracranial aneurysms: rebleeding rates during the acute and long term period and implication for surgical management. *Clin Neurosurg* 1977; **24**: 176–84.

236 Jenkins A, Maxwell WL, Graham DI. Experimental intracerebral haematoma in the rat: sequential light microscopical changes. *Neuropathol Appl Neurobiol* 1989; **15**: 477–86.

237 Jenkins LW, Povlishock JT, Lewelt W et al. The role of postischemic recirculation in the development of ischemic neuronal injury following complete cerebral ischemia. Acta Neuropathol 1981; **55**: 205–20.

238 Jennette JC, Falk RJ, Milling DM. Pathogenesis of vasculitis. Semin Neurol 1994; **14**: 291–306.

239 Jensson O, Gudmundsson G, Arnason A et al. Hereditary cystain C (γ-trace) amyloid angiopathy of the CNS causing cerebral hemorrhage. Acta Neurol Scand 1987; **76**: 102–14.

240 Johnston SC, Halbach VV, Smith WS, Gress DR. Rapid development of giant fusiform cerebral aneurysms in angiographically normal vessels. Neurology 1998; **50**: 1163–6.

241 Johshita H, Asano T, Hanamura T et al. Effect of indomethacin and a free radical scavenger on cerebral blood flow and edema after cerebral artery occlusion in cats. Stroke 1989; **20**: 788–94.

241a Jørgensen L, Torvik A. Ischemic cerebrovascular diseases in an autopsy series. Part 2: Prevalence, location, pathogenesis and clinical course of cerebral infarcts. J Neurol Sci 1969; **9**: 285–320.

242 Joutel A, Andreux F, Gaulis S et al. The ectodomain of the Notch3 receptor accumulates within the cerebrovasculature of CADASIL patients. J Clin Invest 2000; **105**: 597–605.

243 Joutel A, Corpechot C, Ducros A et al. Notch3 mutations in CADASIL, a hereditary late-onset condition causing stroke and dementia. Nature 1996; **383**: 707–10.

244 Joutel A, Vahedi K, Corpechot C et al. Strong clustering and stereotyped nature of Notch3 mutations in CADASIL patients. Lancet 1997; **350**: 1511–15.

245 Juvela S, Hillbom M, Numminen H, Koskinen P. Cigarette smoking and alcohol consumption as risk factors for aneurysmal subarachnoid hemorrhage. Stroke 1993; **24**: 639–46.

246 Juvela S. Minor leak before rupture of an intracranial aneurysm and subarachnoid hemorrhage of unknown etiology. Neurosurgery 1992; **30**: 7–11.

247 Juvela S. Rebleeding from ruptured intracranial aneurysms. Surg Neurol 1989; **32**: 323–6.

248 Juvela S, Kaste M. Reduced platelet aggregability and thromboxane release after rebleeding in patients with subarachnoid hemorrhage. J Neurosurg 1991; **74**: 21–6.

249 Juvela S, Kaste M, Hillbom M. Platelet thromboxane release after subarachnoid hemorrhage and surgery. Stroke 1990; **21**: 566–71.

250 Juvela S, Porras M, Heiskanen O. Natural history of unruptured intracranial aneurysms: a long-term follow-up study. J Neurosurg 1993; **79**: 174–82.

251 Kaku DA, Lowenstein DH. Emergence of recreational drug abuse as a major risk factor for stroke in young adults. Ann Intern Med 1990; **113**: 821–7.

252 Kalimo H, Garcia JH, Kamijyo Y et al. The ultrastructure of 'brain death'. II. Electron microscopy of feline cortex after complete ischemia. Virchows Arch Cell Pathol 1977; **25**: 207–20.

253 Kalimo H, Viitanen M, Amberla K et al. CADASIL: hereditary disease of arteries causing brain infarcts and dementia. Neuropathol Appl Neurobiol 1999; **25**: 257–65.

254 Kamenar E, Burger PC. Cerebral fat embolism: a neuropathological study of a microembolic state. Stroke 1980; **11**: 477–84.

255 Kannel WB, Gordon T, Wolf PA, McNamara P. Hemoglobin and the risk of cerebral infarction: the Framingham Study. Stroke 1972; **3**: 409–20.

256 Karhunen PJ. Neurosurgical vascular complications associated with aneurysm clips evaluated by postmortem angiography. Forensic Sci Int 1991; **51**: 13–22.

257 Karhunen PJ, Männikkö A, Penttilä A, Liesto K. Diagnostic angiography in postoperative autopsies. Am J Forensic Med Pathol 1989; **10**: 303–9.

258 Kase CS. Cerebral amyloid angiopathy. In: Kase CS, Caplan LR eds. Intracerebral hemorrhage. Boston, MA: Butterworth Heinemann, 1994: 179–200.

259 Kase CS, Mohr JP, Caplan LR. Intracerebral hemorrhage. In: Barnett HJM, Mohr JP, Stein BM, Yatsu FM eds. Stroke. Pathophysiology, diagnosis, and management 2nd edn. New York: Churchill Livingstone, 1992: 561–616.

260 Kase CS, Norrving B, Levine SR et al. Cerebellar infarction. Clinical and anatomic observations in 66 cases. Stroke 1993; **24**: 76–83.

261 Kassell NF, Sasaki T, Colohan ART, Nazar G. Cerebral vasospasm following aneurysmal subarachnoid hemorrhage. Stroke 1985; **16**: 562–72.

262 Kassell NF, Torner JC. Aneurysmal rebleeding: a preliminary report from the Cooperative Aneurysm Study. Neurosurgery 1983; **13**: 479–81.

263 Kassell NF, Torner JC. The international cooperative study on timing of aneurysm surgery – an update. Stroke 1984; **15**: 566–70.

264 Kasuya H, Shimizu T. Activated complement components C3a and C4a in cerebrospinal fluid and plasma following subarachnoid hemorrhage. J Neurosurg 1989; **71**: 741–46.

265 Kataoka K, Taneda M, Asai T et al. Structural fragility and inflammatory response of ruptured cerebral aneurysms. A comparative study between ruptured and unruptured cerebral aneurysms. Stroke 1999; **30**: 1396–401.

266 Kaufman HH. Treatment of deep spontaneous intracerebral hematomas. Stroke 1993; **24** (Suppl I): I-101–6.

267 Kay AC, Solberg LAJ, Nichols DA, Petitt RM. Prognostic significance of computed tomography of the brain in thrombotic thrombocytopenic purpura. Mayo Clin Proc 1991; **66**: 602–7.

268 Kay R, Woo J, Kreel L et al. Stroke subtypes among Chinese living in Hong Kong. The Shatin Stroke Registry. Neurology 1992; **42**: 985–7.

269 Kidwell CS, Saver JL, Mattiello J et al. Thrombolytic reversal of acute human cerebral ischemic injury shown by diffusion/perfusion magnetic resonance imaging. Ann Neurol 2000; **47**: 462–9.

270 Kiessling M, Hossmann K-A. Focal cerebral ischemia: molecular mechanisms and new therapeutic strategies. Brain Pathol 1994; **4**: 21–2.

271 Kim JS, Lee JH, Lee MC. Small primary intracerebral hemorrhage. Clinical presentation of 28 cases. Stroke 1994; **25**: 1500–6.

272 Kingman TA, Mendelow AD, Graham DI, Teasdale GM. Experimental intracerebral mass: time-related effects on local cerebral blood flow. J Neurosurg 1987; **67**: 732–8.

273 Kitahara T, Ariga N, Yamura A et al. Familial occurrence of moyamoya disease. Report of three Japanese families. J Neurol Neurosurg Psychiatry 1979; **42**: 208–14.

274 Kitanaka C, Tanaki J, Kuwahara M et al. Nonsurgical treatment of unruptured intracranial vertebral artery dissection with serial follow-up angiography. J Neurosurg 1994; **80**: 667–74.

275 Kittner SJ, Gorelick PB. Antiphospholipid antibodies and stroke: an epidemiological perspective. Stroke 1992; **23** (Suppl I): I-19–22.

276 Kiuru S, Salonen O, Haltia M. Gelsolin-related spinal and cerebral amyloid angiopathy. Ann Neurol 1999; **45**: 305–11.

277 Kondo S, Hashimoto N, Kikuchi H et al. Apoptosis of medial smooth muscle cells in the development of saccular cerebral aneurysms in rats. Stroke 1998; **29**: 181–8.

278 Konishi Y, Hieshima GB, Hara M et al. Congenital fistula of the dural carotid-cavernous sinus: case report and review of the literature. Neurosurgery 1990; 27: 120–6.

279 Korean Neurological Association. Epidemiology of cerebrovascular disease in Korea – a Collaborative Study, 1989–1990. Korean Neurological Association. J Korean Med Sci 1993; 8: 281–9.

280 Kosierkiewicz TA, Factor SM, Dickson DW. Immunocytochemical studies of atherosclerotic lesions of cerebral berry aneurysms. J Neuropathol Exp Neurol 1994; 53: 399–406.

281 Kovanen P, Carpen O, Lassila R, Kaste M. Carotid plaques and stenosis: molecular mechanisms affecting the development of symptomatic lesions. In: Fieschi C, Fisher M eds. Prevention of ischemic stroke. London: Martin Dunitz, 1999: 194–216.

282 Kovanen PT. Atheroma formation: defective control in the intimal round-trip of cholesterol. Eur Heart J 1990; 11: 238–46.

283 Krayenbuhl H. Cerebral venous and sinus thrombosis. Clin Neurosurg 1967; 14: 1–24.

284 Krayenbuhl H. Cerebral venous thrombosis. The diagnostic value of cerebral angiography. Schweiz Arch Neurol Neurochir Psychiatry 1954; 74: 261–87.

285 Kreel L, Kay R, Woo J et al. The radiological (CT) and clinical sequelae of primary intracerebral haemorrhage. Br J Radiol 1991; 64: 1096–100.

286 Krendel DA, Ditter SM, Frankel MR. Biopsy-proven cerebral vasculitis associated with cocaine abuse. Neurology 1990; 40: 1092–4.

287 Kristensen B, Malm J, Nilsson TK et al. Increased fibrinogen levels and acquired hypofibrinolysis in young adults with ischemic stroke. Stroke 1998; 29: 2261–7.

288 Kubes P, Ward PA. Leukocyte recruitment and the acute inflammatory response. Brain Pathol 2000; 10: 127–35.

289 Kudo T. Spontaneous occlusion of circle of Willis. A disease apparently confined to Japanese. Neurology 1968; 18: 458–96.

290 Kuivaniemi H, Prockop DJ, Wu Y et al. Exclusion of mutations in the gene for type III collagen (COL3A1) as a common cause of intracranial aneurysms or cervical artery dissections. Neurology 1993; 43: 2652–8.

291 Kuller L, Reisler DM. An explanation for variations in distribution of stroke and arteriosclerotic heart disease among populations and racial groups. Am J Epidemiol 1971; 93: 1–9.

292 Kunz U, Mauer U, Waldbaur H, Oldenkott P. Früh- und Spätkomplikationen nach Schädel-Hirn Trauma. Chronisches Subduralhämatom/Hygrom, Karotis-Sinus-cavernous-Fistel, Abszedierung, Meningitis und Hydrozephalus. Unfallchirurgie 1993; 96: 595–603.

293 Labauge P, Enjolras O, Bonerandi JJ et al. An association between autosomal dominant cerebral cavernomas and a distinctive hyperkeratotic cutaneous vascular malformation in 4 families. Ann Neurol 1999; 45: 250–4.

294 Lammie GA, Brannan F, Wardlaw JM. Incomplete lacunar infarction (type Ib lacunes). Acta Neuropathol 1998; 96: 164–71.

295 Lassen NA, Agnoli A. The upper limit of autoregulation of cerebral blood flow: on the pathogenesis of hypertensive encephalopathy. J Clin Lab Invest 1973; 30: 113–16.

296 Leadbetter WF, Burkland CE. Hypertension in unilateral renal disease. J Urol 1938; 39: 611–26.

297 Leblanc R. The minor leak preceding subarachnoid hemorrhage. J Neurosurg 1987; 66: 35–9.

298 Lechat P, Mas JL, Lascault G et al. Prevalence of patent foramen ovale in patients with stroke. N Engl J Med 1988; 318: 1148–52.

299 Ledingham JGG, Rajagopalan B. Cerebral complications in the treatment of accelerated hypertension. Q J Med 1979; 48: 25–41.

300 Levine SR, Brey RL, Joseph CLM, Havstad S. Risk of recurrent thromboembolic events in patients with focal cerebral ischemia and antiphospholipid antibodies. Stroke 1992; 23 (Suppl I): I-29–32.

301 Levine SR, Brust JCM, Futrell N. A comparative study of the cerebrovascular complications of cocaine: alkaloidal versus hydrochloride – a review. Neurology 1991; 41: 1173–7.

302 Levine SR, Twyman RE, Gilman S. The role of anticoagulation in cavernous sinus thrombosis. Neurology 1988; 38: 517–22.

303 Levy E, Carman MD, Fernandez Madrid IJ et al. Mutation of the Alzheimer's disease amyloid gene in hereditary cerebral hemorrhage, Dutch type. Science 1990; 248: 1124–6.

304 Levy E, Lopez-Otin C, Ghiso J et al. Stroke in Icelandic patients with hereditary amyloid angiopathy is related to a mutation in a cystatin C gene, an inhibitor of cysteine proteases. J Exp Med 1989; 169: 1771–8.

305 Li Y, Chopp M, Jiang N et al. Temporal profile of in situ DNA fragmentation after transient middle cerebral artery occlusion in the rat. J Cereb Blood Flow Metab 1995; 15: 389–97.

306 Lie JT. Primary (granulomatous) angiitis of the central nervous system: a clinicopathologic analysis of 15 new cases and a review of the literature. Hum Pathol 1992; 23: 164–71.

307 Lie JT. Systemic and isolated vasculitis. A rational approach to classification and pathologic diagnosis. In: Rosen PP, Fechner RE eds. Pathology annual Vol 24, Part 1. Norwalk, CT: Appleton & Lange, 1989: 25–114.

308 Lie JT. The classification and diagnosis of vasculitis in large and medium-sized blood vessels. In: Rosen PP, Fechner RE eds. Pathology annual Vol 22, Part 1. Norwalk, CT: Appleton-Century-Crofts, 1987: 125–62.

309 Little JR, Dial B, Belanger G, Carpenter S. Brain hemorrhage from intracranial tumor. Stroke 1979; 10: 283–8.

310 Little JR, StLouis P, Weinstein M, Dohn DF. Giant fusiform aneurysms of the cerebral arteries. Stroke 1982; 12: 183–8.

311 Lo EH. A haemodynamic analysis of intracranial arteriovenous malformations. Neurol Res 1993; 15: 51–5.

312 Lodder J, Bamford JM, Sandercock PA et al. Are hypertension or cardiac embolism likely causes of lacunar infarction? Stroke 1990; 21: 375–81.

313 Lodder J, Krijne KB, Broekman J. Cerebral hemorrhagic infarction at autopsy: cardiac embolic cause and the relationship to the cause of death. Stroke 1986; 17: 626–9.

314 Loes DJ, Biller J, Yuh WTC et al. Leukoencephalopathy in cerebral amyloid angiopathy: MR imaging in four cases. Am J Neuroradiol 1990; 11: 485–8.

315 Love PE, Santoro SA. Antiphospholipid antibodies: anticardiolipin and the lupus anticoagulant in systemic lupus erythematosus (SLE) and in non-SLE disorders. Ann Intern Med 1990; 112: 682–98.

316 Lüscher TF, Lie JT, Stanson AW et al. Arterial fibromuscular dysplasia. Mayo Clin Proc 1987; 62: 931–52.

317 Luyendijk W, Bots GT, Vegter-van der Vlis M et al. Hereditary cerebral haemorrhage caused by cortical amyloid angiopathy. J Neurol Sci 1988; 85: 267–80.

318 McCormick WF, Acosta-Rua GJ. The size of intracranial saccular aneurysms: an autopsy study. J Neurosurg 1970; 33: 422–7.

319 Macdonald RL, Weir BKA. A review of hemoglobin and the pathogenesis of cerebral vasospasm. Stroke 1991; 22: 971–82.

320 Mackay KB, Kusumoto K, Graham DI, McGulloch J. Effect of the kappa-1 opioid agonist CI-977 on ischemic brain damage and cerebral blood flow after middle cerebral artery occlusion in the rat. *Brain Res* 1993; **629**: 10–18.

321 MacKenzie ET, Strandgaard S, Graham DI et al. Effects of acutely induced hypertension in cats on pial arterial calibre, local cerebral blood flow and the blood–brain barrier. *Circ Res* 1976; **39**: 33–9.

322 Mackenzie RA, Ryan P, Karnes WE, Okazaki H. Herpes zoster arteritis: pathological findings. *Clin Exp Neurol* 1986; **23**: 219–24.

323 Maeda A, Yamada M, Itoh Y et al. Computer-assisted three-dimensional image analysis of cerebral amyloid angiopathy. *Stroke* 1993; **24**: 1857–64.

324 Maggioni AP, Franzosi MG, Santoro E. The risk of stroke in patients with acute myocardial infarction after thrombolytic and antithrombotic treatment. *N Engl J Med* 1992; **327**: 1–6.

325 Malinski T, Bailey F, Zhang ZG, Chopp M. Nitric oxide measured by a porphyrinic microsensor in rat brain after transient middle cerebral artery occlusion. *J Cereb Blood Flow Metab* 1993; **13**: 355–8.

326 Mandybur TI. Cerebral amyloid angiopathy: the vascular pathology and complications. *J Neuropathol Exp Neurol* 1986; **45**: 79–90.

327 Mandybur TI. Intracranial hemorrhage caused by metastatic tumors. *Neurology* 1977; **27**: 650–5.

328 Marchal G, Serrati C, Rioux P et al. PET imaging of cerebral perfusion and oxygen consumption in acute ischaemic stroke: relation to outcome. *Lancet* 1993; **341**: 925–7.

329 Massaro AR, Sacco LR, Mohr JP et al. Clinical discriminators of lobar and deep hemorrhage: the Stroke Data Bank. *Neurology* 1991; **41**: 1881–5.

330 Matsell DG, Keene DL, Jimenez C, Humphreys P. Isolated angiitis of the central nervous system in childhood. *Can J Neurol Sci* 1990; **17**: 151–4.

331 Matsuda M, Shiino A, Handa J. Sequential changes of cerebral blood flow after aneurysmal subarachnoid haemorrhage. *Acta Neurochir* 1990; **105**: 98–106.

332 Mayer SA, Lin J, Homma S et al. Myocardial injury and left ventricular performance after subarachnoid hemorrhage. *Stroke* 1999; **30**: 780–6.

333 Mayer SA, Sacco RL, Shi T, Mohr JP. Neurologic deterioration in noncomatose patients with supratentorial intracerebral hemorrhage. *Neurology* 1994; **44**: 1379–84.

334 Mead S, James-Galton M, Revesz T et al. Familial British dementia with amyloid angiopathy: early clinical, neuropsychological and imaging findings. *Brain* 2000; **123**: 975–9.

335 Meissner I, Whisnant JP, Garraway WM. Hypertension management and stroke recurrence in a community (Rochester, Minnesota, 1950–1979). *Stroke* 1988; **19**: 459–63.

336 Mendelow AD. Mechanisms of ischemic brain damage with intracerebral hemorrhage. *Stroke* 1993; **24** (Suppl I): I-115–17.

337 Menghini VV, Brown RD Jr, Sicks JD et al. Incidence and prevalence of intracranial aneurysms and hemorrhage in Olmstead County, Minnesota, 1965 to 1995. *Neurology* 1998; **51**: 405–11.

338 Metz RJ, Bogousslavsky J. Lacunar stroke. In: Fisher M, Bogousslavsky J eds. *Current review of cerebrovascular disease* 3rd edn. Boston, MA: Butterworth Heinemann, 1999: 93–105.

339 Meurers B, Kohlhepp W, Gold R et al. Histopathological findings in the central and peripheral nervous systems in neuroborreliosis. A report of three cases. *J Neurol* 1990; **237**: 113–16.

340 Meyer FB, Anderson RE, Yaksh TL et al Effect of nimodipine on intracellular brain pH, cortical blood flow, and EEG in experimental focal cerebral ischemia. *J Neurosurg* 1986; **64**: 617–26.

341 Meyer JS, Gilroy J, Barnhart MI, Johnson JF. Therapeutic thrombolysis in cerebral thromboembolism. *Neurology* 1963; **13**: 927–37.

342 Meyohas MC, Roullet E. Cerebral venous thrombosis and dual primary infection with human immunodeficiency virus and cytomegalovirus. *J Neurol Neurosurg Psychiatry* 1989; **52**: 1010–16.

343 Michaeli J, Mittelman M, Grisaru D, Rachmilewitz EA. Thromboembolic complications in beta thalassaemia. *Acta Haematol* 1992; **87**: 71–4.

344 Mies G, Ishimaru S, Xie Y et al. Ischemic thresholds of brain protein synthesis and energy state following middle cerebral artery occlusion in rat. *J Cereb Blood Flow Metab* 1991; **11**: 753–61.

345 Mies G, Kohno K, Hossmann K-A. Prevention of periinfarct direct current shifts with glutamate antagonist NBQX following occlusion of the middle cerebral artery in the rat. *J Cereb Blood Flow Metab* 1994; **14**: 802–7.

346 Milandre L, Brosset C, Gouirand R, Khalil R. Pure cerebellar infarction. Thirty cases. *Presse Med* 1992; **21**: 1562–5.

347 Millikan C, Futrell N. The fallacy of the lacune hypothesis. *Stroke* 1990; **21**: 1251–7.

348 Millikan CH, McDowell F, Easton JD. *Stroke*. Philadelphia, PA: Lea & Febiger, 1987.

349 Miyasaka Y, Yada K, Ohwada T et al. An analysis of the venous drainage system as a factor in hemorrhage from arteriovenous malformations. *J Neurosurg* 1992; **76**: 239–43.

350 Mizukami M, Tazawa T. Theoretical background for surgical treatment in hypertensive intracerebral hemorrhage. In: Mizukami M, Kanaya H, Kogure K, Yamori Y eds. *Hypertensive intracerebral hemorrhage*. New York: Raven Press, 1983: 239–47.

351 Mohamed AA, Gotoh O, Graham DI et al. Effect of pretreatment with the calcium antagonist nimodipide on local cerebral blood flow and histopathology after middle cerebral artery occlusion. *Ann Neurol* 1985; **18**: 705–11.

352 Mohr JP. Lacunes. In: Barnett HJM, Mohr JP, Stein BM, Yatsu FM eds. *Stroke. Pathophysiology, diagnosis, and management* 2nd edn. New York: Churchill Livingstone, 1992: 539–60.

353 Molinari GF, Smith L, Goldstein MN, Satran R. Pathogenesis of cerebral mycotic aneurysms. *Neurology* 1973; **23**: 325–32.

354 Moore P, Calabrese LH. Neurologic manifestations of systemic vasculitides. *Semin Neurol* 1994; **14**: 300–6.

355 Moore PM. Diagnosis and management of isolated angiitis of the central nervous system. *Neurology* 1989; **39**: 167–73.

356 Moossy J. Pathology of cerebral atherosclerosis. Influence of age, race, and gender. *Stroke* 1993; **24** (Suppl): I-22–23.

357 Mori E, del Zoppo GJ, Chambers JD et al. Inhibition of polymorphonuclear leukocyte adherence suppresses no-reflow after focal cerebral ischemia in baboons. *Stroke* 1992; **23**: 712–18.

358 Moschowitz E. An acute febrile pleiochromic anemia with hyaline thrombosis of the terminal arterioles and capillaries. *Arch Intern Med* 1925; **36**: 89–93.

359 Moulin T, Tatu L, Vuillier F et al. Role of a stroke data bank in evaluating cerebral infarction subtypes: patterns and outcome of 1,776 consecutive patients from the Besancon stroke registry. *Cerebrovasc Dis* 2000; **10**: 261–71.

360 Moutsopoulos HM, Sarmas JH, Talal N. Is central nervous system involvement a systemic manifestation of primary

Sjögren's syndrome? *Rheum Dis Clin North Am* 1993; **19**: 909–12.

361 Müller C, Rahn BA, Pfister U, Meinig RP. The incidence, pathogenesis, diagnosis, and treatment of fat embolism. *Orthopaed Rev* 1994; **23**: 107–17.

362 Naff NJ, Wemmer J, Hoenig-Rigamonti K, Rigamonti DR. A longitudinal study of patients with venous malformations: documentation of a negligible hemorrhage risk and benign natural history. *Neurology* 1998; **50**: 1709–14.

363 Nass R, Hays A, Chutorian A. Intracranial dissecting aneurysms in childhood. *Stroke* 1982; **13**: 204–7.

364 Nath FP, Kelly PT, Jenkins A *et al.* Effects of experimental intracerebral hemorrhage on blood flow, capillary permeability, and histochemistry. *J Neurosurg* 1987; **66**: 555–62.

365 Natte R, de Boer WI, Maat-Schieman ML *et al.* Amyloid beta precursor protein-mRNA is expressed throughout cerebral vessel walls. *Brain Res* 1999; **828**: 179–83.

366 Nedergaard M. Neuronal injury in the infarct border: a neuropathological study in the rat. *Acta Neuropathol* 1987; **73**: 267–74.

367 Nehls DG, Mendelow AD, Graham DI *et al.* Experimental intracerebral hemorrhage: progression of hemodynamic changes after production of a spontaneous mass lesion. *Neurosurgery* 1988; **23**: 439–44.

368 Nencini P, Baruffi MC, Abbate R *et al.* Lupus anticoagulant and anticardiolipin antibodies in young adults with cerebral ischemia. *Stroke* 1992; **23**: 189–93.

369 Niazi GA, Awada A, al Rajeh S, Larbi E. Hematological values and their assessment as risk factor in Saudi patients with stroke. *Acta Neurol Scand* 1994; **89**: 439–45.

370 Nishimoto A, Takeuchi S. Abnormal cerebrovascular network related to the internal carotid arteries. *J Neurosurg* 1968; **29**: 255–60.

371 Nobili F, Rodriguez G, Marenco S *et al.* Regional cerebral blood flow in chronic hypertension. A correlative study. *Stroke* 1993; **24**: 1148–53.

372 Nordborg C, Fredriksson K, Johansson BB. Internal carotid and vertebral arteries of spontaneously hypertensive and normotensive rats. A morphometric study on extracranial, intraosseous and intracranial arterial segments. *Acta Pathol Microbiol Immunol Scand A* 1985; **93**: 153–8.

373 Nordborg C, Fredriksson K, Johansson BB. The morphometry of consecutive segments in cerebral arteries of normotensive and spontaneously hypertensive rats. *Stroke* 1985; **16**: 313–20.

374 Nowak-Gottl U, Strater R, Heinecke A *et al.* Lipoprotein (a) and genetic polymorphisms of clotting factor V, prothrombin, and methylenetetrahydrofolate reductase are risk factors of spontaneous ischemic stroke in childhood. *Blood* 1999; **94**: 3678–82.

375 O'Connell BK, Towfighi J, Brennan RW *et al.* Dissecting aneurysms of head and neck. *Neurology* 1985; **35**: 993–7.

376 Oder W, Kollegger H, Zeiler K *et al.* Subarachnoid hemorrhage of unknown etiology: early prognostic factors for long-term functional capacity. *J Neurosurg* 1991; **74**: 601–5.

377 Ogata J, Masuda J, Yutani C. Rupture of atheromatous plaque as a cause of thrombotic occlusion of stenotic internal carotid artery. *Stroke* 1990; **21**: 1740–5.

378 Ogata J, Okayama M, Goto I *et al.* Primary familial amyloidosis with vitreous opacities. Report of an autopsy case. *Acta Neuropathol* 1978; **42**: 766–7.

379 Öhman J, Servo A, Heiskanen O. Risk factors for cerebral infarction in good-grade patients after aneurysmal subarachnoid hemorrhage and surgery: a prospective study. *J Neurosurg* 1991; **74**: 14–20.

380 Okada Y, Copeland BR, Mori E *et al.* P-selectin and intercellular adhesion molecule-1 expression after focal brain ischemia and reperfusion. *Stroke* 1994; **25**: 202–11.

381 Okayama M, Goto I, Ogata J *et al.* Primary amyloidosis with familial vitreous opacities. An unusual case and family. *Arch Intern Med* 1978; **138**: 105–11.

382 Okazaki H, Reagan TJ, Campbell RJ. Clinocopathological studies of primary cerebral amyloid angiopathy. *Mayo Clin Proc* 1979; **54**: 22–31.

383 Oksi J, Kalimo H, Marttila RJ *et al.* Intracranial aneurysms in three patients with disseminated Lyme borreliosis: cause or chance association? *J Neurol Neurosurg Psychiatry* 1998; **64**: 636–42.

384 Oppenheimer BS, Fishberg AM. Hypertensive encephalopathy. *Arch Intern Med* 1928; **41**: 264–78.

385 Osborne AG, Anderson RE. Angiographic spectrum of cervical and intracranial fibromuscular dysplasia. *Stroke* 1977; **8**: 617–26.

386 Østergaard JR. Risk factors in intracranial saccular aneurysms. Aspects on the formation and rupture of aneurysms and development of cerebral vasospasm. *Acta Neurol Scand* 1989; **80**: 81–98.

387 Østergaard JR, Høg E. Incidence of multiple intracranial aneurysms. Influence of arterial hypertension and gender. *J Neurosurg* 1985; **63**: 49–55.

388 Ott E. Hyperviscosity syndromes. In: Toole JF ed. *Handbook of clinical neurology* Vol 11, Part III. Amsterdam: Elsevier, 1989: 483–92.

389 Palsdottir A, Abrahamson M, Thorsteinsson L *et al.* Mutation in cystatin C gene causes hereditary brain haemorrhage. *Lancet* 1988; **ii**: 603–4.

390 Park CK, Nehls DG, Graham DI *et al.* The glutamate antagonist MK801 reduces focal ischaemic brain damage in the rat. *Ann Neurol* 1988; **24**: 543–51.

391 Parker F, Healey LA, Wilske KR, Odland GF. Light and electron microscopic studies on human temporal arteries with special reference to alterations related to senescence, atherosclerosis and giant cell arteritis. *Am J Pathol* 1975; **79**: 57–80.

392 Parlea L, Fahrig R, Holdsworth DW, Lownie SP. An analysis of the geometry of saccular intracranial aneurysms. *Am J Neuroradiol* 1999; **20**: 1079–89.

393 Paschall FE. Thrombotic thrombocytopenic purpura: the challenges of a complex disease process. *AACN Clin Issues Crit Care Nurs* 1993; **4**: 655–63.

394 Pendlebury WW, Iole ED, Tracy RP, Dill BA. Intracerebral hemorrhage related to cerebral amyloid angiopathy and t-PA treatment. *Ann Neurol* 1991; **29**: 210–13.

395 Pessin M. Hemorrhagic transformation in the natural history of acute embolic stroke. In: Hacke W, del Zoppo GJ, Hirschberg M eds. *Thrombolytic therapy in acute ischemic stroke*. Berlin: Springer, 1991: 67–74.

396 Pessin MS, Adelman LS, Barbas NR. Spontaneous intracranial carotid artery dissection. *Stroke* 1989; **20**: 1100–3.

397 Pessin MS, Chimowitz MI, Levine SR *et al.* Stroke in patients with fusiform vertebrobasilar aneurysms. *Neurology* 1989; **39**: 16–21.

398 Pessin MS, Lathi ES, Cohen MB *et al.* Clinical features and mechanism of occipital infarction. *Ann Neurol* 1987; **21**: 290–9.

399 Peterson JW, Kwun BD, Hackett JD, Zervas NT. The role of inflammation in experimental cerebral vasospasm. *J Neurosurg* 1990; **72**: 767–74.

400 Petty GW, Brown RD Jr, Whisnant JP *et al.* Ischemic stroke subtypes: a population-based study of incidence and risk factors. *Stroke* 1999; **30**: 2513–16.

401 Piette JC, Wechsler B, Vidailhet M. Idiopathic intracranial hypertension: don't forget cerebral venous thrombosis. *Am J Med* 1994; **97**: 200.

402 Plant GT, Revesz T, Barnard RO *et al.* Familial cerebral amyloid angiography with nonneuritic amyloid plaque formation. *Brain* 1990; **113**: 721–47.

403 Plate KH. Mechanisms of angiogenesis in the brain. *J Neuropathol Exp Neurol* 1999; **58**: 313–20.

404 Poirier J, Gray F, Gherardi R, Derouesne C. Cerebral lacunae: a new neuropathological classification. *J Neuropathol Exp Neurol* 1985; **44**: 312.

405 Pozzati E, Padovani R, Fabrizi A *et al.* Benign arterial dissections of the posterior circulation. *J Neurosurg* 1991; **75**: 69–72.

406 Provenzale JM, Heinz ER, Ortel TL *et al.* Antiphospholipid antibodies in patients without systemic lupus erythematosus: neuroradiologic findings. *Radiology* 1994; **192**: 531–7.

407 Quinn MT, Parthasarathy S, Fong LG, Steinberg D. Oxidatively modified low density lipoproteins: a potential role in recruitment and retention of monocyte/macrophages during atherogenesis. *Proc Natl Acad Sci USA* 1987; **84**: 2995–8.

408 Rådberg JA, Olsson JE, Rådberg CT. Prognostic parameters in spontaneous intracerebral hematomas with special reference to anticoagulant treatment. *Stroke* 1991; **22**: 571–6.

409 Rahman NU, al Tahan AR. Computed tomographic evidence of an extensive thrombosis and infarction of the deep venous system. *Stroke* 1993; **24**: 744–6.

410 Rail DL, Perkin GD. Computerized tomographic appearance of hypertensive encephalopathy. *Arch Neurol* 1980; **37**: 310–11.

411 Reed DM, Resch JA, Hayashi T *et al.* A prospective study of cerebral artery atherosclerosis. *Stroke* 1988; **19**: 820–5.

412 Reuner KH, Ruf A, Grau A *et al.* Prothrombin gene G20210→A transition is a risk factor for cerebral venous thrombosis. *Stroke* 1998; **29**: 1765–9.

413 Ribes MF. Des recherches faites sur la phlébite. *Revue Médicale Francaise et Etrangère et Journal de Clinique de l'Hôtel-Dieu et de la Charité de Paris* 1825; **3**: 5–41.

414 Ricci S, Celani MG, LaRosa F *et al.* SEPIVAC: a community-based study of stroke incidence in Umbria, Italy. *J Neurol Neurosurg Psychiatry* 1991; **54**: 695–8.

415 Richards A, Graham D, Bullock R. Clinicopathological study of neurological complications due to hypertensive disorders of pregnancy. *J Neurol Neurosurg Psychiatr* 1988; **51**: 416–21.

416 Rigamonti D, Hadley MN, Drayer BP *et al.* Cerebral cavernous malformations: incidence and familial occurrence. *N Engl J Med* 1988; **319**: 343–7.

417 Rinkel GJ, Djibuti M, van Gijn J. Prevalence and risk of rupture of intracranial aneurysms: a systematic review. *Stroke* 1998; **29**: 251–6.

418 Rinkel GJ, Wijdicks EF, Vermeulen M *et al.* Nonaneurysmal perimesencephalic subarachnoid hemorrhage: CT and MR patterns that differ from aneurysmal rupture. *Am J Neuroradiol* 1991; **12**: 829–34.

419 Rinkel GJ, Wijdicks EF, Vermeulen M *et al.* The clinical course of perimesencephalic nonaneurysmal subarachnoid hemorrhage. *Ann Neurol* 1991; **29**: 463–8.

420 Rinne J, Hernesniemi J, Puranen M, Saari T. Multiple intracranial aneurysms in a defined population: prospective angiographic and clinical study. *Neurosurgery* 1994; **35**: 803–8.

421 Risau W. Mechanisms of angiogenesis. *Nature* 1997; **386**: 671–4.

422 Rissanen A. Cerebrovascular disease in the Jyväskylä region, Central Finland. University of Kuopio, 1992.

423 Romanul FCA. Examination of the brain and spinal cord. In: Tedeschi CG ed. *Neuropathology. Methods and diagnosis* 1 edn. Boston, MA: Little, Brown & Co., 1970: 131–214.

424 Ronkainen A, Hernesniemi J. Subarachnoid haemorrhage of unknown aetiology. *Acta Neurochir* 1992; **119**: 29–34.

425 Ronkainen A, Hernesniemi J, Puranen M *et al.* Familial intracranial aneurysms. *Lancet* 1997; **349**: 380–4.

426 Ronkainen A, Hernesniemi J, Tromp G. Special features of familial intracranial aneurysms: report of 215 familial aneurysms. *Neurosurgery* 1995; **37**: 43–7.

427 Ropper AH. Lateral displacement of the brain and level of consciousness in patients with an acute hemispheral mass. *N Engl J Med* 1986; **314**: 953–8.

428 Rosenblum WI. Miliary aneurysms and 'fibrinoid' degeneration of cerebral blood vessels. *Hum Pathol* 1977; **8**: 133–9.

429 Rosenblum WI. The importance of fibrinoid necrosis as the cause of cerebral hemorrhage in hypertension. Commentary. *J Neuropathol Exp Neurol* 1993; **52**: 11–13.

430 Rosenørn J, Eskesen V, Schmidt K, Rønde F. The risk of rebleeding from ruptured intracranial aneurysms. *J Neurosurg* 1987; **67**: 329–32.

431 Ross R. Atherosclerosis – an inflammatory disease. *N Engl J Med* 1999; **340**: 115–26.

432 Ross Russell RW, Enevoldson TP. Unusual types of ischemic stroke. In: Fisher M, Bogousslavsky J eds. *Current review of cerebrovascular disease* 1st edn. Philadelphia, PA: Current Medicine, 1993: 63–77.

433 Roubey RA, Hoffman M. From antiphospholipid syndrome to antibody-mediated thrombosis. *Lancet* 1997; **350**: 1491–3.

434 Rubin LA, Urowitz MB, Gladman DD. Mortality in systemic lupus erythematosus: the bimodal pattern revisited. *Q J Med* 1985; **55**: 87–98.

435 Ruchoux MM, Maurage CA. CADASIL: cerebral autosomal dominant arteriopathy with subcortical infarcts and leukoencephalopathy. *J Neuropathol Exp Neurol* 1997; **56**: 947–64.

436 Russell RWR, Wade JPH. Haematological causes of cerebrovascular disease. In: Toole JF ed. *Handbook of clinical neurology Vol 11 Vascular disease* Part III. Amsterdam: Elsevier, 1989: 463–81.

437 Sacco RL. Classification of stroke. In: Fisher M ed. *Clinical atlas of cerebrovascular disorders*. London: Wolfe, 1994: 2.2–2.25.

438 Sacco RL. Current epidemiology of stroke. In: Fisher M, Bogousslavsky J eds. *Current review of cerebrovascular disease* 1 edn. Philadelphia, PA: Current Medicine, 1993: 3–14.

439 Sacco RL. Frequency and determinants of stroke. In: Fisher M ed. *Clinical atlas of cerebrovascular disorders*. London: Wolfe, 1994: 1.2–1.16.

440 Sacco RL, Hauser WA, Mohr JP. Hospitalized stroke incidence in blacks and hispanics in northern Manhattan. *Stroke* 1991; **22**: 1491–6.

441 Sagoh M, Hirose Y, Murakami H *et al.* Late hemorrhage from persistent pseudoaneurysm in vertebral artery dissection presenting with ischemia: case report. *Surg Neurol* 1999; **52**: 480–3.

442 Sahoo T, Johnson EW, Thomas JW *et al.* Mutations in the gene encoding KRIT1, a Krev-1/rap1a binding protein, cause cerebral cavernous malformations. *Hum Mol Genet* 1999; **8**: 2325–33.

443 Sajanti J, Björkstrand AS, Finnilä S *et al.* Increase of collagen synthesis and deposition in the arachnoid and the dura following subarachnoid hemorrhage in the rat. *Biochim Biophys Acta* 1999; **1454**: 209–16.

444 Samson D, Batjer HH, Bowman G et al. A clinical study of the parameters and effects of temporary arterial occlusion in the management of intracranial aneurysms. *Neurosurgery* 1994; **34**: 22–8.

445 Sarti C, Tuomilehto J, Salomaa V et al. Epidemiology of subarachnoid hemorrhage in Finland from 1983 to 1985. *Stroke* 1991; **22**: 848–53.

446 Sasaki O, Ogawa H, Koike T et al. A clinicopathological study of dissecting aneurysms of the intracranial vertebral artery. *J Neurosurg* 1991; **75**: 874–82.

447 Sauron B, Chiras J, Chain G, Castaigne P. Thrombophlébite cérébelleuse chez un homme porteur d'un déficit familial en antithrombine III. *Rev Neurol (Paris)* 1982; **138**: 685.

448 Savoiado M. The vascular territories of the carotid and vertebrobasilar system. *Ital J Neurol Sci* 1986; **7**: 405–9.

449 Schievink WI, Katzmann JA, Piepgras DG. Alpha-1-antitrypsin deficiency in spontaneous intracranial artery dissections. *Cerebrovasc Dis* 1998; **8**: 42–4.

450 Schievink WI, Parisi JE, Piepgras DG, Michels VV. Intracranial aneurysms in Marfan's syndrome: an autopsy study. *Neurosurgery* 1997; **41**: 866–70.

451 Schievink WI, Piepgras DG, Earnest FIV, Gordon H. Spontaneous carotid-cavernous fistulae in Ehlers–Danlos syndrome type IV. Case report. *J Neurosurg* 1991; **74**: 991–8.

452 Schievink WI, Puumala MR, Meyer FB et al. Giant intracranial aneurysm and fibromuscular dysplasia in an adolescent with alpha 1-antitrypsin deficiency. *J Neurosurg* 1996; **85**: 503–6.

453 Schievink WI, Torres VE, Wiebers DO, Huston J III. Intracranial arterial dolichoectasia in autosomal dominant polycystic kidney disease. *J Am Soc Nephrol* 1997; **8**: 1298–303.

454 Schievink WI, Wijdicks EF, Michels VV et al. Heritable connective tissue disorders in cervical artery dissections: a prospective study. *Neurology* 1998; **50**: 1166–9.

455 Schutta HS, Williams EC, Baranski BG, Sutula TP. Cerebral venous thrombosis with plasminogen deficiency. *Stroke* 1991; **22**: 401–5.

456 Schütz H, Bodeker R-H, Damian M et al. Age-related spontaneous intracerebral hematoma in a German community. *Stroke* 1990; **21**: 1412–18.

457 Schweitzer JS, Chang BS, Madsen P et al. The pathology of arteriovenous malformations of the brain treated by embolotherapy. II. Results of embolization with multiple agents. *Neuroradiology* 1993; **35**: 468–74.

458 Sheffield EA, Weller RO. Age changes at cerebral artery bifurcations and the pathogenesis of berry aneurysms. *J Neurol Sci* 1980; **46**: 341–52.

459 Shi FL, Hart RG, Sherman DG, Tegeler CH. Stroke in the People's Republic of China. *Stroke* 1989; **20**: 1581–5.

460 Shinton R, Beevers G. Meta-analysis of the relation between cigarette smoking and stroke. *BMJ* 1989; **298**: 789–94.

461 Siesjö BK. Pathophysiology and treatment of focal cerebral ischemia. Part I: Pathophysiology. *J Neurosurg* 1992; **77**: 169–84.

462 Siesjö BK, Agardh CD, Bengtsson F. Free radicals and brain damage. *Cerebrovasc Brain Metab Rev* 1989; **1**: 165–211.

463 Sigal LH. The neurologic presentation of vasculitic and rheumatologic syndromes. A review. *Medicine* 1987; **66**: 157–80.

464 Sloan MA. Cerebrovascular disorders associated with licit and illicit drugs. In: Fisher M, Bogousslavsky J eds. *Current review of cerebrovascular disease* 1st edn. Philadelphia, PA: Current Medicine, 1993: 48–62.

465 Sloan MA, Price TR, Foulkes MA et al. Circadian rhythmicity of stroke onset. Intracerebral and subarachnoid hemorrhage. *Stroke* 1992; **23**: 1420–6.

466 Smith SE, Meldrum BS. Cerebroprotective effect of lamotrigine after focal ischemia in rats. *Stroke* 1995; **26**: 117–22.

467 Sokrab T-EO, Johansson BB, Kalimo H, Olsson Y. A transient hypertensive opening of the blood–brain barrier can lead to brain damage. Extravasation of serum proteins and cellular changes in rats subjected to aortic compression. *Acta Neuropathol* 1988; **75**: 557–65.

468 Solberg LA, Eggen DA. Localization and sequence of development of atherosclerotic lesions in the carotid and vertebral arteries. *Circulation* 1971; **43**: 711–24.

469 Somer T, Finegold SM. Vasculitides associated with infections, immunization, and antimicrobial drugs. *Clin Infect Dis* 1995; **20**: 1010–36.

470 Sourander P, Wålinder J. Hereditary multi-infarct dementia. *Acta Neuropathol* 1977; **39**: 247–54.

471 Spangler KM, Challa VR, Moody DM, Bell MA. Arteriolar tortuosity of the white matter in aging and hypertension. A microradiographic study. *J Neuropathol Exp Neurol* 1994; **53**: 22–6.

472 Stanley JC, Gewertz BL, Bove EL et al. Arterial fibrodysplasia: histopathologic character and current etiologic concepts. *Arch Surg* 1975; **110**: 561–6.

473 Steel JG, Thomas HA, Strollo PJ. Fusiform basilar aneurysm as a cause of embolic stroke. *Stroke* 1982; **13**: 712–16.

474 Stehbens WE. Etiology of intracranial berry aneurysms. *J Neurosurg* 1989; **70**: 823–31.

475 Steiger HJ. Pathophysiology of development and rupture of cerebral aneurysms. *Acta Neurochir* 1990; **48** (Suppl): 1–57.

476 Stein BM, Wolpert SM. Arteriovenous malformations of the brain. I. Current concepts and treatment. *Arch Neurol* 1980; **37**: 1–5.

477 Stein BM, Wolpert SM. Arteriovenous malformations of the brain. II. Current concepts and treatment. *Arch Neurol* 1980; **37**: 69–75.

478 Steinberg D, Parthasarathy S, Carew TE et al. Beyond cholesterol. Modifications of low-density lipoprotein that increase its atherogenicity. *N Engl J Med* 1989; **320**: 915–24.

479 Suzuki J, Kodama N. Moya disease – a review. *Stroke* 1983; **14**: 104–9.

480 Suzuki J, Takaku A. Cerebrovascular 'moyamoya– disease. Disease showing abnormal net-like vessels in base of brain. *Arch Neurol* 1969; **20**: 288–99.

481 Suzuki K, Vutsuzawa T, Takita K et al. Clinico-epidemiologic study of stroke in Akita, Japan. *Stroke* 1987; **18**: 402–6.

482 Szer IS, Miller JH, Rawlings D et al. Cerebral perfusion abnormalities in children with central nervous system manifestations of lupus detected by single photon emission computed tomography. *J Rheumatol* 1993; **20**: 2143–8.

483 Takashima S, Becker LE. Neuropathology of cerebral arteriovenous malformation in children. *J Neurol Neurosurg Psychiatry* 1980; **43**: 380–5.

484 Takasugi S, Ueda S, Matsumoto K. Chronological changes in spontaneous intracerebral hematoma – An experimental and clinical study. *Stroke* 1985; **16**: 651–8.

485 Takebayashi S, Kaneko M. Electron microscopic studies of ruptured arteries in hypertensive intracerebral hemorrhage. *Stroke* 1983; **14**: 28–36.

486 Takeya Y, Popper JS, Shimizu Y et al. Epidemiologic studies of coronary heart disease and stroke in Japanese men living in Japan, Hawaii and California: incidence of stroke in Japan and Hawaii. *Stroke* 1984; **15**: 15–23.

487 Tanne D, Triplett DA, Levine SR. Antiphospholipid-protein antibodies and ischemic stroke: not just cardiolipin any more. *Stroke* 1998; **29**: 1755–8.

488 Tardy B, Page Y, Convers P et al. Thrombotic thrombocytopenic purpura: MR findings. Am J Neuroradiol 1993; **14**: 489–90.

489 Tarras S, Gadia C, Mester L. Homozygous protein C deficiency in a newborn. Clinicopathologic correlation. Arch Neurol 1988; **45**: 214–20.

490 Tatlisumak T, Fisher M. Hematologic disorders associated with ischemic stroke. J Neurol Sci 1996; **140**: 1–11.

491 Tell GS, Crouse JR, Furberg CD. Relation between blood lipids, lipoproteins, and cerebrovascular atherosclerosis: a review. Stroke 1988; **19**: 423–30.

492 Terent A. Stroke morbidity. In: Whisnant JP ed. Stroke: populations, cohorts, and clinical trials. Oxford: Butterworth Heinemann, 1993: 37–58.

493 Terent A, Marke LA, Asplund K, Norrving B, Jonsson E, Wester PO. Costs of stroke in Sweden. A national perspective. Stroke 1994; **25**: 2363–9.

494 Thomas WS, Mori E, Copeland BR et al. Tissue factor contributes to microvascular defects after focal cerebral ischemia. Stroke 1993; **24**: 847–54.

495 Thorsteinsson L, Georgsson G, Asgeirsson B et al. On the role of monocytes/macrophages in the pathogenesis of central nervous system lesions in hereditary cystatin C amyloid angiopathy. J Neurol Sci 1992; **108**: 121–8.

496 Thron A, Wessel K, Linden D. Superior sagittal sinus thrombosis: neuroradiological evaluation and clinical findings. J Neurol 1986; **233**: 283–8.

497 Tohgi H, Yamanouchi H, Murakami M, Kameyama M. Importance of the hematocrit as a risk factor in cerebral infarction. Stroke 1978; **9**: 369–74.

498 Tokuda T, Ikeda S, Yanagisawa N et al. Re-examination of ex-boxers' brains using immunohistochemistry with antibodies to amyloid β-protein and tau protein. Acta Neuropathol 1991; **82**: 280–5.

499 Tomonaga M. Cerebral amyloid angiopathy in the elderly. J Am Geriatr Soc 1981; **24**: 151–7.

500 Toole JF. Cerebrovascular disorders 4th edn. New York: Raven Press, 1990.

501 Torvik A, Svindland A. Is there a transitional zone between brain infarcts and the surrounding brain? A histological study. Acta Neurol Scand 1986; **74**: 365–70.

502 Toschi V, Motta A, Castelli C et al. Prevalence and clinical significance of antiphospholipid antibodies to non-cardiolipin antigens in systemic lupus erythematosus. Haemostasis 1993; **23**: 275–83.

503 Toschi V, Motta A, Castelli C et al. High prevalence of antiphosphatidylinositol antibodies in young patients with cerebral ischemia of undetermined cause. Stroke 1998; **29**: 1759–64.

504 Tournier-Lasserve E, Joutel A, Melki J et al. Cerebral autosomal dominant arteriopathy with subcortical infarcts and leukoencephalopathy maps to chromosome 19q12. Nat Genet 1993; **3**: 256–9.

505 Travers RL, Allison DJ, Brettle RP, Hughes GR. Polyarteritis nodosa: a clinical and angiographic analysis of 17 cases. Semin Arthritis Rheum 1979; **8**: 184–99.

506 Tuominen S, Juvonen V, Amberla K et al. The phenotype of a homozygous CADASIL patient in comparison to nine age-matched heterozygous patients with the same R133C Notch3 mutation. Stroke 2001; **32**: 1764–74.

507 Tzourio C, Tehindrazanarivelo A, Iglesias S et al. Case–control study of migraine and risk of ischaemic stroke in young women. BMJ 1995; **310**: 830–3.

508 Uchida K, Nakayama H, Goto N. Pathological studies on cerebral amyloid angiopathy, senile plaques and amyloid deposition in visceral organs in aged dogs. J Vet Med Sci 1991; **53**: 1037–42.

509 Ueda K, Omae T, Hirota Y et al. Decreasing trend in incidence and mortality from stroke in Hisayama residents, Japan. Stroke 1981; **12**: 154–60.

510 Ueda T, Hatakeyama T, Kumon Y et al. Evaluation of risk of hemorrhagic transformation in local intra-arterial thrombolysis in acute ischemic stroke by initial SPECT. Stroke 1994; **25**: 298–303.

511 Uglietta JP, O'Connor CM, Boyko OB. CT patterns of intracranial hemorrhage complicating thrombolytic therapy for acute myocardial infarction. Radiology 1991; **181**: 555–9.

512 Uno H, Walker LC. The age of biosenescence and the incidence of cerebral beta-amyloidosis in aged captive rhesus monkeys. Ann N Y Acad Sci 1993; **695**: 232–5.

513 Ushiyama M, Ikeda S, Yanagisawa N. Transthyretin-type cerebral amyloid angiopathy in type I familial amyloid polyneuropathy. Acta Neuropathol 1991; **81**: 524–8.

514 van Dam AP. Diagnosis and pathogenesis of CNS lupus. Rheumatol Int 1991; **11**: 1–11.

515 van't Hooft FM, von Bahr SJ, Silveira A et al. Two common, functional polymorphisms in the promoter region of the beta-fibrinogen gene contribute to regulation of plasma fibrinogen concentration. Arterioscler Thromb Vasc Biol 1999; **19**: 3063–70.

516 Vermeulen M, Lindsay KW, Murray GD et al. Antifibrinolytic treatment in subarachnoid hemorrhage. N Engl J Med 1984; **311**: 432–7.

517 Vermeulen M, van Gijn J. The diagnosis of subarachnoid haemorrhage. J Neurol Neurosurg Psychiatry 1990; **53**: 365–72.

518 Vermylen J, Badenhorst PN, Deckmyn H, Arnout J. Normal mechanisms of platelet function. Clin Haematol 1983; **12**: 107–51.

519 Vidal R, Frangione B, Rostagno A et al. A stop-codon mutation in the BRI gene associated with familial British dementia. Nature 1999; **399**: 776–81.

520 Vidal R, Revesz T, Rostagno A et al. A decamer duplication in the 3′ region of the BRI gene originates an amyloid peptide that is associated with dementia in a Danish kindred. Proc Natl Acad Sci USA 2000; **97**: 4920–5.

521 Vinters HV. Cerebral amyloid angiopathy. A critical review. Stroke 1987; **18**: 311–24.

522 Vinters HV, Gilbert JJ. Cerebral amyloid angiopathy: incidence and complications in the aging brain. II. The distribution of amyloid vascular changes. Stroke 1983; **14**: 924–8.

523 Vinters HV, Secor DL, Pardridge WM, Gray F. Immunohistochemical study of cerebral amyloid angiopathy. III. Widespread Alzheimer A4 peptide in cerebral microvessel walls colocalizes with gamma trace in patients with leucoencephalopathy. Ann Neurol 1990; **28**: 34–42.

524 Vonsattel JPG, Myers RH, Hedley-Whyte ET et al. Cerebral amyloid angiopathy without and with cerebral hemorrhages: a comparative histological study. Ann Neurol 1991; **30**: 637–49.

525 Wakabayashi S, Ohno K, Shishido T et al. Marked growth of a cerebral arteriovenous malformation: case report and review of the literature. Neurosurgery 1991; **29**: 920–3.

526 Wakai S, Kumakura N, Nagai M. Lobar intracerebral hemorrhage. A clinical, radiographic, and pathological study of 29 consecutive operated cases with negative angiography. J Neurosurg 1992; **76**: 231–8.

527 Wakai S, Nagai M. Histological verification of microaneurysm as a cause of cerebral haemorrhage in surgical specimens. J Neurol Neurosurg Psychiatry 1989; **52**: 595–9.

528 Walker LC, Masters C, Beyreuther K, Price DL. Amyloid in the brains of aged squirrel monkeys. Acta Neuropathol 1990; **80**: 381–7.

529 Wardlaw JM, del Zoppo G, Yamaguchi T. Thrombolysis for acute ischaemic stroke. *Cochrane Database Syst Rev* 2000; No. 2: CD000213.

530 Wardlaw JM, Warlow CP. Thrombolysis in acute ischemic stroke: does it work? *Stroke* 1992; **23**: 1826–39.

531 Warlow CP. Epidemiology of stroke. *Lancet* 1998; **352** (Suppl III): 1–4.

532 Weir B. *Aneurysms affecting the nervous system.* Baltimore, MD: Williams & Wilkins, 1987.

533 Weir B. The clinical problem of intracerebral hematoma. *Stroke* 1993; **24** (Suppl I): I-93.

534 Welch GN, Loscalzo J. Homocysteine and atherothrombosis. *N Engl J Med* 1998; **338**: 1042–50.

535 Weller RO, Massey A, Newman TA *et al*. Cerebral amyloid angiopathy. Amyloid beta accumulates in putative interstitial fluid drainage pathways in Alzheimer's disease. *Am J Pathol* 1998; **153**: 725–33.

536 Westergaard E, van Deurs S, Böndstad HE. Increased vesicular transfer of horseradish peroxidase across cerebral endothelium, evoked by acute hypertension. *Acta Neuropathol* 1977; **37**: 141–52.

537 Wiebers DO, Adams HP Jr, Whisnant JP. Animal models of stroke: are they relevant to human disease? *Stroke* 1990; **21**: 1–3.

538 Wiebers DO, Whisnant JP, Sundt TM Jr, O'Fallon WM. The significance of unruptured intracranial saccular aneurysms. *J Neurosurg* 1987; **66**: 23–9.

539 Wienhard K, Dahlbom M, Eriksson L *et al*. The ECAT EXACT HR: performance of a new high resolution positron scanner. *J Comput Assist Tomogr* 1994; **18**: 110–18.

540 Wilkins RH. Attempts at prevention or treatment of intracranial arterial spasm: an update. *Neurosurgery* 1986; **18**: 808–25.

541 Wilkinson IMS, Russell RWR. Arteries of the head and neck in giant cell arteries. A pathological study to show the pattern of arterial involvement. *Arch Neurol* 1972; **27**: 378–91.

542 Wolf PA. An overview of the epidemiology of stroke. *Stroke* 1990; **21** (Suppl II): II4–6.

543 Wolf PA, Cobb JL. Epidemiology of stroke. In: Barnett JP, Mohr JP, Stein BM, Yatsu FM eds. *Stroke. Pathophysiology, diagnosis, and management* 2nd edn. New York: Churchill Livingstone, 1992: 3–27.

544 Wong V, Yu YL, Liang RH *et al*. Cerebral thrombosis in beta thalassemia/hemoglobin E disease. *Stroke* 1990; **21**: 812–16.

545 Woolfenden AR, Albers GW. Cardioembolic stroke. In: Fisher M, Bogousslavsky J eds. *Current review of cerebrovascular disease* 3rd edn. Boston, MA: Butterworth Heinemann, 1999: 93–105.

546 Worster-Drought C, Greenfield JG, McMenemey WH. A form of familial presenile dementia with spastic paralysis. *Brain* 1940; **63**: 237–54.

547 Yamamura A. Diagnosis and treatment of vertebral aneurysms. *J Neurosurg* 1988; **69**: 345–9.

548 Yamashita M, Oka K, Tanaka K. Histopathology of the brain vascular network in moyamoya disease. *Stroke* 1983; **14**: 50–8.

549 Yang GY, Chan PH, Chen J *et al*. Human copper-zinc superoxide dismutase transgenic mice are highly resistant to reperfusion injury after focal cerebral ischemia. *Stroke* 1994; **25**: 165–70.

550 Yao H, Ginsberg MD, Eveleth DD *et al*. Local cerebral glucose utilization and cytoskeletal proteolysis as indices of evolving focal ischemic injury in core and penumbra. *J Cereb Blood Flow Metab* 1995; **15**: 398–408.

551 Ylä-Herttuala S, Palinski W, Rosenfeld MR *et al*. Evidence for the presence of oxidatively modified low density lipoprotein in atherosclerotic lesions of rabbit and man. *J Clin Invest* 1989; **84**: 1086–95.

552 Yonas H, Sekhar L, Johnson DW, Gur D. Determination of irreversible ischemia by xenon-enhanced computed tomographic monitoring of cerebral blood flow in patients with symptomatic vasospasm. *Neurosurgery* 1989; **24**: 368–72.

553 Yong WH, Robert ME, Secor DL *et al*. Cerebral hemorrhage with biopsy-proved amyloid angiopathy. *Arch Neurol* 1992; **49**: 51–8.

554 Zanette EM, Roberti C, Mancini G *et al*. Spontaneous middle cerebral artery reperfusion in ischemic stroke. A follow-up study with transcranial Doppler. *Stroke* 1995; **26**: 430–3.

555 Zhang F, White JG, Iadecola C. Nitric oxide donors increase blood flow and reduce brain damage in focal cerebral ischemia: evidence that nitric oxide is beneficial in the early stages of cerebral ischemia. *J Cereb Blood Flow Metab* 1994; **14**: 217–26.

556 Zuccarello M, Mandybur TI, Tew JJ, Tobler WD. Acute effect of the Nd:YAG laser on the cerebral arteriovenous malformation: a histological study. *Neurosurgery* 1989; **24**: 328–33.

7

Malformations

BRIAN N. HARDING AND ANDREW J. COPP

INTRODUCTION

Malformations of the central nervous system (CNS) are of major clinical importance, leading to considerable mortality and morbidity, both prenatally and postnatally. The birth prevalence of CNS malformations is between 5 and 10 per 1000 births, and appears to have remained fairly stable over the past 50 years.[475,648] Data collected from Europe and the USA, between 1940 and 1990, show that 8–10% of stillbirths and 5–6% of early neonatal deaths are caused primarily by malformation of the CNS.[475] Moreover, CNS malformations are present in around 15% of infants dying from causes associated with birth defects.[974]

These figures probably underestimate the prevalence of the most severe, and the least severe, malformations. Defects such as anencephaly, which have a higher prevalence among spontaneous abortions than term pregnancies,[183] are probably more common than is suggested by the epidemiological data, which are based predominantly on liveborn infants and stillbirths. By contrast, subtle malformations such as neuronal migration defects are often not recognized at birth or in the first year of life, and so also may not be included in the epidemiological surveys. The most common CNS malformations, according to the epidemiological studies, in declining order of prevalence, are: microcephaly, hydrocephaly, macrocephaly, myelomeningocele, anencephaly and encephalocele.

The disease spectrum includes gross structural malformations such as anencephaly and myelomeningocele (spina bifida) that threaten life directly, more subtle structural defects such as lissencephaly and micrencephaly in which epilepsy and mental retardation are common con-

sequences, and functional brain deficits that cause learning difficulties and behavioural disturbance. In this chapter on CNS malformations, principles that are emerging from contemporary studies of the genetic, molecular, cellular and developmental biology of nervous system development, in both man, and animal models will be reviewed. This will be followed by detailed consideration of the neuropathology of the main classes of malformation in the light of the main embryonic and fetal events of CNS development.

PRINCIPLES OF NERVOUS SYSTEM DEVELOPMENT

The causal factors (aetiology) and the embryonic and fetal processes (pathogenesis) that underlie the development of malformations of the CNS are the subjects of an extremely rapidly growing area of research. To gain an appreciation of the improved understanding that has emerged over the past few years, it is necessary to consider some of the major advances which have included the isolation of causative genes and the elucidation of cellular and molecular mechanisms of embryonic and fetal development. These advances provide a starting point for understanding how genes and environmental factors can disrupt embryonic development to yield CNS malformations. Defining the scientific basis of CNS malformations is important, not only as an adjunct to the pathological analysis of the defects (see section on pathology of malformations), but also as a preliminary to developing improved diagnostic techniques and, ultimately, for primary prevention of the malformations.

Aetiology

Both genetic and environmental factors have been implicated in the aetiology of CNS malformations. Although, for convenience, these categories are considered separately, it is important to bear in mind that, in reality, there is a combination of factors acting in concert to cause most birth defects (see section on environmental factors).

GENES

Rapid progress has been made over the past decade in determining the genetic basis of single-gene disorders in man. Attention is now beginning to turn to those conditions, quantitatively more important, in which polygenic control is implicated. Table 7.1 lists the main diseases and syndromes that involve CNS malformations, including those for which a gene has been mapped or cloned. Three complementary strategies have contributed to this progress in identifying disease genes: positional cloning, analysis of candidate genes and use of animal models.

Positional cloning

The discovery of large numbers of highly polymorphic DNA markers that can be readily analysed by techniques such as Southern blot hybridization and the polymerase chain reaction (PCR)[940] has made it possible to construct detailed genetic maps of all the human chromosomes. This massive research effort, embodied in the international Human Genome Project, has recently come to fruition with the publication of comprehensive genetic and physical maps of the entire genome,[227] and the announcement in June 2000 of the preparation of a nearly complete DNA sequence, which comprises an ordering of the six billion nucleotides in the human genome. This enormous technological achievement will rapidly enable the identification of the majority of transcribed genes in the genome, although it stops short of defining the functions of the genes.[425]

Disease loci can be located from the chromosomal maps by conventional mendelian linkage analysis provided that a sufficient number of informative families is available. The ideal situation is to have access both to patients with chromosomal deletions, which provide a ready means of obtaining an initial chromosomal localization of the gene, and to patients with point mutations or translocation breakpoints, whose DNA is valuable in the later stages of fine mapping and in identifying candidate gene sequences. Once the map position of a disease gene has been determined, its cloning can be attempted using the molecular biological strategy shown in Fig. 7.1. A list of human disease genes identified by positional cloning can be found at http://genome.nhgri.nih.gov/clone/. Examples of the use of positional cloning to identify novel genes implicated in CNS malformations include Kallman syndrome,[538] the aniridia–Wilms' association,[893] Miller–Dieker lissencephaly[748] and X-linked lissencephaly.[242,343]

Candidate genes

The catalogue of mapped and cloned genes is growing rapidly, and it is often possible to draw up a list of candidate genes for a given genetic disease, based on either the putative function of the disease gene or its map position, or preferably both. The candidacy of genes can then be assessed by genetic mapping (finding genetic recombinations between the gene and the disease locus usually rules out its candidacy), or by searching for mutations in the coding region of the gene in patients with the disease. A lack of coding region mutations does not disprove candidacy since regulatory mutations may be located at a considerable distance from the coding region. A full evaluation of a candidate gene may also require, therefore, evaluation of gene expression at the level of messenger RNA (mRNA), by Northern blotting, reverse-transcription PCR and *in situ* hybridization. A candidate gene approach was used to identify *fibroblast growth factor receptor 2* as the gene mutated in Apert's syndrome[943] and to implicate the *sonic hedgehog* gene in holoprosencephaly (HPE3).[63,769]

Animal models

An alternative approach to the isolation of human disease genes is to progress from an animal model and clone the human gene by homology. This is especially useful where informative human families are not readily available. In the case of diseases controlled by multiple genes, or poorly penetrant genes, the analysis of animal models may have special advantages.[167] A large number of homologous loci have been identified in man and mouse,[217,814] some of which cause diseases involving CNS malformations when they are mutated (Table 7.2). The strategy for cloning mouse genes is essentially that outlined for human genes, but with the added advantage that the number of informative individuals that can be scored in the linkage analysis is almost unlimited, thereby permitting more rapid and precise genetic location of genes. An important further advantage of using animal models is the possibility of performing detailed descriptive and experimental analysis of the pathogenesis of the disease phenotype, particularly at prenatal stages when human embryonic and fetal material is not generally available for study (see Pathogenesis section below). Animal models that have aided our understanding of the genetic basis of human CNS disease include the *jimpy* mouse, which led to the identification of the *Proteolipid Protein* (PLP) gene as mutated in Pelizaeus–Merzbacher disease,[658,961] and the *splotch* mouse, which implicated the *Pax3* gene in Waardenburg syndrome types I and III.[35,883]

In recent years, the development of gene targeting techniques has led to a new strategy for the isolation and characterization of genes that control CNS development and which are implicated in the aetiology of CNS malformations.[125,780] In this technique, a cloned gene is the starting

Table 7.1 *Single-gene disorders and other syndromes involving CNS malformations*

Disease or locus name	CNS malformations involved	Gene name	Function of gene product	Chromosome location	OMIM number[a]	Mouse model or homologue
Aicardi's syndrome	Agenesis of corpus callosum, cerebral heterotopias	ND	ND	Xp22	304050	ND
Angelman's syndrome	Microcephaly and cerebellar atrophy	UBE3A	E6-associated protein ubiquitin-protein ligase. Expressed in brain only after maternal transmission	15q11	105830	Deletions or uniparental inheritance of imprinted region[323,901,975]
Aniridia	Severe cerebral neuronal migration disorders in homozygotes	PAX6	Nuclear transcription factor	11p13	106210	sey (small eye) mutant
Apert's syndrome	Cerebellar anomalies, agenesis of corpus callosum, limbic defects	FGFR2 (fibroblast growth factor receptor 2)	Cell surface receptor for fibroblast growth factors	10q25-26	101200	ND
Fukuyama's congenital muscular dystrophy	Polymicrogyria, type II lissencephaly	FCMD (gene encoding fukutin, interrupted by retrotransposon insertion)	Fukutin, a secreted protein, possibly a component of the extracellular matrix	9q31	253800	ND
Holoprosencephaly 1	Alobar holoprosencephaly	ND	ND	21q22.3	236100	ND
Holoprosencephaly 2	Alobar or semilobar holoprosencephaly	SIX3 (homologue of the sine oculis gene of *Drosophila*)	Homeobox-containing transcription factor	2p21	157170	ND
Holoprosencephaly 3	Holoprosencephaly	SHH (sonic hedgehog)	Secreted signalling molecule; neural inducer	7q36	142945	Targeted mutation of *Shh* gene[132]
Holoprosencephaly 4	Holoprosencephaly	ND	ND	18p11.3	142946	ND
Holoprosencephaly 5 (13q32 deletion syndrome)	Holoprosencephaly, exencephaly	ZIC2 (homologue of odd paired gene of *Drosophila*)	Transcription factor	13q32	603073	Targeted mutation of *Zic2* gene
Joubert's syndrome	Aplasia of cerebellar vermis	ND	ND	9q34.3	213300	ND

Table 7.1 (Continued)

Disease or locus name	CNS malformations involved	Gene name	Function of gene product	Chromosome location	OMIM number[a]	Mouse model or homologue
Kallmann's syndrome	Agenesis of olfactory lobes, absence of GnRH-secreting neurons	KAL1	Secreted protein with similarity to cell adhesion molecules	Xp22.3	308700	ND
Lissencephaly with cerebellar hypoplasia (Norman-Roberts syndrome)	Lissencephaly, cerebellar hypoplasia	RELN (reelin)	Extracellular matrix – associated signalling protein	7q22	257320	Reeler mutant mice exhibit disrupted cerebral and cerebellar lamination
Meckel–Gruber syndrome (Meckel's syndrome type 1)	Occipital encephalocele, microcephaly, cerebral and cerebellar hypoplasia, Dandy–Walker syndrome	ND	ND	17q21-24	249000	ND
Meckel syndrome type 2	Occipital meningoencephalocele	ND	ND	11q13	603194	ND
Miller–Dieker syndrome	Lissencephaly, cerebral heterotopias	LIS1 (PAFAH1B1; brain platelet-activating factor acetyl hydrolase)	Non-catalytic subunit of brain PAFAH	17p13.3	247200	Targeted loss of function alleles of Pafah1b1 gene[421]
Neu-Laxova syndrome	Microcephaly, lissencephaly, agenesis of corpus callosum, atrophy of cerebrum, cerebellum and pons, absence of olfactory bulbs	ND	ND	ND	256520	ND
Pallister–Hall syndrome	Hypothalamic hamartoblastoma	GLI3 (frameshift mutations)	Transcription factor in the Sonic hedgehog signalling pathway	7p13	146510	Gli3 mutation in the extra toes (Xt) mutant[892]
Pelizaeus–Merzbacher syndrome	Dysmyelination of corticospinal tracts	Proteo-lipid protein (PLP)	Myelination component	Xq21.3-22	312080	jp (jimpy) mutant mouse[658]
Pettigrew's syndrome	Dandy–Walker malformation, basal ganglia anomalies	ND	ND	Xq25-27	304340	ND

Table 7.1 (*Continued*)

Disease or locus name	CNS malformations involved	Gene name	Function of gene product	Chromosome location	OMIM number[a]	Mouse model or homologue
Prader–Willi syndrome	Microcephaly	Contiguous gene syndrome of (1) SNRPN (small nuclear ribonucleo protein polypeptide N) and (2) Necdin	(1) SNRPN: participates in pre-mRNA splicing. (2) Necdin: interacts with cell cycle proteins	15q11	176270	Targeted mutation of the Necdin gene does not recapitulate the features of Prader–Willi syndrome[335,900]
Sacral agenesis (Currarino's triad)	Meningocele	HLXB9	Homeobox-containing transcription factor, coding. for HB9 protein	7q36	176450	Targeted mutation of the Hlxb9 gene[396,548]
Septo-optic dysplasia	Hypoplastic optic nerves, absent septum pellucidum, hypoplasia of hypothalamic nuclei, agenesis of the corpus callosum	HESX1	Paired-like homeodomain protein expressed in embryonic forebrain	3p21.2-p21.1	182230	Targeted mutation of the Hesx1 gene[209]
Smith–Lemli–Opitz syndrome	Microcephaly, holoprosencephaly	DHCR7 (sterol delta-7-reductase)	Conversion of 7-dihydrocholesterol to cholesterol	11q12-q13	270400	Teratogenic effects of cholesterol biosynthesis inhibitors
Thanatophoric dysplasia, types I and II	Temporal lobe dysplasia, polymicrogyria	FGFR3 (fibroblast growth factor receptor 3)	Cell surface receptor for fibroblast growth factors	4p16.3	187600	Targeted mutation of the Fgfr3 gene[450]
Tuberous sclerosis	Hamartomas of CNS and other tissues	TSC1	ND	9q34	191100	ND
		TSC2	Encodes tuberin, with similarity to GTPase binding protein	16p13.3	191092	ND
Waardenburg's syndrome type I	Neural crest disorders, myelomeningocele in homozygous individuals	PAX3	Nuclear transcription factor	2q35	193500	Sp (splotch) mutant
Walker–Warburg syndrome	Agyria, type II lissencephaly, cerebellar dysplasia and vermal agenesis, hydrocephaly, occipital encephalocele	ND	ND	ND	236670	Targeted mutation of presenilin-1 gene produces a model of type II lissencephaly[399]

Table 7.1 (*Continued*)

Disease or locus name	CNS malformations involved	Gene name	Function of gene product	Chromosome location	OMIM number[a]	Mouse model or homologue
X-Linked hydrocephalus	Stenosis of aqueduct of Sylvius, agenesis of corpus callosum and septum pellucidum, fusion of thalami, hypoplasia of corticospinal tracts	*L1*	Cell adhesion molecule, expressed especially on migrating neurons	Xq28	308840	Targeted mutation of the *L1* gene[158,199,310]
X-Linked lissencephaly	Lissencephaly with agenesis of the corpus callosum in males; subcortical band heterotopia in females	*DCX* (doublecortin)	Microtubule associated protein that interacts with non-receptor tyrosine kinases including Abl	Xq22.3-q23	300067	ND
X-Linked periventricular heterotopia	Periventricular nodular heterotopia with epilepsy	*FLNA* (*Filamin-1*)	Actin-binding protein associated with cytoskeleton	Xq28	300049	ND
Zellweger's syndrome	Microgyria, polymicrogyria	*PEX* gene family members	Proteins participating in peroxisome function	Various loci	214100	Targeted mutation of *Pex2* and *Pex5* genes[31,288]

[a]Catalogue number in On-line Mendelian Inheritance in Man (http://www3.ncbi.nlm.nih.gov/Omim), which includes further details on data in this table.
ND, not determined.

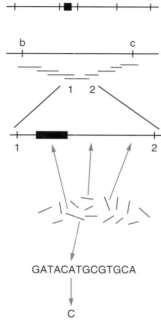

(1) Analyse family pedigrees for recombination events

(2) Map gene on chromosome

(3) Create genomic DNA 'contig' between flanking genetic markers

(4) Refine map using new markers derived from the DNA contig

(5) Screen libraries of cDNA fragments to isolate genes present in the mapped region

(6) Evaluate candidate genes by mutation screening, database sequence analysis, expression pattern, transgenic rescue, etc.

GATACATGCGTGCA

C

Figure 7.1 *Diagram illustrating the principles of positional cloning to identify disease genes. (1) Linkage analysis is performed in one or more family pedigrees to identify recombinant genotypes that can be used to identify a chromosomal location for the disease gene. (2) Polymorphic DNA markers are positioned to identify DNA markers that map closely on either side of the gene. The aim is to define genetically a fragment of DNA that contains the gene of interest and which is sufficiently small to be able to search realistically for candidate coding sequences within it. In practice, this amounts to identifying flanking markers that are no more than 1–2 cM apart (1 cM is defined as 1% genetic recombination, roughly amounting to 1 million nucleotide base pairs of human DNA). (3) Genomic DNA fragments are isolated, from libraries in yeast artificial chromosomes (YACs) or bacterial artificial chromosomes (BACs), which span the region between the flanking markers. Such an overlapping set of YAC or BAC inserts is known as a genomic 'contig'. (4) The genetic map is refined by generating new DNA markers from the genomic fragments. (5) Nucleotide sequences are sought that encode proteins within the genomic contig. (6) Each identified sequence is evaluated as a candidate for the gene of interest. Features that characterize protein coding sequences include evolutionary conservation and association with DNA motifs called CpG islands.[182] Moreover, gene coding sequences can be isolated by selecting for DNA fragments containing splice donor/acceptor sites which are normally found in association with protein coding sequences, a technique called 'exon trapping'.[116] The most*

(Figure 7.1 Continued.)
conclusive demonstration that a gene has been isolated comes from the finding of a pattern of tissue- and stage-specific expression appropriate for the disease phenotype, and the demonstration of mutations, predicted to cause a change in gene function, in patients with the disease. Rescue of a mutant mouse model, by transgenic insertion of the wild-type gene sequence, is a further demonstration that the gene has been cloned.

point and mutations are introduced with the aim of defining the mutant phenotype. This strategy has been used extensively to create null (i.e. loss of function) mutations in a wide range of previously cloned genes (listed at http://research.bmn.com/mkmd). This 'gene knockout' resource provides a range of mouse models that are proving invaluable in determining the function of specific genes during development.

The next phase in development of this technology is now underway with the elaboration of 'conditional' gene targeting approaches.[341] These enable gene mutations to be engineered and expressed in specific tissues or at particular stages of development. This can be achieved either by use of a chemically inducible promoter controlling the gene of interest, or by use of the bacterial enzyme Cre to activate a latent form of the targeted gene, via removal of loxP-flanked sequences. If Cre is expressed in a tissue-specific manner, the activation of the latent targeted gene is similarly tissue specific, generating an animal that is a mosaic of expressing and non-expressing tissues. An important aspect of this innovation is that gene mutations which are lethal to embryos, when expressed throughout the embryo from the stage of fertilization onwards, can be limited in their effects, thus enabling mutant individuals to proceed to later stages of development. This facilitates the analysis of gene function at all periods of prenatal and postnatal development.

An increasing number of malformations and disease phenotypes is being produced by gene targeting, some of which include CNS malformations (Table 7.2). The combination of improved gene cloning, starting from patients or animal models with a particular malformation, and gene targeting is rapidly providing new information on the genetic basis of CNS malformations.

INHERITANCE OF MUTANT GENES

While many genetic diseases conform to the rules of mendelian inheritance, several variations on the theme have been highlighted by recent studies. Certain syndromes appear to result from simultaneous loss of two or more genes that are located adjacent to each other in the genome. These contiguous gene deletions may represent a combination of the effects of loss of function of each gene individually or could result from a defect in an interaction between the gene products which is required for normal development (see section on environmental factors below). A dominant form of hydrocephaly has

Table 7.2 *Mouse mutations producing CNS malformations*

Malformation	Mutations, not yet cloned	Mutations, gene cloned	Gene knockouts
Anencephaly	cranioschisis (crn), open brain (opb), exencephaly (xn)	extra-toes (Xt; mutation of Gli3 gene)	Apolipoprotein B, twist, MARCKS, noggin and others
Arrhinencephaly	ND	polydactyly Nagoya (pdn; mutation of the S100β protein)	NCAM
Basal ganglia	ND	ND	Nkx2.1, Dlx1/2
Cerebellum: agenesis, generalized defects	fidget (fi), lurcher (lc), nervous (nr), cerebellar deficient folia (cdf)	swaying (sw; mutation of Wnt-1 gene), Snell dwarf (Pit1dw; mutation of the Pit1 gene)	Wnt-1, En-1, ErbB3, BDNF, Gbx2, Zic1
Cerebellum: vermis defects	ND	ND	L1
Cerebellum: granule cell anomalies	ND	staggerer (sg; mutation in the RORα gene), weaver (wv; mutation of the Girk2 gene)	Math1, cyclin D, NeuroD
Cerebellum: Purkinje cell anomalies	agitans (ag), purkinje cell degeneration (pcd), stumbler (stu)	ND	ND
Corpus callosum defects	absent corpus callosum (ac), ataxia (ax)	ND	Mrp, Emx-1, Nfia
Cranial nerves, ganglia and hindbrain defects	ND	kreisler (kr, mutation in a novel leucine zipper protein)	Krox20, Hoxa1, Hoxb1
Craniorachischisis	ND	Loop-tail (Lp; mutation of Lpp1 gene)	ND
Encephalocele	brain hernia (bh)	ND	ND
Generalized or multiple defects	teetering (tn)	ND	Brain-derived neurotrophic factor receptor (trkB); Retinoblastoma
Hydrocephalus	brain hernia (bh), congenital hydrocephalus (ch), obstructive hydrocephalus (oh)	ND	Apolipoprotein B, Otx2, NCAM, E2F-5, L1, Nfia
Myelination defects	ducky (du), grey tremor (gy), quaking (qk)	jimpy (jp; mutation of Plp gene encoding myelin proteolipid protein), shiverer (shi; mutation of myelin basic protein gene)	GFAP
Myelomeningocele (open spina bifida)	axial defects (Axd), bent tail (Bn), curly tail (ct), vacuolated lens (vl)	splotch (Sp; mutation of Pax3 gene)	Mrp, noggin, Zic2
Neuronal migration defects	hippocampal lamination defect (Hld)	small eye (sey; mutation of Pax6 gene); reeler (rl; mutation of reelin gene), scrambler & yotari (dbl; mutation of the disabled gene), dreher (dr; mutation of Lmx1a gene)	Pafah1b, cdk5, p35, Dlx1/2, MARCKS, Pex2, Presenilin-1, Emx2

Further details on data in this table can be found at http://www.informatics.jax.org/ and from the following review articles: Hatten et al.,[402] Copp and Harding[172] and Juriloff and Harris.[472] ND, not determined.

been suggested to form part of a contiguous gene deletion syndrome on chromosome 8q.[926]

A second principle governing the inheritance of some genetic diseases is the role of genomic imprinting. This refers to the observation that the parent of origin of a mutation can determine the nature of the disease phenotype observed. Imprinting involves the inactivation by chemical modification, probably involving DNA methylation, of gene sequences as a result of passage through either the male or female germ line.[745] Angelman syndrome results from loss of function of *UBE3A*, a gene on chromosome 15q11 that is active in the brain only after maternal transmission. The disease appears either when both copies of *UBE3A* are inherited from the father (i.e. uniparental disomy) or when a deletion encompassing *UBE3A* is transmitted through the maternal line. Prader–Willi syndrome was originally linked to the same region of chromosome 15q11-q13 as Angelman syndrome, although the two conditions have quite different phenotypes. In Prader–Willi, a contiguous gene syndrome has been described, involving the *SNRPN* and *necdin* genes, which have proven to be active only after paternal transmission. Maternal uniparental disomy or paternal transmission of a 15q11 deletion leads to this disease.[667]

LOSS AND GAIN OF FUNCTION MUTATIONS

It has been traditional to distinguish between dominant and recessive mutations. As individual genes are studied in greater detail, however, it is often found that recessive mutations have minor effects in the heterozygous state, whereas dominant genes may produce additional phenotypes when homozygous. A more useful distinction may be between mutations that act through loss or gain of function. Loss of function mutations abolish normal function of the gene product, as is seen in gene deletions or in cases where single base changes truncate, or otherwise inactivate, the gene product. If halving the gene dosage is not limiting, then the mutation appears recessive, whereas if the gene product is needed in full dose then the gene is said to exhibit haploinsufficiency and the mutation acts as a dominant, for instance as in Miller–Dieker lissencephaly. Gain of function mutations impart a novel function to the mutant gene product, as is seen in Apert's syndrome where mutations confer constitutive ('always on') function to fibroblast growth factor receptor-2 (FGFR-2). Dominant negative mutations involve alterations of the gene product causing an inhibitory effect that overcomes function of the product of the normal allele, as is seen in the *jimpy* mouse model of Pelizaeus–Merzbacher disease, where a wild-type transgene is unable to overcome the mutant phenotype.[808]

CHROMOSOMAL DISORDERS

In addition to the submicroscopic chromosomal alterations discussed above, several large-scale chromosomal anomalies cause CNS malformations as part of their phenotype (Table 7.3). In these cases, it is usually not possible to attribute specific features of the phenotype to particular genes since large parts of the genome are present in either increased or decreased copy number. However, progress is being made towards delineating the features of Down's syndrome that result from trisomy of particular regions of chromosome 21, permitting a more concentrated search for candidate genes.[407] The recent development of techniques for constructing and maintaining artificial mammalian chromosomes[821,980] promises imminent advances in our understanding of aneuploidy as a cause of CNS malformation.

ENVIRONMENTAL FACTORS

The action of exogenous influences in perturbing development *in utero*, leading to congenital malformations, has been studied for many decades under the broad umbrella of developmental toxicology and teratology. Research has been aimed at identifying teratogenic factors, evaluating their risk for human pregnancies and determining the mechanisms of teratogen action. In view of the public health implications, particularly in the aftermath of the thalidomide episode, the identification of teratogens has taken highest priority. This is perpetuated today by the increasing confinement of developmental toxicological research to the industrial pharmaceutical sector where commercial pressures demand efforts aimed mainly at the production of safe new products, rather than the mechanistic evaluation of teratogenic agents. Thus, our understanding of the mechanisms of action of teratogenic drugs and other environmental factors has not increased at the same rate as progress in understanding the genetic aetiology of malformations. Nevertheless, significant progress has been made in understanding the molecular basis of action of a small number of teratogenic agents (see section on molecular pathogenetic events, below). Table 7.4 lists some of the teratogenic agents that are known, or suspected, to cause malformations of the CNS in man and experimental animals.

GENE–GENE AND GENE–ENVIRONMENT INTERACTIONS

The concentration of research studies on the identification of single genes, or the testing of single environmental factors in the aetiology of malformations, tends to obscure the important principle that CNS defects probably always result from complex interactions between factors. As an example, Fig. 7.2 illustrates how such interactions determine the propensity of mouse embryos to develop neural tube defects (NTDs). Three types of interaction may be considered.

- *Major genes*, which cause NTDs when homozygous, can interact with each other in doubly heterozygous individuals. These are called epistatic interactions (see section on Cascades of developmental events, below).

Table 7.3 *Chromosomal disorders involving CNS malformations*

Chromosome	Excess	Deficiency
4	4p+ **Microcephaly**, agenesis of corpus callosum	4p- **Microcephaly**
5		5p- (Cri du chat syndrome) **Microcephaly**
8	8+ **Microcephaly**, agenesis of corpus callosum	
9	9+ **Microcephaly**, meningocele	Ms9p **Microcephaly**
	9p+ **Macrocephaly**, hydrocephaly	
13	13+ (Patau's syndrome) **Holoprosencephaly**, agenesis of corpus callosum, hydrocephaly, fusion of basal ganglia, cerebellar hypoplasia, myelomeningocele	13q- **Microcephaly, holoprosencephaly**
18	18+ (Edwards' syndrome) **Microcephaly**, microgyria, cerebellar hypoplasia, agenesis of corpus callosum, hydrocephaly, myelomeningocele	18p- **Microcephaly**, holoprosencephaly, arrhinencephaly 18q- **Microcephaly**
20	20p+ **Hydrocephaly**	
21	21+ (Down's syndrome) **Microcephaly**	
X	XXXY, XXXXY, XXXX, XXXXX **Microcephaly**	XO (Turner's syndrome) Defects of cerebellum, basal ganglia
Triploidy (often mosaic)	**Holoprosencephaly, hydrocephaly, Arnold–Chiari malformation, microcephaly**, myelomeningocele	

Malformations in bold type are present in the majority of cases. Those in normal type are present in a minority of cases. For further details see Ref. 835.

Interactions of this type between non-allelic mutations in man could yield a relatively high frequency of malformations even in the presence of low carrier gene frequencies.

- Expression of major genes is modulated in incidence and severity by *modifier genes* which, by themselves, do not produce NTDs. Recent studies of inbred mouse strains, with differing susceptibility to a genetically determined cranial NTD (anencephaly), identified a strain-to-strain variation in the precise rostrocaudal position at which the neural tube closes in the mouse brain (Fig. 7.3). Susceptibility to anencephaly is determined by where along the body axis this closure event occurs. Strains which initiate closure at a caudal position, within the midbrain, are resistant to anencephaly, whereas those that begin brain closure rostrally, within the forebrain, are relatively susceptible.[301] The genes that control this variation in brain development in the mouse are predicted to have homologues that determine the risk of anencephaly in man.

- As well as interactions between genes, *environmental factors* interact with both major and modifier genes, a reflection of the principle elaborated by Wilson[948] that teratogenesis depends on both maternal and embryonic genotype. Gene–environment interactions can be either exacerbating or ameliorating with respect to the incidence and severity of the malformations induced. Examples of ameliorating effects

include folic acid, which can prevent NTDs in man and in the *splotch* mouse,[302,933] and *myo*-inositol, which reduces the frequency of NTDs in the folate-resistant *curly tail* mouse.[359]

This interacting model of CNS malformation aetiology fits well with the observed multifactorial causation of conditions such as human NTDs.[127] Diseases that show a more closely mendelian transmission, or a more strict dependence on the action of a teratogen, may also be usefully viewed within this framework since interactions with subsidiary aetiological factors can account for variations in the penetrance and severity of the defects observed.

Pathogenesis

The completion of the Human Genome Project, with the decoding of the genetic material, heralds the start of the post-genomic era. Attention now turns from merely identifying genes to the more difficult task of determining their function. When applied to the study of CNS malformations, the challenge becomes one of understanding the molecular and cellular mechanisms that underlie CNS development which, when disturbed by a genetic or an environmental perturbation, yield a malformation phenotype. Hence, the elucidation of pathogenic mechanisms becomes the focus of research. This is not solely to satisfy scientific curiosity. A thorough knowledge of the mol-

Table 7.4 *Teratogens known or suspected to produce CNS malformations in man*

Teratogenic agent	Malformations
Alcohol	Microcephaly, occasional meningomyelocele and hydrocephaly
Carbamazepine	Myelomeningocele
Cytomegalovirus	Hydrocephalus, microencephaly with cortical microgyria, occasional cerebellar microgyria
Diabetes mellitus (maternal)	Neural tube defects: elevated incidence
Herpes simplex	Microcephaly, hydranencephaly
Hyperthermia	Neuronal heterotopias, microcephaly, possible neural tube defects
Methyl mercury	Microcephaly
Phenylketonuria (maternal)	Microcephaly
Phenytoin	Microcephaly, holoprosencephaly
Retinoids	Hydrocephaly, microcephaly, neuronal migration defects, cerebellar agenesis/hypoplasia
Rubella	Microcephaly, occasional hydrocephalus and agenesis of corpus callosum
Toxoplasmosis	Necrotizing meningoencephalitis leading to hydrocephalus and calcification. Polymicrogyria and hydranencephaly in some cases
Valproic acid	Myelomeningocele
Varicella	Necrotizing encephalitis with polymicrogyria
Warfarin	Microcephaly, hydrocephalus, Dandy–Walker cyst, agenesis of corpus callosum
X-irradiation	Microcephaly, pachygyria, cerebellar microgyria

Further details on data in this table can be found in Refs 101, 476, 514, 515, 836 and 923.

ecular pathogenesis of a disease process provides opportunities to develop interventional approaches to primary prevention, as exemplified by the use of folic acid to prevent NTDs.

CASCADES OF DEVELOPMENTAL EVENTS

The pathogenesis of a CNS malformation can be viewed as a cascade of events (Fig. 7.4a), in which aetiological factors, either genetic or environmental, initiate a sequence of molecular, cellular and tissue alterations, culminating

in the development of a pathological phenotype. The resulting pathogenic cascade is a variant of the normal developmental programme: a CNS component is generally formed, but with anomalous structure or function. The grouping of molecular events into developmental cascades has been placed on a firm foundation in recent years by the emergence of a new type of genetic analysis, called epistasis. In this experimental procedure, two distinct but related genetic defects are combined in the same individual to determine whether the genetic lesions summate (i.e. the resulting phenotype is more severe than with either lesion alone) or whether one lesion dominates (i.e. is epistatic) over the other. Summation is evidence that the two lesions operate in distinct pathways, whereas epistasis suggests a single pathway involving both genes. Originally developed in lower organisms such as *Drosophila* and the nematode *Caenorhabditis elegans*,[30] epistatic analysis is now being applied increasingly to mammalian development. For instance, a mutation in the gene *bcl-x* causes increased death of postmitotic neurons by

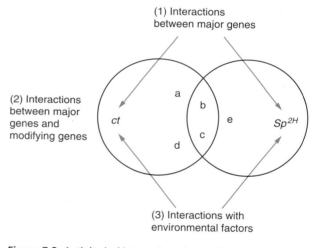

Figure 7.2 *Aetiological interactions during the development of neural tube defects in the mouse. Three types of interaction have been demonstrated. (1) Interactions between major genes. The mutant genes curly tail (ct) and splotch (Sp²ᴴ) each cause spina bifida when homozygous. Embryos that carry both mutations are more severely affected than those that are mutant at only one of the genetic loci,*[281] *demonstrating a summation of the effects of these non-allelic mutations. (2) Interactions between major and modifying genes. Each of the major genes is expressed differently, with varying incidence and severity of defects, on different inbred genetic backgrounds. This demonstrates the existence of a varying complement of polymorphic modifying genes in the different inbred strains. Some of these modifying genes have been mapped.*[664] *(3) Interactions between major genes and environmental factors. Exogenous agents such as folic acid and myo-inositol interact with the mutant genes to modify the incidence and severity of defects. For instance, myo-inositol reduces the frequency of spinal neural tube defects in curly tail mouse embryos,*[359] *while folic acid is effective in preventing neural tube defects in splotch mutant mice.*[302]

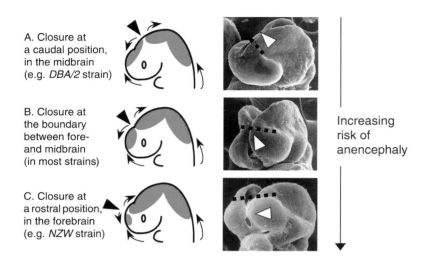

Figure 7.3 *Neural tube closure. Variations in the pattern of neural tube closure in the brain of different mouse strains, as shown diagrammatically (left) and in scanning electron micrographs (right). This variation determines susceptibility to anencephaly, as shown on the right side. Arrowheads mark the site where brain closure begins (closure 2). In the diagrams, green and red shading indicate open regions of neural tube situated rostral and caudal, respectively, to the closure point. Arrows show the directions in which closure spreads throughout the brain. Dotted lines mark the boundary between the forebrain and midbrain. DBA/2 and NZW are inbred mouse strains that exhibit resistance and susceptibility, respectively, to anencephaly. Reproduced with modification from Fleming and Copp.[301]*

apoptosis in the mouse brain,[637] whereas inactivation of the *caspase-3* gene has the opposite effect, reducing neuronal death.[507] Despite the contrasting phenotypes of these knockout mice, the brain phenotype of mice lacking both *bcl-x* and *caspase-3* is similar to the *caspase-3* mutant alone, indicating an epistatic relationship between the genes. *Caspase-3* appears to act downstream of *bcl-x* in the pathway regulating neuronal cell death.[782]

Pathogenic cascades have so far been defined for very few CNS malformations. Usually, only fragmentary information is available on one or more aspects of the molecular and morphogenetic processes. For this reason, the following discussion will consider pathogenic events at the molecular and cellular/tissue levels separately, citing instances in which particular malformations are known to involve a disturbance of a particular developmental process.

MOLECULAR PATHOGENIC EVENTS

Figure 7.4b is a schematic summary of the main molecular components of intercellular and intracellular signalling systems. Pathways of this basic type are being found to play a central role in a wide variety of normal and pathological cellular processes, including development of the nervous system.

Genetic mechanisms

Once a novel gene has been identified as the likely cause of a CNS birth defect, the putative function of the protein product can often be predicted from its amino acid structure. For instance, transmembrane receptors have multiple hydrophobic amino acid stretches that span the lipid bilayer, whereas transcription factors have characteristic DNA-binding motifs. This information enables a schematic depiction of the position in the cell signalling scheme occupied by the various genes that cause CNS malformations (Fig. 7.4b, right side).

Extracellular signalling molecules can be freely diffusible (e.g. nerve growth factor), diffusible but requiring association with the extracellular matrix for their function (e.g. Wnt-1, Sonic hedgehog), or part of the extracellular matrix (e.g. reelin). Mutations in the mouse *Wnt-1* gene lead to faulty specification of the developing brain, so that the posterior midbrain and anterior hindbrain fail to develop (Fig. 7.5). *Sonic hedgehog* function is necessary for correct specification of the telencephalic vesicles, leading to holoprosencephaly when deficient,[132] while reelin, the protein product of the gene mutated in the *reeler* mouse, is required for the normal migration of neuroblasts during formation of the laminated structure of the cerebral cortex.[208,422]

Cell-surface receptors act as conduits, transmitting extracellular signals into the cell. Mutations in the *trkB* gene, which acts as a receptor for brain-derived neurotrophic factor (BDNF), produce abnormalities of cranial motor neurons, ganglia and cerebral cortex.[841] Fibroblast growth factor (FGF) receptors transduce signals from the large number of FGF ligands, and are required for normal skull and brain development. FGFR-2 mutations have been identified in Apert's syndrome.[943]

Inside the cell, a large number of proteins participate in the transduction of extracellular signals. The *mdab1* gene encodes an adaptor protein that binds non-receptor

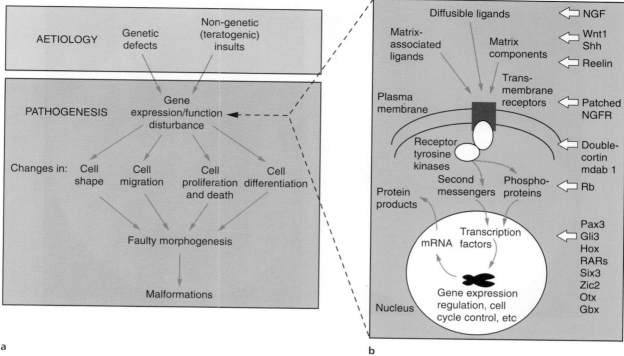

a

b

Figure 7.4 *Cascades of pathogenic events leading to CNS malformations. (a) Relationship between aetiology and pathogenesis, with a schematic representation of the molecular, cell/tissue and morphogenetic levels of organization. (b) Stylized representation of the main categories of molecular signalling event that mediate development of the nervous system. The sites of action of some genetic and environmental insults that cause CNS malformations, as discussed elsewhere in this chapter, are indicated on the right. Cells signal to each other via molecules that may be freely diffusible, associated with the extracellular matrix or part of the extracellular matrix. Receptors for these signalling ligands are connected, directly or indirectly, to intracellular signalling systems that transduce the extracellular signal and alter cellular metabolism and/or gene expression. Protein kinases are enzymes located on the cytoplasmic surface of the plasma membrane which typically operate as dimers. They have been found to mediate a variety of extracellular signals, via protein phosphorylation. A series of phosphorylation events ensues, yielding second messenger molecules (e.g. inositol phosphates) that have the ability to alter gene expression patterns within the cell. A number of genes that are regulated by activation of the signal transduction systems encodes protein products, termed transcription factors, that serve to regulate the expression of other genes, so yielding cascades of gene regulation events.*

tyrosine kinases such as Abl and Fyn. It appears to participate in the *reelin* pathway.[195] The retinoblastoma gene (*Rb*), encodes a nuclear protein the function of which is regulated by phosphorylation events contingent on activation of cell-surface receptors: *Rb* regulates progression through the cell cycle;[151] its loss of function leads to massive cell death in the developing hindbrain, dorsal root ganglia and spinal cord.[535]

Still further downstream are the nuclear transcription factors that control the expression of other genes. Heterozygotes for mutations in the transcription factor *PAX3* develop Waardenburg syndrome types I and III in which disturbance of neural crest development is a prominent feature.[35,883] In the mouse, loss of *Pax3* function yields the *splotch* phenotype, comprising anencephaly, myelomeningocele and neural crest defects.[627] Disturbance of *GLI3* function has been implicated in both Greig's cephalopolysyndactyly and Pallister–Hall syndrome.[480] The *Gli3* transcription factor functions as part of the *Sonic hedgehog* signalling pathway, with loss of function mutations

in the mouse producing anencephaly and forebrain disorders.[311]

Teratogenic mechanisms

As we learn more about the molecular basis of teratogen action, it is becoming apparent that exogenous agents, like genetic lesions, can disrupt key signalling events to produce CNS malformations. For example, retinoic acid (RA) was previously considered to exert its teratogenic effect by direct disruption of plasma membrane function, owing to its lipophilic nature. However, RA is now considered to be an endogenous molecule that initiates a complex signalling pathway that is of key importance in embryonic development. Retinol, the principal dietary retinoid, interacts during normal development with the cytoplasmic retinol binding protein (CRBP) during its metabolism by retinaldehyde dehydrogenase to the metabolically active all-trans-RA. The latter is then bound by cellular retinoic acid binding protein (CRABP), which presents it to

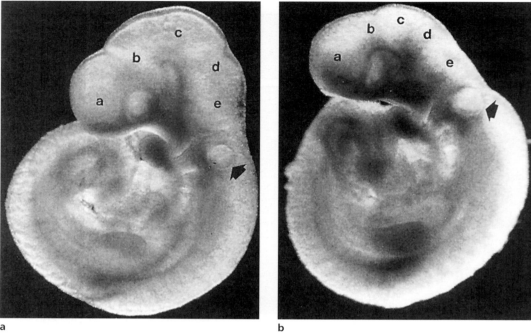

Figure 7.5 *Hypoplasia of midbrain and rostral hindbrain. Midbrain and rostral hindbrain hypoplasia in the mouse resulting from a targeted mutation in the Wnt-1 gene. Mouse embryos at 10.5 days of gestation (27 somite stage) from a mating between* Wnt-1 +/− *heterozygotes. The regions of the developing brain are indicated: a, telencephalon; b, diencephalon; c, mesencephalon; d, metencephalon; e, myelencephalon.* **(a)** Wnt-1 +/− *embryo with normal appearance;* **(b)** Wnt-1 −/− *mutant embryo showing hypoplasia of midbrain and metencephalic region of the hindbrain. Magnification = approximately ×20. Reproduced by permission from Ref. 583.*

nuclear receptors. Two classes of receptor exist: retinoic acid receptors (RARs), which bind all-trans-RA most avidly, and retinoid X receptors (RXRs), which have greater affinity for another retinoid, 9-cis retinoic acid. Occupancy of the receptors by their ligands stimulates them to act as transcription factors, regulating the expression of other genes which contain retinoic acid response elements (RAREs) in their promoter regions, thus initiating cascades of molecular events. While the physiological roles of retinoids in development are not fully understood, it is becoming clear that excess RA produces malformations by a mechanism that involves upregulation of the expression of RARs, especially the β-isoform,[466] presumably leading to supranormal stimulation of RAR pathways. Conversely, retinol deficiency is teratogenic by depleting the developing embryo of activity within this important signalling pathway. Thus, the teratogenic action of an important class of CNS teratogens is becoming understood in terms of the intracellular molecular mechanisms.

Another class of teratogenic agent the function of which has recently come under scrutiny comprises the *Veratrum* alkaloids cyclopamine and jervine, which inhibit cholesterol biosynthesis. When applied to experimental animals these agents produce forebrain defects resembling human holoprosencephaly (HPE). The significance of this finding has come into focus following the discovery of mutations in the *Sonic hedgehog* gene in patients with HPE.[769] Cholesterol substitution of the N-terminal cleav-

age fragment of the Sonic hedgehog protein is essential for its function, and a proportion of patients with Smith–Lemli–Opitz syndrome, in which cholesterol biosynthesis is disturbed, also develop HPE.[484] Although the *Veratrum* alkaloids do not appear to interfere with the cholesterol modification of the Sonic hedgehog protein, they may inhibit the response of the Patched receptor through its 'sterol-sensing domain',[165] thereby inhibiting transmission of the Sonic hedgehog signal.

PATHOGENESIS AT THE CELLULAR AND TISSUE LEVELS

Most CNS malformations result from abnormalities of morphogenesis, the term given to alterations in morphology that accompany embryonic development. In normal CNS development, the molecular signalling events (see section on molecular pathogenic events, above) regulate and co-ordinate a series of cellular changes (Fig. 7.4a), the net effect of which is embryonic shaping. Some key cellular events are: (1) cell shape change, for instance as occurs during the bending of the neuroepithelium as the neural tube closes; (2) cell migration, as in the migration of neuroblasts during the generation of the layered structure of the cerebral cortex; (3) cell proliferation, as occurs in the ventricular zone of the developing brain and spinal cord; (4) programmed cell death, which is responsible for removal of transient CNS structures, such as the

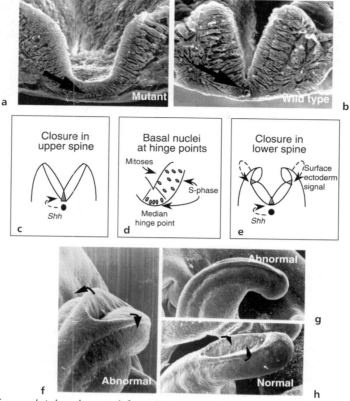

Figure 7.6 *Pathogenesis of neural tube closure defects in two genetic mouse models. At upper spinal levels, bending at the midline of the neural plate (**b, c**) is achieved by concentration of cells with basally located nuclei (**d**). In the loop-tail mutant mouse, an excessively broad midline region is formed (compare arrows in **a** and **b**), preventing apposition of the neural folds in the dorsal midline, and leading to the development of craniorachischisis.[360] Lower spinal levels depend on bending at dorsolaterally positioned locations (**e**). In the curly tail mutant, excessive ventral curvature of the body axis (**g**; see also Fig. 7.7) inhibits the formation of dorsolateral hinge points (**f**), leading to the development of myelomeningocele.[918] Normal embryos achieve apposition of the neural folds in the caudal region, as a result of dorsolateral bending (**h**). Reproduced from Van Straaten et al.[918] and Greene et al.[360] with modification.*

subplate neurons that participate in early cortical neurogenesis; and (5) cell differentiation, the process responsible for the generation of the diverse types of neuron and glia in the CNS. This section provides examples of each of these cellular/tissue events, to illustrate how their disturbance may contribute to the pathogenesis of CNS malformations.

Cell shape change

The conversion of part of the primitive neuroepithelium (the neural plate) into active bending sites is a key feature of the closure of the neural folds during neurulation (Fig. 7.6). Bending occurs in midline neuroepithelial cells (the median hinge point), under the influence of Sonic hedgehog protein produced by the underlying notochord, and at paired dorsolateral hinge points, under the influence of unidentified signals from the overlying surface (epidermal) ectoderm (Fig. 7.6c, e). Bending at these sites is achieved by an interruption of the basal to apical to basal progression of nuclear translocation, which occurs as

neuroepithelial cells progress through the cell cycle.[839] Cells with basally located nuclei accumulate, leading to bending via a local reduction in the apical surface area of the neuroepithelium (Fig. 7.6d). The folded configuration of the bending neural plate is further stabilized by contraction of apically arranged actin microfilaments.[976]

Failure of neural tube closure leads to the appearance of NTDs (anencephaly and myelomeningocele; see section on neural tube defects: dysraphic disorders, below). Although the underlying cellular pathogenesis of human NTDs has not been determined, NTDs in mice are known to result from disturbance of the bending sites in the folding neural plate. For instance, pathological enlargement of the median hinge point in the *loop-tail* mutant interrupts the initiation of closure in the upper spine,[360] leading to the severe NTD craniorachischisis (Fig. 7.6a, b), whereas excessive ventral curvature of the caudal embryonic region inhibits formation of dorsolateral hinge points,[826] thereby disturbing low spinal closure in the *curly tail* mutant, leading to myelomeningocele (Fig. 7.6f–h). The enhanced curvature of the body axis in *curly tail*

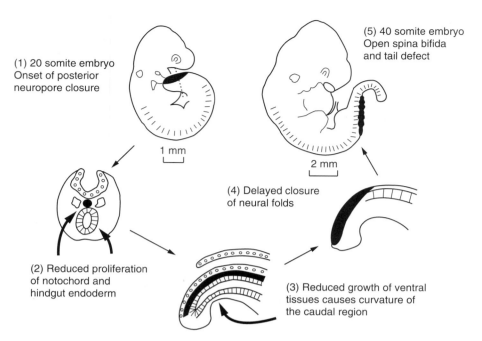

Figure 7.7 *Spina bifida. Experimental analysis of the pathogenic sequence of events underlying spina bifida in the mutant* curly tail *mouse. This mutation causes lumbosacral spina bifida and/or tail flexion defects in around 50% of homozygotes. The defects result from an imbalance of cell proliferation in the caudal embryonic region where growth of certain non-neural tissues, the notochord and hindgut endoderm, is reduced in affected embryos, whereas the neuroepithelium is unimpaired in its rate of proliferation. The notochord and hindgut are midline structures firmly attached to the ventral surface of the neuroepithelium. Their slow proliferation produces a mechanical distortion of the body axis which curves ventrally, thereby opposing dorsolateral bending and inhibiting closure of the neuropore. Spina bifida can be prevented in this mutant either by correcting the cell proliferation imbalance, by inserting a splint into the caudal embryonic region to prevent the development of ventral curvature, or by treating embryos during neuropore closure with* myo-inositol.[107,171,359]

embryos results from defective cell proliferation in non-neural tissues, the notochord and hindgut epithelium (Fig. 7.7), emphasizing the principle that CNS malformations may derive from cellular abnormalities outside the neural tube.

Cell migration

The stratified structures of the cerebral cortex and cerebellum arise through a process of tightly regulated migration of postmitotic neuroblasts from the inner ventricular zone towards more superficial regions of the primitive neural tube (see section on migration and differentiation of neuroblasts). Radial migration of neuroblasts, along radial glial fibres, appears to be the mechanism mainly responsible for the generation of pyramidal neurons in the cerebral cortex, whereas tangential migration from the medial and lateral ganglionic eminence provides many of the non-pyramidal neurons.[702] Defective migration, particularly along radial glial fibres, has been identified as a pathogenic mechanism underlying disturbed lamination of the cerebral cortex and cerebellum in mice homozygous for the *reeler* mutation. Strikingly, the mutant phenotype involves an apparent reversal of the polarity of the normal cortical layers. *Reeler* neuroblasts begin their centrifugal migration along the

radial glial fibres, but they are unable to pass postmigratory neurons in the deeper cortical layers.[724] *Reeler* mice lack an extracellular matrix molecule, named reelin,[208] which exhibits similarities to molecules involved in cell-matrix adhesion, such as tenascin. Reelin is expressed by neuronal cells but not radial glial cells, supporting the idea that the *reeler* phenotype results from a defect in adhesion between early postmigratory neurons. Other proteins that participate in the reelin pathway have recently been identified. Mice with mutations in the *mdab1* gene, and those with mutations in both very low-density lipoprotein (VLDL) receptor and apolipoprotein E (ApoE) receptor-2, develop very similar phenotypes to *reeler*. Molecular studies have shown that VLDL receptor and ApoE receptor-2 bind the reelin protein, whereas the mdab1 protein acts intracellularly to transduce the reelin signal.[207,412] Hence, reelin appears to regulate an important genetic pathway controlling neuroblast migration during CNS development.

Cell proliferation

CNS development occurs against a backdrop of a massive expansion in cell numbers. Cells pass through multiple rounds of proliferation within the ventricular and subventricular zones of the brain and spinal cord, exiting the cell cycle as they embark upon their migration to the cortical plate or mantle layer. In recent years, the molecular machinery that regulates the cell cycle has been elucidated in great detail.[778] Key roles are played by the cyclins, proteins that vary in abundance at specific phases of the cell cycle, the cyclin-dependent kinases, which are activated by specific interactions with cyclins, and cell cycle phase-specific inhibitors, which can induce cells to exit the cell cycle to become quiescent. Null mutations in these 'cell cycle machinery' genes may produce early embryonic lethality, as with the cyclin A2 gene,[646] presumably indicating the essential general requirement of this gene for embryonic cell cycling. Alternatively, there may be no discernible effect on development, as in the case of the G_1 checkpoint inhibitor p21[CIP1/WAF1],[234] perhaps suggesting an overlapping function with another gene that plays a compensatory role. A third type of outcome is the causation of specific CNS defects, as when the gene encoding cyclin D2 is inactivated. Null mutants develop specific abnormalities of cerebellar development, with reduced numbers of granule cells and stellate interneurons.[439] Although these gene targeting experiments confirm the key role played by the cell cycle in development, it remains to be determined whether modulation of cell proliferation may primarily underlie CNS defects such as microcephaly and megalencephaly.

Programmed cell death

Programmed or physiological cell death is the phenomenon in which cells die during normal development. It is an expression of terminal differentiation, involves new gene expression, and is usually equated with the morphological process of apoptosis, in which cells die by nuclear condensation and fragmentation into membrane-bound bodies without release of cytoplasmic contents. This contrasts with necrosis, a pathological process, in which cells rupture and cytoplasmic contents are released. All cells are probably programmed to die by apoptosis, being kept alive only by the constant present of survival factors in the extracellular environment.[452] Moreover, teratogenic agents such as ethanol, which are capable of inducing CNS defects, appear to trigger the apoptotic pathway by inhibiting neurotransmitter receptors.[446]

The genes that specify which cells are destined to die or to survive during development were identified initially in the nematode worm *C. elegans*.[274] A number of corresponding mammalian genes have now been found to participate in the regulation of apoptosis. For instance, the *bcl-2* and *bcl-x* genes encode proteins that inhibit execution of the apoptotic pathway, by preventing the activation of downstream apoptotic enzymes called caspases.[795] The action of these genes is opposed by pro-apoptotic genes including *Bad* and *Bax*. When overexpressed, *bcl-2* can prevent the degeneration of neurons in response to deprivation of neurotrophic factors *in vitro*[14] or cutting their axons *in vivo*,[257] although *bcl-x*

seems likely to play a more important role than *bcl-2* in protecting neurons from programmed cell death *in vivo*.[348] Conversely, disruption of the *caspase3* gene in mice leads to decreased apoptosis, producing heterotopic neuronal masses in the developing cerebral cortex.[507] Hence, details are emerging of the intracellular regulation of programmed cell death, and the ways in which this pathway is integrated into normal CNS development (see also Chapter 1, this Volume).

Cell differentiation and regional patterning

Coincident with the morphogenetic events of CNS development, the various regions of the presumptive brain and spinal cord become regionally specified. As gastrulation proceeds, the neuroepithelium is induced from naive ectoderm through interactions with underlying chordamesoderm and by the transmission of inductive signals in the plane of the neural plate.[485] Bone morphogenetic proteins (BMPs) induce an epidermal default state, while molecules such as chordin and noggin antagonize BMP action and promote a neural differentiative fate.[719,949,982] The newly induced neuroepithelium rapidly becomes regionally specified in both the anteroposterior (i.e. rostrocaudal) and dorsoventral axes, so that subsequent cellular differentiation occurs appropriate to the position within the CNS.

Anteroposterior axis

Neuroepithelial cells at different levels of the body axis express different combinations of homeobox genes, which encode transcription factors bearing the characteristic homeodomain DNA-binding motif. In the hindbrain and spinal cord, a particular class of homeobox genes, the *Hox* genes, play a key role in specifying regional identity. The combination of *Hox* genes expressed in each hindbrain segment, or rhombomere, determines the developmental character of that segment, a mechanism referred to as the *Hox* code.[443] Treatment of gastrulation-stage mouse embryos with retinoic acid alters the pattern of *Hox*-gene expression, causing cells of rhombomeres 2 and 3 to express *Hoxb1*, which is normally expressed only by cells of rhombomeres 4 and 5. The regional character of rhombomeres 2 and 3 is altered so that they now give rise to a nerve resembling cranial nerve VII (facial) rather than cranial nerve V (trigeminal) as would normally occur. Thus, the facial nerve is duplicated in the retinoic acid-treated embryos.[600] Different classes of homeobox genes impart regional identity to the midbrain and forebrain, a topic that is discussed further in the section on disorders of forebrain induction, below.

Dorsoventral axis

Specification of neuronal cell types along the dorsoventral axis of the brain and spinal cord depends on mutually antagonistic signals emanating from the mid-ventral region (initially the notochord, subsequently the floor-plate) and the dorsal midline (initially the apical ectoderm, subsequently the roof-plate). Sonic hedgehog (Shh) is the ventral signal, and the manner in which this extracellular signalling molecule specifies cell identity in the dorsoventral axis is now understood in considerable detail.[279,447] A proteolytic N-terminal fragment of the Shh protein (Shh-N) is the active signal, requiring cholesterol addition for its activity. Shh-N interacts with a transmembrane receptor, encoded by the *Patched* gene which, in the absence of bound Shh ligand, serves to repress an intracellular pathway that is activated by the membrane-bound product of the *smoothened* gene. Binding of Shh-N to Patched de-represses the pathway, enabling the activation of downstream signalling, in which Gli proteins play an important role. The central significance of the Shh pathway is evident from the striking developmental abnormalities that result from loss of function of the mouse genes, and from the association of genes in the pathway with human developmental disease: *SHH* mutants develop holoprosencephaly in both man and mice, *PATCHED* mutants develop Gorlin syndrome in humans and severe CNS defects in mice, while *GLI3* mutations are implicated in Greig cephalopolysyndactly and Pallister–Hall syndrome in humans and brain abnormalities in mice.

The protein Shh exerts a concentration-dependent influence over the differentiative fate of cells in the spinal cord, with high concentrations promoting the formation of ventral neuronal types while low concentrations promote the differentiation of more dorsal cell types. Precisely how this concentration dependence is achieved appears to involve the regulation by Shh of the expression of a series of homeobox-containing genes that constitute a combinatorial code, analogous to the Hox code. Each neuronal type in the ventral spinal cord develops from cells that express a unique combination of these spinal cord homeobox genes.[102] Dorsal neuronal types are known to be specified by signals belonging to the *BMP* and *Wnt* gene families, with important roles for BMP antagonists, such as *noggin*,[591,843] although the details of this dorsal specification process are less well understood than in the ventral neural tube.

THE QUESTION OF CELL AUTONOMY IN PATHOGENESIS

It is often important to ask through which cell type a defect of morphogenesis is mediated. A cell autonomous defect is one in which function of the mutated gene is required within the cell type(s) principally affected. In the converse situation (a non-cell autonomous defect), the mutated gene is required in cells other than those exhibiting overt pathology. Making the distinction between cell autonomy and non-autonomy is useful as it points the investigator towards the precise location of the pathogenic alteration. For instance, non-autonomous defects indicate

a possible defect in an extracellular signal or a survival factor.

A functional approach to this question is provided by the analysis of chimaeras or mosaics, individuals in which cells of two different genotypes coexist. Chimaeras are individuals derived from two or more original zygotes, usually as a result of experimental interventions such as aggregating a pair of preimplantation embryos, or injecting early embryonic cells into another embryo. Mosaics are individuals in which genotypically different cells arise through somatic recombination or X-chromosome inactivation.

Chimaeric studies in animal models

The chimaeric approach has been used, for instance, to investigate the development of defects of Purkinje cell development in the mouse mutants *purkinje cell degeneration* (*pcd*) and *reeler*, in which cerebellar Purkinje cells exhibit reduced survival and abnormal position, respectively.[639] Chimaeric individuals containing both mutant and normal cells show that *pcd* Purkinje cells die irrespective of whether wild-type cells are also present in the developing cerebellum, indicating that the *pcd* defect is cell autonomous. In contrast, positioning of both wild-type and *reeler* Purkinje cells is abnormal in chimaeras,[887] indicating that the *reeler* defect is expressed outside the Purkinje cell (i.e. a non-cell autonomous defect). This finding is consistent with the recent observation that reelin, the product of the *reeler* gene, is not expressed in Purkinje cells.[806]

Mosaic studies in man

The neuronal migration defect present in individuals with X-linked *doublecortin* mutations has been suggested to be cell autonomous, based on the finding of both normal-migrating and abnormal-migrating neurons in the brains of *doublecortin* heterozygous females. In contrast, all neurons appear to be affected in hemizygous males. Female cells inactivate an X chromosome at random during development, so that females heterozygous for X-linked diseases are mosaic, with some cells expressing the normal allele while others express the mutant allele.[571] The normal cortical band in *doublecortin* females may arise solely from cells expressing the wild-type allele, whereas the heterotopic band may comprise cells expressing the mutant allele. Such a cell-autonomous defect would be consistent with the intracellular localization of the protein encoded by the *doublecortin* gene.[242,343]

A GUIDE TO INTERPRETING THE PATHOGENESIS OF MALFORMATIONS

For the neuropathologist faced with the variety and complexity of malformations of the CNS, the challenge is not only one of description, and perhaps diagnosis, but also the urgent, practical task of providing accurate and useful information for genetic counselling. Malformations, resulting from primary disturbance of embryonic and fetal development, need to be distinguished from disruptions and deformations, where there is secondary compromise of development owing to factors such as vascular interruption, necrosis caused by infectious agents, or compression of the embryo or fetus by external mechanical influences. Experimental studies in laboratory animals have demonstrated the capacity of vascular disruptions to produce birth defects that mimic primary malformations. Interest in this aetiology for human defects has been raised by the association between chorionic villus sampling (CVS) performed earlier than 10 weeks after the last menstrual period and a variety of limb and craniofacial defects.[297] Moreover, mechanical trauma, for instance inflicted by amniotic bands, can produce a range of human birth defects.[413] It is of great importance for purposes of genetic counselling that secondary defects are distinguished from primary malformations, since only the latter should have a significant risk of recurrence. To this end, detailed methods of fetal post-mortem analysis are being developed[483] that can provide a rational basis for deciding whether a particular defect is a primary malformation or a secondary disruption or deformation.

In practice, however, the distinction between primary malformations and secondary disruptions is far from simple. This applies particularly to the CNS, for a variety of interrelated reasons which depend ultimately on the extended organogenesis of the brain, which continues right through intrauterine life and, at least for myelination and for the late-migrating granule cells of the cerebellum and temporal lobe, well into postnatal existence. This extended period of brain development is marked not only by rapid structural change, but also by changes in the individual selective vulnerabilities of cells and tissues and in the form of the repair mechanisms that can be mounted by microglia and neuroglia to any deleterious influence. Macrophage responses appear considerably to antedate recognizable astrocytic responses, and so resorption of necrotic tissue may occur without trace of glial repair. Kershman[489] observed macrophages in human brain as early as 11 weeks, and immunohistochemical methods have demonstrated them early in the second trimester.[354] By contrast, astrocytosis was first detected at 20–23 weeks of gestation.[770] Consequently, the morphological end-result of any given noxious influence can vary greatly, depending on the time of its operation, which may be brief, prolonged or repetitive. Moreover, the repertoire of responses is limited. Circumstantial clinical evidence and experimental manipulations indicate that the same

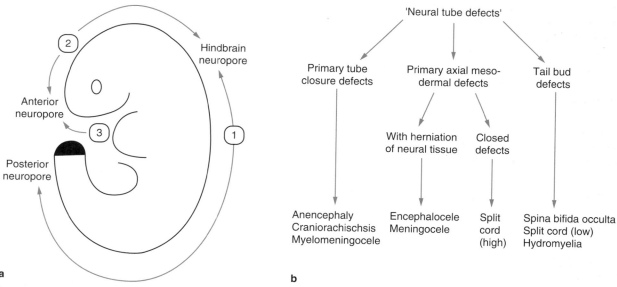

a

b

Figure 7.8 *Stages of neurulation and classification of neural tube defects. (a) Stages of neurulation as demonstrated for the mouse[345] and inferred for man.[915] Primary neural tube closure is initiated at the cervical/hindbrain boundary (closure site 1) and separately, soon afterwards, at the boundary between the future mesencephalon and prosencephalon (closure site 2) and at the rostral extremity of the future prosencephalon (closure site 3). Fusion spreads bidirectionally between closures 1 and 2, and between closures 2 and 3, completing cranial neural tube formation at the hindbrain neuropore and anterior neuropore, respectively. While cranial neural tube formation is occurring, neurulation progresses from the point of closure 1 in a caudal direction, through the spinal region, with completion of closure at the posterior neuropore, which is situated in the future upper sacral region. Below this level, secondary neurulation occurs with formation of all non-epidermal tissues from a multipotential stem cell population in the tail bud (shaded). (b) A classification of neural tube defect malformations based on the embryonic tissue that appears primarily affected. See text for explanation. (a) Modified after Copp et al.[170] and Copp and Bernfield.[167]*

anomaly can be produced by several different causes, both genetic and environmental. Viewed from another standpoint, there appear to be temporal (or perhaps temporospatial) windows when development appears particularly at risk, and consequently particular types of structural anomaly tend to be grouped together, for instance midline malformations or neuronal migration defects. These various lines of argument underscore the importance of the dynamic aspects of the immature nervous system for a proper understanding of developmental neuropathology.

PATHOLOGY OF MALFORMATIONS

Neural tube defects: dysraphic disorders

These disorders must be set in the context of the normal development of (1) the neural tube, the progenitor of the entire central nervous system, and (2) the axial skeleton, which becomes modelled around the neural tube.

Neurulation can be divided broadly into primary and secondary phases. In primary neurulation, which occurs throughout the future brain and spinal cord down to the upper sacral level, the neural tube is formed by neural folding. Secondary neurulation, which produces the neural tube in the lower sacral and coccygeal regions, occurs by a quite different process involving canalization of a solid cord of cells rather than neural folding.[539]

Primary neurulation begins with neural induction leading to the appearance of the neural plate, a thickened dorsal midline ectodermal structure. The lateral edges of the neural plate then elevate, beginning at about 17–18 days postfertilization, defining a longitudinal neural groove that deepens with progressive elevation of the sides of the neural plate. The neural folds converge towards the midline and fuse, forming the neural tube, beginning at the future cervical/occipital boundary (designated closure site 1, Fig. 7.8a) on day 22. Fusion proceeds in cranial and caudal directions from this level. Studies in the mouse have shown that fusion occurs separately, soon after this initial closure, at two other sites within the developing brain. Closure of the cranial neural tube then proceeds in a discontinuous, bidirectional fashion (Fig. 7.8a). Fusion spreads simultaneously along the future spinal region from closure site 1, being completed with closure of the posterior neuropore in the upper sacral region around days 26–28. This multisite closure process has been suggested also to occur in human embryos, since it can explain the variation in level of the body axis affected by neural tube defects in different individuals.[915] By contrast, direct studies of neurulation-stage embryos are equivocal about the precise details of the sequence of closure events in man.[654,687,871,915] Studies of neural tube defects in the mouse show that each element of the neural tube closure sequence has its own distinct requirement for

gene expression, so that mutations in different genes specifically disturb different events during neural tube closure.[166]

Axial skeletal development begins when the sclerotomal component of the mesodermal somites migrates to surround the neural tube, soon after its closure has been completed. In the cranial region, only the vault of the skull is formed by axial mesoderm, whereas the skull base and facial skeleton are derived from the neural crest.[888] By contrast, in the occipital and spinal regions, sclerotomal cells undergo skeletal differentiation to form the entire vertebrae. At the lowest spinal levels, an apparently multipotential population of cells, the tail bud, is the sole source of all non-epidermal tissues including the neural tube and vertebrae. Therefore, anomalies of the sacral and coccygeal regions are often found to embrace several tissue types.

Studies in the mouse have shown that different genes are implicated in the development of open NTDs versus axial mesodermal defects.[169,502] In terms of pathogenic mechanisms, therefore, it is important to distinguish between axial malformations that result from (1) failure of neural tube closure, in which secondary bony defects occur owing to faulty skeletal modelling around the malformed neural tube (e.g. anencephaly, craniorachischisis, myelomeningocele), and (2) lesions that result principally from bony defects that reflect primary abnormalities of axial mesodermal development, without a persistently open neural tube (Fig. 7.8b). This latter group comprises two subgroups: those defects in which there is herniation of the neural tube through the bony defect (e.g. encephalocele, meningocele) and 'closed' defects that are invariably skin covered (e.g. spina bifida occulta, diastematomyelia).

NEURAL TUBE CLOSURE DEFECTS

Craniorachischisis

Craniorachischisis is the most severe form of dysraphism. Brain and spinal cord are exposed to the surrounding amniotic fluid, resulting in necrosis, degeneration or angioma-like formations. It is noticeable that many cases of craniorachischisis exhibit a relatively well-developed optic system and a similar finding has been reported for a mouse model of craniorachischisis, the *loop-tail* (*Lp*) mutant. In this mouse, neural tube fusion fails at closure site 1 (Fig. 7.8a), resulting in the severe dysraphic disorder, but fusion occurs normally in the cranial region, at closure sites 2 and 3,[170] yielding a relatively well-formed prosencephalon and optic vesicles.

Exencephaly

Exencephaly and anencephaly are different stages of the same developmental anomaly. Exencephaly has been rarely described in human fetal pathology,[595] probably because of the rapid necrosis of brain tissue exposed to amniotic

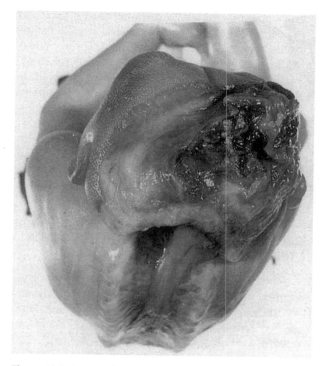

Figure 7.9 *Anencephaly with complete rachischisis. Oblique view from above and behind.*

fluid, leading to anencephaly. This phenomenon has been demonstrated directly in the retinoic acid-treated rat, where an initially exencephalic appearance is converted to anencephaly by late gestation.[960] The degenerative process is not rapid, however, as demonstrated by a study of surgically created neural tube lesions in the sheep, which can be corrected by a skin flap covering several weeks later in gestation, with only minimal functional deficit at birth.[613]

Anencephaly

Anencephaly was known in Egyptian antiquity, and in 1761 Morgagni compared the human monster to a toad. It was also described by Geoffroy Saint-Hilaire early in the nineteenth century.[331,332] The calvaria is hypoplastic or absent, the base of the skull is thick and flattened, and there is a constant anomaly of the sphenoid bone resembling 'a bat with folded wings'.[596] The orbits are shallow, causing protrusion of the eyes. Attached to the skull base is a dark reddish irregular mass of vascular tissue with multiple cavities containing cerebrospinal fluid (CSF), the area cerebrovasculosa. The mass is cystic with a midline dorsal aperture opening to the exterior. No recognizable neural tissue can be found in the anterior and middle fossae except for the trigeminal ganglia and limited lengths of the second to fifth cranial nerves. A hypoplastic anterior pituitary is present in a shallow sella, but the intermediate and posterior lobes are missing. The residual amount of brain tissue varies. If the foramen magnum is intact, a considerable proportion of the medulla is visi-

ble. Usually the foramen is deficient with cervical spina bifida, short neck and deformed pinnae; then only the caudal part of the medulla is present along with the distal parts of the lower cranial nerves. The pons, the cerebellum and the midbrain are grossly absent, although microscopic fragments of cerebellar folia may be seen.[62] Spinal involvement varies from non-fusion of the upper cervical arches without accompanying skull defect to complete rachischisis (Fig. 7.9).[51]

There is controversy regarding the histological interpretation of the area cerebrovasculosa, which includes irregular masses of neural tissue, mainly glia with some neuroblasts or neurons, ependyma and tufts of choroid plexus and numerous thin-walled blood vessels. While some consider that this tissue bears no resemblance to forebrain,[342] others[62] studying well-orientated sections observed vascular meninges surrounding a bilaterally symmetrical cavity, interpreted as forebrain ventricles, containing choroid plexus, and its walls composed of gliovascular tissue and lined partly by ependyma. Covering the cystic area cerebrovasculosa is non-keratinizing squamous epithelium which is laterally continuous with normal skin.

The medulla may be reasonably well preserved but, as with the spinal cord, there is aplasia of descending tracts. The spinal leptomeninges are excessively vascular and contain islands of heterotopic neuroglial tissue.[60]

The absence of neurohypophysis and hypothalamus is associated with a hypoplastic adrenal cortex.[24,904] Various other visceral abnormalities have been reported in cases of anencephaly,[651] a large thymus and hypoplastic lungs being the most frequent. Polyhydramnios is observed in about half of the cases but its pathogenesis is unclear.

Epidemiological studies have shown a high incidence of anencephaly in Ireland and in Wales, 1–6 per 1000 livebirths compared with about 0.5–2 per 1000 in the USA and 0.5 in France.[665] Females are affected more frequently than males. Anencephaly is the most common congenital malformation of the brain in human fetuses. Familial cases of anencephaly and/or spina bifida have been observed, but transmission is poorly understood. The role of diet and social class is still debated.

Early prenatal detection of NTDs is performed routinely by estimation of α-fetoprotein (AFP) in the amniotic fluid.[104] This protein is present in the fetal choroid plexus,[451] in addition to the fetal liver, and its elevated level in the amniotic fluid probably reflects direct leakage from the CSF. AFP can also be measured in maternal serum and this now forms the basis of prenatal screening for NTDs. Increasingly, ultrasound is also being used to identify NTDs early in pregnancy.[194]

Myelomeningocele

This is a severe malformation in which both meninges and spinal cord herniate through a large vertebral defect. The fluctuant mass consists of a distended meningeal sac which

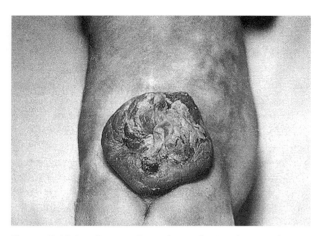

Figure 7.10 *Lumbar myelomeningocele. Lumbar myelomeningocele, showing ulceration of the surface, in an infant with hydrocephalus and paraplegia.*

is filled with CSF and covered by a thin membrane or by skin (Fig. 7.10). The spinal cord may be closed, floating on the posterior surface of the arachnoid cyst. The central canal is often dilated and the posterior part herniates with the meninges. In other cases, often referred to as myelocele, the malformation appears as a flat, open lesion with CSF leaking on to the exposed area. The spinal cord at the site of the bony defect forms a flat, discoidal, highly vascular mass, the area medullovasculosa, which becomes epithelialized after birth. The posterior surface of the spinal cord is open and the central canal blends into the skin. Peripheral nerves end blindly within the vascular mass, which comprises highly vascular connective tissue and islands of CNS including neurons, glia and ependyma.

Hydrocephalus occurs in many infants with one of these defects, usually in association with Arnold–Chiari (Chiari type II) malformation (see below). In addition, anomalies in the spinal cord above the myelomeningocele are common and include syringomyelia, hydromyelia, diastematomyelia, a double or multiple central canal and diplomyelia.[276]

The level of the defect has been the subject of particular attention for a number of reasons. Neurological disturbance depends largely on the level of defect and the latter has been used as a prognostic indicator in terms of both the likely benefit of caesarean delivery before the onset of labour, which has been demonstrated to be beneficial in cases of relatively low, mild lesions,[567] and the outcome of surgery to close the defect in the neonatal period.[236,529,561] Recently, the first cases of myelomeningocele closure *in utero* have been described, with apparently improved neurological function, and a decreased requirement for postnatal hydrocephalic shunting.[2,115]

Epidemiologically, high and low defects show marked differences with, for instance, lesions above T12 exhibiting frequent association with malformations in other systems and a female preponderance, whereas low lesions are more often solitary malformations that have a more equal sex incidence or even a male preponderance. This led to the hypothesis that high and low defects arise by pathogenic mechanisms, involving neural folding (primary neurulation) and canalization (secondary neurulation), respectively.[167] However, this hypothesis appears unlikely in the light of findings that the transition from primary to secondary neurulation occurs in the upper sacral region of the embryo,[168,640] indicating that the vast majority of cases of myelomeningocele, both high and low, arise from disturbance of primary neurulation. The epidemiological differences between high and low lesions almost certainly result from heterogeneity in the mechanism of primary neurulation along the body axis (see Fig. 7.8a).

AXIAL MESODERMAL DEFECTS WITH HERNIATION OF THE NEURAL TUBE

Encephalocele and cranial meningocele consist of a protrusion of brain or meninges through a cranial defect. They occur most frequently in the occipital region, with 75–80% of cases occurring there, while the frontal and lateral parts of the skull are affected much less often.

Occipital encephalocele

The herniation occurs through the occipital bone, with or without involvement of the foramen magnum. The mass of tissue is often voluminous (Fig. 7.11), attached to one of the cerebral hemispheres by a narrow pedicle, and partially covered with normal skin and hair. Ulceration of the skin and secondary infection are frequent. Smaller encephaloceles may only contain fragments of disorganized CNS tissue, glia and ependyma. Larger herniations may include large portions of the cerebral hemispheres with ventricular cavities,[129,481] as well as parts of the brainstem and cerebellum.

In the series of Karch and Urich[481] the herniation was always asymmetrical (Fig. 7.12) and although the gross convolutional pattern was normal and the cortex apparently not malformed, there was severe distortion, displacement and asymmetry of the basal ganglia. Other features included anomalies of the hippocampi and commissural system, aberrant neural tissue in the cavity of the ventricles, distortion of the brainstem and agenesis of cranial nerve nuclei, absence of the vermis and near or complete absence of the cerebellar hemispheres. Karch and Urich drew particular attention to the presence of a persistent fetal vasculature in the form of an extensive plexus of thin-walled sinusoidal blood vessels in the leptomeninges. Similar abnormalities are present in the authors' material, but in addition on several occasions the cerebral cortex has shown polymicrogyria (Fig. 7.13).

Meckel's syndrome

Occipital encephalocele is an important component of the Meckel–Gruber syndrome, a lethal autosomal recessive

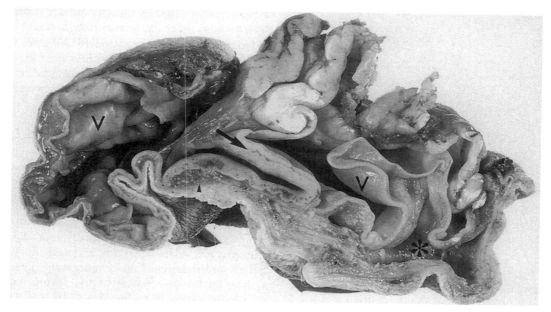

Figure 7.11 *Encephalocele. Cut surface of a large surgical specimen. In this example the two attenuated occipital lobes have herniated with their ventricular cavities (V). The cortex varies in thickness and is partly fused (arrow). Between brain and skin there is vascular meningeal tissue (arrowhead) and a cystic space (*).*

disorder with a characteristic phenotype including sloping forehead, occipital encephalocele, polydactyly, polycystic kidneys and hepatic fibrosis with bile-duct proliferation.[6] The variability of neuropathological findings among the mass of case reports has prompted two extended series in an attempt to define a consistent pattern of abnormality. From observations in 59 cases, and detailed neuropathology in ten, Paetau *et al.*[691] noted encephalocele in 90%, other prominent features being olfactory aplasia, midline defects and migration disorders such as polymicrogyria. Another autopsy study of seven fetal or neonatal cases[6] revealed a consistent pattern of malformations: (1) prosencephalic dysgenesis, arhinencephaly–holoprosencephaly and other midline anomalies; (2) occipital exencephalocele taking the form of extrusion of parts of the rhombic roof through the posterior

fontanelle; and (3) rhombic dysgenesis, notably supracerebellar cyst, vermal agenesis, stenosis of the aqueduct, and flattening and dysplasia of the brainstem.

Parietal encephalocele or meningocele

Parietal encephalocele or meningocele occurs only occasionally.[581] Deformities of the brain are usually present and are not confined to the ipsilateral hemisphere. They include asymmetry, distortion of the ventricular walls, agenesis of the corpus callosum and hydrocephalus.

Anterior encephalocele

Anterior encephalocele (Fig. 7.14) is most commonly found at the frontoethmoidal junction. It is usually visible at the bridge of the nose (in 60% of cases) as a bulging

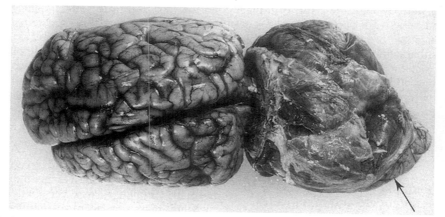

Figure 7.12 *Occipital encephalocele. There is asymmetrical herniation of the cerebral hemispheres, almost half of one hemisphere being displaced into the hernial sac (arrow). The constriction indicates the position of the occipital bone of the skull.*

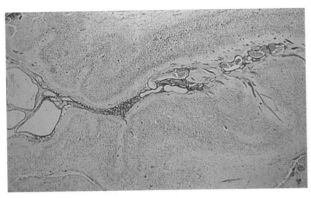

Figure 7.13 *Microscopy of a surgically excised encephalocele. A malformed polymicrogyric cortex and persistent fetal vasculature in the leptomeninges are seen. (Luxol fast blue–cresyl violet.)*

subcutaneous nodule and mild hypertelorism or as a mass of brain tissue. The encephalocele may expand into the nasal cavity (30% of cases), ethmoidal or sphenoidal air sinuses, pharynx or orbit.[983] The abnormal mass may contain disorganized brain tissue or gliotic cerebral cortex. As with occipital encephaloceles, the cerebral hemispheres within the intracranial cavity may be markedly skewed with non-register of the basal ganglia and commissural anomalies. The clinical diagnosis may be difficult if only the meninges protrude through the cribriform plate of the ethmoid bone. CSF passing into the nasal cavity is indicative of a free communication between the subarachnoid space and the encephalocele.

Because frontoethmoidal meningocele and encephalocele are rare in western Europe but relatively common in south-east Asia, genetic and geographical factors may be of importance in their aetiology.[300,873]

Meningocele

This is usually classified as a variant of spina bifida cystica, in which there is a vertebral defect combined with a cystic lesion of the back, most often in the lumbosacral region. Both the dura and arachnoid herniate through a vertebral defect, the spinal cord remaining in a normal

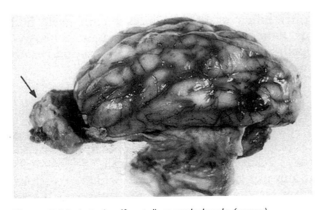

Figure 7.14 *Anterior (frontal) encephalocele (arrow).*

position in the spinal canal, although it may show hydromyelia, diastematomyelia or tethering. The cyst is covered by skin which has atrophic epidermis and lacks rete pegs and skin appendages. The wall of the cyst contains thin-walled blood vessels and islands of arachnoidal tissue, a narrow channel connecting the cyst with the vertebral canal.

SPINA BIFIDA OCCULTA: DEFECTS OF TAIL BUD DEVELOPMENT

This is the least severe group of NTDs, which are sometimes grouped together under the general term occult spina bifida. Although the spinal cord abnormality may be a prominent feature, there are often accompanying defects of skeletal (e.g. sacral agenesis), anorectal and urogenital systems. The spinal cord abnormalities may comprise overdistension of the central canal (hydromyelia), longitudinal duplication or splitting of the spinal cord (diplomyelia, diastematomyelia) and tethering of the lower end of the cord. The defects are most often located in the low lumbar and sacral regions, broadly corresponding to the region of secondary neurulation. Since neural folding is not involved at this level, the defects are always of the closed type. All of the abnormalities can be traced to a disturbance of development of the embryonic tail bud. Defective separation of neuroepithelial and mesodermal tissues during differentiation of the tail bud in animal models commonly yields a split cord.[152,256] Similarly, tethering of the cord within the vertebral canal probably represents the incomplete separation of neural from mesodermal components. The association of low spinal lesions with sacrococcygeal teratoma and lipoma is another manifestation of aberrant differentiation of the tail bud, which comprises a multipotential cell population.[880]

Occurrence of split cord at higher levels seems most likely to reflect secondary injury to the closed neural tube from malformed vertebral elements, as evidenced by the frequent association of diastematomyelia with a bony spur. These higher defects should probably be considered a malformation of axial mesodermal differentiation.

Hydromyelia

Overdistension of the central canal can result either from incomplete fusion of the posterior columns[853] or as a persistence of the primitive large canal of the embryo. The dilatation may be focal and is often more pronounced in the lumbar region. In the neonate, isolated hydromyelia is usually asymptomatic and is an incidental finding at autopsy. It may be found only on serial slices of the spinal cord.[64] Hydromyelia may also be one anomaly in a more complex syndrome. It is, for instance, associated with the Arnold–Chiari malformation in approximately 40% of cases.[580] The central canal may be lined by normal ependyma, which becomes replaced by glial tissue (Fig. 7.15).

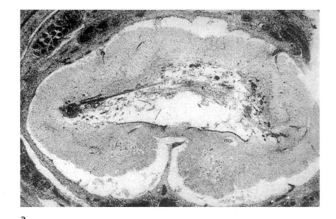

a

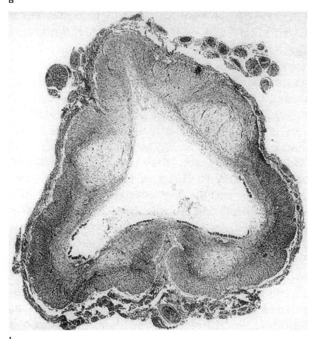

b

Figure 7.15 *Hydromyelia. (a) In a case with myelomeningocele and Arnold–Chiari malformation, the ependyma is intact anteriorly but posteriorly is partially destroyed by necrosis and haemorrhage. Fragments of gauze in the cavity are derived from dressings over the ulcerated meningomyelocele nearby. (b) In a newborn child with an Arnold–Chiari malformation early gliosis replaces the ependymal lining in the posterior half of the cavity.*

Split cord

Although diplomyelia (duplication of the cord) and diastematomyelia (coexistence of two hemicords) are often distinguished (Fig. 7.16), Pang *et al.*[700] proposed an alternative classification based on whether the hemicords have separate dural sacs, separated by a rigid osseocartilaginous septum (split cord malformation type I) or whether the hemicords coexist within a single dural sac, separated only by a non-rigid fibrous median septum (split cord malformation type II). Both types of lesion can occur, in

tandem, in the same patient. Split cord is more likely to be symptomatic in adults than children[698] and, in neonates, may be an incidental finding.

Tethered cord

Defects of the spinal cord can be associated with tethering within the vertebral canal, whatever the level of cord affected as, for instance, in cervical myelomeningocele.[699] However, the tethered cord syndrome is usually reserved for lumbosacral defects in which there are variable combinations of thickening of the filum terminale, low or dilated conus medullaris, spinal lipoma, dermoid cyst, split cord, hydromyelia and sacral agenesis. Clinical signs associated with cord tethering include lower limb motor and sensory deficits and neuropathic bladder. The severity of symptoms increases with age and patients are frequently treated surgically by untethering of the cord. Follow-up studies to determine the long-term effects of surgery have shown a good outcome in terms of maintained cord mobility, and symptomatic improvement in some cases, in terms of resolution of upper motor neuron signs and enhanced bladder function.[175,305]

PREVENTION OF NEURAL TUBE DEFECTS

The prospect for primary prevention of neural tube defects by folic acid was raised by a randomized controlled clinical trial conducted by the Medical Research Council (MRC) in the UK.[933] This study demonstrated a 70% reduction in the recurrence of NTDs, after periconceptional supplementation with 4 mg folic acid per day. Evidence has also accumulated to suggest a preventive effect of folic acid on the first occurrence of NTDs.[70,197] Although 70% of defects were prevented by folic acid in the MRC trial, up to 30% of defects appeared resistant.

Mothers of affected fetuses either have normal red cell and serum folate levels, or are mildly deficient, whereas mildly elevated levels of homocysteine are present in maternal blood and in the amniotic fluid of defective fetuses.[622,857] This finding suggests a key role for the enzyme methionine synthase, which catalyses the remethylation of homocysteine. Indeed, Kirke *et al.*[496] showed that folate

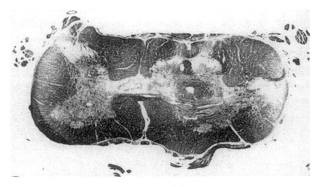

Figure 7.16 *Partial duplication of the spinal cord. Courtesy of Dr C Keohane University of Cork, Ireland.*

and vitamin B_{12} levels are independent risk factors for NTDs. Alternatively, elevated homocysteine could reflect subnormal function of the enzyme 5,10-methylene-tetrahydrofolate reductase (MTHFR), which catalyses the production of 5-methyltetrahydrofolate, the methyl donor in the methionine synthase reaction. Cases of NTDs and their parents are more likely to possess a polymorphic, thermolabile variant of MTHFR than normal controls,[917] suggesting that the MTHRF polymorphism is a genetic risk factor for neural tube defects.

Mouse models of neural tube defect fall into two groups with respect to prevention by folic acid. *Splotch* mice develop anencephaly and myelomeningocele which are preventable by folic acid treatment of embryos either *in vivo* or *in vitro*.[302] During neurulation, *splotch* embryos exhibit a decreased supply of folate-related metabolites for pyrimidine synthesis, which can be ameliorated by administration of folic acid or thymidine, but not by methionine. *Curly tail* mutant mice, in contrast, are resistant to folic acid but low spinal defects in this system can be prevented by another vitamin-like molecule, myo-inositol, administered either *in vivo* or *in vitro*.[359] Myo-inositol exerts its effect via stimulation of the enzyme protein kinase C and upregulation of the gene *retinoic acid receptor-β*. The possibility arises that myo-inositol may be a useful adjunct to folic acid therapy, perhaps allowing prevention of a larger proportion of NTDs than is possible with folic acid alone.

Chiari malformations

In 1891 Chiari defined three types of cerebellar deformity associated with hydrocephalus.[134] In a subsequent paper he added a fourth type, cerebellar hypoplasia,[133] which most authors now regard as a separate entity. The pathogenic relationship among Chiari's three types is controversial, but the morphological classification remains valid.

CHIARI TYPE I

In Chiari's original description, conical elongations of the tonsils and neighbouring parts of the cerebellar hemispheres extend into the vertebral canal. These prolongations could be histologically normal, 'softened' or sclerosed, while the medulla was either unchanged or flattened by the cerebellar tongues. His index case was a girl aged 17 years, asymptomatic during life, in whom there was some widening of the lateral and third ventricles but without enlargement of the head. Chiari stated that he had never found the type I anomaly in the absence of hydrocephalus. Since this was prior to our modern appreciation of the relationships between raised intracranial pressure and tonsillar herniation and our understanding of the causes of hydrocephalus, it has been argued that the term 'Chiari type I' is a misnomer, many alleged cases being

merely examples of chronic tonsillar herniation resulting from space-occupying lesions or chronic hydrocephalus.[318] On this basis Friede and Roessmann[318] proposed the alternative term 'chronic tonsillar herniation' to denote tonsillar herniation alone in the absence of space-occupying lesions, but endeavoured to differentiate this from cases with additional hindbrain herniation and deformation, which they somewhat confusingly call the adult form of Arnold–Chiari malformation. Whether the latter is more closely aligned morphologically and pathogenetically with Chiari type I or type II remains uncertain: spina bifida, for example, is not usually present The issue is further clouded by unilateral tonsillar protrusion mimicking vermal herniation at surgery, and the use of such terms as 'Arnold–Chiari type I'. But there is no need to abandon the term Chiari type I if it is applied

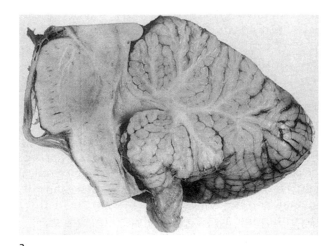

a

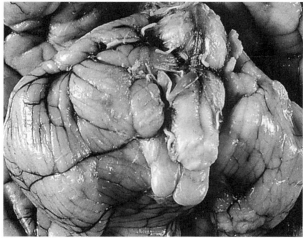

b

Figure 7.17 *Chiari-type I malformation. (a) Chiari type I malformation. Mid-sagittal section through the hindbrain. The peg-like protrusion of the cerebellar hemisphere is quite separate from the normal vermis. (b) Chiari type I malformation in a 10-month-old child presenting with polydactyly, hemihypertrophy and hemimegalencephaly. A bifid tongue of tonsillar tissue extended to 2.5 cm below the olivary bulge.*

to cerebellar herniation restricted solely to the tonsils (Fig. 7.17a, b), which may be atrophic, sclerotic and connected by fibrous adhesions to the sides and back of the slightly elongated medulla. The course of the upper cervical roots has been disputed, but in several cases examined at the National Hospital for Neurology and Neurosurgery, London, upper cervical roots were angled in an upward direction (Fig. 7.18). This has also been the conclusion in some surgical series.[37]

Although often asymptomatic, Chiari type I is a not uncommon cause of late-onset hydrocephalus, with adult patients presenting with cerebellar ataxia, neck pain, pyramidal syndrome, or dissociated sensory loss indicative of syringomyelia. It is increasingly recognized in the paediatric age group, owing to the increased availability of non-invasive neuroimaging, notably magnetic resonance imaging (MRI). In young infants of 2 years or under, presenting symptoms include headache and neck pain,[211] or apnoeic episodes including near-miss sudden infant death syndrome;[264] by contrast, older children exhibit scoliosis and motor weakness associated with syringomyelia.[211] An MRI study of 16 such children aged under 15 years showed an asymmetry of the syrinx towards the convex side of the scoliosis,[449] suggesting that asymmetric damage to the anterior horn may be the pathological substrate for the unbalanced strength of the paravertebral muscles responsible for scoliosis. Lower cranial nerve palsies[267] may lead to sleep apnoea and vocal cord paralysis,[789] or speech defects associated with velopharyngeal insufficiency.[334] For neuropathologists, a further important presentation is in connection with sudden unexpected death in childhood. Friede and Roessmann[318] collected seven cases, aged from 7 months to 17 years, who prior to death were without neurological deficit. Recent personal experience includes two such instances of sudden death associated with Chiari type I in the contexts of craniodiaphyseal dysplasia (Fig. 7.19) and hemimegalencephaly (Fig. 7.17b).

The relationship of type I anomaly to syringomyelia is close: half the patients in clinical series of type I[37,258,630,816] have syringomyelia, whereas about 90% of patients with idiopathic syringomyelia have a Chiari anomaly.[28,330,823] Familial occurrence of syringomyelia and Chiari type I has also been reported.[340] An association with craniocervical bony malformations has been increasingly recognized, notably the presence of platybasia, basilar impression, suboccipital dysplasia and Klippel–Feil anomaly,[29,37,214,544,630,706,816] but Chiari type I may also occur in conjunction with craniosynostosis[318] (Fig. 7.19).

Using detailed measurements of lateral skull radiographs, Shady et al.[816] demonstrated occipital dysplasia in over two-thirds of a large series of adult Chiari type I patients, diagnosed by supine myelography, surgery and computed tomographic (CT) scans. The posterior fossa in these patients was significantly smaller than in controls and there was an inverse relationship between the size of the posterior fossa and the degree of cerebellar herniation. The small size of the posterior fossa was also a notable feature in the family described by Coria et al.:[173] autosomal dominant occipital dysplasia with or without Chiari type

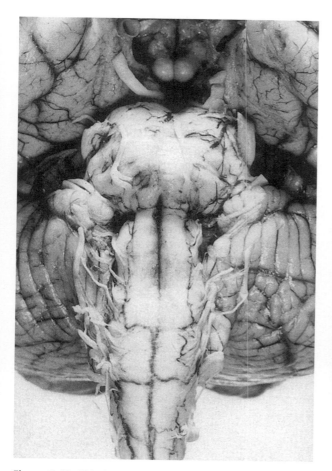

Figure 7.18 *Chiari-type I malformation. Chiari type I malformation showing upwardly directed cervical spinal roots.*

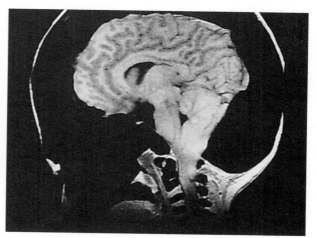

Figure 7.19 *Chiari type I malformation. MRI showing tonsillar herniation to C2 in a patient with massive skull thickening due to craniometaphyseal dysplasia. Courtesy of Dr K Chong, Great Ormond Street Hospital, London.*

I anomaly affected three generations. These studies suggest a primary role for occipital dysplasia in the pathogenesis of the Chiari type I malformation, a hypothesis that parallels that derived from the experimental model of Arnold–Chiari malformation.[597]

CHIARI TYPE II

Cleland[149] first recorded herniation of the vermis combined with deformities of the medulla and tectal plate in an infant with a meningocele, now generally known as the Arnold–Chiari malformation.[812] It has been the subject of numerous pathological studies.[61,122–124,205,338,710,711] Most commonly found in infants in association with myelomeningocele and hydrocephalus, its essential components are elongation of the inferior vermis and brainstem and their displacement into the cervical spinal canal (Fig. 7.20).

Bony and dural anomalies are characteristic and important for radiological diagnosis. Craniolacunia (Fig. 7.21), irregular patches of thinning or complete erosion of the cranial vault, is frequent; in one radiological study[875] it was present in 90% of neonates with Arnold–Chiari and myelomeningocele. The falx is short and fenestrated.[123] The posterior fossa is shallow, the torcula low, and the clivus concave and thinned. The tentorial hiatus is widened but the tentorial insertion is low, near the edge

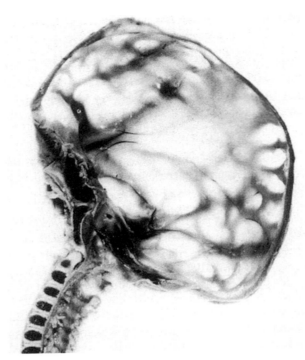

Figure 7.21 *Craniolacunia. Craniolacunia of the skull from an infant with Arnold–Chiari malformation.*

of an enlarged foramen magnum. The herniated cerebellar tissue varies from a short peg to a long tail and involves nodulus, pyramis and uvula in that order.[205] It may extend down as far as the upper dorsal vertebral segments. Rarely, there is no cerebellar displacement, or the herniated tissue includes tonsils as well as vermis. The elongated tongue of flattened whitish cerebellar vermis, often associated with choroid plexus, lies on the dorsal surface of the lower medulla and cord, firmly bound to them by fibrous meningeal adhesions. Its upper end is often grooved by the edge of the foramen magnum. The brainstem, particularly the medulla, the fourth ventricle and its choroid plexus, are elongated and displaced caudally. The cerebellar tail may cover the roof of the ventricle or may be intraventricular. In 50% of cases, just caudal to the ventricle, the lower medulla below the gracile and cuneate nuclei forms an S-shaped curve or kink over the cervical cord (Figs 7.22, 7.23).

Microscopically, the herniated cerebellar tissue shows Purkinje and granule cell depletion with shrinkage and gliosis of the folia and absence of myelin. The presence of focal cortical dysplasia and grey heterotopias in the hemispheric white matter is well recognized, as well as distortion of brainstem tracts and nuclei. Gilbert *et al.*[338] recently called attention to hypoplasia or agenesis of cranial nerve nuclei, olivary nuclei and pontine nuclei in their series of young infants. Additional abnormalities are numerous. The cerebellar hemispheres are often asymmetrical and flattened dorsally; the vermis may be buried between the hemispheres which can extend around the brainstem over its ventral surface, sometimes meeting in

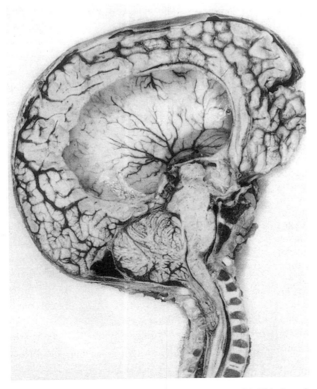

Figure 7.20 *Arnold–Chiari malformation. Arnold–Chiari malformation (Chiari type II) and hydrocephalus in a 7-week-old infant. Note the downward displacement of the cerebellar vermis and tonsils through the foramen magnum into the spinal canal and the beak-like deformity of the quadrigeminal plate.*

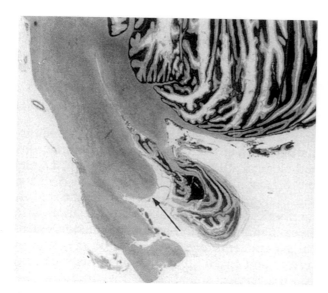

Figure 7.22 *Arnold–Chiari malformation. Sagittal section of brainstem and cerebellum in the Arnold–Chiari malformation. The herniated cerebellar tissue lies posterior to the S-shaped kink (arrow) at the junction of the medulla and spinal cord.*

the midline.[205] The pontomedullary junction is ill defined with an elongated rod-shaped pons. Also common is a beak-like deformity of the corpora quadrigemina which is directed backwards and downwards to a point formed by the fusion of the inferior colliculi.[149] The upper four to six cervical spinal roots are angled upwards towards their intervertebral foramina; lower roots are normally placed. Other frequently described anomalies are subependymal nodular grey heterotopias in the lateral ventricles and thickening of the massa intermedia. Spina bifida is almost invariably present; exceptions are exceedingly rare.[712] Myelomeningocele is more common than meningocele and typically occurs at lumbar or lumbosacral level. Other associated spinal anomalies include hydromyelia, usually at C8,[580] syringomyelia just below the cervicomedullary junction, diastematomyelia and diplomyelia.[338]

Hydrocephalus is usually present and may be due to obstruction of the aqueduct or at the foramen magnum. Aqueduct atresia, forking and gliosis have been described.[123,577] In Emery's series[275] obstruction was never complete, and the shortening and angulation of the aqueduct suggested a valve-like mechanism. Another hypothesis is that the deformed hindbrain may plug the foramen magnum, and, because the exit foramina are situated within the spinal canal, CSF is prevented from reaching the intracranial subarachnoid space. The resultant hydrocephalus is communicating in type; ascending spinal meningitis may thus produce a pyocephalus whilst the cerebral subarachnoid space is spared. The dilated cerebral hemispheres often show an abnormal convolutional pattern consisting of an excessive number of small gyri and shallow sulci, most appropriately termed

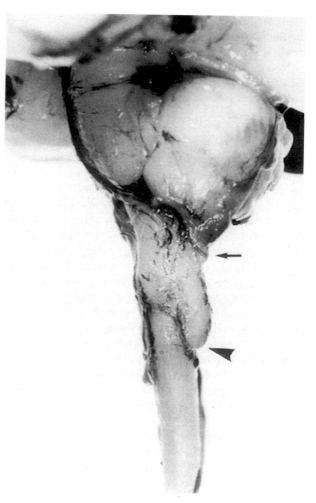

Figure 7.23 *Arnold–Chiari malformation. Arnold–Chiari malformation in a 20-week fetus. Lateral aspect of the hindbrain showing only slight cerebellar herniation (arrow), but marked elongation of the brain stem with a prominent S-shaped curve over the upper cervical cord (arrowhead).*

polygyria since usually the normal cytoarchitecture is preserved, unlike the laminar abnormalities present in polymicrogyria, although several authors have also described true polymicrogyria.[275,710] McLendon et al.[582] carried out a quantitative study on a series of 15 cases of Arnold–Chiari and hydrocephalus; all had polygyria macroscopically, a significant increase in sulcal length per unit area of cortex compared with controls and histologically normal lamination. By contrast, more than half of the 25 cases discussed by Gilbert et al.[338] showed disordered cortical lamination, with polymicrogyria in 40%, a result that may reflect the particular population examined, comprising infants dying before the age of 2 years.

Conflicting theories abound concerning the pathogenesis of Chiari type II, not surprisingly in view of the multiplicity of associated anomalies and the need for any satisfactory theory to explain the almost constant association of spina bifida. The earliest theories invoked pressure from above[133] in the form of hydrocephalus forcing the hindbrain downwards. Gardner[328] suggested that a primary malformation of the fourth ventricle led to hydrocephalus and, subsequently, rupture of the already closed neural tube, while Cameron[122,123] proposed that the hydrocephalus was secondary to failure of neural tube closure, excessive drainage of CSF and apposition then fusion of the ependyma resulting in aqueduct stenosis. Against such theories are the absence of hydrocephalus in some fetal cases[61] and in calves with Arnold–Chiari.[135] Traction from below was seen by Lichtenstein[549] as a consequence of cord tethering by the meningocele. Against this hypothesis are the normal alignment of lower cervical and thoracic roots,[50] the S-shape deformity of the lower brainstem and the rare examples of Arnold–Chiari anomaly without dysraphism.[259,712] Developmental arrest of the pontine flexure was proposed by Daniel and Strich[205] and Peach,[711] but the expected disorganization of the topography of the brainstem nuclei does not occur.

A disproportion between the growth of the posterior fossa and its contents has been the focus of many recent theories. Barry et al.[50] thought that the cerebellum had overgrown, but others have noted reduced cerebellar weights[20,919] and also a reduction in volume of the posterior fossa.[105] The smallness of the posterior fossa is the basis of the hypothesis proposed by Marin-Padilla and Marin-Padilla.[597] Using an experimental model induced by vitamin A administration to pregnant hamsters, they have shown that the basichondrocranium is shorter than normal, causing a reduction in size of the posterior fossa. All the neurological anomalies are considered to be secondary to the skeletal defects. Compression of the developing medulla within a small posterior fossa causes the abnormalities of the pontine and cervical flexures, while the relatively late growth spurt of the cerebellum means that it is neither pushed nor pulled but required to grow into the spinal canal. This explanation would be consistent with observations in early human fetuses. Evidence from the literature[50,61,259] and personal experience (see Fig. 7.23) indicate that in the second trimester the cerebellar herniation is slight, even when the medullary abnormality is extensive.

CHIARI TYPE III

This is very rare.[133,710] It comprises an occipitocervical or a high cervical bony defect with herniation of cerebellum through the bony defect into the encephalocele. Other features may include beaking of the tectum, elongation and kinking of the brainstem and lumbar spina bifida (Fig. 7.24).

Disorders of forebrain induction

The various disorders of telencephalic evagination, cleavage and commissure formation are associated with

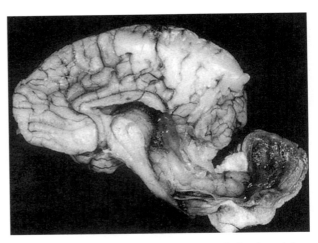

Figure 7.24 *Chiari type III malformation. Cerebellar tissue is herniated into an occipitocervical encephalocele. Also present in this 5-day-old neonate was a lumbosacral meningomyelocele and a thoracic syrinx.*

a number of distinctive clinical syndromes. Their complex terminology, overlapping morphological features and close association with craniofacial anomalies present a particular challenge to the neuropathologist. However, recent advances in genetics and developmental biology have provided important insights into the early embryonic events of forebrain formation and the pathogenesis of holoprosencephaly and associated conditions. Hence, we are beginning to appreciate how the spectrum of forebrain malformations may arise during development, an advance that should provide a more rational basis for the classification and understanding of these conditions in future.

INDUCTION AND EARLY DEVELOPMENT OF THE FOREBRAIN

Before closure of the cranial neural tube, in the third week of gestation, formation of the prosencephalic neural plate is induced in the naive neuroepithelium by interaction with the prechordal plate, a region of underlying midline mesoderm and endoderm that represents a rostral continuation of the notochord above the dorsal lip of the foregut. *Sonic hedgehog* (*Shh*) is the key signalling molecule in this inductive interaction,[787] probably via the stimulation of another signalling molecule, bone morphogenetic protein 7 (BMP7).[200] *Shh* induces the formation of ventral midline cells in the forebrain primordium, a region that appears to grow slowly compared with more dorsolateral regions. Hence, the midline exerts a mechanical constraint on the rapid growth of the forebrain, resulting in its cleavage to form the paired telencephalic vesicles. The effect is not solely mechanical, however, as the influence of *Shh* also induces division of the single optic primordium, which initially spans the midline, into paired structures either side of the midline.

Mutations in the mouse *Shh* gene, produced by gene targeting, have yielded a phenotype resembling holoprosencephaly with cyclopia, with failure of division of the forebrain vesicle and development of a single eye structure.[132] Moreover, mutations at the human HPE3 locus, a cause of holoprosencephaly in man, have been found to disrupt the human *SHH* gene.[769] Interestingly, heterozygosity for *SHH* mutation in man yields holoprosencephaly, albeit towards the mild end of the pathological spectrum, whereas heterozygous *Shh* mutant mice are normal, with only homozygotes exhibiting the holoprosencephalic phenotype. The reason for the haploinsufficiency of *SHH* mutation in man but not mice is unknown. Recently, two other genes have been implicated in the aetiology of holoprosencephaly in man (Table 7.1): the homeobox-containing gene *SIX3* is mutated in HPE2, while the zinc finger-containing transcription factor *ZIC2* appears to be responsible for holoprosencephaly in patients with deletions of 13q32 (HPE5). Although both genes are expressed in the early cranial neural plate, it has not yet been determined precisely how they are involved in forebrain development.

PATTERNING THE FOREBRAIN ALONG THE ANTEROPOSTERIOR AXIS

Other signalling centres, apart from the prechordal plate, are essential for normal development and patterning of the forebrain. A diffusible signalling molecule, fibroblast growth factor-8 (FGF8), is produced by the anterior tip of the neural plate (the anterior neural ridge) and also by the isthmus, a signalling centre at the boundary between the midbrain and hindbrain.[192] FGF8 appears to induce competence within the neural plate to respond to the Shh signal, thereby ensuring the orderly formation of forebrain and midbrain regions. For instance, FGF8 primes the anterior-most neural plate to respond to Shh by expressing brain factor 1 (BF1), which is essential for formation of the cerebral hemispheres, as evidenced by a lack of these forebrain structures in mice without BF1 function.[964] As with the hindbrain, there is also an important role for homeobox-containing genes in specification of the forebrain and midbrain (see also section on pathogenesis at the cellular and tissue levels, above). Genes belonging to the *Otx* family are required for formation of both forebrain and midbrain: mice lacking *Otx2* function exhibit a deficiency in both structures. The caudal boundary of Otx2 expression appears to define the position of the isthmus.[103] More caudally, the homeobox gene *Gbx2* appears essential for midbrain specification.[621] Hence, the subdivision of the primitive brain neural tube is achieved by signals emanating from the underlying prechordal plate and from within the neural plate itself, which serve to induce region-specific expression of homeobox genes that impose and maintain identity within the anteroposterior axis of the brain.

LATER DEVELOPMENT OF THE FOREBRAIN

Concomitant with closure of the neural tube in the prosencephalic region, the paired optic vesicles begin their outgrowth and, shortly afterwards, around 4–5 weeks, the lateral evagination of the paired cerebral or telencephalic vesicles from the single prosencephalic cavity becomes visible. The olfactory vesicles appear as paired outgrowths from the base of the brain at 6 weeks. They are induced to differentiate into olfactory bulbs and tracts by contact with nerve fibres from the olfactory placode which have grown towards them through a perforant zone in the developing ethmoid bone. The anterior wall of the prosencephalon is relatively inert, so exerting a midline constraint on the rapid growth of the telencephalic vesicles and resulting in their apparent cleavage. Around week 7 the choroid plexus invaginates each lateral vesicle, and gradually the broad connections into the central cavity narrow to become the foramina of Monro, while the central telencephalic cavity becomes the third ventricle. The commissures arise from the anterior wall of this central structure, the telecephalon medium. It stretches in the midline dorsally from the chiasmatic plate to the paraphysis. Its ventral portion, the lamina terminalis, remains thin, becoming the anterior wall of the third ventricle. The cellular and thickened dorsal portion, the lamina reuniens, has two parts.[741] Ventrally, the area precommissuralis will form the septal area and anterior commissure; dorsally, there is an area of complex growth and infolding which is the anlage of the fornix, hippocampus, psalterium, corpus callosum and septum pellucidum. As early as 9–10 weeks' gestation the precursor fibres of the anterior commissure meet and decussate in the ventral part of the lamina reuniens, and the bilateral primordia of the fornices appear in the dorsal part of the lamina reuniens and grow dorsally towards the primordia of the hippocampi, which are by now clearly demarcated from the hemispheric isocortex in the medial walls of the hemispheres. By median infolding of the dorsal lamina reuniens a groove develops, the sulcus medianus telencephali medii (SMTM), in the floor of the interhemispheric fissure. The banks of the groove fuse to form the massa commissuralis, into which the fibres of the hippocampal commissure grow at about 10–11 weeks, and dorsal to them the anlage of the corpus callosum at 11–12 weeks, possibly guided by a preformed glial sling.[830] The corpus callosum grows caudally with the growth of the hemisphere; beneath it and between the banks of the SMTM a pocket appears at around 13–14 weeks. Eventually, the anteroventral extension of the rostrum of the corpus callosum seals this pocket, forming the cavum, while its walls and the banks of the SMTM become elongated and thinned into the leaflets of the septum pellucidum by the rapid growth of hemispheres and callosum. The hippocampus also extends backwards and rotates with the growth of the hemispheres, then anteroventrally into the temporal lobe, but its rostral part regresses into a vestigial remnant, the induseum griseum. From this synopsis it will be readily appreciated that a large variety of anomalies may result, depending on the timing and extent of the growth disturbance within the anterior wall of the telencephalon, and particularly in the midline.[537]

HOLOPROSENCEPHALY

Anomalies of prosencephalic outgrowth and cleavage form a wide spectrum, from cyclopia to unilateral olfactory agenesis. Kundrat[508] used the term 'arhinencephaly' considering the absence of olfactory structures to be the cardinal feature of this group of disorders, but this has since been criticized for placing undue emphasis on a relatively minor and variable component of these anomalies. Hence various alternatives have been proposed: holotelencephaly,[966] telencephalosynapsis[229] and holoprosencephaly.[232] The last has found most favour as it underscores the failure of cleavage of both telencephalon and diencephalon. The term arhinencephaly still persists as a generic term or in the more restricted sense of absence of olfactory bulbs, tracts and tubercles, for which the term 'olfactory aplasia' seems preferable.[314]

In holoprosencephaly, the degree of failure of hemispheric cleavage is very variable, but pathological observations are biased towards the most severe forms, and the more subtle variants are less frequently documented. Nevertheless, De Myer and Zeman[232] were able to subdivide holoprosencephaly into alobar, semilobar and lobar types. (For further more recent reviews see Refs 157, 537, 735 and 828.)

Alobar holoprosencephaly

Alobar holoprosencephaly, the most severe form, denotes a very small brain with monoventricular forebrain, a 'holosphere' undivided into hemispheres or lobes and with a bizarre convolutional pattern. The holosphere may be spherical or more flattened into a helmet or pancake shape. It can be tilted forwards within the cranial cavity or retroverted like the uterus.[232,497] Seen from below, the orbital/ventral surface of the holosphere is smooth or shows abnormally wide, rudimentary gyri (Fig. 7.25) with an anomalous vascular pattern (see below). The interhemispheric fissure and gyri recti are absent and there is aplasia of olfactory bulbs, tracts and tubercles and, depending on the state of the eyes, optic nerve hypoplasia or unilateral aplasia. Viewed from above and behind, the dorsal surface of the holosphere and its convolutions appear roughly horseshoe shaped. Attached to its distal edge and extending backwards towards the tentorium is a membrane with associated choroid plexus which partly roofs the single ventricular cavity. This membranous roof, thought to be evaginated tela choroidea,[551,558] often balloons out into a dorsally situated cyst (Fig. 7.26), its thin and diaphanous wall easily torn by the prosector to reveal the single ventricular cavity of the holosphere, in its floor the fused basal ganglia and thalami, and from their lateral edges, running in a complete arch beneath the attachment of the roof membrane to the holosphere, the hippocampal formation (Fig. 7.27). Behind the thalami is the opening

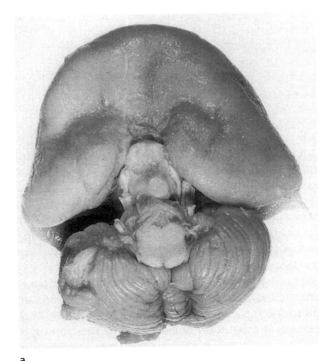

a

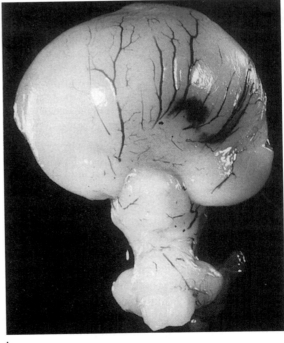

b

Figure 7.25 *Alobar holoprosencephaly. (a) Inferior view of the brain of an 18-month-old child with normal chromosomes. Single fused holosphere without interhemispheric fissure and olfactory aplasia. Anterior and middle cerebral arteries are in shallow gutters over the surface. (b) Fetus of 17 weeks. The horseshoe-shaped holosphere seen from below shows olfactory aplasia and an aberrant vascular pattern.*

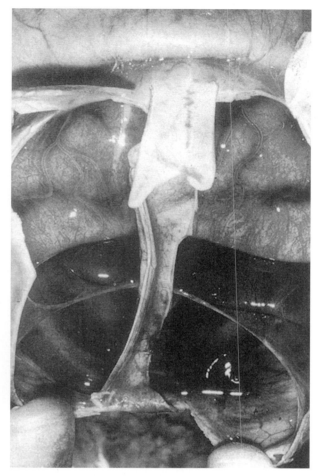

Figure 7.26 *Holoprosencephaly. The delicate roofing membrane of the single ventricle has been photographed in situ within the skull to preserve its integrity. The membrane is continuous with the posterior part of the holosphere. The head is viewed from above.*

into the aqueduct. There is no corpus callosum or septum, and on sectioning the pallium usually consists of cortex and only a thin layer of white matter. Additional abnormalities may include absent corpora striata, fused mamillary bodies or a single cerebral peduncle, and there are occasional reports of associated glioependymal cysts,[781] and aqueductal atresia.[928]

At first sight it might appear that the parietal and occipital cortex are missing, but a cytoarchitectonic analysis by Yakovlev[966] suggested the opposite, i.e. a loss of frontal cortex. In an extensive study of serial section of prosencephalic brains, he demonstrated a concentric arrangement of cortical zones radiating out from the ventricular cavity: first prepyriform and Ammon's horn, then entorhinal and presubicular cortex, surrounded again by limbic (cingulate) cortex and insula. The motor cortex occupied an anteromedian position in the holosphere, and granular type sensory cortex occupied the ventroposterior borders. Between them the parietotemporal association cortex was represented bilaterally by two small areas on

the orbital surface, but the premotor frontal cortex was entirely missing. From this viewpoint holoprosencephaly is not simply a failure of hemispheric cleavage but also a severe hypoplasia of the neopallium. The small size of holoprosencephalic brains is especially notable in fetal cases. An extreme example of holoprosencephalic microcephaly is shown in Fig. 7.28a, b: at 20 weeks' gestation the brain weight was only 7 g (normal being 50 g), the tiny globular forebrain exhibiting a rostral and central mass of heterotopic grey matter, basal polymicrogyria, bilateral hippocampal formations, and a horizontal slit-like ventricle with recognizable temporal horns communicating via two lateral apertures with a delicate cyst lined by ependyma and choroid plexus.

Growth failure in holoprosencephaly is further indicated by abnormalities of cortical structure and paralleled by aberrations of the circle of Willis. Yakovlev's[966] cases in the main had well-preserved cytoarchitecture, but not infrequently holospheric cortex shows various forms of disorganized cortical lamination including polymicrogyria (Fig. 7.29), or periventricular and leptomeningeal heterotopia.[460,625,626,735] In six alobar cases Mizuguchi and Morimatsu[626] demonstrated abnormally thick cortex and disturbed neuronal migration, including segmentation of superficial neurons into irregular groups and deeply

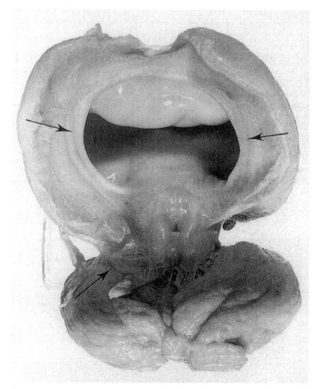

Figure 7.27 *Alobar holoprosencephaly (same case as Fig. 7.25) viewed from behind. Rupture of the cystic posterior roof of the holosphere (arrowhead) reveals the single ventricular cavity, midline fusion of basal ganglia and thalamus and the arch-like hippocampal formation running around the ventricular aperture (arrows).*

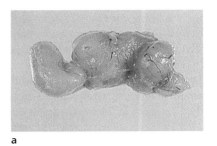
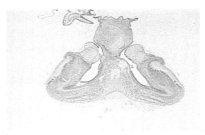
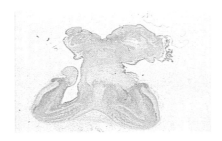

a   b

Figure 7.28 *Holoprosencephaly. Extreme microcephaly with holoprosencephaly at 20 weeks of gestation (see text). (**a**) The 7 g brain viewed from its lateral aspect, anterior to the left. (**b**) Adjacent coronal sections showing bilateral hippocampal formations and temporal horns which communicate (left figure) with a (disrupted) cyst lined by ependyma and choroid plexus (right figure). (H&E.)*

placed glomerular structures devoid of nerve cells and composed of thin dendrites and axons: similar findings were also observed by the authors (Fig. 7.30). In a recent detailed analysis of basal arterial patterns, normal circles of Willis were noted in arhinencephaly (olfactory aplasia), contrasting with eight cases of holoprosencephaly in which the anterior part of the circle was lacking while the posterior part appeared normal. The anterior and middle cerebral arteries were replaced by anteriorly directed branches from either one or both internal carotid arteries and very large-calibre choroidal arteries supplied the wall of markedly vascular dorsal cysts.[688] These anomalous patterns appear to reflect the developmental stage reached before normal development ceased and the further functional demands imposed by the later modified growth pattern of the brain.[688]

Semilobar holoprosencephaly

Semilobar holoprosencephaly is intermediate in severity, with less reduction in brain weight, rudimentary lobar structure and partial formation of a shallow interhemispheric fissure, usually most preserved occipitally. However, the cortex is broadly continuous across the midline (Fig. 7.31). Olfactory structures are usually, but not invariably, absent.[551]

Lobar holoprosencephaly

Despite almost normal brain size, lobar differentiation and separation of the hemispheres, there is midline continuity of the cerebral cortex, at the frontal pole, of the orbital surface or over the corpus callosum (cingulosynapsis).[164,303,655] The state of the olfactory system is variable, the corpus callosum is absent or hypoplastic, and there is often heterotopic grey matter in the roof of the ventricle (Fig. 7.32). De Myer and Zeman[232] included in the lobar group patients with olfactory aplasia and callosal agenesis but with completely separated hemispheres. This is terminologically confusing, and such cases are probably best categorized as commissural defects.

Holoprosencephaly is usually sporadic, but familial cases including affected twins have been documented.[117,232,415,490,766] Estimates for incidence vary from 1 in 31 000 births[319] to 1 in 16 000 livebirths and 1:250 abortions.[154] Increasingly, intrauterine diagnosis is made by ultrasound.[907] Severe forms of holoprosencephaly are often stillborn, while surviving infants present with facial dysmorphism, varying degrees of psychomotor retardation, spasticity, apnoeic attacks and disturbance of temperature regulation.

So frequent is the association of certain craniofacial malformations with holoprosencephaly that De Myer

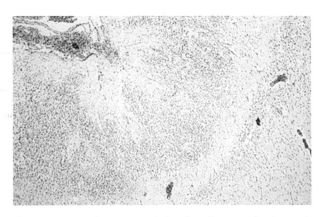

Figure 7.29 *Holoprosencephaly. Four-layer polymicrogyric cortex in alobar holoprosencephaly. Case of trisomy 13. (Cresyl violet.)*

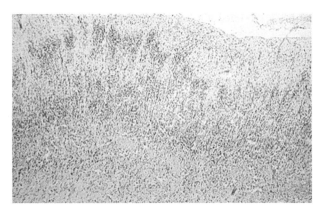

Figure 7.30 *Holoprosencephaly. Abnormal cortex comprising segmentation of superficial layers and deeply placed paucicellular 'glomeruli'. (Cresyl violet.)*

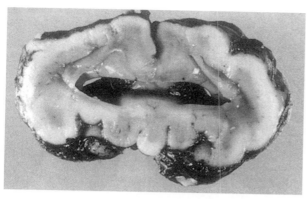

Figure 7.31 *Holoprosencephaly. Semilobar holoprosencephaly in a 32-week fetus. There is a suggestion of lobar organization and partial separation of the hemispheres by a shallow interhemispheric fissure, although the orbital surface is completely fused.*

et al.[233] wrote, 'The face predicts the brain', but there are always exceptions.[705] The development of prechordal mesoderm and forebrain are intimately related, and consequently midfacial hypoplasia is a regular concomitant of holoprosencephaly (Fig. 7.33). The most severe anomaly is cyclopia, fusion of the orbits with a single eye or two eyes close together or fused. A small nasal protuberance or proboscis projects above the orbits; there may be absence of the jaw (agnathia) and fusion of the ears under the eye (synotia, otocephaly). Half the reported cases of agnathia show holoprosencephaly, and there is also an association with situs inversus.[536,707] Lesser deformities include closely spaced orbits (hypotelorism), microphthalmia, a flattened nose with single nostril (cebocephaly) or a proboscis (ethmocephaly).

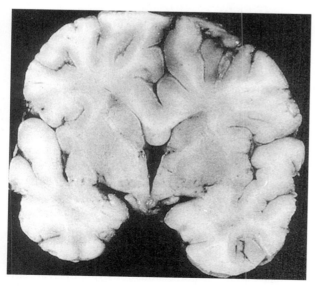

Figure 7.32 *Lobar holoprosencephaly. The two hemispheres are well formed but the cingulate cortex is continuous across the interhemispheric fissure. Note the heterotopic grey matter in the roof of the ventricle. Courtesy of Professor S Love, Frenchay Hospital, Bristol, UK.*

Other anomalies include cleft lip or palate, and sometimes trigonocephaly in which premature closure of the metopic suture produces a narrow pointed forehead, triangular from above. Occasional patients even have hypertelorism,[783] although frontonasal dysplasia (median cleft face syndrome), which includes hypertelorism, a broad nasal ridge, median cleft lip, nose or palate and cranium bifidum occultum, is generally associated with normal mental development and not with holoprosencephaly.[231] Usually in alobar or semilobar holoprosencephaly the skull base is short and narrow, crista galli and lamina cribrosa are absent, the sella turcica is absent or shallow, and there may be varying degrees of hypoplasia of nasal bones (see Fig. 7.33). The falx and sagittal sinus are also usually missing. Anomalies of other organs have been described, but these are quite variable and seem to be more prominent in patients with chromosome anomalies: notable are pituitary aplasia and thyroid or adrenal hypoplasia.

Aetiology of holoprosencephaly

This is heterogeneous. Well-known environmental causes include an increased incidence of holoprosencephaly in the offspring of maternal diabetics[48,155,219,474] and a notable association with maternal toxoplasmosis, syphilis and rubella. Fetal alcohol syndrome has also been implicated.[178] In animals, holoprosencephaly can be induced experimentally by a variety of mechanical and chemical techniques;[157,504,772] the most well-known teratogenic incident concerned ewes grazing in Idaho, USA, which ingested *Veratrum californicum*[80] (see also Teratogenic mechanisms, above). The analysis of families with autosomal recessive, autosomal dominant and X-linked pedigrees[41,154,157,643] has culminated in the identification of several genes responsible for particular forms of holoprosencephaly (see Table 7.1 and Induction and early development of the forebrain, above). Chromosomal aberrations, although common, are not invariable: about half the cases have normal karyotype.[623] The most frequent is trisomy 13;[704,705,766,842] holoprosencephaly is present in 70% of individuals with trisomy 13, but it has also been associated with trisomy 18[119,269,766] and triploidy. Several structural anomalies are non-randomly associated with holoprosencephaly, including del(18p), del(7)(q36), dup(3)(p24-pter), del(2)(21) and del(21)(q22.3).[644]

OLFACTORY APLASIA

Absence of olfactory bulbs, tracts, trigone and anterior perforated substance may occur in isolation, an incidental post-mortem finding unsuspected in life. Anomalies of the orbital frontal convolutions, especially absence of the normal gyrus rectus, are a useful confirmation that the olfactory tract has not been inadvertently avulsed at autopsy. Olfactory aplasia may also be associated with callosal agenesis or septo-optic dysplasia (see Fig. 7.40), is present in Kallman syndrome (Table 7.1) and is frequent

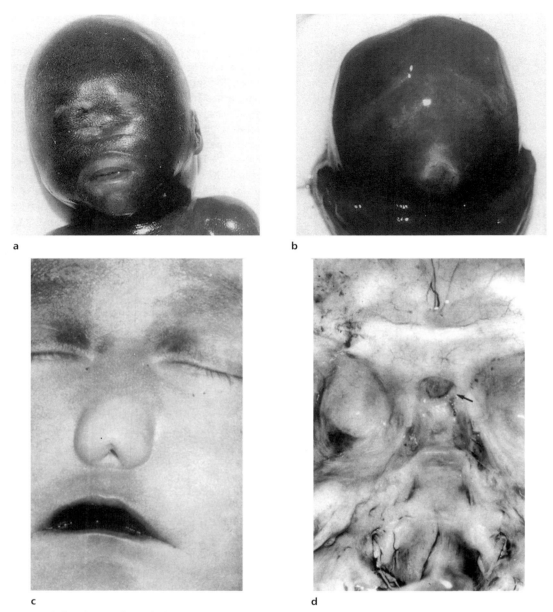

Figure 7.33 *Craniofacial anomalies in holoprosencephaly. (**a**, **b**) Cyclopia. (**a**) Externally no eyes are visible and a central slit replaces the nose. (**b**) Removing the scalp reveals a single midline orbit. (**c**) Hypotelorism and cebocephaly. The base of the skull in this patient (**d**) is without an ethmoid plate. Optic nerves (arrow) are hypoplastic.*

in Meckel's syndrome.[691] A neonate with Apert's syndrome showed absent olfactory bulbs and tracts, fusion of the olfactory tubercles and dysplasia of the hippocampus.[585] Bilateral olfactory aplasia is not so uncommon, but unilateral arhinencephaly is exceptional[12] (Fig. 7.34).

ATELENCEPHALY/APROSENCEPHALY

First described by Iivanainen *et al.*[445] and Garcia and Duncan,[326] the exact nosological position of this rare and extreme form of microcephaly, which has features in common with both anencephaly and holoprosencephaly, is still in question. There are now about a dozen published clinical or morphological observations[206,395,492,566,603,829,894]

together with two personally studied cases. Forebrain structures such as the cerebral cortex, basal ganglia and ventricles are virtually absent in atelencephaly, but in contradistinction to anencephaly the calvaria is intact and slopes sharply to a pointed vertex. Brain weights are some of the lowest on record; for example, 8 g at 35 weeks' gestation and 105 g at 13 months postpartum. In some patients diencephalic structures, including the eyes, optic nerves, mamillary bodies, hypothalamus and hypophysis, are also affected,[566,603] and in these cases the term 'aprosencephaly' has been deemed appropriate. Facial dysmorphism has similarities with holoprosencephaly, including hypertelorism or hypotelorism and cyclopia, and there may be extracranial anomalies of genitalia and limbs.[566] The tiny globular (Fig.

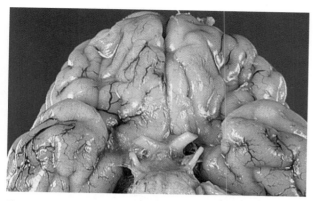

Figure 7.34 *Unilateral olfactory aplasia. The right olfactory bulb, tract and sulcus are absent and the orbital surface has an anomalous gyral pattern in contrast to the normal left side.*

7.35) or multinodular forebrain remnant comprises disorganized grey and white matter and prominent leptomeningeal gliomesodermal proliferation with calcifications, and even calcific vasculopathy,[492] arguing for a destructive basis for the disorder. Some cases also show a residual bilaterality,[894] ependymal-lined tubules or spaces,[445,894] and disorganized or polymicrogyric cortex[326] (Fig. 7.36). In one case there were also three intracranial cysts: an ependymal cyst, a pigmented epithelial cyst and a Rathke's cleft cyst.[492] The hindbrain is largely preserved, although cerebellar hypoplasia has been reported.[492] Given the severity of the malformation it is not surprising that lifespan is short (less than 2 years), but seizures have been recorded in several patients despite the lack of forebrain. The aetiology is unknown: all cases so far have been sporadic. In one infant Towfighi *et al.*[894] demonstrated a chromosomal deletion within 13q, and numerous eosinophilic cytoplasmic inclusions in Purkinje cells.

AGENESIS OF THE CORPUS CALLOSUM

Agenesis of the corpus callosum may form part of a more extensive malformation complex, such as holoprosencephaly, or the callosum may be totally or partially absent or hypoplastic in an otherwise normal brain. For extensive descriptions and reviews see Refs 230, 295, 459, 460, 463, 557, 558, 592 and 703. In partial agenesis the posterior portion is usually missing, while the rostrum and genu remain. Wherever the callosum is absent, the medial interhemispheric surface has an abnormal gyral pattern. There is no cingulate gyrus and the gyri have a radiating pattern extending perpendicularly to the roof of the third ventricle (Fig. 7.37). On coronal sections of the brain no structure seems to separate the lateral ventricles in the midline. The lateral ventricles have a membranous roof and upturned pointed corners, often compared to a bat's wing. A prominent bundle of fibres, the Probst bundle,[685,736] is situated usually in the lateral part of this roof near to the apex of the ventricle (Fig. 7.38a), but occasionally is more medial. It runs in a longitudinal direction, is myelinated at the time when the corpus callosum should be myelinated, and is thought to include the misdirected callosal fibres, although its volume is considerably less than the normal callosum. Experimental studies in acallosal mice would support this contention.[831] The membranous roof of the third ventricle is often distended and bulges into the interhemispheric

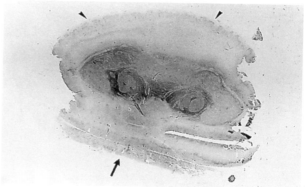

a

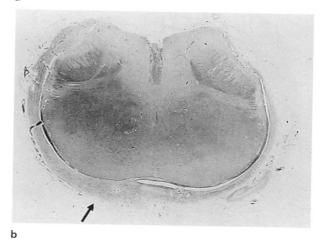

b

Figure 7.36 *Atelencephaly. Low-power microscopy of coronal sections at (a) anterior and (b) posterior levels through the forebrain. Note the near symmetry, the thick meningeal cuff of gliomesodermal tissue (arrow) and the thin undulating cortex (arrowhead). (Luxol fast blue–cresyl violet.)*

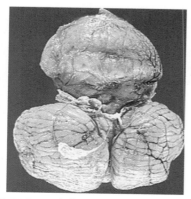

Figure 7.35 *Atelencephaly. A 9-month-old infant with total brain weight of only 95 g, olfactory aplasia, and a tiny, uncleaved, globular forebrain without ventricular cavity.*

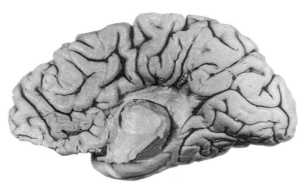

Figure 7.37 *Agenesis of the corpus callosum. Note the radiating pattern of gyri and sulci.*

fissure, displacing the fornices laterally. The septum pellucidum may appear to be absent, but Loeser *et al.*[558] demonstrated that its widely separated leaves do not run vertically but incline laterally from the fornices to the Probst bundles. The occipital horns are often markedly dilated (Fig. 7.38b). Regarding the other commissures, the posterior commissure is always present and the psalterium absent, but the anterior commissure is variable.

Rarely, a local callosal defect is associated with a midline mass: meningioma, cyst,[661] hamartoma or, more often, a lipoma.[554] Interhemispheric lipomata and callosal defects may be closely contiguous, a dorsal lipoma overlying a hypoplastic callosum, wrapping round it or associating with partial agenesis (Fig. 7.39), and both are regularly associ-

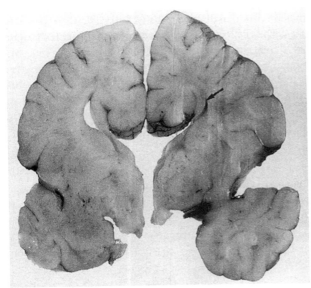

a

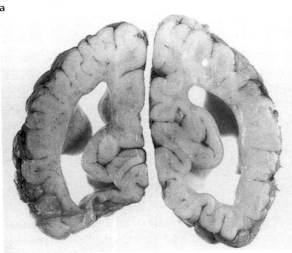

b

Figure 7.38 *Agenesis of the corpus callosum. Agenesis of the corpus callosum in a 3-month-old child with maple syrup urine disease and a cardiomyopathy. (a) Coronal section showing absence of corpus callosum, midline septum and anterior commissure, the characteristic bat's wing-shaped lateral ventricles and Probst's bundles (arrow). (b) Markedly dilated occipital horns.*

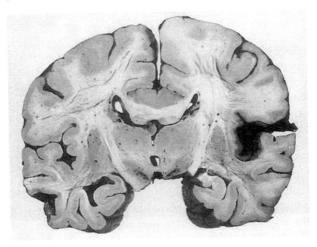

a

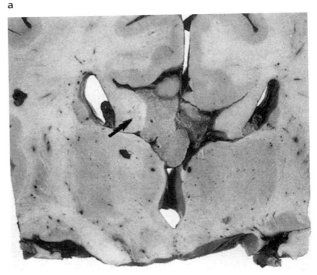

b

Figure 7.39 *Partial callosal agenesis and lipoma. Partial callosal agenesis associated with a lipoma in an asymptomatic adult. (a) At the anterior thalamic level the thin callosum is closely adherent to the lipoma on both dorsal and ventral surfaces. (b) A little further posterior the callosum is completely interrupted by lipomatous tissue and small longitudinal Probst bundles can be discerned (arrow). Courtesy of Dr C Torre, Rome, Italy.*

ated with intraventricular choroid plexus lipoma.[912] It has been suggested that rests of residual meningeal tissue differentiate into adipose tissue and cause mechanical obstruction to the growth of the corpus callosum.[899,977]

Patients with agenesis of the corpus callosum have a high incidence of associated anomalies, both cerebral and visceral. Of 11 cases reported by Parrish et al.,[703] nine had cerebral malformations, while in eight there were malformations in the rest of the body. These findings were confirmed and extended in a larger series in which hydrocephalus, migration defects and rhinencephalic defects were especially frequent.[460]

Agenesis of the corpus callosum may be sporadic or familial.[650] In addition to the associated anomalies described above, there are now several well-defined syndromes in which callosal agenesis is an important feature. In the X-linked dominant Aicardi's syndrome,[11,437,751] it is combined with infantile spasms, chorioretinopathy and depigmented lacunae, mental retardation and vertebral anomalies; polymicrogyria and cerebral heterotopias are also prominent features.[79,292] Menkes et al.[612] described an autosomal recessive syndrome in which seizures were a prominent early feature. Andermann et al.[22] described an autosomal recessive disorder of callosal agenesis, sensorimotor neuropathy and dysmorphic features in a large kindred in Quebec, Canada. Acrocallosal syndrome[661,807] includes polydactyly, macrocephaly and mental retardation. Pineda et al.[723] described two siblings with callosal agenesis, hypothermia and apnoeic spells, and reviewed five further sporadic cases. Finally, defects of midline commissures are common in Meckel's syndrome[691] and hydrolethalus syndrome.[794]

Clinical symptomatology varies, and may largely depend on associated malformations. Agenesis of the corpus callosum can be entirely asymptomatic[98] (Fig. 7.39), and subtle perceptual deficits may only come to light with sophisticated psychological testing.[352,458] The diagnosis is readily confirmed radiologically[495] or by fetal ultrasound.[368]

ANOMALIES OF THE SEPTUM PELLUCIDUM

True primary agenesis of the septum pellucidum must be distinguished from secondary destruction, resulting from inflammation or hydrocephalus, when a fenestrated septum or small fragments of tissue remain attached beneath the corpus callosum. Absence of the septum may be the only abnormality in a brain,[251,314] or it may be associated with callosal agenesis, holoprosencephaly or other complex syndromes. One suggested association, with porencephaly, microgyria and heterotopias,[9,365] does not seem to be genetically determined.[314]

Septo-optic dysplasia

This name was first used by De Morsier[228] in a case report and review of patients with optic hypoplasia and septal aplasia. It is now recognized that hypopituitarism is an equally important component of the syndrome.[438] Judging by the many clinical and radiological reports, the syndrome is not rare, but clinical manifestations are variable and often one part of the clinical triad is missing; in particular, the septum is present in many cases.[855] Neuropathological studies are very few and mostly incomplete. Roessmann et al.[771] reported three cases: in all there was optic nerve and lateral geniculate hypoplasia and dysplasia of hypothalamic nuclei, but only one was without a septum. Olfactory aplasia was noted in two of their cases, and other findings included posterior pituitary hypoplasia, cerebral heterotopias and cerebellar dysplasias. Similarly, in a personally examined case, in addition to the full triad of septal, optic and hypothalamic involvement, there was widespread

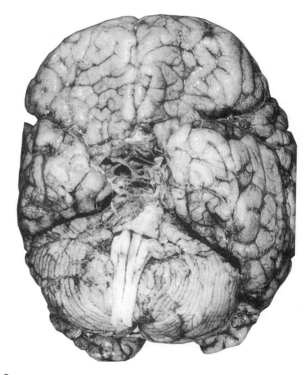

a

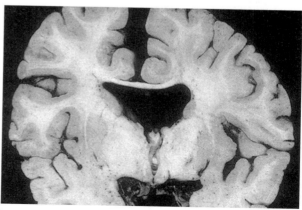

b

Figure 7.40 Septo-optic dysplasia. (a) Base of the brain showing olfactory aplasia and hypoplastic optic nerves and chiasm. (b) Coronal section showing absence of the septum pellucidum. The corpus callosum is thin and has a smooth ventricular surface.

polymicrogyria and olfactory aplasia (Fig. 7.40). Recent molecular analysis has identified mutations of the *HESX1* gene in patients with septo-optic dysplasia, and demonstrated a comparable phenotype in mice with *Hesx1* gene knockouts.[209] Environmental aetiologies also seem likely, in view of the report by Coulter *et al.* of septo-optic dysplasia in combination with fused frontal lobes (semilobar holoprosencephaly) in a $2\frac{1}{2}$-month-old girl exposed to maternal binge alcohol abuse during the first trimester.[178]

Cavum septi pellucidi and cavum vergae

Sometimes misnamed the fifth and sixth ventricles,[203] these midline cavities are bounded above by the corpus callosum and laterally by the two leaves of the septum pellucidum and the fornices. Anteriorly, the cavum septi pellucidi (Fig. 7.41) lies between the transverse fibres of the genu of the corpus callosum and the anterior commissure. As the corpus callosum develops caudally, the cavity stretches backwards. Its posterior limit is ill defined and there is considerable individual variation. At times it is prolonged posteriorly by another cavity, the less common cavum vergae (Fig. 7.42), which in neonates often bulges below the splenium of the corpus callosum. The cavum septi pellucidi and cavum vergae usually communicate freely but may be separated by a bridge of cerebral tissue. The cavum septi pellucidi is a constant feature in the human fetus but tends to become obliterated towards term.[521,819] In adults the cavity is found in about 20% of brains studied at autopsy.[813] The cavum vergae has never been described alone.

The walls of the cavities are lined by neuroglial tissues without a definite epithelial structure. At times, macrophages are found in the walls or within the lumen. Under normal conditions the cavity does not communicate with the lateral ventricles. In premature infants presenting with germinal layer and intraventricular haemorrhage, the veins of the septum are often overdistended and blood may be found in the cavum.

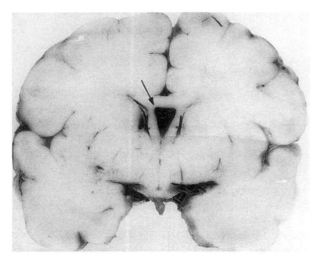

Figure 7.41 *Cavum septi pellucidi (arrow) in a coronal section of a neonatal brain.*

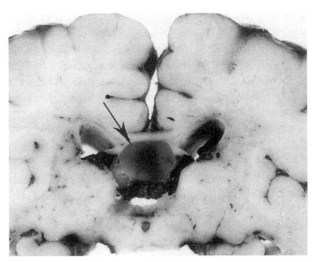

Figure 7.42 *Cavum vergae (arrow) in a neonatal brain.*

Cavum septi pellucidi and cavum vergae have been demonstrated *in utero* by ultrasound as early as 16 weeks.[890] In premature and full-term infants the midline cavities are readily detectable on CT scan and ultrasound.[578]

Cavum veli interpositi

Although this structure is not a commissural formation but a leptomeningeal cistern of minor importance, it seems appropriate to describe it here because of its relationship with the cavum vergae. This cistern, well known when pneumoencephalograms were commonly used, is normally patent in premature infants and becomes progressively sealed off. Sandwiched between the floor of the cavum vergae above and the roof of the third ventricle below, it communicates posteriorly with the cistern of the great vein of Galen. On X-ray it is difficult to distinguish it from a cavum vergae.[521] Occasionally, haemorrhage has been described in this area, collecting over the roof of the third ventricle and leading to obstructive hydrocephalus.[563]

Neuronal migration disorders

The process by which the mitotically active pseudostratified neuroepithelium of the 4-week-old neural tube is transformed into the mature cerebral cortex is a complex morphogenetic process that has been the subject of intense study for decades. The events of neuronal migration have been described in detail anatomically, but recent advances in molecular genetics and developmental biology have added a new dimension to our knowledge of neuronal migration and its pathology.

MIGRATION AND DIFFERENTIATION OF NEUROBLASTS

Between 4 and 6 weeks of gestation, postmitotic neuroblasts begin to migrate across the pallium so that from 6 weeks a three-layered structure is evident: outer margin-

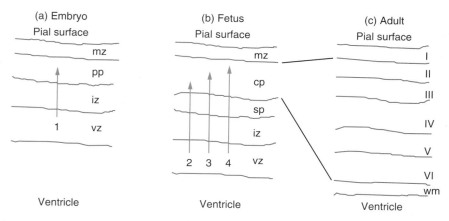

Figure 7.43 *Main stages in the formation of the layered structure of the cerebral cortex. (a) The earliest migrating post-mitotic neuroblasts (1) leave the ventricular zone (vz), crossing the intermediate zone (iz) to form the preplate (pp). (b) The preplate is subsequently split by the settling of later migrating neuroblasts. Successive waves of centrifugally migrating neuroblasts (2–4) establish the 'inside–out' structure of the cortical plate (cp), situated between the subplate (sp), the remnant of the inner aspect of the preplate and the marginal zone. (c) Mature layered structure of the cerebral cortex, demonstrating the origin of layers II–VI from the cortical plate, whereas layer I (marginal zone) Cajal–Retzius neurons derive largely from the outer portion of the preplate.*

al, intermediate and inner ventricular zones. Much of the early neuroblast migration is guided by radial glial processes stretching from the ventricle to the pial surface, although recent research has identified the importance of tangential migration as an additional source of neuroblasts within the cerebral hemispheres (see Pathogenesis at the cellular and tissue levels, above).

PREPLATE AND SUBPLATE

The earliest migrating neuroblasts form a transient subpial structure, the preplate, also called the primitive plexiform layer[594] (Fig. 7.43a). With progression of neuroblast migration, the preplate splits into two components, an outer portion closely related to the marginal zone, and an inner portion designated the subplate (Fig. 7.43b). The neurons of both regions ultimately undergo programmed cell death (apoptosis) in large numbers, although some outer preplate cells survive as Cajal–Retzius cells of the marginal zone. The subpial granular layer is a transient structure that appears in basal allocortex at around 12 weeks, migrates over the cortical surface and disappears by 24 weeks.[111] It may correspond to the outer portion of the preplate. During its brief existence, the subplate appears to subserve several important functions, for instance forming some of the earliest functioning neuronal connections, including the formation of pioneer corticothalamic axons. Moreover, subplate neurons serve as early targets for thalamocortical afferents, anticipating the maturation of layer IV.[13]

CORTICAL PLATE

The splitting of the preplate is achieved by the settling of later-migrating neuroblasts that form the definitive cortical plate, the precursor of the six-layered cerebral cor-

tex. The process of cortical plate formation begins around 7 weeks of human embryonic development and continues until approximately 20 weeks. Successive waves of neuroblasts migrate past their predecessors, through an increasingly cellular environment, to take up progressively more superficial positions in the cortical plate (Fig. 7.43c). Although most neuroblast proliferation is finished by 16 weeks, and migration is largely completed by 20 weeks, some cells continue to migrate until several months after birth. The inside–out pattern of neuronal migration, in which the earliest generated neurons come to occupy the deepest layer,[26,737] is central to the development of the cortical plate and is frequently disrupted in the diverse range of neuropathological conditions grouped under the general term neuronal migration disorders.

DIFFERENTIATION OF NEURONAL AND GLIAL CELL TYPES

Different cortical layers are characterized by neurons of different types, and the layer in which a migrating neuroblast settles appears to be determined even before the parent cell exits the ventricular zone, before the onset of its migration.[575] A 'clock' seems to be running in the ventricular zone, closely related to the cell cycle, so that later-emerging postmitotic neuroblasts 'know' intrinsically that they are destined to settle in more superficial layers of the cortex than earlier-emerging neuroblasts. The fate of neuroblasts, with respect to their pathway of differentiation into neuronal or glial lineages, also appears to be determined while they are still resident in the ventricular zone.[366] Hence, defects involving abnormal cell types present in the cerebral cortex (dysplasia) may arise very early in the process of neuronal migration.

PATHOGENIC MECHANISMS UNDERLYING NEURONAL MIGRATION DISORDERS

Classification of the spectrum of human neuronal migration disorders is controversial. One approach is to distinguish between the different types of pathogenic mechanism that appear to underlie the malformations.

Disruption of neuronal migration

Defective neuronal migration is present in several human conditions for which a genetic causation has recently been identified. Lissencephaly, involving a major disruption of neuroblast migration during development of the cerebral cortex, occurs in patients with mutations of the *LIS1* gene, which has been identified as the non-catalytic subunit of platelet-activating factor acetyl hydrolase (PAFAH).[403,560] Lissencephaly also occurs in males with mutations in the X-linked gene *doublecortin*, whereas heterozygous females exhibit subcortical band heterotopia, with an apparently normal cortical ribbon and an additional abnormal grey matter zone in the subcortical white matter.[242,343] Periventricular heterotopias are found in patients with mutations of another X-linked gene *filamin-1*,[308] whereas heterotopic neurons in the marginal zone are found as part of the phenotype of Fukuyama muscular dystrophy, a condition resulting from a retrotransposal integration into the gene encoding a novel protein, named fukutin.[500] Several distinct types of pathology can be discerned amongst these different neuronal migration disorders.

Large-scale disturbance of neuronal migration

Although the pathogenic defects leading to lissencephaly are not understood in detail, the molecular nature of the gene products involved provides important clues. Both *doublecortin* and *mdab1*, a gene in the *reeler* pathway, appear to function as adapter molecules that interact with Abl, a non-receptor tyrosine kinase,[242,343,757] a finding that may indicate the participation of *doublecortin* in the *reeler* pathway. The role of *PAFAH* mutations in causing lissencephaly is well established, following the demonstration of similar abnormalities in mice with targeted mutations of the *Pafah1b1* gene.[421] Microtubule function is stabilized by platelet-activating factor (PAF),[798] while interference with PAF *in vitro* can disrupt neuronal migratory activity,[1,82] suggesting a mechanism in which *PAFAH* mutations may disrupt the intrinsic ability of neurons to migrate.

Localized defects of neuronal migration

Neurons can either fail to initiate migration, as in periventricular heterotopia, or overmigrate, as in conditions characterized by the presence of heterotopic cells in the marginal zone. X-Linked periventricular heterotopia results from mutations in the gene encoding *filamin-1*, an actin-cross-linking phosphoprotein that is required for actin reorganization following receptor activation, and which is required for locomotion of many cell types.[308]

This suggests that the basic defect in periventricular heterotopia may be a cell-autonomous inability of mutant cells to migrate, although it does not explain why some neurons in patients with *filamin-1* mutations appear to migrate to their normal positions. Overmigration of neurons destined for layers II and III, to populate the marginal zone, appears to be a relatively common pathogenic mechanism that may arise as a result of a disturbance of the interaction between the end-feet of the radial glial fibres and the extracellular matrix of the glial limiting membrane (GLM). Marginal zone heterotopias are seen in primary generalized epilepsy,[608] developmental dyslexia[325] and Fukuyama muscular dystrophy. In the latter, abnormalities of the GLM have been described,[971] although the role of fukutin, the secreted protein product of the gene mutated in this condition, is unknown. Animal models provide further evidence for a role of the GLM in the pathogenesis of marginal zone heterotopias. Breaches of the GLM are present in mice with autoimmune conditions predisposing to marginal zone heterotopias,[822] and in mice with targeted mutations of the *Macs* gene, in which leptomeningeal heterotopias are observed.[83] Similar GLM defects have recently been described in the *dreher* mouse, in which mutations of the *Lmx1a* gene lead to a phenotype including marginal zone heterotopias. In this case, birth-dating studies have demonstrated that the heterotopic neurons, which are mainly confined to the marginal zone, closely resemble layer II and III cells, pointing to overmigration as a pathogenic mechanism.[172]

Disturbance of programmed cell death

Anomalies of programmed cell death (apoptosis) have been implicated in the pathogenesis of certain types of neuronal migration disorder, particularly heterotopias.[773,930] These suggestions followed the demonstration that early migrating preplate neuroblasts die by apoptosis during brain development.[13,733] Support for this idea comes from the finding of heterotopic neuronal masses in the cerebral cortex of mice with a targeted mutation in *caspase 3*, a critical gene in the molecular pathway leading to programmed cell death.[507] Thus, persistence of cells that normally die during brain development can yield neuronal heterotopias. Such apoptosis-related heterotopias may be difficult to distinguish from those arising as a result of disturbed neuronal migration, and it is unclear to what extent failure of programmed cell death should be considered a critical pathogenetic event in the origin of human neuronal migration disorders.

Abnormalities of cytodifferentiation

The lesions of focal cortical dysplasia show clear morphological signs of disturbed cytodifferentiation, with aberrant expression of markers of neuronal and glial differentiation in dysplastic lesions. It is possible that dysplastic lesions are generated when neuroepithelial cells become arrested at various stages in the progression towards increasing cell specialization. The early stage at which determination of cell lineage appears to occur, for instance between neuronal and glial differentiation, among cells of the ventricular zone,[366] suggests that dysplastic lesions containing cells with intermediate neuronal/glial characteristics must have a very early origin during prenatal development. However, putative stem cells have been identified in the postnatal nervous system that retain the ability to differentiate along either neuronal or glial lineages,[579] raising the possibility that dysplastic lesions can arise at almost any stage of development, as a result of the aberrant differentiation of groups of previously multipotential stem cells.

A further possible mechanism of cortical dysplasia is the occurrence of genetic change in otherwise normally differentiated cortical cells. This could account for the finding that cells within dysplastic lesions often re-express genes normally only expressed by cells at an earlier stage of differentiation, or in a different cell lineage. Somatic mutation is commonly observed in the generation of various tumours,[499] and has also been inferred from the finding of 'loss of heterozygosity' for polymorphic DNA markers in the lesions of tuberous sclerosis.[358] It remains to be determined whether somatic mutation or chromosomal damage, followed by clonal expansion, may play a significant role in the development of dysplastic cortical lesions.

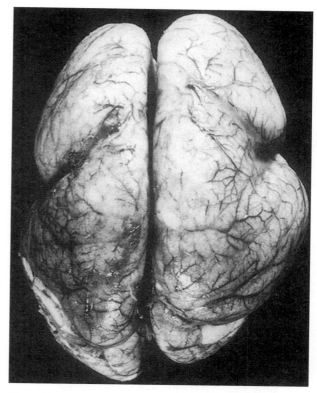

Figure 7.44 *Agyria in a case of Miller–Dieker syndrome.*

AGYRIA (LISSENCEPHALY) AND PACHYGYRIA

Agyria and pachygyria denote macroscopic abnormalities of the cortical surface associated microscopically with a thickened cortical ribbon. The term macrogyria is used in the neuroradiological literature to denote reduced numbers of widened convolutions,[44,368,369,510] but is of little value in neuropathology in view of its non-specificity. Various histological patterns, including polymicrogyria, pachygyria and cortical dysplasia, may contribute to such a macroscopic appearance, and despite recent developments in neuroimaging techniques, differentiation between these patterns is still at the limit of resolution, especially in early life.[7] Friede[314] considered 'agyria' preferable to 'lissencephaly', a term devised by Owen[689] to denote the smooth brains of lower mammalian species. Agyria implies absence of gyri and pachygyria reduced numbers of broadened gyri; the difference is one of degree. However, complete absence of gyri is very rare in practice and the use of these terms is subjective. Reviews and case reports include Refs 52, 187, 202, 243, 249, 461, 506, 671, 708, 709 and 864.

In agyria/pachygyria the calvaria is usually small, misshapen and thickened, and the brain smaller and lighter than normal, but on rare occasions it may be excessively heavy.[23] The agyric brain (Fig. 7.44) is almost completely smooth with no primary sulci, and only poorly defined rolandic and sylvian fissures, and there is a complete failure of opercularization or demarcation of the insula. In pachygyria there are abnormally few widened convolutions and shallow sulci (Fig. 7.45). Occasionally, pachygyria is combined with polymicrogyria (see Fig. 7.64). On coronal sectioning (Fig. 7.46) the cortical ribbon is usually greatly thickened and the underlying white matter markedly reduced. The claustrum and extreme capsule are absent while the lateral ventricles are enlarged (sometimes described as colpocephaly), often with nodules of heterotopic grey matter in the ventricular wall.

The most characteristic histological appearance is a four-layered cortex overlying a thin periventricular rim of white matter in which there are numerous grey heterotopias. The four-layer cortex[187] comprises a molecular layer, a relatively thin superficial neuron layer and a sparsely cellular layer with a tangential myelin fibre plexus, beneath which is a thick neuronal layer which may break up into bands or plumes of cells descending into the white matter (Fig. 7.47). At transitions with normally laminated cortex only the two superficial layers coalesce with the normal cortical ribbon.[187] A radial alignment of neurons in columns is often evident, but the four-layer arrangement may not always be discernible. Neonates lack the tangential myelin fibres and show a single widened band of grey matter, and more complex horizontal lamination (Fig. 7.48) has also been described.[461,642] Inferior olivary heterotopia (see Fig. 7.118) and hypoplasia of the pyramidal tracts are frequent associated findings, while dentate dysplasia, cerebellar heterotopia and granule cell ectopia are less common.

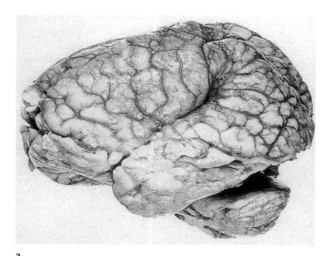

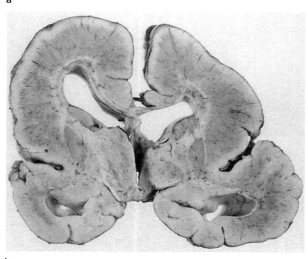

Figure 7.45 *Agyria/pachygyria. The difference between agyria and pachygyria is one of degree. This brain of an 8-month-old boy weighed 500 g. (a) While most of the frontal and parietal lobes are smooth, (b) a coronal section shows shallow cingulate and temporal sulci. Note the great thickness of the cortical ribbon, and the very thin subjacent white matter and corpus callosum.*

Bielschowsky[73] first proposed that agyria was the result of arrested neuroblast migration, and several authors have suggested that the second wave of neuroblast migration is interrupted.[377] Stewart *et al.*[864] postulated that a zone of tissue destruction, indicated by the third cell-free layer of the agyric cortex, occurs at about the fourth fetal month, preventing late migration of neuroblasts or causing their degeneration. Jellinger and Rett's findings concur with this view, their dating for agyria being weeks 11–13, in keeping with the regular association of olivary heterotopia and, in one of their cases, callosal agenesis.[461]

Agyria may be sporadic or familial. Several familial syndromes have been described, the best delineated being Miller–Dieker syndrome.[210,243,249,619] Clinical features comprise microcephaly, bitemporal hollowing, small jaw, diminished spontaneous activity, profound mental and motor retardation, feeding problems, early hypotonia, later hypertonia and seizures. More than 90% of patients with Miller–Dieker syndrome have a visible or submicroscopic deletion in a critical 350 kilobase region in chromosome 17p13.3;[534] recently the gene has been cloned and designated *lissencephaly-1* (*LIS-1*).[748] Smaller deletions in this region with sporadic occurrence give rise to a more retricted phenotype known as the lissencephaly sequence.[249] A personal case of Miller–Dieker syndrome with the deletion resulting from a ring chromosome 17 is illustrated in Figs 7.44, 7.46 and 7.118).[817]

An X-linked form of lissencephaly occurring in male progeny of mothers exhibiting band or laminar heterotopia has now been mapped to Xq22; the gene has been cloned and named *doublecortin* (*DCX*) (see below). Morphological study in one 2-year-old boy revealed a smooth brain and an excessively thick cortex, which microscopically was partly four-layered and partly without laminations.[69] Simplified discontinuous olives and dysplastic dentate nuclei were also reported. In a comparative imaging study of children with *LIS-1* and *DCX*-lissencephaly there were opposing gradients of severity with *LIS-1* associated with more severe malformation posteriorly and *DCX*-lissencephaly worse anteriorly.[250]

Other families with agyria have been reported with slightly different dysmorphology, severe microcephaly[52,671,708] and probable autosomal recessive inheritance. A lethal syndrome combining pachygyria, joint contractures and facial abnormalities was described by Winter *et al.*,[950] followed by two further similar clinical reports.[903] Morphological findings are only available for the index case,[950] a 430-g brain of 38 weeks' gestation showing extreme brachycephaly and broad, simplified (macrogyric) convolutions which histologically had an abnormally thick cortex expanded by one or two poorly cellular layers (Fig. 7.48). The olives were not dysplastic.

A familial lissencephaly with unlayered pachygyric cortex, in combination with cleft palate and extreme cerebellar hypoplasia with brainstem disorganization, has also been reported recently.[488]

CEREBRO-OCULAR DYSPLASIAS

Another group of agyric brains is characterized histologically by a quite distinctive form of cerebral cortical dysplasia, first described in detail by Walker[934] and more recently termed lissencephaly type II.[202] In Europe and the USA these cases fall into several rare and overlapping familial syndromes, combining complex cerebral and ocular malformations and muscular dystrophy. A subtly different disorder, known as Fukuyama congenital muscular dystrophy,[322] is the next most common form of muscular dystrophy in Japan after Duchenne dystrophy.

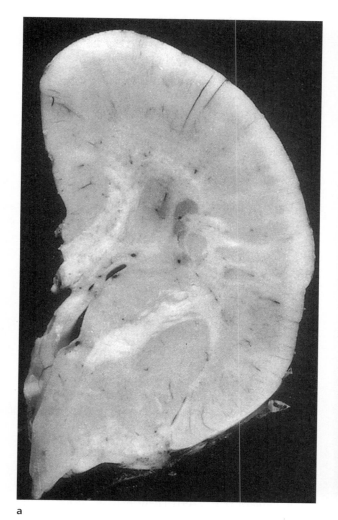

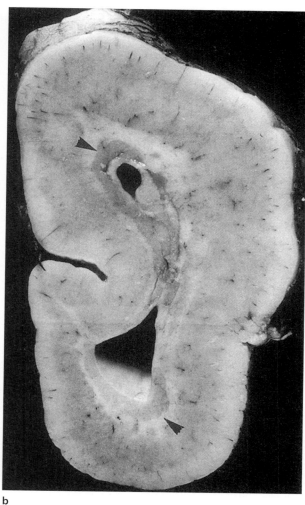

a   b

Figure 7.46 *Agyria. (a) Frontal and (b) occipital coronal sections of the brain depicted in Fig. 7.44. The cortical ribbon is three times the normal thickness and in the small residuum of white matter there are numerous grey heterotopias (arrowheads) which are subependymal and almost continuous around the occipital horn.*

Patients with Walker–Warburg syndrome, also known mnemonically as HARD+E syndrome (**h**ydrocephalus, **a**gyria, **r**etinal **d**ysplasia, **e**ncephalocele),[693,935] show profound psychomotor retardation and hydrocephalus from birth, and a variety of ocular anomalies and developmental defects, dying in infancy. The cerebro-ocular dysplasia–muscular dystrophy syndrome (COD-MD)[896] has closely comparable clinical features with the addition of muscular disease as shown by a sharply rising creatinine phosphokinase and electromyographic evidence of a myopathy. Many cases have now been reported,[93,130,333,525,617,851,876,934,947] with increasing recognition that these two syndromes may be identical,[248] for muscle disease is always present when it is sought. In a review of over 60 patients, the most consistent abnormalities were type II lissencephaly, cerebellar malformation, retinal malformation and congenital muscular dystrophy.[248] A further variant with possibly milder

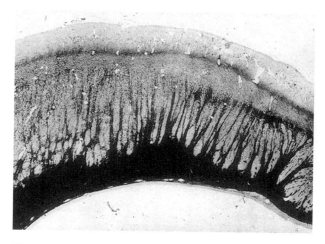

Figure 7.47 *Agyria. Section through the hemispheric wall showing the plume-like radial fibres traversing the deeper layer of the grey matter. (Kultschitsky–Pal method.)*

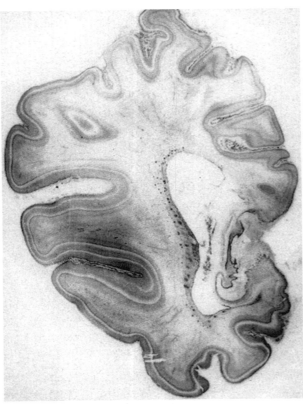

Figure 7.48 *Pachygyria. Coronal section in a neonatal brain. The thick cortex has a varied laminar pattern with either one or two cell-poor layers. (Cresyl violet.)*

phenotype has also been reported as muscle–eye–brain disease.[545–547,797,913]

In COD-MD, ocular abnormalities affect both anterior and posterior chambers, and include central corneal opacity, abnormalities of the iris, cataract, retinal detach-

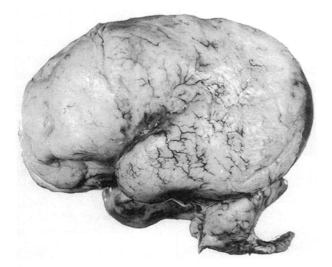

Figure 7.49 *Cerebro-ocular dysplasia. The smoothness of the agyric hemispheres is accentuated by the thickened leptomeninges. Note the short, shallow sylvian fissure and the small, flattened cerebellum.*

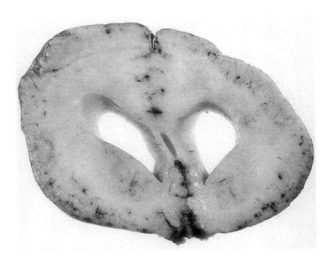

Figure 7.50 *Cerebro-ocular dysplasia. Coronal section at the level of the striatum showing enlarged ventricles, smooth cortical surface and shallow interhemispheric fissure beneath which the medial frontal lobes are interdigitated and fused. The cortical ribbon is abnormally thick but poorly demarcated from the white matter.*

ment and retinal dysplasia. Occipital meningocele or encephalocele is frequent. Skeletal muscle changes are those of a dystrophy with variability of fibre size, marked endomysial fibrosis, fibre degeneration and regeneration, as well as inflammatory infiltrates in some cases. Usually the cerebral hemispheres are enlarged, but microcephaly has also been recorded. The brain is nearly always agyric, its smoothness accentuated by adherent thick white leptomeninges (Fig. 7.49). There may be fusion of the medial parts of the frontal lobes and absent or hypoplastic olfactory bulbs and tracts (Fig. 7.50). Optic nerves and chiasm are usually thin and grey. The cerebellum is small and flattened, its surface coarsely nodular without discernible folia; the vermis is usually partially or completely absent (Fig. 7.51). On sectioning, hydrocephalus is marked, even massive, the aqueduct patent or dilated and the fourth ventricle enlarged (see Fig. 7.50). The corpus callosum is thin or not identified.

Histologically, the leptomeninges show a remarkable mesodermal proliferation with extensive glioneuronal heterotopia, obliterating the subarachnoid space (Fig. 7.52) and fusing with the poorly cellular superficial layer of the cerebral cortex, the most likely cause of hydrocephalus.[947] The cortical ribbon varies: in places it is thin and undulating, somewhat like polymicrogyria (Fig. 7.53a), notably on the medial surface and where hemispheric fusion occurs, but for the most part it is markedly thickened and disorganized (Fig. 7.53b). There appears to be an important direct association between the overlying abnormal leptomeningeal proliferation and the underlying thickened and dysplastic cortex. Squier[851] demonstrated an abrupt transition between normal and thickened meninges in register with the subjacent normal and abnormal cortical plate. From the surface, fibrovascular septa, which are well demonstrated on reticulin preparations,[851] extend inwards and separate the cortical neurons into irregular groups and clusters; areas of greater and lesser cell density can give a wave-like appearance at low magnification (Fig. 7.53c). Normal lamination is absent: larger neurons have a tendency to be rather more superficial than expected but radial alignment can be discerned in some places. Beneath these thicker areas of cortical plate there is usually a narrow, poorly cellular zone and then an archipelago-like arrangement of heterotopic grey matter running parallel with the cortical surface[333,851] (Fig. 7.53b, c; see Fig. 7.56a), which can give a

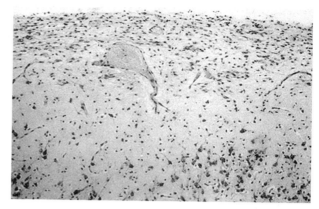

Figure 7.52 *Cerebro-ocular dysplasia. Microscopic section of superficial cortex. The subarachnoid space is obliterated by diffuse glioneuronal heterotopia.*

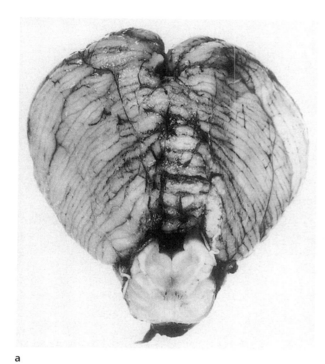

a

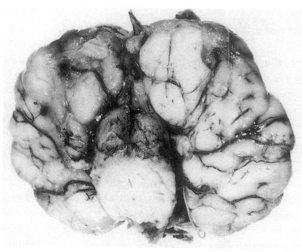

b

Figure 7.51 *Cerebro-ocular dysplasia. Superior view of the hindbrain (b) compared with normal control (a). The vermis is absent. The hemispheres are flattened and irregular with a coarse knobbly surface devoid of folia.*

striking 'double cortical layer' appearance on MRI.[970] These ectopic grey islands are often roughly semicircular with a rounded deeper edge, and a linear upper surface, with tangentially aligned thin-walled blood vessels on its superficial aspect[333] (see Fig. 7.56b). Several observers[333,851] have noted migrating neurons in fetal cases streaming through the gaps between these islands where the tangential blood vessels appear absent (for a similar personal observation see Fig. 7.56b).

In the cerebellum, cortical dysplasia is normally very extensive (see Fig. 7.121), with numerous neuronal heterotopias in the white matter, and simplification or fragmentation of the dentate nuclei. The optic nerves are hypoplastic and the lateral geniculate nuclei disorganized and not laminated. The brainstem is hypoplastic and invested by a thick mantle of fibrous and glial tissue, which is particularly prominent over the midbrain tectum (Fig. 7.54). Pyramidal tracts are virtually absent: small aberrant bundles are sometimes present laterally in the tegmentum of the midbrain. The inferior olives are usually dysplastic and poorly convoluted.

Analysis of the multiplicity of malformations suggests a prolonged disruptive process active during the second and third trimesters. Early authors[130,947] favoured a chronic fetal meningoencephalitis, the infective agent being transmitted transplacentally through consecutive pregnancies, but the frequency of familial cases[93,248] including affected cousins[617] has become compelling evidence for autosomal recessive inheritance. Ultrasound evidence of hydrocephalus and encephalocele are specifically sought in siblings of known affected cases, leading to diagnosis in the second trimester; indeed, affected abortuses as young as 18 weeks' gestation (Fig. 7.55) show evidence of type II lissencephaly and cerebellar cortical dysplasia.[387,851] The availability of such fetal cases has led to several detailed reports attempting to analyse the pathogenesis of the cortical disturbance. Miller *et al.*,[617] Squier[851] and Larroche and Nessmann[525] all considered the tangential blood vessels overlying the deeper neuronal heterotopic clusters to be of

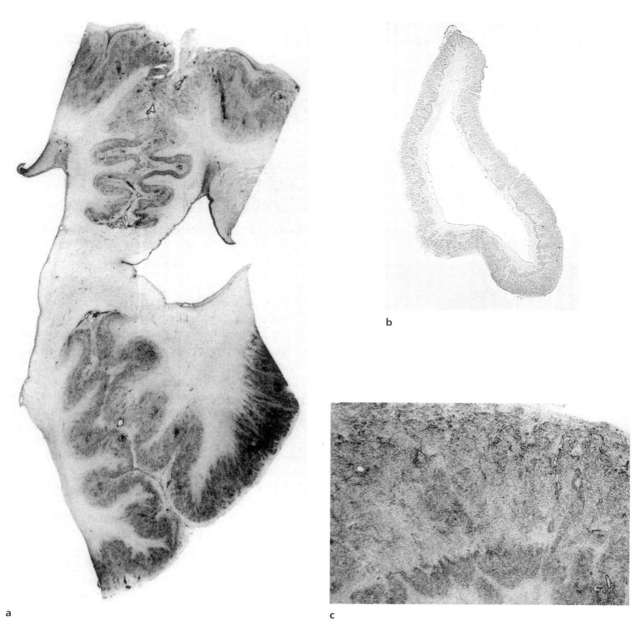

a

b

c

Figure 7.53 *Cerebro-ocular dysplasia. Same case as Figs 7.49 and 7.50. Low-power microscopy. (a) The cortex of the medial walls of the frontal lobes is thin, undulating and fused, while more laterally it is abnormally thick and disorganized. (Luxol fast blue–cresyl violet.) (b) In the occipital lobe an extensive linear array of heterotopias lies beneath the thickened agyric cortex. (Luxol fast blue–cresyl violet.) (c) Higher power of (b). Varying cell density in lissencephaly II cortex gives a wave-like appearance. Deeply placed semicircular heterotopias are separated by a narrow paucicellular zone from the bulk of the cortex.*

meningeal origin, and the disorganized cortex a consequence of massive overmigration of neuronoglial precursors through a disrupted pial–glial barrier. According to Squier, the blood vessels just above the deeply placed heterotopias marked the pial–glial boundary and these deep clusters became less numerous with increasing gestational age as the more superficial disorganized cortical ribbon became more prominent, a view contrary to personal observations (Fig. 7.53) and those of Gelot *et al.*[333] indicating persistence of prominent deeply placed heterotopias well into postnatal life. For Gelot the poorly cellular layer above the heterotopias which selectively stains with glial fibrillary

acidic protein (GFAP) represents subcortical white matter, and the tangential thin-walled blood vessels just superficial to the heterotopias, while reminiscent of the normal horizontal plexus seen in the deep white matter from mid-gestation, are abnormally large and appear to be an obstacle to migration (Fig. 7.56b). In Gelot's view the pathogenesis of lissencephaly type II is more complex and involves two distinct developmental events. An early disruption of radial migration and hypermigration into the meninges, due to both a disrupted pial–glial barrier and an abnormal deep tangential vascular plexus, is followed by a later disturbance in the growth of the cerebral surface with meningeal pro-

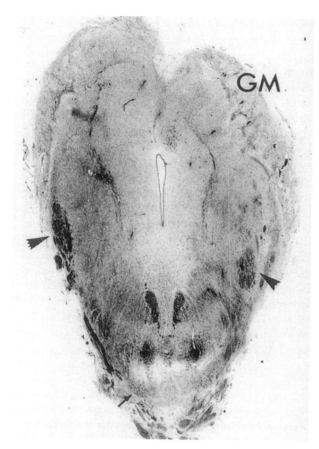

Figure 7.54 *Cerebro-ocular dysplasia. Horizontal section of the midbrain which is severely distorted as well as hypoplastic and surrounded by a thick cuff of gliomesodermal tissue (GM). Cerebral peduncles are absent from their normal position anterior to the substantia nigra (arrow); ectopic fibre bundles are present dorsolaterally (arrowheads). Dorsal to the aqueduct is a focus of neuroblastic tissue. (Luxol fast blue–cresyl violet.)*

liferation and fibrovascular invasion of the cortical plate causing progressive fragmentation, burying and fusion of the surface. All these mechanisms in Gelot's hypothesis can be ascribed to a primary meningeal abnormality.

In Fukuyama congenital muscular dystrophy,[322,525] cerebral malformations are similar but less severe: there is micro-

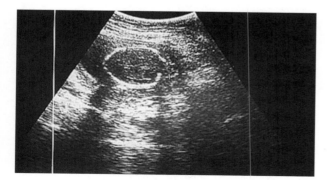

Figure 7.55 *Lissencephaly type II in a fetal brain of 18 weeks' gestation. Ultrasound showing hydrocephaly and encephalocele.*

cephaly with large areas of unlayered polymicrogyria and smaller areas of type II lissencephaly;[877] the survival is generally longer while hydrocephalus and ocular abnormalities are less prominent.

NEU–LAXOVA SYNDROME

Neu–Laxova syndrome is a rare lethal autosomal recessive syndrome comprising severe intrauterine growth retardation, microcephaly, characteristic grotesque facies, flexion deformities of the limbs, skin dysplasia and hypoplasia of various organs.[271,530,532,663] Several family studies have reported normal karyotype. The longest survivor was 7 weeks old. Neuropathological changes are prominent but thus far have received relatively limited study. Microcephaly is extreme; total brain weight as low as 10 g was recorded for a 37-week fetus.[641] Most reports mention lissencephaly, agenesis of the corpus callosum and cerebellar hypoplasia. There are two recent brief reports: one describes lissencephalic brains with evidence of abnormal migration and excessive neuronal loss suggested to result from a defect in lipid metabolism,[196] while the other reports polymicrogyria and growth failure of

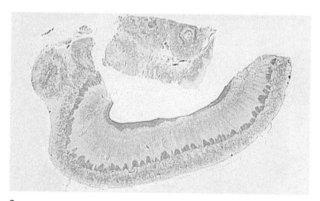

a

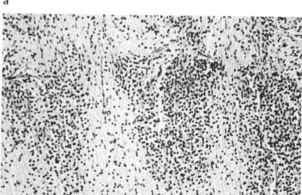

b

Figure 7.56 *Lissencephaly type II. (a) Low-power microscopy of the same case as Fig. 7.55. Lissencephalic cortex with prominent deeply placed heterotopias. (H&E.) (b) At higher magnification, neuroblasts can be seen streaming through a gap between the deep heterotopias; above these islands there are prominent tangential blood vessels. (H&E.)*

cortical neurons in neonates as well as excessive cell death in the ventricular matrix zone in a 14-week fetus.[673]

POLYMICROGYRIA

The term, derived from Bielschowsky,[74] denotes multiple malformed convolutions; it should not be confused with polygyria (see Fig. 7.161), i.e. excessive superficial sulcation with normal microscopic architecture associated with hydrocephalus. The surface configuration of polymicrogyric cortex may belie its convolutional complexity. The miniature gyri are fused together or piled one above the other, producing a smooth or irregularly bumpy surface, like cobblestones or morocco leather (Fig. 7.57), covering broad irregular convolutions which may simulate pachygyria. Coronal sections reveal the heaped up or submerged gyri which contribute to a thickening of the cortical ribbon (Fig. 7.58).

Polymicrogyria is not rare. Crome identified 27 examples out of 500 severely subnormal patients[190] and 50 examples were found over a 15-year period in the Neuropathology Department at The Great Ormond Street Hospital for Children, London.

The extent of the lesion varies greatly, and with it the degree of neurological disability. Widespread involvement of both hemispheres usually accompanies microcephaly and profound psychomotor retardation, while involvement of the centrosylvian cortex results in hypoplastic pyramidal tracts and spastic diplegia. A developmental form of Foix–Chavany–Marie syndrome, or faciopharyngo-glossomasticatory diplegia, has been shown to result from anterior opercular or perisylvian polymicrogyria.[59,824] In recent years several clinical and radiological studies of epileptic subjects have documented a congenital bilateral perisylvian syndrome, in which pseudobulbar palsy and mental retardation are combined with various types of seizure disorder. Initial MRI studies demonstrated a central 'macrogyria' which most investigators now accept to be due to polymicrogyria,[509] a malformation also reported in some autistic individuals.[725]

Polymicrogyria may be bilateral and symmetrical and may correspond to a particular arterial territory, especially the middle cerebral. However, unilateral or markedly asymmetrical lesions are also known and can give rise to hemiplegia and epilepsy necessitating hemispherectomy (see below). The cingulate and striate cortices and the hippocampus are spared. Polymicrogyric cortex also often surrounds porencephalic or hydranencephalic defects[220] (Fig. 7.59 and see Fig. 7.85). Small foci of polymicrogyria may be incidental findings in neurologically normal individuals (Fig. 7.60) and not infrequently are hidden in the depths of the insula (Fig. 7.61). Associated anomalies include neuronal heterotopia in the cerebral and cerebellar white matter (Fig. 7.58) and cerebellar cortical dysplasia. On occasion, polymicrogyria and pachygyria may occur together.

Polymicrogyria has a variety of histological patterns, but in essence the cortical ribbon is abnormally thin and laminated, is excessively folded and shows fusion of adjacent

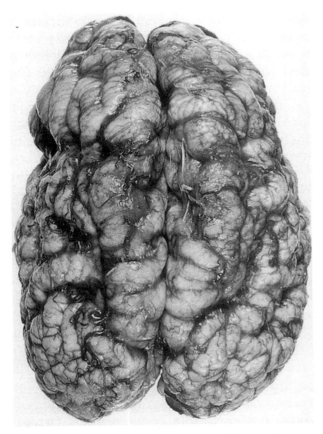

Figure 7.57 *Polymicrogyria affecting most of the cortex but particularly obvious in the frontal lobe. The broad convolutions have a bumpy or cobblestone-like surface.*

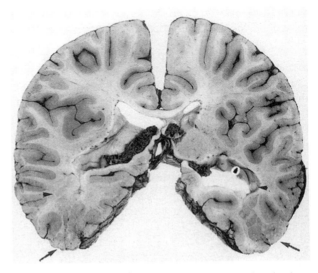

Figure 7.58 *Polymicrogyria. Bilateral symmetrical polymicrogyria (arrows) in the inferior parts of the temporal lobes. The cortical ribbon appears irregularly thickened because of the piling up of mini-convolutions. Nearby are nodular grey heterotopias (arrowheads), one of which is bulging into the ventricular cavity. The asymmetry of the ventricular system has resulted from surgical shunting for chronic hydrocephalus.*

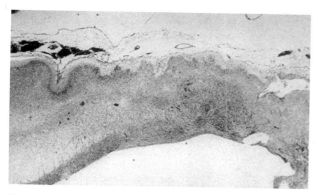

Figure 7.59 *Polymicrogyria. Early stage of polymicrogyria in the cortex adjoining a hydranencephalic cyst in a fetus of 22 weeks' gestation. Note the abrupt transition from the normal cortex to the thin and undulating polymicrogyric ribbon. (H&E.)*

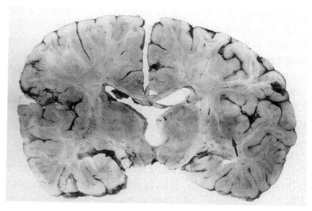

Figure 7.61 *Polymicrogyria hidden beneath the insular cortex (arrow).*

gyri. The most common arrangement, unlayered polymicrogyria,[79,290,454] is a thin, undulating ribbon composed only of a molecular layer and a neuronal layer without laminar organization. The molecular layers between adjacent mini-convolutions appear fused, and median blood vessels suggest an apparent line of fusion (Fig. 7.62 and see Fig. 7.13). These structures form cell-sparse fingers pointing perpendicularly away from the surface into the grey matter, or several may radiate out like the fingers of a glove from a narrow surface zone. More complex pseudoglandular arrangements may arise as these molecular layer stalks branch and rejoin with adjacent stalks to produce completely submerged gyri or a map-like pattern of irregular neuronal clusters and cell-free areas. The undulating cell ribbon has no defined laminae, and neurons are often immature with little cytoplasm. An abnormal tangential layer of myelin fibres may run superficially in the molecular layer and, as with many malformed brains, patches of ectopic glioneuronal tissue may thicken the overlying leptomeninges.

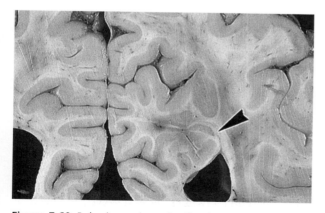

Figure 7.60 *Polymicrogyria and callosal agenesis. Incidental findings in a 57-year-old who died of AIDS were callosal agenesis and polymicrogyria (arrowhead) in the right occipital lobe adjacent to the striate cortex. Courtesy of the Department of Neuropathology, National Hospital for Neurology and Neurosurgery, London, UK.*

A different pattern, sometimes coexistent with that previously described, is the four-layer polymicrogyric cortex[74,185,742] (Fig. 7.63). Many authors have pronounced it the most typical pattern[284,314] and it has been the subject of much pathogenic discussion, but it is relatively uncommon, being present in only one out of ten examples in the collection of the Great Ormond Street Hospital for Children, London. The four layers comprise a molecular layer and two layers of neurons separated by an intermediate layer of few cells and myelinated fibres. This cortex is thinner than normal but at its usually abrupt transition with normal cortex the outer cell layer may be seen to be continuous with normal laminae II, III and IV, the cell-sparse zone with layer V and the inner layer with lamina VI.[71,223,454,668] This four-layer cortex is also abnormally folded but to a variable degree, in some cases only the superficial cell layer being markedly undulating and overlying a relatively flat deep cell layer; alternatively, the whole thickness of the ribbon shows marked perturbations.

The aetiology of polymicrogyria is heterogeneous: it includes examples of intrauterine ischaemia, a close relation with encephaloclastic lesions and twinning, and intrauterine infection, with cytomegalovirus (CMV),[77,189,317,593,599] toxoplasmosis,[223,284] syphilis[284] and varicella-zoster[389] (Fig. 7.63). However, polymicrogyria is not only sporadic: it occurs in a number of familial syndromes and metabolic diseases. Unlayered polymicrogyria and subcortical heterotopias are prominent in Aicardi's syndrome,[11] an X-linked dominant disorder. Other familial occurrences of polymicrogyria, relatively few in number, are probably autosomal recessive. There is a single report of dermatomyositis and polymicrogyria in two mentally retarded sisters,[216] and personal experience includes three sibling pairs with polymicrogyria, two showing prominent intracranial calcification.[42,118,746]

The occurrence of polymicrogyria has been reported in Pelizaeus–Merzbacher disease,[679,697] glutaric acidaemia type II,[88,160] maple syrup urine disease[602] and histidinaemia,[174] in association with Leigh's syndrome and mitochondrial respiratory chain deficiency,[796] and in two

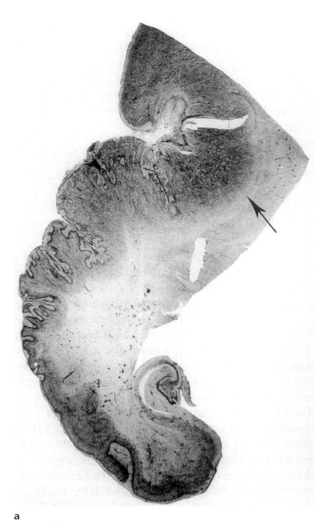
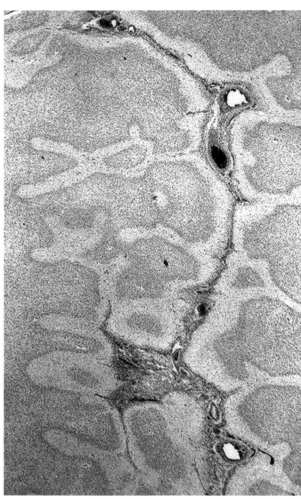

a   b

Figure 7.62 *Unlayered polymicrogyria. (a) Irregularly branching fingers of molecular layer point perpendicularly away from the surface into the cortical grey matter which can appear thickened by the piling up of completely submerged convolutions (arrow). (b) Complex branching of the aberrant molecular layer with median blood vessels suggesting fusion of adjacent convolutions.*

peroxisomal diseases, Zellweger's cerebrohepatorenal syndrome and neonatal adrenoleukodystrophy. Whereas in neonatal adrenoleukodystrophy several authors have described polymicrogyria and subcortical heterotopias,[453,730,910] Zellweger's syndrome regularly shows a more complex malformation involving pachygyria and polymicrogyria (Fig. 7.64) and grey-matter heterotopias,[4,283,931] as well as olivary dysplasia (see Fig. 7.128). Cytoarchitectonic studies suggest a partial disturbance of migration of multiple neuronal classes throughout the greater part of the migratory epoch.[283] Disturbed migration was apparent in fetuses of 14 and 22 weeks' gestation,[732] the abnormality being limited to a wide region of the lateral parietal, frontal and temporal convexity.

The pathogenesis and time of occurrence of polymicrogyria have excited considerable debate, and a diversity of causation has been proposed. Bielschowsky[74] favoured an arrest of migration but his hypothesis fails because it is based upon the now superseded idea of sequential migration, i.e. superficial layers first. More recent theories largely fall into two groups: interference with migration[572] or postmigrational necrosis.[758] Only rarely is there accurate timing of a catastrophic intrauterine event, such as maternal splenic rupture at 16 weeks,[153] or two incidents of maternal coal gas poisoning in the fifth month[374] and at 24 weeks[39] which resulted in large cerebral defects fringed by polymicrogyria. However, early stages of four-layer polymicrogyria have been described in fetuses of 27 weeks[572,758] and unlayered polymicrogyria has been observed at 26 weeks' gestation,[669] both twin fetuses of 25 weeks[95] and 24 weeks,[314] and in a personal case of 22 weeks (Fig. 7.59). Norman's case[669] was one of twins; circumstantial evidence of maternal bleeding at 12 weeks and the age of the dead co-twin (17 weeks) suggest the onset of polymicrogyria to be in the third to fourth month, supported by a similar personal case. This timing suggests that polymicrogyria may result from an interference with the later stages of migration, a view supported by an experimental model of four-layer polymicrogyria in rats produced by contact freezing of the cortical surface.[265,266] Golgi

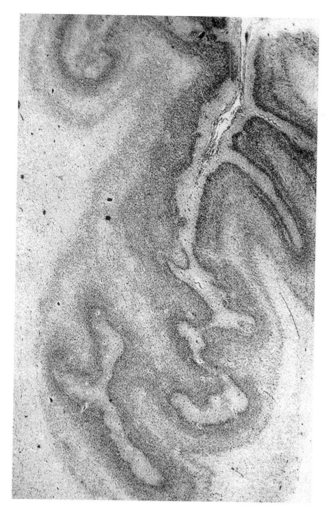

Figure 7.63 *Four-layered polymicrogyria. Varicella-zoster embryopathy. (Luxol fast blue–cresyl violet.)*

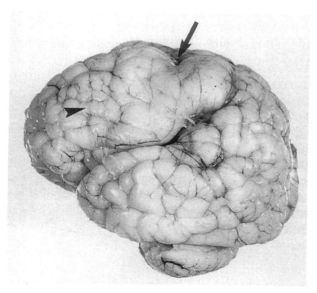

Figure 7.64 *Zellweger's syndrome. Abnormal convolutional pattern in a 1-month-old child. Note areas of both polymicrogyria (arrowhead) and pachygyria (arrow).*

studies by Ferrer and co-workers[290–292] of unlayered polymicrogyrias associated with porencephaly and in Aicardi's syndrome are consistent with this concept. Although cell bodies and dendrites were abnormally orientated, the different neuronal types were situated at their appropriate cortical levels, suggesting that a partial necrosis of the cortical plate had occurred just before the end of the fifth month. However, another Golgi study in Aicardi's syndrome gave somewhat divergent findings. Billette de Villemeur *et al.*[79] also observed a disorientated dendritic tree with apical dendrites bent tangential to the surface, towards and across the perpendicular fingers of fused molecular layers; in their three cases, however, each neuronal type, including the large pyramidal cells, was present through the whole thickness of the cortex, suggesting a severe disturbance of the migratory process. The added presence of numerous nodular subcortical and periventricular heterotopias was further evidence for interference with migration.

An opposing and widely held hypothesis is that polymicrogyria is the result of a postmigrational destructive event.[220,223,454,570] Using cytoarchitectonic analysis and Golgi preparations, Caviness and his associates[542,758,946] demonstrated that, within the four-layer cortex, cells of layers II, III, IV and VI are present in their normal postmigrational positions, while only occasional layer V pyramidal cells can be found in the cell-sparse third layer. This organization implies that migration has been completed and that polymicrogyria is the result of postmigrational midcortical destruction. The laminar nature and topographical arrangement of the lesions, the frequency of bilateral symmetry, with middle cerebral artery distribution or juxtaposition to porencephaly, as well as historical data, suggest a hypoxic–ischaemic pathogenesis or transient intrauterine perfusion failure. As an adjunct to this hypothesis, Richman *et al.*[759] developed a mechanical model of convolutional folding which predicts the excessive buckling of the polymicrogyric cortex.

CHONDRODYSPLASIAS

Abnormal gyral patterns including polymicrogyria are a feature of certain forms of chondrodysplasia. Thanatophoric dwarfism,[598] a lethal congenital chondrodysplasia, is characterized by micromelia, narrow thorax and a large head with or without trilobed skull (clover-leaf) anomaly. Diagnostic neurological findings include flattened vertebral bodies, widened intervertebral disk spaces, thinning of the metaphyses of long bones and 'telephone receiver' femora. Neuropathological findings have been described by a number of authors.[177,356,424,431,958] Principal features include megalencephaly, sometimes with mild hydrocephalus, posterior fossa hypoplasia and, in particular, convolutional anomalies and cortical dysplasia in the temporal lobes. The last are abnormally protuberant with broad gyri and deep sulci (Fig. 7.65). Histologically, there is polymicrogyria with leptomeningeal glioneuronal heterotopia and complete disorganization of Ammon's horns. Dysplastic thalamic and caudate nuclei and hyperconvoluted dentate and olivary nuclei are other findings. Mutations in *fibroblast growth factor receptor-3* (*FGFR3*) were recently identified in patients with thanatophoric dysplasia types I and II.[885]

A still more bizarre convolutional pattern occurs in some cases of short rib polydactyly syndrome. In a personal case, the cerebral hemispheres of an 18-week fetus were distorted by numerous deep irregular clefts (Fig. 7.66), the cerebral mantle was severely disorganized and there was hippocampal dysplasia and olivary heterotopia.

NEURONAL HETEROTOPIAS WITHIN THE CEREBRAL WHITE MATTER

These take three separate forms, classified descriptively into diffuse, nodular and laminar, which may occur separately or together, and both with and without other cerebral malformations. Published clinicopathological data have until recently been sparse, for these lesions are associated with a low mortality, but modern non-invasive investigative techniques for epilepsy are beginning to redress this situation.

Diffuse neuronal heterotopia

Ectopic neurons scattered haphazardly through the gyral and central white matter require cautious interpretation, particularly in early life when modest numbers are a normal occurrence, especially just beneath the cortex.[314] Slightly excessive numbers (compared with controls) have

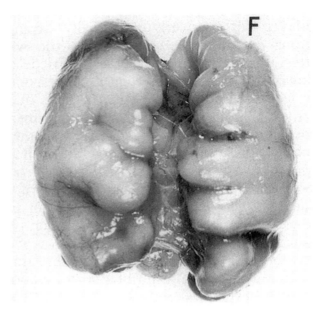

Figure 7.66 *Short rib polydactyly syndrome in an 18-week fetus. The cerebral hemispheres, viewed from above, have lost their normal smooth contours and are deeply indented by irregular clefts. F, frontal.*

been reported in epileptic subjects and termed microdysgenesis (see below). Obviously excessive numbers of neurons scattered diffusely through the cerebral white matter are occasionally associated with nodular heterotopias and other cerebral malformations. There are also rare reports of diffuse neuronal heterotopia as the principal finding in infants with early myoclonic epilepsy. In Spreafico's cases,[850] many of these ectopic cells were large fusiform spiny neurons, immunohistochemically negative to antiglutamic acid decarboxylase antibody, and were interpreted as abnormally persistent interstitial or subplate neurons,[144] suggesting a failure of programmed cell death. Other pathological features were megalencephaly and olivary dysplasia. A similar situation is illustrated in Fig. 7.67.

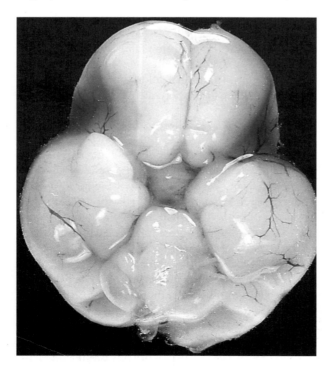

Figure 7.65 *Thanatophoric dysplasia in a 20-week fetus. Note the abnormally large and hyperconvoluted temporal lobes.*

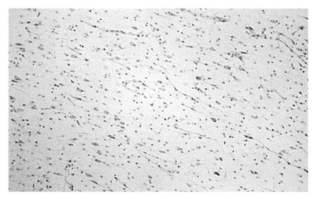

Figure 7.67 *Neuronal heterotopia. Diffuse neuronal heterotopia in a 2-month-old child with congenital nephrotic syndrome. Large numbers of mature neurons are scattered through the white matter. (Luxol fast blue–cresyl violet.)*

Nodular heterotopia

Nodular masses of ectopic grey matter are found in a wide range of pathological and clinical situations, and their occurrence in epileptic subjects is increasingly recognized.[743] Heterotopic nodules can be sited deep within the centrum semiovale or within gyral cores, but more usually are found close to the wall of the ventricle, often bulging into its cavity (Figs 7.58, 7.68). They may occur singly or in large groups and vary in size from small discrete neuronal clusters to large multinodular conglomerates or extensive irregularly serpiginous bands (Fig. 7.69). The histological composition of nodular heterotopias is very variable. Some are simple collections of neurons with apparently random orientation and size distribution, while others exhibit a patterning suggestive of cortical lamination,[79,388] for example a bullseye appearance of a central, poorly cellular molecular zone surrounded by concentric rings of smaller, then larger nerve cells (Fig. 7.70). Some functional aspects of nodular heterotopias in children were addressed in a recent study by Hannan *et al.*[380] Calretinin- and neuropeptide Y-positive interneurons were present in the nodules and were clustered abnormally in the overlying cortex, while fibre tracing using DiI demonstrated fibres exiting the nodules and one example of connectivity between nodules.

Directly correlative clinicopathological observations regarding the occurrence, detailed structure and topography of nodular heterotopia are rare. A retrospective review of autopsy material in the Department of Neuropathology, Great Ormond Street Hospital for Children, London, covering a 15-year period (1975–1990), retrieved 25 autopsy reports of nodular heterotopia in fetuses and children aged from 18 weeks' gestation to 14 years of age.[388] Surveying the available clinical data, there is a 2:1 excess of both females and epileptic subjects. Clinicopathological diagnoses included: (1) aetiological-

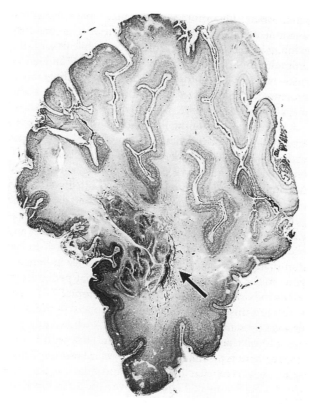

Figure 7.69 *Neuronal heterotopia. Within the fused frontal lobes of a 1-week-old child with a huge occipital encephalocele and arhinencephaly there is a large heterotopia forming a serpiginous grey band (arrow). (Luxol fast blue–cresyl violet.)*

ly specific peroxisomal, mitochondrial and chromosomal disorders, such as Zellweger, Miller–Dieker and cerebral lactic acidosis due to PDH deficiency; (2) well-characterized dysmorphic syndromes, for example Meckel's syndrome and septo-optic dysplasia; and (3) known associations, such as with familial nephrotic syndrome.[694] Some patients had no significant preterminal neurological

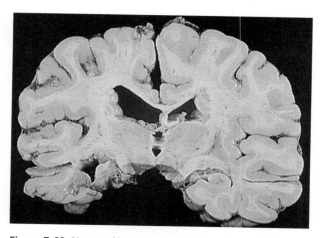

Figure 7.68 *Neuronal heterotopia. Nodular subependymal heterotopias bulging into the frontal horns. A 51-year-old female with a 30-year history of epilepsy. Courtesy of the Department of Neuropathology, National Hospital for Neurology and Neurosurgery, London, UK.*

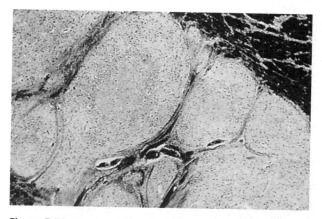

Figure 7.70 *Neuronal heterotopia. Nodular grey heterotopias showing a simple radial organisation of neurons around a central cell-poor zone. (Luxol fast blue–cresyl violet.)*

signs, their heterotopias apparently incidental and unconnected with the terminal illness. The majority exhibited extensive CNS malformations, while in some the only additional abnormality was microcephaly and in two cases nodular heterotopia was the only malformation present. Microcephaly was significant in 14 cases and megalencephaly in three.

The female predominance is even more striking in recent clinical reports linking subependymal heterotopia with epilepsy (Fig. 7.68). Raymond and colleagues[743] reported 13 patients, 12 of them female with normal developmental milestones and normal intelligence, and onset of epilepsy predominantly in the second decade. The subependymal heterotopias were single nodules or coalesced into lumpy bands around the ventricle: trigones and occipital horns were most frequently involved. X-linked dominant inheritance with prenatal lethality in hemizygous males has been suggested in familial pedigrees of subependymal periventricular heterotopia.[444,479] The locus for this disorder has been mapped to Xq28 in females presenting only with epilepsy,[272] while a duplication of Xq28 has been demonstrated in a boy with a more severe phenotype including mental retardation, epilepsy, syndactyly, cerebellar hypoplasia and bilateral periventricular heterotopia.[296] The defective gene is *filamin 1*, the downstream effects of which on actin reorganization are important for cell locomotion and probably therefore cell migration.[308]

This is entirely consistent with earlier hypotheses that heterotopias probably result from a disruption of neuroblast migration. Since they contain neurons of various types (i.e. cells of different 'birthdays') when examined conventionally or with Golgi impregnation,[79,292] there must be a fundamental fault in the migratory process or an early focal insult to the germinal zone. Extrinsic insults associated with neuronal ectopia include sustained maternal hyperthermia in the first trimester,[726] fetal exposure to methyl mercury poisoning,[137] and the atomic bomb at Nagasaki in a survivor who received an estimated dose of 1.57. Gy in the third week of gestation.[662] Experimental induction in rats has been achieved using X-irradiation.[294,761]

Laminar heterotopia

Laminar or band heterotopia consists of extensive plates or bands of grey matter situated between cortex and ventricle but well separated from both. Only a very few neuropathological reports are available in archival German and Italian literature,[455,605,924,941] but modern MRI investigations of epileptic subjects have discovered a 'double cortex syndrome,[45,556,695,696,756] and a genetic disorder has been elaborated.

Personal observations are of three autopsy cases, all female: epilepsy began in the second decade, intellectual deterioration varied from minimal to severe, and in two of them, there was a family history of siblings with epilepsy. The remarkably consistent findings were a normal sur-

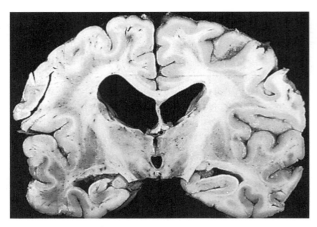

Figure 7.71 *Laminar heterotopia. Coronal slice at mid-thalamic level in a 37-year-old female with a 27-year history of epilepsy. Bilateral, almost symmetrical bands of ectopic grey matter extend widely through the frontal and temporal lobes, sparing medial temporal areas. A well-defined zone of white matter separates the heterotopia from the overlying macroscopically normal cortex.*

face convolutional pattern, and on coronal slices bilateral, roughly symmetrical and very extensive bands of heterotopic grey matter, involving most cortical regions (Fig. 7.71) but sparing the striate (Fig. 7.72), cingulate, fusiform and medial temporal gyri. The heterotopic bands were situated just beneath, running parallel with the cortex, but separated from it by a narrow but well-defined layer of white matter. They ranged in shape from a thin strip, through archipelago-like clusters to thick wedge-like sheets. The overlying cortex and deep grey nuclei appeared normal, except for the claustrum which was incorporated into the heterotopia.

Histologically, the cerebral cortex in these three cases appeared qualitatively normal, but stereological measurements in one indicated an excessively thick cortex of increased neuronal number.[386] This cortex overlay a vari-

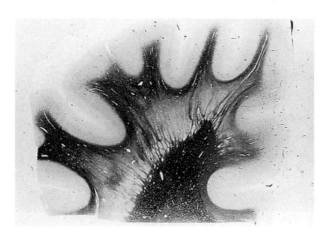

Figure 7.72 *Laminar heterotopia: low-power microscopic section from the frontal lobe. There is a tendency for the ectopia to fragment into islands in its deepest part. (Luxol fast blue–cresyl violet.)*

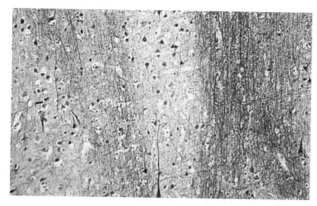

Figure 7.73 *Laminar heterotopia. There is a suggestion of columnar organization in the deeper parts of the ectopic grey matter. (Bielschowsky's silver impregnation.)*

able but substantial zone of well-myelinated white matter including U-fibres, while the heterotopia gradually emerged from beneath the deepest part of this white matter. Neurons were arranged haphazardly in the outer, superficial zone of the heterotopia, but gave the impression of a columnar organization in the deeper part (Fig. 7.73), emphasized by thin, radially arranged bundles of myelinated fibres running through it. Many of the nerve cells were pyramidal, but generally smaller and more loosely scattered than those in the true cortex, and some appeared upside down. Closer to the ventricle, the heterotopia in some areas fragmented into islands separated by thicker bands of white matter (Fig. 7.72). Between the heterotopias and the lateral ventricle there was yet another broad zone of white matter. These observations are broadly in agreement with previous reports.[455,605,924,941] However, the cortex overlying the heterotopia is in some cases normal, and in others[455,941] pachygyric.

All autopsy reports and most MRI studies of laminar heterotopias are in female patients. Families are recorded where mothers and daughters present with laminar heterotopia while sons show lissencephaly.[722] This syndrome has been mapped to Xq22.3-Xq23,[242,343] and this mutation has also been demonstrated in a sporadic occurrence in a boy with laminar heterotopia.[721] The gene encodes doublecortin, a postulated signalling protein.[343]

MICRODYSGENESIS

Subtle structural abnormalities of cortical architecture have been highlighted by several authors studying autopsy material[609,610,920] and temporal lobe specimens[385] from epileptic subjects. The suggestion that these abnormalities may have functional significance in seizure genesis[609] has proved controversial, since some of the abnormalities are present in normal non-epileptic brains.[569] However, large-scale observations with numerous controls have provided some evidence for the pathological relevance of these morphological changes.[610] Nonetheless, precise definitions of microdysgenesis vary. Meenke's compre-

hensive description[610] includes neuronal ectopias in the molecular layer and subcortical white matter, undulations of the second layer and architectural disturbances in deeper cortical layers: these were particularly prominent in subjects with primary generalized epilepsy and were also present in Lennox–Gastaut syndrome. Hardimann *et al.*,[385] in a study of 50 lobectomy specimens resected for intractable temporal lobe epilepsy and 33 carefully age- and sex-matched controls, defined microdysgenesis in terms of (1) severe neuronal ectopia in the subcortical white matter (>8 neurons/2 mm^2) or (2) neuronal clusters (≥ 3 cells) neighbouring bare areas without nerve cells. Present in 42% and 28% of the epilepsy specimens, respectively, but not in controls, these morphological changes showed a statistically significant positive correlation with a favourable clinical outcome following surgery.

CORTICAL DYSPLASIA–HEMIMEGALENCEPHALY

'Cortical dysplasia', a somewhat unsatisfactory term presently used for a characteristic combination of disturbed neuronal migration and abnormal neuronoglial differentiation, occurs in three distinctive clinicopathological settings. The restricted lesions of localized cortical dysplasia are described in Chapter 15 in this volume; a diffuse and multifocal form associated with systemic hamartomata is seen in tuberous sclerosis (see below). In this section discussion is confined to a distinctive form of hemimegalencephaly with the cytoarchitectural changes of cortical dysplasia originally described in isolated post-mortem case studies[78,201,215,252,528,590,891,897] but now, as a result of improved neurosurgical techniques and advances in neuroimaging also in extensive resections, either complete or functional hemispherectomy or multilobar resection of epileptogenic tissue.[237,238,263,286,494,762,925,927]

Cortical dysplasia–hemimegalencephaly in the absence of hemihypertrophy or viscerocutaneous stigmata of phakomatosis is sporadic, the patients presenting with intractable seizures in early life. In the past, the long-term outlook was bleak, but early results with hemispherectomy are encouraging.

Recorded brain weights vary widely from well below to well above the normal. One hemisphere is considerably larger than the other (Fig. 7.74a), usually although not quite always the pathological one (Fig. 7.75a), and this may involve all or some of the lobes (Fig. 7.74a). Gyri are greatly expanded and very firm; after peeling off the meninges the surface appears finely pitted, like orange skin. The convolutional pattern may be relatively preserved, or coarse and macrogyric. Unilateral enlargement of the olfactory tract has also been reported[215] (Fig. 7.74a). On coronal sectioning the abnormal hemisphere shows irregular thickening of the cortical ribbon but with poor demarcation from the underlying white matter. The centrum semiovale is expanded, as well as the basal ganglia in some cases (Fig. 7.74b).

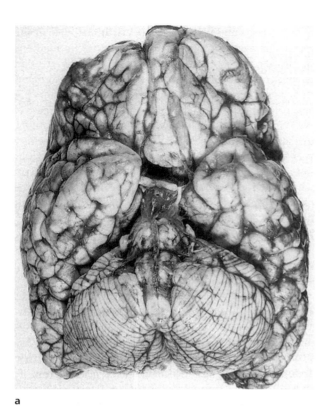

a

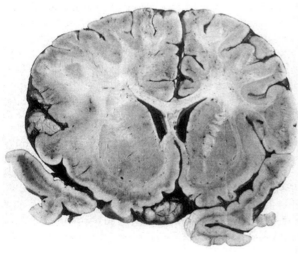

b

Figure 7.74 *Hemimegalencephaly with cortical dysplasia. (a) Inferior view of the brain showing left-sided asymmetrical enlargement of the frontal lobe and olfactory tract. (b) Coronal section showing expanded convolutions with loss of demarcation between grey and white matter on the left side. The striatum is also greatly expanded and its white matter poorly defined.*

Histologically, sulcation can vary from nearly normal to lissencephalic, and the transition from normal to abnormal cortex may be quite abrupt (Fig. 7.76). The abnormal cortical ribbon is widened, although in many cases there is poor or non-existent demarcation (Fig. 7.76) from

the pathological subcortical 'white matter'. There is complete loss of horizontal cortical lamination, and on rare occasions an undulating pattern of the superficial part of the cortical plate indented by stubby fingers of paucicellular molecular layer, slightly reminiscent of polymicrogyria (Fig. 7.77). Neuronal density appears qualitatively reduced,[765] although morphometric analyses are inconclusive, since both decreased[891] and normal[238] cell density has been reported. Particularly striking are the cytological abnormalities of neurons and astrocytes, which may also be present in the basal ganglia, the brainstem and the olfactory tract. Many authors have noted the considerable numbers of abnormally large neurons, some larger than Betz cells, scattered through the cortex and present ectopically in the subcortical white matter (Fig. 7.76). Hippocampal pyramidal cells and granule cells may also show neuronal cytomegaly[765] (Fig. 7.78). Formal morphometry has confirmed these observations.[238,765] Nerve cells are misaligned, often bizarrely shaped, globose or multipolar, sometimes with multilobed or multiple nuclei, occasionally even vacuolated. The nucleus is usually central, often partly outlined by a crescentic condensation of Nissl stain, contrasting with a central chromatolysis-like clearing of the Nissl substance. Using Golgi impregnation, Robain *et al.*[762] demonstrated increased size and complex recurrent branching of the dendritic tree, suggesting that the hypertrophic neurons are both deafferented and polyploid, in keeping with quantitative estimates of increased nuclear DNA.[78,590] Vinters' group has emphasized the cytoskeletal abnormalities in the giant neurons,[238,286,927] which react intensively with silver impregnations and immunomarkers for various neurofilament epitopes, and show tau- and ubiquitin-positive tangle-like formations reminiscent of Alzheimer tangles, except for the absence, both immunologically and ultrastructurally, of paired helical filaments.[263] Personal experience in both biopsy and autopsy specimens, including a neonate of 38 weeks' gestation (Figs 7.75b and 7.79), who also showed olivary dysplasia, supports these observations.

Glial involvement varies from minimal to massive, even tumour-like on occasion,[897] but usually swollen astrocytes are scattered individually or disposed in clusters in both cortex and white matter. They are large, with glassy cytoplasm, and round eccentrically placed, often nucleolated, nuclei, while multinucleated cells are common. Astrocytosis may be intense. Rosenthal fibres have been noted in the affected white matter;[494,752,762] rarely their presence in very large numbers is associated with cystic rarefaction[752] (Fig. 7.80), which could be confused by the unwary with Alexander's disease. Perhaps more common are focal or perivascular calcifications. An important feature of the dysplasia is large globular or 'balloon' cells, of indeterminate phenotype (Fig. 7.81), with round nucleolated nuclei, lacking Nissl substance but having a variable reaction to GFAP. Immunohistochemical colocalization of both GFAP and vimentin[238] and GFAP and synapto-

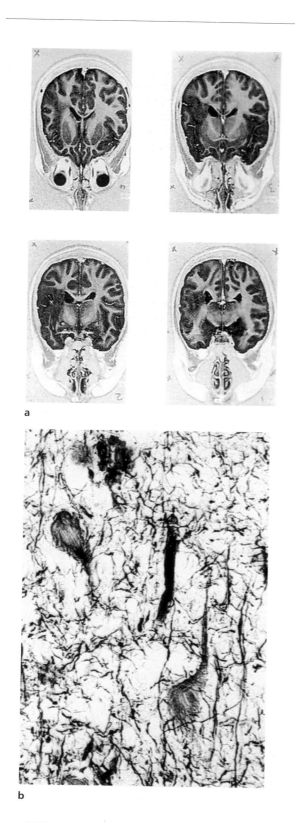

physin[927] has been demonstrated in these cells. A morphometric study using silver impregnation for nuclear organizer regions and PCNA immunohistochemistry suggested that balloon cells are unlikely to be undergoing proliferative activity.[237]

Thus, there are many cytological similarities between this form of hemimegalencephaly and the more restricted lesions of focal cortical dysplasia,[456,886] as well as tuberous sclerosis, the genes for which have now been mapped.[282,358] A further variant which appears to be a transition between the focal and hemimegalencephalic forms has recently been delineated by MRI as focal transmantle dysplasia.[46]

LEPTOMENINGEAL GLIONEURONAL HETEROTOPIA

Isolated islands of CNS tissue, including neurons and glia, within the leptomeninges, or focal protrusions of similar tissue from the surface into the meninges, are a common finding in brains harbouring a great variety of malformations, but especially in holoprosencephaly and migration defects, and are particularly extensive in cerebro-ocular dysplasias and atelencephaly. Indeed, the frequency of these lesions may have deterred investigators from establishing their incidence. However, in a recent study Hirano et al.[419] observed leptomeningeal glioneuronal heterotopia in 31% of 129 autopsied infants, 7 months of age or younger. Significantly, they were present in 65% of individuals with CNS malformations including meningocele and holoprosencephaly, but especially polymicrogyria and neuronal heterotopia. They also occurred in 8% of those with only extra-CNS malformations, and in 4% of infants without any other congenital anomalies.

Hypotheses of pathogenesis include excessive proliferation of the superficial granular layer,[314] glial proliferation resulting from external stimulation such as meningeal inflammation[634] and implantation of germinal cells in the leptomeninges.[881] Disruption of the pial–glial barrier has been postulated[333,851] as the cause of the massive leptomeningeal heterotopia which is such a prominent feature in cerebro-ocular dysplasias and type II lissencephaly. The importance of the pial–glial barrier is further emphasized by Choi and Matthias[138] in an elegant study of an unusual cortical dysplasia in which numerous focal extrusions of neural tissue into the meninges occurred through multiple glial bridges overlying narrow strips of dysplastic cortex.

BRAIN WARTS: NODULAR CORTICAL DYSPLASIA

This is an uncommon anomaly with confusing terminology, including names such as status verrucosus,[742] also being used for polymicrogyria. The best accounts are those of Jakob[454] and Crome[184] (brain warts), and Morel and Wildi;[635] (dysgénésie nodulaire disséminée de l'écorce). These superficial cortical nodules, 1–5 mm in diameter,

Figure 7.75 Cortical dysplasia. Unilateral cortical dysplasia in a 15-year-old girl presenting with intractable seizures. **(a)** MRI shows an extensive unilateral abnormality, but unusually this is in the smaller hemisphere. **(b)** Histology of the functional hemispherectomy specimen shows tangle formation within large dysplastic neurons in the cortex. (Bielschowsky's silver impregnation.)

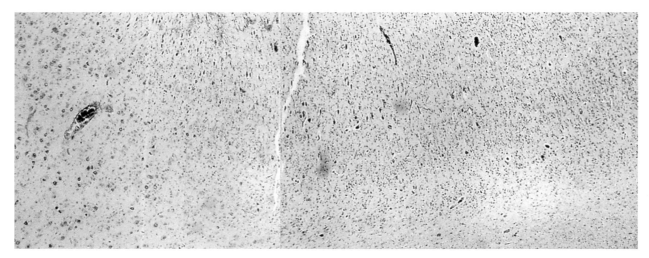

Figure 7.76 *Cortical dysplasia. Hemimegalencephaly with cortical dysplasia: the sharp transition from normal to dysplastic cortex is demonstrated in this low-power montage. Normal cortex is present on the right, the central part of the field contains scattered large dysplastic neurons, while on the left the cortex is completely replaced by abnormal cells. (Luxol fast blue–cresyl violet.)*

are scattered over the surface of the hemispheres, anything from two to 16 per brain, with a predilection for the frontal lobe. The overlying pia mater is often adherent to the nodule, which is usually situated on the crown of a gyrus or bank of a sulcus. Histological examination shows the nodule to be a herniation of laminae II and III through the molecular layer, which is thin or absent. Neurons of varying size are grouped around a radial bundle of myelinated fibres sometimes with a central blood vessel. Nodules can be found in an otherwise normal cortex, but occasionally are present in microcephalic brains with polymicrogyria.[71,184] Cortical nodules have been produced experimentally in rats by freezing the cortex.[266] The pathogenesis of the deformity is not clear, but the associated vascular pattern suggests a close relationship between vascular and tissue dysplasia.

STATUS VERRUCOSUS SIMPLEX OR STATUS PSEUDOVERRUCOSUS

Not to be confused with macroscopic artefacts such as that caused by fixing fetal brains in a gauze bag,[865] or by peeling off the leptomeninges before fixation, which appears as a fine shrinkage of the surface of the brain, status verrucosus simplex[753] is found only on microscopic examination in the brains of some fetuses of about 20 weeks' gestation and may be either a transient stage of development or a malformation. The second layer of the cortex forms irregular protrusions into the molecular layer, the external surface remaining smooth. In Larroche's experience this appearance, although present in fetal brains of 10–28 weeks' gestation, is not sufficiently constant a finding to be regarded as a normal stage of migration. She further remarks that it is severe and diffuse in macerated brains, but that it is not associated with other cortical anomalies.[523] The case illustrated in Fig. 7.82, where status verrucosus simplex occurs adjacent to polymicrogyria, and

a few others in the authors' material, might suggest otherwise.

HIPPOCAMPAL ANOMALIES

Malformations of the hippocampus occur in a variety of clinicopathological settings. Hypoplasia with a dysplastic dentate gyrus is common in trisomy 18.[616,872] Severe disorganization of the medial temporal lobe is well known in thanatophoric dysplasia and includes hypoplasia or aplasia of the dentate gyrus.[177,424,431,958]

Houser and colleagues[434,435] have described various degrees of dispersion of the granular layer of the dentate gyrus, including a bilaminar organization, in a series of patients with severe temporal lobe epilepsy and a history of febrile convulsions early in life. Migration of granule cells occurs late in development, continuing over a relatively long period and even postnatally,[25] so Houser suggests that severe seizures early in life could conceivably

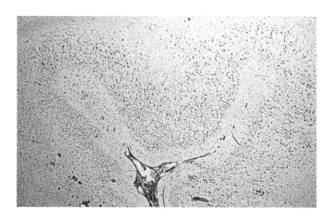

Figure 7.77 *Cortical dysplasia. An undulating cortical ribbon with fused and buried gyri is a rare finding in cortical dysplasia. (Luxol fast blue–cresyl violet.)*

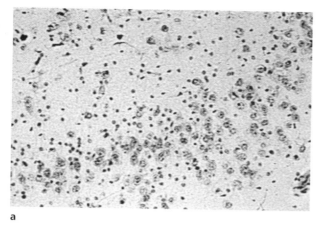

a

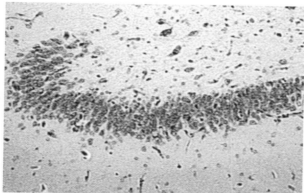

b

Figure 7.78 *Cortical dysplasia. Hemimegalencephaly with cortical dysplasia: involvement of the granule cells from the dentate fascia. Compare their large size and dispersion (a) with a normal age-matched control (b).*

disturb this late migration. Indeed, granule cell dispersion has been produced in a pilocarpine model of experimental epilepsy in rats.[611] However, dispersion or duplication of the dentate gyrus is not confined to classical temporal lobe epilepsy. It has been observed in association with dysem-

bryoplastic neuroepithelial tumour in the temporal lobe,[744] and by the author in microdysgenesis, Sturge–Weber syndrome, and migrational errors and infarcts responsible for extratemporal seizures, as well as on three occasions as a bilateral anomaly (Fig. 7.83) at autopsy with and without epilepsy.[392a]

Encephaloclastic defects

The lesions discussed in this section exemplify the uncertain dividing line between true or 'primary' malformations – defects resulting from an intrinsically abnormal developmental process[849] – and disruptions or 'secondary' malformations. Encephaloclastic processes occurring in the first half of gestation may result in smooth-walled cavities masquerading at birth as primary malformations. This is because macrophage responses in the fetal brain mature long before reactive

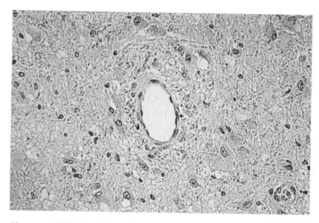

Figure 7.80 *Hemimegalencephaly with cortical dysplasia. Rosenthal fibres abundantly scattered in abnormal white matter and clustered around blood vessels are somewhat reminiscent of Alexander's disease. (H&E.)*

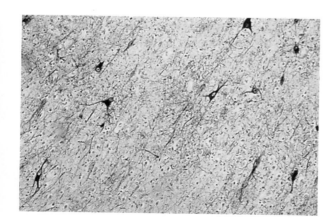

Figure 7.79 *Cortical dysplasia. Upregulation of neurofilament antibody in large dysplastic neurons present diffusely in the cortex of a neonatal brain. Case referred by Dr R Janzer, Lausanne, Switzerland.*

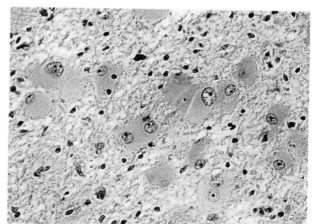

Figure 7.81 *Hemimegalencephaly with cortical dysplasia. Large globular balloon cells of indeterminate phenotype in gliotic demyelinated white matter. (H&E.)*

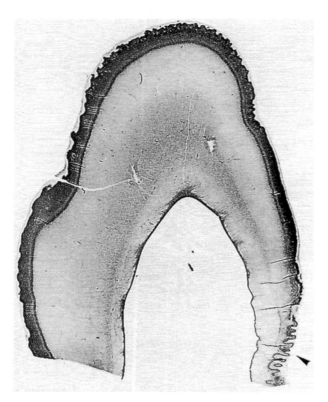

Figure 7.82 *Status verrucosus. Fetus of 24 weeks' gestation. The cortex shows status verrucosus over the vertex, while polymicrogyria is evident on the medial surface (arrowhead). (Luxol fast blue–cresyl violet.)*

astrocytosis becomes detectable. Confusion is further compounded because there is often evidence of deranged development with disturbed neuronal migration near these lesions. However, in the interests of accu-

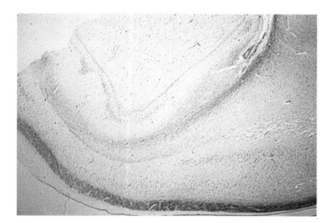

Figure 7.83 *Duplication of the dentate fascia. This $2\frac{1}{2}$-year-old boy presented with global developmental delay, and seizures beginning at $6\frac{1}{2}$ months, and in addition to bilateral hippocampal sclerosis and duplication of the dentate fascia, there were nodular heterotopias in the temporal and insular white matter, cerebellar heterotopia, subtle tract anomalies in the brainstem and unilateral olfactory hypoplasia. (Luxol fast blue–cresyl violet.)*

rate genetic counselling, it is essential to recognize the true nature of these acquired lesions. Series of cases have been described.[186,191,220,317,375,517,570,638,968,969]

PORENCEPHALY

Under this heading Heschl[409,410] described defects in the wall of the cerebral hemisphere communicating between the ventricle and the surface. He considered them to be congenital, the result of destructive processes occurring during fetal life, and differing only in extent from hydranencephaly. Unfortunately, the term came to be applied indiscriminately, particularly in the clinical and radiological literature, along with its corruption, polyporencephaly. There has now been a return, following Friede,[314] to a more precise definition close to Heschl's original concept. Thus, a porus is best defined as a circumscribed hemispheric defect originating during fetal life and antedating the acquisition of a mature astroglial response or completion of convolutional development. Clinical manifestations are varied: some patients survive into adult life but most exhibit severe mental retardation, blindness and sometimes epilepsy, tetraplegia or even decerebrate rigidity. The incidence is difficult to ascertain: one study, from the University of Colorado, USA, accumulated 11 examples out of 18 000 patients with seizure disorder or neurodevelopmental delay investigated with cranial CT over a 3-year period, an incidence of 1 per 1650 patients.[618] Whereas diagnosis used to rely on pneumonencephalography it is now readily attainable with MRI.[47]

Porencephalic defects are always smooth walled and surrounded by an abnormal gyral pattern, but vary considerably in extent and depth, from small indentations (Fig. 7.84) to deep clefts (Fig. 7.85) which may only be separated from the ventricular cavity by a thin layer of tissue, or extensive defects through the full thickness of the hemispheric wall (Fig. 7.84), which very rarely may approach the extent of hydranencephaly.[638] The most typical porus is a full-thickness defect with no inner membrane walling off the ventricle but its exterior closed over by a delicate membrane, often torn during autopsy. Pori are commonly bilateral, roughly symmetrical and centred around the sylvian fissures or central sulci. When the defect is unilateral (Fig. 7.84) there may be a convolutional abnormality, particularly polymicrogyria, in a topographically congruent part of the contralateral hemisphere. Occasionally a porus is parasagittal,[220] orbital or occipital (Fig. 7.84). Around the edge of a porus the convolutional pattern is abnormal; sometimes the gyri form a radiating pattern.

Microscopically, the cortical ribbon is disorganized, either into irregular islands of grey matter or as polymicrogyria (Fig. 7.85). This abnormal cortex extends over the edge of the porus and descends into the cleft where it is co-terminus with the ventricular wall which extends up into the cleft to meet it. This junction

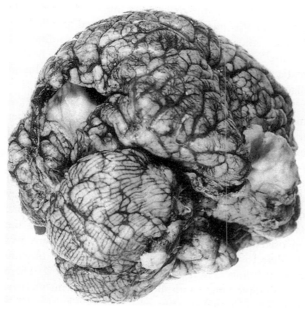

Figure 7.84 *Porencephaly. Two defects are present: a shallow dimple on the orbital surface, and a porus in the occipital lobe allowing communication between the ventricle and subarachnoid space.*

has been termed a pia-ependymal seam, but this is a misnomer because the ventricular surface is largely devoid of ependyma and instead is covered by a thick glial feltwork which may extend for a short length over the abutting cortex before contributing to the inner part of the covering membrane, the outside being arachnoid.

Nodular grey heterotopias are often present beneath the ventricular wall, especially near the cortical junction. Elsewhere in the brain there may be large areas of polymicrogyria. The septum pellucidum is usually absent or

at least partially deficient.[9] The basal ganglia may show focal scarring and mineralization but are usually normal, as are the brainstem and the cerebellum, but the thalamus is small owing to atrophy or hypoplasia of the cortical projection nuclei.[867]

BASKET BRAIN

When bilateral porencephalic defects are very extensive, only a thin central arch of tissue, residual cingulate and adjacent gyri may connect the occipital and frontal parts of the brain, giving the appearance of a basket with a high handle.[682] Similar 'basket brains' have been described by many authors,[159,317,681,682,968,969] and they are best considered as intermediate between porencephaly and hydranencephaly.

HYDRANENCEPHALY

Cruveilhier[193] first described fluid-filled bubble-like hemispheres, or hydranencephaly.[517,936] Most of the cerebral mantle is replaced by a thin, partly translucent membrane without a surface convolutional pattern. Although the inferior parts of the temporal and occipital lobes are often preserved, and sometimes also the orbital frontal area (Fig. 7.86), on occasion only the hippocampi remain intact. The membrane consists of an outer connective tissue layer overlying an irregular patchy layer of glial fibres with occasional residual neurons, mineralized debris and collections of haemosiderin-laden macrophages. Rarely is there recognizable ependyma. At its insertion into the surviving cerebral mantle, the glial layer fuses with the molecular layer of the adjacent cortex, covering it for a variable distance. The cortex may show normal lamination or polymicrogyria. The deep grey masses are often rotated outwards: the thalamic relay nuclei are hypoplastic,

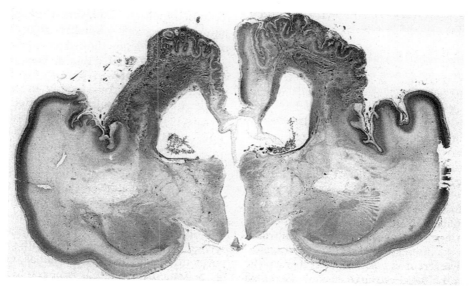

Figure 7.85 *Porencephaly. Bilateral clefts with disorganized neuroblasts in their depths, surrounded by undulating polymicrogyric cortex. Twin of 32 weeks' gestation. Co-twin deceased at 19 weeks. (Luxol fast blue–cresyl violet.)*

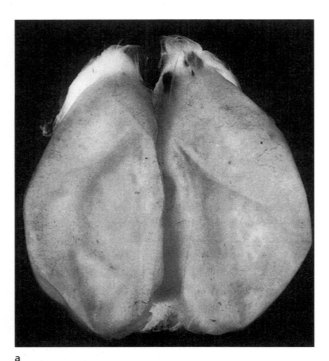

a

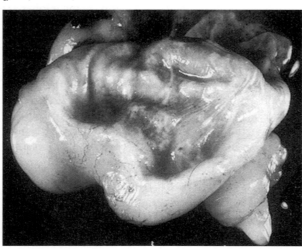

b

Figure 7.86 *Hydranencephaly in a twin of 22 weeks' gestation. Estimated age of deceased co-twin was 17 weeks. (a) Bubble-like hemispheres photographed under water and viewed from above. (b) Lateral view. The cyst has collapsed out of water. Note the preservation of orbital frontal, and inferior temporal and occipital cortex.*

whereas the basal ganglia may be normal, disorganized or show focal destruction. There is also aplasia of the corticospinal tracts.

Clinical manifestations vary: major involvement of the basal ganglia and hypothalamus causes severe impairment of thermoregulation, sleep pattern, sucking and swallowing, so survival is rarely for more than a few weeks. If the deep nuclei are preserved, lifespan may be prolonged for several years but there is spasticity, epilepsy and minimal psychomotor development. Head size is normal at birth but increases over the first few months. This increasing hydrocephalus has been variously ascribed to aqueduct atresia, gliosis or stenosis of the foramina of Monro.[191,517,936] Transillumination may occasionally be dramatic (Fig. 7.87), but MRI is now of particular value in diagnosis,[379] even *in utero*.[5]

The pathogenesis of these lesions has excited much argument. Heschl[409,410] favoured a destructive process rather than an aplastic one. Yakovlev and Wadsworth,[968,969] in an extensive study of bilateral clefts and full-thickness porencephaly, coined the term schizencephaly to embody their concept of a failure of growth and differentiation of circumscribed areas of the cerebral wall, occurring, they believed, during the first 2 months of intrauterine life. However, their interpretation of the structure of the apposed walls of the cleft and the bridging membrane over the defect is no longer convincing, although for obscure reasons it lingers in the radiological literature.[47,618] There is now ample clinical, morphological and experimental evidence favouring a destructive origin for these lesions. Their timing is suggested by the coincident polymicrogyria to be between the fourth and sixth months; indeed, they have been observed as early as 24 and 26 weeks of gestation[314,669] and even at 22 weeks of gestation (see Figs 7.59, 7.86). The topography and symmetry of porencephaly and hydranencephaly and their preference for the territories of the carotid or the anterior and middle cerebral arteries[220,517] suggest ischaemia and infarction as a likely pathogenic mechanism. Hydranencephaly has been produced in animal experiments by blocking or ligating the carotid arteries,[58,647] but in man the major arteries are usually patent, suggesting that perfusion failure rather than arterial insufficiency is responsible. The porus can be perceived as the epicentre of the disturbance, with the surrounding polymicrogyria reflecting less intense ischaemia.[542,570] Norman's case[669] is instructive in this regard: bilateral symmetrical fissures in a twin of 26 weeks' gestation had at their centres completely disorganized groups of neuroblasts mixed with macrophages and a focus of calcification, while the edges of the lesion showed polymicrogyria in the formative stage. A personal case shows similar appearances at 32 weeks of gestation (see Fig. 7.85).

Various aetiological factors have been proposed. In early series a high incidence of illegitimate births and attempted abortion was noted;[220,517] porencephaly has recently been documented following intramuscular injection of benzol as an attempted abortifacient in the first trimester.[96] Case reports of hydranencephaly include clinical histories of maternal poisoning or attempted suicide with domestic gas at 24 weeks, butane at 27 weeks and oestrogen ingestion at 18 weeks.[39,85,289] The evolution of porencephaly has been examined in sequential ultrasound scans following an episode of severe maternal hypoxia at 20 weeks.[349] Multicystic encephalomalacia (see below) has also been reported after attempted suicide with butane gas at 30 weeks[350] and following maternal bee sting anaphylaxis at 35 weeks of gestation.[278]

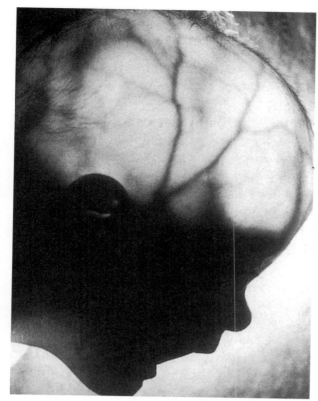

Figure 7.87 *Hydrancephaly. Transillumination of the head of a hydrancephalic infant.*

There is an undoubted association between encephaloclastic lesions and twinning, particularly monozygotic, monochorionic twins,[10,471,522] often but not always in a twin to a macerated fetus[10,522,669] (Figs 7.85, 7.86). Intrauterine death of one twin, and the appearance of multicystic encephalopathy (see below), have been documented in serial CT scans.[440] Most of the suggested mechanisms are based on the twin-to-twin transfusion syndrome, because of the high incidence of interfetal vascular anastomoses in monochorionic twins.[522,574] Following the intrauterine death of a donor twin, in whom the stigmata of ischaemic damage may occasionally be found,[522] embolization of necrotic tissue or transfer of thromboplastin-rich blood from a dead to a surviving recipient twin may cause disseminated intravascular coagulopathy[68,633] and bring in its wake multiple organ infarction.[298] Alternatively, massive blood loss from the surviving (recipient) twin into the tissues of the dead co-twin may have similar consequences. In other cases it is the smaller, presumed donor twin who is affected.[589,838] In a personally examined case, unilateral multicystic encephalopathy was present in one of a pair of conjoined twins who had shared a common pericardial cavity.

Another association is with fetal infection, especially toxoplasmosis and CMV, but other viruses and even intrauterine purulent meningitis are occasionally implicated.[317,432] Similar lesions in animals have been reported in association with intrauterine viral infection.[398]

Persistent or recurrent infection was also postulated by Bordarier and Robain[94] to explain the occurrence of encephaloplastic lesions in two siblings, the first showing hydranencephaly, polymicrogyria and subcortical heterotopias, the second only polymicrogyria and heterotopias. However, recent clinical and neuroimaging reports without pathological confirmation of familial porencephaly[414,433,768] and familial schizencephaly[357] have suggested a genetic abnormality. In the latter a germline mutation of the homeobox gene *EMX2* was demonstrated in two brothers. Mutant mice lacking the homologous *Emx2* gene show impaired reelin signalling, abnormal radial glia and defective neuronal migration.[588]

Finally, it should be stressed that Fowler's familial hydranencephaly syndrome, although indistinguishable macroscopically and ultrasonographically from encephaloclastic hydranencephaly, is easily recognizable on histological examination (see below).

MULTICYSTIC ENCEPHALOPATHY

Although sharing the same clinical antecedents, and probably the same pathogenesis as the smooth-walled porencephalic defects described above, these lesions originating during the third trimester are, by contrast, ragged, irregular and without accompanying cortical malformation[186,293] (Fig. 7.88). The white matter and deep cortical layers of large parts of both hemispheres may be destroyed and replaced by a sponge-like arrangement of myriad glial-lined cysts intersected by thin gliovascular strands enmeshing collections of lipid-containing macrophages. Unilateral lesions can also occur.[253] The basal ganglia and the brainstem may be normal but often show extensive bilateral cystic necrosis[838] (Fig. 7.88). Similar pathology may also occur at or after birth: the often very severe destruction (Fig. 7.89) has been termed global hemispheric necrosis.[314,552,565,938] It is known to occur postnatally in the clinical context of hyperpyrexia and sudden collapse, can be followed in sequential neuroradiological studies and is an important consideration in the legal minefield surrounding claims for inadequate obstetric care.

Microcephaly

Etymologically, 'microcephaly' means a small head, therefore to describe a small brain, the term 'micrencephaly' would be more appropriate. However, because brain and skull usually grow in parallel the term 'microcephaly' is generally used to indicate smallness of the brain, occurring usually as a malformation. Normative data are available for head circumference from birth to adulthood,[270,660] and for brain weight during fetal[367,524,729] and postnatal life.[221] Figures of 2 or more standard deviations below the mean are abnormal. Using this definition, microcephaly is a common but not invariable occurrence in malformed brains.

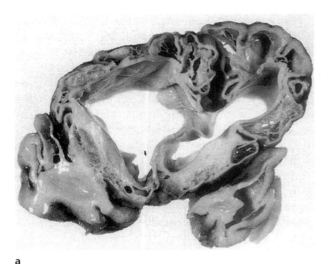

a

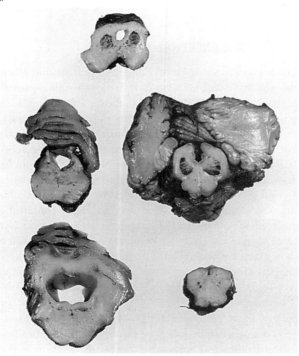

b

Figure 7.88 *Multicystic encephalomalacia. (a) White matter and deeper parts of the cortex as well as basal ganglia are transformed into a gliovascular meshwork. (b) Bilateral symmetrical cystic necrosis extending through the hindbrain.*

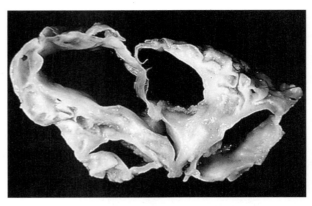

Figure 7.89 *Global hemispheric necrosis following severe birth asphyxia. Courtesy of Dr T Moss, Frenchay Hospital, Bristol, UK.*

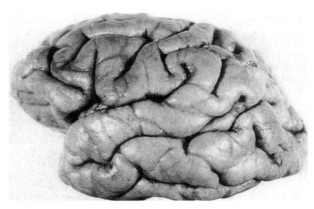

Figure 7.90 *Familial microcephaly. Note the simple convolutional pattern formed by the relatively broad gyri.*

Familial cases[767] may show severe cortical anomalies (Fig. 7.90), but most cases of recessive microcephaly do not. In the neonatal period, sporadic microcephaly without associated malformations should arouse suspicion of intrauterine infection.[383,749]

CHROMOSOMAL DISORDERS

Trisomy 21: Down's syndrome

The external appearance of a Down's syndrome brain is much more diagnostic than are the microscopic findings. The weight of the fully grown brain seldom exceeds 1200 g and is usually nearer 1000 g. The brain is abnormally rounded and short with a steeply rising, almost vertical, occipital contour. The convolutional pattern usually shows no gross departure from normality, but there may be asymmetries on the two sides, a poverty of secondary sulci and exposure of the insula. Very characteristic in Down's although not peculiar to it, is narrowness of the superior temporal gyrus (Fig. 7.91). The anomaly is often bilateral and is present in about half the cases. Conspicuous smallness of the cerebellum and brainstem in comparison with the cerebrum as a whole is also a common feature.[188] Benda[65] proposed that most of these

Microcephaly is a purely descriptive term and does not refer to a particular aetiology; classification is therefore difficult. Ross *et al.*[777] proposed two large groups, with or without associated malformations. Microcephaly with associated malformations includes genetic disorders (chromosomal or single gene defects), environmental causes and cases of unknown aetiology. Microcephaly without associated malformations includes primary microcephaly of proven or possible genetic transmission due to inborn errors of metabolism, is caused by environmental factors or the aetiology remains unknown.

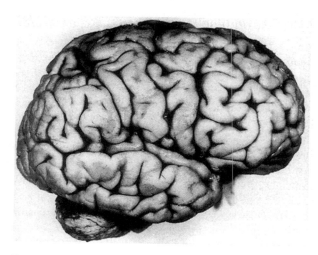

Figure 7.91 *Down's syndrome. Right hemisphere of the brain in Down's syndrome. The cerebellum is small and the occipital contour flatter than normal. The frontal lobe is reduced in its anteroposterior diameter and the superior temporal gyrus is poorly developed.*

abnormalities of shape have been impressed on the developing brain by the retarded growth of the skull and pointed out that the crowns of gyri may be flattened, that the sagittally arranged sulci may show S-shaped distortion and that fibrous union may bind contiguous parts of the convolutions together.

Many microscopic anomalies have been described in the syndrome, but they are not specific. Davidoff[212] reported patchy cerebral calcifications and a poverty of nerve cells in the third cortical layer (Fig. 7.92). This finding is not very common, but irregularities of grouping certainly occur and so relatively acellular areas adjoin those which display an increased density due to the presence of clusters of small nerve cells. Systematic cell counts in random sections indicate that the nerve cells are, in fact, often increased on the average per unit area. This seeming paradox may be related to the small size of the brain as a whole, since, as a general rule, the more underdeveloped the state of the brain, the closer together are the cortical neurons. Active destruction of nerve cells associated with anoxia and oedema takes place in Down's patients dying in infancy.[65] Several more recent morphometric studies have shown a marked reduction in neuron numbers, up to 50% compared with controls, from birth onwards, but not in fetal life,[162,953] which particularly seems to involve granule layers.[779] The Golgi method has shown changes in dendritic arborization and decreased spine numbers of neonatal and infantile Down's subjects, while fetal cases appeared normal.[878]

Benda[65] also emphasized the poor myelination of the grey and white matter and demonstrated a striking poverty of myelin in the U-fibres. Meyer and Jones[614] were the first to demonstrate a conspicuous fibrillary gliosis of the central white matter in many, but by no means all, cases. There was often no corresponding pallor in myelin prepa-

rations, although patchy areas of demyelination were sometimes seen, as they were in Davidoff's cases. Benda also reported frequent minor malformations in the spinal cord including fusion of the columns of Clarke, so the nerve cells occupy a strip of grey matter lying behind the central canal. Except for undoubted signs of retarded or mildly perverted development, the brain thus shows a few pathological changes that cannot be explained on the basis of intercurrent disease. Whether such fortuitous lesions are in some way related to abnormal constitutional factors, such as general circulatory embarrassment or endocrine anomalies, has not been precisely determined. Certainly the frequent association of congenital heart disease is an important factor. Arterial and venous thromboses are well-known complications of Fallot's teratology, as are embolism and cerebral abscess due to detachment of vegetations from congenitally malformed or infected valves. The important influence of congenital heart disease on myelination was also emphasized in the large series of Wisniewski and Schmidt-Sidor.[954] Myelination was not delayed in fetuses but of 129 cases, from birth to 6 years, 23% showed myelination delay compared with controls. In Down's infants with congenital heart disease this figure rose to 48%.

Middle-aged Down's patients often show clinical signs of premature senility, and this may be reflected in the brain by the presence of senile plaques and Alzheimer's

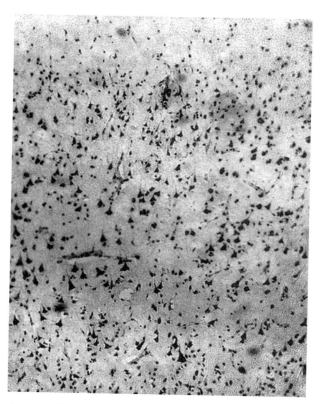

Figure 7.92 *Down's syndrome. Section of the angular gyrus in Down's syndrome showing diffuse loss of neurons in the third layer. (Cresyl violet.)*

neurofibrillary change.[464,684,844] In Malamud's series[586] the brains of all those dying over the age of 40 years showed lesions of this type in various degrees of severity. Ultrastructurally the neurofibrillary tangles are identical with those seen in typical cases of Alzheimer's disease[809] (see also Chapter 4, Volume II).

Three types of chromosomal abnormality are responsible for Down's syndrome: trisomy 21 (in 95% of cases), translocations (< 5%) or mosaicism (< 1%). The relative incidence of different chromosomal types has been remarkably constant in recorded series. The incidence of trisomy increases with advancing maternal age, while a higher proportion of translocations occurs in children of younger mothers. Most familial cases are associated with translocations. The pathogenesis of the condition, or the mechanism by which an additional chromosome which in 95% is maternal in origin can cause a wide range of abnormalities with variable expressivity, has been the subject of abundant speculation, yet remains obscure. Recent work has focused on the effects of free radicals in trisomic cell metabolism. Several studies have shown increased levels of the free radical scavenging enzyme CuZn superoxide dismutase within cell lines from patients with both trisomy 21 and Alzheimer's disease. Free radicals have been implicated in the ageing process and suggested to promote paired helical filament formation.[979] A profound deficiency of repair of Down's cells after X-ray damage has also been reported.[811]

Trisomy 13: Patau's syndrome

Holoprosencephaly and arhinencephaly occur in about two-thirds of cases.[370] Cyclopia and microcephaly are other features. Cerebellar heterotopias and excessive numbers of neuroblasts in dentate and cochlear nuclei are also notable.

Trisomy 18: Edwards' syndrome

Studies by Sumi[872] and Michaelson and Gilles[616] documented a variety of abnormalities in addition to microcephaly, particularly anomalies of the gyral pattern, dysplasia of the hippocampus, disorganization of the lateral geniculate nucleus and olivary dysplasia. Cerebellar heterotopias are less extensive than in trisomy 13.

Deletions

Deletions of part of one chromosome are often associated with mental subnormality and microcephaly; examples include 5p− in the cri du chat syndrome, 4p− in the Wolf–Hirschhorn syndrome associated with convolutional defects, heterotopias, dysplasia of the lateral geniculate, dentate and olivary nuclei and hyperplasia of the corpus callosum,[353] and 17p13− in Miller–Dieker syndrome[534] (described above).

Fragile X syndrome

Fragile X syndrome is now accepted as the second most frequent chromosomal disorder associated with developmental disability. An estimated incidence of 1 in 1000 liveborn males makes it the most common familial form of mental retardation. The fragile X site at position Xq27 can be induced in cells cultured at low folic acid and thymidine concentrations.[686] Distinguishing features are macroorchidism and a long face with prominent forehead and large ears. The scanty neuropathological information available includes microcephaly, neuronal heterotopias,[262] and in one autopsied case studied by light and electron microscopy dendritic spine abnormalities associated with synaptic immaturity.[788]

Environmental factors (see also Table 7.4)

Microcephaly may be associated with intrauterine growth retardation,[519,524] a heterogeneous condition with diverse associations such as malformation (visceral and/or cerebral) and infections, multiple pregnancy, and placental insufficiency with maternal toxaemia or renal diseases. Hypotrophic infants usually have a large brain in relation to body weight and within normal limits for gestational age. However, in only a very few cases of a large series of infants showing retarded intrauterine growth was the brain weight 2 standard deviations below the mean, i.e. microcephalic by definition. The external configuration of the brain corresponds to gestational age, and cytoarchitecture and myelination are not significantly modified in the neonatal period. Placental deficiency, which usually develops during the second half of pregnancy, probably does not affect the number of neurons but may possibly damage glial cells and impair subsequent myelination, which could play a part in the pathogenesis of so-called minimal brain damage. Dobbing and Sands[247] emphasized the vulnerability of the fetal brain at certain periods of its development, and it is possible that microcephaly may be induced by undernutrition. In multiple pregnancies, fetal brain growth may be more retarded than body weight.[427] This may be very pronounced in cases of monochorionic placenta with the twin-to-twin transfusion syndrome.

Offspring of women with phenylketonuria are often microcephalic (Fig. 7.93), mentally retarded and of low birthweight,[309] and this may occur even if a low phenylalanine diet is started during the first trimester.[837] In a recent international collaborative study, only those infants whose mothers were on a strict diet at the time of conception were normocephalic.[255] Histological examination of the microcephalic brain is usually unrewarding,[837] but abnormalities of pyramidal cells have been described in a Golgi study of a 4-month infant.[511]

Microcephaly is also an important feature of the fetal alcohol syndrome, along with a wide variety of other

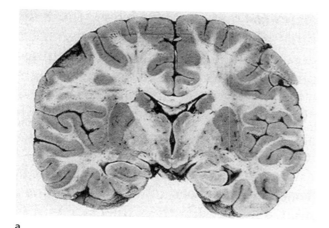

a

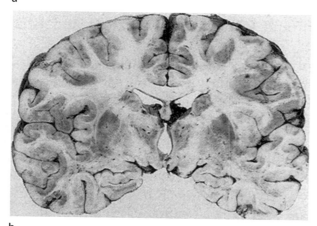

b

Figure 7.93 *Microcephaly. Brain weight at 15 months was 700 g. (a) Coronal slice. Compare with age-matched control (b) of normal size. Maternal phenylketonuria: diet began at 8 weeks' gestation.*

anomalies, including leptomeningeal glioneuronal heterotopias, agenesis of the corpus callosum, lissencephaly and various migration disorders of cerebrum and hindbrain.[147,717,952] Septo-optic dysplasia and holoprosencephaly has recently been documented in a 2½-month-old girl exposed to maternal binge alcohol abuse in the first trimester.[178]

Irradiation

Deep X-ray therapy to the pelvis during the first 4 months of pregnancy has produced many cases of microcephaly. Anomalies of the eye (optic atrophy, choroidoretinitis, abnormal retinal pigmentation) are much more common in these cases than in micrencephaly of genetic origin. Four histologically examined cases in which therapeutic irradiation had been carried out during pregnancy were quoted by Cowen and Geller.[181] Various anomalies of the eyes, cerebral hemispheres and thalamus were present in Johnson's[467] cases. Courville and Edmondson[180] reported microcephaly with diffuse loss of cortical nerve cells. Cerebellar microgyria with some structural disorientation was

the main feature of the cases of Miskolczy[624] and van Bogaert and Radermecker.[87] At autopsy three of these brains exhibited meningoencephalitis. To these cases may be added that of Uiberrack,[908] which showed pachygyria of the cerebral cortex and defective development of the vermis. Studies on children exposed *in utero* to the atomic explosions at Hiroshima and Nagasaki revealed a relatively high incidence of microcephaly and mental retardation, but no specific malformations,[620,727,959,973] apart from one report of periventricular heterotopia in a microcephalic individual whose mother was located 1147 m from the hypocentre of the Nagasaki atomic bomb in the third gestational week.[662]

MATERNAL INFECTION

The deleterious effects of maternal viral infection have become well recognized since Gregg's[362] original observations on the adverse effects of rubella. Intrauterine viral infection can result in two different but sometimes overlapping types of pathological sequel: necrosis and inflammation on the one hand, and developmental interference, i.e. reduced brain growth or malformation, on the other.

Rubella

CNS involvement is common in clinical series, as high as 80%.[240] In addition to ocular defects including cataracts, pigmentary retinopathy and microphthalmos[362,785,957] and sensorineural deafness,[713] neuropathological findings include chronic meningoencephalitis,[240] microcephaly,[649] and retarded myelination and cytoarchitectonic development,[486,775] although the evidence for a causal relationship with specific malformations remains inconclusive.

Cytomegalovirus

The reported incidence of intrauterine CMV infection varies from 0.4 to 2.4%,[518,854] but infection may not result in overt disease. Less than 5% of infected neonates have a rapidly fatal systemic disorder, with involvement of the brain reported in 10–80%.[382,383,576,860,939] Common clinical findings are microcephaly, mental retardation, epilepsy, diplegia, chorioretinitis and intracerebral calcification. Neuropathologically, there is often microcephaly, and sometimes hydrocephalus. Severe necrotizing lesions of the ependyma and periventricular tissue are notable,[405,607] and may form cavitating lesions, such as porencephaly or hydranencephaly.[189,244,659] Intracytoplasmic viral inclusions may be very sparse, but their identification is assisted by immunocytochemistry or *in situ* hybridization. Perivascular calcifications are usually found in periventricular tissue but may be present in the cortex and basal ganglia. The association of intrauterine CMV infection with malformations, notably polymicrogyria and cerebellar cortical dysplasia, is now well accepted.[77,189,317,593,599]

Other viruses

In one series, herpes simplex infection was associated with chorioretinitis, microcephaly, hydranencephaly and microphthalmia. Maternal varicella-zoster infection in the first or second trimester may on some occasions produce a characteristic embryopathy involving skin, muscle, eye and brain.[260] The dermatomal distribution of cutaneous scarring and other various anomalies suggest a fetal zoster, and there is electrophysiological and neuropathological evidence of cord and dorsal root ganglion involvement.[389,852] A few autopsy studies have described severe destruction of the brain, and one personal case, in addition to a widespread necrotizing encephalitis, showed polymicrogyria bilaterally in the insular cortex (Fig. 7.63).[389]

Other organisms

Fetal infection with toxoplasmosis causes a necrotizing meningoencephalitis which results in hydrocephalus and widespread calcification. As with CMV, polymicrogyria and cortical defects such as hydranencephaly have also been recorded. An early stage of hydranencephaly was the result of a rare case of intrauterine purulent encephalitis.[432]

Megalencephaly

The accepted definition of megalencephaly is a brain weight 2.5 standard deviations above the mean for the age and sex. Various descriptive terms have been used, such as cerebral gigantism and macrocephaly. Megalencephaly includes a variety of clinical and pathological conditions and no classification is entirely satisfactory.[235,306,674]

Dekaban and Sakuragawa[222] subdivided the megalencephalies into three main categories and various subgroups, based on their own and previously reported cases: primary and secondary megalencephaly, and hemimegalencephaly. Primary megalencephaly may be an isolated finding or associated with achondroplasia and endocrine disorders, or it may be familial. Males are affected twice as often as females, and in the majority of patients the large head is noticed within the first year of life. In about 25% of the cases there was no obvious abnormality of the brain other than its size, and of the remainder half showed some cytoarchitectonic or neuronal abnormalities, and the other half severe macroscopically visible malformations (Fig. 7.94). Mental retardation and neurological disorders of some sort were present in the majority of patients. Personal observations in several autistic subjects have disclosed megalencephaly as well as olivary heterotopia.[32] Secondary megalencephaly is associated with genetic disorders, such as the sphingolipidoses and mucopolysaccharidoses, and with various leukodystrophies (including Alexander's and Canavan's diseases) and neurocutaneous syndromes. Megalencephaly may be present at birth or may become manifest during the early postnatal years.

A particular form of megalencephaly described as cerebral gigantism was reported by Sotos *et al.*[846] Evident at birth are large hands, feet and cranium with moderate prognathism, and advanced osseous maturation for the age. There have been sporadic as well as familial cases,[381] and autosomal dominant inheritance has been described.[984] Moderate to severe mental retardation is present. In a detailed clinical study of 22 patients,[955] CT scan abnormalities included ventricular dilatation, midline cava and widening of the sylvian fissures.

Hemimegalencephaly

This term denotes manifest asymmetrical enlargement, particularly but not exclusively of one cerebral hemisphere. The nosology is unclear although there is considerable overlap with neurocutaneous disorders. Indeed, hemimegalencephaly may be a feature of tuberous sclerosis[465] and linear sebaceous naevi of Jadassohn (Solomon's) syndrome.[53,978] In an autopsy study of one such patient, Choi and Kudo[136] observed asymmetry of the limbs, extensive skin lesions, and hemimegalencephaly histologically characterized by disturbed neuronal migration, abnormal cortical architecture and glial proliferation. Somewhat similar is a small group of patients in whom hemimegalencephaly is associated with ipsilateral hemihypertrophy, multiple haemangiomas and vascular naevi, the Klippel–Trenaunay–Weber syndrome. In a 17-year-old girl the right cerebral and cerebellar hemispheres and the right side of the pons were enlarged, possibly resulting from an absolute increase in neuronal numbers,[606] but no malformations were found.

With recent advances in MRI and surgical management of intractable epilepsy in the paediatric population,

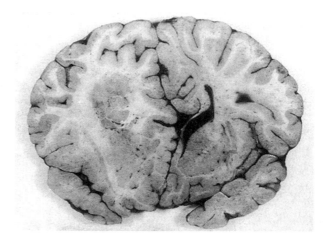

Figure 7.94 *Megalencephaly with multiple cerebral anomalies, including absence of corpus callosum and an abnormal gyral pattern. A child aged 3 years with total brain weight of 1554 g. Coronal section showing a large collection of heterotopias in the white matter on the left and longitudinal callosal (Probst) bundle on the right.*

neuropathologists are increasingly faced with resections (partial or total) of asymmetrically large hemispheres. Morphological findings are quite varied, and include polymicrogyria, pachygyria and cortical dysplasia.[238,765]

Anomalies of the wall of the lateral ventricles

Adhesions between two facing ventricular walls have been described under various names such as coarctation[213] or coaptation[56] of the walls, goniosynapses[176] and transventricular adhesions.[678] The sites of adhesion are between the caudate nucleus and the corpus callosum, or between opposing walls of the anterior horn of the lateral ventricle or, less often, of the occipital and temporal horns. The affected ventricle may be reduced in size and the contralateral cavity enlarged. The pathogenesis is obscure, although a developmental impairment, taking place between weeks 9 and 15 of gestation, has been implicated.[213] However, in two children aged 9 months and 13 years, presenting with transventricular adhesions, Norman and McMenemey[678] described haemosiderin-laden macrophages in the ependymal wall and the caudate

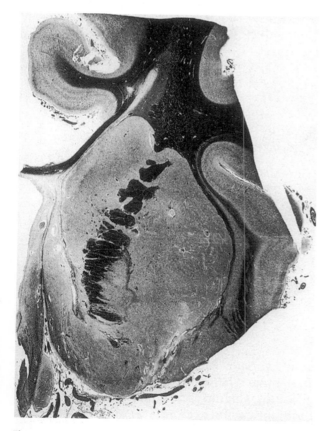

Figure 7.95 *Anomaly of the lateral ventricle. Coronal section of the striatum and frontal lobe showing obliteration of the frontal horn and body of the lateral ventricle with adhesion between the corpus callosum and head of the caudate nucleus. (Luxol fast blue–cresyl violet.)*

nucleus, suggestive of birth injury with residual haemorrhage and scarring. Similar conclusions can be inferred from the case (Fig. 7.95) of a 2-year-old girl, born prematurely at 34 weeks of gestation with a complex congenital heart defect, rapidly progressive postnatal hydrocephalus and evidence of intraventricular haemorrhage. In the line of obliteration of the ventricle astrocytosis, fibrillary gliosis, ependymal tubules and iron-laden macrophages were observed.

THIRD VENTRICULAR OBLITERATION

Neonatal-onset hydrocephalus in association with congenital fusion of the thalamus is extremely rare: it has been reported in two siblings,[143] and in a 6-month-old boy with a unique combination of anomalies including atresia of the aqueduct and upper fourth ventricle and rhomboencephalosynapsis.[487]

Malformations of the cerebellum

The classification of cerebellar anomalies remains difficult and the literature confused. The tendency is to follow phylogenetic principles, but this approach cannot always encompass the great variety of transitional forms that straddle the normally accepted categories. Moreover, the correlation between phylogenetic and morphological subdivision is not very precise. Additional complications are the heterogeneity of associated malformations, the multiplicity of postulated aetiological factors and, most importantly, the very prolonged development of the cerebellum, which extends well into postnatal life. The dividing line between malformative and degenerative processes becomes increasingly blurred in the later stages of gestation. Noxious agents that would be purely destructive elsewhere in the brain may influence granule cell proliferation, differentiation and the late growth spurt of the cerebellum; conversely, secondary atrophy in the wake of perinatal hypoxic–ischaemic embarrassment, epilepsy or consequent anticonvulsant therapy may contribute significantly to the final morphological result. A brief embryological summary is pertinent to the discussion; for detailed reviews and experimental studies see Refs 15, 17–19, 313, 526, 540, 615 and 827.

During gestational week 4, with the closure and segmentation of the neural tube, the rhombencephalon becomes temporarily the largest part of the brain. Differential growth in the rhombencephalon during week 5 of gestation results in formation of the pontine flexure, widening the neural tube at this point with thinning of its roof, which becomes transversely creased. Within this crease, or plica choroidea, the choroid plexus will develop, while caudal to it the membranous roof of the fourth ventricle forms a pouch-like evagination in many species,[84] and in man this perforates forming the foramen of Magendie by 12 weeks,[105] while the foramina of Luschka open later, probably around 16 weeks. The roof rostral to the plica, the anterior membranous area, becomes briefly permeable to CSF and is later incorporated into the developing vermis. Also anterior to the plica, the lateral parts of the alar plates undergo intense neuroblastic proliferation, enlarging to form the rhombic lips, the paired primordia of the cerebellum which gradually extend dorsomedially, meeting the roof of the fourth ventricle at around 6 weeks of gestation and then fusing together in the midline during month 3. Cerebellar growth which has been entirely intraventricular now becomes extraventricular and the various subdivisions begin to appear: first the posterolateral or flocculonodular fissure at 9 weeks, demarcating the vestibular or archicerebellum from the rest, then at 12 weeks the primary fissure separating anterior from posterior lobes, the spinocerebellum or paleocerebellum from the pontocerebellum or neocerebellum. It is this last, phylogenetically youngest, portion of the cerebellum that becomes predominant in mammals and its various fissures form 4–8 weeks after those of the vermis and flocculonodular lobes. The neurons of the cerebellar cortex and deep nuclei as well as the pontine and inferior olivary nuclei all derive from the alar plates: ventral migrations into the pontine grey and olivary ribbons, and lateral migration into the rhombic lips from where there are two divergent pathways, inwards through the cerebellar plate for the Purkinje cells and deep nuclei, and outwards guided by pial basal lamina[404] over the surface of the developing cerebellum forming the external granular layer. This rapidly proliferating layer first appears in week 9, covers the whole surface by 14 weeks, reaches maximum thickness at 24 weeks, persists until the third postnatal month and then disappears quickly, usually by the end of the first year. It is the major influence on folial development, giving rise to the neurons and glia of the molecular and internal granular layers, and in particular the granule cells, the inward growth of which across the molecular layer is directed by a scaffold of radial glial processes.[738]

CEREBELLAR AGENESIS

Total absence of the cerebellum is rare. Early reports, such as that of Combette[163] in a severely retarded epileptic 11-year-old child, and of Priestley[734] in a spastic hydrocephalic infant of 4 months with spina bifida, were without histological verification. Stewart[863] and later Macchi and Bentivoglio,[573] reviewing the literature, pointed out that in most cases some remaining cerebellar tissue, especially the flocculonodular lobe, could be demonstrated[27] (Fig. 7.96). In addition, related structures such as the pontine nuclei and inferior olives are hypoplastic or dysplastic. Ricardi and Marcus[755] reported two brothers with congenital hydrocephalus who died early in infancy: autopsy of one child showed cerebellar agenesis. Larroche's case (Fig. 7.97) was a male stillborn premature infant with hydrocephalus; a large arachnoid cyst filled the interhemispheric fissure, and

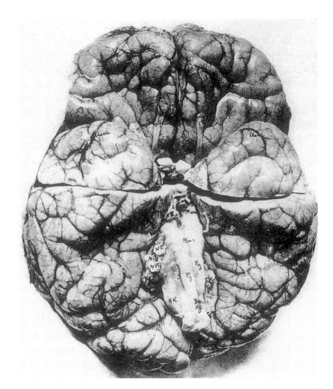

Figure 7.96 *Cerebellar agenesis. Case of Anton and Zingerle.*[27]

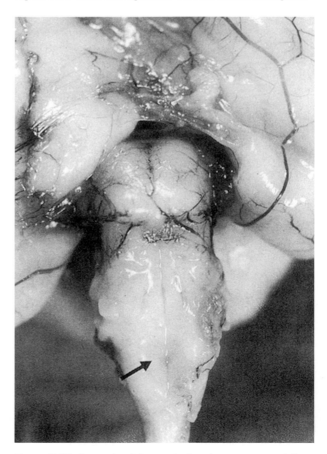

Figure 7.97 *Agenesis of the cerebellum in a premature infant. The floor of the fourth ventricle (arrow) is exposed by the total absence of cerebellar tissue.*

the corpus callosum and septum pellucidum were absent. Patients with total or near-total absence of the cerebellum are usually mentally and physically handicapped, but the cerebellar defect may not be suspected during life.[786,862] Individuals or total agenesis of the cerebellum is also a feature of large occipital encephaloceles.[481] Absence of one hemisphere is much less rare[868] (Fig. 7.98)

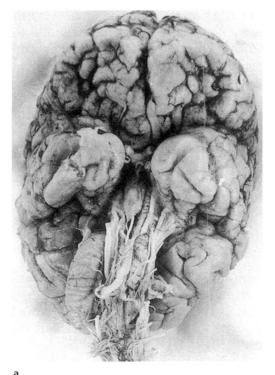

a

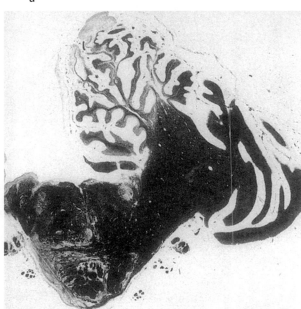

b

Figure 7.98 *Malformation of the cerebellum. Absence of the left cerebellar hemisphere and middle cerebellar peduncle and marked reduction in the size of the contralateral pontine nuclei.*

and is associated with changes in the contralateral inferior olive and pons, which may take the form of secondary atrophy rather than maldevelopment.[550,573]

APLASIA OF THE VERMIS

Developmental defects of the palaeocerebellum, which predominantly involve the vermis, occur in a variety of disorders. The Dandy–Walker and Joubert's syndromes are the best known, but several others will be briefly mentioned. The clinical and radiological diagnosis of these syndromes and the complexities of their differential diagnosis are reviewed by Bordarier and Aicardi.[92] In tectocerebellar dysraphia with occipital encephalocele[315,541,690,840] the three principal features are partial or total vermal agenesis, a severe deformation of the midbrain tectum and a cerebelloencephalocele. Rhomboencephalosynapsis[364,448,487,802] is a rare form of cerebellar hypoplasia in which the hemispheres and underlying dentate nuclei are fused across the midline in the absence of a vermis (Fig. 7.99). Other structures are absent or dysplastic, including the palaeocerebellar roof nuclei, dorsal accessory olive and inferior olive. The cerebellar anomaly may be combined with other midline anomalies, septo-optic dysplasia,[802] commissural abnormalities[364] and fusion of the thalami.[487] Partial or complete absence of the vermis is also a feature of the Walker–Warburg syndrome (see above and Fig. 7.51).

Dandy–Walker syndrome

Case studies by Dandy and Blackfan[204] and Taggart and Walker[874] were amalgamated into the well-known eponym by Benda.[66] For large series and general reviews see Refs 109, 198, 337, 397 and 879. There are three essential elements for diagnosis: agenesis of the vermis, cystic

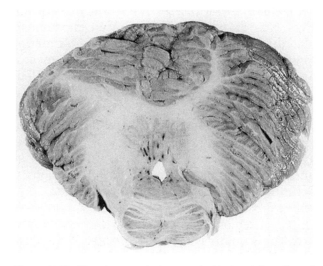

Figure 7.99 *Rhomboencephalosynapsis. Horizontal section of the hindbrain showing absence of the vermis and fusion of the hemispheric cortex and dentate nuclei. Courtesy of Dr PV Best, Aberdeen, UK.*

dilatation of the fourth ventricle and enlargement of the posterior fossa. Hydrocephalus is a frequent but not constant accompaniment.

In a minority of patients the vermis is completely absent, but in most the superior part remains, usually anteriorly rotated, and becomes attenuated inferiorly, where it blends with the membranous roof of the cystic fourth ventricle (Figs 7.100, 7.101). This is often enormously dilated, its cystic roof sometimes herniating upwards through the tentorial hiatus towards the splenium of the corpus callosum. The diaphanous roof membrane (Fig. 7.102), too readily torn by the prosector, is attached laterally to the cerebellar hemispheres and caudally to the medulla. Histologically, it comprises an outer layer of leptomeningeal fibrous tissue and an inner layer of glia including ependyma, and occasionally including cerebellar remnants (Fig. 7.103). The inner aspects of the cerebellar hemispheres, deep white matter overlaid by attenuated ependyma, form the smooth white lateral walls of the cyst, the floor of which is the dorsum of the brainstem. The choroid plexus is abnormally positioned in the lateral recesses and bordering the medullary insertion of the roof membrane. The patency of the fourth ventricle foramina has been much argued over, but in a majority of cases they are patent.[198,397] Enlargement of the posterior fossa is important diagnostically: the skull is characteristically dolichocephalic[66] with an occipital bulge, the attachment of the tentorium is high and almost vertical, while the lateral sinuses and torcula are abnormally elevated.

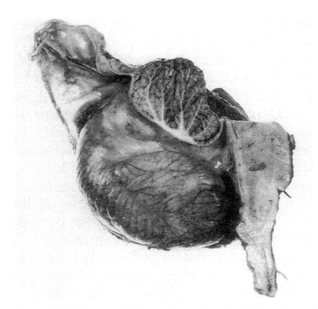

Figure 7.101 *Dandy–Walker malformation. Sagittal section of brain stem and cerebellum showing preservation of the superior vermis and incorporation of the rudimentary inferior vermis into the cyst wall.*

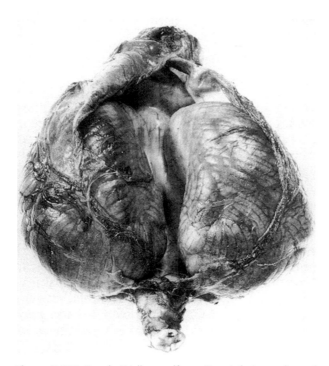

Figure 7.100 *Dandy–Walker malformation. Inferior surface of the cerebellum showing the defect in the vermis and the line of attachment of the tent-like cyst.*

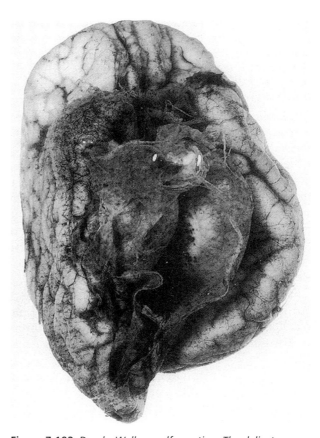

Figure 7.102 *Dandy–Walker malformation. The delicate membrane of the posterior fossa cyst readily ruptures during the dissection. Here it is demonstrated by photography under water.*

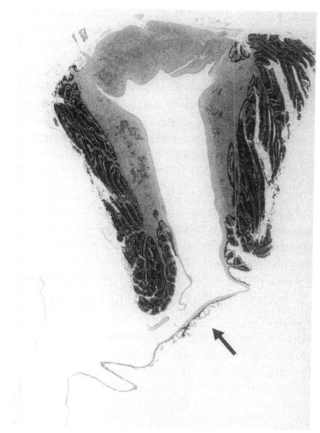

Figure 7.103 *Dandy–Walker malformation. Horizontal section of brainstem and cerebellum. There is complete absence of the vermis and remnants of cerebellar tissue (arrow) are incorporated into the cyst wall.*

Presentation in adulthood is also described,[327] as well as asymptomatic cases found incidentally post-mortem.[553]

CT scan has now superseded contrast ventriculography as the single most useful diagnostic procedure. Skull X-ray will demonstrate the elevated venous sinuses[287] and angiography the downward displacement, hypoplasia or absence of the cerebellar arteries.[527] Diagnosis *in utero* is possible with ultrasound.[401,666] Differentiation must be made from Arnold–Chiari malformation, in which the posterior fossa is small and the tentorial insertion low, and from retrocerebellar arachnoid cysts, which compress the brainstem but do not communicate with the fourth ventricle.

Various pathogenic theories have been advanced. Early workers attached great importance to foraminal atresia, believing that this caused hydrocephalus and subsequent bulging of the anterior membranous area. There are two insurmountable objections: the fourth ventricle foramina are more often patent, and embryologically they become patent only after the paired cerebellar primordia fuse and the anterior membranous area becomes incorporated into the vermis. A more acceptable explanation is a developmental arrest of the hindbrain, which would also account for the atretic foramina as well as the associated brainstem anomalies and the occasional involvement of the cerebellar hemispheres. This would also be in keeping with more widespread evidence of arrested development in the CNS and elsewhere. All of this suggests that the Dandy–Walker malformation originates before the third month. There is also supporting experimental evidence from the hydrocephalic mouse[89,106] in

Apart from hydrocephalus and polygyria (see Fig. 7.161), a great variety of neural and non-neural malformations is associated with the Dandy–Walker syndrome. In the series of Hart *et al.*,[397] two-thirds had other anomalies of the CNS and one-quarter systemic defects. Callosal agenesis is particularly common,[198,397,879] and other anomalies include cerebral cortical dysplasias, polymicrogyria and pachygyria, microcephaly, aqueduct stenosis, infundibular hamartomata, syringomyelia and occipital meningocele. Also important are other hindbrain abnormalities (Fig. 7.104): cerebellar hypoplasia,[457] cerebellar heterotopias, cerebellar cortical dysplasia,[874] dentate dysplasia, olivary dysplasia and heterotopia,[66,378] and anomalies of pyramidal tract decussation.[198,512] Systemic malformations include polydactyly and syndactyly, cleft palate, Klippel–Feil and Cornelia di Lange syndromes, polycystic kidneys and spina bifida.

The usual clinical presentation is early in life with hydrocephalus and a prominent occiput which may be transilluminable posteriorly. Poor head control, motor retardation, spasticity and respiratory failure also occur. Clinical signs in older children, nystagmus and ataxia, simulate those of a posterior fossa space-occupying lesion.

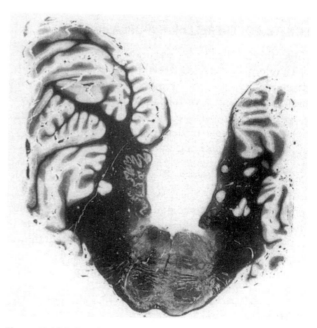

Figure 7.104 *Dandy–Walker malformation. Horizontal section of the hindbrain showing absence of vermis, and hypoplastic right cerebellar hemisphere and dentate nucleus. (Luxol fast blue–cresyl violet.)*

which the anterior membranous area persists and expands between the vermis and the choroid plexus, comparable to the Dandy–Walker cyst. Galactoflavin administration to mice induced a similar defect and callosal agenesis.[477] The aetiology of the human malformation is unknown, but there are occasional reports in siblings[66,198] and identical twins.[462]

Joubert's syndrome

A familial syndrome of episodic hyperpnoea, abnormal eye movements, ataxia and mental retardation, associated with agenesis of the vermis, was first recognized by Joubert et al.[470] At least 40 clinical cases have now been reported,[981] but only seven have been studied postmortem.[121,128,316,393,470,493] On this evidence the cerebral hemispheres are largely unaffected. The ventricular system may be moderately dilated, including the fourth ventricle, although this is slight compared with the cystic dilatation in the Dandy–Walker malformation. The vermis is either completely absent or represented by a few rudimentary folia, but histologically the cerebellar cortex is normal. In the subcortical and deep cerebellar white matter there are numerous heterotopias of large nerve cells, the dentate nucleus is dysplastic and segmented, and the roof nuclei cannot be found. In the medulla, olivary dysplasia, in the form of a C-shaped band, and anomalies of the pyramidal tracts and cranial nerve nuclei have been described.[316,393,493] In one case the midbrain tegmentum was unsegmented.[121] Other features include occipital meningocele,[393,470,493] cystic kidneys and retinal dysplasia.[8,493]

PONTONEOCEREBELLAR HYPOPLASIA

Under this title Brun,[112–114] as part of a larger study of cerebellar anomalies, described two microcephalic and severely retarded children of 11 months and 15 months who showed rudimentary cerebellar hemispheres with relatively well-preserved palaeocerebellum; a peculiar segmentation of the dentate nucleus, severely hypoplastic nuclei pontis, absent arcuate nuclei and hypoplastic inferior olives. A small number of later case reports confirmed these findings[54,76,108,324,482,503,601,718,764] and, with three personally studied cases,[54] form the basis of the following account.

Microcephaly is notable in most of these patients and may be profound,[764] although there are no corresponding histological abnormalities. Even so, the hindbrain is disproportionately small, often 3% or less of the total weight, on account of the slender brainstem (particularly the pons) and extremely small cerebellar hemispheres. The surface of the lateral lobes may be reduced to a few coarse convolutions or be virtually smooth, while the vermis and flocculonodular lobes are more nearly normal in size and foliation (Fig. 7.105a, b).

Histologically, the cortex, associated white matter and roof nuclei of vermis and archicerebellum are normal. In the hypoplastic cerebellar hemispheres, the cortex varies from virtual normality, through modest neuronal depletion to complete absence of Purkinje and granule cells and associated fibre plexuses with, in their stead, a loose gliotic tissue (Fig. 7.106); both forms may coexist closely, with either a gradual transition or a sharp boundary between them, and there may also be foci of dysplastic cortex. The central white matter is very small and poorly myelinated. The dentate nuclei in all these cases are grossly disorganized, lacking their normal undulating ribbon, hilum or proper amiculum. The reduced neuronal population is gathered into small nests (Fig. 7.107), islands of neuropil embedded in a meshwork of myelin fibres, or small groups of neurons rimmed by glial cells. Sometimes the neurons appear rather large and rounded. The superior and middle cerebellar peduncles are thin and poorly myelinated, while the restiform bodies are usually better preserved. The pontine base is very shallow with few transverse fibres and markedly hypoplastic nuclei pontis, often without significant gliosis (see Fig. 7.105c). The inferior olives may be mildly hypoplastic or dysplastic (see Fig. 7.105d) with a variable amount of cell loss and fibrillary gliosis, but the arcuate nuclei are usually absent.

Clinical abnormality is present from birth with microcephaly, severe psychomotor retardation, feeding difficulties, choreiform and other abnormal movements, myoclonic jerks and seizures. Death usually occurs before the age of 2 years, although one of the authors' cases survived until 9 years (see Fig. 7.105a). The aetiology is still a mystery; most cases are sporadic but familial examples (Fig. 7.105) are known.[54,391,601] Most authors agree that the disparity between neocerebellar and palaeocerebellar cortex suggests a developmental disturbance at the end of the third month, but the widespread involvement of other anatomically connected structures has excited considerable debate. Brun[112–114] believed that the 'string of beads' arrangement of the dentate indicated an arrest at an early stage of development, but this is not borne out by developmental studies or personal experience.[76,324,645] Biemond[76] considered the dentate anomaly to be the primary malformation from which all else followed, but more recent authors explain dentate and brainstem changes as secondary linked atrophy, both anterograde and retrograde, after initial interference with neocerebellar cortical development.[54,482,764] Whether anterograde transneuronal degeneration in early life could bring about such a radical transformation of the dentate nucleus is still an open question.

OTHER EXAMPLES OF CEREBELLAR HYPOPLASIA

These are more difficult to classify. One example is the first case of Norman and Urich,[680] discussed and illustrated in previous editions of this book,[911] in which the crenated outline of the dentate ribbon and its amiculum are preserved. In Rubinstein and Freeman's patient,[786] remarkable clinically for his longevity of 72 years and lack of

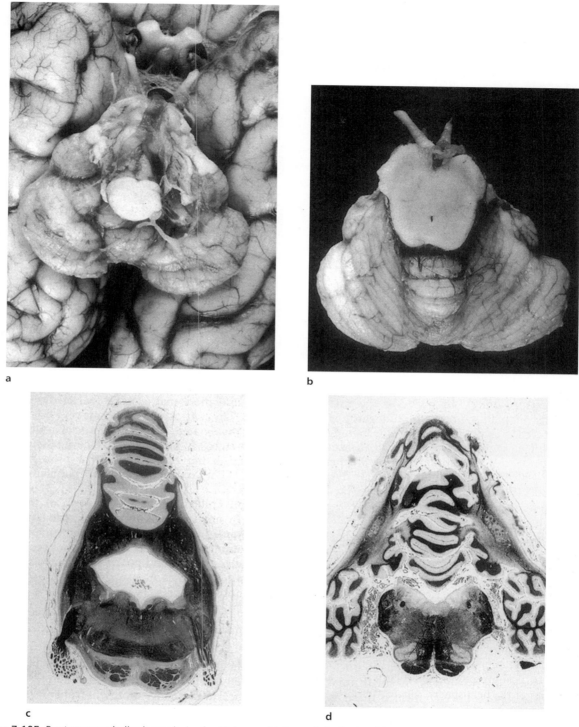

Figure 7.105 *Pontoneocerebellar hypoplasia: familial case. (a) Base of the brain; (b) superior surface of the cerebellum. The tiny cerebellar hemispheres have few, rudimentary folia, while the vermis and flocculi are much better preserved. (c, d) Horizontal sections of the hindbrain. Note the disparity between neocerebellum and vermis and flocculi, the hypoplastic middle cerebellar peduncles and basis pontis, the dentate nuclei broken into islands and the simplified olives. (Luxol fast blue–cresyl violet.)*

cerebellar signs, the vermis and hemispheres were both severely hypoplastic while dentate and olivary nuclei were rudimentary. In case 1 of Vogt and Astwaraturow,[929] the vermis and neocerebellar cortex were both hypoplastic, but cerebellar white matter was well preserved and small, although properly convoluted dentate ribbons were clearly recognizable, accompanied by very large grey matter heterotopias. The example shown in Fig. 7.108 sim-

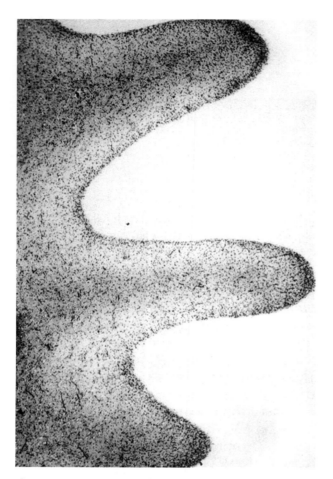

Figure 7.106 *Pontoneocerebellar hypoplasia. Hypoplastic cerebellar folia are devoid of nerve cells. (Luxol fast blue–cresyl violet.)*

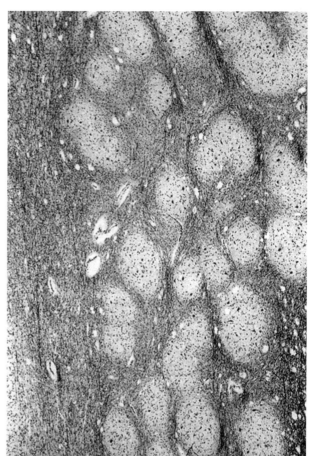

Figure 7.107 *Pontoneocerebellar hypoplasia. The dentate nucleus is broken up into small islands of nerve cells. (Luxol fast blue–cresyl violet.)*

ilarly shows palaeocerebellar and neocerebellar hypoplasia: rudimentary segmented dentate nuclei and large heterotopias are present in the cerebellar white matter and the olivary nuclei are irregularly thickened arcs.

Cerebellar hypoplasia can also present in combination with anterior horn cell degeneration resembling Werdnig–Hoffmann disease.[224,355,478,929,937] In these infants, hypoplasia affects the hemispheres and vermis to a much more equal extent than in pontoneocerebellar hypoplasia, and secondary cortical atrophy is particularly severe in the inferior parts of the hemispheres (Fig. 7.109). The dentate nuclei may be simplified but not segmented, and the olives dysplastic. A sibship of three affected children[355] suggests autosomal recessive inheritance, but all other cases have been sporadic.

Another group of infants with a clinical illness resembling Werdnig–Hoffmann disease showed cerebellar atrophy rather than hypoplasia.[224,355] The nosological position of this disorder remains to be clarified, but it seems both clinically and pathologically district from Fazio–Londe disease, which encompasses cerebellar atrophy, although this is overshadowed by bulbospinal motor neuron degeneration.[584]

GRANULAR LAYER APLASIA

The development of the external granular layer occurs relatively late in fetal life. Granular layer aplasia, a direct consequence of interference with external granule cell proliferation or migration, thus stands uniquely among malformations at the interface between primary maldevelopment and secondary atrophy. It is rare and the small literature is far outweighed by the numerous experimental animal models that simulate the human disorder.

The first description of granular layer aplasia was in a litter of cats,[408] followed by human cases.[87,416,676,799,909] The brain is usually small, but the gyral pattern and histology of the cerebrum are unremarkable. The brainstem has a relatively normal appearance, while the cerebellum is greatly reduced in size: its overall convolutional pattern is retained but individual folia are shrunken and sclerotic (Fig. 7.110). Parts of the vermis or flocculi may appear to be better preserved.

Histologically, the short, stubby folia are composed of a thin molecular layer overlying a rather crowded line of Purkinje cells and virtually no internal granular layer (Fig. 7.111). Many Purkinje cells are scattered ectopically

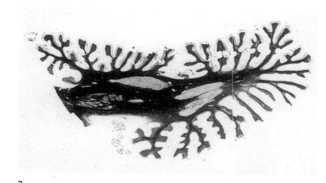

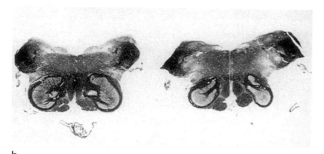

Figure 7.108 *Cerebellar hypoplasia. (a) There is global cortical hypoplasia. Note the rudimentary dentate nucleus and larger grey matter heterotopias as well as (b) olivary dysplasia in the medulla. (Luxol fast blue–cresyl violet.)*

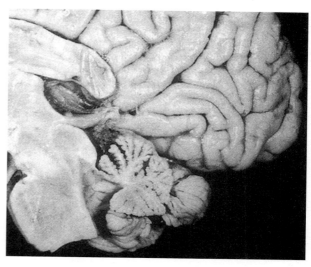

Figure 7.110 *Granular layer aplasia. Mid-sagittal section showing small cerebellum and shrinkage of the superior vermis.*

through the molecular layer, 'tout à fait au hazard, mais le plus souvent jetées comme un paquet de grains'.[87] These dislocated Purkinje cells are abnormally shaped with 'weeping willow' or more horizontal dendritic arborization, and striking cactus-like expansions of terminal dendrites covered in fine spikes (Fig. 7.112). They lack distinct pericellular baskets and their axons, which may run horizontally rather than perpendicular to the surface, often have numerous torpedo expansions. In young infants the external granular layer is severely deficient, while in older patients small foci of the external granular layer may per-

sist. More striking, however, are groups of ectopic granule cell somata stranded at any level in the molecular layer, hanging below the thin external granular layer or just above the Purkinje layer or scattered at random. In one personal case, these cells almost fill the molecular layer apart from a narrow acellular zone just above the Purkinje layer (Fig. 7.113). A diffuse fibrillary gliosis extends through cortex and white matter, although there is minimal myelin depletion. Dentate and olivary neurons are usually preserved within a gliotic neuropil.

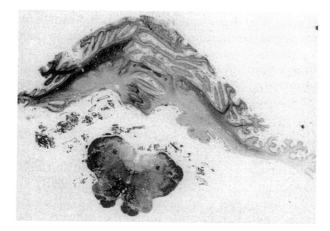

Figure 7.109 *Cerebellar hypoplasia accompanying anterior horn cell degeneration. Horizontal section of hindbrain.*

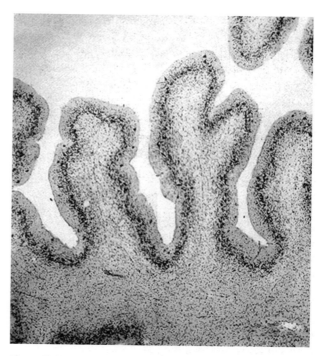

Figure 7.111 *Granular layer aplasia. Atrophy of the granule cell layer and preservation of the Purkinje cells, many of which are present in the molecular layer. (Cresyl violet.)*

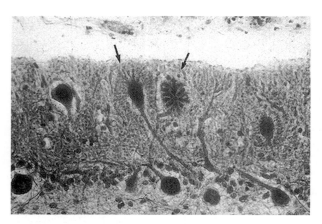

Figure 7.112 *Granular layer aplasia. Dendritic expansion with fine terminal brushwork of fibres. (Bielschowsky's silver method.)*

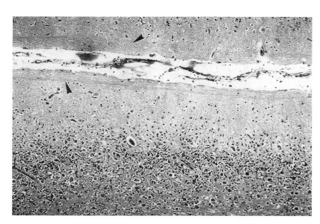

Figure 7.114 *GM2 gangliosidosis. Cerebellar involvement includes granule cell hypoplasia and a dense layer of horizontal fibres superficial to the molecular layer (arrow). (H&E.)*

The main clinical features, severe mental retardation and cerebellar ataxia, present early but remain stationary, with some patients surviving well into adult life. Norman's cases[676] were familial, but all others have been sporadic. The mother of van Bogaert and Radermaker's patient received radium treatment for cancer between months 5 and 6 of gestation,[87] a remarkably close parallel to the irradiation experiments that are discussed next.

Our understanding of the pathogenesis of granular layer aplasia has been greatly assisted by numerous experimental models. In various animals the superficial granular layer can be destroyed and granule cell ectopia produced by neonatal X-irradiation,[16,19] or by exposure to various antimitotic agents.[420,657,825,972] Intrauterine viral infection can also effect the same result.[491] The regenerative capacity of the fetal granular layer is such that a single destructive dose is insufficient and multiple doses must be given.[16] With prolonged dosing, Purkinje cell heterotopia may be produced; allowing regeneration after a few days causes granule cell ectopia. Another intensively studied model is the mutant mouse *weaver* (*wv*), in which a very small cerebellum, granule layer aplasia and ectopic Purkinje and granule cells have been shown to result from both an abnormality of the Bergmann glia and a failure of granule cell migration.[739,740] Functional mossy fibre terminals abnormally situated on Purkinje dendrites have been demonstrated in *wv* cerebellum,[845] and in man a similar phenomenon has been suggested by the abnormal distribution of synaptophysin immunostaining in the molecular layer.[351] In many respects the weaver model is closer to the human situation than the irradiation one, which by contrast shows a layer of tightly packed horizontal fibres superficial to the molecular layer, into which Purkinje dendrites do not penetrate. This is not found in pure granular layer aplasia, but is present in some cases of GM2 gangliosidosis (Fig. 7.114).[75,312] Coincidental granule layer aplasia has also been described in Pelizaeus–Merzbacher disease.[245,805,889]

CROSSED CEREBELLAR ATROPHY

Unilateral cerebellar atrophy (Fig. 7.115), usually observed many years after an extensive lesion in the contralateral cerebral hemisphere, is a capricious, variable and contentious condition. It is capricious in its unpredictability, variable in histological appearance, and despite an extensive case literature it still excites considerable debate. The initial cerebral injury usually occurs in infancy or childhood, but there are occasional observations of initial cerebral damage occurring well into adult life.[57] In addition, the destruction may be intrauterine (Fig. 7.115).

Urich and colleagues have provided a helpful critique of the pathogenic basis of crossed cerebellar atrophy,[866,882] and have defined three types of lesion. The first, reduced size of the cerebellar hemisphere without histological changes to the cortex, results from transneuronal atrophy of the nuclei pontis and thence the middle cerebellar peduncle following on from lesions to the fronto-

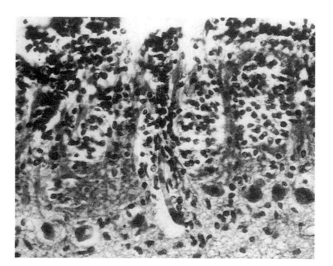

Figure 7.113 *Granular layer aplasia. Ectopic granule cells filling the molecular layer.*

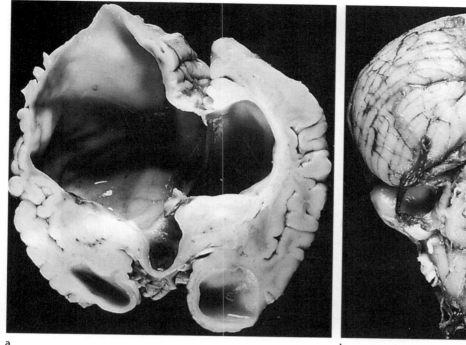
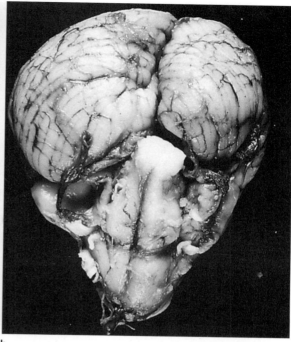

a

b

Figure 7.115 *Crossed cerebellar atrophy in a 5-month-old infant, a twin noted to have ventriculomegaly at 32 weeks' gestation. There is massive old destruction of the left cerebral hemisphere and thalamus (**a**), ipsilateral atrophy of the pontine base and contralateral cerebellar atrophy (**b**). Case referred by Dr PJ Luthert, Institute of Ophthalmology, London, UK.*

pontine and temporopontine tracts. The second pattern, in which granular layer degeneration predominates, is considered to be the result of anterograde transneuronal degeneration, since it is associated with atrophy of the contralateral nuclei pontis.[866] Alternatively, in a few cases, cerebellar cortical degeneration has been linked with retrograde transneuronal degeneration (thalamus, red nucleus, superior cerebellar peduncle, dentate and Purkinje cells).[145,559] A last pattern is lobular sclerosis, for which pathological and circumstantial evidence strongly implicates epileptic seizures as the principal pathogenic factor.[882]

CEREBELLAR HETEROTOPIAS

Foci of ectopic grey matter within the cerebellar white matter are relatively frequent incidental findings in infants. More common in the hemispheres than in the vermis, they vary in size from just a few cells to large islands or sheets of grey matter (Fig. 7.116; see also Figs 7.107, 7.123). Two forms occur: clusters of large cells reminiscent of Purkinje or dentate neurons surrounded by a thin corona of neuropil, and islands of heterotopic cortex, the individual layers being more or less well organized. Heterotopias are notably common in trisomy 13,[675] cerebellar hypoplasias (see Fig. 7.108) and brainstem dysplasias, and in conjunction with other migration disorders. However, ectopic neuronal clusters are relatively frequent in normal infants: the incidence may be over 50%,[774] and roughly equivalent in infants with non-neural mal-

formations. Ectopic neurons are rarely observed in adults (Fig. 7.116b), implying either sampling error or involution.

CEREBELLAR CORTICAL DYSPLASIA

Brun's[112–114] term 'heterotaxia' for disorganized cortical tissue within the cerebellar cortex has not been universally accepted, but other proffered titles such as polymicrogyria and pachygyria are equally unsuitable. Small foci of dysplastic cortex are not rare; occurring for example in 14% of 147 normal infants[774] in the flocculonodular lobes and tonsils and adjacent to the cerebellar peduncles. Cerebellar cortical dysplasia is notable in postencephalitic porencephaly,[223,317] but by far the most extensive examples, replacing most of the normal cortex, are found in the cerebro-ocular dysplasias (Figs 7.51, 7.117). The folial pattern is completely obliterated, with a smooth or irregularly fissured surface, which on sectioning is a very thick grey layer. Microscopically, the cortical layers are in correct register but the folia are scrambled together with an apparent fusing of apposed molecular layers (Fig. 7.117). Deeper parts of the cortex may be spared. In a quantitative study of three examples, Schalch and Friede[803] found a relative excess of granule cells and a deficit of Purkinje cells, suggesting damage to the Purkinje cells before the formation of the external granular layer. In a fourth lesion, however, the internal granular layer was deficient, an observation similar to that of De León *et al.*,[226] who concluded that a relatively late interference with the external gran-

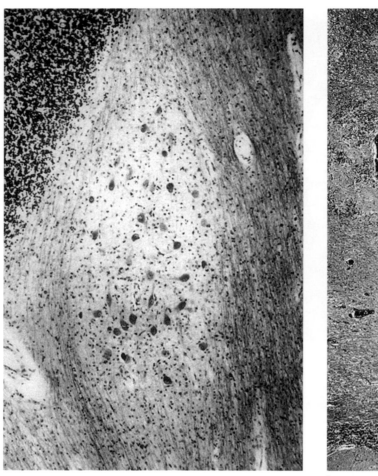

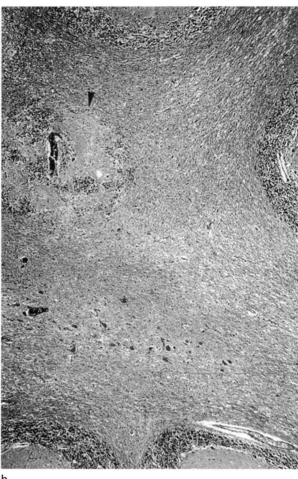

a   b

Figure 7.116 *Cerebellar heterotopias. (a) Small circumscribed collection of large neurons in the folial white matter of a cerebellar hemisphere. (Luxol fast blue–cresyl violet.) (b) Two small heterotopias are incidental findings in an adult: one is a collection of large neurons, the other is an island of heterotopic cortex. (H&E.)*

ular layer was responsible. Superficial destruction might be expected in inflammatory cases, an idea that receives support from experiments in rats and hamsters, where selective destruction of cerebellar meningeal cells by 6-hydroxydopamine appears to destabilize the surface, disrupt the glial scaffold and give rise to cerebellar cortical dysplasia.[498]

Brainstem malformations

OLIVARY HETEROTOPIA

Ectopic segments of inferior olivary nucleus may be found anywhere along the migration route taken by their neuroblastic precursors from the rhombic lip to the ventral medulla.[423] Single or multiple, they comprise small groups of typical olivary neurons and surrounding neuropil, which may also be folded and ensheathed by myelinated fibres in a manner reminiscent of the normal nucleus (Fig. 7.118), although the main part of the nucleus may be dysplastic. Most heterotopias occur laterally,

near the inferior cerebellar peduncle, but some are more medially placed near the rootlets of the hypoglossal nucleus (Fig. 7.119). Autoradiographical studies in the rat[273] demonstrate the majority of olivary neurons to originate laterally in the alar plate, but some arise more medially in the basal plate, which accounts for the medially placed heterotopias. It is presumed that arrested migration leaves stranded precursors to differentiate in an ectopic site. Because migration takes place before the end of the third month,[280] it is not surprising that olivary heterotopias regularly associate with agyria or pachygyria[187,210,243,619,671] (Fig. 7.118), rather than polymicrogyria. Other associations are with the Dandy–Walker syndrome,[378] with cerebral lactic acidosis due to pyruvate dehydrogenase deficiency,[141] and with three cases of megalencephaly, two of trisomy 13, and one with chondrodysplasia and a bizarre gyral pattern (personal observations).

OLIVARY AND DENTATE DYSPLASIAS

In view of their common ancestry from the rhombic lip, it is predictable that malformations of the dentate and the

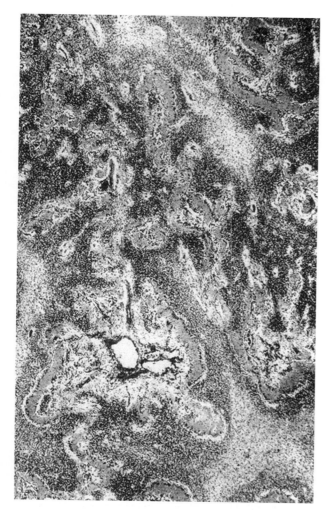

Figure 7.117 *Cerebellar cortical dysplasia in an infant with cerebro-ocular dysplasia. Despite the chaotic appearance of the cortex and lack of foliation the individual layers remain correctly positioned with one another and adjacent molecular layers seem to be fused. (Luxol fast blue–cresyl violet.)*

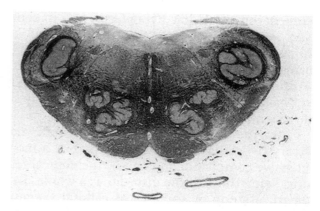

Figure 7.118 *Miller–Dieker syndrome. Horizontal section of the medulla showing multiple olivary heterotopias. Their folded shape and myelin fibre sheaths are reminiscent of the normal nucleus. Here the inferior olives are small and dysplastic. (Luxol fast blue–cresyl violet.)*

these features are combined with an overall C shape and dorsal thickening in several personally studied Zellweger brains (Fig. 7.121). Other varieties of olivary dysplasia include complete disorganization into a group of unconnected segments[815,934] (Fig. 7.122), a solid mass of cells (Fig. 7.123a) and a horseshoe band resembling the initial stage of fetal development (Fig. 7.124a).

As far as the dentate nucleus is concerned, it also can be hyperconvoluted in thanatophoric dysplasia, and simplified or broken into islands or segments in cerebellar hypoplasias and in some cases of trisomy 13[675] and 18.[616] Occasionally, it forms a thick plate without convolution[645] or with interconnected bands and masses of cells (Fig. 125b), or may be unrecognizable (Fig. 123b).

Thus, dentate and olivary dysplasias are often only part of a more extensive complex of anomalies, the clinical

inferior olivary nuclei tend to occur together, to form dentato-olivary dysplasia, but each may also occur separately. The terminology offered is far from satisfactory; terms such as pachygyria and polymicrogyria are quite unsuited to this particular context, necessitating simple description.

The olive may be hyperconvoluted, as in thanatophoric dysplasia,[424,958] or hypoconvoluted, as in cerebellar aplasia or hypoplasia (see above). It may form a simple C-shaped band without folds as described in Joubert's syndrome.[316] Alternatively, the dorsal part of the C may be greatly thickened, sometimes with a peripheral capsule of neurons, a finding noted in trisomy 18[872] and in a personal observation of C trigonocephaly syndrome with callosal agenesis and polymicrogyria (Fig. 7.120). Olivary dysplasia is particularly prominent in Zellweger syndrome. Poverty of convolutions, peripheral margination of neurons and fragmentation of the nucleus have been described in neonates[225,283,931] and in fetal brains.[731] All

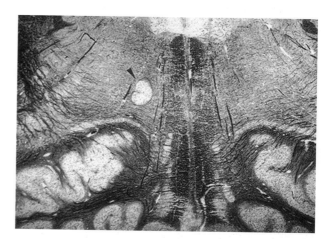

Figure 7.119 *Olivary heterotopia. Ectopic inferior olivary tissue in the medial part of the medullary tegmentum. Case of trisomy 13. Courtesy of Drs RO Barnard and T Revesz, National Hospital for Neurology and Neurosurgery, London, UK. (Luxol fast blue–cresyl violet.)*

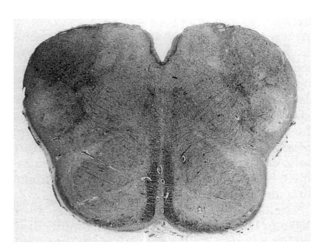

Figure 7.120 *Olivary heterotopia. Olivary dysplasia in a patient with C trigonocephaly syndrome. The olivary nucleus is C shaped, its dorsal part greatly thickened. (Luxol fast blue–cresyl violet.)*

features being those of the disorder as a whole. In a review of 50 cases of callosal agenesis collected over 40 years, Jellinger[460] observed four examples of dentato-olivary dysplasia, but detailed descriptions were not given. Sometimes, however, dentato-olivary dysplasia is the sole significant morphological finding. A remarkably stereotyped dentato-olivary dysplasia has been observed in five children presenting with intractable seizures from early infancy.[100,390] There was severe developmental delay and a variety of seizures occurred, with tonic seizures predominating: the severely abnormal electroencephalograms (EEGs) showed a burst-suppression pattern in the early months of life. Typically, the inferior olives are hook shaped, coarse and lacking undulations, while the dentate nuclei form a compact or club-shaped mass of interconnected grey islands irregularly separated by myelin fibres (Fig. 7.125). Another similar case has since been reported by Robain and Dulac,[763] and three further autopsied examples of this association have been examined, one of whom has a younger sister presenting a strikingly similar clinical picture, suggesting autosomal inheritance.[603a]

The pathogenesis of these lesions is obscure. For some types there is evidence for developmental arrest in the second trimester (Fig. 7.124). In the only detailed study of normal development Murofushi[645] demonstrated the metamorphosis of these nuclei from a hook-shaped plate (olive) or diffuse mass of cells (dentate) at $3\frac{1}{2}$ months of gestation into their typically folded conformations by about 7 months.

MÖBIUS' SYNDROME

Congenital facial diplegia with bilateral abducens palsies[628] produces a striking clinical picture in the neonate: a mask-like, expressionless face with internal strabismus. Other

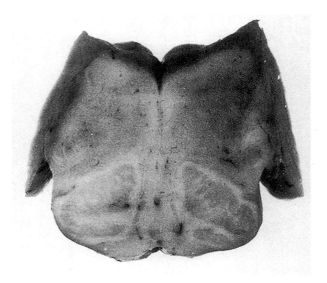

a

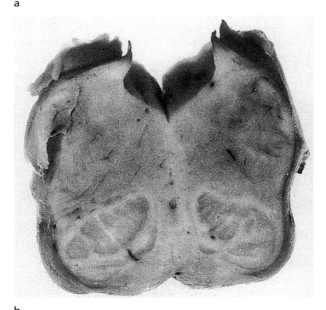

b

Figure 7.121 *Zellweger's syndrome. Adjacent horizontal sections through the medulla (**a, b**). The inferior olivary nuclei are poorly convoluted and fragmented but their basic shape is a dorsally thickened C.*

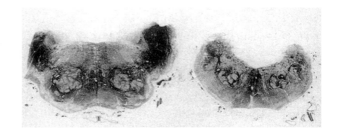

Figure 7.122 *Olivary dysplasia. Horizontal sections of upper and lower medulla. Both inferior olives are broken into a series of convoluted fragments. (Luxol fast blue–cresyl violet.)*

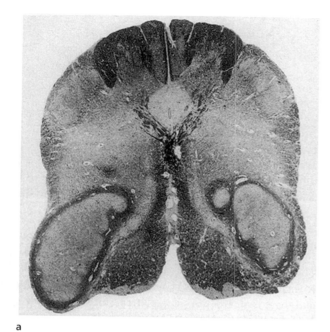

a

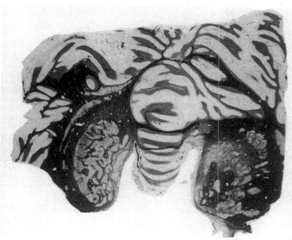

b

Figure 7.123 *Dentato-olivary dysplasia. Identical malformations were present in identical twins suffering a rapidly fatal seizure disorder beginning at 5 months. Another sibling has since presented with a similar clinical disorder. Horizontal sections of medulla (a) and cerebellum (b). The inferior olives are replaced by elliptical masses, while the dentate nucleus is completely disorganized. (Luxol fast blue–cresyl violet.)*

peripheral nerve involvement; focal necrosis and calcification in brainstem nuclei, possibly secondary to fetal infection or anoxia; and myopathy. In the first group, lack of necrosis or evidence of degenerative change, and the presence of other brainstem anomalies such as olivary dysplasia, are strong evidence for a primary malformation.[411,760] Two further autopsied cases have been described briefly by Sudarshan and Goldie;[870] one showed brainstem necrosis, and the other brainstem hypoplasia. In two personally examined cases demonstrating aplasia of nuclei of cranial nerves VII and XII there was olivary dysplasia in one and olivary heterotopia in the other; in a third patient a circumscribed area of old necrosis and calcification involved the brainstem tegmentum including VIth, VIIth, Xth and XIIth cranial nerve nuclei and reticular formation (Fig. 7.126), ultimately leading to sudden death through sleep apnoea.

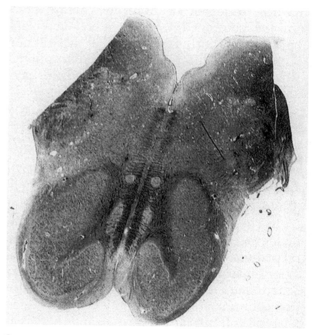

a

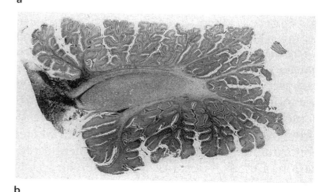

b

Figure 7.124 *Dentato-olivary dysplasia in a neonate. Sections of medulla (a) and cerebellar hemisphere (b). The conformation of both olivary and dentate nuclei is reminiscent of that found in a second trimester fetus. (Luxol fast blue–cresyl violet.)*

oculomotor nerves and lower cranial nerves including the XIIth may also be involved. Skeletal abnormalities, absent muscles and mental retardation are also described:[406] Poland's anomaly (absent pectoralis muscle and symbrachydactyly) is a well-known association. Towfighi *et al.*[895] reported one autopsied case and reviewed 14 others, concluding that Möbius' syndrome was pathologically heterogeneous. They classified the available morphological reports into four groups: aplasia or hypoplasia of cranial nerve nuclei; primary

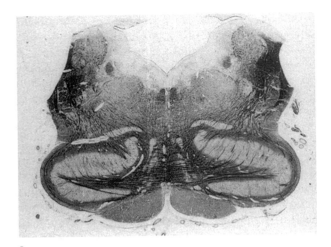

a

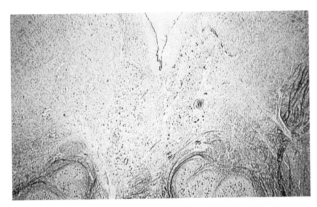

Figure 7.126 *Möbius' syndrome. There is atrophy, gliosis and calcification in the medullary tegmentum. (Luxol fast blue–cresyl violet.)*

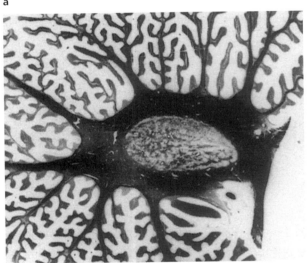

b

Figure 7.125 *Dentato-olivary dysplasia. Sections of medulla (a) and cerebellar hemisphere (b). This particular combination of coarse, hook-shaped olive and apparently solid dentate nucleus lacking a hilum is associated with intractable seizure disorder.[390]*

Harbord *et al.*[384] give a clinical and MRI description of an infant in whom Möbius' syndrome combined with unilateral cerebellar hypoplasia: the authors suggest that these abnormalities could result from a vascular disruption in the basilar artery at between 33 and 40 days of gestation.

ABNORMALITIES OF THE PYRAMIDAL TRACTS

Absence of the corticospinal tracts is usual in anencephaly, holoprosencephaly, porencephaly and hydranencephaly, and an important association has been reported with X-linked congenital aqueduct stenosis.[142] The cerebral peduncles and basis pontis are small, and the inferior olivary nuclei form the ventral border of the medulla (Fig. 7.127). In the spinal cord the dorsal columns are lateral-

ly rotated, the ventral and lateral columns are very small and there is an accessory dorsolateral sulcus.

Unilateral hypertrophy is rare.[36,110,701,800,921,922] Unilateral lesions of the sensorimotor cortex and/or internal capsule in early life may lead to unilateral hypotrophy of the ipsilateral corticospinal tract and hypertrophy of the contralateral fibre bundles. There is obvious asymmetry of the pyramidal tracts throughout the brainstem which continues into the spinal cord, while in the medulla the abnormally large pyramid may displace the inferior olive dorsally (Fig. 7.128). Fibre counts suggest that fibre number rather than size is increased in the hypertrophic tract.[314,800]

Fasciculation of the pyramids into discrete bundles is also occasionally present in malformed brains, as illustrated from a case of polymicrogyria, olivary dysplasia and asymmetry of the pyramidal tracts (Fig. 7.129).

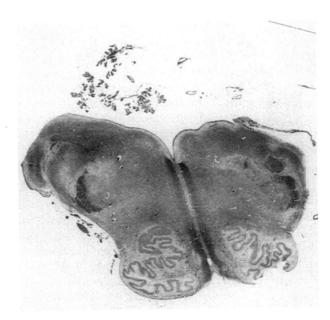

Figure 7.127 *Absence of the pyramids in a case of X-linked hydrocephalus. (Luxol fast blue–cresyl violet.)*

Malformations of the spinal cord

In addition to the severe gross malformations described above under the heading of dysraphic states and usually obvious in the neonatal period, other, less severe, abnormalities may not be suspected on gross examination. Histological examination at many levels of the cord may be required for their identification. These anomalies, usually described in the adult, also raise the question as to whether they are primary malformations or acquired lesions.

SYRINGOMYELIA

The term syringomyelia denotes tubular cavitation of the spinal cord extending over many segments. It may be impossible even at autopsy to distinguish syringomyelia from hydromyelia, although the distinction may have important aetiological implications. Cavities situated in the medulla, syringobulbia, are often associated with syringomyelia. Rarely, cavitation extends into the pons, and exceptionally may reach the midbrain and even the internal capsule.[848]

Clinically, the disease usually begins during the second and third decades and is slowly progressive, or the symptoms may increase at first rapidly and then more slowly. They may cease to progress at any time. Unless associated with bulbar symptoms, the disease rarely causes death directly, but considerable disability is produced by the weakness of limbs and trunk and by the almost invariable spinal deformity. Syringomyelia is usually encountered in

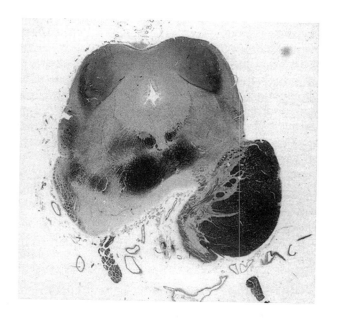
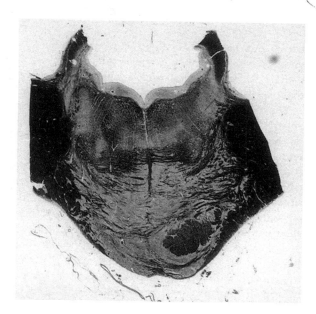
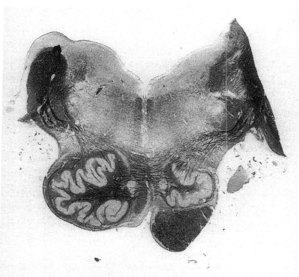
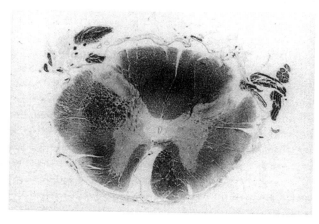

Figure 7.128 *Unilateral hypertrophy of the corticospinal tracts. Horizontal sections of the brainstem and spinal cord. (Luxol fast blue–cresyl violet.)*

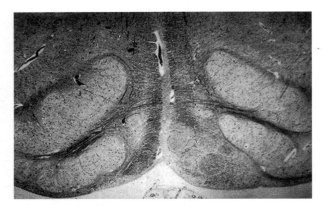

Figure 7.129 *Abnormality of the corticospinal tracts. Section through the ventral part of the medulla showing fasciculation and asymmetry of the pyramids. (Luxol fast blue–cresyl violet.)*

adults but has occasionally occurred in infants, the youngest reported being 5 weeks old.[261] About 90% of patients with idiopathic syringomyelia have Chiari type I malformation.[823]

When exposed at operation or autopsy the spinal cord appears swollen and tense in the cervical region and may fill the spinal canal, an enlargement readily demonstrable radiologically. Externally, apart from the swelling, the spinal cord appears normal and there is no leptomeningeal thickening. The syrinx is filled with a clear fluid,[329] usually of a similar composition to CSF or yellow with a high protein content. When at autopsy the fluid within the syrinx is allowed to escape, the cord becomes flattened, most often in its anteroposterior diameter. A thorough examination of the syrinx may require many transverse sections. The cavity is usually found to be largest in the cervical region but is often absent from the first cervical segment. The syrinx commonly extends through the upper thoracic segments for a varying distance, but the lumbosacral enlargement is rarely involved. In typical cases the cavity in the cervical enlargement extends transversely across the cord, involving the more posterior parts of the ventral horns and passing across the midline behind the central canal. It often extends also into the posterior horns (Fig. 7.130a). When very large, it occupies most of the cross-sectional area of the cord; the more anterior groups of motor nerve cells lie in front of it but otherwise little grey matter remains, and the lateral and posterior white columns are reduced by compression to a narrow zone of fibres (Fig. 7.130b). Extensions in the midline, or more laterally into the posterior columns, are common and the anterior white commissure is often destroyed either by pressure or by a midline anterior extension of the cavity. In the thoracic cord the cavity commonly lies in the posterior horns and is often unilateral. When bilateral, the cavities may be separate or may be joined in the region of the grey commissure and so form a single U-shaped cavity. Serial sections show that cavities that are double at one level usually join into a single cavity at some point above, and it is usual for the cavity on one

side to end at a higher level than the other. More rarely, two cavities join in the lower thoracic region. Although the grey matter is the common site of cavitation, extensions into the posterior or lateral columns or across the white commissure are not unusual, and the cavity may reach the pial surface at the tips of the dorsal horns at any level.

The walls of the cavity vary greatly in character, especially from case to case but also in different parts of the same cavity. Greenfield believed that these variations depended on the age of the cavity and the degree of tension within it. Where there is recent extension the wall is irregular and consists of degenerated neuroglial and neural elements. Myelinated nerve fibres enclosed by sheaths of Schwann cells are commonly found in the wall of the syrinx and have been thought[441] to arise by regeneration from damaged posterior nerve roots. The myelin around the syrinx stains poorly, as it does in the oedematous white matter, and the appearances suggest tearing of the tissues and transudation of serous fluid into them. When the cavity has been established for a long time there is surrounding astrocytic hyperplasia with large fibre-forming astrocytes lying chiefly in a tangential direction to form a dense concentric wall up to 1–2 mm in thickness. It is common to find a thin layer of collagen covering some part of the wall. Thicker strands of colla-

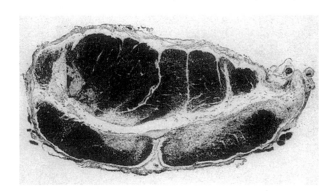

a

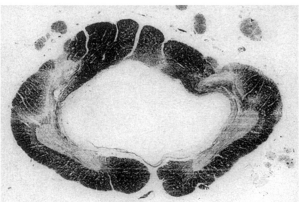

b

Figure 7.130 *Syringomyelia. Transverse sections of the spinal cord stained to demonstrate myelin. (a) Cervical level: the slit-like cavity extends into both posterior horns. (b) Thoracic level: the cavity merges with the central canal. (Loyez's method.)*

gen, or blood vessels with hyalinized walls, may be seen passing across the cavity from one wall to another. Where the cavity communicates with the central canal, as it not uncommonly does, especially in the cervical region, part of the central wall of the cavity is lined with ependymal cells, but in most places these do not take part in the formation of the wall, a feature distinguishing syringomyelia from hydromyelia. When in syringomyelia there is a lining of ependyma, the layer of glial tissue which is deep to the ependymal layer is usually thinner than that surrounding the rest of the cavity.

Syringobulbia

Slit-like cavities in the medulla usually lie in one of three positions.[469]

- The most common is a slit running out in an antero-lateral direction from the floor of the fourth ventricle external to the hypoglossal nucleus. It may communicate with the cavity of the ventricle but sometimes begins anterior to this. It passes outwards and forwards for a variable distance towards the descending tract of the trigeminal nerve, usually destroying the fasciculus solitarius and the fibres that pass dorsally from the nucleus ambiguus to join those arising in the dorsal vagal nucleus (Fig. 7.131c). A cavity in this position is most commonly limited to the lower half or two-thirds of the medulla where it interrupts the fibres passing from the gracile and cuneate nuclei to form the decussation of the medial lemniscus. It may also descend low enough to interrupt many of the decussating pyramidal fibres (Fig. 7.131d). At this level it extends transversely from the grey matter lateral to the central canal to a position anterior to the substantia gelatinosa and the descending tract of the trigeminal nerve. Cavities in this position usually have thin walls of neuroglial tissue.

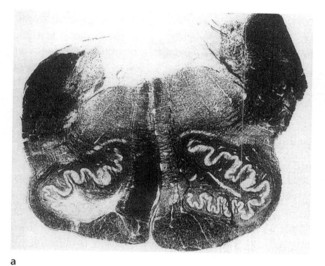

a

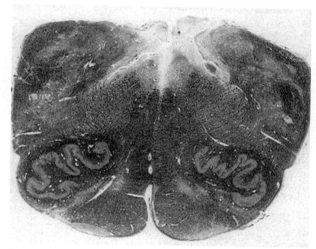

b

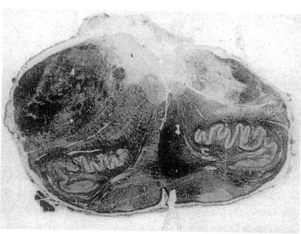

c

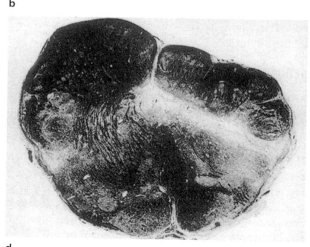

d

Figure 7.131 *Syringobulbia. Transverse sections of medulla. (a) Case with ventral slit between olive and pyramid and dorsolateral slit at a lower level which has produced degeneration of the contralateral medial lemniscus. (b) Case with bilateral dorsolateral and dorsomedial slits. (c) Case with dorsolateral slit producing degeneration of the medial lemniscus. (d) Section at the level of the pyramidal decussation. The lateral extension of the cavity has destroyed the crossed pyramidal fibres. (Loyez's method for myelin.)*

Occasionally the slit is replaced by a neuroglial scar which interrupts the fibre system as completely as a slit or cavity. Such appearances are not uncommon at the upper and lower ends of a cavity, and may arise from secondary fusion of its walls. These cavities are usually unilateral, but may be bilateral and roughly symmetrical (Fig. 7.131b), although extending over differing levels of the cord.

- Almost equally common is an extension of the fourth ventricle along the median raphe for a variable distance. This is usually lined by ependyma, but occasionally is replaced by a neuroglial scar containing ependymal cells or small ependyma-lined tubules, like those seen in atresia of the aqueduct (Fig. 7.131b). By interrupting the decussation of fibres passing from the descending vestibular nucleus to the median longitudinal fasciculus these slits may cause nystagmus, but are otherwise asymptomatic. When this median extension is small and is not associated with other cavitation in the medulla, it scarcely merits the name of syringobulbia.

- A rarer position for a cavity is between the pyramid and the inferior olive, where it interrupts the emerging fibres of the hypoglossal nerve (Fig. 7.131a). These cavities are usually unilateral; in Spiller's case[848] they were bilateral, although only one was large enough to cause atrophic palsy of the tongue. A cavity in this situation may also damage the anteromedian part of the olive or the posterior part of the pyramid.

Cavities in the pons usually lie in the tegmentum, where they may destroy the fibres of the VIth or VIIth cranial nerves, or the central tegmental tract. They may pass down posterior to the olive for a short distance. Extensions of the cavity to a higher level are extremely rare. In Spiller's case the cavity in one pyramid passed up among the corticospinal fibres, destroying also the substantia nigra, and ended in the internal capsule and the caudate and lentiform nuclei.

SECONDARY DEGENERATIONS

Secondary degenerations follow destruction of tracts and fibre systems both in syringomyelia and in syringobulbia. The pyramidal tracts may be pressed on by an anterior cavity between the pyramid and medullary olive, or a slit at a lower level may interrupt pyramidal fibres during their decussation. In the latter case there is commonly some retrograde degeneration of the pyramidal fibres in the medulla. Alternatively, a large cavity in the cervical region may destroy much of the pyramidal tract by compression. The spinocerebellar tracts may degenerate owing to destruction of their cells of origin in the grey matter of the cord or of the fibres leaving these. The fibres passing in the posterior columns may be compressed or destroyed by extensions of the cavity in the cord. In cases of syringobulbia the fibres relayed to the thalamus from the gracile and cuneate nuclei are commonly destroyed as they pass towards the decussation of the medial lemniscus, so there is more or less complete absence of the medial lemniscus on the side opposite to the lesion (Fig. 7.131a, c); retrograde degeneration occurs in the nerve cells of these nuclei. Fibres passing to the spinothalamic tracts are very commonly involved either at or near their cells of origin in the posterior horns or as they cross the midline in the central commissure. The dorsolateral cavities in the medulla commonly interrupt some of the fibres passing inwards from the descending trigeminal nucleus to the medial lemniscus.

A great variety of clinical signs is associated with these lesions. Wasting of the muscles of the hands and forearms, dissociated or complete anaesthesia, paralysis of the lower cranial nerves and facial or corneal analgesia, oculomotor palsies and nystagmus occur depending on the level and extent of the lesions.

SECONDARY SYRINGOMYELIA

This term should be reserved for longitudinal cysts secondary to clearly evident causes. Tumours, trauma, adhesive arachnoiditis, haematomyelia and vascular lesions account for most cases. Most of the cysts are small, but in tumours the associated cystic lesion may be extensive and progressive. Post-traumatic syringomyelia is dealt with in Chapter 14, this Volume.

AETIOLOGY AND PATHOGENESIS

The inclusion of syringomyelia in the large group of spinal cord malformations appears justified at first sight on anatomical grounds, but this may not be correct and brings us little nearer to an understanding of its cause. One difficulty is the distinction of syringomyelia from hydromyelia. Gardner[329] summarized his conclusions in the statement that 'syringomyelia is symptomatic hydromyelia'. This view was derived from the finding of a malformation of the hindbrain obstructing the foramen of Magendie in a large proportion of cases. Gardner proposed that this obstruction causes distension initially of the central canal which may then rupture, allowing CSF to escape into the substance of the spinal cord. In hydromyelia there is an undoubted association with neural tube malformations. It is also possible in some cases to trace the development of a syringomyelic cavity from hydromyelia; for example, in cases of Chiari's malformation in the adult, but this is true for only a minority of cases. Syringomyelia is only occasionally familial.

Several different factors may be combined in the pathogenesis of cavitation in syringomyelia. (1) Instability in the lines of junction of the alar and basal laminae with each other is suggested by the position of the cavities, particularly in the medulla, along lines of fusion which occur relatively late in fetal life. (2) The constant movements of flexion and torsion to which the cervical cord and lower medulla are exposed when the neck is bent or the head is turned[804] must impose stresses which may well cause small tears of the tissue in the centre of the cord, explaining the tendency for cavities to begin and attain greatest size in the cervical region. (3) Once cavitation in the spinal cord has begun, it may be enlarged by transudation of fluid into it under pressure. This expansion is more likely to occur in the grey matter than in the firmer columns of white matter and, owing to the restricting investment of pia mater, must take place chiefly upwards and downwards. It is favoured by anything that increases venous congestion in the body cavity, such as muscular effort, since there are no valves on the veins draining the spinal cord. The fact that a syringomyelic cavity usually ceases at the C2 level and has no communications with the fourth ventricle may also be of considerable importance.[848]

ASYMMETRY OF CROSSING OF THE CORTICOSPINAL TRACTS

Failure to decussate is rare,[922] but asymmetrical decussation is a not uncommon finding in neonates (Fig. 7.132). The classic concept of the decussation of the pyramidal tract and of anterior (direct) and lateral (crossed) fibres was revised by Yakovlev,[965] who studied fetal and neonatal brains in serial sections stained for myelin. The pyramidal tracts are readily identified in the spinal cord of the very young because they are poorly myelinated and their size and shape can be studied more easily than in adults. Most frequently, the fibres of the left pyramidal tract cross the midline first, and pass anteriorly to those of the right.

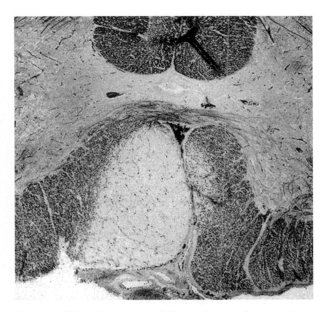

Figure 7.132 *Malformation of the corticospinal tracts. Transverse section of cervical spinal cord. There is marked asymmetry of the direct pyramidal tracts (unmyelinated in the neonate and therefore pale in section stained for myelin).*

Moreover, the cord is usually asymmetric. Nathan *et al.*[656] found three-quarters of these asymmetric cords to be larger on the right side owing to a greater number of corticospinal fibres crossing to the right. Crossing from left to right occurs at a more cranial level than the reverse. Two other rare anomalies have been described: a superficially placed lateral tract[314,922] and fibres crossing into the dorsal columns[922] where they are normally found in rodents.

ARTHROGRYPOSIS MULTIPLEX CONGENITA

The clinical presentation of multiple congenital contractures can result from a multiplicity of prenatal disorders that cause fetal hypokinesia.[629] Clinicopathological studies of large series of cases[38,373] indicate most to be neurogenic, and fewer myopathic. Neurogenic causes include many examples of developmental brain disease, either acquired destructive lesions or malformation syndromes (trisomy 18, Arnold–Chiari, Meckel–Gruber, Marden–Walker or Möbius). Anterior horn cell degeneration is a frequent cause, but morphological studies suggest subtle differences from Werdnig–Hoffmann disease.[148] It is also important to distinguish the cerebral and spinal pathology of Pena–Shokeir syndrome, an autosomal recessive lethal condition, which comprises camptodactyly, multiple ankyloses, facial dysmorphism, polyhydramnios, fetal growth retardation and pulmonary hypoplasia.[372]

Vascular malformations

ANEURYSMAL MALFORMATION OF THE VEIN OF GALEN

This is the most frequent form observed in the neonate. The first recognition of the abnormality is attributed to Wohak.[956] More than 100 cases have been reviewed by Lagos.[513] The malformation is not a true aneurysm but an arteriovenous fistula, the vein of Galen undergoing aneurysmal dilatation.[417] The dilated vein of Galen (Fig. 7.133) is generally fed by blood from one or both posterior cerebral arteries or one of their branches (Fig. 7.134), and less frequently from small posterior branches of the middle cerebral arteries. The aneurysm may also be fed by anomalous branches of the carotid and/or basilar circulation.[555] The blood vessels may have a normal architecture, but more often a lace-like network of tortuous vessels empties into the saccular vein of Galen, which may be up to several centimetres in diameter. The entire venous system, including transverse and straight sinuses, is dilated. If the shunt is large, clinical signs may develop soon after birth or within a few weeks. Silverman *et al.*[832] and Pollock and Laslett[728] were the first to point out that cerebral arteriovenous fistula can lead to cardiomegaly and congestive cardiac failure in the newborn, and many cases have since been recognized.[347,428,562]

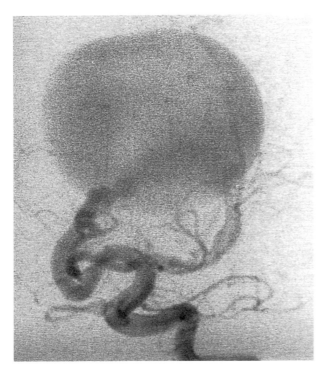

Figure 7.133 *Aneurysm of the great vein of Galen. This angiogram demonstrates at least two fistulae from the markedly hypertrophic posterior choroidal arteries. Courtesy of Dr W Taylor. National Hospital for Neurology and Neurosurgery, London, UK.*

The differential diagnosis from congenital heart defect is important. In arteriovenous fistula, auscultation over the surface of the skull may reveal a continuous murmur, indicating the flow of blood through the fistula;[543,562] this sign may be found in 80% of cases.[428] In addition, twitching or generalized tonic convulsions[146] and hydrocephalus may occur as a result of compression of the aqueduct.[150,632,791]

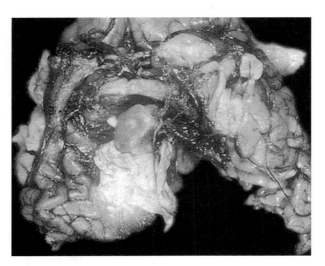

Figure 7.134 *Aneurysm of the vein of Galen. The hemispheres are splayed apart to reveal the aneurysm and its feeding blood vessels from the posterior cerebral artery.*

Various cerebral lesions, either in the territory of the corresponding arteries or elsewhere, have been described in association with this vascular malformation, including periventricular infarction and intraventricular haemorrhage due to compression by the tumour-like vascular mass[670,810] and periventricular calcification.[715] In addition, the aneurysm itself may become calcified[834] or thrombosed.[531]

Other arteriovenous malformations may be located elsewhere. In the neonate, communication between the anterior or middle cerebral arteries and the sagittal sinus[861] or between a branch of the middle cerebral artery and the lateral sinus[126] have been described. An arteriovenous malformation involving cerebellar veins and arteries in a complicated network of blood vessels over the vermis was found in a premature infant.[33] These vascular malformations probably result from failure of the primitive capillary plexus to differentiate into mature arterial and venous channels.

STURGE–WEBER SYNDROME (ENCEPHALOFACIAL ANGIOMATOSIS)

This neurocutaneous syndrome, characterized by naevus formation in the skin in the territories of the sensory branches of the Vth cranial nerve, and by ocular angioma, was first described clinically by Sturge in 1879.[869] In 1897 Kalischer demonstrated the meningeal angiomatosis[473] and in 1923 Dimitri described skull calcification on X-ray, later shown to be intracerebral.[246] There is excessive vascularity of the meninges, the small veins being tortuous and increased in number, giving a dark purple colour to the cerebral surface. On sectioning the brain, calcification may be readily visible beneath the hypervascularized meninges in the outer cortical layers. On microscopic examination (Fig. 7.135), the walls of the blood vessel are encrusted with deposits of iron and calcium, and calcific granular deposits of varying size lie freely in the parenchyma. Polymicrogyria and heterotopias may also be found in the cerebrum and cerebellum. The port-wine stain of the face is present at birth, as is buphthalmos in 70% of cases.[914] Intracranial calcification has exceptionally been reported in neonates[820] and diagnosed on CT scan.[683]

Focal neurological signs and cerebral atrophy may be evident at birth, but most of the symptoms such as hemiparesis, hemiplegia, epilepsy and mental retardation begin within the first year of life[856] or in early childhood.[140,363] The pathogenesis of the disease is not known, but incomplete involution of the embryonal vasculature has been proposed.[140] Although familial cases have been reported, there is no clear evidence for hereditary transmission.

FOWLER'S SYNDROME: PROLIFERATIVE VASCULOPATHY AND HYDRANENCEPHALY–HYDROCEPHALY

It is most important to differentiate between this rare familial syndrome, first described in five siblings by

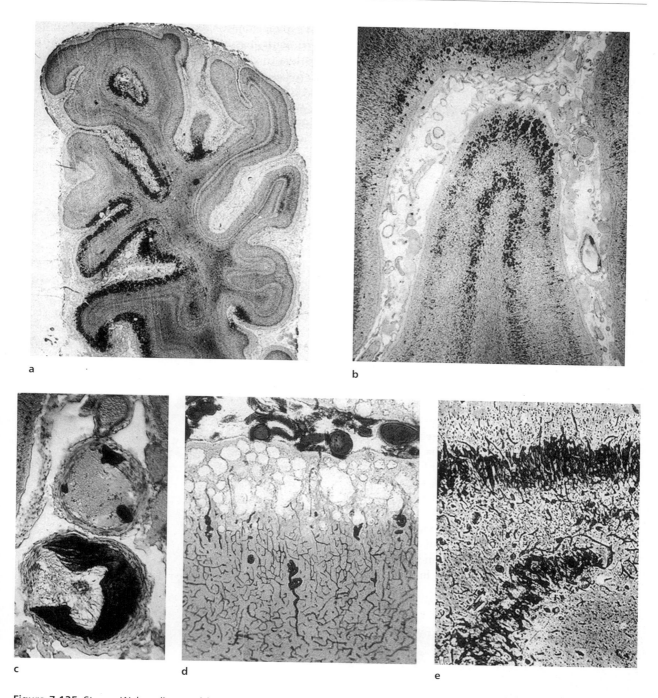

Figure 7.135 *Sturge–Weber disease. (a) Low-power view of section through the occipital pole showing the meningeal venous angioma and the darkly stained dense calcification mainly in the outer layers of the cortex. (Carbol azure.) (b) A higher power view of the meninges and cortex of the occipital pole. The calcification affects deeper as well as superficial layers of the cortex. (Carbol azure.) (c) Calcified meningeal arteries. (Carbol azure.) (d) Abnormal convoluted blood vessels in the non-calcified layer of the cerebral cortex. (Masson's trichrome.) (e) Adventitial fibrosis occasionally found in areas of laminar calcification. The calcium deposits are peculiarly dense and powdery in these areas. (Gomori's reticulin.)*

Fowler, and the more typical sporadically occurring encephaloclastic form of hydranencephaly from which it is ultrasonographically and macroscopically indistinguishable. To date there have been four published reports.[307,392,394,672]

Clinical and pathological findings are remarkably consistent. Recurrent intrauterine death or therapeutic interruption of pregnancy following ultrasound demonstration of 'hydranencephaly' as early as 13 weeks' gestation reveals an abortus with severe arthrogryposis,

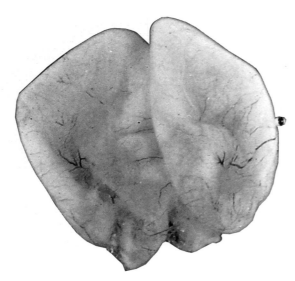

Figure 7.136 *Fowler's syndrome, or proliferative vasculopathy and hydranencephaly–hydrocephaly. Cystic cerebral hemispheres in a 17-week fetus. Reproduced by permission from J Neuropathol Appl Neurobiol.*[392]

pterygia and muscular hypoplasia, and massive cystic dilatation of the ventricles (Fig. 7.136). Although extremely attenuated, the cerebral wall retains some degree of normal organization with a thin but recognizable ventricular zone and persistence of radial glia.[392] However, the cortical plate is very thin, interrupted or folded; there is a greatly reduced population of neurons, scattered calcospherites, and a most remarkable and pathognomonic glomeruloid vascular proliferation (Fig. 7.137). These striking vascular structures, composed of inclusion-bearing endothelial cells[392] (Fig. 7.138a), are found in all parts of the CNS including the germinal matrix and the spinal cord (Fig. 7.138b), and in Fowler's case also in the retina, but

not in the leptomeninges or other tissues. Calcifications are particularly massive near the ventricular surface of the basal ganglia and only here is there minor evidence of necrosis.

The presence of pterygia[672] and ultrasound evidence of well-established hydranencephaly by 13 weeks of gestation[392] date the onset of this autosomal recessive disorder to the first trimester; Norman and McGillivray[672] considered a primary failure of neuroectodermal proliferation to occur before the seventh week. Alternatively,

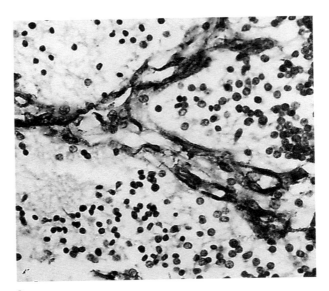

a

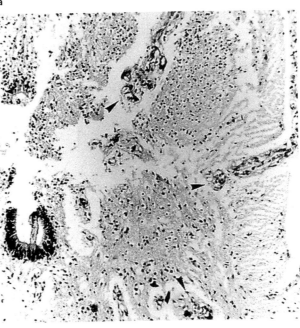

b

Figure 7.138 *Same case as Fig. 7.140. (a) The constituent cells of the glomeruli are decorated by antibodies to the endothelial marker,* Ulex europaeus *lectin. (b) Vascular glomeruloids are widespread in CNS tissue: several (arrowheads) are shown in the spinal cord.*

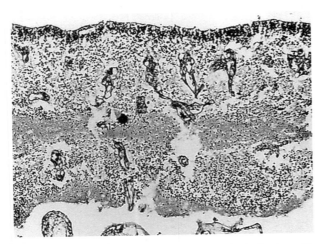

Figure 7.137 *Same case as Fig. 7.140. Histologically the pallium is severely attenuated and contains numerous glomeruloid vascular structures. (Gordon and Sweet silver impregnation for reticulin fibres.)*

since vascular channels first appear in the pallium at about the time when neuronal migration begins, and may be critical to the survival of neuronoglial precursors, it could be argued that glomeruloid changes set in train a destructive process.[392] Massive cystic ventricular dilatation could then be a consequence of an altered hydrodynamic equilibrium between CSF pressure and the attenuated and weakened cerebral wall, since CSF pressure is known to exert a powerful effect on embryonic brain enlargement.[241]

DIFFUSE MENINGOCEREBRAL ANGIODYSPLASIA AND RENAL AGENESIS

This rare association has been documented in three isolated reports[120,501,914] and a fourth example is depicted in Fig. 7.139. All were premature stillbirths with bilateral renal agenesis and other features typical of the oligohydramnios sequence, namely Potter's facies, contraction deformities of the limbs and bilateral pulmonary hypoplasia. A diffuse angiodysplasia, of dilated and thrombosed capillaries and venules, involves the leptomeninges and parenchyma of the cerebral hemispheres, and is associated with extensive infarction and calcification.

Arachnoid cysts

Arachnoid cysts have been the subject of an abundant literature.[820] However, there seems to be some confusion concerning the definition itself as well as the pathogenesis of the lesions. Anomalies as diverse as dilated cisterns, ependymal cysts of the cavum vergae, diverticula of the ventricles and cysts of neural origin have been described under the term 'congenital arachnoid cyst'. Strictly speaking, the so-called primary arachnoid cyst should be regarded as a developmental abnormality of the arachnoid.[363,683,856] Ultrastructural studies[140,750,801] have demon-

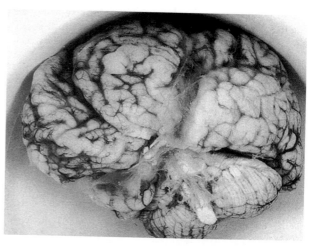

Figure 7.140 *Arachnoid cysts. Bilateral sylvian fissure arachnoid cysts in a 9-month-old child. (Photographed in water.)*

strated that the cyst is formed by splitting of the arachnoid membrane, which is reinforced by a thick layer of collagen. The wall of the cyst is totally independent of the inner layer of the dura mater. The fine structure of the cells is similar to that of normal trabecular arachnoid cells.

In more than 200 cases of arachnoid cyst the distribution of the cysts was: sylvian fissure 49% (Fig. 7.140), cerebellopontine angle 11%, supracollicular area 10%, vermis 9%, interhemispheric fissure 5%, cerebral convexity 4%, and the clival and interpeduncular area 3%.[750]

Arachnoid cysts are rare in neonates. Larroche[520] found five in about 3000 consecutive fetal and neonatal autopsies: two extended over the convexity of the hemispheres (Fig. 7.141a) or filled the interhemispheric fissure (Fig. 7.141b) (in one there was an associated absence of the septum pellucidum), one occurred over the temporal pole, and two occurred in the posterior fossa over a cerebellar hemisphere, clearly differing from a Dandy–Walker malformation. Other types of cyst have been reported in the neonatal period. Loeser and Alvord[557] described a cluster of interhemispheric cysts attached to the falx, with absence of the corpus callosum. These were lined by ependyma and contained choroid plexus, features that might be found in diverticula of the third ventricle. A dilated cavum veli interpositi may be mistaken for a cyst or a posterior fossa tumour.[884] Haemorrhage in this area with secondary hydrocephalus due to compression of the aqueduct of Sylvius was reported by Lourie and Berne,[563] and a paracollicular plate cyst described in a baby born after a difficult labour and containing stigmata of old haemorrhage[505] may represent a link between primary and secondary arachnoid cysts. The possibility exists that the anomalies may be overlooked at autopsy in fetuses and neonates, or certain cysts may develop and become symptomatic only after birth. Occasional cases have been diagnosed in neonates by CT scan[400] and by ultrasound.[578]

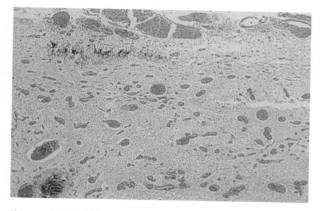

Figure 7.139 *Diffuse meningocerebral angiodysplasia and renal agenesis. Leptomeninges (arrowhead) and cerebral parenchyma are studded with numerous dilated and thrombosed capillaries. Infarction and calcification ensue. (H&E.)*

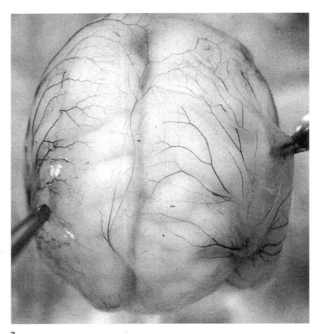

a

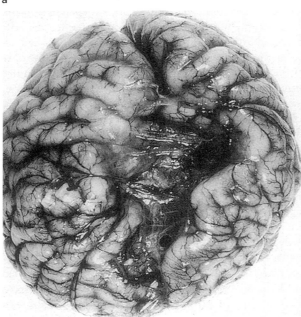

b

Figure 7.141 *Arachnoid cysts. (a) Cystic dilatation of sub-arachnoid space extending over the convexities of both hemispheres in a neonatal brain. (b) Arachnoid cyst in the interhemispheric fissure.*

Phakomatosis

TUBEROUS SCLEROSIS (BOURNEVILLE'S DISEASE)

This complex disorder of protean manifestations was first described by von Recklinghausen[747] in a neonate with cardiac rhabdomyomata, but the name tuberous sclerosis was invoked by Bourneville[99] in a 3-year-old girl with mental retardation, seizures and facial angiofibromas.[91] Recent clinical and morphological reviews include that of Fryer and Osborne[321] and the monograph edited by Gomez.[346]

The brain is the most frequently affected organ in tuberous sclerosis. Brain weights, although usually normal, can range widely from microcephalic to megalencephalic. The characteristic lesions are cortical tubers, subependymal nodules and heterotopias in the white matter, all of which have been recorded in fetuses as early as 28 weeks of gestation.[139,818] In the unfixed brain, cortical tubers are readily recognizable as firm nodules projecting slightly above the surface of the cortex, but they are even more striking after the leptomeninges have been stripped (Figs 7.142, 7.143). In fetal and neonatal brains tubers are not so visually prominent but are obvious on palpation. Varying in size from millimetres to several centimetres, tubers are rounded or wart-like protrusions of single or adjacent

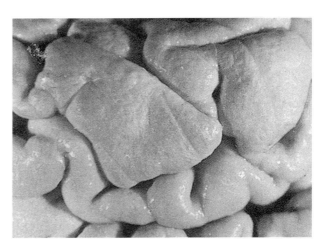

Figure 7.142 *Tuberous sclerosis. A cortical tuber (Pellizzi type 1) is shown as a widened and flattened region of a gyrus. The surface is slightly granular and the tuber is pale and firm to the touch. The leptomeninges have been stripped off.*

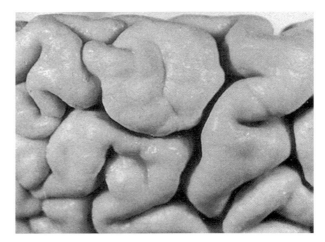

Figure 7.143 *Tuberous sclerosis. A cortical tuber (Pellizzi type 2) appears as a rounded flattened nodule with a rough dimpled surface. The tuber is elevated above the surrounding brain, from which it is demarcated by a sulcus.*

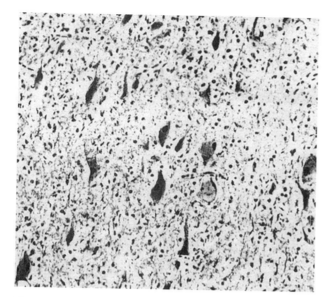

Figure 7.144 *Tuberous sclerosis. Section of a cortical tuber showing giant cells. (Hortega's silver carbonate method for astrocytes.)*

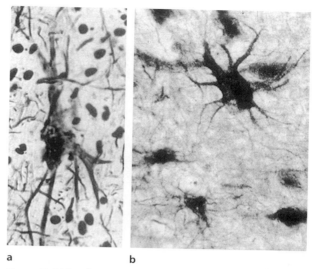

Figure 7.146 *Tuberous sclerosis. Giant cells of astrocytic type in a cortical tuber. (a, Hortega's method; b, Cajal's gold sublimate method.)*

gyri, very firm to the touch and pale in colour. They may be wide and flat or round and dimpled (Figs 7.142, 7.143).[714] Scattered randomly over the cortical surface, up to 40 have been observed in a single brain. On coronal section, tubers greatly expand the gyri and blur the margin between grey and white matter; they may also be present in the depths of sulci. Histologically, the normal cortical architecture is effaced by collections of large, bizarre cells with stout processes, peripheral vacuolation, prominent nucleoli and sometimes multiple nuclei (Figs

7.144–7.147). With conventional stains they may be characterized as atypical astrocytes or abnormal malorientated neurons, but many are indeterminate. Neurofibrillary tangles, argentophilic globules and granulovacuolar degeneration have also been described.[418] Clusters of these abnormal cells may also be found widely scattered in the deep white matter and macroscopically normal cortex. The tuber may show a marked fibrillary gliosis, particularly in the subpial zone where fibres are condensed into sheaf-like structures (Fig. 7.148). In older individuals myelin staining stops abruptly like a flat plate beneath the abnormal cortex, while the gyral core is depleted of myelin and is gliotic (Fig. 7.149). Tubers may calcify and multiple 'brain stones' can be seen radiologically.[967] Tubers are occasionally present in the cerebellum;[86] disorganized cortex, abnormal astrocytes and Purkinje cells and calcification are the main features (Fig. 7.150).

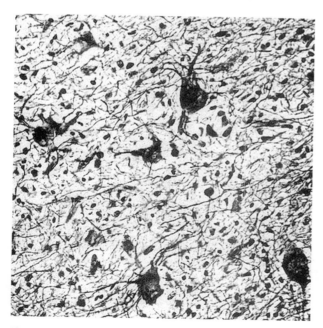

Figure 7.145 *Tuberous sclerosis. A group of large abnormal cells in a cortical tuber. They are stained by Bielschowsky's silver method, suggesting a neuronal phenotype.*

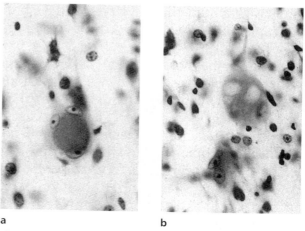

Figure 7.147 *Tuberous sclerosis. (a) Multinucleated cell in a tuber. (Carbol azure.) (b) Large cells with vacuolated cytoplasm. (Carbol azure.)*

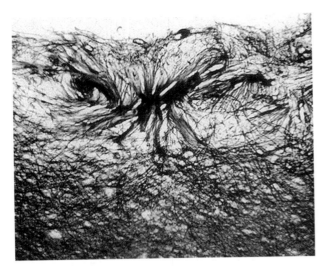

Figure 7.148 *Tuberous sclerosis. Sheaf-like bundles of neuroglial fibres in the superficial part of a cortical tuber. (Holzer's method.)*

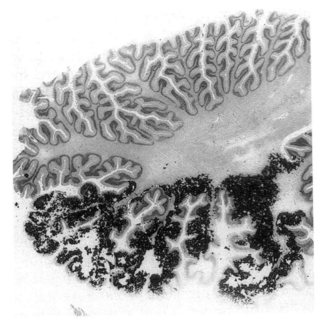

a

Subependymal nodules may occur in the third and fourth ventricles, even the aqueduct, but most are found in the lateral ventricles, particularly near the sulcus terminalis with their deeper parts embedded in the caudate nucleus or thalamus. They are firm, or stony hard due to calcification, and form round or elongated protrusions into the ventricles, either singly or in rows, when they have been likened to candle gutterings (Fig. 7.151). Nodules at the foramen of Monro are of particular clinical importance because they may obstruct the foramen to cause hydrocephalus. Histologically (Fig. 7.152), beneath a covering layer of ependyma there is a mixture of elongated or markedly swollen glial cells and their processes, giant or multinucleated cells, and often marked calcium deposition, while in neonates there may be scattered clusters

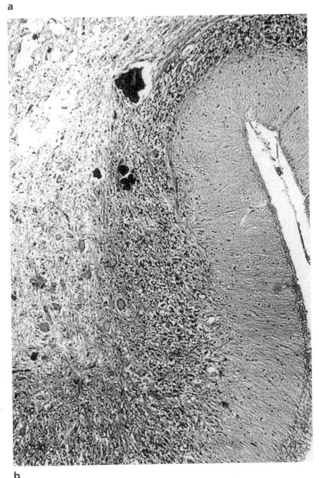

b

Figure 7.150 *Tuberous sclerosis. (a) A cerebellar tuber with extensive calcification in the inferior part of the hemisphere. (b) Higher magnification shows disorganized cortex and destruction of the white matter. There are large astrocytes and calcospherites. (H&E.)*

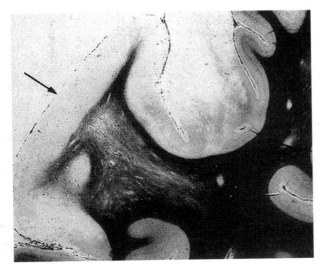

Figure 7.149 *Tuberous sclerosis. A cortical tuber (arrow) overlies the flat margin of the central core of white matter which shows a paucity of myelin and is also gliosed. (Heidenhain's method for myelin.)*

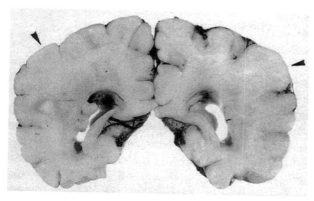

Figure 7.151 *Tuberous sclerosis. Tuberous sclerosis in a premature infant. There are multiple subependymal nodules and cortical tubers (arrowheads).*

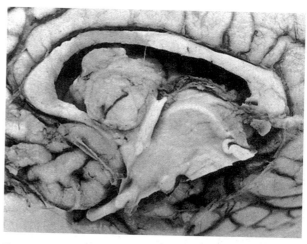

Figure 7.153 *Tuberous sclerosis. A large tumour arises from a subependymal nodule over the caudate nucleus in an adult case of tuberous sclerosis.*

of neuroblasts. A sequential CT study[636] has documented the gradual progression of a subependymal nodule into a subependymal giant cell astrocytoma (Fig. 7.153) (see also Chapter 11, Volume II). Histologically, the distinction between the two is far from clear, but for the clinician signs of raised intracranial pressure herald the presence of a tumour with enhanced growth potential and a potentially lethal location.

Much discussion has attended the ontogenesis of the bizarre giant cells in tuberous sclerosis. Ultrastructural studies have indicated both astrocytic and neuronal features.[67,218,754,833,898] Several immunohistochemical studies, however,[90,139,653,818,859] have shown a paucity of staining for GFAP in the subependymal giant cells (Fig. 7.154), and some authors have noted a high proportion of GFAP-positive cells in subcortical lesions and cortical tubers, suggesting that acquisition of GFAP is associated with migration.[139,818] Concomitant expression of neurofilament[90,139] and galactocerebroside[139] has also been reported. It seems that both migration and differentiation are disturbed in these apparently pluripotential cells.

There is a high incidence of seizures in patients with tuberous sclerosis and they usually commence within the first few months of life when their significance may be underestimated in the absence of skin signs.[346,631] Mental retardation is the second most common neurological manifestation. Evidence of raised intracranial pressure is found in about 5% of cases. Behavioural problems are common and include hyperactivity, screaming, destructiveness, aggression, sleeplessness, self-mutilation and autism.

Skin manifestations, the most common clinical findings in tuberous sclerosis, are of five types. Hypomelanotic

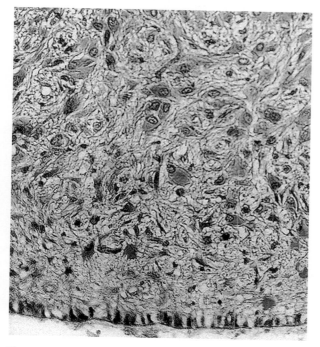

Figure 7.152 *Tuberous sclerosis. Subependymal nodule in a neonatal case of tuberous sclerosis. The cells are large with a single rounded nucleus and abundant eosinophilic cytoplasm, and are intermingled with leashes or whorls of glial fibres.*

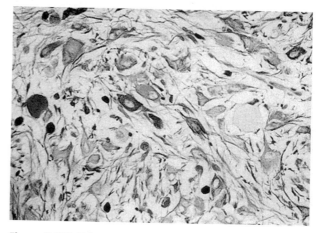

Figure 7.154 *Tuberous sclerosis. Subependymal nodule. Immunohistochemistry for GFAP shows marked variation in reactivity. Only a minority of giant cells are strongly positive.*

macules, 1–3 cm in diameter, are present in 90% of patients, but may only be visible under Wood's light and may not be found in early life. Facial angiofibromas (adenoma sebaceum) form a butterfly rash over the cheeks, nose, lower lip and chin, and appear at between 2 and 5 years of age. Periungual or subungual fibromas, more often on toes than on fingers, rarely occur before puberty, and may be the sole manifestation of the disease. Shagreen patches, which are fibrous hamartomas of dorsal surfaces, are rarely seen before puberty, whereas fibrous plaques on the forehead and scalp can be the earliest skin sign. Poliosis and leucotrichia are also common.

In the Mayo Clinic series[346] 50% of patients had ocular involvement. The characteristic lesion is the retinal giant cell astrocytoma, but other diagnostically significant lesions include hypopigmented iris spots, white eyelashes and hamartomata of the eyelids and conjunctivae.

Cardiac rhabdomyoma, whether single or multiple are common: *in vivo* studies using two-dimensional echocardiography found an incidence of 50% in the population attending a paediatric neurology clinic,[55] and 64% in a combined child and adult population.[336] Rhabdomyomata have been reported in a fetus of 6 months' gestation,[533] and in several other fetal cases presenting with hydrops.[139] In general, these tumours are slow growing and asymptomatic, but may cause obstruction to flow, myocardial dysfunction, cardiac arrhythmias and sudden death.[131,902,916] The tumours grow within the ventricular walls and, although not encapsulated, are sharply demarcated from surrounding myocardium. Some form large pedunculated masses which protrude into the chambers of the heart, obstructing flow (Fig. 7.155). Histologically, the tumour cells are large, up to 20 μm in diameter, with eccentrically placed single or multiple nuclei, and vacuolated glycogen-containing cytoplasm with fine cytoplasmic strands (spider cells) (Fig. 7.156).

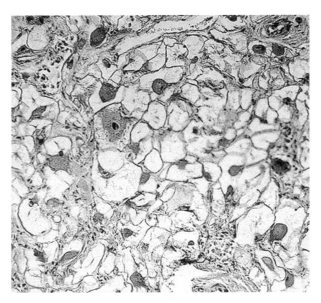

Figure 7.156 *Tuberous sclerosis. Typical microscopic appearance of one of the multiple rhabdomyomatous nodules found in the tuberous sclerosis complex. (H&E.)*

In the Mayo Clinic series[346] 55% of living patients had renal lesions. Angiomyolipomas, usually multiple, are the most common, but they are rare under 10 years of age. Renal cysts are less frequent, but may present in infancy. The lungs, liver, adrenals, thyroid, gonads, teeth, gums and bones may also be affected.

In recent years there has been increased recognition of milder forms of tuberous sclerosis, and older prevalence figures have been radically revised: the Oxford prevalence study suggested that the true prevalence for 0–5 years could be as high as 1 in 10 000.[442] Tuberous sclerosis is inherited as an autosomal dominant trait with very high penetrance.[43] It had been thought that the large number of new cases was explicable in terms of a high mutation rate, but studies of asymptomatic family members with cranial CT scanning have identified a significant proportion with abnormalities.[304]

Linkage studies have shown locus heterogeneity with disease-determining genes mapped to chromosome 9q34 (designated *TSC1* gene) and 16p13.3 (*TSC2* gene).[282,320] Allele loss (i.e. loss of heterozygosity) for 16p13.3 has recently been demonstrated in hamartomas, a cortical tuber and a giant cell astrocytoma from patients with tuberous sclerosis, consistent with the hypothesis that *TSC2* acts as a tumour suppressor gene.[358]

HYPOMELANOSIS OF ITO

This rare neurocutaneous syndrome has a variable phenotype.[344] The few neuropathological reports indicate some similarities with tuberous sclerosis and cortical dysplasia, although the process extends more widely and shows a lesser degree of cytological dysplasia.[587,776] Megalencephaly, firm macrogyric convolutions, loss of cortical

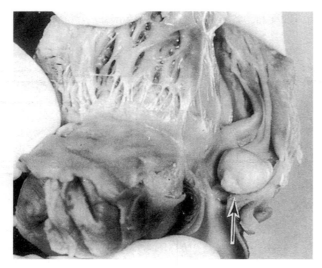

Figure 7.155 *Tuberous sclerosis. Dissection of the heart of a neonate with tuberous sclerosis. A large rhabdomyoma obstructs the left ventricular outflow tract (arrow).*

layering and widespread neuronal heterotopia, with reactive (not giant) astrocytes and Rosenthal fibres, are the chief morphological features.

VON RECKLINGHAUSEN'S DISEASE

See Chapter 11, Volume II.

Hydrocephalus

An overview of the causes of hydrocephalus in childhood is given in Table 7.5; the content of this section will roughly follow this plan. However, since general aspects of the subject are dealt with in Chapter 4, this Volume, only developmental lesions producing hydrocephalus will be described here, concentrating on those lesions not covered earlier in the chapter.

IMBALANCE BETWEEN PRODUCTION AND DRAINAGE OF CSF

Most frequently this results from obstruction to the flow of CSF:[790] extrinsic tumours may compress the ventricular system, while intraventricular tumours, malformations, haemorrhage and inflammation directly impede flow.

Obstruction to the foramina of Monro

This is usually the result of neoplasia, neonatal meningitis and ventriculitis or the aftermath of intraventricular haemorrhage, but there are rare reports of unilateral hydrocephalus secondary to membranous obstruction of one foramen,[942] including intrauterine diagnosis by ultrasound at 29 weeks of gestation.[652] In one case, the obstructive glial–ependymal membrane and other subtle anomalies suggested an early developmental onset.[716]

Obliteration of the third ventricle

This is exceptional. Fusion of the thalami has been demonstrated post-mortem in one of two siblings presenting with neonatal hydrocephalus,[143] and in a unique association with aqueductal atresia and rhombo-encephalosynapsis.[487]

Connatal obstruction of the aqueduct of Sylvius

Russell[790] emphasized the importance of the aqueduct, the narrowest part of the ventricular system, as a site of maldevelopmental causes of hydrocephalus, but her attempts to define clear-cut categories for the lesions, stenosis, forking (atresia) and septum formation which she regarded as malformative, in contrast to gliotic lesions which were considered a sequel to acquired inflammation, have excited much controversy. Subsequent investigators have varied in their use of this terminology, and individual cases may defy simple categorization.[254] Several considerations necessitate modification of her schema. It has become increasingly realized that the distinction between congenital and acquired

Table 7.5 *A scheme for hydrocephalus in childhood*

(A) Imbalance between production and drainage of CSF
   (1) Overproduction of CSF: choroid plexus papilloma
   (2) Interference with CSF movement
      (a) Reduced propulsion: ciliary dysplasia
      (b) Physical block to flow
         (i) Ventricular system
            Tumours
               Intrinsic block
               Extrinsic compression
            Malformation
               Membranous obstruction to the foramen of Monro
               Obliteration of the third ventricle
               Connatal obstruction of the aqueduct of Sylvius (atresia, stenosis, vascular anomaly)
               Obstruction to foramina of Luschka and Magendie (atresia, Dandy–Walker, arachnoid cyst)
            Inflammation and haemorrhage and their consequences
               Adhesions in lateral ventricle, obliteration of foramen of Monro
               Gliosis or septum of aqueduct
               Gliosis or fibrosis of fourth ventricle outlets
         (ii) Subarachnoid space
            Chiari malformation at foramen magnum
            Diffuse obliteration: cerebro-ocular dysplasias
            Fibrosis: after haemorrhage, meningitis, mucopolysaccharidosis
   (3) Failure of absorption
            Absence of arachnoid granulations and cilia
             Functional changes: cranial dysplasias

(B) Developmental abnomalies: ventriculomegaly of uncertain pathogenesis

(C) Following destruction or degeneration of brain tissue
            Hypoxic–ischaemic (prenatal or postnatal)
             Degenerative (grey or white matter)

(D) Mixed due to (A) and (C)

lesions is somewhat artificial. The aqueduct develops as a gradual narrowing of the neural tube[905] which has *ab initio* a lumen, so all obstructions are, strictly speaking, acquired. Furthermore, absence of gliosis does not militate against an infectious aetiology, as demonstrated by experimental induction of aqueduct stenosis in hamsters inoculated with mumps virus.[468] Finally, aqueduct stenosis may be the result, rather than the cause of hydrocephalus. From a study of resin casts of the aqueduct in children with spina bifida, Williams[945] postulated that the tectal plate was compressed by the expanding hydrocephalic hemispheres. There is experimental support for this idea. Communicating hydrocephalus followed by stenosis of the aqueduct was described in the hydrocephalic mutant mouse *oh*.[97] Masters *et al*.[604] demonstrated in mice inoculated with Reovirus that hydrocephalus was related to the degree of inflammation and fibrosis within CSF pathways, and aqueduct stenosis was a secondary consequence of midbrain compression. Findings in X-linked hydrocephalus in man would also favour this concept (see below).

Stenosis

To substantiate a diagnosis of aqueduct stenosis, that is, a greatly reduced lumen in the absence of significant histological abnormality or gliosis (Fig. 7.157), serial sections may be required. The aqueduct is a curved irregular tube which varies in calibre along its length, having two constrictions either side of a central ampulla. In adults the narrowest part ranges in area from 0.4 to 1.5 mm^2.[962] Emery and Staschak[277] found a wide range of calibre in normal children: the mean diameter at the narrowest point was 0.5 mm^2. A rare form of X-linked recessive hydrocephalus and aqueduct stenosis was first described by Bickers and Adams.[72] Perhaps 2% of all cases of congenital hydrocephalus are of this type.[41] Some 30 families have now been reported.[269,361,516] Hydrocephalus affects boys only, who are usually stillborn or show neonatal

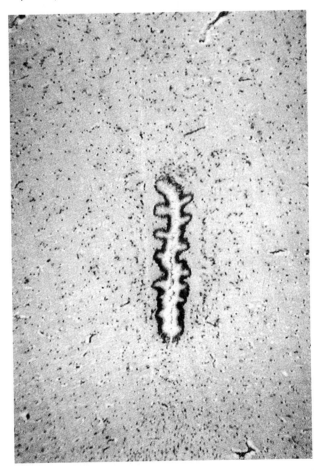

Figure 7.157 *Aqueduct stenosis. Note the lack of histological abnormality in the adjacent neuropil. (H&E.)*

macrocephaly, but there is considerable variability of expression within families, with some male siblings showing more subtle changes in head circumference, mental retardation and survival into adult life.[268,944] Adduction–flexion deformity of the thumbs is present in about 25% of cases.[285] Neuropathological examination revealed a very narrow stenotic aqueduct in some cases[269,430] but a normally patent aqueduct in others,[376,516,944] leading to the suggestion that aqueduct stenosis was a secondary phenomenon. Congenital absence of the pyramids is an important association.[142,269,516] A very rare autosomal recessive form of aqueduct stenosis has also been reported.[436]

Atresia/forking

Both terms have their detractors: 'atresia' was unacceptable to Russell[790] because a small lumen was always present; 'forking' was abandoned by Friede[314] because of confusion with normal anatomical variation and embryological inconsistency. Baker and Vinters[34] made the suggestion of 'aqueductal dysgenesis', which also carries pathogenetic implications that may not prove to be justified. In view of our knowledge of experimental virally induced aqueduct block, the term 'obliteration' seems more appropriate at present.

A variable portion of the aqueduct may be invisible to the naked eye, but histologically there are groups of ependymal cells forming small rosettes or tiny ependymal canals irregularly scattered across the midbrain tegmentum (Fig. 7.158). The normal outline of the aqueduct cannot be discerned, but there is no gliosis surrounding the aqueductules. Aqueduct atresia may be associated with Arnold–Chiari malformation, hydranencephaly and cases of craniosynostosis,[34] or may occur in isolation. Mumps infection is a possible aetiological factor in view of the histological similarity of experimentally induced aqueduct atresia[468] and reports of aqueduct stenosis in children following mumps meningoencephalitis.[81,847]

Gliosis

By contrast with atresia, in aqueductal gliosis the contours of the aqueduct remain recognizable as an interrupted ring of ependymal cells, rosettes and tubules. Dense fibrillary subependymal gliosis surrounds this ring and largely fills the area within it. There may be one or two small central channels but they are without ependymal lining. Widespread ependymitis, especially of the fourth ventricle, suggests that the lesion is either postinflammatory or posthaemorrhagic; proliferation of the subependymal glia and organization of pus or haematoma blocking the aqueductal lumen are possible mechanisms.[314] Such cases are characterized clinically by the gradual onset of hydrocephalus in early childhood, or occasionally in adult life.

Septum

Occlusion of the aqueduct by a thin septum is rare. Turnbull and Drake[906] described four cases and reviewed 12 oth-

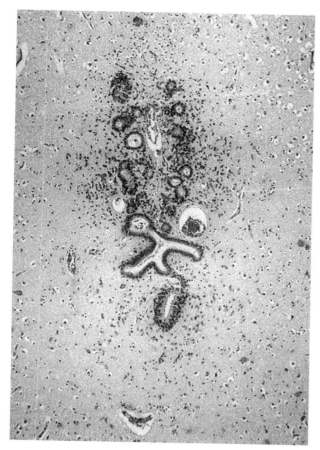

Figure 7.158 *Aqueduct atresia. Small tubules and tiny ependymal canals are irregularly disposed in the expected position for the aqueduct in the midbrain tegmentum. (H&E.)*

ers: one was 4 months old, and the others ranged in age from 2 to 46 years. A thin translucent membrane interrupts the aqueduct at its lower end (Fig. 7.159a) and sometimes there is a pinhole opening. Histologically, the membrane is composed of loose fibrillary glial tissue. Turnbull and Drake[906] suggested that the membrane was derived from a glial plug at the caudal end of the aqueduct which had become attenuated by prolonged pressure from above. The notion that septum formation is a variant of aqueductal gliosis is supported by several personal observations in which the thin glial membrane is surrounded almost completely by a ring of ependymal tissue (Fig. 7.159b).

Vascular malformation

The aqueduct may be compressed by an aneurysm of the great vein of Galen situated over the quadrigeminal plate[791] or can be directly blocked by a vascular malformation.[179,784]

Fourth ventricular foramina

Vuia[932] and Friede[314] have drawn an important distinction between the Dandy–Walker malformation (see above), in which the fourth ventricular foramina may or may not be closed, and rare reports of atresia of these foramina and

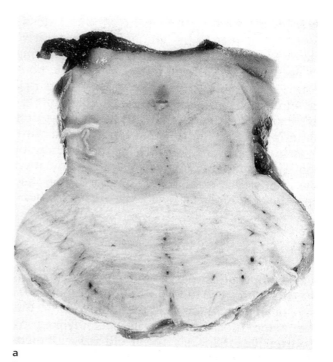

a

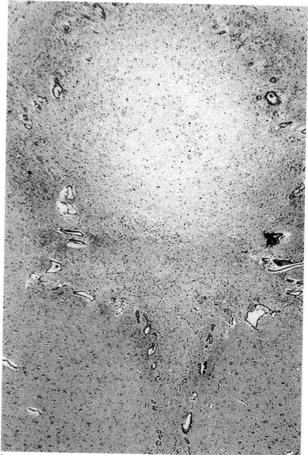

b

Figure 7.159 *Occlusion of the aqueduct by a membranous septum. (a) Section through the junction of midbrain and pons. (b) The membrane comprises loose glial tissue surrounded by a ring of ependymal canals. (H&E.)*

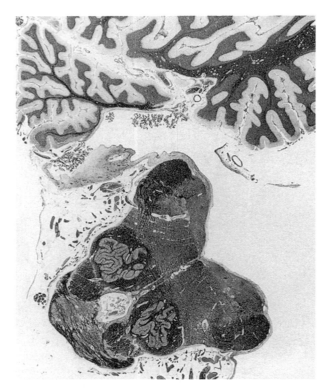

Figure 7.160 *Atresia of the foramina of Luschka. Note the choroid plexus within the widened foramina, which are closed over with glial membranes.*

hydrocephalus without vermal aplasia. Each outlet is more than sufficient for CSF drainage,[49] so all three must be obstructed to produce hydrocephalus. Several authors have described membranous pouches closing over the foramina. Histologically, either the membrane is fibroblastic, suggesting a haemorrhagic or inflammatory causation,[21] or it consists of a delicate glial membrane lined on the inside by ependyma[429] (Fig. 7.160).

Arachnoid granulations

Congenital aplasia of arachnoid granulations has been rarely described in hydrocephalic children.[339,371] Hydrocephalus complicating certain forms of cranial dysplasia, craniosynostosis, achondroplasia, and Apert's, Crouzon's and Pfeiffer's syndromes may be related to functional changes in CSF absorption by arachnoid granulations.[156,161,299,426,951] Physiological studies in such patients, simultaneously recording pressures in the lateral ventricle, superior sagittal sinus and jugular vein while manipulating the intracerebral pressure, suggest that the superior sagittal sinus venous pressure resulting from anatomical obstruction is increased independently of changes in intracranial pressure and is the cause of the hydrocephalus.[720,792]

REDUCED PROPULSION OF CSF

Bulk flow of CSF in man is the result of both continuous secretion from the choroid plexus and the cervical pres-

sure wave; a contributory role for the beating of ependymal cilia is less certain.[963] There are, however, rare reports of hydrocephalus in children associated with primary ciliary dyskinesia related ultrastructurally to absence of the outer dynein arms of each cilium,[361] and with ciliary aplasia.[239] There is also a mutant mouse (*hpy/hpy*) that shows a generalized disorder of cilia and hydrocephalus.[3]

DEVELOPMENTAL ABNORMALITIES IN WHICH VENTRICULOMEGALY IS AN ESSENTIAL FEATURE BUT OF UNCERTAIN PATHOGENESIS

Hydrocephalus is a cardinal feature of the hydrolethalus syndrome, an autosomal recessive lethal disorder, largely confined to Finland where it was first recognized in the course of a large-scale study of Meckel's syndrome.[793,794] The complex phenotype includes micrognathia, polydactyly, congenital heart defects and genitourinary anomalies. A preliminary neuropathological report on eight cases[692] showed a keyhole-shaped foramen magnum, hypoplastic hindbrain, arhinencephaly, midline dysgenesis and fusion of the thalami. The widely separated hemispheres sit in the base of the skull covered by a distended and torn arachnoid membrane allowing communication of the large ventricles with the subarachnoid space, the result of a massive intracranial accumulation of CSF.

Hydrocephalus is also present in severe forms of Smith–Lemli–Opitz syndrome,[564] X-linked orofacial–digital syndrome,[40] occasionally in Meckel's syndrome (see above), and in a rare malformation syndrome associated with congenital cerebral lactic acidosis and pyruvate dehydrogenase deficiency, characterized morphologically by microcephaly, hypoplastic pyramids, olivary heterotopia and hydrocephalus.[141]

GENERAL ASPECTS

The distended hemispheres are fragile and easily torn postmortem, and collapse when CSF escapes. In many cases, however, even after complete draining of CSF, the brain is heavier than that of an infant of the same age. This may be due to infiltration of fluid into the brain tissue. In addition, the external surface of the brain may show increased numbers of small gyri and shallow sulci without any underlying cytoarchitectonic abnormality, best termed polygyria (Fig. 7.161). Postnatal growth of the cortical surface seems to proceed normally in spite of the expanding hydrocephalus, and Friede[314] suggested that with the abnormal distension of the hemisphere a great portion of intrasulcal cortex is exposed, resulting in redundant gyration.

Sections of the brain show the enlarged cavities, a grossly distended infundibulum (Fig. 7.162) reduced to a thin transparent membrane, and a fenestrated or absent septum pellucidum. The corpus callosum becomes extremely thin. The anterior horns of the ventricles are usually less dilated than the temporal and occipital horns, where the cerebral mantle may be reduced in thickness to

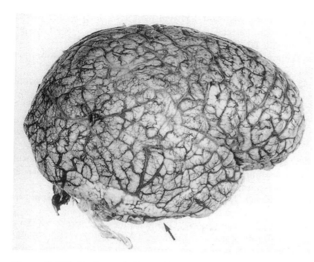

Figure 7.161 *Hydrocephalus with polygyria, i.e. increased numbers of normal but small convolutions. Note the marked contrast between the polygyria which involves most of the surface of the hemisphere and a small area of polymicrogyria affecting the inferior part of the temporal and occipital lobes (arrow).*

a few millimetres. While the cortex is relatively well preserved, the white matter is severely reduced in amount. Degenerative changes may be due to the stretching and tearing of nerve fibres, diffusion of CSF into the periventricular white matter causing interstitial oedema or chronic compression. Remarkable re-expansion of the cerebral mantle may occur after shunting, suggesting that

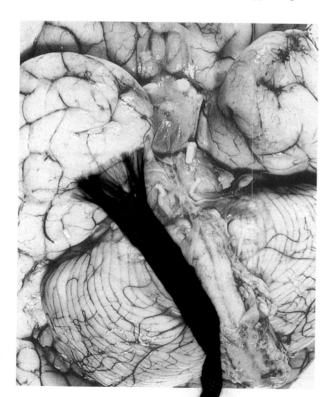

Figure 7.162 *Hydrocephalus. Close-up of the base of the brain showing cystic distension of the infundibulum.*

a mechanical cause is at least partly responsible for the thinning of the white matter. On microscopic examination the ventricular walls are denuded and the ependyma is replaced by a layer of glial tissue.

REFERENCES

1 Adachi T, Aoki J, Manya H *et al*. PAF analogues capable of inhibiting PAF acetylhydrolase activity suppress migration of isolated rat cerebellar granule cells. *Neurosci Lett* 1997; **235**: 133–6.

2 Adzick NS, Sutton LN, Crombleholme TM, Flake AW. Successful fetal surgery for spina bifida. *Lancet* 1998; **352**: 1675–6.

3 Afzelius BA. The immotile cilia syndrome and other ciliary diseases. *Int Rev Exp Pathol* 1979; **19**: 1–43X.

4 Agamanolis DP, Patre S. Glycogen accumulation in the central nervous system in cerebro-hepatorenal syndrome. Report of a case with ultrastructural studies. *J Neurol Sci* 1979; **41**: 325–42.

5 Aguirre-Villa-Coro A, Dominguez R. Intrauterine diagnosis of hydranencephaly by magnetic resonance. *Magn Res Imag* 1989; **7**: 105–7.

6 Ahdab-Barmada M, Claassen D. A distinctive triad of malformations of the central nervous system in the Meckel–Gruber syndrome. *J Neuropathol Exp Neurol* 1990; **49**: 610–20.

7 Aicardi J. The agyria–pachygyria complex: a spectrum of cortical malformations. *Brain Dev* 1991; **13**: 1–8.

8 Aicardi J, Castello-Branco M, Roy C. Le syndrome de Joubert. A propos de cinq observations. *Arch Fr Pediatr* 1983; **40**: 625–9.

9 Aicardi J, Goutières F. The syndrome of absence of the septum pellucidum with porencephalies and other developmental defects. *Neuropediatrics* 1981; **12**: 319–29.

10 Aicardi J, Goutières F, Verbois AH de. Multiple encephalomalacia of infants and its relationship to abnormal gestation and hydranencephaly. *J Neurol Sci* 1972; **15**: 357–73.

11 Aicardi J, Lefebvre J, Lerique-Koechlin A. A new syndrome: spasms in flexion, callosal agenesis, ocular abnormalities. *Electroencephalogr Clin Neurophysiol* 1965; **19**: 609–10.

12 Aleksic S, Budzilovich G, Reuben R *et al*. Unilateral arhinencephaly in Goldenhar–Gorlin syndrome. *Dev Med Child Neurol* 1975; **17**: 498–504.

13 Allendoerfer KL, Shatz CJ. The subplate, a transient neocortical structure: its role in the development of connections between thalamus and cortex. *Annu Rev Neurosci* 1994; **17**: 185–218.

14 Allsopp TE, Wyatt S, Paterson HF, Davies AM. The proto-oncogene *bcl-2* can selectively rescue neurotrophic factor-dependent neurons from apoptosis. *Cell* 1993; **73**: 295–307.

15 Altman J. Autoradiographic and histological studies of postnatal neurogenesis. II. A longitudinal investigation of the kinetics, migration and transformation of cells incorporation tritiated thymidine in infant rats, with special reference to postnatal neurogenesis in some brain regions. *J Comp Neurol* 1966; **128**: 431–74.

16 Altman J, Anderson WJ. Experimental reorganization of the cerebellar cortex. II. Effects of elimination of most microneurons with prolonged X-irradiation started at four days. *J Comp Neurol* 1973; **149**: 123–52.

17 Altman J, Anderson WJ, Bayer SA. Embryonic development of the rat cerebellum. III. Regional differences in the time of origin, migration and settling of Purkinje cells. *J Comp Neurol* 1985; **231**: 42–65.

18 Altman J, Anderson WJ, Bayer SA. Prenatal development of the cerebellar system in the rat. I. Cytogenesis and histogenesis of the deep nuclei and the cortex of the cerebellum. *J Comp Neurol* 1978; **179**: 23–48.

19 Altman J, Anderson WJ, Wright KA. Reconstitution of the external granular layer of the cerebellar cortex in infant rats after low-level X-irradiation. *Anat Rec* 1969; **163**: 453–72.

20 Alvord EC Jr, Fields WS, Desmond MM eds. *The pathology of hydrocephalus*. Springfield, IL: CC Thomas, 1961.

21 Amacher AL, Page LK. Hydrocephalus due to membranous obstruction of the fourth ventricle. *J Neurosurg* 1971; **35**: 672–6.

22 Andermann E, Andermann F, Bergeron D et al. Familial agenesis of the corpus callosum with sensori-motor neuronopathy; genetic and epidemiological studies of over 170 patients. *Can J Neurol Sci* 1979; **6**: 400.

23 Andrews PI, Hulette CM. An infant with macrocephaly, abnormal neuronal migration and persistent olfactory ventricles. *Clin Neuropathol* 1993; **12**: 13–18.

24 Angevine DM. Pathologic anatomy of hypophysis and adrenals in anencephaly. *Arch Pathol* 1938; **26**: 507–18.

25 Angevine JB. Time of neuron origin in the hippocampal region: an autoradiographic study in the mouse. *Exp Neurol* 1965; **13**(Suppl 2): 1–70.

26 Angevine JB, Sidman RL. Autoradiographic study of cell migration during histogenesis of cerebral cortex in the mouse. *Nature* 1961; **192**: 766–8.

27 Anton G, Zingerle H. Gename Beschreibung eines Falles von beiderseitigem Kleinhirnmangel. *Arch Psychiat Nervenkrankheit* 1914; **54**: 8–75.

28 Appleby A, Foster JB, Hankinson J, Hudgson P. The diagnosis and management of the Chiari anomalies in adult life. *Brain* 1968; **91**: 131–40.

29 Archer CR, Horenstein S, Sudaram M. The Arnold–Chiari malformation presenting in adult life. A report of 13 cases and review of the literature. *J Chronic Dis* 1977; **30**: 369–82.

30 Avery L, Wasserman S. Ordering gene function: The interpretation of epistasis in regulatory hierarchies. *Trends Genet* 1992; **8**: 312–16.

31 Baes M, Gressens P, Baumgart E et al. A mouse model for Zellweger syndrome. *Nat Genet* 1997; **17**: 49–57.

32 Bailey A, Luthert P, Bolton P et al. Autism and megalencephaly. *Lancet* 1993; **341**: 1225–6.

33 Baird WF, Stitt D. Arteriovenous aneurysm of the cerebellum in a premature infant. *Pediatrics* 1959; **24**: 455–7.

34 Baker DW, Vinters HV. Hydrocephalus with cerebral aqueductal dysgenesis and craniofacial anomalies. *Acta Neuropathol (Berl)* 1984; **63**: 170–3.

35 Baldwin CT, Hoth CF, Amos JA et al. An exonic mutation in the *HuP2* paired domain gene causes Waardenburg's syndrome. *Nature* 1992; **355**: 637–8.

36 Balthasar K, Schlagenhauff R. Unilateral agenesis of pyramidal system. *Vth International Congress of Neuropathology*. Zurich, Switzerland, 1965: 881–7.

37 Banerji NK, Millar JHD. Chiari malformation presenting in adult life. Its relationship to syringomyelia. *Brain* 1974; **97**: 157–68.

38 Banker BQ. Neuropathologic aspects of artherogryposis multiplex congenita. *Clin Orthopaed* 1985; **144**: 30–43.

39 Bankl H, Jellinger J. Zentralnervöse Schäden nach fätaler Kohlenoxydvergiftung. *Beitr Pathol Anat Pathol* 1967; **135**: 350–76.

40 Baraitser M. Syndrome of the mouth: the orofaciodigital syndromes. *J Med Genet* 1986; **23**: 116–19.

41 Baraitser M. *The genetics of neurological disorders* 2nd edn. Oxford: Oxford University Press, 1990.

42 Baraitser M, Brett EM, Piesowicz AT. Microcephaly and intracranial calcification in two brothers. *J Med Genet* 1983; **20**: 210–12.

43 Baraitser M, Patton MA. Reduced prevalance in tuberous sclerosis. *J Med Genet* 1985; **22**: 29–31.

44 Barkovich AJ, Chuang SH, Norman D. MR of neuronal migration anomalies. *Am J Neuroradiol* 1987; **8**: 1009–17.

45 Barkovich AJ, Jackson DE, Boyer RS. Band heterotopias: a newly recognised neuronal migration anomaly. *Radiology* 1989; **171**: 455–8.

46 Barkovich AJ, Kuzniecky RI, Bollen AW, Grant PE. Focal transmantle dysplasia: a specific malformation of cortical development. *Neurology* 1997; **49**: 1148–52.

47 Barkovich AJ, Norman D. MR imaging of schizencephaly. *Am J Neuroradiol* 1988; **9**: 297–302.

48 Barr M Jr, Hansen JW, Currey K et al. Holoprosencephaly in infants of diabetic mothers. *J Pediatr* 1983; **102**: 565–8.

49 Barr ML. Observations on the foramen of Magendie in a series of human brains. *Brain* 1948; **71**: 281–9.

50 Barry A, Patten BM, Stewart BH. Possible factors in the development of the Arnold–Chiari malformation. *J Neurosurg* 1957; **14**: 285–301.

51 Barson AJ. Spina bifida: the significance of the level and extent of the defect to the morphogenesis. *Dev Med Child Neurol* 1970; **12**: 129–44.

52 Barth PG, Mullaart R, Stam FC, Sloof JL. Familial lissencephaly with extreme neopallial hypoplasia. *Brain Dev* 1982; **4**: 145–51.

53 Barth PG, Valk J, Kalsbeek GL, Blom A. Organoid nevus syndrome (linear nevus sebaceous of Judassohn). Clinical and radiological study of a case. *Neuropediatrics* 1977; **8**: 418–28.

54 Barth PG, Vrensen GFJM, Uylings HBM et al. Inherited syndrome of microcephaly, dyskinesia and pontocerebellar hypoplasia: a systemic atrophy with early onset. *J Neurol Sci* 1990; **97**: 25–42.

55 Bass JL, Breningstall GN, Swaiman KF. Echocardiographic evidence of cardiac rhabdomyoma in tuberous sclerosis. *Am J Cardiol* 1985; **55**: 1379–82.

56 Bates JI, Netsky MG. Developmental anomalies of the horns of the lateral ventricles. *J Neuropathol Exp Neurol* 1995; **14**: 316–25.

57 Baudrimont M, Gray F, Meininger V, Escourolle R, Castaine P. Atrophie cérébelleuse croisée après lésion hémisphérique survenue à l'âge adulte. *Rev Neurol* 1983; **139**: 485–9.

58 Becker H. Über Hirngefässausschaltungen II. Intrakranielle Gefässverschlüssw. Über experimentelle Hydranencephalie (Blasenhirn). *Dtsch Z Nervenheilkunde* 1949; **161**: 446–505.

59 Becker PS, Dixon AM, Troncoso JC. Bilateral opercular polymicrogyria. *Ann Neurol* 1989; **25**: 90–2.

60 Bell JE, Gordon A, Maloney AFJ. Abnormalities of the spinal meninges in anencephalic fetuses. *J Pathol* 1981; **133**: 131–44.

61 Bell JE, Gordon A, Maloney AFJ. The association of hydrocephalus and Arnold–Chiari malformation with spina bifida in the fetus. *Neuropathol Appl Neurobiol* 1980; **6**: 29–39.

62 Bell JE, Green RJL. Studies on the area cerebrovasculosa of anencephalic fetuses. *J Pathol* 1982; **137**: 315–28.

63 Belloni E, Muenke M, Roessler E et al. Identification of *Sonic hedgehog* as a candidate gene responsible for holoprosencephaly. *Nat Genet* 1996; **14**: 353–6.

64 Benda CE. Dysraphic states. *J Neuropathol Exp Neurol* 1959; **18**: 56–74.

65 Benda CE. *Mongolism and cretinism*. New York: Grune and Stratton, 1947.

66 Benda CE. The Dandy–Walker syndrome or the so-called atresias of the foramen of Magendie. *J Neuropathol Exp Neurol* 1954; **13**: 14–29.

67 Bender BL, Yunis EJ. Central nervous system pathology of tuberous sclerosis in children. *Ultrastruct Pathol* 1980; **1**: 287–99.

68 Benirschke K. Twin placenta in perinatal mortality. *NY J Med* 1961; **61**: 1499–508.

69 Berg MJ, Schifitto G, Powers JM *et al*. X-linked female band heterotopia–male lissencephaly syndrome. *Neurology* 1998; **50**: 1143–6.

70 Berry RJ, Li Z, Erickson JD *et al*. China–US Collaborative Project Neu. Prevention of neural-tube defects with folic acid in China. *N Engl J Med* 1999; **341**: 1485–90.

71 Bertrand I, Gruner J. The status verrucosus of the cerebral cortex. *J. Neuropathol Exp Neurol* 1955; **14**: 331–47.

72 Bickers DS, Adams RD. Hereditary stenosis of the aqueduct of Sylvius as a cause of congenital hydrocephalus. *Brain* 1949; **72**: 246–62.

73 Bielschowsky M. Über die Oberflächengestaltung des Grosshirnmantels bei Pachgyrie, Mikrogyrie und bei normaler Entwicklung. *J Psychol Neurol* 1923; **30**: 29–76.

74 Bielschowsky M. Über Mikrogyrie. *J Psychol Neurol* 1916; **22**: 1–47.

75 Bielschowsky M. Zur Histopathologie und Pathogenese der amaurotischen Idiotie mit besonderer Berücksichtigung der zerebellären Veränderungen. *J Psychol Neurol* 1920; **26**: 123–244.

76 Biemond A. Hypoplasia ponto-neocerebellaris, with malformation of the dentate nucleus. *Folia Psychiat Neurol Neurochirung Neerland* 1955; **58**: 2–7.

77 Bignami A, Appicciutoli L. Micropolygyria and cerebral calcification in cytomegalic inclusion disease. *Acta Neuropathol (Berl)* 1964; **4**: 127–37.

78 Bignami A, Palladini G, Zappella M. Unilateral megalencephaly with nerve cell hypertrophy. An anatomical and quantitative histochemical study. *Brain Res* 1968; **9**: 103–14.

79 Billette de Villemeur T, Chiron C, Robain O. Unlayered polymicrogyria and agenesis of the corpus callosum: a relevant association? *Acta Neuropathol (Berl)* 1992; **83**: 265–70.

80 Binns W, James LF, Shupe JL, Thacker EJ. Cyclopian-type malformation in lambs. *Arch Environ Hlth* 1962; **5**: 106–8.

81 Bistrian B, Phillips CA, Kaye IS. Fatal mumps meningoencephalitis. Isolation of virus premortem and postmortem. *JAMA* 1972; **222**: 478–9.

82 Bix GJ, Clark GD. Platelet-activating factor receptor stimulation disrupts neuronal migration *in vitro*. *J Neurosci* 1998; **18**: 307–18.

83 Blackshear PJ, Silver J, Nairn AC *et al*. Widespread neuronal ectopia associated with secondary defects in cerebrocortical chondroitin sulfate proteoglycans and basal lamina in MARCKS-deficient mice. *Exp Neurol* 1997; **145**: 46–61.

84 Blake JA. The roof and lateral recesses of the fourth ventricle, considered morphologically and embryologically. *J Comp Neurol* 1900; **10**: 79–108.

85 Blanc JF, Lapillonne A, Pouillaude JH, Badinand N. Hydranencephaly and ingestion of estrogens during pregnancy. Fetal cerebral vascular complication? *Arch Fr Pediatr* 1988; **45**: 483–5.

86 Bogaert L van, Paillas JE, Berard-Badier M, Payan H. Etude sur la sclérose tubéreuse de Bourneville a forme cérébelleuse. *Rev Neurol* 1958; **98**: 673–89.

87 Bogaert L van, Radermecker MA. Une dysgénésie cérébelleuse chez un enfant du radium. *Rev Neurol* 1955; **93**: 65–82.

88 Böhm N, Uy J, Kiessling M, Lehnert W. Multiple acyl-CoA dehydrogenase deficiency (glutaric acidemia type II), congenital polycystic kidneys and symmetrical warty dysplasia of the cerebral cortex in two newborn brothers. II Morphology and pathogenesis. *Eur J Pediatr* 1982; **139**: 60–5.

89 Bonnevie K, Brodal A. Hereditary hydrocephalus in the house mouse. IV. The development of the cerebeller anomalies during fetal life with notes on the normal development of the mouse cerebellum. *Skrifter utgitt av det Norske Videnkapsakademi i Oslo* 1946; I. Mat-Nat. Kl, No. 4.

90 Bonnin JM, Rubinstein LJ, Papasozomenos SCh, Marangos PJ. Subependymal giant cell astrocytoma. Significance and possible cytogenic implications of an immunohistochemical study. *Acta Neuropathol (Berl)* 1984; **62**: 185–93.

91 Borberg A. Clinical and genetic investigations into tuberous sclerosis and Recklinghausen's neurofibromatosis. *Acta Psychol Neurol Scand* 1951; **71**(Suppl): 11–239.

92 Bordarier C, Aicardi J. Dandy–Walker syndrome and agenesis of the cerebellar vermis: diagnostic problems and genetic counselling. *Dev Med Child Neurol* 1990; **32**: 285–94.

93 Bordarier C, Aicardi J, Goutières F. Congenital hydrocephalus and eye abnormalities with severe developmental brain defects: Warburg's syndrome. *Ann Neurol* 1984; **16**: 60–5.

94 Bordarier C, Robain O. Familial recurrence of prenatal encephaloclastic damage: anatomo-clinical report of two cases. *Neuropediatrics* 1989; **20**: 103–6.

95 Bordarier C, Robain O. Microgyric and necrotic cortical lesions in twin fetuses: original cerebral damage consecutive to twinning? *Brain Dev* 1992; **14**: 174–8.

96 Bordarier C, Robain O, Ponsot G. Bilateral porencephalic defect in a newborn after injection of benzol during pregnancy. *Brain Dev* 1991; **13**: 126–9.

97 Borit A, Sidman RL. New mutant mouse with communicating hydrocephalus and secondary aqueductal stenosis. *Acta Neuropathol (Berl)* 1972; **21**: 316–31.

98 Bossy JG. Morphological study of a case of complete, isolated and asymptomatic agenesis of the corpus callosum. *Arch Anat Histol Embryol* 1970; **53**: 289–340.

99 Bourneville DM. Sclérose tubéreuse des circonvolutions cérébrales: idiotie et épilepsie hémiplégique. *Arch Neurol* 1880; 1: 81–91.

100 Boyd SG, Harding BN. Intractable seizures, intermittent EEG activity and dentato-olivary dysplasia. *Electroencephalogr Clin Neurophysiol* 1991; **78**: 85P.

101 Brent RL. Radiation teratogenesis. *Teratology* 1980; **21**: 281–98.

102 Briscoe J, Pierani A, Jessell TM, Ericson J. A homeodomain protein code specifies progenitor cell identity and neuronal fate in the ventral neural tube. *Cell* 2000; **101**: 435–45.

103 Broccoli V, Boncinelli E, Wurst W. The caudal limit of *Otx2* expression positions the isthmic organizer. *Nature* 1999; **401**: 164–8.

104 Brock DJH, Sutcliffe RG. Alpha-fetoprotein in the antenatal diagnosis of anencephaly and spina bifida. *Lancet* 1972; ii: 197–8.

105 Brocklehurst G. The development of the human cerebrospinal fluid pathway with particular reference to the roof of the fourth ventricle. *J Anat* 1969; **105**: 467–75.

106 Brodal A, Bonnevie K, Harkmark W. Hereditary hydrocephalus in the house mouse. II. The anomalies of the cerebellum, and partial defective development of the vermis. *Skrifter utgitt av det Norske Videnkapsakademi i Oslo* 1944; I. Mat-Nov. K2, No. 8.

107 Brook FA, Shum AS, Van Straaten HW, Copp AJ. Curvature of the caudal region is responsible for failure of neural tube closure in the curly tail (ct) mouse embryo. *Development* 1991; **113**: 671–8.

108 Brouwer B. Hypoplasia ponto-neocerebellaris. *Psychiat Neurol Bladen* 1924; **6**: 461–9.

109 Brown JR. The Dandy–Walker syndrome. In: Vinken PJ, Bruyn GW eds. *Handbook of clinical neurology*. Amsterdam: North-Holland, 1977: 623–46.

110 Bruggen J van der. Über Ersatz der Pyramidenbahnfunktion. *Disch Z Nervenheilkunde* 1930; **113**: 250–77.

111 Brun A. Marginal glioneural heterotopias of the central nervous system. *Acta Pathol Microbiol Scand* 1965; **65**: 221–33.

112 Brun R. Zur Kenntnis der Bildungsfehler des Kleinhirns. *Schweizer Arch Neurol Psychiatrie* 1917; **1**: 61–123.

113 Brun R. Zur Kenntnis der Bildungsfehler des Kleinhirns. *Schweizer Arch Neurol Psychiatrie* 1918; **2**: 48–105.

114 Brun R. Zur Kenntnis der Bildungsfehler des Kleinhirns. *Schweizer Arch Neurol Psychiatrie* 1918; **3**: 13–88.

115 Bruner JP, Tulipan N, Paschall RL *et al*. Fetal surgery for myelomeningocele and the incidence of shunt-dependent hydrocephalus. *JAMA* 1999; **282**: 1819–25.

116 Buckler AJ, Chang DD, Graw SL *et al*. Exon amplification: a strategy to isolate mammalian genes based on RNA splicing. *Proc Natl Acad Sci USA* 1991; **88**: 4005–9.

117 Burk U, Hayek HW, Zeider U. Holoprosencephaly in monozygotic twins – clinical and computed tomographic findings. *Am J Med Genet* 1981; **9**: 13–17.

118 Burn J, Wickramasinghe T, Harding BN, Baraitser M. A syndrome of intracerebral calcification and microcephaly in 2 siblings, resembling intrauterine infection. *Clin Genet* 1986; **30**: 112–16.

119 Butler LJ, Snodgrass G, France N *et al*. Trisomy syndrome. Analysis of 13 cases. *Arch Dis Child* 1965; **40**: 600–11.

120 Byrnes RL, Boellaard JW. Renal agenesis and meningocerebral angiomatosis. *Arch Pathol* 1958; **66**: 23–31.

121 Calogero JA. Vermian agenesis and unsegmented midbrain tectum. *J Neurosurg* 1977; **47**: 605–8.

122 Cameron AH. Malformations of the neuro-spinal axis, urogenital tract and foregut in spina bifida attributable to disturbances of the blastopore. *J Pathol Bacteriol* 1957; **73**: 213–21.

123 Cameron AH. The Arnold–Chiari and the neuroanatomical malformations associated with spina bifida. *J Pathol Bacteriol* 1957; **73**: 195–211.

124 Cameron AH, Jones EL, Smith WT, Wood BSB. Combined hepatic and cerebral degeneration in infancy. *J Pathol Bacteriol* 1968; **96**: 227–30.

125 Capecchi MR. Altering the genome by homologous recombination. *Science* 1989; **244**: 1288–92.

126 Carrea R, Girado JM. In: Angiomatous and fistulous arteriovenous aneurysm in children. Luyendijk W eds. *Progress in brain research*. Amsterdam: Elsevier, 1968: 433–9.

127 Carter CO. Clues to the aetiology of neural tube malformations. *Dev Med Child Neurol* 1974; **16** (Suppl 32): 3–15.

128 Casaer P, Ules JSH, Devlieger H *et al*. Variability of outcome in Joubert syndrome. *Neuropediatrics* 1985: **16**: 43–5.

129 Caviness VS Jr, Evrard P. Occipital encephalocele: a pathologic and anatomic analysis. *Acta Neuropathol (Berl)* 1975; **32**: 245–55.

130 Chan CC, Egbert PR, Herrick MK, Urich H. Oculocerebral malformations. A reappraisal of Walker's 'lissencephaly'. *Arch Neurol* 1980; **37**: 104–8.

131 Chan HSL, Sonley JJ, Moës CAF *et al*. Primary and secondary tumours of childhood involving the heart, pericardium and great vessels. *Cancer* 1985; **56**: 825–36.

132 Chiang C, Litingtung Y, Lee E *et al*. Cyclopia and defective axial patterning in mice lacking *Sonic hedgehog* gene function. *Nature* 1996; **383**: 407–13.

133 Chiari H. Über die Veränderungen des Kleinhirns, des Pons, und der Medulla oblongata infolge von congenitaler Hydrocephalie des Grosshirns. *Denkschr Akad Wissenchaft Wien* 1896; **63**: 71–116.

134 Chiari H. Über Veränderungen des Kleinhirns, des Pons und der Medulla oblongata infolge von congenitaler Hydrocephalie des Grosshirns. *Dtsch Med Wochenschr* 1891; **27**: 1172–5.

135 Cho DY, Leipold HW. Arnold–Chiari malformation and associated anomalies in calves. *Acta Neuropathol (Berl)* 1977; **39**: 129–34.

136 Choi BH, Kudo M. Abnormal neuronal migration and gliomatosis cerebri in epidermal nevus syndrome. *Acta Neuropathol (Berl)* 1981; **53**: 319–25.

137 Choi BH, Lapham LW, Amin-Zaki L, Saleem T. Abnormal neuronal migration, deranged cerebral cortical organization, and diffuse white matter astrocytosis of human fetal brain; a major effect of methylmercury poisoning *in utero*. *J Neuropathol Exp Neurol* 1978; **37**: 719–33.

138 Choi BH, Matthias SC. Cortical dysplasia associated with massive ectopia of neurons and glial cells within the subarachnoid space. *Acta Neuropathol (Berl)* 1987; **73**: 105–9.

139 Chou TM, Chou SM. Tuberous sclerosis in the premature infant: a report of a case with immunohistochemistry on the CNS. *Clin Neuropathol* 1989; **8**: 45–52.

140 Choux M, Raybaud C, Puisard N *et al*. Intracranial supratentorial cysts in children excluding tumour and parasitic cysts. *Childs Brain* 1978; **4**: 15–32.

141 Chow CH, Anderson RM, Kelly GCT. Neuropathology in cerebral lactic acidosis. *Acta Neuropathol (Berl)* 1987; **74**: 393–6.

142 Chow CH, Halliday JL. Anderson RM *et al*. Congenital absence of pyramids and its significance in genetic diseases. *Acta Neuropathol (Berl)* 1985; **65**: 313–17.

143 Chow CW, McKelvie PA, Anderson RM *et al*. Autosomal recessive hydrocephalus with third ventricle obstruction. *Am J Med Genet* 1990; **35**: 310–13.

144 Chun JJM, Shatz CJ. Interstitial cells of the adult neocortical white matter are the remnant of the early generated subplate neuron population. *J Comp Neurol* 1989; **282**: 555–69.

145 Chung HD. Retrograde crossed cerebellar atrophy. *Brain* 1985; **108**: 881–95.

146 Claireaux ER, Newman CGH. Arterio-venous fistula (aneurysm) of the great vein of Galen with heart failure in the neonatal period. *Arch Dis Child* 1960; **35**: 605–12.

147 Clarren SK, Alvord EC Jr, Sumi SM *et al*. Brain malformations related to prenatal exposure to alcohol. *J Pediatr* 1978; **92**: 64–7.

148 Clarren SK, Hall JG. Neuropathologic findings on the spinal cords of 10 infants with arthrogryposis. *J Neurol Sci* 1983; **58**: 89–102.

149 Cleland J. Contribution to the study of spina bifida, encephalocele and anencephalus. *J Anat Physiol* 1883; **17**: 257–92.

150 Clément R, Gerbeaux J, Combes-Hamelle A *et al*. Anévrysmes arterio-veineux de l'ampoule de Galien chez le nourrisson. Leur rôle dans l'hydrocéphalie communicante. *Presse Med* 1954; **62**: 658–61.

151 Cobrinik D, Dowdy SF, Hinds PW *et al*. The retinoblastoma protein and the regulation of cell cycling. *Trends Biochem Sci* 1992; **17**: 312–5.

152 Cogliatti SB. Diplomyelia: caudal duplication of the neural tube in mice. *Teratology* 1986; **34**: 343–52.

153 Cohen M, Roessmann U. *In utero* brain damage: relationship of gestational age to pathological consequences. *Dev Med Child Neurol* 1994; **36**: 263–8.

154 Cohen MM Jr. Perspectives on holoprosencephaly: Part I. Epidemiology, genetics, and syndromology. *Teratology* 1989; **40**: 211–35.

155 Cohen MM Jr. Perspectives on holoprosencephaly: Part III. Spectra, distinctions, continuities and discontinuities. *Am J Med Genet* 1989; **34**: 271–88.

156 Cohen MM Jr, Kreiborg S. The central nervous system in Apert syndrome. *Am J Med Genet* 1990; **35**: 36–45.

157 Cohen MM Jr, Sulik KK. Perspectives on holoprosencephaly: Part II. Central nervous system, craniofacial anatomy, syndrome commentary, diagnostic approach, and experimental studies. *J Craniofac Genet Dev Biol* 1992; **12**: 196–244.

158 Cohen NR, Taylor JSH, Scott LB et al. Errors in corticospinal axon guidance in mice lacking the neural cell adhesion molecule L1. *Curr Biol* 1998; **8**: 26–33.

159 Cohn R, Neumann MA. Porencephaly. A clinicopathologic study. *J Neuropathol Exp Neurol* 1946; **5**: 257–70.

160 Colevas AD, Edwards J, Hruban RH et al. Glutaric acidemia type II. Comparison of pathologic features in two infants. *Arch Pathol Lab Med* 1988; **112**: 1133–9.

161 Collmann H, Sörensen N, Krauss J, Mühling J. Hydrocephalus in craniosynostosis. *Childs Nerv Syst* 1988; **4**: 279–85.

162 Colon EY. The structure of the cerebral cortex in Down's syndrome: quantitative analysis. *Neuropediatrics* 1972; **3**: 362–76.

163 Combette M. Absence complète du cervelet, des pédoncules postérieurs et de la protubérance cérébrale chez une jeune fille morte dans sa onzième année. *Bull Soc Anat Paris* 1831; **5**: 148–53.

164 Constantinidis J. Cingulosynapsis (continuité interhémisphérique du cortex cingulaire). *Arch Suisse Neurol Neurochurg Psychiatry* 1969; **104**: 137–49.

165 Cooper MK, Porter JA, Young KE, Beachy PA. Teratogen-mediated inhibition of target tissue response to *Shh* signaling. *Science* 1998; **280**: 1603–7.

166 Copp AJ. Genetic models of mammalian neural tube defects. In: Bock G, Marsh J eds. *Neural tube defects* (Ciba Foundation Symposium 181). Chichester: John Wiley, 1994: 118–34.

167 Copp AJ, Bernfield M. Etiology and pathogenesis of human neural tube defects: insights from mouse models. *Curr Opin Pediatr* 1994; **6**: 624–31.

168 Copp AJ, Brock FA. Does lumbosacral spina bifida arise by failure of neural folding or by defective canalisation? *J Med Genet* 1989; **26**: 160–6.

169 Copp AJ, Brook FA, Estibeiro P et al. The embryonic development of mammalian neural tube defects. *Prog Neurobiol* 1990; **35**: 363–403.

170 Copp AJ, Checiu I, Henson JN. Developmental basis of severe neural tube defects in the *loop-tail* (*Lp*) mutant mouse: use of microsatellite DNA markers to identify embryonic genotype. *Dev Biol* 1994; **165**: 20–9.

171 Copp AJ, Crolla JA, Brook FA. Prevention of spinal neural tube defects in the mouse embryo by growth retardation during neurulation. *Development* 1988; **104**: 297–303.

172 Copp AJ, Harding BN. Neuronal migration disorders in humans and in mouse models – an overview. *Epilepsy Res* 1999; **36**: 133–41.

173 Coria F, Quintana F, Rebollo M et al. Occipital dysplasia and Chiari type I deformity in a family. *J Neurol Sci* 1983; **62**: 147–58.

174 Corner BD, Holton JB, Norman RM, Williams PM. A case of histidinemia controlled with a low histidine diet. *Pediatrics* 1968; **41**: 1074–81.

175 Cornette L, Verpoorten C, Lagae L et al. Tethered cord syndrome in occult spinal dysraphism – timing and outcome of surgical release. *Neurology* 1998; **50**: 1761–5.

176 Costoulas G. Un type peu connu d'anomalies des ventricules cérébraux: les goniosynapses (étude anatomo-clinique et statistique). *Ann Anat Pathol* 1958; **3**: 268–83.

177 Coulter CL, Leech RW, Brumback RA, Bradley Schaefer G. Cerebral abnormalities in thanatophoric dysplasia. *Childs Nerv Syst* 1991; **7**: 21–6.

178 Coulter CL, Leech RW, Schaefer GB et al. Midline cerebral dysgenesis, dysfunction of the hypothalamic–pituitary axis, and fetal alcohol effects. *Arch Neurol* 1993; **50**: 771–5.

179 Courville CB. Obstructive internal hydrocephalus incidental to small vascular anomaly of the midbrain. *Bull LA Neurol Soc* 1961; **26**: 41–5.

180 Courville CB, Edmondson HA. Mental deficiency from intrauterine exposure to radiation. *Bull LA Neurol Soc* 1958; **23**: 11–20.

181 Cowen D, Geller LM. Long-term pathological effects of prenatal X-irradiation on the central nervous system of the rat. *J Neuropathol Exp Neurol* 1960; **19**: 488–527.

182 Craig JM, Bickmore WA. The distribution of CpG islands in mammalian chromosomes. *Nat Genet* 1994; **7**: 376–82.

183 Creasy MR, Alberman ED. Congenital malformations of the central nervous system in spontaneous abortions. *J Med Genet* 1976; **13**: 9–16.

184 Crome L. Brain warts. *J Ment Def Res* 1969; **13**: 360–5.

185 Crome L. Microgyria. *J Pathol Bacteriol* 1952; **64**: 479–95.

186 Crome L. Multilocular cystic encephalopathy of infants. *J Neurol Neurosurg Psychiatry* 1958; **21**: 146–52.

187 Crome L. Pachygyria. *J Pathol Bacteriol* 1956; **71**: 335–52.

188 Crome L, Cowie V, Slater RE. A statistical note on cerebellar and brain-stem weight in mongolism. *J Ment Def Res* 1966; **10**: 69–72.

189 Crome L, France N. Microgyria and cytomegalic inclusion disease in infancy. *J Clin Pathol* 1959; **12**: 427–34.

190 Crome L, Stern J. *Pathology of mental retardation* 2nd edn. Edinburgh: Churchill Livingstone, 1972.

191 Crome L, Sylvester PE. Hydranencephaly (hydrencephaly). *Arch Dis Child* 1958; **33**: 235–45.

192 Crossley PH, Martinez S, Martin GR. Midbrain development induced by FGF8 in the chick embryo. *Nature* 1996; **380**: 66–8.

193 Cruveilhier J. *Anatomie pathologique du corps humain*. Paris: Baillière, 1829.

194 Cuckle HS. Screening for neural tube defects. In: Bock G, Marsh J eds. *Neural tube defects* (Ciba Foundation Symposium 181). Chichester: John Wiley, 1994: 253–66.

195 Curran T, D'Arcangelo G. Role of reelin in the control of brain development. *Brain Res Rev* 1998; **26**: 285–94.

196 Curtis MT, Furth EE, Rorke LB. Cortical dysplasia and lipids in Neu–Laxova syndrome. *Brain Pathol* 1994; **4**: 456.

197 Czeizel AE, Dudás I. Prevention of the first occurrence of neural-tube defects by periconceptional vitamin supplementation. *N Engl J Med* 1992; **327**: 1832–5.

198 D'Agostino AN, Kernohan JN, Brown JR. The Dandy–Walker syndrome. *J Neuropathol Exp Neurol* 1963; **22**: 450–70.

199 Dahme M, Bartsch U, Martini R et al. Disruption of the mouse *L1* gene leads to malformations of the nervous system. *Nat Genet* 1997; **17**: 346–9.

200 Dale JK, Vesque C, Lints TJ et al. Cooperation of BMP7 and SHH in the induction of forebrain ventral midline cells by prechordal mesoderm. *Cell* 1997; **90**: 257–69.

201 Dambska M, Wisniewski K, Sher JH. An autopsy case of hemimegalencephaly. *Brain Dev* 1984; **6**: 60–4.

202 Dambska M, Wisniewski K, Sher JH. Lissencephaly: two distinct clinico-pathological types. *Brain Dev* 1983; **5**: 302–10.

203 Dandy WE. Congenital cerebral cysts of the cavum septi pellucidi (fifth ventricle) and cavum vergae (sixth ventricle). *Arch Neurol Psychiatry* 1931; **25**: 44–66.

204 Dandy WE, Blackfan KD. Internal hydrocephalus, an experimental clinical and pathological study. *Am J Dis Child* 1914; **8**: 406–82.

205 Daniel PM, Strich SJ. Some observations on the congenital deformity of the central nervous system known as the Arnold–Chiari malformation. *J Neuropathol Exp Neurol* 1958; **17**: 255–66.

206 Danner R, Shewmon DA, Sherman MP. Seizures in an atelencephalic infant: is the cortex essential for neonatal seizures? *Arch Neurol Psychiatry* 1985; **42**: 1014–16.

207 D'Arcangelo G, Homayouni R, Keshvara L *et al*. Reelin is a ligand for lipoprotein receptors. *Neuron* 1999; **24**: 471–9.

208 D'Arcangelo G, Miao GG, Chen S-C *et al*. A protein related to extracellular matrix proteins deleted in the mouse mutant reeler. *Nature* 1995; **374**: 719–23.

209 Dattani MT, Martinez-Barbera JP, Thomas PQ *et al*. Mutations in the homeobox gene *HESX1/Hesx1* associated with septo-optic dysplasia in human and mouse. *Nat Genet*, 1998; **19**: 125–33.

210 Daube JR, Chou SM. Lissencephaly. Two cases. *Neurology* 1966; **16**: 179–91.

211 Dauser RC, DiPietro MA, Venes JL. Symptomatic Chiari I malformation in childhood: a report of 7 cases. *Pediatr Neurosci* 1984; **14**: 184–90.

212 Davidoff LM. Brain in mongolian idiocy; report of 10 cases. *Arch Neurol Psychiatry* 1928; **20**: 1229–57.

213 Davidoff LM. Coarctation of the walls of the lateral angles of the lateral cerebral ventrices. *J Neurosurg* 1946; **3**: 250–6.

214 Davies WW. Radiological changes associated with Arnold–Chiari malformation. *Br J Radiol* 1967; **40**: 262–9.

215 Davis RL, Nelson E. Unilateral ganglioglioma in a tuberosclerotic brain. *J Neuropathol Exp Neurol* 1961; **21**: 571–81.

216 De Bleecker J, De Reuck J, Martin JJ *et al*. Autosomal recessive inheritance of polymicrogyria and dermatomyositis with paracrystalline inclusions. *Clin Neuropathol* 1990; **9**: 299–304.

217 DeBry RW, Seldin MF. Human/mouse homology relationships. *Genomics* 1996; **33**: 337–51.

218 De Chadarevian JP, Hollenberg RD. Subependymal giant cell tumor of tuberose sclerosis; a light and ultrastructural study. *J Neuropathol Exp Neurol* 1979; **38**: 419–33.

219 Dekaban A. Arhinencephaly in an infant born to a diabetic mother. *J Neuropathol Exp Neurol* 1959; **18**: 620–6.

220 Dekaban A. Large defects in cerebral hemispheres associated with cortical dysgenesis. *J Neuropathol Exp Neurol* 1965; **24**: 512–30.

221 Dekaban AS, Sadowsky D. Changes in brain weights during the span of human life: relation of brain weights to body heights and body weights. *Ann Neurol* 1978; **4**: 345–56.

222 Dekaban AS, Sakuragawa N. Megalencephaly. In: Vinken PJ, Bruyn GW eds. *Handbook of clinical neurology*. Amsterdam: North-Holland, 1977: 647–60.

223 De Leon G. Observations on cerebral and cerebellar microgyria. *Acta Neuropathol (Berl)* 1972; **20**: 278–87.

224 De Leon GA, Grover WD, D'Cruz CA. Amyotrophic cerebellar hypoplasia. A specific form of infantile spinal atrophy. *Acta Neuropathol (Berl)* 1984; **63**: 282–6.

225 De Leon GA, Grover WD, Huff DS *et al*. Globoid cells, glial nodules and peculiar fibrillary changes in the cerebro-hepa-

to-renal syndrome of Zellweger. *Ann Neurol* 1977; **2**: 473–84.

226 De León GA, Grover WD, Mestre GM. Cerebellar microgyria. *Acta Neuropathol (Berl)* 1976; **35**: 81–5.

227 Deloukas P, Schuler GD, Gyapay G *et al*. A physical map of 30,000 human genes. *Science* 1998; **282**: 744–6.

228 De Morsier G. Agénésie du septum lucidum avec malformations du tractus optique – la dysplasie septo-optique. *Schweizer Arch Neurol Psychiatrie* 1956; **77**: 267–92.

229 De Morsier G. Études sur les dysraphies crânioencéphaliques. VI. Télencéphalosynapsis: hémisphères cérébraux incomplètement séparés. *Psychiat Neurol Basel* 1961; **141**: 239–79.

230 De Morsier G, Mozer JJ. Agénésie compleète de la commissure calleuse et troubles du développement de l'héisphère gauche avec hémiparesie droite et intégrité mentale. (Le syndrome embryonnaire précoce de l'artère cérébrale antérieure.) *Schweizer Arch Neurol Psychiatrie* 1935; **35**: 64–95.

231 De Myer W. The median cleft face syndrome. *Neurology* 1967; **17**: 961–71.

232 De Myer W, Zeman W. Alobar holprosencephaly (arhinencephaly) with median cleft lip and palate: clinical, electroencephalographic and nosologic considerations. *Confinia Neurol Basel* 1963; **23**: 1–36.

233 De Myer W, Zeman W, Palmer C. The face predicts the brain; diagnostic significance of median facial anomalies for holoprosencephaly (arhinencephaly). *Pediatrics* 1964; **34**: 256–63.

234 Deng CX, Zhang PM, Harper JW *et al*. Mice lacking p21$^{CIP1/WAF1}$ undergo normal development, but are defective in G1 checkpoint control. *Cell* 1995; **82**: 675–84.

235 Dennis JP, Rosenberg HS, Alvord EC Jr. Megalencephaly, internal hydrocephalus and other neurological aspects of achondroplasia. *Brain* 1961; **84**: 427–45.

236 Deonna T. Prognostic des myeloméningocèles. *J Gynecol Obstet Biol Reprod* 1981; **10**: 181–4.

237 De Rosa MJ, Farrell MA, Burke MM *et al*. An assessment of the proliferative potential of 'balloon cells' in focal cortical resections performed for childhood epilepsy. *Neuropathol Appl Neurobiol* 1992; **18**: 566–74.

238 De Rosa MJ, Secor DL, Barsom M *et al*. Neuropathologic findings in surgically treated hemimegalencephaly: immunohistochemical, morphometric, and ultrastructural study. *Acta Neuropathol (Berl)* 1992; **84**: 250–60.

239 De Santi MM, Magni A, Valletta EA *et al*. Hydrocephalus bronchiectasis and ciliary aplasia. *Arch Dis Child* 1990; **65**: 543–4.

240 Desmond M, Wilson G, Melnick J *et al*. Congenital rubella encephalitis. *J Pediatr* 1967; **71**: 311–31.

241 Desmond ME, Jacobson AG. Embryonic brain enlargement requires cerebrospinal fluid pressure. *Dev Biol* 1977; **57**: 188–98.

242 Des Portes V, Pinard JM, Billuart P *et al*. A novel CNS gene required for neuronal migration and involved in X-linked subcortical laminar heterotopia and lissencephaly syndrome. *Cell* 1998; **92**: 51–61.

243 Dieker H, Edwards RH, ZuRhein G *et al*. The lissencephaly syndrome. *Birth Defects Original Articles Series* 1969; **5**: 53–64.

244 Diezel P. Mikrogyrie infolge cerebraler Speicheldrüsen-virusinfektion im Rahmen einer generalisierten Cytomegalie bei einem Säugling zugleich ein Beitrag zur Theorie der Windungsbildung. *Virchows Arch Pathol Anat* 1954; **325**: 109–30.

245 Diezel PB, Fritsch H, Jakob H. Leukodystrophie mit orthochromatischen Abbaustoffen. Ein Beitrag zur Pelizaeus-Merzbacherschen Krankheit. *Virchows Arch (A)* 1965; **338**: 371–94.

246 Dimitri V. Tumor cerebral congénito (angioma cavernoso). *Revista del Asociacion Medica Argentina* 1923; **36**: 1029.

247 Dobbing J, Sands J. Vulnerability of developing brain. IX. The effect of nutritional growth retardation on the timing of the brain growth spurt. *Biol Neonate* 1971; **19**: 363–78.

248 Dobyns WB, Pagon RA, Armstrong D et al. Diagnostic criteria for Walker–Warburg syndrome. *Am J Med Genet* 1989; **32**: 145–210.

249 Dobyns WB, Stratton RF, Greenberg F. Syndromes with lissencephaly: I Miller–Dieker and Norman–Roberts syndromes. *Am J Med Genet* 1984; **18**: 509–26.

250 Dobyns WB, Truwit CL, Ross ME et al. Differences in the gyral pattern distinguish chromosome 17-linked and X-linked lissencephaly. *Neurology* 1999; **53**: 270–7.

251 Dolgopol VB. Absence of the septum pellucidum as the only anomaly in the brain. *Arch Neurol Psychiatry* 1938; **40**: 1244–8.

252 Dom R, Brucher JM. Hamartoblastome (gangliocytome diffuse) unilateral de l'écorce cérébrale. *Rev Neurol* 1969; **120**: 307–18.

253 Doornik MC van, Hennekam RCM. Hemihydranencephaly with favourable outcome. *Dev Med Child Neurol* 1992; **34**: 454–8.

254 Drachman DA, Richardson EP Jr. Aqueductal narrowing congenital and acquired. *Arch Neurol* 1961; **5**: 552–9.

255 Droghari E, Smith I, Beaseley M, Lloyd JK. Timing of strict diet in relation to fetal damage in maternal phenylketonuria. *Lancet* 1987; **ii**: 927–30.

256 Dryden RJ. Duplication of the spinal cord: a discussion of the possible embryogenesis of diplomyelia. *Dev Med Child Neurol* 1980; **22**: 234–43.

257 Dubois-Dauphin M, Frankowski H, Tsujimoto Y et al. Neonatal motoneurons overexpressing the bcl-2 protooncogene in transgenic mice are protected from axotomy-induced cell death. *Proc Natl Acad Sci USA* 1994; **91**: 3309–13.

258 Du Boulay G, Shah JH, Currie JC, Logue V. The mechanism of hydromyelia in Chiari I malformations. *Br J Radiol* 1974; **47**: 579–87.

259 Duckett S. Foetal Arnold–Chiari malformation. *Acta Neuropathol (Berl)* 1966; **7**: 175–9.

260 Dudgeon JA. Varicella-zoster infections. In: Dudgeon JA, Marshall WC eds. *Viral diseases of the fetus and newborn* 2nd edn. Philadelphia, PA: WB Saunders, 1985: 161–74.

261 Duffy PE, Ziter FA. Infantile syringobulbia: a study of its pathology and a proposed relationship to neurogenic stridor in infancy. *Neurology* 1964; **14**: 500–9.

262 Dunn HG, Renpenning H, Gerrard JW et al. Mental retardation as a sex-linked defect. *Am J Ment Def* 1963; **64**: 827–48.

263 Duong T, De Rosa MJ, Poukens V et al. Neuronal cytoskeletal abnormalities in human cerebral cortical dysplasia. *Acta Neuropathol (Berl)* 1994; **87**: 493–503.

264 Dure LS, Percy AK, Cheek WR, Laurent JP. Chiari type I malformation in children. *J Pediatr* 1989; **15**: 573–6.

265 Dvorák K, Feit J. Migration of neuroblasts through partial necrosis of the cerebral cortex in newborn rats. Contribution to the problems of morphological development and developmental period of cerebral microgyria. *Acta Neuropathol (Berl)* 1977; **38**: 203–12.

266 Dvorák K, Feit J, Juránková Z. Experimentally induced focal microgyria and status verrucosus deformity in rats – pathogenesis and interrelations. Histological and autoradiological study. *Acta Neuropathol (Berl)* 1978; **44**: 121–9.

267 Dyste GN, Menezes AH. Presentation and management of pediatric Chiari malformations without myelodysplasia. *Neurosurgery* 1988; **23**: 589–97.

268 Edwards JH. The syndrome of sex-linked hydrocephalus. *Arch Dis Child* 1961; **36**: 486–93.

269 Edwards JH, Norman RM, Roberts JM. Sex-linked hydrocephalus: report of a family with 15 affected members. *Arch Dis Child* 1961; **36**: 481–5.

270 Eichorn DH, Bayley N. Growth in head circumference from birth through young adulthood. *Child Dev* 1962; **33**: 257–71.

271 Ejeckam GG, Wadhwa JK, Williams JP, Lacson AG. Neu–Laxova syndrome: report of two cases. *Pediatr Pathol* 1986; **5**: 195–306.

272 Eksioglu YZ, Scheffer IE, Cardenas P et al. Periventricular heterotopia: an X-linked dominant epilepsy locus causing aberrant cerebral cortical development. *Neuron* 1996; **16**: 77–87.

273 Ellenberger C Jr, Hanaway J, Netsky MG. Embryogenesis of the inferior olivary nucleus in the rat: a radiographic study and a re-evaluation of the rhombic lip. *J Comp Neurol* 1969; **137**: 71–87.

274 Ellis HM, Horvitz HR. Genetic control of programmed cell death in the nematode C. elegans. *Cell* 1986; **44**: 817–29.

275 Emery JL. Deformity of the aqueduct of Sylvius in children with hydrocephalus and myelomeningocoele. *Dev Med Child Neurol* 1974; **16**(Suppl 32): 40–8.

276 Emery JL, Lendon RG. The local cord lesion in neurospinal dysraphism (meningomyelocele). *J Pathol* 1973; **110**: 83–96.

277 Emery JL, Staschak MC. The size and form of the cerebral aqueduct in children. *Brain* 1972; **95**: 591–8.

278 Erasmus C, Blackwood W, Wilson J. Infantile multicystic encephalomalacia after maternal bee sting anaphylaxis during pregnancy. *Arch Dis Child* 1982; **57**: 785–7.

279 Ericson J, Briscoe J, Rashbass P et al. Graded sonic hedgehog signaling and the specification of cell fate in the ventral neural tube. *Cold Spring Harbor Symp Quant Biol* 1997; **62**: 451–66.

280 Essick CR. The development of the nuclei pontis and nucleus arcuatus in man. *Am J Anat* 1912; **13**: 25–54.

281 Estibeiro JP, Brook FA, Copp AJ. Interaction between splotch (Sp) and curly tail (ct) mouse mutants in the embryonic development of neural tube defects. *Development* 1993; **119**: 113–21.

282 European Chromosome 16 Tuberous Sclerosis Consortium. Identification and characterization of the tuberous sclerosis gene on chromsome 16. *Cell* 1993; **75**: 1305–15.

283 Evrard P, Caviness VS, Prats-Vinas J, Lyon G. The mechanism of arrest of neuronal migration in the Zellweger malformation: an hypothesis based upon cytoarchitectonic analysis. *Acta Neuropathol (Berl)* 1978; **41**: 109–17.

284 Evrard P, Saint-Georges P de, Kadhim HJ et al. Pathology of prenatal encephalopathies. In: French JH, Hard S, Casaer P eds. *Child neurology and developmental disabilities.* Baltimore, MD: Paul H Brookes, 1989; 153–76.

285 Faivre J, Lemarec B, Bretagne J, Pecker J. X-linked hydrocephalus, aqueductal stenosis, mental retardation, and adduction–flexion deformity of the thumbs. Report of a family. *Child's Brain* 1976; **2**: 226–33.

286 Farrell MA, DeRosa MJ, Curran JG et al. Neuropathologic findings in cortical resections (including hemispherectomies) performed for the treatment of intractable childhood epilepsy. *Acta Neuropathol (Berl)* 1992; **83**: 246–59.

287 Fauré C, Lepintre J, Lyon G. Étude radiologique du syndrome de Dandy–Walker. *Acta Radiol* 1963; **1**: 843–56.

288 Faust PL, Hatten ME. Targeted deletion of the PEX2 peroxisome assembly gene in mice provides a model for Zellweger syndrome, a human neuronal migration disorder. *J Cell Biol* 1997; **139**: 1293–305.

289 Fernandez F, Perez-Higueras A, Hernandez R *et al*. Hydranencephaly after maternal butane-gas intoxication. *Dev Med Child Neurol* 1986; **28**: 361–3.

290 Ferrer I. A Golgi analysis of unlayered polymicrogyria. *Acta Neuropathol (Berl)* 1984; **65**: 69–76.

291 Ferrer I, Catala I. Unlayered polymicrogyria: structural and developmental aspects. *Anat Embryol* 1991; **184**: 517–28.

292 Ferrer I, Cusi MV, Liarte A, Campistol J. A Golgi study of the polymicrogyric cortex in Aicardi syndrome. *Brain Dev* 1986; **8**: 518–25.

293 Ferrer I, Navarro C. Multicystic encephalomalacia of infancy. Clinico-pathological report of 7 cases. *J Neurol Sci* 1978; **38**: 179–89.

294 Ferrer I, Xumeira A, Santamaria J. Cerebral malformation induced by prenatal X-irradiation: an autoradiographic and Golgi study. *J Anat* 1984; **138**: 81–93.

295 Field M, Ashton R, White K. Agenesis of the corpus callosum; report of two preschool children and review of the literature. *Dev Med Child Neurol* 1978; **20**: 47–61.

296 Fink JM, Dobyns WB, Guerrini R, Hirsch BA. Identification of a duplication of Xq28 associated with bilateral periventricular nodular heterotopia. *Am J Hum Genet* 1997; **61**: 379–87.

297 Firth HV, Boyd PA, Chamberlain P *et al*. Severe limb abnormalities after chorion villus sampling at 56–66 days' gestation. *Lancet* 1991; **337**: 762–3.

298 Fisher JE, Siongco A. Complications from *in utero* death of a monozygous co-twin. *Pediatr Pathol* 1989; **9**: 765–71.

299 Fishman MA, Hogan GR, Didge PR. The concurrence of hydrocephalus and craniosynostosis. *J Neurosurg* 1971; **34**: 621–9.

300 Flatz G, Sukthomya C. Fronto-ethmoidal encephalomeningoceles in the population of northern Thailand. *Humangenetik* 1970; **11**: 1–9.

301 Fleming A, Copp AJ. A genetic risk factor for mouse neural tube defects: defining the embryonic basis. *Hum Mol Genet* 2000; **9**: 575–81.

302 Fleming A, Copp AJ. Embryonic folate metabolism and mouse neural tube defects. *Science* 1998; **280**: 2107–9.

303 Fleming GWTH, Norman RM. Arhinencephaly with incomplete separation of the cerebral hemispheres. *J Ment Sci* 1942; **88**: 341–3.

304 Fleury P, Groot WP de, Delleman JW *et al*. Tuberous sclerosis: the incidence of sporadic cases versus familial cases. *Brain Dev* 1979; **2**: 107–17.

305 Fone PD, Vapnek JM, Litwiller SE *et al*. Urodynamic findings in the tethered spinal cord syndrome: does surgical release improve bladder function. *J Urol* 1997; **157**: 604–9.

306 Fontan A, Battin JJ. La Mégalencéphalie primitive. *Arch Fr Pediatr* 1965; **22**: 521–9.

307 Fowler M, Dow R, White TA, Greer CH. Congenital hydrocephalus-hydranencephaly in five siblings with autopsy studies: a new disease. *Dev Med Child Neurol* 1972; **14**: 173–88.

308 Fox JW, Lamperti ED, Eksioglu YZ *et al*. Mutations in filamin 1 prevent migration of cerebral cortical neurons in human periventricular heterotopia. *Neuron* 1998; **21**: 1315–25.

309 Frankenberg WK, Duncan BR, Coffelt RW *et al*. Maternal phenylketonuria: implications for growth and development. *J Pediatr* 1968; **75**: 560–70.

310 Fransen E, D'Hooge R, Van Camp G *et al*. L1 knockout mice show dilated ventricles, vermis hypoplasia and impaired exploration patterns. *Hum Mol Genet* 1998; **7**: 999–1009.

311 Franz T. Extra-toes (Xt) homozygous mutant mice demonstrate a role for the Gli-3 gene in the development of the forebrain. *Acta Anat* 1994; **150**: 38–44.

312 Friede RL. Arrested cerebellar development. A type of cerebellar degeneration in amaurotic idiocy. *J Neurol Neurosurg Psychiatry* 1964; **27**: 41–5.

313 Friede RL. Dating the development of the human cerebellum. *Acta Neuropathol (Berl)* 1973; **23**: 48–58.

314 Friede RL. *Developmental neuropathology* 2nd edn. Berlin: Springer, 1989.

315 Friede RL. Uncommon syndromes of cerebellar vermis aplasia. II: Tecto-cerebellar dysplasia with occipital encephalocele. *Dev Med Child Neurol* 1978; **20**: 764–72.

316 Friede RL, Boltshauser E. Uncommon syndromes of cerebellar vermis aplasia. I. Jourbert syndrome. *Dev Med Child Neurol* 1978; **20**: 758–63.

317 Friede RL, Mikolasek J. Postencephalitic porencephaly hydranencephaly or polymicrogyria. A review. *Acta Neuropathol (Berl)* 1978; **43**: 161–8.

318 Friede RL, Roessmann S. Chronic tonsillar herniation. An attempt at clarifying chronic herniations at the foramen magnum. *Acta Neuropathol (Berl)* 1986; **34**: 219–35.

319 Frutiger P. Zur Frage der Arhinencephalie. *Acta Anat* 1969; **73**: 410–30.

320 Fryer AE, Chalmers A, Connor JM *et al*. Evidence that the gene for tuberous sclerosis is on chromosome 9. *Lancet* 1987; **i**: 659–61.

321 Fryer AE, Osborne JP. Tuberous sclerosis. A clinical appraisal. *Pediatr Res Commun* 1987; **1**: 239–55.

322 Fukuyama Y, Osawa M, Suzuki H. Congenital progressive muscular dystrophy of the Fukuyama type – clinical, genetic and pathological considerations. *Brain Dev* 1981; **3**: 1–29.

323 Gabriel JM, Merchant M, Ohta T *et al*. A transgene insertion creating a heritable chromosome deletion mouse model of Prader–Willi and Angelman syndromes. *Proc Natl Acad Sci USA* 1999; **96**: 9258–63.

324 Gadisseux JF, Rodriguez J, Lyon G. Pontoneocerebellar hypoplasia. A probable consequence of prenatal destruction of the pontine nuclei and a possible role of phenytoin intoxication. *Clin Neuropathol* 1984; **3**: 160–7.

325 Galaburda AM. Neuroanatomic basis of developmental dyslexia. *Neurol Clin* 1993; **11**: 161–73.

326 Garcia CA, Duncan C. Atelencephalic microphaly. *Dev Med Child Neurol* 1977; **19**: 227–32.

327 Gardner E, O'Rahilly R, Prolo D. The Dandy–Walker and Arnold–Chiari malformations: clinical developmental and teratological considerations. *Arch Neurol* 1975; **32**: 393–407.

328 Gardner WJ. Rupture of the neural tube. The cause of myelomeningocele. *Arch Neurol* 1961; **4**: 1–7.

329 Gardner WJ. *The dysraphic states*. Amsterdam: Excerpta Medica, 1973.

330 Gardner WJ, Karnosh LJ, Angel L. Syringomyelia: a result of embryonal atresia of foramen of Magendie. *Trans Am Neurol Assoc* 1957; **82**: 144–5.

331 Geoffroy Saint-Hilaire I. *Histoire générale et particulière des anomalies de l'organisation chez l'homme et les anomaux*. Paris: JB Bailière, 1832.

332 Geoffroy Saint-Hilaire I. Sur de nouveaux anencéphales humains confirmant par leur fait d'organisation la derniére théorie sur les monstres. *Mém Muséum d'Hist Nat (Paris)* 1825; **12**: 233–56.

333 Gelot A, Billette de Villemeur T, Bordarier C *et al*. Developmental aspects of type II lissencephaly. Comparative study of dysplastic lesions in fetal and post-natal brains. *Acta Neuropathol (Berl)* 1995; **89**: 72–84.

334 Gerard CL, Dugas M, Narcy P, Hertz-Pannier J. Chiari malformation Type I in a child with velopharyngeal insufficiency. *Dev Med Child Neurol* 1992; **34**: 174–6.

335 Gerard M, Hernandez L, Wevrick R, Stewart CL. Disruption of the mouse necdin gene results in early post-natal lethality. *Nat Genet* 1999; **23**: 199–202.

336 Gibbs JL. The heart and tuberous sclerosis. *Br Heart J* 1985; **54**: 596–9.

337 Gibson JB. Congenital hydrocephalus due to atresia of the foramen of Magendie. *J Neuropathol Exp Neurol* 1955; **14**: 244–62.

338 Gilbert JN, Jones KC, Rorke LB *et al*. Central nervous system anomalies associated with meningomyelocele, hydrocephalus and the Arnold–Chiari malformations: reappraisal of thesis regarding the pathogenesis of posterior neural tube closure defects. *Neurosurgery* 1986; **18**: 559–63.

339 Gilles FH, Davidson RI. Communicating hydrocephalus associated with deficient dysplastic parasagittal arachnoidal granulations. *J Neurosurg* 1971; **35**: 421–6.

340 Gimenez-Roldani S, Benito C, Mateo D. Familial communicating syringomyelia. *J Neurol Sci* 1987; **36**: 135–46.

341 Gingrich JR, Roder J. Inducible gene expression in the nervous system of transgenic mice. *Annu Rev Neurosci* 1998; **21**: 377–405.

342 Giroud A. Causes and morphogenesis of anencephaly. In: Wolstenholme GEW, O'Connor eds. *Congenital malformations*. London: Churchill, 1960: 199–212.

343 Gleeson JG, Allen KM, Fox JW *et al*. Doublecortin, a brain-specific gene mutated in human X-linked lissencephaly and double cortex syndrome, encodes a putative signaling protein. *Cell* 1998; **92**: 63–72.

344 Glover MT, Brett EM, Atherton DJ. Hypomelanosis of Ito: spectrum of the disease. *J Pediatr* 1989; **115**: 75–80.

345 Golden JA, Chernoff GF. Intermittent pattern of neural tube closure in two strains of mice. *Teratology* 1993; **47**: 73–80.

346 Gomez MR ed. *Tuberous sclerosis*. New York: Raven Press, 1979.

347 Gomez MR, Whitten CF, Nolke A *et al*. Aneurysmal malformation of the great vein of Galen causing heart failure in early infancy: report of 5 cases. *Pediatrics* 1963; **31**: 400–11.

348 González-García M, García I, Ding L *et al*. bcl-x is expressed in embryonic and postnatal neural tissues and functions to prevent neuronal cell death. *Proc Natl Acad Sci USA* 1995; **92**: 4304–8.

349 Goodlin RC, Heidrick WP, Papenfuss HL, Kubitz RL. Fetal malformations associated with maternal hypoxia. *Am J Obstet Gynecol* 1984; **49**: 228–9.

350 Gosseye S, Golaire M, Larroche JC. Cerebral, renal and splenic lesions due to fetal anoxia and their relationship to malformations. *Dev Med Child Neurol* 1982; **24**: 510–18.

351 Goto S, Hirano A, Rojas-Corona RR. A comparative immunocytochemical study of human cerebellar cortex in X-chromosome-linked copper malabsorption (Menkes-kinky hair disease) and granule cell type cerebellar degeneration. *Neuropathol Appl Neurobiol* 1989; **15**: 419–31.

352 Gott PS, Saul RE. Agenesis of the corpus callosum: limits of functional compensation. *Neurology* 1978; **28**: 1272–9.

353 Gottfried M, Lavine L, Roessmann U. Neuropathological findings in Wolf–Hirschhorn (4p-) syndrome. *Acta Neuropathol (Berl)* 1981; **55**: 163–5.

354 Gould S, Howard S. An immunohistological study of macrophages in the human fetal brain. *Neuropathol Appl Neurobiol* 1990; **16**: 261–2.

355 Goutières F, Aicardi J, Farkas E. Anterior horn cell disease associated with pontocerebellar hypoplasia in infants. *J Neurol Neurosurg Psychiatry* 1977; **40**: 370–8.

356 Goutières F, Aicardi J, Farkas-Bargeton E. Une malformation cérébrale particulière associée au nanisme thanatophore. *Rev Neurol* 1971; **125**: 435–46.

357 Granata T, Farina L, Faiella A *et al*. Familial schizencephaly associated with EMX2 mutation. *Neurology* 1997; **48**: 1403–6.

358 Green AJ, Smith M, Yates JRW. Loss of heterozygosity on chromosome 16p13.3 in hamartomas from tuberous sclerosis patients. *Nat Genet* 1994; **6**: 193–6.

359 Greene NDE, Copp AJ. Inositol prevents folate-resistant neural tube defects in the mouse. *Nat Med* 1997; **3**: 60–6.

360 Greene NDE, Gerrelli D, Van Straaten HWM, Copp AJ. Abnormalities of floor plate, notochord and somite differentiation in the *loop-tail (Lp)* mouse: a model of severe neural tube defects. *Mech Dev* 1998; **73**: 59–72.

361 Greenstone MA, Jones RWA, Dewar A *et al*. Hydrocephalus and primary ciliary dyskinesia. *Arch Dis Child* 1984; **59**: 481–2.

362 Gregg NM. Congenital cataract following German measles in the mother. *Trans Ophthalmol Soc Austral* 1941; **3**: 35–46.

363 Grollmus JM, Wilson CB, Newton TH. Paramesencephalic arachnoid cysts. *Neurology* 1976; **26**: 128–34.

364 Gross H. Die Rhombencephalosynapsis, eine systemisierte Kleinhirnfehlbildung. *Arch Psychiat Nervenkrankheit* 1959; **199**: 537–52.

365 Gross H, Hoff H. Sur les dysraphies cranioencéphaliques. In: Heuyer G, Feld M, Gjuner J. eds. *Malformations congénitales du cerveau*. Paris: Masson, 1959: 287–96.

366 Grove EA, Williams BP, Li D-Q *et al*. Multiple restricted lineages in the embryonic rat cerebral cortex. *Development* 1993; **117**: 553–61.

367 Gruenwald P, Minh H. Evaluation of body and organ weights in perinatal pathology. I. Normal standard derived from autopsies. *Am J Clin Pathol* 1960; **39**: 247–53.

368 Guerrini R, Dravet C, Raybaud C *et al*. Epilepsy and focal gyral anomalies detected by MRI: electroclinico-morphological correlations and follow-up. *Dev Med Child Neurol* 1992; **34**: 706–18.

369 Guerrini R, Dravet C, Raybaud C *et al*. Neurological findings and seizure outcome in children with bilateral opercular macrogyric-like changes detected by MRI. *Dev Med Child Neurol* 1992; **34**: 694–705.

370 Gullotta F, Rehder H, Gropp A. Descriptive neuropathology of chromosomal disorders in man. *Hum Genet* 1981; **57**: 337–44.

371 Gutierrez Y, Friede RL, Kaliney WJ. Agenesis of arachnoid granulations and its relationship to communicating hydrocephalus. *J Neurosurg* 1975; **43**: 553–8.

372 Hageman G, Willemse J, Ketel BA van *et al*. The heterogeneity of the Pene–Shokeir syndrome. *Neuropaediatrics* 1987; **45**: 18–50.

373 Hageman G, Willemse J, Ketel BA van, Verdonck AFMM. The pathogenesis of fetal hypokinesia: a neurological study of 72 cases of congenital contractures with emphasis on cerebral lesions. *Neuropediatrics* 1987; **18**: 22–33.

374 Hallervorden J. Über eine Kohlenoxydvergiftung im Fötalleben mit Entwicklungstörung der Hirnrinde. *Allg Z Psychiatrie* 1949; **124**: 289–98.

375 Halsey JH, Allen N, Chamberlin HR. The morphogenesis of hydranencephaly. *J Neurol Sci* 1971; **12**: 187–217.

376 Hanau J, Franc B, Faivre J, Foncin JF. Hydrocéphalie genetique liée au sexe. Étude anatomique. *Rev Neurol* 1978; **134**: 437–42.

377 Hanaway J, Lee SI, Netsky MG. Pachygyria: relation of findings to modern embryological concepts. *Neurology* 1968; **18**: 791–9.

378 Hanaway J, Netsky M. Heterotopias of the inferior olive: relation to Dandy–Walker malformation and correlation with experimental data. *J Neuropathol Exp Neurol* 1968; **30**: 380–9.

379 Hanigan WC, Aldrich WM. MRI and evoked potentials in a child with hydranencephaly. *Pediatr Neurol* 1988; **4**: 185–7.

380 Hannan AJ, Servotte S, Katsnelson A et al. Characterization of nodular neuronal heterotopia in children. *Brain* 1999; **122**: 219–38.

381 Hansen FJ, Friis B. Familial occurrence of cerebral gigantism. Sotos– syndrome. *Acta Paediatr Scand* 1976; **65**: 387–9.

382 Hanshaw JB. Congenital and acquired cytomegalovirus infection. *Pediatr Clin North Am* 1966; **13**: 279–93.

383 Hanshaw JB, Dudgeon JA, Marshall WC. *Viral diseases of the fetus and newborn* 2nd edn. Philadelphia, PA: WB Saunders, 1985.

384 Harbord MG, Finn JP, Hall-Craggs MA et al. Moebius syndrome with unilateral cerebellar hypoplasia. *J Med Genet* 1989; **26**: 579–82.

385 Hardimann O, Burke T, Phillips J et al. Microdysgenesis in resected temporal neocortex: incidence and clinical significance in focal epilepsy. *Neurology* 1988; **38**: 1041–7.

386 Harding B. Laminar heterotopia: a possible failure of programmed cell death? *J Neuropath exp Neurol* 1996; **55**: 1.

387 Harding BN. Cerebro-ocular dysplasia with muscular dystrophy. *Neuropathol Appl Neurobiol* 1988; **14**: 258.

388 Harding BN. Gray matter heterotopia. In: Guerrini R, Pfanner P, Roger J et al. eds. *Dysplasias of cerebral cortex in childhood-onset epilepsy*. Philadelphia, PA: Lippincott-Raven, 1996: 81–8.

389 Harding BN, Baumer JA. Congenital varicellazoster: a serologically proven case with necrotizing encephalitis and malformation. *Acta Neuropathol (Berl)* 1988; **76**: 311–15.

390 Harding BN, Boyd S. Intractable seizures from infancy can be associated with dentato-olivary dysplasia. *J Neurol Sci* 1991; **104**: 157–65.

391 Harding BN, Erdohazi M. Cerebellar disease in childhood: pontoneocerebellar hypoplasia. *Neuropathol Appl Neurobiol* 1989; **15**: 294.

392 Harding BN, Ramani P, Thurley P. The familial syndrome of proliferative vasculopathy and hydranencephaly–hydrocephaly: immunocytochemical and ultrastructural evidence for endothelial proliferation. *Neuropathol Appl Neurobiol* 1995; **21**: 61–7.

392a Harding B, Thom M. Bilateral hippocampal granule cell dispersion: autopsy study of 3 infants. *Neuropathol Appl Neurobiol* 2001; **27**: 245–51.

393 Harmant-van Rijckevorsel G, Aubert-Tulkens G, Moulin D, Lyon G. Le Syndrome de Jourbert. Étude clinique et anatome-pathologique. *Rev Neurol* 1983; **139**: 715–24.

394 Harper C, Hockey A. Proliferative vasculopathy and an hydranencephalic–hydrocephalic syndrome: a neuropathological study of two siblings. *Dev Med Child Neurol* 1983; **25**: 232–9.

395 Harris CP, Townsend JJ, Norman MG et al. Atelencephalic aprosencephaly. *J Child Neurol* 1994; **9**: 412–16.

396 Harrison KA, Thaler J, Pfaff SL et al. Pancreas dorsal lobe agenesis and abnormal islets of Langerhans in *Hlxb9*-deficient mice. *Nat Genet* 1999; **23**: 71–5.

397 Hart MN, Malamud N, Ellis WG. The Dandy–Walker syndrome. A clinicopathological study based on 28 cases. *Neurology* 1972; **22**: 771–80.

398 Hartley WJ, Saram WG de, Della-Porta AJ et al. Pathology of congenital bovine epizootic arthrogyposis and hydranencephaly and its relationship to Akabane virus. *Austral Vet J* 1977; **53**: 319–25.

399 Hartmann D, De Strooper B, Saftig P. Presenilin-1 deficiency leads to loss of Cajal–Retzius neurons and cortical dysplasia similar to human type 2 lissencephaly. *Curr Biol* 1999; **9**: 719–27.

400 Harwood-Nash DC, Fitz CR. *Neuroradiology in infants and children* 3rd edn. St Louis; MO: Mosby, 1976: 1026 pp.

401 Hatjis CG, Horber JD, Anderson GG. The *in utero* diagnosis of a posterior fossa intracranial cyst (Dandy–Walker cyst). *Am J Obstet Gynecol* 1981; **140**: 473–4.

402 Hatten ME, Alder J, Zimmerman K, Heintz N. Genes involved in cerebellar cell specification and differentiation. *Curr Opin Neurobiol* 1997; **7**: 40–7.

403 Hattori M, Adachi H, Tsujimoto M et al. Miller–Dieker lissencephaly gene encodes a subunit of brain platelet-activating factor. *Nature* 1994; **370**: 216–18.

404 Hausmann B, Sievers J. Cerebellar external granule cells are attached to the basal lamina from the onset of migration up to the end of their proliferative activity. *J Comp Neurol* 1985; **241**: 50–62.

405 Haymaker W, Girdany BR, Stephens G et al. Cerebral involvement with advanced periventricular calcification in generalised cytomegalic inclusion disease in the newborn. *J Neuropathol Exp Neurol* 1954; **13**: 562–86.

406 Henderson JL. The congenital facial diplegia syndrome: clinical features, pathology and etiology. *Brain* 1939; **62**: 381–403.

407 Hernandez D, Fisher EMC. Down syndrome genetics: unravelling a multifactorial disorder. *Hum Mol Genet* 1996; **5**: 1411–16.

408 Herringham WP, Andrewes FW. Two cases of cerebellar disease in cats, with staggering. *St Bartholomews Hosp Rep* 1888; **24**: 241–8.

409 Heschl R. Ein neuer Fall von Porencephalie. *Vierteljahrschrift für praktikale Heilkunde Prague* 1861; **72**: 102–4.

410 Heschl R. Gehirndefect und Hydrocephalus. *Vierteljahrschrift für praktikale Heilkunde Prague* 1959; **61**: 59–74.

411 Heubner O. Ueber angeborene Kernmangel (infantiler Kernschwund, Moebius). *Charitéannalen* 1900; **25**: 211–43.

412 Hiesberger T, Trommsdorff M, Howell BW et al. Direct binding of Reelin to VLDL receptor and ApoE receptor 2 induces tyrosine phosphorylation of disabled-1 and modulates tau phosphorylation. *Neuron* 1999; **24**: 481–9.

413 Higginbottom MC, Jones KL, Hall BD, Smith DW. The amniotic band disruption complex: timing of amniotic rupture and variable spectra of consequent defects. *J Pediatr* 1979; **95**: 544–9.

414 Hilburger AC, Willis JK, Bouldin E, Henderson-Tilton A. Familial schizencephaly. *Brain Dev* 1993; **15**: 234–6.

415 Hintz RL, Menking M, Sotos JF. Familial holoprosencephaly with endocrine dysgenesis. *J Pediatr* 1968; **72**: 81–7.

416 Hirano A, Dembitzer HM, Ghatak NKI, Zimmerman HM. On the relationship between human and experimental granule cell type cerebellar degeneration. *J Neuropathol Exp Neurol* 1973; **32**: 493–502.

417 Hirano A, Solomon S. Arteriovenous aneurysm of the vein of Galen. *Arch Neurol* 1960; **3**: 589–93.

418 Hirano A, Tuazon R, Zimmerman HM. Neurofibrillary changes, granulovacuolar bodies and argentophilic globules observed in tuberous sclerosis. *Acta Neuropathol (Berl)* 1968; **11**: 257–61.

419 Hirano S, Houdou S, Hasegawa M et al. Clinicopathologic studies on leptomeningeal glioneuronal heterotopia in congenital anomalies. *Pediatr Neurol* 1992; **8**: 441–4.

420 Hirono I, Shibuya C, Hayashi K. Induction of a cerebellar disorder with cycasin in newborn mice and hamsters. *Proc Soc Exp Biol Med* 1969; **131**: 593–600.

421 Hirotsune S, Fleck MW, Gambello MJ et al. Graded reduction of Pafah1b1 (Lis1) activity results in neuronal migration defects and early embryonic lethality. Nat Genet 1998; 19: 333–9.

422 Hirotsune S, Takahara T, Sasaki N et al. The reeler gene encodes a protein with an EGF-like motif expressed by pioneer neurons. Nat Genet 1995; 10: 77–83.

423 His W. Die Entwicklung des menschlichen Rautenhirns vom Ende des ersten bis zum Beginn des dritten Monats. I Verlängstes Mark. Abhandlungen des Königlich Sächsischen Gesellschaft der Wissenschaften Leipzig 1891; 29: 1–74.

424 Ho KL, Chang CH, Yang SS, Chason JL. Neuropathologic findings in thanatophoric dysplasia. Acta Neuropathol (Berl) 1984; 63: 218–28.

425 Hochgeschwender U, Brennan MB. The impact of genomics on mammalian neurobiology. BioEssays 1999; 21: 157–63.

426 Hoffman HJ, Hendrick EB. Early neurosurgical repair in craniofacial dysmorphism. J Neurosurg 1979; 51: 769–803.

427 Hofman MA. Energy metabolism and relative brain size in human neonates from single and multiple gestations: an allometric study. Biol Neonate 1984; 45: 157–64.

428 Holden AM Jr, Fyler DC, Shillito J, Nadas AS. Congestive heart failure from intracranial arteriovenous fistula in infancy. Pediatrics 1972; 49: 30–9.

429 Holland HC, Graham WL. Congenital atresia of the foramina of Luschka and Magendie with hydrocephalus. Report of a case in an adult. J Neurosurg 1958; 15: 688–94.

430 Holmes L, Nash A, Zu Rhein G et al. X-linked aqueductal stenosis: clinical and morphological findings in two families. Pediatrics 1973; 51: 697–704.

431 Hori A, Friede RL, Fischer G. Ventricular diverticles with localised dysgenesis of the temporal lobe in cloverleaf skull anomaly. Acta Neuropathol (Berl) 1983; 60: 132–6.

432 Hori A, Minwegen J. Intrauterine purulent encephalitis with early stage of hydranencephaly. Case report. Acta Neuropathol (Berl) 1984; 64: 72–4.

433 Hosley MA, Abroms IF, Ragland RL. Schizencephaly: case report of familial incidence. Pediatr Neurol 1992; 8: 148–50.

434 Houser CR. Granule cell dispersion in the dentate gyrus of humans with temporal lobe epilepsy. Brain Res 1990; 535: 195–204.

435 Houser CR, Swartz BE, Walsh GO et al. Granule cell dispersion in the dentate gyrus: possible alterations of neuronal migration in human temporal lobe epilepsy. In: Engel JJ, Wasterlain C, Cavalheiro EA et al. eds Molecular biology of epilepsy. Amsterdam: Elsevier, 1992: 41–9.

436 Howard FH, Till K, Carter CO. A family study of hydrocephalus resulting from aqueduct stenosis. J Med Genet 1981; 18: 252–5.

437 Hoyt CS, Billson F, Ouvrier R, Wise G. Ocular features of Aicardi's syndrome. Arch Ophthalmol 1978; 96: 291–5.

438 Hoyt WF, Kaplan SL, Grumbach MM, Glaser JS. Septo-optic dysplasia and pituitary dwarfism. Lancet 1970; i: 893–4.

439 Huard JMT, Forster CC, Carter ML et al. Cerebellar histogenesis is disturbed in mice lacking cyclin D2. Development 1999; 126: 1927–35.

440 Hughes HE, Miskin M. Congenital microcephaly due to vascular disruption: in utero documentation. Pediatrics 1986; 78: 85–7.

441 Hughes JT, Brownell B. Aberrant nerve fibres within the spinal cord. J Neurol Neurosurg Psychiatry 1963; 26: 528–34.

442 Hunt A, Lindenbaum RH. Tuberous sclerosis: a new estimate of prevalence within the Oxford region. J Med Genet 1984; 21: 272–7.

443 Hunt P, Krumlauf R. Hox codes and positional specification in vertebrate embryonic axes. Annu Rev Cell Biol 1992; 8: 227–56.

444 Huttenlocher RR, Taravath S, Mojtahedi S. Periventricular heterotopia and epilepsy. Neurology 1994; 44: 51–5.

445 Iivanainen M, Haltia M, Lydecken K. Atelencephaly. Dev Med Child Neurol 1977; 19: 663–8.

446 Ikonomidou C, Bittigau P, Ishimaru MJ et al. Ethanol-induced apoptotic neurodegeneration and fetal alcohol syndrome. Science 2000; 287: 1056–60.

447 Ingham PW. Transducing hedgehog: the story so far. EMBO J 1998; 17: 3505–11.

448 Isaac M, Best P. Two cases of agenesis of the vermis of cerebellum, with fusion of the dentate nuclei and cerebellar hemispheres. Acta Neuropathol (Berl) 1987; 74: 278–80.

449 Isu T, Chono Y, Iwasaki Y et al. Scoliosis associated with syringomyelia presenting in children. Childs Nerv Syst 1992; 8: 97–100.

450 Iwata T, Chen L, Li CI et al. A neonatal lethal mutation in FGFR3 uncouples proliferation and differentiation of growth plate chondrocytes in embryos. Hum Mol Genet 2000; 9: 1603–13.

451 Jacobsen M, Jacobsen GK, Clausen PP et al. Intracellular plasma proteins in human fetal choroid plexus during development. II. The distribution of prealbumin, albumin, α-fetoprotein, transferrin, IgG, IgA, IgM, and alpha$_1$-antitrypsin. Dev Brain Res 1982; 3: 251–62.

452 Jacobson MD, Weil M, Raff MC. Programmed cell death in animal development. Cell 1997; 88: 347–54.

453 Jaffe R, Crumrine P, Hashida Y, Moser HW. Neonatal adenoleukodystrophy. Clinical, pathological and biochemical delineation of a syndrome affecting both males and females. Am J Pathol 1982; 108: 100–11.

454 Jakob H. Die feinere Oberflächengestaltung der Hirnwindungen, die Hirnwarzenbildung und die Mikropolygrie. Z Neurol Psychiatrie 1940; 170: 64–84.

455 Jakob H. Faktoren bei der Entstehung der normalen und der entwicklungs-gestörten Hirnrinde. Z Neurol Psychiatrie 1936; 155: 1–39.

456 Janota I, Polkey CE. Cortical dysplasia in epilepsy – a study of material from surgical resections for intractable epilepsy. In: Pedley TA, Meldrum BS eds. Recent advances in epilepsy 5th edn. London: Churchill Livingstone, 1992: 37–49.

457 Janzer RC, Friede RL. Dandy–Walker syndrome with atresia of the fourth ventricle and multiple rhombencephalic malformations. Acta Neuropathol (Berl) 1982; 58: 81–6.

458 Jeeves MA. Agenesis of the corpus callosum. In: Boller F, Grafman J eds. Handbook of neuropsychology 4th edn. New York: Elsevier, 1990: 99–114.

459 Jellinger K, Gross H. Congenital telencephalic midline defects. Neuropädiatrie 1973; 4: 446–52.

460 Jellinger K, Gross H, Kaltenbäck E, Grisold W. Holoprosencephaly and agenesis of the corpus callosum; frequency of associated malformations. Acta Neuropathol (Berl) 1981; 55: 1–10.

461 Jellinger K, Rett A. Agyria–pachygyria (lissencephaly syndrome). Neuropädiatrie 1976; 7: 66–91.

462 Jenkyn LR, Roberts DW, Merlis AL et al. Dandy–Walker malformation in identical twins. Neurology 1981; 31: 337–41.

463 Jeret JS, Serur D, Wisniewski KE. Lubin RA. Clinicopathological findings associated with agenesis of the corpus callosum. Brain Dev 1987; 9: 255–64.

464 Jervis GA. Early senile dementia in mongoloid idiocy. Am J Psychiatry 1948; 105: 102–6.

465 Jervis GA. Spongioneuroblastoma and tuberous sclerosis. *J Neuropathol Exp Neurol* 1954; **13**: 105–16.

466 Jiang H, Gyda M III, Harnish DC *et al*. Teratogenesis by retinoic acid analogs positively correlates with elevation of retinoic acid receptor-β2 mRNA levels in treated embryos. *Teratology* 1994; **50**: 38–43.

467 Johnson FE. Injury of the child by Roentgen ray during pregnancy. Report of a case. *J Pediatr* 1938; **13**: 894–901.

468 Johnson RT, Johnson K. Hydrocephalus following virus infection: the pathology of aqueductal stenosis developing after experimental mumps virus infection. *J Neuropathol Exp Neurol* 1968; **27**: 591–606.

469 Jonesco-Sisesti N. *La syringobulbie*. Paris: Masson, 1932.

470 Joubert M, Eisenring JJ, Robb JP, Andermann F. Familial agenesis of the cerebellar vermis. A syndrome of episodic hyperpnea, abnormal eye movements, ataxia and retardation. *Neurology* 1969; **19**: 813–25.

471 Jung JH, Graham JM Jr, Schultz N, Smith DW. Congenital hydranencephaly/porencephaly due to vascular disruption in monozygotic twins. *Pediatrics* 1984; **73**: 467–9.

472 Juriloff DM, Harris MJ. Mouse models for neural tube closure defects. *Hum Mol Genet* 2000; **9**: 993–1000.

473 Kallischer S. Demonstration des Gehirns eines Kindes mit Telangectasie der links-seitigen Gesicht und Kopfhaut und der Hirnoberfläche. *Kindische Wochenschrift* 1897; **34**: 1059.

474 Kalter H. Case reports of malformations associated with maternal diabetes: history and critique. *Clin Genet* 1993; **43**: 174–9.

475 Kalter H. Five-decade international trends in the relation of perinatal mortality and congenital malformations: stillbirth and neonatal death compared. *Int J Epidemiol* 1991; **20**: 173–9.

476 Kalter H. *Teratology of the central nervous sytem*. Chicago, IL: University of Chicago Press, 1968.

477 Kalter H, Warkany J. Congenital malformations – etologic factors and their role in prevention. *N Engl J Med* 1983; **308**: 424–31.

478 Kamoshita S, Takei Y, Miyao M *et al*. Pontocerebellar hypoplasia associated with infantile motor neuron disease (Norman's disease). *Pediatr Pathol* 1990; **10**: 133–42.

479 Kamuro K, Tenokuchi Y. Familial periventricular nodular heterotopia. *Brain Dev* 1993; **15**: 237–41.

480 Kang S, Graham JM Jr, Olney AH, Biesecker LG. GLI3 frameshift mutations cause autosomal dominant Pallister–Hall syndrome. *Nat Genet* 1997; **15**: 266–8.

481 Karch SB, Urich H. Occipital encephalocele: a morphological study. *J Neurol Sci* 1972; **15**: 89–112.

482 Kawagoe T, Jacob H. Neocerebellar hypoplasia with systemic combined olivo-ponto-dentatal degeneration in a 9-day-old baby: contribution to the problem of relations between malformation and systemic degeneration in early life. *Clin Neuropathol* 1986; **5**: 203–8.

483 Keeling JW, Kjær I. Diagnostic distinction between anencephaly and amnion rupture sequence based on skeletal analysis. *J Med Genet* 1994; **31**: 823–9.

484 Kelley RI, Roessler E, Hennekam RCM *et al*. Holoprosencephaly in RSH/Smith–Lemli–Opitz syndrome: does abnormal cholesterol metabolism affect the function of *Sonic Hedgehog*. *Am J Med Genet* 1996; **66**: 478–84.

485 Kelly OG, Melton DA. Induction and patterning of the vertebrate nervous system. *Trends Genet* 1995; **11**: 273–8.

486 Kemper TL, Lecours AR, Gates MG, Yakovlev PI. Retardation of the myelo- and cyto-architectonic maturation of the brain in the congenital rubella syndrome in early development. *Res Publ Pub Assoc Res Nerv Ment Dis* 1973; **51**: 23–62.

487 Kepes JJ, Clough C, Villanueva A. Congenital fusion of the thalami (atresia of the third ventricle) and associated anomalies in a 6 month old infant. *Acta Neuropathol (Berl)* 1969; **13**: 97–104.

488 Kerner B, Graham JM Jr, Golden JA *et al*. Familial lissencephaly with cleft palate and severe cerebellar hypoplasia. *Am J Med Genet* 1999; **87**: 440–5.

489 Kershman J. Genesis of microglia in the human brain. *Arch Neurol Psychiatry* 1939; **41**: 24–50.

490 Khan M, Rozdilsky B, Gerrard JW. Familial holoprosencephaly. *Dev Med Child Neurol* 1970; **12**: 71–6.

491 Kilham L, Margolis G. Cerebellar ataxia in hamsters inoculated with rat virus. *Science* 1964; **143**: 1047–8.

492 Kim TS, Cho S, Dickson DW. Aprosencephaly: review of the literature and report of a case with cerebellar hypoplasia, pigmented epithelial cyst and Rathke's cleft cyst. *Acta Neuropathol (Berl)* 1990; **79**: 424–31.

493 King MD, Dudgeon J, Stephenson JBP. Joubert's syndrome with retinal dysplasia: neonatal tachypnoea as the clue to a genetic brain–eye malformation. *Arch Dis Child* 1984; **59**: 709–18.

494 King MD, Stephenson JBP, Ziervogel M *et al*. Hemimegalencephaly – a case for hemispherectomy. *Neuropediatrics* 1985; **16**: 46–55.

495 Kingsley DPE. Neuro-imaging. In: Brett EM ed. *Paediatric neurology*. London: Churchill Livingstone, 1991: 836–7.

496 Kirke PN, Molloy AM, Daly LE *et al*. Maternal plasma folate and vitamin B_{12} are independent risk factors for neural tube defects. *Q J Med* 1993; **86**: 703–8.

497 Kitanaka C, Iwasaki Y, Yamada H. Retroflexion of holoprosencephaly: report of two cases. *Childs Nerv Syst* 1992; **8**: 317–21.

498 Knebel-Doeberitz C, Sievers J, Sadler M *et al*. Destruction of meningeal cells in the newborn hamster cerebellum with 6 hydroxydopamine prevents foliation and lamination in the rostral cerebellum. *Neurosci* 1986; **17**: 409–26.

499 Knudson AJ. Genetics of human cancer. *Annu Rev Genet* 1986; **20**: 231–51.

500 Kobayashi K, Nakahori Y, Miyake M *et al*. An ancient retrotransposal insertion causes Fukuyama-type congenital muscular dystrophy. *Nature* 1998; **394**: 388–92.

501 Köhler U. Sturge-Webersche Krankheit bei einer Frühgeburt. *Zentralblatt Allg Pathol Anat* 1940; **75**: 81–5.

502 Koseki H, Wallin J, Wilting J *et al*. A role for *Pax-1* as a mediator of notochordal signals during the dorsoventral specification of vertebrae. *Development* 1993; **119**: 629–60.

503 Koster S. Two cases of hypoplasia pontoneocere bellaris. *Acta Psychiat Kobenhavn* 1926; **1**: 47–76.

504 Kotzot D, Weigl J, Huk W, Rott HD. Hydantoin syndrome with holoprosencephaly: a possible rare teratogenic effect. *Teratology* 1993; **48**: 15–19.

505 Kruyff E. Paracollicular plate cysts. *Am J Roentgenol* 1965; **95**: 899–916.

506 Kuchelmeister K, Bergmann M, Gullotta F. Neuropathology of lissencephalies. *Childs Nerv Syst* 1993; **9**: 394–9.

507 Kuida K, Zheng TS, Na SQ *et al*. Decreased apoptosis in the brain and premature lethality in CPP32-deficient mice. *Nature* 1996; **384**: 368–72.

508 Kundrat H. *Arhinencephalie als typische Art von Missbildung*. Graz: Luschner and Lubensky, 1882.

509 Kuznicky R, Andermann F, Guerrini R. The epileptic spectrum in the congenital bilateral perisylvian syndrome. CBPS Multicenter Collaborative Study. *Neurology* 1994; **44**: 379–85.

510 Kuznicky R, Andermann F, Tampieri D *et al*. Bilateral central macrogyria: epilepsy, pseudobulbar palsy, and mental retardation – a recognizable neuronal migration disorder. *Ann Neurol* 1989; **25**: 547–54.

511 Lacey DJ, Terplan K. Abnormal cerebral cortical neurons in a child with maternal PKU syndrome. *J Child Neurol* 1987; **2**: 201–4.

512 Lagger RL. Failure of pyramidal tract decussation in the Dandy–Walker syndrome. Report of two cases. *J Neurosurg* 1979; **50**: 382–7.

513 Lagos JC. Congenital aneurysms and arteriovenous malformations. In: Vinken PJ, Bruyn GW eds. *Handbook of clinical neurology*. Amsterdam: North-Holland, 1977: 137–209.

514 Lammer EJ, Chen DT, Hoar RM *et al*. Retinoic acid embryopathy. *N Engl J Med* 1985; **313**: 837–41.

515 Lammer EJ, Sever LE, Oakley GP. Teratogen update: valproic acid. *Teratology* 1987; **35**: 465–73.

516 Landrieu P, Ninane J, Ferrière G, Lyon G. Aqueductal stenosis in X-linked hydrocephalus: a secondary phenomenon? *Dev Med Child Neurol* 1979; **21**: 637–52.

517 Lange-Cosack H. Die Hydranencephalie (Blasenhirn) als Sonderform der Grosshirnlosigkeit. *Arch Psychiat Nervenkrankheit* 1944; **117**: 1–51.

518 Larke RPB, Wheatley E, Saroj S, Chernesky M. Congenital cytomegalovirus infection in an urban Canadian community. *J Infect Dis* 1980; **142**: 647–53.

519 Larroche J. *Developmental pathology of the neonate*. Amsterdam: Excepta Medica, 1977.

520 Larroche J. Malformations of the nervous system. In: Hume Adams J, Corsellis JAN, Duchen LW eds. *Greenfield's neuropathology* 4th edn. London: Edward Arnold, 1984: 385–450.

521 Larroche JC, Baudey J. Cavum septi lucidi, cavum vergae, cavum veli interpositi: cavités de la ligne médiane (étude anatomique et pneumoencephalographique dans la période néonatale). *Biol Neonate* 1961; **3**: 193–236.

522 Larroche JC, Droulle P, Delezoide AL *et al*. Brain damage in monozygous twins. *Biol Neonate* 1990; **57**: 261–78.

523 Larroche JC, Encha-Razavi F. The central nervous system. In: Wigglesworth JS, Singer DB eds. *Textbook of fetal and perinatal pathology*. Oxford: Blackwell, 1991: 778–842.

524 Larroche JC, Maunoury T. Analyse statistique de la croissance pondérale des foetus et des viscères pendant la vie intrautérine. *Arch Fr Pediatr* 1973; **30**: 927–49.

525 Larroche JC, Nessmann C. Focal cerebral anomalies and retinal dysplasia in a 23–24-week-old fetus. *Brain Dev* 1993; **15**: 51–6.

526 Larsell O. The development of the cerebellum in man in relation to its comparative anatomy. *J Comp Neurol* 1947; **87**: 85–129.

527 La Torre E, Fortuna A, Occhipinti E. Angiographic differentiation between Dandy–Walker cyst and arachnoid cyst of the posterior fossa in newborn infants and children. *J Neurosurg* 1973; **38**: 298–308.

528 Laurence KM. A case of unilateral megalencephaly. *Dev Med Child Neurol* 1964; **6**: 585–90.

529 Laurence KM, Tew BJ. Follow-up of 65 survivors from the 425 cases of spina bifida born in South Wales between 1956 and 1962. *Dev Med Child Neurol* 1967; **13** (Suppl): 1–13.

530 Laxova R, O'Hara PT, Timothy JAD. A further example of a lethal autosomal recessive condition in sibs. *J Ment Def Res* 1971; **16**: 139–43.

531 Lazar ML. Vein of Galen aneurysm: successful excision of a completely thrombosed aneurysm in an infant. *Surg Neurol* 1974; **2**: 22–4.

532 Lazjuk GI, Lurie IW, Ostrowskaja TI *et al*. Brief clinical observations: the Neu–Laxova syndrome – a distinct entity. *Am J Med Genet* 1979; **3**: 261–7.

533 Leach WB. Primary neoplasms of the heart. *Acta Pathol* 1947; **44**: 198–204.

534 Ledbetter SA, Kuwano A, Dobyns WB, Ledbetter DH. Microdeletions of chromosome 17p13 as a cause of isolated lissencephaly. *Am J Hum Genet* 1992; **50**: 182–9.

535 Lee EY-HP, Chang C-Y, Hu N *et al*. Mice deficient for Rb are nonviable and show defects in neurogenesis and haematopoiesis. *Nature* 1992; **359**: 288–94.

536 Leech RW, Bowlby LS, Brumback RA, Schaefer GB Jr. Agnathia, holoprosencephaly and situs inversus. Report of a case. *Am J Med Genet* 1988; **29**: 483–90.

537 Leech RW, Shuman RM. Holoprosencephaly and related midline cerebral anomalies: a review. *J Child Neurol* 1986; **1**: 3–18.

538 Legouis R, Hardelin J-P, Levilliers J *et al*. The candidate gene for the X-linked Kallman syndrome encodes a protein related to adhesion molecules. *Cell* 1991; **67**: 423–35.

539 Lemire RJ. Variations in development of the caudal neural tube in human embryos (Horizons XIV–XXI). *Teratology* 1969; **2**: 361–70.

540 Lemire RJ, Loeser JD, Leech RW *et al*. *Normal and abnormal development of the human nervous system*. Hagerstown, MD: Harper & Row, 1975.

541 Leong ASY, Shaw CM. The pathology of occipital encephalocele and a discussion of the pathogenesis. *Pathology* 1979; **11**: 223–34.

542 Levine DN, Fisher MA, Caviness VS. Porencephaly with microgyria: a pathological study. *Acta Neuropathol (Berl)* 1974; **29**: 99–113.

543 Levine OR, Jameson A, Nellhaus G, Gold AP. Cardiac complications of cerebral arterio-venous fistula in infancy. *Pediatrics* 1962; **30**: 563–75.

544 Levy WS, Mason L, Hahn JF. Chiari malformation presenting in adults: a surgical experience in 127 cases. *Neurosurgery* 1983; **12**: 377–89.

545 Leyten QH, Gabreels FJ, Renier WO *et al*. Congenital muscular dystrophy with eye and brain malformations in six Dutch patients. *Neuropediatrics* 1992; **23**: 316–20.

546 Leyten QH, Renkawek K, Renier WO. Neuropathological findings in muscle–eye–brain disease (MEB-D). Neuropathological delineation of MEB-D from congential muscular dystrophy of Fukuyama type. *Acta Neuropathol (Berl)* 1999; **83**: 55–60.

547 Leyten QH, Renkawek K, Renier WO *et al*. Neuropathological findings in muscle–eye–brain disease (MEB-D). Neuropathological delineation of MEB-D from congenital muscular dystrophy of the Fukuyama type. *Acta Neuropathol (Berl)* 1991; **83**: 55–60.

548 Li H, Arber S, Jessell TM, Edlund H. Selective agenesis of the dorsal pancreas in mice lacking homeobox gene *Hlxb9*. *Nat Genet* 1999; **23**: 67–70.

549 Lichtenstein BW. Distant neuroanatomic complications of spina bifida (spinal dysraphism). *Arch Neurol Psychiatry* 1942; **47**: 195–214.

550 Lichtenstein BW. Maldevelopments of the cerebellum. *J Neuropathol Exp Neurol* 1943; **2**: 164–77.

551 Lichtenstein BW, Maloney JE. Malformation of the forebrain with comments on the so-called dorsal cyst, the corpus callosum and the hippocampal structures. *J Neuropathol Exp Neurol* 1954; **13**: 117–28.

552 Lindenberg R, Swanson PD. Infantile hydranencephaly. A report of five cases of infarction of both cerebral hemispheres in infancy. *Brain* 1967; **90**: 839–50.

553 Lipton HL, Prezios TJ, Moses H. Adult onset of the Dandy–Walker syndrome. *Arch Neurol* 1978; **35**: 672–4.

554 List CF, Holt JE, Everett M. Lipoma of the corpus callosum – a clinicopathological study. *Am J Radiol* 1946; **55**: 125–34.

555 Litvak J, Yahr MD, Ransohoff J. Aneurysms of great vein of Galen and midline cerebral arteriovenous anomalies. *J Neurosurg* 1995; **17**: 945–54.

556 Livingston JH, Aicardi J. Unusual MRI appearances of diffuse subcortical heterotopia or 'double cortex' in two children. *J Neurol Neurosurg Psychiatry* 1990; **53**: 617–20.

557 Loeser JD, Alvord EC. Clinicopathological correlation in agenesis of the corpus callosum. *Neurology* 1968; **18**: 745–56.

558 Loeser JD, Ellsworth CA, Alvord EC. Agenesis of the corpus callosum. *Brain* 1968; **91**: 533–70.

559 Loiseau P, Vital C, DeBoucard P *et al*. Étude anatomo-clinique d'un cas d'hémiplégie–épilepsie avec mouvements anormaux. Atrophie cérébelleuse croisée. *Rev Neurol* 1968; **118**: 77–82.

560 Lo Nigro C, Chong CS, Smith AC *et al*. Point mutations and an intragenic deletion in LIS1, the lissencephaly causative gene in isolated lissencephaly sequence and Miller–Dieker syndrome. *Hum Mol Genet* 1997; **6**: 157–64.

561 Lorber J. Results of treatment of myelomeningocele. An analysis of 524 unselected cases, with special reference to possible selection for treatment. *Dev Med Child Neurol* 1971; **13**(Suppl 25): 279.

562 Loth P, Casasoprana A, Thibert M. Une cause rare de défaillance cardiaque néonatale: l'anévrysme arterio-veineux intracranien. *Arch Fr Pediatr* 1972; **24**: 255–68.

563 Lourie H, Berne A. A contribution on the etiology and pathogenesis of congenital communicating hydrocephalus. *Biol Neonate* 1961; **15**: 815–22.

564 Lowry RB. Variability in the Smith–Lemli–Opitz syndrome: overlap with the Meckel syndrome. *Am J Med Genet* 1983; **14**: 429–33.

565 Lumsden CE. Multiple cystic softening of the brain in the newborn. *J Neuropathol Exp Neurol* 1950; **9**: 119–37.

566 Lurie IW, Nedzved MK, Lazjuk GI *et al*. Aprosencephaly–atelencephaly and the aprosencephaly (XK) syndrome. *Am J Med Genet* 1979; **3**: 303–9.

567 Luthy DA, Wardinsky T, Shurtleff DB *et al*. Cesarean section before the onset of labor and subsequent motor function in infants with meningomyelocele diagnosed antenatally. *N Engl J Med* 1991; **324**: 662–6.

568 Lynn RB, Buchanan DG, Fenichel GM, Freeman FR. Agenesis of the corpus callosum. *Arch Neurol* 1980; **37**: 444–5.

569 Lyon G, Gastaut H. Considerations on the significance attributed to unusual cerebral histological findings recently described in eight patients with primary generalised epilepsy. *Epilepsia* 1985; **26**: 365–7.

570 Lyon G, Robain O. Étude comparative des encéphalopathies circulatoires prénatales et paranatales (hydranencéphalies, porencéphalies et encéphalomalacias kystiques de la substance blanche). *Acta Neuropathol (Berl)* 1967; **9**: 79–98.

571 Lyon MF. Some milestones in the history of X-chromosome inactivation. *Annu Rev Genet* 1992; **26**: 17–28.

572 McBride MC, Kemper TL. Pathogenesis of fourlayered microgyric cortex in man. *Acta Neuropathol (Berl)* 1982; **57**: 93–8.

573 Macchi G, Bentivoglio M. Agenesis or hypoplasia of cerebellar structures. In: Vinken PJ, Bruyn G eds. *Handbook of clinical neurology*. Amsterdam: Elsevier, 1977: 367–93.

574 Machin GA. Twins and their disorders. In: Reed GB, Claireaux AE, Cockburn F eds. *Diseases of the fetus and newborn. Pathology, imaging, genetics and management* 2nd edn. London: Chapman & Hall, 1995: 201–25.

575 McConnell SK, Kaznowski CE. Cell cycle dependence of laminar determination in developing neocortex. *Science* 1991; **254**: 282–5.

576 McCracken G, Shinefield H, Cobb K *et al*. Congenital cytomegalic inclusion disease. *Am J Dis Child* 1969; **117**: 522–39.

577 MacFarlane A, Maloney AFJ. The appearance of the aqueduct and its relationship to hydrocephalus in the Arnold–Chiari malformation. *Brain* 1957; **80**: 479–91.

578 Mack LD, Rumack CM, Johnson ML. Ultrasound evaluation of cystic intracranial lesions in the neonate. *Radiology* 1980; **37**: 451–55.

579 McKay R. Stem cells in the central nervous system. *Science* 1997; **276**: 66–71.

580 MacKenzie NG, Emery JL. Deformities of the cervical cord in children with neurospinal dysraphism. *Dev Med Child Neurol* 1971; **13**(Suppl 25): 58–61.

581 McLaurin RL. Parietal cephaloceles. *Neurology* 1964; **14**: 764–74.

582 McLendon RE, Crain BJ, Oakes WJ, Burger PC. Cerebral polygyria in the Chiari type II (Arnold–Chiari) malformation. *Clin Neuropathol* 1985; **4**: 200–5.

583 McMahon AP, Bradley A. The Wint-I (*int-I*) proto-oncogene is required for development of a large region of the mouse brain. *Cell* 1990; **62**: 1073–85.

584 McShane MA, Boyd S, Harding B *et al*. Progressive bulbar paralysis of childhood: a reappraisal of Fazio–Londe disease. *Brain* 1992; **115**: 1889–900.

585 Maksem A, Roessmann U. Apert's syndrome with central nervous system anomalies. *Acta Neuropathol (Berl)* 1979; **48**: 59–61.

586 Malamud N, Gaitz CM eds. Neuropathology of organic brain syndromes associated with aging. In: *Aging and the brain*. New York: Plenum Press, 1972: 63–87.

587 Malherbe V, Pariente D, Tardieu M *et al*. Central nervous system lesions in hypomelanosis of Ito: an MRI and pathological study. *J Neurol* 1993; **240**: 302–4.

588 Mallamaci A, Mercurio A, Muzio L *et al*. The lack of Emx2 causes impairment of Reelin signalling and defects of neuronal migration in the developing cerebral cortex. *J Neurosci* 2000; **20**: 1109–19.

589 Manterola A, Towbin A, Yakovlev PI. Cerebral infarction in the human fetus near term. *J Neuropathol Exp Neurol* 1966; **25**: 471–88.

590 Manz HJ, Phillips TM, McCullough DC, Rowden G. Unilateral megalencephaly, cerebral cortical dysplasia, neuronal hypertrophy, and heterotopia. Cytomorphometric, fluorometric cytochemical, and biochemical analyses. *Acta Neuropathol (Berl)* 1979; **45**: 97–103.

591 Manzanares M, Krumlauf R. Developmental biology – raising the roof. *Nature* 2000; **403**: 720–21.

592 Marburg O. So-called agenesis of the corpus callosum (callosal defect). *Arch Neurol Psychiatry* 1949; **61**: 297–312.

593 Marie J, See G, Gruner J *et al*. Manifestations cérébrales de la maladie des inclusions cytomégaliques. *Ann Pediatr* 1957; **25**: 248–56.

594 Marín-Padilla M. Cajal–Retzius cells and the development of the neocortex. *Trends Neurosci* 1998; **21**: 64–71.

595 Marin-Padilla M. Morphogenesis of anencephaly and related malformations. *Curr Topics Pathol* 1970; **51**: 145–74.

596 Marin-Padilla M. Study of the skull in human cranioschisis. *Acta Anat* 1965; **62**: 1–20.

597 Marin-Padilla M, Marin-Padilla TM. Morphogenesis of experimentally induced Arnold–Chiari malformation. *J Neurol Sci* 1981; **50**: 29–55.

598 Maroteaux P, Lamy M. Robert JM. La nanisme thanatophore. *Presse Med* 1967; **75**: 2519–24.

599 Marques Dias MJ, Harmant-van Rijckevorsel G, Landrieu P, Lyon G. Prenatal cytomegalovirus disease and cerebral microgyria: evidence for perfusion failure, not disturbance of his-

togenesis, as the major cause of fetal cytomegalovirus encephalopathy. *Neuropediatrics* 1984; **15**: 18–24.

600 Marshall H, Nonchev S, Sham MH *et al.* Retinoic acid alters hindbrain *Hox* code and induces transformation of rhombomeres 2/3 into a 4/5 identity. *Nature* 1992; **360**: 737–41.

601 Martin F. Ueber eine vestibulo-cerebelläre Entwicklungshemmung im Rahmen ausgedehnter osteo-neuraler Dysgenesien. *Acta Psychiat Neurol Scand* 1949; **24**: 207–22.

602 Martin JK, Norman RM. Maple syrup urine disease in an infant with microgyria. *Dev Med Child Neurol* 1967; **9**: 152–9.

603 Martin RA, Carey JG. A review and case report of aprosencephaly and the XK aprosencephaly syndrome. *Am J Med Genet* 1982; **11**: 369–71.

603a Martland BN, Harding RE, Morton, Young I. Dentato-olivary dysplasia in sibs: an autosomal recessive disorders? Anonymous. Anonymous. *J Med Genetics* 1997; **34**: 1021–3.

604 Masters C, Alpers M, Kakulas B. Pathogenesis of Reovirus type 1 hydrocephalus in mice. Significance of aqueductal changes. *Arch Neurol* 1977; **34**: 18–28.

605 Matell M. Ein Fall von Heterotopie der grauen Substanz in den beiden Hemisphären des Grosshirns. *Arch Psychiat Nervenkrankheit* 1893; **25**: 124–36.

606 Matsubara O, Tanaka M, Ida T, Okeda R. Hemimegalencephaly with hemihypertrophy (Klippel–Trénaunay–Weber syndrome). *Virchows Arch Pathol Anat* 1983; **400**: 155–62.

607 Mediaris DN. Cytomegalic inclusion disease. An analysis of the clinical features based on the literature and six additional cases. *Pediatrics* 1957; **19**: 466–80.

608 Meencke HJ. Neuron density in the molecular layer of the frontal cortex in primary generalized epilepsy. *Epilepsia* 1985; **26**: 450–4.

609 Meencke HJ, Janz D. Neuropathological findings in primary generalised epilepsy: a study of eight cases. *Epilepsia* 1984; **25**: 8–21.

610 Meencke HJ, Veith G. Migration disturbances in epilepsy. In: Engel JJ, Wasterlain C, Cavalheiro EA *et al.* eds. *Molecular biology of epilepsy*. Amsterdam: Elsevier, 1992: 31–40.

611 Mello LEAM, Cavalheiro EA, Tan AI *et al.* Granule cell dispersion in relation to mossy fiber sprouting, hippocampal loss, silent period and seizure frequency in the pilocarpine model of epilepsy. In: Engel JJ, Wasterlain C, Cavalheiro EA *et al.* eds. *Molecular biology of epilepsy*. Amsterdam: Elsevier, 1992: 51–60.

612 Menkes JH, Philippart M, Clark DE. Hereditary partial agenesis of the corpus callosum. *Arch Neurol* 1964; **11**: 198–208.

613 Meuli M, Meuli-Simmen C, Hutchins GM *et al.* In utero surgery rescues neurological function at birth in sheep with spina bifida. *Nat Med* 1995; **1**: 342–7.

614 Meyer A, Jones TB. Histological changes in brain in mongolism. *J Ment Sci* 1939; **85**: 206–21.

615 Miale IL, Sidman RL. An autoradiographic analysis of histogenesis in the mouse cerebellum. *Exp Neurol* 1961; **4**: 277–96.

616 Michaelson PS, Gilles FH. Central nervous system abnormalities in trisomy E (17–18) syndrome. *J Neurol Sci* 1972; **15**: 193–208.

617 Miller G, Ladda RL, Towfighi J. Cerebro-ocular dysplasia–muscular dystrophy (Walker–Warburg) syndrome. Findings in a 20 week fetus. *Acta Neuropathol (Berl)* 1991; **82**: 234–8.

618 Miller GM, Stears JC, Guggenheim MA, Wilkening GN. Schizencephaly: a clinical and CT study. *Neurology* 1984; **34**: 997–1001.

619 Miller J. Lissencephaly in two siblings. *Neurology* 1963; **13**: 841–50.

620 Miller RW. Effects of ionizing radiation from the atomic bomb on Japanese children. *Pediatrics* 1968; **41**: 257–63.

621 Millett S, Campbell K, Epstein DJ *et al.* A role for *Gbx2* in repression of *Otx2* and positioning the mid/hindbrain organizer. *Nature* 1999; **401**: 161–4.

622 Mills JL, McPartlin JM, Kirke PN *et al.* Homocysteine metabolism in pregnancies complicated by neural-tube defects. *Lancet* 1995; **345**: 149–51.

623 Ming PL, Goodner DM, Park TS. Cytogenetic variants in holoprosencephaly. Report of a case and review of the literature. *Am J Dis Child* 1976; **130**: 864–7.

624 Miskolczy D. Ein Fall von Kleinhirnmissbildung. *Arch Psychiat Nervenkrankheit* 1931; **93**: 596–615.

625 Mizuguchi M, Maekawa S, Kamoshita S. Distribution of leptomeningeal glioneuronal heterotopia in alobar holoprosencephaly. *Arch Neurol* 1994; **51**: 951–4.

626 Mizuguchi M, Morimatsu Y. Histopathological study of alobar holoprosencephaly. 1. Abnormal laminar architecture of the telencephalic cortex. *Acta Neuropathol (Berl)* 1989; **78**: 176–82.

627 Moase CE, Trasler DG. Splotch locus mouse mutants: models for neural tube defects and Waardenburg syndrome type I in humans. *J Med Genet* 1992; **29**: 145–51.

628 Möbius PJ. Ueber angeborene doppelseitige Abducens-Facialis-Lähmung. *Münchner Med Wochenschr* 1888; **35**: 108–11.

629 Moessinger AC. Fetal akinesia deformation sequence: an animal model. *Pediatrics* 1983; **72**: 857–63.

630 Mohr PD, Strang FA, Sambrook MA, Bodie HG. The clinical and surgical features of 40 patients with primary cerebellar ectopia (adult Chiari malformation). *Q J Med* 1977; **181**: 85–96.

631 Monaghan HP, Krafchik BR, Macgregor DL, Fitz CR. Tuberous sclerosis complex in children. *Am J Dis Child* 1981; **135**: 912–17.

632 Montoya G, Dohn DF, Mercer RD. Arteriovenous malformation of the vein of Galen as a cause of heart failure and hydrocephalus in infants. *Neurology* 1971; **21**: 1054–8.

633 Moore CM, McAdams AJ, Sutherland J. Intrauterine disseminated intravascular coagulation: a syndrome of multiple pregnancy with a dead twin fetus. *J Pediatr* 1969; **74**: 523–8.

634 Moore GR, Raine CS. Leptomeningeal and adventitial gliosis as a consequence of chronic inflammation. *Neuropathol Appl Neurobiol* 1986; **12**: 371–8.

635 Morel F, Wildi E. Dysgénésie nodulaire disséminée de l'écorce frontale. *Rev Neurol* 1952; **87**: 251–70.

636 Morimoto K, Mogami H. Sequential CT study of subependymal giant-cell astrocytoma associated with tuberous sclerosis. *J Neurosurg* 1986; **65**: 874–7.

637 Motoyama N, Wang F, Roth KA *et al.* Massive cell death of immature hematopoietic cells and neurons in Bcl-x-deficient mice. *Science* 1995; **267**: 1506–10.

638 Muir CS. Hydranencephaly and allied disorders. A study of cerebral defect in Chinese children. *Arch Dis Child* 1959; **34**: 231–46.

639 Mullen RJ, Herrup K. Chimeric analysis of mouse cerebellar mutants. In: Breakfield XO ed. *Neurogenetics: genetic approaches to the nervous system*. New York: Elsevier, 1979: 173–96.

640 Müller F, O'Rahilly R. The development of the human brain, the closure of the caudal neuropore, and the beginning of secondary neurulation at stage 12. *Anat Embryol* 1987; **176**: 413–30.

641 Muller LM, De Jong G, Mouton SCE *et al.* A case of Neu–Laxova syndrome: prenatal ultrasound monitoring in the third trimester and the histopathological findings. *Am J Med Genet* 1987; **26**: 421–9.

642 Münchoff C, Noetzel H. Ueber eine nahezu totale Agyrie bei einem 6 Jahre alt gewordenen Knaben. *Acta Neuropathol (Berl)* 1965; **4**: 469–75.

643 Münke M. Clinical, cytogenetic, and molecular approaches to the genetic heterogeneity of holoprosencephaly. *Am J Med Genet* 1989; **34**: 237–45.

644 Münke M, Emanuel BS, Zackai EH. Holoprosencephaly: association with interstitial deletion of 2p and review of the cytogenetic literature. *Am J Med Genet* 1988; **30**: 929–38.

645 Murofushi K. Normalentwicklung und Dysgenesien von Dentatum und Oliva inferior. *Acta Neuropathol (Berl)* 1974; **27**: 317–28.

646 Murphy M, Stinnakre MG, Senamaud-Beaufort C *et al.* Delayed early embryonic lethality following disruption of the murine cyclin A2 gene. *Nat Genet* 1997; **15**: 83–6.

647 Myers RE. Brain pathology following fetal vascular occlusion: an experimental study. *Invest Ophthalmol* 1969; **8**: 41–50.

648 Myrianthopoulos NC. Our load of central nervous system malformations. *Birth Defects* 1979; **15**: 1–18.

649 Naeye RL. Brain stem and adrenal abnormalities in the sudden infant death syndrome. *Am J Clin Pathol* 1966; **66**: 526–39.

650 Naiman J, Frazer FC. Agenesis of the corpus callosum. *Arch Neurol Psychiatry* 1955; **74**: 182–5.

651 Nakado KK. Anencephaly: a review. *Dev Med Child Neurol* 1973; **15**: 383–400.

652 Nakamura S, Makiyama H, Miyagi A *et al.* Congenital unilateral hydrocephalus. *Childs Nerv Syst* 1989; **5**: 367–70.

653 Nakamura Y, Becker LE. Subependymal giant-cell tumour: astrocytic or neuronal? *Acta Neuropathol (Berl)* 1983; **60**: 271–7.

654 Nakatsu T, Uwabe C, Shiota K. Neural tube closure in humans initiates at multiple sites: evidence from human embryos and implications for the pathogenesis of neural tube defects. *Anat Embryol* 2000; **201**: 455–66.

655 Nathan PW, Smith MC. Normal mentality associated with a maldeveloped 'rhinencephalon'. *Neurol Neurosurg Psychiatry* 1950; **13**: 191–7.

656 Nathan PW, Smith MC, Deacon P. The corticospinal tracts in man: course and location of fibres at different segmental levels. *Brain* 1990; **113**: 303–24.

657 Nathanson N, Cole G, Van der Loos H. Heterotopic cerebellar granule cells following administration of cyclophosphamide to suckling rats. *Brain Res* 1969; **15**: 532–6.

658 Nave KA, Lai C, Bloom FE, Milner RJ. Jimpy mutant mouse: a 74-base deletion in the mRNA for myelin proteolipid protein and evidence for a primary defect in RNA splicing. *Proc Natl Acad Sci USA* 1986; **83**: 9264–8.

659 Navin JJ, Angevine JM. Congenital cytomegalic inclusion disease with porencephaly. *Neurology* 1968; **18**: 470–2.

660 Nellhaus G. Head circumference from birth to eighteen years. Practical composite international and interracial graphs. *Pediatrics* 1968; **41**: 106–19.

661 Nelson MM, Thompson AJ. The acrocallosal syndrome. *Am J Med Genet* 1982; **12**: 195–9.

662 Neriishi S, Matsumura H. Morphological observation of the central nervous system in an *in utero* exposed autopsy case. *J Radiat Res* 1983; **24**: 18.

663 Neu RL, Kajii T, Gardner LI *et al.* A lethal syndrome of microcephaly with multiple congenital anomalies in three siblings. *Pediatrics* 1971; **47**: 610–12.

664 Neumann PE, Frankel WN, Letts VA, Coffin JM, Copp AJ, Bernfield M. Multifactorial inheritance of neural tube defects: localization of the major gene and recognition of modifiers in ct mutant mice. *Nat Genet* 1994; **6**: 357–62.

665 Nevin NC, Johnston WP, Merrett JD. Influence of social class on the risk of recurrence of anencephalus and spina bifida. *Dev Med Child Neurol* 1981; **23**: 155–9.

666 Newman GCI, Buschi A, Sugg NK *et al.* Dandy–Walker syndrome diagnosed *in utero* by ultrasonography. *Neurology* 1982; **32**: 180–4.

667 Nicholls RD, Saitoh S, Horsthemke B. Imprinting in Prader–Willi and Angelman syndromes. *Trends Genet* 1998; **14**: 194–200.

668 Nieuwenhuijse P. Zur Kenntnis der Mikrogyrie. *Psychiat Neurog Bladen Amsterdam* 1913; **17**: 9–53.

669 Norman MG. Bilateral encephaloclastic lesions in a 26 week gestation fetus: effect on neuroblast migration. *Can J Neurol Sci* 1989; **7**: 191–4.

670 Norman MG, Becker LE. Cerebral damage in neonates resulting from arterio-venous malformations of the vein of Galen. *J Neurol Neurosurg Psychiatry* 1974; **37**: 252–8.

671 Norman MG, Becker LE, Sirois J, Tremblay LJM. Lissencephaly. *Can J Neurol Sci* 1976; **3**: 39–46.

672 Norman MG, McGillivray B. Fetal neuropathology of proliferative vasculopathy and hydranencephaly–hydrocephaly with multiple limb pterygia. *Pediatr Neurosci* 1988; **14**: 301–6.

673 Norman MG, White VA, Dimmick JE. Pathology of Neu–Laxova syndrome. *Brain Pathol* 1994; **4**: 394.

674 Norman RM. Cerebral birth injury. In: Greenfield JG, Norman RM *et al.* eds. *Greenfield's neuropathology*. London: Edward Arnold, 1958: 354–68.

675 Norman RM. Neuropathological findings in trisomies 13–15 and 17–18 with special reference to the cerebellum. *Dev Med Child Neurol* 1966; **8**: 170–7.

676 Norman RM. Primary degeneration of the granular layer of the cerebellum; an unusual form of familial cerebellar atrophy occurring in early life. *Brain* 1940; **63**: 365–79.

677 Norman RM, Kay JM. Cerebello-thalamo-spinal degeneration in infancy: an unusual variant of Werdnig–Hoffmann disease. *Arch Dis Child* 1965; **40**: 302–8.

678 Norman RM, McMenemey WH. Transventricular adhesion in association with birth injury of the caudate nucleus. *J Neuropathol Exp Neurol* 1955; **14**: 85–91.

679 Norman RM, Tingey AH, Harvey PW, Gregory AM. Pelizaeus–Merzbacher disease; a form of sudanophil leukodystrophy. *J Neurol Neurosurg Psychiatry* 1966; **29**: 521–9.

680 Norman RM, Urich H. Cerebellar hypoplasia associated with systemic degeneration in early life. *J Neurol Neurosurg Psychiatry* 1958; **21**: 159–66.

681 Norman RM, Urich H, Woods GE. The relationship between prenatal porencephaly and the encephalomalacias of early life. *J Ment Sci* 1958; **104**: 758–71.

682 Obersteiner H. Ein porencephalisches Gehirn. *Arbeit Neurol Inst Wien* 1902; **8**: 1–66.

683 Oliver LC. Primary arachnoid cysts. Report of two cases. *B M J* 1958; **2**: 1147–9.

684 Olson MI, Shaw CM. Presenile dementia and Alzheimer's disease in mongolism. *Brain* 1969; **92**: 147–56.

685 Onufrowicz W. Das balkenlose Microcephalengehirn Hofmann. Ein Beitrag zur pathologischen und normalen Anatomie des menschlichen Gehirnes. *Arch Psychiat Nervenkrankheit* 1887; **18**: 305–28.

686 Opitz JM, Sutherland GR. Conference report: International workshop on the fragile X and X-linked mental retardation. *Am J Med Genet* 1984; **17**: 5–94.

687 O'Rahilly R, Muller F. Bidirectional closure of the rostral neuropore in the human embryo. *Am J Anat* 1989; **184**: 259–68.

688 Overbeeke JJ van, Hillen B, Vermeij-Keers C. The arterial pattern at the base of arhinencephalic and prosencephalic brains. *J Anat* 1994; **185**: 51–63.

689 Owen C. *On the anatomy of the vertebrates*. London: Longmans & Green, 1868.

690 Padget DH, Lindenberg R. Inverse cerebellum morphogenetically related to Dandy–Walker and Arnold–Chiari syndromes: bizarre malformed brain with occipital encephalocele. *Johns Hopkins Med J* 1972; **131**: 228–46.

691 Paetau A, Salonen R, Haltia M. Brain pathology in the Meckel syndrome: a study of 59 cases. *Clin Neuropathol* 1985; **4**: 56–62.

692 Paetau A, Salonen R, Herva R. Neuropathology of hydrolethalus syndrome (Abstract). *Brain Pathol* 1994; **4**: 392.

693 Pagon RA, Chandler JW, Collie WR et al. Hydrocephalus, agyria, retinal dysplasia, encephalocele (HARD±E) syndrome: an autosomal recessive condition. *Birth Defects* 1995; **14**: 233–41.

694 Palm L, Hägerstrand I, Kristoffersson U et al. Nephrosis and disturbances of neuronal migration in male siblings – new hereditary disorder? *Arch Dis Child* 1986; **61**: 545–8.

695 Palmini A, Andermann F, Aicardi J et al. Diffuse cortical dysplasia, or the 'double cortex– syndrome: the clinical and epileptic spectrum in 10 patients. *Neurology* 1991; **41**: 1656–62.

696 Palmini A, Andermann F, Grissac H de et al. Stages and patterns of centrifugal arrest of diffuse neuronal migration disorders. *Dev Med Child Neurol* 1993; **35**: 331–9.

697 Pamphlett R, Silberstein P. Pelizaeus–Merzbacher disease in a brother and sister. *Acta Neuropathol (Berl)* 1986; **69**: 343–6.

698 Pang D. Split cord malformation: Part II: Clinical syndrome. *Neurosurgery* 1992; **31**: 481–500.

699 Pang D, Dias MS. Cervical myelomeningoceles. *Neurosurgery* 1993; **33**: 363–73.

700 Pang D, Dias MS, Ahab-Barmada M. Split cord malformation: Part I: A unified theory of embryogenesis for double spinal cord malformations. *Neurosurgery* 1992; **31**: 451–80.

701 Papez JW, Vonderahe AR. Infantile cerebral palsy of hemiplegic type. *J Neuropathol Exp Neurol* 1947; **6**: 244–52.

702 Parnavelas JG. The origin and migration of cortical neurones: new vistas. *Trends Neurosci* 2000; **23**: 126–31.

703 Parrish ML, Roessmann U, Levinsohn MW. Agenesis of the corpus callosum: a study of the frequency of associated malformations. *Ann Neurol* 1979; **6**: 349–54.

704 Patau K, Smith DW, Therman E et al. Multiple congenital anomaly caused by an extra autosome. *Lancet* 1960; **i**: 790–3.

705 Patel H, Dolman CL. Byrne MA. Holoprosencephaly with median cleft lip. *Am J Dis Child* 1972; **124**: 217–21.

706 Paul K, Lye RH, Strang FA, Dutton J. Arnold–Chiari malformation: review of 71 cases. *J Neurosurg* 1983; **58**: 183–7.

707 Pauli RM, Graham JM, Barr M. Agnathia, situs inversus, and associated malformations. *Teratology* 1981; **23**: 85–93.

708 Pavone L, Gullotta F, Incorpora G et al. Isolated lissencephaly: report of four patients from two unrelated families. *J Child Neurol* 1990; **5**: 52–9.

709 Pavone L, Rizzo R, Dobyns WB. Clinical manifestations and evaluation of isolated lissencephaly. *Childs Nerv Syst* 1993; **9**: 387–90.

710 Peach B. Arnold–Chiari malformation. Anatomic features of 20 cases. *Arch Neurol* 1965; **12**: 613–21.

711 Peach B. Arnold–Chiari malformation: morphogenesis. *Arch Neurol* 1965; **12**: 527–35.

712 Peach B. Arnold–Chiari malformation with normal spine. *Arch Neutrol* 1964; **10**: 497–501.

713 Peckham CS, Martin JAM, Marshall WC, Dudgeon JA. Congenital rubella deafness: a preventable disease. *Lancet* 1978; **i**: 258–61.

714 Pelizzi GB. Contributo allo studio dell'idiozia. *Rivista Spermentali di Freniatria e Medicina Legale delle Alienazioni Mentale* 1901; **27**: 265–9.

715 Perez-Fontan JJ, Herrera M, Fina A, Peguero G. Periventricular calcifications in a newborn associated with aneurysm of the great vein of Galen. *Pediatr Radiol* 1982; **12**: 249–51.

716 Pfeiffer G, Friede RL. Unilateral hydrocephalus from early developmental occlusion of one foramen of Monro. *Acta Neuropathol (Berl)* 1984; **64**: 75–7.

717 Pfeiffer J, Majewski F, Fischbach H et al. Alcohol embryopathy and fetopathy: neuropathology of 3 children and 3 fetuses. *J Neurol Sci* 1979; **41**: 125–37.

718 Pfeiffer J, Pfeiffer RA. Hypoplasia ponto-neocerebellaris. *J Neurol* 1977; **215**: 241–51.

719 Piccolo S, Sasai Y, Lu B, De Robertis EM. Dorsoventral patterning in *Xenopus*: inhibition of ventral signals by direct binding of Chordin to BMP-4. *Cell* 1996; **86**: 589–98.

720 Pierre-Kahn A, Hirsch J, Renier D et al. Hydrocephalus and achondroplasia. A study of 25 observations. *Child's Brain* 1981; **7**: 205–19.

721 Pilz DT, Kuc J, Matsumoto N et al. Subcortical band heterotopia in rare affected males can be caused by missense mutations in DCX (XLIS) or LIS-1. *Hum Mol Genet* 1999; **8**: 1757–60.

722 Pinard JM, Motte J, Chiron C et al. Subcortical laminar heterotopia and lissencephaly in two families: a single X linked dominant gene. *J Neurol Neurosurg Psychiatry* 1994; **57**: 914–20.

723 Pineda M, Gonzalez A, Fabreques I et al. Familial agenesis of the corpus callosum with hyperthermia and apnoeic spells. *Neuropediatrics* 1984; **15**: 63–7.

724 Pinto-Lord MC, Evrard P, Caviness VS Jr. Obstructed neuronal migration along radial glial fibers in the neocortex of the reeler mouse: a Golgi-EM analysis. *Dev Brain Res* 1982; **4**: 379–93.

725 Piven J, Berthier ML, Starkstein SE et al. Magnetic resonance imaging evidence for a defect of cerebral cortical development in autism. *Am J Psychiatry* 1990; **147**: 734–9.

726 Pleet H, Graham JM Jr, Smith DW. Central nervous system and facial defects associated with maternal hyperthermia at four to 14 weeks gestation. *Pediatrics* 1981; **67**: 785–9.

727 Plummer C. Anomalies occurring in children exposed *in utero* to atomic bomb in Hiroshima. *Pediatrics* 1952; **10**: 687–93.

728 Pollock AQ, Laslett PA. Cerebral arteriovenous fistula producing cardiac failure in the newborn infant. *J Pediatr* 1958; **53**: 731–6.

729 Potter EL, Potter EL, Craig JM eds. *Pathology of the fetus and infant* 3rd edn. Chicago, IL: Year Book, 1976.

730 Powers JM. Adreno-leukodystrophy (adreno-testiculo-leuko-myelo-neuropathic complex). *Clin Neuropathol* 1985; **4**: 181–99.

731 Powers JM, Moser HW, Moser AB et al. Fetal cerebrohepatorenal (Zellweger) syndrome: dysmorphic, radiologic, biochemical, and pathologic findings in four affected fetuses. *Hum Pathol* 1985; **16**: 610–20.

732 Powers JM, Tummons RC, Caviness VS et al. Structural and chemical alteration in the cerebrohepato-renal (Zellweger) syndrome. *J Neuropathol Exp Neurol* 1989; **48**: 270–89.

733 Price DJ, Aslam S, Tasker L, Gillies K. Fates of the earliest generated cells in the developing murine neocortex. *J Comp Neurol* 1997; **377**: 414–22.

734 Priestley DB. Complete absence of the cerebellum. *Lancet* 1920; **ii**: 1302–17.

735 Probst FP. *The prosencephalies*. Berlin: Springer, 1979.

736 Probst M. Über den Bau des vollständig balkenlosen Grosshirns sowie über Mikrogyrie und Heterotopie der grauen Substanz. *Arch Psychiat Nervenkrankheit* 1901; **34**: 709–86.

737 Rakic P. Mode of cell migration to the superficial layers of fetal monkey neocortex. *J Comp Neurol* 1972; **145**: 61–84.

738 Rakic P. Neuron–glia relationship during granule cell migration in developing cerebellar cortex. A Golgi and electron microscopic study in Macacus rhesus. *J Comp Neurol* 1971; **141**: 283–312.

739 Rakic P, Sidman RL. Organization of cerebellar cortex secondary to deficit of granule cells in weaver mutant mice. *J Comp Neurol* 1973; **152**: 133–62.

740 Rakic P, Sidman RL. Sequence of developmental abnormalities leading to granule cell deficit in cerebellar cortex of weaver mutant mice. *J Comp Neurol* 1973; **152**: 103–32.

741 Rakic P, Yakovlev PI. Development of the corpus callosum and cavum septi in man. *J Comp Neurol* 1968; **132**: 45–72.

742 Ranke O. Beiträge zur Kenntnis der normalen und pathologischen Hirnrindenbildung. *Beit Pathol Anat Pathol* 1910; **47**: 51–125.

743 Raymond AA, Fish DR, Stevens JM *et al.* Subependymal heterotopia: a distinct neuronal migration disorder associated with epilepsy. *J Neurol Neurosurg Psychiatry* 1994; **57**: 1195–202.

744 Raymond AA, Halpin SFS, Alsanjari N *et al.* Dysembryoplastic neuroepithelial tumour. Features in 16 patients. *Brain* 1994; **117**: 461–75.

745 Razin A, Cedar H. DNA methylation and genomic imprinting. *Cell* 1994; **77**: 473–6.

746 Reardon W, Hockey A, Silberstein P *et al.* Autosomal recessive congenital intrauterine infection-like syndrome of microcephaly, intracranial calcification and CNS disease. *Am J Med Genet* 1994; **52**: 58–65.

747 Recklinghausen F von. *Über die multiplen Fibrome der Haut und ihre Beziehung zu den multiplen Neuromen* 20th edn. Berlin: Hirschwald, 1882.

748 Reiner O, Carrozzo R, Shen Y *et al.* Isolation of a Miller–Dieker lissencephaly gene containing G protein beta-subunit-like repeats. *Nature* 1993; **364**: 717–21.

749 Remington JS, Klein JO. *Infectious disease of the fetus and newborn infant*. Philadelphia, PA: WB Saunders, 1976.

750 Rengachary SS, Watanabe I. Ultrastructure and pathogenesis of intracranial arachnoid cysts. *J Neuropathol Exp Neurol* 1982; **40**: 61–83.

751 Renier W, Gabreels FJM, Mol L, Korten J. Agenesis of the corpus callosum, chorioretinopathy and infantile spasms (Aicardi syndrome). *Psychiat Neurol Neurochirurg* 1973; **76**: 39–45.

752 Renowden SA, Squier MV. Unusual magnetic resonance and neuropathological findings in hemimegalencephaly: report of a case following hemispherectomy. *Dev Med Child Neurol* 1994; **36**: 357–69.

753 Retzius G, quoted by Streeter L ed. In: *Das Menschenhird*. Stockholm: 1895.

754 Ribadeau-Dumas JL, Poirier J, Escourolle R. Etude ultrastructurale des lésions cérébrales de la sclérose tubéreuse de Bourneville. *Acta Neuropathol (Berl)* 1973; **25**: 259–70.

755 Riccardi VM, Marcus ES. Congenital hydrocephalus and cerebellar agenesis. *Clin Genet* 1978; **13**: 443–7.

756 Ricci S, Cusmai R, Fariello G *et al.* Double cortex: a neuronal migration anomaly as a possible cause of Lennox Gastaut syndrome. *Arch Neurol* 1992; **49**: 61–4.

757 Rice DS, Curran T. Mutant mice with scrambled brains: understanding the signaling pathways that control cell positioning in the CNS. *Genes Dev* 1999; **13**: 2758–73.

758 Richman DP, Stewart RM, Caviness VS. Cerebral microgyria in a 27 week fetus: an architectonic and topographic analysis. *J Neuropathol Exp Neurol* 1974; **33**: 374–84.

759 Richman DP, Stewart RM, Hutchinson JW, Caviness VS. Mechanical model of brain convolutional development. *Science* 1975; **189**: 18–21.

760 Richter RB. Unilateral congenital hypoplasia of the facial nucleus. *J Neuropathol Exp Neurol* 1960; **19**: 33–41.

761 Riggs HE, McGrath JJ, Schwarz HP. Malformation of the adult brain (albino rat) resulting from prenatal irradiation. *J Neuropathol Exp Neurol* 1956; **15**: 432–47.

762 Robain O, Chiron C, Dulac O. Electron microscopic and Golgi study in a case of hemimegalencephaly. *Acta Neuropathol (Berl)* 1989; **77**: 664–6.

763 Robain O, Dulac O. Early epileptic encephalopathy with suppression bursts and olivary-dentate dysplasia. *Neuropaediatrics* 1992; **23**: 162–4.

764 Robain O, Dulac O, Lejeune J. Cerebellar hemispheric agenesis. *Acta Neuropathol (Berl)* 1987; **74**: 202–6.

765 Robain O, Floquet C, Heldt N, Rozenberg F. Hemimegalencephaly: a clinicopathological study of four cases. *Neuropathol Appl Neurobiol* 1988; **14**: 125–35.

766 Robain O, Gorce F. Arhinencéphalie. *Arch Fr Pediatr* 1972; **29**: 861–79.

767 Robain O, Lyon G. Les micrencéphalies familiales par malformations cérébrales. *Acta Neuropathol (Berl)* 1972; **20**: 96–109.

768 Robinson RO. Familial schizencephaly. *Dev Med Child Neurol* 1991; **33**: 1010–12.

769 Roessler E, Belloni E, Gaudenz K *et al.* Mutations in the human *Sonic Hedgehog* gene cause holoprosencephaly. *Nat Genet* 1996; **14**: 357–60.

770 Roessmann U, Gambetti P. Astrocytes in the developing human brain. *Acta Neuropathol (Berl)* 1986; **70**: 309–13.

771 Roessmann U, Velasco ME, Small EJ, Hori A. Neuropathology of 'septo-optic dysplasia' (de Morsier syndrome) with immunohistochemical studies of the hypothalamus and pituitary gland. *J Neuropathol Exp Neurol* 1987; **46**: 597–608.

772 Rogers KT. Experimental production of perfect cyclopia in chick by means of LiCl with a survey of the literature on cyclopia produced experimentally by various means. *Dev Biol* 1963; **8**: 129–50.

773 Rorke LB. The role of disordered genetic control of neurogenesis in the pathogenesis of migration disorders. *J Neuropath Exp Neurol* 1994; **53**: 105–17.

774 Rorke LB, Fogelson MH, Riggs H. Cerebellar heterotopia in infancy. *Dev Med Child Neurol* 1968; **10**: 644–50.

775 Rorke LB, Spiro AJ. Cerebral lesions in congenital rubella syndrome. *J Pediatr* 1967; **70**: 243–55.

776 Ross DL, Liwnicz BH, Chun RWM, Gilbert E. Hypomelanosis of Ito (incontinentia pigmenti achromians) – a clinicopathologic study: macrocephaly and gery matter heterotopias. *Neurology* 1982; **32**: 1013–16.

777 Ross JJ, Frias JL, Vinken PJ, Bruyn GW eds. Microcephaly. In: *Handbook of clinical neurology*. Amsterdam: North-Holland, 1977: 507–24.

778 Ross ME. Cell division and the nervous system: regulating the cycle from neural differentiation to death. *Trends Neurosci* 1996; **19**: 62–8.

779 Ross MH, Galaburda AM, Kemper TL. Down's syndrome: is there a decreased population of neurons? *Neurology* 1984; **34**: 909–16.

780 Rossant J. Manipulating the mouse genome: implications for neurobiology. *Neuron* 1990; **4**: 323–34.

781 Rossing R, Friede RL. Holoprosencephaly with retroprosencephalic extracerebral cyst. *Dev Med Child Neurol* 1992; **34**: 177–81.

782 Roth KA, Kuan CY, Haydar TF et al. Epistatic and independent functions of Caspase-3 and Bcl-X$_L$ in developmental programmed cell death. Proc Natl Acad Sci USA 2000; 97: 466–71.

783 Roubicek M, Spranger J, Wende S. Frontonasal dysplasia as an expression of holoprosencephaly. Eur J Pediatr 1981; 137: 229–31.

784 Rowbotham GF. Small aneurysm completely obstructing lower end of aqueduct of Sylvius. Arch Neurol Psychiatry 1938: 40: 1241–3.

785 Roy FH, Hiatt RL, Korones SB, Roane J. Ocular manifestations of congenital rubella syndrome. Arch Ophthalmol 1966; 75: 601–7.

786 Rubinstein HS, Freeman W. Cerebellar agenesis. J Nerv Ment Dis 1940; 92: 489–502.

787 Rubenstein JLR, Beachy PA. Patterning of the embryonic forebrain. Curr Opin Neurobiol 1998; 8: 18–26.

788 Rudelli RD, Brown WT, Wisniewski K et al. Adult fragile X syndrome: clinico-neuropathologic findings. Acta Neuropathol 1985; 67: 289–95.

789 Ruff ME, Oakes WJ, Fisher SR, Spock A. Sleep apnea and vocal cord paralysis secondary to type I Chiari malformation. Pediatrics 1987; 80: 231–4.

790 Russell D. Observations on the pathology of hydrocephalus. MRC Special Report Series No. 265. London: HMSO, 1949.

791 Russell DS, Nevin S. Aneurysm of the great vein of Galen causing internal hydrocephalus: report of two cases. J Pathol Bacteriol 1940; 51: 375–83.

792 Sainte-Rose LH, LaCombe J, Pierre-Khan A et al. Intracranial venous sinus hypertension: cause or consequence of hydrocephalus in infants. J Neurosurg 1984; 60: 727–36.

793 Salonen R, Herva R. Hydrolethalus syndrome. J Med Genet 1990; 27: 756–9.

794 Salonen R, Herva R, Norio R. The hydrolethalus syndrome: delineation of a 'new' lethal malformation syndrome based on 28 patients. Clin Genet 1981; 19: 321–30.

795 Salvesen GS, Dixit VM. Caspases: intracellular signaling by proteolysis. Cell 1997; 91: 443–6.

796 Samsom JF, Barth PG, Vries JIP de et al. Familial mitochondrial encephalopathy with fetal ultrasonographic ventriculomegaly and intracerebral calcifications. Eur J Pediatr 1994; 153: 510–16.

797 Santavuori P, Somer H, Saino K. Muscle–eye–brain disease (MEB). Brain Dev 1989; 11: 147–53.

798 Sapir T, Elbaum M, Reiner O. Reduction of microtubule catastrophe events by LIS1, platelet-activating factor acetylhydrolase subunit. EMBO J 1997; 16: 6977–84.

799 Sarnat HB, Alcala H. Human cerebellar hypoplasia. A syndrome of diverse causes. Arch Neurol 1980; 37: 300–5.

800 Scales DA, Collins GH. Cerebral degeneration with hypertrophy of the contralateral pyramid. Arch Neurol 1972; 26: 186–90.

801 Schachenmayr W, Friede RL. Fine structure of arachnoid cysts. J Neuropathol Exp Neurol 1979; 38: 434–46.

802 Schachenmayr W, Friede RL. Rhombencephalosynapsis: a Viennese malformation? Dev Med Child Neurol 1982; 24: 178–82.

803 Schalch E, Friede RL. A quantitative study of the composition of cerebellar cortical dysplasias. Acta Neuropathol (Berl) 1979; 47: 67–70.

804 Schaltenbrandt G. Die Nervenkrankheiten. Stuttgart: G Thieme, 1951.

805 Scheffer IE, Baraitser M, Wilson J et al. Pelizaeus–Merzbacher disease: classical or connatal? Neuropediatrics 1991; 22: 71–8.

806 Schiffmann SN, Bernier B, Goffinet AM. Reelin mRNA expression during mouse brain development. Eur J Neurosci 1997; 9: 1055–71.

807 Schinzel A, Schipke R, Riege D, Scoville WB. Postaxial polydactyly, hallux duplication, absence of the corpus callosum, macrencephaly and severe mental retardation: a new syndrome? Acute subdural haemorrhage at birth. Helv Paediatr Acta 1954; 14: 468–73.

808 Schneider A, Griffiths IR, Readhead C, Nave K-A. Dominant-negative action of the jimpy mutation in mice complemented with an autosomal transgene for myelin proteolipid protein. Proc Natl Acad Sci USA 1995; 92: 4447–51.

809 Schochet SS, Lampert PW, McCormick WF. Neurofibrillary tangles in patients with Down's syndrome: a light and electron-microscopic study. Acta Neuropathol (Berl) 1973; 23: 342–6.

810 Schum TR, Meyer GA, Gransz JP, Glaspey JC. Neonatal intraventricular hemorrhage due to an intracranial arteriovenous malformation: a case report. Pediatrics 1979; 64: 242–4.

811 Schwaiger H, Weirich HG, Brunner P et al. Radiation sensitivity of Down's syndrome fibroblasts might be due to overexpressed Cu/Zn-superoxide dismutase. Eur J Cell Biol 1989; 48: 79–87.

812 Schwalbe E, Gredig M. Über Entwicklungstörungen des Kleinhirns, Hirnstamms and Halsmarks bei Spina Bifida (Arnold'sche und Chiari'sche Missbildung). Beit Pathol Anat 1907; 40: 132–94.

813 Schwidde JT. Incidence of cavum septi pellucidi and cavum vergae in 1032 human brains. Arch Neurol Psychiatry 1952; 67: 625–32.

814 Searle AG, Edwards JH, Hall JG. Mouse homologues of human hereditary disease. J Med Genet 1994; 31: 1–19.

815 Sees JN, Towfighi J, Robins DB, Ladda RL. 'Marden–Walker syndrome': neuropathologic findings in two siblings. Pediatr Pathol 1990; 10: 807–18.

816 Shady W, Metcalfe RA, Butler P. The incidence of craniocervical bony anomalies in the adult Chiari malformation. J Neurol Sci 1987; 82: 193–203.

817 Sharief N, Craze J, Summers D et al. Miller–Dieker syndrome with ring chromosome 17. Arch Dis Child 1991; 667: 10–12.

818 Sharp D, Robertson DM. Tuberous sclerosis in an infant of 28 weeks gestational age. Can J Neurol Sci 1983; 10: 59–62.

819 Shaw CM, Alvord EC. Cava septi pellucidi et vergae: their normal and pathological states. Brain 1969; 92: 213–24.

820 Shaw CM, Alvord EC. 'Congenital arachnoid' cysts and their differential diagnosis. In: Vinken PJa, Bruyn GW eds. Handbook of clinical neurology. Amsterdam: North-Holland, 1977: 75–135.

821 Shen MH, Yang J, Loupart ML et al. Human mini-chromosomes in mouse embryonal stem cells. Hum Mol Genet 1997; 6: 1375–82.

822 Sherman GF, Morrison L, Rosen GD et al. Brain abnormalities in immune defective mice. Brain Res 1990; 532: 25–33.

823 Sherman JL, Barkovich AJ, Citrin CM. The MR appearances of syringomyelia: new observations. Am J Neuroradiol 1986; 7: 985–95.

824 Shevell MI, Carmant L, Meagher Villemure K. Developmental bilateral perisylvian dysplasia. Pediatr Neurol 1992; 8: 299–302.

825 Shimada M, Langman J. Repair of the external granular layer of the hamster cerebellum after prenatal and postnatal administration of methylazoxymethanol. Teratology 1970; 3: 119–39.

826 Shum ASW, Copp AJ. Regional differences in morphogenesis of the neuroepithelium suggest multiple mechanisms of spinal neurulation in the mouse. Anat Embryol 1996; 194: 65–73.

827 Sidman RL, Rakic P. Neuronal migration, with special reference to the developing human brain: a review. Brain Res 1973; 62: 1–35.

828 Siebert JR, Cohen MM Jr, Sulik KK *et al. Holoprosencephaly. An overview and atlas of cases.* New York: Wiley-Liss, 1990: 48–93.

829 Siebert JR, Warkany J, Lemire RJ. Atelencephalic microcephaly in a 21 week human fetus. *Teratology* 1986; **34**: 9–19.

830 Silver J, Lorenz SE, Wahlstein D, Coughlin J. Axonal guidance during development of the great cerebral commissures: descriptive and experimental studies, *in vivo*, on the role of preformed glial pathways. *J Comp Neurol* 1982; **210**: 10–29.

831 Silver J, Ogawa MY. Postnatally induced formation of the corpus callosum in acallosal mice on glia-coated cellulose bridges. *Science* 1983; **220**: 1067–9.

832 Silverman BK, Brechx T, Craig J, Nadas A. Congestive failure in the newborn, caused by cerebral arterio-venous fistula. *AM J Dis Child* 1955; **89**: 539–43.

833 Sima AAF, Robertson DM. Subependymal giant-cell astrocytoma. Case report with ultrastructural study. *J Neurosurg* 1979; **50**: 240–5.

834 Siqueira EB, Murray KJ. Calcified aneurysms of the vein of Galen: report of a presumed case and review of the literature. *Neurochirurgia* 1972; **15**: 106–12.

835 Smith DW. *Recognizable patterns of human malformations: Genetic, embryologic and clinical aspects.* Philadelphia: WB Saunders, 1988.

836 Smith DW. The fetal alcohol syndrome. *Hosp Pract* 1979; October: 121–8.

837 Smith I, Erdohazi M, Macartney FJ *et al.* Fetal damage despite low-phenylalanine diet after conception in a phenylketonuric woman. *Lancet* 1979; **i**: 17–19.

838 Smith JF, Rodeck C. Multiple cystic and focal encephalomalacia in infancy and childhood with brain stem damage. *J Neurol Sci* 1975; **25**: 377–88.

839 Smith JL, Schoenwolf GC. Role of cell-cycle in regulating neuroepithelial cell shape during bending of the chick neural plate. *Cell Tissue Res* 1988; **252**: 491–500.

840 Smith MT, Huntington HW. Inverse cerebellum and occipital encephalocele: a dorsal fusion defect uniting the Arnold–Chiari and Dandy–Walker spectrum. *Neurology* 1977; **27**: 246–51.

841 Snider WD. Functions of the neurotrophins during nervous system development: What the knockouts are teaching us. *Cell* 1994; **77**: 627–38.

842 Snodgrass G, Butler J, France N *et al.* The 'D' (13–15) trisomy syndrome: an analysis of 7 examples. *Arch Dis Child* 1966; **42**: 250–61.

843 Sokol SY. Wnt signaling and dorso-ventral axis specification in vertebrates. *Curr Opin Genet Dev* 1999; **9**: 405–10.

844 Solitare GB, Lamarche JB, Solt LC *et al.* Alzheimer's disease and senile dementia as seen in mongoloids: neuropathological observations. Interhemispheric cyst of neuroepithelial origin in association with partial agenesis of the corpus callosum. Case report and review of the literature. *Am J Ment Def* 1980; **52**: 399–403.

845 Sotelo C. Anatomical physiological and biochemical studies of the cerebellum from mutant mice. II. Morphological study of cerebellar cortical neurons and circuits in the Weaver mouse. *Brain Res* 1975; **94**: 19–44.

846 Sotos JF, Dodge PR, Muirhead D *et al.* Cerebral gigantism in childhood. *N Engl J Med* 1964; **271**: 109–16.

847 Spataro RF, Lin SR, Horner FA *et al.* Aqueductal stenosis and hydrocephalus: rate sequelae of mumps virus infection. *Neuroradiology* 1976; **12**: 11–13.

848 Spiller WG. Syringomyelia, extending from the sacral region of the spinal cord through the medulla oblongata, right side of the pons and right cerebral peduncle to the upper part of the right internal capsule (syringobulbia). *B M J* 1906; **2**: 1017–21.

849 Spranger JJ, Benirschke K, Hall JG *et al.* Errors of morphogenesis concepts and terms. Recommendations of an international working group. *J Pediatr* 1982; **100**: 160–5.

850 Spreafico R, Angelini L, Binelli S *et al.* Burst suppression and impairment of neocortical ontogenesis: electroclinical and neuropathological findings in two infants with early myoclonic encephalopathy. *Epilepsia* 1993; **34**: 800–8.

851 Squier MV. Fetal type II lissencephaly: a case report. *Childs Nerv Syst* 1993; **9**: 400–2.

852 Srabstein JC, Morris N, Larke RPB *et al.* Is there a congenital varicella syndrome? *J Pediatr* 1974; **84**: 239–43.

853 Staemmler M. *Hydromyelie, Syringomyelie und Gliose.* Berlin: Springer, 1942.

854 Stagno S, Reynolds DW, Huang E *et al.* Congenital cytomegalovirus infection: occurrence in an immune population. *N Engl J Med* 1977; **296**: 1254–8.

855 Stanhope R, Preece MA, Brook CGD. Hypoplastic optic nerves and pituitary dysfunction. A spectrum of anatomical and endocrine abnormalities. *Arch Dis Child* 1984; **59**: 111–14.

856 Starkman SP, Brown TC, Linell EA. Cerebral arachnoid cysts. *J Neuropathol Exp Neurol* 1958; **17**: 484–500.

857 Steegers-Theunissen RPM, Boers GHJ, Trijbels FJM, Eskes TKAB. Neural-tube defects and derangement of homocysteine metabolism. *N Engl J Med* 1991; **324**: 199–200.

858 Steimann GS, Rorke LB, Brown MJ. Infantile neuronal degeneration masquerading as Werdnig–Hoffmann disease. *Ann Neurol* 1980; **8**: 317–24.

859 Stephansson K, Wollmann R. Distribution of glial fibrillary acidic protein in central nervous system lesions of tuberous sclerosis. *Acta Neuropathol (Berl)* 1980; **52**: 135–40.

860 Stern H, Elek SD, Booth JC, Fleck DG. Microbial causes of mental retardation. The role of prenatal infection with cytomegalovirus, rubella virus and toxoplasma. *Lancet* 1969; **ii**: 443–8.

861 Stern L, Ramos AD, Wigglesworth FW. Congenital heart failure secondary to cerebral arteriovenous aneurysm in the newborn infant. *Am J Dis Child* 1968; **115**: 581–7.

862 Sternberg C. Ueber vollständigen Defekt des Kleinhirnes. *Verhandlungen Dtsch Pathol Ges* 1912; **15**: 353–9.

863 Stewart RM. Cerebellar agenesis. *J Ment Sci* 1956; **102**: 67–77.

864 Stewart RM, Richman DP, Caviness VS Jr. Lissencephaly and pachygyria, an architectonic and topographical analysis. *Acta Neuropathol (Berl)* 1975; **31**: 1–12.

865 Streeter G. The cortex of the brain in the human embryo during the fourth month with special reference to the so-called 'papillae of Retzius'. *Am J Anat* 1912; **7**: 337–44.

866 Strefling AM, Urich H. Crossed cerebellar atrophy: an old problem revisited. *Acta Neuropathol (Berl)* 1982; **57**: 197–202.

867 Strefling AM, Urich H. Prenatal porencephaly: the pattern of secondary lesions. *Acta Neuropathol (Berl)* 1986; **71**: 171–5.

868 Strong OS. A case of unilateral cerebellar agenesia. *J Comp Neurol* 1915; **25**: 361–74.

869 Sturge WA. A case of partial epilepsy, apparently due to a lesion of one of the vasomotor centres of the brain. *Trans Clin Soc Lond* 1879; **12**: 162–7.

870 Sudarshan A, Goldie WD. The spectrum of congenital facial diplegia (Moebius syndrome). *Pediatr Neurol* 1985; **1**: 180–4.

871 Sulik KK, Zuker RM, Dehart DB *et al.* Normal patterns of neural tube closure differ in the human and the mouse. *Proc Greenwood Genet Center* 1998; **18**: 129–30.

872 Sumi SM. Brain malformations in the trisomy 18 syndrome. *Brain* 1970; **93**: 821.

873 Suwanwela C, Suwanwela N. A morphological classification of sincipital encephalomeningoceles. *J Neurosurg* 1972; **36**: 201–11.

874 Taggart JK, Walker AE. Congenital atresia of the foramina of Luschka and Magendie. *Arch Neurol Psychiatry* 1942; **48**: 583–612.

875 Tajima M, Yamada H, Kageyama N. Craniolacunia in newborn with myelomeningocele. *Childs Brain* 1977; **3**: 297–303.

876 Takada K, Becker LE, Takashima S. Walker–Warburg syndrome with skeletal muscle involvement. A report of three patients. *Pediatr Neurosci* 1987; **13**: 202–9.

877 Takada K, Nakamura H, Takashima S. Cortical dysplasia in Fukuyama congenital muscular dystrophy (FCMD): a Golgi and angioarchitectonic analysis. *Acta Neuropathol (Berl)* 1988; **76**: 170–8.

878 Takashima S, Becker LE, Armstrong DL, Chan F. Abnormal neuronal development in the visual cortex of the human fetus and infant with Down's syndrome: a quantitative and qualitative Golgi study. *Brain Res* 1981; **225**: 1–21.

879 Tal Y, Freigung B, Dunn HG *et al*. Dandy–Walker syndrome analysis of 2 cases. *Dev Med Child Neurol* 1980; **22**: 184–201.

880 Tam PPL. The histogenetic capacity of tissues in the caudal end of the embryonic axis of the mouse. *J Embryol Exp Morphol* 1984; **82**: 253–66.

881 Tamagawa K, Scheidt P, Friede RL. Experimental production of leptomeningeal heterotopias from dissociated fetal tissue. *Acta Neuropathol (Berl)* 1989; **78**: 153–8.

882 Tan N, Urich H. Postictal cerebral hemiatrophy: with a contribution to the problem of crossed cerebellar atrophy. *Acta Neuropathol (Berl)* 1984; **62**: 332–9.

883 Tassabehji M, Read AP, Newton VE *et al*. Waardenburg's syndrome patients have mutations in the human homologue of the *Pax-3* paired box gene. *Nature* 1992; **355**: 635–6.

884 Taveras JM, Poser CM. Roentgenologic aspects of cerebral angiography in children. *Am J Roentgenol* 1959; **82**: 371–91.

885 Tavormina PL, Shiang R, Thompson LM *et al*. Thanatophoric dysplasia (types I and II) caused by distinct mutations in fibroblast growth factor receptor 3. *Nat Genet* 1995; **9**: 321–8.

886 Taylor DC, Falconer MA, Bruton CJ, Corsellis JAN. Focal dysplasia of the cerebral cortex in epilepsy. *J Neurol Neurosurg Psychiatry* 1971; **34**: 369–87.

887 Terashima T, Inoue K, Inoue Y *et al*. Observations on the cerebellum of normal–reeler mutant mouse chimera. *J Comp Neurol* 1986; **252**: 264–78.

888 Thorogood P. Differentiation and morphogenesis of cranial skeletal tissues. In: Hanken J, Hall BK eds. *The skull*. Chicago: University of Chicago Press, 1994: 113–52.

889 Thulin B, McTaggart D, Neuberger KT. Demyelinating leukodystrophy with total cortical cerebellar atrophy. *Arch Neurol* 1968; **18**: 113–22.

890 Timor-Tritsch IE, Monteagudo A, Warren WB. Transvaginal ultrasonographic definition in CNS in first and early second trimester. *Am J Obstet Gynecol* 1991; **164**: 497–503.

891 Tjiam AT, Stefanko S, Schenk VMD, Vlieger M. Infantile spasms associated with hemihypsarrhthmia and hemimegalencephaly. *Dev Med Child Neurol* 1978; **20**: 779–98.

892 Tole S, Ragsdale CW, Grove EA. Dorsoventral patterning of the telencephalon is disrupted in the mouse mutant *extra-toes*. *Dev Biol* 2000; **217**: 254–65.

893 Ton CCT, Hirvonen H, Miwa H *et al*. Positional cloning and characterization of a paired box- and homeobox-containing gene from the aniridia region. *Cell* 1991; **67**: 1059–74.

894 Towfighi J, Ladda RL, Sharkey FE. Purkinje cell inclusions and 'atelencephaly' in 13q-chromosomal syndrome. *Arch Pathol Lab Med* 1987; **111**: 146–50.

895 Towfighi J, Marks K, Palmer E, Vannucci R. Moebius syndrome. Neuropathologic observations. *Acta Neuropathol (Berl)* 1979; **48**: 11–17.

896 Towfighi J, Sassani JW, Suzuki K, Ladda RL. Cerebro-ocular dysplasia–muscular dystrophy (COD-MD) syndrome. *Acta Neuropathol (Berl)* 1984; **65**: 110–23.

897 Townsend JJ, Nielsen SL, Malamud N. Unilateral megalencephaly: hamartoma or neoplasm? *Neurology* 1975; **25**: 448–53.

898 Trombley IK, Mirra SS. Ultrastructure of tuberous sclerosis: cortical tuber and subependymal tumor. *Ann Neurol* 1981; **9**: 174–81.

899 Truwit CL, Barkovich AJ. Pathogenesis of intracranial lipoma: an MR study in 42 patients. *Am J Neuroradiol* 1987; **11**: 665–74.

900 Tsai TF, Armstrong D, Beaudet AL. Necdin-deficient mice do not show lethality or the obesity and infertility of Prader–Willi syndrome (Letter). *Nat Genet* 1999; **22**: 15–16.

901 Tsai TF, Jiang YH, Bressler J *et al*. Paternal deletion from *Snrpn* to *Ube3a* in the mouse causes hypotonia, growth retardation and partial lethality and provides evidence for a gene contributing to Prader–Willi syndrome. *Hum Mol Genet* 1999; **8**: 1357–64.

902 Tsarkraklides V, Burke B, Mastri A *et al*. Rhabdomyomas of the heart. *Am J Dis Child* 1974; **128**; 639–46.

903 Tsukahara M, Sugio Y, Kajii T *et al*. Pachygyria, joint contractures, and facial abnormalities: a new lethal syndrome. *J Med Genet* 1990; **27**: 532.

904 Tuchmann-Duplessis H, Larroche JC. Anencéphalie et atrophie cortico-surrénale. *C R Soc Biol* 1958; **152**: 300–2.

905 Turkewitsch N. La constitution anatomique de l'Aquaeductus cerebri de l'homme. *Arch Anat Histol Embryol* 1936; **21**: 323–57.

906 Turnbull IM, Drake CG. Membranous occlusion of the aqueduct of Sylvius. *J Neurol* 1966; **24**: 24–33.

907 Twining P, Zuccollo J. The ultrasound markers of chromosomal disease: a retrospective study. *Br J Radiol* 1993; **66**: 408–14.

908 Uiberrack F. Demonstration eines Falles von Ganglienzellerkrankung bei einem Fötus nach Röntgenbestrahlung der Mutter. *Zentralblatt Allg Pathol Pathol Anat* 1942; **80**: 187.

909 Ule G. Kleinhirnrindenatrophie vom Körnertyp. *Dtsch Z Nervenheilkunde* 1952; **168**: 195–226.

910 Ulrich J, Herschkowitz N, Heitz P *et al*. Adenoleukodystrophy: preliminary report of a connatal case: light and electron microscopical, immunohistochemical and biochemical findings. *Acta Neuropathol (Berl)* 1978; **43**: 77–83.

911 Urich H. Malformations of the nervous system. In: Blackwood W, Corsellis JAN eds. *Greenfield's neuropathology* 3rd edn. London: Edward Arnold, 1977: 361–469.

912 Vade A, Horowitz SW. Agenesis of the corpus callosum and intraventricular lipomas. *Pediatr Neurol* 1992; **8**: 307–9.

913 Valanne L, Pihko H, Katevuo K *et al*. MRI of the brain in muscle–eye–brain (MEB) disease. *Neuroradiology* 1994; **36**: 473–6.

914 Valdivieso EMB, Scholtz CL. Diffuse meningocerebral angiodysplasia. *Pediatr Pathol* 1986; **6**: 119–26.

915 Van Allen MI, Kalousek DK, Chernoff GF *et al*. Evidence for multi-site closure of the neural tube in humans. *Am J Med Genet* 1993; **47**: 723–43.

916 Van der Hauwaert LG. Cardiac tumours in infancy and childhood. *Br Heart J* 1971; **33**: 125–32.

917 Van der Put NMJ, Eskes TKAB, Blom HJ. Is the common 677C→T mutation in the methylenetetrahydrofolate reductase gene a risk factor for neural tube defects? A meta-analysis. *Q J Med* 1997; **90**: 111–15.

918 Van Straaten HWM, Hekking JWM, Consten C, Copp AJ. Intrinsic and extrinsic factors in the mechanism of neurulation: effect of curvature of the body axis on closure of the posterior neuropore. *Development* 1993; **117**: 1163–72.

919 Variend S, Emery JL. The weight of the cerebellum in children with myelomeningocele. *Dev Med Child Neurol* 1973; **15**(Suppl 29): 77–83.

920 Veith G, Wicke R. *Cerebrale Differenzierungsstörungen bei Epilepsie Jahrbuch 1968*. Köln-Opladen: Westdeutscher, 1968.

921 Verhaart W. Hypertrophy of peduncle and pyramid as a result of degeneration of contralateral corticofugal fiber tracts. *J Comp Neurol* 1950; **19**: 1–15.

922 Verhaart W, Kramer W. The uncrossed pyramidal tract. *Acta Psychiat Neurol Scand* 1952; **27**: 181–200.

923 Vestermark V. Teratogenicity of carbamazepine: a review of the literature. *Dev Brain Dysfunct* 1993; **6**: 266–78.

924 Viani F, Strada GP, Riboldi A et al. Aspetti neuropatologici della sindrome di Lennox-Gastaut: considerazioni su tue casi. *Riv Neurol* 1977; **4**: 413–52.

925 Vigevano F, Bertini E, Boldrini R et al. Hemimegalencephaly and intractable epilepsy. Benefits of hemispherectomy. *Epilepsia* 1989; **30**: 833–43.

926 Vincent C, Kalatzis V, Compain S et al. A proposed new contiguous gene syndrome on 8q consists of branchio-oto-renal (BOR) syndrome, Duane syndrome, a dominant form of hydrocephalus and trapeze aplasia; implications for the mapping of the BOR gene. *Hum Mol Genet* 1994; **3**: 1859–66.

927 Vinters HV, Fisher RS, Cornford ME et al. Morphological substrates of infantile spasms: studies based on surgically resected cerebral tissue. *Childs Nerv Syst* 1992; **8**: 8–17.

928 Vogel H, Gessaga EC, Horoupian DS, Urich H. Aqueductal atresia as a feature of arhinencephalic syndromes. *Clin Neuropathol* 1990; **9**: 191–5.

929 Vogt H, Astwaraturow M. Ueber angeborene Kleinhirnerkrankungen mit Beiträgen zur Entwicklungsgeschichte des Kleinhirns. *Arch Psychiat Nervenkrankheit* 1912; **49**: 175–203.

930 Volpe JJ. Subplate neurons – missing link in brain injury of the premature infant. *Pediatrics* 1996; **97**: 112–13.

931 Volpe JJ, Adams RD. Cerebro-hepatorenal syndrome of Zellweger: an inherited disorder of neuronal migration. *Acta Neuropathol (Berl)* 1972; **20**: 175–98.

932 Vuia O. Malformation of the paraflocculus and atresia of the foramina Magendie and Luschka in a child. *Psychiat Neurol Neurochirurg Amsterdam* 1973; **76**: 261–6.

933 Wald N, Sneddon J, Densem J et al. MRC Vitamin Study Research Group. Prevention of neural tube defects: results of the Medical Research Council Vitamin Study. *Lancet* 1991; **338**: 131–7.

934 Walker AE, Lissencephaly. *Arch Neurol Psychiatry* 1942; **48**: 13–29.

935 Warburg M. Hydrocephaly, congenital retinal nonattachment and congenital falciform fold. *Am J Ophthalmol* 1978; **85**: 88–94.

936 Watson EH. Hydranencephaly. Report of two cases which combine features of hydrocephalus and anencephaly. *Am J Dis Child* 1944; **67**: 282–7.

937 Weinberg AG, Kirkpatrick JB. Cerebellar hypoplasia in Werdnig–Hoffmann disease. *Dev Med Child Neurol* 1975; **17**: 511–16.

938 Weiss MH, Young HF, McFarland DE. Hydranencephaly of postnatal origin. *J Neurosurg* 1970; **32**: 715–20.

939 Weller TH, Macauley JC, Craig JH, Wirth P. Isolation of intranuclear inclusion producing agents from infants with illnesses resembling cytomegalic inclusion disease. *Proc Sec Exp Biol NY* 1957; **94**: 4–12.

940 Wicking C, Williamson B. From linked marker to gene. *Trends Genet* 1991; **7**: 288–93.

941 Wiest WD, Hallerworden J. Migrationshemmung in Gross- und Kleinhirn. *Dtsch Z Nervenheilkunde* 1958; **178**: 244–38.

942 Wilberger JE Jr, Vertosick FT Jr. Vries JK. Unilateral hydrocephalus secondary to congenital atresia of the foramen of Monro. Case report. *J Neurosurg* 1983; **59**: 899–901.

943 Wilkie AOM, Slaney SF, Oldridge M et al. Apert syndrome results from localized mutations of *FGFR2* and is allelic with Crouzon syndrome. *Nat Genet* 1995; **9**: 165–72.

944 Willems PJ, Brouwer OF, Dijkstra I, Wilminik J. X-linked hydrocephalus. *Am J Med Genet* 1987; **27**: 921–8.

945 Williams B. Is aqueduct stenosis a result of hydrocephalus? *Brain* 1973; **93**: 399–412.

946 Williams RS, Ferrante RJ, Caviness VS. The cellular pathology of microgyria. *Acta Neuropathol (Berl)* 1976; **36**: 269–83.

947 Williams RS, Swisher CN, Jennings M et al. Cerebro-ocular dysgenesis (Walker–Warburg syndrome): neuropathologic and etiologic analysis. *Neurology* 1984; **34**: 1531–41.

948 Wilson JG. *Environment and birth defects*. New York: Academic Press, 1973: 11–34.

949 Wilson PA, Hemmati-Brivaniou A. Induction of epidermis and inhibition of neural fate by Bmp-4. *Nature* 1995; **376**: 331–3.

950 Winter RM, Harding BN, Hyde J. Unknown syndrome: pachygyria, joint contractures, and facial abnormalities. *J Med Genet* 1989; **26**: 788–9.

951 Wise BL, Sondheimer F, Kaufman S. Achondroplasia and hydrocephalus. *Neuropediatrics* 1971; **3**: 106–13.

952 Wisniewski K, Dambska M, Sher JH, Qazi Q. A clinical neuropathological study of the fetal alcohol syndrome. *Neuropaediatrics* 1995; **14**: 197–201.

953 Wisniewski KE, Laure-Kamionowska M, Wisniewski HM. Evidence of arrest of neurogenesis and synaptogenesis in Down syndrome brains. *N Engl J Med* 1984; **311**: 1187–8.

954 Wisniewski KE, Schmidt-Sidor B. Postnatal delay of myelin formation in brains from Down syndrome infants and children. *Clin Neuropathol* 1989; **8**: 55–62.

955 Wit JM, Beemes FE, Barth FC et al. Cerebral gigantism (Sotos syndrome). Compiled data of 22 cases. Analysis of clinical features, growth, and palsma somatomedin. *Eur J Pediatr* 1985; **144**: 131–40.

956 Wohak H. Ein Fall von Varix der Vena magna Galeni bei einem Neugeborenen. *Virchows Arch Pathol Anat* 1923; **242**: 58–68.

957 Wolf SM. The ocular manifestations of congenital rubella. A prospective study of 328 cases of congenital rubella. *Pediatr Ophthalmol* 1973; **10**: 101–41.

958 Wongmongkolrit T, Bush M, Roessmann U. Neuropathological findings in thanatophoric dysplasia. *Arch Pathol Lab Med* 1983; **107**: 132–5.

959 Wood JW, Johnson KG, Omori Y. *In utero* exposure to the Hiroshima atomic bomb. An evaluation of head size and mental retardation twenty years later. *Pediatrics* 1967; **39**: 385–92.

960 Wood LR, Smith MT. Generation of anencephaly: 1. Aberrant neurulation and 2. Conversion of exencephaly to anencephaly. *J Neuropathol Exp Neurol* 1984; **43**: 620–33.

961 Woodward K, Malcolm S. Proteolipid protein gene: Pelizaeus–Merzbacher disease in humans and neurodegeneration in mice. *Trends Genet* 1999; **15**: 125–8.

962 Woollam DHM, Millen JW. Anatomical considerations in the pathology of stenosis of the cerebral aqueduct. *Brain* 1953; **76**: 104–12.

963 Worthington WC, Cathcart RS. Ciliary currents on ependymal surfaces. *Ann N Y Acad Sci* 1965; **130**: 944–50.

964 Xuan S, Baptista CA, Balas G *et al*. Winged helix transcription factor BF-1 is essential for the development of the cerebral hemispheres. *Neuron* 1995; **14**: 1141–52.

965 Yakovlev PI. A proposed definition of the limbic system. In: Hockman CH ed. *Limbic system mechanisms and autonomic function*. Springfield, IL: CC Thomas, 1972: 241–83.

966 Yakovlev PI. Pathoarchitectonic studies of the cerebral malformations. III. Arhinencephalies (holotelencephalies). *J Neuropathol Exp Neurol* 1959; **18**: 22–55.

967 Yakovlev PI, Corwin W. Roentgenographic sign in cases of tuberous sclerosis of the brain (multiple 'brain stones'). *Arch Neurol Psychiatry* 1939; **40**: 1030–7.

968 Yakovlev PI, Wadsworth RC. Schizencephalies. A study of the congenital clefts in the cerebral mantle. I. Clefts with fused lips. *J Neuropathol Exp Neurol* 1946; **5**: 116–30.

969 Yakovlev PI, Wadsworth RC. Schizencephalies. A study of the congenital clefts in the cerebral mantle. II. Clefts with hydrocephalus and lips separated. *J Neuropathol Exp Neurol* 1946; **5**: 169–206.

970 Yamaguchi E, Hayashi T, Kondoh H *et al*. A case of Walker–Warburg syndrome with uncommon findings. Double cortical layer, temporal cyst and increased serum IgM. *Brain Dev* 1993; **15**: 61–5.

971 Yamamoto T, Toyoda C, Kobayashi M *et al*. Pial–glial barrier abnormalities in fetuses with Fukuyama congenital muscular dystrophy. *Brain Dev* 1997; **19**: 35–42.

972 Yamano T, Shimada M, Abe Y *et al*. Destruction of external granular layer and subsequent cerebellar abnormalities. *Acta Neuropathol (Berl)* 1983; **59**: 41–7.

973 Yamazaki JN, Wright SW, Wright PM. Outcome of pregnancy in women exposed to atomic bomb in Nagasaki. *Am J Dis Child* 1954; **87**: 448–63.

974 Yang QH, Khoury MJ, Mannino D. Trends and patterns of mortality associated with birth defects and genetic diseases in the United States, 1979–1992: an analysis of multiple-cause mortality data. *Genet Epidemiol* 1997; **14**: 493–505.

975 Yang T, Adamson TE, Resnick JL *et al*. A mouse model for Prader–Willi syndrome imprinting-centre mutations. *Nat Genet* 1998; **19**: 25–31.

976 Ybot-Gonzalez P, Copp AJ. Bending of the neural plate during mouse spinal neurulation is independent of actin microfilaments. *Dev Dyn* 1999; **215**: 273–83.

977 Yock DH Jr. Choroid plexus lipomas associated with lipoma of the corpus callosum. *J Comput Assist Tomogr* 1980; **4**: 678–82.

978 Zaremba J, Wislawski J, Bidzinsky J *et al*. Jadassohn's naevus phakomatosis: a report of two cases. *J Ment Def* 1978; **22**: 91–102.

979 Zemlan FP, Thienhaus OJ, Bosmann HB. Superoxide dismutase activity in Alzheimer's disease: possible mechanism for paired helical filament formation. *Brain Res* 1989; **476**: 160–2.

980 Zheng BH, Sage M, Cai WW *et al*. Engineering a mouse balancer chromosome. *Nat Genet* 1999; **22**: 375–8.

981 Ziegler AL, Deonna T, Calame A. Hidden intelligence of a multiple handicapped child with Joubert syndrome. *Dev Med Child Neurol* 1990; **32**: 261–6.

982 Zimmerman LB, De Jesús-Escobar JM, Harland RM. The Spemann organizer signal noggin binds and inactivates bone morphogenetic protein 4. *Cell* 1996; **86**: 599–606.

983 Ziter F, Bramwit D. Nasal encephaloceles and gliomas. *Br J Radiol* 1970; **43**: 136.

984 Zonana J, Sotos JF, Romshe CA *et al*. Dominant inheritance of cerebral gigantism. *J Pediatr* 1977; **91**: 251–6.

8

Metabolic and neurodegenerative diseases of childhood

B.N. HARDING AND R. SURTEES

INTRODUCTION

In this chapter primarily childhood disorders which do not fit neatly into other chapters in this book will be reviewed. They are paediatric neurometabolic degenerations which are not strictly organelle related or still have an undefined pathogenesis even as the genetic defects begin to be deciphered. The chapter has three parts: grey-matter disorders, leukoencephalopathies and systemic metabolic defects. The biochemical and molecular understanding of neurological disease in children is rapidly expanding, and of necessity a rather selective approach, biased towards those conditions more likely to present to the neuropathologist, has been adopted.

GREY-MATTER DISORDERS

Alpers–Huttenlocher syndrome (progressive neuronal degeneration of childhood with liver disease)

This autosomal recessive disorder presents usually in the first 2 years of life. The onset is usually insidious with seizures and developmental stagnation, although presentation with generalized or focal status epilepticus can occur. As the disease progresses, epilepsy becomes prominent with myoclonus and other seizure types, especially partial continuous epilepsy. Dementia, blindness and spasticity develop and, usually late in the course of the disease, liver involvement which ends in terminal liver failure. The electroencepholagram (EEG) is often helpful, with large slow waves and asymmetrical runs of polyspikes. Visual evoked potentials (VEPs) can often be asymmetrical early in the disease. Neuroimaging shows progressive cerebral atrophy, especially of the occipital lobes, without signal change.[89,178,231,262,268]

PATHOLOGY

The distinctive pattern of cerebrohepatic pathology originally described in paediatric cases does not differ significantly in the young adult patients more recently reported.

Systemic pathology

Hepatic disease (Fig. 8.1) is constant: at least in a small minority of patients there is only fatty change, occasionally mid-zonal necrosis,[92] but most have a characteristic pathology. Severe and diffuse microvesicular fatty change, portal inflammation, hepatocyte necrosis and collapse of liver cell plates, massive haphazard bile-duct proliferation or transformation and bridging fibrosis result in disorganization of the lobular architecture. In many cases supervening regeneration leads to nodular cirrhosis. Oncocytic change, that is an intense eosinophilia suggesting a superfluity of mitochondria, is sometimes observed in groups of hepatocytes and its sharp contrast with adjacent groups of pale fat-laden cells produces a characteristic motheaten appearance to the regenerative nodules. In some instances, however, there is merely destruction and fibrosis and an end-stage hepatic remnant of bile ductules and dense connective tissue. Examination of sequential biopsies followed by autopsy in the same

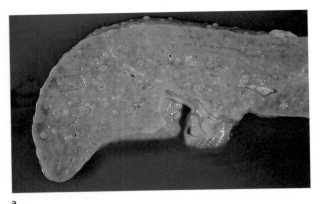

a

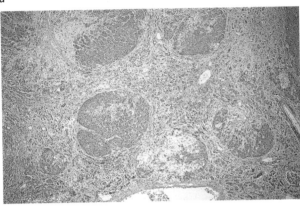

b

Figure 8.1 *Hepatic disease of Alpers' disease (PNDC). (a) Nodular cirrhosis in a post-mortem specimen. (b) Histological features include architectural disarray, bile-duct proliferation, nodular regeneration and fat deposition, which often gives a motheaten appearance to the cirrhotic nodules. (H&E.)*

patient has demonstrated progression of hepatopathy, from focal necrosis, inflammation and fatty change through nodule formation to the full-blown cirrhosis, bile-duct proliferation and fat accumulation.[88] In the right clinical context (i.e. including typical visual evoked responses or suggestive neuroimaging) liver biopsy may significantly aid diagnosis.

Similar pathological changes occur irrespective of treatment with sodium valproate. This is important because there is still considerable confusion in the literature regarding the relationship of valproate to hepatic disease. Examples with typical hepatic changes long antedate the use of valproate as an anticonvulsant therapy.[29] Indeed, clinical and biochemical evidence of hepatopathy may be adduced before any anticonvulsant therapy is commenced.[63] Moreover, some cases of progressive neuronal degeneration of childhood (PNDC) may have inadvertently been reported as apparent idiosyncratic drug reactions without realization of the interdependence of the hepatic and cerebral disease processes.[209,217] It has also been suggested that exposure to valproate may exacerbate the disease, hastening its progression,[72] but this is not the experience of the present authors. Acute pancreatitis with fat necrosis has occurred in a few patients.

Neuropathology

Macroscopic appearances may be disconcertingly normal even on close examination, but characteristically there are patches of thinned, granular discoloured cortex, and sometimes laminar disruption. Selective involvement of the medial occipital lobe, especially the calcarine cortex, is typical (Fig. 8.2). Cerebral white-matter and deep grey nuclei are usually unremarkable, but circumscribed softening of the occipital white matter has been documented in one adult patient.[89] In one extreme example global cerebral atrophy was present.

Microscopic changes (Fig. 8.3), usually more widespread than naked-eye appearances suggest, are patchy and do not respect vascular territories or sulcal topography. The pathological process, devoid of specific cytological markers or inflammatory changes, has the appearance of a graded intensification and extension through the depth of the cortical ribbon. The mildest lesions are a superficial astrocytosis, but more severely affected areas show increasing vacuolation, neuronal loss and astrocytosis spreading down through the ribbon until the whole cortex is thin, with nerve cells and neuropil replaced by hypertrophic astrocytes, glial fibres and prominent capillaries. In the end there is a gliomesodermal scar often demonstrating considerable neutral fat in frozen sections. If liver failure is present, Alzheimer type II astrocytes may be prominent.

The striate cortex seems to bear the brunt of the damage: in a personal series the visual cortex in 17 of 22 cases showed complete devastation, and in only three was it less severely affected than other cortical areas.[88] The two hemispheres need not be equally affected. White-matter changes, by contrast, are usually slight. Neuronal loss, vacuolation and astrocytosis can be notable in the thalamus and the lateral geniculate body, and may also affect the amygdala, the substantia nigra and the dentate nuclei. Hippocampal sclerosis and focal or diffuse cerebellar cortical lesions are common, while neuronal loss in the brainstem and tract degeneration in the spinal cord are occasional findings.

Pathogenesis

Although the disease mechanism of PNDC remains uncertain, there is general agreement that the stereotyped clinical and pathological features of developmental delay, seizures, neurological decline and liver failure in combination with cerebral destruction biased towards the medial occipital lobe represent a homogeneous nosological entity. Various authors have noted some histological similarities with transmissible spongiform encephalopathies,[54,116] and a single report of a successful transmission experiment using brain tissue from an affected 2½-year-old girl inoculated into hamsters[167] has not so far been replicated. Equally, immunohistochemistry for prion proteins has been negative.[268]

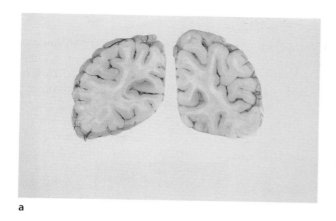

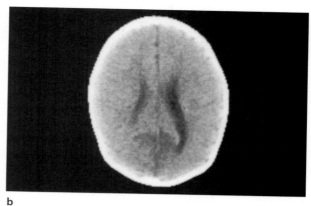

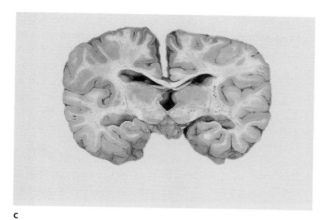

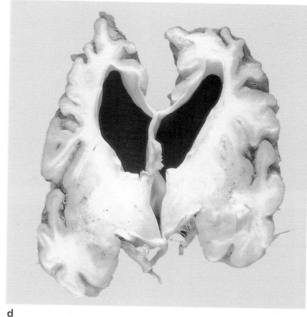

Figure 8.2 *Alpers' disease (PNDC): macroscopic features. (a) In coronal sections patches of granular and brown shrunken cortex most characteristically involve medial (calcarine) cortex in the occipital lobes. (b) CT scan demonstrating similar anatomical changes. (c) Patchy lesions involving the frontal cortex. (d) A rare case showing global cortical destruction.*

The many instances of sibling involvement (12 out of 26 families in Harding's series,[88] including one pair of twins and two sets of three siblings), suggest autosomal recessive inheritance and therefore implicate a metabolic error as originally suggested[258] and later confirmed.[108] The hypothesis of a mitochondrondrial disorder is attractive but the evidence is inconclusive. Some reports of associated lactic acidaemia[97,225] or respiratory chain abnormalities[200–203] can be disputed on neuropathological grounds,[88] while ultrastructural changes in mitochondria[213,239] have not been readily reproducible. Moreover, evidence for raised cerebrospinal fluid (CSF) lactates was lacking. More recently, however, two bona fide cases, one in an infant[178] and the other in a young adult,[268] both with raised CSF lactates,

were reported to have complex IV deficiency from biochemical studies of muscle biopsy tissue which did not show ragged red fibres or cytochrome oxidase abnormality on histochemistry. Mitochondrial DNA (mtDNA) analysis excluded pathogenic mutations. In addition, Naviaux *et al.*[182] described mtDNA depletion and mtDNA polymerase γ deficiency in one familial infantile case of PNDC. Liver pathology present in the well-recognized hepatic form of mitochondrial depletion syndrome is identical to that present in PNDC but the cerebral changes are lacking. It remains likely that PNDC is the phenotypic endpoint of a variety of rare, probably mitochondrially related disorders, a situation somewhat similar to the better understood Leigh's syndrome.

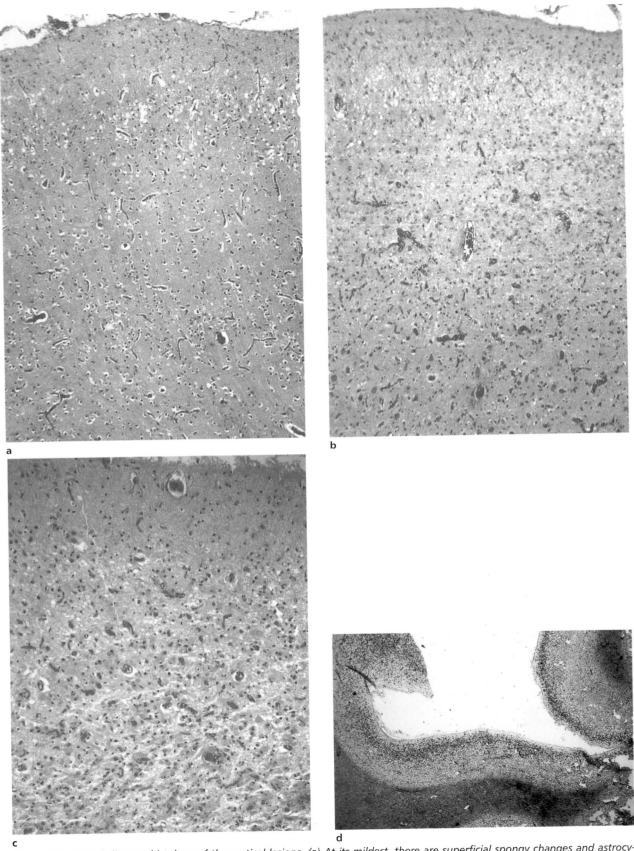

Figure 8.3 *Alpers' disease: histology of the cortical lesions. (a) At its mildest, there are superficial spongy changes and astrocytosis in layers I and II. (H&E.) (b) Neuronal loss spreads gradually more deeply into the cortical laminae (H&E), until (c) the whole cortical ribbon is affected (H&E), and (d) sudanophilic lipid is readily demonstrated in frozen sections.*

Rett's syndrome

This disorder almost exclusively affects girls.[107,155,192] While early development is not entirely normal, first symptoms are usually noticed between 6 and 18 months of age and consist of developmental stagnation, muscular hypotonia, retarded head growth and disinterest. This phase is followed after a few months by rapid regression with irritability, the loss of purposeful hand movements and the development of hand stereotypies (e.g. 'knitting' movements, fingers to mouth) and loss of communication (language and social). After a few weeks of regression, girls enter a more stable stage that lasts for several years with severe learning difficulties, retarded head growth (or frank microcephaly), hand stereotypies, ataxia or apraxia and an abnormal respiratory pattern; they often develop epilepsy and scoliosis. The final stage of Rett's disorder develops after the age of 10 years. It consists of the development of upper and lower motor neuron signs, decreased motility, a progressive scoliosis and often reduced seizures.

Approximately three-quarters of patients with Rett's disorder, typical or atypical (retained speech or without microcephaly), have new mutations in the *MECP2* gene, making this an X-linked dominant disorder. *MECP2* encodes a methyl-CpG-binding protein that recruits histone deacetylase to repress gene transcription. Whilst *MECP2* is expressed in all tissues, expression is enhanced during the differentiation and maturation of the hippocampus.

PATHOLOGY

Morphological abnormalities in Rett's syndrome are subtle. They have been extensively reviewed by Armstrong.[13] The most obvious changes are in somatic and brain growth. Decreased head growth is observed in the first few months of life, followed by slowing of body growth in terms of both height and weight. Particularly small feet in girls with Rett's syndrome have been attributed to autonomic dysfunction. All organs except for the adrenal glands weigh less than in normal age-matched controls but in relation to body length only the brain is small, around 900 g and static, for there is not a significant increase or progressive decline after 4 years of age.[14]

Jellinger and Seitelberger[119] in the first neuropathological examination of a Rett brain noted reduced melanin in the pars compacta of the substantia nigra. Neither gliosis nor pigmentary incontinence is seen,[117] but tyrosine hydroxylase staining is reported to be diminished.[132] Studies of the cerebral cortex have indicated reduced neuronal size and packing density,[24] reductions in dendritic spines, in the numbers of afferent axons and in synaptophysin expression.[27] A significant reduction in dendritic branching in frontal motor and temporal cortex, even greater than that seen in brains in Down's syndrome,[12] has been reported. Other findings include a variable gliosis in the basal ganglia,[117] progressive loss of cerebellar Purkinje cells,[189] which may begin before birth,[24] and changes in the olive.[189] Corticospinal tract degeneration has been reported by some[24] and gliosis by others,[12] as well as a distal peripheral neuropathy.[118] Although there is clinical evidence of autonomic dysfunction the pathology remains to be determined. In a study of the cardiac conducting system, Kearney et al.[127] described an immature dispersed arrangement of cardiac muscle fibres.

Infantile neuroaxonal dystrophy (INAD)

The onset of this disorder is usually early in the second year of life. Development stagnates, severe truncal hypotonia develops and a squint or visual failure appears. The disorder then progresses with dementia, visual failure, spastic tetraparesis and areflexia, and amyotrophy developing before 4 years of age. Seizures are not a prominent feature. In some patients the course is not so rapid and cerebellar signs can be demonstrated in later childhood. Neurophysiology is helpful in the diagnosis, with the EEG showing fast rhythms and the electromyogram (EMG) showing signs of denervation. Magnetic resonance imaging (MRI) shows early cerebellar atrophy, followed by cerebral atrophy and secondary white-matter changes. Late in the disease signal changes in the basal ganglia may become evident.[110,129,165,181] The disorder is autosomal recessive. The metabolic defect is not known. However, a small subgroup (Schindler's disease) has α-N-acetylgalactosaminidase deficiency which otherwise causes angiokeratosis without neurological involvement.

Hallervorden–Spatz syndrome (neuroaxonal dystrophy with iron deposition or neurodegeneration with brain iron accumulation type I)

This disorder comprises progressive dystonia with an akinetic–rigid syndrome and pyramidal tract involvement. There may also be dementia, optic atrophy, retinitis pigmentosa, seizures and acanthocytosis. Characteristic is the demonstration of iron storage in the globus pallidus and in the pars reticularis of the substantia nigra with MRI or pathologically. The post-infantile variant has an onset between 7 and 15 years of age and runs a progressive course with death occurring some 15–20 years after onset. There is also an infantile variant with onset before 6 years of age with death occurring around 8 years after onset. Adult-onset cases have also been described but these are clinically and pathologically variable and seem to encompass distinct subgroups.[8,82,84,166,191,214,244]

PATHOLOGY

Dystrophic axonal swellings with distinctive ultrastructural appearances, known also as spheroids, occur in the central and peripheral nervous systems (CNS and PNS) under many conditions, both physiological as part of the normal ageing process in the gracile and cuneate nuclei, the substantia nigra and pallidum, and pathological, either as the core feature or as a secondary reactive phenomenon associated with another disease[222] (see also Chapter 6, Volume II). In the context of this chapter, diffuse occurrence of pathological axonal swellings in childhood is relevant in relation to infantile neuroaxonal dystrophy, or Seitelberger's disease, its later-onset variants and juvenile-onset Hallervorden–Spatz disease.

The axonal swellings (Fig. 8.4) on which diagnosis depends range in diameter from 20 to 120 µm, are round, oval or elongated in outline, and stain quite variably with eosin from a subtle or granular pallor to a dense eosinophilia. Sometimes a dense core and peripheral pallor, or a narrow cleft can be seen. Silver methods such as Bodian or Glees readily demonstrate the spheroids, but with irregular intensity, vacuolation or whorling. The histochemical method for non-specific esterase in frozen tissue[64,206] is useful in diagnostic brain biopsies (now rarely performed) since the rather small cortical spheroids are elusive on conventional light microscopy. Spheroids are immunoreactive with anti-neurofilament and ubiquitin antibodies, although larger swellings (>30 µm) are unreactive.[176] Contradictory results have been reported with the use of α-synuclein.[183,256]

With electron microscopy (Fig. 8.5) the swellings, which appear to develop preferentially in terminal axons and presynaptic endings, are filled with various organelles to include synaptic vesicles, but most characteristically granulovesicular and tubulomembranous material, sometimes with a paracrystalline appearance, often with a central cleft.[152,206] This is the method of choice for definitive diagnosis from various tissues including the brain, peripheral nerve, muscle, conjunctiva, rectum and skin (for preference near sweat glands where nerve terminals are plentiful).[10,64,69,70,78,131,169,194,206,263]

In INAD, macroscopic appearances (Fig. 8.6) vary from normal to severe cerebral atrophy, but cerebellar atrophy is common. Histologically, axon spheroids are present widely in the brain, the spinal cord and the PNS, but are particularly abundant in the brainstem tegmentum, the posterior columns and the spinal grey matter, the cerebellar grey and white matter, the pallidum, thalamus, the substantia nigra, the hypothalamus and the cerebral

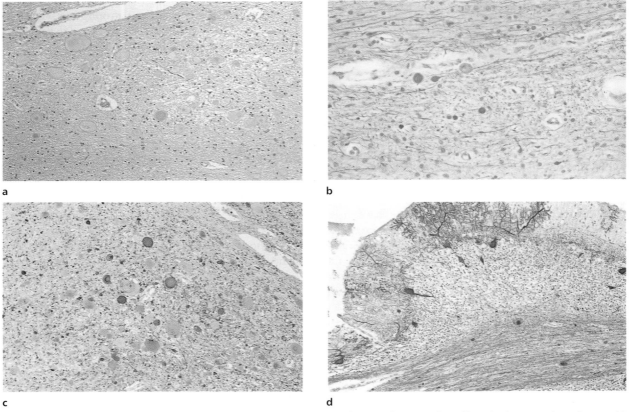

a   b   c   d

Figure 8.4 *Infantile neuroaxonal dystrophy. Microscopic appearances of dystrophic axonal swellings in the posterior columns. (a) H&E. (b) Glees silver method. (c) Immunohistochemistry with anti-neurofilament antibody (note that large swellings >35 µm in diameter stain only irregularly). (d) In the cerebellum anti-neurofilament antibody demonstrates both Purkinje torpedo swellings in the cortex and dystrophic axons in the deep white matter.*

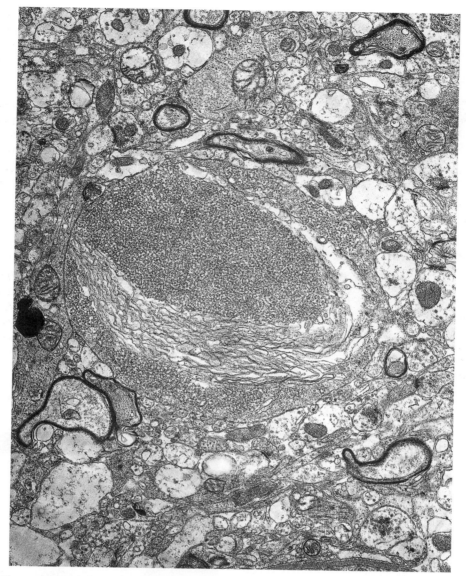

Figure 8.5 *Infantile neuroaxonal dystrophy. Electron micrograph of cerebral biopsy. The axonal spheroid is bound by a single membrane and packed with tubules cut in the transverse or longitudinal plane.*

cortex. Cerebellar cortical atrophy and myelin pallor are other features. Cases with neonatal onset may show preferential involvement of the cerebellum[124,240] or brainstem.[115] Autosomal recessive lysosomal α-*N*-acetyl-galactosaminidase deficiency has been reported in two German brothers in association with typical morphological features of INAD in brain and rectal biopsies,[219,265] and similar findings in a further Dutch sibship have been recorded.[121] Enzyme studies in some other patients with INAD are normal. An autosomal dominant form with extensive demyelination of cerebral white matter has been termed neuroaxonal leukodystrophy or leukoencephalopathy.[16,137,175]

Instances of neuroaxonal dystrophy with late infantile or juvenile onset cause nosological difficulties, particularly as in many the preferential involvement of the pallidum

and substantia nigra, and the presence of iron-containing pigment in addition to spheroids suggests a close similarity to more typical cases of Hallervorden–Spatz disease (Fig. 8.7).

LEUKOENCEPHALOPATHY

Alexander's disease

This disorder is characterized pathologically by a diffuse or focal demyelination and the presence of astrocytic inclusions, Rosenthal fibres. These are formed by intermediate filaments composed of glial fibrillary acidic protein (GFAP) conjugated with abnormally

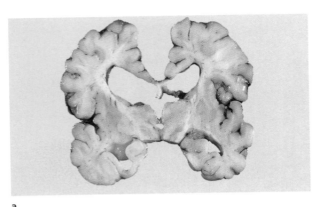

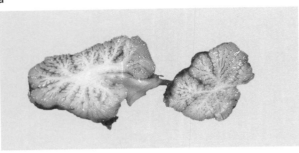

Figure 8.6 *Infantile neuroaxonal dystrophy. (a) Marked cerebral cortical atrophy and ventriculomegaly, with (b) striking shrinkage of cerebellar folia.*

phosphorylated and partly ubiquitinated heat-shock proteins α-B-crystallin and hsp 27. Recent work suggests that most pathologically proven cases of Alexander's disease are associated with *de novo* dominant gain-of-function mutations in the gene encoding GFAP.[36,42,43,58,168,242]

PATHOLOGY

In this rare disease, morphological description relies upon individual case reports following Alexander's original observation,[6] a few reviews[35,204,212] and personal experience. Macroscopic findings may be misleading. Megalencephaly, a characteristic presenting sign in early infancy, may have given way to atrophy by the time of autopsy several years later. Macroscopic changes may be minimal, particularly in cases of juvenile onset dominated by bulbar signs, but infantile examples usually present varying degrees of ventricular dilatation and white-matter atrophy or destruction (Fig. 8.8a). Hydrocephalus may be striking in younger patients and related to aqueduct compression.[226,248] The cerebral white matter appears granular, yellow, sunken-in or cavitated (Fig. 8.8a); this may be very extensive or more confined to anterior parts of frontal and temporal lobes. Grey-matter and hindbrain structures are usually unremarkable.

The principal microscopic feature is the extensive accumulation of Rosenthal fibres (Fig. 8.8b) throughout the brain. Demyelination is variable, being most extensive in infantile cases where it largely parallels in intensity the

degree of Rosenthal fibre formation in the white matter. Macrophages accumulating neutral fat, cyst formation, occasional perivascular lymphocytic cuffs or calcospherites may also occur. Demyelination is less prominent in the cerebrum of juvenile cases. With conventional stains the rod and club-shaped hyaline eosinophil structures isolated from cell bodies and identical to those first described by Rosenthal in 1898,[211] differ only in degree and extent from those found in many other lesions including low-grade tumours, chronic demyelination and inflammation, and cortical dysplasia. Ultrastructurally, they comprise amorphous osmiophilic granular material surrounded by 10-nm filaments; immunocytochemistry demonstrates peripheral staining with antibodies to GFAP, α-B crystallin, 27-kDa heat-shock protein and ubiquitin,[159] while the centre is left unstained. In Alexander's disease the accumulation of Rosenthal fibres is most intense in subependymal, subpial and perivascular locations (Fig. 8.8b), with marked involvement of cerebral white matter, thalamus and basal ganglia, while the cerebral cortex is largely spared. Rosenthal fibre formation may be very intense in brainstem nuclei and tracts as well as the cerebellar white matter and dentate nucleus, but usually the cerebellar cortex is spared. Illustrated in Fig. 8.8(e) is a rare exception where Rosenthal fibres develop in the cerebellar cortex and penetrate the leptomeninges.

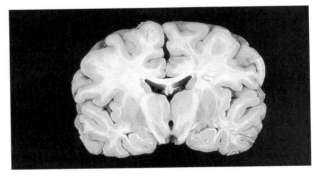

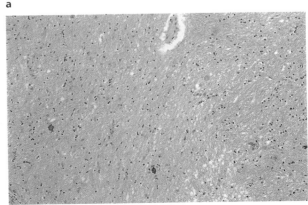

Figure 8.7 *Hallervorden–Spatz disease. (a) Characteristic yellow–brown discoloration and atrophy of globus pallidus. (b) Axon spheroids, calcospherites and brown pigment deposits in the globus pallidus.*

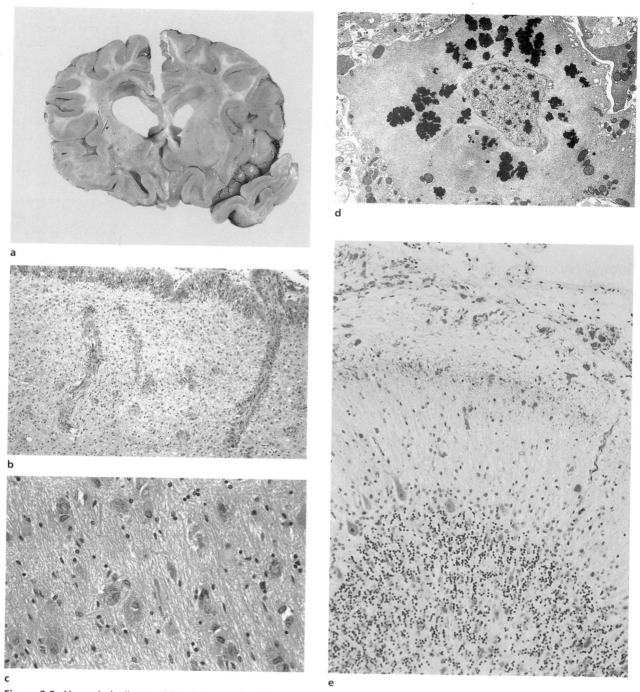

Figure 8.8 *Alexander's disease. (a) Gelatinous dissolution and cavitation of the frontal white matter. (b) Microscopy of the midbrain tegmentum showing myriad Rosenthal fibres beneath the pia and surrounding blood vessels. (H&E.) (c) In younger patients typical Rosenthal fibres may be lacking, but eosinophilic granules fill the juxtanuclear cytoplasm. (H&E.) (d) Ultrastructurally, these intracytoplasmic structures are osmiophilic densities coated with intermediate filaments, i.e. miniature Rosenthal bodies. (e) Very unusual involvement of the cerebellar cortex with massive deposition of Rosenthal fibres in the cortex and the leptomeninges. (H&E.)*

Rosenthal fibre formation is also notable in the proximal parts of the optic nerves and both grey and white matter of the spinal cord.

In general, neurons are preserved even in severely affected areas, but cerebellar degeneration has been described. An important feature in infantile cases is the presence of swollen astrocytes containing small hyaline granules within their cell bodies, sometimes forming a peripheral ring in the cytoplasm (Fig. 8.8c), and identical ultrastructurally (Fig. 8.8d) to Rosenthal fibres. These cells can show nuclear atypia and mitotic activity suggesting a neoplasm, particularly in a biopsy.

Pathogenesis

It has long been suspected that Alexander's disease is a disorder of astrocytes,[35,99] but its genetic status has been uncertain since all cases, with one exception,[264] have been sporadic. However, very recently Messing's group has demonstrated Alexander's disease to be the first example of a primary genetic disease in astrocytes.[36,174] Following on from the observation that overexpression of human GFAP in a transgenic mouse is lethal and produces inclusion bodies indistinguishable from Rosenthal fibres, direct sequence analysis of DNA from patients with Alexander's disease has identified non-conservative *de novo* dominant gain-of-function mutations in the gene encoding GFAP.

Spongy leukodystrophy (Canavan's or van Bogaert–Bertrand disease)

The onset of this autosomal recessive disorder is normally in the first 6 months of life, although exceptionally may be later. First symptoms are usually non-specific with poor visual fixation, irritability and poor sucking. Developmental stagnation (or loss of developmental skills), nystagmus and macrocephaly develop during the first year of life in the majority of patients. Epilepsy usually manifests later.

The disorder is caused by deficiency of aspartoacylase, an enzyme necessary for the catabolism of *N*-acetylaspartate and *N*-acetylaspartoglutamate. The pathogenesis of the leukodystrophy is unclear.[40,126,171,224]

PATHOLOGY

In the typical infantile form brain weight is usually increased by 50% in the first 2 years of life but later decreases to normal levels as cerebral atrophy progresses. Little myelin is evident in coronal sections, and the loss of U-fibres blurs the cortical grey–white junction. The white matter appears grey, gelatinous and sunken in; occasionally there is cystic breakdown (Fig. 8.9a). The capsules and callosum are also affected. The cortex, basal ganglia and brainstem appear normal but the white matter of the cerebellar and spinal cord are soft, retracted and grey.

Histologically, a fine vacuolization with myriad optically empty, histochemically negative, spaces up to 200 μm in diameter extensively involves the white matter of the cerebral hemispheres (Fig. 8.9b) including the callosum, capsules and fornix, the optic nerves, cerebellum and long tracts of the brainstem and spinal cord. Myelin staining is not seen, but immunohistochemistry has demonstrated myelin basic protein lining the vacuoles.[75] Sudanophilia is not usually present but there is astrocytosis including both Alzheimer type I and Alzheimer type II glia. Oligodendroglia are present until quite late in the process. Axons are largely preserved but axon swellings have been demonstrated.[125] Rarely, in the authors' experience, the

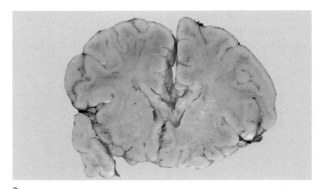

a

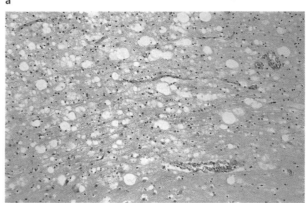

b

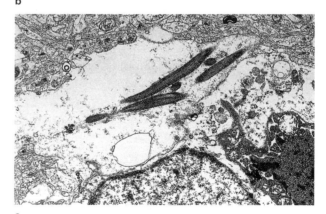

c

Figure 8.9 *Canavan's disease. (a) Coronal section through the frontal lobes from a 6-month-old child showing extensive lack of myelin, brown discoloration and 'softening' involving cerebral white matter and U-fibres, as well as the corpus callosum and internal capsule. (b) The cerebral white matter and especially the U-fibres are demyelinated and finely vacuolated. (Luxol fast blue.) (c) Electron microscopy of a swollen astrocytic process in the cortex containing extremely elongated mitochondria with abnormally structured cristae.*

central parts of the cerebral and cerebellar white matter are replaced by a loose mass of astrocytes, macrophages and capillaries. Vacuole formation is particularly intense at the cortical grey–white junction and spreads into the deeper layers of the cortex, where reactive astrocytes and Alzheimer II glia are present but neurons are spared. Alzheimer II glia are also notable in the basal ganglia.

Another zone of prominent spongy change is the boundary between the molecular and granule cell layers in the cerebellum which may result in a line of cleavage between the layers, with Purkinje cells and Bergmann glia clinging to the molecular layer. Ultrastructural studies have shown that the vacuoles in the white matter correspond to large electron-lucent spaces surrounded by myelin leaflets which appear to be formed by splitting of myelin lamellae at the intraperiod line. In the cortex cell bodies and processes of astrocytes are markedly swollen, and their watery cytoplasm contains extremely elongated mitochondria, 12–15 μm in length, with a diagnostically characteristic structure of central crystalline cores surrounded by a ladder-like array of abnormal cristae (Fig. 8.9c).

Pelizaeus–Merzbacher disease

In contrast to the above, this X-linked disorder is a dysmyelinating condition where normal myelin is not formed owing to an increase in oligodendrocyte death. Boys present with nystagmus, hypotonia, progressive spastic paraparesis and movement disorder in the first year of life, without evidence of peripheral demyelination. Thereafter, the disorder is variable with a progressive motor disorder, mental retardation and often dementia. MRI of the brain shows an absence of normal myelin formation in the cerebral hemispheres, although some myelin may be present subtentorially. Lifespan is shortened and appears to be determined by the severity of the disorder.

There are many other dysmyelinating disorders. Some, such as 18q-syndrome, 3-phosphoglycerate dehydrogenase deficiency and merosin-deficient congenital muscular dystrophy, are part of recognized diseases, whereas others are of unknown aetiology. Children of either sex with the clinical and neuroradiological features of Pelizaeus–Merzbacher disease (PMD) are often designated as having a PMD-like disorder.[33,76,101,180,266,267]

PATHOLOGY

In the past PMD was subtyped on a morphological and clinical basis into connatal, transitional and classical variants.[223] Recent progress in the understanding of myelin biochemistry and the molecular genetics of the X-chromosome have rendered the old classification redundant. In PMD there are mutations in the proteolipid protein,[141] the chief structural protein of central compact myelin. In one-third of patients there are point mutations and deletions, and in two-thirds of patients duplications of the gene at Xq21-22.[81,93,270] The essential pathological process is very similar in all cases. Although the clinical onset is almost always in the first year of life, the rate of progression is variable, and not surprisingly the degree of myelin loss and subsequent astrocytosis reflects this. A possible genetic basis for these differences remains to be determined.

The brain is usually small, and below normal weight by one-third to one-half. On sectioning the grey matter appears intact, and ventricular dilatation is proportionate to the loss of white matter. The central and digitate white matter, callosum, capsules, commissures and fornix are grey–brown, gelatinous or firm and sunken in (Fig. 8.10a). There may be patchy sparing of the U-fibres and sometimes streaks of whiteness in the centrum semiovale. The optic nerves and chiasm are grey and thin, white other cranial nerves are normal. The cerebellar white matter and brainstem and cord tracts are shrunken grey and gelatinous, in contrast to the plump and white cranial and spinal nerve roots (Fig. 8.10b).

Histology confirms the preserved grey matter apart from cerebellar cortical atrophy with either predominant granule or Purkinje cell degeneration. Polymicrogyria has occasionally been reported.[195,223] In the hemispheres white matter varies from almost complete absence of myelin, particularly when death occurs in infancy, to the classical tigroid or discontinuous pattern with preserved perivascular islets when the clinical course is more protracted (Fig. 8.10d). Oligodendrocytes are markedly reduced in number or absent. There is astrocytosis, fibrillary gliosis and usually only sparse sudanophilic lipid in perivascular macrophages. Axons are preserved, and while most are naked, myelin discontinuities can be observed ultrastructurally (Fig. 8.10e). Spinal and cranial nerve roots with a different myelin structural protein (PMP-22) are normally myelinated (Fig. 8.10c). In well-orientated sections individual axons can be followed in continuity from an unmyelinated state centrally through the root transition zone into the normally myelinated root.

Cockayne's syndrome

This disorder is characterized by poor growth, dysmorphism, sensitivity of the skin to the sun and neurological abnormalities. The latter are normally apparent after the first year, although some can be present from birth, and consist of microcephaly, structural ocular abnormalities, cataracts, pigmentary retinopathy, deafness, a peripheral neuropathy, and progressive pyramidal tract and cerebellar signs secondary to a leukodystrophy. Neuroimaging shows brain atrophy and calcification of the basal ganglia. Unlike other sun-sensitive conditions, tumour formation is not a feature. It is inherited in an autosomal recessive manner and at least three different gene defects are responsible.

The defect causing the syndrome is believed to be failure of transcription-coupled repair of oxidized DNA bases. Because neurons are rapidly metabolizing cells that produce high levels of reactive oxygen species, this eventually causes a general failure of DNA transcription with reduced messenger RNA (mRNA) formation and a strong proapoptotic signal.[17,31,45,49,50,74,111,120,149,179,193,243]

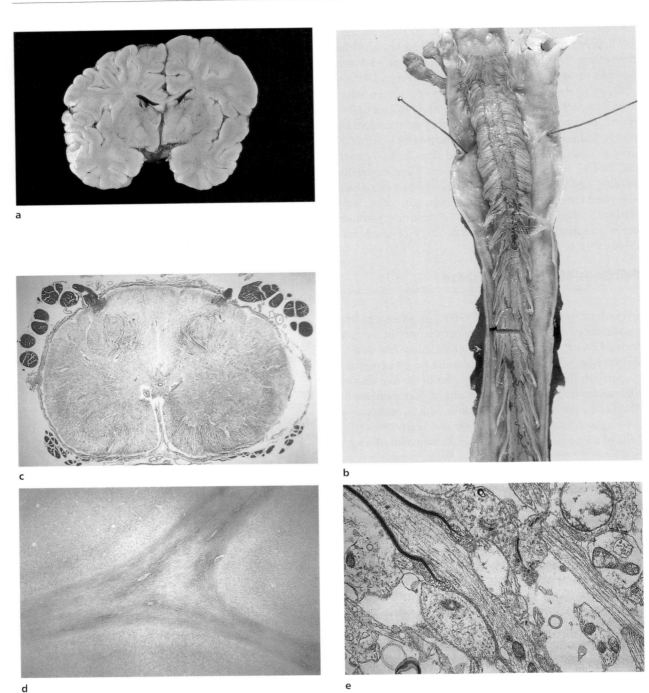

Figure 8.10 *Pelizaeus–Merzbacher disease. (a) Coronal section of the frontal lobes in a 9-month-old boy. There is not any normal white matter, but central and digitate white matter, corpus callosum and capsules are grey–brown and sunken in. (b) Anterior aspect of the spinal cord. There is a striking disparity between the normal bulk and whiteness of the spinal roots and the grey unmyelinated spinal cord. (c) The central white matter of the cord is completely unstained by Luxol fast blue, while peripheral myelin in the spinal nerve roots stains normally. (d) Preserved perivascular myelin islets in cerebral white matter (Luxol fast blue). (e) Electron micrograph of a biopsy in which there is discontinuous myelination as the myelin sheath stops abruptly at a heminode, leaving the naked axon to continue through the neuropil.*

PATHOLOGY

Various case reports have been reviewed by Nance and Berry.[179] Microcephaly and cerebral atrophy are very marked. The brain weight is half that expected for age, but the hindbrain is even smaller. The cortex looks normal but the lateral ventricles are greatly enlarged while the central white matter is considerably reduced in volume and has a striking appearance of alternating grey and white patches[196] (Fig. 8.11a), which also involves the corpus callosum, capsules and optic nerves. There may be thalamic atrophy and visible calcifications in the deep grey matter. The brainstem is shrunken and the cerebellar folia are often atrophied, while their white matter is narrow and grey. The principal histological features are discontinuous demyelination (Fig. 8.11b) with gliosis throughout the supratentorial and infratentorial white matter, and numerous mulberry-like calcific concretions affecting both the grey and white matter (Fig. 8.11c), and sometimes also the walls of blood vessels and Purkinje cell bodies and dendritic trees. Cerebellar cortical degeneration may be prominent, producing a plethora of Purkinje axon torpedoes and dendritic asteroid expansions. Other occasional findings are multinucleated neurons[147] and neurofibrillary tangles.[241]

Aicardi–Goutières leukoencephalopathy

This disorder is a familial syndrome of calcification of the basal ganglia and cerebral white matter, diffuse demyelination, brain atrophy and a mild CSF pleocytosis. Its onset is in the first 4 months of life in most patients,

with microcephaly developing in the first year. Development stagnates, there is hypotonia punctuated by opisthotonus and the children become decerebrate over a few years. Even within the same family, there is considerable variation in the symptoms and rate of evolution of the brain calcification and atrophy.[5,22,69,79,163,254]

The disorder is thought to arise from the overproduction of α-interferon within the CNS. Raised α-interferon in the CSF may constitute a biochemical marker for the disorder.

PATHOLOGY

The original case reports of Aicardi and Goutières[4] did not include morphological studies, but the pathology can be inferred from other publications, notably those of Razavi-Encha[207] and Troost.[249] Several similar cases have been examined by the authors. Microcephaly is striking, brain weights being two-thirds to one-half that expected, but the hindbrain is disproportionately smaller. Coronal sections demonstrate atrophic convolutions with a crumbly consistency, pronounced ventricular dilatation, shrunken central white matter, thin corpus callosum, and atrophic

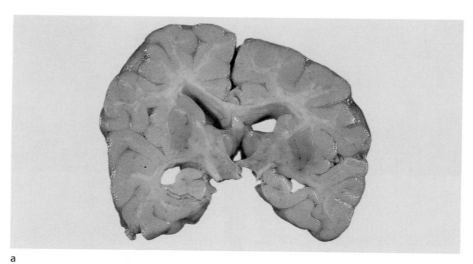

a

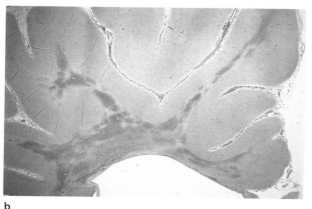

b

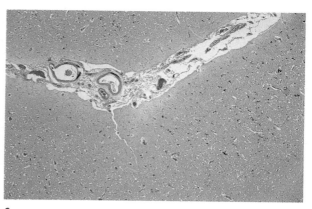

c

Figure 8.11 *Cockayne's syndrome. (a) Central white matter and corpus callosum are reduced in volume and have a mottled appearance. (b) Tigroid demyelination in a section from the frontal lobe. (Luxol fast blue.) (c) There are small calcospherites in the atrophied cortex and linear calcification in leptomeningeal vessel walls.*

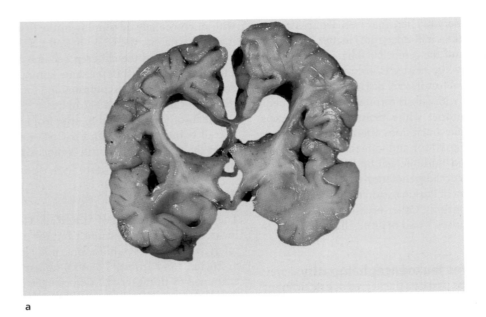

a

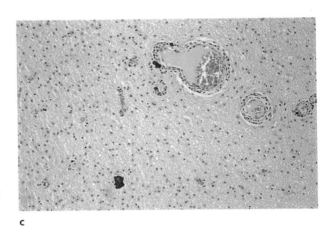

b

c

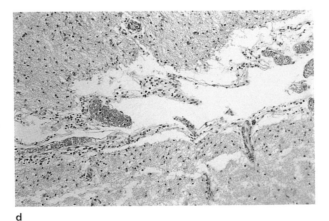

d

Figure 8.12 *Aicardi–Goutières leukoencephalopathy. (**a**) Profound grey- and white-matter atrophy in a 2-year-old boy. (**b**) Low-power view of the thalamus and temporal lobe. The shrunken white matter is without myelin, the cortex and thalamus are severely atrophied, and there are central mineralizations in the thalamus. (Luxol fast blue–cresyl violet.) (**c**) Calcospherites and thin perivascular lymphocytic cuffs in the white matter. (H&E.) (**d**) Slight lymphocytic infiltrate in the leptomeninges with calcospherites near vessels. (H&E.)*

basal ganglia and thalamus (Fig. 8.12a, b). The brainstem is slender and firm and the cerebellum small with marked cortical atrophy.

Microscopic calcification is widespread (Fig. 8.12c): slight in the cortex, and more severe in white matter, the basal ganglia, thalamus and cerebellum. Spherical lamellated periodic acid–Schiff (PAS)-, iron- and calcium-positive concretions are scattered freely in the parenchyma or cluster around blood vessels. Mineralization is intramural in the basal ganglia and affects the dendritic tree of cerebellar Purkinje cells. Hemispheric and cerebellar white matter and brainstem tracts are greatly reduced in volume (Fig. 8.12b) and show a diffuse lack of myelin staining or fragmentation of myelinated fibres. Oligodendroglial populations are preserved but there is marked fibrillary gliosis and astrocytosis; many hypertrophic astrocytes show intracytoplasmic neutral lipid. In the cerebral grey matter, neuronal loss parallels the degree of calcification. Other features include hippocampal sclerosis, cerebellar cortical degeneration involving Purkinje cells with axonal torpedoes and dendritic asteroid deformities, and destruction and calcification of the olivary and dentate nuclei. Scanty lymphocytic infiltrates can be found in the leptomeninges and sometimes the parenchyma (Fig. 8.12c, d).

Megalencephalic cystic leukoencephalopathy

In this macrocephaly develops during the first year of life, but without other symptoms. Neuroimaging at this stage will reveal a diffuse abnormality of cerebral hemispheric white matter, and there may already be cysts in the temporal and parietal lobes. Onset of a spastic–ataxic motor disorder usually occurs by the fifth year of life but may exceptionally be later. The motor disorder is progressive, and seizures and dementia develop later, usually in the teenage years. The disorder is inherited in an autosomal recessive manner and one responsible gene has recently been identified. Distinction from other, recently reported, cystic leukoencephalopathies is made on clinical grounds.[138,190]

PATHOLOGY

At present knowledge of the neuropathology of this condition is limited to two biopsy reports. A spongiform leukoencephalopathy with gliosis, intact myelinated fibres and many oil red O-positive macrophages was described by van der Knaap et al.[135] Ultrastructurally, there were many vacuoles containing some debris and surrounded by five-layered membranes equivalent to myelin lamellae; splitting of myelin at the intraperiod line and vacuolation in the outer part of the myelin sheath was also observed. By contrast, in a biopsy from one of two affected siblings[87] the white matter was rarefied and pale staining but not spongy, corresponding

with electron microscopy to a hugely increased extracellular space and abnormally thin myelin surrounding swollen axons.

Childhood ataxia with central hypomyelination (CACH) syndrome/vanishing white-matter disease

This autosomal recessive disorder is characterized by the onset of neurological symptoms following a minor head injury or incidental infections and a diagnostic MRI appearance. Early development is normal and the first symptoms usually develop between 18 months and 5 years of age. Exceptionally, middle-aged adults may develop symptoms. The initial neurological feature is that of a progressive ataxic–spastic disorder, later bulbar involvement and optic atrophy and occasionally epilepsy. Although difficult to assess, intellect appears to be preserved.

MRI shows diffuse lesion of the cerebral white matter with variable brainstem involvement in presymptomatic individuals. Once symptoms develop, there is progression of the white-matter changes with areas having the signal intensity of CSF and involvement of the dentate nucleus.[134,136,139,148]

PATHOLOGY

Brief biopsy and autopsy descriptions accompany the original clinical delineation of this white-matter disorder,[134,218] but detailed morphological studies of similar cases pre-date them by 30 years. The eye-catching cavitations have been described not only in children,[57] including three siblings, but also in adults.[77,257] Indeed, van der Knaap et al.[136] expanded the phenotype to include onset later in childhood, in adolescence and even early adulthood. Personal experience with autopsied cases of both childhood and adolescent onset support the proposition of a single entity with an extended spectrum of age. The most detailed recent histological, ultrastructural and biochemical report is that of Rodriguez et al.[208] Linkage to chromosome 3q27 has recently been demonstrated.[148]

Significant atrophy or reduction in brain weight is not usually present, but an undue softness on palpation evidently results from the remarkable cavitation of the hemispheric white matter (Fig. 8.13a). Cortex and basal ganglia are unaffected and the lateral ventricles are only slightly enlarged, but much of the cerebral white matter is cavitated and gelatinous or has the appearance of a greyish, lacey cobweb punctuated by yellow–white spots. Subcortical U-fibres are only partially spared, while the corpus callosum, capsules and commissures are affected to a variable extent. The cerebellar cortex is normal or slightly atrophied but its white matter is diffusely grey. The brainstem is also shrunken and its

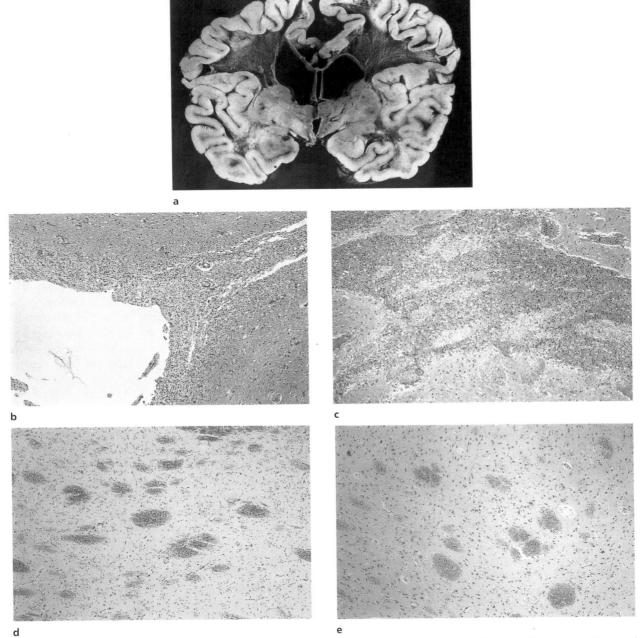

Figure 8.13 *Childhood ataxia with central hypomyelination syndrome/vanishing white-matter disease. (a) Extreme cavitation of the frontal white matter. (b) At the edge of the cavity the white matter is hypercellular with increased numbers of oligodendroglia. (H&E.) (c) Increased density of oligodendrocytes in the internal capsule. (H&E.) (d) Compare the hypercellularity due to oligodendrocytes in the pencil fibres of the basal ganglia with the age-matched control to the right (e). (Luxol fast blue–cresyl violet.)*

white-matter tracts are diffusely grey, but in some cases focal spots of chalky whiteness stand out in the pontine tegmentum.

Microscopic examination confirms the preservation of grey structures in general, with the exception of the cerebellar cortex which is subject to Purkinje cell degeneration and depletion. The large cavities in the centrum semi-ovale are surrounded by cellular tissue in which there are many naked axons, few myelin fragments with nor-

mal staining characteristics, reactive astrocytes but only modest gliosis, macrophages containing sudanophilic material and in particular oligodendrocytes which appear increased in density (Fig. 8.13b–d). Demyelination extends well beyond the area of cavitation to include digitate white matter, capsules callosum, commissures, fornix and cerebral peduncles as well as the cerebellum; in these areas oligodendrocyte numbers are clearly increased. However, myelin loss in the brainstem tracts and spinal cord is apparently not accompanied by an increase in oligodendrocytes. Sheets of lipid phagocytes in the pontine tegmentum correspond to the discrete lesions observed macroscopically.[208] These are the presumed morphological correlate of symmetrical foci of high signal intensity on MRI, characteristic of this disorder.[134]

The oligodendrocyte population has been repeatedly shown to have normal ultrastructural, histochemical and immunohistochemical properties without increased mitotic or proliferative activity, and the morphological and biochemical properties of the myelin are also normal.[208] According to Rodriguez et al.[208] the abundant organelle-rich cytoplasm of the oligodendrocytes, reminiscent of myelinating glia, suggests abnormal maturation which is also observed in the rumpshaker mouse mutant. This has a point mutation in the *PLP* gene, but molecular analysis including sequencing in their patient has not so far revealed any *PLP* abnormality.

Pigmentary type of orthochromatic leukodystrophy

One of the rarest forms of orthochromatic, sudanophilic leukodystrophy is that described by van Bogaert and Nissen.[32] In total, there are about two dozen post-mortem descriptions of both sporadic and familial cases (for recent references see Refs 26, 80, 188, 221 and 250). Onset is between the second and fourth decades; early clinical signs are emotional lability and abnormal behaviour, followed by progressive intellectual deterioration, frontal lobe syndrome, motor signs, rigidity, seizures, tetraparesis, incontinence, mutism and decerebration. Seiser's sporadic case[221] differed in its particularly protracted course: there was retarded motor development from birth with ataxic gait, but progressive mental and neurological deterioration only from the age of 13, with death at 26 years. The only truly paediatric example of this condition was reported in a 12-year-old African–American whose seizural disorder began in infancy; a brother and sister were similarly affected.[90] Brain weights vary from normal to profoundly reduced. The surface of the fresh brain may have a greenish tinge. On sectioning the lateral ventricles are dilated and the hemispheric white matter is shrunken and grey–brown (Fig. 8.14a). Subcortical U-fibres, optic nerves, cortex, deep grey matter, cerebellum and brainstem all appear normal.

Microscopic demyelination is extensive, sparing only the U-fibres (Fig. 8.14b), optic nerves and hindbrain. Areas of complete myelin loss show severe gliosis and few macrophages; axons are relatively spared but there are frequent axonal swellings. In other areas demyelination is not complete and there are large numbers of globular macrophages containing dark yellow–brown pigment which is autofluorescent, birefringent, non-metachromatic, sudanophilic and positively stained by Luxol-fast blue, PAS, Masson Fontana for melanin, Schmorl, and in some cases Perls' iron stain (Fig. 8.14c). Similar pigment is present in astrocytes and in the authors' case was observed in microglial cells. All recent authors have carried out electron-microscopic studies to similar effect. Cytoplasmic inclusions of two types, some membrane bound, are present in macrophages, astrocytes and oligodendroglia. There are mixed structures invoking lipofuscin, and fingerprint or multilamellar bodies interpreted as ceroid pigment (Fig. 8.14d). Okeda et al.[188] observed similar inclusions in the peripheral nerve of one patient but without evidence of hypomyelination.

INBORN ERRORS OF INTERMEDIARY METABOLISM

The hyperphenylalaninaemic syndromes

The hyperphenylalaninaemic syndromes comprise of L-phenylalanine 4-mono-oxygenase (phenylalaninehydroxylase) deficiency, and deficiency of its essential cofactor tetrahydrobiopterin (Fig. 8.15).[18,19,47,48,59,102,161,162,229,237,246,247,259]

Phenylketonuria (phenylalanine 4-mono-oxygenase deficiency)

Phenylketonuria (PKU) is caused by deficiency of the hepatic enzyme phenylalanine mono-oxygenase. The biochemical consequences of this are the accumulation of phenylalanine and its metabolites in the blood and a relative deficiency of tyrosine, which becomes an essential amino acid. However, the main impact of the disease is upon the brain, which normally does not contain phenylalanine mono-oxygenase. Untreated, the early manifestations of PKU are microcephaly, severe mental retardation and epilepsy and, in the second or third decade, there is the emergence or progression of a motor disorder.

Severe neurological disability in PKU can largely be prevented by a strict reduced phenylalanine diet started in early infancy. Despite such treatment, patients with PKU are of lower intelligence, may have neuropsychological or neurological abnormalities and have abnormalities of cerebral white matter. There is also the risk of late motor and cognitive decline in adults who have relaxed their diet. Untreated maternal PKU leads to severe teratogenic effects.

Current understanding of the biochemical pathogenesis of the neurological consequences of PKU is that these are secondary to the accumulation of phenylalanine in the blood. This causes an increase in brain phenylalanine concentration and deficiencies of the other large neutral amino acids (importantly tyrosine and methionine). As a consequence of these changes, brain protein synthesis, myelin turnover and biogenic amine neurotransmission are all disturbed.

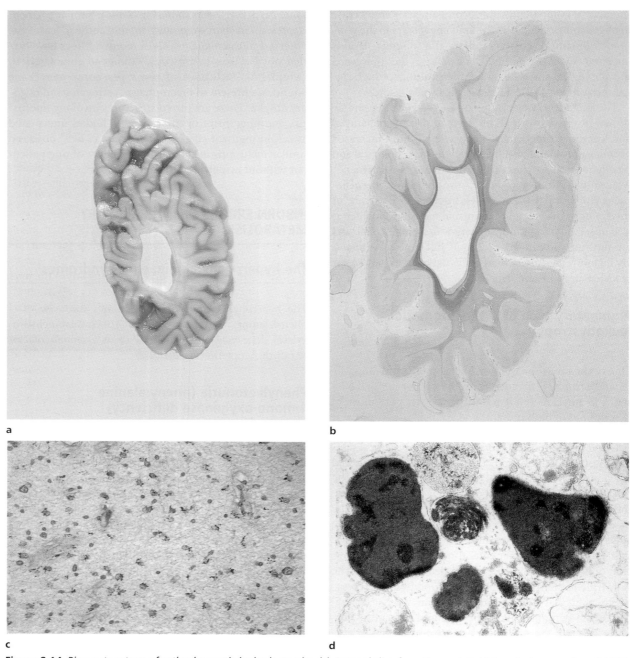

Figure 8.14 *Pigmentary type of orthochromatic leukodystrophy. (a) Coronal slice from the occipital lobe of a teenage boy. (b) Diffuse demyelination of the white matter. (Luxol fast blue.) (c) Pigment in astrocytes and microglia is present throughout the white matter. (Masson–Fontana.) (d) Electron microscopy shows multilamellar inclusions and fingerprint inclusions in glial cells and macrophages.*

PATHOLOGY

Significant morphological findings in untreated patients are microcephaly and variable degrees of white-matter disturbance ranging from spongiosis and delayed myelination in younger children to focal myelin pallor or even breakdown with accumulation of neutral fat in adults.[170] There is some evidence for a biochemical disturbance of myelin.[172] Three profoundly retarded adults studied by Bauman and Kemper[23] showed, in addition to myelin pallor in hemispheric association fibres, non-specific thalamic radiations and brainstem reticular formation, subtle developmental anomalies, increased packing density of cortical neurons, reduced neuronal size and Nissl content, and poorly developed dendritic trees and spines. Similar abnormalities have been documented in experimental animal models of PKU.[52,106]

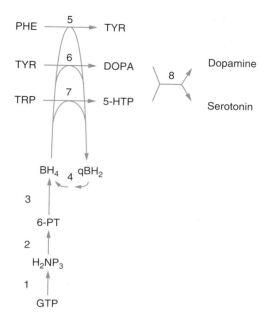

Figure 8.15 *Pterin and aromatic amino acid metabolism. GTP, guanosine triphosphate; H₂NP₃, dihydroneopterin triphosphate; 6-PT, 6-pyruvyltetrahydropterin; BH₄, tetrahydrobiopterin; qBH₂, quinonoid dihydrobiopterin; PHE, phenylalanine; TYR, tyrosine; TRP, tryptophan, DOPA, dihydroxyphenylalanine; 5-HTP, 5-hydroxytryptophan. 1, GTP cyclohydrolase I; 2, 6-pyruvyltetrahydropterin synthetase; 3, sepiapterin reductase; 4, dihydropteridine reductase; 5, phenylalanine 4-mono-oxygenase; 6, tyrosine 4-mono-oxygenase; 7, tryptophan 5-mono-oxygenase; 8, aromatic amino acid decarboxylase.*

Despite effective treatment with tight dietary control, the offspring of mothers with PKU are at increased risk of microcephaly (see Fig. 7.93 in Chapter 7, this Volume), mental retardation, impaired growth and cardiac anomalies: they develop the maternal PKU syndrome.[156,230] Head circumference and brain weight appear to be inversely related to the maternal plasma concentration of phenylalanine.

Tetrahydrobiopterin deficiencies

Tetrahydrobiopterin is the cofactor for phenylalanine, tyrosine and tryptophan mono-oxygenases and nitric oxide synthase. Severe forms (recessively inherited) present in infancy with hyperphenylalaninaemia and infantile parkinsonism–dystonia (due to dopamine and serotonin deficiency). These are caused by pterin-4-α-carbinolamine and dihydropteridine reductase deficiencies, which prevent the recycling of tetrahydrobiopterin, and by guanosine triphosphate (GTP)-cyclohydrolase, 6-pyruvoyltetrahydropterin synthase and, in theory, sepiapterin reductase deficiencies, which are defects of tetrahydrobiopterin synthesis. A dominantly inherited, less severe, form of GTP-cyclohydrolase-I deficiency may present later in life with symptoms of dopamine deficiency alone (dopa-responsive dystonia). Infantile parkinsonism–dystonia can also be caused by aromatic amino acid decarboxylase deficiency, and both infantile parkinsonism–dystonia and dopa-responsive dystonia can be caused by tyrosine 4-mono-oxygenase deficiency.

Non-ketotic hyperglycinaemia

Non-ketotic hyperglycinaemia is a recessively inherited disorder caused by deficiency of the intramitochondrial enzyme complex the glycine cleavage system.[34,86,144,160] The vast majority of the patients present with the severe neonatal-onset form, although milder disease can present later in infancy or even in childhood. The phenotype appears to breed true in individual families. In the neonatal-onset form, most babies develop symptoms in the first 2 days of life, becoming profoundly hypotonic (with preserved or brisk tendon reflexes) and lethargic with abnormalities of eye movement. The encephalopathy progresses to coma with the development of segmental myoclonic jerks, hiccups and apnoea. The EEG at this stage shows bursts of spike-wave complexes without normal background activity. Many babies will die at this stage. Survivors regain respiration at around 3 weeks of age: intractable epilepsy develops after about 3 months and the infants and children become profoundly mentally retarded with no adaptive or social behaviour. MRI of the brain at this stage of the disease shows a severe leukoencephalopathy. Glycine accumulates in all body fluids, but is preferentially elevated in the CSF. A CSF to plasma glycine ratio of greater than 0.08 is considered diagnostic of non-ketotic hyperglycinaemia. The normal physiological hyperglycinuria of the newborn renders urinary glycine difficult to interpret.

The current understanding of the pathogenesis of non-ketotic hyperglycinaemia involves the neurotransmitter and cotransmitter roles of glycine and the supply of single carbon units to brain metabolism. The early vegetative symptoms can be understood as arising from excessive stimulation of brainstem inhibitory glycine receptors. The later symptoms are thought to arise from excessive stimulation of excitatory glutamate *N*-methyl-ᴅ-aspartate (NMDA) receptors, which require glycine as a coagonist. Later still, the reduced supply of single carbon groups to brain metabolism might result in myelin abnormalities. This schema underlies current therapeutic approaches. Glycine can be reduced in body fluids by the administration of sodium benzoate that binds to glycine to form sodium hippurate, which is readily excreted in urine. Glutamate secretion can be reduced by the use of antiepileptic drugs such as lamotrigine, and ketamine or dextromethorphan can block the NMDA receptor. Single carbon groups can be supplied as folinic acid, betaine or choline. Despite such therapeutic endeavours, outcome remains disappointingly poor.

PATHOLOGY

Abnormalities of myelination and malformations are frequent. Two-thirds of Dobyns' cases[60] showed anomalies of gyration, callosal agenesis and cerebellar hypoplasia. In the 3-year-old child studied by Shuman et al.,[227] cerebral white matter and brainstem tracts stained poorly for myelin and were gliotic, the centrum semi-ovale being severely vacuolated.

Agamanolis et al.[3] described spongy myelopathy in a series of neonates; while the amount of myelin did not differ from normal controls, all areas had a spongy appearance, but the cerebellar white matter, corticospinal and optic tracts were particularly affected. Neuronal ferrugination and leukomalacia were noted in some patients. Ultrastructurally, the vacuoles were lined by myelin and appeared to form by intraperiod splitting. Defective glycine–serine interconversion reducing the availability of one-carbon units could be the pathogenic basis for dysmyelination.[98]

The homocystinurias

The homocystinurias comprise classical homocystinuria (cystathionine β-synthase deficiency) and the remethylation defects (inborn errors of cobalamin and folate metabolism that prevent the recycling of homocysteine to methionine). They are characterized by the excretion of homocystine in the urine and by increased homocysteine in the plasma. In cystathionine β-synthase deficiency plasma methionine is raised, whereas in the remethylation defects it is reduced (Fig. 8.16).[7,9,15,61,65,96,109,133,158,210,234,252,260,261,269,272]

Cystathionine β-synthase deficiency

Cystathionine β-synthase deficiency is a multisystem disorder with ocular, skeletal, vascular and CNS involvement. It often presents with high myopia or lens dislocation. The skeletal abnormalities become more obvious around puberty with arachnodactyly, dolichostenomelia and enlargement of both metaphyses and epiphyses. Most patients will have CNS manifestations including mental retardation, epilepsy or psychiatric disturbance. The possibility of a thromboembolic event increases with age. These are more commonly venous than arterial, although both may occur. Thromboembolism in childhood is commonly precipitated by an intercurrent illness that causes dehydration.

Approximately half of the patients with cystathionine β-synthase deficiency respond to pharmacological doses of pyridoxine (the coenzyme for cystathionine β-synthase) and subsequently do well. The other patients are more difficult to treat and often require dietary restriction of methionine and an alternative methyl group donor such as betaine; their outcome is less good. Patients detected at birth and prospectively treated do not develop the complications.

The ocular, skeletal and vascular complications of cystathionine β-synthase deficiency appear to be secondary to the accumulation of homocysteine. The pathogenesis of the neural complications is less clear, but involves metabolic mechanisms as well as cerebrovascular disease.

Remethylation defects

The remethylation defects consist of three groups of disorder: inborn errors of cobalamin metabolism termed cobalamine mutant (cbl), causing actual (cblG) or functional (cblE) deficiency of methionine synthase; inborn errors of cobalamin metabolism causing combined functional deficiency of methionine synthase and methylmalonyl coenzyme A (CoA) mutase (cblC, cblD and cblF); and 5,10-methylenetetrahydrofolate reductase deficiency. Each group has similar clinical features that vary according to the age of onset (and presumably the severity of the defect).

In the early infantile-onset remethylation defects, symptoms start in the first 3 months of life. After a period of well-being, the babies develop non-specific symptoms of lethargy and poor feeding. After a few days, rapidly progressive neurological symptoms occur leading to coma. Infants with inborn errors of cobalamin metabolism can also present with a micro-angiopathy with widespread organ involvement.

In the late infantile early childhood-onset remethylation defects, symptoms start between 3 months and 10 years of age. These are usually neurological and consist of slowing of brain growth and development followed by progressive neurological disorder resembling leukodystrophies. During the progressive phase, the children dement, may develop an ataxic–spastic or extrapyramidal movement disorder and often have signs of a peripheral neuropathy. Characteristically there may be bouts of unexplained lethargy and coma.

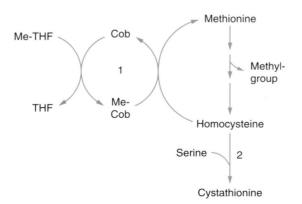

Figure 8.16 *Simplified scheme of homocysteine metabolism. THF, tetrahydrofolate; Me, methyl; Cob, cobalamin; 1, methionine synthase; 2, cystathionine β-synthase.*

In late childhood/adult-onset remethylation defects, symptoms start after the age of 10 years and may present in a similar way to those in the younger patient. However, there may be asymptomatic siblings, stroke, unexplained psychosis and symptoms of subacute combined degeneration.

The inborn errors of cobalamin metabolism may be accompanied by a macrocytic anaemia. A high index of suspicion and a raised plasma total homocysteine and a reduced (or low normal) plasma methionine concentration are the initial pointers to a remethylation defect. Treatment of the remethylation defects generally gives a disappointing neurological outcome. A good biochemical and haematological response to pharmacological doses of hydroxycobalamin is seen in inborn errors of cobalamin metabolism. 5,10-Methylenetetrahydrofolate reductase generally does not respond well to pharmacological doses of folinic acid, and treatment with the methyl donor betaine is becoming the preferred choice.

PATHOLOGY

In homocystinuria, the principal lesions are ischaemic: thromboembolic occlusive vascular disease in arteries, veins and dural sinuses leads to cerebral, cerebellar, thalamic and midbrain infarcts. Degenerative changes in vascular muscle and elastic coats and intimal thickening are prominent, but the underlying pathogenesis is unknown.

Appearances suggestive of subacute combined degeneration have been reported in a patient with an inborn error of cobalamin metabolism,[56] although the spinal cord was not examined. A similar diffuse leukoencephalopathy of focal perivascular demyelination coalescing into a large area of myelin loss in the centrum semi-ovale combined with typical changes of subacute combined degeneration throughout the cord has been observed by the author in two patients with 5,10-methylenetetrahydrofolate reductase deficiency (Fig. 8.17).[46]

Organic acid disorders

Organic acid disorders are a group of individually rare, recessively inherited disorders where there is accumulation of an organic acid in body fluids due to a defect in its catabolism (Fig. 8.18). Here, only three organic acid

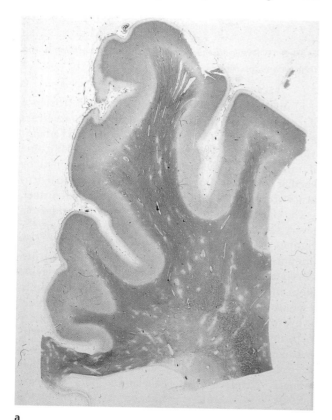

a

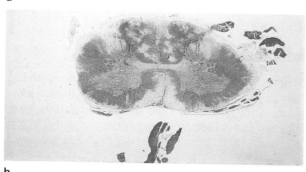

b

Figure 8.17 *5,10-Methylenetetrahydrofolate reductase deficiency. (a) Multiple foci of perivascular demyelination in the cerebral white matter. (b) Subacute combined degeneration of the spinal cord.(Hexol fast blue–acryl violet.)*

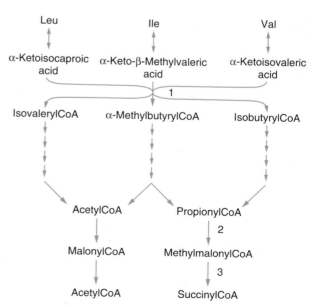

Figure 8.18 *Branched chain amino acid catabolism. Leu, leucine; Ile, isoleucine; Val, valine. 1, branched chain ketoacid decarboxylase; 2, propionylCoA carboxylase; 3, methylmalonylCoA mutase.*

disorders are discussed, all involving defects in the catabolism of branched chain amino acids: propionic acidaemia, methylmalonic aciduria and maple syrup urine disease. Each presents in one of two ways, each is treated by dietary protein restriction with appropriate amino acid, mineral and vitamin supplementation, and each has a disappointing long-term neurological outcome.[25,28,30,37,44,73,85,100,122,142,146,150,153,154,184,186,197,205,220,238,253,255]

Propionic acidaemias

Accumulation of propionic acid and its metabolites in body fluids is caused by actual or functional deficiency of propionylCoA carboxylase. Functional deficiency of propionylCoA carboxylase is caused by inborn errors of biotin metabolism, or very rarely biotin deficiency, and is not considered further here. Most children with propionic acidaemia present in the early neonatal period with a relentlessly progressive encephalopathy resulting in coma with variable muscle tone and myoclonus. Later-onset forms are usually characterized by episodes of acute encephalopathy on a background of anorexia, failure to thrive and developmental delay. Investigation reveals neutropenia and thrombocytopenia with acidosis, ketosis, hyperammonaemia, mild or moderate hyperglycinaemia, reduced free carnitine and raised propionylcarnitine, and the excretion of propionylglycine and methylcitrate in the urine (especially during an acute episode). Despite treatment with protein restriction and carnitine, the outlook for the neonatal-onset form is poor, with mental retardation, chorea and early death. The outlook for the later-onset forms with treatment is better, although a high proportion of the children develop a disabling movement disorder (mainly generalized chorea) following a further episode of acute encephalopathy.

PATHOLOGY

Spongy degeneration of the white matter and especially of the globus pallidus are the chief findings in patients with neonatal onset and death during infancy.[104,227,235] However, spongiosis is not present in the later-onset group, where pathology centres on the basal ganglia: this includes perivascular rarefaction in the caudate,[235] bilateral symmetrical encephalomalacia in the lentiform nucleus,[228] both striatal and pallidal neuronal loss and gliosis, or even bilateral marbling (Fig. 8.19).[95] These changes correspond to computed tomographic (CT) lucencies seen in the basal ganglia during episodic decompensation and underlie the severe movement disorder commonly present in this group.[238]

Methylmalonic acidaemias

Accumulation of methylmalonic acid in body fluids is caused by actual (mut^0 or mut^-) or functional deficien-

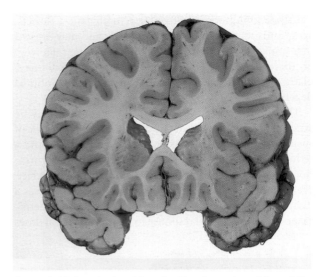

Figure 8.19 *Propionic acidaemia. Atrophy and marbling of the striatum are apparent.*

cy of methylmalonylCoA mutase. Functional deficiency of methylmalonylCoA mutase is caused by inborn errors of cobalamin metabolism affecting its coenzyme adenosylcobalamin (*cblA*, *cblB* and *cblH*). Because the outcome of methylmalonic acidaemia is partly determined by whether it is cobalamin responsive or not, functional deficiency of methylmalonylCoA mutase is considered further.

The clinical presentation of methylmalonic acidaemia is very similar to that of propionic acidaemia, as are the findings on investigation, with the exception that large amounts of methylmalonic acid are excreted in the urine. Once started on a protein-restricted diet and receiving supplemental carnitine, it is mandatory that cobalamin responsiveness is assessed by giving pharmacological doses of hydroxycobalamin for 5 days to see whether urinary methylmalonic acid excretion is at least halved. The neurological outcome of methylmalonic acidaemia is determined by the age at onset and the cobalamin responsiveness. Neonatal-onset cobalamin non-responsive patients have mental retardation and neurological complications (dystonia and spasticity) and die early. Cobalamin-responsive and late-onset cobalamin non-responsive patients have a better outcome.

PATHOLOGY

Neuropathological changes (Fig. 8.20) are non-specific. Dave *et al.*[55] describe multiple small cerebellar haemorrhages, while Adams and Lyon[1] noted neuronal loss in the putamen and pallidum of one patient.

Maple syrup urine disease (branched chain oxo-acid dehydrogenase complex deficiency)

The clinical presentation of maple syrup urine disease is similar to that of methylmalonic and propionic acidaemias

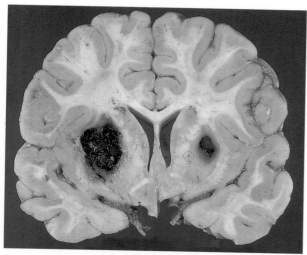

Figure 8.20 *Methyl malonic acidaemia. There are bilateral putaminal haemorrhages.*

with severe neonatal-onset and less severe later-onset forms. There is also an extremely rare thiamine-responsive form. With the development of neurological symptoms the infants emit a sweet, caramel-like smell (similar to maple syrup or fenugreek), caused by the accumulation of sotolone. Unlike methylmalonic and propionic acidaemias, dehydration and a pronounced metabolic acidosis are not features of acute metabolic decompensation. The branched chain oxo-acid dehydrogenase complex consists of three catalytic components, one of which (E_3 component, dihydrolipoyl dehydrogenase) is shared with pyruvate dehydrogenase and combined defects occur rarely. Investigation shows raised plasma concentrations of the branched chain amino acids with a disproportionate increase in leucine and the presence of alloisoleucine, and urinary excretion of 2-oxo acids, in particular α-hydroxyisovaleric acid.

Treatment of maple syrup urine disease is by protein restriction with sufficient amino acid supplementation to allow for normal growth and development. Long-term neurological outcome is poor, with mental retardation, abnormal neurological signs and early death in a proportion of patients. Outcome in the neonatal-onset form appears to depend upon the delay between onset of symptoms and treatment, with better outcomes the earlier the treatment.

PATHOLOGY

Neuropathological observations from fatalities in early infancy include widespread sponginess in the white matter, with loss of myelin sheaths and oligodendroglia, astrocytosis and retarded myelination,[53] but usually there is no evidence of myelin destruction. Grey structures are unaffected. Lipid patterns in the white matter at this early stage are normal,[173] but in untreated older patients cerebrosides and proteolipid protein are markedly reduced[199] compared with the normal levels present in treated

patients. Experimental studies of myelinating cerebellar cultures[228] have suggested that the metabolite α-keto-isocaproic acid is an inhibitor of myelination and is toxic to glial cells. There is a single report of abnormal dendritic development in a 6-year-old mildly retarded patient with maple syrup urine disease.[123]

Glutaric aciduria type 1

Glutaric aciduria type 1 is a recessively inherited disorder caused by deficiency of glutarylCoA dehydrogenase.[20,103,145,157,177,220] During the first year of life, infants may show mild developmental delay and be irritable and develop macrocephaly. At this stage, neuroimaging shows characteristic frontotemporal atrophy. Clear symptoms of the disease develop towards the end of the first year of life. Approximately two-thirds of the patients will develop an encephalitic crisis (often mistaken for encephalitis) and recover from this with a complex movement disorder consisting of dystonia and chorea. The other third develops an insidiously progressive dystonia without an encephalitic crisis. Neuroimaging at this stage will show basal ganglia lesions in addition to the frontotemporal atrophy. Thereafter, there may be further encephalitic crises resulting in an increasingly severe movement disorder, spasticity, mental retardation and epilepsy, or these may develop insidiously. Rarely, infants can present with acute subdural haemorrhage, which is often misdiagnosed as child abuse. The children excrete excessive amounts of glutaric and 3-hydroxyglutaric acids in the urine, while plasma free carnitine is reduced and glutarylcarnitine is raised. Fibroblast glutarylCoA dehydrogenase activity is reduced. Treatment of glutaric aciduria type 1 is by protein restriction and carnitine supplementation. If treatment is started before any encephalitic crisis, the outcome is good.

PATHOLOGY

There are a few neuropathological reports, all of which describe striatal degeneration,[130,151,232] but additional features include frontotemporal atrophy and status spongiosus of the white matter (Fig. 8.21).

Urea cycle disorders

These comprise five disorders (each with considerable phenotypic variability) affecting the five reactions of the urea cycle: carbamoylphosphate synthetase deficiency, ornithine carbamoyltransferase deficiency, citrullinaemia, arginosuccinic aciduria and arginase deficiency (Fig. 8.22). Ornithine carbamoyltransferase deficiency is the most common and is X-linked with manifesting heterozygotes. The others are all recessively inherited.[38,41,68,140,164,185,187,198,233,245,251]

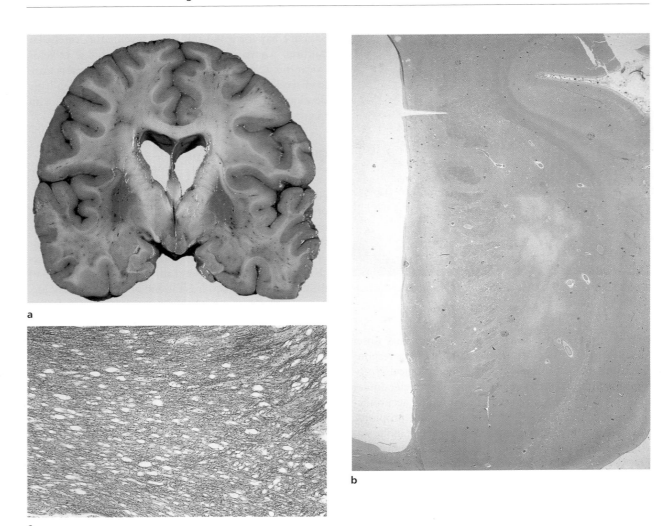

c

Figure 8.21 *Glutaric acidaemia type I. (a) The caudate and putamen are shrunken and grey. (b) Linear gliotic scars are seen in the atrophied striatal nuclei. (H&E.) (c) Status spongiosus in the optic nerve. (Luxol fast blue.)*

With the exception of arginase deficiency, approximately two-thirds of the urea cycle disorders present in the neonatal period. The other third presents later, even in adulthood. Again excluding arginase deficiency, urea cycle disorders present with symptoms of hyperammonaemic encephalopathy with loss of appetite, vomiting, lethargy, ataxia, coma and seizures. There may be hepatomegaly. In the later-onset forms, there is often a preceding history of protein avoidance, vomiting, failure to thrive and mental retardation. Children with arginosuccinic aciduria will develop brittle hair with trichorrhexis nodosa. Whilst children with arginase deficiency can have episodes of acute hyperammonaemic encephalopathy, most present with a progressive diplegia and dementia; dystonia, ataxia and seizures also commonly develop. The key investigations are plasma ammonia and amino acids, and urinary orotic acid. These determine the severity of hyperammonaemia (and therefore the acute management) and will point towards the site of the defect. Depending upon the disease, the diagnosis is confirmed enzymatically or by mutation analysis.

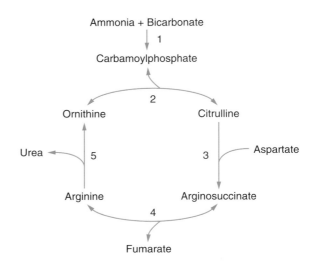

Figure 8.22 *The urea cycle. 1, carbamoylphosphate synthase; 2, ornithine carbamoyltransferase; 3, arginosuccinate synthetase; 4, arginosuccinate lyase; 5, arginase.*

The principles of the long-term treatment of urea cycle disorders are the restriction of dietary protein intake, promoting nitrogen excretion via alternative pathways utilizing sodium benzoate and sodium phenylbutyrate, and supplementation of arginine which, excepting arginase deficiency, becomes an essential amino acid. Outcome data are generally only available for ornithine carbamoyltransferase deficiency. Here, neonatal forms, especially in boys, do badly with early death and a high rate of neurological handicap. Later-onset forms have a better prognosis, but there is still a high incidence of learning difficulties and focal neurological abnormalities.

PATHOLOGY

Autopsy studies in newborns dying rapidly from fulminant hyperammonaemia show relatively non-specific findings: brain swelling, spongy changes in white matter and basal ganglia, and cortical nerve cell loss.[62,143] A more specific and frequent, although by no means consistent observation is the presence of Alzheimer type II astrocytes which appear to correlate with the level of hyperammonaemia. Massive cystic destruction of the cerebral hemispheres, producing a 'walnut' brain or ulegyria (Fig. 8.23), and mineralization of neurons in deep grey matter have been described in several severely affected girls with

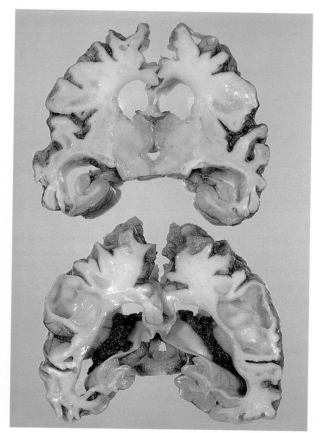

Figure 8.23 *Ornithine carbamyl transferase deficiency. Global cystic destruction has resulted in a walnut brain with gliotic knife-edge gyri.*

X-linked ornithine carbamoyl transferase deficiency surviving beyond the neonatal period[39,94,143] and in a girl with carbamoylphosphate synthetase deficiency.[62] The relative contributions of hypotension and cardiac arrest to the pathogenesis of these lesions are disputed but it is notable that the Ammon's horn and cerebellum may be spared.[62,143] The occurrence in some cases of hypomyelination and cerebellar heterotopias as well as very early pathological or CT observations of cystic necrosis suggests that damage may begin in fetal life.[71,94]

CONGENITAL DISORDERS OF GLYCOSYLATION

These are a recently described class of inherited disorders affecting the assembly or processing of the carbohydrate moiety of glycoconjugates. The field is rapidly expanding. Congenital disorders of glycosylation (CDG) are subclassified into two types: CDG-I in which the defect lies in the assembly of the *N*-glycan in the cytosol and endoplasmic reticulum; and CDG-II in which the defect lies in the processing of the *N*-glycan moiety of the glycoconjugate in the Golgi apparatus. Recently described defects in *O*-glycan assembly in the Golgi apparatus are included in CDG-II. The biochemical bases of at least six CDG-I and at least two of CDG-II are now known. However, only two will be discussed here.[11,21,83,112–114,128,216,271]

CDG-Ia (phosphomannomutase deficiency)

This recessively inherited multisystem disorder usually has severe CNS involvement. In infancy, developmental delay, rolling eye movements and an alternating squint, hypotonia and depressed reflexes develop. Later, ataxia and moderate to severe mental retardation become evident. In childhood, retinitis pigmentosa, stroke-like episodes and epilepsy may occur, but dementia is not evident. Mild facial dysmorphism, abnormal subcutaneous fat distribution on the buttocks and inverted nipples may be apparent early. There is great variability in the involvement of other organs, even between siblings. Investigation shows abnormalities in many glycoproteins such as thyroid binding globulin, coagulation factors, lysosomal enzymes and hormones. Neuroradiology shows marked cerebellar atrophy of early onset. The diagnosis is suspected from abnormalities of serum transferrin isoelectric focusing and confirmed on leukocyte phosphomannomutase activity. There is no effective treatment.

CDG-IIa (N-acetylglucosaminyltransferase II deficiency)

This recessively inherited multisystem disorder also usually has severe CNS involvement. However, there

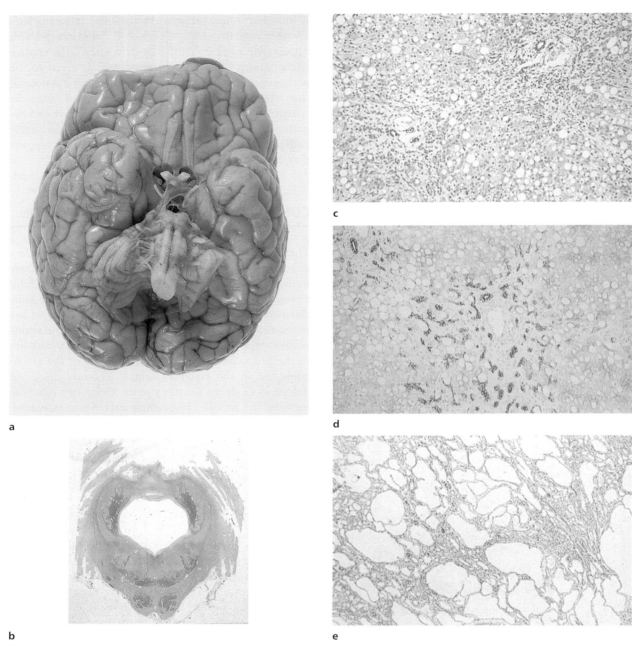

Figure 8.24 *Congenital disorders of glycosylation. CDG-Ia. (a) The cerebellum is small with prominent folia and the pontine base is narrow and scalloped. (b) A horizontal section through the hindbrain shows massive global atrophy of cerebellar folia and white matter, and loss of middle cerebellar peduncles, transverse fibres and nuclei pontis from the shallow pons, but the dentate ribbon and its hilar outflow are spared. (Luxol fast blue–cresyl violet.) (c) The liver shows prominent steatosis (H&E) and (d) abnormal bile duct plates. (e) In the kidney there is pronounced cystic dilation of tubules and collecting ducts (H&E) (immunoperoxidase for CAM 5.2).*

is a pronounced dysmorphism with brachycephaly, hypertelorism, a broad nose with upturned nostrils, a broad mouth and large, abnormally formed ears. There may also be skeletal involvement. There is severe mental retardation and generalized hypotonia, but tendon reflexes are preserved. Investigation also shows abnormalities in many glycoproteins. Neuroradiology shows cerebral atrophy with secondary white-matter involvement.

PATHOLOGY

Not surprisingly our knowledge of the pathology[2,51,91,105,236] is limited to infants with a severe and early presentation when mortality is highest. Two early descriptions[2,91] pre-date the discovery of the metabolic error, although it was retrospectively confirmed in the second study. Systemic abnormalities include pronounced pleural and pericardial effusions, marked thickening of the cardiac ventricular wall, cystic dilatation of renal tubules and collecting ducts, hepatic steatosis, ductal plate abnormality, portal fibrosis and ascites (Fig. 8.24c–e). Degeneration of retinal photoreceptors and pigment epithelium has also been described. The brain shows severe olivopontocerebellar atrophy (Fig. 8.24a, b) with minimal changes elsewhere: global subtotal Purkinje and granule cell depletion with rare torpedo swellings and asteroid dendritic expansions, atrophy of the cerebellar white matter but relative sparing of the dentate neuronal ribbon, and devastation of the pontine nuclei, inferior olives and the middle and inferior cerebellar peduncles. Lysosomal inclusions have been described in Schwann cells and hepatocytes of some patients, and in one atypical infantile case without cerebellar disturbance ballooned spinal anterior horn cells showed lysosomal membranous cytoplasmic bodies on ultrastructural examination.[66]

REFERENCES

1 Adams RD, Lyon G. *Neurology of hereditary metabolic diseases of children*. New York: McGraw-Hill, 1982.

2 Agamanolis DP, Naito HK, Robinson HB et al. Lipoprotein disorder, cirrhosis, and olivopontocerebellar degeneration in two siblings. *Neurology* 1986; **36**: 674–81.

3 Agamanolis DP, Potter JL, Herrick MK, Sternberger NH. The neuropathology of glycine encephalopathy: a report of five cases with immunohistochemical and ultrastructural observations. *Neurology* 1982; **32**: 975–85.

4 Aicardi J, Goutières F. A progressive familial encephalopathy in infancy with calcifications of the basal ganglia and chronic cerebrospinal fluid lymphocytosis. *Ann Neurol* 1984; **15**: 49–54.

5 Akwa Y, Hassett DE, Eloranta ML et al. Transgenic expression of IFN-alpha in the central nervous system of mice protects against lethal neurotropic viral infection but induces inflammation and neurodegeneration. *J Immunol* 1998; **161**: 5016–26.

6 Alexander WS. Progressive fibrinoid degeneration of fibrillary astrocytes associated with mental retardation in a hydrocephalic infant. *Brain* 1943; **72**: 373–81.

7 Andersson HC, Shapira E. Biochemical and clinical response to hydroxocobalamin versus cyanocobalamin treatment in patients with methylmalonic acidemia and homocystinuria (cblC). *J Pediatr* 1998; **132**: 121–4.

8 Angelini L, Nardocci N, Rumi V et al. Hallervorden–Spatz disease: clinical and MRI study of 11 cases diagnosed in life. *J Neurol* 1992; **239**: 417–25.

9 Anonymous. Disorders of homocysteine metabolism: from rare genetic defects to common risk factors. Proceedings of an international symposium. Fulda, Germany, 20–22 November 1996. *Eur J Pediatr* 1998; **157** (Suppl 2): S39–142.

10 Anonymous. Pathology of skeletal muscle and intramuscular nerves in infantile neuroaxonal dystrophy. *Acta Neuropathol* 1986; **69**: 1–2.

11 Antoun H, Villeneuve N, Gelot A et al. Cerebellar atrophy: an important feature of carbohydrate deficient glycoprotein syndrome type 1. *Pediatr Radiol* 1999; **29**: 194–8.

12 Armstrong D. The neuropathology of Rett syndrome. *Brain Dev* 1992; **14** (Suppl): S89–98.

13 Armstrong DD. Review of Rett syndrome. *J Neuropathol Exp Neurol* 1997; **56**: 843–9.

14 Armstrong DD, Dunn JK, Schultz RJ et al. Organ growth in Rett syndrome: a postmortem examination analysis. *Pediatr Neurol* 1999; **20**: 125–9.

15 Augoustides SP, Mylonas I, Sewell AC, Rosenblatt DS. Reversible dementia in an adolescent with cblC disease: clinical heterogeneity within the same family. *J Inherit Metab Dis* 1999; **22**: 756–8.

16 Axelsson R, Roytta M, Sourander P et al. Hereditary diffuse leucoencephalopathy with spheroids. *Acta Psychiatr Scand Suppl* 1984; **314**: 1–65.

17 Balajee AS, Bohr VA. Genomic heterogeneity of nucleotide excision repair. *Gene* 2000; **250**: 15–30.

18 Bandmann O, Nygaard TG, Surtees R et al. Dopa-responsive dystonia in British patients: new mutations of the GTP-cyclohydrolase I gene and evidence for genetic heterogeneity. *Hum Mol Genet* 1996; **5**: 403–6.

19 Bandmann O, Valente EM, Holmans P et al. Dopa-responsive dystonia: a clinical and molecular genetic study. *Ann Neurol* 1998; **44**: 649–56.

20 Baric I, Zschocke J, Christensen E et al. Diagnosis and management of glutaric aciduria type I. *J Inherit Metab Dis* 1998; **21**: 326–40.

21 Barone R, Pavone L, Fiumara A et al. Developmental patterns and neuropsychological assessment in patients with carbohydrate-deficient glycoconjugate syndrome type IA (phosphomannomutase deficiency). *Brain Dev* 1999; **21**: 260–3.

22 Barth PG, Walter A, van Gelderen I. Aicardi–Goutières syndrome: a genetic microangiopathy? *Acta Neuropathol Berl* 1999; **98**: 212–16.

23 Bauman ML, Kemper TL. Morphologic and histoanatomic observations of the brain in untreated human phenylketonuria. *Acta Neuropathol* 1982; **58**: 55–63.

24 Bauman ML, Kemper TL, Arin DM. Microscopic observations of the brain in Rett syndrome. *Neuropediatrics* 2001; **26**: 105–9.

25 Baumgarter ER, Viardot C. Long-term follow-up of 77 patients with isolated methylmalonic acidaemia. *J Inherit Metab Dis* 1995; **18**: 138–42.

26 Belec L, Gray F, Louarn F et al. Pigmentary orthochromatic leukodystrophy. Van Bogaert and Nyssen disease. *Rev Neurol Paris* 1988; **144**: 347–57.

27 Belichencko PA, Hagberg B, Dahlstrom A. A morphological study of cortical areas in Rett syndrome. *Acta Neuropathol* 1997; **93**: 50–61.

28 Bergman AJ, Knaap MS van der, Smeitink JA et al. Magnetic resonance imaging and spectroscopy of the brain in propionic acidemia: clinical and biochemical considerations. *Pediatr Res* 1996; **40**: 404–9.

29 Blackwood W, Buxton PH, Cumings JN et al. Diffuse cerebral degeneration in infancy (Alpers' disease). *Arch Dis Child* 1963; **38**: 193–204.

30 Bodemer C, De Prost Y, Bachollet B et al. Cutaneous manifestations of methylmalonic and propionic acidaemia: a description based on 38 cases. *Br J Dermatol* 1994; **131**: 93–8.

31 Boer J de, Hoeijmakers JH. Nucleotide excision repair and human syndromes. *Carcinogenesis* 2000; **21**: 453–60.

32 Bogaert L van, Nissen R. Le type tardif de la leucodystrophie progressive familiale. *Rev Neurol* 1936; **65**: 21–45.

33 Boespflug TO, Mimault C, Melki J et al. Genetic homogeneity of Pelizaeus–Merzbacher disease: tight linkage to the proteolipoprotein locus in 16 affected families. PMD Clinical Group. *Am J Hum Genet* 1994; **55**: 461–7.

34 Boneh A, Degani Y, Harari M. Prognostic clues and outcome of early treatment of nonketotic hyperglycinemia. *Pediatr Neurol* 1996; **15**: 137–41.

35 Borrett D, Becker LE. Alexander's disease; a disease of astrocytes. *Brain* 1985; **108**: 367–85.

36 Brenner M, Johnson AB, Boespflug-Tanguy O *et al*. Mutations in GFAP, encoding glial fibrillary acidic protein, are associated with Alexander disease. *Nat Genet* 2001; **27**: 117–20.

37 Brismar J, Ozand PT. CT and MR of the brain in the diagnosis of organic acidemias. Experiences from 107 patients. *Brain Dev* 1994; **16** (Suppl): 104–24.

38 Brusilow SW, Maestri NE. Urea cycle disorders: diagnosis, pathophysiology, and therapy. *Adv Pediatr* 1996; **43**: 127–70.

39 Bruton CJ, Corsellis JAN, Russell A. Hereditary hyperammonaemia. *Brain* 1970; **93**: 423–34.

40 Burlina AP, Ferrari V, Divry P *et al*. N-Acetylaspartylglutamate in Canavan disease: an adverse effector? *Eur J Pediatr* 1999; **158**: 406–9.

41 Butterworth RF. Effects of hyperammonaemia on brain function. *J Inherit Metab Dis* 1998; **21** (Suppl 1): 6–20.

42 Castellani RJ, Perry G, Brenner DS, Smith MA. Alexander disease: Alzheimer disease of the developing brain? *Alzheimer Dis Assoc Disord* 1999; **13**: 232–5.

43 Castellani RJ, Perry G, Harris PL *et al*. Advanced glycation modification of Rosenthal fibers in patients with Alexander disease. *Neurosci Lett* 1997; **231**: 79–82.

44 Chuang DT. Maple syrup urine disease: it has come a long way. *J Pediatr* 1998; **132**: S17–23.

45 Citterio E, Rademakers S, Horst GT van der *et al*. Biochemical and biological characterization of wild-type and ATPase-deficient Cockayne syndrome B repair protein. *J Biol Chem* 1998; **273**: 11844–51.

46 Clayton PT, Smith I, Harding BN *et al*. Subacute combined degeneration of the cord, dementia and Parkinsonism due to an inborn error of folate metabolism. *J Neurol Neurosurg Psychiatry* 1986; **49**: 920–7.

47 Cleary MA, Walter JH, Wraith JE *et al*. Magnetic resonance imaging of the brain in phenylketonuria. *Lancet* 1994; **344**: 87–90.

48 Cleary MA, Walter JH, Wraith JE *et al*. Magnetic resonance imaging in phenylketonuria: reversal of cerebral white matter change. *J Pediatr* 1995; **127**: 251–5.

49 Cleaver JE, Thompson LH, Richardson AS, States JC. A summary of mutations in the UV-sensitive disorders: xeroderma pigmentosum, Cockayne syndrome, and trichothiodystrophy. *Hum Mutat* 1999; **14**: 9–22.

50 Colella S, Nardo T, Botta E *et al*. Identical mutations in the CSB gene associated with either Cockayne syndrome or the DeSanctis-cacchione variant of xeroderma pigmentosum. *Hum Mol Genet* 2000; **9**: 1171–5.

51 Conradi N, vos R de, Jaeken J *et al*. Liver pathology in the carbohydrate-deficient glycoprotein syndrome. *Acta Paediatr Scand* 1990; Suppl **375**: 50–4.

52 Cordero ME, Trejo M, Colombo M, Aranda V. Histological maturation of the neocortex in phenylketonuric rats. *Early Hum Dev* 1983; **8**: 157–73.

53 Crome L, Dutton G, Ross CF. Maple syrup urine disease. *J Pathol Bacteriol* 1961; **81**: 379–84.

54 Crompton MR. Alpers' disease – variant of Creutzfeldt–Jakob disease and subacute spongiform encephalopathy. *Acta Neuropathol* 1968; **10**: 99–104.

55 Dave P, Curless RG, Steinman L. Cerebellar hemorrhage complicating methylmalonic and propionic acidemia. *Arch Neurol* 1984; **41**: 1293–6.

56 Dayan AD, Ramsey RB. An inborn error of vitamin B_{12} metabolism associated with cellular deficiency of coenzyme forms of the vitamin. Pathological and neurochemical findings in one case. *J Neurol Sci* 1974; **23**: 117–28.

57 Deisenhammer E, Jellinger K. Cavitating neutral fat leukodystrophy with recurrent course. *Neuropaediatrie* 1976; **7**: 111–21.

58 Deprez M, D'Hooge M, Misson JP *et al*. Infantile and juvenile presentations of Alexander's disease: a report of two cases. *Acta Neurol Scand* 1999; **99**: 158–65.

59 Diamond A. Evidence for the importance of dopamine for prefrontal cortex functions early in life. *Phil Trans R Soc Lond B Biol Sci* 1996; **351**: 1483–93.

60 Dobyns WB. Agenesis of the corpus callosum and gyral malformations are frequent manifestations of non-ketotic hyperglycinemia. *Neurology* 1989; **39**: 817–20.

61 Doshi SN, Goodfellow J, Lewis MJ, McDowell IF. Homocysteine and endothelial function (Editorial; Comment). *Cardiovasc Res* 1999; **42**: 578–82.

62 Ebels EJ. Neuropathological observations in a patient with carbamylphosphate-synthetase deficiency and in two sibs. *Arch Dis Child* 1972; **47**: 47–51.

63 Egger J, Harding BN, Boyd SG *et al*. Progressive neuronal degeneration of childhood (PNDC) with liver disease. *Clin Pediatr* 1987; **26**: 167–73.

64 Elleder M, Jirasek A. New enzymatic findings in infantile neuroaxonal dystrophy. *Acta Neuropathol* 1983; **60**: 153–5.

65 Enns GM, Barkovich AJ, Rosenblatt DS *et al*. Progressive neurological deterioration and MRI changes in cblC methylmalonic acidaemia treated with hydroxocobalamin. *J Inherit Metab Dis* 1999; **22**; 599–607.

66 Eyskens F, Ceuterick C, Martin JJ *et al*. Carbohydrate-deficient glycoprotein syndrome with previously unreported features. *Acta Paediatr* 1994; **83**: 892–6.

67 Faure S, Bordelais I, Marquette C *et al*. Aicardi–Goutières syndrome: monogenic recessive disease, genetically heterogeneous disease, or multifactorial disease? *Clin Genet* 1999; **56**: 149–53.

68 Feillet F, Leonard JV. Alternative pathway therapy for urea cycle disorders. *J Inherit Metab Dis* 1998; **21** (Suppl 1): 101–11.

69 Ferreira RC, Mierau GW, Bateman JB. Conjunctival biopsy in infantile neuroaxonal dystrophy. *Am J Ophthalmol* 1997; **123**: 264–6.

70 Ferrer I, Fabreques I, Pineda M *et al*. Diagnosis of infantile neuro-axonal dystrophy by conjunctival biopsy. *Neuropaediatrics* 1983; **14**: 53–5.

71 Filloux F, Townsend JJ, Leonard C. Ornithine transcarbamylase deficiency: neuropathologic changes acquired *in utero*. *J Pediatr* 1986; **108**: 942–5.

72 Fink JM, Dobyns WB, Guerrini R, Hirsch BA. Identification of a duplication of Xq28 associated with bilateral periventricular nodular heterotopia. *Am J Hum Genet* 1997; **61**: 379–87.

73 Fowler B. Genetic defects of folate and cobalamin metabolism. *Eur J Pediatr* 1998; **157** (Suppl 2): S60–6.

74 Francis MA, Bagga PS, Athwal RS, Rainbow AJ. Incomplete complementation of the DNA repair defect in cockayne syndrome cells by the *denV* gene from bacteriophage T4 suggests a deficiency in base excision repair. *Mutat Res* 1997; **385**: 59–74.

75 Friede RL. *Developmental neuropathology* 2nd edn. Berlin: Springer, 1989.

76 Garbern J, Cambi F, Shy M, Kamholz J. The molecular pathogenesis of Pelizaeus–Merzbacher disease. *Arch Neurol* 1999; **56**: 1210–14.

77 Gautier JC, Gray F, Awanda A, Escourolle R. Cavitary orthochromatic leukodystrophy in the adult. Oligodendroglial proliferation and inclusions. *Rev Neurol Paris* 1984; **140**: 493–501.

78 Goebel HH, Kohlschutter A, Schulte FJ. Rectal biopsy findings in infantile neuroaxonal dystrophy. *Neuropediatrics* 1980; **11**: 388–92.

79 Goutières F, Aicardi J, Barth PG, Lebon P. Aicardi–Goutières syndrome: an update and results of interferon-alpha studies. *Ann Neurol* 1998; **44**: 900–7.

80 Gray F, Destee A, Bourre JM et al. Pigmentary type of orthochromatic leukodystrophy (OLD): a new case with ultrastructural and biochemical study. *J Neuropathol Exp Neurol* 1987; **46**: 585–96.

81 Griffiths IR, Montague P, Dickinson P. The proteolipid protein gene. *Neuropathol Appl Neurobiol* 1995; **21**: 85–96.

82 Grimes DA, Lang AE, Bergeron C. Late adult onset chorea with typical pathology of Hallervorden–Spatz syndrome. *J Neurol Neurosurg Psychiatry* 2000; **69**: 392–5.

83 Grunewald S, Matthijs G. Congenital disorders of glycosylation (CDG): a rapidly expanding group of neurometabolic disorders (Editorial; Comment). *Neuropediatrics* 2000; **31**: 57–9.

84 Halliday W. The nosology of Hallervorden–Spatz disease. *J Neurol Sci* 1995; **134** (Suppl): 84–91.

85 Hamilton RL, Haas RH, Nyhan WL et al. Neuropathology of propionic acidemia: a report of two patients with basal ganglia lesions. *J Child Neurol* 1995; **10**: 25–30.

86 Hamosh A, Maher JF, Bellus GA et al. Long-term use of high-dose benzoate and dextromethorphan for the treatment of nonketotic hyperglycinemia. *J Pediatr* 1998; **132**: 709–13.

87 Harbord MG, Harden A, Harding BN et al. Megalencephaly with dysmyelination, spasticity, ataxia, seizures and distinctive neurophysiological findings in two siblings. *Neuropediatrics* 1990; **21**: 164–8.

88 Harding BN. Progressive neuronal degeneration of childhood with liver disease (Alpers–Huttenlocher syndrome) – a personal review. *J Child Neurol* 1990; **5**: 273–87.

89 Harding BN, Alsanjari N, Smith SJM et al. Progressive neuronal degeneration of childhood with liver disease (Alpers' disease) presenting in young adults. *J Neurol Neurosurg Psychiatry* 1995; **58**: 320–5.

90 Harding BN, Donley D, Wilson ER. Pigmentary orthochromatic leucodystrophy: a new familial case with onset in early infancy (Abstract). *Neuropathol Appl Neurobiol* 1990; **16**: 270–1.

91 Harding BN, Dunger DB, Grant DB, Erdohazi M. Familial olivopontocerebellar atrophy with neonatal onset a recessively inherited syndrome with systemic and biochemical abnormalities. *J Neurol Neurosurg Psychiatry* 1988; **51**: 385–90.

92 Harding BN, Egger J, Portmann B, Erdohazi M. Progressive neuronal degeneration of childhood with liver disease. A pathological study. *Brain* 1986; **109**: 181–206.

93 Harding BN, Ellis D, Malcolm S. Pelizaeus–Merzbacher disease can be associated with increased proteolipid protein gene dosage (Abstract). *Neuropathol Appl Neurobiol* 1995; **21**: 148.

94 Harding BN, Leonard JV, Erdohazi M. Ornithine transcarbamylase deficiency. *Eur J Pediatr* 1984; **141**: 215–20.

95 Harding BN, Leonard JV, Erdohazi M. Propionic acidaemia: a neuropathological study of two patients presenting in infancy. *Neuropathol Appl Neurobiol* 1991; **17**: 133–8.

96 Harrison DA, Mullaney PB, Mesfer SA et al. Management of ophthalmic complications of homocystinuria. *Ophthalmology* 1998; **105**: 1886–90.

97 Hart ZH, Chang CH, Perrin EVD et al. Familial poliodystrophy, mitochondrial myopathy, and lactate acidemia. *Arch Neurol* 1977; **34**: 180–5.

98 Hayasaka K, Tada K, Fueki N et al. Nonketotic hyperglycinemia: analysis of glycine cleavage system in typical and atypical cases. *J Pediatr* 1987; **110**: 873–7.

99 Herndon RM, Rubinstein LJ. Leucodystrophy with Rosenthal fibers (Alexander's disease): a histochemical and electron microscopic study. *Neurology* 1968; **18**: 300.

100 Hilliges C, Awiszus D, Wendel U. Intellectual performance of children with maple syrup urine disease. *Eur J Pediatr* 1993; **152**: 144–7.

101 Hodes ME, Zimmerman AW, Aydanian A et al. Different mutations in the same codon of the proteolipid protein gene, PLP, may help in correlating genotype with phenotype in Pelizaeus–Merzbacher disease/X-linked spastic paraplegia (PMD/SPG2). *Am J Med Genet* 1999; **82**: 132–9.

102 Hoffmann GF, Surtees RA, Wevers RA. Cerebrospinal fluid investigations for neurometabolic disorders. *Neuropediatrics* 1998; **29**: 59–71.

103 Hoffmann GF, Zschocke J. Glutaric aciduria type I: from clinical, biochemical and molecular diversity to successful therapy. *J Inherit Metab Dis* 1999; **22**: 381–91.

104 Hommes FA, Kuipers JRG, Elema JD et al. Propionic acidemia, a new inborn error of metabolism. *Pediatr Res* 1968; **2**: 519–24.

105 Horslen SP, Clayton PT, Harding BN et al. Neonatal onset olivopontocerebellar atrophy and disialotransferrin deficiency syndrome. *Arch Dis Child* 1991; **66**: 1027–32.

106 Huether G, Neuhoff V, Kaus R. Brain development in experimental hyperphenylalaninaemia: disturbed proliferation and reduced cell numbers in the cerebellum. *Neuropediatrics* 1983; **14**: 12–19.

107 Huppke P, Laccone F, Kramer N et al. Rett syndrome: analysis of MECP2 and clinical characterization of 31 patients. *Hum Mol Genet* 2000; **9**: 1369–75.

108 Huttenlocher RR, Solitare GB, Adams G. Infantile diffuse cerebral degeneration with hepatic cirrhosis. *Arch Neurol* 1976; **33**: 186–92.

109 Isherwood DM. Homocystinuria (Editorial; Comment). *BMJ* 1996; **313**: 1025–6.

110 Itoh K, Negishi H, Obayashi C et al. Infantile neuroaxonal dystrophy – immunohistochemical and ultrastructural studies on the central and peripheral nervous systems in infantile neuroaxonal dystrophy. *Kobe J Med Sci* 1993; **39**: 133–46.

111 Itoh M, Hayashi M, Shioda K et al. Neurodegeneration in hereditary nucleotide repair disorders. *Brain Dev* 1999; **21**: 326–33.

112 Jaeken J, Carchon H. What's new in congenital disorders of glycosylation? *Eur J Paediatr Neurol* 2000; **4**: 163–7.

113 Jaeken J, Matthijs G, Barone R, Carchon H. Carbohydrate deficient glycoprotein (CDG) syndrome type I. *J Med Genet* 1997; **34**: 73–6.

114 Jaeken J, Schachter H, Carchon H et al. Carbohydrate deficient glycoprotein syndrome type II: a deficiency in Golgi localised N-acetyl-glucosaminyltransferase II. *Arch Dis Child* 1994; **71**: 123–7.

115 Janota I. Neuroaxonal dystrophy in the neonate. *Acta Neuropathol* 1979; **46**: 151–4.

116 Janota I. Spongy degeneration of grey matter in three children: neuropathological report. *Arch Dis Child* 1974; **49**: 571–5.

117 Jellinger K, Armstrong D, Zoghbi HY, Percy AK. Neuropathology of Rett syndrome. *Acta Neuropathol* 1988; **76**: 142–58.

118 Jellinger K, Griswold W, Armstrong D, Rett A. Peripheral nerve involvement in the Rett syndrome. *Brain Dev* 1990; **12**: 109–14.

119 Jellinger K, Seitelberger F. Neuropathology of Rett syndrome. *Am J Med Genet* 1986; **24**: 259–88.

120 Johnson RT, Squires S. The XPD complementation group. Insights into xeroderma pigmentosum, Cockayne's syndrome and trichothiodystrophy. *Mutat Res* 1992; **273**: 97–118.

121 Jong J de, Berg C van den, Wijburg H *et al*. Alpha-*N*-acetyl-galactosaminidase deficiency with mild clinical manifestations and difficult biochemical diagnosis. *J Pediatr* 1994; **125**: 385–91.

122 Jouvet P, Rustin P, Felderhoff U *et al*. Maple syrup urine disease metabolites induce apoptosis in neural cells without cytochrome *c* release or changes in mitochondrial membrane potential. *Biochem Soc Trans* 1998; **26**: S341.

123 Kamei A, Takashima S, Chan F, Becker LE. Abnormal dendritic development in maple syrup urine disease. *Pediatr Neurol* 1992; **8**: 145–7.

124 Kamoshita S, Neustein HB, Landing BH. Infantile neuroaxonal dystrophy with neonatal onset. *J Neuropathol Exp Neurol* 1968; **27**: 300–23.

125 Kamoshita S, Reed GB, Aguilar MJ. Axonal dystrophy in a case of Canavan's spongy degeneration. *Neurology* 1967; **17**: 895–8.

126 Kaul R, Balamurugan K, Gao GP, Matalon R. Canavan disease: genomic organization and localization of human ASPA to 17p13-ter and conservation of the ASPA gene during evolution. *Genomics* 1994; **21**: 364–70.

127 Kearney D, Armstrong D, Glaze D. The conduction system in Rett syndrome (Abstract). *Hand in hand with Rett syndrome*, 1996.

128 Keir G, Winchester BG, Clayton P. Carbohydrate-deficient glycoprotein syndromes: inborn errors of protein glycosylation. *Ann Clin Biochem* 1999; **36**: 20–36.

129 Keulemans JL, Reuser AJ, Kroos MA *et al*. Human alpha-*N*-acetylgalactosaminidase (alpha-NAGA) deficiency: new mutations and the paradox between genotype and phenotype. *J Med Genet* 1996; **33**: 458–64.

130 Kimura S, Hara M, Nezu A *et al*. Two cases of glutaric aciduria type 1: clinical and neuropathological findings. *J Neurol Sci* 1994; **123**: 38–43.

131 Kimura S, Sasaki Y, Warlo I, Goebel HH. Axonal pathology of the skin in infantile neuroaxonal dystrophy. *Acta Neuropathol Berl* 1987; **75**: 212–15.

132 Kitt CA, Troncoso JC, Price DL *et al*. Pathological changes in substantia nigra and basal forebrain neurons in Rett syndrome. *Ann Neurol* 1990; **28**: 416–17.

133 Kluijtmans LA, Boers GH, Kraus JP *et al*. The molecular basis of cystathionine beta-synthase deficiency in Dutch patients with homocystinuria: effect of CBS genotype on biochemical and clinical phenotype and on response to treatment. *Am J Hum Genet* 1999; **65**: 59–67.

134 Knaap MS van der, Barth PG, Gabreels FJ *et al*. A new leukoencephalopathy with vanishing white matter. *Neurology* 1997; **48**: 845–55.

135 Knaap MS van der, Barth PG, Vrensen GF, Valk J. Histopathology of an infantile-onset spongiform leukoencephalopathy with a discrepantly mild clinical course. *Acta Neuropathol Berl* 1996; **92**: 206–12.

136 Knaap MS van der, Kamphorst W, Barth PG *et al*. Phenotypic variation in leukoencephalopathy with vanishing white matter. *Neurology* 1998; **51**: 540–7.

137 Knaap MS van der, Naidu S, Kleinschmidt DB *et al*. Autosomal dominant diffuse leukoencephalopathy with neuroaxonal spheroids. *Neurology* 2000; **54**: 463–8.

138 Knaap MS van der, Valk J, Barth PG *et al*. Leukoencephalopathy with swelling in children and adolescents: MRI patterns and differential diagnosis. *Neuroradiology* 1995; **37**: 679–86.

139 Knaap MS van der, Wevers RA, Kure S *et al*. Increased cerebrospinal fluid glycine: a biochemical marker for a leukoencephalopathy with vanishing white matter. *J Child Neurol* 1999; **14**: 728–31.

140 Kobayashi K, Sinasac DS, Iijima M *et al*. The gene mutated in adult-onset type II citrullinaemia encodes a putative mitochondrial carrier protein. *Nat Genet* 1999; **22**: 159–63.

141 Koeppen AH, Ronca NA, Greenfield EA, Hans MB. Defective biosynthesis of proteolipid protein in Pelizaeus–Merzbacher disease. *Ann Neurol* 1987; **21**: 159–70.

142 Korein J, Sansaricq C, Kalmijn M *et al*. Maple syrup urine disease: clinical, EEG, and plasma amino acid correlations with a theoretical mechanism of acute neurotoxicity. *Int J Neurosci* 1994; **79**: 21–45.

143 Kornfeld M, Woodfin BM, Papile L *et al*. Neuropathology of ornithine carbamyl transferase deficiency. *Acta Neuropathol Berl* 1985; **65**: 261–4.

144 Kure S, Rolland MO, Leisti J *et al*. Prenatal diagnosis of non-ketotic hyperglycinaemia: enzymatic diagnosis in 28 families and DNA diagnosis detecting prevalent Finnish and Israeli–Arab mutations. *Prenat Diagn* 1999; **19**: 717–20.

145 Kyllerman M, Skjeldal OH, Lundberg M *et al*. Dystonia and dyskinesia in glutaric aciduria type I: clinical heterogeneity and therapeutic considerations. *Mov Disord* 1994; **9**: 22–30.

146 Larnaout A, Mongalgi MA, Kaabachi N *et al*. Methylmalonic acidaemia with bilateral globus pallidus involvement: a neuropathological study. *J Inherit Metab Dis* 1998; **21**: 639–44.

147 Leech RW, Brumback RA, Miller RH *et al*. Cockayne syndrome: clinicopathologic and tissue culture studies of affected siblings. *J Neuropathol Exp Neurol* 1985; **44**: 507–19.

148 Leegwater PA, Konst AA, Kuyt B *et al*. The gene for leukoencephalopathy with vanishing white matter is located on chromosome 3q27. *Am J Hum Genet* 1999; **65**: 728–34.

149 Lehmann AR, Thompson AF, Harcourt SA *et al*. Cockayne's syndrome: correlation of clinical features with cellular sensitivity of RNA synthesis to UV irradiation. *J Med Genet* 1993; **30**: 679–82.

150 Lehnert W, Sperl W, Suormala T, Baumgartner ER. Propionic acidaemia: clinical, biochemical and therapeutic aspects. Experience in 30 patients. *Eur J Pediatr* 1994; **153**: S68–80.

151 Leibel RL, Shih VE, Goodman SI *et al*. Glutaric acidemia: a metabolic disorder causing progressive choreoathetosis. *Neurology* 1980; **30**: 1163–8.

152 Leon GA de, Mitchell MH. Histological and ultrastructural features of dystrophic isocortical axons in infantile neuroaxonal dystrophy (Seitelberger's disease). *Acta Neuropathol Berl* 1985; **66**: 89–97.

153 Leonard JV. Stable isotope studies in propionic and methylmalonic acidaemia. *Eur J Pediatr* 1997; **156** (Suppl 1): S67–9.

154 Leonard JV. The management and outcome of propionic and methylmalonic acidaemia. *J Inherit Metab Dis* 1995; **18**: 430–4.

155 Leontovich TA, Mukhina JK, Fedorov AA, Belichenko PV. Morphological study of the entorhinal cortex, hippocampal formation, and basal ganglia in Rett syndrome patients. *Neurobiol Dis* 1999; **6**: 77–91.

156 Levy HL, Lobbregt D, Barnes PD, Poussaint TY. Maternal phenylketonuria: magnetic resonance imaging of the brain in offspring. *J Pediatr* 1996; **128**: 770–5.

157 Liesert M, Zschocke J, Hoffmann GF *et al*. Biochemistry of glutaric aciduria type I: activities of *in vitro* expressed wild-type and mutant cDNA encoding human glutaryl-CoA dehydrogenase. *J Inherit Metab Dis* 1999; **22**: 256–8.

158 Lipton SA, Kim WK, Choi YB et al. Neurotoxicity associated with dual actions of homocysteine at the *N*-methyl-D-aspartate receptor. *Proc Natl Acad Sci USA* 1997; **94**: 5923–8.

159 Lowe J, Mayer RJ, Landon M. Ubiquitin in neurodegenerative diseases. *Brain Pathol* 1993; **3**: 55–65.

160 Lu FL, Wang PJ, Hwu WL et al. Neonatal type of nonketotic hyperglycinemia. *Pediatr Neurol* 1999; **20**: 295–300.

161 Ludecke B, Knappskog PM, Clayton PT et al. Recessively inherited L-DOPA-responsive parkinsonism in infancy caused by a point mutation (L205P) in the tyrosine hydroxylase gene. *Hum Mol Genet* 1996; **5**: 1023–8.

162 McCombe PA, McLaughlin DB, Chalk JB et al. Spasticity and white matter abnormalities in adult phenylketonuria. *J Neurol Neurosurg Psychiatry* 1992; **55**: 359–61.

163 McEntagart M, Kamel H, Lebon P, King MD. Aicardi–Goutières syndrome: an expanding phenotype. *Neuropediatrics* 1998; **29**: 163–7.

164 Maestri NE, Clissold D, Brusilow SW. Neonatal onset ornithine transcarbamylase deficiency: a retrospective analysis. *J Pediatr* 1999; **134**; 268–72.

165 Malandrini A, Cavallaro T, Fabrizi GM et al. Ultrastructure and immunoreactivity of dystrophic axons indicate a different pathogenesis of Hallervorden–Spatz disease and infantile neuroaxonal dystrophy. *Virchows Arch* 1995; **427**: 415–21.

166 Malandrini A, Fabrizi GM, Bartalucci P et al. Clinicopathological study of familial late infantile Hallervorden–Spatz disease: a particular form of neuroacanthocytosis. *Childs Nerv Syst* 1996; **12**: 155–60.

167 Manuelidis EE, Rorke LB. Transmission of Alpers' disease (chronic progressive encephalopathy) produces experimental Creutzfeldt–Jakob disease in hamsters. *Neurology* 1989; **39**: 615–21.

168 Martidis A, Yee RD, Azzarelli B, Biller J. Neuro-ophthalmic, radiographic, and pathologic manifestations of adult-onset Alexander disease. *Arch Ophthalmol* 1999; **117**: 265–7.

169 Martin JJ, Martin L. Infantile neuroaxonal dystrophy. *Eur Neurol* 1972; **8**: 239–50.

170 Martin JJ, Schlote W. Central nervous system lesions in disorders of amino-acid metabolism. *J Neurol Sci* 1972; **15**: 49–76.

171 Matalon R, Michals K, Kaul R. Canavan disease: from spongy degeneration to molecular analysis. *J Pediatr* 1995; **127**: 511–17.

172 Menkes JH. Cerebral proteolipids in phenylketonuria. *Neurology* 1968; **18**: 1003–8.

173 Menkes JH, Phillipart M, Fiol RE. Cerebral lipids in maple syrup urine disease. *J Pediatr* 1965; **66**: 584.

174 Messing A, Head MW, Galles K et al. Fatal encephalopathy with astrocyte inclusions in GFAP transgenic mice. *Am J Pathol* 1998; **152**: 391–8.

175 Minagawa M, Maeshiro H, Kato K, Shioda K. A rare case of leucodystrophy–neuroaxonal leucodystrophy (Seitelberger) (Author's transl). *Seishin Shinkeigaku Zasshi* 1980; **82**: 488–503.

176 Moretto G, Sparaco M, Monarco S et al. Cytoskeletal changes and ubiquitin expression in dystrophic axons of Seitelberger's disease. *Clin Neuropathol* 1993; **12**: 34–7.

177 Morris AA, Hoffmann GF, Naughten ER et al. Glutaric aciduria and suspected child abuse. *Arch Dis Child* 1999; **80**: 404–5.

178 Morris AA, Singh KR, Perry RH et al. Respiratory chain dysfunction in progressive neuronal degeneration of childhood with liver disease. *J Child Neurol* 1996; **11**: 417–19.

179 Nance MA, Berry SA. Cockayne syndrome: review of 140 cases. *Am J Med Genet* 1992; **42**: 68–84.

180 Nance MA, Boyadjiev S, Pratt VM et al. Adult-onset neurodegenerative disorder due to proteolipid protein gene mutation in the mother of a man with Pelizaeus–Merzbacher disease. *Neurology* 1996; **47**: 1333–5.

181 Nardocci N, Zorzi G, Farina L et al. Infantile neuroaxonal dystrophy: clinical spectrum and diagnostic criteria. *Neurology* 1999; **52**: 1472–8.

182 Naviaux RK, Nyhan WL, Barshop BA et al. Mitochondrial DNA polymerase gamma deficiency and mtDNA depletion in a child with Alpers' syndrome. *Ann Neurol* 1999; **45**: 54–8.

183 Newell KL, Boyer P, Gomez TE et al. Alpha-synuclein immunoreactivity is present in axonal swellings in neuroaxonal dystrophy and acute traumatic brain injury. *J Neuropathol Exp Neurol* 1999; **58**: 1263–8.

184 Nicolaides P, Leonard J, Surtees R. Neurological outcome of methylmalonic acidaemia. *Arch Dis Child* 1998; **78**: 508–12.

185 Nicolaides P, Liebsch D, Dale N et al. The neurological outcome of patients with ornithine carbamoyltransferase deficiency. *Arch Dis Child* 2001 (in press).

186 Nyhan WL, Rice KM, Klein J, Barshop BA. Treatment of the acute crisis in maple syrup urine disease. *Arch Pediatr Adolesc Med* 1998; **152**: 593–8.

187 Oechsner M, Steen C, Sturenburg HJ, Kohlschutter A. Hyperammonaemic encephalopathy after initiation of valproate therapy in unrecognised ornithine transcarbamylase deficiency. *J Neurol Neurosurg Psychiatry* 1998; **64**: 680–2.

188 Okeda R, Matsuo T, Kawahara Y et al. Adult pigment type (Peiffer) of sudanophilic leukodystrophy. Pathological and morphometrical studies on two autopsy cases of siblings. *Acta Neuropathol Berl* 1989; **78**: 533–42.

189 Oldfors A, Sourander P, Armstrong D et al. Rett syndrome: cerebellar pathology. *Pediatr Neurol* 1990; **6**: 310–14.

190 Olivier M, Lenard HG, Asku F, Gartner J. A new leukoencephalopathy with bilateral anterior temporal lobe cysts. *Neuropediatrics* 1998; **29**: 225–8.

191 Orrell RW, Amrolia PJ, Heald A et al. Acanthocytosis, retinitis pigmentosa, and pallidal degeneration: a report of three patients, including the second reported case with hypoprebetalipoproteinemia (HARP syndrome). *Neurology* 1995; **45**: 487–92.

192 Orrico A, Lam C, Galli L et al. MECP2 mutation in male patients with non-specific X-linked mental retardation. *FEBS Lett* 2000; **481**: 285–8.

193 Ozdirim E, Topcu M, Ozon A, Cila A. Cockayne syndrome: review of 25 cases. *Pediatr Neurol* 1996; **15**: 312–16.

194 Ozmen M, Caliskan M, Goebel HH, Apak S. Infantile neuroaxonal dystrophy: diagnosis by skin biopsy. *Brain Dev* 1991; **13**: 256–9.

195 Pamphlett R, Silberstein P. Pelizaeus–Merzbacher disease in a brother and sister. *Acta Neuropathol Berl* 1986; **69**: 343–6.

196 Patton MA, Giannelli F, Francis AJ et al. Early onset Cockayne's syndrome: case reports with neuropathological and fibroblast studies. *J Med Genet* 1989; **26**: 154–9.

197 Podebrad F, Heil M, Reichert S et al. 4,5-Dimethyl-3-hydroxy-2[^{5}H]-furanone – the odour of maple syrup urine disease. *J Inherit Metab Dis* 1999; **22**: 107–14.

198 Prasad AN, Breen JC, Ampola MG, Rosman NP. Argininemia: a treatable genetic cause of progressive spastic diplegia simulating cerebral palsy: case reports and literature review. *J Child Neurol* 1997; **12**: 301–9.

199 Prensky AL, Carr S, Moser HW. Development of myelin in inherited disorders of amino-acid metabolism. A biochemical investigation. *Arch Neurol* 1968; **19**: 552–8.

200 Prick MJJ, Gabreels FJM, Renier WO et al. Pyruvate dehydrogenase deficiency restricted to the brain. Neurology 1981; 31: 398–404.

201 Prick MJJ, Gabreels FJM, Renier WO et al. Progressive infantile poliodystrophy. Association with disturbed pyruvate oxidation in muscle and liver. Arch Neurol 1981; 38: 767–72.

202 Prick MJJ, Gabreels FJM, Renier WO et al. Progressive infantile poliodystrophy (Alpers' disease) with a defect in citric acid cycle activity in liver and fibroblasts. Neuropediatrics 1982; 13: 108–11.

203 Prick MJJ, Gabreels FJM, Janssen AJM et al. Progressive poliodystrophy (Alpers') disease with a defect in cytochrome aa3 in muscle: a report of two unrelated patients. Clin Neurol Neurosurg 1983; 85: 57–70.

204 Pridmore CL, Baraitser M, Harding B et al. Alexander's disease: clues to diagnosis. J Child Neurol 1993; 35: 727–41.

205 Raby RB, Ward JC, Herrod HG. Propionic acidaemia and immunodeficiency. J Inherit Metab Dis 1994; 17: 250–1.

206 Ramaekers VT, Lake BD, Harding BN et al. Diagnostic difficulties in infantile neuroaxonal dystrophy: a clinicopathological study of eight cases. Neuropediatrics 1987; 18: 170–5.

207 Razavi EF, Larroche JC, Gaillard D. Infantile familial encephalopathy with cerebral calcifications and leukodystrophy. Neuropediatrics 1988; 19: 72–9.

208 Rodriguez D, Gelot A, Della GB et al. Increased density of oligodendrocytes in childhood ataxia with diffuse central hypomyelination (CACH) syndrome: neuropathological and biochemical study of two cases. Acta Neuropathol Berl 1999; 97: 469–80.

209 Rolles CJ. Hepatic injury with sodium valproate: a reappraisal with special reference to children. Br J Clin Pract 1983; 27: (Suppl): 72–8.

210 Rosenblatt DS, Whitehead VM. Cobalamin and folate deficiency: acquired and hereditary disorders in children. Semin Hematol 1999; 36: 19–34.

211 Rosenthal W. Uber eine eigentumlicher, mit Syringomyelie komplizierte Geschwulst des Ruckenmarks. Beitrage Pathol Anat 1898; 23: 111–43.

212 Russo LS, Aron A, Anderson PJ. Alexander's disease: a report and reappraisal. Neurology 1976; 26: 607–14.

213 Sandbank U, Lerman P. Progressive cerebral poliodystrophy: Alpers' disease: disorganized giant neuronal mitochondria on electron microscopy. J Neurol Neurosurg Psychiatry 1972; 35: 749–55.

214 Savoiardo M, Halliday WC, Nardocci N et al. Hallervorden–Spatz disease: MR and pathologic findings. AJNR Am J Neuroradiol 1993; 14: 155–62.

215 Schadewaldt P, Wendel U. Metabolism of branched-chain amino acids in maple syrup urine disease. Eur J Pediatr 1997; 156 (Suppl 1): S62–6.

216 Schaftingen E van, Jaeken J. Phosphomannomutase deficiency is a cause of carbohydrate-deficient glycoprotein syndrome type I. FEBS Lett 1995; 377: 318–20.

217 Scheffner D, König St, Rauterberg-Ruland I et al. Fatal liver failure in 16 children with Valproate therapy. Epilepsia 1988; 29: 530–42.

218 Schiffmann R, Moller JR, Trapp BD et al. Childhood ataxia with diffuse central nervous system hypomyelination. Ann Neurol 1994; 35: 331–40.

219 Schindler D, Bishop DF, Wolfe DE et al. Neuroaxonal dystrophy due to lysosomal alpha-N-acetylgalactosaminidase deficiency. N Engl J Med 1989; 320: 1735–40.

220 Schwartz M, Christensen E, Superti FA, Brandt NJ. The human glutaryl-CoA dehydrogenase gene: report of intronic sequences and of 13 novel mutations causing glutaric aciduria type I. Hum Genet 1998; 102: 452–8.

221 Seiser A, Jellinger K, Brainin M. Pigmentary type of orthochromatic leukodystrophy with early onset and protracted course. Neuropediatrics 1990; 21: 48–52.

222 Seitelberger F. Neuroaxonal dystrophy: its relation to aging and neurological diseases. In: Vinken PJ, Bruyn G, Klawans H eds. Handbook of Annual Neurology Vol. 49. Extrapyramidal disorders. Amsterdam: Elsevier, 1986: 391–415.

223 Seitelberger F. Pelizaeus–Merzbacher disease. In: Vinken PJ, Bruyn G eds. Handbook of clinical neurology. Amsterdam: North Holland, 1970: 150–202.

224 Shaag A, Anikster Y, Christensen E et al. The molecular basis of canavan (aspartoacylase deficiency) disease in European non-Jewish patients. Am J Hum Genet 1995; 57: 572–80.

225 Shapira Y, Cederbaum SD, Cancilla PA et al. Familial poliodystrophy, mitochondrial myopathy, and lactate acidemia. Neurology 1975; 25: 614–21.

226 Sherwin RM, Berthong M. Alexander's disease with sudanophilic leukodystrophy. Arch Pathol 1970; 89: 321–8.

227 Shuman RM, Leech RW, Scott CR. The neuropathology of the nonketotic and ketotic hyperglycinemias: three cases. Neurology 1978; 28: 139–46.

228 Silberberg DH. Maple syrup urine disease metabolites studies in cerebellum cultures. J Neurochem 1969; 16: 1141–6.

229 Smith I, Beasley MG, Ades AE. Intelligence and quality of dietary treatment in phenylketonuria. Arch Dis Child 1990; 65: 472–8.

230 Smith I, Erdohazi M, Macartney FJ et al. Fetal damage despite low-phenylalanine diet after conception in a phenylketonuric woman. Lancet 1979; i: 17–19.

231 Smith JK, Mah JK, Castillo M. Brain MR imaging findings in two patients with Alpers' syndrome. Clin Imaging 1996; 20: 235–7.

232 Soffer D, Amir N, Elpeleg ON et al. Striatal degeneration and spongy myelinopathy in glutaric acidemia. J Neurol Sci 1992; 107: 199–204.

233 Sperl W, Felber S, Skladal D, Wermuth B. Metabolic stroke in carbamyl phosphate synthetase deficiency. Neuropediatrics 1997; 28: 229–34.

234 Steen C, Rosenblatt DS, Scheying H et al. Cobalamin E (cblE) disease: a severe neurological disorder with megaloblastic anaemia, homocystinuria and low serum methionine. J Inherit Metab Dis 1997; 20: 705–6.

235 Steinman L, Clancy RR, Cann H, Urich H. The neuropathology of propionic acidemia. Dev Med Child Neurol 1983; 25: 87–94.

236 Stromme P, Maehlen J, Strom EH, Torvik A. Postmortem findings in two patients with the carbohydrate-deficient glycoprotein syndrome. Acta Paediatr Scand 1991; Suppl 375: 55–62.

237 Surtees R, Clayton P. Infantile parkinsonism–dystonia: tyrosine hydroxylase deficiency. Mov Disord 1998; 13: 350.

238 Surtees RAH, Matthews EE, Leonard JV. Neurologic outcome of propionic acidemia. Pediatr Neurol 1992; 8: 333–7.

239 Suzuki K, Rapin I. Giant neuronal mitochondria in an infant with microcephaly and seizure disorder. Arch Neurol 1969; 20: 62–72.

240 Tachibana H, Hayashi T, Kashi T. Neuroaxonal dystrophy of neonatal onset with unusual clinicopathological findings. Brain Dev 1986; 8: 605–9.

241 Takada K, Becker LE. Cockayne's syndrome: report of two autopsy cases associated with neurofibrillary tangles. Clin Neuropathol 1986; 5: 64–8.

242 Takanashi J, Sugita K, Tanabe Y, Niimi H. Adolescent case of Alexander disease: MR imaging and MR spectroscopy. *Pediatr Neurol* 1998; **18**: 67–70.

243 Tantin D. RNA polymerase II elongation complexes containing the Cockayne syndrome group B protein interact with a molecular complex containing the transcription factor IIH components xeroderma pigmentosum B and p62. *J Biol Chem* 1998; **273**: 27794–9.

244 Taylor TD, Litt M, Kramer P *et al*. Homozygosity mapping of Hallervorden-Spatz syndrome to chromosome 20p12.3-p13 (published erratum appears in *Nat Genet* 1997; **16**: 109). *Nat Genet* 1996; **14**: 479–81.

245 Thoene JG. Treatment of urea cycle disorders. *J Pediatr* 1999; **134**: 255–6.

246 Thompson AJ, Smith I, Brenton D *et al*. Neurological deterioration in young adults with phenylketonuria. *Lancet* 1990; **336**: 602–5.

247 Thompson AJ, Tillotson S, Smith I *et al*. Brain MRI changes in phenylketonuria. Associations with dietary status. *Brain* 1993; **116**: 811–21.

248 Townsend JJ, Wilson JF, Harris T *et al*. Alexander's disease. *Acta Neuropathol* 1985; **67**: 163–6.

249 Troost D, Rossum A van, Veiga PJ, Willemse J. Cerebral calcifications and cerebellar hypoplasia in two children: clinical, radiologic and neuropathological studies – a separate neurodevelopmental entity. *Neuropediatrics* 1984; **15**: 102–9.

250 Tunon T, Ferrer I, Gallego J *et al*. Leucodystrophy with pigmented glial and scavenger cells (pigmentary type of orthochromatic leucodystrophy). *Neuropathol Appl Neurobiol* 1988; **14**; 337–44.

251 Uchino T, Endo F, Matsuda I. Neurodevelopmental outcome of long-term therapy of urea cycle disorders in Japan. *J Inherit Metab Dis* 1998; **21** (Suppl 1): 151–9.

252 Ueland PM, Refsum H, Beresford SA, Vollset SE. The controversy over homocysteine and cardiovascular risk. *Am J Clin Nutr* 2000; **72**: 324–32.

253 Ugarte M, Perez CC, Rodriguez PP *et al*. Overview of mutations in the PCCA and PCCB genes causing propionic acidemia. *Hum Mutat* 1999; **14**: 275–82.

254 Verrips A, Hiel JA, Gabreels FJ *et al*. The Aicardi–Goutières syndrome: variable clinical expression in two siblings. *Pediatr Neurol* 1997; **16**: 323–5.

255 Wajner M, Vargas CR. Reduction of plasma concentrations of large neutral amino acids in patients with maple syrup urine disease during crises (Letter). *Arch Dis Child* 1999; **80**: 579.

256 Wakabayashi K, Yoshimoto M, Fukushima T *et al*. Widespread occurrence of alpha-synuclein/NACP-immunoreactive neuronal inclusions in juvenile and adult-onset Hallervorden–Spatz disease with Lewy bodies. *Neuropathol Appl Neurobiol* 1999; **25**: 363–8.

257 Watanabe I, Muller J. Cavitating diffuse sclerosis. *J Neuropathol Exp Neurol* 1967; **26**: 437–55.

258 Wefring KW, Lamvik JO. Familial progressive poliodystrophy with cirrhosis of the liver. *Acta Paediatr Scand* 1967; **56**: 295–300.

259 Weglage J, Pietsch M, Funders B *et al*. Neurological findings in early treated phenylketonuria. *Acta Paediatr* 1995; **84**: 411–15.

260 Wilcken DE, Wilcken B. The natural history of vascular disease in homocystinuria and the effects of treatment. *J Inherit Metab Dis* 1997; **20**: 295–300.

261 Wilson A, Leclerc D, Saberi F *et al*. Functionally null mutations in patients with the cblG-variant form of methionine synthase deficiency. *Am J Hum Genet* 1998; **63**: 409–14.

262 Wilson DC, McGibben D, Hicks EM, Allen IV. Progressive neuronal degeneration of childhood (Alpers' syndrome) with hepatic cirrhosis. *Eur J Pediatr* 1993; **152**: 260–2.

263 Wisniewski K, Wisniewski HM. Diagnosis of infantile neuroaxonal dystrophy by skin biopsy. *Ann Neurol* 1980; **7**: 377–9.

264 Wohlwill FS, Bernstein J, Yakovlev PI. Dysmyelinogenic leukodystrophy. *J Neuropathol Exp Neurol* 1959; **18**: 359–83.

265 Wolfe DE, Schindler D, Desnick RJ. Neuroaxonal dystrophy in infantile alpha-*N*-acetylgalactosaminidase deficiency. *J Neurol Sci* 1995; **132**: 44–56.

266 Woodward K, Kirtland K, Dlouhy S *et al*. X inactivation phenotype in carriers of Pelizaeus–Merzbacher disease: skewed in carriers of a duplication and random in carriers of point mutations. *Eur J Hum Genet* 2000; **8**: 449–54.

267 Woodward K, Malcolm S. Proteolipid protein gene: Pelizaeus–Merzbacher disease in humans and neurodegeneration in mice. *Trends Genet* 1999; **15**: 125–8.

268 Worle H, Kohler B, Schlote W *et al*. Progressive cerebral degeneration of childhood with liver disease (Alpers Huttenlocher disease) with cytochrome oxidase deficiency presenting with epilepsia partialis continua as the first clinical manifestation. *Clin Neuropathol* 1998; **17**: 63–8.

269 Yap S, Naughten E. Homocystinuria due to cystathionine beta-synthase deficiency in Ireland: 25 years' experience of a newborn screened and treated population with reference to clinical outcome and biochemical control. *J Inherit Metab Dis* 1998; **21**: 738–47.

270 Yool DA, Edgar JM, Montague P, Malcolm S. The proteolipid protein gene and myelin disorders in man and animal models. *Hum Mol Genet* 2000; **9**: 987–92.

271 Young G, Driscoll MC. Coagulation abnormalities in the carbohydrate-deficient glycoprotein syndrome: case report and review of the literature. *Am J Hematol* 1999; **60**: 66–9.

272 Zittoun J. Congenital errors of folate metabolism. *Baillieres Clin Haematol* 1995; **8**: 603–16.

9

Perinatal neuropathology

HANNAH C. KINNEY AND DAWNA DUNCAN ARMSTRONG

INTRODUCTION

Perinatal neuropathology merits special consideration because the patterns of injury in the perinatal brain differ significantly from those in the mature brain. At its broadest level, perinatal neuropathology reflects cellular and tissue reactions brought about by a complex interplay of developmental and pathological processes, encompassing central nervous system (CNS) disorders that occur in the premature (less than 37 weeks of gestation) and term newborn, and the infant within the first 2 years of life. This age span corresponds to a critical period in human brain growth that begins after the embryonic and early fetal periods when the fundamental structure of the CNS is established, and ends at the beginning of the third postnatal year when the brain has attained 80% of the adult weight. From midgestation through infancy, brain growth reflects synaptogenesis, dendritic arborization and spine formation, axonal elongation and collateral formation, myelination, gliogenesis, and neurotransmitter and vascular development. In the embryonic period, CNS inborn or acquired lesions result in malformations or, if severe enough, miscarriage. In the adult brain, structure is relatively set, such that cellular and tissue reactions generally reflect the pathological and reparative processes together. During the perinatal period, however, the neuropathology of the developing brain is characterized not only by the disease and reparative processes, but also by

their effects upon multiple developmental programmes. Patterns of injury in the perinatal period are modified by the degree of the underlying anatomical, cellular, neurochemical and vascular maturity of the brain at successive stages of development. Moreover, the plasticity of the human brain appears to be at its peak during the critical growth period from midgestation through infancy. When the brain is damaged, normal regressive events may be modified, and overabundant synapses, dendrites and/or axonal collaterals destined for elimination may be preserved for function; in addition, during this period, the brain still has the capacity to develop new projections in response to injury.

In a landmark study of perinatal injury in the developing human brain, Marin-Padilla[428] showed that primarily undamaged cortical regions adjacent to injured sites (e.g. microgyrias, ulegyrias, leptomeningeal heterotopias, multicystic encephalopathies, porencephalies and hydranencephalies) survive, retain their intrinsic vasculature, and undergo progressive postinjury transformations (acquired cortical dysplasia) which affect the structural and functional organization of developing neurons, fibres, glial elements and microvasculature (Fig. 9.1). In general, undamaged cortical regions adjacent to an injured site are characterized by cytoarchitectural disorganization (neuronal hypertrophy, atrophy), abnormal dendritic orientation, partial obliteration of laminations, grey- and white-matter attenuations, macrophage infiltration, gliosis, including layer I and grey-matter/white-matter border gliosis, and/or mineralization.[428] Marin-Padilla speculated that eventually, these progressive postinjury transformations influence the neurological and cognitive maturation of affected children, and play a crucial role in the pathogenesis of ensuing neurological and cognitive disorders, e.g. epilepsy, cerebral palsy, dyslexia, cognitive impairment and poor school performance.

In this chapter, the spectrum of perinatal lesions is highlighted, emphasizing the special features that separate perinatal lesions from those in the mature brain. The pathology of malformations, perinatal degenerative disorders and inborn errors of metabolism is considered elsewhere (see Chapters 7, 8, 11 and 12, this Volume). A timetable of the approximate peak occurrences of common perinatal brain lesions is provided (Fig. 9.2).

BRAIN GROWTH

The growth of the fetus depends upon the availability of oxygen and nutrients and the appropriate growth factors operating according to a genetic plan under the influence of the maternal environment. The fetus gains 5 g/day until 15 weeks' gestation, and then 30 g/day until 34 weeks,

when there is a decrease in weight gain until 40 weeks, after which there is no gain and may be weight loss. At birth the infant is classified according to weight as: appropriate for gestational age, small for gestational age (if less than the 10th percentile), and intrauterine growth restricted or retarded (IUGR, if less than the 3rd percentile). The IUGR is classified as symmetrical if the head circumference and body weight are both small, and asymmetrical IUGR if the head circumference is relatively spared.[626] Alterations in growth and fetal malnutrition are related to specific conditions.[271] Growth is less than expected in twin pregnancies and sometimes in maternal hypertension, and greater than normal in infants of diabetic mothers. Growth is also decreased in fetal infections, in fetuses within mothers who smoke[607] and in association with malformations. In some cases of isoimmunization and in infants of diabetic mothers the brain weight is decreased. In infants of diabetic mothers the brain weight is decreased, not only in relationship to the abnormally high body weight, but also in relation to gestational age. In the brains of growth-retarded infants the markers of maturation are appropriate for the gestational age.[607] Studies of the neurodevelopmental outcome of children with intrauterine growth retardation suggest that the children

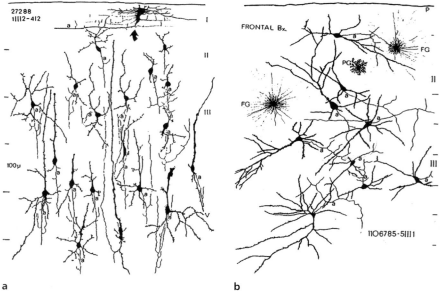

a   b

Figure 9.1 *Neuronal anomalies and organization. (a) Perinatally acquired microgyria and primarily undamaged cortical region (b) adjacent to a small marginal (layer I) heterotopia. (a) Detail of the dysplastic cortex of a microgyrus with neuronal disorganization, poor neuronal development (atrophy) and dendritic alterations suggesting degenerative changes. Some neurons are transformed into small stellate cells postinjury, others show alterations suggesting centripetal dendritic reabsorption, while still other neurons appear to be pyramidal cells which have lost their contact with layer I, perhaps by progressive distal reabsorption. Many of these postinjury transformed neurons have intracortically distributed axons (a) with ascending collaterals. The surviving Cajal–Retzius cells (arrow) have retained their typical morphological features and long horizontal axons which are recognized throughout the affected microgyrical cortex. (b) Detail of a primarily undamaged cortex adjacent to a small marginal (layer I) heterotopia showing laminar obliteration, neuronal disorganization, and marked disorientation of dendrites of many neurons, which seem to have lost their normal orientation to layer I. This dendritic disorientation is considered to be acquired postinjury to alterations of the region's intrinsic circuitry and to the lack of response to layer I developmental cues altered by the marginal heterotopia. This primarily undamaged cortex also shows a mild increase in the number of reactive astroyctes (FG) as well as non-reactive protoplasmic astrocytes (PG). (Rapid Golgi preparations; camera lucida drawings.) From Marin-Padilla.*[428]

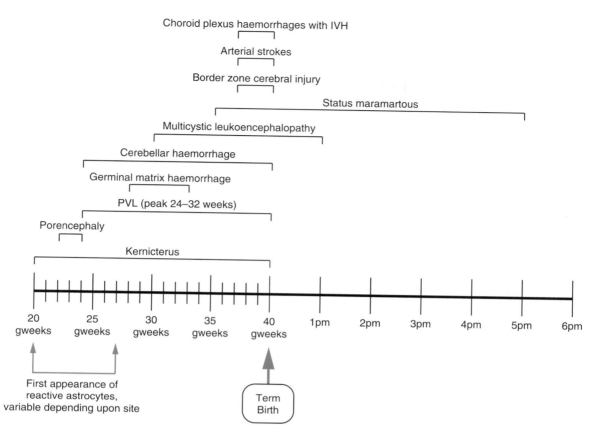

Figure 9.2 *Timetable of the approximate peak occurrences of common perinatal brain lesions of note, PVL may originate in term infants and the first few postnatal months. g, Gestational; pm, postnatal month; IVH, intraventricular haemorrhage.*

are at greater risk than controls for developmental disabilities, especially if there are perinatal complications.[199] Charts of normal perinatal brain growth by age are provided in Tables 9.1 and 9.2.

CELLULAR REACTIONS IN THE DEVELOPING HUMAN CNS

Neurons

The growth and differentiation of neurons change in different brain regions at different times and rates. Neuronal proliferation and migration occur in the first and early second trimester. The peak period for neuronal proliferation is 2–4 months of gestation, and for neuronal migration 3–5 months of gestation.[679] Perinatal neuropathology is concerned mainly with the organizational events in brain growth and maturation that follow upon neuronal proliferation and migration. These organizational events occur from approximately the fifth gestational month until several years after birth, and probably continue for many years. Organizational events include the establishment, differentiation and cell death of subplate neurons; the alignment, orientation and layering of neurons; the determination of neuronal number, density, size, differentiation and final

position; axonal outgrowth (Fig. 9.3), collateralization and establishment of synaptic contacts; development of the cytoskeleton; formation and arborization of dendrites and the formation of spines; synaptogenesis; cell death (apoptosis) and selective elimination of neuronal processes and synapses; and the synthesis of neurotransmitters and the formation of the cellular apparatus for their function. The postmitotic neuron develops from an undifferentiated cell into a polarized cell with a complex shape characterized by a dendritic tree and an axon with collateralization. Neurons are postulated to be committed to a particular phenotype when they are in the ventricular zone.[551] Experimentally, however, there is a period in the cell cycle (late S-phase to mitosis) when neuroblasts are susceptible to environmental cues, and can be induced to alter their programmed phenotype, laminar position and possibly even their subcortical connections.[418]

The cytoskeleton of the neuron maintains its shape and polarity, with the elaboration of a dendritic tree to receive impulses, and of an axon for the transfer of information. The polarity of the neuron is reflected in differences between the morphology of dendrites and axons, the organization of the cytoskeleton and membrane specializations, and the absence of protein synthesis in the axon. During development the dendrites and axons grow out in a predetermined manner, but the initiation of this is influenced by variable

Table 9.1 (a) *Fresh brain weight, fixed brain weight, infratentorial weight and percentage of infratentorial weight/total brain weight in relation to age*

Age (weeks)	Fresh brain weight (n = 175)	Fixed brain weight (n = 298)	Infratentorial weight (n = 114)	% Infratentorial/total brain weight (n = 113)
8–9	—	0.80 (1)	—	—
10–11	—	1.20 (1)	—	—
12–13	—	5.87 (1)	—	—
14–15	15.45 ± 1.20 (2)	14.40 ± 3.34 (6)	0.76 ± 0.14 (4)	5.91 ± 0.62 (4)
16–17	21.17 ± 1.05 (3)	21.49 ± 5.34 (10)	1.21 ± 0.19 (8)	5.37 ± 0.78 (8)
18–19	37.33 ± 8.17 (10)	38.75 ± 9.52 (22)	2.19 ± 0.7 (16)	4.88 ± 0.50 (16)
20–21	52.19 ± 7.23 (15)	55.38 ± 10.18 (22)	2.81 ± 0.42 (10)	4.98 ± 0.49 (10)
22–23	75.01 ± 17.76 (9)	78.15 ± 14.37 (30)	3.71 ± 0.74 (14)	4.54 ± 4.41 (13)
24–25	101.53 ± 18.75 (9)	111.97 ± 17.30 (22)	5.23 ± 0.70 (12)	4.61 ± 0.29 (12)
26–27	130.62 ± 17.38 (21)	146.21 ± 21.69 (31)	6.95 ± 1.41 (8)	4.52 ± 0.32 (8)
28–29	169.22 ± 19.11 (18)	184.62 ± 26.40 (29)	7.63 ± 0.79 (6)	4.76 ± 0.46 (6)
30–31	203.02 ± 25.99 (21)	229.54 ± 29.84 (26)	12.25 ± 2.02 (4)	5.24 ± 0.35 (4)
32–33	234.98 ± 28.24 (13)	266.00 ± 32.78 (13)	14.00 (1)	5.18 (1)
34–35	280.3 ± 28.19 (14)	309.32 ± 47.04 (19)	15.75 ± 3.18 (2)	5.58 ± 0.41 (2)
36–37	325.83 ± 40.75 (6)	366.00 ± 50.27 (11)	21.43 ± 3.36 (6)	6.07 ± 0.66 (6)
38–39	391.69 ± 41.39 (10)	433.30 ± 56.89 (20)	26.93 ± 4.70 (10)	6.27 ± 0.56 (10)
40–41	409.63 ± 37.55 (17)	455.27 ± 53.66 (33)	29.05 ± 4.04 (13)	6.68 ± 0.65 (13)

Data are means ± SD (number of cases in parentheses).
Data from Guihart-Costa and Larrode.[276]

extrinsic conditions, including adhesion molecules, extracellular matrix molecules, and growth factors produced by glial cells, blood vessels and axonal targets. It is beyond the scope of this chapter to discuss details of the neuronal organizational events, thus here only selected events will be discussed.

LAMINATION

Lamination, the proper alignment, orientation and layering of cortical neurons, is one of the earliest cortical organizational events and occurs as neuronal migration ceases. For the neocortex, the initial cortical plate appears at 7–10 weeks of gestation, and condensation into a six-layered cortex occurs at approximately 16 weeks of gestation.[451] With lamination, neurite outgrowth progresses, with the elaboration of dendritic and axonal ramifications. These major neuronal changes are demonstrated in the developing visual cortex (Fig. 9.4). Trisomy 21 exemplifies organizational disorders that result in defective lamination. Golden and Hyman[254] showed that the lamination is abnormal in the superior temporal neocortex in trisomy 21 (Fig. 9.5). This altered cortical maturation may reflect an abnormality in axonal and dendritic arborization.

Table 9.1 (b) *Percentiles of brain weights in relation to gestational age*

Gestational age (weeks)	Percentile				
	10	25	50	75	90
26–27	94	102	110	120	120
28–29	125	135	147	160	170
30–31	170	180	190	203	217
32–33	190	201	210	234	252
34–35	226	240	251	280	287
36–37	280	295	311	328	346
38–37	317	332	356	328	346
40–41	370	400	420	440	463

Adapted from Larroche.[389]

Table 9.2 *Brain weight in infants in relation to age and length*

Age	Body length (cm)	Brain weight (g)
Birth to 3 days	49	335
3–7 days	49	358
1–3 weeks	52	382
3–5 weeks	52	413
5–7 weeks	53	422
7–9 weeks	55	489
3 months	56	516
4 months	59	540
5 months	61	644
6 months	62	660
7 months	65	691
8 months	65	714
9 months	67	750
10 months	69	809
11 months	70	852
12 months	73	925
14 months	74	944
16 months	77	1010
18 months	78	1042
20 months	79	1050
22 months	82	1059
24 months	84	1064

Adapted from Sanderman and Boerner.[578]

SYNAPTOGENESIS

During development, synapses are eliminated as remodelling of cortical connections progresses. This elimination occurs via several mechanisms, including competition for trophic substances and increased electrical activity. The elimination of synapses in infancy has been reported in the human visual cortex.[331] Multiple disorders of dendrites and/or spines, e.g. abnormal density and/or shape in Down's syndrome (Fig. 9.6), are recognized in the perinatal period and beyond (Table 9.3). For example, in Rett's syndrome, there is selective abnormality of dendrites in the motor, frontal and limbic cortices (Fig. 9.7).[28] Because the quantitative differences are non-progressive in Rett's syndrome, an arrest of dendritic development rather than degeneration has been suggested.

Historically, synapses have been examined with Golgi impregnation techniques which define spines and axonal boutons, and with electron microscopy, using sections stained with ethanolic phosphotungstic acid for visualizing synaptic junctions. Both of these techniques depend upon very short post-mortem intervals. The discovery of synapse-associated molecules provides an alternative means for studying human synapses, allowing for immunocytochemical labelling in tissue sections with realistic post-mortem intervals. The molecules include GAP-43, synapsin I and II, and synaptophysin. GAP-43 is a synapse-related molecule that is a neuronal membrane phosphoprotein.[367] Because its expression occurs maximally during periods of growth and change, markers for GAP-43 or its messenger RNA (mRNA) can be highly informative regarding the temporospatial patterns of synaptogenesis *in vivo*. Although the precise mechanisms by which GAP-43 influences neuronal growth are unclear, a linkage to the submembrane actin cytoskeleton seems likely.[54] During development, the highest levels of GAP-43 appear along the entire length of the axon as it is elongating, then in preterminal branches and their growth cones in the period in which end arbors are being elaborated. After the establishment of stable synapses, most neurons cease expressing GAP-43 at high levels. In certain regions, however, high GAP-43 levels persist into adulthood, e.g. in the limbic and associative regions of the forebrain. These presynaptic terminals in which GAP-43 remains high may represent sites that can undergo functional and possibly even structural changes in response to physiological activity throughout life.[367] GAP-43 immunostaining has been used to delineate the sequences of synaptogenesis and fibre tract elongation in the human brainstem (Fig. 9.8).[367] The establishment of timetables of synaptogenesis across the forebrain is now feasible by the temporospatial mapping of the expression of the various synapse-related molecules.

NEUROTRANSMITTERS AS NEURONAL GROWTH FACTORS

At various stages of development, neurons are supported by different growth factors that promote neuronal survival and stimulate axonal and dendritic growth Neurotransmitters, e.g. acetylcholine, serotonin (5-hydroxytryptamine, 5-HT), glutamate and opioids, probably act as growth factors early in development.[411] The neurotransmitters interact via their respective receptors to influence neurite outgrowth and neuronal survival and differentiation. The implications of neurotransmitter–receptor interactions in the growth and maturation of the brain are considerable. During gestation, drugs ingested by the mother can cross the placenta and interact with the fetal

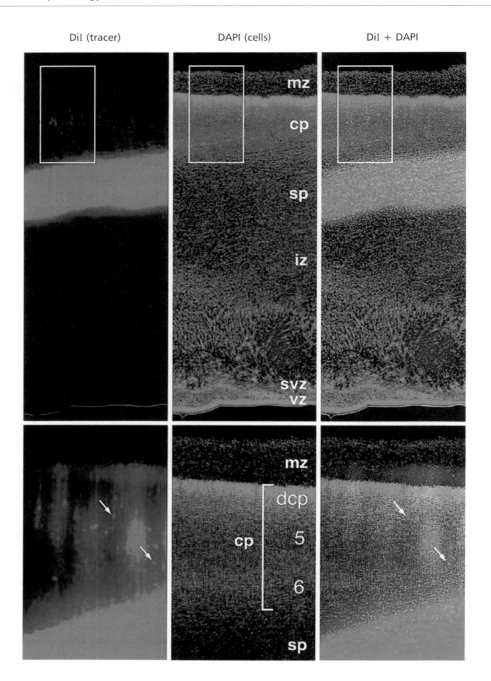

Figure 9.3 *Human visual cortex (area 17): development of cortical connections at mid-gestation. DiI was injected into the optic radiations between the lateral geniculate nucleus and visual cortex in a fixed brain. Labelled thalamocortical axons project heavily into the subplate (sp), a transient cellular compartment where thalamocortical axons 'wait' for the arrival of layer IV neurons. At this age, the cortical plate (cp) contain only neurons belonging to layers V and VI, and a dense cortical plate (dcp) containing newly migrated neurons. Superficial cortical layers are 'born' later than deep layers, thus corticogenesis proceeds in an 'inside–out' gradient. The cerebral wall also consists of a ventricular zone (vz) and a subventricular zone (svz), where neurons and glia proliferate; an intermediate zone (iz), where neurons migrate and axonal pathways develop; and a marginal zone (mz), precursor of cortical layer I. At higher magnifications (bottom panels), the cortical plate is seen to contain some retrogradely labelled neurons (arrows), corresponding to corticobulbar and corticospinal projections from layer V, and corticothalamic projections from layer VI. After layer IV neurons arrive and differentiate , the thalamocortical axons will invade the cortical plate and synapse in layer IV. This experiment exemplifies the dynamic processes of cortical cell proliferation, migration, and axon growth and pathfinding which are susceptible to insults during fetal life. (Fluorescent axons tracer DiL, counterstained with DAPI, a fluorescent DNA-binding molecule.) From Hevner.[309a]*

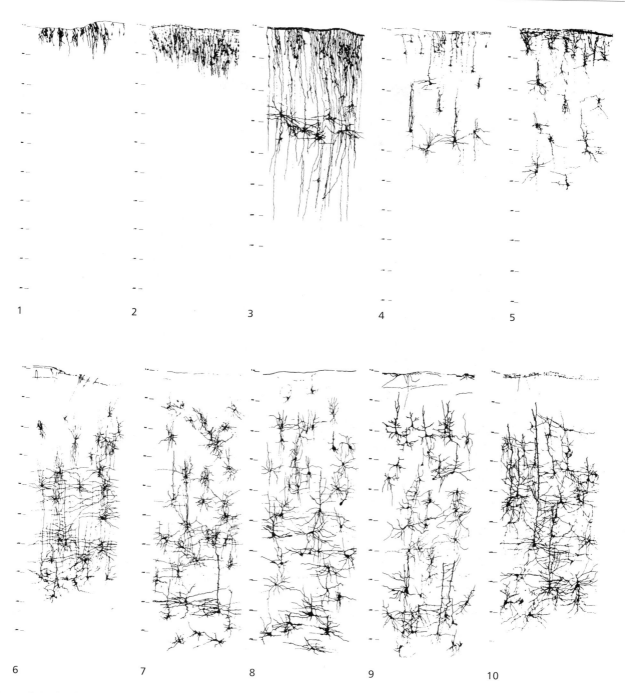

Figure 9.4 *Visual cortex of human fetus and infant. Camera lucida drawings at: (1) 14, (2) 20, (3) 28, (4) 30, (5) 35, and (6) 40 gestational weeks; and at: (7) 1, (8) 2, (9) 4, and (10) 6 postnatal months. (Rapid Golgi preparations; camera lucida drawings.) Courtesy of F Chan, Hospital for Sick Children, Toronto, Canada.*

brain's endogenous receptors to affect growth processes adversely. For example, cocaine may adversely affect brain development *in utero* by interfering with the maturation of neuronal pathways or neurons that utilize monoamines as neurotransmitters, or that are the targets of neurons that use monoamines as neurotransmitters. There are mono-aminergic systems originating in the brainstem that have widely distributed projections to the cerebral cortex, thalamus, hypothalamus, basal ganglia and the basal forebrain.

In experimental animals, pharmacological and structural lesions in these developing systems can result in subtle developmental abnormalities in neuronal differentiation, lamination, dendritic arborization and spine density. Postnatal rats, for example, deprived of noradrenaline from the locus coeruleus develop elongated apical dendrites without branches in layer VI of the neocortex.[422] Cocaine has the potential to interact with the developing monoaminergic systems in several ways: it impairs the reuptake of

Normal   Trisomy 21

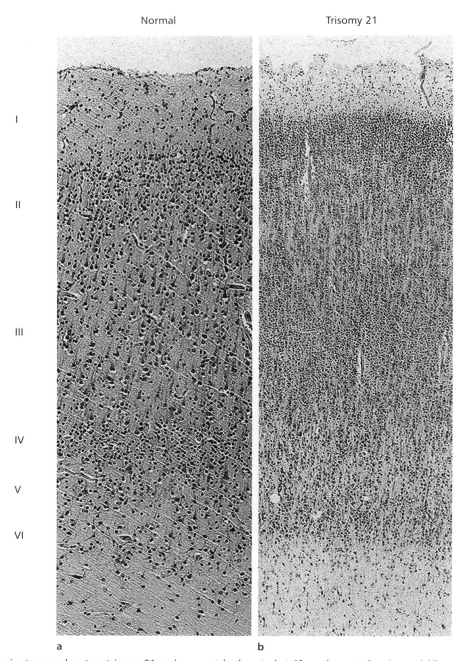

I

II

III

IV

V

VI

a   b

Figure 9.5 *Superior temporal cortex: trisomy 21 and age-matched control at 40 weeks gestation. Layers I–VI are easily identified and have been labelled in the age-matched control cortex (a). The cortex in cases of trisomy 21 (b) revealed a normal layer I and the cortical thickness was preserved. However, layers II–VI are difficult to elucidate in the trisomy 21 cortex and there appears to be many more cells in the cortex confirmed by cell counting.[254] The cellularity resembles that of a more immature brain. From Golden and Hyman.[254]*

noradrenaline and adrenaline by presynaptic nerve endings, impairs the reuptake of dopamine by binding to the transporter that mediates dopamine uptake, and impairs the homeostasis of 5-HT by blocking the uptake of tryptophan, its precursor, and of 5-HT itself.[676] This potential for trophic-regulated abnormalities is supported by a study of cerebral cortical development in the rat: in the adult cortex subtle abnormalities of neuronal lamination and organization after prenatal exposure to cocaine have been reported.[268] Animal data provide further compelling evi-

dence that the early appearance of monoamine systems plays a role in neural development. In animals with intrauterine exposure to cocaine, specific alterations are seen in dopamine-rich areas of the cerebral cortex, such as the anterior cingulate cortex: D_1-receptor–G-protein coupling is greatly reduced, the γ-aminobutyric acidergic (GABAergic) system is altered and pyramidal dendrites undergo excessive growth (as reviewed by Levitt *et al.*).[406] In a transgenic mouse line in which the gene that encodes monoamine oxidase A is disrupted and excessively high 5-

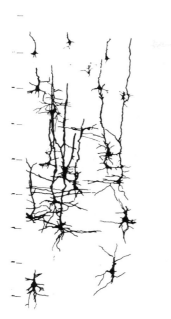

Figure 9.6 *Trisomy 21, age 2 years, occipital lobe. There is a decreased number and length of dendrites, decreased spines, and obscure lamination. (Rapid Golgi; camera lucida drawings.) F Chan, Hospital for Sick Children, Toronto, Canada.*

HT levels result, barrels fail to form in the developing somatosensory cortex.[99,100]

The adverse effects upon neural development by heroin via endogenous opioid receptors[359] and by nicotine via cholinergic nicotinic receptors and maternal cigarette smoking[367] (Fig. 9.9) have similarly been postulated. A high level of [^{3}H]nicotine binding, for example, has been reported in the human brainstem tegmentum at midgestation, with a rapidly changing profile over late gestation.[367] This dynamic change suggests that mid-to-late gestation is a developmental period during which this region is likely to be most vulnerable to the harmful effects of nicotine in maternal cigarette smoke during pregnancy. Animal and tissue culture studies indicate that acetylcholine can act as a growth factor and influence the development of neurons and cholinergic pathways via interactions with nicotinic receptors (see review in Ref. 367). At midgestation in the human fetus, when [^{3}H]nicotine binding is very high in the brainstem tegmental nuclei (Fig. 9.9), exogenous nicotine from maternal cigarette smoke may cause over-stimulation of the nicotinic receptors, thereby exacerbating acetylcholine's growth-related effects upon the targeted neuronal populations. Alternatively, exogenous nicotine may desensitize the nicotinic receptors, thereby rendering them non-responsive to acetylcholine. Either way, exogenous nicotine may adversely affect brainstem cholinergic development *in utero* via interactions mediated by endogenous nicotinic receptors. Subtle abnormalities in neuronal proliferation, migration and/or differentiation may require sensitive immunocytochemical, Golgi, cellular quantitative and neuropharmacological techniques for detection of abnormalities in the perinatal human brain.

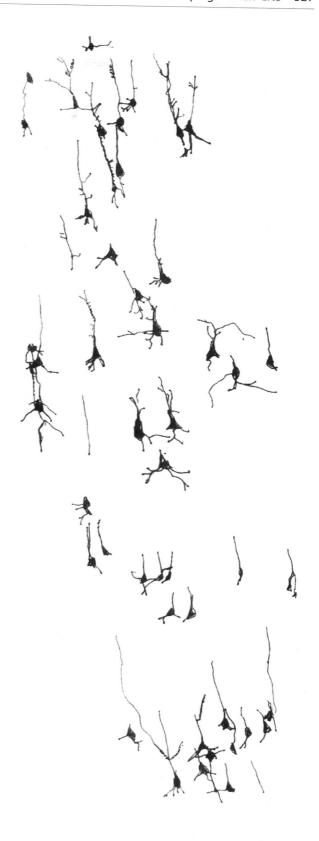

Figure 9.7 *Rett's syndrome: cerebral cortex. The apical and basalar dendrites are reduced in length and in branching number compared with non-Rett controls. (Golgi preparation; camera lucida drawings.) From Armstrong et al.[28]*

Table 9.3 *Human perinatal brain disorders with abnormalities of dendrites and/or spines*

Abnormality	Type	Lesion	References
Malformation	Trisomy 21	Short basal dendrites	Takashima et al.[634]
		Decreased spines	
		Spine dysgenesis	
	Trisomy 13–15	Spine dysgenesis	Marin-Padilla[431]
	Microgyria	Dendrite alignment	Williams et al.[696]
	Lissencephaly	Dendrite alignment	Jagadha and Becker[340]
		Decreased spines	
	Lhermitte–Duclos	Dendrite dysgenesis	Ferrer et al.[201]
Storage/metabolic	Ceroid lipofuscinosis	Enlarged proximal axon	Williams et al.[697]
		Meganeurites	Paula-Barbosa et al.[521]
	GM2 gangliosidosis	Meganeurites	Purpura[543]
	Sanfilippo's	Meganeurites	Jagadha and Becker[340]
	Leukodystrophy	Decreased dendrites	Becker and Takashima[50]
		Decreased spines	
	Menkes'	Purkinje cell sprouts	Pupura et al.[544]
	Phenylketonuria	Decreased dendrites	Bauman and Kemper[49]
		Decreased spines	
	Zellweger	Heterotopic neurons	Della Giustina et al.[142]
Infection	Cytomegalovirus	Dysplastic ectopic neurons	Kristt[376]
Miscellaneous	Mental retardation (unspecified)	Decreased dendrites	Huttenlocher[330]
		Decreased spines	
	Tuberous sclerosis	Short dendrites	Blake et al.[67]
		Decreased spines	
	SIDS	Immature dendrites	Quattrochi et al.[546]
		Increased spines	
	Rett's syndrome	Selective decreased dendrites	Armstrong et al.[28]

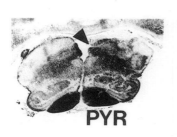
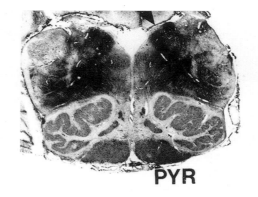
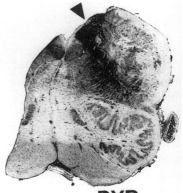

a   b   c

Figure 9.8 *Development of GAP-43 expression in human mid-medulla. (**a**) Fetus; (**b**) infant; (**c**) adult. The most striking change is a decrease in staining intensity in the corticospinal tract in the pyramid across development. Staining is intense in the fetal pyramid at 21 gestational weeks. In the infant pyramid (**b**), staining is still visually detectable, but substantially reduced; in the adult pyramid (**c**), however, staining is negligible. Intense immunostaining is notable in the autonomic-related nuclei (nucleus of the solitary tract and dorsal motor nucleus of the vagus) beyond infancy and into adulthood (arrow). (GAP-43 immunostaining.) From Kinney et al.*[367]

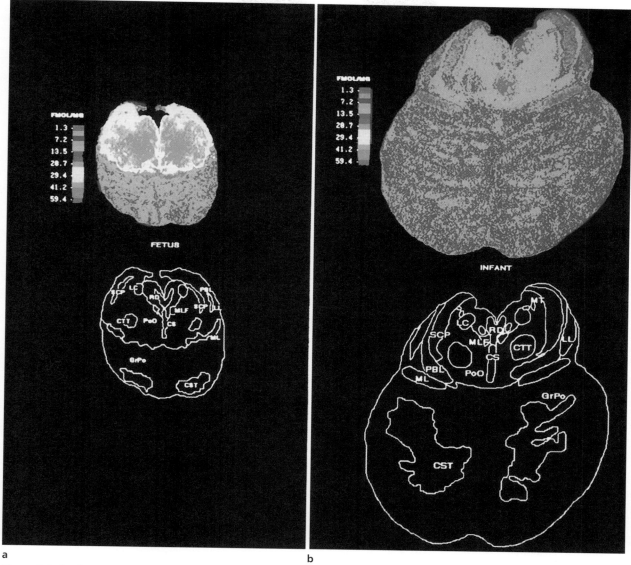

Figure 9.9 *Fetal pons and infant pons at matched levels. The sections, shown at the same scale, are from fetal and infant cases at (a) 21 gestational weeks and (b) 53.5 postconceptional weeks, respectively. The top figure is the computer-generated, colour-coded specific activity mosaic in fmol/mg; the bottom figure demonstrates the anatomical boundaries of brainstem nuclei and fibre tracts. The colour scale with specific activity levels is shown in the accompanying scale. A marked decrease in [³H]nicotine binding occurs in the nucleus pontis oralis, locus coeruleus and nucleus parabrachialis lateralis from the fetal to the infant period. In contrast, binding remains constant in the griseum pontis. ([³H]Nicotine binding.) From Kinney et al.[367]*

Astrocytes

Radial glial cells are the first of the telencephalic glial cell sublineages to be morphologically and immunologically identified. Radial glial cells express glial fibrillary acidic protein (GFAP), the definitive marker of the astrocytic phenotype. They span the entire cerebral wall prior to the first migration of postmitotic neurons, and are thought to organize the cerebral cortex by providing contact guidance to the migrating neurons.[94] They are transient, disappearing at the end of neuronal migration, and transforming into fibrillary or protoplasmic astrocytes.[112,132,674]

Little is known about the cellular or molecular events underlying this transformation. Marin-Padilla[430] studied the prenatal development of astrocytes in the cerebral cortex using the rapid Golgi technique and identified three glial precursors. The first is derived from the original neuroectodermal cells which retain a nucleus above the primordial plexiform layer. This layer I astrocyte is involved in the maintenance of the external glial limiting membrane. The second glial precursor cell is the type I radial glial cell which retains connections with the ependyma and the pia, and functions as a guide for migrating neuroblasts and glial cells. The third glial precursor is a radial glial cell that loses its pial attachment and then its ependymal attachment, and migrates to become the fibre-forming fibrous astrocyte of the white matter. Its relationship to the oligodendrocyte is not defined. After the cortex has formed, additional layer I astrocyte precursors migrate up the radial glia to layer I, contribute to the maintenance of the external glial-limiting membrane and, according to Marin-Padilla, become the subpial granular layer of Ranke.[430] From 15 weeks onwards, the layer I astrocytes begin to send processes towards the developing cortical blood vessels and gradually transform into protoplasmic astrocytes of the grey matter.

In the human fetus, radial glial processes are present by 12 weeks of gestation, and mature GFAP-positive astrocytes are present in the brainstem at 15 weeks and increase until 20 weeks.[564] At 17 weeks they are detected in the hilus of the dentate gyrus[564] and at 18 weeks there is GFAP-positive staining of tanycytes and cells in the germinal matrix. The more posterior germinal matrix matures first, whereas the most anterior portions do not express GFAP reactivity until after 35 weeks of gestation.[259] At 20 weeks of gestation GFAP-positive astrocytes are present in the neocortical plate, and at 28–30 weeks the astrocytes of the outer molecular layer are prominent.[564] Takashima et al.[635] identified GFAP-positive glia in the deep white matter of the cerebral hemispheres by 28 weeks which increase in number until after birth.[259] There is a similar increase in the GFAP-positive glia in the intermediate and subcortical zones of the cerebral white matter, with the deeper layers beginning first and the most superficial beginning last.[630] Takashima and Becker also demonstrated that myelin basic protein (MBP) immunoreactivity lags behind the GFAP immunoreactivity in these regions of the white matter.[630] The distal processes of radial glial fibres disappear from 20–28 weeks of gestation, possibly marking the time when migration on glial guides ceases.[429]

Radial glial cells and layer I astrocyte precursors transform into astrocytes between 21 and 40 weeks of gestation.[347]

In human fetal brain, astrocytes appear to multiply and differentiate independently of, and in many areas well before, myelinogenesis.[564] The capacity of astrocytes to 'react' with proliferation and hypertrophy develops after the first half of gestation. Gliosis is first detectable with GFAP-positive immunostaining around 20 weeks, and gemistocytic morphology is recognized around 23 weeks (Fig. 9.10).[565] Hypertrophied astrocytes are not found in normal myelinating telencephalic white matter.[234] The immature astrocyte responds with less fibre formation than the astrocyte in the older brain. This restricted response creates problems in distinguishing reactive astrocytes from myelination glia (Fig. 9.10). The reactive astrocyte, in haematoxylin and eosin (H&E) preparations, has a pale vesicular nucleus with a rim of irregular smooth eosinophilic cytoplasm. Myelination glia have a smaller, denser nuclei with a 'flag' of cytoplasm on one side of the nucleus. The reactive astrocyte is situated in an abnormal neuropil; myelination glia are found in white matter which appears cellular but orderly, i.e. normal neuropil. The astrocyte of the immature brain can also respond to cellular derangements by increasing the size and pallor of the nucleus. There is a debate as to whether this represents an Alzheimer type 2 astrocyte. Astrocytes in the adult brain play a role in detoxification, remodelling of the extracellular matrix, inflammatory/immune phenomena and production of various trophic factors in response to CNS injury.[492] The developmental profile of these processes in human astrocytes is not known, although there is some knowledge of glutamate receptors in glial cells in immature animals.[621]

Oligodendrocytes and CNS myelination

Human CNS myelination progresses in predictable sequences from caudal (spinal cord and brainstem) to rostral (telencephalon).[79,210,233,236,361,704] It begins at least as early as 12–13 gestational weeks in the spinal cord,[688] and continues at least into the third decade in intracortical fibres of the cerebral cortex.[704] The most rapid changes, however, occur between midgestation and the end of the second postnatal year.[79,361] During development, myelin is produced by the oligodendrocyte as a flattened cytoplasmic process that is elaborated around the axon and becomes compacted to form a tightly wound, membranous sheath. Myelination can be viewed as preceding through two, partially overlapping stages: stage 1, a period of oligodendrocyte proliferation and differentiation, and stage 2, a period of rapid myelin synthesis and deposition. Oligodendrocytes arise and proliferate as precursor cells amid the subependymal zone of the lateral ventricles and are generated over a short period, during late gestation and the early postnatal period.[15,301,402,554]

The analysis of oligodendrocyte maturation has been facilitated by the characterization of sequentially expres-

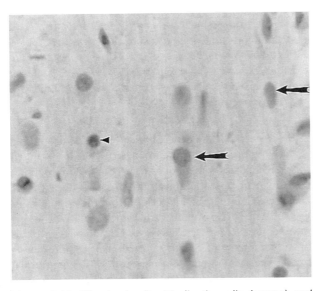

Figure 9.10 *Oligodendroglia. Myelination glia (arrows) and mature oligodendroglia (arrowhead) in the white matter of the cerebrum. (H&E.)*

sed oligodendrocyte cell-specific glycolipids and protein and the development of cell-type-specific antibodies.[227,548] Cell-specific antibodies identify defined phenotypes in the oligodendrocyte lineage. In brief, antibodies to the gangliosides A2B5 and G_{D3} identify the bipotential cell from which all neurons and macroglia are derived. An intermediate stage is identified by immunoreactivity to O4: the mouse monoclonal antibody O4 [immunoglobulin M (IgM)] recognizes the glycolipids sulfatide and seminolipid. This is followed by the acquisition of O1 and 2'3'-cyclic-nucleotide-3'-phosphohydrolase (CNPase) antigens, then proteolipid protein (PLP) and finally MBP. Mouse monoclonal antibody O1 (IgM) reacts with galactocerebroside (GalC), myelin associated glycoprotein (MAG), and less strongly with psychosine, and is a reliable indicator of surface GalC expression. The appearance of O1 and CNPase appears to correlate with terminal progression into the oligodendrocyte lineage.[227]

The regulation of oligodendrocyte number appears to be dependent upon a network of growth factors and associated receptor components coupled to second messenger systems.[256] The role of these factors is relevant in understanding the mechanisms underlying recovery from oligodendrocyte loss in pathological conditions. The success of the reparative process depends, at least in part, upon the regeneration and/or survival of a critical mass of oligodendrocytes in white-matter disorders. Some of the growth factors involved in the control of oligodendrocyte number are platelet-derived growth factor (PDGF) and insulin-like growth factor-I (IGF-I). The role of PDGF upon oligodendrocyte development is two-fold: (1) to stimulate proliferation of O-2A cells until termination by an intrinsic clock; and (2) to stimulate chemotaxis.[491,540,555] IGF-I, a member of the insulin gene family, induces oligodendrocyte proliferation, differentiation and myelin synthesis in cultured glial cells.[421,464] The role of IGF-I in myelination *in vivo* is suggested by the observation that transgenic mice overexpressing IGF-I have increased myelin content.[436] PDGF and IGF-I appear to influence oligodendrocyte survival during development *in vitro* and *in vivo*. Whereas IGF-I increases the survival of both O-2A progenitor cells and mature oligodendrocytes *in vitro*, PDGF increases survival of O-2A cells and only those mature oligodendrocytes which retain PDGF receptors.[46] Competition for survival factors may adjust the number of oligodendrocytes to the number of axons requiring myelination, ensuring even spacing of oligodendrocytes along the length of axons, with death occurring in regions of oligodendrocyte crowding.[46]

The cellular sequences of myelination have been determined in the mid- and late gestational human fetus in the parietal white matter.[38] Myelination is initiated at a restricted number of neurofilament protein-positive axons along which selected oligodendrocyte processes are longitudinally aligned. A discrete population of immature oligodendrocytes (O4+O1+MBP−) displays such initiator morphology and generate 'premyelin tubules' that label for

O4 and O1, but not MBP. A quiescent population of immature oligodendrocytes is detected at 18 gestational weeks, at least 3 months before the onset of myelin sheath synthesis at 30 gestational weeks. At 30 gestational weeks, these immature cells display a complex arbor of processes, which contact multiple axons, and individual processes commonly divide to generate more than one segment of premyelin. At sites of premyelin formation, distal oligodendrocyte processes typically divide into an array of finer processes that span the longitudinal extent of the axon segment. Premyelin tubules are localized together with a transitional population of myelin tubules that label for O4, O1 and MBP, as well as a third population that labels for MBP, but not for O4 or O1. These observations support three sequential phases of myelinogenesis: (1) the initial ensheathment of axons by premyelin tubules generated by immature oligodendrocytes (O4+O1+MBP−); (2) the insertion of MBP into transitional early myelin; and (3) the generation of mature, fully compacted myelin.

The regional sequences of human myelination have been determined in the mid- and late gestational fetus, neonate and infant.[79,210,233,236,361,704] Myelination is rapid from midgestation through the second postnatal year, and is detected in histological sections stained for myelin, e.g. with H&E/Luxol fast blue (LFB) during this period. Gilles *et al.*[236] established the anatomical sequences of human CNS myelination from midgestation to birth. A postnatal study defined the degree of myelination (0–4) in standardized sites based upon the visual intensity of blue LFB staining compared with an internal standard of 'mature myelin' (degree 3) in the inferior cerebellar peduncle.[79,361] Myelination begins in different sites at different times. By birth, the brainstem and cerebellum contain well-myelinated tracts (degree 3), whereas the forebrain almost completely lacks myelin. In the forebrain, only the posterior limb of the inter-

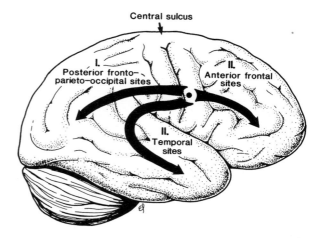

Figure 9.11 *Pattern of myelination. Progression of myelination in telencephalic sites from the central sulcus outward to the poles, with the posterior sites preceding the anterior fronto-temporal sites. The occipital pole (primary visual) myelinates slightly earlier than the posterior parietal (association) white matter. Reproduced by permission from Kinney* et al.[361]

nal capsule, corona radiata, optic tract and chiasm, ansa lenticularis, and pallidal and precommissural fibres contain microscopical myelin (degree 1) at birth. Myelination in telencephalic sites progresses from the central sulcus outward towards all poles: the occipital pole myelinates before the frontal pole which in turn myelinates before the temporal pole (Fig. 9.11). The posterior hemispheres (posterior fronto-parieto-occipital regions) myelinate earlier and more rapidly than the anterior frontotemporal regions. Other sequences in telencephalic myelination follow this general principle, so that the posterior limb myelinates earlier and more rapidly than the anterior limb of the internal capsule and the body and splenium of the corpus, callosum, interconnecting the posterior frontal and parieto-occipital hemispheres, myelinate earlier and more rapidly than the rostrum, interconnecting the frontal poles.

The rate of myelination in a particular pathway or region may change across time, such that the onset of myelination before or at birth is not necessarily associated with early myelin maturation, as indicated by distinct time-related patterns of myelination (Tables 9.4, 9.5). White matter sites fall into eight subgroups based upon: (1) the presence or absence of microscopic myelin (degree 1) at birth (group A or group B, respectively); and (2) the age at which mature myelin (degree 3) is reached in 50% of the cases (Tables 9.4, 9.5). The sites attain myelin maturity within closely related time intervals which are called early (by 6 postnatal months), intermediate (between 7 and 15 months), late (between 18 and 23 months) and very late (after 23 months) (Tables 9.4, 9.5). The proximal and dis-

tal components of an axonal system do not necessarily myelinate simultaneously or even at the same rate. For example, the component fibre tracts of functional systems, e.g. visual system, fall into different subgroups of myelination patterns, in contrast to Flechsig's concept that functional systems myelinate simultaneously. In all projection systems (e.g. visual and auditory pathways, pyramidal system) the proximal components myelinate earlier and more rapidly than the distal components, and the more proximal the component of the system, the shorter its myelination interval. These data indicate considerable variability in myelination within and across multiple axonal systems, and suggest that the molecular and cellular signals which control the timing and synchronization of myelination are likely to be quite complex.

The major lipid components of CNS myelin include cholesterol, galactolipids (cerebrosides and sulfatides), phospholipids and sphingomyelin. The major CNS myelin proteins are PLP and MBP, and the minor ones are myelin-associated glycoprotein (MAG) and CNPase. PLP and MBP are necessary for CNS myelination, probably for membrane compaction. In addition to coding for proteins, the *MBP* and *PLP* genes encode for signals regulating oligodendrocyte number, amount of myelin and other aspects of oligodendrocyte behaviour. Biochemical sequences, as manifested by the appearance of the myelin-associated lipid and myelin-specific proteins, closely follow previously described anatomical sequences both temporally and by region.[366] Sphingomyelin is followed simultaneously by cerebrosides, MBP, PLP and non-hydroxysulfatide, followed by

Table 9.4 White matter sites in Group A

	A-1 (≤68 weeks)	A-2 (70–107 weeks)	A-3 (119–14 weeks)	A-4 (>144 weeks)
Sensory system	Optic tract Optic chiasm			
Auditory			Brachium inferior colliculus	
Other				Tractus solitarius
Pyramidal system	Posterior limb Midbrain CST Pons CST	Pyramid	Cervical CST Thoracic CST Lumbar CST	
Extrapyramidal system	Hilus inferior olive Amiculum inferior Capsule red nucleus Peridentate Middle-cerebellar peduncle	Dentate hilus Ansa lenticularis Pontocerebellar fibres Cerebellum lateral hemisphere	Globus pallidus	Central tegmental tract
Central white matter				
Commissures and capsules	Posterior limb Central corona radiata			
Limbic system		Stria medullaris thalami		Anterior commissure outer

hydroxysulfatide.[366] Cholesterol ester is transiently elevated during late gestation and early infancy, before and around the time of the appearance of cerebrosides, sulfatides, PLP and MPB. The onset and tempo of the expression of individual constituents, however, are quite variable among sites (Fig. 9.12), suggesting a wide differential in vulnerable periods to insult in biochemically specific pathways in early life. The biochemical heterogeneity among myelinating sites is likely to contribute substantially to the regional variability and complexity of the histopathology of many inborn and acquired disorders of CNS white matter in the fetal, perinatal and infant periods.

Microglia

In the immature and mature CNS, microglia are primarily immune effector cells that, as the resident macrophages, play major roles in the defence and repair of CNS tissues in response to injury. In the resting state, microglia form a network which covers much of the CNS parenchyma and probably play a role in tissue homoeostasis. The nature of this role is unknown. During embryonic development, bone marrow-derived monocytes enter the retina and brain and differentiate into microglia through a series of morphological transitions.[138,529] Macrophages in the parenchyma of the developing brain have a different morphology from those in the adult brain, and in animal studies express different surface antigens.[138,529,644] Ameboid microglia cells, a transient population, transform into ramified (resting) microglia cells which persist throughout adulthood and are capable of conversion into active macrophages. Most microglia precursors appear to migrate into the brain during development, before and during the formation of the blood–brain barrier (BBB). The cells become trapped following formation of the BBB and remain as permanent residents in CNS tissues. Subsequent increases in microglial result from their proliferation. Microglia have immunophenotypic properties of monocytes and macrophages. Reactive microglia are distinguished from resting microglia by a change in morphology and of regulation of monocyte–macrophage molecules. A number of monocyte–macrophage antibodies and reagents identify microglia, but microglia-specific antibodies are not yet available.

Animal studies suggest that the stimulus for the entry of monocytes into the developing nervous system and their differentiation to form macrophages and microglia is the programmed death of neurons.[529,530] Dying cells are postulated to act as chemotactic signals for monocytes, and to stimulate monocytic recruitment for phagocytosis and removal of cellular debris. Macrophages make their appearance in developing mouse retina, for example, during the phases of cell death in the ganglion cell and inner nuclear layers where they are seen closely apposed to degenerating neurons.[327] In this way, the monocyte–macrophage–microglia system is thought to participate in the remodelling of the CNS during development. Macrophages are also known to secrete a variety of cytokines and growth factors, including interleukin-1 (IL-1) and tumour necrosis

Table 9.5 White matter sites in Group B

	B-1 (≤68 weeks)	B-2 (70–109 weeks)	B-3 (119–42 weeks)	B-4 (>144 weeks)
Sensory system				
Visual	Optic radiation proximal Optic radiation distal	SAF calcarine cortex		Stripe of Gennari
Auditory	Auditory radiation proximal	Heschl's gyrus		
Other			Lateral olfactory stria	
Pyramidal				
Extrapyramidal system		Lateral crus Pedunculi	Medial crus pedunculi	
Central white matter		Distal radiation to precentral gyrus Posterior frontal Posterior parietal Occipital pole	Putaminal pencils Temporal lobe at LGN Temporal pole Frontal pole SAF all sites	
Commissures and capsules	Corpus callosum body Splenium	Rostrum Anterior limb External capsule	Anterior commissure inner	Extreme capsule
Limbic system		Cingulum	Mammillothalamic tract Alveus, fimbria	Medial fornix Lateral fornix

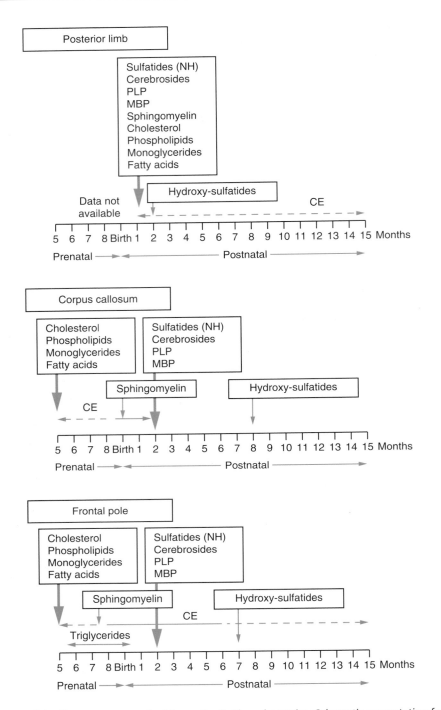

Figure 9.12 *Sequences of the first appearance of white-matter lipids and proteins. Schematic presentation for the posterior limb of the internal capsule ('early' myelinating site), body of the corpus callosum ('intermediate' myelinating site), and frontal pole ('late' myelinating site). Biochemical sequences are identical in the different sites, although they occur at different times. For cholesterol ester (CE), trace amounts are indicated by the dotted line, and more than trace by the solid line. From Kinney et al.*[366]

factor (TNF), that can stimulate angiogenesis and glial proliferation.[243,244,370,399,529] Thus, it is postulated that macrophages contribute to angiogenesis and gliogenesis in the developing CNS.

The timing of microglial histogenesis and migration has been studied in the developing human CNS with monoclonal antibodies having a high specificity for human tissue macrophages, and with lectins, *Ricinus communis* agglutinin-1 (RCA-1) and tomato lectin (TL), *Lycopersicon esculentum*, which recognize macrophages and microglia.[22] Lectin-positive cells are observed at 4.5 gestational weeks, the youngest age examined. They are detected in the leptomeninges around the neural tube, and only rarely in the CNS parenchyma. At 5.5 gestational weeks, lectin-positive cells are present throughout the CNS parenchyma, and a portion of these cells also label with antibody to the macrophage antigen CD68. In subsequent weeks, both types of cells, lectin-positive and CD68[+]/lectin[+] cells, coexist in the CNS parenchyma. Additional immunocytochemical studies with appropriate markers exclude the possibility that any of the cells described with lectins are astrocytes, oligodendrocytes, endothelial cells or neurons. The finding that one class of cells can be labelled early only with lectins, before vascularization, while another can be labelled with both lectins and CD 68 macrophage antibody, and coincides with the development of vascularization in the brain and bone marrow production of monocytes, may reflect a different origin of microglia in the early embryonic CNS compared with the fetal stages. The lectin-positive cells may consist of primitive/fetal macrophages which originate in the yolk sac and colonize the CNS early in development; the lectin[+]/CD68[+] cells may be monocyte-derived macrophages and arise in sites of haemopoiesis (the liver, with shift to the bone marrow later in gestation).[22] Immunohistochemical reactions for macrophages, microglia and human leukocyte antigen (HLA)-DR antigens have been tested on frozen sections of autopsy brain tissue from 20 fetuses and infants ranging in age from 18 weeks to 8 postnatal months.[190] Macrophages are detected at all of these ages, in the germinal matrix and subependymal zones, in perivascular spaces throughout the brain, and in the leptomeninges. Well-differentiated microglia are present after 35 gestational weeks; less well-ramified forms are seen at earlier stages. HLA-DR antigens are detected on a small number of chiefly perivascular macrophages, in almost all cases analysed.[190] The fewest reactive cells and the weakest reactions occur in the youngest fetuses. The microglia–monocyte–macrophage system appears to mature earlier than astroglia because removal of necrotic tissue by macrophages is detected in the fetal brain when the astrocytic response is still minimal.

The ependyma

In the developing nervous system the first structure to differentiate is the floor plate, a specialized ependyma in the midline of the neural tube. The floor plate secretes retinoic acid and sonic hedgehog glycoprotein, and has a ventralizing influence on the neural tube.[705] The immature ependyma is a pseudostratified secretory epithelium, which produces glycosaminoglycans and proteoglycans which repel growth cones, and netrin and S-100, which attract growing axons.[352] The immature ependyma differentiates in a precise spatial and temporal pattern beginning in the floor plate at 3 weeks of gestation and covering the entire surface of the lateral ventricles by 22 weeks of gestation. The pseudostratified epithelium gradually becomes thinned to a single layer of cells with ciliated microvilli on the surface. The mature

cells cannot undergo mitosis. The mature ependymal cells function as regulators of the transport of fluid, ions and small molecules between cerebrospinal fluid (CSF) and brain parenchyma.

TOXIC AND METABOLIC DAMAGE

Hypoxia–ischaemia

Hypoxic–ischaemic brain injury is a major neurological disorder of the perinatal period. The incidence has been reported in various series to range from 1.8 per 1000 to 47 per 1000.[29] Neurological deficits in survivors of perinatal hypoxic–ischaemic encephalopathy include mental retardation, seizures, and cerebral palsy with ataxia, spasticity and choreoathetosis. The neuropathology of hypoxic–ischaemic damage is complex, and there is no single presentation. Rather, in the human infant, the type and extent of hypoxic–ischaemic damage are affected by many structural and functional variables which influence the reaction to injury of the developing CNS.

The fundamental abnormality in hypoxic–ischaemic encephalopathy is a deficit of oxygen supply. Two mechanisms are operative: hypoxaemia, defined as a diminished amount of oxygen in the blood supply; and ischaemia, a diminished amount of blood perfusing the brain. Experimental and clinical data suggest that ischaemia is the more important.[679] Moreover, the period of reperfusion has been shown to be the time of occurrence of many of the harmful consequences of ischaemia on brain metabolism.[677] During the perinatal period, hypoxaemia and/or ischaemia result most commonly from asphyxia, which refers to respiratory dysfunction that causes hypoxaemia, carbon dioxide retention and acidosis. Thus, the entity of hypoxic–ischaemic brain injury has been used synonymously with asphyxia. Asphyxia is followed by a series of metabolic and biochemical reactions that can cause brain injury, lesions of other organs, hypotension, hypoglycaemia and coagulopathy. Each of these insults has potential deleterious effects on the developing CNS, and for each of these, the gestational age of the infant and duration of insult influence the damage inflicted upon the brain. The asphyxia or therapy directed towards its correction can also affect the heart and lungs, and/or central respiratory control circuits, so that there may be continuing insult to the immature nervous system.

Multiple pathological entities have become associated with perinatal asphyxia, including periventricular leukomalacia, status marmoratus and multicystic encephalopathy. A comment about the relationship of such lesions to the clinical diagnosis of cerebral palsy is warranted. Cerebral palsy is defined clinically as a non-progressive motor deficit sustained in the perinatal period. The neuropathology of cerebral palsy is complex, including not only hypoxic–ischaemic encephalopathy in the perinatal period, but also malformations, traumatic lesions, infections and inborn metabolic disorders.[481] The clinicopathological associations of cerebral palsy were examined in the National Perinatal Collaborative Project in the USA, a study of 54 000 pregnancies. This study concluded that perinatal factors, including birth asphyxia, contributed very little to the overall incidence of cerebral palsy; rather, factors operating before birth were responsible for most cases.[480] This observation has been supported by other studies.[651] With such information it is imperative that neuropathologists consider carefully the relationship of cerebral palsy to perinatal asphyxial lesions, as only 12–23% cases can be related to intrapartum asphyxia.[480] That is not to say, however, that intrapartum asphyxia is not important.[263,482] Indeed, a large number of experimental, clinical and brain imaging studies clearly show that brain injury occurs intrapartum in a large number of absolute cases.[679] The Collaborative Perinatal Project showed that one-third of newborns with intrapartum asphyxia had some type of congenital malformation, suggesting that prenatal disorders could predispose to perinatal hypoxia–ischaemia.[480]

The clinical diagnosis of perinatal asphyxia is suspected when there are problems before or during labour, at delivery or immediately after. Fetal asphyxia is associated with meconium staining of amniotic fluid, heart rate above 170 or below 120 beats/min, or irregular heart rate. At delivery the signs suggesting asphyxia include maternal shock, severe antepartum haemorrhage, infarction of the placenta, cord tightly around the neck, prolapse of cord, Apgar at 1 min less than 3, at 5 min less than 5, the need for intermittent positive pressure ventilation, severe postpartum respiratory distress, arterial pH 7.2 or less, or carbon dioxide tension (PCO_2) greater than 60 mmHg. In the neonatal period, the signs suggestive of asphyxia are apnoea, cyanosis, seizures, hypothermia, cerebral cry, feeding difficulties, persistent vomiting and hypotonia. None of the perinatal behavioural or physical indicators of asphyxia can be taken as definitive predictors of eventual outcome, and for each condition an aetiology other than asphyxia may be operating.

GREY-MATTER LESIONS

Hypoxic–ischaemic neuronal cell injury

Most of the energy requirements of the brain are obtained from the oxidation of glucose. Neither oxygen nor glucose is stored in the brain, so that their deprivation, even for only a few minutes, will cause neuronal energy depletion and death. The pathophysiology of hypoxic–ischaemic brain damage is complex and multifactorial, involving vascular and metabolic factors, and is reviewed elsewhere in this book (Chapters 6 and 8, Volume I) and in several recent other sources.[141,398,452,535,639,663,679] An abbreviated outline of the possible sequence of events leading to neuronal damage in the perinatal brain is provided here.

Hypoxia–ischaemia initially depresses adenosine triphosphate (ATP) synthesis with failure of ion pumps, as well as of the energy-dependent glutamate uptake mechanisms in presynaptic nerve terminals and in astrocytes. Extracellular glutamate accumulates and prolongs the stimulation of the N-methyl-D-aspartate (NMDA), kainate and α-amino-3-hydroxy-5-methyl-4-isoxazole (AMPA) receptors. Calcium and sodium enter the neuron through the open NMDA-receptor channels, and sodium enters through open AMPA and kainate-receptor channels. Increases in intracellular sodium and water cause neuronal swelling and 'rapid cell death' via kainate and AMPA receptors. Until a few years ago, the NMDA receptor was the only glutamate receptor subtype known to have an associated calcium channel. Recent studies, however, suggest that the non-NMDA receptors are also associated with calcium channels and influx. In the newborn striatum, loss of glutamate transporters accompanies neuronal loss after hypoxia–ischaemia, suggesting that reduced uptake of glutamate could reflect altered expression of glutamate transporter proteins.[438]

Increased cytosolic calcium plays a pivotal role in the mediation of 'delayed cell death', with multiple deleterious effects. Given that calcium is toxic at high intracellular concentrations, the normal cell contains multiple mechanisms to maintain free calcium concentrations within non-toxic levels. The failures of these protective mechanisms occur during hypoxia–ischaemia. Insufficient adenosine 5'-triphosphate, for example, contributes to calcium accumulation in the cytosol.[141] Increased cytosolic calcium activates numerous lipases, proteases and endonucleases that attack the structural integrity of the neuron, degrading phospholipids, proteins and DNA. Activated phospholipases rapidly hydrolyse membrane phospholipids, releasing free fatty acids. Activated phospholipase A₂ generates arachidonic acid, which mediates injury by several mechanisms, including the uncoupling of oxidative phosphorylation, inactivation of membrane Na/K-ATPase, and stimulation of the release and inhibition of the reuptake of glutamate. Activated calcium-dependent proteases degrade cytoskeletal and regulatory proteins. The prevention of glutamate accumulation in the synaptic cleft and of calcium accumulation in the cytosol are major therapeutic strategies in perinatal hypoxic–ischaemic brain injury. Evidence is mounting that neurotrophic factors are neuroprotective. In a neonatal rat model of hypoxia–ischaemia, prior to hypoxia–ischaemia, postnatal day 7 rat pups received an intracerebral injection of nerve growth factor (NGF): NGF was markedly neuroprotective when the brains were assessed 2 weeks later.[32] While the precise mechanism (or mechanisms) of neuroprotection of NGF is unknown, it may involve upregulation or release of other trophic factors, alterations in free radical detoxification systems (see below) and alterations in response to glutamate-receptor stimulation.[32]

Hypoxic–ischaemic injury generates free radicals in fetal and neonatal tissues during and after the insult, and these in turn perpetuate more tissue and cellular injury. Free radicals are molecular species with an unpaired electron in the outer orbit with a tendency to initiate chain reactions that result in lipid membrane peroxidation and disruption, DNA oxidation and cell damage. Normally, greater than 80% of the oxygen consumed by the cell is reduced by cytochrome oxidase without production of oxygen free radicals.[141,218] The remaining 10–20% follows other oxidation–reduction reactions in the cytoplasm and mitochondria that produce the superoxide anion radical.[141,623] To protect against the deleterious effects of oxygen free radicals, cells possess multiple enzymatic (catalases, peroxidases and dismutases) and non-enzymic (glutathione, cholesterol, ascorbic acid and tocopherol) defences.[141,549] Hypoxic–ischaemic injury generates free radicals that overwhelm these endogenous antioxidant systems. During hypoxic–ischaemic injury, one source of free radicals is the reaction of free ferric iron with peroxide that generates the potent hydroxyl radical. A second source of free radicals is nitric oxide from the activation of nitric oxide synthase and from the infiltration of neutrophils and microglia. In rat cortical neuron cultures, rat hippocampal slices, and in rats *in vivo* in the neonatal period, nitric oxide behaves as a mediator of glutamate toxicity: the neurotoxic effect of NMDA receptors is blocked by nitric oxide synthetase inhibitors. Additional sources of free radicals include increased intracellular calcium and mitochondrial injury, activation of proteases leading to conversion of xanthine dehydrogenase to xanthine oxidase, and activation of phospholipase A_2 leading to increased generation of oxygen free radicals from cyclooxygenase and lipoxygenase pathways. Free radical injury is the critical component of reperfusion injury: when oxygen is reintroduced into hypoxic–ischaemic tissues, the massive production of oxygen free radicals results, producing reperfusion injury over and above the damage already produced during the hypoxia. Several clinical and experimental studies have examined the possibility of reducing neurological morbidity in perinatal hypoxic–ischaemic brain injury by delivering antioxidants and reducing the effects of oxidative stress to the fetal and newborn brain.[582,638]

Hypoxic–ischaemic injury in the grey matter of human newborns,[177,721] as well as perinatal animal models,[541,720] is now known to result in two distinct forms of cell death, necrosis and apoptosis, which are distinguished on the basis of biochemical and morphological criteria. The recognition that apoptosis, as well as necrosis, occurs in perinatal hypoxic–ischaemic brain injury has important implications, as neuroprotective strategies are being developed that may prevent injured cells from committing to apoptotic cell death.[110] Necrosis is characterized by cellular swelling, disintegration of cell membranes and an inflammatory cellular response. Apoptosis is considered a result of an active, intrinsic and delayed programme of cell death, that requires time, energy and, in some instances, gene transcription and translation. It is characterized by cellular and nuclear shrinkage, chromatin condensation and DNA fragmentation ('laddering' by activated endonucleases). As in *C. elegans* where the cysteine protease ced-3 is absolutely required for programmed cell death, the mammalian homologues of ced-3, the caspase family proteases, now are considered the central players in all apoptotic events in mammals.[120] Apoptosis is a result of the proteolysis of various cellular components initiated by activated caspases. *In vitro* abnormalities of mitochondrial morphology and function precede caspase 3 activation, suggesting a role for mitochondria in the cell death cascade. In a rat model of neonatal hypoxic–ischaemic brain injury, caspase activation followed a delayed time-course after hypoxia–ischaemia, and systemic injections of a caspase inhibitor given later resulted in significant neuroprotection.[110] The *bcl-2* family of proto-oncogenes encodes specific proteins which regulate programmed cell death in different physiological and pathological conditions.[77] Several *in vitro* systems have shown that the ratio of the pro-apoptosis protein BAX and the anti-apoptosis proteins Bcl-2 and Bcl-x(l) is critical in determining cell survival. The *bcl-2* family of genes is expressed within the mitochondrial matrix. Measurements of bcl-2, BAX and Bcl-x expression following hypoxia–ischaemia in the infant rat brain are unrevealing, suggesting that bcl-2, BAX, and Bcl-x do not play a leading role in the fate of damaged neurons following a severe hypoxic–ischaemic insult in the developing brain.[202] The mechanism by which hypoxia–ischaemia induces apoptosis is not clear, and many involve several different or overlapping pathways, including free radical damage and increase in concentration of intracellular calcium.[176] Survival signals may be reduced by impaired secretion from injured cells, damage to membrane receptors or interruption of intracellular signalling pathways.[176] Known agents of hypoxia–ischaemia damage, e.g. glutamate and nitric oxide, can induce apoptosis under some conditions.[176]

In tissue sections of perinatal human brains, the conventional morphological criteria for apoptosis are: intense, uniform nuclear basophilia; chromatin condensation with nuclear shrinkage (pyknosis) or fragmentation of the nucleus into several rounded and uniformly dense basophilic masses (karyorrhexis) (Fig. 9.13); or the formation of apoptotic bodies.[177] Cells are considered necrotic if they have intensely eosinophilic cytoplasm, pyknotic or karyorrhectic nuclei, breakdown of the nuclear and plasma membranes, and cell swelling.[177] The ISEL (*in situ* end labelling) and TUNEL (terminal deoxytransferase-mediated dUTP-biotin nick end labelling) methods (based upon the incorporation of labelled oligonucleotides into cleaved fragments of DNA) are frequently used to detect apoptotic cells in tissue sections.

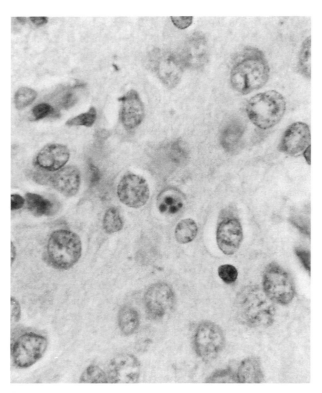

Figure 9.13 *Neuronal karyorrhexis. Immature cerebral cortex. (H&E.)*

These techniques are based upon the incorporation of labelled oligonucleotides into cleaved fragments of DNA. There are several reasons, however, why these techniques should not be regarded as standard for detecting apoptosis, including the observation that DNA fragmentation resulting in the formation of nucleosome ladders has been reported in cells undergoing necrosis, and apoptosis can occur without DNA cleavage.[720] Electron-microscopic criteria are considered the standard for apoptosis but are difficult to meet in human perinatal autopsy material with unavoidably long post-mortem intervals (>2 h) and on a large scale. Immunocytochemical markers for caspase expressions (activation) are considered reliable indicators of cells undergoing apoptosis, particularly when combined with the TUNEL method that identifies dying cells.[478]

Several factors are likely to influence whether a cell undergoes apoptosis or necrosis after hypoxic–ischaemic injury, including the type of initiating insult, the severity of injury, and perhaps the stage of cell maturation and cell type, as well as yet unknown factors. The predominant form of cell death is determined by the dose and the duration of the insult: the same cell type can be triggered to undergo apoptosis following mild injury, but necrosis if the damage is severe. This has now been demonstrated in several *in vitro* systems (see review in Ref. 639). In terms of the stage of cell maturation, it has been speculated that in the fetal and newborn brain developmental processes that involve the apoptotic death of redundant cells are at

their peak or near peak, and therefore immature cell types may be particularly vulnerable to apoptotic cell death triggered by hypoxia–ischaemia at that age. In support of this idea, cerebellar Purkinje cells differentiate early in brain development. In the piglet model of perinatal hypoxic–ischaemia injury, these cells are very sensitive indicators of hypoxia–ischaemia and undergo only necrosis, never apoptosis; in contrast, cerebellar granule cells, which continue to divide and migrate after birth, undergo apoptosis following hypoxic–ischaemic injury.[720] With regard to cell type, it has been suggested that, for as yet unknown reasons, certain cells, e.g. hippocampal pyramidal neurons, necrosis, whereas other cells, e.g. hippocampal dentate gyral cells, only undergo apoptosis.[720] A major criticism of the interpretation of these observations is that the cells considered destined for apoptosis have essentially no cytoplasm in their adult forms, e.g. internal granule cells in the cerebellum, or hippocampal dentate gyral cells. When these cells die by either necrosis or apoptosis, they have a pyknotic nucleus. Moreover, in the premature brain, neuronal necrosis may likewise be characterized by nuclear and cellular pyknosis, as in apoptosis, and recognition of both necrosis and apoptosis amongst normal immature neurons by conventional light microscopy can be difficult since the latter are densely packed, lack cytoplasm and Nissl substance, and have no distinct nucleolus. In contrast, in necrosis in the term neonate and infant, the neuronal cytoplasm becomes hypereosinophilic, the Nissl substance is lost, and the nucleus becomes pyknotic, karyorrhectic or disintegrates. Necrosis is further distinguished in both the preterm and term brain by inflammation: microglia become reactive, and 3–5 days after the insult hypertrophic astrocytes appear. Macrophages phagocytose the necrotic debris and glial scars form; severe lesions may result in cavity formation, especially in the cerebral cortex. Thus, in the fetal brain, in which immature neurons have no cytoplasm, and in the neonatal brain, in which certain mature cell types have little or no cytoplasm, the form of cell death can be difficult to ascertain by conventional microscopy in regions in which there are pyknotic cells without inflammation. Until better markers are available to label apoptotic cells in tissue sections on a large scale (e.g. caspase immunocytochemistry combined with TUNEL technique),[478] the conservative approach may be to diagnose such pyknotic cells simply as 'dying' cells in perinatal brains, without reference to the mode of cell death. Portera-Cailliau *et al.*[536] maintain that neurons injured by excitotoxins in the newborn brain can undergo morphological changes not encountered in similarly injured neurons in the adult brain. They suggest that the morphology of cell death of postmitotic neurons is dependent on maturation. Moreover, the excitotoxic neuronal death in the newborn rat brain model is a morphological continuum, ranging from apoptosis to necrosis, with overlapping morphologies, and this degenerative morphology is dependent on cell type, location and maturation.[536]

FACTORS CONTRIBUTING TO NEURONAL VULNERABILITY TO HYPOXIA–ISCHAEMIA IN THE PERINATAL BRAIN

Passive-pressure circulation

The cascade leading to excitotoxic death of neurons is the same in the immature and mature nervous systems;[717] however, there are several features which are unique to the newborn that contribute to hypoxic–ischaemic damage. Loss of cerebrovascular autoregulation occurs in asphyxiated infants and is a major factor in perinatal hypoxic–ischaemic injury.[267,679] Cerebral blood flow increases with postnatal age, coinciding with an increase in cerebral metabolic activity and demand. Autoregulation is the ability of brain blood vessels to maintain a constant cerebral blood flow in spite of fluctuations in the cerebral perfusion pressure, which depends upon the systemic blood pressure. Autoregulation is maintained by changes in the resistance of cerebral arterioles, the regulation of which depends upon constriction of smooth muscle in vascular walls, oxygen, carbon dioxide, pH, and the sympathetic and cholinergic nervous system, prostaglandins, arginine vasopressin and vasointestinal polypeptide.[398] In newborns, particularly preterm infants, cerebral circulation is very sensitive to minimal fluctuations in blood pressure. In the preterm infant, the range of autoregulation is especially small in the upper limit of the curve, producing a risk for congestion and haemorrhage with modest hypertension.[398] In preterm infants, the mean arterial pressure (which decreases with gestational age) is only slightly above the lower limit of the curve of autoregulation, producing increased vulnerability to ischaemic brain injury with modest hypotension.[398] Moreover, the mechanism of autoregulation is itself sensitive to hypoxemia and hypercarbia in the preterm infant, so that persistent or severe asphyxia causes loss of autoregulation and the cerebral blood flow becomes passive to the changes in blood pressure.[398]

Glutamate receptors

A developmental vulnerability to hypoxia–ischaemia in different regions of the brain has been linked (by animal data) to age-related, transient elevations in glutamate receptors. The neurotoxicity of NMDA in the hippocampus, striatum and neocortex is maximal in the immature rat brain, peaking at postnatal day 6–7.[45] Enhanced sensitivity of the immature brain to glutamate-induced toxicity could reflect increased receptor density, altered receptor sensitivity (due to age-related differences in the molecular constitution of glutamate receptors), or differences in modulatory or compensatory mechanisms.[45] Autoradiographical receptor binding studies in rats indicate that in certain regions, e.g. hippocampus and basal ganglia, the immature brain has a higher density of both NMDA and non-NMDA receptors than the adult brain.[335,419,447,652] Ligand affinities at recombinant NMDA receptors depend upon subunit composition, and there are marked developmental changes in the three major molecular subunits in the NMDA receptor [NMDAR1 (NR1), NMDAR2 (NR2A-B) and NMDAR3] in experimental animals.[391] Ontogenetic peaks, however, of glutamate receptor density and vulnerability to hypoxia–ischaemia do not always parallel one another. Discrepancies are partly explained by simultaneous changes in factors that contribute to excitotoxicity other than the density of glutamate receptors. Some immature neurons, for example, may not be able to buffer glutamate-induced increases in intracellular calcium because they have not yet produced the calcium binding protein calbindin D_{28k}.[45]

Studies of glutamate receptor subtypes have been performed in a limited number of perinatal human brains,[165,394,534] but a comprehensive and systematic mapping throughout the vulnerable period to perinatal hypoxia–ischaemia has not been performed. The developmental profile of glutamate receptor subtypes has been mapped in the human brainstem using tissue autoradiography from midgestation to early infancy, and compared with the adult as the index of maturity.[511,512] There is virtually no NMDA receptor binding in the human fetal brainstem at midgestation, suggesting that the vulnerability of the fetal brainstem to hypoxia–ischaemia is due to the high concentrations of kainate/AMPA, and not NMDA receptors at that age. NMDA receptors appear around birth and thereafter in infancy, whereas AMPA receptor binding sharply declines to significantly low levels thereafter. The finding that NMDA receptor/channel binding is virtually undetectable in all regions of the human fetal brainstem at midgestation is unexpected, given the trophic role for NMDA in early CNS maturation in experimental animals. The brainstem data also suggest a differential development of components of the NMDA receptor/channel complex across early development.[513] Kainate binding is transiently elevated in the fetal and/or infant periods in the basis pontis, the inferior olive, the reticular core and the inferior colliculus, regions all thought to be particularly vulnerable to perinatal, but not to adult, hypoxia–ischaemia (Fig. 9.14).

Antioxidant systems

The newborn human infant, especially the premature infant, may be particularly susceptible to free radical injury in hypoxia–ischaemia because of a relative developmental deficiency in the brain's antioxidants, including the enzymes superoxide dismutase (SOD) and glutathione peroxidase.[334,487] The premature infant also has low circulating levels of glutathione and a relative inability to sequester iron because of low transferrin levels.[610]

NEUROPATHOLOGY OF NEURONAL INJURY IN PERINATAL HYPOXIA–ISCHAEMIA

Neuronal necrosis may occur in a widespread distribution, or in particular combinations of sites, e.g. thalamus–brainstem pattern, pontosubicular pattern, in the perinatal

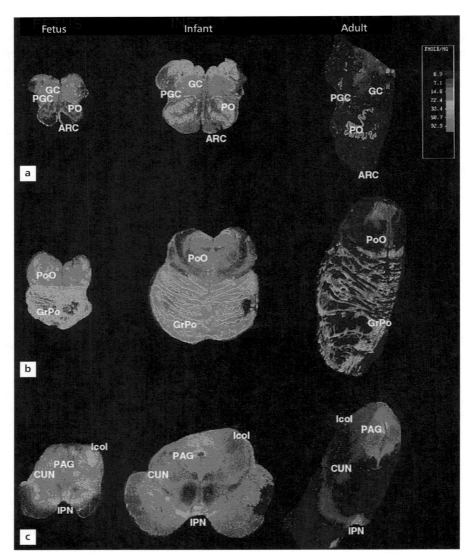

Figure 9.14 *Development in the human brainstem. Relative distribution of [³H]kainate binding in colour-coded, specific activity mosaics across development in the human brainstem at three levels. Three cases are represented: fetus, 21 gestational weeks; infant, 47 postconceptional weeks; and adult, 52 years. The colour scale with specific activity levels in fmol/mg tissues is shown. (a) Rostral medulla: [³H]kainate binding is transiently elevated in the principal inferior olive (PO) in the infant period compared with the fetal and mature periods. Binding is not substantially different between the fetal and infant rostral reticular core nucleus paragigantocellularis lateralis (PLG) and nucleus gigantocellularis (GC), but decreases to low levels by maturity. (b) Rostral pons: the most dramatic change is decreased [³H]kainate binding in the griseum pontis (GrPo) between infancy and maturity (poO, nucleus pontis oralis). (c) Caudal midbrain: there is a substantial decrease in [³H]kainate binding in the inferior colliculus (Icol) between early life and maturity. In contrast, binding in the interpeduncular nucleus (IPN), nucleus raphé dorsalis and periaqueductal grey (PAG) are comparable between infancy and maturity (CUN, nucleus cuneiformis). ([³H]kainate binding.) From Panigraphy et al.[513]*

brain. Neuronal necrosis often coexists with other lesions, such as germinal matrix haemorrhages and periventricular leukomalacia (PVL). Although all neuronal populations are vulnerable to perinatal hypoxia–ischaemia, including the cerebral cortex, the thalamus, the caudate putamen, the globus pallidus, the hippocampus, the cerebellum and the brainstem, neuronal necrosis may occur in these regions in isolation or in overlapping, characteristic patterns. Some of the patterns of injury are seen only in the perinatal period and not in the mature brain, such as thalamic–brainstem injury, pontosubicular necrosis and status marmoratus.

The underlying molecular and cellular basis for the different patterns of neuronal injury in the perinatal brain in response to hypoxia–ischaemia is poorly understood. The reasons for selective vulnerability are likely to be multifactorial. Circulatory factors play a role, as evidenced by selective neuronal necrosis in vascular border zones. There

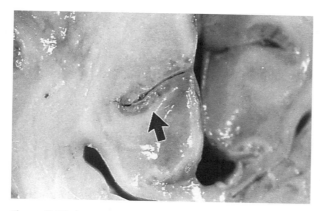

Figure 9.15 *Acute necrosis of the cerebral cortex. The necrotic cingulate cortex in a term neonate is granular (arrow).*

are other factors: differences in regional metabolism that predispose to hypoxic cell death have been identified in experimental systems, e.g. differences in anaerobic glycolytic capacity, energy requirements, lactate accumulations, calcium influx, and free radical formation and scavenging capacity, regional distribution of glutamate receptors, and the regional accumulation of excitotoxic amino acids.[679]

Cerebral cortex

Cortical neuronal necrosis may be focal, bilateral, symmetrical or diffuse (Fig. 9.15). With severe injury, the entire cortex may be involved. Necrosis may be limited to border zone regions between the arterial distribution of major blood vessels: here lesions are thought to result from hypotension and consequent decreased perfusion of tissues served by end branches of major blood vessels. In term newborn and infant brains with cortical lesions, the only gross abnormality may be cerebral swelling, manifested by diffuse widening and flattening of cerebral gyri and partial obliteration of sulci. Cerebral oedema is rarely severe enough to cause bilateral uncal and parahip-

pocampal herniation in the newborn with open fontanelles, and sectioning reveals slit-like ventricles. The 'ribbon effect' may be present: the accentuation of cortical pallor against the congested, red–brown white matter. Total cerebral cortical necrosis results in severe brain 'softening', with fragmentation of the cerebrum upon removal at autopsy.

The microscopic features of acute cortical necrosis vary with the extent of damage. Initially, in preparations stained with H&E or cresyl violet, there is tissue pallor characterized at low power by irregular, sharply delineated zones. The appearance of the necrotic neurons varies with the degree of maturation of the infant (see above). With organization, macrophages phagocytose debris, and endothelial cell swell and proliferate (Fig. 9.16). Neurons in the area of necrosis or at the edge may retain their shape, become encrusted with granular periodic acid-Schiff (PAS)-positive material and occasionally stain for calcium or iron salts (ferrugination of neurons). The capillary bed within or adjacent to the areas of necrosis may also be ferruginized.

In the chronic phase after severe cortical neuronal necrosis, the brain weight may be reduced, and there is a discrepancy between the relative sizes of the cerebrum and cerebellum. Severely damaged cerebral gyri are narrowed, sclerotic, cystic and/or whiter than adjacent intact cortex. Subcortical and/or deep white matter is reduced in volume, sclerotic or cystic. Damaged gyri may have a mushroom appearance termed ulegyria. Ulegyria develops when damage has been most severe at the depth of the sulcus, and when this portion of the gyrus becomes cystic or sclerotic, leaving the more intact wide crown. Sclerotic gyri may contain few or no neurons; the cortical ribbon is replaced by hypertrophic astrocytes and macrophages, producing linear scars of variable sizes and lengths. With survival, astrocytes become fibrillary, with small nuclei and a network of fibres with rare Rosenthal fibres. Macrophages may cluster in the neuropil or in Virchow–Robin spaces.

Hippocampus

The hippocampus of infants is susceptible to hypoxic–ischaemic injury, but this rarely occurs as an isolated lesion. Pathology of the infant hippocampus is difficult to interpret because it is partially immature at birth. Neurons of CA2, CA3 and the endplate have visually matured, but neurons of Sommer's sector (CA1), which is vulnerable to hypoxia–ischaemia, do not appear mature until 2 years of age.[219] Thus, the interpretation of necrosis in Sommer's sector must be made cautiously, evaluating the distinction between immature and pyknotic neurons.[219]

Basal ganglia

The neurons of the infant caudate putamen and the globus pallidus are frequently damaged by hypoxia–ischaemia.

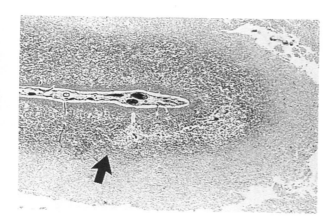

Figure 9.16 *Necrosis of the cerebral cortex. Necrosis in depths of the sulcus extending the width of the cerebral cortex (arrow) in a term neonate.*

In some extensive injuries, a marked gliosis occurs and, if the brain is actively forming myelin in that region, hypermyelination of the area with aberrant myelination of astrocytic processes occurs.[60] There is frequently neuronal loss and mineralization of residual neurons. The resulting white, firm, marbled-appearing lesion is called 'status marmoratus'.[24] It most frequently involves the caudate nucleus and the putamen, and the thalamus in 80–90% of cases,[221] and, less often, the globus pallidus. Status marmoratus is thought to occur if an hypoxic–ischaemic insult occurs before the age of 6–9 months (Fig. 9.2) and the period of active myelination. It has been associated with complicated parturitions or acute febrile illness during the first year of life. Lesions in the basal ganglia occurring after the period of active myelination exhibit only gliosis associated with neuronal loss.

Thalamus

Thalamic neurons are consistently affected in hypoxic–ischaemic injury in the premature and term newborn.[701] They are also vulnerable to damage during fetal life: thalamic lesions have been found in infants whose mothers inhaled household gas or experienced some other catastrophic cardiorespiratory event during gestation. Severe damage to the thalamic nuclei usually accompanies other lesions of the CNS. Histological features of the acute and subacute lesions include neuronal necrosis and neuronophagia, with or without axonal spheroids. The neuropil often demonstrates spongiform change. Chronic lesions are characterized by atrophy, firmness and a chalk-white appearance secondary to gliosis. The third ventricle may be especially dilated owing to thalamic atrophy. There is neuronal loss, gliosis and mineralization of neurons (Fig. 9.17). Walls of blood vessels are occasionally thickened or encrusted with basophilic material.

Cerebellum

Diffuse or isolated foci of cerebellar cortical necrosis are less common than cerebral cortical necrosis, and they most frequently coexist with hypoxic–ischaemic lesions elsewhere. The cerebellum, however, may escape damage altogether in infants with severe cerebral necrosis secondary to perinatal asphyxia. Selective necrosis of mature Purkinje cells does occur, usually in infants beyond 36 gestational weeks,[568] but it is uncommon. Selective granule cell necrosis occurs infrequently in the postnatal period.[568] It also occurs *in utero*: the vulnerability of the cells may in part be due to their high metabolic rate. Immature neurons which form the external granular layer retain their capacity to undergo mitosis after they have migrated and are thus metabolically active cells. This appears to increase their vulnerability to hypoxia[568] (Fig. 9.18). Experimental studies indicate that hypoxia inhibits proliferative activity of the external granule cells and retards development of neuronal processes.[568,718] If destruction of the external granule cells is sufficiently severe, cerebellar hypoplasia can result. Longstanding, diffuse damage of the cerebellum consists grossly of atrophy; there is partial or complete loss of Purkinje cells, variable decrease in granule cells, little or no residual external granular layer, tissue mineralization and proliferation of Bergmann glia. White matter may have a sclerotic appearance with gliosis and little or no myelin.

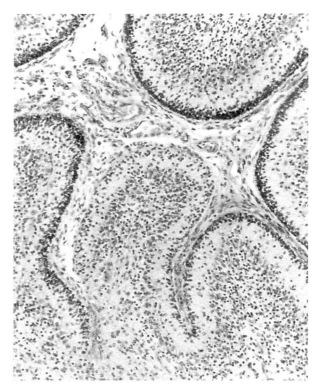

Figure 9.18 *Selective damage to external granular cell layer. One folium in the cerebellum in a fetus at 32 gestational weeks. (H&E.)*

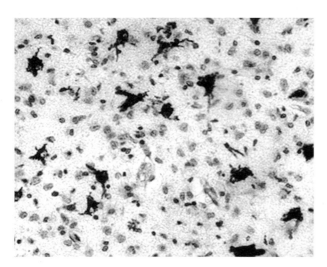

Figure 9.17 *Thalamus. There are darkly staining fossilized neurons and gliosis. (H&E.)*

Brainstem

Involvement of the brainstem is particularly characteristic of hypoxic–ischaemic encephalopathy in the newborn. Selective necrosis of brainstem nuclei is a recognized complication of asphyxia in experimental animals.[472,473,702] In man, the structures most consistently and severely injured include the inferior colliculus, the nuclear populations in the tegmentum at all levels, the basis pontis, the inferior olive, and the gracile and cuneate nuclei. Isolated damage to the brainstem is rarely seen in the perinatal period; selective brainstem neuronal necrosis generally occurs in combination with lesions elsewhere in the neuroaxis.

Pontosubicular necrosis consists of neuronal necrosis (identified by nuclear karyorrhexis and cytoplasmic shrinking) in the basis pontis and the subiculum.[6,220,456] Macrophages appear after 3–5 days and astrocytes proliferate without cavitation. Axonal spheroids are present. Pontine changes vary from a few karyorrhectic cells to subtotal necrosis. Neuronal necrosis in the subiculum may extend into the adjacent Sommer's sector and entorhinal cortex. After several months of survival, pontine atrophy may be seen grossly; microscopically there is neuronal loss and gliosis. The lesion develops from 22 gestational weeks to 2 postnatal months, and is postulated to reflect a response of pontine and subicular neurons in a critical window of development. Although it has been suggested that pontosubicular necrosis represents a distinct form of hypoxic–ischaemic encephalopathy and can occur in isolation, it typically coexists with other forms of perinatal damage, including intraventricular haemorrhages and PVL. An association between pontosubicular necrosis and hyperoxaemia has been suggested.[6]

Spinal cord

Spinal cord neurons undergo necrosis along with neurons of the rostral neuroaxis in severe asphyxia and hypotension. Necrosis of the ventral horn is a typical component of the encephalopathy after cardiac arrest.

WHITE-MATTER LESIONS

Periventricular leukomalacia

PVL is a developmental lesion of the cerebral white matter characterized by focal necrosis in the periventricular region. It is typically associated with diffuse white matter injury, characterized by pyknotic glial nuclei and gliosis. Impaired myelination is a consequence of perinatal cerebral white matter injury, and has been postulated to underlie, at least in part, cerebral palsy in survivors of premature intensive care nurseries. Two widely held (but not mutually exclusive) potential aetiologies for PVL are ischaemia–reperfusion and cytotoxic cytokines released during infection or ischaemia. In addition, a complex interplay of vascular factors predisposes to human periventricular white-matter injury, including the presence of vascular end-zones and a propensity for the sick premature infant to exhibit a pressure-passive circulation reflecting disturbance of cerebral autoregulation. The greatest period of risk for PVL is in the premature infant during mid to late gestation (24–32 weeks) (Fig. 9.2), although it also occurs in full-term neonates. Thus, perinatal cerebral white-matter injury coincides with the period before active myelin synthesis in the cerebral hemispheres, suggesting that oligodendroglial precursors play a key role in the developmental vulnerability of cerebral white matter to injury. Oligodendrocyte differentiation is critical for myelin formation, and sequential stages in oligodendrocyte maturation have been identified experimentally with antibodies to cell-specific markers. The period of risk for perinatal cerebral white-matter injury occurs before active myelin synthesis and the presence of mature, myelin-forming oligodendrocytes in telencephalic white matter. Ischaemic or other insults preferentially to oligodendrocyte precursors could result in their death, with the consequence of a lack of mature, myelin-producing oligodendrocytes and impaired myelination.

OLIGODENDROCYTE INJURY IN PERINATAL CEREBRAL WHITE-MATTER DAMAGE

PVL consists of sharply circumscribed foci in the periventricular regions of the lateral ventricles (Fig. 9.19). These foci measure 2–6 mm in diameter and are within 15 mm of the ventricular wall. The most common locations are anterior to the frontal horn, lateral corners of the lateral ventricles at the level of the foramen of Monro, and lateral regions of the trigone and occipital horn, including the optic radiations. The evolution of PVL begins with coagulation necrosis within 3–8 h of the insult: this consists of nuclear pyknosis, tissue vacuolation (indicative of oedema), staining changes with increased eosinophilia, and acutely necrotic, swollen axons (spheroids). Necrosis of all cellular elements, i.e. oligodendrocyte precursors, astrocytes, blood vessels and axons, occurs in the periventricular foci. Within 12 h, marginal astrocytic proliferation and capillary hyperplasia develop, and within a week, microglia proliferate and lipid-laden cells accumulate (Fig. 9.20). In contrast to coagulative necrosis in systemic tissues, neutrophils do not enter the site of injury in PVL. Reactive astrocytes delineate PVL in its organizing stages, and the swollen axons mineralize, staining for calcium and/or iron (Fig. 9.21). Cavitation occurs within a few weeks (Fig. 9.22); alternatively, the focal necrosis heals with a solid glial scar. The healed lesions stain palely for myelin (e.g. with Luxol fast blue or immunocytologically with antibodies against MBP) as myelin-producing oligodendrocytes are not present within the lesion. In some instances, widespread necrosis of the cerebral white matter occurs,[396] with dif-

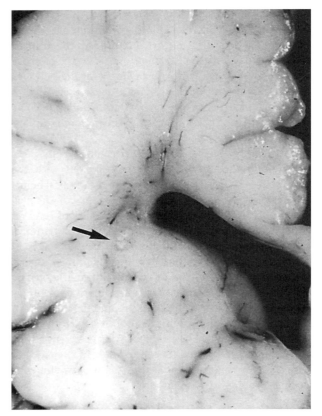

Figure 9.19 *Periventricular leukomalacia. Neonatal brain (arrow).*

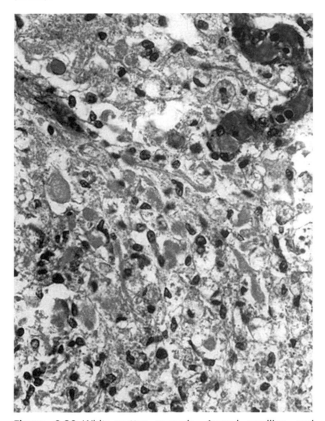

Figure 9.20 *White-matter necrosis. Axonal swelling and bulbs, lipid-laden macrophages and astrocytes. (H&E.)*

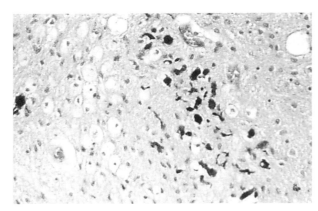

Figure 9.21 *Periventricular leukomalacia. The lesion is characterized by macrophages, reactive astrocytes and mineralized axonal processes.*

fuse damage to all cellular elements, including oligodendrocytes. The relationship of this widespread lesion to PVL (i.e. sharply circumscribed, small necrotic foci in the periventricular region) is unclear, but it may represent the most severe end of a continuum of periventricular white-matter damage. In these extreme cases, necrotic foci extend from the periventricular sites for a variable distance into the centrum semiovale, rarely as far as the subcortical white matter (Fig. 9.23); in the chronic stage, the entire white

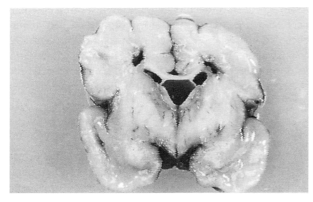

Figure 9.22 *Periventricular leukomalacia. Bilateral cavities are present in the periventricular white matter at the angles of the lateral ventricles.*

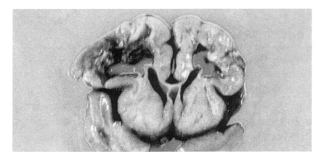

Figure 9.23 *Bilateral cavitation of the cerebral white matter. The lesion involves the periventricular, central and subcortical white matter.*

matter becomes cavitated. When perinatal white-matter damage is severe or longstanding, there may be an overall reduction in cerebral white-matter volume, ventriculomegaly (hydrocephalus *ex vacuo*) and thinning of the corpus callosum.[146]

CEREBRAL WHITE-MATTER GLIOSIS

Diffuse gliosis in the cerebral white matter beyond the territory of focal necrosis is commonly associated with PVL. Hypertrophic astrocytes (defined morphologically in H&E-stained sections by pale, vesicular nuclei and eosinophilic, irregular, hyaline cytoplasm) are present throughout the periventricular, central and intragyral white matter. Their cell bodies stain positively for GFAP, thereby establishing their astrocytic phenotype (Fig. 9.24). In chronic damage, the white matter is markedly decreased in volume relative to the cerebral cortex and the corpus callosum is thin, and ventriculomegaly develops.[146] There are no recognized clinical manifestations of diffuse white-matter gliosis in the perinatal period, nor are there radiographical correlates in the acute phases. Periventricular leukomalacia and diffuse gliosis are postulated to represent a continuum of ischaemic damage to cerebral white matter in the perinatal period. At the most severe end of the continuum is diffuse necrosis extending beyond the periventricular region into central and subcortical white matter, followed by PVL and diffuse gliosis combined, then PVL alone and, at the least severe end, white-matter gliosis alone. Perinatal white-matter damage may coexist with a variety of other CNS lesions. Many of these lesions, like PVL, are considered to be related to hypoxia–ischaemia and include germinal matrix haemorrhage, thalamic infarcts and pontosubicular necrosis. Although the cerebral cortex is typically spared in perinatal white-matter damage, widespread neuronal necrosis may occur. Thus, cerebral white matter damage in the perinatal period occurs neither in isolation nor to the exclusion of grey-matter lesions.

The question is whether the reactive astrocytes in perinatal cerebral white-matter damage are stimulated by diffuse injury to oligodendrocyte precursors in white matter surrounding foci of necrosis (PVL), and/or to axons coursing through the white matter. In the diffusely gliotic white matter, glial nuclei are often pyknotic, 'acutely damaged glia', because injury causes morphological change and thereby precludes their identification as astrocytes or oligodendrocytes.[236] Gilles and Leviton suggested that acutely damaged glia may represent a response of 'pluripotential glial cells' in the telencephalic white matter of newborns to an acute insult.[236] These acutely damaged glia probably include oligodendrocyte precursors, but a specific oligodendrocytic marker that simultaneously labels the damaged cell is needed for certainty. It is possible that the acutely damaged glia may be oligodendrocyte precursors dying by apoptosis complicating ischaemia and free radical attack (see below). Apoptosis is marked by (non-specific) nuclear pyknosis (condensation of chromatin), and is associated with shrinkage of the nucleus and cytoplasm, histological features of the acutely damaged glia. In this regard, apoptosis, demonstrated by light and electron microscopy and the ISEL method, has been reported in the cerebral periventricular white matter of a piglet model of hypoxia–ischaemia; the cell type (astrocyte or oligodendrocyte) undergoing apoptosis was not identified with specific cell markers.[720] Leviton and Gilles[403] suggest that PVL, hypertrophic astrocytes, globules and acutely damaged glia, the major features of perinatal white-matter damage, are all manifestations of the same entity, i.e. acquired perinatal telencephalic leukoencephalopathy (PTL), because of the similarities in their risk-factor profiles, either alone or in combination. Amphophilic globules, located in vessel walls, perivascular spaces or, rarely, extravascular parenchyma, are postulated to represent mineralized-plasma proteins leaked through damaged vascular endothelium.

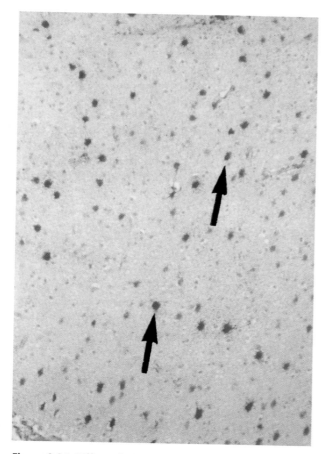

Figure 9.24 *Diffuse gliosis in the cerebral white matter. In the perinatal brain it is characterized by GFAP-positive astrocytes with hypertrophied cytoplasm (arrows). (GFAP immunostaining.)*

OLIGODENDROCYTE INJURY IN PVL

Support for the idea that oligodendrocyte precursors are the main target in perinatal cerebral white-matter injury comes in part from radiographical studies demonstrating hypomyelination or delayed myelination in the telencephalic white matter of survivors beyond the neonatal period.[73,149,166,211,212,699] In a study of premature infants with cystic periventricular leukomalacia analysed in the neonatal period and between 9 and 16 months of age, De Vries et al.[149] reported that magnetic resonance imaging (MRI) scans at 9 months or longer showed dilated occipital horns and delayed myelination in contrast to age-matched controls, most marked in the occipitothalamic radiation in five of six infants; on subsequent scanning in four infants, there was 'good progress in myelination'. Dubowitz et al.[166] reported the evolution of severe PVL by ultrasonography in the perinatal period and by MRI in the postnatal period in three infants who survived the perinatal period. These investigators described the development and subsequent resolution of cysts, followed by the appearance of ventricular enlargement and delayed myelination.[166] The delay was most noticeable in the opticothalamic region, the site of the most extensive lesions observed on ultrasonography. Progress in myelination was observed in one infant in whom a repeat scan was performed, although the degree of myelination was still less than expected for age. In a study of seven very preterm infants with PVL at 44 postconceptional weeks, van de Bor et al.[73] used a myelin grading score in MRI and found impaired myelination compared with age-matched controls. In a study of 15 infants with spastic diplegia or quadriplegia and a history of premature birth who were analysed at a mean age of 17 months, Flodmark et al.[211] found that all computed tomographic (CT) scans showed evidence of reduction of periventricular white matter and ventriculomegaly; in some cases the reduction was so severe that the periventricular white matter was absent and grey matter abutted directly onto the ventricle. A primary loss of axons, as well as hypomyelination, is likely to underlie this severe radiographical abnormality (see below).

Reports of survivors beyond the neonatal period with documented PVL have also been observed at autopsy to have gross and/or histological evidence of impaired myelination. DeVries et al.,[149] for example, reported two infants with PVL documented by ultrasound at 4 weeks and 10 days, respectively, who lived to 7 months and 3 years: at autopsy, the brains were remarkable for ventricular dilatation, gliosis and a generalized lack of white matter (hypomyelination); and periventricular cystic cavities, seen on ultrasound in the perinatal period, had disappeared. Rorke[568] reported anatomical evidence of retarded myelination in telencephalic white matter in 19 autopsied high-risk infants, 15 (79%) of whom had gliosis in the white matter. Almost all of the infants had serious cardiorespiratory dysfunction associated with congenital heart disease, respiratory distress syndrome with bronchopulmonary dysplasia, or repeated episodes of unexplained cyanosis. According to Rorke,[568] 'myelination glia' (oligodendrocyte precursors) are frequently incon-

spicuous in diffuse white-matter gliosis, but this observation has not been confirmed by finding labelled oligodendrocyte precursors by quantitation, a formidable task given the difficulties in labelling oligodendrocyte precursors with immunocytochemical markers in formalin-fixed, paraffin-embedded tissue. Iida et al.[332] addressed the question of delayed myelination in PVL with an immunocytochemical study: antibodies to MBP, a marker of myelinated fibres, and to ferritin, a marker of oligodendrocytes (but not specific to oligodendrocytes), were used. Semi-quantitative assessment did not reveal any difference in these markers between nine infants with only focal PVL (35 gestational weeks to 10 postnatal months at death) and 23 control infants without neuropathological lesions (23 gestational weeks to 12 postnatal months). In contrast, myelination was considered impaired in four of nine patients with widespread necrotic foci or marked gliosis (29 gestational weeks to 10 postnatal months at death): the degree of myelination was decreased relative to controls in the internal capsule and the deep, intermediate and subcortical white matter of the precentral gyrus in Luxol fast blue-stained sections more strongly than MBP-immunostained sections. Hypomyelination was not found by either method in the optic radiation or corpus callosum. In the focal PVL brains, the number and shape of ferritin-containing cells in non-necrotic areas were similar to those in controls; in contrast, in some (one to three) of the nine brains with widespread foci of necrosis or diffuse gliosis, the number of ferritin-containing cells appeared decreased in number. This study suggests that myelination is not affected in focal PVL, but is affected in at least some brains in which there is severe, diffuse damage. Hence, radiographical and pathological studies of PVL support a developmental vulnerability of the white matter to injury: this injury may reflect diffuse death to oligodendrocyte precursors, the predominate oligodendroglial cell type at the age of vulnerability.

AXONAL INJURY IN PVL

The question of primary diffuse axonal damage in perinatal cerebral white-matter injury is not completely resolved, and the possibility exists that ventricular enlargement and decreased white-matter volume, as well as neurological handicaps, in survivors beyond the neonatal period are due, at least in part, to such injury. Axonal injury in focal PVL occurs, without question, as a component of the focal coagulative necrosis, and is identified histologically by swollen axons (spheroids). Recently, Arai et al.[26] demonstrated human Aβ precursor protein (APP) immunoreactivity in spheroids around the edges of the necrotic foci of PVL. In the peripheral and central nervous system, APP undergoes fast axonal transport and is expressed in dystrophic axonal swellings; it is considered a marker of damaged axons in traumatic axonal injury.[228] Arai et al.[26] speculated that intra-axonal accumulation of APP at the periphery of the PVL lesion may be due to disturbances in axoplasmic transport at the lesion sites. In extensive white-matter injury with widespread cavitation (see above), axons are obviously destroyed, as detected in standard histological preparations. A study of subtle axonal injury in the white matter adjacent to foci of PVL and associated with diffuse gliosis is needed using specific markers for axons.

LONG-TERM CONSEQUENCES OF PERINATAL WHITE-MATTER DAMAGE

The long-term consequences of perinatal white matter damage are considered to be hypomyelination due to death of oligodendrocyte precursors, probably at a vulnerable age to hypoxia–ischaemia. The impairment in myelination is responsible for the spastic motor deficits of cerebral palsy. Yet, the question arises: what accounts for the cognitive and attentional deficits, school failure and seizures also found in premature infants? According to the analysis of Golgi preparations of the overlying cerebral cortex of white-matter necrosis, Marin-Padilla[427] found that the subsequent differentiation of the cerebral cortex may be deprived of afferent terminals from corticopetal and association fibres severed by the underlying white-matter lesion. Moreover, some of the neurons will fail to reach their targets because their axons (corticofugal fibres)

have also been destroyed by the underlying white-matter lesion. Consequently, the postinjury structural differentiation and functional maturation of the partially isolated grey matter will be altered, resulting in a variety of acquired cytoarchitectural alterations. Axotomized pyramidal cells, for example, are transformed from long-projecting neurons into local-circuit interneurons with an intracortical distribution of their axonal. Some deep-sited axotomized pyramidal neurons develop long horizontal axonic collaterals that expand above the border of the necrotic zone (Fig. 9.25). In this regard, Marin-Padilla[427] proposed that the neurological sequelae (e.g. epilepsy and cerebral palsy) after perinatal white-matter lesions are a direct consequence of postinjury grey-matter transformations. Further, Volpe proposed that white-matter lesions in the premature infant are likely to disrupt the subplate neurons or their axonal collaterals to subcortical or cortical sites, and thereby interfere with their critical functions in cortical development, with an enormous impact upon cortical neuronal development and a variety of cortical projection systems.[680] This hypothesis could be tested by analysis of subplate neurons in premature infant brains with special methods in neuropathology, e.g. lipophilic dyes, Golgi stains and immunocytochemistry. The idea of impaired cerebral cortical development in PVL in the premature infant is supported by a recent study using an advanced quantitative three-dimensional MRI

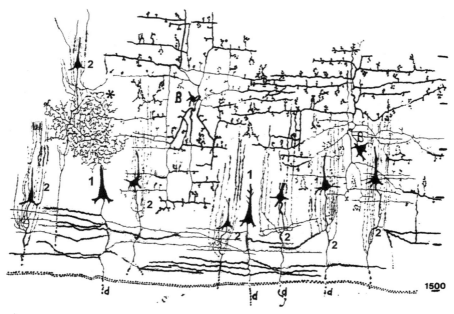

Figure 9.25 *Grey matter overlying subcortical white-matter lesion. Composite figure illustrating some postinjury neuronal alterations. The following grey-matter elements are illustrated: the axonal profiles of two axotomized pyramidal neurons (1) with long horizontal collaterals bordering the necrotic zone (n); the axonal profiles of seven axotomized pyramidal neurons (2) with several long ascending (arcuate) collaterals; the axonal profiles of two large (hypertrophic) basket cells (B) with long horizontal collaterals and numerous terminal pericellular nests; and the complex axonal profiles (*) of unidentified local circuit interneurons. The upper border of the necrotic (n) zone has been marked with a double ink line. The retrograde degeneration (d) and axonal fragmentation of some projecting neurons are illustrated within the necrotic zone. The cortical depth of these GM elements can be estimated by the right scale. (Golgi preparations; camera lucida drawings.) From Marin-Padilla.[427]*

technique: premature infants with PVL had a marked reduction in cerebral cortical grey matter at term compared with either premature infants without PVL or normal term infants.[334]

OLIGODENDROCYTES AND ISCHAEMIA

Current data strongly implicate ischaemia as a major cause of perinatal cerebral white-matter damage.[675] In addition to vascular factors, intrinsic factors related to developing white-matter itself are likely to be important. The temporal association of PVL and diffuse white-matter gliosis with the first stage in telencephalic myelination, i.e. the differentiation and proliferation of oligodendrocyte (premyelinating) precursors, supports the idea that an intrinsic vulnerability of these cell types predisposes them preferentially to ischaemic insult. In the mature brain, it is well recognized that the oligodendrocyte is sensitive to hypoxia–ischaemia and undergoes necrosis to a degree secondary only to the neuron.[416] Potentially major mechanisms underlying the oligodendrocyte injury in ischaemia include glutamate toxicity, free radical injury and cytokine damage mediated by macrophages accompanying ischaemia-induced inflammation.

A role for glutamate toxicity in perinatal cerebral white-matter injury is suggested by the observation that PVL is characterized by coagulative necrosis and disruption of axonal cylinders, thereby raising the possibility that the damaged axons release glutamate extracellularly with toxic effects upon surrounding oligodendrocytes analogous to glutamate's toxic effects upon neurons. In cell culture, Oka et al.[502] showed that oligodendrocytes are vulnerable to micromolar concentrations of glutamate. Moreover, the peak period of glutamate-induced cell death corresponded with the period in which immature oligodendrocytes (O1$^+$, MBP$^-$) dominate the culture, suggesting that glutamate toxicity preferentially involves immature oligodendrocytes.[502] The mechanism of the glutamate-induced oligodendrocyte cell death involves both non-receptor- and receptor-mediated mechanisms. The receptor-independent mechanism involves glutamate transport into cells via glutamate–cystine exchange, depletion of intracellular cystine, a precursor for glutathione, and thereby depletion of glutathione, a key scavenger of oxygen free radicals, and finally death by intracellular oxygen free radicals.[502,710] Oligodendrocyte precursors exposed to gradual hypoxia in culture die because of free radical-induced damage to which they are exquisitively sensitive.[329] The role of free radical toxicity in triggering the death of immature oligodendrocytes is supported by the cytoprotection provided by structurally distinct free radical scavengers, including ascorbate, α-tocopherol and idebenone, despite glutamate uptake into the cell and glutathione depletion.[502] It has been suggested that the mechanism of cell death in free radical attack is apoptosis, as studies of oligodendrocytes subjected to free radical attack in culture show features indica-

tive of apoptosis, e.g. delayed temporal course of cell death (over 12–24 h), ultrastructural changes, the occurrence of oligonucleosomal fragmentation (TUNEL method) and the prevention of cell death by inhibitors of protein or RNA synthesis.[40] Energy failure complicating hypoxia–ischaemia could cause derangements in glutamate uptake and thereby render the oligodendrocyte vulnerable to free radical injury.

Recently, it has been shown that glutamate-induced toxicity to oligodendrocytes is also receptor mediated.[438,714] Cultured oligodendrocytes isolated from perinatal rat optic nerves express AMPA receptor subunits GluR3 and GluR4 and the kainate receptor subunits GluR6, GluR7, KA1 and KA2.[438] Acute and chronic exposure to kainate causes extensive oligodendrocyte death in culture.[438] This effect is partially prevented by the AMPA receptor antagonist GYKI 522466 and is completely abolished by the non-NMDA receptor antagonist 6-cyano-7-nitroquinoxaline-2,3-dione (CNQX), suggesting that both AMPA and kainate receptors mediate the observed kainate toxicity.[438] Chronic application of kainate to optic nerves in vivo results in massive oligodendrocyte cell death which is prevented by simultaneous infusion of the toxin and CNQX.[438] Oligodendrocyte vulnerability to AMPA and kainate receptor activation is fully prevented by removal of calcium from the culture medium, indicating that it is triggered by the influx of this cation through the plasma membrane.[438] Studies are needed to determine whether receptor-mediated glutamate toxicity is cell-stage specific in the oligodendrocyte lineage.

What are the mechanisms underlying the maturation-dependent vulnerability of oligodendrocyte precursors to free radical attack? One possible answer is that a rise in free radicals exceeds the capacity of antioxidant enzymes in the oligodendrocyte precursor to handle the free radicals.[37] The primary antioxidant enzymes required by most cell types to inactivate free radicals are copper- and zinc-containing superoxide dismutase (CuZnSOD), manganese-containing superoxide dismutase (MnSOD), catalase and glutathione perioxidase. CuZnSOD and MnSOD reduce superoxide anion radical (O$_2^-$) to hydrogen peroxide (H$_2$O$_2$); intracellularly, H$_2$O$_2$ is reduced to H$_2$O by catalase and peroxidases. In cell culture exogenous catalase protects against oligodendrocyte cell death induced by free radicals.[355] It is postulated that antioxidant enzymes may be normally upregulated during the course of oligodendrocyte development to prevent toxicity from free radicals generated during the active lipid metabolism of myelin synthesis in the second stage of myelination.[37] Arnold and Holtzman[32] showed an increase in the population of microperoxisomes (which produce catalase) simultaneously with the onset of myelination and their abundance in the oligodendroglial cells during myelination in the rat brain. Adamo et al.[1] reported that catalase activity in oligodendroglial cells, isolated from total rat brain at different ages, increased with maturation. The vulnerability of oligodendrocyte precursors to oxidative stress may in part be due to a lack of or imbalance in the expression of antioxidant enzymes early in development, prior to active myelin synthesis.[37] In a study of six fetuses, seven infants and two adults, Houdou et al.[321] reported that catalase immunoreactive glial cells are not present in cerebral white-matter from midgestation until 31–32 postconceptional weeks, at which time they are first visualized in the deep white-matter; by term, all regions of the cerebral white-matter (deep, intermediate and superficial) contain catalase-positive glia. Takashima et al. reported in a study of ten fetuses (earliest age, 17 weeks' gestation), six children and two adults that SOD-1 immunoreactive glial cells appear in cerebellar white-matter at 25–26 weeks of gestation, and in temporal white-matter at 31–32 weeks of gestation.[636] It is suggested that the catalase- and SOD-1-positive glia are 'myelination glia', i.e. oligodendrocyte precursors, based upon morphological criteria ('eccentric cytoplasm'), but double immunolabelling of catalase- or SOD-1-positive cells with astrocytic (GFAP) or oligodendrocyte precursor (O4 O1) markers was not performed. These human studies suggest that antioxidant enzymes are not produced, or are just beginning to be produced, in telencephalic white-matter in the period of greatest risk for PVL, before active myelin synthesis (less than 35–37 weeks of gestation). Quantitative studies of antioxidant enzymes in developing human brain are needed, as well as cell-specific analysis of CuZnSOD, MnSOD, catalase and gluthionine peroxidase in oligodendrocyte precursors.

Although it is currently unknown which free radical species may be toxic to oligodendrocytes, it may be important that iron is a major source of oxygen free radicals, and that the oligodendrocyte is one of the primary reservoirs of iron within the human brain.[229] The oligodendrocyte transports the protein transferrin, and its storage protein ferritin, suggesting that this cell type may be the mediator of CNS iron metabolism.[124] However, iron, ferritin and/or transferrin also localize to microglia, and to astrocytes in some pathological conditions.[123,125] The peak utilization of iron appears to occur with the onset of myelin formation.[37] Iron is required for cholesterol and lipid synthesis, both of which are abundant in myelin; iron-containing enzymes leading to lipid synthesis (fatty acid desaturase) and degradation (lipid dehydrogenases) are enriched in oligodendrocytes.[123] During development, a variety of free radicals may be normally produced as a byproduct of iron-requiring metabolic processes that are activated near the onset of myelin formation.[37] Iron storage by ferritin is observed in white-matter as early as 19 weeks of gestation in human fetal brainstem, a period when active myelin synthesis is beginning in that region.[458] Ferritin-positive oligodendrocytes (identified by morphological criteria, 'small cells with prominent, rounded nuclei and no or few processes') appear at 25 weeks of gestation in subcortical and periventricular white-matter in frontal and occipital lobes and increase

with age, starting around birth (37–40 weeks of gestation).[509] Supporting a role for iron in triggering free radical-mediated oligodendrocyte injury, cystine deprivation-induced death of oligodendrocyte precursors (see above) is prevented by pretreatment with the iron chelator desferrioxamine.[710] A photochemically induced rise in reactive oxygen species is also prevented in oligodendrocytes by desferrioxamine.[648] The hydroxyl radical, which is generated when H_2O_2 reacts with ferrous ions via the Fenton reaction, is highly toxic to cells.[292]

OLIGODENDROCYTE CELL LINEAGE AND PVL

Given the possibility that an increased susceptibility of oligodendrocyte precursors to death from oxidative stress might contribute directly to the pathogenesis of PVL, the timing of oligodendrocyte lineage progression in human cerebral white-matter is of importance, particularly if oligodendrocyte precursors peak during the known developmental window of vulnerability for PVL (24–32 weeks). Back et al.[39] using double-immunocytochemical methods to co-localize anti-NG2, O4, O1 and anti-MBP antibodies, in a study of parietal white-matter in human fetuses and premature infants, defined three successive oligodendrocyte stages in 26 brains between 18 and 41 weeks of gestation.[39] The successive stages are: the early oligodendrocyte progenitor, the late oligodendrocyte progenitor or preoligodendrocyte, the immature oligodendrocyte, and the mature oligodendrocyte (see above). The chondroitin sulfate proteoglycan NG2 is a marker for rat oligodendrocyte progenitors and preoligodendrocytes. Between 18 and 27 weeks, $NG2^+O4^+$ preoligodendrocytes were the major oligodendrocyte stage present. Between 28 and 41 weeks there was a three-fold increase in immature oligodendrocytes that comprised 32% of the total oligodendrocytes. However, $O4^+$ preoligodendrocytes were still the major oligodendrocyte population. The approach of term gestation was accompanied by a progressive increase in MBP^+ myelin tubules. Thus, the developmental window for periventricular white-matter injury coincides with a period before the onset of myelination. This period is dominated by one major population of pre-oligodendrocytes and identifies these cells as a potential target for injury in PVL (Fig. 9.26).

SUSCEPTIBILITY TO ISCHAEMIA AND VASCULAR ZONES

The susceptibility of developing white-matter to ischaemia has been attributed to vascular zones. Although the presence of arterial border zones has been controversial, some argue that PVL occurs in areas that represent arterial border or end zones.[146,567,631] The blood vessels penetrating the brain from the pial surface, the long and short penetrators, are derived from the middle cerebral artery, and to a lesser extent, from the posterior and anterior cerebral arteries: the putative blood vessels supplying the immediate periventricular area are derived from the

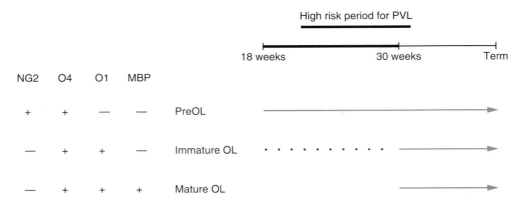

Figure 9.26 *Sequence of oligodendrocyte (OL) maturation in the human brain. Note that the high-risk period for periventricular leukomalacia (PVL) in the human parietal white matter is 24–32 weeks' gestation. From Back* et al.[39]

lenticulostriate arteries and other basal penetrating and choroidal arteries.[567] Ventriculofugal arteries in the human brain are said to run from the lateral ventricle to terminate in deep white-matter. A putative vascular border zone between ventriculopetal arteries of long medullary arteries and ventriculofugal arteries is postulated to explain how hypoperfusion of the fetal brain produced periventricular lesions: the arterial border zones represent distal fields which are the most susceptible to a fall in perfusion pressure and cerebral blood flow. Independent studies have demonstrated the existence of ventriculofugal arteries in fetal and neonatal brains.[631,661,692] Several studies, however, deny the existence of ventriculofugal arteries and a border zone between ventriculofugal and ventriculopedal arteries in developing brain.[379,459] However, a major vascular contribution to white-matter injury is the propensity for the sick premature neonate to exhibit a pressure-passive circulation reflecting a disturbance of cerebral autoregulation,[236] such that decreases in cerebral blood flow accompany decreases in arterial pressure.

OLIGODENDROCYTES AND INFECTION

A causal role for infection in PVL is suggested by several lines of evidence: (1) neonates with bacteraemia[403] or those born to mothers with chorioamnionitis or premature rupture of membranes[526] are at risk for PVL; (2) PVL occurs in a kitten model of *Escherichia coli* endotoxin-induced injury;[235,237] (3) cerebral white-matter lesions occur in fetal rabbits after the induction of maternal intrauterine infection;[711] and (4) elevation in umbilical cord blood of the proinflammatory cytokine Il-6 is associated with an increased risk of PVL.[713] Infectious, inflammatory and coagulation pathways are considered mutually interactive, and neonatal cytokines, chemokines, interferons and coagulation factors have been found elevated in children with cerebral palsy.[483] Higher concentrations, for example, of IL-1, -8 and -9, and TNF-α are observed in neonates on day 3 of life who progressed to childhood cerebral palsy than in any control child.[483] A criticism of the animal model studies is the lack of detailed monitoring for adverse

systemic reactions to infection (endotoxin), including hypotension and failure of autoregulation. Studies in rabbit pups[23] and neonatal dogs[716] demonstrate that cerebral white-matter lesions occur within 1–3 days of endotoxin exposure in the setting of transient acute arterial hypotension. As discussed above, organizing PVL is characterized by infiltrates of macrophages and reactive astrocytes. Of critical importance in understanding the pathogenesis of PVL is information about the cellular mediators of this inflammatory response, particularly in regard to the role of cytokines. Cytokines are a heterogeneous group of polypeptide mediators that have been associated with the activation of the immune response and inflammatory responses.[319] In the CNS, microglia induce reactive astrocytosis via release of TNF, IL-1, IL-6 and interferon-γ (IFN-γ).[492,592] Of relevance to perinatal white-matter injury, these cytokines are soluble and diffusible, suggesting that they play a role, at least in part, in triggering the diffuse reactive gliosis adjacent to focal PVL, the immediate site of inflammation. Microglia are potently stimulated by endotoxin to produce IL-1β, which secondarily stimulates astrocytic expression of both TNF-α and IL-6.[395] *In vitro* studies indicate that TNF-α and IFN-γ have toxic effects upon mature oligodendrocytes.[415,445,559,591,665] TNF causes oligodendrocyte cell death by apoptosis.[420]

In an immunocytochemical study of human perinatal brain tissues, Yoon *et al.*[711] reported the expression of TNF-α, IL-1β or IL-6 in 15 out of 17 cases with and in three out of 17 of cases without PVL ($p < 0.001$). The cytokines were expressed mainly in hypertrophic astrocytes and microglial cells, as demonstrated by double-labelling immunocytochemistry. The expression of TNF-α, IL-1β and IL-6 was identified in 14 out of 17, five out of 17, and 12 out of 17 of cases of PVL, respectively.[711] These findings support the idea that cytokines play a role in the pathogenesis of PVL. Yoon *et al.* proposed that microbial products in PVL stimulate fetal microglia to produce TNF-α, IL-1β and IL-6; TNF-α in turn provides a mitogenic stimulus for astrocytes and is responsible for astrocytic hypertrophy: the white-matter damage of PVL may be the result of a direct cytotoxic effect of TNF on oligodendrocytes.[711] However, that cytokines are part of the inflammatory response, whether induced by infection, ischaemia or other insults, and their presence in microglia and reactive astrocytes in PVL do not prove an infectious aetiology, nor exclude a causal role for ischaemia. More information is needed concerning the cytotoxic effects of proinflammatory cytokines upon immature oligodendrocytes, the predominant cell type of the oligodendrocyte lineage during the greatest period of risk.

COMBINED GREY- AND WHITE-MATTER LESIONS

Parasagittal cerebral injury

This parasagittal cerebral injury refers to necrosis of the cerebral cortex and subjacent white-matter in the parasagittal region with or without haemorrhage. It is characteristic of the full-term infant with perinatal asphyxia (Fig. 9.2). This lesion is most likely to be due to a disturbance in cerebral perfusion: the necrotic areas are in border zones between the end fields of the major cerebral arteries. The most marked injury occurs in the posterior cerebrum and the border zone of all three major cerebral blood vessels. Parasagittal cerebral injury typically does not occur in the premature infant; this is possibly related to the immaturity of the cerebral vasculature and different border zone patterns.[679]

Neonatal 'stroke'

There are two types of thromboembolic stroke in the neonatal period: arterial infarcts, typically in the distribution of the middle cerebral artery,[150,372] and venous sinus thrombosis.[558] Arterial infarcts are seen more commonly in full-term infants (Fig. 9.2) and rarely in premature infants, whereas venous sinus thrombosis occurs in infants of all gestations. Neonatal thromboembolic 'stroke' is a known cause of cerebral palsy. The incidence of arterial stroke in full-term infants is rare, estimated at 1 in 10 000 births. It is relatively common, however, in children born at term with hemiplegic cerebral palsy (22%), and among full-term infants with neonatal seizures (18%). The incidence of venous sinus thrombosis is unknown. The neonate with an arterial infarct may present with seizures, apnoea, lethargy or focal weakness. Alternatively, the patient may present during early childhood with focal weakness and cerebral palsy. Little is known about the risk of recurrence in the patient or in subsequent pregnancies. The aetiology of neonatal 'stroke' is incompletely understood and the majority of cases remain idiopathic with the infant born after an apparently uncomplicated pregnancy, labour and delivery. Some cases are associated with dehydration or congenital heart defects (embolism). Coagulation defects have been implicated in the pathogenesis of neonatal infarction,[284] including genetic abnormalities, e.g. factor V Leiden mutation,[647,664] prothrombin G20210 variant A, methyltetrahydrofolate c677T mutation, elevation of lipoprotein (a) and deficiencies of protein C, protein S, antithrombin III and plasmogen. Acquired prothrombotic conditions also increase the risk of 'stroke', e.g. the presence of antiphospholipid (anticardiolipin) antibodies.[9] Nevertheless, the incidence of coagulation defects in neonatal 'stroke' remains unknown, as does their interaction with various factors, e.g. infection, hypoxic–ischaemic encephalopathy, to increase risk for 'stroke'. The role of maternal autoimmune coagulation abnormalities in neonatal 'stroke' also needs to be elucidated.

Porencephaly

Porencephaly is a circumscribed area of hemispheric necrosis resulting in a smooth-walled cyst which communicates between the ventricle and subarachnoid space. It has minimal scarring and abnormally formed gyri (micropolygyria), or radial gyri situated around the cyst. It is frequently bilateral. Porencephaly is considered to develop as a result of an ischaemic injury to the brain *in utero*, before the mature cortex has developed (Fig. 9.2). The cyst forms because the immature brain has a propensity to cavitate rapidly in areas of necrosis.

Multicystic encephalopathy

Multicystic encephalopathy refers to lesions composed of large septated cavities throughout the cerebral cortex and white-matter of both hemispheres (Fig. 9.27). The cavities are variable in distribution, with a relative, but not total, sparing of the temporal lobe, basal ganglia and brainstem. Most lesions are thought to develop as the

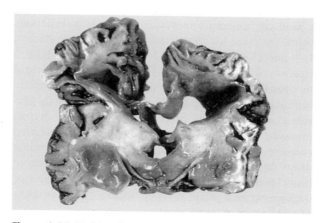

Figure 9.27 *Multicystic encephalopathy. There are large septated cavities throughout the central cortex and white matter of both cerebral hemispheres.*

result of an hypoxic–ischaemic insult near the end of gestation or in the early post-natal period (Fig. 9.2).[688] However, multicystic encephalopathy is not specific for hypoxic–ischaemic damage but can occur in other settings, e.g. herpes viral infection.[688]

Prenatal exposure to maternal cocaine and intrauterine brain lesions

Cocaine impairs the reuptake of noradrenaline and adrenaline by presynaptic nerve endings leading to the activation of the adrenergic system with tachycardia, hypertension and vasoconstriction in the mother, placenta and fetus. These changes are postulated to lead to vascular-related lesions in the fetal brain, including intraventricular and intraparenchymal haemorrhages, large blood vessel cerebral infarcts and PVL.[106,323,676] Many infants exposed to cocaine in utero have been reported with cerebral infarction in the distribution of major cerebral arteries, usually the middle cerebral artery.[163] Based on radiographical and clinical criteria, the timing of the infarcts has varied from hours to months before delivery. Porencephaly has been reported in cocaine-exposed infants,[307] compatible with an intrauterine event occurring early in gestation (Fig. 9.2). In a prospective longitudinal study, three cocaine exposure groups were defined by maternal report and infant meconium assay: unexposed, heavier cocaine exposure, or lighter cocaine exposure.[217] After controlling for infant gender, gestational age, birth weight, maternal parity, blood pressure in labour, ethnicity, and use of cigarettes, alcohol and marijuana during pregnancy, the more heavily cocaine-exposed infants were more likely to show subependymal haemorrhages in the caudothalamic groove than the unexposed infants.[217] The precise incidence of vascular-related lesions in cocaine-exposed infants is controversial, however, and varies considerably in reported series.

The most common teratogenic effect, i.e. effect on brain development, of cocaine is an impairment of intrauterine brain growth, manifested as microcephaly (defined as a head circumference more than 2 standard deviations below the mean for gestational age). In two large studies, 16% and 21.4% of newborns exposed to cocaine in utero (compared with 6% and 3.5%, respectively, of control newborns) had microcephaly, as well as systemic intrauterine growth retardation.[281,294] Microcephaly persists as an intrauterine effect of cocaine when such confounding variables as maternal nutrition, maternal smoking, intrauterine infection and use of other illicit drugs during pregnancy are controlled for. Reports of more severe CNS malformations are rare in intrauterine cocaine-exposed infants. They include a study of a selected group of seven infants with varying combinations of agenesis of the corpus callosum, absence of the septum pellucidum, septo-optic dysplasia, schizencephaly, neuronal heterotopias and optic nerve hypoplasia.[163]

Approximately 10–15% of cocaine-exposed infants demonstrate genitourinary anomalies, most commonly hydronephrosis. Concerning the pathogenesis of the microcephaly and impairment of intrauterine brain growth, cocaine administration to neonatal rats results in inhibition of DNA synthesis in brain regions, raising the possibility of direct toxic effects.[21] Evidence from animal data that prenatal cocaine exposure disrupts the influence of monoamine systems on early neural development is discussed above. Cognitive and neurodevelopmental studies in infants and school-age children exposed to cocaine in utero have revealed no gross intellectual deficits such as mental retardation, but rather subtle deficits in behaviour especially valuable in the classroom, e.g. concentrating for long periods, blocking out distractions, and controlling impulsivity, anxiety, aggression and depression (for review see Ref. 671).

Extracorporeal membrane oxygenation (ECMO) and vascular-related lesions

ECMO, a temporary life-support treatment for neonates with severe cardiorespiratory failure, is the standard of care for neonatal cardiorespiratory failure in many paediatric centres. ECMO has been used in newborns with congenital diaphragmatic hernia, meconium aspiration syndrome, severe pneumonia and septic shock with myocardial dysfunction, with an aggregate survival of >83% in a population with an estimated mortality of 80%.[349] ECMO involves a membrane oxygenator and non-pulsatile blood-flow system. The procedure involves the insertion of cannulaes into the right common carotid artery and internal jugular vein with ligation of the cephalic ends of the two blood vessels. Veno-venous ECMO has recently been introduced and is seen as advantageous to veno-arterial ECMO by preserving the right common carotid artery.[7] Systemic anticoagulation is required.

The neuropathology of ECMO-treated patients suggests hypoxic–ischaemic damage and may be related to the condition of the critically ill infant before, during or after the procedure. Neuropathology includes multifocal cerebral cortical infarcts, neuronal necrosis of the cerebral cortex and other regions, thalamic damage with infarcts, parenchymal haemorrhages, PVL, and pontine and olivary necrosis and/or gliosis.[342,383,640] Infarcts may be associated with the ligation of the carotid artery for cannula placement, although infarcts or haemorrhages do not always lateralize to the right side.[342] Disseminated intravascular coagulation has been associated with multiple, small cerebral infarcts and haemorrhages.[342] Infarcts associated with aluminium emboli were described in the initial period of ECMO use, but are essentially eliminated now by the correction of heat exchangers that utilized aluminium tubes.[672] The systemic heparinization of ECMO-treated infants exacerbates bleeding that frequently occurs during reperfusion in areas that have been ischaemic.

In ECMO survivors, both short- and long-term, neurological complications are predominately related to severe intracranial haemorrhage and cerebral infarction. The absence of intracranial haemorrhage and cerebral infarction before, during and after ECMO has been associated with near-normal short-term outcome.[269] Several ECMO centres have reported that 70–80% of ECMO survivors have normal growth and development.[316,587] There are studies suggestive of poorer neurocognitive or growth outcomes in patients with congenital diaphragmatic hernia surviving ECMO.[7,624]

Congenital heart disease and vascular-related lesions

CNS lesions are frequent complications of congenital heart disease.[75,219,246,643] These lesions include ischaemic or haemorrhagic cerebral infarcts that are the result of thromboemboli from the heart, or paradoxically from the peripheral circulation. Polycythaemia with an increased tendency for local thrombus formation may be responsible for infarcts. Cerebral abscesses occur, particularly with cyanotic congenital heart disease, that permit the mixture of arterial and venous blood, bypassing the pulmonary capillaries.[219] The sources of infection include the respiratory tract and pharynx. Most abscesses are solitary, with a predilection for the cerebral hemispheres, thalamus or cerebellum. *Streptococcus* and mixed organisms are the most common causative agents. In considering congenital heart disease and neurological disease, it is noteworthy that certain cardiac malformations are associated with malformations of the brain. Indeed, the prevalence at autopsy of associated dysgenesis in infants with congenital heart disease ranges from 10 to 29%.[214] Table 9.6 summarizes some of the combined cardiac and brain malformative disorders.

Advances in cardiac surgery since the 1980s have facilitated repair of congenital heart disease in increasingly younger patients, and in many centres, neonatal repair of congenital heart disease is now commonplace.[214,345] Remarkable achievements in neonatal cardiac repair include low-flow cardiopulmonary bypass (CPB) and deep hypothermic circulatory arrest (DHCA) that allow access to a relatively bloodless surgical field. Hypothermia is neuroprotective, by suppressing metabolism, increasing cerebral high-energy phosphates and intracellular pH, decreasing glutamate release and inhibiting excitotoxicity.[345] As surgical and support techniques improve, attention is increasingly focused upon the neurological outcome of survivors and the prevention of preoperative, intraoperative and/or postoperative hypoxic–ischaemic brain injury that may result in life-long cognitive disturbances, seizures and motor disorders.[52,214,345,485] Postoperative infants with congenital heart disease who come to autopsy reveal a diverse spectrum of grey- and white-matter CNS lesions due to hypoxia–ischaemia of varying severity. In one extensive autopsy survey, virtually all brains had some evidence of hypoxic–ischaemic injury, however minor, reinforcing the vulnerability of the perinatal brain to hypoxia–ischaemia.[511] The most frequent types of hypoxic–ischaemic CNS lesions in neonates and infants with surgically corrected congenital heart disease (all surgical modalities combined) in this

Table 9.6 *Examples of combined cardiac and brain malformative disorders*

Disorder	Cardiac malformation	Brain malformation	References
Hypoplastic left heart syndrome	Hypoplastic left heart syndrome	Microcephaly, agenesis of the corpus callosum, microdysgenesis, holoprosencephaly	Glauser et al.[246]
Trisomy 21	Endocardial cushion defect	Microcephaly, foreshortened frontal poles, dendritic and spine abnormalities, altered myelination	Chapter 7, this Volume
Trisomy 13	Ventricular septal defect, patent ductus arteriosus	Holoprosencephaly	Chapter 7, this Volume
Trisomy 18	Ventricular septal defect, patent ductus arteriosus	Neuronal migration defects, olivary anomalies	Chapter 7, this Volume
Catch 22[a], including the diGeorge syndrome and velo-cardio-facial (VCF) syndrome	Conotruncal cardiac malformation (diGeorge syndrome); ventricular septal defect, tetrology of Fallot (VCF syndrome)	Small cerebellar vermis, cysts adjacent to frontal horns, small posterior fossa, myelomeniongocele (VCF syndrome)	Demczuk et al.[143] Mitnick et al.[583] Nickel et al.[486]

[a]Catch 22: cardiac defect, abnormal facies, thymic hypoplasia, cleft palate, hypocalcaemic, chromosome 22q11 deletions; a term used to designate clinical spectrum which includes diGeorge syndrome and VCF or Shprintzen syndrome. Both of these syndromes may present in the newborn period with hypocalcaemic seizures.

series were inferior olivary gliosis, diffuse gliosis of the cerebral white-matter, cerebral cortical injury, hippocampal injury (CA1–4), PVL and brainstem neuronal injury.[511] Diffuse lesions in the basal ganglia, the thalamus and the cerebellum, as well as focal infarcts in the cerebral cortex, the thalamus and the cerebellum, also occurred, albeit to a lesser degree. Taken together, these lesions probably account for most of the diverse neurological handicaps in survivors of cardiac surgery, including cognitive deficits, seizures and motor dysfunction. In this study, there was no correlation between the overall severity of hypoxic–ischaemic brain injury and the length of CPB and DHCA or significant age-related pattern of hypoxic–ischaemic injury in the narrow age window studied.[511] Finally, there were no significant differences in the types of hypoxic–ischaemic lesion among congenital heart disease infants with closed heart surgery without CPB or DHCA; CPB alone; and both CPB and DHCA.[511] Thus, specific types of hypoxic–ischaemic lesions were not restricted to a particular surgical support technique.

No differences in neuroradiological hypoxic–ischaemic abnormalities, as visualized by MRI, have been detected between patients whose surgery was performed using predominantly low-flow CPB, compared with predominantly DHCA.[52] In a clinical trial comparing predominantly low-flow CPB and predominantly DHCA, for example, there were no differences in MRI abnormalities, including PVL and selective neuronal necrosis, in infants of 1 year of age after cardiac surgery.[52] It is difficult, however, to distinguish between the cerebral effects of DHCA and CPB, as CPB is always combined with DHCA. While the neurodevelopment of infants randomly assigned to DHCA was worse than that of infants assigned to predominantly low-flow CPB, both groups had outcomes that were considerably below normal.[52] The study by Glauser et al.[246] found a higher prevalence of acquired neuropathology in infants with hypoplastic left heart syndrome, whose hypothermic arrest time exceeded 40 min. In a study of 40 infants with hypoplastic left heart syndrome coming to autopsy, about half of the infants were free of acquired brain lesions (although microscopic examination was not performed in all grossly normal cases).[246] The other 45% had combinations of hypoxic–ischaemic lesions and intracranial haemorrhage. CNS perfusion and glucose-oxygen delivery appeared to be important factors in the occurrence of hypoxic–ischaemic lesions or intracranial haemorrhage, whereas acidosis and hypercarbia were not.[246]

The postcardiac chorea syndrome is a movement disorder that is seen as a rare complication of CPB surgery accompanied by induced hypothermia during total circulatory arrest time.[703] This procedure enhances tissue preservation while providing a bloodless operative field. The postcardiac chorea syndrome is characterized by chorea and ballismus, and accompanied by hypotonia, tonic conjugate deviations of the eyes, tongue thrusting and inability to swallow.[317] The syndrome has been described in infants and in children as old as 12 years of age, but it occurs predominantly in infants between 9 months and 2 years of age at the time of surgery, and does not occur in neonates. Autopsy cases have demonstrated isolated lesions in the globus pallidus consisting of neuronal loss, reactive gliosis and degeneration of myelinated fibres.[382] In most cases there is a paucity of other lesions despite the dramatic illness. The mechanism for pallidal damage is unknown, but the lack of tissue necrosis in the globus pallidus and the sparing of other brain regions usually susceptible to hypoxic–ischaemic damage suggests either that hypothermia significantly ameliorates the tissue reaction to such damage or that a mechanism other than hypoxia–ischaemia is responsible: the patient's age, rate of cooling and rewarming, presence of pulmonary congestion and management of pH during CPB may influence the outcome. Greeley et al.[264] presented evidence for impaired cerebral autoregulation and cerebral reperfusion during rewarming of infants and children treated with hypothermia and cardiac arrest. It is likely that hypothermia produces brain damage through hypoxic–ischaemic mechanisms by affecting cerebral perfusion rather than by the effects of hypothermia per se.

Kernicterus

Kernicterus, meaning yellow nuclei, was described by Schmorl, who observed yellow staining in specific nuclei in the brains of infants who died with severe neonatal jaundice. The term is also used in clinical medicine for cases with evidence of 'bilirubin encephalopathy': poor feeding, feeble suck, lethargy, high-pitched cry, hypertonia/hypotonia, decerebrate/opisthotonic posturing, seizures, sensorineural hearing loss, incomplete Moro reflex, thermal instability, fever, motor delay, choreoathetosis, asymmetrical spasticity, paresis of upward gaze, dental dysplasia and cognitive dysfunction. All neonates are at risk for increased serum levels of free bilirubin and jaundice.[260] Bilirubin from the breakdown of blood is normally conjugated by the liver to form bilirubin diglucuronide, which is carried into the bile and then deconjugated in the intestine. Here, bacterial flora convert it to urobilinogens and urobilins which are excreted in the faeces. Neonates have immaturity of the enzymes required for bilirubin conjugation so they have more unconjugated bilirubin. They also lack intestinal flora, so that more free bilirubin is absorbed from the intestine. The meconium of the neonate also contains bilirubin and β-glucuronidase, which contributes to the increased level of unconjugated bilirubin in the intestine and serum. In any condition that stresses this immature conjugation and elimination system (prematurity, increased production of bilirubin in haemolytic disease, haematomas, polycythaemia, haemoglobinopathies, hepatic disease, bowel disease with decreased emptying time, cholestatic syndromes and obstruction of the biliary tree), the level of serum unconjugated bilirubin may be increased and cause jaundice, with the possibility of kernicterus. There are additional risk factors, e.g. drugs that displace unconjugated bilirubin from binding proteins in the serum, deficiency of hepatic glucuronyl transferase activity,[219] glucose-6-phosphate deficiency, breast milk[260] and possibly sepsis.[174]

The pathogenesis of the cytotoxic lesions of kernicterus is poorly understood. Bilirubin has been shown to alter the electrophysiology of nervous tissue *in vitro*.[297] Unconjugated bilirubin is lipid soluble and can pass through the BBB. Normally unconjugated bilirubin is bound to serum protein, particularly albumin, but serum pH and drugs competing for the protein binding sites (such as sulfonamides) can increase the amount of unbound unconjugated serum bilirubin and increase its entrance into the brain. Once the bilirubin has entered the brain, there is poor understanding of its specificity for certain groups of neurons and for its mode of cellular injury. It may inhibit oxidative phosphorylation[189] by altering mitochondria.[588] A role for glutamate transport has been postulated in bilirubin encephalopathy on the basis of observations that unconjugated bilirubin in cultured rat cortical astrocytes inhibits glutamate transport.[605] The effect was observed at unbound unconjugated bilirubin concentrations of about 600 nm, similar to the level found in jaundiced newborns.[518] Thus, at least part of the neuronal injury in bilirubin encephalopathy might be due to excitotoxcity caused by the blockade of glutamate transport.

The gross lesions of kernicterus consist of symmetrical bright yellow coloration (due to unconjugated bilirubin) of selective neuronal groups (Fig. 9.28). These, in the term infant, are the globus pallidus, the subthalamus and Ammon's horn. Less common sites are the thalamus, the striatum, the cranial nerve nuclei, the dentate nucleus, the reticular formation, the substantia nigra and the spinal cord. In premature infants tissue coloration is prominent in the lateral thalamus, the locus coeruleus and the Purkinje cells.[5,600] The early microscopic lesions consist of vacuolization of neuronal cytoplasm with eosinophilic change, chromatolysis and spongy neuropil. The coloration of neurons may be observed in frozen sections, but formalin fixation will cause fading of the colour. In subacute lesions there is a loss of neurons and astrocytosis with macrophages. The characteristic sites of these lesions are the subthalamic nucleus, the globus pallidus and, unlike in hypoxia–ischaemia, the resistant sector of Ammon's horn. In the dentate nucleus in kernicterus, dendritic swellings and eosinophilic bodies positive for synaptophysin and neurofilament antibodies have been described.[381] Kernicterus frequently occurs in clinical settings predisposing to hypoxic–ischaemic insults, so that both lesions may be present. Kernicterus is rare if hyperbilirubinaemia can be anticipated, treated or prevented. There has been a concern that, because hyperbilirubinaemia develops after 24 h, the practice of early hospital discharge of mothers and term neonates may increase the incidence of dangerous levels of bilirubin.[260] Preterm infants remain at risk because of their immature livers and intestines.

HYPOGLYCAEMIA

Glucose is essential for brain metabolism. Its homoeostasis is complex, and the effects of hypoglycaemia on the developing fetus and the neonate are not readily identified. Ogata reviewed some of the issues.[498] Before birth the fetus derives its glucose from the mother who, during the first half of gestation, sustains fetal growth and increases her own deposits of fat and glucose. During the second half of gestation maternal catabolism increases, making more fuel available to the fetus. During this time the fetus increases the glycogen reserve in the liver. Thus, conditions associated with maternal hypoglycaemia and ketogenesis (diabetes, fasting, starvation) may have profound effects on fetal growth and the development of the brain and other organs. Altered glucose states in the mother have been related to the health of the infant in later life.[659] In the neonate the development of glycoregulatory capabilities is in a state of change, as enzyme induction continues in the liver and as glycoregulatory hormones (insulin, glucagon) mature in the pancreas. At the time of birth, or prenatally, if the fetus is stressed, elevation of catecholamines will affect gluconeogenesis and the action of insulin. Some of the primary causes of hyperinsulinism in the neonate are being defined[619] and include mutations of the potassium channel in the plasma membrane of pancreatic β-cells, and adenomatous lesions of the pancreas associated with mutations of the sulfonylurea receptor (SUR-1). Glucose production and brain glucose utilization are linked and glucose requirements for the newborn exceed those of adult. The relationship between glucose production and utilization in the brain has been expressed as a ratio of brain to body mass: this ratio is greatest in the premature infant and least in the adult.

The chemical definition of hypoglycaemia has been problematic. The value is less for low birth-weight infants than for term infants. A value of 40–45 mg/dl of serum has been proposed as a safe definition.[589] The difficulties of defining a specific value relate to fluctuations

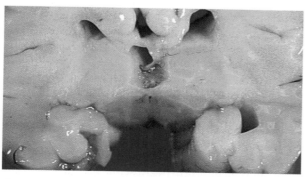

Figure 9.28 *Kernicterus. There is symmetrical, bright yellow coloration of the thalamus. Photograph by Dr H Vogel, Texas Children's Hospital, Houston, TX, USA.*

in glucose levels, differences between blood and serum values, and the state of health of the infant. For example, the small for gestational age (SGA) infant will have less hepatic reserve than that of the appropriate for gestational age (AGA) infant. In this regard, the ratio of the brain weight to liver weight (normal = 3) has been used as an index of the infant's nutritional status at autopsy.[20]

The incidence of neonatal hypoglycaemia is reported to be 1.3–4.4 cases per 1000 full-term births and 15–55 cases per 1000 premature births.[56] The symptoms of hypoglycaemia are not specific and, of particular concern, the newborn may be asymptomatic. The following symptoms have been identified: 'jitteriness', tremors, cyanosis, apnoea, limpness, lethargy, feeding difficulty and seizures. Infants at risk for hypoglycaemia are those with limited glycogen stores, hyperinsulinism and diminished glucose production. Those with limited glycogen stores are: premature infants, infants with perinatal stress and those with glycogen storage disease. Those with hyperinsulinism include infants of diabetic mothers, those with nesidioblastosis/pancreatic islet adenoma, Beckwith–Wiedemann syndrome, erythroblastosis fetalis/change transfusion, and maternal drugs such as chlorpropamide or benzothiazides. Infants with diminished glucose production are SGA infants and those with rare inborn errors of metabolism.

Anderson et al.[20] reported the effects of neonatal hypoglycaemia on the nervous system in six infants. In three untreated cases they observed abnormalities which were diffuse and widespread, affecting large and small neurons. In the small neurons, there were indistinct or absent nuclear membranes and chromatin clumping. In some cells the nucleus was broken into uniform fragments, while in others there was a pyknotic nuclear mass. In large neurons the nuclei were shrunken, opaque and stippled, with chromatolysis. Motor neurons of cranial nerve nuclei and spinal cord contained vacuoles. Nuclei of glial cells were pyknotic in two of three cases. The classic ischaemic neuronal changes (eosinophilic cytoplasm with an irregular pyknotic nucleus) rarely occurred. The authors excluded post-mortem autolysis as the cause of these morphological alterations. The changes developed throughout the brain but did not affect immature cells in germinal areas. The occipital region of the cortex and the insula were the most extensively involved. There was selective vulnerability identified with reference to cortical layers, boundary zones or sulcus versus crest of gyri. The authors considered that the reserves of glycogen in the infant heart preserved its function so that the effects of ischaemia were not involved in the location of the lesions in hypoglycaemia. The infants who received treatment for their hypoglycaemia did not show these lesions, attesting to the importance of treating perinatal hypoglycaemia. The cellular changes of hypoglycaemia in the adult brain are similar to those in the infant but affect the outer layers of the cerebral cortex, the putamen and the caudate, without the involvement of the brainstem and the spinal cord, as in the infant.[392]

The effects of hypoglycaemia per se are difficult to determine because of the additional complications which attend the sick neonate. Functional studies of infants who have survived perinatal hypoglycaemia suggest that the brain may be affected. In a prospective study of SGA preterm infants, recurrent episodes of hypoglycaemia were associated with persistent neurodevelopmental and physical growth deficits until 5 years of age.[172] A retrospective examination of cranial MRI studies of eight children who had severe neonatal hypoglycaemia revealed abnormal signals in the deep white-matter of the parietal–occipital lobes and cortical atrophy, primarily in the occipital lobes. These children were abnormal, exhibiting multiple deficits including clumsiness, quadriplegia, epilepsy and microencephaly. Four children had visual impairment correlating with the occipital lobe lesions,[471] underscoring the importance of visual evaluations in children with neonatal hypoglycaemia. A prospective study using cerebral MRI and ultrasonography of 18 full-term infants with treated perinatal hypoglycaemia (transient perinatal hypoglycaemia) revealed abnormalities in the occipital region and thalamus four times more often than in healthy controls. Fortunately, most of these lesions resolved after 2 months.[356] There are few documented studies of infants with uncomplicated hypoglycaemia who have had functional and morphological long-term evaluations. The availability of excellent imaging technology should allow future meaningful correlations. The present information suggests that treatment of neonatal hypoglycaemia is essential.

The mechanisms of cell injury in hypoglycaemia are complex. Studies in infant rats subjected to a daily episode of hypoglycaemia for 18 days resulted in diminution of brain weight, cellularity and protein content.[105] Auer and Siesjo[35] compared the effects of hypoglycaemia with those of ischaemia and epilepsy. They observed that hypoglycaemia specifically involves the excitotoxin aspartate and that neuronal death occurring in 1–8 h involves the superficial cortical neurons, the middle region of CA1 and the medial subiculum. These hypoglycaemic lesion sites differed from those in ischaemia and epilepsy. There is a cumulative effect of hypoglycaemia when added to ischaemia, hypoxaemia and asphyxia, and an excitotoxic mechanism of cellular injury appears to be operative.[677] Hypoglycaemia is associated with increased extracellular glutamate concentrations, presumed to be due to a combination of increased glutamate release from presynaptic neurons and decreased ATP-dependent glutamate uptake by glial cells.[412] The observed increase in intracellular free calcium during hypoglycaemia is largely mediated by ionotropic glutamate receptors, particularly the NMDA receptor. Increased activation of the NMDA receptor is associated with both acute and delayed neuronal injury. In cell culture, hypoglycaemic neuronal injury is reduced in the presence of NMDA receptor antagonists.[109] In the adult rat, administration of dizocilpine maleate (MK-801), a specific non-competitive NMDA receptor–ion channel antagonist, reduces neuronal necrosis following severe hypoglycaemia in the hippocampus and striatum, but not in the cortex.[514] In contrast, other studies do not demonstrate a neuroprotective effect of MK-801 during severe hypoglycaemia.[724] While changes in NMDA receptor function and neuronal cytoplasmic free calcium concentrations appear to be one mechanism leading to neuronal injury during hypoglycaemia, other mechanisms are likely to be involved. Studies of the pathology of neonatal hypoglycaemia revealed the serious effects of untreated hypoglycaemia.[430]

CEREBRAL HAEMORRHAGES

Intraventricular haemorrhage

Intraventricular haemorrhage (IVH) is the most common intracerebral haemorrhage in the premature infant, with an incidence around 40% in very low birth-weight infants.[691] It causes neurological deficits or death in its most severe forms. Although the incidence of IVH has decreased in recent years, the increasing survival of the smallest premature infants indicates that the lesion will be a continuing problem in intensive care nurseries. Most of the affected babies have been artificially ventilated because of respiratory distress, and perinatal asphyxia may be present.[248] The site of origin of the IVH is usually the germinal matrix which lines the immature ventricles and is thickest in the lateral wall of the lateral ventricle, particularly at the germinal eminence between the head of the caudate and the thalamus (Figs 9.29, 9.30). In the germinal matrix progenitor cells give rise to immature neurons of the caudate, putamen and amygdala between 10 and 20 weeks of gestation, and in the third trimester to immature glial cells. The matrix cells are densely packed immature cells with bare nuclei, associated with thin-walled blood vessels with relatively large lumina.[273] These matrix capillaries are considered to be in border zones in the end field of the striate and the thalamic arteries,[679] which form a fine network of anastomosing arterioles.

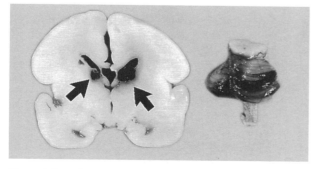

Figure 9.29 *Bilateral germinal matrix haemorrhage. Blood passes through the ventricular system (arrows) and collects over the cerebellum in the posterior fossa.*

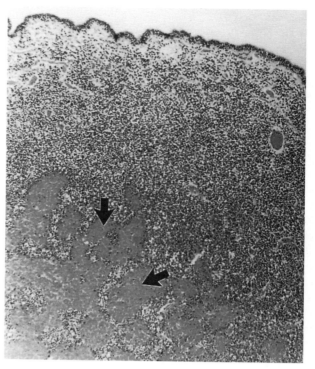

Figure 9.30 *Subependymal, germinal matrix haemorrhage. (Arrows point to blood.)*

Venules of the matrix drain into subependymal veins of the deep venous system converging with the medullary, thalamostriate and choroidal veins as they form the terminal vein, the internal cerebral vein and the vein of Galen.[477]

The blood vessels of the matrix are unusual and may be particularly vulnerable to rupture and haemorrhage, as they are in a state of involution, and excessive fibrinolytic activity has been defined around them in the periventricular germinal matrix regions of the immature human brain.[238] The source of this activity is not known but may reflect the proteolytic action of the plasmin-generating system, and fibrinolysis is one action of the proteolytic system which is found in developing remodelling systems.[679] The end-field architecture of blood vessels of the germinal matrix makes them vulnerable to hypoxic–ischaemic injury, and rupture and the convergence of its veins makes them vulnerable to overloading in conditions where there is venous pressure elevation.

IVH may present as a sudden clinical deterioration with bulging fontenelle, hypotension, seizures, coma and apnoea. It may be protracted over several days or it may be asymptomatic.[517] It is usually diagnosed with cranial ultrasound and graded as follows: grade 1, in the germinal matrix haemorrhage is blood limited to the germinal matrix; grade 2, blood filling the lateral ventricles without distension; grade 3, blood filling and distending the ventricular system; and grade 4, haemorrhage with parenchymal involvement. The definition of grade 4 'IVH' is controversial, because haemorrhage in the periventricular

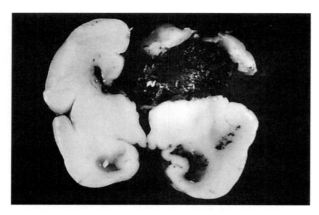

Figure 9.31 *Cerebral parenchymal haemorrhage. Note associated intraventricular haemorrhage.*

white-matter may occur without IVH.[510] In about 15% of cases of IVH there is an intraparenchymal lesion characterized by haemorrhagic necrosis in the periventricular white-matter, lateral and dorsal to the external angle of the lateral ventricles (Fig. 9.31). The lesion is typically asymmetrical, with 67% being unilateral.[679] Approximately half of these lesions are huge, extending from the frontal to the parietal and occipital lobes. They are considered to be venous infarctions related to obstruction of the terminal veins by the large IVH. These may be classified as grade 4 haemorrhages.

Recent studies of the blood vessels of the germinal matrix in preterm neonates have identified a venous origin for most haemorrhages.[230] In serial sections, germinal matrix haemorrhages are small, multifocal and caused by direct injury to the vascular endothelium.[426] The central, often large or dilated, blood vessel (venule) of practically every haemorrhagic focus shows focal endothelial cell necrosis, rupture of the vascular wall and focal thrombosis. The injured blood vessel shows focal cytoplasmic and nuclear fragmentation of a few endothelial cells intermingled with fibrin products, while the remaining vessel wall is unaffected. These small haemorrhagic foci have a tendency to coalesce, thus evolving rapidly into larger destructive lesions. Marin-Padilla[426] argues that by the time most germinal matrix haemorrhages are studied histologically, it is already too late to demonstrate these early vascular changes. Moreover, to demonstrate early vascular changes it is necessary to study serial sections.

SEQUELAE OF IVH

Blood from the germinal matrix haemorrhage enters the ventricular system and subarachnoid space where it may initiate a reactive process in the cerebral aqueduct, meninges or arachnoid granulations, contributing to the development of posthaemorrhagic hydrocephalus, one of the causes of ventricular enlargement in the premature infant.[577] Destruction of the germinal matrix by haemorrhage can lead to cyst formation within the germinal matrix with haemosiderin-laden macrophages, iron and

reactive astrocytes (Fig. 9.32).[128] The reduction of progenitor cells in the germinal matrix has been hypothesized to contribute to the decrease of white-matter seen in infants with ventricular enlargement.[405] In periventricular haemorrhagic injury, Golgi preparations[428] indicate that the local destruction of radial glia stops cellular migration above the lesion (Fig. 9.33), and the precursor cells already travelling in damaged radial glia stop their migration, miss their target and form acquired heterotopias. The thickness of the neocortex overlying a repaired germinal matrix haemorrhage or a posthaemorrhagic hydrocephalus is reduced, and the cytoarchitecture of the maturing grey matter may be secondarily altered (acquired neocortical dysplasia). These cytoarchitectural alterations include displacement and disorientation of neurons, abnormal (atrophic and hypertrophic) neurons, laminar disorganization, anomalies in local circuitry, vascular anomalies, focal heterotopias, microgyria and leptomeningeal heterotopias. These alterations are the result of various factors. Since radial glial fibres (still used in cellular migration) are destroyed throughout the haemorrhagic site, all cellular migration will cease above the haemorrhage and many cells will miss their targets. However, the subsequent degeneration of the ascending radial glial fibres will stop the migration of any undiffer-

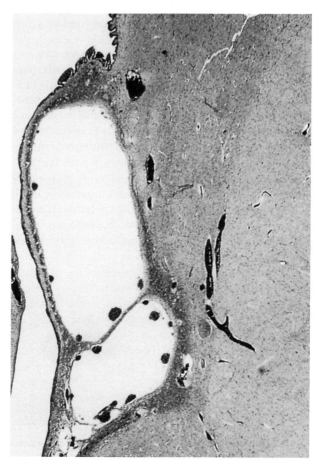

Figure 9.32 *Germinal matrix cyst.*

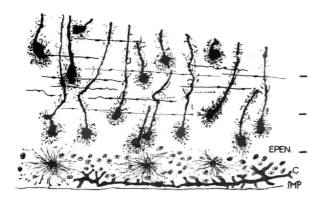

Figure 9.33 *Periventricular haemorrhage. Lesion (EPEN) showing degenerating radial glial fibres damaged (severed) by the haemorrhage with retractile heads, proliferation of fibre-forming astrocytes, haemosiderin-laden macrophages, and postinjury revascularization (C) of the region. From Marin-Padilla.*[426]

entiated cell still being carried by them, resulting in focal heterotopias at any level of the cortex. Any of these posthaemorrhagic grey-matter changes may play a role in the pathogenesis of neurological sequelae.[426]

IVH is rarely an isolated lesion at autopsy; choroid plexus haemorrhage, PVL, necrosis of the basis pontis (pontine necrosis), subicular necrosis or cerebellar necrosis may also occur.[30] The associated brain lesions may contribute to the suboptimal outcome in survivors of severe IVH (motor handicap, hearing impairment, vision loss, seizure disorders[673] and ocular morbidity)[532] and should be considered in attempts to prevent IVH.

AETIOLOGY OF IVH

The aetiology of IVH is multifactorial, and risk factors are defined for various gestations and times of presentation, e.g. prenatal, early postnatal premature, late postnatal premature and mature. IVH has been reported to occur prenatally.[667] A review of all antepartum fetal intracranial haemorrhages identified certain maternal risk factors: alloimmune and idiopathic thrombocytopenia, Van Willebrand's disease, warfarin, cocaine, seizures, severe abdominal trauma, amniocentesis, cholestasis of pregnancy and febrile disease. Fetal risk factors included congenital factor X and factor V deficiencies, haemorrhage into congenital tumours, twin–twin transfusions, demise of co-twin and fetomaternal haemorrhage associated with anaemia.[95,599]

Early-onset IVH in the premature infant occurs within the first day of life, with 50% in the first 12 h. These early haemorrhages are more likely to progress and become a higher grade than are late-onset haemorrhages. The early-onset haemorrhage is associated with lower gestational age, lower birth weight, fetal distress, fetal acidosis, vaginal delivery, vertex presentation, resuscitation and mechanical ventilation.[691] Inflammation of the amnion has been identified as a risk factor,[576] as well as premature rupture of membranes and premature labour.[668] Low

serum thyroxine on initial newborn screening is associated with IVH and death in very low birth-weight infants.[520] One study demonstrated elevation of umbilical cord blood IL-6 in premature neonates who subsequently developed IVH.[687] Antenatal steroids reduce the risk of severe IVH in very immature infants.[107,595] There is an association between pregnancy-induced hypertension and a reduced risk for IVH.[162]

The late-onset haemorrhages are those occurring after the first 24 h. The risk factors are respiratory distress syndrome, vigorous neonatal resuscitation, hypoxemia, suctioning, acidosis, pneumothorax, bicarbonate administration, seizures, hypothermia, heparin use, hypercarbia and blood-pressure fluctuation.[673,691] Indomethacin use may be protective.[691] Most IVH in preterm infants occurs before 5 days of age, irrespective of the gestational age.[443] This may be related to postnatal maturation of the germinal matrix blood vessels. IVH is rare in term infants in whom several clinical presentations have been recorded: apnoea in infants of diabetic mothers, hypoxic–ischaemic encephalopathy and respiratory distress.[295] In 32 cases studied the choroid plexus and germinal matrix were the source of the haemorrhage. In their series, in addition to pulmonary disease, congenital heart defects were common clinical associations.

The final common pathway to rupture of germinal matrix blood vessels may be related to alterations in cerebral blood flow. In ventilated preterm infants with respiratory distress syndrome, Doppler studies[525] have determined that there is a marked continuous alteration in velocity of systolic and diastolic flow, related to the mechanics of ventilation. Serial cranial ultrasound studies have demonstrated the relationship between fluctuating patterns of blood-flow velocity and the subsequent development of IVH.[678] Both increases and decreases in cerebral blood flow are likely to play a pathogenic role in IVH. Sick premature infants are at risk from harmful elevations in cerebral blood flow because there is a limited range of autoregulation and a pressure passive state regulates flow.[679] Increased flow, with resulting vascular congestion, may also occur with hypercapnia. Decreased flow, which can accompany asphyxia and hypotension, may injure the walls of blood vessel, causing then to rupture on reperfusion. Complex alterations in flow and pressure associated with pain[19] or ECMO[299] may be related to IVH.

CHOROID PLEXUS HAEMORRHAGES

In term infants, the majority of IVH arises from bleeding in the choriod plexus, particularly the glomus. In a minority of term infants with IVH, the site of origin is the residual germinal matrix overlying the caudate in the caudate–thalamic groove, the last part of the matrix to involute. Many of the factors relative to cerebral blood flow, venous pressure and vascular integrity that are operative in IVH in the premature infant are also involved in

IVH of the full-term infant. Trauma, however, appears to play a larger role. One-third of cases with adequate perinatal histories have experienced difficult deliveries due to forceps rotations and breech extractions.[679] Approximately 25% of term infants with IVH, however, have no definable pathogenic factors.[679]

CEREBELLAR HAEMORRHAGES

Cerebellar haemorrhages are more common in premature than term infants, with an incidence of 15–25% of premature infants less than 32 weeks of gestation and/or with a birth weight of 1500 g.[274,435,516] The haemorrhages occur in the clinical setting of a difficult delivery, but in a minority of cases there is no obvious predisposing factor. Clinical signs include apnoea, bradycardia, skew deviation of eyes, intermittent tonic extension of limbs and flaccid quadriparesis; the fontanelles are full and the sutures separate owing to obstruction of the flow of CSF.

Cerebellar haemorrhages occur either in isolation or in association with haemorrhage or other lesions elsewhere. They are located in the cortex or subcortical white-matter; they may be multiple and petechial, or focal and large with contiguous blood in the subarachnoid space (Fig. 9.34). Their pathogenesis is probably multifactorial. Particular importance, however, has been attributed to traumatic delivery with breech or forceps extraction, to hypoxic events, especially respiratory distress syndrome, and to prematurity. The compliant skull of the premature has been cited: external pressures, such as associated with breech and difficult forceps extractions, are likely to cause forward movement of the upper part of the squamous portion of the occipital bone under the parietal bones, distorting the venous sinuses at the torcula and increasing venous pressure. Similar pathogenic mechanisms have been suggested in patients with intracerebellar haemorrhage who receive positive pressure ventilation via a face mask with an occipital band.[516] The band causes occipital moulding, resulting in obstruction of major venous sinuses.[516] It is important that cerebellar haemorrhages have been documented by ultrasound before the onset of labour, so that antenatal factors must be considered in their pathogenesis.[282]

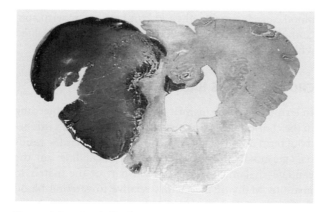

Figure 9.34 *Cerebellar haemorrhage in a premature infant.*

INTRACEREBRAL HAEMORRHAGE

Other causes of intracranial haemorrhage in the perinatal infant include trauma, haemorrhagic infarction (secondary to embolic arterial occlusion, venous thrombosis or arterial thrombosis) coagulation defects (thrombocytopenia, vitamin K deficiency), vascular defects (congenital arterial aneurysm, arteriovenous malformation)[92] and haemorrhage into a cerebral tumour (congenital glioma, cavernous haemangioma, haemangiopericytoma). In the fetus the intracerebral or intraparencymatous haemorrhage has a poor prognosis in 90% of cases, whereas the infants with grade 1 and 2 IVH have a much better outcome.[667] Neonatal haemorrhage is a recognized complication of the maternal administration of anticonvulsant drugs, including hydantoins, barbiturates and primidone (metabolized to phenobarbitol *in vivo*).[126,127,139] Intracranial haemorrhage has been reported in 20–25% of cases in which there is a depression of cord levels of vitamin K, as well as the vitamin K-dependent clotting factors.

INFECTION

In the perinatal period, bacterial, viral, protozoal and fungal organisms infect the CNS. Infections may originate during gestation, intrapartum, or in the first postnatal days or weeks. The pattern of brain injury depends upon the age of the infant. Teratogenic effects arise in the embryonic period when the basic structure of the CNS is under formation. Inflammatory destructive processes tend to occur from the second half of gestation onwards, after formation of the CNS, and when cellular responses to injury, e.g. gliosis, are appropriately developed. There is definite overlap between teratogenic and inflammatory destructive lesions, as destructive processes affecting the developing brain after the first trimester often cause tissue loss and subsequent maldevelopment at the cellular and tissue levels.[679] In the microgyria seen with fetal cytomegalic infection, it has been suggested that the microgyria are not the consequence of a disturbance of neurogenesis or neuronal migration caused by a selective cytopathic effect of the virus on germinal cells, but the result of perfusion failure of the brain.[432] The microbiological aspects of infections have been reviewed elsewhere in this book (Chapters 1–3, Volume II), and are also discussed in other sources.[515] The emphasis of the following discussion is upon the morphological aspects of perinatal infection.

Neonatal meningitis

This term applies to the onset of meningitis in the first 30 days of life. Bacterial meningitis is the most common and serious type of neonatal intracranial bacterial infection.[679] It is more common in premature than full-term infants, and in the first months of life than in any suc-

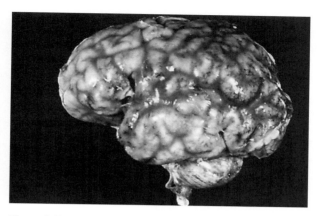

Figure 9.35 *Neonatal bacterial meningitis. The leptomeninges are cloudy and congested.*

ceeding months. Significant host factors are present in the neonatal period that underlie the vulnerability to neonatal meningitis. These include developmental deficiencies in immunity (e.g. immature leukocyte chemotaxis and phagocytosis, deficiencies of IgM and IgG classes of antibodies). The major organisms associated with neonatal meningitis in the order of frequency are: group B *Streptococcus*, *E. coli* (Fig. 9.35) and *Listeria monocytogenes*. Remaining cases are secondary to other streptococcal and staphylococcal species, other Gram-negative enteric bacilli and various unusual organisms. The prognosis for neonatal bacterial meningitis depends upon the microorganism, and the rapidity of diagnosis and therapy. For group B *Streptococcus*, the overall fatality rate is 25%; 50% of survivors are normal and 21% have severe neurological deficits.[178] For Gram-negative organisms, the rates are roughly comparable, with a mortality rate of 17% and a normal outcome of 44%.[216,324,657] During the 1990s, there has been a sharp decrease in the mortality rate for Gram-negative organisms.[216,324,657]

Two patterns of neonatal meningitis are differentiated by their times of onset.[324,527,657,690] Early-onset meningitis begins during the first week postpartum, usually in newborns with a history of complications during labour and delivery. The infection is acquired just before or during delivery, and the responsible organisms are almost always group B *Streptococcus* or *E. coli*. Late-onset meningitis is due to postnatal contamination: it may begin as early as the fourth postpartum day, but usually occurs after the first week. A variety of organisms (e.g. *Staphylococcus*, *Pseudomonas* and *Klebsiella*) have been implicated, in addition to *E. coli* and group B *Streptococcus*. Since bacteraemia virtually always precedes meningitis, a close association exists between the causes and rates of neonatal sepsis and meningitis. Septic dissemination may result from pneumonia, gastroenteritis, umbilical or skin infections, or other systemic infections.

The study of cases of neonatal meningitis with variable lengths of survival has led to a basic understanding of its pathogenesis.[57,72] Bacteria invade the CNS via the blood.

They appear to localize first in the choroid plexus and cause choroid plexitis, with entrance of bacteria into the ventricular system and subsequent movement to the leptomeninges via CSF flow. Ventriculitis, i.e. inflammation of the ventricle and its lining, is a particularly common feature of neonatal meningitis (Fig. 9.36). In the acute phase, i.e. the first week, the predominating cells in the subarachnoid space and ventricles are polymorphonuclear leukocytes (PMNs), with scattered monocytes. Inflammatory infiltrate extends into the Virchow–Robin space. Bacteria are detectable free and within PMNs and macrophages. At the cellular level, certain components of the bacteria incite meningeal inflammation, e.g. lipopolysaccharides (endotoxins) of Gram-negative bacterial cell membranes. The permeability of the BBB is increased and the inflammatory response, with the synthesis and secretion of cytokines, is induced. The CSF culture may be positive, with little or no evidence of leptomeningeal inflammation at autopsy, particularly with early-onset group B streptococcal infections: this discrepancy may reflect the rapidity of death or the immaturity of host responses.

In the second and third weeks, the proportion of PMNs decreases to comprise approximately 25% of the cells. Lymphocytes and plasma cells are present in relatively small numbers. Cranial nerves are infiltrated by exudate. An active ependymitis occurs and glial bridges may develop. After the third week, the exudate decreases and consists mainly of mononuclear cells, including macrophages. The exudate becomes organized, with proliferation of arachnoidal fibroblasts and formation of collagen strands. Dense fibrosis in the leptomeninges and ventricular system obstruct CSF flow and cause hydrocephalus. Vasculitis occurs from the first week with involvement of arteries and veins developing as an extension of the inflammatory reaction in the leptomeninges. Thrombosis with infarction may occur as early as the first week; the lesions are usually related to venous occlusion and may be haemorrhagic. The site of infarction is most often the cerebral cortex and subjacent white-matter, although

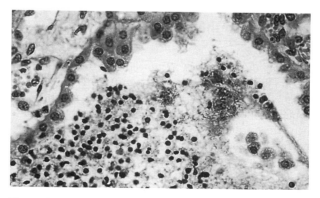

Figure 9.36 *Ventriculitis. Case of neonatal bacterial meningitis. The inflammatory cells are in the ventricle adjacent to the glomus of the choroid plexus.*

subependymal and deep white-matter infarction may occur. Cerebral oedema in the acute phase is common. Its cause is unknown, although it may relate to the vasculitis and increased permeability of blood vessels. This vasogenic component may be complicated by a cytotoxic component when parenchymal infarction occurs. Distensibility of the neonatal skull is likely to account for the low incidence of transtentorial or tonsillar herniation in neonatal meningitis.

Diffuse gliosis occurs in the molecular layer of the cerebral and cerebellar cortex, marginal white-matter of the brainstem and spinal cord, and subependymal regions. This lesion has been postulated to underlie an 'associated encephalopathy' of neonatal meningitis involving the brain parenchyma.[679] This gliosis occurs in regions subjacent to the inflammatory exudate and presumably reflects injury to the superficial regions by toxic and metabolic factors associated with the bacterial meningitis. Other parenchymal lesions include neuronal loss and PVL. These lesions may reflect secondary damage from inflammation. For example, cytokines activate arachidonic acid metabolism. The byproducts of this metabolism include free radicals, platelet activating factor, prostaglandins, thromboxanes and leukotrienes.[545] These products are postulated to lead to neuronal injury. Neuronal loss and PVL may also result from complicating hypoxia–ischaemia, induced by septic shock and systemic hypotension. In addition, cerebrovascular autoregulation is impaired.

The two major neuropathological sequelae of bacterial meningitis in the neonate are hydrocephalus secondary to leptomeningeal or ventricular fibrosis, and multicystic encephalopathy secondary to hypoxia–ischaemia and infarction. Cerebral cortical and white matter atrophy may also occur, secondary to the neuronal loss, PVL and other damage of the 'associated encephalopathy'. More refined techniques, e.g. quantitative Golgi analysis, may reveal subsequent aberrations of brain development, as suggested by experimental data in infant rats in which meningitis was associated with disturbances of subsequent dendritic arborization and synaptogenesis in neurons.[36]

Meningitis in the infant

Haemophilus influenzae, *Meningococcus* and *Pneumococcus* are the most common micro-organisms at 1–2 postnatal years of age. The changes in susceptibility are explained in part by changes in antibody formation in the neonate. Antibodies to *Haemophilus*, for example, readily cross the placenta and grant passive immunity to the newborn; immunity subsides with the expected turnover and decay of antibodies. A lack of immunity between approximately the second month and the second year corresponds to the peak occurrence of *Haemophilus* meningitis. A vaccine has been developed for immunization of infants against *H. influenzae*.

Fungal infections

The most common disseminated fungal infection in the neonate, particularly the premature infant, is with *Candida albicans*. *Mucor*, *Cryptococcus*, *Coccidioides* and *Aspergillus* have rarely caused meningitis and/or abscess in the newborn and infant.[11,219,337,433] The sick, premature newborn in the intensive care unit is particularly vulnerable to disseminated *Candida* and other fungal infections for the following reasons: developmental immune deficiencies, presence of prolonged indwelling vascular catheters and endotracheal tubes (breakdown of anatomical barriers to infection), and the use of multiple courses of broad-spectrum antibiotics (disruption of microbial flora). At least one-third of cases of systemic candidiasis in premature infants exhibit CNS involvement.[192,193] In a study population of 358 premature infants (less than 1500 g) hospitalized for more than 3 days, 4.5% developed invasive candidiasis.[193] The CNS manifestations of candidiasis are purulent leptomeningitis with ventriculitis and hyphae in a granulocytic and lymphocytic exudate, and/or invasion of the brain parenchyma with a widespread necrotizing encephalitis with microabscesses. There are large areas of necrosis, massive granulocytic infiltrates, gliosis and a granulomatous tissue response, often with giant cells. Fungus (yeast spores and mycelial forms) is present in the necrotic areas and the adjacent tissue. Previously, affected infants with CNS involvement were first detected at autopsy or died before therapy could be started. Now, with prompt diagnosis and antifungal therapy, approximately 50% of premature infants have survived without sequelae.[679]

TORCH infections

The major non-bacterial infections of the perinatal CNS are due to viruses, *Toxoplasma* and *Treponema*. The infections of this group are frequently designated by the term TORCH syndrome [T, toxoplasmosis; O, others, e.g. syphilis; R, rubella; C, cytomegalovirus (Figs 9.37, 9.38); and H, herpes simplex (Fig. 9.39) and, more recently,

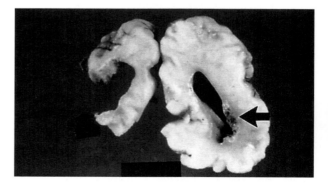

Figure 9.37 *Periventricular calcification. Neonatal brain with cytomegalic viral infection (arrow).*

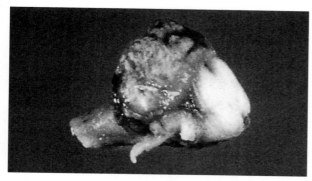

Figure 9.38 *Cerebellar hypoplasia. Neonatal brain with cyto-megalic viral infection. Histologically, the cerebellar tissue was destroyed and extensively calcified.*

human immunodeficiency virus (HIV)]. The TORCH acronym is useful, for it focuses attention upon similarities in the clinical presentation of perinatal infections caused by different agents, and the necessity of diagnostic tests for multiple pathogens in the evaluation of suspected perinatal infection.[368] It also underscores the possibility that clinically silent infection in the neonatal period is associated with dehabilitating long-term effects, and that maternal infections from these agents are usually asymptomatic.[368] The list of other infections now includes not only syphilis, but also tuberculosis, *L. monocytogenes*, leptospirosis, hepatitis B, enteroviruses, adenoviruses, Varicella-zoster virus and Epstein–Barr virus.

Critical pathological features of the TORCH infections are summarized in Table 9.7. Most of these infections result from the transplacental route. Herpes simplex infection, however, is an exception: most cases are contracted around the time of birth, as an ascending infection prior to birth or during passage through an infected birth canal. Neonates with TORCH infections demonstrate a wide spectrum of clinical symptoms, ranging from asymptomatic to severe. Herpes simplex is rarely asymptomatic in the neonatal period.

Neurological manifestations of HIV are rare in the newborn period and do not present until later in infancy.[590] In approximately 85% of paediatric cases of the acquired immunodeficiency syndrome (AIDS), HIV infection appears to be vertically transmitted from mother to infant during gestation or the perinatal period, with blood transfusion accounting for most of the remaining cases.[102] Abuse of intravenous drugs by the mother, in turn, accounts for most cases of maternal infection.[102] HIV has been isolated from fetal tissues, including the CNS, as early as 15 weeks of gestation.[417,616] Longitudinal studies in children have documented neurological abnormalities in approximately 90% of patients, mostly due to a direct HIV infection of the CNS, whereas a spectrum of opportunistic disorders accounts for a high percentage of neurological disease in adults.[91] Neurological manifestations of direct HIV infection in infants and young children include primary HIV encephalopathy, with microcephaly in the congenital cases, pyramidal tract abnormalities, and cognitive impairment characterized by loss of language and social skills. Morphologically, there is cerebral parenchymal atrophy, symmetrical ventricular dilatation, calcification in the walls of blood vessels of the basal ganglia and white matter of frontal lobe, myelin alterations (broad, ill-defined areas of pallor in cerebral white matter to more discrete, well-defined areas of demyelination), white-matter gliosis and scattered macrophages, and inflammatory infiltrates with perivascular microglial nodules and multinucleated giant cells. Cerebral cortical alterations include neuronal depopulation, astrogliosis and scattered multinucleated giant cells. Spinal cord abnormalities include symmetrical pallor of the corticospinal tract.[152] Vacuolar myelopathy, reported in adults, is rare in children. In congenital cases, HIV encephalopathy is associated with microcephaly, but small brain size may be due to secondary destructive effects of the virus, rather than a primary teratogenic effect upon growth. The pathogenesis of neurological manifestations of HIV infection is discussed in detail in Chapter 1, Volume II.

TRAUMA

Birth trauma

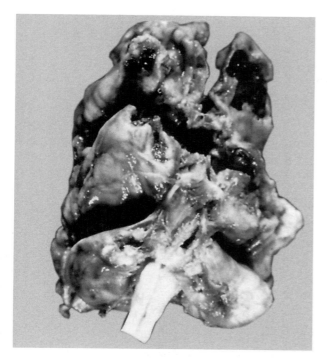

Figure 9.39 *Herpes encephalitis perinatal type II HSE. Acquired during delivery in a term infant. There is generalized cortical necrosis, collapse and haemorrhage.*

Birth trauma refers to injury of the CNS or peripheral nervous system (PNS) in the premature or full-term newborn caused by mechanical factors during labour or delivery.

Table 9.7 *Critical pathological features of the TORCH infections*

Infection	Organisms	Major route of infection	Typical timing of infection	Neuroimaging	Eye	CNS inflammation	CNS teratogenic effects	Late secondary effects
Toxoplasmosis	*Toxoplasma gondii*, protozoan parasite; free, intracellular, or encysted organisms in tissue	Transplacental	Trimesters 1 and 2	Diffuse and periventricular calcifications; calcification of the basal ganglia	Chorioretinitis	Meningoencephalitis with multifocal, necrotizing granulomas; perivascular infiltrates with eosinophils; multifocal and diffuse necrosis of brain parenchyma; miliary granulomas with large, epithelioid cells; organisms in tissue	Porencephaly, hydranencephaly	Hydrocephalus; secondary aqueductal block; microcephaly; secondary tissue destruction
Rubella	Rubella	Transplacental	Trimester 1	Focal calcifications; focal areas of ischaemic necrosis	Chorioretinitis, cataracts, microphthalmia	Meningoencephalitis; necrosis of brain parenchyma; vasculopathy with focal ischaemic necrosis; vascular deposits of amorphous granular material	Microcephaly	Microcephaly; secondary to tissue destruction; delayed myelination; late progressive panencephalitis; hearing loss; secondary cochlear injury
Cytomegalovirus	Cytomegalovirus	Transplacental	Trimesters 1 and 2	Periventricular calcification	Chorioretinitis, cataracts	Meningoencephalitis; parenchymal necrosis; predilection for periventricular region of lateral ventricles; cytomegalic cells; intranuclear inclusions	Microcephaly; polymicrogyria, lissencephaly; pachygyria, neuronal heterotopias	Microcephaly; secondary tissue destruction; cerebellar hypoplasia
Acquired immunodeficiency syndrome (AIDS)	Human immunodeficiency virus (HIV)	Intrapartum; transplacental; postnatal (breast feeding)	Trimester 2 when transplacental; intrapartum (most important)	Difficult detection in neonate; basal ganglia and cerebral calcifications; cerebral and white-matter atrophy		Meningoencephalitis months or years after infection; multinucleated giant cells; diffuse or focal myelin loss; calcific vasculopathy in basal ganglia and cerebral cortex; CNS lymphoma; secondary infection with CMV, fungus or toxoplasmosis; ischaemic and haemorrhagic infarcts; secondary arteriopathy	Microcephaly	Cerebral atrophy; secondary loss of neurons of cerebral cortex and basal ganglia; myelin loss; microcephaly

Infection	Agent	Transmission	Timing	Brain findings	Eye	Pathology		Clinical features
Varicella	Varicella zoster	Transplacental	Congenital Trimesters 1, 2, 3	Dilated lateral ventricles, suggesting loss of cerebral tissue	Chorioretinitis; cataracts; optic atrophy; Horner's syndrome	Meningoencephalitis, myelitis, dorsal root ganglioneuritis, anterior horn cell involvement, segmental muscle denervation, ependymitis		Atrophy or hypoplasia of limb muscle, associated usually with deformity, e.g. talipes equinovarus, hypoplasia of facial, neck or abdominal muscles
Enteroviruses	Coxsackie A and B; echovirus; polio	Transplacental, intrapartum, postnatal infant–infant transmission	Fetal, intrapartum, postpartum	No findings	None	Aseptic meningitis; primary encephalitis (Coxsackie B); neuronophagia of motor neurons	None	Post-poliomyelitis syndrome (adults)
Syphilis	Treponema pallidum	Transplacental	Trimesters 2 and 3		Chorioretinitis, cataracts	Early stage (first two years of life): acute and subacute meningitis, mononuclear inflammation with lymphocytes, plasma cells and macrophages; basal meninges; superficial cortex involved; chronic meningitis most marked in basal meninges; vasculitis with cerebral infarction, rarely aneurysm and haemorrhage	None	Cranial nerve abnormalities; secondary chronic basal meningitis (e.g. optic atrophy); hydrocephalus; secondary chronic arachnoiditis; juvenile general paresis and tabes dorsalis at 10–15 years of age
Herpes simplex	75% caused by herpes simplex type 2 (infects maternal genitalia most); herpes simplex type 1 (infects non-genital sites)	Acquired during passage through infected birth canal; ascending infections near time of birth; uncommon transplacental or postnatal acquisition	Intrapartum		Eye vesicles	Meningoencephalitis; multifocal parenchymal necrosis, occasionally haemorrhagic; brain swelling; Cowdry type A intranuclear inclusions in neurons, astrocytes and oligodendrocytes	Fetal (transplacental) infection: microphthalmia, microcephaly	Microcephaly; secondary tissue destruction; multicystic encephalomalacia; hydranencephaly

The occurrence of traumatic injuries has dropped significantly with improved obstetrical care, notably in the use of Caesarean section. These lesions have been reviewed elsewhere.[219,679] Haematomas of the perinatal period, and injuries to peripheral nerves and spinal cord will be discussed because of their clinical and pathological importance. The finding of a subdural haematoma in an infant raises the possibility of the shaken baby syndrome and child abuse: it is however, important to keep perinatal trauma in the differential diagnosis.

Caput succedaneum is a common lesion consisting of localized haemorrhagic oedema of the subcutaneous tissue in the presenting part of the head. It resolves without problems.

Subgaleal haemorrhage refers to the collection of blood above the periosteum and below the aponeurosis of the scalp. This is not common and is related to trauma which tears the emissary veins connecting dural sinuses to scalp veins.[25] It is sometimes in association with coagulation abnormalities.[563] The blood may dissect into the neck and the infant must be observed for effects of serious blood loss during the first 2 weeks of life.[679]

Cephalhaematoma is a collection of blood between the periosteum and the outer surface of the skull, limited by the suture lines. It is associated with skull fracture in 25% of cases.[351] Its incidence increases with the use of forceps[116] and it resolves usually without problems.

Epidural haematomas, blood between the skull and the periosteum on its inner aspect, are usually related to trauma. These are rare in infancy[308] and require surgical removal.

Subdural haematoma, blood between the dura and the leptomeninges, typically occurs in the full-term infant, although the relative proportion of affected premature infants has increased because of advances in obstetrical management of difficult full-term deliveries.[679] The source of haemorrhage may be: (1) rupture of bridging superficial cerebral veins; (2) cerebellar tentorial laceration with rupture of the straight sinus, transverse sinus, vein of Galen or smaller infratentorial veins;[679] (3) occipital osteodiastasis with rupture of the occipital sinus; or (4) laceration of the falx with rupture of the inferior sagittal sinus. According to Volpe[679] subdural haemorrhage is more likely to occur when: the infant is relatively large, and the birth canal relatively small; the skull is unusually compliant, as in premature infants; the pelvic structures are unusually rigid, as in primigravidas or older multiparous mothers; the duration of the labour is unusually brief, not allowing the enough time for dilatation of the pelvic structures, or unusually long, subjecting the head to prolonged compression and moulding; or there is breech or footling presentation, or face or brow presentation necessitating difficult forceps extraction, vacuum extraction or rotational manoeuvres. In these circumstances, there is excessive vertical moulding and frontal–occipital elongation or oblique expansion of the head. Extreme vertical moulding appears to underlie most tears

of the superficial cerebral veins and the formation of convexity subdural haematomas. A tear of the falx occurs particularly with face or brow presentations. Occipital osteodiastasis refers to traumatic separation of the cartilaginous joint between the squamous and lateral portion of the occipital bone, and typically occurs with a breech delivery. The injury occurs if there is suboccipital pressure when the head is trapped beneath the symphysis and is hyperextended. Occipital osteodiastasis can result in a posterior fossa subdural haematoma and laceration of the cerebellum. This bony lesion can be missed at autopsy if not specifically considered. Subdural haematoma in the newborn infant is not always associated with a clinical traumatic delivery. There are reports of prenatal or intrauterine subdural haematomas secondary to maternal abuse,[622] severe factor V deficiency,[179] high-dose aspirin in the mother, medulloblastoma with haemorrhage, and neonatal vitamin K deficiency.[528]

Skull fractures may be linear, depressed or occipital osteodiastasis. Fractures may resolve without difficulty; however, they may be associated with growing skull fractures caused when the dura is damaged and the subarachnoid space communicates with the surrounding extraosseous tissue, producing a leptomeningeal cyst which expands and prevents the fracture from healing. This rare complication of skull fracture occurs only in children. It has been reported in association with vacuum extraction.[326] Intraosseous haematoma of the skull has been reported as a complication of skull trauma at birth.[719]

Nerve injury

The incidence of birth injury to the head and neck in a USA tertiary medical facility was reported to be 0.82%, so that peripheral or cranial nerve injury needs to be considered in neonates with stridor, respiratory distress, feeding difficulty, facial deformity, or altered Moro or grasp reflexes.[325] Laryngeal nerve injury may present as stridor, airway obstruction, dysphonia, dysphagia and aspiration. If the injury is bilateral, tracheostomy is usually required.[479] Facial nerve injury results from compression by forceps or the maternal sacral promontory. This paralysis must be differentiated from developmental facial paralysis.[194,325] Brachial plexus injury occurred in 0.15% of 1 094 298 deliveries in 300 California hospitals. The potential causes were shoulder dystocia, other malpresentations, diabetes and operative vaginal delivery.[231] Erb's palsy involves C5–6; Klumpke's paralysis involves C5–7 and Horner's syndrome (ptosis, miosis and anhidrosis) results from injury to the T1 root sympathetic fibres.[325] Phrenic nerve injury is usually associated with brachial plexus injury and may present with respiratory distress on the first day of life after some delay. It is frequently associated with pulmonary infection.[325,586] Radial nerve injury has been reported in cases of failed progression of labour with prolonged radial nerve compression.[306]

Nerve injury is defined as neurapraxia when there is transient conduction block due to ischaemia or acute demyelination, axonotmesis when there is disruption of the axon with maintenance of the connective tissue skeleton of the nerve, and neuronotmesis when there is an interruption of the nerve axons associated with connective tissue damage.[583] In most injuries there is a spontaneous recovery; however, when avulsion and complete severance occur, immediate surgery may be indicated. Definitive determination of the degree of nerve injury requires electromyography, nerve conduction and myelogram studies. After the injury varying amounts of motor, sensory and autonomic abnormalities develop, including muscle wasting and contractures, pain and dysaesthesias, altered sweating and vasomotor responses, and trophic changes in the skin and nails.[583] Neuropathology specimens obtained during nerve exploration and repair exhibit traumatized nerves with evidence of haemorrhage, demyelination, and eventually neuroma formation in which there is proliferation of displaced nerve fibres, Schwann cells and connective tissue septa.

Spinal cord injury

Injury to the infant's spinal cord during delivery results from excessive traction or rotation, unlike the usual compression injury characteristic of cord injuries in older patients. The anatomy of the newborn accounts for these differences. The bony vertebral column is nearly entirely cartilaginous and elastic, as are the ligaments, and the muscles are relatively hypotonic, the latter partially related to maternal drugs and anaesthesia. The vertebral facet joints are more horizontal in newborns and are thus more mobile and less stable. The spinal cord is less elastic, anchored above by the medulla and roots of the brachial plexus and below by the cauda equina. With longitudinal traction and hyperextension, as in breech deliveries, the cord moves less than the spine and the cord 'ruptures' at its mobile sites, the lower cervical to upper thoracic levels. The spine may not show radiological evidence of injury.[401] In cephalic deliveries, the relatively heavy head with poor muscle tone places strain on the cervical cord. When forceps produce excessive rotational manipulation, the infant's immature flat uncinate processes fail to limit flexion–rotational forces which tear the less mobile spinal cord in the upper cervical regions. The clinical symptoms include hypotonia, loss of reflexes in the extremities, apnoea and early flaccidity which may change to spasticity. The various clinical presentations of perinatal spinal cord injury have been described in classic papers.[129,130,215]

The acute lesion of traumatic spinal cord injury is intraspinal haemorrhagic necrosis, particularly involving the dorsal and central grey matter. The chronic lesion exhibits cystic cavitation with disruption of cord architecture and fibrous adhesions between the dura, the leptomeninges and the cord. Vascular occlusions, perhaps developing as a post-traumatic event, may cause infarction of cord segments caudal to the level of the primary lesion. Lesions of the vertebral column are uncommon, consisting of fractures, or dislocations and separation of the vertebral epiphysis.

Spinal cord injury may be difficult to diagnose, and has to be differentiated from cerebral anoxia (which may also affect the cord),[117] spinal muscular atrophy, muscular dystrophies, myelodysplasia and congenital intraspinal tumours. Brachial plexus injury may accompany spinal cord injury and confuse the clinical presentation.[570] Moreover, in a retrospective survey of spinal cord insults in the prenatal, perinatal and neonatal periods, the aetiology was unknown in 24 of 51 cases.[571]

CHILD ABUSE

The typical battered or abused child is an infant, undernourished with or without other external signs of neglect (uncleanliness, sores from inadequate sanitation, napkin rashes, insect bites, inadequate clothing) and/or multiple injuries (burns, cuts, lacerations, 'patterned' injuries related to the injuring object, genital and anal injuries).[397] It is estimated that approximately 10 in 1000 children in the USA are subjected to abuse; 50% are under 3 years of age and 25% are under 1 year of age.[506] Child abuse ranks second only to sudden infant death syndrome (SIDS) as the leading cause of death in infants under 1 year of age,[506] and it is most common cause of serious head injury in infants. The incidence of non-accidental head trauma in children is not known, but in fatal child-abuse injuries the rate of head trauma is approximately 60%.[506] The American Academy of Pediatrics Committee on Child Abuse and Neglect emphasizes the need for medical presumption of physical abuse when a child younger than 1 year of age has intracranial injury.[378] In a population-based study of subdural haemorrhages in children under 2 years of age in south Wales and south-west England, Jayawant et al.[343] found that subdural haemorrhage was usually due to child abuse, and that three-quarters of the infants died or had profound disablement. They recommend that clinical investigation of infants with subdural haemorrhages should include multidisciplinary social assessment, ophthalmic examination, skeletal survey supplemented with bone scan or a skeletal survey repeated after 10 days, coagulation screen, and CT or MRI.[291] The multidisciplinary approach to the clinical investigation of suspected child abuse is of utmost importance, because there is not one pathognomonic sign of child abuse, as well as controversial issues pertaining to the pathoaetiology of several of the lesions found in child abuse. These issues are clearly defined by Wilkins.[695] The following discussion will consider the injuries to the head and nervous system.

Head injuries in child-abuse cases are considered to be caused by direct impact, by shaking, or by both.[397] In an impact injury there may be skin bruises or contusion, indicating the site at which the head was struck or where it impacted after a fall. These changes must be interpreted with caution.[700] The galea of the reflected scalp and the soft tissues beneath the skin must be carefully examined for bruises or haemorrhages. It is of particular importance to examine the cervical region, soft tissues and spinal cord (C1–4).[170]

Shaking injuries, first described by John Caffey in 1972, are produced by the infant being grabbed around the thorax and shaken to and fro, causing the head to 'whip' back and forth with accelerations and decelerations presumably producing injuries in the brain, meninges and eyes. Caffey's whiplash shaken baby syndrome included a constellation of findings in infants 6–8 months of life, with retinal haemorrhages and intracranial injury (subdural and/or subarachnoid haemorrhage with little or no evidence of external head trauma). The infants head is relatively heavy and immobile, with poor neck muscle tone: it produces little resistance to the forces produced by shaking. Guthkelch[277] postulated that subdural haemorrhages are caused by tearing of the bridging cortical veins by the acceleration–decleration forces. Duhaime et al.,[171] in a study based on an experimental model for brain injury, considered that shaking alone cannot produce the force required to cause subdural and diffuse brain injury. They have shown that subgaleal injury is present in most cases of shaken baby syndrome, and proposed that the additional impact injury is necessary to produce the force required for serious brain injury. They suggest the name shaking-impact syndrome. There is, however, some controversy about this conclusion.[13,239]

The historical, clinical, laboratory and radiographical aspects of non-accidental head injury have been clearly defined.[170] There is a history of trauma, the details of which may vary with repeated tellings, and which is inconsistent with the degree of injury observed. The signs and symptoms range in severity from irritability, lethargy, meningismus, seizures, tone alterations, altered consciousness, vomiting, poor feeding, breathing abnormalities, apnoea and unresponsiveness, to a moribund state. Retinal haemorrhages may be seen in 65–95% of cases (with optimal examination). They may be unilateral or bilateral with retinal folds or detachments. They are not, however, specific for abuse and are seen in accidental trauma, after resuscitation, in papilloedema, and in 40% of newborns delivered vaginally, until 1 month of age. They may be seen in association with subarachnoid haemorrhage, coagulopathy, galactosaemia and hypertension. There may be skin bruises, burns or marks, or these may not be apparent. Lumbar puncture reveals bloody fluid. CT studies reveal subdural or subarachnoid haemorrhage, often posteriorly in the interhemispheric fissures. There may be poor definition of the grey–white-matter margins and a diffuse hypodensity, except for the basal ganglia and posterior fossa structures. The timing of these changes is addressed by Dias et al.[151] MRI will define parenchymal

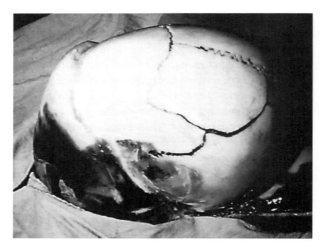

Figure 9.40 *Non-accidental injury. Skull fracture in infant due to physical abuse. Photograph by Dr B Blackbourne, San Diego Medical Examiner's Office, San Diego, CA, USA.*

lesions, whereas plane films will optimally define skull fractures. A skeletal survey will identify extracranial injury, such as rib fractures or metaphyseal fractures, in 30–70% of cases. Repeated or delayed scans or radionucleotide bone scans may show subtle lesions.[170]

The autopsy may reveal external injuries,[170] usually in the head and neck, in 85% of cases. Scalp trauma may require head shaving; fractures are present in 25% of cases and are usually posterior parietal or occipital. In accidental skull fractures the fractures are usually single, simple and linear, compared with the multiple and complex fractures seen in victims of child abuse (Fig. 9.40).[313] A recent survey of head-injured infants revealed that the significant scalp haematoma is a useful indicator of intracranial injury in otherwise asymptomatic infants.[266]

The neuropathological injuries seen in child abuse are retinal haemorrhages (Fig. 9.41), epidural and subdural

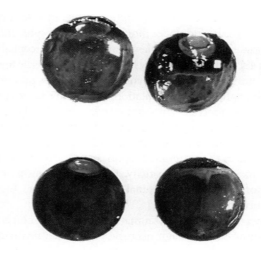

Figure 9.41 *Non-accidental injury. Retinal haemorrhages in infant due to physical abuse. Photograph Dr B Blackbourne, San Diego Medical Examiner's Office, San Diego, CA, USA.*

haemorrhage, subarachnoid haemorrhage, cerebral contusions, white-matter injury and diffuse axonal injury. The retinal haemorrhages in 12 cases were recent, preretinal, intraretinal or subretinal, predominantly in the superficial retinal layers and subsensory retinal space.[468] The haemorrhages were most prominent in the posterior pole. Epidural haemorrhage is caused by bleeding into the epidural space from branches of the torn middle meningeal artery or from major veins or sinuses. A linear skull fracture and cephalohaematoma may be present in the parietal or temporal regions. The volume of blood in the haematoma may be dangerously large.[114] Subdural haemorrhages are usually at the parieto-occipital junction or posterior interhemispheric fissure. The dura of the young infant is adherent to the inner skull, so that veins leading to the dural sinuses are easily disrupted by tearing injuries. Acute subdural haematomas appear liquid or as 'currant jelly', and are not usually of a sufficient volume to produce a threatening mass. The age of the subdural haematoma has been defined histologically by Hirsh,[312] but Duhaime et al.[170] caution about the various factors limiting this method. Membranes will be present in old haematomas; however, because newly formed subdural membranes may be related to causes in addition to non-accidental trauma these need to be interpreted in conjunction with all other observations.[566] Subarachnoid haemorrhage may result from the tearing of a subarachnoid vein. It may be seen alone or together with subdural haematomas. In infants and children there are many causes of subarachnoid haemorrhage to consider: coagulopathy such as vitamin K deficiency, leukaemia, thrombocytopenia and, rarely, rupture of a congenital vascular malformation.[611] Cerebral contusion, foci of necrosis and haemorrhage, are most often in the olfactory bulb and tracts and gyrus rectus, or appear as slit-like tears in the subcortical white matter.[170,408] Gliding contusions are seen in the corpus callosum.

Diffuse axonal injuries are considered to be very important contributors to the patient's clinical state after head injury. They have been described variously as shearing injuries, diffuse damage to white matter of the immediate impact type, diffuse white-matter shearing injury, and inner cerebral trauma. They reflect a process that begins at the time of the shearing, rotational or acceleration–deceleration injury and are described in detail in Chapter 14, this Volume. The microscopic axonal bulbs (Fig. 9.42) are brought about by extrusion of axoplasm from anterograde axoplasmic flows, and classically are reported to take 12–18 h to develop. They can be seen in the absence of haemorrhage and may be seen in H&E sections, but are better defined by silver impregnation, or antibodies to neurofilaments or to APP.[247] Axonal β-amyloid precursor protein reactivity can be seen 2 h after injury, but it will not detect diffuse axonal injury if survival is less than 2 h, if cerebral perfusion has not been adequate to ensure function of axonal transport system, if the time from injury is excessive, or if inadequate numbers of brain regions (corpus callosum, brainstem) are sampled.[247] However, axonal injury detected by APP is not specific for trauma and can also be seen in infarcts and in areas near haematomas where axons have been disrupted. In a study of shaken baby syndrome using brains of infants with hypoxic–ischaemic injury as controls, Shannon et al.[596] demonstrated axonal injury in the cerebral white matter, midbrain and medulla in all cases, but in the white matter of the cervical cord, axonal injury was only seen in the abuse cases. It was postulated that the flexion extension injury of the cervical spinal cord in shaken baby syndrome was responsible for this specific site of axonal injury. Axonal injury has been graded: in grade 1 injury there is microscopic evidence of axonal injury in the white matter of the cerebral hemispheres, corpus callosum, brainstem and sometimes the cerebellum; in grade 2 there are gross focal lesions in the corpus callosum; and in grade 3 injury there are focal lesions in the dorsolateral sector of the rostral brainstem.[2]

The infant brain exhibits a diffuse parenchymal response to injury. Gilles and Nelson[232] evaluated the CT patterns of cerebral parenchymal injury in 14 children with non-accidental head injury. All had acute subdural haematomas; the youngest patients (mean age 5 months) had diffuse hypoattenuation, whereas the older patients (mean age 19 months) had focal hypoattenuation. All of these children then developed CT evidence of infarction. The aetiology for diffuse brain swelling in the younger brain is not known: immature biomechanical properties, autoregulation, vasoreactivity and ischaemic tolerance, as well as postinjury apnoea and hypotension, are suggested. Similarly, in the older patients with an acute subdural haematoma, the aetiology of hemispheric swelling and secondary necrosis is not understood; ischaemia, local pressure and excitatory amino acids are suggested. Strangulation with carotid injury has to be considered. It has been demonstrated in rat brains that there is much more apoptotic neurodegeneration following trauma in 3–7-day-old animals than in older animals, suggesting a special vulnerability of the immature brain.[66]

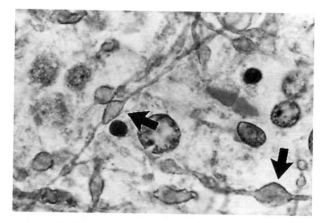

Figure 9.42 *Traumatic brain injury. Diffuse axonal injury in cerebral white matter of infant due to physical abuse. The axons contain focal swellings (arrows). Photograph by Dr H Wilson, Department of Pathology, El Paso, TX, USA.*

Clinical sequelae of non-accidental head injuries include cognitive delay, cortical visual loss and other focal neurological deficits. Micrencephaly develops in up to 73% of survivors. Haviland and Russell[305] report similarly poor outcomes with two deaths out of 15 patients with non-accidental trauma, and major neurological handicap in 69% of survivors. This was compared with the outcome in ten patients with accidental trauma, in which 67% of survivors were normal.

NEOPLASIA

In congenital brain tumours, the unique host situation of the neonate and young infant is dramatically underscored: the rapidly growing brain is an environment for proliferating tumour cells which have escaped factors regulating normal growth. Several unusual biological aspects of brain tumours in the fetus and infant under 2 years of age have been emphasized.[241] The first is their supratentorial sites, particularly along the midline in phylogenetically older brain structures (Fig. 9.43). Guiffre[241] suggests that several factors may influence this location of brain tumours, such as site-specific cellular factors, or circulatory factors carrying carcinogens. A second unique feature of congenital tumours is their histopathology. The incidence of teratomas is high in the fetus, but after 1 year of life the primitive neuroectodermal tumours (PNETs)/medulloblastomas become the most common tumour type. High-grade astrocytomas and ependymomas are more common in infants less than 2 years than in older children.[69,169,556] In all children both PNETs and mixed tumours (Fig. 9.44) are common, differing from the glial tumours composed of one cell type which constitute the most common type in adults. In infancy a given tumour type may have unusual biological behaviour. For example, some malignant tumours (medulloblastoma, ependymoma)[122] are more aggressive in infancy than in older children, while others (optic nerve glioma) are more benign. Moreover, a recent study

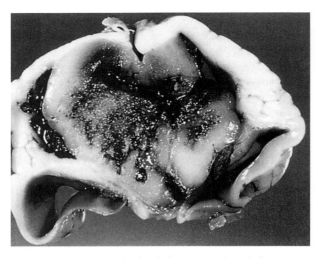

Figure 9.44 *Congenital mixed glioma. Newborn infant.*

demonstrated enhanced chemosensitivity of malignant glial tumours in infants than in adults.[169]

The clustering of certain immature tumour types, such as teratoma and primitive neuroectodermal tumours, in the infantile period has been interpreted to result from an interruption of normal cellular development. Such tumours may therefore parallel the molecular biology of normal brain development, expressing similar proteins.[654] Some of these proteins are used to identify tumour types, e.g. vimentin, GFAP or synaptophysin. There is some evidence for a genetic predisposition to congenital brain tumours in Li–Fraumeni cancer family syndrome, neurofibromatosis (types 1 and 2), tuberous sclerosis, nevoid basal cell carcinoma syndrome, familial polyposis, von Hippel–Lindau disease[70] and Gorlin syndrome[191] (see also Chapter 11, Volume II). In spite of these demonstrated genetic associations with some congenital brain tumours, most are considered to be sporadic. Epidemiological studies have investigated teratogens, irradiation and some infectious agents (toxoplasmosis, chicken pox, simian virus 40). Maternal vitamins during pregnancy may be protective.[439]

The precise definition of congenital tumours is problematic because several ages have been applied to the description of 'congenital', 'infantile' or 'perinatal'. These include tumours diagnosed during the first 60 days,[33,88] the first year,[161,280] the first 18 months[198] or within the first 24 months.[650] Solitaire and Krigman[612] defined congenital tumours according to onset of symptoms as definitely congenital (symptoms present at birth), probably congenital (symptoms within first week of life) and possibly congenital (symptoms in the first month of life). Examinations with ultrasound have made it possible to diagnose intracranial neoplasms before birth in fetuses.[296,407,674] The numerous definitions of congenital tumours explain their varying relative incidence, ranging from 0.5–1.9%[88] through 1.4–8.5%[280] to 16% of paediatric brain tumours.[161] There is also a discrepancy in the reported incidence of congenital tumours in Eastern and

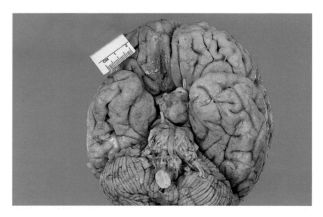

Figure 9.43 *Hypothalamic hamartoma. Congenital tumour in newborn extends from the hypothalamus to the interpenduncular fossa.*

Table 9.8 *Congenital brain tumours, sites and types*

Location	Tumour type	References
Third ventricle	Teratoma	Sakamoto et al.,[575] Wakai et al.[681]
	Craniopharyngioma	Sakamoto et al.[575]
	Choroid plexus papilloma	Wakai et al.[68]
Third suprasellar	Gliosarcoma	Tomita and McLone[650]
	Ependymoblastoma	Sato et al.[581]
	Craniopharyngioma	Kane et al.[348]
Fourth ventricle	Subependymoma	Wakai et al.[681]
	Sarcoma	Arnstein et al.[33]
	Astrocytoma	Sakamoto et al.[575]
	Cerebellar neurocytoma	Brandis et al.[76]
	Choroid plexus carcinoma	Shinoda et al.[602]
Hypothalamus	Hamartoma	Sakamoto et al.[575]
	Astrocytoma	Tomita and McLone[650]
Corpus callosum	Lipoma	Sakamoto et al.[575]
Pineal region	Medulloblastoma	Sakamoto et al.[575]
	Teratoma	Wakai et al.[681]
	Medulloepithelioma	Tomita and McLone[650]
	Pineoblastoma	Arnstein et al.[33]
	ATT/RT	Hilden et al.[311]
Brainstem	Glioblastoma multiforme	Sakamoto et al.[575]
	Astrocytoma	Wakai et al.[681]
	Teratoma	Takaku et al.[628]
	Malignant astrocytoma	Tomita and McLone[650]
Cerebellopontine angle	'Glioblastoma/ medulloblastoma'	Takaku et al.[628]
Lateral ventricle	Astrocytoma	Sakamoto et al.[575]
	Ependymoma	Sakamoto et al.[575]
	Choroid plexus papilloma	Sakamoto et al.[575]
	Teratoma	Wakai et al.[681]
	Dermoid	Arnstein et al.[33]
	Choroid plexus carcinoma	Shinoda et al.[602]
	Congenital subependymal giant-cell astrocytoma	Mirkin et al.[450]
Temporal lobe	Glioblastoma	Sakamoto et al.[575]
	Sarcoma	Sato et al.[581]
Cerebellum	Medulloblastoma	Sakamoto et al.[575]
	Ependymoma	Tomita and McLone[650]
	Astrocytoma	Tomita and McLone[650]
	Ependymoblastoma	Tomita and McLone[650]
	Immature teratoma	Tomita and McLone[650]
	Haemangioblastoma	Tomita and McLone[650]
	Metastatic sarcoma	Tomita and McLone[650]
Cerebral hemisphere	Astrocytoma	Tomita and McLone[650]
	Malignant astrocytoma	Tomita and McLone[650]
	PNET	Tomita and McLone[650]
	Giant cell astrocytoma	Tomita and McLone[650]
	Gliosarcoma Angiosarcoma	Arnstein et al.[33]

Table 9.8 *Continued*

Location	Tumour type	References
	Ganglioglioma	Price et al.[537]
	Glioblastoma multiforme	Mazewski et al.[439]
Skull Supratentorial	Desmoblastic cerebral glioblastoma	Al Sarraj and Bridges[14]
	Melanotic progonoma	Sakamoto et al.[575]
	Huge, brain-replacing teratoma	Wakai et al.[681]
Supratentorial and infratentorial	Teratoma	Lipman et al.[410]
Supratentorial not otherwise specified	Germinoma	Buetow et al.[88]
	Astrocytoma	Buetow et al.[88]
	Glioblastoma multiforme	Buetow et al.[88]
	Choroid plexus papilloma	Buetow et al.[88]
	Papillary ependymoma	Buetow et al.[88]
	PNET	Buetow et al.[88]
	Medulloblastoma	Buetow et al.[88]
	Medulloepithelioma	Buetow et al.[88]
	Angioblastic meningioma	Buetow et al.[88]
	Teratoma	Buetow et al.[88]
	Choroid plexus carcinoma	Wakai et al.[681]
	Pineoblastoma	Wakai et al.[681]
	Sarcoma	Wakai et al.[681]
Infratentorial not otherwise specified	Astrocytoma	Buetow et al.[88]
	PNET	Buetow et al.[88]
	Medulloblastoma	Buetow et al.[88]
	Medulloepithelioma	Buetow et al.[88]
	Teratoma	Buetow et al.[88]
	Oligodendroglioma	Wakai et al.[681]
	Mixed glioma	Wakai et al.[681]
	Sarcoma	Wakai et al.[681]
	ATT/RT	Hilden et al.[311]
Meninges	Angioblastic meningioma	Buetow et al.[88]
	Sarcoma	Russell and Ellis[572]

ATT/RT, atypical teratoid tumour/rhabdoid tumour; PNET, primitive neuroectodermal tumour.

Western countries. Di Rocco et al.[161] report no difference, whereas Oi et al.[501] report fewer congenital brain tumours in Japan. Giuffre[241] observed that the USA, some Scandinavian countries, Israel and New Zealand had the highest incidence of childhood brain tumours, whereas Japan, some Latin American countries, Nigeria, Czechoslovakia, Hungary, Singapore and Bombay had the lowest. He also reported that of the six main groups of childhood tumours (CNS tumours, leukaemias, Hodgkin's disease, non-Hodgkin lymphomas, renal and ocular tumours) only brain tumours show a steady rise

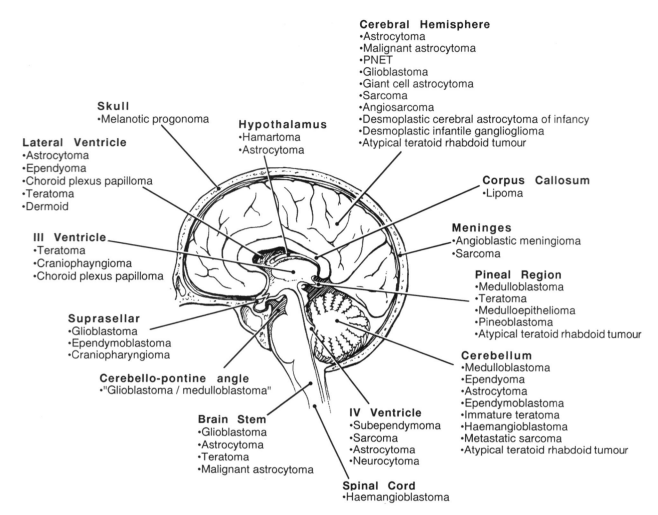

Skull
•Melanotic progonoma

Lateral Ventricle
•Astrocytoma
•Ependyoma
•Choroid plexus papilloma
•Teratoma
•Dermoid

III Ventricle
•Teratoma
•Craniophayngioma
•Choroid plexus papilloma

Suprasellar
•Glioblastoma
•Ependymoblastoma
•Craniopharyngioma

Cerebello-pontine angle
•"Glioblastoma / medulloblastoma"

Brain Stem
•Glioblastoma
•Astrocytoma
•Teratoma
•Malignant astrocytoma

Hypothalamus
•Hamartoma
•Astrocytoma

Cerebral Hemisphere
•Astrocytoma
•Malignant astrocytoma
•PNET
•Glioblastoma
•Giant cell astrocytoma
•Sarcoma
•Angiosarcoma
•Desmoplastic cerebral astrocytoma of infancy
•Desmoplastic infantile ganglioglioma
•Atypical teratoid rhabdoid tumour

Corpus Callosum
•Lipoma

Meninges
•Angioblastic meningioma
•Sarcoma

Pineal Region
•Medulloblastoma
•Teratoma
•Medulloepithelioma
•Pineoblastoma
•Atypical teratoid rhabdoid tumour

Cerebellum
•Medulloblastoma
•Ependyoma
•Astrocytoma
•Ependymoblastoma
•Immature teratoma
•Haemangioblastoma
•Metastatic sarcoma
•Atypical teratoid rhabdoid tumour

IV Ventricle
•Subependymoma
•Sarcoma
•Astrocytoma
•Neurocytoma

Spinal Cord
•Haemangioblastoma

Figure 9.45 *Congenital CNS-associated tumours. Congenital tumours reported in infants under 24 months of age with sites and types of tumour indicated.*

in incidence that can be only partially explained by diagnostic awareness.[353] Brain tumours are the second most common neoplasm causing perinatal death and account for 7.2% of all neonatal cancer.[439] In many reports, infant boys and girls have a similar incidence of brain tumours.[161,198,501,575,612] Although some series[88,550] report a slight male predominance, others[388,650,681] report more tumours in girls. Haddad *et al.*[280] observed that girls had twice as many astrocytomas and PNETs as boys, and Fessard[203] reported more choroid plexus tumours, astrocytomas and medulloblastomas in boys under 2 years of age.

The signs and symptoms of perinatal brain tumours are not specific, and include vomiting, large head, seizures and, less often, cranial nerve signs,[161] failure-to-thrive, congenital malformation,[280] visual changes, hemiparesis and skull fracture.[88] It has been stressed that the clinical presentations of neonatal tumours are quite subtle and non-specific because of the infants' capacity to accommodate the expanding intracranial mass owing to open sutures.[439] In one series, one-fifth of the cases were diagnosed clinically as meningitis.[257]

Most tumour types have been reported in the perinatal period. Figure 9.45 and Table 9.8 show tumour types at the sites at which they have been described. In the report

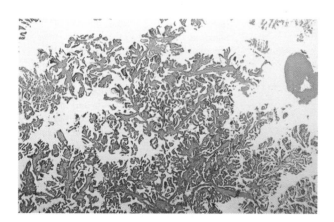

Figure 9.46 *Choroid plexus papilloma. The tumour is papillary with a single layer of benign epithelium and a fibrovascular core. (H&E.)*

of Di Ricco *et al.*[161] of 886 tumours diagnosed during the first year of life, astrocytomas, including pilocytic astrocytomas,[576] medulloblastomas, ependymomas and choroid plexus papillomas (Fig. 9.46), were the most common, followed by teratomas and meningiomas. In their series, 63% were supratentorial and 29.6% were infratentorial; in 1.3% both compartments were involved. Several other series of perinatal tumours reveal similar observations, e.g. Wakai *et al.*,[681] Buetow *et al.*,[88] Lipman *et al.*[410] and Richert *et al.*[556]

In 1996, Rorke *et al.*[569] drew attention to a highly malignant tumour of the infantile period, the atypical teratoid/rhabdoid tumour (Fig. 9.47). In the original description it occurred in infants and children ranging in age from *in utero* to 14.9 years, but with three-quarters in children under 3 years of age. The details of the morphology of this tumour, together with two other unique tumours encountered in this extended perinatal period, the desmoplastic infantile ganglioglioma and the desmoplastic astrocytoma of infancy,[594] are presented in Chapter 11, Volume II.

The treatment of congenital brain tumours is surgical, sometimes preceded by a shunt and followed by chemotherapy. Radiation is usually avoided because of its possible deleterious effect on the developing brain, the spinal cord and the vertebrae. The outcome is related to the tumour type and site, but aggressive therapy is always a consideration because of the infantile brain's capacity to compensate for large resections.[161] The complications and sequelae of brain tumour therapy are a matter of concern.[208] Cognitive deficits are reported in 40–100% of long-term survivors. Younger children undergoing radiotherapy or methotrexate chemotherapy are most at risk.[245] The deficits are possibly related to vascular lesions or demyelination.[121,454] Secondary brain tumours may occur after high-dose cranial radiation and include most commonly aggressively behaving meningiomas and gliomas. Lymphoproliferative disorders and 'stroke' have also been reported after cranial irradiation.[454] There are deleterious effects of the therapeutic modalities on other systems: neuroendocrine, skeletal, cardiac, pulmonary, renal and reproductive. The roles of radiation, chemotherapy, immune suppression and genetic susceptibility are all factors which need to be considered in the pathogenesis of these devastating lesions which may develop after the treatment of childhood brain tumours. In spite of these serious concerns, there has been an improvement in the overall 5-year survival of infants under 1 year of age with intracranial neoplasms.[348]

Brain malformation may be associated with brain tumours: frontonasal dysplasia, lipoma of the corpus callosum,[441] hydranencephaly,[666] vascular malformations[175,448] and craniosynostosis.[103] Wakai *et al.*[681] found anomalies (brain or elsewhere) in 18 of 193 cases of neonatal brain tumours. These observations serve to emphasize the importance of the biology of the developing brain and its response to pathogenic mechanisms during its critical period of development.[169]

MUSCULOSKELETAL DISORDERS

In the perinatal period, pathology of the lower motor unit presents conspicuously as hypotonia with weakness. The differential diagnosis of such motor disability is extensive, including, in addition to the neuromuscular conditions, diseases of the CNS,[580] and endocrine, chromosomal and metabolic disorders.[47,449] The skeletal muscle of the infant is frequently biopsied in multisystem disorders, cardiomyopathies and encephalomyopathies. The neuromuscular disease entities are discussed in detail in Chapter 10, Volume II and are tabulated here (Table 9.9) to emphasize their importance in the neuropathology of the perinatal period. In the series of Fardeau *et al.*,[196] comprising 250 cases of severe perinatal hypotonia, the disorders were 20% undetermined, 18% metabolic myopathies, 14% congenital myopathies, 14% myotonic dystrophy, 12% spinal muscular atrophy, 8% CNS disease, 6% malformations or chromosomal disorders, 6%

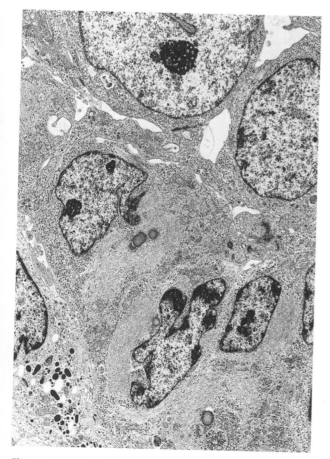

Figure 9.47 *Atypical teratoid/rhabdoid tumour. Electron micrograph of rhabdoid cells in an atypical teratoid/rhabdoid tumour showing pleomorphic nuclei and collections of intermediate filaments adjacent to the nuclei.*

Table 9.9 *Spinal muscular and neurogenic atrophies*

Site of lesion	Clinical feature	Genetics	Subtypes	References
Spinal cord				Modified from DeVisser et al.[147] Brzustowicz et al.[86]
	Proximal spinal muscular atrophy	Autosomal recessive inheritance (gene at 5q11.2-13-3)		
			Acute spinal muscular atrophy	Byers and Banker[93]
			Intermediate spinal muscular atrophy	Byers and Banker[93]
			Chronic spinal muscular atrophy	Byers and Banker[93]
			X Chromosome recessive	Greenberg et al.[265] Pearn[523]
	Proximal spinal muscular atrophy	Autosomal dominant		
	Distal spinal muscular atrophy			Harding and Thomas[300]
		Autosomal recessive Autosomal dominant		Bertini et al.[58]
Brainstem	Progressive bulbar palsy			Londe,[414] Alexander et al.[12]
	Miscellaneous		Polio	Price and Plum[538]
			Cervical cord trauma	Haldeman et al.[285]
			Infantile neuroaxonal dystrophy	Berard-Badier et al.[55]
			Schindler's (*N*-acetylgalactosaminidase deficiency)	Schindler et al.[584]
			Infantile neuronal degeneration	Steiman et al.[620]
Peripheral neuropathy		Hereditary sensory and autonomic neuropathy		Dyke[173]
			Type II	Ohta et al.[507]
			Type III (familial dysautonomia)	Aguayo et al.[4]
			Type IV (absent unmyelinated fibres)	Swanson et al.[627]
			With neurotrophic keratitis	Goebel et al.[253] Donaghy et al.[164]
		Hereditary motor and sensory neuropathies		Dyke[173]
			Type I, hypertrophic, rare symptoms in infancy	Hamiel et al.[293]
			Type III, with onion bulbs	
			Congenital hypomyelination neuropathy	Guzzetta et al.[278]
			Congenital hypomyelination with axonopathy	Vital et al.[670]
	Metabolic neuropathies		Metachromatic leukodystrophy	Bardosi et al.[44]
			Globoid leukodystrophy	Bischoff and Ulrich[65]
			Respiratory enzyme Complex I deficiency	Petty et al.[531]
			Leigh's disease	Goebel et al.,[251] Jacobs et al.[338]
			Hereditary tyrosinaemia	Mitchell et al.[453]
	Inflammatory neuropathies		Guillain–Barré syndrome	Gilmartin and Ch'ien[240]
			Chronic relapsing polyneuropathy	Pasternak et al.[519]
	Miscellaneous		Giant axonal neuropathy	Ouvrier et al.[508]
			Neuroaxonal dystrophy	

Table 9.10 *Classification of congenital myopathies*

Type	Site	Disease	References
Structural congenital myopathies	Involving the sarcomere	Central core disease	Shy and Magee[603]
		Multicore disease	Engel et al.[187]
		Minicore disease	Currie et al.[133]
		Myofibrillar lysis myopathy	Cancilla et al.[96]
		Selective myosin degeneration myopathy	Yarom and Shapira[709]
		Cap disease	Fidzianska et al.[204]
	Involving the Z-disc	Trilaminar fibre myopathy	Ringel et al.[557]
		Nemaline/rod myopathy	Shy et al.[604]
		Desmin-related forms	
		Cytoplasmic body myopathy	Goebel et al.[252]
	Involving the nucleus	Mallory body myopathy	Fidzianska et al.[204]
		Myotubular myopathy	Spiro et al.[615]
		Centronuclear myopathy	Sher et al.[518]
		Sex-linked myotubular myopathy	van Wijmgaarten et al.[694]
	With abnormal inclusions	Mixed myopathies (a,b,c)	Dubowitz[168]
		Fingerprint body myopathy	Engel et al.[186]
		Zebra body myopathy	Lake and Wilson[386]
		Reducing body myopathy	Brooke and Neville[84]
		Tubular aggregate[a]	Bodensteiner[68]
	Abnormalities of organelles	Sarcotubular myopathy	Jerusalem et al.[344]
		Rimmed vacuole myopathy	Argov and Yarom[27]
	Miscellaneous	Type I atrophy and subsarcolemmal bodies	Sahgal and Sahgal[573]
		Type I hypotrophy and central nuclei	Bender and Bender[53]
Unstructured congenital myopathies		Congenital fibre type disproportion	Brooke[81]
		Uniform type I fibre myopathy	Oh and Danon[499]
		Microfibre myopathy	Hanson et al.[298]
		Type II muscle fibre hypoplasia	Gallanti et al.[226]
		Type I myofibre hypotrophy	Prince et al.[539]
		Type I fibre predominance	Brooke[82]

Modified from Goebel and Lenard.[250]
[a]Not a specific entity.

arthrogryposis, 2% congenital muscular dystrophy, < 1% myasthenic syndromes and < 1% peripheral neuropathy. For the majority of these disorders muscle and/or nerve biopsy is a diagnostic necessity.

Congenital myopathies

The congenital myopathies (Table 9.10) are muscle disorders in which characteristic morphological features other than those of denervation or dystrophy are identified by light or electron microscopy or immunocytochemistry. The morphological features include alterations in muscle fibre structure, size or enzyme histochemistry (Figs 9.48, 9.49). A congenital myopathy is diagnosed when a majority of the following clinical features is present: infantile or early childhood onset, slow or no progression,[10] generalized or proximal weakness of varying degrees of severity,[309,656] atrophy, hypotonia,

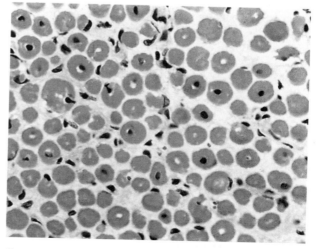

Figure 9.48 *Central nuclear myopathy. This muscle biopsy in a term newborn infant shows variation in fibre diameter and central nuclei in > 40% of the fibres. (H&E.)*

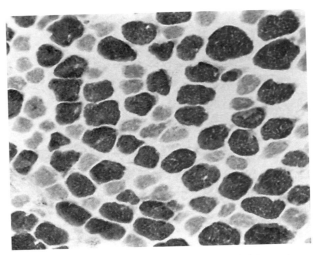

Figure 9.49 *Fibre type disproportion. This muscle biopsy shows large type II fibres and atrophic type 1 fibres. (Myosin ATPase, pH 9.4.)*

contractures, dysmorphism and family history. There is an associated normal or slightly elevated creatine phosphokinase (CPK) and normal or myopathic electromyogram (EMG).[82,195,250] Adverse reactions to anaesthesia are reported in some congenital myopathies.[371,413] Table 9.10 reflects the diversity of the congenital myopathies, but three conditions are considered to be the classic congenital myopathies: nemaline, central core and centronuclear myopathies. The genetics of these entities are complicated. For central core myopathy, genetic linkage has defined 9q13.1[279] to be a locus for some cases. This is the site of the ryanodine receptor-1 gene, which is related to malignant hyperthermia.[725] For the autosomal dominant form of nemaline myopathy, a locus has been identified at 1q21-q23,[384] where the disease gene has been identified as α-tropomyosin.[385] For the autosomal recessive form of nemaline myopathy, a locus has been identified at 2q21.2-2q22.[684] In X-linked centronuclear myopathy the gene has been localized to Xq28.[136] The identification of non-classic congenital myopathies increases yearly with overlapping observations, so that the distinctions between the various structural entities is becoming more complex. Some biopsies show combined lesions,[43,115,336,339,354,374,495,500,553,645] several entities accumu-

Table 9.11 *Congenital myasthenic syndromes*

Type	Example
Presynaptic defects	Familial infantile myasthenia
Postsynaptic or synaptic defects	Endplate acetylcholinesterase deficiency
Classic slow channel syndrome	Increased response to acetylcholine
Congenital acetylcholine receptor deficiency	

late the same proteins, and there is some overlap with some other types of muscle disorder. The reviews by Goebel,[249] Engel[185] and Darras[137] describe the complexities of classifying and understanding these disorders.

Myasthenic syndromes

The myasthenic syndromes (Table 9.11) are rare diseases which may occur in early life. They have been classified by Engel[182,184] transient neonatal myasthenia (produced by transplacental antiacetylcholine receptor antibodies from the mother to the fetus), or congenital myasthenic syndromes with genetic defects that impair neuromuscular transmission.[137] Precise diagnosis requires correlation of clinical, electrophysiological, morphological and molecular genetic studies.[183]

Metabolic myopathies

The metabolic myopathies (Table 9.12) may be suspected clinically when there is episodic exacerbation of weakness with exercise, diet or infection (Fig. 9.50), or lactic acidosis. In most conditions there is involvement of other organ systems,[425,490] particularly the brain, the liver or the heart,[608] so that the hypotonia or weakness may not be a predominant symptom. The classification of these disorders, which may involve several components of the lower motor unit, is in rapid evolution, and molecular studies are defining increasing numbers of sites where defects may cause disease (e.g. assembly genes may produce respiratory chain enzyme defects).[148] The investigation of the metabolic myopathies is often complex, requiring integrated interpretation of clinical, biochemical, morphological and molecular investigations.[156]

Muscular dystrophies

The muscular dystrophies have a characteristic histological appearance, with increased endomysial connective tissue, degeneration, regeneration and variation in fibre size (Fig. 9.51). They occur in the infantile period, and recent clinical and molecular analyses have identified that dystrophin and the dystrophin-related proteins are defective in many of the dystrophies of early life (Table 9.13). Dystrophin protein (with its gene located at Xp21) is absent in Duchenne's dystrophy and abnormal in size or quantity in Becker's dystrophy. An autosomal recessive limb girdle dystrophy of early onset and rapid progression is associated with deficiency of α-sarcoglycan, also called adhalin.[533] Other dystrophies have been recorded with abnormalities in γ-, β- and δ-sarcoglycans.[346] Moreover, a relatively large number of patients with classic congenital muscular dystrophy have been found to have a deficiency of α₂-laminin (or merosin) with its gene located

Table 9.12 *Classification of metabolic myopathies*

Morphological abnormality	Deficiency/defect	Type	References
Disorders of glycogen metabolism	Acid maltase deficiency (glycogenosis type II)	Infantile acid maltase deficiency (Pompe's)	DiMauro[155]
		Childhood acid maltase deficiency	Engel et al.[188]
	Brancher deficiency (glycogenosis type IV)		Fernandes and Huijing[200]
	Myophosphorylase deficiency (glycogenosis type V)		DiMauro and Hartlage[157]
	Phosphorylase B kinase deficiency (type VIII)		Van den Berg[660]
	Phosphofructokinase deficiency (type VII)		Guibaud et al.[275]
	Uncharacterized glycogenoses	Cardiomyopathy, mental retardation, myopathy	Danon et al.[134]
Disorders of lipid metabolism	Primary systemic carnitine deficiency		Stanley et al.[619]
	Secondary carnitine deficiency	From total parenteral nutrition	Engel[181]
		From valproate therapy	DiDonato et al.[153]
	Myopathic carnitine deficiency		DiDonato et al.[153]
	Long-chain acyl-CoA dehydrogenase deficiency		Stanley[618]
	Short-chain acyl-CoA dehydrogenase deficiency		Coates et al.[119]
	Long-chain 3-hydroxyacyldehydrogenase deficiency		Glasgow et al.[244]
	Triglyceride storage disease		Chanarin et al.[104] DiDonato et al.[154]
Mitochondrial diseases (a) Defects of substrate transport–nuclear DNA	Carnitine deficiency		DiMauro et al.[160] Stanley[618]
(b) Defects of substrate utilization–nuclear DNA	Defects in β-oxidation (see above)		
	Defects in pyruvate dehydrogenase complex		
	Pyruvate decarboxylase deficiency	Neonatal (fatal) Infantile (Leigh's syndrome) Benign form	Robinson[560]
	Dihydrolipoyl dehydrogenase deficiency		Robinson et al.[562]
	Dihydrolipoyl transacetylase deficiency		Robinson et al.[561]
	Pyruvate dehydrogenase phosphatase deficiency		Robinson[560]
	Defects of pyruvate carboxylase		Robinson[560]
Defects in Krebs cycle–nuclear DNA	α-Ketoglutarate dehydrogenase deficiency		Robinson et al.[562]
	Fumarase deficiency		Zinn et al.[727]

(Continued over page.)

Table 9.12 (Continued)

Morphological abnormality	Deficiency/defect	Type	References
Defects in the respiratory chain–nuclear or mitochondrial DNA	Complex I deficiency	Fatal multisystem disorder	Moreadith et al.[461]
		Ocular motor apraxia	Punal et al.[542]
		Myopathy	Morgan-Hughes et al.[462]
		Encephalomyopathy	Morgan-Hughes et al.[462]
	Complex II deficiency	Leigh's with leukodystrophy	DiMauro and Moraes[159]
			Sengers et al.[593]
			Birch-Machin et al.[62]
	Complex III deficiency	Infantile encephalomyopathy	Birch-Machin et al.[63]
	Complex IV deficiency	Fatal infantile myopathy	Bresolin et al.[78]
		Benign infantile myopathy	DiMauro et al.[158]
		Leigh's syndrome	DiMauro et al.[158]
			Tiranti et al.[649]
		MNGIE (myoneurogastrointestinal encephalopathy)	Bardosi et al.[44]
		POLIP	Blake et al.[67]
	Complex V deficiency		Schotland[585]
	Combined defects of respiratory chain		Zheng et al.[726]
Defects of mtDNA	Deletions and duplications	Kearns–Sayre syndrome	DiMauro and Morales[159]
		Leber hereditary optic atrophy	Mrak et al.[466]
	Point mutations	MERFF	Wallace et al.[683]
		MELAS	
		ATPase-6 mutation syndrome	Holt et al.[318]
		Fatal infantile myopathy and cardiopathy	Zeviani et al.[723]
		Multiple mtDNA deletions	Zeviani et al.[723]
		Cardiomyopathy and/or skeletal myopathy	Bruno et al.[85]
Defects of communication with nuclear and mitochondrial genome		Severe depletion	Boustany et al.[74]
			Moraes et al.[460]
Depletion of mtDNA		Partial depletion	Tritschler et al.[653]
			Arnaudo et al.[31]

Modified from DiMauro et al.[160]

on chromosome 6q2. These patients with merosin-negative congenital dystrophy also have a leukodystrophy. It should be noted that some merosin-negative muscle biopsies, because of prominent lymphocytic infiltrates, have been confused with the inflammatory myopathies.[465] The merosin-positive congenital muscular dystrophy in which a defect has not yet been identified does not have an associated leukodystrophy, but one recent report has identified mental retardation.[489] Because the muscle

membrane proteins are functionally related, abnormalities in one protein may cause secondary reductions in others, so that the analysis and identification of the primary defect must be rigorous.

Emery Dreifuss muscular dystrophy, which is associated with contractures and heart disease, has a complex inheritance. An X-linked form is related to a defect in *emerin* (gene on Xq28), a nuclear membrane protein,[346] and an autosomal dominant form is related to a defect in

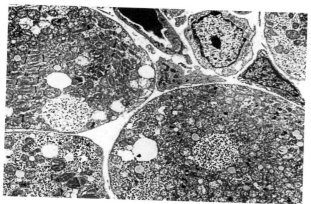

Figure 9.50 *Cytochrome c oxidase deficiency. The ultrastructural abnormalities of the muscle biopsy consist of variation in fibre diameter and increased glycogen, lipid and mitochondria.*

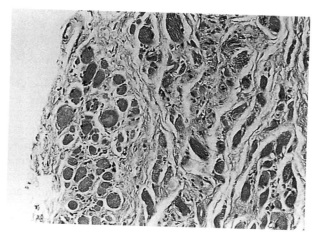

Figure 9.51 *Congenital muscular dystrophy. This muscle biopsy shows variation in fibre diameter, a rare degenerating fibre and marked endomysial fibrosis. (H&E.)*

lamin A/C.[71] There are three disorders with infantile muscular dystrophy which are associated with CNS abnormalities, in addition to merosin-negative congenital muscular dystrophy. These have been called the eye, brain and muscle disorders. The best studied is Fukuyama muscular dystrophy.[574,706,707] The defective gene, *fukutin*, has been identified at 9q31. Fukuyama muscular dystrophy is associated with microencephaly, cerebral pachygyria, cerebellar polymicrogyria, heterotopias, subpial gliosis and hydrocephalus *ex vacuo*.[137] Patients with the Walker–Warburg syndrome present with neonatal weakness, hydrocephalus, macrocephaly and eye abnormalities. The cerebral cortex exhibits type 2 lissencephaly, with cerebellar hypoplasia, Dandy–Walker malformation, small optic nerves, absent corpus callosum, encephalocele and heterotopias. The genetic defect is not known. Eye–muscle–brain disease resembles Walker–Warburg syndrome but is much less severe and the genetic defect is 1p32-p32. Brain imaging has been useful in identifying the CNS lesions in these complex disorders.[369] A congenital muscular dystrophy associated with rigid spine has been recently mapped to 1p35-36.[209] Prenatal diagnosis is available for those dystrophies for which a gene locus is known, i.e. Becker's, Duchenne,[8] Emery-Dreifuss[314] and myotonic dystrophy.[34] Linkage analysis for fascioscapulohumeral dystrophy, which does not have an infantile presentation, has been related by linkage analysis to the long arm of chromosome 4.[693]

Inflammatory myopathies

Inflammatory myopathies (Table 9.14) occurring before or soon after birth are rare, and may be associated with arthrogryposis. Their aetiologies are not well proven, but

Table 9.13 *Muscular dystrophies present in the first 2 years*

Class of dystrophy	Types	References
Dystrophinopathies	Duchenne's dystrophy	Hoffman et al.[315]
	Becker's dystrophy[a]	Specht and Shapiro[614]
Myotonic dystrophy	Congenital with defective myotonin protein kinase	Vanier[662]
		Brook et al.[80]
Early-onset autosomal dominant limb girdle dystrophy[a]		Bethlem and Wijngaarden[59]
Congenital muscular dystrophies		
	Congenital muscular dystrophy	Banker[43]
	Fukuyama's congenital muscular dystrophy	Batten[48]
	Walker–Warberg congenital muscular dystrophy	Fukuyama et al.[222]
	Eye, muscle, brain	Walker[682]
	Santavuori congenital muscular dystrophy	Pavone et al.[522]
	Rigid spine syndrome	Santavuori et al.[579]
		Dubowitz[167]

[a]Rare in infancy.

Table 9.14 *Inflammatory myopathies present in the first 2 years*

Type	References
Congenital inflammatory myopathy	Shevell et al.[601]
Infantile myositis	Thompson[646]

intrauterine infections and autoimmune processes have been suggested.[476,601,646] There are reports of merosin-deficient congenital muscular dystrophy, with a marked lymphocytic infiltrate, being misinterpreted as an inflammatory myopathy.[465]

SPINAL MUSCULAR AND NEUROGENIC ATROPHIES

The 'neurogenic' causes of perinatal neuromuscular diseases (Table 9.9) may be situated in the motor nuclei of the brainstem, the anterior horn of the spinal cord, nerve roots or peripheral nerves. In generalized metabolic diseases, such as acid maltase deficiency, the weakness may be related to abnormalities affecting neurons at all levels of the neuroaxis. In infants with hypoxic–ischaemic brain injury, abnormal neuromuscular activity can be induced by CNS lesions which extend beyond the motor unit, so that the muscle biopsy shows only non-specific type II fibre atrophy.[83] Nevertheless, the examination of the muscle and/or nerve can often be an essential part of the diagnostic armentarium for the neonatologist or paediatrician dealing with problematic hypotonia or weakness.

The spinal muscular atrophies (SMAs) are associated with 'degenerations' of the anterior horn neurons and bulbar motor neurons, usually without pyramidal or sensory system involvement. The diagnosis is suggested by the clinical appearance of the hypotonic alert infant, by EMG

findings[87] of spontaneous activity, fibrillation potentials, and increased amplitude and duration of motor unit potentials, and by muscle biopsy. The muscle biopsy reveals groups of small, round fibres and groups of type I hypertrophied fibres (Fig. 9.52). The spinal cord shows subtle degeneration with loss of large and small neurons in the anterior horns. Some neurons of the lower cranial nerve motor nuclei are also involved. Neurons may be in various stages of degeneration, with swelling of cytoplasm and shrinkage of neurons, or associated with microglia exhibiting neuronophagia or astrogliosis. There is spinal cord gliosis and atrophy of the ventral roots (Fig. 9.53). Rare degeneration of the dorsal root ganglion cells and sensory columns,[303] and loss of neurons in the posteroventral nucleus of the thalamus[272] have also been reported.

SMA has three presentations: a severe infant form, before 6 months, a moderately severe form presenting after 6 months of age, and a childhood form.[495] In the infants there is a progressive deterioration with a delay in motor milestones, a weakening of suck, dysphagia, frequent aspiration and laboured breathing. Evidence of progressive denervation may be seen in fasciculating muscles, especially the tongue. The weakness and loss of reflexes are most marked initially in the proximal lower limb, but spread to involve both limbs, distal limb and neck muscles. The diaphragm is usually spared, although it may be involved initially in some infants with severe respiratory distress.[442] Death occurs within the first 2 years in the acute form and within the first two decades in the intermediate form.

The SMAs are relatively common causes of neonatal weakness, but can be diagnostic problems for several reasons. First, the anterior horn neurons can be involved in other degenerative or aplastic diseases of the nervous system that affect more than the motor neurons of the spinal cord and brainstem. There are multisystem diseases, for example, which involve the spinal cord, the cerebellum, the pons, the thalamus and peripheral nerves,[113,620] and the spinal cord, the pons and the cerebellum.[113,261,400,493,689] Secondly, genetic testing has expanded the phenotype of SMAs. The majority of SMA patients have deletions in 5q11.2-13-3,[469] and are identified as one of three clinical forms: severe, intermediate and mild. The candidate genes in this region are the survival motor neuron gene (SMN),[90,494] the neuronal apoptosis inhibitory protein

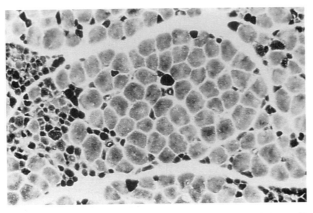

Figure 9.52 *Spinal muscular atrophy, type I, Werdnig–Hoffmann disease. There is hypertrophy of type I fibres and atrophy of type I and type II fibres. (Myosin ATPase, pH 9.4.)*

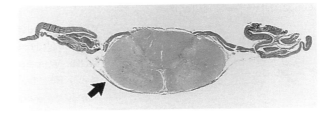

Figure 9.53 *Spinal muscular atrophy, type I, Werdnig–Hoffmann disease. There is atrophy of the anterior roots (arrow).*

(NAIP) gene, and the *p44* gene.[64] In the past, guidelines based on clinical examination defined criteria for the diagnosis of SMAs.[470] There are now reports of cases, however, which exhibit SMN deletions, but which clinically demonstrate some of the exclusion criteria. There are cases of SMA with arthrogryposis,[61] uncharacteristic muscle biopsies,[658] axonal neuropathy,[373] and atypical muscle and nerve biopsies.[505] The genetic–clinical characterization of SMAs is also complicated by the involvement of other chromosomes. An X-linked form of SMA[265] associated with joint deformities has been reported, and there are other cases suggesting possible X-linked inheritance.[350,484] A form of SMA with severe respiratory distress has been linked to 11q13-q21.[270] There are reports of cases of SMAs associated with other conditions, e.g. oral–facial–digital syndrome[304] and Arnold–Chiari malformation with juvenile distal SMA.[101] It is therefore essential that genetic testing be performed to verify typical and atypical cases of SMA, to assist in the understanding of the pathogenesis of these disorders, and to provide up-to-date genetic information and counselling.

The peripheral neuropathies presenting in the infantile period include various hereditary motor and sensory neuropathies, congenital dysmyelinopathies, inflammatory polyneuropathies and neuropathies associated with various metabolic diseases of the nervous system. Their identification requires nerve conduction studies, nerve biopsies (Fig. 9.54) and careful family histories.[17] The genetic abnormalities of the hereditary neuropathies are becoming defined so that more precise molecular diagnoses can be made, but our understanding of the clinical correlations with the molecular defects and the pathogenesis of the lesions is incomplete. The most common hereditary neuropathy in childhood is Charcot–Marie–Tooth type I (HMSN-I, a demyelinating hypertrophic neuropathy with onion skins), although the clinical presentation rarely begins in infancy. Several genetic abnormalities have been identified, which are also observed in other infantile neuropathies. In HMSN-Ia

there is duplication of the peripheral myelin protein (PMP-22) gene or a point mutation in *PMP-22*. In HMSN-Ib, there are mutations in myelin protein zero (P0), and in the X-linked HMSN-I there are mutations in the connexin 32 gene. There is a neuronal form of Charcot–Marie–Tooth disease (HMSN-II), which is less common and associated with abnormalities of chromosome 1. HSMN-III or Déjeriné Sotas disease is a severe disorder which has also been associated with mutations in *P0* and *PMP-22* genes. It is classified as a congenital dysmyelinating neuropathy.[223,446] Other examples of this type of neuropathy presenting in infancy are listed in Table 9.9. The peripheral nerve is involved in the diseases associated with abnormal DNA repair, metabolic abnormalities and inflammatory neuropathies, many of which present in infancy and early childhood. The neuropathology of these entities is described in Chapters 9 and 14, Volume II.

ARTHROGRYPOSIS MULTIPLEX CONGENITA

Arthrogryposis multiplex congenita (AMC) is a syndrome characterized by congenital fixation of multiple joints. There are numerous diseases associated with AMC, each of which presumably interferes with the movement of skeletal muscle *in utero*. Hall[286] considers that webbing will develop if the restriction of movement occurs around 14 weeks of gestation, but that akinesia developing after 20 weeks will not be associated with skin webs at the abnormal joints. The prognosis for an infant with congenital contractures depends upon the diagnosis associated with AMC. In Hall's 1985 survey,[288] a specific diagnosis could not made in 20% of cases. Most infants with AMC will survive, but cases with CNS involvement are more likely to be fatal and to recur in subsequent pregnancies. Banker[41,42] has identified numerous conditions associated with AMC and has observed that each exhibits lesions in some component of the motor system: anterior horn neurons, nerve roots, peripheral nerves, end-plate, muscle or the CNS. Other authors have observed lesions involving the sensory system.[214] The conditions associated with arthrogryposis, based primarily on Banker's observations, are listed in Table 9.15. In most of the diseases associated with AMC, the lesions of the CNS and PNS are static, with the exception of the rare examples of SMAs and muscular dystrophies.

Many aetiologies and patterns of inheritance (Table 9.16) are associated with AMC. The clinical presentations are frequently complicated, exhibiting lesions and malformations in other systems. One of these complicated, multisystem entities associated with AMC was described in 1974 by Pena and Shokeir:[524] a particular clinical constellation of campodactyly, facial anomalies and pulmonary hypoplasia in two sisters with AMC. Other reports[108,310,409,440] described somewhat similar conditions, but included a variety of other organ anomalies,

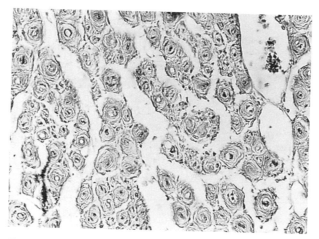

Figure 9.54 *Hypertrophic neuropathy. There is onion bulb formation in the peripheral nerve.*

Table 9.15 *Aetiology for arthrogryposis multiplex congenita according to site of lesion*

Site	Type	References
Neurogenic disease: motor lesion	Muscle fibre type predominance or disproportion	
	Dysgenesis of motor nuclei or spinal cord and brainstem[a]	Clarren and Hall[118]
	Dysgenesis of brain	Mulliez et al.[467]
	Dysgenesis of CNS: abnormal chromosome 18	
	Arthrogryposis and trisomy 21	
	Dysgenesis of motor nuclei of brainstem and cord in Pierre–Robin syndrome	
	Dysgenesis of motor nuclei of brainstem and cord in Mobius' syndrome	
	Dysgenesis of spinal cord and prune belly syndrome	
	Craniocarpotarsal (Freeman–Sheldon) syndrome	
	Arrhinencephaly, encephalocele; Meckel–Gruber syndrome, dysgenesis of anterior horns	
	Anencephaly with dysgenesis of anterior horn neurons	
	Microcephaly alone and with Marden–Walker and Bowen–Conradi syndrome	Hageman et al.[283]
	Arnold–Chiari syndrome	
	Caudal regression syndrome	
	Arthrogryposis and Potter sequence	Hageman et al.[283]
	Cerebrohepatorenal (Zellweger's) syndrome	
	X-linked spinal muscular atrophy	Greenberg et al.[265]
	Type I spinal muscular atrophy[b]	
Neurogenic disease: secondary neural disease	Congenital infection	Hageman et al.[283]
	Toxaemia	Hageman et al.[283]
Neurogenic disease	Posterior column and peripheral neuropathy	Folkerth et al.[214]
Myopathic disease	Congenital muscular dystrophy	
	Congenital myotonic dystrophy	
	Central core disease[b]	
	Nemaline myopathy[b]	Lammens et al.[387]
	Myopathy with cortex deficiency	Vielhaber et al.[669]
	Myopathy[c] with increased glycogen	Lebenthal et al.[393] Darin et al.[135]
	Myopathy with contractures	Lammens et al.[387]
	Ophthalmophegia with rimmed vacuole	
	Muscle fibrosis in congenital torticollis	
	Phosphofructokinase deficiency	Nowak et al.[495]
Motor endplate disease	Maternal autoimmune myasthenia gravis	Moutard-Codou et al.[463]
	Congenital myasthenic syndrome	Smit and Barth[609]
	Curare induced	Jago[341]
Unknown	Isolated club foot	

Modified from Banker.[41,42]

[a]Amyoplasia, described by Hall et al.[289] as a common sporadic condition with congenital contractures, may fall into this category.

[b]Rare in this condition.

[c]Banker[42] suggests that this may be a neurogenic type based on the report of Krugliak et al.[377]

Table 9.16 *Inheritance of arthrogryposis multiplex congenita*

Source	Type	References
Chromosomal	Trisomy 18, 21	
	Trisomy 8 mosiacism	
	Turner's syndrome	
Autosomal dominant	Distal arthrogryposis multiplex congenita	Hall *et al.*[290]
	Craniocarpotarsal (Freeman–Shelton) syndrome	
	Pterygoarthro-myodysplasia	Krieger and Espiritu[375]
	Congenital myotonic dystrophy	
	Marfan's syndrome	Reeve *et al.*[552]
Autosomal recessive	Cerebrohepatorenal (Zellweger) syndrome	
	Spinal muscular atrophy[a]	
	Congenital muscular dystrophy	
	Lethal pterygium syndrome	
	Multiple pterygium syndrome	Hall *et al.*[290]
	Pena–Shokeir	Pena and Shokeir[524]
Sex-linked	Lethal CNS dysgenesis and arthrogryposis, multifactorial	Mulliez *et al.*[467]
	Dysraphic conditions with arthrogryposis	

From Hall *et al.*[290] and Banker.[42]
[a]Rare in this condition.

histopathological findings, and patterns of inheritance. Hall[286] analysed the reports of the Pena–Shokeir phenotype, and recognized a pattern of morphological anomalies that had been produced experimentally by Moessinger.[457] He curarized fetal rats to decrease movements *in utero* and developed in them a predictable sequence of secondary anomalies referred to as the fetal akinesia deformation sequence. The phenotype is tabulated in Table 9.17. Hall[286] considers that the human fetal akinesia deformation sequence, with its wide spectrum of clinical and pathological lesions, reflects degrees of severity of outcomes from intrauterine immobilization caused by neurogenic (upper and/or lower motor neuron), myopathic or possibly constricting skin lesions. These conclusions are an expansion of Banker's explanation of the pathogenesis of AMC. Hall[287] and Gordon[258] have summarized the current literature pertaining to classification of genetics and approaches to diagnosis.[287]

Table 9.17 *Fetal akinesia deformity sequence (phenotype of Pena–Shokeir syndrome)*[296]

Deformity	Features
Intrauterine growth retardation	
Craniofacial anomalies	Ocular hypertelorism, micrognathia, short neck, low-set ears, depressed nasal tip
Limb anomalies	Lack of growth, limited movement of joints, abnormal shape, abnormal position, decreased calcification of bone
Pulmonary hypoplasia	
Short umbilical cord	
Polyhydramnios	

SUDDEN INFANT DEATH SYNDROME

SIDS is defined as 'the sudden death of an infant under one year of age which remains unexplained after a thorough case investigation, including performance of a complete autopsy, examination of the death scene, and review of the clinical history'.[698] SIDS is temporally associated with sleep, leading to the premise that it occurs during sleep or transitions between sleep and waking. SIDS peaks at 2–4 months of age, and 90% of cases occur under 6 months of age. The time-frame of SIDS coincides with the period in which dramatic and rapid changes occur as the newborn adapts to extrauterine life.[363] Despite a dramatic 38% fall in the incidence of SIDS in the USA following the 1994 national recommendation for the supine sleeping position, SIDS remains the leading cause of postneonatal infant mortality, with an overall incidence of 0.7 per 1000 live births. The mechanism that underlies the increased risk for SIDS from the prone sleeping position is unknown, but may involve rebreathing of expired gases with hypoxia, hypercapnia or asphyxia, upper airway obstruction, impaired arousal thresholds in the prone position that hamper effects to turn the head, compromised upper airway reflexes; hyperthermia due to heat trapping in the face-down position, or altered sensory/vestibular influences on blood pressure.[302] All of these mechanisms potentially involve the brainstem.

In order to conceptualize SIDS, a triple-risk model has been proposed.[205] According to this model, SIDS occurs when three factors impinge simultaneously upon the infant: (1) an underlying vulnerability in the infant's homoeostatic control; (2) a critical developmental period in autonomic and respiratory control and state maturation; and (3) an exogenous stressor, e.g. hypoxia, hypercapnia, asphyxia or reflex apnoea from the prone sleep position, or hyperthermia from overbundling (Fig. 9.55). Only when these three factors come together will a SIDS death occur. The underlying vulnerability explains why not all babies die when placed prone: healthy babies do not die of SIDS. The exogenous stressor explains why the Back-to-Sleep risk reduction campaign has been successful, although the causes of SIDS are not known: by removing the exogenous stressor, the vulnerable infant is known to pass through the critical developmental period unharmed. According to this model, there may be several causes of SIDS, with different underlying vulnerabilities.

An underlying vulnerability in the infant as a risk factor for SIDS is supported by four lines of evidence: (1) subtle CNS and/or systemic abnormalities in cases of SIDS, detected by quantitative methods at autopsy; (2) neonatal abnormalities in neurological or autonomic function in at least some infants who subsequently die of SIDS; (3) postneonatal abnormalities in crying, cardiac and ventilatory patterns, and state organization in cases that subsequently die of SIDS; and (4) maternal and pregnancy-related factors associated with increased SIDS risk.[363] Epidemiological risk factors include prematurity, low birth weight, young maternal age, maternal anaemia, maternal cocaine and heroin abuse during pregnancy, and maternal cigarette smoking during pregnancy. Together, these risk factors point to a suboptimal intrauterine environment, and suggest that the mechanisms for risk of SIDS develop in fetal life. A variety of autonomic, respiratory and state irregularities have been reported in infants at increased epidemiological risk for SIDS and/or infants who subsequently die of SIDS, strengthening the possibility of a primary defect in autonomic, respiratory and/or sleep–waking state regulation. These irregularities include higher heart rates, reduced heart-rate variability, increased incidence of tachycardic episodes, fewer apnoeic pauses, and reduced minute-by-minute correlations between cardiac and respiratory measures.[363] Many of these differences become apparent only during particular sleep–waking states, underscoring the possibility of central neural dysfunction. Cases of SIDS show greater amounts of rapid eye movement (REM) and non-REM (NREM) sleep and reduced amounts of waking relative to controls during the early morning, the time when SIDS deaths occur. Some infants at increased epidemiological risk for SIDS have also been found to have diminished ventilatory responsiveness and/or impaired arousal to hypercarbia or hypoxia.[328] Analysis of cardiorespiratory recordings of the time of death in home-monitored SIDS and other infants show a profound bradycardia.[444] In addition, such recordings indicate terminal gasping in most cases, suggesting that failure to autoresuscitate may be an important contributing factor in these deaths.[444] Cranial Doppler sonography in nine out of 39 infants with apparent life-threatening events showed a reduction in blood flow in the basilar artery caused by compression of the contralateral vertebral artery at the craniocervical junction.[140]

The concept of a vulnerable infant is supported by reports of neuropathological abnormalities in cases of SIDS, including increased brain weight,[597] subtle brainstem scarring,[362,475,496,625,632] altered dendritic and spine density development in the brainstem,[547,629,637] increased synaptic density in the central reticular nucleus of the medulla,[503] altered brainstem neurotransmitter levels,[98,111,144,145,424,497] subtle hypomyelination within and rostral to the brainstem,[97,360] cerebral white-matter gliosis,[18,496] PVL,[360,496,632] increased neuropil in the hypoglossal nucleus,[504] increased ALZ-50-reactive neurons in the hippocampus,[613] increased lipid-containing cells in the cerebral white matter,[190,224] olivary gliosis,[362,625] apoptosis,[685] delay in the maturation of the external granular layer of the cerebellum[131] and increased substance P in trigeminal fibres.[708] These findings are non-specific, and it is not clear which, if any, are directly related to the pathogenesis of sudden death. Several of these findings (cerebral white-matter gliosis, olivary gliosis, PVL, apoptosis) are considered secondary, for example, to hypoxia–ischaemia, including

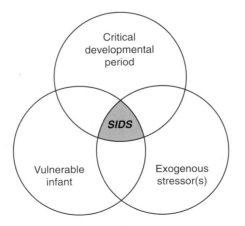

Figure 9.55 *Sudden infant death syndrome. According to the triple-risk model, SIDS occurs when three factors impinge upon the infant simultaneously: (1) an underlying vulnerability; (2) the critical developmental period; and (3) an exogenous stressor. From Filiano and Kinney.*[205]

prenatal hypoxia–ischaemia, and implicate hypoxia–ischaemia in the pathogenesis of SIDS. Other findings (e.g. delayed myelination, delayed cerebellar granule cell maturation, altered dendrite spine development) suggest abnormalities in developmental programmes involving neurons and oligodendrocytes. It is not clear how these findings relate to one another because they have generally been analysed in separate studies and not within the same brains. Any of these abnormalities may represent the neuropathology of an underlying metabolic defect that results in sudden death and coincident subtle brain pathology.

One neural hypothesis is that SIDS, or a subset, results from a failure of the ventral medulla in mediating homoeostatic responses to life-threatening challenges (e.g. asphyxia, hypoxia, hypercapnia) during sleep, as the vulnerable infant passes through the critical developmental period (triple-risk model).[363] The ventral medulla is composed of neurons and glia along the ventral and ventrolateral rim, which is involved in chemoreception, respiratory drive, upper airway reflexes and blood-pressure responses.[655] In a comparative anatomical study of the ventral surface of the cat and human infant, homologous cell populations between the two species were defined based upon cytoarchitecture and three-dimensional distribution, and the arcuate nucleus along the ventral medullary surface was proposed to be cytologically homologous to components of the respiratory fields of the cat ventral surface.[207] Severe hypoplasia of the arcuate nucleus hypoplasia has been reported in a subset of SIDS.[206,380,424,437] The idea that the arcuate nucleus is involved in central chemosensitivity is strengthened by the report of an infant with clinically recognized insensitivity to carbon dioxide, sudden death and absence of the arcuate nucleus at autopsy.[213] DiI labelling studies in human midgestational fetuses demonstrated connections between the arcuate nucleus and the caudal raphé, suggesting a potential functional link between these two regions. This is of special interest in SIDS given the well-defined role of the caudal raphé in respiration, chemoreception, blood pressure regulation and upper airway control.[722] Subsequent neurotransmitter receptor-binding studies were undertaken between 1985 and 1997.[365] (The majority of the cases were collected before the risk reduction campaign.) These studies, involving 19 brainstem regions and six neurotransmitter systems, demonstrated isolated decreased muscarinic and kainate receptor binding in the arcuate nucleus.[364,512] Perhaps most significantly, these studies demonstrated serotonergic binding deficiencies in cases of SIDS in the caudal raphé (nucleus raphé obscurus) and five other functionally and developmentally related components of the medulla [including the arcuate nucleus, nucleus paragigantocellularis lateralis, nucleus gigantocellularis, lateral reticular zone (homologous to the gasping centre in experimental animals) and the inferior olive], all regions critically involved in chemoreception, respiratory drive, blood-pressure responses, upper airway reflexes and/or thermoregulation (Fig. 9.56).[365,511] Four of the six regions, including the nucleus raphé obscurus, arcuate nucleus, inferior olive and nucleus paragigantocellularis lateralis, are considered derivatives of a common embryonic anlage, the rhombic lip, and five of the six regions, including the nucleus raphé obscurus, arcuate nucleus, nucleus paragigantocellularis lateralis, nucleus gigantocellularis and lateral reticular zone, contain serotonergic neurons in the developing human brainstem. Taken together, these findings suggest a primary defect in serotonergic neurons, derived at least in part from the rhombic lip, in cases of SIDS, resulting from a failure of cell division, migration and/or differentiation. These studies

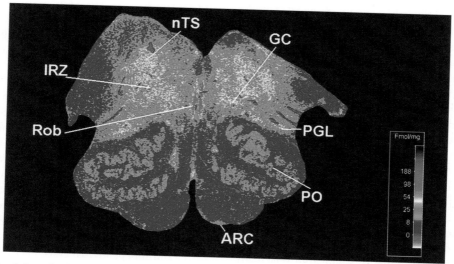

Figure 9.56 *Sudden infant death syndrome. Serotonergic receptors in the medulla of the human infant. Binding was decreased in SIDS cases compared with controls in the nucleus raphé obscurus (ROb), nucleus paragigantocellularis lateralis (PGL), nucleus gigantocellularis (GC), intermediate reticular zone (IRZ), principal inferior olive (PO) and arcuate nucleus (ARC). Binding did not differ in the nucleus of the solitary tract (NTS). ([³H]LSD binding.) From Panigraphy et al.[511]*

have led to an expanded hypothesis: the medullary serotonergic deficiency hypothesis in SIDS: SIDS, or a subset of SIDS, is due to a developmental abnormality of medullary neurons composed of (at least in part) rhombic lip-derived, serotonergic neurons of the ventral medulla, and this abnormality results in a failure of protective responses to life-threatening challenges during sleep as the infant passes through a critical period in homoeostatic control.

NEUROPATHOLOGY OF THE STILLBORN

There has been increased attention focused upon the neuropathology of the stillborn since 1986 when Nelson and Ellenberg revealed in the National Collaborative Perinatal Project (NCPP) data (gathered between 1959 and 1966) that birth asphyxia and postnatal factors contributed very little to the overall incidence of cerebral palsy. In this landmark article factors operating before birth were identified as being responsible for most cases.[480] This paper prompted systematic studies of the stillborn brain to determine the types of injuries to which it was susceptible, and from which cerebral palsy might develop in postpartum survivors. In the stillborn, intrapartum, neonatal and early postnatal factors are eliminated as causes of brain damage. The practising neuropathologist is frequently called upon to determine whether brain pathology is the cause of death in a stillborn, e.g. a large germinal matrix with intraventricular haemorrhage, or to explain the significance of brain pathology, e.g. cerebral white-matter gliosis. The definition of a stillborn varies among states and countries and depends upon the defined cut-off age for abortions. In America a recent definition[423] is 'an infant born with no sign of life between 20 weeks' gestation and term'.

The causes of stillbirth include placental failure, major malformations, bleeding, isoimmunization, severe chorioamnionitis, tumours and cervical cord necrosis. In a survey of 243 cases, Hovatta et al.[322] found that the major cause of stillbirth (approximately 60% of cases) is placental failure, e.g. abruption of the placenta, placental infarction and cord complication. A second leading cause (17% of cases) is major malformations (types not specified in this series).[322] In another report major malformations included the CNS lesions of anencephaly and hydrocephalus.[89] Other causes (11%) include unexplained asphyxia, isoimmunization, fetal bleeding (e.g. fetofetal transfusion, fetomaternal transfusion) and severe chorioamniotis.[322] Approximately 9% of the cases of stillbirth are unexplained,[322] a point of interest in the possible relationship to SIDS. CNS pathology, excluding the major malformations, is not the primary cause of stillbirth in very many cases. However, global (asphyxial) destruction of the CNS of a type seen with anoxia and circulatory failure in children and adults does occur in stillborns, even without recognized changes in the maternal circulation.[3] It has been

associated at birth with clinical and electrographical criteria of brain death.[3] Germinal matrix haemorrhages with dissemination into the ventricular system are found in stillborns at autopsy[617] and, if large, are considered the cause of death. There are rare reports of neoplasm as the cause of fetal demise, in particular extremely large tumours, e.g. the case report of a congenital craniopharyngioma, 10 cm in its widest diameter, in a full-term male stillborn infant.[686] In addition, CNS infections have rarely been reported as the cause of stillbirth, e.g. a 35 week stillborn with purulent meningitis associated with cocci on tissue stains caused by amniochorionitis via the umbilical route.[320] Intrauterine cord necrosis was reported in a liveborn female who was born in the breech position with hyperextension of the neck; she died at 26 h of respiratory failure and intractable bradycardia.[715] At autopsy she had intrauterine necrosis of the upper cervical cord and lung hypoplasia, the latter suggesting chronic and inadequate innervation to the muscles of respiration. Dislocation of the upper cervical vertebrae from the hyperflexed breech position can cause decreased blood flow, resulting in upper cervical cord necrosis, respiratory failure and death.[715]

Although they are not considered the primary cause of death, virtually all types of neuropathology have been reported in case reports or surveys of the stillborn. These include malformations, grey-matter necrosis or neuronal loss involving the cerebral cortex, hippocampus and subiculum, thalamus, basal ganglia, cerebellum and brainstem,[89,255] PVL,[617] choroid plexus, germinal matrix, petechial, subarachnoid and intraparenchymal haemorrhages,[255,617] haemorrhagic necrosis,[255] cerebral white-matter gliosis,[617] pontosubicular necrosis,[456] hypotensive brainstem necrosis,[641] neoplasms, bacterial, viral and protozoal infections, chromosomal disorders (e.g. Down's syndrome), degenerative disorders, metabolic disorders and genetic diseases. The white-matter lesions of Krabbe leukodystrophy, for example, are seen in utero: typical globoid cells containing tubular inclusions are found in the spinal tracts of fetuses at 18–23 gestational weeks, a time when comparable changes are not seen in the non-myelinating cerebral hemispheres.[180,197,434] Tubers have been reported in the brain of a stillborn at 36 gestational weeks with tuberous sclerosis, cardiac rhabdomyomas and multicystic kidneys.[488] Non-immune hydrops fetalis can result in stillbirth and intrauterine brain damage.[390] The neuropathological changes include PVL, white-matter gliosis, microcalcifications and microthromboses (probably secondary to blood dyscrasias); anoxic neuronal damage involving the cerebral cortex, basal ganglia, dentate nucleus and subiculum is less common. Miscellaneous lesions include isolated thalamic infarct, germinal matrix infarct and subependymal cysts. Larroche et al.[390] speculate that anaemia, hypoproteinaemia and cardiac failure with hypotension, which often occur in hydrops fetalis, account for brain perfusion failure and hypoxic-ischaemic changes in this condition.

Surveys of the stillborn brain have been prompted by a consideration of the relationship between antepartum brain injury and cerebral palsy. One of the largest systematic studies to examine the antecedents of cerebral palsy was the prospective NCPP of the National Institute of Neurological and Communicative Disorders and Stroke in 12 university hospitals. The neuropathology studies of the NCPP[236] collated and defined the high prevalence of perinatal white-matter damage, i.e. perinatal telencephalic leukoencephalopathy (PTL), a brain lesion of infants between 28 gestational weeks and 4 postnatal months.[234] This entity is characterized by four histological features: foci of necrosis (PVL), hypertrophic (reactive) astrocytes, perivascular amphophilic globules (considered to be mineralized extravasated vascular proteins reflecting endothelial vascular damage) and cells described as acutely damaged glia. These glia may reflect injured oligodendrocyte and/or astrocytic precursors that are pyknotic and therefore morphologically indistinguishable as to their cell of origin; some investigators suggest that they are oligodendrocyte precursors that are apoptotic secondary to free radical injury complicating ischaemia/reperfusion.[357] Because of similarities in the risk factors of each histological feature and of a cluster of features, they have been regarded as components of one entity, PTL.[236,403] The entity is common: in a sample of autopsied newborns enrolled in the NCPP, 56% had some combination of the features of PTL.[403] It is now well recognized that PVL, white-matter gliosis, decreased white-matter volume, delayed myelination or hypomyelination, thinned corpus callosum and hydrocephalus *ex vacuo* (ventriculomegaly) are the major underlying substrates of cerebral palsy in premature infants surviving the neonatal intensive care nursery (see review in Ref. 357). Gilles proposed that perinatal white-matter damage may interfere with normal myelination by diverting glial stem cells into reactive astrocytes and thus reducing the population of mature oligodendrocytes available to synthesize myelin, thereby causing hypomyelination, the correlate of some cases of cerebral palsy in later life.[236]

The aetiology for these various white-matter pathologies is being defined and the neuropathological observations in particular were critical in the formation of the endotoxin/infection/cytokine hypothesis for PVL in the premature infant,[403] an active area of cerebral palsy research today. In the NCPP, indicators of presumed endotoxin exposure were identified as risk factors for PTL. These indicators included neonatal bacteraemia and maternal urinary tract infection, especially when accompanied by fever. However, the associations between maternal infection and infant brain pathology are not straightforward. For example, chorioamnionitis was associated with a decreased risk of both hypertrophic astrocytes and foci of necrosis in the univariate analyses. The NCPP provided epidemiological evidence that amniotic fluid infections were associated with psychomotor dysfunction in survivors.[474]

A second major hypothesis about the cause and mechanism of PVL and hypertrophic astrocytes (reactive gliosis) and its relationship to cerebral palsy, based primarily upon the studies of other investigators,[679] implicates ischaemia/reperfusion. In the NCPP, obvious correlates and/or measures of hypoxia, such as low Apgar scores, were not identified as risk factors for any of the histological features of PTL, including PVL; however, blood gases and blood pressures were not included in the data file. In an analysis of the brains of 165 stillbirths in the NCPP, 35% had hypertrophic astrocytes, 26% had amphophilic globules, 16% had acutely damaged glia and 4% had focal necrosis (PVL).[403] The fact that PTL occurs in the stillborn and prior to the influences of labour and delivery is directly relevant to the epidemiological findings in the NCPP suggesting that cerebral palsy is more likely to be due to antenatal factors. Studies of the stillborn have attempted to provide links between neuropathological findings, particularly focal necrosis (PVL) and white-matter gliosis, and infectious and/or vascular risk factors in the fetus and/or placenta.

In 1967, Terplan[642] described the neuropathology of 1152 perinatal and infant deaths, including 66 stillborns. Of the stillborns, 11% had germinal matrix haemorrhages, 15% had white-matter necrosis (five preterm, five full-term) and 21% had cortical neuronal injury. Sims et al.[606] examined 433 autopsies of stillborns and found periventricular/intraventricular haemorrhage in 15 (five with parenchymal haemorrhage), five with parenchymal haemorrhage alone and five with white-matter gliosis. (CNS malformations were excluded from the survey.) Squier and Keeling[617] reported the brain findings in 39 stillborns: ten cases had white-matter damage, including diffuse gliosis and focal necrosis, two had germinal matrix haemorrhage and intraventricular rupture, and five had germinal matrix haemorrhage in association with gliosis or necrosis of adjacent white-matter. In this series, although Squier and Keeling were proponents of the hypothesis that the white-matter damage was ischaemic in origin and 'related to circulatory disorders', they did not provide supporting clinical or pathological data. In a study of the clinical associations of prenatal ischaemic white-matter injury, Gaffney et al.[225] performed neuropathological examinations on 274 cases of intrauterine death or neonatal death at or before 3 days after birth. Fifty-six (20%) of the cases had evidence of prenatal ischaemic brain damage. There was an increased incidence of intrauterine growth retardation and oligohydramnios, but not maternal infection (including urinary tract infection) in cases with prenatal white-matter damage. The association of intrauterine growth retardation and white-matter damage remained after excluding fetuses with a major congenital anomaly. The findings were interpreted as chronic intrauterine hypoxia (leading to intrauterine growth retardation) being associated with damage to cerebral white-matter among fetuses and infants who die. Gaffney et al. further speculated that such hypoxic damage may also affect developing oligodendrocytes and result in decreased mature, myelin-producing cell numbers, thereby resulting in delayed or hypomyelination in infants who survive the neonatal period and potentially resulting in cerebral palsy.[225]

Rare studies have combined stillborn neuropathology with placental analysis to help to determine the causes of the antenatal brain damage.[51,89] Bejar et al.[51] reported that 10% of the preterm infants they had studied had evidence of antenatal white-matter necrosis. Placental vascular anatomoses in multiple pregnancies, purulent amnionic fluid and funisitis were the only variables with significant associations with the white-matter necrosis. After excluding stillbirths with major cerebral malformations, Burke and Tannenberg[89] studied the brains of 175 cases and the corresponding placentas in 165 cases. Seventy of the 175 brains (40%) showed microscopic evidence of ischaemic white-matter gliosis; in 62 of these 70 brains, the periventricular white-matter was the main site of damage. Three of these brains showed focal white-matter necrosis. Eight brains showed diffuse neuronal necrosis. Forty-six (28%) of the corresponding 165 placentas showed macroscopic and microscopic evidence of infarction, 39 of which were associated with ischaemic cerebral lesions. Burke and Tannenberg[89] concluded that placental infarcts are commonly associated with prenatal cerebral ischaemic lesions, and they speculated that stillborn white-matter lesions are correlated with reduced uteroplacental blood flow and are due to circulatory disturbances.

Grafe[262] undertook a study to determine whether correlations exist between specific types of placental pathology and prenatal brain injury. Ninety-eight stillborns and livebirths with < 1 h survival and complete placental and neuropathological examinations were reviewed. Most brain damage was in three categories: germinal matrix/intraventricular haemorrhage, white-matter gliosis/necrosis and neuronal necrosis. Neuropathological changes were seen in 43% of all cases: white-matter injury was the most frequent type of prenatal brain injury, present in 28% of all fetuses and 63% of those with brain injury. Neuronal necrosis was seen in six cases (6%), four of which also had white-matter gliosis. Neuronal injury was seen in the subiculum (not the hippocampus), basis pontis, caudate-putamen, cerebellum and spinal motor neurons, but not the cerebral cortex. Statistical analysis showed significant associations of white-matter necrosis with placental chronic vascular changes, umbilical cord problems, old infarction/abruptio and meconium staining of the placenta. Associations were found between neuronal necrosis and placental chronic vascular changes, old surface blood-vessel thrombosis and old infarction/abruptio. Germinal matrix haemorrhage was associated with funisitis, but no other factors. Grafe points out that chronic placental vascular problems, including umbilical cord problems, surface blood-vessel thrombosis and old infarcts, were significantly associated with brain injury in

this study. It is speculated that these placental findings could either produce or reflect chronic hypoxia or ischaemia in the fetus. The underlying aetiologies behind chronic placental vascular problems are numerous and include, but are not limited to, maternal and fetal factors such as pregnancy-induced hypertension, lupus anticoagulant, infections, coagulation disorders, maternal heart disease, maternal diabetes and hypotension.[262] White-matter injury was also associated with meconium on or in the placenta. The meconium-induced vein constriction demonstrated by Altshuler and Hyde[16] provides a potential mechanism for fetal hypoxic–ischaemic injury in this situation. No significant associations were seen between chorioamniotis and any form of brain injury. Previous investigators have reported associations between white-matter necrosis and chorioamniotis[51] or infection in the infant.[236,403,404] Grafe suggests that the previous studies involved infants who survived for various postnatal intervals, while in her study, the time between an insult and fetal death may not have been sufficient for morphological changes to develop in all cases. Grafe[262] concludes that it is likely that certain types of placental pathology can be correlated with prenatal injury in liveborn infants, and examination of the placenta may indicate which infants are at greater risk for neurological injury.

The finding of germinal matrix and intraventricular haemorrhages and white-matter necrosis and gliosis in the brains of stillborns indicates that the pathogenesis of these lesions does not need to include birth and postnatal factors. In the germinal matrix haemorrhage, for example, fluctuating cerebral blood flow has been implicated in the pathogenesis, with altered regulation in the blood flow, pressure and volume in the microvascular bed of the germinal matrix (see above). The cause of fluctuations in both the cerebral and systemic circulations has been related to intrapartum and extrauterine factors such as labour and delivery, respiratory distress syndrome, tracheal suctioning, rapid infusion of colloid and exchange transfusion.[679] The occurrence of the germinal matrix haemorrhage in the stillborn shows that fluctuations must occur in the cerebral circulation in the fetal brain that are unrecognized clinically and can have devastating consequences.

The question arises of whether the pathological features in the stillborn brain, e.g. white-matter gliosis, focal necrosis and neuronal necrosis, are age dependent? In the NCPP, all four histological features of PTL were found in fetal brains from 20 to 44 gestational weeks, with a striking peak of PVL (11% of cases) between 32 and 35 gestational weeks compared with 2–3% of cases at all other fetal and neonatal age groups studied. In addition, there was a peak of hypertrophic astrocytes (68% of cases) at 36–44 gestational weeks, compared with 45–49% of cases between 28 and 35 gestational weeks, and 11% of cases at 20–27 gestational weeks.[403] These observations suggest that 32–35 gestational weeks is a period of vulnerability to PVL, and that attention should be focused upon delineating the factors that place the prenatal brain at risk for this lesion during this period (see discussion about PVL above). The progressive increase in reactive astrocytosis with increasing gestational age is consistent with the observation that astrocytes obtain the capability to become hypertrophic in the early part of the second trimester (see above). In a study of fetal brains from stillborns and liveborns of very low birth weight (500–1500 g), Golden et al.[255] examined neuropathological findings in each gestational age group from < 24 weeks to ≥ 30 weeks (total n = 67) (Table 9.18). Choroid plexus haemorrhages, thought to be a lesion of the full-term infant, were found in 13% of fetuses of < 24 gestational weeks. Hypertrophic astrocytes increased progressively with age from 13% at < 24 gestational weeks to 100% (n = 4) at ≥ 30 gestational weeks. PVL peaked at 75% (n = 3) at ≥ 30 gestational weeks, the oldest age group studied (Table 9.18). In this study, acutely damaged glia were not appreciated until ≥ 30 gestational weeks.

In considering the neuropathology of the stillborn, there is always a certain percentage in which no cause of death is found after a complete autopsy.[322,423] This observation has intrigued SIDS researchers, who have raised the possibility that some of these stillborn deaths, particularly those at or close to term, may represent late gestational SIDS. The link between SIDS and stillbirth is strengthened by epidemiological data that have found a two-fold risk for SIDS in mothers who have delivered a stillborn. As discussed above, SIDS, or a subset of SIDS, has been widely considered to be a neurological disorder. It is of particular interest in regard to antenatal brain injury and SIDS that PVL,[360,633] subtle white-matter gliosis[358] and subtle hypomyelination[360] have been reported in varying proportions of SIDS brains, e.g. PVL in 25% of SIDS victims.[360] Moreover, antenatal factors, some of which are associated with placental vascular compromise, e.g. maternal cigarette smoking during pregnancy, are strong risk factors for SIDS. In the myelin study, involvement of white-matter sites that initiate myelination before birth and myelinate rapidly and early (by 6 postnatal months) suggested that the insults affecting myelination in SIDS infants began before birth.[360] No study has correlated cerebral white-matter findings with brainstem findings in the same SIDS cases, with the hypothesis that white-matter lesions are markers of antenatal hypoxic–ischaemic injury, with similar injury to the brainstem that leads to lethal homoeostatic control in a critical period of postnatal development.

A final consideration in the neuropathology of the stillborn is the examination of the macerated stillborn brain. This is a difficult task and a recent paper by Magee[423] discusses the appropriate techniques for this important examination. Before fixation genetic and microbiological specimens should be gathered. Macroscopic examination of the brain can reveal large subarachnoid, parenchymal, plexal, germinal and intraventricular haemorrhages, as well as pus. Microscopic examination can reveal, in addition to the autolysis, PVL, microcalcification, neuronal injury, storage material and inflammation.

Table 9.18 *Distribution neuropathological findings in each gestational age group*

Neuropathological finding	Gestational age (weeks)				
	<24	24–26	27–29	≥ 30	Total
Germinal matrix haemorrhage	12 (80)	25 (69)	6 (50)	2 (50)	45 (67)
Intraventricular haemorrhage	8 (53)	16 (44)	8 (67)	1 (25)	33 (49)
Subarachnoid haemorrhage	12 (80)	13 (36)	7 (58)	1 (25)	33 (49)
Parenchymal haemorrhage	7 (47)	15 (42)	3 (25)	0	25 (37)
Petechial haemorrhage	3 (20)	15 (42)	5 (42)	2 (50)	25 (37)
Choroid plexus haemorrhage	2 (13)	1 (3)	0	1 (25)	5 (6)
Moderate/severe ventriculomegaly	5 (33)	6 (17)	3 (25)	0	14 (21)
Axon retraction balls	0	1 (3)	0	1 (25)	2 (3)
Rarefaction	2 (13)	7 (19)	5 (42)	1 (25)	15 (22)
Neuronal loss	0	2 (6)	0	0	2 (3)
Amphophilic globules	0	5 (14)	4 (33)	2 (50)	11 (16)
Hypertrophic astrocytes	2 (13)	11 (31)	5 (42)	4 (100)	22 (33)
Acutely damaged glia	0	0	0	1 (25)	1 (1)
Microglial nodules	0	0	1 (8)	1 (25)	2 (3)
Macrophage focus	1 (7)	3 (8)	2 (17)	1 (25)	7 (10)
Coagulative necrosis	1 (7)	10 (28)	6 (50)	3 (75)	20 (30)
Haemorrhagic necrosis	0	4 (11)	1 (8)	1 (25)	6 (9)
Karyorrhexis	0	2 (6)	0	0	2 (3)
Total	15	36	12	4	67

Data are shown as number (%).
From Golden et al.[255]

REFERENCES

1 Adamo AM, Aloise PA, Pasquini JM. A possible relationship between concentration of microperoxisomes and myelination. *Int J Dev Neurosci* 1986; **4**: 6513–17.

2 Adams JH, Doyle D, Ford I *et al*. Diffuse axonal injury in head injury: definition, diagnosis and grading. *Histopathology* 1989; **15**: 49–59.

3 Adams RD, Prod'hom LS, Rabinowicz T. Intrauterine brain death. Neuraxial reticular core necrosis. *Acta Neuropathol (Berl)* 1977; **40**: 41–9.

4 Aguayo AJ, Nair CP, Bray GM. Peripheral nerve abnormalities in the Riley–Day syndrome. Findings in a sural nerve biopsy. *Arch Neurol* 1971; **24**: 106–116.

5 Ahdab-Barmada M, Moossy J. The neuropathology of kernicterus in the premature neonate: diagnostic problems. *J Neuropathol Exp Neurol* 1984; **43**: 45–56.

6 Ahdab-Barmada M, Moossy J, Painter M. Pontosubicular necrosis and hyperoxemia. *Pediatrics* 1980; **66**: 840–7.

7 Ahmad AE, Gangitano RM, Odell R *et al*. Survival, intracranial lesions and neurodevelopmental outcome in infants with congenital diaphragmatic hernia treated with extracorporeal membrane oxygenation. *J Perinatol* 1999; **19**: 436–40.

8 Ahn AH, Kunkel LM. The structural and functional diversity of dystrophin. *Nat Genet* 1993; **3**: 283–91.

9 Akanli LF, Trasi SS, Thuraisamy K *et al*. Neonatal middle cerebral artery infarction: association with elevated maternal anticardiolipin antibodies. *Am J Perinatol* 1998; **15**: 399–402.

10 Akiyama C, Nonaka I. A follow-up study of congenital nonprogressive myopathies. *Brain Dev* 1996; **18**: 404–8.

11 Akkoyunlu A, Yucel FA. Aspergillose bronchopulmonaire et encephalo-meningee chez un nouveau-né de 20 jour. *Arch Fr Pediatr* 1957; **14**: 615–22.

12 Alexander MP, Emery ES III, Koerner FC. Progressive bulbar paresis in childhood. *Arch Neurol* 1976; **33**: 66–8.

13 Alexander R, Sato Y, Smith W, Bennett T. Incidence of impact trauma with cranial injuries ascribed to shaking. *Am J Dis Child* 1990; **144**: 724–6.

14 Al Sarraj ST, Bridges LR. Desmoplastic cerebral glioblastoma of infancy. *Br J Neurosurg* 1996; **10**: 215–19.

15 Altman J. Proliferation and migration of undifferentiated precursor cells in the rat during postnatal gliogenesis. *Exp Neurol* 1996; **16**: 263–78.

16 Altshuler G, Hyde S. Meconium-induced vasocontraction: a potential cause of cerebral and other fetal hypoperfusion and of poor pregnancy outcome. *J Child Neurol* 1989; **4**: 137–42.

17 Alvarez E, Ferrer T, Perez-Conde C *et al*. Evaluation of congenital dysautonomia other than Riley–Day syndrome. *Neuropediatrics* 1996; **27**: 26–31.

18 Ambler MW, Neave C, Sturner WQ. Sudden and unexpected death in infancy and childhood: neuropathological findings. *Am J Forensic Med Pathol* 1981; **2**: 23–30.

19 Anand KJ. Clinical importance of pain and stress in preterm neonates. *Biol Neonate* 1998; **73**: 1–9.

20 Anderson JM, Milner RD, Strich SJ. Effects of neonatal hypoglycaemia on the nervous system: a pathological study. *J Neurol Neurosurg Psychiatry* 1967; **30**: 295–310.

21 Anderson-Brown T, Slotkin TA, Seidler FJ. Cocaine acutely inhibits DNA synthesis in developing rat brain regions: evidence for direct actions. *Brain Res* 1990; **537**: 197–202.

22 Andjelkovic AV, Nikolic B, Pachter JS, Zecevic N. Macrophages/microglial cells in human central nervous system during development: an immunohistochemical study. *Brain Res* 1998; **814**: 13–25.

23 Ando M, Takashima S, Mito T. Endotoxin, cerebral blood flow, amino acids and brain damage in young rabbits. *Brain Dev* 1988; **10**: 365–70.

24 Anton G. Ueber die Betheiligung der basalen Gehirnganglien bei Bewegongsstörungen und is sbesondere bei der chorea; mit Demonstrationen von Gehirnschnitten. *Wien Klin Wochenschr* 1893; **6**: 859–61.

25 Anton J, Pineda V, Martin C *et al*. Posttraumatic subgaleal hematoma: a case report and review of the literature. *Pediatr Emerg Care* 1999; **15**: 347–9.

26 Arai Y, Deguchi K, Mizuguchi M, Takashima S. Expression of beta-amyloid precursor protein in axons of periventricular leukomalacia brains. *Pediatr Neurol* 1995; **13**: 161–3.

27 Argov Z, Yarom R. 'Rimmed vacuole myopathy' sparing the quadriceps. A unique disorder in Iranian Jews. *J Neurol Sci* 1984; **64**: 33–43.

28 Armstrong D, Dunn JD, Antalffy B, Trivedi R. Selective dendritic alterations in the cortex of Rett syndrome. *J Neuropathol Exp Neurol* 1995; **54**: 195–201.

29 Armstrong DD. Neonatal encephalopathies. In: Duckett S ed. *Pediatric neuropathology*. Baltimore, MD: Williams & Wilkins, 1995: 334–5.

30 Armstrong DL, Sauls CD, Goddard-Finegold J. Neuropathologic findings in short-term survivors of intraventricular haemorrhage. *Am J Dis Child* 1987; **141**: 617–21.

31 Arnaudo E, Dalakas M, Shanske S *et al*. Depletion of muscle mitochondrial DNA in AIDS patients with zidovudine-induced myopathy. *Lancet* 1991; **337**: 508–10.

32 Arnold G, Holtzman E. Microperoxisomes in the central nervous system of the postnatal rat. *Brain Res* 1978; **155**: 1–17.

33 Arnstein LH, Boldrey E, Naffziger HC. A case report and survey of brain tumors during the neonatal period. *J Neurosurg* 1951; **8**: 315–90.

34 Aslanidis C, Jansen G, Amemiya C *et al*. Cloning of the essential myotonic dystrophy region and mapping of the putative defect. *Nature* 1992; **355**: 548–51.

35 Auer RN, Siesjo BK. Biological differences between ischemia, hypoglycemia, and epilepsy. *Ann Neurol* 1988; **24**: 699–707.

36 Averill DR Jr, Moxon ER, Smith AL. Effects of *Haemophilus influenzae* meningitis in infant rats on neuronal growth and synaptogenesis. *Exp Neurol* 1976; **50**: 337–45.

37 Back SA, Volpe JJ. Cellular and molecular pathogenesis of periventricular white matter injury. *Ment Retard Dev Dis* 1997; **3**: 96–207.

38 Back SA, Borenstein NS, Luo NL *et al*. Cellular sequences of prenatal myelinogenesis in human cerebral white matter. Submitted for publication.

39 Back SA, Luo NL, Borenstein NS *et al*. Late oligodendrocyte progenitors coincide with the developmental window of vulnerability for human perinatal white matter injury. *J Neurosci* 2001; **21**: 1302–12.

40 Back SA, Yonezawa M, Gan X *et al*. Oligodendrocyte death induced by cystine deprivation occurs by apoptosis. *Soc Neurosci Abst* 1995; **21**.

41 Banker BQ. Congenital deformities. In: Engel AG, Franzini-Armstrong C eds. *Myology* 2nd edn. New York: McGraw-Hill, 1994: 1905–37.

42 Banker BQ. The congenital muscular dystrophies. In: Engel AG, Franzini-Armstrong C eds. *Myology* 2nd edn. New York: McGraw-Hill, 1994: 1275–89.

43 Banwell BL, Becker LE, Jay V *et al*. Cardiac manifestations of congenital fiber-type disproportion myopathy. *J Child Neurol* 1999; **14**: 83–7.

44 Bardosi A, Friede RL, Ropte S, Goebel HH. A morphometric study on sural nerves in metachromatic leucodystrophy. *Brain* 1987; **110**: 683–94.

45 Barks JD, Silverstein FS. Excitatory amino acids contribute to the pathogenesis of perinatal hypoxic–ischemic brain injury. *Brain Pathol* 1992; **2**: 235–43.

46 Barres BA, Hart IK, Coles HS *et al*. Cell death in the oligo-dendrocyte lineage. *J Neurobiol* 1992; **23**: 1221–30.

47 Barth PG, Wanders RJ, Vreken P. X-linked cardioskeletal myopathy and neutropenia (Barth syndrome)-MIM 302060 (Editorial; Comment). *J Pediatr* 1999; **135**: 273–6.

48 Batten FE. Three cases of myopathy, infantile type. *Brain* 1903; **26**: 147–9.

49 Bauman ML, Kemper TL. Morphologic and histoanatomic observations of the brain in untreated human phenylke-tonuria. *Acta Neuropathol (Berl)* 1982; **58**: 55–63.

50 Becker LE, Takashima S. Dendritic structure in leukodys-trophies: a Golgi study analysis of metachromatic leuko-dystrophy, adrenoleukodystrophy, Cockayne's disease and Pelizaeus–Merzbacher disease. Kyoto, 1981: 37–52.

51 Bejar R, Wozniak P, Allard M *et al*. Antenatal origin of neurologic damage in newborn infants. I. Preterm infants. *Am J Obstet Gynecol* 1988; **159**: 357–63.

52 Bellinger DC, Jonas RA, Rappaport LA *et al*. Developmental and neurologic status of children after heart surgery with hypothermic circulatory arrest or low-flow cardiopulmo-nary bypass. *N Engl J Med* 1995; **332**: 549–55.

53 Bender AN, Bender MB. Muscle fiber hypotrophy with intact neuromuscular junctions. A study of a patient with congenital neuromuscular disease and ophthalmoplegia. *Neurology* 1977; **27**: 206–12.

54 Benowitz LI, Routtenberg A. GAP–43: an intrinsic deter-minant of neuronal development and plasticity. *Trends Neurosci* 1997; **20**: 84–91.

55 Berard-Badier M, Gambarelli D, Pinsard N *et al*. Infantile neuroaxonal dystrophy or Seitelberger's disease. II. Peri-pheral nerve involvement: electron microscopic study in one case. *Acta Neuropathol (Berl)* 1971; **5**: 30–9, Suppl 9.

56 Berkenbaugh JT, Wright CM. Glucose hemeostasis. In: Merenstein GB, Gardner SL eds. *Handbook of neonatal intensive care*. St. Louis, MO: Mosby, 1993: 169–85.

57 Berman PH, Banker BQ. Neonatal meningitis. A clinical and pathological study of 29 cases. *Pediatrics* 1966; **38**: 6–24.

58 Bertini E, Gadisseux JL, Palmieri G *et al*. Distal infantile spinal muscular atrophy associated with paralysis of the diaphragm: a variant of infantile spinal muscular atrophy. *Am J Med Genet* 1989; **33**: 328–35.

59 Bethlem J, Wijngaarden GK. Benign myopathy, with auto-somal dominant inheritance. A report on three pedigrees. *Brain* 1976; **99**: 91–100.

60 Bignami A, Ralston HJ, III. Myelination of fibrillary astroglial processes in long term Wallerian degeneration. The possible relationship to 'status marmoratus'. *Brain Res* 1968; **11**: 710–13.

61 Bingham PM, Shen N, Rennert H *et al*. Arthrogryposis due to infantile neuronal degeneration associated with deletion of the SMNT gene. *Neurology* 1997; **49**: 848–51.

62 Birch-Machin MA, Marsac C, Ponsot G, *et al*. Biochemical investigations and immunoblot analyses of two unrelated patients with an isolated deficiency in complex II of the mitochondrial respiratory chain. *Biochem Biophys Res Com-mun* 1996; **220**: 57–62.

63 Birch-Machin MA, Shepherd IM, Watmough NJ *et al*. Fatal lactic acidosis in infancy with a defect of complex III of the respiratory chain. *Pediatr Res* 1989; **25**: 553–9.

64 Biros I, Forrest S. Spinal muscular atrophy: untangling the knot? *J Med Genet* 1999; **36**: 1–8.

65 Bischoff A, Ulrich J. Peripheral neuropathy in globoid cell leukodystrophy (Krabbe's disease). Ultrastructural and his-tochemical findings. *Brain* 1969; **92**: 861–70.

66 Bittigau P, Sifringer M, Pohl D *et al*. Apoptotic neurode-generation following trauma is markedly enhanced in the immature brain. *Ann Neurol* 1999; **45**: 724–35.

67 Blake D, Lombes A, Minetti C *et al*. MINGIE syndrome: report of 2 new patients (Abstract). *Neurology* 1990; Suppl 40: 294.

68 Bodensteiner JB. Congenital myopathies. *Muscle Nerve* 1994; **17**: 131–44.

69 Bognar L. Brain tumors during the first year of life. *Ann NY Acad Sci* 1997; **824**: 148–55.

70 Bondy M, Wiencke J, Wrensch M, Kyritsis AP. Genetics of primary brain tumors: a review. *J Neurooncol* 1994; **18**: 69–81.

71 Bonne G, Di Barletta MR, Varnous S *et al*. Mutations in the gene encoding lamin A/C cause autosomal dominant Emery–Dreifuss muscular dystrophy. *Nature Genetics* 1999; **21**: 285–8.

72 Bortolussi R, Krishnan C, Armstrong D, Tovichayathamrong P. Prognosis for survival in neonatal meningitis: clinical and pathologic review of 52 cases. *Can Med Assoc J* 1978; **118**: 165–8.

73 Bor M van de, Guit GL, Schreuder AM *et al*. Early detec-tion of delayed myelination in preterm infants. *Pediatrics* 1989; **84**: 407–11.

74 Boustany RN, Aprille JR, Halperin J *et al*. Mitochondrial cytochrome deficiency presenting as a myopathy with hypotonia, external ophthalmoplegia, and lactic acidosis in an infant and as fatal hepatopathy in a second cousin. *Ann Neurol* 1983; **14**: 462–70.

75 Bozoky B, Bara D, Kertesz E. Autopsy study of cerebral com-plications of congenital heart disease and cardiac surgery. *J Neurol* 1984; **231**: 153–61.

76 Brandis A, Heyer R, Hori A, Walter GF. Cerebellar neurocy-toma in an infant: an important differential diagnosis from cerebellar neuroblastoma and medulloblastoma? *Neuro-pediatrics* 1997; **28**: 235–8.

77 Bredesen DE. Neural apoptosis. *Ann Neurol* 1995; **38**: 839–51.

78 Bresolin N, Zeviani M, Bonilla E *et al*. Fatal infantile cyto-chrome *c* oxidase deficiency: decrease of immunologically detectable enzyme in muscle. *Neurology* 1985; **35**: 802–12.

79 Brody BA, Kinney HC, Kloman AS, Gilles FH. Sequence of central nervous system myelination in human infancy. I. An autopsy study of myelination. *J Neuropathol Exp Neurol* 1987; **46**: 283–301.

80 Brook JD, Mc Currach ME, Harley HG *et al*. Molecular basis of myotonic dystrophy: expansion of a trinucleotide (CTG) repeat at the 3′ end of a transcript encoding a protein kinase family member (published erratum appears in *Cell* 1992; **69**: 385). *Cell* 1992; **68**: 799–808.

81 Brooke MH. Congenital fiber type disproportion. In: Kaku-las BA ed. *Clinical studies in myology* 2nd edn. Amsterdam: Excepta Medica, 1973: 147–59.

82 Brooke MH. Congenital (more or less) muscle diseases. A clinician's view of neuromuscular diseases. In: Brook MH ed. *A clinician's view of neuromuscular diseases* 2nd edn. Baltimore, MD: Williams & Wilkins, 1986: 36–80.

83 Brooke MH, Engel WK. The histographic analysis of human muscle biopsies with regard to fiber types. 4. Children's biopsies. *Neurology* 1969; **19**: 591–605.

84 Brooke MH, Neville HE. Reducing body myopathy. *Neurol-ogy* 1972; **22**: 829–40.

85 Bruno C, Kirby DM, Koga Y *et al*. The mitochondrial DNA C3303T mutation can cause cardiomyopathy and/or skele-tal myopathy. *J Pediatr* 1999; **1**: 197–202.

86 Brzustowicz LM, Lehner T, Castilla LH *et al*. Genetic map-ping of chronic childhood-onset spinal muscular atrophy to chromosome 5q11.2-13.3. *Nature* 1990; **344**: 540–1.

87 Buchthal F, Olsen PZ. Electromyography and muscle biopsy in infantile spinal muscular atrophy. *Brain* 1970; **93**: 15–30.

88 Buetow PC, Smirniotopoulos JG, Done S. Congenital brain tumors: a review of 45 cases. *Am J Roentgenol* 1990; **155**: 587–93.

89 Burke CJ, Tannenberg AE. Prenatal brain damage and placental infarction – an autopsy study. *Dev Med Child Neurol* 1995; **37**: 555–62.

90 Burlet P, Huber C, Bertrandy S *et al*. The distribution of SMN protein complex in human fetal tissues and its alteration in spinal muscular atrophy. *Hum Molec Genet* 1998; **7**: 1927–33.

91 Burns DK. The neuropathology of pediatric acquired immunodeficiency syndrome. *J Child Neurol* 1992; **7**: 332–46.

92 Burrows PE, Robertson RL. Neonatal central nervous system vascular disorders. *Neurosurg Clin N Am* 1998; **9**: 155–80.

93 Byers RK, Banker BQ. Infantile muscular atrophy. *Arch Neurol* 1961; **5**: 140–64.

94 Cameron RS, Rakic P. Glial cell lineage in the cerebral cortex: a review and synthesis. *Glia* 1994; **4**: 124–37.

95 Canapicchi R, Cioni G, Strigini FA *et al*. Prenatal diagnosis of periventricular haemorrhage by fetal brain magnetic resonance imaging. *Childs Nerv Syst* 1998; **14**: 689–92.

96 Cancilla PA, Kalyanaraman K, Verity MA *et al*. Familial myopathy with probable lysis of myofibrils in type I fibers. *Neurology* 1971; **21**: 579–85.

97 Carey EM, Foster PC. The activity of 2′,3′-cyclic nucleotide 3′-phosphohydrolase in the corpus callosum, subcortical white matter, and spinal cord in infants dying from sudden infant death syndrome. *J Neurochem* 1984; **42**: 924–9.

98 Carpentier V, Vaudry H, Mallet E *et al*. Increased density of somatostatin binding sites in respiratory nuclei of the brainstem in sudden infant death syndrome. *Neuroscience* 1998; **86**: 159–66.

99 Cases O, Seif I, Grimsby J *et al*. Aggressive behavior and altered amounts of brain serotonin and norepinephrine in mice lacking MAOA. *Science* 1995; **268**: 1763–6.

100 Cases O, Vitalis T, Seif I *et al*. Lack of barrels in the somatosensory cortex of monoamine oxidase A-deficient mice: role of a serotonin excess during the critical period. *Neuron* 1996; **16**: 297–307.

101 Celebisoy N, Uludag B, Yunten N. Juvenile distal spinal muscular atrophy: a case with Arnold–Chiari malformation (Letter). *J Neurol* 1998; **245**: 561–2.

102 Centers for Disease Control. *HIV/AIDS Surveillance Report*. Atlanta, GA: Centers for Disease Control, 1992.

103 Chadduck WM, Boop FA, Blankenship JB, Husain M. Meningioma and sagittal craniosynostosis in an infant: case report. *Neurosurgery* 1992; **30**: 441–2.

104 Chanarin I, Patel A, Slavin G *et al*. Neutral-lipid storage disease: a new disorder of lipid metabolism. *BMJ* 1975; **i**: 553–5.

105 Chase HP, Marlow RA, Dabiere CS, Welch NN. Hypoglycemia and brain development. *Pediatrics* 1973; **52**: 513–20.

106 Chasnoff IJ, Bussey ME, Savich R, Stack CM. Perinatal cerebral infarction and maternal cocaine use. *J Pediatr* 1986; **108**: 456–9.

107 Chen B, Basil JB, Schefft JL *et al*. Antenatal steroids and intraventricular haemorrhage after premature rupture of membranes at 24–28 weeks' gestation. *Am J Perinatol* 1997; **14**: 171–6.

108 Chen H, Blumberg B, Immken L *et al*. The Pena–Shokeir syndrome: report of five cases and further delineation of the syndrome. *Am J Med Genet* 1983; **16**: 213–24.

109 Cheng B, Mattson MP. IGF-I and IGF-II protect cultured hippocampal and septal neurons against calcium-mediated hypoglycemic damage. *J Neurosci* 1992; **12**: 1558–66.

110 Cheng Y, Deshmukh M, D'Costa A *et al*. Caspase inhibitor affords neuroprotection with delayed administration in a rat model of neonatal hypoxic-ischemic brain injury. *J Clin Invest* 1998; **101**: 1992–9.

111 Chigr F, Najimi M, Jordan D *et al*. Immunohistochemical absence of adrenergic neurons in the dorsal part of the solitary tract nucleus in sudden infant death. *C R Acad Sci III* 1989; **309**: 543–9.

112 Choi BH, Kim RC, Lapman LW. Do radial glia give rise to both astroglial and oligodendroglial cells. *Dev Brain Res* 1983; **8**: 119–30.

113 Chou SM, Gilbert EF, Chun RW *et al*. Infantile olivopontocerebellar atrophy with spinal muscular atrophy (infantile OPCA + SMA). *Clin Neuropathol* 1990; **9**: 21–32.

114 Choux M, Lena G, Gentori L. Intracranial hematomas. In: Raimondi AJ, Choux M, DiRocco C eds. *Head injuries in the newborn and infant*. New York: Springer, 1986: 203–16.

115 Chudley AE, Rozdilsky B, Houston CS *et al*. Multicore disease in sibs with severe mental retardation, short stature, facial anomalies, hypoplasia of the pituitary fossa, and hypogonadotrophic hypogonadism. *Am J Med Genet* 1985; **20**: 145–58.

116 Churchill JA, Stevenson L, Habhab G. Cephalhematoma and natal brain injury. *Obstet Gynecol* 1966; **27**: 580–4.

117 Clancy RR, Sladky JT, Rorke LB. Hypoxic–ischemic spinal cord injury following perinatal asphyxia. *Ann Neurol* 1989; **25**: 185–9.

118 Clarren SK, Hall JG. Neuropathologic findings in the spinal cords of 10 infants with arthrogryposis. *J Neurol Sci* 1983; **58**: 89–102.

119 Coates PM, Hale DE, Finocchiaro G *et al*. Genetic deficiency of short-chain acyl-coenzyme A dehydrogenase in cultured fibroblasts from a patient with muscle carnitine deficiency and severe skeletal muscle weakness. *J Clin Invest* 1988; **81**: 171–5.

120 Cohen GM. Caspases: the executioners of apoptosis. *Biochem J* 1997; **326**: 1–16.

121 Cohen ME, Duffner PK eds. *Brain tumors in children: principles of diagnosis and treatment* 2nd edn. New York: Raven Press, 1994.

122 Comi AM, Backstrom JW, Burger PC, Duffner PK. Clinical and neuroradiologic findings in infants with intracranial ependymomas. Pediatric Oncology Group. *Pediatr Neurol* 1998; **18**: 23–9.

123 Connor JR, Benkovic SA. Iron regulation in the brain: histochemical, biochemical, and molecular considerations. *Ann Neurol* 1992; **32** (Suppl): S51–61.

124 Connor JR, Menzies SL. Relationship of iron to oligodendrocytes and myelination. *Glia* 1996; **17**: 83–93.

125 Connor JR, Menzies SL, St. Martin SM, Mufson EJ. Cellular distribution of transferrin, ferritin, and iron in normal and aged human brains. *J Neurosci Res* 1990; **27**: 595–611.

126 Cornelissen M, Steegers-Theunissen R, Kollee L *et al*. Supplementation of vitamin K in pregnant women receiving anticonvulsant therapy prevents neonatal vitamin K deficiency. *Am J Obstet Gynecol* 1993; **168**: 884–8.

127 Cornelissen M, Steegers-Theunissen R, Kollee L *et al*. Increased incidence of neonatal vitamin K deficiency resulting from maternal anticonvulsant therapy. *Am J Obstet Gynecol* 1993; **168**: 923–8.

128 Craver RD. The cytology of cerebrospinal fluid associated with neonatal intraventricular haemorrhage. *Pediatr Pathol Lab Med* 1996; **16**: 713–19.

129 Crouthers B. Injury of the spinal cord in breech extraction as an important cause of fetal death and of paraplegia in childhood. *Am J Med Sci* 1923; **165**: 94–110.

130 Crouthers B, Putman MC. Obstetrical injuries of the spinal cord. *Medicine* 1927; **6**: 41–126.

131 Cruz-Sanchez FF, Lucena J, Ascaso C *et al*. Cerebellar cortex delayed maturation in sudden infant death syndrome. *J Neuropathol Exp Neurol* 1997; **56**: 340–6.

132 Culican SM, Baumrind NL, Yamamoto M, Pearlman AL. Cortical radial glia: identification in tissue culture and evidence for their transformation to astrocytes. *J Neurosci* 1990; **10**: 684–92.

133 Currie SM, Noronha M, Harriman D. 'Minicore' disease. In: *Abstracts of papers presented at the 3rd International Congress in Muscle Diseases*, Newcastle upon Tyne. Amsterdam: Excerpta Medica ICS, 1974: 12.

134 Danon MJ, Oh SJ, DiMauro S *et al*. Lysosomal glycogen storage disease with normal acid maltase. *Neurology* 1981; **31**: 51–7.

135 Darin N, Kyllerman M, Wahlstrom J *et al*. Autosomal dominant myopathy with congenital joint contractures, ophthalmoplegia, and rimmed vacuoles. *Ann Neurol* 1998; **44**: 242–8.

136 Darnfors C, Larsson HE, Oldfors A *et al*. X-linked myotubular myopathy: a linkage study. *Clin Genet* 1990; **37**: 335–40.

137 Darras BT. Neuromuscular disorders in the newborn. *Clin Perinatol* 1997; **24**: 827–44.

138 Davis EJ, Foster TD, Thomas WE. Cellular forms and functions of brain microglia. *Brain Res Bull* 1994; **34**: 73–8.

139 Deblay MF, Vert P, Andre M, Marchal F. Transplacental vitamin K prevents haemorrhagic disease of infant of epileptic mother (Letter). *Lancet* 1982; **i**: 1247.

140 Deeg KH, Alderath W, Bettendorf U. Basilar artery insufficiency – a possible cause of sudden infant death? Results of a Doppler ultrasound study of 39 children with apparent life-threatening events. *Ultraschall Med* 1998; **19**: 250–8.

141 Delivoria-Papadopoulos M, Mishra OP. Mechanisms of cerebral injury in perinatal asphyxia and strategies for prevention. *J Pediatr* 1998; **132**: S30–4.

142 Della Giustina E, Goffinet AM, Landrieu P, Lyon G. A Golgi study of the brain malformation in Zellweger's cerebro-hepato-renal disease. *Acta Neuropathol (Berl)* 1981; **55**: 23–8.

143 Demezuk S, Levy A, Aubry M *et al*. Excess of deletions of maternal origin in the DiGeorge/velo-cardio-facial syndromes. A study of 22 new patients and review of the literature. *Hum Genet* 1995; **96**: 9–13.

144 Denoroy L, Gay N, Gilly R *et al*. Catecholamine synthesizing enzyme activity in brainstem areas from victims of sudden infant death syndrome. *Neuropediatrics* 1987; **18**: 187–90.

145 Denoroy L, Kopp N, Gay N *et al*. Activities des enzymes de synthese des catecholamines dans des regions du tronc cerebral au cours de la mort subite du nourrisson. *C R Acad Sci (D)* 1980; **291**: 245–8.

146 DeReuck J, Chattha AS, Richardson EP Jr. Pathogenesis and evolution of periventricular leukomalacia in infancy. *Arch Neurol* 1972; **27**: 229–36.

147 DeVisser M, Boljuis PA, Barth PG. Differential diagnosis of spinal muscular atrophies and other disorders of motor neurons with infantile or juvenile onset. In: deJong JMBV ed. *Handbook of clinical neurology: Diseases of the motor system*. New York: Elsevier, 1991: 367–82.

148 De Vivo DC. Solving the COX puzzle (Editorial; Comment). *Ann Neurol* 1999; **46**: 142–3.

149 De Vries LS, Connell JA, Dubowitz LM *et al*. Neurological, electrophysiological and MRI abnormalities in infants with extensive cystic leukomalacia. *Neuropediatrics* 1987; **18**: 61–6.

150 De Vries LS, Groenendaal F, Eken P *et al*. Infarcts in the vascular distribution of the middle cerebral artery in preterm and fullterm infants. *Neuropediatrics* 1997; **28**: 88–96.

151 Dias MS, Backstrom J, Falk M, Li V. Serial radiography in the infant shaken impact syndrome. *Pediatr Neurosurg* 1998; **29**: 77–85.

152 Dickson DW, Belman AL, Kim TS *et al*. Spinal cord pathology in pediatric acquired immunodeficiency syndrome. *Neurology* 1989; **39**: 227–35.

153 Di Donato S, Garavaglia B, Rimolki M. Clinical and biomedical phenotypes of carnitine deficiencies. In: Ferrari R, DiMauro S, Sherwood G eds. *L-Carnitine and its role in medicine: from function to therapy*. London: Academic Press, 1992: 81–98.

154 Di Donato S, Garavaglia B, Strisciuglio P *et al*. Multisystem triglyceride storage disease is due to a specific defect in the degradation of endocellularly synthesized triglycerides. *Neurology* 1988; **38**: 1107–10.

155 DiMauro S. Metabolic myopathies. In: Vinkin PJ, Bruyn GW, Ringel SP, Klawans HL eds. *Handbook of clinical neurology: Diseases of muscle, Part II*. Amsterdam: North-Holland, 1979: 175–234.

156 DiMauro S, Andreu AL. Mutations in mtDNA: are we scraping the bottom of the barrel? *Brain Pathol* 2000; **10**: 431–41.

157 DiMauro S, Hartlage PL. Fatal infantile form of muscle phosphorylase deficiency. *Neurology* 1978; **28**: 1124–9.

158 DiMauro S, Lombes A, Nakase H *et al*. Cytochrome *c* oxidase deficiency. *Pediatr Res* 1990; **28**: 536–41.

159 DiMauro S, Moraes CT. Mitochondrial encephalomyopathies. *Arch Neurol* 1993; **50**: 1197–208.

160 DiMauro S, Tonin P, Servidei S. Metabolic myopathies. In: Vinkin PJ, Bruyn GW, Klawans HL *et al*. eds. *Handbook of clinical neurology: Myopathies*. New York: Elsevier, 1992: 479–526.

161 Di Rocco C, Iannelli A, Ceddia A. Intracranial tumors of the first year of life. A cooperative survey of the 1986–1987 Education Committee of the ISPN. *Childs Nerv Syst* 1991; **7**: 150–3.

162 DiSalvo D. The correlation between placental pathology and intraventricular haemorrhage in the preterm infant. The Developmental Epidemiology Network Investigators (published erratum appears in *Pediatr Res* 1998; **43**: 570). *Pediatr Res* 1998; **43**: 15–19.

163 Dominguez R, Aguirre Vila-Coro A, Slopis JM, Bohan TP. Brain and ocular abnormalities in infants with *in utero* exposure to cocaine and other street drugs. *Am J Dis Child* 1991; **145**: 688–95.

164 Donaghy M, Hakin RN, Bamford JM *et al*. Hereditary sensory neuropathy with neurotrophic keratitis. Description of an autosomal recessive disorder with a selective reduction of small myelinated nerve fibres and a discussion of the classification of the hereditary sensory neuropathies. *Brain* 1987; **110**: 563–83.

165 D'Souza SW, McConnell SE, Slater P, Barson AJ. *N*-Methyl-D-aspartate binding sites in neonatal and adult brain (Letter). *Lancet* 1992; **339**: 1240.

166 Dubowitz LM, Bydder GM, Mushin J. Developmental sequence of periventricular leukomalacia. Correlation of ultrasound, clinical, and nuclear magnetic resonance functions. *Arch Dis Child* 1985; **60**: 349–55.

167 Dubowitz V. Pseudomuscular dystrophy. In: Dubowitz V. *Research in muscular dystrophy. Proceedings of the 3rd Symposium*. London: Pitman, 1965.

168 Dubowitz V. *The floppy infant* 2nd edn. Philadelphia, PA: Lippincott, 1980.

169 Duffner PK, Krischer JP, Burger PC *et al*. Treatment of infants with malignant gliomas: the Pediatric Oncology Group experience. *J Neurooncol* 1996; **28**: 245–56.

170 Duhaime AC, Christian CW, Rorke LB, Zimmerman RA. Nonaccidental head injury in infants – the 'shaken-baby syndrome'. *N Engl J Med* 1998; **338**: 1822–9.

171 Duhaime AC, Gennarelli TA, Thibault LE *et al*. The shaken baby syndrome. A clinical, pathological, and biomechanical study. *J Neurosurg* 1987; **66**: 409–15.

172 Duvanel CB, Fawer CL, Cotting J *et al*. Long-term effects of neonatal hypoglycemia on brain growth and psychomotor development in small-for-gestational-age preterm infants. *J Pediatr* 1999; **134**: 492–8.

173 Dyke PJ. Inherited neuronal degeneration and atrophy affecting peripheral motor, sensory and autonomic neurons. In: Dyck PJ, Thomas PK, Lambert EH, Bunge RP eds. *Peripheral neuropathy*. Philadelphia, PA: WB Saunders, 1984.

174 Ebbesen F, Knudsen A. The risk of bilirubin encephalopathy, as estimated by plasma parameters, in neonates strongly suspected of having sepsis. *Acta Paediatr* 1993; **82**: 26–9.

175 Ecklund J, Schut L, Rorke L. Associated vascular malformations and neoplasms in children. *Pediatr Neurosurg* 1993; **19**: 196–201.

176 Edwards AD, Mehmet H. Apoptosis in perinatal hypoxic-ischaemic cerebral damage. *Neuropathol Appl Neurobiol* 1996; **22**: 494–8.

177 Edwards AD, Yue X, Cox P *et al*. Apoptosis in the brains of infants suffering intrauterine cerebral injury. *Pediatr Res* 1997; **42**: 684–9.

178 Edwards MS, Rench MA, Haffar AA *et al*. Long-term sequelae of group B streptococcal meningitis in infants. *J Pediatr*. 1985; **106**: 717–22.

179 Ehrenforth S, Klarmann D, Zabel B *et al*. Severe factor V deficiency presenting as subdural haematoma in the newborn (Letter). *Eur J Pediatr* 1998; **157**: 1032.

180 Ellis WG, Schneider EL, McCulloch JR *et al*. Fetal globoid cell leukocystrophy (Krabbe disease). Pathological and biochemical examination. *Arch Neurol* 1973; **29**: 253–7.

181 Engel AG. Carnitine deficiency syndromes and lipid storage myopathies. In: Engel AG, Banker BQ eds. *Myology: basic and clinical*. New York: McGraw-Hill, 1986: 1663–96.

182 Engel AG. Congenital myasthenic syndromes. *J Child Neurol* 1988; **3**: 233–46.

183 Engel AG. Congenital myasthenic syndromes. *J Child Neurol* 1999; **14**: 38–41.

184 Engel AG. Myasthenic syndromes. In: Engel AG, Franzini-Armstrong C eds. *Myology* 2nd edn. New York: McGraw-Hill, 1994: 1798–835.

185 Engel AG. Myofibrillar myopathy (Editorial; Comment). *Ann Neurol* 1999; **46**: 681–3.

186 Engel AG, Angelini C, Gomez MR. Fingerprint body myopathy, a newly recognized congenital muscle disease. *Mayo Clin Proc* 1972; **47**: 377–88.

187 Engel AG, Gomez MR, Groover RV. Multicore disease. A recently recognized congenital myopathy associated with multifocal degeneration of muscle fibers. *Mayo Clin Proc* 1971; **46**: 666–81.

188 Engel AG, Gomez MR, Seybold ME, Lambert EH. The spectrum and diagnosis of acid maltase deficiency. *Neurology* 1973; **23**: 95–106.

189 Ernster L. The mode of action of bilirubin on mitochondria. In: Sass-Korsak A ed. *Kernicterus*. Toronto: University of Toronto Press, 1961: 174–85.

190 Esiri MM, Urry P, Keeling J. Lipid-containing cells in the brain in sudden infant death syndrome. *Dev Med Child Neurol* 1990; **32**: 319–24.

191 Evans DG, Farndon PA, Burnell LD *et al*. The incidence of Gorlin syndrome in 173 consecutive cases of medulloblastoma. *Br J Cancer* 1991; **64**: 959–61.

192 Faix RG. Systemic *Candida* infections in infants in intensive care nurseries: high incidence of central nervous system involvement. *J Pediatr* 1984; **105**: 616–22.

193 Faix RG, Kovarik SM, Shaw TR, Johnson RV. Mucocutaneous and invasive candidiasis among very low birth weight (less than 1,500 grams) infants in intensive care nurseries: a prospective study. *Pediatrics* 1989; **83**: 101–7.

194 Falco NA, Eriksson E. Facial nerve palsy in the newborn: incidence and outcome. *Plast Reconstruct Surg* 1990; **85**: 1–4.

195 Fardeau M, Tome FM. Congenital myopathies. In: Engel AG, Franzini-Armstrong C eds. *Myology* 2nd edn. New York: McGraw-Hill, 1994: 1487–532.

196 Fardeau M, Tome FM, Derambure S. Familial fingerprint body myopathy. *Arch Neurol* 1976; **33**: 724–5.

197 Farrell DF, Sumi SM, Scott CR, Rice G. Antenatal diagnosis of Krabbe's leucodystrophy: enzymatic and morphological confirmation in an affected fetus. *J Neurol Neurosurg Psychiatry* 1978; **41**: 76–82.

198 Farwell JR, Dohrmann GJ, Flannery JT. Intracranial neoplasms in infants. *Arch Neurol* 1978; **35**: 533–7.

199 Fattal-Valevski A, Leitner Y, Kutai M *et al*. Neurodevelopmental outcome in children with intrauterine growth retardation: a 3-year follow-up. *J Child Neurol* 1999; **14**: 724–7.

200 Fernandes J, Huijing F. Branching enzyme-deficiency glycogenosis: studies in therapy. *Arch Dis Child* 1968; **43**: 347–52.

201 Ferrer I, Isamat F, Acebes J. A Golgi and electron microscopic study of a dysplastic gangliocytoma of the cerebellum. *Acta Neuropathol (Berl)* 1979; **47**: 163–5.

202 Ferrer I, Pozas E, Lopez E, Ballabriga J. Bcl-2, Bax and Bcl-x expression following hypoxia–ischemia in the infant rat brain. *Acta Neuropathol (Berl)* 1997; **94**: 583–9.

203 Fessard C. Cerebral tumors in infancy. 66 clinicoanatomical case studies. *Am J Dis Child* 1968; **115**: 302–8.

204 Fidzianska A, Badurska B, Ryniewicz B, Dembek I. 'Cap disease': new congenital myopathy. *Neurology* 1981; **31**: 1113–20.

205 Filiano JJ, Kinney HC. A perspective on neuropathologic findings in victims of the sudden infant death syndrome: the triple-risk model. *Biol Neonate* 1994; **65**: 194–7.

206 Filiano JJ, Kinney HC. Arcuate nucleus hypoplasia in the sudden infant death syndrome. *J Neuropathol Exp Neurol* 1992; **51**: 394–403.

207 Filiano JJ, Choi JC, Kinney HC. Candidate cell populations for respiratory chemosensitive fields in the human infant medulla. *J Comp Neurol* 1990; **293**: 448–65.

208 Fisher PG. Rethinking brain tumors in babies and more (Editorial; Comment). *Ann Neurol* 1998; **44**: 300–2.

209 Flanigan KM, Kerr L, Bromberg MB *et al*. Congenital muscular dystrophy with rigid spine syndrome: a clinical, pathological, radiological, and genetic study. *Ann Neurol* 2000; **47**: 152–61.

210 Flechsig PE. *Anatomic des menschlichen gehrins and ruckenmarks auf myelogenetischer gundlange*. Vol. 1. Leipzig: Thieme, 1920.

211 Flodmark O, Lupton B, Li D *et al*. MR imaging of periventricular leukomalacia in childhood. *Am J Roentgenol* 1989; **152**: 583–90.

212 Flodmark O, Roland EH, Hill A, Whitfield MF. Periventricular leukomalacia: radiologic diagnosis. *Radiology* 1987; **162**: 119–24.

213 Folgering H, Kuyper F, Kille JF. Primary alveolar hypoventilation (Ondine's curse syndrome) in an infant without external arcuate nucleus. Case report. *Bull Eur Physiopathol Respir* 1979; **15**: 659–65.

214 Folkerth RD, duPlessis A, Jones HR Jr. Arthrogryposis multiplex congenital and congenital peripheral neuropathy. *J Neuropathol Exp Neurol* 1992; **51**: 347.

215 Ford FR. Breech delivery in its possible relations to injury of the spinal cord. With special reference to infantile paraplegia. *Arch Neurol Psychiatry* 1925; **14**: 742–50.

216 Franco SM, Cornelius VE, Andrews BF. Long-term outcome of neonatal meningitis. *Am J Dis Child* 1992; **146**: 567–71.

217 Frank DA, McCarten KM, Robson CD et al. Level of *in utero* cocaine exposure and neonatal ultrasound findings. *Pediatrics* 1999; **104**: 1101–5.

218 Fridovich I. The biology of oxygen radicals. *Science* 1978; **201**: 875–80.

219 Friede RL. Hemorrhages in asphyxiated premature infants. In: Friede RL ed. *Developmental neuropathology* 2nd edn. Berlin: Springer, 1989: 44–58.

220 Friede RL. Ponto-subicular lesions in perinatal anoxia. *Arch Pathol* 1972; **94**: 343–54.

221 Friede RL, Schachenmayr W. Early stages of status marmoratus. *Acta Neuropathol (Berl)* 1977; **38**: 123–7.

222 Fukuyama Y, Kawazura M, Haruna H. A peculiar form of congenital progressive muscular dystrophy: report of fifteen cases. *Paediatrics (Univ Tokyo)* 1960; **4**: 5–8.

223 Gabreels-Festen A, Gabreels F. Hereditary demyelinating motor and sensory neuropathy. *Brain Pathol* 1993; **3**: 135–46.

224 Gadsdon DR, Emery JL. Fatty change in the brain in perinatal and unexpected death. *Arch Dis Child* 1976; **51**: 42–8.

225 Gafney G, Squier M, Johnson A et al. Clinical associations of prenatal ischemic white matter injury. *Arch Dis Child* 1994; **70**: F101–6.

226 Gallanti A, Prelle A, Chianese L et al. Congenital myopathy with type 2A muscle fiber uniformity and smallness. *Neuropediatrics* 1992; **23**: 10–13.

227 Gard AL, Pfeiffer SE. Two proliferative stages of the oligodendrocyte lineage (A2B5$^+$O4$^-$ and O4$^+$GalC$^-$) under different mitogenic control. *Neuron* 1990; **5**: 615–25.

228 Gentleman SM, Nash MJ, Sweeting CJ et al. Beta-amyloid precursor protein (beta APP) as a marker for axonal injury after head injury. *Neurosci Lett* 1993; **160**: 139–44.

229 Gerber MR, Connor JR. Do oligodendrocytes mediate iron regulation in the human brain? *Ann Neurol* 1989; **26**: 95–8.

230 Ghazi-Birry HS, Brown WR, Moody DM et al. Human germinal matrix: venous origin of haemorrhage and vascular characteristics. *Am J Neuroradiol* 1997; **18**: 219–29.

231 Gilbert WM, Nesbitt TS, Danielsen B. Associated factors in 1611 cases of brachial plexus injury. *Obstet Gynecol* 1999; **93**: 536–40.

232 Gilles EE, Nelson MD Jr. Cerebral complications of nonaccidental head injury in childhood. *Pediatr Neurol* 1998; **19**: 119–28.

233 Gilles FH. Myelination in the neonatal brain. *Hum Pathol* 1976; **7**: 244–8.

234 Gilles FH, Murphy SF. Perinatal telencephalic leucoencephalopathy. *J Neurol Neurosurg Psychiatry* 1969; **32**: 404–13.

235 Gilles FH, Averill DR Jr, Kerr CS. Neonatal endotoxin encephalopathy. *Ann Neurol* 1977; **2**: 49–56.

236 Gilles FH, Leviton A, Dooling EC eds. *The Developing human brain: growth and epidemiologic neuropathology*. Boston, MA: John Wright-PSG, 1983.

237 Gilles FH, Leviton A, Kerr CS. Endotoxin leucoencephalopathy in the telencephalon of the newborn kitten. *J Neurol Sci* 1976; **27**: 183–91.

238 Gilles FH, Price RA, Kevy SV, Berenberg W. Fibrinolytic activity in the ganglionic eminence of the premature human brain. *Biol Neonate* 1971; **18**: 426–32.

239 Gilliland MG, Folberg R. Shaken babies – some have no impact injuries. *J Forensic Sci* 1996; **41**: 114–16.

240 Gilmartin RC, Ch'ien LT. Guillain-Barre syndrome with hydrocephalus in early infancy. *Arch Neurol* 1977; **34**: 567–9.

241 Giuffre R. Biological aspects of brain tumors in infancy and childhood. *Childs Nerv Syst* 1989; **5**: 55–9.

242 Giulian D, Baker TJ. Peptides released by ameboid microglia regulate astroglial proliferation. *J Cell Biol* 1985; **101**: 2411–15.

243 Giulian D, Lachman LB. Interleukin-1 stimulation of astroglial proliferation after brain injury. *Science* 1985; **228**: 497–9.

244 Glasgow AM, Engel AG, Bier DM et al. Hypoglycemia, hepatic dysfunction, muscle weakness, cardiomyopathy, free carnitine deficiency and long-chain acylcarnitine excess responsive to medium chain triglyceride diet. *Pediatr Res* 1983; **17**: 319–26.

245 Glauser TA, Packer RJ. Cognitive deficits in long-term survivors of childhood brain tumors. *Childs Nerv Syst* 1991; **7**: 2–12.

246 Glauser TA, Rorke LB, Weinberg PM, Clancy RR. Congenital brain anomalies associated with the hypoplastic left heart syndrome. *Pediatrics* 1990; **85**: 984–90.

247 Gleckman AM, Bell MD, Evans RJ, Smith TW. Diffuse axonal injury in infants with nonaccidental craniocerebral trauma: enhanced detection by beta-amyloid precursor protein immunohistochemical staining. *Arch Pathol Lab Med* 1999; **123**: 146–51.

248 Goddard-Finegold J. Periventricular, intraventricular hemorrhages in the premature newborn. Update on pathologic features, pathogenesis, and possible means of prevention. *Arch Neurol* 1984; **41**: 766–71.

249 Goebel HH. Congenital myopathies. *Semin Pediatr Neurol* 1996; **3**: 152–61.

250 Goebel HH, Lenard HG. Congenital myopathies. In: Rowland LP, DiMauro S eds. *Handbook of clinical neurology: Myopathies*. New York: Elsevier, 1992: 331–67.

251 Goebel HH, Bardosi A, Friede RL et al. Sural nerve biopsy studies in Leigh's subacute necrotizing encephalomyelopathy. *Muscle Nerve* 1986; **9**: 165–73.

252 Goebel HH, Schloon H, Lenard HG. Congenital myopathy with cytoplasmic bodies. *Neuropediatrics* 1981; **12**: 166–80.

253 Goebel HH, Veit S, Dyck PJ. Confirmation of virtual unmyelinated fiber absence in hereditary sensory neuropathy type IV. *J Neuropathol Exp Neurol* 1980; **39**: 670–5.

254 Golden JA, Hyman TH. Development of the superior temporal neocortex is anomalous in trisomy 21. *J Neuropathol Exp Neurol* 1995; **53**: 513–20.

255 Golden JA, Gilles FH, Rudelli R, Leviton A. Frequency of neuropathological abnormalities in very low birth weight infants. *J Neuropathol Exp Neurol* 1997; **56**: 472–8.

256 Goldman JE. Regulation of oligodendrocyte differentiation. *Trends Neurosci* 1992; **15**: 359–62.

257 Gordon GS, Wallace SJ, Neal JW. Intracranial tumours during the first two years of life: presenting features. *Arch Dis Child* 1995; **73**: 345–7.

258 Gordon N. Arthrogryposis multiplex congenita. *Brain Dev* 1998; **20**: 507–11.

259 Gould SJ, Howard S. Glial differentiation in the germinal layer of fetal and preterm infant brain: an immunocytochemical study. *Pediatr Pathol* 1988; **8**: 25–36.

260 Gourley GR. Bilirubin metabolism and kernicterus. *Adv Pediatr* 1997; **44**: 173–229.

261 Goutieres F, Aicardi J, Farkas E. Anterior horn cell disease associated with pontocerebellar hypoplasia in infants. *J Neurol Neurosurg Psychiatry* 1977; **40**: 370–8.

262 Grafe MR. The correlation of prenatal brain damage with placental pathology. *J Neuropathol Exp Neurol* 1994; **53**: 407–15.

263 Granet KM. Cerebral palsy (Letter; Comment). *N Engl J Med* 1994; **330**: 1760.

264 Greeley WJ, Ungerleider RM, Smith LR, Reves JG. The effects of deep hypothermic cardiopulmonary bypass and total circulatory arrest on cerebral blood flow in infants and children. *J Thorac Cardiovasc Surg* 1989; **97**: 737–45.

265 Greenberg F, Fenolio KR, Hejtmancik JF *et al.* X-linked infantile spinal muscular atrophy. *Am J Dis Child* 1988; **142**: 217–19.

266 Greenes DS, Schutzman SA. Clinical indicators of intracranial injury in head-injured infants. *Pediatrics* 1999; **104**: 861–7.

267 Greisen G. Effect of cerebral blood flow and cerebrovascular autoregulation on the distribution, type and extent of cerebral injury. *Brain Pathol* 1992; **2**: 223–8.

268 Gressons P, Kosofsky BE, Evrard P. Cocaine-induced disturbances of corticogenesis in the developing murine brain. *Neurosci Lett* 1992; **140**: 113–16.

269 Griffin MP, Minifee PK, Landry SH *et al.* Neurodevelopmental outcome in neonates after extracorporeal membrane oxygenation: cranial magnetic resonance imaging and ultrasonography correlation. *J Pediatr Surg* 1992; **27**: 33–5.

270 Grohmann K, Wienker TF, Saar K *et al.* Diaphragmatic spinal muscular atrophy with respiratory distress is heterogeneous, and one form is linked to chromosome 11q13-q21 (Letter). *Am J Hum Genet* 1999; **65**: 1459–62.

271 Gruenwald P. Growth of the human fetus. II. Abnormal growth in twins and infants of mothers with diabetes, hypertension, or isoimmunization. *Am J Obstet Gynecol* 1966; **94**: 1120–32.

272 Gruner JE, Bargeton E. Lesions thalamiques dans la myatonie du nourrisson. *Rev Neurol* 1952; **86**: 236–42.

273 Grunnet ML. Morphometry of blood vessels in the cortex and germinal plate of premature neonates. *Pediatr Neurol* 1989; **5**: 12–16.

274 Grunnet ML, Shields WD. Cerebellar haemorrhage in the premature infant. *J Pediatr* 1976; **88**: 605–8.

275 Guibaud P, Carrier H, Mathieu M *et al.* Familial congenital muscular dystrophy caused by phosphofructokinase deficiency. *Arch Fr Pediatr* 1978; **35**: 1105–15.

276 Guihard-Costa AM, Larroche JC. Differential growth between the fetal brain and its infratentorial part. *Early Hum Dev* 1990; **23**: 27–40.

277 Guthkelch AN. Infantile subdural haematoma and its relationship to whiplash injuries. *BMJ* 1971; **ii**: 430–1.

278 Guzzetta F, Ferriere G, Lyon G. Congenital hypomyelination polyneuropathy. Pathological findings compared with polyneuropathies starting later in life. *Brain* 1982; **105**: 395–416.

279 Haan EA, Freemantle CJ, McCure JA *et al.* Assignment of the gene for central core disease to chromosome 19. *Hum Genet* 1990; **86**: 187–90.

280 Haddad SF, Menezes AH, Bell WE *et al.* Brain tumors occurring before 1 year of age: a retrospective reviews of 22 cases in an 11-year period (1977–1987). *Neurosurgery* 1991; **29**: 8–13.

281 Hadeed AJ, Siegel SR. Maternal cocaine use during pregnancy: effect on the newborn infant. *Pediatrics* 1989; **84**: 205–10.

282 Hadi HA, Finley J, Mallette JQ, Strickland D. Prenatal diagnosis of cerebellar haemorrhage: medicolegal implications. *Am J Obstet Gynecol* 1994; **170**: 1392–5.

283 Hageman G, Willemse J, Ketel van BA, Verdonck AF. The pathogenesis of fetal hypokinesia. A neurological study of 75 cases of congenital contractures with emphasis on cerebral lesions. *Neuropediatrics* 1987; **18**: 22–33.

284 Hajnal BL, Sahebkar-Moghaddam F, Barnwell AJ *et al.* Early prediction of neurologic outcome after perinatal depression. *Pediatr Neurol* 1999; **21**: 788–93.

285 Haldeman S, Fowler GW, Ashwal S, Schneider S. Acute flaccid neonatal paraplegia: a case report. *Neurology* 1983; **33**: 93–5.

286 Hall JG. Analysis of Pena Shokeir phenotype. *Am J Med Genet* 1986; **25**: 99–117.

287 Hall JG. Arthrogryposis multiplex congenita: etiology, genetics, classification, diagnostic approach, and general aspects. *J Pediatr Orthop B* 1997; **6**: 159–66.

288 Hall JG. Genetic aspects of arthrogryposis. *Clin Orthopaed Relat Res* 1985; **194**: 44–53.

289 Hall JG, Reed SD, Driscoll EP. Part I. Amyoplasia: a common, sporadic condition with congenital contractures. *Am J Med Genet* 1983; **15**: 571–90.

290 Hall JG, Reed SD, Greene G. The distal arthrogryposes: delineation of new entities – review and nosologic discussion. *Am J Med Genet* 1982; **11**: 185–239.

291 Haller JP, Kleinman PK, Merten DF *et al.* American Academy of Pediatrics. Section on Radiology: Diagnostic imaging of child abuse. *Pediatrics* 1991; **87**: 262–4.

292 Halliwell B, Gutteridge J. Oxygen radicals and nervous system. *Trends Neurosci* 1985; **7**: 22–6.

293 Hamiel OP, Raas-Rothschild A, Upadhyaya M *et al.* Hereditary motor-sensory neuropathy (Charcot–Marie–Tooth disease) with nerve deafness: a new variant. *J Pediatr* 1993; **123**: 431–4.

294 Handler A, Kistin N, Davis F, Ferre C. Cocaine use during pregnancy: perinatal outcomes. *Am J Epidemiol* 1991; **133**: 818–25.

295 Hanigan WC, Powell FC, Miller TC, Wright RM. Symptomatic intracranial haemorrhage in full-term infants. *Childs Nerv Syst* 1995; **11**: 698–707.

296 Hanquinet S, Christophe C, Rummens E *et al.* Ultrasound, computed tomography and magnetic resonance of a neonatal ganglioglioma of the brain. *Pediatr Radiol* 1986; **16**: 501–3.

297 Hansen TW. Bilirubin in the brain. Distribution and effects on neurophysiological and neurochemical processes. *Clin Pediatr (Phila)* 1994; **33**: 452–9.

298 Hanson PA, Mastrianni AF, Post L. Neonatal ophthalmoplegia with microfibers: a reversible myopathy? *Neurology* 1977; **27**: 974–80.

299 Hardart GE, Fackler JC. Predictors of intracranial haemorrhage during neonatal extracorporeal membrane oxygenation. *J Pediatr* 1999; **134**: 156–9.

300 Harding AE, Thomas PK. Hereditary distal spinal muscular atrophy. A report on 34 cases and a review of the literature. *J Neurol Sci* 1980; **45**: 337–48.

301 Hardy R, Reynolds R. Proliferation and differentiation potential of rat forebrain oligodendroglial progenitors both *in vitro* and *in vivo*. *Development* 1991; **111**: 1061–80.

302 Harper RM, Kinney HC, Fleming PJ, Thach BT. Sleep influences on homeostatic functions: implications for the sudden infant death syndrome. *Respir Physiol* 2001; **119**: 123–32.

303 Harriman DGF. Disease of muscle. In: Adams JH, Duchen LW eds. *Greenfield's neuropathology*. New York: Oxford University Press, 1992: 1447–93.

304 Hashimoto Y, Kashiwagi T, Takahashi H, Iizuka H. Oral–facial–digital syndrome (OFDS) type I in a patient with Werdnig–Hoffman disease. *Int J Dermatol* 1998; **37**: 45–8.

305 Haviland J, Russell RI. Outcome after severe non-accidental head injury. *Arch Dis Child* 1997; **77**: 504–7.

306 Hayman M, Roland EH, Hill A. Newborn radial nerve palsy: report of four cases and review of published reports. *Pediatr Neurol* 1999; **21**: 648–51.

307 Heier LA, Carpanzano CR, Mast J *et al.* Maternal cocaine abuse: the spectrum of radiologic abnormalities in the neonatal CNS. *AJNR Am J Neuroradiol* 1991; **12**: 951–6.

308 Hendrick EB, Harwood-Hash DC, Hudson AR. Head injuries in children: a survey of 4465 consecutive cases at the hospital for sick children, Toronto, Canada. *Clin Neurosurg* 1964; **11**: 46–65.

309 Herman GE, Finegold M, Zhao W, Gouyon B de, Metzenberg A. Medical complications in long-term survivors with X-linked myotubular myopathy. *J Pediatr* 1999; **134**: 206–14.

309a Hevner RF. Development of connections in the human visual system during fetal mid-gestation: a DiI-tracing study. *J Neuropathol Exp Neurol* 2000; **59**: 385–92.

310 Herva R, Leisti J, Kirkinen P, Seppanen U. A lethal autosomal recessive syndrome of multiple congenital contractures. *Am J Med Genet* 1985; **20**: 431–9.

311 Hilden JM, Watterson J, Longee DC *et al.* Central nervous system atypical teratoid tumor/rhabdoid tumor: response to intensive therapy and review of the literature. *J Neurooncol* 1998; **40**: 265–75.

312 Hirsch CS. Craniocerebral trauma. In: Froede RC ed. *Handbook of forensic pathology*. Northfield: College of American Pathologists, 1990: 182–90.

313 Hobbs CJ. Skull fracture and the diagnosis of abuse. *Arch Dis Child* 1984; **59**: 246–52.

314 Hodgson S, Boswinkel E, Cole C *et al.* A linkage study of Emery–Dreifuss muscular dystrophy. *Hum Genet* 1986; **74**: 409–16.

315 Hoffman EP, Brown RH Jr, Kunkel LM. Dystrophin: the protein product of the Duchenne muscular dystrophy locus. *Cell* 1987; **51**: 919–28.

316 Hofkosh D, Thompson AE, Nozza RJ *et al.* Ten years of extracorporeal membrane oxygenation: neurodevelopmental outcome. *Pediatrics* 1991; **87**: 549–55.

317 Holden KR, Sessions JC, Cure J *et al.* Neurologic outcomes in children with post-pump choreoathetosis. *J Pediatr* 1998; **132**: 162–4.

318 Holt IJ, Harding AE, Petty RK, Morgan-Hughes JA. A new mitochondrial disease associated with mitochondrial DNA heteroplasmy. *Am J Hum Genet* 1990; **46**: 428–33.

319 Hopkins SJ, Rothwell NJ. Cytokines and the nervous system. I: Expression and recognition. *Trends Neurosci* 1995; **18**: 83–8.

320 Hori A, Fischer G. Intrauterine purulent leptomeningitis. *Acta Neuropathol (Berl)* 1982; **58**: 78–80.

321 Houdou S, Kuruta H, Hasegawa M *et al.* Developmental immunohistochemistry of catalase in the human brain. *Brain Res* 1991; **556**: 267–70.

322 Hovatta O, Lipasti A, Rapola J, Karjalainen O. Causes of stillbirth: a clinicopathological study of 243 patients. *Br J Obstet Gynaecol* 1983; **90**: 691–6.

323 Hoyme HE, Jones KL, Dixon SD *et al.* Prenatal cocaine exposure and fetal vascular disruption. *Pediatrics* 1990; **85**: 743–7.

324 Hristeva L, Booy R, Bowler I, Wilkinson AR. Prospective surveillance of neonatal meningitis. *Arch Dis Child* 1993; **69** (Special Issue): 14–18.

325 Hughes CA, Harley EH, Milmoe G *et al.* Birth trauma in the head and neck. *Arch Otolaryngol Head Neck Surg* 1999; **125**: 193–9.

326 Huisman TA, Fischer J, Willi UV *et al.* 'Growing fontanelle': a serious complication of difficult vacuum extraction. *Neuroradiology* 1999; **41**: 381–3.

327 Hume DA, Perry VH, Gordon S. Immunohistochemical localization of a macrophage-specific antigen in developing mouse retina: phagocytosis of dying neurons and differentiation of microglial cells to form a regular array in the plexiform layers. *J Cell Biol* 1983; **97**: 253–7.

328 Hunt CE. Impaired arousal from sleep: relationship to sudden infant death syndrome. *J Perinatol* 1989; **9**: 184–7.

329 Husain J, Juurlink BH. Oligodendroglial precursor cell susceptibility to hypoxia is related to poor ability to cope with reactive oxygen species. *Brain Res* 1995; **698**: 86–94.

330 Huttenlocher PR. Dendritic development in neocortex of children with mental defect and infantile spasms. *Neurology* 1974; **24**: 203–10.

331 Huttenlocher PR, Courten C de, Garey LJ, Van Der Loos H. Synaptogenesis in human visual cortex – evidence for synapse elimination during normal development. *Neurosci Lett* 1982; **33**: 247.

332 Iida K, Takashima S, Ueda K. Immunohistochemical study of myelination and oligodendrocyte in infants with periventricular leukomalacia. *Pediatr Neurol* 1995; **13**: 296–304.

333 Inder TE, Graham P, Sanderson K, Taylor BJ. Lipid peroxidation as a measure of oxygen free radical damage in the very low birthweight infant. *Arch Dis Child Fetal Neonatal Ed* 1994; **70**: F107–11.

334 Inder TE, Huppi PS, Warfield S *et al.* Periventricular white matter injury in the premature infant is followed by reduced cerebral cortical gray matter volume at term. *Ann Neurol* 1999; **46**: 755–60.

335 Insel TR, Miller LP, Gelhard RE. The ontogeny of excitatory amino acid receptors in rat forebrain – I. *N*-Methyl-D-aspartate and quisqualate receptors. *Neuroscience* 1990; **35**: 31–43.

336 Itakura Y, Ogawa Y, Murakami N, Nonaka I. Severe infantile congenital myopathy with nemaline and cytoplasmic bodies: a case report. *Brain Dev* 1998; **20**: 112–15.

337 Iyer S. Two cases of aspergillus infection of the central nervous system. *J Neurol Neurosurg Psychiatry* 1952; **15**: 152–63.

338 Jacobs JM, Harding BN, Lake BD *et al.* Peripheral neuropathy in Leigh's disease. *Brain* 1990; **113**: 447–62.

339 Jadro-Santel D, Grcevic N, Dogan S *et al.* Centronuclear myopathy with type I fibre hypotrophy and 'fingerprint' inclusions associated with Marfan's syndrome. *J Neurol Sci* 1980; **45**: 43–56.

340 Jagadha V, Becker LE. Dendritic pathology: an overview of Golgi studies in man. *Can J Neurol Sci* 1989; **16**: 41–50.

341 Jago RH. Arthrogryposis following treatment of maternal tetanus with muscle relaxants. *Arch Dis Child* 1970; **45**: 277–9.

342 Jarjour IT, Ahdab-Barmada M. Cerebrovascular lesions in infants and children dying after extracorporeal membrane oxygenation. *Pediatr Neurol* 1994; **10**: 13–19.

343 Jayawant S, Rawlinson A, Gibbon F *et al.* Subdural haemorrhages in infants: population based study. *BMJ* 1998; **317**: 1558–61.

344 Jerusalem F, Engel AG, Gomez MR. Sarcotubular myopathy. A newly recognized, benign, congenital, familial muscle disease. *Neurology* 1973; **23**: 897–906.

345 Jonas RA, Newburger JW, Volpe JJ. *Brain injury and pediatric cardiac surgery*. Boston, MA: Butterworth-Heinemann, 1996.

346 Jones KJ, North KN. Recent advances in diagnosis of the childhood muscular dystrophies. *J Paediatr Child Health* 1997; **33**: 195–201.

347 Kadhim HJ, Gadisseux JF, Evrard P. Topographical and cytological evolution of the glial phase during prenatal development of the human brain: histochemical and electron microscopic study. *J Neuropathol Exp Neurol* 1988; **47**: 166–88.

348 Kane PJ, Phipps KP, Harkness WF, Hayward RD. Intracranial neoplasms in the first year of life: results of a second cohort of patients from a single institution. *Br J Neurosurg* 1999; **13**: 294–8.

349 Kanto WP Jr. A decade of experience with neonatal extracorporeal membrane oxygenation. *J Pediatr* 1994; **124**: 335–47.

350 Kelly TE, Amoroso K, Ferre M *et al.* Spinal muscular atrophy variant with congenital fractures. *Am J Med Genet* 1999; **87**: 65–8.

351 Kendall N, Wolochin H. Cephalhematoma associated with fracture of the skull. *J Pediatr* 1952; **41**: 125.

352 Kennedy TE, Serafini T, Torre de la JR, Tessier-Lavigne M. Netrins are diffusible chemotropic factors for commissural axons in the embryonic spinal cord. *Cell* 1994; **78**: 425–35.

353 Kenney LB, Miller BA, Ries LA *et al.* Increased incidence of cancer in infants in the US: 1980–1990. *Cancer* 1998; **82**: 1396–400.

354 Kim JJ, Armstrong DD, Fishman MA. Multicore myopathy, microcephaly, aganglionosis, and short stature. *J Child Neurol* 1994; **9**: 275–7.

355 Kim YS, Kim SU. Oligodendroglial cell death induced by oxygen radicals and its protection by catalase. *J Neurosci Res* 1991; **29**: 100–6.

356 Kinnala A, Rikalainen H, Lapinleimu H *et al.* Cerebral magnetic resonance imaging and ultrasonography findings after neonatal hypoglycemia. *Pediatrics* 1999; **103**: 724–9.

357 Kinney HC, Back SA. Human oligodendroglial development: relationship to periventricular leukomalacia. *Semin Pediatr Neurol* 1998; **5**: 180–9.

358 Kinney HC, Filiano JJ. Brain research in the sudden infant death syndrome. In: Kraus HF, Byard RW eds. *Sudden infant death syndrome: a diagnostic approach*. London: Chapman and Hall, in press.

359 Kinney HC, White WF. Opioid receptors localize to the external granular cell layer of the developing human cerebellum. *Neuroscience* 1991; **45**: 13–21.

360 Kinney HC, Brody BA, Finkelstein DM *et al.* Delayed central nervous system myelination in the sudden infant death syndrome. *J Neuropathol Exp Neurol* 1991; **50**: 29–48.

361 Kinney HC, Brody BA, Kloman AS, Gilles FH. Sequence of central nervous system myelination in human infancy. II. Patterns of myelination in autopsied infants. *J Neuropathol Exp Neurol* 1988; **47**: 217–34.

362 Kinney HC, Burger PC, Harrell FE Jr, Hudson RP Jr. 'Reactive gliosis' in the medulla oblongata of victims of the sudden infant death syndrome. *Pediatrics* 1983; **72**: 181–7.

363 Kinney HC, Filiano JJ, Harper RM. The neuropathology of the sudden infant death syndrome. A review. *J Neuropathol Exp Neurol* 1992; **51**: 115–26.

364 Kinney HC, Filiano JJ, Sleeper LA *et al.* Decreased muscarinic receptor binding in the arcuate nucleus in sudden infant death syndrome. *Science* 1995; **269**: 1446–50.

365 Kinney HC, Filiano JJ, White WF. Deficits in the medullary serotonergic network in the sudden infant death syndrome. Review of a 15-year study of a single data set. *J Neuropathol Exp Neurol* 2001; **60**: 228–47.

366 Kinney HC, Karthigasan J, Borenshteyn NI *et al.* Myelination in the developing human brain: biochemical correlates. *Neurochem Res* 1994; **19**: 983–96.

367 Kinney HC, O'Donnell TJ, Kriger P, White WF. Early developmental changes in [^{3}H]nicotine binding in the human brainstem. *Neuroscience* 1993; **55**: 1127–38.

368 Kinney JS, Kumar ML. Should we expand the TORCH complex? A description of clinical and diagnostic aspects of selected old and new agents. *Clin Perinatol* 1988; **15**: 727–44.

369 Knaap MS van der, Smit LM, Barth PG *et al.* Magnetic resonance imaging in classification of congenital muscular dystrophies with brain abnormalities. *Ann Neurol* 1997; **42**: 50–9.

370 Knighton DR, Hunt TK, Scheuenstuhl H *et al.* Oxygen tension regulates the expression of angiogenesis factor by macrophages. *Science* 1983; **221**: 1283–5.

371 Koch BM, Bertorini TE, Eng GD, Boehm R. Severe multicore disease associated with reaction to anesthesia. *Arch Neurol* 1985; **42**: 1204–6.

372 Koelfen W, Freund M, Varnholt V. Neonatal stroke involving the middle cerebral artery in term infants: clinical presentation, EEG and imaging studies, and outcome. *Dev Med Child Neurol* 1995; **37**: 204–12.

373 Korinthenberg R, Sauer M, Ketelsen UP *et al.* Congenital axonal neuropathy caused by deletions in the spinal muscular atrophy region. *Ann Neurol* 1997; **42**: 364–8.

374 Kornfeld M. Mixed nemaline–mitochondrial 'myopathy'. *Acta Neuropathol (Berl)* 1980; **51**: 185–9.

375 Krieger I, Espiritu CE. Arthrogryposis multiplex congenita and the Turner phenotype. *Am J Dis Child* 1972; **123**: 141–4.

376 Kristt DA. Impaired neuronal migration in cytomegalic inclusion disease: a Golgi analysis (Abstract). *J Neuropathol Exp Neurol* 1976; **35**: 369.

377 Krugliak L, Gadoth N, Behar AJ. Neuropathic form of arthrogryposis multiplex congenita. Report of 3 cases with complete necropsy, including the first reported case of agenesis of muscle spindles. *J Neurol Sci* 1978; **37**: 179–85.

378 Krugman RD. Child abuse and neglect. Follow-up. *Am J Dis Child* 1993; **147**: 517.

379 Kuban KC, Gilles FH. Human telencephalic angiogenesis. *Ann Neurol* 1985; **17**: 539–48.

380 Kubo S, Orihara Y, Gotohda T *et al.* Immunohistochemical studies on neuronal changes in brainstem nucleus of forensic autopsied cases. II Sudden infant death syndrome. *Jpn J Legal Med* 1998; **52**: 350–4.

381 Kumada S, Hayashi M, Umitsu R *et al.* Neuropathology of the dentate nucleus in developmental disorders. *Acta Neuropathol (Berl)* 1997; **94**: 36–41.

382 Kupsky WJ, Drozd MA, Barlow CF. Selective injury of the globus pallidus in children with post-cardiac surgery choreic syndrome. *Dev Med Child Neurol* 1995; **37**: 135–44.

383 Kupsky WJ, Kinney HC, Lidov HGW *et al.* Neuropathology of infants dying after extracorporal membrane oxygenation (ECMO). *J Neuropathol Exp Neurol* 1989; **48**: 307–70.

384 Laing NG, Majda BT, Akkari PA *et al.* Assignment of a gene (NEMI) for autosomal dominant nemaline myopathy to chromosome I. *Am J Hum Genet* 1992; **50**: 576–83.

385 Laing NG, Wilton SD, Akkari PA *et al.* A mutation in the alpha tropomyosin gene TPM3 associated with autosomal dominant nemaline myopathy (published erratum appears in *Nat Genet* 1995; **10**: 249). *Nat Genet* 1995; **9**: 75–9.

386 Lake BD, Wilson J. Zebra body myopathy. Clinical, histochemical and ultrastructural studies. *J Neurol Sci* 1975; **24**: 437–46.

387 Lammens M, Moerman P, Fryns JP *et al.* Fetal akinesia sequence caused by nemaline myopathy. *Neuropediatrics* 1997; **28**: 116–19.

388 Lapras C, Guilburd JN, Guyotat J, Patet JD. Brain tumors in infants: a study of 76 patients operated upon. *Childs Nerv Syst* 1988; **4**: 100–4.

389 Larroche JC. *Developmental pathology of the neonate*. Amsterdam: Excerpta Medica, 1977: 1–21.

390 Larroche JC, Aubry MC, Narcy F. Intrauterine brain damage in nonimmune hydrops fetalis. *Biol Neonate* 1992; **61**: 273–80.

391 Laurie DJ, Bartke I, Schoepfer R *et al*. Regional, developmental and interspecies expression of the four NMDAR2 subunits, examined using monoclonal antibodies. *Brain Res Mol Brain Res* 1997; **51**: 23–32.

392 Lawrence RD, Meyer S, Nevin S. The pathological changes in the brain in fatal hypoglycemia. *Q J Med* 1942; **11**: 181–202.

393 Lebenthal E, Shochet SB, Adam A *et al*. Arthrogryposis multiplex congenita: twenty-three cases in an Arab kindred. *Pediatrics* 1970; **46**: 891–9.

394 Lee H, Choi BH. Density and distribution of excitatory amino acid receptors in the developing human fetal brain: a quantitative autoradiographic study. *Exp Neurol* 1992; **118**: 284–90.

395 Lee SC, Liu W, Dickson DW *et al*. Cytokine production by human fetal microglia and astrocytes. Differential induction by lipopolysaccharide and IL-1 beta. *J Immunol* 1993; **150**: 2659–67.

396 Leech RW, Alvord EC Jr. Morphologic variations in periventricular leukomalacia. *Am J Pathol* 1974; **74**: 591–602.

397 Leestma J. Forensic neuropathology. In: Duckett S ed. *Pediatric neuropathology*. Baltimore, MD: Williams & Wilkins, 1995.

398 Legido A. Pathophysiology of perinatal hypoxic–ischemic encephalopathy. *Acta Neuropediatr* 1994; **1**: 97–110.

399 Leibovich SJ, Polverini PJ, Shepard HM *et al*. Macrophage-induced angiogenesis is mediated by tumour necrosis factor-alpha. *Nature* 1987; **329**: 630–2.

400 Leon GA de, Grover WD, D'Cruz CA. Amyotrophic cerebellar hypoplasia: a specific form of infantile spinal atrophy. *Acta Neuropathol (Berl)* 1984; **63**: 282–6.

401 Leventhal HR. Birth injuries of the spinal cord. *J Pediatr* 1960; **56**: 447–53.

402 LeVine SM, Goldman JE. Spatial and temporal patterns of oligodendrocyte differentiation in rat cerebrum and cerebellum. *J Comp Neurol* 1988; **277**: 441–55.

403 Leviton A, Gilles FH. Acquired perinatal leukoencephalopathy. *Ann Neurol* 1984; **16**: 1–8.

404 Leviton A, Gilles FH. An epidemiologic study of perinatal telencephalic leucoencephalopathy in an autopsy population. *J Neurol Sci* 1973; **18**: 53–66.

405 Leviton A, Gilles F. Ventriculomegaly, delayed myelination, white matter hypoplasia, and 'periventricular' leukomalacia: how are they related? *Pediatr Neurol* 1996; **15**: 127–36.

406 Levitt P, Harvey JA, Friedman E *et al*. New evidence for neurotransmitter influences on brain development. *Trends Neurosci* 1997; **20**: 269–74.

407 Lilue RE, Jequier S, O'Gorman AM. Congenital pineoblastoma in the newborn: ultrasound evaluation. *Radiology* 1985; **154**: 363–5.

408 Lindenberg R, Freytag E. Morphology of brain lesions from blunt trauma in early infancy. *Arch Pathol* 1969; **87**: 298–305.

409 Lindhout D, Hageman G, Beemer FA *et al*. The Pena–Shokeir syndrome: report of nine Dutch cases. *Am J Med Genet* 1985; **21**: 655–68.

410 Lipman SP, Pretorius DH, Rumack CM, Manco-Johnson ML. Fetal intracranial teratoma: US diagnosis of three cases and a review of the literature. *Radiology* 1985; **157**: 491–4.

411 Lipton SA, Kater SB. Neurotransmitter regulation of neuronal outgrowth, plasticity, and survival. *Trends Neurosci* 1989; **12**: 265–70.

412 Lipton SA, Rosenberg PA. Excitatory amino acids as a final common pathway for neurologic disorders. *N Engl J Med* 1994; **330**: 613–22.

413 Loke J, MacLennan DH. Malignant hyperthermia and central core disease: disorders of Ca^{2+} release channels. *Am J Med* 1998; **104**: 470–86.

414 Londe P. Paralysie bulbaire: progressive infantile and familiale. *Rev Med (Paris)* 1992; **13**: 1020–30.

415 Louis JC, Magal E, Takayama S, Varon S. CNTF protection of oligodendrocytes against natural and tumor necrosis factor-induced death. *Science* 1993; **259**: 689–92.

416 Ludwin SK. The pathobiology of the oligodendrocyte. *J Neuropathol Exp Neurol* 1997; **56**: 111–24.

417 Lyman WD, Kress Y, Kure K *et al*. Detection of HIV in fetal central nervous system tissue. *AIDS* 1990; **4**: 917–20.

418 McConnell SK, Kaznowski CE. Cell cycle dependence of laminar determination in developing neocortex. *Science* 1991; **254**: 282–5.

419 McDonald JW, Johnston MV, Young AB. Differential ontogenic development of three receptors comprising the NMDA receptor/channel complex in the rat hippocampus. *Exp Neurol* 1990; **110**: 237–47.

420 McLaurin J, D'Souza S, Stewart J *et al*. Effect of tumor necrosis factor alpha and beta on human oligodendrocytes and neurons in culture. *Int J Dev Neurosci* 1995; **13**: 369–81.

421 McMorris FA, Dubois-Dalcq M. Insulin-like growth factor I promotes cell proliferation and oligodendroglial commitment in rat glial progenitor cells developing *in vitro*. *J Neurosci Res* 1988; **21**: 199–209.

422 Maeda T, Tohyama M, Shimizu N. Modifications of post natal development of neocortex in rat brain with experimental deprivation of locus ceruleus. *Brain Res* 1974; **70**: 515–20.

423 Magee JF. Investigation of stillbirth. *Pediatr Dev Pathol* 2001; **4**: 1–22.

424 Mallard C, Tolcos M, Leditschke J *et al*. Reduction in choline acetyltransferase immunoreactivity but not muscarinic-m2 receptor immunoreactivity in the brainstem of SIDS infants. *J Neuropathol Exp Neurol* 1999; **58**: 255–64.

425 Marin-Garcia J, Ananthakrishnan R, Goldenthal MJ *et al*. Skeletal muscle mitochondrial defects in nonspecific neurologic disorders. *Pediatr Neurol* 1999; **21**: 538–42.

426 Marin-Padilla M. Developmental neuropathology and impact of perinatal brain damage. I: Hemorrhagic lesions of neocortex. *J Neuropathol Exp Neurol* 1996; **55**: 758–73.

427 Marin-Padilla M. Developmental neuropathology and impact of perinatal brain damage. II: White matter lesions of the neocortex. *J Neuropathol Exp Neurol* 1997; **56**: 219–35.

428 Marin-Padilla M. Developmental neuropathology and impact of perinatal brain damage. III: gray matter lesions of the neocortex. *J Neuropathol Exp Neurol* 1999; **58**: 407–29.

429 Marin-Padilla M. Prenatal and early postnatal ontogenesis of the human motor cortex: a Golgi study. I. The sequential development of the cortical layers. *Brain Res* 1970; **23**: 167–83.

430 Marin-Padilla M. Prenatal development of fibrous (white matter), protoplasmic (gray matter) and layer I astrocytes in the human cerebral cortex: a Golgi study. *J Comp Neurol* 1995; **357**: 554–72.

431 Marin-Padilla M. Structural abnormalities of the cerebral cortex in human chromosomal aberrations: a Golgi study. *Brain Res* 1972; **44**: 625–9.

432   Marques Dias MJ, Harmant-van Rijckevorsel G, Landrieu P, Lyon G. Prenatal cytomegalovirus disease and cerebral microgyria: evidence for perfusion failure, not disturbance of histogenesis, as the major cause of fetal cytomegalovirus encephalopathy. *Neuropediatrics* 1984; **15**: 18–24.

433   Martin FP, Lukeman JM, Ranson RF, Geppert LJ. Mucormycosis of the central nervous system associated with thrombosis of the internal carotid artery. *J Pediatr* 1954; **44**: 437–42.

434   Martin JJ, Leroy JG, Ceuterick C *et al.* Fetal Krabbe leukodystrophy. A morphologic study of two cases. *Acta Neuropathol (Berl)* 1981; **53**: 87–91.

435   Martin R, Roessmann U, Fanaroff A. Massive intracerebellar haemorrhage in low-birth-weight infants. *J Pediatr* 1976; **89**: 290–3.

436   Mathews LS, Hammer RE, Behringer RR *et al.* Growth enhancement of transgenic mice expressing human insulin-like growth factor I. *Endocrinology* 1988; **123**: 2827–33.

437   Matturri L, Biondo B, Mercurio P, Rossi L. Severe hypoplasia of medullary arcuate nucleus: quantitative analysis in sudden infant death syndrome. *Acta Neuropathol (Berl)* 2000; **99**: 371–5.

438   Matute C, Sanchez-Gomez MV, Martinez-Millan L, Miledi R. Glutamate receptor-mediated toxicity in optic nerve oligodendrocytes. *Proc Natl Acad Sci USA* 1997; **94**: 8830–5.

439   Mazewski CM, Hudgins RJ, Reisner A, Geyer JR. Neonatal brain tumors: a review. *Semin Perinatol* 1999; **23**: 286–98.

440   Meese AD, Yeatman GW, Pettet G. A syndrome of ankylosis, facial anomalies, and pulmonary hypoplasia secondary to fetal neuromuscular dysfunction. In: Bergsma D ed. *Cytogenetics, environmental and malformation syndromes*. New York: Alan Liss for The National Foundation March of Dimes, 1976: 193–200.

441   Meguid NA. Frontonasal dysplasia, lipoma of the corpus callosum and tetralogy of Fallot. *Clin Genet* 1993; **44**: 95–7.

442   Mellins RB, Hays AP, Gold AP *et al.* Respiratory distress as the initial manifestation of Werdnig–Hoffmann disease. *Pediatrics* 1974; **53**: 33–40.

443   Ment LR, Oh W, Ehrenkranz RA *et al.* Risk period for intraventricular haemorrhage of the preterm neonate is independent of gestational age. *Semin Perinatol* 1993; **17**: 338–41.

444   Meny RG, Carroll JL, Carbone MT, Kelly DH. Cardiorespiratory recordings from infants dying suddenly and unexpectedly at home. *Pediatrics* 1994; **93**: 44–9.

445   Merrill JE. Effects of interleukin-1 and tumor necrosis factor-alpha on astrocytes, microglia, oligodendrocytes, and glial precursors *in vitro*. *Dev Neurosci* 1991; **13**: 130–7.

446   Midrone G, Bilbao JM eds. *Biopsy diagnosis of peripheral neuropathy*. Boston, MA: Butterworth-Heinemann, 1995.

447   Miller LP, Johnson AE, Gelhard RE, Insel TR. The ontogeny of excitatory amino acid receptors in the rat forebrain–II. Kainic acid receptors. *Neuroscience* 1990; **35**: 45–51.

448   Miller PD, Albright AL. Posterior dural arteriovenous malformation and medulloblastoma in an infant: case report. *Neurosurgery* 1993; **32**: 126–30.

449   Miller SP, Riley P, Shevell MI. The neonatal presentation of Prader–Willi syndrome revisited. *J Pediatr* 1999; **134**: 226–8.

450   Mirkin LD, Ey EH, Chaparro M. Congenital subependymal giant-cell astrocytoma: case report with prenatal ultrasonogram. *Pediatr Radiol* 1999; **29**: 776–80.

451   Mischel PS, Nguyen LP, Vinters HV. Cerebral cortical dysplasia associated with pediatric epilepsy. Review of neuropathologic features and proposal for a grading system. *J Neuropathol Exp Neurol* 1995; **54**: 137–53.

452   Mishra OP, Delivoria-Papadopoulos M. Cellular mechanisms of hypoxic injury in the developing brain. *Brain Res Bull* 1999; **48**: 233–8.

453   Mitchell G, Larochelle J, Lambert M *et al.* Neurologic crises in hereditary tyrosinemia. *N Engl J Med* 1990; **322**: 432–7.

454   Mitchell WG, Fishman LS, Miller JH *et al.* Stroke as a late sequela of cranial irradiation for childhood brain tumors. *J Child Neurol* 1991; **6**: 128–33.

455   Mitnick RJ, Bello JA, Shprintzen RJ. Brain anomalies in velo-cardio-facial syndrome. *Am J Med Genet* 1994; **54**: 100–6.

456   Mito T, Kamei A, Takashima S, Becker LE. Clinicopathological study of pontosubicular necrosis. *Neuropediatrics* 1993; **24**: 204–7.

457   Moessinger AC. Fetal akinesia deformation sequence: an animal model. *Pediatrics* 1983; **72**: 857–63.

458   Mollgard K, Dziegielewska KM, Saunders NR *et al.* Synthesis and localization of plasma proteins in the developing human brain. Integrity of the fetal blood–brain barrier to endogenous proteins of hepatic origin. *Dev Biol* 1988; **128**: 207–21.

459   Moody DM, Bell MA, Challa VR. Features of the cerebral vascular pattern that predict vulnerability to perfusion or oxygenation deficiency: an anatomic study. *Am J Neuroradiol* 1990; **11**: 431–9.

460   Moraes CT, Shanske S, Tritschler HJ *et al.* mtDNA depletion with variable tissue expression: a novel genetic abnormality in mitochondrial diseases. *Am J Hum Genet* 1991; **48**: 492–501.

461   Moreadith RW, Batshaw ML, Ohnishi T *et al.* Deficiency of the iron–sulfur clusters of mitochondrial reduced nicotinamide-adenine dinucleotide-ubiquinone oxidoreductase (complex I) in an infant with congenital lactic acidosis. *J Clin Invest* 1984; **74**: 685–97.

462   Morgan-Hughes JA, Schapira AH, Cooper JM, Clark JB. Molecular defects of NADH-ubiquinone oxidoreductase (complex I) in mitochondrial diseases. *J Bioenerg Biomembr* 1988; **20**: 365–82.

463   Moutard-Codou ML, Delleur MM, Dulac O *et al.* Myasthenie neonatale severe avex arthrogyrpose. *Presse Med* 1987; **16**: 615–18.

464   Mozell RL, McMorris FA. Insulin-like growth factor I stimulates oligodendrocyte development and myelination in rat brain aggregate cultures. *J Neurosci Res* 1991; **30**: 382–90.

465   Mrak RE. The pathologic spectrum of merosin deficiency. *J Child Neurol* 1998; **13**: 513–15.

466   Mrak RE, Lange B, Brodsky MC. Broad A bands of striated muscle in Leber's congenital amaurosis: a new congenital myopathy? *Neurology* 1993; **43**: 838–41.

467   Mulliez N, Roux CH, Loterman OV *et al.* Microcéphalie, arthrogryposes. Syndrome létal récessif autosomique. *Arch Fr Pediatr* 1980; **37**: 591–6.

468   Munger CE, Peiffer RL, Bouldin TW *et al.* Ocular and associated neuropathologic observations in suspected whiplash shaken infant syndrome. A retrospective study of 12 cases. *Am J Forensic Med Pathol* 1993; **14**: 193–200.

469   Munsat TL. Infantile scapuloperoneal muscular atrophy. *Neurology* 1968; **18**: 285.

470   Munsat TL, Davies KE. International SMA Consortium Meeting, 26–28 June 1992. Bonn, Germany: Neuromuscular Diseases, 1992; 423–8.

471   Murakami Y, Yamashita Y, Matsuishi T *et al.* Cranial MRI of neurologically impaired children suffering from neonatal hypoglycaemia. *Pediatr Radiol* 1999; **29**: 23–7.

472   Myers RE. Experimental models of perinatal brain damage: relevance to human pathology. In: Gluck L ed. *Intrauterine asphyxia and the developing fetal brain*. Chicago, IL: Year Book Medical Publishers, 1977: 37–97.

473 Myers RE. Four patterns of perinatal brain damage and their conditions of occurrence in primates. *Adv Neurol* 1975; **10**: 223–34.

474 Naeye RL. Amniotic fluid infections, neonatal hyperbilirubinemia, and psychomotor impairment. *Pediatrics* 1978; **62**: 497–503.

475 Naeye RL. Brain-stem and adrenal abnormalities in the sudden-infant-death syndrome. *Am J Clin Pathol* 1976; **66**: 526–30.

476 Nagai T, Hasegawa T, Saito M et al. Infantile polymyositis: a case report. *Brain Dev* 1992; **14**: 167–9.

477 Nakamura Y, Okudera T, Hashimoto T. Vascular architecture in white matter of neonates: its relationship to periventricular leukomalacia. *J Neuropathol Exp Neurol* 1994; **53**: 582–9.

478 Namura S, Zhu J, Fink K et al. Activation and cleavage of caspase-3 in apoptosis induced by experimental cerebral ischemia. *J Neurosci* 1998; **18**: 3659–68.

479 Narcy P, Contencin P, Viala P. Surgical treatment for laryngeal paralysis in infants and children. *Ann Otol Rhinol Laryngol* 1990; **99**: 124–8.

480 Nelson KB, Ellenberg JH. Antecedents of cerebral palsy. Multivariate analysis of risk. *N Engl J Med* 1986; **315**: 81–6.

481 Nelson KB, Ellenberg JH. *The pathology of cerebral palsy*. Springfield, IL: Charles C Thomas, 1960.

482 Nelson KB, Leviton A. How much of neonatal encephalopathy is due to birth asphyxia? *Am J Dis Child* 1991; **145**: 1325–31.

483 Nelson KB, Dambrosia JM, Grether JK, Phillips TM. Neonatal cytokines and coagulation factors in children with cerebral palsy. *Ann Neurol* 1998; **44**: 665–75.

484 Nevo Y, Kramer U, Legum C et al. SMA type 2 unrelated to chromosome 5q13. *Am J Med Genet* 1998; **75**: 193–5.

485 Newburger JW, Jonas RA, Wernovsky G et al. A comparison of the perioperative neurologic effects of hypothermic circulatory arrest versus low-flow cardiopulmonary bypass in infant heart surgery. *N Engl J Med* 1993; **329**: 1057–64.

486 Nickel RE, Pillers DA, Merkens M et al. Velo-cardio-facial syndrome and DiGeorge sequence with meningomyelocele and deletions of the 22q11 region. *Am J Med Genet* 1994; **52**: 445–9.

487 Nishida A, Misaki Y, Kuruta H, Takashima S. Developmental expression of copper, zinc-superoxide dismutase in human brain by chemiluminescence. *Brain Dev* 1994; **16**: 40–3.

488 Nishimura M, Takashima S, Takeshita K, Tanaka J. Immunocytochemical studies on a fetal brain of tuberous sclerosis. *Pediatr Neurol* 1985; **1**: 245–8.

489 Nishino I, Kobayashi O, Goto Y et al. A new congenital muscular dystrophy with mitochondrial structural abnormalities. *Muscle Nerve* 1998; **21**: 40–7.

490 Nissenkorn A, Zeharia A, Lev D et al. Multiple presentation of mitochondrial disorders. *Arch Dis Child* 1999; **81**: 209–14.

491 Noble M, Murray K, Stroobant P et al. Platelet-derived growth factor promotes division and motility and inhibits premature differentiation of the oligodendrocyte/type-2 astrocyte progenitor cell. *Nature* 1988; **333**: 560–2.

492 Norenberg MD. Astrocyte responses to CNS injury. *J Neuropathol Exp Neurol* 1994; **53**: 213–20.

493 Norman RM, Urich H. Cerebellar hypoplasia associated with systemic degeneration in early life. *J Neurol Neurosurg Psychiatry* 1958; **21**: 159–66.

494 Novelli G, Calza L, Amicucci P et al. Expression study of survival motor neuron gene in human fetal tissues. *Biochem Mol Med* 1997; **61**: 102–6.

495 Nowak KJ, Wattanasirichaigoon D, Goebel HH et al. Mutations in the skeletal muscle alpha-actin gene in patients with actin myopathy and nemaline myopathy. *Nat Genet* 1999; **23**: 208–12.

496 Obonai T, Takashima S. *In utero* brain lesions in SIDS. *Pediatr Neurol* 1998; **19**: 23–5.

497 Obonai T, Yasuhara M, Nakamura T, Takashima S. Catecholamine neurons alteration in the brainstem of sudden infant death syndrome victims. *Pediatrics* 1998; **101**: 285–8.

498 Ogata ES. Carbohydrate metabolism in the fetus and neonate and altered neonatal glucoregulation. *Pediatr Clin North Am* 1986; **33**: 25–45.

499 Oh SJ, Danon MJ. Nonprogressive congenital neuromuscular disease with uniform type 1 fiber. *Arch Neurol* 1983; **40**: 147–50.

500 Ohkubo M, Ino T, Shimazaki S et al. Multicore myopathy associated with multiple pterygium syndrome and hypertrophic cardiomyopathy. *Pediatr Cardiol* 1996; **17**: 53–6.

501 Oi S, Kokunai T, Matsumoto S. Congenital brain tumors in Japan (ISPN Cooperative Study): specific clinical features in neonates. *Childs Nerv Syst* 1990; **6**: 86–91.

502 Oka A, Belliveau MJ, Rosenberg PA, Volpe JJ. Vulnerability of oligodendroglia to glutamate: pharmacology, mechanisms and prevention. *J Neurosci* 1993; **13**: 1441–53.

503 O'Kusky JR, Norman MG. Sudden infant death syndrome: increased synaptic density in the central reticular nucleus of the medulla. *J Neuropathol Exp Neurol* 1994; **53**: 263–71.

504 O'Kusky JR, Norman MG. Sudden infant death syndrome: postnatal changes in the numerical density and total number of neurons in the hypoglossal nucleus. *J Neuropathol Exp Neurol* 1992; **51**: 577–84.

505 Omran H, Ketelsen UP, Heinen F et al. Axonal neuropathy and predominance of type II myofibers in infantile spinal muscular atrophy. *J Child Neurol* 1998; **13**: 327–31.

506 Ophoven JJ. Forensic pathology. In: Stocker JT, Dehner LP eds. *Pediatric Pathology*. Philadelphia, PA: JP Lippincott, 1992: 257–323.

507 Ota M, Ellefson RD, Lambert EH, Dyck PJ. Hereditary sensory neuropathy, type II. Clinical, electrophysiologic, histologic and biochemical studies of a Quebec kinship. *Arch Neurol* 1973; **29**: 23–37.

508 Ouvrier RA, Prineas J, Walsh JC et al. Giant axonal neuropathy – a third case. *Proc Aust Assoc Neurol* 1974; **11**: 137–44.

509 Ozawa H, Nishida A, Mito T, Takashima S. Development of ferritin-positive cells in cerebrum of human brain. *Pediatr Neurol* 1994; **10**: 44–8.

510 Paneth N. Classifying brain damage in preterm infants (Editorial; Comment). *J Pediatr* 1999; **134**: 527–9.

511 Panigraphy A, Filiano J, Sleeper LA et al. Decreased serotonergic receptor binding in rhombic lip-derived regions of the medulla oblongata in the sudden infant death syndrome. *J Neuropathol Exp Neurol* 2000; **59**: 377–84.

512 Panigraphy A, Filiano J, Sleeper LA et al. Decreased kainate receptor binding in the arcuate nucleus of the sudden infant death syndrome. *J Neuropathol Exp Neurol* 1997; **56**: 1253–61.

513 Panigraphy A, Rosenberg PA, Assmann S et al. Differential expression of glutamate receptor subtypes in hyman brainstem sites involved in perinatal hypoxia–ischemia. *J Comp Neurol* 2001; **427**: 196–208.

514 Papagapiou MP, Auer RN. Regional neuroprotective effects of the NMDA receptor antagonist MK-801 (dizocilpine) in hypoglycemic brain damage. *J Cereb Blood Flow Metab* 1990; **10**: 270–6.

515 Papasian CJ, Parker JC. Bacterial and fungal infections. In: Duckett S ed. *Pediatric neuropathology*. Baltimore, MD: Williams & Wilkins, 1995: 352–73.

516 Pape KE, Armstrong DL, Fitzhardinge PM. Central nervous system pathology associated with mask ventilation in the very low birthweight infant: a new etiology for intracerebellar hemorrhages. *Pediatrics* 1976; **58**: 473–83.

517 Papile LA, Burstein J, Burstein R, Koffler H. Incidence and evolution of subependymal and intraventricular haemorrhage: a study of infants with birth weights less than 1,500 gm. *J Pediatr* 1978; **92**: 529–34.

518 Pascolo L, Del Vecchio S, Koehler RK *et al*. Albumin binding of unconjugated [³H]bilirubin and its uptake by rat liver basolateral plasma membrane vesicles. *Biochem J* 1996; **316**: 999–1004.

519 Pasternak JF, Fulling K, Nelson J, Prensky AL. An infant with chronic, relapsing polyneuropathy responsive to steroids. *Dev Med Child Neurol* 1982; **24**: 504–24.

520 Paul DA, Leef KH, Stefano JL. Bartoshesky L. Low serum thyroxine on initial newborn screening is associated with intraventricular haemorrhage and death in very low birth weight infants. *Pediatrics* 1998; **101**: 903–7.

521 Paula-Barbosa MM, Tavares MA, Silva CA *et al*. Axo-dendritic abnormalities in a case of juvenile neuronal storage disease. *J Submicrosc Cytol Pathol* 1981; **13**: 657–65.

522 Pavone L, Gullotta F, Grasso S, Vannucchi C. Hydrocephalus, lissencephaly, ocular abnormalities and congenital muscular dystrophy. A Warburg syndrome variant? *Neuropediatrics* 1986; **17**: 206–11.

523 Pearn J. Autosomal dominant spinal muscular atrophy: a clinical and genetic study. *J Neurol Sci* 1978; **38**: 263–75.

524 Pena SD, Shokeir MH. Syndrome of camptodactyly, multiple ankyloses, facial anomalies, and pulmonary hypoplasia: a lethal condition. *J Pediatr* 1974; **85**: 373–5.

525 Perlman JM, McMenamin JB, Volpe JJ. Fluctuating cerebral blood-flow velocity in respiratory-distress syndrome. Relation to the development of intraventricular haemorrhage. *N Engl J Med* 1983; **309**: 204–9.

526 Perlman JM, Risser R, Broyles RS. Bilateral cystic periventricular leukomalacia in the premature infant: associated risk factors. *Pediatrics* 1996; **97**: 822–7.

527 Perlman JM, Rollins N, Sanchez PJ. Late-onset meningitis in sick, very-low-birth-weight infants. Clinical and sonographic observations. *Am J Dis Child* 1992; **146**: 1297–301.

528 Perrin RG, Rutka JT, Drake JM *et al*. Management and outcomes of posterior fossa subdural hematomas in neonates. *Neurosurgery* 1997; **40**: 1190–9.

529 Perry VH, Gordon S. Macrophages and microglia in the nervous system. *Trends Neurosci* 1988; **11**: 273–7.

530 Perry VH, Hume DA, Gordon S. Immunohistochemical localization of macrophages and microglia in the adult and developing mouse brain. *Neuroscience* 1985; **15**: 313–26.

531 Petty RK, Harding AE, Morgan-Hughes JA. The clinical features of mitochondrial myopathy. *Brain* 1986; **109**: 915–38.

532 Phillips J, Christiansen SP, Ware G, Landers S, Kirby RS. Ocular morbidity in very low birth-weight infants with intraventricular haemorrhage. *Am J Ophthalmol* 1997; **123**: 218–23.

533 Piccolo F, Roberds SL, Jeanpierre M *et al*. Primary adhalinopathy: a common cause of autosomal recessive muscular dystrophy of variable severity (published erratum appears in *Nat Genet* 1995; **11**: 104). *Nat Genet* 1995; **10**: 243–5.

534 Piggot MA, Perry EK, Perry RH, Scott D. *N*-Methyl-D-asparate (NMDA) and non-NMDA binding sites in developing human frontal cortex. *Neurosci Res Commun* 1993; **12**: 9–16.

535 Plessis AJ du, Johnston MV. Hypoxic–ischemic brain injury in the newborn. Cellular mechanisms and potential strategies for neuroprotection. *Clin Perinatol* 1997; **24**: 627–54.

536 Portera-Cailliau C, Price DL, Martin LJ. Excitotoxic neuronal death in the immature brain is an apoptosis–necrosis morphological continuum. *J Comp Neurol* 1997; **378**: 70–87.

537 Price DB, Miller LJ, Drexler S, Schneider SJ. Congenital ganglioglioma: report of a case with an unusual imaging appearance. *Pediatr Radiol* 1997; **27**: 748–9.

538 Price RW, Plum F. Poliomyelitis. In: Vinkin PJ, Bruyn GW eds. *Infections of the nervous system*. Amsterdam: North-Holland, 1978: 93–132.

539 Prince AD, Engel WK, Warmolts JR. Type 1 myofiber smallness without central nuclei or myotonia. *Neurology* 1972; **22**: 401.

540 Pringle N, Collarini EJ, Mosley MJ *et al*. PDGF A chain homodimers drive proliferation of bipotential (O-2A) glial progenitor cells in the developing rat optic nerve. *EMBO J* 1989; **8**: 1049–56.

541 Pulera MR, Adams LM, Liu H *et al*. Apoptosis in a neonatal rat model of cerebral hypoxia–ischemia. *Stroke* 1998; **29**: 2622–30.

542 Punal JE, Rodriguez E, Pintos E *et al*. Congenital ocular motor apraxia associated with myopathy, external hydrocephalus and NADH dehydrogenase deficiency (published erratum appears in *Brain Dev* 1998; **20**: 547). *Brain Dev* 1998; **20**: 175–8.

543 Purpura DP. Ectopic dendritic growth in mature pyramidal neurones in human ganglioside storage disease. *Nature* 1978; **276**: 520–1.

544 Purpura DP, Hirano A, French JH. Polydendritic Purkinje cells in X-chromosome linked copper malabsorption: a Golgi study. *Brain Res* 1976; **117**: 125–9.

545 Quagliarello V, Scheld WM. Bacterial meningitis: pathogenesis, pathophysiology and progress. *N Engl J Med* 1992; **327**: 864–72.

546 Quattrochi JJ, Baba N, Liss L, Adrion W. Sudden infant death syndrome (SIDS): a preliminary study of reticular dendritic spines in infants with SIDS. *Brain Res* 1980; **181**: 245–9.

547 Quattrochi JJ, McBride PT, Yates AJ. Brainstem immaturity in sudden infant death syndrome: a quantitative rapid Golgi study of dendritic spines in 95 infants. *Brain Res* 1985; **325**: 39–48.

548 Raff MC, Mirsky R, Fields KL *et al*. Galactocerebroside is a specific cell-surface antigenic marker for oligodendrocytes in culture. *Nature* 1978; **274**: 813–16.

549 Raichle ME. The pathophysiology of brain ischemia. *Ann Neurol* 1983; **13**: 2–10.

550 Raimondi AJ, Tomita T. Brain tumors during the first year of life. *Childs Brain* 1983; **10**: 193–207.

551 Rakic P. Specifications of cerebral cortical areas. *Science* 1988; **241**: 170–6.

552 Reeve R, Silver HK, Ferrier P. Marfan's syndrome (arachnodactyly) with arthrogryposis (amyoplasia congenita). *Am J Dis Child* 1960; **99**: 101–6.

553 Reichmann H, Goebel HH, Schneider C, Toyka KV. Familial mixed congenital myopathy with rigid spine phenotype. *Muscle Nerve* 1997; **20**: 411–17.

554 Reynolds R, Wilkin GP. Development of macroglial cells in rat cerebellum. II. An *in situ* immunohistochemical study of oligodendroglial lineage from precursor to mature myelinating cell. *Development* 1988; **102**: 409–25.

555 Richardson WD, Pringle N, Mosley MJ *et al*. A role for platelet-derived growth factor in normal gliogenesis in the central nervous system. *Cell* 1988; **53**: 309–19.

556 Rickert CH, Probst-Cousin S, Gullotta F. Primary intracranial neoplasms of infancy and early childhood. *Childs Nerv Syst* 1997; **13**: 507–13.

557 Ringel SP, Neville HE, Duster MC, Carroll JE. A new congenital neuromuscular disease with trilaminar muscle fibers. *Neurology* 1978; **28**: 282–9.

558 Rivkin MJ, Anderson ML, Kaye EM. Neonatal idiopathic cerebral venous thrombosis: an unrecognized cause of transient seizures or lethargy. *Ann Neurol* 1992; **32**: 51–6.

559 Robbins DS, Shirazi Y, Drysdale BE *et al.* Production of cytotoxic factor for oligodendrocytes by stimulated astrocytes. *J Immunol* 1987; **139**: 2593–7.

560 Robinson BH. Lactic acidemia. In: Schriver CR, Beaudet AL, Sly WS, Valle D. *The metabolic basis of inherited disease.* New York: McGraw-Hill, 1989: 869–88.

561 Robinson BH, MacKay N, Petrova-Benedict R *et al.* Defects in the E2 lipoyl transacetylase and the X-lipoyl containing component of the pyruvate dehydrogenase complex in patients with lactic acidemia. *J Clin Invest* 1990; **85**: 1821–4.

562 Robinson BH, Taylor J, Sherwood WG. Deficiency of dihydrolipoyl dehydrogenase (a component of the pyruvate and alpha-ketoglutarate dehydrogenase complexes): a cause of congenital chronic lactic acidosis in infancy. *Pediatr Res* 1977; **11**: 1198–202.

563 Robinson RJ, Rossiter MA. Massive subaponeurotic haemorrhage in babies of African origin. *Arch Dis Child* 1968; **43**: 684–7.

564 Roessmann U, Gambetti P. Astrocytes in the developing human brain. An immunohistochemical study. *Acta Neuropathol (Berl)* 1986; **70**: 308–13.

565 Roessmann U, Gambetti P. Pathological reaction of astrocytes in perinatal brain injury. Immunohistochemical study. *Acta Neuropathol (Berl)* 1986; **70**: 302–7.

566 Rogers CB, Itabashi HH, Tomiyasu U, Heuser ET. Subdural neomembranes and sudden infant death syndrome. *J Forensic Sci* 1998; **43**: 375–6.

567 Rorke LB. Anatomical features of the developing brain implicated in pathogenesis of hypoxic–ischemic injury. *Brain Pathology* 1992; **2**: 211–21.

568 Rorke LB. *Pathology of the perinatal brain injury.* New York: Raven Press, 1982.

569 Rorke LB, Packer RJ, Biegel JA. Central nervous system atypical teratoid/rhabdoid tumors of infancy and childhood: definition of an entity. *J Neurosurg* 1996; **85**: 56–65.

570 Rossitch E Jr, Oakes WJ. Perinatal spinal cord injury: clinical, radiographic and pathologic features. *Pediatr Neurosurg* 1992; **18**: 149–52.

571 Ruggieri M, Smarason AK, Pike M. Spinal cord insults in the prenatal, perinatal, and neonatal periods. *Dev Med Child Neurol* 1999; **41**: 311–17.

572 Russell DS, Ellis RWB. Circumscribed cerebral tumors in young infants. *Arch Dis Child* 1933; **8**: 329–42.

573 Sahgal V, Sahgal S. A new congenital myopathy. *Acta Neuropathol (Berl)* 1977; **37**: 225–30.

574 Saito K, Kondo-Iida E, Kawakita Y *et al.* Prenatal diagnosis of Fukuyama type congenital muscular dystrophy in eight Japanese families by haplotype analysis using new markers closest to the gene. *Am J Med Genet* 1998; **77**: 310–16.

575 Sakamoto K, Kobayashi N, Ohtsubo H, Tanaka Y. Intracranial tumors in the first year of life. *Childs Nerv Syst* 1986; **2**: 126–9.

576 Salafia CM, Minior VK, Rosenkrantz TS *et al.* Maternal, placental, and neonatal associations with early germinal matrix/intraventricular haemorrhage in infants born before 32 weeks– gestation. *Am J Perinatol* 1995; **12**: 429–36.

577 Saliba E, Bertrand P, Gold F *et al.* Area of lateral ventricles measured on cranial ultrasonography in preterm infants: association with outcome. *Arch Dis Child* 1990; **65** (Special Issue): 1033–7.

578 Sanderman FW, Boerner F. *Normal values in clinical medicine.* Philadelphia, PA: WB Saunders, 1949.

579 Santavuori P, Leisti J, Kruus S. Muscle, eye and brain disease. *Neuropediatrics* 1977; **8** Suppl: 553.

580 Sasaki K, Suga K, Tsugawa S *et al.* Muscle pathology in Marinesco–Sjogren syndrome: a unique ultrastructural feature. *Brain Dev* 1996; **18**: 64–7.

581 Sato O, Tamura A, Sano K. Brain tumors in early infants. *Childs Brain* 1975; **1**: 121–5.

582 Saugstad OD. Mechanisms of tissue injury by oxygen radicals: implications for neonatal disease. *Acta Paediatr* 1996; **85**: 1–4.

583 Schaumberg HH. Disorders of peripheral nerves. In: Schaumberg HH, Spencer PS, Thomas PK eds. *Contemporary neurology series.* Philadelphia, PA: Davis, 1983: 187–95.

584 Schindler D, Bishop DF, Wolfe DE *et al.* Neuroaxonal dystrophy due to lysosomal alpha-*N*-acetylgalactosaminidase deficiency. *N Engl J Med* 1989; **320**: 1735–40.

585 Schotland DL, DiMauro S, Bonilla E *et al.* Neuromuscular disorder associated with a defect in mitochondrial energy supply. *Arch Neurol* 1976; **33**: 475–9.

586 Schullinger JN. Birth trauma. *Pediatr Clin North Am* 1993; **40**: 1351–8.

587 Schumacher RE, Palmer TW, Roloff DW *et al.* Follow-up of infants treated with extracorporeal membrane oxygenation for newborn respiratory failure. *Pediatrics* 1991; **87**: 451–7.

588 Schutta HS, Johnson L, Neville HE. Mitochondrial abnormalities in bilirubin encephalopathy. *J Neuropathol Exp Neurol* 1970; **29**: 296–305.

589 Schwartz RP. Neonatal hypoglycemia: how low is too low? (Editorial; Comment). *J Pediatr* 1997; **131**: 171–3.

590 Scott GB. Natural history of HIV infection in children. HRS-D-MC-87. US Department of Health and Human Services. Report of the Surgeon General's Workshop in Children with HIV Infection and Their Families, 1987: 1900.

591 Selmaj KW, Raine CS. Tumor necrosis factor mediates myelin and oligodendrocyte damage *in vitro*. *Ann Neurol* 1988; **23**: 339–46.

592 Selmaj KW, Farooq M, Norton WT *et al.* Proliferation of astrocytes *in vitro* in response to cytokines. A primary role for tumor necrosis factor. *J Immunol* 1990; **144**: 129–35.

593 Sengers RC, Fischer JC, Trijbels JM *et al.* A mitochondrial myopathy with a defective respiratory chain and carnitine deficiency. *Eur J Pediatr* 1983; **140**: 332–7.

594 Setty SN, Miller DC, Camras L *et al.* Desmoplastic infantile astrocytoma with metastases at presentation. *Mod Pathol* 1997; **10**: 945–51.

595 Shankaran S, Bauer CR, Bain R *et al.* Relationship between antenatal steroid administration and grades III and IV intracranial haemorrhage in low birth weight infants. The NICHD Neonatal Research Network. *Am J Obstet Gynecol* 1995; **173**: 305–12.

596 Shannon P, Smith CR, Deck J *et al.* Axonal injury and the neuropathology of shaken baby syndrome. *Acta Neuropathol (Berl)* 1998; **95**: 625–31.

597 Shaw CM, Siebert JR, Haas JE, Alvord EC Jr. Megalencephaly in sudden infant death syndrome. *J Child Neurol* 1989; **4**: 39–42.

598 Sher JH, Rimalovski AB, Athanassiades TJ, Aronson SM. Familial centronuclear myopathy: a clinical and pathological study. *Neurology* 1967; **17**: 727–42.

599 Sherer DM, Anyaegbunam A, Onyeije C. Antepartum fetal intracranial haemorrhage, predisposing factors and prenatal sonography: a review. *Am J Perinatol* 1998; **15**: 431–41.

600 Sherwood AJ, Smith JF. Bilirubin encephalopathy. *Neuropathol Appl Neurobiol* 1983; **9**: 271–85.

601 Shevell M, Rosenblatt B, Silver K *et al.* Congenital inflammatory myopathy. *Neurology* 1990; **40**: 1111–14.

602 Shinoda J, Kawaguchi M, Matsuhisa T *et al.* Choroid plexus carcinoma in infants: report of two cases and review of the literature. *Acta Neurochir* 1998; **140**: 557–63.

603 Shy GM, Magee KR. A new congenital nonprogressive myopathy. *Brain* 1956; **79**: 610–21.

604 Shy GM, Engel WK, Somers JE, Wanko T. Nemaline myopathy: a new congenital myopathy. *Brain* 1963; **86**: 793–810.

605 Silva R, Mata LR, Gulbenkian S *et al.* Inhibition of glutamate uptake by unconjugated bilirubin in cultured cortical rat astrocytes: role of concentration and pH. *Biochem Biophys Res Commun* 1999; **265**: 67–72.

606 Sims ME, Turkel SB, Halterman G, Paul RH. Brain injury and intrauterine death. *Am J Obstet Gynecol* 1985; **151**: 721–3.

607 Singer DB, Sung CJ, Wigglesworth JS. Fetal growth and maturation: with standards for body and organ development. In: Wigglesworth JS, Singer DB eds. *Textbook of fetal and perinatal pathology*. Boston, MA: Blackwell, 1991: 3–47.

608 Skyllouriotis ML, Marx M, Skyllouriotis P *et al.* Nemaline myopathy and cardiomyopathy. *Pediatr Neurol* 1999; **20**: 319–21.

609 Smit LM, Barth PG. Arthrogryposis multiplex congenita due to congenital myasthenia. *Dev Med Child Neurol* 1980; **22**: 371–4.

610 Smith CV, Hansen TN, Martin NE *et al.* Oxidant stress responses in premature infants during exposure to hyperoxia. *Pediatr Res* 1993; **34**: 360–5.

611 Smith JF. *Pediatric Neuropathology*. New York: McGraw-Hill, 1974.

612 Solitare GB, Krigman MR. Congenital intracranial neoplasms. A case report and review of the literature. *J Neuropathol Exp Neurol* 1964; **23**: 280–92.

613 Sparks DL, Hunsaker JC III. Increased ALZ-50-reactive neurons in the brains of SIDS infants: an indicator of greater neuronal death? *J Child Neurol* 1991; **6**: 123–7.

614 Specht L, Shapiro F. Boys with Duchenne and Becker muscular dystrophy are clinically indistinguishable at present (Abstract). *Ann Neurol* 1990; **28**: 443.

615 Spiro AJ, Shy GM, Gonatas NK. Myotubular myopathy. Persistence of fetal muscle in an adolescent boy. *Arch Neurol* 1966; **14**: 1–14.

616 Sprecher S, Soumenkoff G, Puissant F, Degueldre M. Vertical transmission of HIV in 15-week fetus (Letter). *Lancet* 1986; **ii**: 288–9.

617 Squier M, Keeling JW. The incidence of prenatal brain injury. *Neuropathol Appl Neurobiol* 1991; **17**: 29–38.

618 Stanley CA. New genetic defects in mitochondrial fatty acid oxidation and carnitine deficiency. *Adv Pediatr* 1987; **34**: 59–88.

619 Stanley CA, DeLeeuw S, Coates PM *et al.* Chronic cardiomyopathy and weakness or acute coma in children with a defect in carnitine uptake. *Ann Neurol* 1991; **30**: 709–16.

620 Steiman GS, Rorke LB, Brown MJ. Infantile neuronal degeneration masquerading as Werdnig–Hoffmann disease. *Ann Neurol* 1980; **8**: 317–24.

621 Steinhauser C, Gallo V. News on glutamate receptors in glial cells. *Trends Neurosci* 1996; **19**: 339–45.

622 Stephens RP, Richardson AC, Lewin JS. Bilateral subdural hematomas in a newborn infant. *Pediatrics* 1997; **99**: 619–21.

623 Stevens MK, Yaksh TL. Systematic studies on the effects of the NMDA receptor antagonist MK-801 on cerebral blood flow and responsivity, EEG, and blood–brain barrier fol-lowing complete reversible cerebral ischemia. *J Cereb Blood Flow Metab* 1990; **10**: 77–88.

624 Stolar CJ, Crisafi MA, Driscoll YT. Neurocognitive outcome for neonates treated with extracorporeal membrane oxygenation: are infants with congenital diaphragmatic hernia different? *J Pediatr Surg* 1995; **30**: 366–71.

625 Storm H, Nylander G, Saugstad OD. The amount of brainstem gliosis in sudden infant death syndrome (SIDS) victims correlates with maternal cigarette smoking during pregnancy. *Acta Paediatr* 1999; **88**: 13–18.

626 Styne DM. Fetal growth. *Clin Perinatol* 1998; **25**: 917–38, vii.

627 Swanson AG, Buchan GC, Alvord EC Jr. Anatomic changes in congenital insensitivity to pain: absence of small primary sensory neurons in ganglia, roots and Lissauer's tract. *Arch Neurol* 1965; **12**: 12–18.

628 Takaku A, Kodama N, Ohara H, Hori S. Brain tumor in newborn babies. *Childs Brain* 1978; **4**: 365–75.

629 Takashima S, Becker LE. Developmental abnormalities of medullary 'respiratory centers' in sudden infant death syndrome. *Exp Neurol* 1985; **90**: 580–7.

630 Takashima S, Becker LE. Developmental neuropathology in bronchopulmonary dysplasia: alteration of glial fibrillary acidic protein and myelination. *Brain Dev* 1984; **6**: 451–7.

631 Takashima S, Tanaka K. Development of cerebrovascular architecture and its relationship to periventricular leukomalacia. *Arch Neurol* 1978; **35**: 11–16.

632 Takashima S, Armstrong D, Becker L, Bryan C. Cerebral hypoperfusion in the sudden infant death syndrome? Brainstem gliosis and vasculature. *Ann Neurol* 1978; **4**: 257–62.

633 Takashima S, Armstrong D, Becker LE, Huber J. Cerebral white matter lesions in sudden infant death syndrome. *Pediatrics* 1978; **62**: 155–9.

634 Takashima S, Becker LE, Armstrong DL, Chan F. Abnormal neuronal development in the visual cortex of the human fetus and infant with down's syndrome. A quantitative and qualitative Golgi study. *Brain Res* 1981; **225**: 1–21.

635 Takashima S, Becker LE, Nishimura M, Tanaka J. Developmental changes of glial fibrillary acidic protein and myelin basic protein in perinatal leukomalacia: relationship to a predisposing factor. *Brain Dev* 1984; **6**: 444–50.

636 Takashima S, Kuruta H, Mito T *et al.* Immunohistochemistry of superoxide dismutase-1 in developing human brain. *Brain Dev* 1990; **12**: 211–13.

637 Takashima S, Mito T, Becker LE. Dendritic development of motor neurons in the cervical anterior horn and hypoglossal nucleus of normal infants and victims of sudden infant death syndrome. *Neuropediatrics* 1990; **21**: 24–6.

638 Tan S, Zhou F, Nielsen VG *et al.* Increased injury following intermittent fetal hypoxia–reoxygenation is associated with increased free radical production in fetal rabbit brain. *J Neuropathol Exp Neurol* 1999; **58**: 972–81.

639 Taylor DL, Edwards AD, Mehmet H. Oxidative metabolism, apoptosis and perinatal brain injury. *Brain Pathol* 1999; **9**: 93–117.

640 Taylor GA, Fitz CR, Kapur S, Short BL. Cerebrovascular accidents in neonates treated with extracorporeal membrane oxygenation: sonographic–pathologic correlation. *Am J Roentgenol* 1989; **153**: 355–61.

641 Taylor SR, Roessmann U. Hypotensive brain stem necrosis in a stillborn. *Acta Neuropathol (Berl)* 1984; **65**: 166–7.

642 Terplan K. Histopathologic brain changes in 1152 cases of perinatal and early infancy period. *Biol Neonate* 1967; **11**: 348–66.

643 Terplan KL. Brain changes in newborns, infants and children with congenital heart disease in association with car-

diac surgery. Additional observations. *J Neurol* 1976; **212**: 225–36.

644 Theele DP, Streit WJ. A chronicle of microglial ontogeny. *Glia* 1993; **7**: 5–8.

645 Thomas C. Nemaline rod and central core disease: a coexisting Z-band myopathy. *Muscle Nerve* 1997; **20**: 893–6.

646 Thompson CE. Infantile myositis. *Dev Med Child Neurol* 1982; **24**: 307–13.

647 Thorarensen O, Ryan S, Hunter J, Younkin DP. Factor V Leiden mutation: an unrecognized cause of hemiplegic cerebral palsy, neonatal stroke, and placental thrombosis. *Ann Neurol* 1997; **42**: 372–5.

648 Thorburne SK, Juurlink BH. Low glutathione and high iron govern the susceptibility of oligodendroglial precursors to oxidative stress. *J Neurochem* 1996; **67**: 1014–22.

649 Tiranti V, Hoertnagel K, Carrozzo R et al. Mutations of SURF-1 in Leigh disease associated with cytochrome c oxidase deficiency. *Am J Hum Genet* 1998; **63**: 1609–21.

650 Tomita T, McLone DG. Brain tumors during the first twenty-four months of life. *Neurosurgery* 1985; **17**: 913–19.

651 Torfs CP, Berg B van den, Oechsli FW, Cummins S. Prenatal and perinatal factors in the etiology of cerebral palsy. *J Pediatr* 1990; **116**: 615–19.

652 Tremblay E, Roisin MP, Represa A et al. Transient increased density of NMDA binding sites in the developing rat hippocampus. *Brain Res* 1988; **461**: 393–6.

653 Tritschler HJ, Andreetta F, Moraes CT et al. Mitochondrial myopathy of childhood associated with depletion of mitochondrial DNA. *Neurology* 1992; **42**: 209–17.

654 Trojanowski JQ, Tohyama T, Lee VM. Medulloblastomas and related primitive neuroectodermal brain tumors of childhood recapitulate molecular milestones in the maturation of neuroblasts. *Mol Chem Neuropathol* 1992; **17**:121–35.

655 Trouth CO, Mills RM, Kiwull-Schoene H, Schlaefke ME eds. *Ventral brainstem mechanisms and control of respiration and blood pressure*. New York: Marcel Dekker, 1995.

656 Tsuji M, Higuchi Y, Shiraishi K et al. Congenital fiber type disproportion: severe form with marked improvement. *Pediatr Neurol* 1999; **21**: 658–60.

657 Unhanand M, Mustafa MM, McCracken GH Jr, Nelson JD. Gram-negative enteric bacillary meningitis: a twenty-one-year experience. *J Pediatr* 1993; **122**: 15–21.

658 Vajsar J, Balslev T, Ray PN et al. Congenital cytoplasmic body myopathy with survival motor neuron gene deletion or Werdnig–Hoffmann disease. *Neurology* 1998; **51**: 873–5.

659 Van Assche FA, Holemans K, Aerts L. Fetal growth and consequences for later life. *J Perinat Med* 1998; **26**: 337–46.

660 Van den Berg I, Berger R. Phosphorylase b kinase deficiency in man: a review. *J Inherit Metab Dis* 1990; **13**: 442–51.

661 Van den Bergh R. Centrifugal elements in the vascular pattern of the deep intracerebral blood supply. *Angiology* 1969; **20**: 88–94.

662 Vanier TM. Dystrophia myotonia in childhood. *BMJ* 1960; **ii**: 1284–8.

663 Vannucci RC, Perlman JM. Interventions for perinatal hypoxic–ischemic encephalopathy. *Pediatrics* 1997; **100**: 1004–14.

664 Varelas PN, Sleight BJ, Rinder HM et al. Stroke in a neonate heterozygous for factor V Leiden. *Pediatr Neurol* 1998; **18**: 262–4.

665 Vartanian T, Li Y, Zhao M, Stefansson K. Interferon-gamma-induced oligodendrocyte cell death: implications for the pathogenesis of multiple sclerosis. *Mol Med* 1995; **1**: 732–43.

666 Velasco ME, Brown JA, Kini J, Ruppert ES. Primary congenital rhabdoid tumor of the brain with neoplastic hydranencephaly. *Childs Nerv Syst* 1993; **9**: 185–90.

667 Vergani P, Strobelt N, Locatelli A et al. Clinical significance of fetal intracranial haemorrhage. *Am J Obstet Gynecol* 1996; **175**: 536–43.

668 Verma U, Tejani N, Klein S et al. Obstetric antecedents of intraventricular haemorrhage and periventricular leukomalacia in the low-birth-weight neonate. *Am J Obstet Gynecol* 1997; **176**: 275–81.

669 Vielhaber S, Feistner H, Schneider W et al. Mitochondrial complex I deficiency in a female with multiplex arthrogryposis congenita. *Pediatr Neurol* 2000; **22**: 53–6.

670 Vital A, Vital C, Coquet M et al. Congenital hypomyelination with axonopathy. *Eur J Pediatr* 1989; **148**: 470–2.

671 Vogel G. Cocaine wreaks subtle damage on developing brains (News). *Science* 1997; **278**: 38–9.

672 Vogler C, Sotelo-Avila C, Lagunoff D et al. Aluminum-containing emboli in infants treated with extracorporeal membrane oxygenation. *N Engl J Med* 1988; **319**: 75–9.

673 Vohr B, Ment LR. Intraventricular haemorrhage in the preterm infant (published erratum appears in *Early Hum Dev* 1996; **5**: 169). *Early Hum Dev* 1996; **44**: 1–16.

674 Voigt T. Development of glial cells in the cerebral wall of ferrets: direct tracing of their transformation from radial glia into astrocytes. *J Comp Neurol* 1989; **289**: 74–88.

675 Volpe JJ. Brain injury in the premature infant: overview of clinical aspects, neuropathology, and pathogenesis. *Semin Pediatr Neurol* 1998; **5**: 135–51.

676 Volpe JJ. Effect of cocaine use on the fetus (published erratum appears in *N Engl J Med* 1992; **327**: 1039). *N Engl J Med* 1992; **327**: 399–407.

677 Volpe JJ. Hypoglycemia and brain injury. In: Volpe JJ ed. *Neurology of the new born* 3rd edn. Philadelphia, PA: WB Saunders, 1995: 467–98.

678 Volpe JJ. Intraventricular haemorrhage in the premature infant – current concepts. Part I. *Ann Neurol* 1989; **25**: 3–11.

679 Volpe JJ. *Neurology of the newborn* 3rd edn. Philadelphia, PA: WB Saunders, 1995.

680 Volpe JJ. Subplate neurons – missing link in brain injury of the premature infant? *Pediatrics* 1996; **97**: 112–13.

681 Wakai S, Arai T, Nagai M. Congenital brain tumors. *Surg Neurol* 1984; **21**: 597–609.

682 Walker AE. Lissencephaly. *Arch Neurol Psychiatry* 1942; **48**: 13–29.

683 Wallace DC, Zheng XX, Lott MT et al. Familial mitochondrial encephalomyopathy (MERRF): genetic, pathophysiological, and biochemical characterization of a mitochondrial DNA disease. *Cell* 1988; **55**: 601–10.

684 Wallgren-Pettersson C, Avela K, Marchand S et al. A gene for autosomal recessive nemaline myopathy assigned to chromosome 2q by linkage analysis. *Neuromusc Disord* 1995; **5**: 441–3.

685 Waters KA, Meehan B, Huang JQ et al. Neuronal apoptosis in sudden infant death syndrome. *Pediatr Res* 1999; **45**: 166–72.

686 Weber F, Mori Y. Congenital craniopharyngioma. *Helv Paediatr Acta* 1976; **31**: 261–70.

687 Weeks JW, Reynolds L, Taylor D et al. Umbilical cord blood interleukin-6 levels and neonatal morbidity. *Obstet Gynecol* 1997; **90**: 815–18.

688 Weidenheim KM, Kress Y, Epshteyn I et al. Early myelination in the human fetal lumbosacral spinal cord: characterization by light and electron microscopy. *J Neuropathol Exp Neurol* 1992; **51**: 142–9.

689 Weinberg AG, Kirkpatrick JB. Cerebellar hypoplasia in Werdnig–Hoffmann disease. *Dev Med Child Neurol* 1975; **17**: 511–16.

690 Weisman LE, Stoll BJ, Cruess DF et al. Early-onset group B streptococcal sepsis: a current assessment. J Pediatr 1992; **121**: 428–33.

691 Wells JT, Ment LR. Prevention of intraventricular haemorrhage in preterm infants. Early Hum Dev 1995; **42**: 209–33.

692 Wigglesworth JS, Pape KE. An integrated model for haemorrhagic and ischaemic lesions in the newborn brain. Early Hum Dev 1978; **2**: 179–99.

693 Wijmenga C, Frants RR, Brouwer OF et al. Location of facioscapulohumeral muscular dystrophy gene on chromosome 4. Lancet 1990; **336**: 651–3.

694 Wijngaarden GK van, Fleury P, Bethlem J, Meijer AE. Familial 'myotubular' myopathy. Neurology 1969; **19**: 901–8.

695 Wilkins B. Head injury – abuse or accident? Arch Dis Child 1997; **76**: 393–6.

696 Williams RS, Ferrante RJ, Caviness VS Jr. The cellular pathology of microgyria. A Golgi analysis. Acta Neuropathol (Berl) 1976; **36**: 269–83.

697 Williams RS, Lott IT, Ferrante RJ, Caviness VS Jr. The cellular pathology of neuronal ceroid-lipofuscinosis. A Golgi–electronmicroscopic study. Arch Neurol 1977; **34**: 298–305.

698 Willinger M, James LS, Catz C. Defining the sudden infant death syndrome (SIDS): deliberations of an expert panel convened by the National Institute of Child Health and Human Development. Pediatr Pathol 1991; **11**: 677–84.

699 Wilson DA, Steiner RE. Periventricular leukomalacia: evaluation with MR imaging. Radiology 1986; **160**: 507–11.

700 Wilson EF. Estimation of the age of cutaneous contusions in child abuse. Pediatrics 1977; **60**: 750–2.

701 Wilson ER, Mirra SS, Schwartz JF. Congenital diencephalic and brain stem damage: neuropathologic study of three cases. Acta Neuropathol (Berl) 1982; **57**: 70–4.

702 Windle WF, Jacobson HN, Ramirez De Arellano MIR de, Combes CM. Structural and functional sequelae of asphyxia neonatorum in monkeys. Res Publ Ass Res Nerv Ment Dis 1962; **39**: 169–82.

703 Wong PC, Barlow CF, Hickey PR et al. Factors associated with choreoathetosis after cardiopulmonary bypass in children with congenital heart disease. Circulation 1992; **86** (Suppl): II118–26.

704 Yakovlev PI, Lecours AR. The myelogenetic cycles of regional maturation of the brain. In: Minkowski A ed. Regional development of the brain in early life. Oxford: Blackwell, 1967: 3–70.

705 Yamada T, Placzek M, Tanaka H et al. Control of cell pattern in the developing nervous system: polarizing activity of the floor plate and notochord. Cell 1991; **64**: 635–47.

706 Yamamoto T, Shibata N, Kanazawa M et al. Localization of laminin subunits in the central nervous system in Fukuyama congenital muscular dystrophy: an immunohistochemical investigation. Acta Neuropathol (Berl) 1997; **94**: 173–9.

707 Yamamoto T, Shibata N, Kanazawa M et al. Early ultrastructural changes in the central nervous system in Fukuyama congenital muscular dystrophy. Ultrastruct Pathol 1997; **21**: 355–60.

708 Yamanouchi H, Takashima S, Becker LE. Correlation of astrogliosis and substance P immunoreactivity in the brainstem of victims of sudden infant death syndrome. Neuropediatrics 1993; **24**: 200–3.

709 Yarom R, Shapira Y. Myosin degeneration in a congenital myopathy. Arch Neurol 1977; **34**: 114–15.

710 Yonezawa M, Back SA, Gan X et al. Cystine deprivation induces oligodendroglial death: rescue by free radical scavengers and by a diffusible glial factor. J Neurochem 1996; **67**: 566–73.

711 Yoon BH, Kim CJ, Romero R et al. Experimentally induced intrauterine infection causes fetal brain white matter lesions in rabbits. Am J Obstet Gynecol 1997; **177**: 797–802.

712 Yoon BH, Romero R, Kim CJ et al. High expression of tumor necrosis factor-alpha and interleukin-6 in periventricular leukomalacia. Am J Obstet Gynecol 1997; **177**: 406–11.

713 Yoon BH, Romero R, Yang SH et al. Interleukin-6 concentrations in umbilical cord plasma are elevated in neonates with white matter lesions associated with periventricular leukomalacia. Am J Obstet Gynecol 1996; **174**: 1433–40.

714 Yoshioka A, Hardy M, Younkin DP et al. Alpha-amino-3-hydroxy-5-methyl-4-isoxazolepropionate (AMPA) receptors mediate excitotoxicity in the oligodendroglial lineage. J Neurochem 1995; **64**: 2442–8.

715 Young RS, Towfighi J, Marks KH. Focal necrosis of the spinal cord in utero. Arch Neurol 1983; **40**: 654–5.

716 Young RS, Yagel SK, Towfighi J. Systemic and neuropathologic effects of E. coli endotoxin in neonatal dogs. Pediatr Res 1983; **17**: 349–53.

717 Younkin DP. Hypoxic–ischemic brain injury of the newborn – statement of the problem and overview. Brain Pathol 1992; **2**: 209–10.

718 Yu MC, Yu WH. Effect of hypoxia on cerebellar development: morphologic and radioautographic studies. Exp Neurol 1980; **70**: 652–64.

719 Yucesoy K, Mertol T, Ozer H, Ozer E. An infantile intraosseous hematoma of the skull. Report of a case and review of the literature. Childs Nerv Syst 1999; **15**: 69–72.

720 Yue X, Mehmet H, Penrice J et al. Apoptosis and necrosis in the newborn piglet brain following transient cerebral hypoxia–ischaemia. Neuropathol Appl Neurobiol 1997; **23**: 16–25.

721 Yue X, Mehmet H, Squier MV et al. Apoptosis and necrosis in the brains of infants dying after birth asphyxia. Pediatr Res 1995; **17**: 187A.

722 Zec N, Filiano JJ, Kinney HC. Anatomic relationships of the human arcuate nucleus of the medulla: a DiI-labeling study (published erratum appears in J Neuropathol Exp Neurol 1997; **56**: 1070). J Neuropathol Exp Neurol 1997; **56**: 509–22.

723 Zeviani M, Servidei S, Gellera C et al. An autosomal dominant disorder with multiple deletions of mitochondrial DNA starting at the D-loop region. Nature 1989; **339**: 309–11.

724 Zhang ET, Hansen AJ, Wieloch T, Lauritzen M. Influence of MK-801 on brain extracellular calcium and potassium activities in severe hypoglycemia. J Cereb Blood Flow Metab 1990; **10**: 136–9.

725 Zhang Y, Chen HS, Khanna VK et al. A mutation in the human ryanodine receptor gene associated with central core disease. Nat Genet 1993; **5**: 46–50.

726 Zheng X, Shoffner JM, Lott MT et al. Evidence in a lethal infantile mitochondrial disease for a nuclear mutation affecting respiratory complexes I and IV. Neurology 1989; **39**: 1203–9.

727 Zinn AB, Kerr DS, Hoppel CL. Fumarase deficiency: a new cause of mitochondrial encephalomyopathy. N Engl J Med 1986; **315**: 469–75.

10

Nutritional and metabolic disorders

CLIVE HARPER AND ROGER BUTTERWORTH

MALNUTRITION

The effects of malnutrition on the central nervous system (CNS) are diverse and are significantly different depending upon the stage of development or maturity of the brain and the severity and specificity of the deficiency state. For example, selective deficiency of one or more essential ingredients of the diet such as vitamins, trace elements or protein will cause quite different clinical syndromes and pathological states. This section deals with the effects of chronic protein–calorie malnutrition (undernutrition). In general, there appear to be adverse effects on the development and function of the nervous system of all animal species studied. During development somatic growth is markedly retarded but there is only a modest decrease in brain weight. There is no definable neuropathology in the traditional sense as a consequence of the nutritional insult, but during development malnutrition can influence cell division, migration of cells and the elaboration of their processes. The bulk of evidence suggests that there are only minimal effects on the nervous system once it has fully developed. Thus, the brains of adults are relatively resistant to the effects of malnutrition, although significant changes on computed tomographic (CT) scans and magnetic resonance imaging (MRI) are the rule in patients with anorexia nervosa.[231] A magnetic resonance spectroscopy study of four patients with anorexia nervosa showed a significant elevation of the phosphodiester peak, suggesting that there may be an abnormality in membrane phospholipid metabolism.[219] However, the sulcal widening and dilatation of the ventricles seen in these cases appear to be reversible once the eating disorder has resolved, suggesting that the changes are not associated with any permanent structural abnormality.[114] Gunston et al.[168] showed

a similar pattern of reversible shrinkage in kwashiorkor using MRI. Twelve children aged 6–37 months who required admission to hospital for treatment of kwashiorkor were evaluated clinically, biochemically and by MRI. Brain shrinkage was noted in every child on admission and white and grey matter appeared to be equally affected. By 30 days there was already some improvement (Fig. 10.1) and at 90 days the cerebral changes had resolved in nine and improved substantially in the remainder. The brain seems to be particularly vulnerable during the fastest growth periods (growth spurts), although in infants it may be difficult to determine the impact of the malnutrition because of associated medical conditions, especially infections, and social and physical deprivation. The overall problem, which predominantly affects people in developing countries, has been reviewed by Udani.[438,439] Infantile malnutrition has been defined in the Jamaica Declaration as either kwashiorkor (oedematous children with a weight for age from 60 to 80% of the standard) or marasmic kwashiorkor (weight for age below 60%).[208] Marasmus results from insufficient intake of protein and calories, usually owing to undernutrition, whereas in kwashiorkor the caloric intake may be sufficient but protein intake is reduced owing to malnutrition. These two conditions are really part of a continuum so that the evaluation of pathogenic factors in the neuropathology of these diseases is difficult. There is general agreement concerning the clinical definition of kwashiorkor, which is graphically depicted in a single case report by Udani.[437] The children have severe generalized oedema, skin lesions (similar to pellagra), hair discoloration and friability, hepatomegaly (fatty liver), hypoproteinaemia and mental changes such as irritability alternating with apathy. Kwashiorkor has been reproduced in a number of experimental animals, but most convincingly by Coward and Whitehead,[97] who fed baboons the same diet that

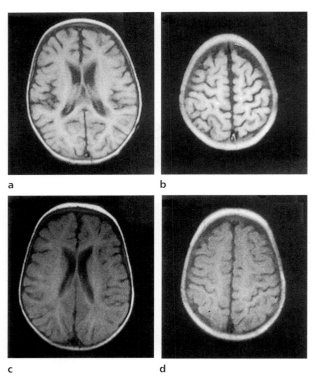

a　　　　　　　　b

c　　　　　　　　d

Figure 10.1 *(a, b) Type MRI changes (mid and high axial views) of cerebral atrophy seen in a young child admitted to hospital for treatment of kwashiorkor. There is widening of cortical sulci, widened interhemispheric fissure and cerebellar folia, and enlarged ventricles and cisterns. (c, d) Improvement was seen by day 30 and there was almost complete resolution by day 90 with refeeding. Reproduced by permission from Gunston* et al.[168]

children with kwashiorkor received in Uganda. Numerous hypotheses including protein deficiency, niacin deficiency, hormonal dysadaptation, aflatoxin intoxication and others have been proposed to explain the more specific entity kwashiorkor.[155] Currently, there is good evidence to suggest that oxidative stress (free radicals) plays an important role.[155] Lipid mediators such as cysteinyl leukotrienes may be involved in the pathophysiology, particularly in oedema formation.[281] Apart from the mental changes, neurological signs are not a prominent feature of kwashiorkor. However a rhythmic coarse tremor, hypotonia and areflexia have been described during the recovery period and these signs usually disappear spontaneously. Udani and Dastur[440] claim that the most common clinical manifestation, seen in between 25 and 30% of children with kwashiorkor, is an apparent lower motor disorder with hypotonia, muscle weakness and absent deep tendon reflexes. The symptoms and signs improve over 6–12 weeks with appropriate treatment. They named this condition 'kwashiorkor myelopathy' and described loss of Nissl substance in anterior horn neurons in the spinal cords of children.[437] Similar changes have been described in experimental animals with kwashiorkor and the authors have likened the change to chromatolysis.[356]

In the animal model there was also an increase in the concentration of neuroglial cells. Given the reversible nature of the clinical syndrome and the fact that associated deficiency states such as pellagra can cause chromatolysis of anterior horn cells, these findings require further investigation. Dastur et al.[108] have detailed the neuropathological changes in skeletal muscle and sural nerves of children with protein calorie malnutrition, but this will not be discussed further.

There is general consensus that severe malnutrition after birth in infants results in smaller-than-normal brains in smaller-than-normal bodies.[55,405] Head circumference is reduced but radiological studies show that this is in part due to thinning of the scalp and skull.[128] Surprisingly, the head size in children with marasmus is smaller than in those with kwashiorkor.[359] In a meticulous study of nine Jamaican infants, five of whom died of malnutrition, Garrow et al. reported lower fresh brain weights than for normal children of the same age.[148] Similar studies have shown the same pattern.[55,70,467] The extent to which prenatal influences, especially maternal malnutrition, have influenced these data is uncertain (see experimental studies).

Studies in humans have demonstrated significant associations between maternal malnutrition and congenital malformations of the CNS such as hydrocephalus, anencephaly, encephalocoele and spina bifida.[21,89,361] This is discussed further in the section dealing specifically with folate deficiency. Neuropathological changes associated with malnutrition have been reviewed by Trowell et al.[436] in their classic paper on kwashiorkor and more recently by Duckett and Winick.[124] Both groups concluded that there is no histological counterpart to the striking mental changes. Duckett and Winick[124] described the neuropathology in two marasmic Guatemalan children aged 1 and 2 years. Macroscopically, the brains were normal and weighed 645 and 720 g, respectively. The cases were widely sampled and a broad range of staining procedures was carried out. The results in both cases were similar, the myelin was normal, there was no gliosis, and lipofuscin granules were present in the cytoplasm of neurons in the inferior olives, basal ganglia and cortex. In the middle layers of the cortex many of the neurons appeared atrophic. The accumulation of lipofuscin in the neurons is interesting given the recent studies suggesting the importance of oxidative stress in kwashiorkor.[155] Several authors have suggested that myelin may be abnormal in some cases of 'malnutrition encephalopathy'. Most of the evidence comes from biochemical analyses of the brains of infants dying with marasmus. It has been shown that reductions in the cerebroside and plasmalogen fractions of the cerebral lipids (essential components of myelin) were especially prominent.[137] In a subsequent study using the same material Fox et al.[141] showed that the composition of the myelin was not altered. In a rat model, Krigman and Hogan[233] showed that there is a greater than 60% deficit in the relatively myelin-specific galactolipids following early undernutrition. Moreover, they noted that the proportion of myelinated axons in the pyramidal tract was reduced and that the myelin sheath was disproportionately reduced relative to axon diameter. This change may relate to abnormal glial function.[113] The question of myelin abnormalities has been addressed in a number of experimental models.[375]

Bedi[39] has presented a detailed review of the neuro-anatomical changes in the CNS following undernutrition in early life. Many of the findings are derived from animal models, most often the laboratory rat. Some of the abnormalities of the brain appear to be permanent and others reversible. Body and brain weight changes replicate the data in man. Undernutrition during the latter half of gestation and/or during the suckling period can cause up to 25% reduction in brain weight.[40] Biochemical estimates of DNA in the brain, which provide a crude measure of total cell number but do not discriminate between cell types, are also reduced in this model.[119] Nayak and Chatterjee showed that there is a decrease in homogenate DNA content in the thalamus, midbrain and cerebellum but not in the cerebrum;[315] however, the concept that some brain regions are more affected than others is refuted by Peeling and Smart.[336] They claim that the 'selective' effect on the cerebellum is not an example of an especially sensitive process but results from expressing the deficits as '% of age control values' and disappear when proper comparisons of growth are made. Most studies have shown that the cerebellum has greater weight deficits than the rest of the brain in rats undernourished during postnatal life.[39,468] Quantitative studies of cerebral cortical thickness are inconsistent but the majority suggests that undernutrition causes reduced cortical depths.[22,166] The deficits disappear after relatively short periods of nutritional rehabilitation.[39] Most studies have shown an increase in the numerical density of cortical neurons, which may relate to reduced cortical volume as a result of reduced dendritic growth.[39] This change also seems to be reversible as rehabilitated animals show no significant differences. After reviewing the current literature and emphasizing the difficulties inherent in quantitative neuropathological studies, Bedi[39] found that the data on glial cell changes related to undernutrition during early life are inconclusive. Some workers have found no change in the numerical density of glial cells,[394] while others have found it to increase or decrease[118] with respect to control animals. In a rat model of the effects of dietary protein restriction initiated at the time of conception there was decreased glial fibrillary acidic protein (GFAP) staining suggesting delayed astrocytogenesis.[166] These authors also showed reduced expression of microtubule-associated protein-5 (MAP-5), increased expression of MAP-1 and increased expression of synaptophysin in the basal ganglia. These parameters normalized (except for MAP-1) as the rats matured.[166] There is an alteration in the neuron-to-glial cell ratios and it is uncertain whether or not this is a permanent change.[39] There are also conflicting data on the numerical density of the cerebellar granule and Purkinje cells following

undernutrition. Bedi[39] reviewed these data and concluded that 'there is considerable evidence to show that undernutrition during early life causes a substantial deficit in the granule-to-Purkinje cell ratio which is permanent'. Golgi studies suggest that there are permanent deficits and alterations in the dendritic network, its branching pattern and spines.[82,286] There are numerous articles on the number and morphology of synapses in undernutrition.[39] Most have shown deficits and abnormal morphology.[214] Some of the changes appear to be partially rectified by nutritional rehabilitation. Bedi et al.[41] showed a deficit in synapse-to-neuron ratio in the frontal cortex and cerebellar granule cell layer. Several experimental studies have shown regional alterations in receptor density[443] and neurotransmitter changes.[79] The implications of these dendritic, synaptic, transmitter and receptor changes are unknown but in man there are many authors who believe that malnutrition during development and in early infancy can result in functional deficits of attentional processes and important interactions which in turn lead to various types of learning disability.[306]

Contrary to these data, many experimental models of life-long food restriction have shown a positive effect with a delay in the 'normal' age-related impairments of cognition and motor performance.[354]

VITAMIN DEFICIENCIES

Vitamin deficiency states can lead to a number of important neurological disorders. The most common disorders are associated with deficiencies of the B group of vitamins, particularly thiamine. Although these disorders are seen in populations suffering from general malnutrition there are specific groups of people who are particularly susceptible to specific deficiencies. For example, thiamine deficiency is frequently seen in alcoholics. This results not only from poor diet, but also from the alcohol interfering with the normal absorption, storage and metabolism of thiamine. The complexity of these types of case can make interpretation of the neuropathology difficult as it may be impossible to determine which pathological changes are caused by the deficiency, toxic or other metabolic state. It has been shown that quantitative morphometry is a more discriminant technique in such studies and subtle neuropathological changes such as proportional neuronal loss can be identified. These types of study, together with molecular pathology, have contributed significantly to the understanding of many of these disorders.

Studies of various deficiency states show that there are significant variations in the prevalence of these disorders in different countries. For example, the highest prevalence of the Wernicke–Korsakoff syndrome (WKS), which is caused by thiamine deficiency, has been reported in Australia.[181,186] In these studies there were no cases of pellagra (caused by a deficiency of niacin), whereas in a study of a similar alcoholic population in France[195] the prevalence of pellagra was very high (approximately 0.3%) and the prevalence of WKS was only 1.3%. The explanation for this apparent discrepancy may rest in the difficulty in diagnosing these conditions or in the diligence of the pathological examinations. However, one should also entertain the possibility that these are real findings which might be explained on the basis of dietary, cultural, racial or other differences. This issue has been addressed in an analysis of the international prevalence rates of WKS.[182] The possibility of multiple vitamin deficiencies should always be kept in mind.

Thiamine

Thiamine is a water-soluble vitamin. The daily requirement in humans is estimated to be 1.0–1.5 mg per day[146] and body stores can be depleted within about 3 weeks. The main role of thiamine is that of a coenzyme in the form of thiamine pyrophosphate. Cerebral thiamine metabolism is rapid and varies from one brain region to another.[365] In the CNS there are four main thiamine-dependent enzymes, each of which largely relates to glucose metabolism: pyruvate dehydrogenase, α-ketoglutarate dehydrogenase, transketolase and branched-chain α-ketoacid dehydrogenase.[197] Thiamine also plays a role in nerve conduction and probably membrane transport, independent of its function as an enzyme cofactor.[197] Although most of the thiamine is found in mitochondrial fractions of brain tissue, thiamine liberation by TPPase comes from the smaller (10%) membrane fraction.[207] Thiamine deficiency may be difficult to assess clinically in those with marginal deficiency but the reliability of the test is improved by using a new age-dependent parameter (modified transketolase activation).[371]

BERIBERI

Rarely encountered in Western countries, beriberi is a disorder with peripheral nervous system and cardiac manifestations.[234] Beriberi is classified as either 'wet' or 'dry' depending on the presence of oedema. Acute, subacute and chronic forms of beriberi have been described. In the infant, beriberi is generally acute and the underlying abnormality may result from combined protein malnutrition and thiamine deficiency.[355] The peripheral neuropathy is generally symmetrical and characterized by weakness, dysaesthesia and cutaneous hyperaesthesia. Cranial nerve involvement may occur and involvement of the vagus nerve may result in dysphonia.[420] The pathology of beriberi neuropathy is one of axonal degeneration with relative sparing of small myelinated and unmyelinated axons.[325] Diameter–frequency histograms of unmyelinated fibres manifest a bimodal distribution suggesting an increase in newly formed small unmyelinated fibres, indicative of regeneration.[415] Segmental demyelination has been reported more proximally, but this is considered to be a secondary phenomenon.[420] In addition, degeneration and neuronal loss in the anterior horn of the spinal cord as well as pallor in the gracile columns are occasionally seen.

WERNICKE–KORSAKOFF SYNDROME

Although WKS is seen most commonly in the alcoholic population there are several other 'at-risk' groups.[185] Most of these are self-evident: patients on starvation diets, gastric stapling, haemodialysis[204] or prolonged intravenous feeding without vitamin supplementation, and other causes of severe malnourishment. There have been reports in patients with the acquired immunodeficiency syndrome (AIDS), but the mechanism is presumed to be the same, that is, cachexia and a severe catabolic state.[63] In the original report of this disease by Wernicke[458] two of the patients were alcoholics and the third was a young woman who developed pyloric stenosis from ingestion of sulfuric acid.

The clinical syndrome is said to be typical in Wernicke's encephalopathy with patients presenting with ophthalmoplegia, nystagmus, ataxia and mental symptoms such as confusion, disorientation and even coma.[445] However, large autopsy studies have shown that the majority of cases do not have the classical clinical triad and many present with changes only in the conscious state.[188,313] The diagnosis is being made more frequently with the aid of neuroimaging techniques in both acute and chronic cases.[27,412] Studies have confirmed the usefulness of measuring mamillary body volumes in the diagnosis of chronic Wernicke's encephalopathy, although there are other causes of shrinkage, such as Alzheimer's disease.[389,412] The clinical diagnosis of Korsakoff's psychosis in alcoholics has only recently been standardized,[66] with the amnestic syndrome characterized by persistent anterograde episodic memory loss and preserved semantic memory, intelligence and learned behaviour.[401] This disease is most likely to be the end-result of repeated episodes of Wernicke's encephalopathy, although some of the episodes may have been subclinical or the diagnosis missed.[264] Korsakoff's psychosis may occur as the result of other diencephalic lesions such as tumours and trauma.[25,449] It should be noted that Korsakoff's psychosis is not inevitable in alcoholics with Wernicke's encephalopathy. Until recently, no consistent differences had been identified in the severity or topography of neuropathological changes in patients with or without amnesia in the Wernicke–Korsakoff syndrome. However, a recent pathological study provided strong evidence that damage to the anterior principal nucleus of the thalamus is more severe in patients with amnesia.[177] A number of reviews have dealt with the clinical and pathological aspects of WKS.[77,190,234,445]

Neuropathological changes

The most characteristic lesions are seen in the mamillary bodies and in the periventricular regions of the third and

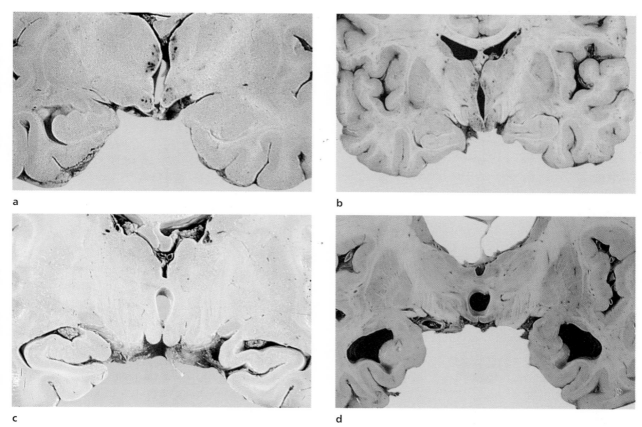

a   b

c   d

Figure 10.2 *(a) Coronal section of the brain showing haemorrhages in the mamillary bodies and walls of the third ventricle in a patient who died suddenly and unexpectedly. The diagnosis of acute Wernicke's encephalopathy was made at autopsy. Reproduced by permission from Harper.[185] (b) Coronal section of the brain showing symmetrical grey–brown zones of necrosis in the walls of the third ventricle and in the medial regions of mamillary bodies. The diagnosis is acute Wernicke's encephalopathy. (c) Coronal section of the cerebral hemispheres at the level of the mamillary bodies. No macroscopic abnormality is noted but histological examination (see Fig. 10.5) confirmed the diagnosis of subacute Wernicke's encephalopathy of 7–10 days duration. (d) Coronal section of the cerebral hemispheres showing brown, shrunken mamillary bodies, characteristic of chronic Wernicke's encephalopathy. This 56-year-old man was a known alcoholic with cirrhosis of the liver. There was also cerebral atrophy with dilatation of the third and lateral ventricles.*

fourth ventricles and aqueduct (Figs 10.2a–d, 10.3). The macroscopic and microscopic features will depend upon the stage and severity of the disease. The stages are gen-

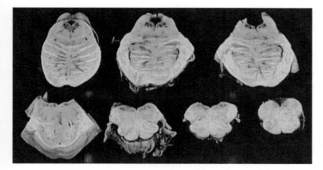

Figure 10.3 *Horizontal sections through the mid-brain, pons and medulla showing, grey–brown discoloration in the peri-aqueductal region and in the floor of the fourth ventricle consistent with haemorrhages and necrosis in acute Wernicke's encephalopathy (same case as shown in Fig. 10.2b).*

erally considered to be acute, subacute or chronic. Repeated episodes are common, so that acute-on-chronic changes are frequently seen. In a study of 131 cases of WKS 17% were acute, 66% chronic and 17% acute-on-chronic.[186] In a Scandinavian study of 45 cases, 53% were acute and 47% chronic.[427] In the absence of visible haemorrhages, which are only seen in about 5% of cases (Fig. 10.2a), it is possible to miss the diagnosis of acute Wernicke's encepthalopathy unless sections are taken for microscopic examination (see Figs 10.2c, 10.4b). Twenty-five per cent of cases can have normal mamillary bodies on macroscopic examination.[186] In some cases of acute Wernicke's encephalopathy there are symmetrical areas of necrosis in the walls of the third ventricle (Figs 10.2b, 10.5), around the aqueduct and in the floor of the fourth ventricle (Fig. 10.3). These necrotic zones may be difficult to detect as they are merely a greyish-brown discoloration (Figs 10.2b, 10.3). Myelin-stained whole mounts of the affected regions highlight the zones of necrosis (Fig. 10.5). The most consistent abnormality in the chronic WKS is

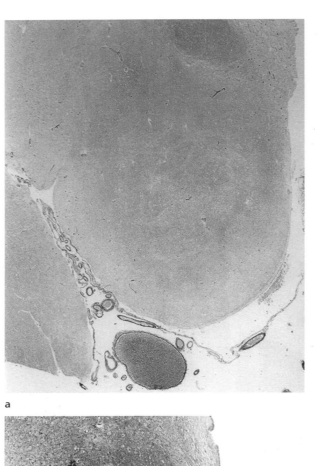

a

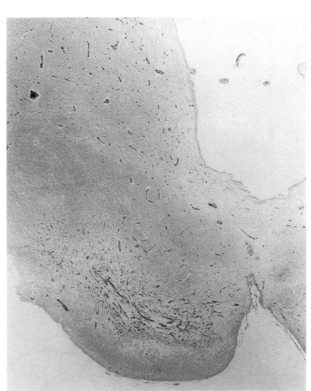

c

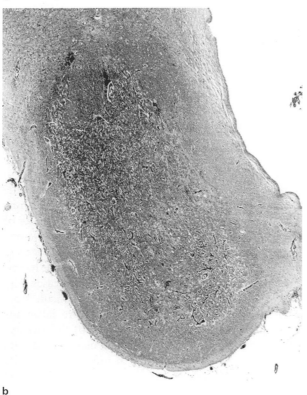

b

Figure 10.4 *Sections of mamillary body showing (a) relative paucity of vessels in a normal case, (b) intense capillary proliferation in a case of subacute Wernicke's encephalopathy (7–10 days' duration; same case as Fig. 10.2c), and (c) the typical features in a case of chronic Wernicke's encephalopathy with an apparent increase in vascularity in a shrunken mamillary body. (Reticulin stains.)*

shrinkage and brown discoloration of the mamillary bodies (Fig. 10.2d). Unilateral mamillary body lesions have been reported but are much more likely to be caused by posterior cerebral artery territory infarction or trans-

neuronal degeneration subsequent to an ipsilateral hippocampal lesion.[182]

Microscopic changes can be related to the duration of the disease (Fig. 10.4a–c). The earliest changes are seen in

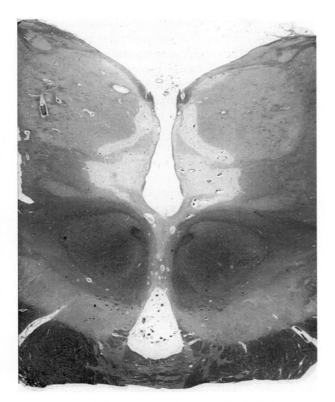

Figure 10.5 *Whole-amount section of walls of third ventricle showing symmetrical zones of necrosis in medial thalamic nuclei in a case of acute Wernicke's encephalopathy. (Weil myelin stain.)*

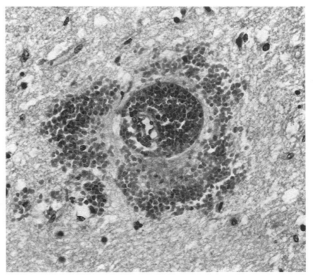

a

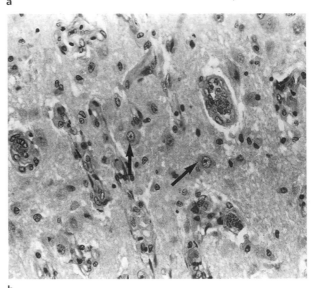

b

Figure 10.6 *(a) Section from mamillary body in acute Wernicke's encephalopathy (1–3 days' duration) showing small ring haemorrhages around blood vessels. (H&E.) (b) Section from mamillary body of case of subacute Wernicke's encephalopathy (7–10 days' duration) showing endothelial hypertrophy and hyperplasia. Note that neurons are relatively preserved (arrows). (H&E.)*

the neuropil and in and around blood-vessel walls. There is oedema and extravasation of red blood cells into the perivascular spaces. In some instances these extend outwards into the parenchyma to form 'ball' micro-haemorrhages (Fig. 10.6a) or macroscopically visible haemorrhages. Within 1–2 days the endothelial cells become hypertrophic and capillary budding commences. These changes are maximal at about 7–10 days (Figs 10.4b, 10.6b). Tissue necrosis is occasionally seen but is more common in the thalamic nuclei and is often symmetrical bilaterally (Fig. 10.5). There is usually sparing of a thin rim of tissue in the subependymal region. Neurons show relatively little change and do not appear to be the principal target of this disease process (Fig. 10.6b). There is relative sparing of neurons even in the chronic WKS. Thalamic and olivary neurons appear to be an exception to this rule, as discussed below.[339] An astrocytic reaction is noted by the third or fourth day. There are increased numbers of nuclei and some of the astrocytes have visible eosinophilic cytoplasm. Myelin and axons are often destroyed and this is most easily recognized when a specific pathway such as the mamillothalamic tract is affected. Apart from occasional histiocytes there is generally no inflammatory reaction.

In chronic lesions, parenchymal elements are lost and reactive changes are largely restricted to increased numbers of astrocytes. There are increased numbers of thin-walled capillaries with normal endothelium (Fig. 10.4c). This is partly due to loss of parenchymal elements and a compaction of surviving elements and partly reflects the vascular proliferation that occurred in the acute stage of the disease. There is a relative preservation of neurons (Fig. 10.6b) but loss of myelin and axons. Haemosiderin-laden macrophages in perivascular spaces are the tombstones of microhaemorrhages. In the most severe cases the mamillary bodies become shrunken and spongy with almost no residual parenchyma (Figs 10.2d, 10.4c).

Table 10.1 *Incidence of thalamic lesions in pathological studies of the Wernicke–Korsakoff syndrome*

	Year	n	Thalamic lesions (%)
Malamud and Skillicorn[273]	1956	70	53
Cravioto and Silberman[99]	1961	28	100
Victor et al.[444]	1971	45	89
Harper[186]	1983	131	61
Torvik[428]	1985	46	69

Changes in other hypothalamic nuclei display a similar pattern of disease but it is usually much less severe and can be quite difficult to identify in chronic Wernicke's encephalopathy. Very occasionally, the lesions may be centred not on the mamillary bodies but on the anterior hypothalamus, and the optic chiasm may be involved.[298] Campbell and Russell noted involvement of the optic nerves.[69] Optic nerve involvement is more common in Leigh's disease, which has a similar topography and microscopic appearance to subacute Wernicke's encephalopathy.

The thalamus appears to be particularly susceptible to damage in WKS. Table 10.1 lists the frequency of observed thalamic lesions in five of the largest pathological studies of the WKS.

The wide range in the proportion of WKS cases with thalamic lesions in these studies (53–100%) may relate to differences in case selection criteria and the detail in which the cases were examined. In the study by Victor et al.[444] the majority of cases had been diagnosed with WKS prior to death. In the study by Harper[186] only 20% of cases had been diagnosed prior to death, with many of the cases having none or only one of the classical clinical signs of WKS.[188] Thus, the pathological changes in this latter group might be expected to be less severe.

From a pathological point of view, the most detailed study was that of Victor et al.,[444] who examined serial sections of the thalamus in 17 cases and multiple representative sections in another 23 cases. They listed the incidence of involvement in 24 different thalamic nuclei. The most frequently affected nuclei were the medial dorsal (88%), submedius and medial ventral (58%), lateral dorsal (68%) and medial pulvinar (85%). Torvik[428] studied 46 cases of WKS but only 21 had step sections through the thalamus. They only commented on four different regions, the medial dorsal nucleus, medial part of lateral nucleus, anterior nucleus and pulvinar, of which the medial dorsal was by far the most commonly affected region (76%).

The distribution of lesions in the thalamus is an important issue as most authors believe that the severe amnestic syndrome which characterizes Korsakoff's psychosis is caused by lesions in specific thalamic and hypothalamic regions.[272,273,284,444] However, there has been debate as to the most relevant thalamic nuclei. Recently, Harding et al.

reported quantitative analyses on thalamic and hypothalamic nuclei from five uncomplicated alcoholics, five cases of Wernicke's encephalopathy and eight cases of Korsakoff's psychosis.[177] The success of this study is in large part due to the careful selection of cases for study using recently standardized clinical criteria for WKS as discussed above.[66] Using 50 μm serial frozen sections of the diencephalon, they showed that neuronal loss in the anterior principal nucleus of the thalamus was present consistently only in alcoholic Korsakoff's psychosis (Fig. 10.7). However, there were changes in the volumes and estimated neuronal numbers of medial mamillary nuclei and medial dorsal nucleus of thalamus in both amnestic and non-amnestic Wernicke cases.[177] There were no significant changes in the uncomplicated alcoholic group studied. These authors also showed that neuronal loss in the anterior principal nucleus occurs in concert with regional atrophy so that changes in neuronal density are minimal and the examination of a single histological section will not enable the pathologist to diagnose accurately Korsakoff's psychosis.

Victor et al.[444] first proposed that damage to the medial dorsal nucleus was correlated with the amnesia. Animal models of WKS also supported this hypothesis in that degeneration of the medial dorsal thalamic nucleus correlates with a loss of spontaneous synchronous bursts of activity in the cortex.[26] However, detailed studies of four autopsied cases of alcoholics with Korsakoff's psychosis showed that there was damage to medial thalamus, but the medial dorsal nucleus was largely spared.[272,284] A thin band of gliosis between the wall of the third ventricle and the medial magnocellular portion of the medial dorsal nucleus was noted. Mair et al.[272] concluded that lesions in this site (paratenial nucleus) can induce memory impairment. This nucleus borders the medial dorsal nucleus and Victor et al.[445] criticized this work, stating that the figure showed lesions extending into the medial dorsal nucleus.

Thalamic lesions appear to differ from those seen in other brain regions (e.g. mamillary bodies) in the same cases. The principal difference is that there is almost a complete loss of neurons in the thalamus compared with relative sparing of neurons elsewhere.[428] In rare cases of WKS symmetrical zones of necrosis are seen in the thalamus (Fig. 10.5). Such lesions are similar to those seen in experimental models of WKS in which thiamine antagonists (e.g. pyrithiamine) are used to induce the disorder.[243] In acute Wernicke's encephalopathy several authors have described neuronal changes in the thalamus and inferior olivary nuclei which are quite different to the more classical vascular and neuropil changes seen in mamillary bodies and other periventricular regions.[65,428] Torvik described eosinophilic change of the neuronal cytoplasm similar to that seen after an hypoxic insult.[428] Byrne et al. showed that there were perineuronal vacuoles and apparent degeneration of the neurons.[65] The latter study used 50 μm frozen sections so that artefactual vacuolation should have been minimal. These findings may have important implications with regard to the pathogenic mechanisms linking thiamine deficiency and tissue damage. There has been a number of reports of neuronal vacuolation and eosinophilic cell change in relation to experimental excitotoxic lesions.[295,326] This issue is discussed in more detail in the section on experimental thiamine deficiency.

The focus on the classical periventricular lesions and a failure to apply quantitative techniques have obscured changes in other regions of the brain in WKS. Four other regions need to be considered: the cerebral cortex, the basal forebrain, the locus coeruleus and the raphe nuclei in the brainstem.

Brain weight and volume studies in alcoholics have shown that there is a significant loss of tissue, particularly in those alcoholics with WKS.[187,429] The loss of tissue is largely from the white matter of the cerebral hemispheres.[112,183] Jernigan et al.[211] analysed MRI scans of patients with WKS and showed a reduction in cerebral cortical volume. There are conflicting data in analyses of cortical neuronal counts in alcoholic cases. Kril and Harper showed a 22% reduction in the number of neurons in the superior frontal cortex (Brodmann's area 8), but no significant change in the primary motor (area 4), frontal cingulate (area 32) or inferior temporal cortex (areas 20 and 36).[236] However, analysis of counts in the different alcoholic groups revealed no significant difference between those alcoholics with WKS or cirrhosis of the liver and the uncomplicated alcoholics.[236] This finding suggests that alcohol abuse is responsible for the neuronal loss in the superior frontal cortex and that the additional complication of WKS, although significantly contributing to the brain shrinkage in alcoholics, does not accentuate neuronal loss. Jensen and Pakkenberg[209] used stereological techniques to make unbiased estimates of total numbers of neurons in the neocortex in 11 alcoholic and 11 control patients. They found no difference between the two groups but cases of WKS were excluded. It must also be said that regional differences, with an apparent selective damage of the superior frontal region, could have been missed using this technique. Kril et al. calculated regional volumes of frontal cortex, medial temporal lobe, deep grey matter and cerebral white matter. Unbiased estimates of neuronal numbers confirmed that there was a selective loss of neurons from the superior frontal association cortex (23%) but no loss from the motor cortex in the uncomplicated alcoholics. The neuronal loss appeared to be confined to non-GABAergic pyramidal neurons.[235] There are clinical and radiological data which support the finding of selective frontal lobe damage in alcoholics.[210,328]

The hippocampus has been relatively poorly studied in alcoholic subjects, despite the fact that pathological changes in the hippocampus have dominated the literature on experimental models of alcohol toxicity.[293,452] Using MRI analysis Sullivan et al.[413] showed a 4–6% reduction in the volume of the hippocampus in non-amnestic alcoholics. The change was greatest in the anterior segment but there was no correlation between alcohol consumption or impaired memory function and the degree of atrophy. Those alcoholics with a history of withdrawal seizures had significantly smaller temporal lobe white matter volumes.[414] There have been three quantitative pathological studies of the hippocampus in alcoholics.[43,178,235] Bengochea and Gonzalo[43] showed that there is an age-related reduction in the density of neurons in alcoholics, whereas the other two studies found no cell loss, even though there were five cases of Korsakoff's psychosis in the study by Harding et al.[178] and Kril et al. studied four cases of Wernicke's encephalopathy and four with Korsakoff's psychosis.[235] However, the latter studies noted a reduction in the volume of the hippocampus in the uncomplicated alcoholics and those with WKS, but this change could be explained on the basis of loss of white matter.[178,235] Apart from cases with hippocampal sclerosis (see below), structural changes to hippocampal neurons in alcoholics have not been documented. However, recent studies have shown that hippocampal-dependent learning is impaired by alcohol in a dose-dependent fashion.[294]

Two quantitative studies of the amygdala are reported in the literature. Kril et al.[235] noted a significant reduction in the volume of the amygdala complex only in those alcoholics with WKS, whereas Alaverez et al. found a significant reduction in neuronal density in alcoholics of all ages.[19]

Epilepsy is a relatively common clinical syndrome in alcoholics. Wilkinson et al.[465] found an incidence of 7.8% in their study of 1000 alcoholics and many of these cases would have hippocampal sclerosis. In a recent study of the prevalence of WKS in forensic autopsies, 25 cases were identified out of 2212 autopsies, a prevalence of 1.1%.[184] There were 130 cases with a history of alcohol-related problems and 12 (9.2%) had sclerosis of the hippocampus.

Several authors have suggested that the amnestic disorder of Korsakoff's psychosis relates to damage of the cholinergic magnocellular neurons in the basal nucleus of Meynert. Arendt et al.[24] compared the pathological changes in the basal nucleus of Meynert in Alzheimer's disease, Parkinson's disease and Korsakoff's psychosis. They calculated numbers of neurons and neuronal population density from serial sections. There was a significant loss of neurons in Alzheimer's disease (30%), Parkinson's disease (23%) and Korsakoff's psychosis (53%). They also studied five alcoholics without dementia and the mean neuronal counts were no different from control data. Mayes et al.[284] studied the basal nucleus of Meynert in two cases of Korsakoff's psychosis using morphometric methods. They were unable to show a reduction in neuronal numbers or nucleolar volume but commented that many of the neurons were shrunken and showed a loss of Nissl substance. In this study, single sections of the nucleus basalis were taken as representative of this complex anatomical structure and this may account for the conflicting data. In a detailed morphometric study of the brains of seven chronic alcoholics, two of whom had well-documented Korsakoff's psychosis, Cullen *et al.*[102] showed a significant loss of neurons from the Ch4 region of the nucleus in both Wernicke's encephalopathy and Korsakoff's psychosis cases (24% and 21%, respectively). There was no difference between the uncomplicated alcoholics and controls. Ch4 cell numbers in all groups were significantly correlated with the volume of this region's major projection target, the cerebral cortex. Although there was no causal relationship between the neuronal loss and the amnesia there appeared to be a relationship with the attentional deficits seen in some patients with Wernicke's encephalopathy and Korsakoff's psychosis.[102] Neurofibrillary tangles have been reported to be common in the magnocellular neurons of the nucleus basalis in alcoholics with WKS, although the number of tangles seen is considerably smaller than in the average case of Alzheimer's disease.[101] There were only occasional tangles in the two uncomplicated alcoholic cases that were examined and there were no tangles or neuritic plaques in the cortex of any of the cases. In all of the WKS cases, and in some of the uncomplicated alcoholics, neurons in the nucleus basalis showed increased peroxidase activity. The authors speculated that neurodegeneration of the nucleus basalis in chronic alcoholics, especially those with additional thiamine deficiency, begins with the formation of neurofibrillary tangles which may be linked to the presence of increased peroxidase.[101]

Brainstem lesions in WKS generally follow the pattern seen elsewhere in the brain. They are in the periventricular and periaqueductal regions, with the exception of the

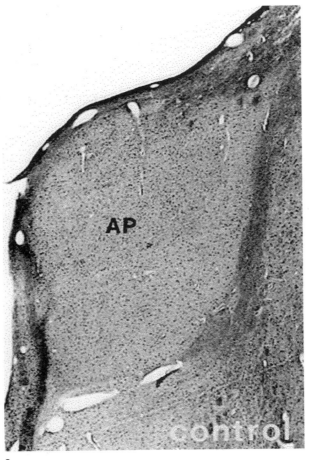
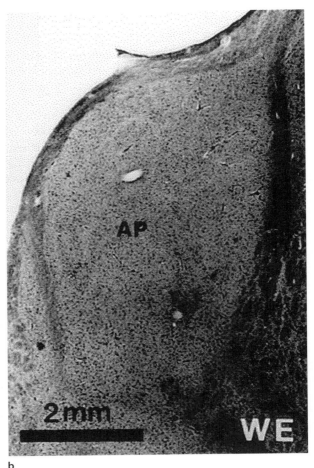

a

b

Figure 10.7 *Photomicrographs of the right anterior principal nucleus of the thalamus (AP). (a)–(c) were all stained with haematoxylin and eosin, and photographed at the same magnification at similar levels. (d)–(f) are higher magnifications of the sections adjacent to (a)–(c), stained with cresyl violet and photographed at the same magnification. (a) Normal architecture of the AP and surrounding structures in a control for comparison with (b) and (c). (b) An alcoholic with Wernicke's encephalopathy. In some alcoholics there were limited changes in the AP. (c) An alcoholic with Korsakoff's psychosis. There were often blood vessel abnormalities, myelin and parenchymal changes, and shrinkage of the AP. (d) Normal neuronal and glial configuration for comparison with (e) and (f). (e) Changes observed in an alcoholic with Wernicke's encephalopathy, including gliosis without apparent neuronal loss. (f) An alcoholic with Korsakoff's psychosis. In most of these alcoholics there was a visible reduction in the number of neurons and a further increase in the density of glia.[177]*

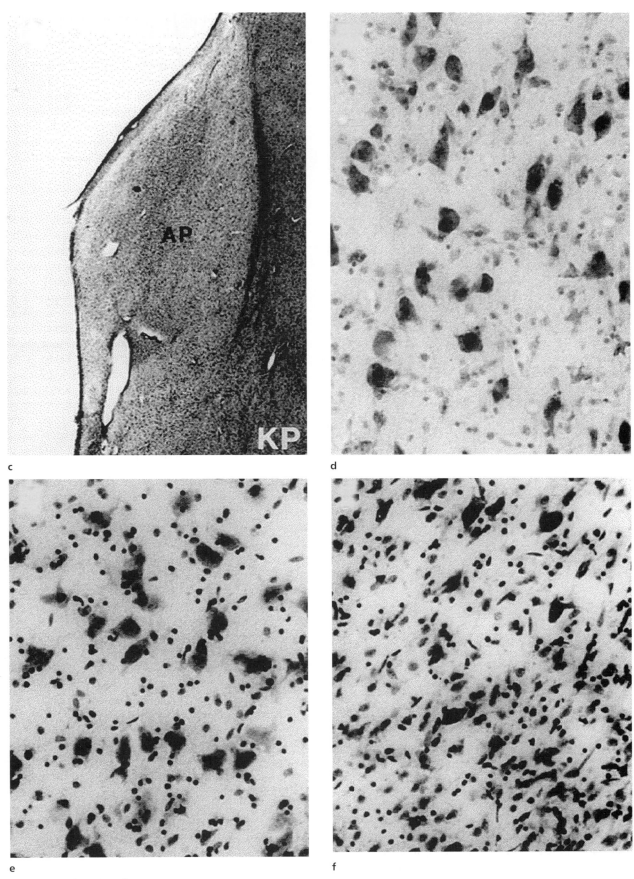

Figure 10.7 *(Continued).*

olivary lesions (discussed below). The pathological changes will depend upon whether the disease is acute or chronic. The incidence of involvement of different nuclei and regions in the brainstem is presented in detail in the monograph by Victor et al.[445] The most common sites of involvement were central superior (70.4%), medial vestibular nuclei (71.1%), interpositus and prepositus (68.2%) and locus coeruleus (67.9%). Data for many other specific nuclei are given in their monograph. Most other authors give figures for more general regions such as midbrain, pons and medulla and highlight specific clinically relevant regions such as oculomotor and vestibular nuclei.[99,186,273,427] Torvik[427] studied 21 cases of WKS by step sections through the brainstem and noted that lesions were far more common in acute than in chronic cases. This is consistent with the clinical observations that ophthalmoplegia and nystagmus are usually quickly reversed in acute WKS after treatment with parenteral thiamine.[346] Several authors have noted that changes in the inferior olives, which are distant from the periventricular tissues, are common and morphologically different.[273,427] The change is characterized by neuronal loss with relative sparing of the neuropil and capillary endothelium. The change has been likened to that in the thalamus, as discussed above. To complicate the issue the olives often show secondary changes resulting from alcoholic cerebellar vermal degeneration. This is presumed to be a transsynaptic degeneration. Other regions which warrant further study include the nucleus and tractus solitarius and ambiguus. These regions are of interest because of their role in cardiorespiratory control. A feature which has tended to be overlooked in cases of WKS is the frequency with which patients die suddenly and unexpectedly. In one study by Harper[181] 32 of 51 WKS cases died in this way and in ten instances there was no evident cause of death at necropsy. Eight of the cases were acute and lesions involving vital cardiorespiratory centres in the brainstem could well have accounted for their sudden death.[185] Autonomic neuropathy could also play a role in sudden unexpected death.

Lesions in the noradrenergic locus coeruleus are said to cause impairment of attention and information processing. There may also be links with learning and memory, as indicated by experimental models.[401] Several groups of workers have emphasized the importance of this nucleus and its noradrenergic pathways in alcoholics with WKS.[272,289] Victor et al.[444] noted abnormalities in the locus coeruleus in 19 of the 28 cases studied (67.9%). They did not provide any details of the pathological changes and no quantification was included. Mayes et al.[284] used quantitative techniques to study the loss of locus coeruleus neurons in two alcoholics with Korsakoff's psychosis. The patient with the more severe amnesia had a significant (19%) loss of neurons. McEntee and Mair[289] used biochemical studies to address the question of abnormalities of noradrenergic pathways. They showed significant reductions in noradrenaline and its metabolites in the cerebrospinal fluid (CSF) of WKS patients. Moreover, there is evidence of memory improvement with noradrenaline replacement therapy.[289] Halliday et al.[172] reported a quantitative study of the locus coeruleus in nine alcoholics with WKS. Four of these cases had the severe amnesia of Korsakoff's psychosis. The data were compared with five age-matched controls. There were no significant differences in the number, morphology or distribution of pigmented locus coeruleus neurons between any of the groups analysed. This study contradicts accounts of substantial cellular damage to this region in an alcoholic[23] and suggests that damage to the locus coeruleus is not responsible for the amnesia in WKS.

The median raphe nucleus is a midline structure in the caudal midbrain and rostral pons. The dorsal raphe nucleus lies dorsal to the median raphe in the ventral part of the central grey matter and is divided from it by the medial longitudinal fasciculus. Together, these two nuclei provide the primary source of serotonergic axons innervating large regions of the forebrain, particularly the cerebral cortex, the limbic system and the hypothalamus.[426] The anatomical location of the dorsal raphe nucleus and its ascending serotonergic fibres is such that it is likely to be damaged by the periventricular lesions which are characteristic of WKS. A quantitative study of dorsal raphe neurones in two alcoholics with WKS found no loss or degenerative changes in the region.[284] Victor et al.[444] did not specifically mention the raphe nuclei in their study of the pathology of WKS, but noted that the 'central grey matter' was involved in 55% of the 40 cases. Of the many other pathological studies of WKS, none has mentioned the raphe nuclei. Biochemical studies have shown abnormally low levels of serotonergic metabolites in the CSF of alcoholics with WKS and drug therapies enhancing serotonergic activity are reported to improve significantly memory performance in such patients.[289]

Halliday et al.[173] completed a quantitative morphometric study of the dorsal and median raphe nuclei in alcoholics. They used immunohistochemistry to identify the serotonergic neurons (PH8 antibody). There were five controls and nine alcoholics with the WKS. Four of these cases had the severe amnesia typical of Korsakoff's psychosis. There was a significant reduction (50%) in the number of serotonergic neurons from dorsal and median raphe nuclei in both the WKS and Korsakoff's psychosis cases compared with controls (Fig. 10.7). The loss was particularly evident in the pons. Thus, it appears that the serotonergic system is disrupted in alcoholics with thiamine deficiency.

There are neuropathological changes in the cortex, white matter, diencephalon, cerebellum and brainstem in WKS. The basal ganglia appear to be spared but Jernigan et al.[211] using MRI, showed reduced volumes of the caudate nuclei. This finding highlights the importance of a multidisciplinary approach to studies of the WKS, each discipline providing new data and ideas which give direction for further research.

EXPERIMENTAL THIAMINE DEFICIENCY

Numerous experimental models in different species have been used to study the structural, biochemical and functional effects of thiamine deficiency on the brain. Although many of the models do not reliably reproduce lesions of a similar nature and distribution to those seen in WKS in man, this does not invalidate their usefulness in understanding the effects of thiamine deficiency on the CNS.

Thiamine deficiency may be induced either by the use of a thiamine-deficient diet or by the use of the central thiamine antagonist, pyrithiamine, either with or without a thiamine-deficient diet. Dietary deficiency alone causes symptoms of neurological impairment in rats in 5–6 weeks. The combination of dietary deficiency and pyrithiamine leads to ataxia, opisthotonus and convulsions within 11–12 days in the mouse[455] and somewhat longer (13–14 days) in the rat.[197] Convulsions are a major problem in this animal model as they may cause significant pathological changes themselves. Cycling experiments, with thiamine supplementation between periods of deficiency, best replicate the chronic form of the disease in man, but these experiments have only been done in primates.[470,471] An additional factor to consider is that the majority of cases of WKS in man are associated with alcoholism.[186] Chronic ethanol treatment in the absence of thiamine deficiency does not result in Wernicke-type brain lesions in rodents. There are important interrelationships between alcohol and thiamine deficiency. Alcohol has been shown to impair thiamine absorption from the gastrointestinal system and to impair the conversion of thiamine to its metabolically active phosphorylated form.[422] It has been noted in an experimental rat model of thiamine deficiency that the clinical symptoms occur earlier and are more severe if the rats are also given alcohol.[480] Reviews of animal models of WKS show comparative tables of the neuroanatomical distribution of lesions in animals with a pyrithamine-induced thiamine deficiency encephalopathy.[197,434] The rat and mouse models appear to be the most useful. The review by Heroux and Butterworth provides detailed protocols of the diet, appropriate control groups, neurological evaluation and sampling techniques for blood and brain tissues.[197] In rats fed a thiamine-deficient diet in addition to administration of pyrithiamine, lesions are seen in the mamillary bodies, thalami, periaqueductal grey matter, superior and inferior colliculi, floor of the fourth ventricle and inferior olives.[434]

Microscopically, the lesions affect the neuropil, myelin and the small blood vessels, with a relative sparing of neuronal elements. However, in a similar rat model Vortmeyer and Colmant[450] showed that there was neuronal damage in the thalamus and olives which has been described in some human cases of acute Wernicke's encephalopathy.[65,428] As stated above, a significant concern with the pyrithiamine model is the occurrence of convulsions, which may modify the pathological and biochemical findings.

Electron-microscopic studies have focused attention upon changes in the glial and neuronal elements of the CNS in experimental thiamine deficiency. Several authors have demonstrated swelling of the cytoplasm of glial cells[91,367,455] together with microglial reaction[423] in the early stages of thiamine deficiency. Later, swelling of the inner loop of the myelin sheath develops.[367] It has been postulated that initially the oedema occurs as a result of defective active transport and a breakdown of the blood–brain barrier (BBB) with enhanced pinocytic transport.[68,275] Neuronal perikarya in certain thalamic nuclei show degenerative changes resembling glutamate-mediated excitotoxic damage in the pyrithiamine rat model,[244] and other changes have been described in the terminal axons and synaptic boutons.[340,419]

An autoradiographic study using the astrocytic mitochondrial ligand PK11195 demonstrated early alterations in the thalamus, inferior colliculus and inferior olivary nucleus of pyrithiamine-treated rats.[256] Whether these changes represent gliosis accompanying neuronal cell loss or primary astrocytic changes due to thiamine deficiency remains to be established.

In their review of the neurochemistry of thiamine deficiency, Heroux and Butterworth[197] outline the complex biochemical changes in the different animal models. Tissue levels of thiamine, the activity of thiamine-dependent enzymes, brain glucose utilization and neurotransmitter synthesis have all been measured. Some of the biochemical changes are more severe in vulnerable regions of the brain. In an attempt to explain the reversibility of the neurological signs in WKS, Butterworth[60,62] proposed a mechanism to explain the 'biochemical lesion'. Thus, decreased brain levels of thiamine pyrophosphate cause decreased activity of α-ketoglutarate dehydrogenase, which cause decreased glucose and pyruvate oxidation, resulting in decreased synthesis of neurotransmitters (GABA, glutamate and acetylcholine).

Mechanisms proposed to explain neuronal cell death in experimental thiamine deficiency include impairment of cerebral energy metabolism and focal lactic acidosis. For example, studies of oxidative phosphorylation in isolated mitochondria from symptomatic thiamine-deficient rats reveal decreased ATP synthesis resulting from depressed activities of thiamine-dependent enzymes.[171] It has been known since the pioneering work of Peters in the 1930s that brain lactate is increased in thiamine deficiency, leading to the suggestion that focal accumulation of lactate and the consequent alterations in cellular pH could contribute to neuronal cell death in thiamine deficiency. In favour of this possibility, an autoradiographic study showed significant acidosis in the mamillary bodies, brainstem and thalamus of thiamine-deficient rats.[196]

Free radical-mediated breakdown of the BBB has also been reported in thiamine deficiency, where it was found to be associated with enhanced expression of endothelial nitric oxide synthase[242] and microglial activation,[242,423] suggesting that these cells were responding to an oxidative challenge. A subsequent study showed that antioxidants are neuroprotective in thiamine deficiency,[425] supporting the oxidative damage hypothesis.

A glutamate [N-methyl-D-aspartate (NMDA) receptor]-mediated excitotoxic mechanism is suggested by the observation that extracellular brain levels of glutamate rise in the medial thalamus during neuronal degeneration in experimental thiamine deficiency.[446] Furthermore, dizocilpine maleate (MK-801), a selective NMDA receptor antagonist, was found to protect against thalamic neuronal loss.[67] However, a subsequent study found that this protective effect was only apparent at late (convulsive) stages of thiamine deficiency,[424] suggesting that excitotoxic mechanisms are late-stage phenomena.

ALCOHOLIC CEREBELLAR DEGENERATION

Atrophy of the cerebellum is commonly associated with alcoholism. It is characterized clinically by ataxia and incoordination of the lower limbs.[444] In a general hospital autopsy study Victor and Laureno[446] found an incidence of 4.1% in patients over 18 years old. The incidence among alcoholics is much greater. Torvik et al.[429] reported that 26.8% of alcoholics and 38.6% of alcoholics with WKS had cerebellar atrophy. Both Harper[186] and Victor et al.[444] studied patients with WKS and found an incidence of cerebellar atrophy of 32% and 36%, respectively. Cerebellar atrophy can also be identified radiologically during life. Cala et al.[67] identified cerebellar atrophy in 63% of their alcoholic patients. In an MRI study, Shear et al. showed significant cerebellar shrinkage in an alcoholic group but were unable to distinguish accurately between amnestic (WKS) and non-amnestic patients.[388]

Macroscopically, the neuropathological findings are of shrinkage of the folia, particularly the anterior superior vermis (Fig. 10.8). A number of volumetric changes have been documented with the aid of stereometry. Phillips et al. showed a reduction in the volume of the molecular and medullary layers in the vermis.[348] More recently, Baker et al. showed that the molecular layer volume in the vermis was reduced by 32% in chronic alcoholics with WKS.[28] A greater loss of white matter from the vermis was noted in those alcoholics with ataxia.[28] In a rat model of alcohol toxicity the volumes of both the molecular and granule cell layers were reduced in female alcohol-non-preferring animals, suggesting a sex difference.[366] Interestingly, the white matter volumes did not change, even after 22 months of alcohol treatment.

Microscopically, there is a loss of Purkinje cells with proliferation of Bergmann glia. Quantitatively, there is a significant reduction in the number and size of Purkinje cells which is most marked in the smaller rostral and caudal lobes of the vermis (lobes I–IV, IX and X).[348,431] Data from a recent quantitative study of the cerebellum

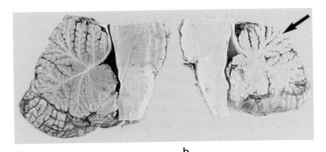

a   b

Figure 10.8 *Sagittal sections of cerebellar hemispheres and brainstem from (a) a normal case and (b) patient with alcoholic cerebellar degeneration. The atrophy is most severe in the anterior superior part of the vermis (arrow).*

revealed that there is no consistent correlation in the number of neurons or the structural volume for any of the cerebellar regions in the uncomplicated chronic alcoholics.[28] This suggests that chronic alcohol consumption per se does not necessarily damage human cerebellar tissue. However, significant changes were noted in alcoholics with WKS. In the cerebellar vermis there was a decrease in Purkinje cell density (reduced on average by 43%),[28] confirming previous findings.[349] The severity of cerebellar damage was correlated with clinical signs: there was a 36% loss of Purkinje cells in the lateral lobes in alcoholics with mental state signs and a 42% atrophy of vermal white matter in ataxic alcoholics.[28] The former correlation is of particular interest given recent evidence showing the importance of the cerebellum in the organization of higher order cerebral functions.[380]

Studies of the dendritic arborization of Purkinje cells using Golgi impregnation techniques have revealed reduced arbor in alcoholics[134] and in rats fed an alcohol-containing diet.[342,418] Pentney reviewed the experimental data on the effects of long-term ethanol consumption on the cerebellum.[341] A reduction in the dendritic arbor of Purkinje cells could explain the documented reduction in the volume of the molecular layer.[28,348] The concept of thiamine deficiency playing the dominant role in causing alcohol-related cerebellar damage is consistent with Adams' description of a disease identical to alcoholic cerebellar degeneration in malnourished individuals without alcoholism.[7] Additional evidence pointing towards the importance of thiamine deficiency as the principal pathogenic factor is that the clinical deficits have been shown to be reversed by the administration of thiamine, even in the presence of continued alcohol consumption.[445]

ALCOHOLIC MYELOPATHY

There are no pathological studies of cases purported to be alcoholic myelopathy. Sage et al.[377] reported five well-nourished alcoholic patients who developed a progressive myelopathy. Abstinence from alcohol halted the progression of the disease but there was no improvement. Most of the previous reports of myelopathy in alcoholics had been linked to cases with severe cirrhosis and portocaval shunts and had been referred to as 'shunt myelopathy'[266,479] (see also section on Post-shunt myelopathy). The five cases studied by Sage et al.[377] did not have severe liver disease or shunts, which led the authors to suggest that alcoholic myelopathy without hepatic encephalopathy may be more common that realized. They suggested that it could be masked by other common neurological complications of alcoholism, especially neuropathy. Until the pathological basis of this condition is clarified it is difficult to speculate further. In vivo studies, particularly MRI, could help in the diagnosis and identification of the site of the lesion(s) and pathologists should try to study the spinal cord of alcoholics at necropsy more frequently.

A common pathological abnormality in the spinal cord of alcoholics is posterior column degeneration. This is best seen in myelin-stained sections of the cord and is an ascending Wallerian degeneration secondary to peripheral neuropathy. This is an extremely common clinical finding in alcoholics.[445]

ALCOHOLIC PERIPHERAL NEUROPATHOLOGY

Alcoholic peripheral neuropathy is one of the most common forms of polyneuropathy. Electromyographic studies reveal abnormalities in 93% of ambulatory alcoholic patients, most of whom showed few clinical signs.[105] Pathological studies of the sural nerve from patients with alcoholic peripheral neuropathy reveal damage to both large- and small-diameter myelinated fibres. The predominant pathological process is considered to be one of axonal degeneration affecting the distal nerve segments (dying-back neuropathy).[453] A high incidence of peripheral neuropathy is encountered in alcoholic patients with WKS.[445] Whether alcoholic peripheral neuropathy is entirely the result of thiamine deficiency, or deficiencies of other water-soluble vitamins, or results from direct toxic effects of ethanol on peripheral nerves has not been definitively established.[106]

ALCOHOLIC AUTONOMIC NEUROPATHY

Peripheral neuropathy is a seen frequently in the alcoholic population and associated autonomic dysfunction is a common complication. In an excellent review of autonomic neuropathies, McDougall and McLeod noted that the most common clinical manifestation in alcoholics is impaired sweating distally, although postural hypotension may occur in severe cases and in alcoholics with associated WKS.[287,288] Abnormalities of cardiovascular parasympathetic control are common, but cardiovascular sympathetic changes are much less frequent. Clinical assessment of 30 alcoholic subjects was carried out by Barter and Tanner[31] using five simple tests of cardiovascular response. There was evidence of parasympathetic

neuropathy alone in 16% of the cases and of combined parasympathetic and sympathetic neuropathy in an additional 20% of cases. Those patients with the autonomic neuropathy were older, and more likely to be female and to have established alcoholic liver disease.[31] In a similar study, 79 male alcoholics were tested for autonomic neuropathy and then followed up for a period of 7 years.[212] On initial testing three groups were identified: 40% had no evidence of a vagal neuropathy, 32% had one abnormal test and 29% had two or more abnormal tests. Based on survival data for these groups, the authors concluded that evidence of vagal neuropathy in chronic alcoholics is associated with a significantly higher mortality.[212] Liver disease, whether induced by alcohol or not, seems to play a role in the pathogenesis of autonomic neuropathy.[138,263]

Pathological studies of the vagus nerve in chronic alcoholic patients show a significant reduction in the density of myelinated fibres in the distal parts of the vagus and carotid sinus nerves.[169,416] This is consistent with the concept that alcohol abuse causes a distal dying-back neuropathy so that the long vagal fibres to the heart are affected first. Teased nerve preparations showed axonal degeneration consistent with the dying-back pathology previously described in this condition.[453] These findings may provide the pathological explanation for some of the clinical manifestations of autonomic dysfunction in chronic alcoholics such as impaired heart-rate responses. It should also be noted that sudden unexpected death occurs commonly in alcoholic patients with WKS[181,185] and there may be a link between this and autonomic dysfunction.[212]

OTHER DISORDERS RELATED TO ALCOHOLISM

Although not the result of thiamine deficiency, two other disorders encountered in chronic alcoholism and associated with malnutrition are central pontine myelinolysis (CPM) and Marchiafava–Bignami (MFB) disease.

Central pontine myelinolysis

CPM is a relatively uncommon disorder which was first described in 1959 by Adams et al. in three alcoholic patients and one patient with malnutrition.[9] Victor et al.[444] found an incidence of 11.8% in their study of 34 cases of WKS, whereas Harper[181] found CPM in only 4% of his 51 cases. The expansive descriptions and figures of the pathological changes in central pontine regions provided by Adams et al.[9] have not been bettered. Although CPM has been described most commonly in alcoholics with WKS many other non-alcoholic groups of patients can be affected. The most common of these are patients with severe liver disease (especially postorthotropic liver transplant),[1,464] severe burns cases,[290] malnutrition, anorexia and severe electrolyte disorders,[228] and most recently cases with advanced human immunodeficiency virus (HIV) infection.[304] In many cases the most important pathogenic factor appears to be a too-rapid correction of a profound hyponatraemia.[296,321] However, some reports have questioned the validity of this mechanism[333,464] and alternative hypotheses have been proposed such as hypophosphataemia.[337] The diagnosis of CPM is being made more frequently with the availability of CT and MRI scans.[116] Initially, patients with CPM were thought to have a very high mortality but CT and MRI scans have permitted the identification of many more cases in the earliest stages of the disease and cases with complete clinical recovery are now being reported.[76,451] The size of the pontine lesion on CT and MRI does not appear to correlate with the severity of the clinical presentation or the final outcome.[246] Moreover, some pontine lesions found incidentally on MRI and diagnosed as CPM have been shown to be caused by ischaemia.[227] In spite of an awareness of possible mechanisms of causation and modifications in clinical management the incidence of asymptomatic CPM, as determined by a study of over 3000 autopsies, has remained steady over the period 1981–1994.[316]

Pathologically, most cases of CPM have a very similar topography. The lesions are usually in the centre of the basis pontis (Fig. 10.9) and extend from just below the midbrain rostrally through the upper two-thirds of the pons. The cross-sectional topography is often triangular or butterfly shaped and is characteristically symmetrical about the midline rostro-caudal axis. The tegmentum of the pons is usually not involved and there is almost always a rim of normal white matter surrounding the central lesion. The diagnosis is not always evident on macroscopic examination of the brainstem and examination with a hand lens or dissecting microscope can be helpful in making the correct diagnosis. Goebel and Zur[154] reported ten cases, three of which were only identified after microscopic examination. The central pontine region is prone to poor fixation and a chalky white central zone can often mimic CPM.

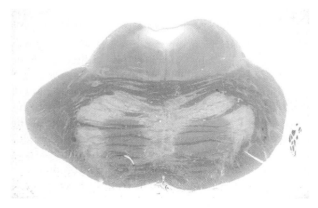

Figure 10.9 *Whole-mount section of mid pons showing a symmetrical, butterfly-shaped area of pallor in the basis pontis which was shown to be demyelination. The features are fairly typical of central pontine myelinolysis, although the zone is often triangular in shape. (H&E.)*

Microscopically, the CPM lesion is recognized easily on the myelin-stained sections in which there is a sharply demarcated area of pallor within the basis pontis. Other microscopic changes will depend upon the age of the lesion. In those cases with a short history there is demyelination with preservation of axons, best seen using silver impregnation techniques. There is usually no inflammatory reaction and neurons in the nuclei of the basis pontis are preserved. There may be reduced numbers of oligodendroglia. As the lesion progresses a proportion of the axons undergo degeneration, and axonal swellings and fragmentation are noted. The transverse ponto-cerebellar fibres are mainly affected, with long rostro-caudal tracts being involved next. In the most severe lesions the central zone can become completely necrotic, although this is uncommon. Macrophages appear after several days and may be a prominent feature, their cytoplasm being filled with myelin debris as the disease progresses. The single most important feature which enables one to distinguish between a central pontine infarct and CPM is the preservation of the neurons in the nuclei pontis; this is a constant feature except in the occasional case with total central necrosis but, even then, in the peripheral zone of demyelination the neurons will be recognized. An immunohistochemical study of CPM showed reduced immunolabelling of GFAP in early CPM and changes which the authors referred to as 'astroglial dystrophy' in older lesions.[153] They suggest that these changes may play a role in the pathogenesis of this disorder.

Extrapontine myelinolytic lesions have been reported in approximately 10% of cases.[472] These authors state that the common sites for extrapontine lesions are the striatum, thalamus, cerebellum and cerebral white matter. Estol et al.,[130] in their study of CPM in 85 liver transplant patients, found 11 cases of CPM, four of whom had extrapontine myelinolysis of the lateral geniculate nuclei. There are relatively few pathological studies of extrapontine myelinolysis and the frequency of occurrence of these lesions should become evident with the use of CT and MRI in clinically diagnosed cases.

Ultrastructural studies in human CPM have been limited by the quality of the preservation of necropsy material. Nevertheless, two studies have shown that the mechanism of myelinolysis consists of intramyelinitic splitting, vacuolization and rupture of the myelin sheaths.[140,358] These changes do not simulate other demyelinating diseases such as multiple sclerosis but, rather, are seen in toxic and metabolic conditions.[358]

Although there is substantial disparity of opinion regarding the management of the hyponatraemia, most authors believe that it is the absolute change in serum sodium rather than the rate of change which is critical. Harris et al. recently suggested that water restriction and diuretic cessation alone may be a reasonable approach in patients with normal renal function.[194]

Marchiafava–Bignami disease

MFB disease is an extremely rare condition which is seen almost exclusively in male alcoholics and was originally described in Italian red-wine drinkers.[276] It has subsequently been described in drinkers with other preferences in alcoholic beverages and occasionally in poorly nourished non-drinkers.[255] In large studies of the neuropathology of alcohol-related disorders in Australia only one case in 10 years (approximately 10 000 brains) has been diagnosed.[190] The incidence seems to be much higher in France, where 17 cases of MFB disease were diagnosed from 8200 necropsies, a prevalence of 0.21%.[195] Nine of the cases were associated with pellagra-like changes in the CNS. MFB disease has also been found in association with Wernicke's encephalopathy,[229] CPM,[151] alcoholic cerebellar atrophy and various combinations of these disorders.[370]

There is no stereotypical clinical presentation of MFB disease, perhaps because of the variable pattern of pathological lesions. However, two major clinical pictures are evident: an acute form, often with seizures, severe neurological disturbances, and disorders of consciousness progressing to death; and a more chronic form with progressive dementia or interhemispheric disconnection syndromes which may last for several years.[249,282] Recovery with good functional outcome has been reported in MFB disease.[149] The diagnosis was often not made until autopsy but more recently cases have been diagnosed during life with CT and MRI and several cases have had serial MRIs which have shown diffuse swelling of the corpus callosum, thought to represent oedema and demyelination, and subsequent atrophy and focal necrosis.[75] These techniques have also demonstrated the wide range of anatomical sites that can be affected in this disease. MFB disease should not be confused with the more diffuse shrinkage of the corpus callosum that has been described in MRI and pathological studies of chronic alcoholics.[189,345]

Macroscopically, MFB disease is characterized by necrotizing, often cystic lesions of the corpus callosum (Figs 10.10, 10.11). Involvement is generally maximal in the genu and body of the corpus callosum. Similar lesions can be seen in the optic chiasm, anterior commissure, centrum semiovale and middle cerebellar peduncles. The more diffuse pathology tends to be associated with the acute form of the disease.

Microscopically, there is predominant demyelination with relative sparing of the axons. In the corpus callosum the central fibres are mainly affected with preservation of thin upper and lower edges. Oligodendrocytes are reduced in number and lipid-laden macrophages are abundant. Astrocytes generally show only mild reactive changes, but they are more prominent in and around necrotizing lesions. Vessels within the region often show proliferation and hyalinization of their walls.

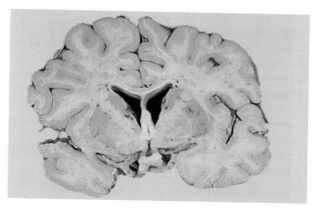

Figure 10.10 *Coronal section of the cerebral hemispheres at the level of the anterior commissure showing grey–brown discoloration of the superior margin of the corpus callosum. The corpus callosum is thinned. The macroscopic features are typical of Marchiafava–Bignami disease.*

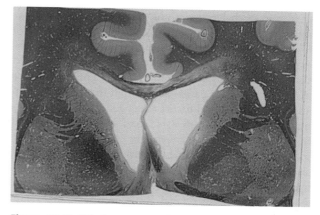

Figure 10.11 *Whole-mount section of corpus callosum (same case as Fig. 10.10) showing extensive demyelination of corpus callosum typical of Marchiafava–Bignami disease. (Luxol fast blue/Nissl stain.)*

The pathogenesis of MFB disease is still unknown but there are similarities in the pathology with experimental cyanide intoxication and some cases of carbon monoxide poisoning.[259]

Fetal alcohol syndrome

Alcohol consumption during pregnancy can cause a variety of CNS abnormalities which range from gross morphological changes with mental retardation [fetal alcohol syndrome (FAS)] to more subtle cognitive and behavioural disorders [fetal alcohol effects (FAE)]. From the point of view of the neuropathology it should be emphasized that, without an adequate history of excessive alcohol intake during pregnancy, and/or evidence of the typical dysmorphic features, it can be extremely difficult to make a diagnosis of FAS. Thus, precise estimates of the incidence and prevalence of the FAS are difficult to determine. Nevertheless, based on a large number of epidemiological studies of FAS, Abel and Sokol[4] estimated the incidence to be 0.33 cases per 1000 live births. Given that the clinical features are difficult to recognize in the neonatal period, and CNS dysfunction may not be identified until several years of age, the true incidence may be much higher.[265] It is thought that FAS is now a more common cause of mental retardation than either Down's syndrome or spina bifida.[5]

The characteristic features of the FAS were described by Jones and Smith[215] and include:

- prenatal and postnatal growth retardation
- facial abnormalities, including short palpebral fissures, epicanthal folds, thin upper lip and growth retardation of jaw
- cardiac defects, mostly septal
- minor joint and limb abnormalities
- delayed development and mental deficiency varying from borderline to severe.

Subsequently, ocular abnormalities,[409] hearing disorders[81] and cerebellar symptoms[277] have been noted in a significant proportion of cases. Clarren[83] provides a long list of other malformations which are seen in FAS with a higher than chance frequency. Follow-up studies have shown that the characteristic facial anomalies of FAS become less distinctive in older patients, although the thin upper lip and narrow palpebral fissures are persistent discriminating features.[408] As well as mental retardation, several important behavioural disorders occur in FAS which include hyperactivity, irritability, delayed development and sleep disorders. Lemoine et al.[254] reported the average intelligence quotient (IQ) for 127 children born to alcoholic mothers to be 70. In general, the degree of mental retardation is positively correlated with the severity of the physical features of FAS.[407] The phenotype of FAS is not specific and is also thought to occur after in utero exposure to other drugs such as hydantoins, and in the children of women with phenylketonuria.[374]

Although heavy drinking during pregnancy increases the risk for FAS in offspring, not all women who drink excessively give birth to children with FAS.[399] Studies suggest that various biological and environmental factors, along with the amount and timing of prenatal alcohol intake, may affect vulnerability to FAS and FAE. Human and animal studies have shown that increasing age and parity of the mother may confer a heightened risk.[3] Differences in maternal metabolism of alcohol may also contribute.[52] Critical periods during the pregnancy, doses and drinking patterns are also very important parameters. Ernhart et al.[129] found that about 30 g of alcohol per day was the conservative threshold for FAS-related neonatal physical abnormalities. Based on experimental models, binge drinking appears to be more harmful than the same amount or more consumed evenly over time.[49] Genetic factors may also play a role, in that certain inbred rodent strains have been shown to be more vulnerable to FAS and FAE given equivalent amounts of alcohol.[156]

Despite the frequency with which this syndrome is diagnosed clinically, the number of neuropathological studies is relatively limited. In a major review by Wisniewski et al.[469] only 16 cases were cited. An additional case was reported by Ferrer and Galfore in 1987.[135] Konovalov et al. studied 44 embryos and three fetuses from mothers who used alcohol during pregnancy. There were features of abnormal brain development in 75.5% of the cases.[230] MRI and position emission tomography (PET) are proving useful in the evaluation of neuroanatomical abnormalities in FAS. Roebuck et al. reviewed recent MRI studies which show corpus callosal, basal ganglia and regional cerebellar abnormalities.[368] Pathological studies show a broad range of abnormalities. The most common abnormalities are cerebellar dysgenesis (reported in 11/17 cases) and heterotopic neuroglial clusters (11/17). The latter are found in the meninges (Fig. 10.12) and less commonly in the periventricular regions.[338] These changes are thought to indicate disordered neuronal and glial migration occurring during the first 3 months of gestation and may be seen in the absence of any other features of FAS.[86] Microcephaly is an important finding and was present in 8 of the 17 cases of FAS. In the most severe cases there may be arrhinencephaly with agenesis of the corpus callosum, porencephaly, Dandy–Walker syndrome, syringomyelia and other dysraphic lesions.[338] Neural tube defects and renal abnormalities have also been described in FAS (see Folic acid deficiency).[457] Brainstem malformations causing hydrocephalus were reported in an early paper by Clarren et al.[86] In three of the six cases described by Peiffer et al.[338] there was spongiosus of the thalamus and/or hypothalamus. Less obvious types of structural change such as dendritic and synaptic abnormalities may also be produced. Ferrer and Galofre[135]

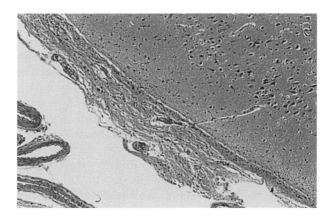

Figure 10.12 *Microscopic section showing heterotopic nests of glial cells in the subarachnoid space of a case of fetal alcohol effects and cerebral dysgenesis. These nests were seen in the region of the tuber cinerum and in the depths of cerebral sulci. (H&E.) Reproduced by permission from Coulter et al.[95]*

showed, in a quantitative study on Golgi-impregnated cortical (layer V) pyramidal neurons, that the number of dendritic spines was significantly reduced and the spines had unusually long, thin pedicles. Dendritic abnormalities have also been recognized in animal models (see experimental section). The neuroanatomical and neurophysiological mechanisms involved in CNS dysfunction by prenatal exposure to alcohol were reviewed by Guerri.[167]

From a general pathological point of view there appears to be a relationship between maternal drinking and spontaneous abortion. Harlap and Shiono[180] reported a doubling of the rate of spontaneous abortion during the second trimester for women drinking one or two drinks per day and consumption of more than this increased the rate 3–5-fold. Other authors have shown a similar relationship.[2] Most studies have failed to show a relationship between maternal alcohol consumption and stillbirths. Similarly, no relationship has been recognized with neonatal mortality.[400] Tolerance and withdrawal can develop in utero.[351] Prenatal and postnatal growth retardation are among the most consistent characteristics of FAE/FAS. Abel[2] reviewed the literature and noted that, in a group of term infants the average birthweight was 1999 g compared with the median birthweight of 3320 g for all children born in the USA during 1975. Even in situations where the mother is not an alcoholic, alcohol consumption decreases birthweight and the extent of this decrease is dose related.

Experimental studies show remarkable similarities to the human material with regard to both the physical abnormalities and behavioural effects.[121] The mouse is said to be the best model[38] although many recent studies have used the innovative 'pup in a cup' method with rats.[461] Advantages of these models include the ability to examine the combined effects of gestational exposure to multiple drugs under controlled circumstances, and some of these studies have suggested that nicotine[253] and cocaine[80] magnify the negative consequences associated with maternal alcohol consumption. Craniofacial changes, resembling those in human FAS, and holoprosencephalic malformations are found in mice exposed to alcohol from day 7 of gestation.[411] Polymicrogyria and neuroglial heterotopias are seen in primate models of FAS.[85] In rat models, neonatal alcohol exposure results in reduced brain growth,[48] brain cell loss,[460] alterations in brain microvasculature[222] and behavioural abnormalities.[30] Prenatal exposure alters the generation, proliferation and migration of cerebral cortical neurons in rats.[301,303] These changes result in abnormal patterns of distribution and organization of neurons in the cortex (Fig. 10.12). Alcohol treatment may also result in neuronal death among more mature populations of cells. For example, there are reduced numbers of neurons in the hippocampus in rats exposed to alcohol at different stages of maturation.[29,462] The cerebellum is especially vulnerable to neuronal depletion.[347] Borges and Lewis[50] showed a sig-

nificant reduction in cerebellar weight and midsagittal cross-sectional area in young rats of mothers given alcohol in their drinking water. There was an increase in the thickness of the external granular layer which persisted beyond the normal time for involution, suggesting retardation of maturation. Alcohol exposure during the period of rapid brain development, which occurs neonatally in the rat, produces Purkinje and granule cell loss.[34,158,350] Using antibodies against MAP-2 West et al.[460] have shown that the cerebellar lobules with Purkinje cells that are in the process of extending their dendrites are more vulnerable. Smith et al.[396] showed that dendritic length and the extent of the dendritic field of cerebellar granule cells were both reduced as a result of fetal alcohol exposure. The same changes have been documented in cortical neurons.[131,175] It appears that some of these changes may revert towards normality in the postnatal period.[268] Granule cell cultures have also been shown to be a useful model in that neuronal numbers are depleted by alcohol in a concentration-dependent and duration-dependent fashion.[332] In a rat model, microcephaly was used as a marker in evaluating the timing of alcohol exposure and the effect on brain development. The whole brain, forebrain and cerebellum to body weight ratios of pups exposed to alcohol during the third trimester showed more significant brain growth deficits than with earlier exposure.[270] However, exposure during all three trimesters resulted in a greater reduction in cerebellar Purkinje cell numbers compared with exposure to alcohol during the third trimester alone.[271]

Ethanol-induced disturbances of gliogenesis have been reported by several authors in a mouse model.[157,302] It has been shown that alcohol induces a premature transformation of the radial glia into astrocytes during neuronal migration and suggested that this might be an explanation for some of the glioneuronal abnormalities reported in FAS.[165] The resulting postmigratory cortex was almost completely devoid of normal vertical columnization (Fig. 10.13). The alcohol also seemed to inhibit late gliogenesis.

Ocular pathology may also be important, as shown in a non-human primate model, in which microphthalmia was noted in three of 26 animals exposed to alcohol and five of the cases (some without microphthalmia) had significant retinal ganglion cell loss.[84] The same animal model was used to look for ultrastructural abnormalities induced by alcohol.[84] Neurons were examined from the caudate nucleus and several abnormalities were described. The cytoplasm of many neurons lacked the usual distribution and number of organelles. The most striking difference was in the endoplasmic reticulum, which showed swollen, distended cisternae. The mitochondria showed loss of cristae, similar to the changes described in rat pups exposed to 20% ethanol solution during gestation.[32] In a review of the neurohistological and neurobiological aspects of the FAS, Volk[448] details the synaptic ultrastructural changes in the cerebellum in a rat

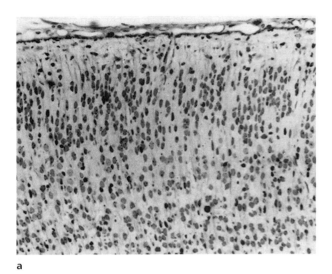

a

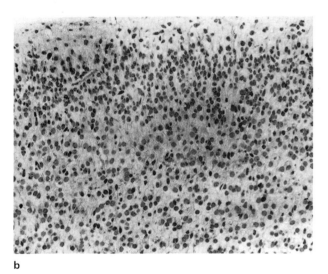

b

Figure 10.13 *Representative sections of identical cortical areas from nine (a) control and (b) in vivo ethanol-treated mice. The ethanol induces a dramatic loss of vertical neuronal organization and a partial neuronal invasion of the marginal layer. Special attention was paid to obtaining a perfectly coronal plane of section in all cases. Reproduced by permission from Gressens et al.[165]*

model and concludes that they may explain some of the neurological deficits of FAS.

Thiamine deficiency during gestation results in intrauterine growth retardation in the rat[369] and alterations in the developmental pattern of thiamine-dependent enzymes in the brains of offspring.[61] It was suggested that, in view of the finding that chronic alcoholism may cause thiamine deficiency, the latter may contribute to the CNS damage encountered in FAS.

In addition to the morphological changes discussed above, alcohol exposure during CNS development can produce a number of neurochemical disturbances. The principal systems affected are monoaminergic. A 30–40% reduction in striatal and cortical dopamine levels, along with a reduction in dopamine uptake sites and a reduction in the number of some receptor sites, was found in rats exposed to alcohol *in utero.*[123] Similarly, decreased levels of serotonin and its major metabolite 5-HIAA have been detected in some regions of the brain.[122] These effects may be particularly important in that these monoamines are not only implicated in a variety of neurobehavioural functions but also thought to play a role in neuronal maturation and differentation.[245,247]

Discussion of the molecular and cellular events that may contribute to the toxic and teratogenic effects of alcohol on the fetus is beyond the scope of this chapter, but was reviewed by Michaelis in 1990.[300] Using differential display to identify markers for FAS, three of 1080 mRNA transcripts were altered in embryos exposed to alcohol; one encoded for heat shock protein 47, one encoded for α-tropomysin and one was novel.[251] West has reviewed possible mechanisms of damage in FAS.[459]

Niacin

Pellagra is a disease caused primarily by niacin (nicotinic acid) deficiency. The amino acid tryptophan is a niacin precursor and dietary deficiency of either or both may produce the syndrome. It is much less common today compared with the 'epidemic' prevalence during the early part of the twentieth century. The diminished incidence is in large part related to public health programmes whereby niacin has been added to staple foods such as flour and bread. Pellagra is most commonly seen in the alcoholic population[205] but also in patients with tuberculosis (TB) being treated with isoniazid[205,206] and other drugs including isonicotinic acid, thiosemicarbizone, 6-mercaptopurine, 5-fluorouracil and puromycin.[404] Isoniazid has a similar structure to niacin and interferes with the conversion of tryptophan to niacin by producing a deficiency in the pyridoxine coenzyme required for the conversion. Deaths attributable to pellagra are said to be twice as high in women than in men and it seems that oestrones inhibit the synthesis of niacin from tryptophan.[390] Pellagra is more likely to occur in patients who are vegetarians or vegans. Defective intestinal absorption of niacin is sometimes the cause of 'secondary' pellagra which may occur even though there is adequate niacin in the diet. Possible causes include dysentry or long-term diarrhoea, or following resection of the stomach or small bowel. Hartnup disease pellagra results from failure of tryptophan absorption.

The characteristic clinical triad in 'endemic' pellagra is dermatitis, diarrhoea and dementia. The skin lesions begin with erythema on the parts of the body exposed to light. This may progress to desquamation, exfoliation and, later, pigmentation and atrophy. Gastrointestinal disturbances include glossitis, anorexia and vomiting, with diarrhoea and weight loss. It is important to note that patients with non-endemic pellagra (the most common form seen in the Western world today) often do not exhibit dermatitis and diarrhoea and the diagnosis can be very difficult to make.[386] In the report by Ishii and Nishihara[205] 20 cases of pellagra were diagnosed at autopsy from 74 chronic alcoholics and the diagnosis had not been made ante-mortem because in the majority there were no skin lesions. Jolliffe et al.[213] suggested that the absence of the classical clinical signs may be due to the severity and rapidity of development of the niacin deficiency.

Neurological signs and symptoms range from disturbances of higher mental function such as insomnia, anxiety, depression, apathy and confusion to more specific features including gait disturbances, extrapyramidal signs and even spastic paraplegia.[205,206] Serdaru et al.[389] emphasized the importance of confusion, clouding of consciousness, 'gegenhalten' and myoclonic jerks in their retrospective review of 22 cases of pellagra in alcoholics. Many patients also have evidence of involvement of peripheral nerves, with a burning sensation in the hands and feet and numbness.

The pathological features of 'endemic' pellagra were described by a number of authors in the late nineteenth and early twentieth centuries. Winkelman, in 1926, found 2000 articles relating to the aetiology, clinical and pathological findings in pellagra.[466] There is consistency in the nature of the neuropathological change seen in all types of pellagra regardless of the underlying cause. The brain is macroscopically normal. Changes are restricted to neurons and the characteristic finding is chromatolysis. There are no associated changes in the glial cells, myelin, blood vessels or meninges. The affected neurons are ballooned, there is loss of Nissl substance and the nuclei are located eccentrically (Fig. 10.14). The changes constitute the classical picture of central chromatolysis seen following axonal damage. However, authors who have examined these cases using techniques to highlight axons have been unable to identify actual changes in the axons and it is thought that the chromatolytic reaction is a primary cytoplasmic lesion.[195] Concerning the recognition of chromatolysis, Hauw et al.[195] warned of three potential errors: (1) some neurons in brainstem and spinal cord structures have eccentrically placed nuclei; (2) excess lipofuscin storage in neurons of, for example, dentate and olivary nuclei can be difficult to distinguish from chromatolysis; and (3) ischaemic neuronal change can mask chromatolysis.

Although chromatolysis is a consistent feature of pellagra there is still debate in the literature concerning the variability in the distribution of lesions throughout the brain depending upon the underlying cause (dietary, alcohol, isoniazid, etc.). In the most recent paper on pellagra in alcoholics, neuronal chromatolysis was seen most commonly in the brainstem, especially in the pontine nuclei

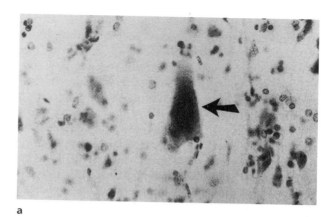

a

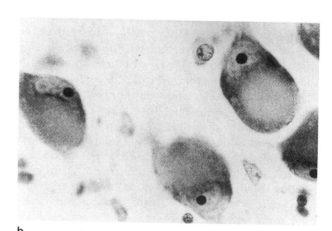

b

Figure 10.14 *Neurons from (a) cerebral cortex (precentral area) and (b) pontine nuclei showing more severe chromatolysis in the pons. Abnormal neurons show nuclear eccentricity and loss of Nissl substance typical of central chromatolysis in pellagra. There is no change in the Betz cell (arrow) in (a). (Celloidin preparation with Nissl stain.) Reproduced by permission from Harper.[195]*

and dentate nuclei of the cerebellum (Fig. 10.14).[195] Nuclei of the cranial nerves (mainly the third, sixth, seventh and eighth), the reticular nuclei, arcuate nuclei and posterior horn cells were also markedly affected. Changes were sometimes seen in the cerebral cortex, the interpeduncular nuclei, the central mesencephalic grey matter, the colliculi, the tenth and 12th cranial nerves and perihypoglossal nuclei, the gracile and cuneate nuclei and anterior horn cells. The main point of debate concerns the topography of the chromatolytic change and the extent of involvement of Betz cells of the motor cortex and other large cortical neurons in the different types of pellagra. Hauw et al.[195] provide an excellent review of the literature and point out that although some of the earliest authors stressed the changes in the cerebral cortex in 'endemic' pellagra,[132] other authors were stressing the lesions in the brainstem and cerebellum in alcoholic patients.[297] In studies of pellagra in alcoholics[205] and tuberculous patients treated with isoniazid, Ishii and Nishihara[206] noted chromatolysis in Betz cells and other large cortical neurons in most of the cases. In other areas of the brain the pattern of involvement was similar to that described above. Other case reports of 'endemic', isoniazid-induced and endogenous pellagra emphasize chromatolytic change in the brainstem nuclei and cortical neurons, especially Betz cells. Most authors have also emphasized the frequency of chromatolysis of spinal cord neurons. Some authors noted changes in anterior horn cells, whereas others noted changes in posterior horns and Clarke's column. In several early studies, degeneration of long tracts was described, but these changes seem to be rare. Hauw et al.[195] noted that the changes in the spinal cord varied in severity from case to case, from one level to another and from one side to another. The lumbar cord was more severely involved than the cervical and changes in the thoracic cord were rare. This variability could account for some of the discrepancies in the literature.

Experimental studies have been unhelpful, although an analogous condition termed 'black tongue' can be produced in dogs by dietary restriction of niacin. Rat and mouse models are not particularly useful as neuronal chromatolysis at the light-microscopic level is seldom recognized, even following axonal transection.[430] However, a mouse model has been developed using 6-aminonicotinamide, an antagonist of niacin.[14] These animals develop skin and gastrointestinal lesions and the anterior horn cells of the spinal cord show ultrastructural features of neuronal chromatolysis.

Vitamin B$_{12}$

Vitamin B$_{12}$ (cobalamin) is a complex organometallic compound, which includes a cobalt atom situated within a corrin ring. Although this structure is similar to porphyrin, unlike the latter, it cannot be synthesized in the human body and must be supplied in the diet. Animal products (meat and dairy foods) are the only dietary source of vitamin B$_{12}$. Castle realized the importance of both intrinsic (gastric) and extrinsic (dietary) factors in the absorption of vitamin B$_{12}$ in 1929.[72] The vitamin is absorbed from the distal ileum by binding to intrinsic factor, a glycoprotein produced by the parietal cells of the stomach. Subsequently, the vitamin was purified and synthesized.[257,364] Vitamin B$_{12}$ deficiency is most common in patients with pernicious anaemia who fail to produce intrinsic factor as a result of autoimmune gastritis. Gastric surgery and diseases of the small intestine such as strictures, fistulae, diverticulae, regional ileitis, tumours, tapeworm infestation, TB, and idiopathic and tropical sprue may also be causative factors. Vitamin B$_{12}$ deficiency of dietary origin is rare but can occur in vegetarians, particularly vegans. Neurological sequelae of dietary deficiency are also rare, but may be seen in infants of vegetarian mothers who are exclusively breastfed.[161,269] Hereditary disorders of cobalamin metabolism may also play a role; Carmel et al.[71] described a case with neurological symptoms resembling those of a patient with vitamin B$_{12}$ deficiency. The 21-year-old patient was shown to have homocystinuria and a cblG mutation. A similar case was also described in a patient with common variable immune deficiency.[477]

The role of vitamin B$_{12}$ in the metabolism of the nervous system remains uncertain. Two vitamin B$_{12}$-dependent enzymes are known to exist in man: methylmalonyl coenzyme A (CoA) mutase, which uses adenosylcobalamin for the degradation of proprionate through methylmalonyl CoA to succinate; and folate-dependent methionine synthetase, which uses methylcobalamin to synthesize methionine from homocystine. Methionine is needed for the production of choline and choline-containing phospholipids as well as for methylation of myelin basic protein. Lack of adenosylcobalamin causes large increases in tissue levels of methylmalonyl CoA and its precursor, propionyl CoA. As a consequence, non-physiological fatty acids containing an odd number of carbon atoms are synthesized and incorporated into neuronal lipids, which are important building blocks of cell membranes and myelin. Both of these biochemical abnormalities may contribute to the neurological manifestations of vitamin B$_{12}$ deficiency. The biochemical basis for the neuropathy of vitamin B$_{12}$ deficiency has recently been reviewed.[456]

Vitamin B$_{12}$ deficiency adversely affects haemopoietic tissue (causing megaloblastic anaemia), epithelial surfaces and the nervous system. Initially, it was thought that the disease was linked to tabes dorsalis because of the similarities in spinal cord pathology, but Lichtheim[261] noted that they differed in several respects. In B$_{12}$ deficiency there was no thickening of the leptomeninges; only slight atrophy of the lumbar dorsal nerve roots, and both the dorsal and anterolateral columns are involved. The first full clinical and pathological description of the neurological consequences of vitamin B$_{12}$ deficiency was published by Russell et al.[376] who coined the term 'subacute degeneration of the spinal cord'.

Clinically, most untreated cases develop functional disturbances which progress to cause severe disability within a few weeks or months; hence the term subacute. The onset is usually heralded by symmetrical sensory disturbances in the distal limbs, with loss of the discriminative modalities of sensation, 'pins and needles' and a feeling of 'walking on cotton wool'. These changes progress to involve the hands and fingers. Subsequently, the legs may become unsteady and limb movements clumsy. In the fully developed case the patient will have ataxia, diminished proprioceptive and vibration sense, positive Rhomberg's sign, spasticity and loss of reflexes. Various mental changes have been observed and range from neuraesthenia, depression and confusional states to amnestic syndromes and dementia ('megaloblastic madness').[203]

Paranoid psychoses have also been documented.[283] Lindenbaum et al.[262] found neuropsychiatric abnormalities in 28% of 141 patients with vitamin B$_{12}$ deficiency but with no anaemia or macrocytosis. Similar results have been documented in other studies.[16] Although the cause of neuropsychiatric symptoms is not known, abnormalities of central myelin probably play a role, a hypothesis supported by a recently documented case of a leukoencephalopathy associated with cobalamin deficiency.[78] Fine and Soria[136] emphasize that any patient presenting with myelopathy, neuropathy, dementia or depression, with or without megaloblastic anaemia, must be screened for vitamin B$_{12}$ deficiency. Some 30% of cases will be missed if the diagnosis is based on abnormal haemoglobin, haematocrit or mean corpuscular volume values.[136]

Recently, several case reports have documented the MRI appearances in the CNS complicating vitamin B$_{12}$ deficiency, the findings correlating closely with the known pathological changes.[33,125,217,220,269]

Pathologically, vitamin B$_{12}$ deficiency is associated with both central and peripheral nerve diseases. Pallis and Lewis[330] claim that the latter is the most common neurological complication, but this issue remains contentious. Neurophysiological studies have shown that 65% of untreated patients have reduced nerve conduction velocities, but it was also noted that thiamine deficiency was present in the majority of cases.[98] Some studies indicate a demyelinating neuropathy,[403,432] whereas others describe predominantly axonal degeneration.[18,232,285]

The brain appears macroscopically normal but the spinal cord may be shrunken and, when cut in the transverse plane, the posterior and lateral columns may appear grey–white in colour and have an almost translucent appearance.

Microscopically, there are multifocal vacuolated and demyelinated lesions in the white matter of the spinal cord, particularly affecting the posterior and lateral columns, but with occasional involvement of the anterior columns (Fig. 10.15). The early lesions consist of swelling of myelin sheaths with little change in the axons. Fibres with the greatest diameter are predominantly affected.[331] The lesions are said to begin as small foci in the centre of the posterior columns and later on the surface of the lateral columns. These tend to become confluent, which creates the erroneous impression that specific tracts (anatomical) are involved. In terms of rostrocaudal involvement, lesions are usually most severe in the mid-thoracic segments, but they can extend rostrally to involve the cervical segments and even the medulla. An early report by Greenfield and O'Flynn[162] commented that the lesions are first seen in a perivenular distribution. As the myelin breaks down foamy macrophages are seen and occasionally there is some perivascular lymphocytic infiltration. The oligodendroglia appear normal. As demyelination and vacuolation increase, axons begin to degenerate but this seems to be a secondary phenomenon. This is supported by examination of upper cervical and

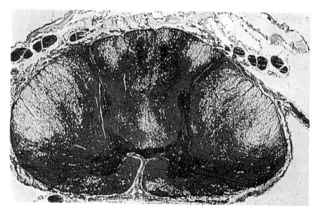

Figure 10.15 *Transverse section of thoracic spinal cord showing spongy vacuolation in posterior and lateral white matter columns consistent with a diagnosis of subacute combined degeneration of the cord. (Loyez myelin stain.)*

lower lumbar segments, which shows a typical wallerian pattern of degeneration, posterior columns and spinocerebellar tracts being abnormal in the cervical region and corticospinal tracts in the lumbar region. Gliosis is a feature of older lesions.

Brain pathology has been reported in a limited number of cases. Typically, lesions are small, perivascular foci of demyelination within the cerebral white matter. Histologically, these foci are similar to those encountered in the spinal cord and consist of swelling of myelin sheaths and axons followed by fibre degeneration.[133] Degeneration of the optic nerves (papillomacular bundles) was described by Adams and Kubik.[8]

Ultrastructural studies are limited to experimental models of vitamin B$_{12}$ deficiency. The definitive work was carried out in rhesus monkeys by Agamanolis et al.[11] although there are similar models using chicks, rats and calves.[15] The pathological changes in the monkeys were indistinguishable topographically and microscopically from those of subacute combined degeneration of the cord in man. The degeneration of myelin is characterized by separation of myelin lamellae and the formation of intramyelinic vacuoles, leading eventually to complete destruction of myelin sheaths. Intramyelin oedema and interstitial oedema are also prominent findings.[433] Later, there is degeneration and loss of axons, and gliosis.[11]

A similar clinical and pathological disorder can be induced in mice[147] and chicks[395] using cycloleucine, which blocks the formation of S-adenosylmethionine and interferes with the biosynthesis of choline, an important constituent of myelin. Lee et al.[250] found that intramyelinic vacuolation in the CNS begins within 12–24 h after the administration of the cycloleucine. Based on the cycloleucine model, Small et al.[395] suggested that inhibition of the methylation of myelin basic protein, required for the process of myelin compaction, may play a role, but Deacon *et al.*[111] showed that methylation of residue 107 (arginine) in myelin basic protein is normal in rat and fruit bat models of vitamin B₁₂ deficiency. Recent studies in rats made vitamin B₁₂ deficient by total gastrectomy have shown that the myelinolytic lesions in the spinal cord are mediated as a result of the production of epidermal growth factor and tumour necrosis factor-α.[58,378]

Chronic exposure to nitrous oxide also produces lesions in the spinal cord similar to those found in human vitamin B₁₂ deficiency.[20,382,441,456] This occurs because nitrous oxide inactivates methionine synthetase, one of the vitamin B₁₂-dependent enzymes. Monkeys can be almost completely protected by the administration of methionine.[382]

During the 1920s and 1930s primates in zoos were fed on a conventional fruit diet and many developed serious vitamin B₁₂ deficiency. The entity was known as 'cage paralysis' and the clinical and pathological features were similar to the disease in man except that the white matter of the cerebral hemispheres showed more myelin loss, especially from the corpus callosum.[343]

A vacuolar myelopathy which resembles subacute combined degeneration has also been reported in a significant proportion of patients with AIDS.[340] These authors described the clinical and pathological features in 20 of 89 patients dying with AIDS. Changes were most severe in the thoracic cord, with vacuolation of the posterior and lateral columns (Fig. 10.16). The presence of macrophages within the vacuoles is required to make the diagnosis, to eliminate the possibility that the changes are artefactual. Electron microscopy showed that the vacuoles were surrounded by a thin myelin sheath and they appeared to have formed by intramyelin swelling. The clinical syndrome also mimics vitamin B₁₂ deficiency. Keating *et al.*[22] investigated whether there is a similar pathogenic mechanism in AIDS myelopathy and subacute combined degeneration of the spinal cord. They measured the CSF levels of *S*-adenosylmethionine and *S*-adenosylhomocysteine and found that there was a significant difference in the methylation ratio, similar to that seen in the nitrous oxide models and in patients with vitamin B₁₂ deficiency. However, they were unable to identify a common mechanism producing the reduced methylation ratio and stated that it was not due to B₁₂ deficiency. In a review, Tan and Guiloff[417] presented a hypothesis for the pathogenesis of vacuolar myelopathy, dementia and peripheral neuropathy in AIDS. They suggested that products derived from macrophages, including cytokines and other substances, may interfere directly with the methyl transfer cycle through the generation of reactive oxygen intermediates and reactions involving nitric oxide and peroxynitrite. These may limit the supply of methionine for the conversion to adenosyl methionine, both by direct interaction and through inhibition of methionine synthetase. They suggested that this mechanism might underlie the pathogenesis of vacuolar myelopathy, dementia, cerebral atrophy and peripheral neuropathy in AIDS, where local factors or differential susceptibility determine whether myelintoxic or neurotoxic processes predominate.

Folic acid

Folate (pteroylglutamic acid) is crucial for the synthesis and methylation of DNA during fetal and early postnatal development.[74] There appears to be a specialized transport system across the BBB for folic acid.[473] Studies of the effects of folate deficiency during pregnancy indicate that there is an increased incidence of fetal malformations and mental retardation.[92] Findings from two multicentre trials have confirmed that folic acid supplements during pregnancy reduce the risk of both occurrent[457] and recurrent[308] neural tube defects in babies. Some antiepileptic drug therapies may increase the risk of neural tube defects, probably because of their antifolate activity.[314] Studies in experimental animals suggest that folate deficiency during gestation and lactation results in alteration of non-hydroxy-fatty acid components of myelin lipids.[200] Studies in the developing rat CNS suggest that folate uptake and storage is related to a folate-binding protein (10-formyltetrahydrofolate dehydrogenase) which is preferentially located in glial cells.[279] Excessive maternal alcohol intake may increase the likelihood of folate deficiency.[202] This is probably as a result of alcohol-induced changes in membrane transport of folate.[292]

Inborn errors of folate absorption and metabolism can cause severe disease of the CNS. Clayton *et al.*[87] reported the case of a 3-year-old girl with 5,10-methylenetetrahydrofolate reductase deficiency who had subacute combined degeneration of the cord and a leukoencephalopathy with foci of perivascular demyelination throughout the white matter. The neuropathological

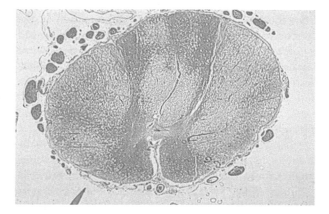

Figure 10.16 *Lower thoracic spinal cord showing marked, confluent vacuolation in the posterior and lateral columns and mild to moderate vacuolation in the anterior columns in a case of AIDS myelopathy. Note the similarity to Fig. 10.15. (H&E.) Reproduced by permission from Petito et al.*[344]

changes were said to be indistinguishable from those found in patients with vitamin B_{12} deficiency. Although less frequent than cord lesions, extensive lesions have been described in vitamin B_{12} deficiency.[8] The metabolic defect affects the formation of 5-methyltetrahydrofolate, a methyl group donor for conversion of homocysteine to methionone. As discussed in the previous section (vitamin B_{12} deficiency), this mechanism may interfere with the production and/or structural integrity of myelin.

Folate deficiency can also result from poor diet or malabsorption and from treatment with anticonvulsant drugs such as phenytoin and primidone or with anti-folate drugs such as methotrexate, trimethoprin and triamterene. The latter drugs inhibit the enzyme dihydrofolate reductase.

The neurological sequelae of folate deficiency are still controversial. Many patients alleged to show involvement of the nervous system from this cause also suffer from other conditions which are likely to produce neurological signs. Low serum folate is not uncommon in elderly patients, but it is difficult to know whether or not the folate deficiency is responsible for the neurological signs and symptoms. Pallis and Lewis[330] reviewed all the available case reports of neurological manifestations of folate deficiency and concluded that it remained uncertain whether or not folate deficiency induces neurological disorders. Other authors have linked folate deficiency to encephalopathy,[406] cerebellar atrophy,[176] myelopathy[13,160,353] and peripheral neuropathy.[115,160,176] Reports of possible associations between folate deficiency and neurological disease continue to appear in the literature. Botez[51] suggested that the 'restless leg' syndrome may sometimes be due to folate deficiency and the evidence for an association with an organic brain syndrome seems reasonably conclusive.[109,127,363] The most recent review of the literature by Parry[334] found that 20 patients fulfilled the following criteria: (1) they presented with appropriate neurological signs for which no other cause could be found; (2) the serum or red cell and/or CSF folate was low; (3) the serum vitamin B_{12} or vitamin B_{12} absorption was normal; and (4) folic acid produced at least a partial response of the neurological disorder or, in cases of subacute combined degeneration of the cord, there was pathological evidence of posterolateral sclerosis at autopsy. There were ten patients with peripheral neuropathy, eight with subacute combined degeneration and two with a myelopathy. Nine had mental symptoms in addition to the neurological disorder. Recent papers suggest that folate deficiency may be related to psychiatric illnesses including depression[17] and schizophrenia.[53,203]

Pyridoxine

In 1942 Snell et al.[397] demonstrated that vitamin B_6 was composed of pyridoxine, pyridoxal and pyridoxamine, each with a phosphorylated form. A comprehensive review of the neurobiology of pyridoxine appeared in 1990.[104] There are over 100 pyridoxal phosphate dependent enzymes, most of which are involved in catabolic reactions of various amino acids. The crucial role played by pyridoxine in the nervous system is evident from the fact that the putative neurotransmitters dopamine, noradrenaline, serotonin, gamma-aminobutyric acid (GABA) and taurine, as well as the sphingolipids and polyamines, are synthesized by pyridoxine phosphate-dependent enzymes. There are different affinities between the respective apoenzmes and the pyridoxal phosphate, so that in partial deficiency states some neurotransmitters will be depleted more than others. This imbalance can lead to a number of disorders which can affect the hypothalamus and pineal gland and their neuroendocrine functions, and can also cause spontaneous or drug-induced seizure activity. This propensity to induce fitting was recognized when an epidemic of nervousness, irritability and seizures occurred in infants fed a canned milk formula which was deficient in pyridoxine.[96,305] It has been shown that similar fitting episodes can develop in infants who have inadequate pyridoxine absorption, either as a result of an inborn error of metabolism or from imperfect artificial feeding.[44] In both cases the seizures can be arrested by giving large doses of pyridoxine. It is thought that patients with pyridoxine-dependent epilepsy (inherited as an autosomal recessive characteristic) have abnormal glutamate decarboxylase (GAD).[239] MRI and PET studies indicate diffuse structural and functional abnormalities with progressive dilatation of the ventricular system and atrophy of the cortex and white matter.[159,391] The clinical syndrome of pyridoxine deficiency was described in 1950 by Mueller and Vilter[310] in eight human subjects treated with desoxypyridoxine and a diet poor in B complex vitamins.[310] Patients developed seborrhoeic dermatitis, glossitis, cheilosis and lymphopenia. In a review of these and 42 other cases Vilter et al.[447] noted that patients also had anorexia, nausea, listlessness, lethargy, conjunctivitis and polyneuropathy. The dermatitis was similar to that seen in pellagra. They concluded that pyridoxine deficiency mimics other B complex deficiency states. The polyneuropathy is the only consistent neurological sign related to pyridoxine deficiency. The pyridoxine antagonist deoxypyridoxine also causes peripheral neuropathy in man which is relieved by treatment with the vitamin.[447] Isoniazid treatment in man may result in peripheral neuropathy and concomitant inhibition of pyridoxine phosphorylation. Similarly, a side-effect of the antihypertensive agent hydralazine may result in pyridoxine deficiency. Pyridoxine deficiency in a rat model resulted in decreased dendritic arborization and reduced numbers of synapses as well as reduced numbers of myelinated axons.[150]

Pyridoxine intoxication can also cause a neurological syndrome. Xu et al.[474] showed that rats given high doses of pyridoxine (600–1200 mg/kg per day) develop a neuronopathy with necrosis of dorsal root ganglia neurons, and a centrifugal axonal atrophy and breakdown of peripheral and central sensory axons. The effect varies from species to species and seems to depend upon body size, with larger mammals being more susceptible. Man appears to be the most sensitive to the neurotoxic effects of pyridoxine, on a dose–weight basis.[474] The mechanism of action is thought to be a dose-dependent interference with neuronal metabolism. Epileptiform electroencephalographic (EEG) discharges can be induced in rats by physiological doses of pyridoxine[442] and excess dietary pyridoxine causes an increase in the concentrations of some amino acids in the serum and caudate nucleus.[379]

Riboflavin

Riboflavin (vitamin B$_2$) is necessary for the synthesis of flavine–adenine dinucleotides and other flavoproteins which play an important role in electron transport and hence oxidative metabolism and the generation of high-energy phosphates. These metabolic pathways are particularly important for the skin and tissues of the nervous system. The term 'aribo flavinosis' was assigned by Sebrell and Butler[384] and an excellent historical review is given in the paper by Stannus in 1944.[402] Deficiency of riboflavin is thought to cause the clinical syndrome of ambylopia, painful neuropathy and orogential dermatitis and has been reported from the West Indies, the Far East and Nigeria.[241,329,402] Studies in developing countries such as India have revealed a very high incidence of riboflavin deficiency, especially in women and children.[240] In the few human autopsy studies of the condition the gracile tracts of the posterior columns of the spinal cord were degenerate and gliotic,[72,364] and the anterolateral tracts may show abnormalities. Ogunleye and Odutuga[324] described the effects of riboflavin deficiency on developing rat brain and showed a reduction in brain weight and in several important components of myelin. Experimental studies in adult rats[387] showed that riboflavin-deficient diets caused degeneration of myelin in peripheral nerves and spinal cord, especially the posterior columns. Treatment of rats with the riboflavin antagonist galactoflavin results in demyelination of sciatic nerves.[323]

SYSTEMIC DISORDERS

Many systemic disorders have adverse effects on CNS function. Medical conditions such as acute or chronic liver failure, diabetes and cardiac failure all have serious repercussions for cerebral function, resulting in the 'metabolic encephalopathies', a series of disorders that, although potentially reversible following appropriate therapy or organ transplantation, may ultimately result in structural CNS changes. The better characterized of these disorders include those associated with liver or kidney failure.

The neuropathology of hypoxia/ischaemia is covered in a separate chapter, as are the CNS complications of viral infections (including AIDS).

Hepatic encephalopathy

Hepatic encephalopathy is a neuropsychiatric syndrome occurring in acute or chronic liver disease. Depending upon the nature and extent of liver damage and of portal-systemic collateral shunting, hepatic encephalopathy may present in one of four distinct forms:

- hepatic encephalopathy in fulminant hepatic failure
- portal–systemic encephalopathy (PSE)
- acquired (non-Wilsonian) hepatocerebral degeneration
- familial hepatolenticular degeneration (Wilson's disease).

HEPATIC ENCEPHALOPATHY IN FULMINANT HEPATIC FAILURE

Fulminant hepatic failure results from severe inflammatory or necrotic liver disease of rapid onset and progression of neurological signs from altered mental status to stupor and coma within hours or days. It is also seen in 'failed' liver transplants. Delerium and mania are encountered and, occasionally, seizures which may be multifocal, prior to coma. Death results in 70–80% of cases which reach grade IV coma and is generally the consequence of cerebellar tonsillar herniation and brainstem compression caused by increased intracranial pressure (ICP) as a result of massive brain swelling.

Brain swelling in fulminant hepatic failure varies according to the aetiology of liver disease, with patients with hepatitis B or non-A, non-B hepatitis having the highest incidence of this complication.[126] If the diagnosis of brain swelling is suspected in patients with fulminant hepatic failure continuous monitoring should be instituted in order to facilitate the early recognition of intracranial hypertension. This will enable treatment to be instituted at a potentially reversible stage. ICP measurements permit the calculation of cerebral perfusion pressure (mean arterial blood pressure minus ICP), which must be maintained at >40 mmHg if adequate brain perfusion is to be maintained and tonsillar herniation prevented.[126] CT scan is of little value in the detection of early brain swelling in patients with fulminant hepatic failure.[312] Clinical symptoms of raised ICP include increased muscle tone in the arms and legs, progressing to full decerebrate posturing with hyperpronation and abduction of the arms. Hyperventilation may be marked and pupils are dilated and react sluggishly to light. As ICP increases, opisthotonus may occur. Failure to arrest the process at this stage invariably leads to tonsillar herniation and respiratory arrest. Absence of the oculovestibular (caloric) reflex is a reliable sign of cerebellar tonsillar herniation.[126]

Macroscopically, the brain appears 'tight', with flattening of gyri, and there may be both tentorial (bilateral) and

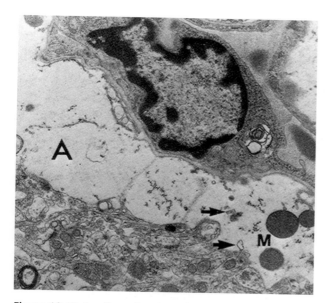

Figure 10.17 *Swelling of perivascular astrocytes (A) in a case of fulminant hepatic failure due to acetaminophen overdose. In addition to marked swelling and the presence of vacuoles, the endoplasmic reticulum is dilated (arrow) and mitochondria (M) are swollen. Reproduced by permission from Kato et al.[218]*

cerebellar tonsillar herniation. The lateral ventricles are compressed in a symmetrical fashion and occasionally there is a greenish hue throughout the cerebral tissue due to a breakdown in the BBB in a jaundiced patient. Secondary (Duret) haemorrhages in the brainstem may occur as a terminal event.

Microscopically, the principal change is the presence of Alzheimer II astrocytes (discussed below). Secondary changes such as hypoxia and haemorrhages (due to a bleeding diathesis) may also be noted. Brain swelling in fulminant hepatic failure appears to be almost exclusively of the cytotoxic type. In a recent study of brain ultrastructure in material from nine patients who died in fulminant hepatic failure (resulting mainly from intentional acetaminophen overdose), swelling of endothelial and perivascular astrocytes was consistently observed.[218] In perivascular astrocytes, mitochondria were swollen and there was marked dilatation of endoplasmic reticulum with small amounts of electron-dense amorphous material (Fig. 10.17).

PORTAL–SYSTEMIC ENCEPHALOPATHY

PSE is the most commonly encountered form of hepatic encephalopathy. PSE accompanies the development of portal–systemic collaterals arising as a result of portal hypertension in liver cirrhosis. Neurologically, PSE develops slowly: the onset is insidious starting with anxiety, restlessness and altered sleep patterns. These symptoms are followed by shortened attention span and muscular incoordination, asterixis and lethargy progressing to stupor and coma. Multiple episodes of PSE

are not uncommon. PSE frequently results from a precipitating factor such as dietary protein overload, constipation or gastrointestinal bleeding. Other conditions such as hypoglycaemia, hypoxia or the use of sedative drugs (particularly benzodiazepines) may also precipitate PSE in cirrhotic patients.

A new approach to the treatment of portal hypertension and the prevention of variceal bleeding in cirrhotic patients makes use of transjugular intrahepatic portal–systemic shunts (TIPS). TIPS are artificial fistulae placed between branches of the portal and systemic venous systems performed via the jugular vein. TIPS is safer and less expensive to perform than portacaval anastomosis surgery and is now finding wide application. However, a major complication of TIPS is PSE, which occurs in over 30% of patients, particularly those over 60 years old.[93]

Macroscopically, the brains are usually normal but quantitative neuropathological studies of brains from patients with non-alcoholic cirrhosis and with alcoholic cirrhosis are of interest. Based on regional cerebral hemisphere volumes there are no significant changes in the brains of the non-alcoholic cirrhotics compared with controls, whereas the alcoholic cirrhotics show a significant white matter shrinkage (Table 10.2). Although this is only a small sample of non-alcoholic cirrhotics the data suggest that cirrhosis per se does not contribute significantly to brain shrinkage. Neuroradiological studies by Lee et al.[252] support this contention, but Acker[6] found a significant correlation between the degree of liver damage and brain shrinkage.

The characteristic neuropathological finding in PSE is the Alzheimer type II astrocyte. These astrocytes have enlarged, pale watery nuclei containing little chromatin, most of which is marginated around the periphery (Fig. 10.18). They often have prominent nucleoli and in long-standing cases of hepatic encephalopathy, glycogen dots, which resemble nucleoli, can be seen. There may be an increase in lipofuscin content. In more severe cases the nuclei become lobulated or bean shaped. Norenberg,[319] in a review of astrocyte responses to CNS injury, claimed that the nuclear lobulation is more prominent in certain brain regions such as the pallidum, substantia nigra and dentate nucleus. There appears to be a relationship between the severity of the astrocytic change and the severity of the hepatic failure, although this has not been well documented scientifically. The Alzheimer type II change is, however, reversible. Paired and triplet forms are commonly encountered and this is thought to reflect astrocyte proliferation, although mitoses are not seen in either man or experimental animals. Diemer[117] found no increase in the total number of glia and whether or not there is a true astrocytosis remains unclear. The Alzheimer type II astrocyte in PSE is more pronounced in the grey matter, particularly in deep layers of the cerebral cortex, striatum, globus pallidus, thalamus, inferior olives and dentate nucleus, as well as in Bergmann glial cells of the cerebellum. Less obvious changes are observed in brainstem, hypothalamus and spinal cord.[64,320]

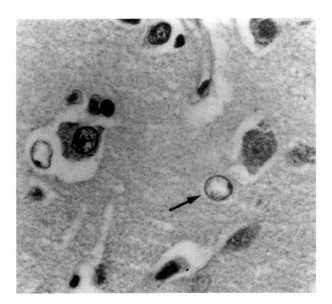

Figure 10.18 *Micrograph of human cerebral cortex showing Alzheimer type II astrocyte (arrow) characterized by vacuolation of nucleus with margination of chromatin. Reproduced by permission from Butterworth et al.[64]*

Electron-microscopic studies of Alzheimer II astrocytes in man are scarce, but one study described cytoplasmic enlargement with increased numbers of ribosomes and glycogen particles.[139] In some mitochondria, increased electron density of the cristae has been reported.[280]

In a study of the basal ganglia, thalamus and cerebral cortex of seven cases of PSE, using the immunohistochemical technique for GFAP, it was reported that, in contrast to age-matched control material, the perikarya and processes of Alzheimer type II astrocytes in the material from PSE patients did not stain for GFAP.[398] A selective instability of GFAP mRNA may be responsible for the observed loss of GFAP in man as well as in ammonia-treated astrocytes in culture.[322] However, the immunocytochemical expression of the S-100 protein, another glial-associated protein, is reportedly unchanged in Alzheimer type II astrocytes in human hepatic encephalopathy.[224] The dissociation between GFAP and S-100 protein expression in Alzheimer type II astrocyes in PSE defines this unique glial reaction and it was suggested that this phenomenon could be referred to as 'gliofibrillary dystrophy'.

Table 10.2 *Brain weight and volume measurements in alcoholic and non-alcoholic patients with cirrhosis of the liver*

	n (%)	Grey matter (%)	White matter (%)
Control	56	54.2 ± 0.4	40.1 ± 0.4
Alcoholic cirrhosis	21	56.4 ± 0.7*	37.1 ± 0.7*
Non-alcoholic cirrhosis	4	54.8 ± 0.7	39.4 ± 0.5

Data are means ± SEM.
*$P < 0.01$.

In contrast to the alterations in astrocytic integrity and in the expression of astrocyte-related proteins in human PSE, there is little convincing evidence to suggest significant neuronal loss in this condition. In studies from different groups of alcoholic patients, analysis of cortical neuronal counts reveals that there is no significant difference between those alcoholics with WKS and those with cirrhosis of the liver. This finding suggests that alcohol abuse is responsible for the neuronal loss in the superior frontal cortex and that the additional complications of WKS and cirrhosis do not accentuate cortical neuronal loss.[236] Other histopathological studies reveal no evidence of neuronal damage, and the measurement of neuronal marker enzymes[248] or specific binding sites for postsynaptic neuronal ligands[60] provides no evidence of neuronal loss.

It should be noted that Alzheimer type II astrocytes are seen in a variety of other metabolic encephalopathies, including uraemia and hypercapnia, and in the early stages of anoxia and hypoglycaemia, especially in infants. The change is common in the setting of elevated brain or blood ammonia.[319]

Studies in experimental PSE

Following construction of an end-to-side portacaval anastomosis in the rat, two distinct types of astrocytic changes are apparent. Starting 1 week postsurgery, there is selective astrocytic swelling.[478] This is accompanied by folding of the capillary basement lamina and an increase in the surface area of astrocytic end-feet. From 4 weeks onwards there is an increase in organelles within astrocytes followed by an increase in astroglial filaments. Degenerative changes may occur simultaneously in myelinated fibres with accumulation of granular and fibrillary material in oligodendroglial cytoplasm. A subsequent study confirmed the findings of astrocytic nuclear swelling as well as swelling of perivascular astrocytic foot processes following portacaval anastomosis in the rat.[352] However, in this latter study, there was no evidence of Alzheimer type II astrocytes and the authors suggested that the change seen in man is a post-mortem artefact. In a rat model of severe PSE produced by feeding ammonia resins to animals following portacaval anastomosis, a progression of astrocytic abnormalities was reported.[318,352] Prior to the onset of coma, astrocytes show marked cytoplasmic enlargement, mitochondrial proliferation and an accumulation of cytoplasmic glycogen (Fig. 10.19). It was suggested that the initial astrocytic hypertrophy following portacaval anastomosis reflects cellular hyperactivity, possibly in response to elevated brain ammonia.[478] The finding of increased mitochondria is paralleled by increases in the activity of mitochondrial enzymes such as glutamate dehydrogenase[320] and by increased densities of mitochondrial (peripheral-type) benzodiazepine receptors (PTBRs).[152] The PTBR is a subclass of benzodiazepine receptor that is not coupled allosterically to the neuronal GABA receptor; rather, it appears to be localized on the astrocytic outer mitochondrial membrane.

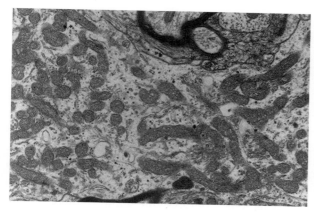

Figure 10.19 *Cerebral cortical astrocyte in early experimental PSE following feeding of ammonia resins to portacaval shunted rats. Note marked enlargement of the cytoplasm with proliferation of mitochondria. Occasional glycogen granules are seen. Reproduced by permission from Norenberg.[318]*

Exposure of cultured glioma cells to ligands for the PTBR results in a proliferative response.[392] Increased densities of PTBRs have been reported in autopsied brain tissue from cirrhotic patients with PSE.[248]

Studies in cultured astrocytes

Exposure of primary cultures of astrocytes to millimolar concentrations of ammonia for 4 days results in cytoplasmic basophilia, vacuolization and dense body formation.[163,164] Longer periods of exposure to ammonia result in degeneration and necrosis resembling Alzheimer type II changes. Ultrastructural studies reveal alterations that are similar to those observed under *in vivo* hyperammonaemic conditions, notably cytoplasmic hypertrophy followed by degenerative changes. These findings strongly suggest that the Alzheimer type II changes observed in PSE are the direct result of ammonia toxicity.

Non-invasive techniques

PET studies using [^{13}N]ammonia for the measurement of brain ammonia utilization and [^{15}O]H$_2$O for the measurement of cerebral blood flow have been performed in patients with mild PSE.[267] Brain ammonia utilization was found to be increased 2–3-fold and the permeability/surface area product (a measure of BBB permeability to ammonia) was found to be increased in PSE patients.

MRI in cirrhotic patients with PSE reveals bilateral signal hyperintensity of T$_1$-weighted images in the globus pallidus.[237] Pallidal hyperintensity was found to correlate with abnormal EEG tracings and with brain manganese concentrations in these patients. More recent studies have revealed a selective loss of dopaminergic D$_2$ (postsynaptic) receptors in the globus pallidus of PSE patients[307] and it was suggested that these findings reflect dopaminergic neuronal dysfunction in the brains of these patients and, as such, could contribute to the extrapyramidal signs encountered in human PSE (Fig. 10.20).

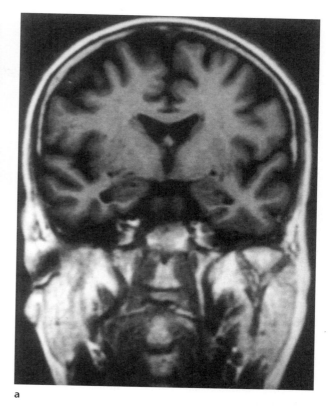

a

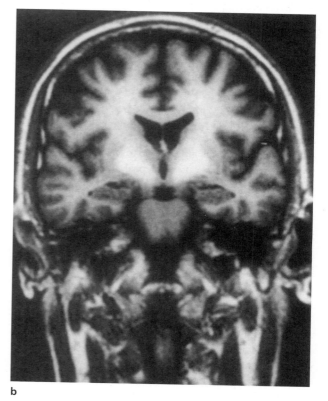

b

Figure 10.20 *Coronal MRI showing (a) the appearance of the basal ganglia in a normal subject and (b) bilateral increase in signal intensity in the globus pallidus (repetition time 1500 ms; echo time 200 ms; inversion time 650 ms). Reproduced by permission from Kulisevsky et al.[237]*

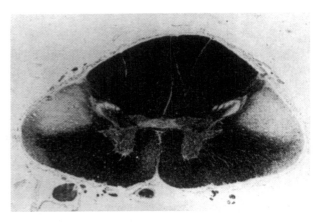

Figure 10.21 *Section of lumbar spinal cord in a case of post-shunt myelopathy showing bilateral degeneration of direct and indirect corticospinal tracts. (Spielmeyer myelin stain.) Reproduced by permission from Bechard* et al.[36]

POST-SHUNT MYELOPATHY

Rarely, following spontaneous or surgical portal–systemic shunting, irreversible spastic paresis or paralysis of the lower extremities develops. Neuropathlogical characteristics include degeneration of anterior and lateral corticospinal tracts (Fig. 10.21). Alzheimer type II astrocytes are frequently observed in the cerebral cortex, basal ganglia and spinal cord of cases of post-shunt myelopathy.[105,385]

POST-TRANSPLANT NEUROPATHOLOGY

Neurological signs and symptoms in patients who underwent orthotopic liver transplantation for end-stage liver disease include hepatic encephalopathy/altered mental status, seizures and stroke. Neuropathological findings in these patients include central pontine myelinolysis, intracerebral haemorrhages and infections.[46]

REYE'S SYNDROME

Reye's syndrome is an acute non-inflammatory encephalopathy that may be precipitated by toxic, infectious or metabolic insults. Although not strictly a hepatic encephalopathy, more than half of all patients show hepatomegaly and pathological studies reveal severe periportal fatty infiltration with areas of necrosis. Onset of clinical symptoms is acute and consists of vomiting, convulsions and coma. Children aged 2–16 years are most susceptible to developing Reye's syndrome, which carries a high mortality and, in many surviving patients, CNS sequellae. The CSF is usually normal apart from a low sugar which is associated with hypoglycaemia, an important clinical feature. The cause of Reye's syndrome is not known. A strong association with viral illness has consistently been observed. Workers using virus mouse models are able to reproduce many clinical and pathological features of Reye's syndrome.[110] Administration of salicylates during viral illness has also been suggested to contribute to the disorder.[174] A trend towards a reduced use of aspirin for children in the USA, UK and Australia has coincided with a dramatic decline in the number of reported cases of Reye's syndrome.[42,179] A percentage of cases which present clinically as Reye's syndrome may have an underlying inherited metabolic defect,[201,223,327] including hereditary organic acidaemias, urea cycle disorders, mitochondrial disorders, fulminant hepatitis and other even rarer conditions. In a 10-year follow-up study of 26 cases, 69% were subsequently diagnosed as having other diseases, the most common being medium-chain acyl-coenzyme dehydrogenase deficiency.[327] These authors emphasized the importance of applying more precise diagnostic criteria to avoid misdiagnosis.

Biochemical findings suggest that mitochondrial dysfunction plays an important pathophysiological role in Reye's syndrome. In a study using rat liver mitochondria, Trost and Lemasters showed that mitochondrial permeability translation (MPT) can be induced by opening a high-conductance, cyclosporin-sensitive pore in the mitochondrial inner membrane.[435] This causes swelling, depolarization and uncoupling of oxidative phosphorylation. The hydrolytic product of aspirin (salicylate) is a potent dose-dependent activator of MPT and it appears that the induction of MPT by these agents is a common pathophysiological mechanism causing mitochondrial injury in Reye's syndrome.[435] Other pathophysiological factors suggested to be involved in Reye's syndrome include hyperammonaemia and alterations of fatty acid metabolism.

Structural changes in mitochondria are apparent on electron-microscopic evaluation. Pleomorphic changes in the mitochondria of the neurons are similar to those seen in liver mitochondria. They have an irregular outline, intact cristae and matrix rarefaction. Swelling of astrocytes and focal ballooning of myelin sheaths have been noted.[54,335] The change is quite different to that seen in hypoxia and there is evidence to suggest that the mitochondrial injury is reversible.[335] MRI studies have shown diffuse cortical and white matter changes, with a definite laminar distribution similar to laminar cortical necrosis in hypoxic brain damage.[226]

Neuropathological findings consist of marked brain oedema in all cases.[274] Oedema is generally cytoxic in nature with marked swelling of astrocytic foot processes.[47] Monitoring of intracranial pressure is important in patients with Reye's syndrome. In addition to brain oedema, other pathological findings include acute, multifocal ischaemic changes, often with a laminar distribution, affecting the cerebral cortex, basal ganglia, diencephalon and brainstem. Hypoxic changes in the cerebral cortex, hippocampus, basal ganglia and cerebellum appear to be secondary.[103]

Uraemic encephalopathy

Uraemic encephalopathy occurs when the glomerular filtration rate declines below 10% of normal. Neuropsychiatric symptoms tend to fluctuate and, although, variable, include disturbances of memory and cognition and may progress to delerium, convulsions, stupor and coma.[59] The pathophysiology of uraemic encephalopathy is complex and probably a multi-factorial process, and may initially reflect a neuro-transmission defect. There is evidence to suggest that parathyroid hormone (PTH) plays a role[143] since, in uraemic patients, both the EEG abnormalities and the neuropsychiatric symptoms are improved by either parathyroidectomy or medical suppression of PTH.[90] The mechanism whereby parathyroid hormone disturbs CNS function is unknown but could relate to the facilitation of Ca^{2+} entry into the cell and consequent cell death.[143]

Pathological studies in over 400 patients who died with chronic renal failure revealed subdural haemorrhages in 1–3% of cases.[145] Generalized but variable neuronal degeneration has been described including perivascular areas of necrosis and demyelination. Brain areas involved include the cerebral cortex, subcortical nuclei, nuclei of the brainstem and cerebellum. Alzheimer II astrocytes are a common finding in uraemic encephalopathy (see Portal–systemic encephalopathy).[319]

Dialysis may be associated with at least three clinical disorders of the CNS: dialysis disequilibrium syndrome, progressive intellectual dysfunction and dialysis dementia.[144] Wernicke's encephalopathy has also been reported in association with haemodialysis.[204] Dialysis disequilibrium syndrome occurs as a consequence of an osmotic gradient which develops between plasma and the brain during rapid dialysis. Dialysis dementia is a progressive, frequently fatal disease seen almost exclusively in patients being treated with chronic haemodialysis. It has been suggested that aluminium neurotoxicity may play a major role in the pathogenesis of dialysis dementia; the frequency of dialysis dementia has reduced with the use of aluminium-free dialysate.[59] Not only is brain aluminium content increased in patients with the condition, but PTH excess may result in increased brain uptake or retention of aluminium. Increased brain aluminium has also been reported in Alzheimer's disease and neuropathological investigation of patients with dialysis dementia has revealed the presence of senile plaques and neurofibrillary tangles similar to those encountered in Alzheimer's disease. Recently, it has been noted that fine, granular, aluminium-containing inclusions are seen in the cytoplasm of cortical neurons and glia in dialysis-associated encephalopathy and that these changes develop via different pathogenic pathways to those in Alzheimer's disease.[362]

INHERITED METABOLIC DEFECTS

Disorder of amino acid metabolism

There have been relatively few recent advances in the neuropathology of amino acidurias since the reviews by Martin and Scholte[278] and Crome and Stern.[100] Nevertheless, considerable progress has been made in understanding the mechanisms, biochemistry and genetics of these disorders[291,383] and the use of animal models holds great promise.[191] Important determinants of the neuropathological changes are the age of the patient (length of survival) and efficacy of treatments such as dietary restriction. In most of the amino acidurias the CNS lesions are non-specific, the most common change being spongiosus or cavitation of the white matter and gliosis. One exception is homocystinuria, in which the lesions are usually ischaemic in type. Disorders of urea cycle enzymes, which cause the accumulation of precursors of urea (ammonia and glutamine), induce widespread transformation of astrocytes to the Alzheimer II type. A number of different mechanisms may play a role in causing the structural and functional deficits in amino acidurias. Some amino acids are neurotransmitters (e.g. glycine) or are required in the formation of neuroactive substances (e.g. tyrosine); others, when present in excessive amounts, can interfere with mitochondrial function; and deficits of others may lead to abnormalities of lipid and protein metabolism. Further, the keto acids or other byproducts (e.g. ammonia) of metabolic failure in amino acid metabolism may induce toxicity by interfering with various cellular functions, including neurotransmission.

Phenylketonuria (PKU) is one form of hyperphenylalaninaemia (defined as a plasma phenylalanine level >0.12 mM/dl) and is associated with impaired cognitive development if not detected and treated during the first few weeks of life. Non-PKU hyperphenylalaninaemia is a benign condition. The different clinical manifestations in two phenotypes suggest that the amount of phenylalanine overburden influences pathogenesis.[383] There is a defect in the hydroxylation of phenylalanine to tyrosine. DNA analysis has identified six mutations, so far, which cause the PKU phenotype.[383] Recent MRI studies suggest that the severity of changes seen on the MRI correlate with phenylalanine concentrations at the time of investigation and the time since dietary treatment had been withdrawn.[421] Moreover, there appears to be a relationship between genotype and biochemical control.[454] There is great geographical and ethnic variation in the incidence of PKU, with 5–190 cases per million births.[373] Scriver et al.[383] state that three pathogenetic elements need to be considered: a putative deficiency of tyrosine, the effect of phenylalanine on transport mechanisms and distribution of metabolites, and secondary effects on neurochemical reactions. However, they concluded that no single process explains the pathology.

Macroscopically, in untreated cases there is usually microcephaly. Fortunately, this is rare as most cases are identified by neonatal urine screening for phenylalanine and early dietary treatment has resulted in a dramatic decrease in the severity of neurological dysfunction. However, MRI studies show white matter changes in a significant proportion of these cases.[421] Microscopically, there is spongiosus of the white matter and gliosis and it has been suggested that there is a delay in myelination. Biochemical studies support the concept of an alteration in myelin. There are diminished levels of cerebral lipids and proteolipids.[278] In severely retarded adults Bauman and Kemper[35] noted a higher density of packing of cortical neurons, which were smaller than normal and few Nissl granules. The dendritic arborization was poorly developed and there were fewer dendritic spines than normal. Experimental studies show abnormalities of both myelin and cortical neurons.[94,198] Since effective dietary control of PKU has been established an important variant, maternal PKU, has been recognized. Damage to the fetus may result in microcephaly, mental retardation, impaired growth and other malformations.[260]

HYPERGLYCINAEMIA

Two distinct types of hyperglycinaemia are recognized and both can present as a life-threatening illness in the newborn period. In ketotic hyperglycinaemia there is a primary metabolic block in the catabolism of some organic acids leading to a severe acidosis and hyperglycinaemia. In the second type, non-ketotic hyperglycinaemia, there is a molecular defect in the glycine cleavage enzyme system. Large amounts of glycine accumulate in body fluids, including CSF. During the first few days of life the infants become lethargic with poor feeding. They may fit and their state of consciousness deteriorates rapidly to deep coma.

In non-ketotic hyperglycinaemia neuropathological changes are similar to those described in other amino acidurias with spongiosus and gliosis of the white matter (spongy myelinopathy). In a study of the brains of three infants Shuman et al.[393] demonstrated a dramatic reduction in the volume of the white matter of the cerebral hemispheres compared with control material (Fig. 10.22). In a study of a 17-year-old patient, Agamanolis et al.[10] found that the myelinopathy appeared to be static compared with neonatal cases, suggesting that the neurological deficits are probably due to neurotransmitter abnormalities rather than damage to myelin. Glycine is the major inhibitory neurotransmitter in the spinal cord and brainstem, but it seems that glycine may also play a role as a transmitter in the cerebral cortex, and the high levels that can be measured in the CNS tissue in this disease may account for the clinical syndrome.[45] Electron microscopy shows that the vacuoles in this condition lie within the myelin sheath.[258] An additional pathological observation is the presence of calcium oxalate crystals throughout the cerebellum, probably derived from the degradation of glycine.[10] Deposits of birefringement crystals have also been noted in the choroid plexus in a long-surviving case of cystinuria.[258]

MAPLE SYRUP URINE DISEASE

Classically, this disease presents as a fulminating neurological disorder with vomiting, lethargy, hypertonicity, convulsions and a peculiar odour (maple syrup) of the urine. It is caused by several different inherited defects in the mitochondrial multienzyme complex branched-chain α-keto acid dehydrogenase.[107] Rapid deterioration may lead to death and longer survival results in mental retardation. The primary approach to therapy is diet and the usual sequelae are reduced if treatment begins in early

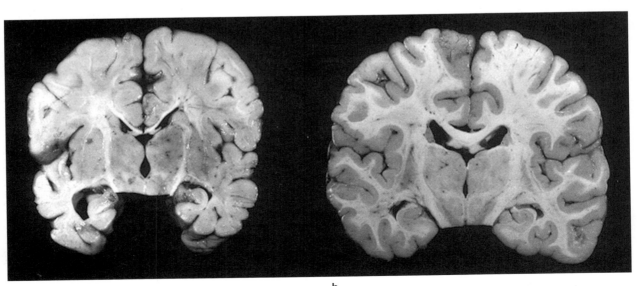

a　　　　　　　　　　　　　　　　　　　b

Figure 10.22 *Comparison of the bulk of cerebral white matter in* (**a**) *a 2-year-old child with non-ketotic hyperglycinaemia with* (**b**) *a control of the same age. Reproduced by permission from Shuman* et al.[393]

life. Neurophysiological and MRI studies in treated cases showed only minor abnormalities.[311] The principal neuropathological finding in untreated cases is spongiosus and gliosis of the white matter. Golgi studies reveal aberant orientation of neurons and abnormalities of dendrites and dendtritic spines.[216] Secondary effects of hypoxia and hypoglycaemia, which may be associated with the classic crises, can complicate the pathological picture. A natural animal model is seen in Poll Hereford calves, which show spongiosus of the white matter with intramyelinic vacuoles (Fig. 10.23a, b) and occasional axonal swellings are seen in longer term cases.[192] The pathogenic mechanism of the encepholopathy in acute bovine maple syrup urine disease appears to be a diminution of GABA-mediated inhibitory neurotransmission.[120]

HOMOCYSTINURIA

Homocystinuria is a disorder of transsulfuration and is most commonly caused by a deficiency of cystathione β-synthase. However, seven different genetic abnormalities are now known to lead to homocystinuria.[309] The clinical syndrome is more complex than the other amino acidurias, with abnormalities of the eye, and the skeletal, central nervous and vascular systems. Although mental retardation is common in infants who are not treated from birth the structural explanation is not evident. The predominant neuropathological lesions relate to thromboembolic disease. Involvement of cerebral vessels

has resulted in infarcts in the cerebrum, cerebellum, midbrain and thalamus.[309] Thrombi in the dural sinuses have also been reported.[88] Arterial walls often have fibrous intimal thickening, even in children.[463] Other amino acidurias such as tyrosinaemia, and disorders of histidine, proline and hydroxyproline metabolism are discussed by Crome and Stern[100] and Martin and Schlote.[278]

UREA-CYCLE DISORDERS

Hyperammonaemia in childhood frequently results from inborn errors of the urea cycle. Ornithine transcarbamylase (OTC) deficiency is probably the most common, but there are four other enzymes which, if defective, result in elevated levels of blood ammonia due to the failure of conversion of ammonia to urea. The other disorders are known as arginaemia, arginosuccinicaciduria, citrullinaemia and hyperornithinaemia. Except for arginaemia, which can present as a progressive tetraplegia and mental retardation, the urea-cycle disorders have a similar clinical presentation. In the neonatal period infants can develop lethargy, hypothermia and apnoea. The clinical syndrome is related to hyperammonaemia. In late infancy they may also present with vomiting and mental changes typical of hyperammonaemia, and in may cases the precipitant is a protein load (e.g. change of diet) or infection. OTC generally has an X-linked mode of inheritance and most males with low residual OTC activity present with severe chronic hyperammonaemia in the

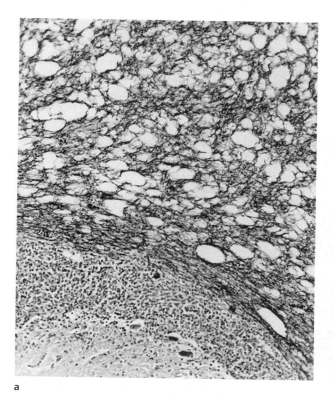

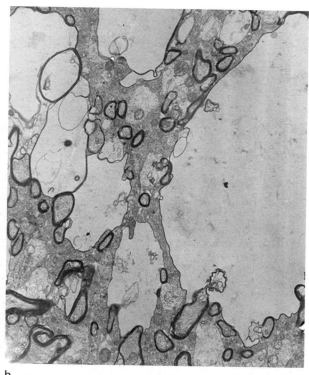

a   b

Figure 10.23 (a) Section of cerebellum from a Poll Hereford calf with maple syrup urine disease. There is spongiosus of the white matter. The granule cell and molecular layers appear normal. (PTAH stain.) Courtesy of Dr PAW Harper.[191] (b) Electron microscopy from specimen in (a) showing that the vacuoles are intramyelinic. Courtesy of Dr PAW Harper.[191]

neonatal period. Female carriers have a milder form of the disease. Dietary protein restriction coupled with treatment using sodium benzoate has extended the lifespan of patients with OTC deficiency.[56] CNS injury in OTC deficiency may occur *in utero*.

Neuropathological findings in congenital OTC deficiency are variable, ranging from a microscopically normal brain with Alzheimer type II astrocytic change to severe damage to the cerebral cortex and deep grey matter structures. For example, Bruton *et al.*[57] described the cerebral hemispheres of a female aged 6 years as 'little more than bags of leptomeninges', whereas her cousin, aged 8 years and affected by the same disorder, had no macroscopic abnormality of her brain. Brusilow and Horwich[56] reviewed the pathological reports and noted that an analysis of the changes is hampered by the heterogeneity of the disorders and complicated by lesions induced by the various agonal states. Fitting is a common occurrence and may well cause some of the more devastating neuropathological damage reported in these disorders. In a natural animal model in Holstein–Friesian calves affected with critrullinaemia due to argininosuccinate synthetase deficiency, there is spongiosus of the cerebrocortical grey matter with vacuolation of the cytoplasm of astroglial cells (Fig. 10.24).[191] The acute clinical encepalopathy is associated with hyperammonaemia and a relative increase in glutamate-mediated excitatory activity.[120]

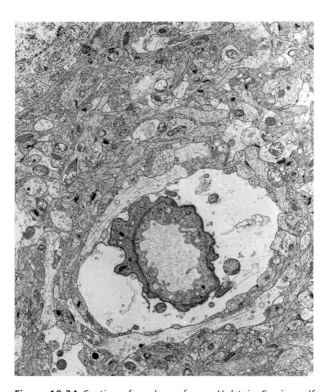

Figure 10.24 *Section of cerebrum from a Holstein–Fresian calf with citrullinaemia. There is expansion of the cytoplasm of the astroglial processes in the neuropil and surrounding blood vessels, with reduced concentrations of organelles. The myelin is normal. Courtesy of Dr PAW Harper.[193]*

The identification of other animal models of amino acidurias and the study of the mechanisms of brain dysfunction may contribute to a better understanding of the relationship between the clinical course, biochemistry and neuropathology of this group of disorders.

Prophyria

Porphyrias are a heterogeneous group of disorders that result from inherited or acquired dysregulation of one of the eight enzymes in the haem biosynthetic pathway.[142] Each of the porphyrias is characterized by a unique pattern of overproduction, accumulation and excretion of intermediates of haem biosynthesis.[317] They are classified as erythropoietic or hepatic in type depending on the primary organ in which excess production takes place. The main clinical manifestations are nervous system dysfunction and/or photosensitivity. The neurological manifestations of porphyria were reviewed by Becker and Kramer in 1977.[37] The most common neurological manifestations are autonomic and peripheral motor neuropathy (see Diseases of the peripheral nerves). Neuropsychiatric symptoms such as anxiety, depression, insomnia, disorientation, hallucinations and paranoia, as well as seizures and cranial nerve neuropathies are also often reported.[170]

Neuropathological studies of the CNS in porphyrias have reported a range of inconsistent findings. Hierons[199] reviewed the literature on the changes in the nervous system in acute porphyria and presented five cases of his own. He and others have concluded that lesions are either minimal or absent, except for those that can be explained on the basis of associated hypoxia.[357] Suarez *et al.* reviewed the literature and correlated the morphological findings of 35 patients with acute intermittent porphyria.[410] They noted that reported cerebral cortex findings have included diffuse neuronal loss, occipital cerebral ischaemia, perivascular pigmentation, diffuse perivascular demyelination, cytolysis of Betz cells and no abnormality. Nuclear chromocytolysis of cranial nerves has been reported, as has Purkinje cell loss, diffuse neuronal loss and no abnormality within the cerebellum. Two reports have documented neuronal loss of the supraoptic and paraventricular nuclei of the hypothalamus together with median eminence cell loss. This has been proposed as a mechanism for the hyponatraemia observed in some porphyric patients.[410] Several recent MRI studies have shown multiple cerebral lesions during attacks of acute porphyria.[12,225,238] In these cases the lesions were multifocal and resolved after several weeks. The authors speculated that the lesions are probably due to transient ischaemic cerebral changes. Kupferschmidt *et al.* hypothesized that because nitric oxide synthetase is a haem protein and nitric oxide is a vasodilator, unopposed cerebral vasoconstriction due to decreased nitric oxide from severe haem deficiency may occur during acute attacks.[238] Rosenbaum[372] stated that similar transient imaging abnormalities are not uncommon in the postictal state and the proposed mechanism is believed to be hyperperfusion and disruption of the BBB. Given the reversibility of these lesions it is not surprising that neuropathological abnormalities are rarely reported and are inconsistent. An alternative explanation for the neurological symptoms is that aminolevulinic acid (one of the early haem precursors) or a deficiency in haem itself may cause neuronal dysfunction.[299]

Chromatolysis of neurons in peripheral ganglia and the spinal cord, particularly the anterior horn cells, is frequently reported.[410] Hierons[199] and other authors[381] agree that the anterior horn cell changes relate to peripheral nerve pathology. Degeneration of various spinal cord tracts and dorsal root ganglia has also been reported.[199,381,476] The peripheral nerves have shown segmental demyelination and axonal swelling and fragmentation.[410,475] This may be related to abnormal activity of haem biosynthetic enzymes in peripheral nerves in porphyria.[476] There is evidence of axonal regeneration and collateral sprouting in the muscles of cases with chronic porphyria.[73] It was suggested by Price et al.[360] that patients with porphyria might develop an associated pyridoxine deficiency which could play a role in the pathology, but treatment with pyridoxine supplements does not alter the course of the disease.

REFERENCES

1 Abbasoglu O, Goldstein RM, Vodapally MS et al. Liver transplantation in hyponatremic patients with emphasis on central pontine myelinolysis. Clin Transplant 1998; 12: 263–9.
2 Abel EL. In utero alcohol exposure and developmental delay of response inhibition. Alcohol Clin Exp Res 1982; 6: 369–76.
3 Abel EL, Dintcheff BA. Factors affecting the outcome of maternal alcohol exposure: II Maternal age. Neurobehav Toxicol Teratol 1985; 7: 263–6.
4 Abel EL, Sokol RJ. A revised conservative estimate of the incidence of FAS and its economic impact. Alcohol Clin Exp Res 1991; 15: 514–24.
5 Abel EL, Sokol RJ. Fetal alcohol syndrome is now leading cause of mental retardation. Lancet 1986; ii: 1222.
6 Acker C. Neuropsychological deficits in alcoholics: the relative contributions of gender and drinking history. Br J Addict 1986; 81: 395–403.
7 Adams RD. Nutritional cerebellar degeneration. Amsterdam: Elsevier, 1976.
8 Adams RD, Kubik CS. Subacute degeneration of the brain in pernicious anaemia. N Engl J Med 1944; 231: 1–9.
9 Adams RD, Victor M, Mancall EL. Central pontine myelinolysis. Arch Neurol Psychiatry 1959; 81: 159–72.
10 Agamanolis DP, Potter JL, Lundgren DW. Neonatal glycine encephalopathy: biochemical and neuropathologic findings. Pediatr Neurol 1993; 9: 140–3.
11 Agamanolis DP, Victor M, Harris JW et al. An ultrastructural study of subacute combined degeneration of the spinal cord in vitamin B_{12} deficient rhesus monkeys. J Neuropathol Exp Neurol 1978; 37: 273–99.
12 Aggarwal A, Quint DJ, Lynch JP. MR imaging of porphyric encephalopathy. Am J Roentgenol 1994; 162: 1218–20.
13 Ahmed M. Neurological disease and folate deficiency. BMJ 1972; i: 181.
14 Aikawa H, Suzuki K. Lesions in the skin, intestine, and central nervous system induced by antimetabolite of niacin. Am J Pathol 1986: 335–42.
15 Alexander WF. Vitamin B_{12} and the intrisic factor. Stuttgart: Theime, 1957.
16 Allen RH, Stabler SP, Lindenbaum J. Relevance of vitamins, homocysteine and other metabolites in neuropsychiatric disorders. Eur J Pediatr 1998; 157: S122–6.
17 Alpert JE, Fava M. Nutrition and depression: the role of folate. Nutr Rev 1997; 55: 145–9.
18 Al-Shubaili AF, Farah SA, Hussein JM et al. Axonal and demyelinating neuropathy with reversible proximal conduction block, an unusual feature of vitamin B_{12} deficiency. Muscle Nerve 1998; 21: 1341–3.
19 Alvarez I, Gonzalo LM, Llor J. Effects of chronic alcoholism on the amygdaloid complex. A study in humans and rats. Histo Histopathol 1989; 4: 183–92.
20 Amess JA, Burman JF, Rees GM et al. Megaloblastica-haemopoiesis in patients receiving nitrous oxide. Lancet 1978; ii: 339–42.
21 Anderson WJR, Baird D, Thomson AM. Epidemiology of stillbirths and infant deaths due to congenital malformation. Lancet 1958; i: 1304–6.
22 Angulo-Colmenares AG, Vaughan DW, Hinds JW. Rehabilitation following early malnutrition in the rat: body weight, brain size and cerebral cortex development. Brain Res 1979; 169: 121–38.
23 Arango V, Underwood MD, Mann JJ. Fewer pigmented neurons in the locus coeruleus of uncomplicated alcoholics. Brain Res 1994; 650: 1–8.
24 Arendt T, Bigl V, Arendt A, Tennstedt A. Loss of neurons in nucleus basalis of Meynert in Alzheimer's disease, paralysis agitans and Korsakoff's disease. Acta Neuropathol 1983; 61: 101–8.
25 Armstrong E. Enlarged limbic structures in the human brain: the anterior thalamus and medial mamillary body. Brain Res 1986; 362: 394–7.
26 Armstrong-James M, Ross DT, Chen F, Ebner FF. The effect of thiamine deficiency on the structure and physiology of the rat forebrain. Metab Brain Dis 1988; 3: 91–124.
27 Ashikaga R, Araki Y, Ono Y et al. FLAIR appearance of Wernicke encephalopathy. Radiat Med 1997; 15: 251–3.
28 Baker KG, Harding AJ, Halliday GM et al. Neuronal loss in functional zones of the cerebellum of chronic alcoholics with and without Wernicke's encephalopathy. Neuroscience 1999; 91: 429–38.
29 Barnes DE, Walker DW. Prenatal ethanol exposure permanently reduces the number of pyramidal neurons in the rat hippocampus. Dev Brain Res 1981; 1: 333–40.
30 Barron S, Riley EP. Passive avoidance performance following neonatal alcohol exposure. Neurotoxicol Teratol 1990; 12: 135–8.
31 Barter F, Tanner AR. Autonomic neuropathy in an alcoholic population. Postgrad Med J 1987; 63: 1033–6.
32 Baruah JK, Kinder D. Mitochondria and fetal alcohol syndrome. Exp Pathol 1987; 32: 187–8.
33 Bassi SS, Bulundwe KK, Greeff GP et al. MRI of the spinal cord in myelopathy complicating vitamin B_{12} deficiency: two additional cases and a review of the literature. Neuroradiology 1999; 41: 271–4.
34 Bauer-Moffett C, Altman J. The effect of ethanol chronically administered to preweaning rats on cerebellar development: a morphological study. Brain Res 1977; 119: 249–68.
35. Bauman ML, Kemper TL. Morphologic and histoanatomic observations of the brain in untreated human phenylketonuria. Acta Neuropathol 1982; 58: 55–63.

36 Bechard M, Freud M, Kott et al. Hepatic cirrhosis with post-shunt myelopathy. *J Neurol Sci* 1970; **11**: 101–7.

37 Becker DM, Kramer S. The neurological manifestations of porphyria: a review. *Medicine* 1977; **56**: 411–22.

38 Becker HC, Randall CL, Middaugh LD. Behavioral teratogenic effects of ethanol in mice. *Ann NY Acad Sci* 1989; **562**: 340–1.

39 Bedi KS. Lasting neuroanatomical changes following undernutrition in early life. In: Dobbing J ed. *Early nutrition and later achievement*. London: Academic Press, 1987: 1–49.

40 Bedi KS. Nutrition, environment and brain development. *Sci Prog* 1986; **70**: 555–70.

41 Bedi KS, Thomas YM, Davies CA, Dobbing J. Synapse-to-neuron ratios of the frontal and cerebellar cortex of 30-day-old and adult rats undernourished during early postnatal life. *J Comp Neurol* 1980; **193**: 49–56.

42 Belay ED, Bresee JS, Holman RC et al. Reye's syndrome in the United States from 1981 through 1997. *N Engl J Med* 1999; **340**: 1377–82.

43 Bengochea O, Gonzalo LM. Effect of chronic alcoholism on the human hippocampus. *Histo Histopathol* 1990; **5**: 349–57.

44 Bessy OA, Adam DJD, Hanson AE. Intake of vitamin B_6 and infantile convulsions: a first approximation of requirements of pyridoxin in infants. *Pediatrics* 1957; **20**: 33–44.

45 Betz H. Glycine receptors: heterogeneous and widespread in the mammalian brain. *Trends Neurosci* 1991; **14**: 458–61.

46 Blanco R, DeGirolami U, Jenkins RL, Khettry U. Neuropathology of liver transplantation. *Clin Neuropathol* 1995; **14**: 109–17.

47 Blisard KS, Davis LE. Neuropathologic findings in Reye syndrome. *J Child Neurol* 1991; **6**: 41–4.

48 Bonthius DJ, West JR. Blood alcohol concentration and microencephaly: a dose–response study in the neonatal rat. *Teratology* 1988; **37**: 223–31.

49 Bonthius DJ, West JR. Alcohol induced neuronal loss in developing rats: increased brain damage with binge exposure. *Alcohol Clin Exp Res* 1990; **14**: 107–18.

50 Borges S, Lewis PD. A study of alcohol effects on the brain during gestation and lactation. *Teratalogy* 1982; **25**: 283–9.

51 Botez MI. Folate deficiency and neurological disorders in adults. *Med Hypotheses* 1976; **2**: 135–40.

52 Brien JF, Loomis CW, Tranmer J, McGrath M. Disposition of ethanol in human maternal venous blood and amniotic fluid. *Am J Obstet Gynecol* 1983; **146**: 181–6.

53 Brown AS, Susser ES, Butler PD et al. Neurobiological plausibility of prenatal nutritional deprivation as a risk factor for schizophrenia. *J Nerv Ment Dis* 1996; **184**: 71–85.

54 Brown JK, Imam H. Interrelationships of liver and brain with special reference to Reye syndrome. *J Inherit Metab Dis* 1991; **14**: 436–58.

55 Brown RE. Organ weight in malnutrition with special reference to brain weight. *Dev Med Child Neurol* 1966; **8**: 512–22.

56 Brusilow SW, Horwich AL. Urea cycle enzymes. In: Scriver CF, Beaudet AL, Sly WS, Valle D eds. *The metabolic basis of inherited disease*. New York: McGraw Hill, 1989: 629–63.

57 Bruton CJ, Corsellis JAN, Russell A. Hereditary hyperammonaemia. *Brain* 1970; **93**: 423–34.

58 Buccellato FR, Miloso M, Braga M et al. Myelinolytic lesions in spinal cord of cobalamin-deficient rats are TNF-alpha-mediated. *FASEB J* 1999; **13**: 297–304.

59 Burn DJ, Bates D. Neurology and the kidney. *J Neurol Neurosurg Psychiatry* 1998; **65**: 810–21.

60 Butterworth RF. Cerebral thiamine-dependent enzyme changes in experimental Wernicke's encephalopathy. *Metab Brain Dis* 1986; **1**: 165–75.

61 Butterworth RF. Maternal thiamine deficiency: a factor in intrauterine growth retardation? *Ann NY Acad Sci* 1993; **678**: 325–9.

62 Butterworth RF. Pathophysiologic mechanisms responsible for the reversible (thiamine-responsive) and irreversible (thiamine non-responsive) neurological symptoms of Wernicke's encephalopathy. *Drug Alcohol Rev* 1993; **12**: 315–22.

63 Butterworth RF, Gaudreau C, Vincelette J et al. Thiamine deficiency and Wernicke's encephalopathy in AIDS. *Metab Brain Dis* 1991; **6**: 207–12.

64 Butterworth RF, Giguere JF, Michaud J et al. Ammonia: key factor in the pathogenesis of hepatic encephalopathy. *Neurochem Pathol* 1987; **6**: 1–12.

65 Byrne C, Halliday G, Ellis J, Harper C. Thalamic vacuolation in acute Wernicke's encephalopathy. *Metab Brain Dis* 1993; **8**: 107–13.

66 Caine D, Halliday GM, Kril JJ, Harper CG. Operational criteria for the classification of chronic alcoholics: identification of Wernicke's encephalopathy. *J Neurol, Neurosurg Psychiatry* 1997; **62**: 51–60.

67 Cala LA, Jones B, Mastaglia FL, Wiley B. Brain atrophy and intellectual impairment in heavy drinkers: a clinical, psychometric computerized tomography study. *Aust NZ J Med* 1978; **8**: 147–53.

68 Calingasan NT, Baker H, Sheu KFR, Gibson GE. Blood–brain barrier abnormalities in vulnerable brain regions in thiamine deficiency. *Exp Neurol* 1995; **134**: 64–72.

69 Campbell ACP, Russell WR. Wernicke's encephalopathy: clinical features and their probable relationship to vitamin B deficiency. *Q J Med* 1941; **34**: 41–64.

70 Canosa CA, Salomon JB, Klein RE. The intervention approach: the Guatemala study. In: Moore WM, Silverberg MM, Read MS eds. *Nutrition, growth and development of North American Indian children*. Washington, DC: Government Printing Office, 1972.

71 Carmel R, Watkins D, Goodman SI, Rosenblatt DS. Hereditary defect of cobalamin metabolism (cblG mutation) presenting as a neurologic disorder in adulthood. *N Engl J Med* 1988; **318**: 1738–41.

72 Castle WB. Extrinsic factor in pernicious anaemia. *Am J Med Sci* 1929; **178**: 748–64.

73 Cavanagh JB. Peripheral neuropathy caused by chemical agents. *CRC Crit Rev Toxicol* 1973; **2**: 365–417.

74 Chanarin I. *Folate deficiency*. New York: John Wiley, 1986.

75 Chang KH, Cha SH, Han MH et al. Marchiafava–Bignami disease: serial changes in corpus callosum on MRI. *Neuroradiology* 1992; **34**: 480–2.

76 Charness ME, Diamond I. Alcohol and the nervous system. In: Appel SH, ed. *Current Neurology*. New York: John Wiley, 1984: 383–422.

77 Charness ME, Simon RP, Greenberg DA. Ethanol and the nervous system. *N Engl J Med* 1989; **321**: 442–54.

78 Chatterjee A. A 44-month clinical-brain MRI follow-up in a patient with B_{12} deficiency (Letter; Comment). *Neurology* 1998; **50**: 1932.

79 Chen JC, Turiak G, Galler J, Volicer L. Postnatal changes of brain monoamine levels in prenatally malnourished and control rats. *Int J Dev Neurosci* 1997; **15**: 257–63.

80 Church MW, Holmes PA, Overbeck GW et al. Interactive effects of prenatal alcohol and cocaine exposure on postnatal mortality, development and behavior in the Long–Evans rat. *Neurotoxicol Teratol* 1991; **13**: 377–86.

81 Church MW, Kaltenbach JA. Hearing, speech, language, and vestibular disorders in the fetal alcohol syndrome: a literature review. *Alcohol Clin Exp Res* 1997; **21**: 495–512.

82 Cintra L, Aguilar A, Granados L et al. Effects of prenatal protein malnutrition on hippocampal CA1 pyramidal cells in rats of four age groups. Hippocampus 1997; 7: 192–203.

83 Clarren SK. Recognition of fetal alcohol syndrome. JAMA 1981; 245: 2436–9.

84 Clarren SK, Astley SJ, Bowden DM et al. Neuroanatomic and neurochemical abnormalities in non-human primate infants exposed to weekly doses of ethanol during gestation. Alcohol Clin Exp Res 1990; 14: 674–83.

85 Clarren SK, Bowden DM. Fetal alcohol syndrome: a new primate model for binge drinking and its relevance to human ethanol teratogenesis. J Pediatr 1982; 101: 819–24.

86 Clarren SK, Smith DW. The fetal alcohol syndrome: a review of the world literature. N Engl J Med 1978; 298: 1063–7.

87 Clayton PT, Smith I, Harding B et al. Subacute combined degeneration of the cord, dementia and parkinsonism due to an inborn error of folate metabolism. J Neurol, Neurosurg Psychiatry 1986; 49: 920–7.

88 Cochran FB. Homocystinuria presenting as sagittal sinus thrombosis. Eur Neurol 1992; 32: 1–3.

89 Coffey VP, Jessop WJE. A three-year study of anencephaly in Dublin. Ir J Med Sci 1958; 6: 391–413.

90 Cogan M, Covey C, Arieff AI et al. Central nervous system manifestations of hyperparathyroidism. Am J Med 1978; 65: 963.

91 Collins GH. Glial cell changes in the brainstem of thiamine deficient rats. Am J Pathol 1967; 50: 791–802.

92 Colman N, Herbert V. Folates and the nervous system. In: Blakley RL, Whitehead VM eds. Folates and pterins, Vol. 3, Nutritional, pharmacological and physiological aspects. New York: John Wiley, 1986.

93 Conn HO. Transjugular intrahepatic portal–systemic shunts: the state of the art. Hepatology 1993; 1: 148–58.

94 Cordero ME, Trejo M, Colombo M, Arenda V. Histological maturation of the neocortex in phenylketonuric rats. Early Hum Dev 1983; 8: 157.

95 Coulter CL, Leech RW, Schaefer GB et al. Midline cerebral dysgenesis, dysfunction of the hypothalamic–pituitary axis, and fetal alcohol effects. Arch Neurol 1993; 50: 771–5.

96 Coursin DB. Convulsive seizures in infants with pyridoxine deficient diet. JAMA 1954; 154: 406.

97 Coward DG, Whitehead RG. Experimental protein-energy malnutrition in baby baboons. Attempts to reproduce the pathological features of kwashiorkor as seen in Uganda. Br J Nutr 1972; 28: 223–37.

98 Cox-Klazinga M, Endtz LJ. Peripheral nerve involvement in pernicious anaemia. J Neurol Sci 1980; 45: 367–71.

99 Cravioto H, Silberman J. Wernicke's encephalopathy. A clinical and pathological study of 28 autopsied cases. Arch Neurol 1961; 4: 510–19.

100 Crome L, Stern J. The pathology of mental retardation 2nd edn. Edinburgh, Churchill Livingstone, 1972.

101 Cullen KM, Halliday GM. Neurofibrillary degeneration and cell loss in the nucleus basalis in comparison to cortical Alzheimer pathology. Neurobiol Aging 1998; 19: 297–306.

102 Cullen K, Halliday G, Caine D. The nucleus basalis in the alcoholic Wernicke-Korsakoff syndrome: cell loss in both amnesic and non-amnesic patients. Brain 1994.

102 Cullen KM, Halliday GM, Caine D, Kril JJ. The nucleus basalis (Ch4) in the alcoholic Wernicke–Korsakoff syndrome: reduced cell number in both amnesic and non-amnesic patients. J Neurol, Neurosurg Psychiatry 1997; 63: 315–20.

103 Cullity GJ, Kakulas BA. Encephalopathy and fatty degeneration of the viscera: an evaluation. Brain 1970; 93: 77–88.

104 Dakshinamurti K, Paulose CS, Viswanathan M et al. Neurobiology of pyridoxine. Ann N Y Acad Sci 1990; 585: 128–44.

105 D'Amour ML, Bruneau J, Butterworth RF. Abnormalities of peripheral nerve conduction in relation to thiamine status in alcoholic patients. Can J Neurol Sci 1991; 18: 126–8.

106 D'Amour ML, Butterworth RF. Pathogenesis of alcoholic peripheral neuropathy: direct effect of ethanol or nutritional deficit? Metab Brain Dis 1994; 9: 133–42.

107 Danner DJ, Elsas LJ. Disorders of branched chain amino acid and keto acid metabolism. In: Schriver CF, Beaudet AL, Sly WS, Valle D eds. The metabolic basis of inherited disease 6th edn. New York: McGraw-Hill, 1989: 671–92.

108 Dastur et al. Nerve and muscle in children with protein calorie malnutrition compared to well nourished children. Xth International Congress of Nutrition, 1973, Kyoto, Japan.

109 Davies-Jones GAB, Preston FE, Timperley WR. Neurological complications in clinical haematology. Oxford: Blackwell, 1980.

110 Davis LE, Blisard KS, Kornfeld M. The influenza B virus mouse model of Reye's syndrome: clinical, virologic and morphologic studies of the encephalopathy. J Neurol Sci 1990; 97: 221–31.

111 Deacon R, Purkiss P, Green R et al. Vitamin B_{12} neuropathy is not due to failure to methylate myelin basic protein. J Neurol Sci 1986; 72: 113–7.

112 De la Monte SM. Disproportionate atrophy of cerebral white matter in chronic alcoholics. Arch Neurol 1988; 45: 990–2.

113 Delaney AL, Samorajski T, Fuller GN, Wiggins RC. A morphometric comparison of central and peripheral hypomyelination induced by postnatal undernourishment of rats. J Nutr 1981; 111: 746–54.

114 Deniker P, Susini JR, Ruyer F, Fredy D. Cerebral x-ray computed tomography in anorexia nervosa. Study of 16 cases. Encephale 1986; 12: 63–70.

115 Derot M, Castaigne P, Morel-Maroger A, Leclercq A. [Complex nutritional neurologic syndrome reversible by administration of folic acid.] Bull Mem Soc Med Hopitaux Paris 1967; 118: 867–74.

116 DeWitt LD, Buonanno FS, Kistler JP et al. Central pontine myelinolysis: demonstration by nuclear magnetic resonance. Neurology 1984; 34: 570–6.

117 Diemer NH. Glial and neuronal changes in experimental hepatic encephalopathy. Acta Neurol Scand 1978; 58 (Suppl 71): 1–144.

118 Dobbing J, Hopewell JW, Lynch A. Vulnerability of developing brain. VII. Permanent deficits of neurons in cerebral and cerebellar cortex following early mild undernutrition. Exp Neurol 1971; 32: 439–47.

119 Dobbing J, Sands J. Vulnerability of developing brain. IX. The effect of nutritional growth retardation on the timing of the brain growth-spurt. Biol Neonate 1971; 19: 363.

120 Dodd PR, Williams SH, Gundlach AL et al. Glutamate and gamma-aminobutyric acid neurotransmitter systems in the acute phase of maple syrup urine disease and citrullinemia encephalopathies in newborn calves. J Neurochem 1992; 59: 582–90.

121 Driscoll CD, Streissguth AP, Riley EP. Prenatal alcohol exposure: comparability of effects in humans and animal models. Neurotoxicol Teratol 1990; 12: 231–7.

122 Druse MJ, Kuo A, Tajuddin N. Effects of in utero ethanol exposure on the developing serotonergic system. Alcohol Clin Exp Res 1991; 15: 678–84.

123 Druse MJ, Tajuddin N, Kuo A, Connerty M. Effects of *in utero* ethanol exposure on the developing dopaminergic system in rats. *J Neurosci Res* 1990; **27**: 233–40.

124 Duckett S, Winick M. *Brain dysfunction in children: etiology, diagnosis, and management*. New York: Raven Press, 1981.

125 Duprez TP, Gille M, Vande Berg BC *et al*. MRI of the spine in cobalamin deficiency: the value of examining both spinal cord and bone marrow. *Neuroradiology* 1996; **38**: 511–15.

126 Ede RJ, Williams R. Hepatic encephalopathy and cerebral edema. *Semin Liver Dis* 1986; **6**: 107–18.

127 Editorial. Folic acid and the nervous system. *Lancet* 1976; ii: 836.

128 Engsner G, Habte D, Sjögren I, Vahlquist B. Brain growth in children with kwashiorkor. *Acta Paediatr Scand* 1974; **63**: 687–94.

129 Ernhart CB, Sokol RJ, Ager JW *et al*. Alcohol related birth defects: assessing the risk. *Ann NY Acad Sci* 1989; **562**: 159–72.

130 Estol CJ, Faris AA, Martinez J, Ahdab-Barmada M. Central pontine myelinolysis after liver transplant. *Neurology* 1989; **39**: 493–8.

131 Fabregues I, Ferrer I, Gairi JM *et al*. Effects of prenatal exposure to ethanol on the maturation of the pyramidal neurons in the cerebral cortex of the guinea pig: a quantitative Golgi study. *Neuropathol Appl Neurobiol* 1985; **11**: 291–8.

132 Faure M. Sur les lesions cellulaires corticales observees dans six cas de troubles mentaux toxi-infectieux: ces lesions sont-elles primitives au secondaires?: etude anatomopathogique. *Rev Neurol (Paris)* 1899; **7**: 932–44.

133 Ferraro A, Arieti S, English WH. Cerebral changes in the course of pernicious anemia and their relationship to psychic symptoms. *J Neuropathol Exp Neurol* 1945; **4**: 217–39.

134 Ferrer I, Fabreques I, Pineda M *et al*. Golgi study of cerebellar atrophy in human chronic alcoholism. *Neuropathol Appl Neurobiol* 1984; **10**: 245–53.

135 Ferrer I, Galofre E. Dendritic spine abnormalities in fetal alcohol syndrome. *Neuropediatrics* 1987; **18**: 161–3.

136 Fine EJ, Soria ED. Myths about vitamin B_{12} deficiency. *South Med J* 1991; **84**: 1475–81.

137 Fishman MA, Prensky AL, Dodge PR. Low content of cerebral lipids in infants suffering from abnormal nutrition. *Nature* 1969; **221**: 552–3.

138 Fleckenstein JF, Frank S, Thuluvath PJ. Presence of autonomic neuropathy is a poor prognostic indicator in patients with advanced liver disease. *Hepatology* 1996; **23**: 471–5.

139 Foncin JF, Nicolaides S. Encephalopathie porto-cave; contribution a la pathologie ultrastructurale de la glie chez l'homme. *Rev Neurol (Paris)* 1970; **123**: 81–7.

140 Forno LS, Rivera L. Central pontine myelinolysis. *J Neuropathol Exp Neurol* 1975; **34**: 77.

141 Fox JH, Fishman MA, Prensky AL, Dodge PR. The effect of malnutrition on human central nervous system myelin. *Neurology* 1972; **22**: 1213.

142 Frank J, Christiano AM. The genetic bases of the porphyrias. *Skin Pharmacol Appl Skin Physiol* 1998; **11**: 297–309.

143 Fraser CL. Neurologic manifestations of the uremic state. In: Arieff AI, Griggs RC eds. *Metabolic brain dysfunction in systemic disorders*. Boston, MA: Little, Brown & Co., 1992: 139–66.

144 Fraser CL, Arieff AI. Metabolic encephalopathy as a complication of renal failure: mechanisms and mediators. *New Horiz* 1994; **2**: 518–26.

145 Fraser CL, Arieff AI. Nervous system complications in uremia. *Ann Intern Med* 1988; **109**: 143.

146 Freeman RM, ed. *Rational use of vitamins in practice*. Toronto: JB Lippincott, 1979.

147 Gandy G, Jacobson W, Sidman R. Inhibition of a transmethylation reaction in the nervous system: an experimental model for subacute combined degeneration of the cord. *J Physiol* 1973; **233**: 1–3P.

148 Garrow JS, Fletcher K, Halliday D. Body composition in severe infantile malnutrition. *J Clin Invest* 1965; **44**: 417.

149 Gass A, Birtsch G, Olster M *et al*. Marchiafava–Bignami disease: reversibility of neuroimaging abnormality. *J Comput Assist Tomogr* 1998; **22**: 503–4.

150 Gerster H. [The importance of vitamin B_6 for development of the infant. Human medical and animal experiment studies.] *Z Ernahrungswiss* 1996; **35**: 309–17.

151 Ghatak NR, Hadfield MG, Rosenblum WI. Association of central pontine myelinolysis and Marchiafava–Bignami disease. *Neurology* 1978; **12**: 1295–8.

152 Giguere JF, Hamel E, Butterworth RF. Increased densities of binding sites for the 'peripheral-type' benzodiazepine receptor ligand 3H-PK11195 in rat brain following portacaval anastomosis. *Brain Res* 1992; **585**: 295–8.

153 Gocht A, Lohler J. Changes in glial cell markers in recent and old demyelinated lesions in central pontine myelinolysis. *Acta Neuropathol* 1990; **80**: 46–58.

154 Goebel HH, Zur PH. Central pontine myelinolysis. A clinical and pathological study of ten cases. *Brain* 1972; **95**: 495–504.

155 Golden MHN, Ramdath D. Free radicals in the pathogenesis of kwashiorkor. *Proc Nutr Soc* 1987; **46**: 53–68.

156 Goodlett CR, Gilliam DM, Nichols JM, West JR. Genetic influences on brain growth restriction induced by developmental exposure to alcohol. *Neurotoxicology* 1989; **10**: 321–34.

157 Goodlett CR, Leo JT, O'Callaghan JP *et al*. Transient cortical astrogliosis induced by alcohol exposure during the neonatal brain growth spurt in rats. *Brain Res Dev Brain Res* 1993; **72**: 85–97.

158 Goodlett CR, Marcussen BL, West JR. A single day of alcohol exposure during the brain growth spurt induces brain weight restriction and cerebellar Purkinje cell loss. *Alcohol* 1990; **7**: 107–14.

159 Gospe SM Jr, Hecht ST. Longitudinal MRI findings in pyridoxine-dependent seizures. *Neurology* 1998; **51**: 74–8.

160 Grant HC, Hoffbrand AV, Wells DG. Folate deficiency and neurological disease. *Lancet* 1965; ii: 763–7.

161 Grattan-Smith PJ, Wilcken B, Procopis PG, Wise GA. The neurological syndrome of infantile cobalamin deficiency: developmental regression and involuntary movements. *Mov Disord* 1997; **12**: 39–46.

162 Greenfield JG, O'Flynn E. Subacute combined degeneration and pernicious anaemia. *Lancet* 1933; ii: 62–3.

163 Gregorios JB, Mozes LW, Norenberg MD. Morphologic effects of ammonia on primary astrocyte cultures. II. Electron microscopic studies. *J Neuropathol Exp Neurol* 1985; **44**: 404–14.

164 Gregorios JB, Mozes LW, Norenberg OB, Norenberg MD. Morphologic effects of ammonia on primary astrocyte cultures. 1. Light microscopic studies. *J Neuropathol Exp Neurol* 1985; **44**: 397–403.

165 Gressens P, Lammens M, Picard JJ, Evrard P. Ethanol-induced disturbances of gliogenesis and neurogenesis in the developing murine brain: an *in vitro* and *in vivo* immunohistochemical and ultrastructural study. *Alcohol Alcohol* 1992; **27**: 219–26.

166 Gressens P, Muaku SM, Besse L *et al*. Maternal protein restriction early in rat pregnancy alters brain development in the progeny. *Brain Res Dev Brain Res* 1997; **103**: 21–35.

167 Guerri C. Neuroanatomical and neurophysiological mechanisms involved in central nervous system dysfunctions induced by prenatal alcohol exposure. *Alcohol Clin Exp Res* 1998; **22**: 304–12.

168 Gunston GD, Burkimsher D, Malan H, Sive AA. Reversible cerebral shrinkage in kwashiorkor: an MRI study. *Arch Dis Child* 1992; **667**: 1030–2.

169 Guo YP, McLeod JG, Baverstock J. Pathological changes in the vagus nerve in diabetes and chronic alcoholism. *J Neurol, Neurosurg Psychiatry* 1987; **50**: 1449–53.

170 Gupta S, Dolwani S. Neurological complications of porphyria. *Postgrad Med J* 1996; **72**: 631–2.

171 Hakim AM. The induction and reversibility of cerebral acidosis in thiamine deficiency. *Ann Neurol* 1984; **16**: 673–9.

172 Halliday G, Ellis J, Harper C. The locus coeruleus and memory: a study of chronic alcoholics with and without the memory impairment of Korsakoff's psychosis. *Brain Res* 1992; **598**: 33–7.

173 Halliday G, Ellis J, Heard R *et al*. Brainstem serotonergic neurons in chronic alcoholics with and without the memory impairment of Korsakoff's psychosis. *J Neuropathol Exp Neurol* 1993; **52**: 567–79.

174 Halpin TJ, Holtzhaner FJ, Campbell RJ *et al*. Reye's syndrome and medication use. *JAMA* 1982; **248**: 687–91.

175 Hammer RP, Scheibel AB. Morphological evidence for a delay of neuronal maturation in fetal alcohol exposure. *Exp Neurol* 1981; **74**: 587–96.

176 Hansen HA, Nordquist P, Sourander P. Megaloblastic anaemia and neurological disturbances combined with folic acid deficiency; observations on an epileptic patient treated with anticonvulsants. *Acta Med Scand* 1964; **176**: 243–51.

177 Harding A, Halliday G, Caine D, Kril J. Degeneration of anterior thalamic nuclei differentiates alcoholics with amnesia. *Brain* 2000; **123**: 141–54.

178 Harding AJ, Wong A, Svoboda M *et al*. Chronic alcoholic consumption does not cause hippocampal neuron loss in humans. *Hippocampus* 1997; **7**: 78–87.

179 Hardie RM, Newton LH, Bruce JC *et al*. The changing clinical pattern of Reye's syndrome 1982–1990. *Arch Dis Child* 1996; **74**: 400–5.

180 Harlap S, Shiono P. Alcohol, smoking and incidence of spontaneous abortions in the first and second trimester. *Lancet* 1980; **ii**: 173–6.

181 Harper C. Wernicke's encephalopathy: a more common disease than realised. *J Neurol, Neurosurg Psychiatry* 1979; **42**: 226–31.

182 Harper C, Fornes P, Duyckaerts C *et al*. An international perspective on the prevalence of the Wernicke-Korsakoff syndrome. *Metab Brain Dis* 1994; **10**: 17–24.

183 Harper C, Kril J. Brain atrophy in chronic alcoholic patients: a quantitative pathological study. *J Neurol, Neurosurg Psychiatry* 1985; **48**: 211–17.

184 Harper C, Sheedy D, Lara A *et al*. Is thiamin supplementation useful in preventing Wernicke's encepholopathy? *Brain Pathol* 1997; **7**: 1253–5.

185 Harper CG. Sudden, unexpected death and Wernicke's encephalopathy. A complication of prolonged intravenous feeding. *Aust NZ J Med* 1980; **10**: 230–5.

186 Harper CG. The incidence of Wernicke's encephalopathy in Australia – a neuropathological study of 131 cases. *J Neurol, Neurosurg Psychiatry* 1983; **46**: 593–8.

187 Harper CG, Blumbergs PC. Brain weights in alcoholics. *J Neurol, Neurosurg Psychiatry* 1982; **45**: 838–40.

188 Harper CG, Giles M, Finlay-Jones R. Clinical signs in the Wernicke–Korsakoff complex – a retrospective analysis of 131 cases diagnosed at autopsy. *J Neurol, Neurosurg Psychiatry* 1986; **49**: 341–5.

189 Harper CG, Kril JJ. Corpus callosum thickness in alcoholics. *Br J Addict* 1988; **83**: 577–80.

190 Harper CG, Kril JJ. Neuropathological changes in alcoholics. In: Hunt WA, Nixon SJ eds. *Alcohol-induced brain damage*. Rockville, MD: U.S. Department of Health and Human Services, 1993: 39–69.

191 Harper PA, Dennis JA, Healy PJ, Brown GK. Maple syrup urine disease in calves: a clinical, pathological and biochemical study. *Aust Vet J* 1989; **66**: 46–9.

192 Harper PA, Healy PJ, Dennis JA. Ultrastructural findings in maple syrup urine disease in Poll Hereford calves. *Acta Neuropathol* 1986; **71**: 316–20.

193 Harper PAW, Healy PJ, Dennis JA. Animal model of human disease, citrullinaemia. *Am J Pathol* 1989; **135**: 1213–15.

194 Harris CP, Townsend JJ, Baringer JR. Symptomatic hyponatraemia: can myelinoysis be prevented by treatment? *J Neurol, Neurosurg Psychiatry* 1993; **56**: 626–32.

195 Hauw J-J, De Baecque C, Hausser-Hauw C, Serdaru M. Chromatolysis in alcoholic encephalopathies. *Brain* 1988; **111**: 843–57.

196 Hazell A, Butterworth R, Hakim A. Cerebral vulnerability is associated with selective increase in extracellular glutamate concentration in experimental thiamine deficiency. *J Neurochem* 1993; **61**: 1155–8.

197 Heroux M, Butterworth R eds. *Animal models of neurological disease,II*. Clifton, NJ: Humana Press, 1992.

198 Heuther G, Kaus R, Neuhoff V. Brain development in experimental hyperphenylalaninaemia: myelination. *Neuropediatrics* 1982; **13**: 177.

199 Hierons R. Changes in the nervous system in acute porphyria. *Brain* 1957; **80**: 176–92.

200 Hirono H, Wada Y. Effects of dietary folate deficiency, a developmental increase of myelin lipids in rat brain. *J Nutr* 1978; **108**: 766–72.

201 Hou JW, Chou SP, Wang TR. Metabolic function and liver histopathology in Reye-like illnesses. *Acta Paediatr* 1996; **85**: 1053–7.

202 Hoyumpa AM. Mechanisms of vitamin deficiencies in alcoholism. *Alcohol Clin Exp Res* 1986; **10**: 573–81.

203 Hutto BR. Folate and cobalamin in psychiatric illness. *Compr Psychiatry* 1997; **38**: 305–14.

204 Ihara M, Ito T, Yanagihara C, Nishimura Y. Wernicke's encephalopathy associated with hemodialysis: report of two cases and review of the literature. *Clin Neurol Neurosurg* 1999; **101**: 118–21.

205 Ishii N, Nishihara Y. Pellagra among chronic alcoholics: clinical and pathological study of 20 necropsy cases. *J Neurol, Neurosurg Psychiatry* 1981; **44**: 209–15.

206 Ishii N, Nishihara Y. Pellagra encephalopathy among tuberculous patients: its relation to isoniazid therapy. *J Neurol, Neurosurg Psychiatry* 1985; **48**: 628–34.

207 Itokawa H, Cooper JR. Ion movements and thiamine. II. The release of the vitamin from membrane fragments. *Biochim Biophys Acta* 1970; **196**: 274–84.

208 Jelliffe DB. *The assessment of the nutritional status of the community*. Geneva: World Health Organization, 1966.

209 Jensen GB, Pakkenberg B. Do alcoholics drink their neurons away? *Lancet* 1993; **342**: 1201–4.

210 Jernigan TL, Butters N, DiTriaglia G *et al*. Reduced cerebral grey matter observed in alcoholics using magnetic resonance imaging. *Alcohol Clin Exp Res* 1991; **15**: 418–27.

211 Jernigan TL, Schafer K, Butters N, Cermak LS. Magnetic resonance imaging of alcoholic Korsakoff's patients. *Neuropsycho-pharmacology* 1991; **4**: 175–86.

212 Johnson RH, Robinson BJ. Mortality in alcoholics with autonomic neuropathy. *J Neurol, Neurosurg Psychiatry* 1988; **51**: 476–80.

213 Jolliffe N, Bowman K, Rosenblum L, Fein H. Nicotinic acid deficiency encephalopathy. *JAMA* 1940; **114**: 307–9.

214 Jones DG, Dyson SE. The influence of protein restriction rehabilitation and changing nutritional status on synaptic development: a quantitative study in rat brain. *Brain Res* 1981; **208**: 97–111.

215 Jones KL, Smith DW. Recognition of fetal alcohol syndrome in early infancy. *Lancet* 1973; ii: 999–1001.

216 Kamei A, Takashima S, Chan F, Becker LE. Abnormal dendritic development in maple syrup urine disease. *Pediatr Neurol* 1992; **8**: 145–7.

217 Karacostas D, Artemis N, Bairactaris C *et al*. Cobalamin deficiency: MRI detection of posterior columns involvement and posttreatment resolution. *J Neuroimaging* 1998; **8**: 171–3.

218 Kato M, Hughes RD, Keays RT, Williams R. Electron microscopic study of brain capillaries in cerebral edema from fulminant hepatic failure. *Hepatology* 1992; **15**: 1060–6.

219 Kato T, Shioiri T, Murashita J, Inubushi T. Phosphorus-31 magnetic resonance spectroscopic observations in 4 cases with anorexia nervosa. *Prog Neuropsychopharmacol Biol Psychiatry* 1997; **21**: 719–24.

220 Katsaros VK, Glocker FX, Hemmer B, Schumacher M. MRI of spinal cord and brain lesions in subacute combined degeneration. *Neuroradiology* 1998; **40**: 716–19.

221 Keating JN, Trimble KC, Mulcahy F *et al*. Evidence of brain methyltransferase inhibition and early brain involvement in HIV-positive patients. *Lancet* 1991; **337**: 935–9.

222 Kelly SJ, Mahoney JC, West JR. Changes in brain microvasculature resulting from early postnatal alcohol exposure. *Alcohol* 1990; **7**: 43–7.

223 Kimura S, Amemiya F. Brain and liver pathology in a patient with carnitine deficiency. *Brain Dev* 1990; **12**: 436–9.

224 Kimura T, Budka H. Glial fibrillary acidic protein and S-100 protein in human hepatic encephalopathy: immuncytochemical demonstration of two glial-associated proteins. *Acta Neuropathol* 1986; **70**: 17–21.

225 King PH, Bragdon AC. MRI reveals multiple reversible cerebral lesions in an attack of acute intermittent porphyria. *Neurology* 1991; **41**: 1300–2.

226 Kinoshita T, Takahashi S, Ishii K *et al*. Reye's syndrome with cortical laminar necrosis: MRI. *Neuroradiology* 1996; **38**: 269–72.

227 Kleinschmidt-DeMasters BK, Anderson CA, Rubinstein D. Asymptomatic pontine lesions found by magnetic resonance imaging: are they central pontine myelinolysis? *J Neurol Sci* 1997; **149**: 27–35.

228 Klineschmidt-DeMasters BK, Norenberg MD. Neuropathologic observations in electrolyte-induced myelinolysis in the rat. *J Neuropathol Exp Neurol* 1982; **41**: 67–80.

229 Koeppen AH, Barron KD. Marchiafava–Bignami disease. *Neurology* 1978; **28**: 290–4.

230 Konovalov HV, Kovetsky NS, Bobryshev YV, Ashwell KW. Disorders of brain development in the progeny of mothers who used alcohol during pregnancy. *Early Hum Dev* 1997; **48**: 153–66.

231 Kornreich L, Shapira A, Horev G *et al*. CT and MR evaluation of the brain in patients with anorexia nervosa. *Am J Neuroradiol* 1991; **12**: 1213–6.

232 Kosik KS, Mullins TF, Bradley WG *et al*. Coma and axonal degeneration in vitamin B_{12} deficiency. *Arch Neurol* 1980; **37**: 590–2.

233 Krigman MR, Hogan EL. Undernutrition in the developing rat: effect upon myelination. *Brain Res* 1976; **107**: 239–55.

234 Kril JJ. Neuropathology of thiamine deficiency disorders. *Metab Brain Dis* 1996; **11**: 9–17.

235 Kril JJ, Halliday GM, Svoboda MD, Cartwright H. The cerebral cortex is damaged in chronic alcoholics. *Neuroscience* 1997; **79**: 983–98.

236 Kril JJ, Harper CG. Neuronal counts from four cortical regions of alcoholic brains. *Acta Neuropathol (Berl)* 1989; **79**: 200–4.

237 Kulisevsky J, Pujol J, Balauzo J *et al*. Pallidal hyperintensity on magnetic resonance imaging in cirrhotic patients: clinical correlations. *Hepatology* 1992; **16**: 1382–8.

238 Kupferschmidt H, Bont A, Schnorf H *et al*. Transient cortical blindness and biooccipital brain lesions in two patients with acute intermittent porphyria. *Ann Intern Med* 1995; **123**: 598–600.

239 Kure S, Sakata Y, Miyabayashi S *et al*. Mutation and polymorphic marker analyses of 65K- and 67K-glutamate decarboxylase genes in two families with pyridoxine-dependent epilepsy. *J Hum Genet* 1998; **43**: 128–31.

240 Lakshmi AV. Riboflavin metabolism: relevance to human nutrition. *Indian J Med Res* 1998; **108**: 182–90.

241 Lane M, Smith FE, Alfrey CP. Experimental dietary and antagonist-induced human riboflavin deficiency. In: Rivlin R ed. *Riboflavin*. New York, 1975: 245–77.

242 Langlais PJ, Mair RG. Protective effects of the glutamate antagonist MK-801 on pyrithiamine-induced lesions and amino acid changes in rat brain. *J Neurosci* 1990; **10**: 1664–74.

243 Langlais PJ, Zhang SX, Savage LM. Neuropathology of thiamine deficiency: an update on the comparative analysis of human disorders and experimental models. *Metab Brain Dis* 1996; **11**: 19–37.

244 Langlais PJ, Zhang SX, Weilersbacher G *et al*. Histamine-mediated neuronal death in a rat model of Wernicke's encephalopathy. *J Neurosci Res* 1994; **38**: 565–74.

245 Lankford KL, DeMello FG, Klein WL. D_1-Type dopamine receptors inhibit growth cone motility in cultured retina neurons: evidence that neurotransmitters act as morphogenic growth regulators in the developing central nervous system. *Proc Natl Acad Sci USA* 1988; **85**: 2839–43.

246 Laubenberger J, Schneider B, Ansorge O *et al*. Central pontine myelinolysis: clinical presentation and radiologic findings. *Eur Radiol* 1996; **6**: 177–83.

247 Lauder JM, Wallace JA, Wilkie MB *et al*. Role for serotonin in neurogenesis. *Monogr Neural Sci* 1983; **9**: 3–10.

248 Lavoie J, Pomier Layargues G, Butterworth RF. Increased densities of 'peripheral-type' benzodiazepine receptors in autopsied brain tissue from cirrhotic patients with hepatic encephalopathy. *Hepatology* 1990; **11**: 874–8.

249 Lechevalier B, Anderson JC, Morin P. Hemispheric disconnection syndrome with a 'crossed avoiding' reaction in a case of Marchiafava–Bignami disease. *J Neurol, Neurosurg Psychiatry* 1977; **40**: 483–97.

250 Lee C, Surtees R, Duchen L. Distal motor axonopathy and central nervous system myelin vacuolation caused by cycloleucine, an inhibitor of methionine adenosyltransferase. *Brain* 1992; **115**: 935–55.

251 Lee IJ, Soh Y, Song BJ. Molecular characterization of fetal alcohol syndrome using mRNA differential display. *Biochem Biophys Res Commun* 1997; **240**: 309–13.

252 Lee L, Hard F, Moller L *et al*. Alcohol-induced brain damage and liver damage in young males. *Lancet* 1979; ii: 759–61.

253 Leichter J. Growth of fetuses of rats exposed to ethanol and cigarette smoke during gestation. *Growth Dev Aging* 1989; **53**: 129–34.

254 Lemoine P, Harouseau H, Borteryu JT, Menuet J-C. Les enfants des parents alcooliques: anomalies observees apropos de 127 cas. *Quest Med* 1968; **21**: 476–82.

255 Leong ASV. Marchiafava–Bignami disease in a non-alcoholic Indian male. *Pathology* 1979; **11**: 241–9.

256 Leong DK, Le O, Oliva L, Butterworth RF. Increased densities of binding sites for the 'peripheral-type' benzodiazepine receptor ligand ^{3}H-PK11195 in vulnerable regions of the rat brain in thiamine deficiency encephalopathy. *J Cerebr Blood Flow Metab* 1994; **14**: 100–5.

257 Lester-Smith E. Purification of antipernicious anaemia factors from liver. *Nature* 1948; **161**: 638–9.

258 Levine S, Paparo G. Brain lesions in a case of cystinosis. *Acta Neuropathol* 1982; **57**: 217–20.

259 Levine S, Stypulkowski W. Experimental cyanide encephalopathy. *Arch Pathol* 1959; **67**: 306–23.

260 Levy HL. Effect of mutation on maternal–fetal metabolic homeostasis: maternal aminoacidopathies. In: Llyord JK, Scriver CR eds. *Genetic and metabolic disease in pediatrics*. London: Butterworths, 1985: 250.

261 Lichtheim H. *Zur Kenntnis der perniciosen Anamie*. 1887.

262 Lindenbaum J, Healton EB, Savage DG et al. Neuropsychiatric disorders caused by cobalamin deficiency in the absence of anaemia or macrocytosis. *N Engl J Med* 1988; **318**: 1720–8.

263 Lindgren S, Lilja B, Verbaan H, Sundkvist G. Alcohol abuse exaggerates autonomic dysfunction in chronic liver disease. *Scand J Gastroenterol* 1996; **31**: 1120–4.

264 Lishman WA. Alcohol and the brain. *Br J Psychiatry* 1990; **156**: 635–44.

265 Little BB, Snell LM, Rosenfeld CR et al. Failure to recognize fetal alcohol syndrome in newborn infants. *Am J Dis Child* 1990; **144**: 1142–6.

266 Liversedge LA, Rawson MD. Myelopathy in hepatic disease and portosystemic venous anastomosis. *Lancet* 1966; **i**: 277–9.

267 Lockwood AH, Yap EWH, Wong WH. Cerebral ammonia metabolism in patients with severe liver disease and minimal hepatic encephalopathy. *J Cereb Blood Flow Metab* 1991; **11**: 337–41.

268 Lopez-Tejero D, Ferrer I, Llobera M, Herrera E. Effects of prenatal ethanol exposure on physical growth, sensory reflex maturation and brain development in the rat. *Neuropathol Appl Neurobiol* 1986; **12**: 251–60.

269 Lovblad K, Ramelli G, Remonda L et al. Retardation of myelination due to dietary vitamin B_{12} deficiency: cranial MRI findings. *Pediatr Radiol* 1997; **27**: 155–8.

270 Maier SE, Chen WJ, Miller JA, West JR. Fetal alcohol exposure and temporal vulnerability regional differences in alcohol-induced microencephaly as a function of the timing of binge-like alcohol exposure during rat brain development. *Alcohol Clin Exp Res* 1997; **21**: 1418–28.

271 Maier SE, Miller JA, Blackwell JM, West JR. Fetal alcohol exposure and temporal vulnerability: regional differences in cell loss as a function of the timing of binge-like alcohol exposure during brain development. *Alcohol Clin Exp Res* 1999; **23**: 726–34.

272 Mair WGP, Warrington GK, Weiskrantz L. Memory disorder in Korsakoff's psychosis. *Brain* 1979; **102**: 749–83.

273 Malamud N, Skillicorn SA. Relationship between the Wernicke and Korsakoff syndrome. *Arch Neurol Psychiatry* 1956; **76**: 585–96.

274 Manz HJ, Colon AR. Neuropathology, pathogenesis and neuropsychiatric sequelae of Reye syndrome. *J Neurol Sci* 1982; **53**: 377–95.

275 Manz HJ, Robertson DM. Vascular permeability to horseradish peroxidase in brainstem lesions of thiamine-deficient rats. *Am J Pathol* 1972; **66**: 565–76.

276 Marchiafava E, Bignami A. Sopra un alterazione del corpo callosa osservata in sogetti alcoolista. *Riv Patol Nerv Mentale* 1903; **8**: 544–9.

277 Marcus JC. Neurological findings in the fetal alcohol syndrome. *Neuropediatrics* 1987; **18**: 158–60.

278 Martin JJ, Schlote W. Central nervous system lesions in disorders of amino-acid metabolism. *J Neurol Sci* 1972; **15**: 49–76.

279 Martinasevic MK, Rios GR, Miller MW, Tephly TR. Folate and folate-dependent enzymes associated with rat CNS development. *Dev Neurosci* 1999; **21**: 29–35.

280 Martinez A. Electron microscopy in human hepatic encephalopathy. *Acta Neuropathol* 1968; **11**: 82–6.

281 Mayatepek E, Becker K, Gana L et al. Leukotrienes in the pathophysiology of kwashiorkor. *Lancet* 1993; **342**: 958–60.

282 Mayer JM, De Liege P, Netter JM et al. Computerized tomography and nuclear magnetic resonance imaging in Marchiafava–Bignami disease. *J Neuroradiol* 1987; **14**: 152–8.

283 Mayer-Gross W, Slater E, Roth M. *Clinical psychiatry*. London: Cassell, 1954.

284 Mayes AR, Meudell PR, Mann D, Pickering A. Locations of the lesions in Korsakoff's syndrome: neuropathological data on two patients. *Cortex* 1988; **24**: 367–88.

285 McCombe PA, McCLeod JG. The peripheral neuropathy of vitamin B_{12} deficiency. *J Neurol Sci* 1984; **66**: 117–26.

286 McConnell P, Berry M. The effects of refeeding after varying periods of neonatal undernutrition on the morphology of Purkinje cells in the cerebellum of the rat. *J Comp Neurol* 1981; **200**: 433–79.

287 McDougall AJ, McLeod JG. Autonomic neuropathy, I. Clinical features, investigation, pathophysiology, and treatment. *J Neurol Sci* 1996; **137**: 79–88.

288 McDougall AJ, McLeod JG. Autonomic neuropathy, II: Specific peripheral neuropathies. *J Neurol Sci* 1996; **138**: 1–13.

289 McEntee WJ, Mair RG. The Korsakoff syndrome: a neurochemical perspective. *Trends Neurosci* 1990; **13**: 340–4.

290 McKee AC, Winkleman MD, Banker BQ. Central pontine myelinolysis in severely burned patients: relationship to serum hyperosmolality. *Neurology* 1988; **38**: 1211–17.

291 McKusick VA. Francomano CA, Antonarakis SE. *Mendelian inheritance in man*. Baltimore, MD: John Hopkins University Press, 1990.

292 McMartin KE, Bates WR, Fortney T, Bhandari SD. *Effect of acute alcohol on membrane transport of folate*. Clifton, NJ: Humana Press, 1989.

293 McMullen PA, Saint-Cyr JA, Carlen PL. Morphological alterations in rat CA1 hippocampal pyramidal cell dendrites resulting from chronic ethanol consumption and withdrawal. *J Comp Neurol* 1984; **225**: 111–18.

294 Meila KR, Ryabinin AE, Corodimas KP et al. Hippocampal-dependent learning and experience-dependent activation of the hippocampus are preferentially disrupted by ethanol. *Neuroscience* 1996; **74**: 313–22.

295 Meldrum B, Garthwaite J. Excitatory amino acid neurotoxicity and neurodegenerative disease. *Trends Pharmacol Sci* 1991; **11** Suppl: 54–62.

296 Messert B, Orrison WMH, M.J., Quaglieri CE. Central pontine myelinolysis. *Neurology* 1979; **29**: 147–60.

297 Meyer A. On parenchymatous systemic degeneration mainly in the central nervous system. *Brain* 1901; **24**: 47–115.

298 Meyer A. The Wernicke syndrome: with special reference to manic syndromes associated with hypothalamic lesions. *J Neurol Psychiatry* 1944; **7**: 66–75.

299 Meyer UA, Schuurmans MM, Lindberg RL. Acute porphyrias: pathogenesis of neurological manifestations. *Semin Liver Dis* 1998; **18**: 43–52.

300 Michaelis EK. Fetal alcohol exposure: cellular toxicity and molecular events involved in toxicity. *Alcohol Clin Exp Res* 1990; **14**: 819–26.

301 Miller MW. Effect of prenatal exposure to ethanol on the development of cerebral cortex: I. Neuronal generation. *Alcohol Clin Exp Res* 1988; **12**: 440–9.

302 Miller MW. Supporting cells as targets of ethanol toxicity: altered regulation of growth factors and extracellular matrix. *Alcohol Clin Exp Res* 1996; **20**: 260–4A.

303 Miller MW, Potempa G. Numbers of neurons and glia in mature rat somatosensory cortex: effects of prenatal exposure to ethanol. *J Comp Neurol* 1990; **293**: 92–102.

304 Miller RF, Harrison MJ, Hall-Craggs MA, Scaravilli F. Central pontine myelinolysis in AIDS. *Acta Neuropathol* 1998; **96**: 537–40.

305 Moloney CJ, Parmalee AH. Convulsions in young infants as a result of pyridoxine (vitamin B_6) deficiency. *JAMA* 1954; **154**: 405.

306 Morgane PJ, Austin-LaFrance R, Bronzino J et al. Prenatal malnutrition and development of the brain. *Neurosci Behav Rev* 1993; **17**: 91–128.

307 Mousseau DD, Perney P, Pomier Layargues G, Butterworth RF. Selective loss of pallidal dopamine D_2 receptor density in hepatic encephalopathy. *Neurosci Lett* 1993; **162**: 192–6.

308 MRC Vitamin Study Research Group. Prevention of neural tube defects: results of the Medical Council Vitamin Study. *Lancet* 1991; **338**: 131–7.

309 Mudd SH, Levy HL, Skovby F. Disorders of transsulfuration. In: Scriver CF, Beaudet AL, Sly WS, Valle D eds. *The metabolic basis of inherited disease* 6th edn. New York: McGraw-Hill, 1989: 693–734.

310 Mueller JF, Vitler RW. Pyridoxine deficiency in human beings induced with desoxypyridoxine. *J Clin Invest* 1950; **29**: 193.

311 Muller K, Kahn T, Wendel U. Is demyelination a feature of maple syrup urine disease? *Pediatr Neurol* 1993; **9**: 375–82.

312 Munoz SJ, Robinson M, Northup B et al. Elevated intracranial pressure and computed tomography of the brain in fulminant hepatocellular failure. *Hepatology* 1990; **13**: 209–12.

313 Naidoo PN, Bramdev A, Cooper K. Wernicke's encepathalopathy and alcohol-related disease. *Postgrad Med J* 1991; **67**: 978–81.

314 Nau H. Valproic acid-induced neural tube defects. *Ciba Found Symp* 1994; **181**: 144–52.

315 Nayak P, Chatterjee AK. Impact of protein malnutrition on subcellular nucleic acid and protein status of brain of aluminum-exposed rats. *J Toxicol Sci* 1998; **23**: 1–14.

316 Newell KL, Kleinschmidt-DeMasters BK. Central pontine myelinolysis at autopsy; a twelve year retrospective analysis. *J Neurol Sci* 1996; **142**: 134–9.

317 Nordmann Y, Puy H, Deybach JC. The porphyrias. *Hepatology* 1999; **30**: 12–16.

318 Norenberg MD. A light and electron microscopic study of experimental portal–systemic (ammonia) encephalopathy. Progression and reversal of the disorder. *Lab Invest* 1977; **36**: 618–27.

319 Norenberg MD. Astrocyte response to CNS injury. *J Neuropathol Exp Neurol* 1994; **53**: 213–20.

320 Norenberg MD. The astrocyte in liver disease. *Adv Cell Neurobiol* 1981; **2**: 303–52.

321 Norenberg MD, Leslie KO, Robertson AS. Association between rise in serum sodium and central pontine myelinolysis. *Ann Neurol* 1982; **11**: 128–35.

322 Norenberg MD, Neary JT, Norenberg LOB, McCarthy M. Ammonia induced decrease in glial fibrillary acidic protein in cultured astrocytes. *J Neuropathol Exp Neurol* 1990; **49**: 399–405.

323 Norton WN, Daskal I, Savage HE et al. Effects of riboflavin deficiency on the ultrastructure of rat sciatic nerve fibres. *Am J Pathol* 1976; **85**: 651–60.

324 Ogunleye AJ, Odutuga AA. The effect of riboflavin deficiency on cerebrum and cerebellum of developing rat brain. *J Nutri Sci Vitaminol* 1989; **35**: 193–7.

325 Ohnishi A, Tsuji S, Igisu H et al. Beriberi neuropathy. Morphometric study of sural nerve. *J Neurol Sci* 1980; **45**: 177–90.

326 Olney J. Excitotoxin-mediated death in youth and old age. *Prog Brain Res* 1990; **86**: 37–51.

327 Orlowski JP. Whatever happened to Reye's syndrome? Did it ever really exist? *Crit Care Med* 1999; **27**: 1582–7.

328 Oscar-Berman M, Hutner N. Frontal lobe changes after chronic alcohol ingestion. In: Hunt WA, Nixon SJ eds. *Alcohol induced brain damage*. Rockville, MD: NIH Publications, 1993: 121–56.

329 Osuntokun BO. Epidemic ataxia in Western Nigeria. *BMJ* 1972; **ii**: 589.

330 Pallis CA, Lewis PD. *The neurology of gastrointestinal disease*. London: Saunders, 1974.

331 Pant SS, Asbury AK, Richardson EPJ. The myelopathy of pernicious anaemia. A neuropathological appraisal. *Acta Med Scand Suppl* 1968; **44**: 1–36.

332 Pantazis NJ, Dohman DP, Goodlett CR et al. Vulnerability of cerebellar granule cells to alcohol induced cell death diminishes with time in culture. *Alcohol Clin Exp Res* 1993; **17**: 1014–21.

333 Papadakis MA, Fraser CL, Arieff AI. Hyponatraemia in patients with cirrhosis. *Q J Med* 1990; **76**: 675–88.

334 Parry TE. Folate responsive neuropathy. *Presse Med* 1994; **23**: 131–7.

335 Partin JS, McAdams AJ, Partin JC et al. Brain ultrastucture in Reye's disease. II. *J Neuropathol Exp Neurol* 1978; **37**: 796–819.

336 Peeling AN, Smart JL. Review of literature showing that undernutrition affects the growth rate of all processes in the brain to the same extent. *Metab Brain Dis* 1994; **9**: 33–42.

337 Peeters A, Van de Wyngaert F, Van Lierde M et al. Wernicke's encephalopathy and central pontine myelinolysis induced by hyperemesis gravidarum. *Acta Neurol Belg* 1993; **93**: 276–82.

338 Peiffer J, Majewski F, Fischbach H et al. Alcohol embryo and fetopathy. *J Neurol Sci* 1979; **41**: 125–37.

339 Pena CE. Wernicke's encepathalopathy: report of seven cases with severe nerve cell changes in the mamillary bodies. *Am J Clin Pathol* 1969; **51**: 603–9.

340 Pena CE, Felter R. Ultrastructural changes of the lateral vestibular nucleus in acute experimental thiamine deficiency. *Z Neurol* 1973; **204**: 263–80.

341 Pentney RJ. Alterations in the structure of the cerebellum after long-term ethanol consumption. In: Hunt WA, Nixon SJ eds. *Alcohol-induced Brain Damage*. Rockville, MD: US Department of Health and Human Services, 1993:249–76.

342 Pentney RJ. Quantitative analysis of ethanol effects on Purkinje cell dendritic tree. *Brain Res* 1982; **249**: 397–401.

343 Perdrau JR. Schilder's encephalitis periaxialis diffusa in rhesus monkey. *J Pathol Bacteriol* 1930; **32**: 991–4.

344 Petito CK, Navia BA, Cho ES et al. Vacuolar myelopathy pathologically resembling subacute combined degeneration in patients with the acquired immunodeficiency syndrome. *N Engl J Med* 1985; **312**: 874–9.

345 Pfefferbaum A, Lim KO, Desmond JE, Sullivan EV. Thinning of the corpus callosum in older alcoholic men: a magnetic resonance imaging study. *Alcohol, Clin Exp Res* 1996; **20**: 752–7.

346 Phillips GB, Victor M, Adams RD. A study of the nutritional defect in Wernicke's syndrome. The effect of a purified diet, thiamine, and other vitamins on the clinical manifestations. *J Clin Invest* 1952; **31**: 859–71.

347 Phillips SC, Cragg BG. A change in susceptibility of rat cerebellar Purkinje cells to damage by alcohol during fetal, neonatal and adult life. *Neuropathol Appl Neurobiol* 1982; **8**: 441–54.

348 Phillips SC, Harper CG, Kril J. A quantitative histological study of the cerebellar vermis in alcoholic patients. *Brain* 1987; **110**: 301–14.

349 Phillips SC, Harper CG, Kril JJ. The contribution of Wernicke's encephalopathy to alcohol-related cerebellar damage. *Drug Alcohol Rev* 1990; **9**: 53–60.

350 Pierce DR, Goodlett CR, West JR. Differential neuronal loss following postnatal alcohol exposure. *Teratology* 1989; **40**: 113–26.

351 Pierog S, Chandavasu O, Wexler I. Withdrawal symptoms in infants with the fetal alcohol syndrome. *J Pediatr* 1977; **90**: 630–3.

352 Pilbeam CM, Anderson RM, Bhthal PS. The brain in experimental portal-systemic encephalopathy. 1. Morphological changes in three animal models. *J Pathol* 1983; **140**: 331–45.

353 Pincus JH, Reynolds EH, Glaser GH. Subacute combined system degeneration with folate deficiency. *JAMA* 1972; **221**: 496–7.

354 Pitsikas N, Carli M, Fidecka S, Algeri S. Effects of life-long hypocaloric diet on age-related changes in motor and cognitive behaviour in a rat population. *Neurobiol Aging* 1990; **11**: 417–23.

355 Platt BS. Clinical features of endemic beriberi. *Fed Proc* 1958; **17**: 8–20.

356 Platt BS, Stewart RJC. Effects of protein calorie deficiency on dogs. 2. Morphological changes on the nervous system. *Dev Med Child Neurol* 1969; **11**: 174–92.

357 Powers JM. Metabolic diseases of the nervous system. In: Rosenberg RN ed. *The clinical neurosciences*. New York: Churchill Livingstone, 1983: 447–94.

358 Powers JM, McKeever PE. Central pontine myelinolysis. An ultrastructural and elemental study. *J Neurol Sci* 1976; **29**: 65–81.

359 Pretorius PJ, Novis H. Nutritional marasmus in Bantu infants in the Pretoria area. II. Clinical and pathological aspects. *South Afr Med J* 1965; **39**: 501.

360 Price JM, Brown RR, Peters HA. Tryptophan metabolism in porphyria, schizophrenia, and a variety of neurologic and psychiatric diseases. *Neurology* 1959; **9**: 456.

361 Ramos M. Vitamin B_{12} deficiency and hydrocephalus. In: Fields WS, Desmond MM, eds. *Disorders of the developing nervous system*. Springfield, IL: Charles C Thomas, 1961: 146.

362 Reusche E. Argyrophilic inclusions distinct from Alzheimer neurofibrillary changes in one case of dialysis-associated encephalopathy. *Acta Neuropathol (Berl)* 1997; **94**: 612–16.

363 Reynolds EH. Neurological aspects of folate and vitamin B_{12} metabolism. *Clin Haematol* 1976; **5**: 661–96.

364 Rickes EL, Brink NG, Konuisky FR *et al*. Vitamin B_{12}, a cobalt complex. *Science* 1948; **108**: 134.

365 Rindi G. Metabolism of thiamine and its phosphoric esters in different regions of the nervous system: a new approach. *Acta Vitaminol Enzymol* 1982; **4**: 59–68.

366 Rintala J, Jaatinen P, Lu W *et al*. Effects of lifelong ethanol consumption on cerebellar layer volumes in AA and ANA rats. *Alcohol Clin Exp Res* 1997; **21**: 311–17.

367 Robertson DM, Wasan SM, Skinner DB. Ultrastructural changes of features of early brainstem lesions in thiamine deficient rats. *Am J Pathol* 1968; **52**: 1081–7.

368 Roebuck TM, Mattson SN, Riley EP. A review of the neuroanatomical findings in children with fetal alcohol syndrome or prenatal exposure to alcohol. *Alcohol Clin Exp Res* 1998; **22**: 339–44.

369 Roecklein B, Levin SW, Comly M, Mukherjee AB. Intrauterine growth retardation induced by thiamine deficiency and pyrithamine during pregnancy in the rat. *Am J Obstet Gynecol* 1985; **151**: 455–60.

370 Romero-Lopez J, Moreno-Carretero MJ, Escriche-Jaime D *et al*. The association of Marchiafava–Bignami disease, cerebral pellagra and cerebellar degeneration in an alcoholic patient. *Rev Neurol* 1997; **25**: 1577–8.

371 Rooprai HK, Pratt OE, Shaw GK, Thomson AD. Thiamine pyrophosphate effect and normalized erythrocyte transketolase activity ratio in Wernicke–Korsakoff patients and acute alcoholics undergoing detoxification. *Alcohol Alcohol* 1996; **31**: 493–501.

372 Rosenbaum DH. MRI in porphyria. *Neurology* 1994; **44**: 1553–4.

373 Rosenberg RN. In: *Neurogenetics: principles and practice*. New York: Raven Press, 1986; 168–82.

374 Rosett HL, Weiner L. *Alcohol and the fetus: a clinical perspective*. New York: Oxford University Press, 1984.

375 Royland J, Klinkhachorn P, Konat G, Wiggins RC. How much undernourishment is required to retard brainmyelin development. *Neurochem Int* 1992; **21**: 269–74.

376 Russell JSR, Batten FE, Collier J. Subacute combined degeneration of the spinal cord. *Brain* 1900; **23**: 39–110.

377 Sage JI, Van Uitert RL, Lepore FE. Alcoholic myelopathy without substantial liver disease. A syndrome of progressive dorsal and lateral column dysfunction. *Arch Neurol* 1984; **41**: 999–1001.

378 Scalabrino G, Nicolini G, Buccellato FR *et al*. Epidermal growth factor as a local mediator of the neurotrophic action of vitamin B_{12} (cobalamin) in the rat central nervous system. *FASEB J* 1999; **13**: 2083–90.

379 Schaeffer MC, Gretz D, Gietzen DW, Rogers QR. Dietary excess of vitamin B_6 affects the concentrations of amino acids in the caudate nucleus and serum and the binding properties of serotonin receptors in the brain cortex of rats. *J Nutr* 1998; **128**: 1829–35.

380 Schmahmann JD, Sherman JC. The cerebellar cognitive affective syndrome. *Brain* 1998; **121**: 561–79.

381 Schwarz GA, Moulton JAL. Porphria. *Arch Intern Med* 1954; **94**: 221–33.

382 Scott JM, Wilson P, Dinn JJ, Weir DG. Pathogenesis of subacute combined degeneration: a result of methyl group deficiency. *Lancet* 1981; **ii**: 334–7.

383 Scriver CR, Kaufman S, Woo SLC. The hyperphenylalaninemias. In: Scriver CF, Beaudet AL, Sly WS, Valle D eds. *The metabolic basis of inherited disease* 6th edn. New York: McGraw-Hill, 1989: 495–546.

384 Sebrell WHJ, Butler RE. Riboflavin deficiency in man (ariboflavinosis). *Public Health Rep* 1939; **54**: 2121–31.

385 Selwa LM, Vanderzant CW, Brunberg JA *et al*. Correlation of evoked potential and MRI findings in Wilson's disease. *Neurology* 1993; **43**: 2059–64.

386 Serdaru M, Hausser-Hauw C, Laplane D *et al*. The clinical spectrum of alcoholic pellagra encephalopathy. *Brain* 1988; **111**: 829–42.

387 Shaw JH, Phillips PH. The pathology of riboflavin deficiency in the rat. *J Nutr* 1941; **22**: 345–58.

388 Shear PK, Sullivan EV, Lane B, Pfefferbaum A. Mammillary body and cerebellar shrinkage in chronic alcoholics with and without amnesia. *Alcohol Clin Exp Res* 1996; **20**: 1489–95.

389 Sheedy D, Lara A, Garrick T, Harper C. The size of the mamillary bodies in health and disease. *Alcohol Clin Exp Res* 1999; **23**: 1624–8.

390 Shibata K, Toda S. Effects of sex hormones on the metabolism of tryptophan to niacin and to serotonin in male rats. *Biosci Biotech Biochem* 1997; **61**: 1200–2.

391 Shih JJ, Kornblum H, Shewmon DA. Global brain dysfunction in an infant with pyridoxine dependency: evaluation with EEG, evoked potentials, MRI, and PET. *Neurology* 1996; **47**: 824–6.

392 Shiraishi T, Black KL, Ikesaki K. Peripheral benzodiazepine receptor ligands induce morphological changes in mitochondria of cultured glioma cells. *J Neurosci Res* 1991; **30**: 463–74.

393 Shuman RM, Leech RW, Scott CR. The neuropathology of the nonketotic and ketotic hyperglycinemias: three cases. *Neurology* 1978; **28**: 139–46.

394 Siassi F, Siassi B. Differential effects of protein–calorie restriction and subsequent repletion on neuronal and non-neuronal components of cerebral cortex in newborn rats. *J Nutr* 1973; **103**: 1625–33.

395 Small DH, Carnegie PR, Anderson RM. Cycloleucine induced vacuolation of myelin is associated with inhibition of protein methylation. *Neurosci Lett* 1981; **21**: 287–92.

396 Smith DE, Foundas A, Canale J. Effect of perinatally administered ethanol on the development of the cerebellar granule cell. *Exp Neurol* 1986; **92**: 491–501.

397 Snell EE, Guirard BM, Williams RJ. Occurrence of natural products of physiologically active metabolite of pyridoxine. *J Biol Chem* 1942; **143**: 519.

398 Sobel RA, DeArmond SJ, Forno LS, Eng LF. Glial fibrillary acidic protein in hepatic encephalopathy: an immunohistochemical study. *J Neuropathol Exp Neurol* 1981; **40**: 625–32.

399 Sokol RJ, Ager J, Martier S *et al*. Significant determinants of susceptibility to alcohol teratogenicity. *Ann NY Acad Sci* 1986; **477**: 87–102.

400 Sokol RJ, Miller SI, Reed G. Alcohol abuse during pregnancy: an epidemiological study. Alcohol Clin Exp Res 1980; **4**: 135–45.

401 Squire LR, Knowlton B, Musen G. The structure and organization of memory. *Annu Rev Psychol* 1993; **44**: 435–95.

402 Stannus HS. Some problems in riboflavin and their deficiencies. *BMJ* 1944; **ii**: 103–5.

403 Steiner I, Kidron D, Soffer D *et al*. Sensory peripheral neuropathy of vitamin B_{12} deficiency: a primary demyelinating disease? *J Neurol* 1988; **235**: 163–4.

404 Still CN. *Nicotinic acid and nicotinamide deficiency: pellagra and related disorders of the nervous system*. Amsterdam: North-Holland, 1976.

405 Stoch MB, Smythe PM. The effects of undernutrition during infancy in subsequent brain growth and intellectual development. *South Afr Med J* 1967; **41**: 1027–30.

406 Strachan RW, Henderson JG. Dementia and folate deficiency. *Q J Med* 1967; **36**: 189–204.

407 Streissguth AP. Psychologic handicaps in children with the fetal alcohol syndrome. *Ann NY Acad Sci* 1976; **273**: 140–5.

408 Streissguth AP, Aase JM, Clarren SK, Randels SP, LaDue RA, Smith DF. Fetal alcohol syndrome in adolescents and adults. *JAMA* 1991; **265**: 1961–7.

409 Stromland K. Ocular involvement in the fetal alcohol syndrome. *Surv Ophthalmol* 1987; **31**: 277–84.

410 Suarez JI, Cohen ML, Larkin J *et al*. Acute intermittent porphyria: clinicopathologic correlation. Report of a case and review of the literature. *Neurology* 1997; **48**: 1678–83.

411 Sulik KK, Lauder JM, Dehort DB. Brain malformations in prenatal mice following acute maternal ethanol administration. *Int J Dev Neurosci* 1984; **2**: 203–14.

412 Sullivan E, Lane B, Deshmukh A *et al*. *In vivo* mamillary body volume deficits in amnesic and nonamnesic alcoholics. *Alcohol Clin Exp Res* 1999; **23**: 1629–36.

413 Sullivan EV, Marsh L, Mathalon DH *et al*. Anterior hippocampal volume deficits in nonamnesic, ageing chronic alcoholics. *Alcohol Clin Exp Res* 1995; **19**: 110–22.

414 Sullivan EV, Marsh L, Mathalon DH *et al*. Relationship between alcohol withdrawal seizures and temporal lobe white matter volume deficits. *Alcohol Clin Exp Res* 1996; **20**: 348–54.

415 Takahashi K, Nakamura H. Axonal degeneration in beriberi neuropathy. *Arch Neurol* 1976; **33**: 836–41.

416 Tamura N, Baverstock J, McLeod J. A morphometric study of the carotid sinus nerve in patients with diabetes mellitus and chronic alcoholism. *J Auton Nerv Syst* 1988; **23**: 9–15.

417 Tan SV, Guiloff RJ. Hypothesis on the pathogenesis of vacuolar myelopathy, dementia, and peripheral neuropathy in AIDS. *J Neurol, Neurosurg Psychiatry* 1998; **65**: 23–8.

418 Tavares MA, Paula-Barbosa MM. Lipofuscin granules in Purkinje cells after long-term alcohol consumption in rats. *Alcohol Clin Exp Res* 1983; **7**: 302–6.

419 Tellez I, Terry RD. Fine structure of the early changes in the vestibular nuclei of the thiamine-deficient rat. *Am J Pathol* 1968; **52**: 777–87.

420 Thomas PK, London DN, King RHM. Diseases of peripheral nerves. In: Adams JH, Corsellis JAN, Duchen LW, eds. *Greenfield's neuropathology* 4th edn. London: Edward Arnold, 1984: 806–920.

421 Thompson AJ, Tillotson S, Smith I *et al*. Brain MRI changes in phenylketonuria. Associations with dietary status. *Brain* 1993; **116**: 811–21.

422 Thomson AD, Jeyasingham MD, Pratt OE, Shaw GK. Nutrition and alcoholic encephalopathies. *Acta Med Scand Suppl* 1987; **717**: 55–65.

423 Todd KG, Butterworth RF. Early microglial response in experimental thiamine deficiency: an immunohistochemical analysis. *Glial* 1999; **25**: 190–8.

424 Todd KG, Butterworth RF. Evaluation of the role of NMDA-mediated excitotoxicity in the selective neuronal loss in experimental Wernicke encephalopathy. *Exp Neurol* 1998; **149**: 130–8.

425 Todd KG, Butterworth RF. Increased neuronal survival after L-Deprenyl treatment in experimental thiamine deficiency. *J Neurosci Res* 1998; **52**: 240–6.

426 Tork I, Hornung J-P. Raphe nuclei and the serotonergic system. In: Paxinos G ed. *The human nervous system*. San Diego, CA: Academic Press, 1990: 1001–22.

427 Torvik A. Topographic distribution and severity of brain lesions in Wernicke's encephalopathy. *Clin Neuropathol* 1987; **6**: 25–9.

428 Torvik A. Two types of brain lesions in Wernicke's encephalopathy. *Neuropathol Appl Neurobiol* 1985; **11**: 179–90.

429 Torvik A, Lindboe CF, Rodge S. Brain lesions in alcoholics. A neuropathological study with clinical correlations. *J Neurol Sci* 1982; **56**: 233–48.

430 Torvik A, Skjorten F. Electron microscopic observations on nerve cell regeneration and degeneration after axon lesions: I. changes in the nerve cell cytoplasm. *Acta Neuropathol (Berl)* 1971; **17**: 248–64.

431 Torvik A, Torp S. The prevalence of alcoholic cerebellar atrophy. A morphometric and histological study of autopsy material. *J Neurol Sci* 1986; **75**: 43–51.

432 Tredici G, Buccellato FR, Braga M et al. Polyneuropathy due to cobalamin deficiency in the rat [published erratum appears in *J Neurol Sci* 1999; **162**: 209]. *J Neurol Sci* 1998; **156**: 18–29.

433 Tredici G, Buccellato FR, Cavaletti G, Scalabrino G. Subacute combined degeneration in totally gastrectomized rats: an ultrastructural study. *J Submicrosc Cytol Pathol* 1998; **30**: 165–73.

434 Troncoso JC, Johnston MV, Hess KM, Price DL. Model of Wernicke's encephalopathy. *Arch Neurol* 1981; **38**: 350–4.

435 Trost LC, Lemasters JJ. The mitochondrial permeability transition: a new pathophysiological mechanism for Reye's syndrome and toxic liver injury. *J Pharmacol Exp Ther* 1996; **278**: 1000–5.

436 Trowell HC, Davies JND, Dean RFA. *Kwashiorkor*. London: Edward Arnold, 1954.

437 Udani PM. Kwashiorkor myelopathy. *Indian J Child Health* 1962; **11**: 498–501.

438 Udani PM. Nutritional problems in developing countries. *Paediatrician* 1979; **8** (Suppl): 48–63.

439 Udani PM. Protein energy malnutrition (PEM), brain and various facets of child development. *Indian J Pediatr* 1992; **59**: 165–86.

440 Udani PM, Dastur DK. Pediatric malnutrition: a global neurological problem. In: Dastur DK, Shahani M, Bharucha EP eds. *Neurological sciences – an overview of current problems*. New Delhi: Interprint, 1989: 251–75.

441 Van der Westhuyzen J, Fernandez-Costa F, Metz J. Cobalamin inactivation by nitrous oxide produces severe neurological impairment in fruit bats. Protection by methionine and aggravation by folates. *Life Sci* 1982; **31**: 2001–10.

442 Veresova S, Kabova R, Velisek L. Proconvulsant effects induced by pyridoxine in young rats. *Epilepsy Res* 1998; **29**: 259–64.

443 Viana GS, Figueiredo RM, Bruno JA. Effects of protein-energy malnutrition on muscarinic receptor density and acetylcholinesterase activity in rat brain. *Ann Nutr Metab* 1997; **41**: 52–9.

444 Victor M, Adams RD, Collins GH. *The Wernicke–Korsakoff syndrome*, 1st edn. Oxford: Blackwell Scientific, 1971.

445 Victor M, Adams RD, Collins GH. *The Wernicke–Korsakoff syndrome*, 2nd edn. Philadelphia, PA: Davis, 1989.

446 Victor M, Laureno R. *Neurologic complications of alcohol abuse: epidemiologic aspects*. New York: Raven Press, 1978.

447 Vitler KLW, Mueller JF, Glazer HS et al. The effect of vitamin B_6 deficiency induced by desoxypyridoxine in human beings. *J Lab Clin Med* 1953; **42**: 335–57.

448 Volk B. *Neurohistological and neurobiological aspects of fetal alcohol syndrome in the rat*. New York: Elsevier Science Publishers, 1984.

449 Von Cramon DY, Hebel N, Schuri U. A contribution to the anatomical basis of thalamic amnesia. *Brain* 1985; **108**: 993–1008.

450 Vortmeyer AO, Colmant HJ. Differentiation between brain lesions in experimental thaimine deficiency. *Virchows Archiv A Pathol Anat Histopathol* 1988; **414**: 61–7.

451 Wakui H, Nishimura S, Watahiki Y et al. Dramatic recovery from neurological deficits in a patient with central pontine myelinolysis following severe hyponatremia. *Jpn J Med* 1991; **30**: 281–4.

452 Walker DW, Barnes DE, Zorneyzer SF et al. Neuronal loss in hippocampus induced by prolonged ethanol consumption in rats. *Science* 1980; **209**: 711–13.

453 Walsh JC, McLeod JG. Alcoholic neuropathy. An electrophysiological and histological study. *J Neurol Sci* 1970; **10**: 459–69.

454 Walter JH, Tyfield LA, Holton JB, Johnson C. Biochemical control, genetic analysis and magnetic resonance imaging in patients with phenylketonuria. *Eur J Pediatr* 1993; **152**: 822–7.

455 Watanabe I, Tomita T, Hung K-S, Iwasaki Y. Edematous necrosis in thiamine-deficient encephalopathy of the mouse. *J Neuropathol Exp Neurol* 1981; **40**: 454–71.

456 Weir DG, Keating S, Molloy A et al. Methylation deficiency causes vitamin B_{12} associated neuropathy in the pig. *J Neurochem* 1988; **51**: 1949–52.

457 Werler MM, Shapiro S, Mitchell AA. Preconceptional folic acid exposure and risk of occurrent neural tube defects. *JAMA* 1993; **269**: 1257–61.

458 Wernicke C. *Der acute haemorrhagische Polioencephalitis superior*. Berlin: Fischer, Kassel, 1881.

459 West JR. Recent findings on the mechanisms by which alcohol damages the developing nervous system. *Alcohol Alcohol* 1994; **2**: 395–9.

460 West JR, Goodlett CR, Bonthius DJ et al. Cell population depletion associated with fetal alcohol brain damage: mechanisms of BAC-dependent cell loss. *Alcohol Clin Exp Res* 1990; **14**: 813–18.

461 West JR, Hamre KM, Pierce DR. Delay in brain development induced by alcohol in artificially reared rat pups. *Alcohol* 1984; **1**: 213–22.

462 West JR, Pierce DR. *Perinatal alcohol exposure and neuronal damage*. New York: Oxford University Press, 1986.

463 White HH, Rowland LP, Araki S et al. Homocystinuria. *Arch Neurol* 1965; **13**: 455.

464 Wijdicks EF, Blue PR, Steers JL, Wiesner RH. Central pontine myelinolysis with stupor alone after orthotopic liver transplantation. *Liver Transplant Surg* 1996; **2**: 14–16.

465 Wilkinson P, Kornaczewski A, Rankin JG, Santamaria JN. Physical disease in alcoholism. Initial survey of 1,000 patients. *Med J Aust* 1971; **1**: 1217–23.

466 Winkelman NW. Beitrage zur Neurohistopathologie der Pellagra. *Z Neurol Psychiat* 1926; **102**: 38.

467 Winick M, Rosso P. The effect of severe early malnutrition on cellular growth of human brain. *Pediatr Res* 1969; **3**: 181.

468 Winick M, Rosso P, Waterlow J. Cellular growth of cerebrum, cerebellum and brain stem in normal and marasmic children. *Exp Neurol* 1970; **26**: 393–400.

469 Wisniewski K, Dambska W, Sher JH, Qazi Q. A clinical neuropathology study of the fetal alcohol syndrome. *Neuropediatrics* 1983; **14**: 197–201.

470 Witt ED, Goldman-Rakic PS. Intermittent thiamine deficiency in the rhesus monkey, I. Progression of neurological signs and neuronanatomical lesions. *Ann Neurol* 1983; **13**: 376–95.

471 Witt ED, Goldman-Rakic PS. Intermittent thiamine deficiency in the rhesus monkey II. Evidence for memory loss. *Ann Neurol* 1983; **13**: 396–401.

472 Wright DG, Laureno R, Victor M. Pontine and extrapontine myelinolysis. *Brain* 1979; **102**: 361–85.

473 Wu D, Pardridge WM. Blood–brain barrier transport of reduced folic acid. *Pharm Res* 1999; **16**: 415–19.

474 Xu Y, Sladky JT, Brown MJ. Dose-dependent expression of neuronopathy after experimental pyridoxine intoxication. *Neurology* 1989; **39**: 1077–83.

475 Yamada K, Shrier DA, Tanaka H, Numaguchi Y. A case of subacute combined degeneration: MRI findings *Neuroradiology* 1998; **40**: 398–400.

476 Yamada M, Kondo M, Tanaka M *et al*. An autopsy case of acute porphyria with a decrease of both uroporphyrinogen I synthetase and ferrochelatase activities. *Acta Neuropathol* 1984; **64**: 6–11.

477 Yousry TA, Strupp M, Bruning R. Common variable immunodeficiency leading to spinal subacute combined degeneration monitored by MRI. *J Neurol, Neurosurg Psychiatry* 1998; **64**: 663–6.

478 Zamora AJ, Cavanagh JB, Kyn MH. Ultrastructural response of the astrocytes to portcaval anastomosis in the rat. *J Neurol Sci* 1973; **18**: 25–45.

479 Zieve L, Mendelson DF, Goepfert M. Shunt encephalopathy. II. Occurrence of permanent myelopathy. *Ann Intern Med* 1960; **53**: 53–63.

480 Zimitat C, Kril J, Harper CG, Nixon PF. Progression of neurological disease in thiamin deficient rats is enhanced by ethanol. *Alcohol* 1990; **7**: 493–501.

11

Lysosomal diseases

KINUKO SUZUKI AND KUNIHIKO SUZUKI

INTRODUCTION

Lysosome is the subcellular membrane-bound organelle containing acid hydrolases responsible for digestion of cellular constituents.[133] Defective catabolic activity of any of these enzymes results in blockage of the intracellular digestive process. As a result, undigested substrate accumulates within the lysosome, forming abnormal intracellular inclusions or storage bodies. In 1963, Hers discovered that type II glycogenosis (Pompe's disease) is caused by the defect of an α-1,4-glucosidase normally present in lysosomes and that glycogen accumulated within vacuoles presumably derived from the lysosomal system, and proposed the concept of inborn lysosomal disorder or lysosomal storage disease.[279,280] This concept included two easily detectable characteristics: (1) a single lysosomal hydrolytic enzyme must be genetically deficient, and (2) as a consequence, the substrate of the defective enzyme accumulates within pathologically altered secondary lysosomes. At least 41 distinct genetic lysosomal disorders have been identified. Many involve the central nervous system (CNS). They are autosomal recessive disorders, with the exceptions of Fabry's disease and Hunter's disease, which are X-linked recessive disorders. Today, the enzyme deficiency underlying the majority of the known lysosomal storage diseases has been elucidated and detection of heterozygotes and prenatal diagnosis has become common practice in medicine. Enzyme activity can be determined on any fresh (or frozen) tissues but leukocyte preparations or cultured fibroblasts are routinely used for the enzymic assay in the clinical setting.

The concept of the genetic lysosomal disease has evolved over the years to include those disorders that are caused by genetic abnormalities of lysosomal proteins that

are not themselves enzymes, such as activator proteins or transporter proteins. Lysosomal storage diseases are traditionally classified according to the nature of the material that accumulates within the cells, such as sphingolipidosis or mucopolysaccharidosis. They are a clinically heterogeneous group of diseases and multiple clinical phenotypes are known in each group of the disease. Although definitive diagnosis depends on enzymic assays and/or molecular analysis, morphological investigation of tissues remains an important diagnostic procedure. Many lysosomal storage diseases affect the nervous system but can be diagnosed by biopsy studies of nonneural tissues.[93,217] In some instances, prenatal diagnosis can be carried out by morphological examination of chorionic villi or cultured amniotic cells.[382]

In this chapter, the focus will be on the morphological and pathological aspects of lysosomal storage diseases. Information on the biochemistry and molecular genetics of the individual diseases will be provided to a limited extent. Readers who wish to learn more on the molecular genetics and biochemical aspects of lysosomal diseases are referred to Scriver *et al.*[598,599]

SPHINGOLIPIDOSES

Sphingolipidoses are a group of lysosomal storage diseases caused by deficient activity of lysosomal enzymes crucial for the degradation of sphingolipids. The enzymatic deficiency causes blockage and excessive storage of the undegraded substrate. This group includes gangliosidoses, Niemann–Pick disease types A and B, Gaucher's disease, Farber's disease, Fabry's disease, metachromatic leukodystrophy, multiple sulfatase deficiency, Krabbe's

Table 11.1 *Major sphingolipidoses*

Clinical diagnosis	Affected lipids	Enzyme defect
GM1 gangliosidosis	GM1 ganglioside, Galactose-rich fragments of glycoproteins	GM1 ganglioside β-Galactosidase
GM2 gangliosidosis Tay–Sachs disease; B variant	GM2 ganglioside	β-Hexosaminidase A
B1 variant	GM2 ganglioside	β-Hexosaminidase (see text)
AB variant	GM2 ganglioside	GM2 activator protein
Sandhoff's disease; O variant	GM2 ganglioside, Asialo GM2 ganglioside, Globoside	β-Hexosaminidase A, B
Niemann–Pick disease (A and B)	Sphingomyelin	Sphingomyelinase
Gaucher's disease	Glucosylceramide Glucosylsphingosine	Glucosylceramidase
Farber's disease	Ceramide	Acid ceramidase
Fabry's disease	Trihexosylceramide	α-Galactosidase A
Metachromatic leukodystrophy	Sulfatide	Arylsulfatase A
Multiple sulfatase deficiency	Sulfatide and other compounds (see text)	Arylsulfatase A, B, C and others (see text)
Globoid cell leukodystrophy (Krabbe's disease)	Galactosylceramide Galactosylsphingosine	Galactosylceramidase
Total SAP deficiency	Multiple sphingolipids (see Ref. 77)	Sphingolipid activator protein
SAP-B deficiency	Sulfatide and others	Sulfatidase activator (SAP-B)
SAP-C deficiency	Glucosylceramide	SAP-C

disease, and sphingolipid activator protein (SAP) deficiency (Table 11.1, Fig. 11.1a).

Gangliosidoses

Gangliosidoses are a group of diseases caused by defective degradation and a consequent excessive accumulation of gangliosides in the CNS and to some extent in the viscera. There are two main groups: GM1 and GM2 gangliosidoses.[235,236,655] A case reported as GM3 gangliosidosis was later retracted when the initial findings could not be confirmed in a sibling who died of a clinically identical disease.[78,416,681]

GM1 GANGLIOSIDOSIS AND MORQUIO'S DISEASE TYPE B

These diseases are allelic in that they are both caused by deficient activity of acid β-galactosidase.[18] GM1 gangliosidosis affects predominantly the CNS but in severe infantile cases additional bony and visceral involvements

are prominent. The clinical phenotype of Morquio's disease type B is similar to Morquio's disease type A (MPS IV), characterized by bony abnormalities and corneal clouding but without CNS involvement. CNS damage may occur only secondarily to bony abnormalities.

History and clinical features

The first detailed report of a probable case of GM1 gangliosidosis is that by Norman *et al.*[478] They reported a 9-month-old male infant who presented with generalized flaccidity with enlargement of the liver, a facies with depressed nasal bones, slight corneal haze and lumbar kyphosis, features suggestive of a mucopolysaccharidosis. Cherry-red spots were present at the macula. Histopathologically, there was a massive neuronal storage and infiltration of foamy macrophages in the bone marrow and visceral organs suggestive of Niemann–Pick disease. However, biochemical analysis revealed a large excess of ganglioside in the brain. Reports of similar cases followed.[117,383] Clinical features of these cases are typical of infantile type of GM1 gangliosidosis. Biochemical

a

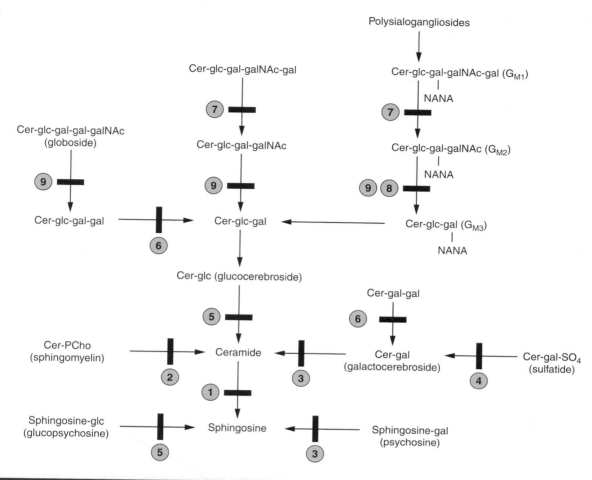

Polysialogangliosides

Cer-glc-gal-galNAc-gal (G$_{M1}$)

| NANA

Cer-glc-gal-galNAc-gal

⑦

Cer-glc-gal-galNAc (G$_{M2}$)

| NANA

Cer-glc-gal-gal-galNAc
(globoside)

Cer-glc-gal-galNAc

Cer-glc-gal-gal (G$_{M3}$)

| NANA

⑨   ⑨   ⑨ ⑧

Cer-glc-gal-gal   Cer-glc-gal

⑥

Cer-glc (glucocerebroside)

Cer-gal-gal

⑤   ⑥

Cer-PCho
(sphingomyelin)   Ceramide   Cer-gal
(galactocerebroside)   Cer-gal-SO$_4$
(sulfatide)

②   ③   ④

①

Sphingosine-glc
(glucopsychosine)   Sphingosine   Sphingosine-gal
(psychosine)

⑤   ③

b

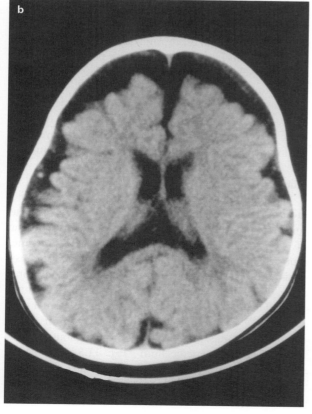

Figure 11.1 (a) Chemical and metabolic relationship among the major sphingolipids. Normal catabolic pathways are indicated by arrows. Biosynthesis of these lipids occurs in the reverse direction. Location of genetic metabolic blocks of known diseases is indicated with a rectangle. The numbers correspond to the following diseases: 1, Farber's disease; 2, Niemann–Pick disease (types A and B); 3, to the globoid cell leukodystrophy (Krabbe's disease); 4, metachromatic leukodystrophy; 5, Gaucher's disease; 6, Fabry's disease; 7, GM1 gangliosidosis; 8, GM2 gangliosidosis (Tay–Sachs disease, B1 variant, AB variant); 9, GM2 gangliosidosis (Sandhoff's disease). (Reproduced from Fig. 41-1, Basic Neurochemistry, 6th edn, Lippincott Williams & Wilkins, by permission of the copyright holder, the American Society for Neurochemistry.) (b) GM1 gangliosidosis, infantile. Axial CT showing diffuse brain atrophy, mildly enlarged lateral ventricles and widened subarachnoid spaces, particularly in the frontal and temporal regions.

characterization that these patients represented an entirely new class of ganglioside storage disease, distinct from the then only known gangliosidosis, Tay–Sachs disease, came a few years later.[229,312,483] Late infantile/juvenile type has a more heterogeneous clinical course, and in some cases the cherry-red spot or visceromegaly may not be apparent. Progressive mental and motor retardation usually begins between 1 and 5 years of age. Dysmorphic features that are pronounced in infantile type are not usually present.[140,214,229,482,560,659,777] Chronic (or adult) type patients have a more slowly progressive pyramidal and extrapyramidal disease without dysmorphic features, visceromegaly or macular cherry-red spot. Intellectual deterioration is usually mild. Dystonia is the most pronounced clinical feature of the adult type of GM1 gangliosidosis.[227,242,464,650,755,785] Morquio's disease type B is primarily a disease of the skeletal system, and neurological manifestations may occur secondarily to bony deformity. All patients with Morquio's disease type B have normal intelligence without any evidence of mental deterioration.

Biochemistry

The cause of GM1 gangliosidosis and Morquio's disease type B is a genetic deficiency of the lysosomal acid β-galactosidase. This enzyme deficiency was first reported in 1967 by Sacrez et al.[571] and by Okada and O'Brien in 1968.[491] In the infantile type, three to five times the normal amounts of total brain ganglioside could be accumulated at the terminal stage. GM1 ganglioside, which constitutes approximately 22–25 molar per cent of total ganglioside in the normal grey matter, is present at 90–95 molar per cent in the grey matter of affected infants. Thus, the increase in GM1 ganglioside itself could be up to 20 times normal in the grey matter.[660] The main storage materials in the systemic organs are heterogeneous, derived from glycoprotein, keratan sulfate and other carbohydrate-containing tissue constituents.[655,667] An abnormal increase in GM1 ganglioside, although the absolute amount is relatively small, is also detected in the visceral organs. In the adult type, an accumulation of GM1 ganglioside is limited to the regions where morphological evidence of neuronal storage is present.[356] All types of GM1 gangliosidosis patients excrete galactose-rich fragments of glycoproteins and keratan sulfate into the urine similar to Morquio's A (MPS IV). Little is known of the analytical chemistry of the brain in Morquio's B.

Molecular genetics

The human β-galactosidase gene is located on chromosome 3.[612] The cDNA coding for the normal human acid β-galactosidase was cloned and many mutations responsible for GM1 gangliosidosis and Morquio's B disease have been identified.[88,655,667] The molecular basis for the distinct phenotypes of GM1 gangliosidosis and Morquio's B disease has not been clarified. However, it is logically spec-

ulated that specific mutations that cause Morquio's B result in altered substrate specificity in such a way that degradation of keratan sulfate is deficient with preserved activity towards GM1 ganglioside.[498]

Neuroimaging

In patients with infantile GM1, computed tomographic (CT) imaging shows increased density in the thalami and low density in the cerebral white matter and, as the disease progresses, diffuse cerebral atrophy is pronounced (Fig. 11.1b). Magnetic resonance imaging (MRI) shows that the thalami may be slightly bright on T_1-weighted images while the basal ganglia are hyperintense on T_2-weighted images.

Pathology

Hepatosplenomegaly, bony abnormalities and facial dysmorphism similar to those found in the mucopolysaccharidoses are usually present in the infantile type.[383] These changes are milder or absent in the late infantile/juvenile type.[777] Visceromegaly and bony changes are not the features of the adult (or chronic) type.[227,650] Histologically, infiltration of storage cells is present in the spleen, in both the red pulp and the lymphoid follicles, in the lymph nodes, in hepatic sinusoids and bone marrow. The storage materials are water soluble and, as a consequence, the cytoplasm of storage cells often appears empty (foamy) on routine histological sections or electron micrographs. The cytoplasm of the renal glomerular epithelium is also often vacuolated.[677] Vacuoles are also found in the sweat gland epithelium, skin fibroblasts and lymphocytes. The storage cells in the hepatic sinusoids stain pale with eosin on routine haematoxylin and eosin (H&E) section (Fig. 11.2) and strongly positive with periodic acid–Schiff (PAS), and are alcian blue positive. Fine filamentous or tubular structures are found within these cytoplasmic vacuoles at the ultrastructural level (Fig. 11.3).[214,522,659] Similar tubular structures are also noted in some adult types.[227] Various degrees of cardiomyopathy with infiltration of storage cells in the myocardium and mitral valve have been reported in some patients with infantile type.[214,249]

The neuropathology of infantile and late infantile/juvenile types of GM1 gangliosidosis is that of typical neuronal storage disease similar to or almost identical to that of GM2 gangliosidosis. The megalencephaly sometimes reported in Tay–Sachs disease (infantile GM2 gangliosidosis), however, has not been reported. At the terminal stage, the brain is diffusely atrophied with dilated ventricles and markedly reduced weight, and may be firmer than normal.[214,659] Histologically, ballooned neurons with cytoplasmic storage materials are seen throughout the cerebrum (Fig. 11.4), cerebellum (Fig. 11.5), brainstem, spinal cord, and even in dorsal root ganglia, peripheral autonomic ganglia and myenteric plexuses in the intestine. On routine paraffin sections, the storage materials in neu-

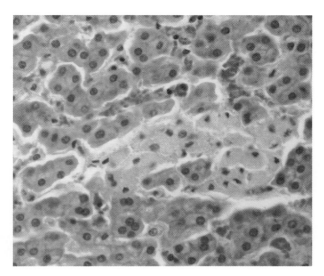

Figure 11.2 *GM1 gangliosidosis, late infantile type. A cluster of macrophages is seen among normal-appearing hepatocytes in liver. (H&E.)*

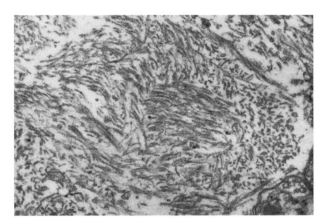

Figure 11.3 *GM1 gangliosidosis, late infantile type. The storage material in the macrophage in the liver consists of fine tubular/filamentous material morphologically totally different from the storage material in neurons. (Electron micrograph.) (From Ref. 649 with permission.)*

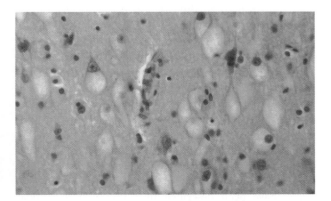

Figure 11.4 *GM1 gangliosidosis, infantile type. Diffuse neuronal storage with swollen perikarya is evident in the cerebral cortex. (H&E.)*

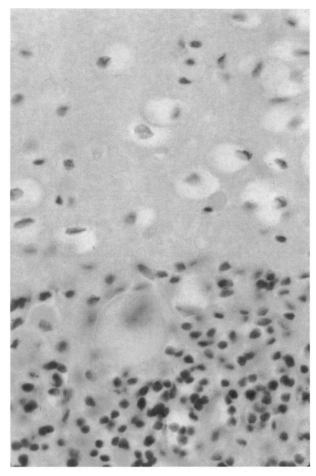

Figure 11.5 *GM1 gangliosidosis, infantile type. In addition to storage in the perikarya of Purkinje cells, many macrophages with storage material are identified in the molecular layer. (H&E.)*

rons are variably and weakly stained with PAS and/or Luxol fast blue (LFB). In contrast, glial cells are strongly positive with the PAS stain. On frozen sections, however, neuronal as well as glial storage materials both stain strongly with PAS (Fig. 11.6) and mildly positive with Sudan black. The storage materials (inclusions) are strongly positive for acid phosphatase activity, indicating their lysosomal nature. The inclusions show the ultrastructural feature of membranous cytoplasmic bodies (MCBs) (Figs 11.7, 11.8).[229,659] The MCBs in GM1 gangliosidosis are indistinguishable from those of GM2 gangliosidosis[690] morphologically, although the major constituent in the former is GM1 ganglioside instead of GM2 ganglioside in the latter.[660] With Golgi preparation, abnormally enlarged axon hillock regions, 'meganeurites', are readily recognized in the cerebral cortical neurons.[536] Notable ocular pathological features are a corneal haze and cherry-red spots in the maculae. The cytoplasm of retinal ganglion cells is filled with MCBs. In the cornea, alcian blue- and colloidal iron-positive materials accumulate, and corneal epithelial cells are vacuolated. This corneal pathology is closely similar to

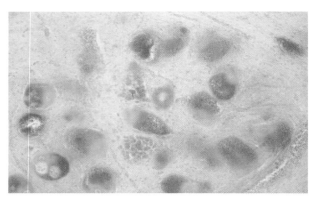

Figure 11.6 *GM1 gangliosidosis, late infantile type. Frozen section histology of anterior horn neurons of the spinal cord. Neuronal storage material stains strongly with PAS stain on frozen section, while no or only faint PAS stain is detected on paraffin-embedded tissue. (PAS.)*

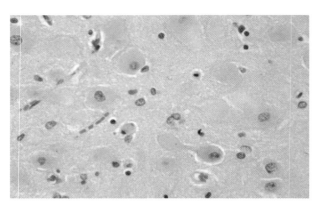

Figure 11.9 *GM1 gangliosidosis, chronic/adult type. Affected neurons in the putamen. (H&E.)*

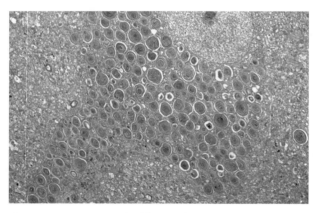

Figure 11.7 *GM2 gangliosidosis, infantile type. Cytoplasm of affected neurons is packed with MCBs. (Electron micrograph.) (From Ref. 536 with permission.)*

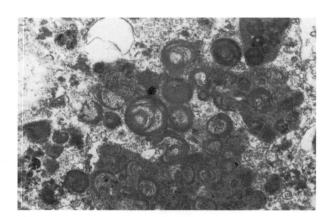

Figure 11.10 *GM1 gangliosidosis, chronic/adult type. Neuronal storage material consists of aggregate of small MCB-like structures and amorphous electron-dense material. (Electron micrograph.)*

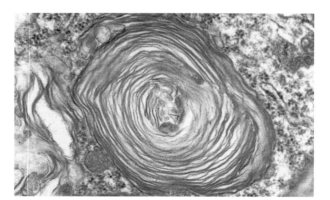

Figure 11.8 *GM2 gangliosidosis. Higher magnification of a MCB, consisting of multilayered concentric lamellae. (Electron micrograph.)*

that seen in mucopolysaccharidosis.[173] The neuropathological investigation of the adult/chronic type of GM1 gangliosidosis is very limited.[227,650,785] However, the pathology of the brain in all reported cases is similar. The brain shows localized atrophy of the caudate nucleus with mild to moderate dilatation of the lateral ventricle. Histologically, ballooned neurons are mainly identified in the basal ganglia regions (Fig. 11.9) (caudate nucleus, putamen and globus pallidus), accompanied by a marked neuronal loss. Storage materials stain positively with anti-GM1 ganglioside antibody.[785] MCBs and other morphologically heterogeneous inclusions are demonstrated ultrastructurally (Fig. 11.10). Meganeurites are noted in some neurons in the basal ganglia[227] but ballooned neurons are rare in the cerebral cortex. Purkinje cells may be moderately reduced in number and some display focal swelling of dendrites with storage materials.[227] MCBs may be present in the neurons in the myenteric plexus.[464,707] MCBs have been described in neurons in the spinal anterior horn, dorsal root ganglion, myenteric plexus and retina of an affected fetus as early as 22–24 weeks of gestational age.[61,783]

The G_{M2} gangliosidoses

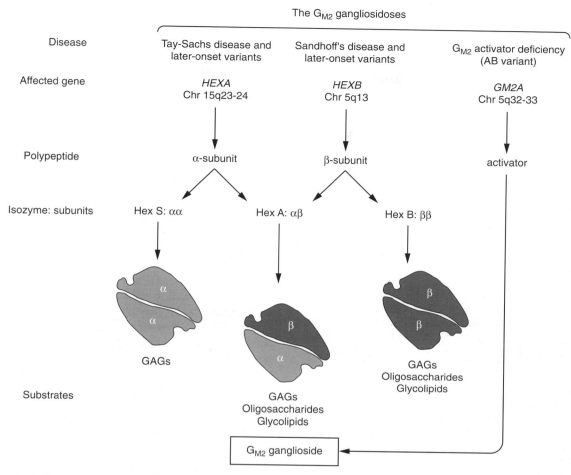

Figure 11.11 *Diagram of GM2 gangliosidosis and the β-hexosaminidase system in man. (From Ref. 654.)*

Animal models

GM1 gangliosidosis is wide spread in the animal kingdom and has been reported in the cat,[535,736] cow[151,604] and dog.[10,558] Neuropathological features are closely similar to those of infantile/late infantile GM1 gangliosidosis in man. The feline model has been used extensively in studies on aberrant dendritogenesis in the neuronal storage diseases.[535,736,743] The extent of the visceral involvement in these models is variable. More recently, with the targeted disruption of the β-galactosidase gene, mouse models of GM1 gangliosidosis were generated independently by two groups.[255,434] The neuropathology of these murine models is that of typical neuronal storage disease. Unlike human and other naturally occurring animal models, however, visceral or bony abnormalities are not apparent in these murine models.

GM2 GANGLIOSIDOSES

Human hexosaminidase system

Three polypeptides in the β-hexosaminidase system are involved in the degradation of GM2 ganglioside *in vivo* (Fig. 11.11). Hexosaminidase A is a heterodimer consist-

ing of the α- and β-subunits (αβ) and hexosaminidase B is a homodimer of two β-subunits (ββ). The minor form, hexosaminidase S, is a homodimer of the α-subunit (αα). The gene for the α-subunit is located on chromosome 15, while the gene for β-subunit is located on chromosome 5. Thus, a genetic defect in either subunit causes a distinct type of GM2 gangliosidoses; hexosaminidase A and S deficiency (Tay–Sachs disease, B variant) or hexosaminidase A and B deficiency (Sandhoff's disease; O variant). In addition, a polypeptide, GM2 activator, is necessary for the degradation of GM2 ganglioside. The gene coding for this peptide is located on chromosome 5 and its primary function is to assist β-hexosaminidase A to degrade GM2 ganglioside *in vivo*. Thus, genetic defects in GM2 activator protein cause conditions similar to the deficiency of β-hexosaminidase A activity, resulting in a clinical disease that closely mimics hexosaminidase A deficiency despite the normal enzyme activity (GM2 activator deficiency, AB variant).[235,236,655]

History and clinical features

The infantile type of hexosaminidase A deficiency, or Tay–Sachs disease, is the prototype of neuronal storage disease in man. This disease was first reported by Tay in 1881 as a case of mental retardation with the macular cherry-red spot,[685] and later widespread neurological manifestations were described by Sachs.[570] The classical infantile Tay–Sachs disease occurs among Ashkenazi Jews with an unusually high frequency. The affected infants appear normal at birth but develop progressive psychomotor retardation several months later. Clinical symptoms are almost exclusively neurological, with poor head control, hypotonia and hyperacusis. Megalencephaly and tonic-clonic or minor motor seizures may occur later in the course of the disease. Death usually results within a few years.[235,655,729] The clinical phenotype of infantile Sandhoff's disease (hexosaminidase B deficiency) is essentially indistinguishable from Tay–Sachs disease. Despite some visceral storage as described below, usually there is no detectable organomegaly or skeletal abnormality. The AB variant is exceedingly rare. The clinical phenotype of reported cases is similar to that of Tay–Sachs disease.[132] Unlike the high frequency of Tay–Sachs disease among Ashkenazi Jews with their ancestors from eastern Poland or western Russia, no ethnic or geographical preponderance has been noted in Sandhoff's disease or AB variant. The clinical signs and symptoms of infantile GM2 gangliosidosis are usually stereotypic but, among late-onset cases, clinical symptoms may vary considerably.[632] The onset can be at any time from the late infantile to the adult age. The onset of the late-infantile type is after 18 months of age with progressive dementia and seizures. The juvenile form becomes symptomatic between the ages of 4 and 6 years with dementia. The first patient described as having juvenile GM2 gangliosidosis[661] was later recognized as having the enzymologically unique B1 variant form as described below.[679] Several additional B1 variant cases have been reported since. All are of juvenile type.[51,225,418]

The chronic or adult form usually develops neurological signs and symptoms in early childhood with a protracted course. As of 1993, approximately 50 patients with late-onset GM2 gangliosidosis had been identified, most of them being Ashkenazi Jews. At least some 35% of these patients had their first symptoms before the age of 10 years. Progression of clinical signs and symptoms is usually slow. In some cases, mentation may be well preserved,[295] but psychosis or depression has been reported.[466] The cherry-red spots are less frequently detected.[546] Dystonia,[266,439,476] choreoathetosis and other extrapyramidal signs, ataxia, the signs that are reminiscent of spinocerebellar degeneration,[295,546] Friedreich's ataxia[768] or motor neuron disease[313,315,316,363,445,507] have been well documented. Parkinsonism has been reported in a patient with adult-onset hexosaminidase deficiency.[302] The clinical features may vary between and within families and classical infantile Tay–Sachs disease has been reported within the families of late-onset adult type.[465] Spinocerebellar and motor neuron phenotypes have been noted within the same families.[19] The majority of these late-onset cases are

B variant or hexosaminidase A deficiency but late-onset Sandhoff's disease with similar clinical phenotypes has also been reported.[68,92,566,593]

Biochemistry

GM2 ganglioside is normally a very minor constituent in the brain. In GM2 gangliosidoses, GM2 ganglioside accumulates in the brain and to a lesser extent in the visceral organs. In the infantile type, the accumulation is massive. Degradation of GM2 ganglioside and related compounds is a complex process (β-hexosaminidase system). As stated above, the β-hexosaminidase system consists of two major isozymes, β-hexosaminidase A and B, one minor isozyme S, and the GM2 activator protein. These isozymes are formed by the different combination of two subunits, α and β. Degradation of GM2 ganglioside *in vivo* requires both β-hexosaminidase A and GM2 activator protein. Since α- and β-subunits and the GM2 activator protein are encoded by three distinct genes, abnormalities in any one of the three genes result in defective catabolism of GM2 ganglioside and related lipids and thus in genetically different forms of GM2 gangliosidosis. In Tay–Sachs disease and its variant cases, hexosaminidase A is genetically absent or defective but hexosaminidase B is intact (B variant).[492,575] In Sandhoff's disease resulting from genetic defect of the β-subunit, activity of both hexosaminidase A and B is deficient (O variant).[575] As a result, no natural sphingolipid and glycolipid substrates can be degraded and other sphingoglycolipids, such as globoside, are additionally accumulated in the systemic organs. The activities of both β-hexosaminidases are normal in the AB variant since this type results from a GM2 activator deficiency.[575] In the B1 variant the α-subunit is defective.[679] As a consequence, hexosaminidase A shows normal activity against the artificial substrate, 4-methylumbelliferyl-2-acetamido-2-deoxy-β-D-glucopyranoside (4MU-GlcNAc) but is defective against its sulfated form (4MU-GlcNAc sulfate) and the natural substrate, GM2 ganglioside.[378] In late-onset cases, GM2 ganglioside accumulation is much less than that in infantile cases.[235,236,655]

Molecular genetics

The gene coding for the α-subunit of β-hexosaminidase is located on chromosome 15. A deletion or mutation of certain segment of this gene causes GM2 gangliosidosis B variant. Numerous disease-causing abnormalities are known in the β-hexosaminidase α-subunit gene.[235,236,328] Some mutations are associated with specific ethnic groups. For example, the specific point mutation that is found in more than 80% of the abnormal alleles among Japanese patients with infantile Tay–Sachs disease has not been reported anywhere else.[680] The point mutation that causes the typical juvenile B1 variant form has been traced to Northern Portugal.[152] In contrast, mutations in the classical infantile Tay–Sachs disease among the Ashkenazi Jewish population turned out to be heterogeneous.[235,236,655] The gene coding for the β-subunit is on chromosome 5 and many disease-causing mutations are being identified. The GM2 activator protein deficiency is exceedingly rare and only several disease-causing mutations have been reported.[576]

Neuroimaging

CT and MRI of patients with infantile GM2 gangliosidosis are very similar to those of infantile GM1 (Fig. 11.1b) and may show bilaterally increased density in the thalami and basal ganglia. These regions may be hyperintense on T_1- and T_2-weighted MR images. The cerebral white matter shows patchy areas of increased T_2 signal intensity. In the late stages of the disease, cerebral atrophy with ventricular enlargement is evident. In late-onset GM2 gangliosidosis, the cerebellum may show atrophy.

Pathology

The pathology of Tay–Sachs disease (B variant) and AB variant is limited to the nervous system. In Sandhoff's disease (O variant), however, visceral pathology such as vacuolation of hepatocytes and pancreatic acinar cells, PAS-positive Kupffer cells in the hepatic sinusoids, and histiocytes in the germinal centres in the spleen are often observed. PAS-positive material is also present in the renal tubular epithelium.[248,663]

The neuropathology of Tay–Sachs disease has been well described by Volk et al.[729] The gross changes of the brain may vary with the duration of the clinical course. During the first 12–14 months, the brain is atrophic with moderately dilated ventricles. The brain weight gradually increases during the period between 15 and 24 months and marked enlargment of the brain occurs in patients who survive beyond the age of 24 months. The brain is rubbery and firm in consistency. With progression of the disease white matter becomes depressed and translucent, and the grey–white junction becomes blurred. The optic nerves, cerebellum and brainstem become atrophic. Histopathologically, neuronal storage is present throughout the CNS (Fig. 11.12) and the normal cytoarchitecture is markedly distorted. The Nissl substance disappears or is pushed to the periphery of the neuronal perikarya and the storage materials show strong PAS positivity on frozen sections (Fig. 11.6). The axon hillocks of the pyramidal neurons are dramatically enlarged by an accumulation of storage materials (meganeurites) (Figs 11.13, 11.14). Normal apical as well as basal dendrites are distorted and atrophied, and aberrant dendrites are formed from meganeurites and make aberrant synaptic formation (ectopic dendritogenesis) (Figs 11.15, 11.16).[534,536] Ultrastructurally, the perikarya of affected neurons are packed with concentrically lamellated lipid inclusions of approximately 1 μm in diameter, termed MCBs (Figs 11.7, 11.8).[690] The MCBs consist of gangliosides (mostly GM2 ganglioside), cholesterol and phospholipids, with minor amounts of proteins. Loss of myelin in the white matter is notable and, in some, demyelination may involve almost

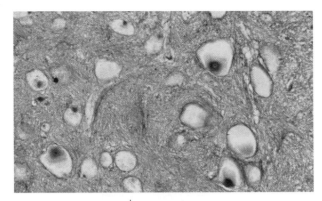

Figure 11.12 *GM2 gangliosidosis, infantile type (Tay–Sachs disease). Affected neurons in the anterior horn of the spinal cord: paraffin section stained with PAS. (Compare with frozen section with PAS stain in Fig. 11.6.)*

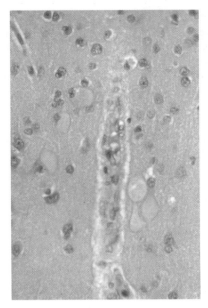

Figure 11.13 *GM2 gangliosidosis, juvenile type. Unlike in infantile type, the extent of neuronal storage in the cerebral cortex varies among individual neurons. Meganeurite is evident in some neurons. (H&E.)*

the entire white matter, resembling leukodystrophy. Astrocytic as well as microglial/ macrophage responses are extensive. Degenerative changes are pronounced in the cerebellum, with loss of the Purkinje and granule cells. The remaining Purkinje cells show distended perikarya and an antler-like expansion of their dendrites from stored materials. Apoptotic neuronal death has been demonstrated by the terminal deoxytransferase-mediated dUTP-biotin nick end labelling (TUNEL) stain in Tay–Sachs and Sandhoff's diseases.[292] Neuronal storage is also noted in the ganglion cells in the retina, in the autonomic ganglia, in the dorsal root ganglia and in the myenteric plexus. The neuropathology of infantile Sandhoff's disease is closely similar to that of Tay–Sachs disease. Neurons contain

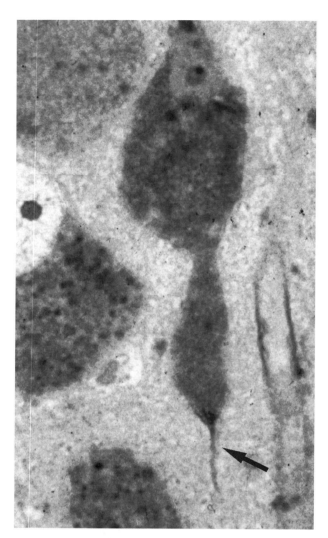

Figure 11.14 *GM1 gangliosidosis (feline). A cerebral cortical neuron stained with ferric ion-ferrocyanide demonstrating stained initial segment (arrow) distal to a meganeurite, indicating that meganeurites are expansions of the axonal hillock proximal to the initial segment and that they are distinct from axonal enlargement. (From Ref. 743 with permission.)*

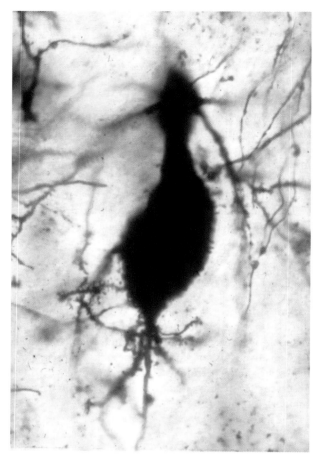

Figure 11.15 *GM2 gangliosidosis, AB variant. Golgi preparation of medium-sized pyramidal neurons in the cerebral cortex. Ectopic dendritic growth from a meganeurite is evident. (From Ref. 534 with permission.)*

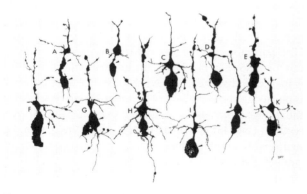

Figure 11.16 *GM2 gangliosidosis, infantile type. Camera lucida drawing of meganeurites in cerebral cortical neurons. (From Ref. 536 with permission.)*

MCBs that are morphologically identical to those seen in Tay–Sachs disease. However, isolated MCBs from the brain of the Sandhoff patient contain a much higher accumulation of ceramide trihexoside than the MCBs of Tay–Sachs disease.[663] The AB variant is extremely rare and neuropathological examination has been carried out on a very limited number of cases. The clinical and biochemical phenotype is very similar to that of Tay–Sachs disease and the neuropathology of the reported case is essentially indistinguishable from that of Tay–Sachs or Sandhoff's disease by light-microscopic examination.[132,228] Progressive formation of the meganeurites with aberrant neurites has been well documented in this variant (Fig. 11.15).[534] Electron-microscopic investigation has shown, in addition to typical MCBs, 'zebra' bodies within the perikarya of some cortical

neurons (Fig. 11.17). Various heterogeneous inclusions have been noted in astrocytes, oligodendroglia and microglia.[132,228] Thus, these fine structural findings appear somewhat different from those of Tay–Sachs or Sandhoff's disease.

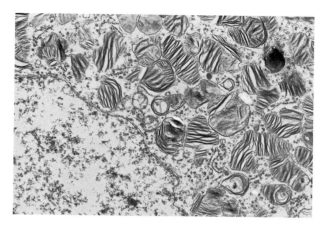

Figure 11.17 *GM2 gangliosidosis, AB variant. A cerebral cortical neuron containing zebra bodies. (Electron micrograph.)*

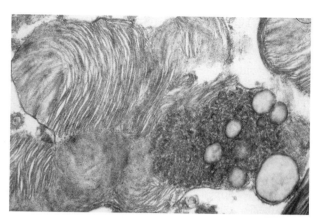

Figure 11.20 *GM2 gangliosidosis, juvenile type. Electron micrograph of a neuron containing MCBs.*

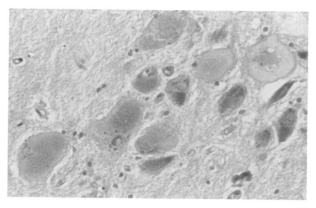

Figure 11.18 *GM2 gangliosidosis, chronic/adult type. Neurons in the substantia nigra, demonstrating heterogeneous neuronal storage materials. (PAS.)*

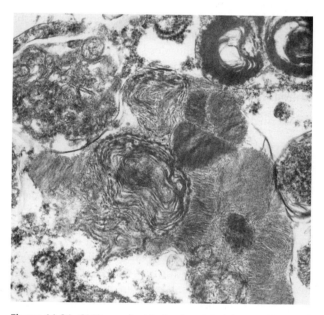

Figure 11.21 *GM2 gangliosidosis, chronic/adult type. Neuronal inclusions consisting of heterogeneous electron-dense conglomerates of storage materials. (Electron micrograph.) (From Ref. 546 with permission.)*

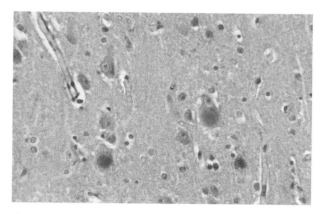

Figure 11.19 *GM2 gangliosidosis, chronic/adult type. Cerebral cortex shows selective neuronal storage of PAS-positive material in pyramidal neurons. (PAS.)*

The neuropathological investigation of late-onset GM2 gangliosidosis is also very limited. In a juvenile B1 variant form of β-hexosaminidase patient, Benninger *et al.* reported an atrophied brain with markedly dilated ventricles. The neurons were moderately to severely ballooned and the perikarya distended by a granular,

strongly LFB-positive stored material, and contained MCB and zebra bodies at the ultrastructural level.[51] Marked cerebral and cerebellar atrophy was present in a 14-year-old patient reported by Suzuki *et al.*[661] Microscopically, neuronal storage is observed throughout the brain but is less than that of the infantile type. Light- and electron-microscopic features of the chronic or adult type are very similar to those of the juvenile type reported by Suzuki *et al.* Neuronal storage material is more heterogeneous, in particular in the deep cerebral nuclei and brainstem (Fig. 11.18), and coarsely granular, showing strong PAS positivity even on paraffin section (Fig. 11.19). The electron-microscopic features of the storage materials are heterogeneous and complex. In addition to MCBs (Fig. 11.20), membranous vesicular bodies and electron-dense conglomerates of morphologically heterogeneous lipofuscin-like materials (Fig. 11.21) are found in many neurons.[313,546,650] The patient reported by Rapin et al. was a 16-year-old female, youngest of three affected siblings with the spinocerebellar phenotype.[546] Jellinger et al. reported a 67-year-old patient whose clinical symptoms were those of chronic neuromuscular disease beginning at the age of 19 years.[313] In both patients, heterogeneous inclusions were found throughout the cerebrum, cerebellum and brainstem. A 44-year-old female reported by Kornfeld had the motor neuron phenotype and, later in her life, developed a peculiar pain syndrome with dysaesthesia, paraesthesia and hyperalgesia affecting most of her body, as well as psychiatric symptoms. In this patient neuronal storage was most extensive in the spinal cord neurons and dorsal root ganglia. There was minimal storage in the cerebrum and cerebellum.[363] Ballooned neurons containing well-formed MCBs were identified in myenteric plexus neurons in all types including adult or chronic type GM2 gangliosidosis (Fig. 11.22), despite heterogeneous clinical phenotypes.[316,465,768]

Animal models

GM2 gangliosidosis has been reported in the dog,[58,125] cat,[113,114,458,469,745] deer[188] and in pig.[365,526] In all species, the typical feature of neuronal storage with swollen neuronal perikarya was noted throughout the brain. The feline models are equivalent to Sandhoff's disease (hexosaminidase β-subunit deficiency) and visceral storage is present. The GM2 gangliosidosis in Muntjak deer is deficient in the activity of β-hexosaminidase A and thus is equivalent to the B variant. Accumulation of GM2 ganglioside is well documented in canine and porcine models, but the data for further classification are not available. Meganeurites as seen in human GM2 gangliosidosis have been reported in the canine[125] and feline[745] models (Fig. 11.13). Walkley and collaborators have been studying aberrant dendritogenesis using feline models and have shown a positive correlation between

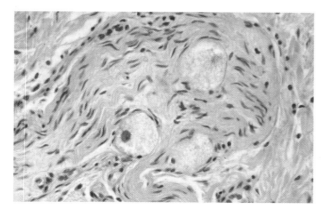

Figure 11.22 GM2 gangliosidosis, chronic/adult type. Affected neurons in the myenteric plexus show marked perikaryal storage as noted in infantile type. (H&E.)

ectopic neurite growth and the accumulation of GM2 ganglioside.[232,618,737,780] Murine models of Tay–Sachs disease, Sandhoff's disease and AB variant have been generated by targeted disruption of the genes for the α-subunit,[105,524,683,780] the β-subunit[524,579] and the GM2 activator protein.[404] Unlike Tay–Sachs disease in man, the mouse model of Tay–Sachs disease lacks a clinical phenotype, and neuronal storage occurs in relatively localized regions. Most notably, there is no or very little evidence of neuronal storage in the cerebellum and spinal cord.[683] Diffuse neuronal storage is present in the murine model of Sandhoff's disease. GM2 activator-deficient mice or murine AB variant show localized neuronal storage in the cerebrum similar to the Tay–Sachs model, but unlike the Tay–Sachs model storage is also present in the cerebellar Purkinje cells. These differences in the pathology of these mutant mice are due to the differences in the ganglioside metabolism between mice and men.[654]

Niemann–Pick disease types A and B

Niemann–Pick disease is a neurovisceral lipid storage disease that had been subclassified into types A, B, C and D (type E was also suggested by some).[119,121] It has been clearly established in the past two decades that, despite some phenotypic resemblance, type A and B on the one hand, and type C and D on the other, represent two totally different and unrelated genetic diseases.[511,520,596] Niemann–Pick disease types C and D will be described separately in this chapter.

History and clinical course

The first patient with Niemann–Pick disease type A was described by the German paediatrician Albert Niemann[472] and the pathological uniqueness of this disease was shown later by Ludwick Pick. The incidence of type A Niemann–pick disease is high in the Ashkenazi Jewish population. The clinical presentation of a type A patient is relatively stereotyped and the patient described by Niemann, an Ashkenazi Jewish infant with massive hepatosplenomegaly and rapidly progressive neurological symptoms who died at age 18 months, was a classic example. About 50% of type A patients may develop cherry-red spots, as noted in Tay–Sachs disease patients, but hyperacusis or macrocephaly apparently does not occur and seizures are rare. In addition to hepatosplenomegaly, a diffuse reticular infiltration is found in the lungs. The majority of type A patients are infantile, but a late infantile and juvenile variant also has been documented.[596,716] In contrast, type B patients present with massive hepatosplenomegaly without any significant neurological abnormalities. The hepatosplenomegaly may be detected within the first year or, more usually, later in childhood, but patients usually survive to adulthood.[121] Pulmonary infiltration is commonly detected radiologically. Although the clinical presentation of Gaucher's and

Niemann–Pick disease is similar, bone involvement is not a serious complication in the latter. Compared with type A, the phenotypic presentation of type B may be more variable. In some cases, macular changes similar to or reminiscent of cherry–red spot with apparently normal intelligence have been well documented.[167,262,401,633] Several cases with some atypical neurological or psychiatric symptoms, suggestive of an intermediate type between A and B, have been reported.[156,170,673]

Biochemistry

In both type A and B Niemann–Pick disease, the lysosomal hydrolase, acid sphingomyelinase, is deficient.[81,592,596] Analysis of the lipid contents in the liver and spleen shows up to 50-fold accumulation of sphingomyelin associated with increases of unesterified cholesterol and other phospholipids. In the brain of type A patients, sphingomyelin is increased five- to ten-fold in the grey matter. The ganglioside pattern in the grey matter is altered, with a significant increase in GM2 and GM3 gangliosides.[331] In the white matter, myelin lipids are reduced in general but sphingomyelin is relatively increased. The lipid profile in the brain of patients with type B is normal, without an increase in sphingomyelin.[559,716] Increased levels of lysosphingomyelin (sphingosylphosphorylcholine) are reported in the liver and spleen in both type A and B patients. Massive accumulation of this lipid is documented in the brain of type A patients.[559] Since lysosphingolipids have been implicated in the biochemical pathogenesis of genetic lysosomal sphingolipidoses,[264,265] this elevation of lysosphingomyelin in type A could play a role in the pathophysiology of brain dysfunction in type A.

Molecular genetics

The type A and B Niemann–Pick disease are allelic in that they are both caused by mutations in the same acid sphingomyelinase gene. The gene is localized to the chromosome region 11p15.1 to 15.4. Many mutations causing Niemann–Pick disease have been identified.[596,716]

Neuroimaging

The imaging findings in patients with Niemann–Pick disease type A are non-specific and similar to those of infantile GM1 and GM2 gangliosidoses. The most common finding is cortical atrophy with enlarged ventricles. In the late stages of the disease the corpus callosum appears thin. The white matter may show patchy areas of increased T_2 signal intensity.

Pathology

Type A is a neurovisceral lipid storage disease, while the storage is limited in the visceral organs in type B. The liver and spleen are grossly enlarged. Histologically, numerous foamy macrophages (Fig. 11.23) are found in many organs, including bone marrow, on routinely processed

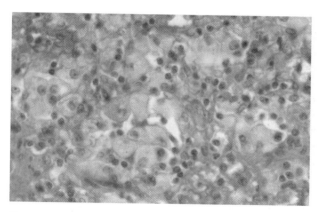

Figure 11.23 *Niemann–Pick disease type A. Macrophages replete with stored material within the liver. (H&E.)*

paraffin sections. Cholesterol is demonstrated in the cytoplasm of these cells by Schultz or perchloric acid naphthoquinone (PAN) stain on frozen sections. Vacuolation in lymphocytes has been reported. The foamy macrophages are usually mononuclear but rarely multinuclear, filling the red pulp of the spleen, hepatic sinusoids, pulmonary alveolar spaces, thymus and lymph nodes. In older patients with type B, macrophages may be less vacuolated and instead their cytoplasm may be filled with small granules staining intensely blue with Giemsa or Wright stain (sea-blue histiocytes). Ultrastructural features of the stored materials are multiple electron-lucent vacuoles and small, concentric, electron-dense lamellar structures. The cytoplasmic granules seen in older patients consist of electron-dense and more tightly packed lamellar or vesicular structures.

The brain of the type A patient is diffusely atrophied. The cerebellum is often severely affected and small. Histopathology is typical of a neuronal storage disease, indistinguishable from that of infantile GM1 or GM2 gangliosidosis (Figs 11.4, 11.5, 11.12). Ballooned neurons with distended perikarya are seen throughout the nervous system, including the autonomic ganglia, dorsal root ganglia and myenteric plexus. The neuronal inclusions closely resemble the MCBs of gangliosidoses but are smaller and less compact. Lamellar membranes are often arranged concentrically around vacuoles or electron-dense small MCB-like structures.[716] In addition to the neuronal storage, lipid storage is conspicuous in macrophages and microglia. Vacuolated macrophages similar to those of visceral organs are also found in the leptomeninges and choroid plexus. The lipid storage is also recognized in the retinal ganglion cells, amacrine and Müller cells, and conjunctival and corneal epithelial cells.[556,716] Peripheral neuropathy with infiltration of foamy macrophages has also been reported.[384]

Animal models

Naturally occurring models of type A Niemann–Pick disease have been described in the poodle dog[85] and

Siamese cat.[754] In a feline model, Walkley and Baker demonstrated meganeurites and aberrant neurite formation, similar to those observed in gangliosidoses, in the affected neurons in the brain.[739] More recently, with targeted disruption of the acid sphingomyelinase gene, murine models of Niemann–Pick disease type A have been generated by two groups.[289,373,374,443,499] The phenotypes of these two murine models appear somewhat different from each other, however. Light- and electron-microscopic features of the pathological processes in these mice closely resemble those of human Niemann–Pick disease type A.[289,373,374]

Niemann–Pick disease types C and D

History and clinical course

In 1961, Crocker classified Niemann–Pick disease into four groups, A, B, C and D, on the basis of clinical phenotypes and biochemical analysis of stored lipids in the tissue.[119] Type C was thought to be a sphingomyelin storage disease with slowly progressive neurological illness, with type D closely resembling type C except that it is a genetic isolate in Nova Scotia. Now it has been clearly established that Niemann–Pick disease type C is not a primary sphingomyelin storage disorder due to genetic acid sphingomyelinase deficiency, but a distinct disease of intracellular cholesterol trafficking abnormalities. Type D is allelic with type C.[511,520,716,717] In contrast to the rather uniform clinical phenotype in types A and B, type C shows heterogeneous clinical manifestations of a progressive neurological disease.[183,716] Because of this heterogeneous clinical presentation without well-defined and specific enzymic or biochemical abnormalities, type C disease, in particular of late-onset and slowly progressive phenotypes, has been described with a multitude of descriptive names in the past, as listed in Table 11.2. The age of presentation may vary considerably and initial manifestation can be hepatic, neurological or psychiatric. The systemic (liver, spleen, lung) involvement and neurological symptoms are not always correlated. Clinically, the disease is classified from the age of onset and presenting neurological symptoms.[183,520,716,720] The most common type of patients (70–80% of cases) are those with late-infantile and juvenile neurological onset forms, with splenomegaly or hepatosplenomegaly, although no clinically detectable organomegaly has been reported in at least 10% of cases. Ataxic gait and poor school performance due to intellectual impairment and impaired fine movement are often the initial presenting symptoms, followed by onset of seizures, cataplexy and supranuclear vertical gaze palsy (downward, upward or both).[564] Prolonged neonatal cholestatic jaundice associated with progressive hepatosplenomegaly is present in nearly half of these patients but usually it is self-limiting and spontaneously resolves by 2–4 months of age. In about 10% of the patients with neonatal jaundice, a rapidly fatal liver fail-

Table 11.2 *Terms associated with Niemann–Pick disease types C and D*

Juvenile dystonic lipidosis
Juvenile dystonic idiocy without amaurosis
Atypical cerebral lipidosis
Atypical juvenile lipidosis
Subacute Niemann–Pick disease
Juvenile Niemann–Pick disease
Ophthalmoplegic lipidosis
Neurovisceral storage disease with visceral supranuclear
    ophthalmoplegia
Neville–Lake syndrome
Neville's disease
Subacute neurovisceral lipidosis
Lactosylceramidosis
Sea-blue histiocyte disease
Chronic reticuloendothelial cell storage disease
Nova Scotian variant of Niemann–Pick disease

Source: Lake BD. *Greenfield's Neuropathology*, 6th edn.

ure may develop, with death before the age of 6 months, but they do not show any neurological symptoms. There is a rare severe infantile form with hepatosplenomegaly and severe neurological symptoms. Hypotonia and delayed developmental milestones are the presenting neurological symptoms around the age of 1–1.5 years and the affected children die before the age of 5 years. This form is more frequent in southern Europe and the Middle East than the USA. A psychosis and/or progressive dementia is a common presentation of the adult-onset patients.[294,615] Visceromegaly is not clinically detectable in nearly half of the patients. Vertical gaze paresis may not be present.

Some children may develop fetal ascites[417] and severe pulmonary involvement.[367]

Biochemistry

Unlike in Niemann–Pick disease types A and B, acid sphingomyelinase is not genetically deficient in type C or D.[592] In type C, endocytosed exogenous cholesterol is sequestered in lysosomes and intracellular transport to the plasma membrane and the endoplasmic reticulum is retarded.[372,517–519] After an addition of low-density lipoprotein (LDL) to the media, the cultured fibroblasts of type C patients accumulate unesterified cholesterol in the perinuclear lysosomes, which is easily detected by filipin stain. Thus, the filipin stain is useful for the diagnosis of Niemann–Pick type C.[628,715] In the liver and spleen, sphingomyelin and cholesterol are moderately (two- to five-fold) increased. An accumulation of *bis*-(monoacylglycero)-phosphate, glucosylceramide, lactosylceramide and, to a lesser extent, other phospholipids and glycolipids is also present. In the brain, however, cholesterol or sphingomyelin is not increased. In the cerebral cortex, the concentrations of total cholesterol, sphingomyelin and gangliosides are within the normal range. In the white matter, loss of galactosylceramide and other myelin lipids (including cholesterol) is extensive in the infantile or late-infantile forms with severe clinical phenotype, while only a slight decrease is noted in the late-onset or chronic form. Glycolipid composition is markedly abnormal. Glucosylceramide and lactosylceramide are significantly increased.[511,714] Normally very minor GM1 and GM2 gangliosides are relatively increased, but only to the extent that is seen non-specifically in many other neurodegenerative disorders including Niemann–Pick type A (see above).[511,714] The storage disease reported by Dawson et al. as lactosylceramidosis because of marked accumulation of lactosylceramide in the brain has been proven to be a case of Niemann–Pick type C, biochemically and by mutation analysis.[130] These changes in glycolipid composition in the brain apparently occur concomitant with the onset of neurological symptoms, in contrast to the earlier accumulation of glycolipid in visceral organs.[714] The quantitative aspects of the brain glycolipid abnormalities must be kept in perspective. The sum of sphingomyelin, galactosylceramide and sulfatide constitutes more than 90% of normal brain sphingolipids, while total gangliosides are less than 5%. The relative 'increase' in GM2 and GM3 is much less than 1% of total brain sphingolipids and even the increase in glucosylceramide and lactosylceramide does not add more than a few percentage to the total sphingolipids. However, owing to significant myelin loss, combined galactosylceramide, sulfatide and sphingomyelin is reduced by one-third or more. Thus, the total quantity of sphingolipids in the whole brain of Niemann–Pick type C is reduced by one-third or more.

Molecular genetics

Niemann–Pick disease type C is panethnic. Genetically, it consists of two distinct groups, NPC1 and NPC2, identified by complementation analysis and chromosomal localization of the respective genes.[511] More than 95% of Niemann–Pick type C patients belong to NPC1. The estimated prevalence of NPC1 is about 1 in 150 000 but the real prevalence could be higher because of difficulty in clinical diagnosis due to the very heterogeneous clinical phenotypes. This type is more common than type A and B combined. A regionally high incidence is reported in Nova Scotia in Canada (formerly type D). The NPC1 gene is located on chromosome 18q11.[90,91] The NPC1 gene has been cloned and over 70 disease-causing mutations have been identified in 2 years. The NPC2 gene has been cloned recently.[464a] The precise physiological function of the NPC1 gene has not been clarified, but the gene contains a region common among genes involved in intracellular cholesterol homoeostasis.

Pathology

Niemann–Pick disease type C is a neurovisceral lipid storage disease. Reflecting clinical heterogeneity, the

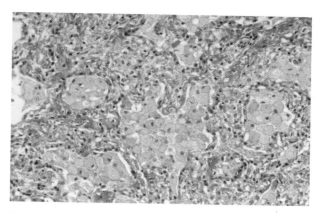

Figure 11.24 *Niemann–Pick disease type C. Massive accumulation of affected macrophages within alveolar spaces in the lung. (H&E.)*

extent of the pathology may differ considerably in individual patients. In general, however, younger patients with an acute clinical course tend to have more severe hepatosplenomegaly and marked neuronal storage than patients with a slowly progressive clinical course. Visceral organs are variously infiltrated with foamy macrophages, and in older patients, macrophages containing basophilic granules (sea-blue histiocytes) are also present. These storage cells tend to be clustered in the red pulp in the spleen, and within the hepatic sinusoids. These histological features of visceral organs are closely similar to those of types A and B Niemann–Pick disease. In early-onset cases, hepatic pathology is usually very conspicuous, with cholestasis and giant cell transformation of hepatocytes, and thus not uncommonly diagnosed as 'giant cell hepatitis'.[307,568,600] In an ultrastructural study of a 20-week fetus, crystalline structures consistent with cholesterol were demonstrated in the Kupffer cells and other macrophages. Large pleomorphic inclusions and hyperplasia of pericanalicular microfilaments in hepatocytes, suggestive of an early feature of cholestasis, were also reported.[157] Severe pulmonary involvement has been reported in some infantile cases (Fig. 11.24).[367,527] Three of these early lethal pulmonary cases belonged to the second, rare genetic complementary group, NPC-2.[594] With ultrastructural investigation, storage material (inclusions) can be detected in cell types other than macrophages; for example, hepatocytes, conjunctival epithelium, endothelial cells, pericytes, keratinocytes, lens epithelial cells, Schwann cells, smooth-muscle cells and fibroblasts.[21,74,504,782] These inclusions are pleomorphic, consisting of various sized electron-lucent vacuoles and electron-dense amorphous or curved short membranous structures (Fig. 11.25).[17,74,212,514]

The brain is usually atrophic. However, the extent of atrophy can be quite variable. Cerebellar atrophy may be particularly pronounced in some cases. Histopathology is that of a neuronal storage disease characterized by swollen perikarya with storage material. The neuronal storage is more extensive and widespread in younger

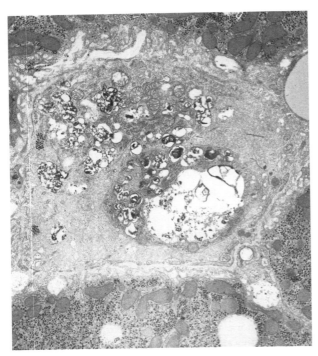

Figure 11.25 *Niemann–Pick disease type C. Macrophage in the liver containing multiple membrane-bound vacuoles and electron-dense membranous structures. (Electron micrograph.)*

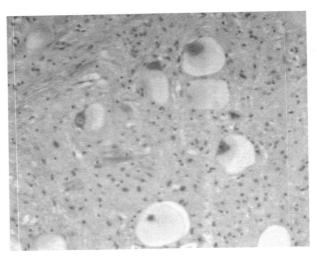

Figure 11.26 *Niemann–Pick disease type C. Ballooned neurons in the anterior horn of the spinal cord. (H&E.)*

patients, with a shorter clinical course than in chronic progressive adult cases. In the latter, neuronal storage may be more localized in the deep cerebral nuclei, brainstem and spinal cord (Fig. 11.26).[653] On H&E sections, the perikarya of affected neurons are packed with fine vacuoles and are variably stained with PAS and/or LFB. On frozen sections, neuronal storage materials stain strongly positive with PAS and to some extent with filipin stain, while other conventional histochemical stains for cholesterol are reported to be negative or only weakly positive.[168,212] The ultrastructural features of the neuronal storage materials closely resemble the MCBs of gangliosidoses but they are smaller and more pleomorphic (Fig. 11.27).[164,212] Swollen axon hillocks (meganeurites) are conspicuous, particularly in infantile cases (Fig. 11.28). Braak and co-workers described isocortical pathology using a combined Golgi–pigmentoarchitectonic technique. They described meganeurites, ectopic neurites and irregular focal dendritic swelling in large pyramidal neurons in the deep cerebral cortex.[76] Focal neuroaxonal dystrophies (Fig. 11.29) (axonal spheroids) are very conspicuous in infantile forms. These spheroids contain many degenerated cellular organelles and neurofilaments in various proportions.[168] The neuroaxonal dystrophy is less common in older patients. In patients with a slowly progressive chronic course, neuroaxonal dystrophy is rarely seen.[652,653] Instead, neurofibrillary tangles (NFTs) are detected consistently in these patients (Figs 11.30,

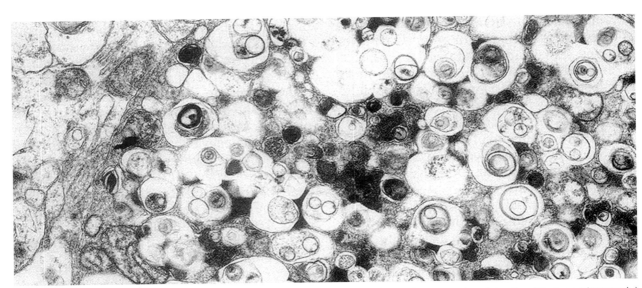

Figure 11.27 *Niemann–Pick disease type C. Neuronal inclusions consist of polymorphous cytoplasmic bodies. (Electron micrograph.)*

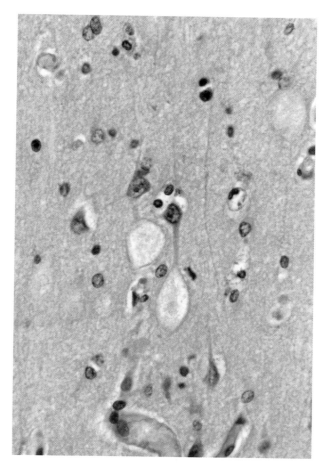

Figure 11.28 *Niemann–Pick disease type C. Ballooned neurons in cerebral cortex (temporal lobe) with meganeurites. (H&E.)*

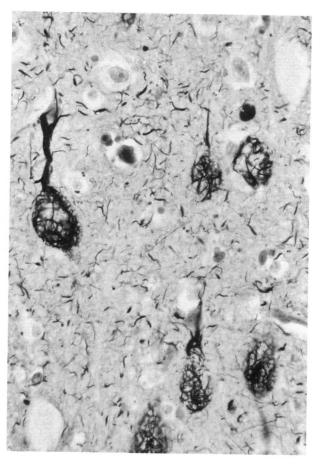

Figure 11.30 *Niemann–Pick disease type C. Affected neurons in the cerebral cortex (temporal lobe), showing neurofibrillary tangles in meganeurites. Numerous threads are present in the neuropil. (Bielschowsky.) (From Ref. 717.)*

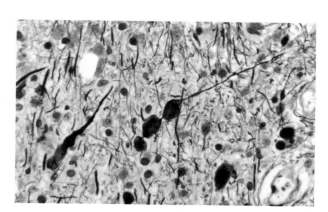

Figure 11.29 *Niemann–Pick disease type C. Neuroaxonal dystrophy with focal axonal swelling. (Bielschowsky.) (From Ref. 717.)*

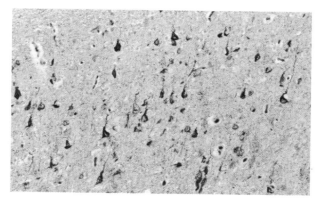

Figure 11.31 *Niemann–Pick disease type C. Cerebral cortex (orbital gyrus) showing many flame-shaped Alzheimer-type neurofibrillary tangles without amyloid deposition. (Bielschowsky.)*

11.31).[115,290,407,606,652,653] These tangles consist of paired helical filaments (PHFs), identical to those found in Alzheimer's disease. By immunocytochemistry and by Western blot analysis, the PHF tau in Niemann–Pick type C disease was shown to be similar to PHF tau in Alzheimer's disease.[27] The variable extent of neuronal loss, in particular loss of Purkinje cells in the cerebellum, is conspicuous in some cases. TUNEL staining shows neuronal as well as glial cell apoptosis (unpublished observation). Combined features of axonal and myelin degeneration with spheroid formation have been reported in the peripheral nerve. Schwann cells contain membrane-bound multilobulated lysosomal inclusions in their distended cytoplasm.[252]

Animal models

A feline model[411,424] and two murine models, C57BL/ KsJ[spm] and BALB/c[nih,282,283,284,682,750] are known. All known animal models are NPC1 equivalents and no NPC2 animal models are known. Light- and electron-microscopic features of these models are closely similar to those of type C patients with an acute or subacute clinical course. Infiltration of lipid-containing foamy macrophages is extensive in the lung,[420] liver, spleen and lymph nodes.[282,284,411] Hepatosplenomegaly is absent in the canine model. Neuroaxonal dystrophy is frequently observed in the feline and murine models but relatively mild in the canine model. Similar to cases in man, meganeurites with aberrant neurite formation are reported in the feline model.[424] In the murine models, cerebral and cerebellar atrophy is pronounced and loss of Purkinje cells is extensive in older mice.[282,682] Peripheral nerve degeneration, as noted in man, is also reported in the murine model.[283]

Gaucher's disease

Gaucher's disease is an autosomal recessive glycolipid storage disorder characterized by an accumulation of glucosylceramide (glucocerebroside) within cells of the monocyte–macrophage system. It is caused by the deficient activity of a lysosomal hydrolase, acid β-glucosidase (glucosylceramidase). It is usually classified into three clinical phenotypes, types I, II and III.[59,79]

History and clinical features

The first description of a patient with 'Gaucher disease' was by Phillipe Charles Ernest Gaucher in 1882. In his doctoral thesis he described a 32-year-old female with massive splenomegaly thought to have a primary splenic neoplasm.[207] This was the first description of what is now known as the adult type or type I (non-neuronopathic) Gaucher's disease. Type II, or the acute neuronopathic type of Gaucher's disease, usually with infantile onset, was described more than two decades later.[369] In 1934 Aghion demonstrated that the major lipid accumulated in Gaucher's disease was a glucosylceramide.[6] In 1959, slowly progressive subacute neuronopathic type III was described and called as the 'Norrbottnian' type because this type of patient was clustered in Norrbotten province in northern Sweden.[285] The deficient activity of β-glucosidase (glucocerebrosidase) was reported in 1965 by two groups as the primary cause of Gaucher's disease.[82,509] The most prominent clinical manifestation of type I is massive hepatosplenomegaly without neurological involvement. Although the majority of this type occurs in adults,

children may also be affected. Children with type I Gaucher's disease usually show massive hepatosplenomegaly with severe hepatic dysfunction and extensive skeletal abnormalities.[298] Neurological symptoms are usually absent but some patients with various neurological manifestations are known.[438,770] Clinical features of type II Gaucher disease are those of severe progressive neurological illness in addition to hepatosplenomegaly. It usually affects infants. Oculomotor abnormalities are often the initial clinical manifestation and the majority of patients die within 2 years.[108,362] The severity of the clinical manifestation in type III is intermediate between that of types II and I. Neurological symptoms occur later and are usually less severe than in type II.[154,174] A severe neonatal form of Gaucher's disease with a rapidly progressive fulminant course has been reported. Infants with this form may exhibit marked ichthyotic skin or hydrops fetalis.[616,644] Patients with genetic deficiency in one of the sphingolipid activator proteins, saposin C (sap-C), show a clinical phenotype similar to that of neuronopathic Gaucher's disease (see below).

Biochemistry

The basic biochemical defect of Gaucher's disease is a deficient activity of acid β-glucosidase (glucocerebrosidase), resulting in massive accumulation of glucocerebroside in cells of the monocyte–macrophage system. Glucocerebroside is markedly increased and a toxic substrate, glucosylsphingosine, is detected in the liver and spleen in all types.[474] The extent of glucocerebroside accumulation in the brain may be quite variable even within the same type. Nilsson et al. analysed glucosylceramide (glucocerebroside) and glucosylsphingosine in two type I patients, 3 and 56 years old. Neither had any clinical or neuropathological evidence of neuronal involvement. While no difference was detected in the extent of glucosylceramide accumulation in the viscera, glucosylceramide accumulation was greater in the brain of the 3-year-old than in the older patient.[473] Concentrations of brain glucocerebroside in types II and III are much higher than in type I, the highest value being found in the most fulminant cases.[108,475] Glucosylsphingosine, never detected in normal brain, was demonstrated in the brains from all types, with a positive correlation with neurological involvement.[338,475] The accumulation of the cytotoxic glucosylsphingosine may be responsible for extensive neuronal degeneration, which is most striking in type II.

Molecular genetics

All types of Gaucher's disease are autosomal recessive caused by mutations in the gene coding for glucocerebrosidase. The gene is localized on chromosome 1q21 and so far more than 60 disease-causing mutations have been identified.[43] Type I occurs frequently in Ashkanazi Jews and the most common mutation in this type is X1226Y. However, this mutation is not found among Gaucher

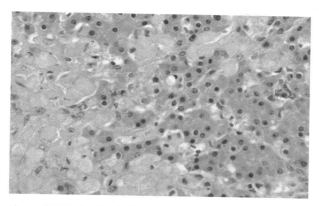

Figure 11.32 *Gaucher's disease, type II. Massive infiltration of Gaucher cells in liver. (H&E.)*

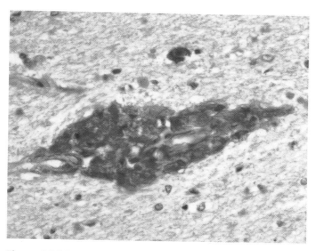

Figure 11.34 *Gaucher's disease in adult type I without neurological signs or symptoms. Perivascular Gaucher cells are strongly stained with PAS in hypothalamic region. (PAS.)*

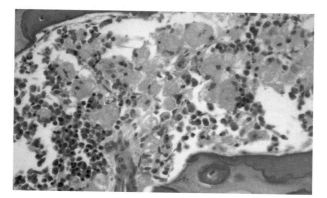

Figure 11.33 *Gaucher's disease, type II. Bone marrow that is almost totally replaced by infiltrating Gaucher cells. (H&E.)*

patients from East Asia.[298] No ethinic predominance is known for type II. A number of mutations has been identified in type II patients. A somewhat common mutation in this type is X1448Y, but this mutation has also been noted in type I, in particular among Japanese type I patients. Type III patients are clustered in northern Sweden and the prevailing mutation is X444Y. However, the same mutation may be detected in any of these three phenotypes. At this time there is no clear explanation for why the same genotype for a disease-causing mutation may express very different clinical phenotypes.[59,298]

Neuroimaging

There are no specific neuroradiological findings in any type of Gaucher's disease. In type I, the vertebrae may show irregular endplates and this finding may simulate diskitis with osteomyelitis. Extramedullary haematopoiesis may lead to thickening of the bones and formation of soft-tissue masses that may compress the spinal cord and occasionally the brain.

Pathology

In all types, massive infiltration of macrophages with glucocerebroside storage (Gaucher cells) is seen in visceral organs. Infiltration is particularly conspicuous in the liver (Fig. 11.32) and spleen, resulting in hepatosplenomegaly. Gaucher cell infiltration in the bone marrow (Fig. 11.33) often causes severe bone disease such as avascular necrosis and pathological fracture.[226,797,801] Severe bone disease appears to be much more frequent in splenectomized patients.[24,562,801] Gaucher cells are characterized by the cytoplasm having a wrinkled appearance. The cytoplasm is PAS positive (Fig. 11.34) in both paraffin and frozen sections. Ultrastructurally, the cytoplasm contains a curved or twisted tubular structure characteristic of glucocerebroside (Figs 11.35, 11.36). The brain of type I patients is grossly normal. However, Gaucher cells have been demonstrated microscopically in the leptomeninges as well as in the perivascular regions (Fig. 11.34) within the brain in association with an intense gliomesodermal reaction.[389,626,770] Some of the patients may have well-documented neurological symptoms, but others are without significant clinical manifestations of CNS involvement. In type II patients with severe neurological symptoms, such as oculomotor apraxia, myoclonus and progressive bulbar signs, marked infiltration of Gaucher cells (Fig. 11.37) with neuronal degeneration and gliosis are well documented. Neuronal loss and degeneration are widespread. The basal ganglia, the thalamus, hypothalamus and brainstem are more severely affected than the cerebral cortex.[338,477] In the cerebellum, the dentate nuclei are often severely involved. In the cerebral cortex, neuronal degeneration and Gaucher cell infiltration are most conspicuous in the occipital cortex.[44,338,389] On rare occasions, neurons contain the typical tubular inclusions as seen in Gaucher cells and also 'membranous cytosomes filled with flat parallel membranes', resembling the zebra bodies in neurons of mucopolysaccharidoses.[5,234] Some patients with type II disease may develop the disease prenatally, neonatally or later during the first year of life, and may have associated hydrops fetalis and/or congenital

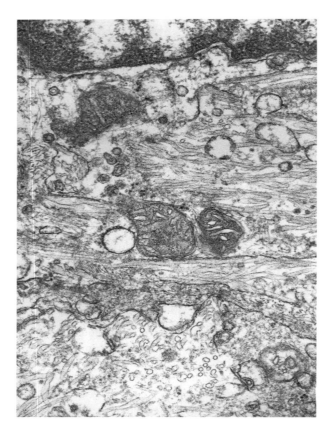

Figure 11.35 *Gaucher's disease, type II. Longitudinal tubular glucocerebroside inclusions within Gaucher cells. (Electron micrograph.)*

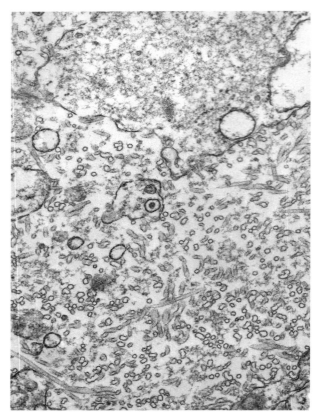

Figure 11.36 *Gaucher's disease, type II. Cross-section of tubular inclusions in a Gaucher cell. (Electron micrograph.)*

ichthyosis.[400,605,616,617,640] In type III patients, neuropathology is essentially similar to but less severe than type II.[109,110,338] Conradi *et al.* reported a child with late-infantile Gaucher's disease with oculomotor apraxia, progressive myoclonus and prominent bulbar signs. In that child, the dentate nuclei were severely involved, consistent with the clinical sign of myoclonus. In addition, there was an extensive band-like intraparenchymal accumulation of Gaucher cells, as noted in infantile type II disease.[108]

Animal models

A naturally occurring canine model has been reported but not propagated.[267] With targeted disruption of the murine glucocerebrosidase gene, a murine model of Gaucher's disease was generated.[703] This mouse was null allele and died within 24 h of birth. These mice had less than 4% of the normal glucosylceramidase activity. There was no hepatosplenomegaly. Accumulation of glucocerebroside was found in the liver, lung, brain and bone marrow biochemically, and glucocerebroside inclusions were identified in macrophages in the liver, spleen and bone marrow at the ultrastructural level.[703,765] The most significant pathology in these mice was abnormally prominent wrinkling with hyperkeratosis in the skin.[616] The phenotype of these mice were similar to that of the

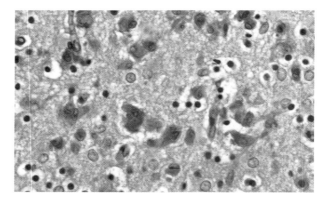

Figure 11.37 *Gaucher's disease, type II neuronopathic form. Individually scattered Gaucher cells with PAS-positive storage material within the occipital cortex. (PAS.)*

severe subtype of type II Gaucher's disease ('collodion' babies).[616,686] Another group had generated mice carrying mutations found among human patients, the RecNeil mutation that can cause type II disease or the L444P mutation associated with type III. Mice homozygous for the RecNeil mutation had a little enzyme activity and accumulated glucocerebroside in the tissues. Mice homozygous for the L444P mutation had a higher level of enzyme activity and there was no detectable accumulation of glucocerebroside in the tissues. These mice with the point mutation of the glucocerebroside gene, however, also died within 48 h of birth, with a clinical phenotype similar to the mice with the null mutation despite detectable residual glucocerebrosidase activities.[405]

Farber's disease

Farber's disease is caused by the deficiency of lysosomal acid ceramidase with a consequent accumulation of ceramide in tissues. This is a very rare, clinically heterogeneous disease.

History and clinical features

In 1952, Farber described three children with disseminated 'lipogranulomatosis'.[178] The patients developed swollen joints and hoarse, weak cries shortly after birth. Joint movements became increasingly limited owing to joint deformities, multiple subcutaneous nodules, particularly over the joints, osteoporosis and erosions of bones.[179] Episodes of fever and dyspnoea, associated with pulmonary infiltration, occurred frequently. The clinical course of the majority of reported cases is similar to that of Farber's original cases. The onset is usually soon after birth, with progressive symptoms and death with intercurrent infection or inanition by 2–3 years of age. Outstanding clinical features are stiff, swollen and painful joints, with amyotrophy and mucocutaneous nodules in the larynx, causing a hoarse or faint voice, and in the scalp and abdominal or thoracic walls. Psychomotor retardation and other signs of neurological manifestations are present in many patients. In some, progression of the disease process may be less aggressive and the patients may survive until adolescence or young adulthood.[120,512] Moser described seven clinical subtypes.[452] Coexistence with congenital hypothyroidism,[162,700] Sandhoff's disease[200] or hydrocephalus[49,542] has been reported.

Biochemistry

All tissues examined show excess of ceramide, and in particular high concentrations of ceramide are found in the subcutaneous nodules and in the kidney.[530,574] In 1972, Sugita et al. demonstrated the deficient activity of an acid ceramidase in the tissue of the patient reported by Prensky.[643] Diagnosis can be made by the assay of this enzyme in cultured fibroblasts and leukocytes. In severely affected patients, an increase of GM1 ganglioside has been reported in the kidney, lymph nodes and subcutaneous nodules.[530]

Molecular genetics

The mode of inheritance is autosomal recessive. The human and mouse acid ceramidase cDNA and gene have been cloned and characterized, and a few disease-causing mutations have been identified.[357,397]

Pathology

The cutaneous nodules are granulomatous lesions containing varying numbers of foam cells. These cells are distended with PAS-positive material. In later stages, fibrosis and infiltration with lymphocytes and plasma cells become apparent. Similar granulomata involve joints, subcutaneous tissue (usually at points that are subjected to pressure, such as knees and elbows), the larynx, the lungs, the kidney and, less commonly, the heart, liver and spleen. Hepatosplenomegaly, conjunctival nodules and macroglossia may be present. In the nervous system, the major pathology is neuronal storage with PAS-positive material. The neuronal storage is most pronounced in anterior horn cells and large neurons in the medulla, pons and cerebellum and least in the cerebral cortex. In the patient reported by Moser et al. loss of neurons and gliosis were prominent in the cerebral cortex, and dying neurons and neuronophagia were noted in the anterior horns.[453] The white matter shows focal myelin degeneration and gliosis. Neuronal storage is also noted in autonomic ganglia and posterior root ganglia. Macular cherry-red spots representing retinal ganglion cell storage may be present.[104,200,453,555,795] Various types of ultrastructural feature have been reported in the storage materials. Short curvilinear tubular bodies are observed mainly in fibroblasts and cells in the monocyte–macrophage system.[2,794] In peripheral nerves, the cytoplasm of Schwann cells is often filled with electron-lucent lysosomal inclusions of various shapes that have well-defined electron-dense rims. They are called 'banana bodies'.[49,513] Loss of large myelinated fibres has been reported.[513] Zebra bodies have been described in the neuronal perikarya.[794] A detailed review of the pathological lesions has been provided by Pellissier et al.[513]

Animal models

There are no known animal models of Farber's disease.

Fabry's disease

Fabry disease is an X-linked recessive disorder caused by the deficiency of α-galactosidase A. Female carriers may be symptomatic. Progressive deposits of neutral glycolipids in the vascular endothelial cells and smooth-muscle cells cause ischaemia and infarction, resulting in the major clinical manifestation of the disease.

History and clinical features

Fabry's disease was originally described as a dermatological disease, angiokeratoma corporis diffusum, independently by two dermatologists, Fabry in Germany and Anderson in England in 1898.[13,177] The X-linked recessive inheritance was first documented by Opitz et al. in 1965.[496] Brady et al.[80] demonstrated deficiency of the enzyme, ceramide trihexosidase (α-galactosidase A) as the cause of the disease. Typical clinical features of hemizygous males with Fabry's disease are the presence of angiokeratoma in the skin, painful peripheral neuropathy, transient ischaemic attacks and/or cerebral infarction (stroke), myocardial infarction (heart attack) and renal failure. Corneal and lenticular opacities are usually detected by slit-lamp examination. These clinical manifestations are due to progressive storage of glycolipid in the vascular endothelial cells, resulting in ischaemia. The onset of these symptoms is usually during childhood or adolescence. Heterozygous females are usually asymptomatic but some symptoms may manifest themselves with increasing age.[141,291] A rare 'cardiac variant' of Fabry's disease has been described in recent years. These patients are usually asymptomatic during most of their lives and are diagnosed only after the later onset of cardiac manifestations such as hypertrophic cardiomyopathy or myocardial infarction.[107,165,460,487,731] Patients with these atypical variants have residual activity of α-galactosidase A consistent with their milder phenotype.

Biochemistry

The enzyme deficient in Fabry's disease is the lysosomal enzyme, α-galactosidase A.[80] Consequently, globotriaosylceramide [ceramide trihexoside (TCH), Gal'-Gal-Glc-ceramide] and galabiosylceramide (Gal-Gal-ceramide) accumulate in the tissue.[670] Classically affected hemizygotes have essentially no demonstrable α-galactosidase A activity. However, residual activity has been detected in an atypical variant form.[66,102,354,561]

Molecular genetics

The α-galactosidase A gene is localized in the q22 region of the X-chromosome. Gene mutations are heterogeneous and most mutations have been private and found only in single pedigrees. Approximately 75% of the mutations causing Fabry's disease are missense or nonsense mutations.

Neuroimaging

In patients with severe CNS involvement, areas of infarction involving both grey and white matter may be seen. The periventricular white matter may be of abnormal signal intensity on T_2-weighted MRI. With time, these abnormal areas of T_2 signal become confluent and the brain becomes atrophic. In female heterozygous patients the imaging findings tend to be subtle.

Pathology

The pathology of Fabry's disease is characterized by widespread tissue deposits of glycosphingolipids that show birefringence with 'Maltese crosses' under polarizing microscopy. Many parenchymal organs, including the

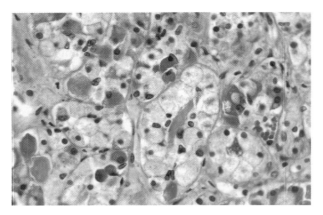

Figure 11.38 *Fabry's disease. Swollen epithelial cells with stored lipid in the anterior lobe of the pituitary gland. (H&E.)*

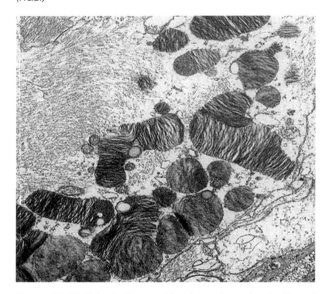

Figure 11.39 *Fabry's disease. Membrane-bound collection of lipid lamellae in an astrocyte. (Electron micrograph.)*

liver, pancreas, testis, thyroid, prostate, urinary bladder, adrenal glands and gastrointestinal tract, are involved. These lipids are preferentially deposited in the endothelial and smooth-muscle cells of the blood vessels, autonomic ganglia and peripheral nerves throughout the body. Lipid storage has been demonstrated in the macrophages in the bone marrow and lymph nodes, epithelial cells of mucous glands, eccrine sweat gland[386] and pituitary gland (Fig. 11.38), and epithelial cells of the glomerulus and tubules of the kidney.[698] Foam cells containing birefringent lipid droplets are frequently detected in the urinary sediment. Ultrastructurally they are found to be composed of electron-dense concentric tightly packed lamellar structures (Fig. 11.39). The swollen vascular endothelial cells, often accompanied by endothelial proliferation, encroach upon the lumen, causing a focal increase of the intraluminal pressure and thrombus formation resulting in ischaemia or infarction.[462] Progressive aneurysmal dilatation of the weakened vascular walls has been well

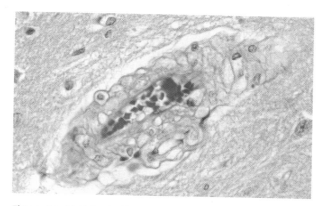

Figure 11.40 *Fabry's disease. Vacuolated smooth-muscle cells are very conspicuous in a cerebral vessel. (H&E.)*

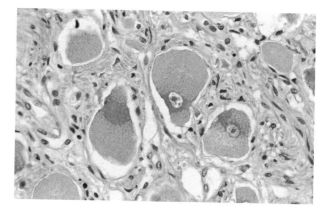

Figure 11.41 *Fabry's disease, neuronal storage in the periaortic sympathetic ganglion. (H&E.)*

documented in the retinal and conjunctival blood vessels and telangiectatic vessels in the skin. In the heart, lipids are deposited within the myocardial cells and many lipid-laden storage cells are found in mitral and tricuspid valves.[141] Vascular involvement is also prominent in the nervous system (Fig. 11.40), often resulting in cerebral ischaemia/infarction or peripheral nerve conduction abnormalities.[607] In a longitudinal MRI study of 50 patients, Crutchfield and co-workers found that all patients with Fabry's disease older than 54 years had typical features of a small-vessel disease.[123] The lipid deposition is also noted in the leptomeningeal cells, neurons of the peripheral and central autonomic nervous system (Fig. 11.41) and primary neurons of somatic afferent pathways.[144,166,488,540,645,671] In the CNS, swollen storage neurons are detected in the amygdala, hypothalamic nuclei, hippocampus, and entorhinal cortex and brainstem nuclei. The storage materials are also detected in astrocytes (Fig. 11.39). They stain positively with LFB and are strongly immunoreactive with antibodies to TCH.[144] A recent proton MRI study indicated a widespread pathological process throughout the brain.[687] In peripheral nerves, loss of myelinated and unmyelinated nerve fibres has been well documented.[198,488,619,697] Lipid deposits in Schwann cells have been also reported in some cases.[619,645]

Animal models

There is no naturally occurring animal model of Fabry's disease. By targeted disruption of the gene, mouse models have been generated independently by two groups.[489,747] These mice are phenotypically normal, although α-galactosidase A activity is undetectable. The lipid inclusions similar to those seen in man are demonstrated in the liver and kidney with the electron microscope as well as with lectin histochemistry with *Griffonia (Bandeiraea) simplicifolia*, which selectively binds to α-D-galactosyl residues. Accumulation of these lipids increases with age.[490] However, unlike in man, lipid accumulation does not occur in the vascular endothelial cells. Correction of enzymatic and lysosomal storage defects in the murine model by adenovirus-mediated gene transfer has been reported.[800] α-Galactosidase A transgenic mice carrying the normal or mutant human α-galactosidase gene have also been generated.[305,609]

Metachromatic leukodystrophy (MLD) and multiple sulfatase deficiency (MSD)

MLD is an autosomal recessive sphingolipid storage disease, characterized by storage of sulfatide in central and peripheral nervous tissues and some visceral organs. The disease is caused by deficiency in the activity of arylsulfatase A. In addition, patients with genetic deficiency of the sulfatide activator protein, saposin B, exhibit a phenotype similar to MLD (see below). These patients show normal activity of arylsulfatase A. MSD is another disorder genetically distinct from MLD. Multiple sulfatases are genetically deficient and patients show a phenotype that is a combination of MLD and mucopolysaccharidoses.[360]

History and clinical course

The heterogeneous clinical types have been classified into three major subtypes, late infantile, juvenile and adult. Rare congenital and infantile types have also been reported.[180,239] In 1925, Scholz reported three children from one family with progressive leukodystrophy of a juvenile type.[595] Later, Peiffer demonstrated striking brown metachromasia in the brain of the patients reported by Scholz[523] using the acetic acid–cresyl violet stain.[730] Thus, the report by Peiffer[523] is the first comprehensive clinicopathological account of MLD. Excessive accumulation of sulfatide in MLD tissues was discovered in 1958[29,310] and the deficiency of arylsulfatase A as the underlying cause of the sulfatide accumulation was reported several years later.[34,311,441] The late infantile type is the most frequent type. Patients have normal early milestones, although neuroimaging studies may detect abnormalities before the clinical onset of the disease. The usual initial clinical presentation is frequent falls with mild spasticity of extremities during the first and the second years. Loss of motor functions and language, spastic quadriplegia and cortical blindness follow rapidly to the point of a vegetative state, and the patients survive only rarely beyond 5 years of age. The juvenile MLD has a more insidious onset between 4 and 12 years, and the clinical signs and symptoms tend to progress more slowly than in the late infantile type.[233] Behavioural abnormalities and slurred speech precede extrapyramidal or motor dysfunction. Adult MLD may occur at any age after puberty. Progress is usually very slow, with changes in personality, decreased mental status or other psychiatric symptoms.[30,47,672] In some patients with the adult type, peripheral neuropathy may be the presenting clinical symptom.[71,191] Patients with MSD show combined features of both late infantile MLD and a mucopolysaccharidosis (MPS). Features of MPS may or may not be evident during the early stages, however. Rare patients with sphingolipid activator protein B (sap B or saposin B deficiency) present an MLD-like clinical phenotype[254,587,603,638,752] (see below).

Biochemistry

The basic genetic defect causing MLD is deficiency of arylsulfatase A, resulting in an accumulation of sulfatide in the tissue. The enzyme activity is extremely low in late infantile type but some residual activity can be detected in late-onset cases.[390] Reflecting the extensive loss of myelin in the white matter, the concentrations of myelin lipids, cholesterol, phospholipids and cerebrosides are markedly decreased in the late-infantile type, while the sulfatide content is increased.[668] Increased sulfatide is also reported in isolated myelin.[480] Sulfatide concentrations are increased in the liver, gall bladder and kidney, and excess amounts of sulfatide are excreted in urine.[360] Rare patients with a deficiency in the cerebroside sulfate activator protein (saposin B; SAP-B) show normal levels of arylsulphatase A activity.[587,603] In patients with MSD, arylsulfatase A, B and C, steroid sulfatases, and various sulfatases related to degradation of mucopolysaccharides are deficient (Table 11.1), resulting in an accumulation of sulfatides and mucopolysaccharides in the brain, liver, kidney and urine.[33,459,543,547] Similar to MLD, the proportion of sulfatide is higher in the myelin and the pattern of gangliosides in the brain is abnormal in MSD patients, with increases in the normally minor monosialogangliosides GM2 and GM3.[175]

Molecular genetics

All forms of MLD – late infantile, juvenile, adult types and MSD – are diseases of autosomal recessive inheritance. Late infantile, juvenile and adult types are all caused by a primary genetic defect in the arylsulfatase A gene on chromosome 22. Polten and co-workers have suggested that there are two distinct types of arylsulfatase A mutation, allele O (or I) and allele A (or R).[335,528] The allele O tends

to be without any functioning gene product and thus is associated with the late infantile type, and the allele A tends to be associated with some residual enzymatic activity and, thus, is found in patients diagnosed as juvenile or adult MLD. Patients heterozygous for both alleles A and O were juvenile MLD.[211] However, Berger et al. stressed the genetic heterogeneity of MLD and indicated that the genotype–phenotype correlation suggested by Polten et al. was not followed in their study.[53] More recently, Qu et al. have documented differences in both molecular weight and electric charges among different types of MLD mutation.[537] One or two per cent of the healthy individual may have arylsulfatase A activity sufficiently low for enzymic diagnosis of MLD (pseudodeficiency). It is important to know the existence of such a condition because individuals with the pseudodeficient allele may be misdiagnosed as MLD or as its carriers.[211,336] In MSD, activities of multiple sulfatases are defective. Schmidt and co-workers recently discovered a novel cotranslational or post-translational modification common to many sulfatases. This modification of a cysteine residue to formyl glycine appears to be a prerequisite for the catalytic activity of many sulfatases. In at least two sulfatases known to be deficient in MSD, this conversion did not take place. Thus a genetic defect in MSD appears to be a deficiency of this conversion mechanism.[588]

Neuroimaging

CT of the brain shows non-specific areas of low density, particularly in the periventricular white matter. These abnormalities tend to be bilateral and fairly symmetrical (Fig 11.42a). Similar findings are seen on MRI. The abnormalities preferentially involve the frontal lobes, but may occur anywhere in the brain. The subcortical U-fibres tend to be spared until late in the disease (Fig. 11.42c). The periventricular lesion extends into the corpus callosum, the internal and external capsules, and into the white matter in the brainstem. MRI also demonstrates increased T_2 signal intensity in the medial aspects of the cerebellum. None of the lesions enhances after intravenous contrast administration. In the advanced and late stages of the disease, cerebral atrophy is prominent.

Pathology

The major pathology of MLD is demyelination in the central (Figs 11.42c and 11.43) and peripheral nervous systems and deposits of metachromatic materials in cells within the nervous system and visceral organs (Figs 11.44–11.46).[776] The metachromatic deposits show pink metachromasia with toluidine blue (Fig. 11.44) and characteristic brown metachromasia with acidic cresyl violet stain (Figs 11.45, 11.46).[730] The metachromatic granules from the brain of an MLD patient were isolated and their composition was characterized. Chemical analysis has shown that the molar ratio of cholesterol to galactolipids

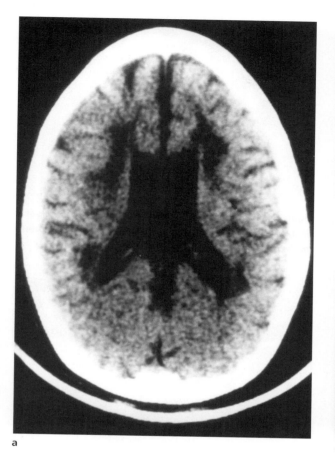

a

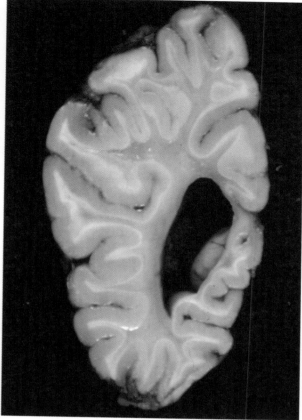

c

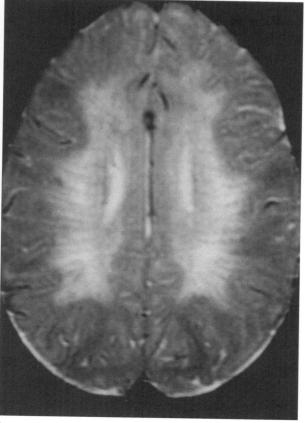

b

Figure 11.42 *Metachromatic leukodystrophy. (a) MLD in an advanced stage. Axial CT shows low-density in the periventricular white matter and diffuse cerebral cortical atrophy. (b) Axial T_2-weighted image shows increased and abnormal signal intensity in the centrum semiovale. (c) Coronal section of the occipital region of a cerebral hemisphere. The demyelinated white matter appears greyish, in contrast to preserved white matter in the subcortical region.*

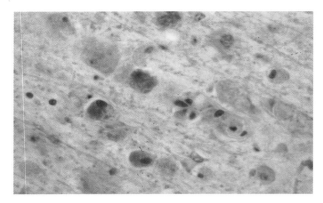

Figure 11.43 *Metachromatic leukodystrophy. Demyelinating white matter with scattered glial cells and macrophages. (H&E.)*

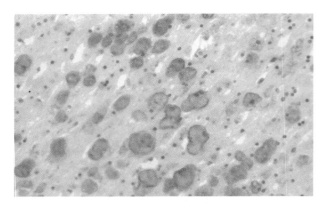

Figure 11.45 *Metachromatic leukodystrophy. Macrophages in demyelinating cerebral white matter demonstrate brown metachromasia on a frozen section. (Acidic cresyl violet.)*

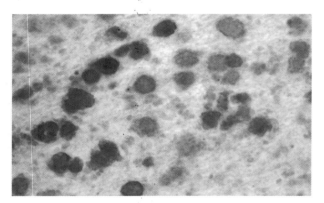

Figure 11.44 *Metachromatic leukodystrophy. The stored material in the macrophages and glial cells of demyelinating white matter shows pink metachromasia on a frozen section. (Toluidine blue.)*

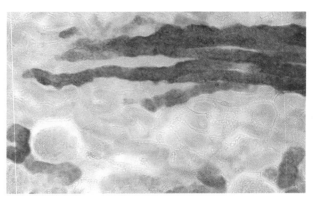

Figure 11.46 *Metachromatic leukodystrophy. Brown metachromasia is also recognized in renal tubules on a frozen section. (Acidic cresyl violet.)*

to phosphatides is 1:1:1. Most of the galactolipids are sulfatides.[657,658] Electron-microscopic studies revealed various morphological features. Prismatic and tuffstone inclusions were especially characteristic (Fig. 11.47).[16,240,241] Herringbone and honeycomb patterns were often well recognized as unique components of the prismatic inclusion (Fig. 11.47). These MLD inclusions can be reproduced *in vivo* or *in vitro* by an overload of sulfatides into the tissue or addition to the culture medium.[16,569] In the adult type, MLD inclusions frequently form composites with lipofuscin.[218,220] In the visceral organs, the metachromatic granules are found in macrophages in lymph nodes and spleen, sweat gland epithelial cells, in Kupffer cells and the bile-duct epithelium in the liver, in the epithelium and stroma of the gall bladder, in the adrenal medulla, and in the islets of Langerhans in the pancreas.[250,776] A rare occurrence of papillomatosis of the gall bladder has been reported.[481] In the kidney, the metachromatic material is present in the epithelial cells of the distal convoluted tubules (Fig. 11.46), the thin limb of the loop of Henle and the collecting tubules. The brains of patients with the late infantile type show extensive demyelination throughout the white

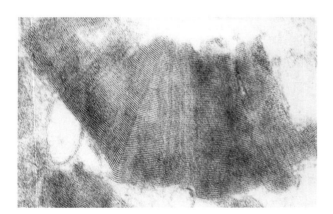

Figure 11.47 *Metachromatic leukodystrophy. Characteristic storage material in macrophage showing alternating fine electron-dense and electron-lucent short prismatic lamellar structures arranged into a herringbone pattern. (Electron micrograph.)*

matter (Fig. 11.42c), which shows grey discoloration and a firm consistency. The cerebellum and brainstem are atrophic. A paucity of myelin with numerous reactive astrocytes and macrophages containing metachromatic granules (Figs 11.43–11.45) are the characteristic

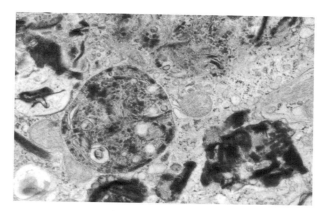

Figure 11.48 *Metachromatic leukodystrophy. Pleomorphic inclusions in glial cells. (Electron micrograph.)*

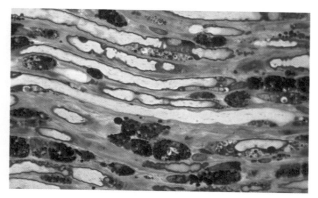

Figure 11.49 *Metachromatic leukodystrophy. Demyelinating nerve fibres and macrophages with stored material of the cauda equina in a 1-μm-thick section. (Toluidine blue.)*

features of MLD. Axons are also decreased. Unlike adrenoleukodystrophy or orthochromic leukodystrophy, the granules in the macrophages are eosinophilic, PAS positive and non-sudanophilic, and show the characteristic brown metachromasia (Fig. 11.45) on frozen sections. Some neurons in the motor cortex, thalamus, hypothalamus, basal ganglia, brainstem, dentate nucleus and the anterior horn of the spinal cord contain inclusions with metachromasia.[3,516] At the ultrastructural level, these neuronal inclusions resemble MCBs of gangliosidoses. In contrast to the relatively uniform neuronal inclusions, inclusions in the glial cells are more pleomorphic (Fig. 11.48).[516] These neuropathological changes are basically similar but milder in juvenile and adult types. Segmental demyelination is found in the peripheral nerves (Fig. 11.49). Large-diameter fibres tend to be affected more severely than the small-diameter fibres. Loss of axons is relatively mild in late infantile or juvenile type but is more pronounced in the adult type, which is often associated with endoneurial fibrosis.[45,191,694] Schwann cells and endoneurial macrophages contain metachromatic granules. The different clinical variants do not show any striking differences in the type of inclusions.[694]

The pathology of MSD is that of a combined metachromatic leukodystrophy and a mucopolysaccharidosis.[244,344] Grossly, the leptomeninges are fibrotic, causing severe obstructive hydrocephalus in a case reported by Kepes et al.,[344] while the case reported by Guerra et al. showed atrophy of both the cerebrum and the cerebellum.[244] Perivascular dilatation as noted in MPS is pronounced in the cerebral white matter. In the distended cortical neurons, zebra bodies similar to those noted in MPS[7] and other types of 'granulo-membrano-vacuolar bodies' are described at the ultrastructural level. The honeycomb structure with a hexagonal configuration as described in MLD is found in glial cells.[547] In a rare patient who had only mild deficiencies of arylsulfatases but with severe deficiencies of iduronate sulfatase and heparan-sulfamidase, pathological changes were closer to MPS, with minimal deposition of metachromatic materials in the white matter.[415]

Animal models

There is no naturally occurring animal model of metachromatic leukodystrophy. Arylsulfatase A-deficient mice, generated by homologous recombination, exhibit significant impairment of neuromuscular co-ordination and hearing. Histological evidence of lipid storage and focal demyelination in the acoustic ganglia are detected. However, unlike human MLD, the mouse model has a normal lifespan and does not develop extensive demyelination.[210,281]

In 2-year-old arylsulfatase A-deficient mice, loss of Purkinje cells and simplified dendritic architecture of Purkinje cells have been reported.[146] In such mice, there is some evidence of peripheral nerve demyelination, but no appreciable demyelination in the CNS.

Krabbe's disease (globoid cell leukodystrophy, GLD)

Krabbe's disease is an autosomal recessive neurological disease caused by the deficiency of galactosylceramidase (galactocerebrosidase β-galactosidase), usually affecting young infants with a rapidly progressive and fatal course. Rare late-onset cases are also known.[359,662,757]

History and clinical course

In 1916, the Danish physician Kund Krabbe described clinical and pathological findings in five infants from two families who died of an 'acute infantile familial diffuse brain sclerosis'.[368] These infants developed fits of violent crying and irritability beginning at the age of 4–6 months, followed by progressive muscular rigidity, and violent tonic spasms evoked by such stimuli as noise, light and touch. Death occurred between 11 months and 1.5 years. The clinical course of these patients is typical of patients with infantile GLD. In 1970, deficiency in the activity of the lysosomal enzyme galactocerebroside β-galactosidase (galactosylceramidase) was identified as the underlying genetic cause.[656] Human galactosylceramidase cDNA was cloned in 1993[96] and more than 40 disease-causing mutations have been identified.[195,753,757] Late-onset juvenile or adult cases with an insidious onset and slower course are also known.[359,361,414] The onset of juvenile type GLD is between 3 and 10 years. A gait disturbance, pes cavus or equinovarus deformity of the feet may be starting symptoms that lead to spastic paraparesis. Visual failure and an intellectual decline develop slowly but progressively.[414] The course of the disease of later onset, however, is less stereotyped than the infantile form, and some may attain close to the normal lifespan.[361] Adult-onset GLD is usually characterized by slowly developing asymmetric limb weakness, a spastic gait, poor co-ordination and balance, and tremors.[353,525,721] Dementia is reported only in rare patients.[124] Although the clinical course of the infantile and late-onset GLD differs significantly, there are no apparent differences in the level of residual activity of galactosylceramidase activity among different types as measured *in vitro*.[414,757]

Biochemistry

The unique biochemical characteristic of the infantile GLD is the lack of abnormal accumulation of galactosylceramide in the brain, despite the fact that galactosylceramide is the primary natural substrate of the genetically deficient degradative enzyme, galactosylceramidase.[669,718,719] This paradoxical phenomenon results from the unique localization of galactosylceramide in the myelin sheath and very rapid and early disappearance of oligodendrocytes. Since oligodendrocytes disappear at a very early stage of myelination and no further synthesis of galactosylceramide occurs, it does not accumulate galactosylceramide beyond the level attained at the early stage of myelination. Instead, however, a related toxic metabolite, psychosine (galactosylsphingosine) does accumulate abnormally and is considered the key compound in the pathogenesis of the disease.[447,713] Galactosylceramide accumulates within the characteristic globoid cells, so termed by Collier and Greenfield[106] by their appearance. Biochemical analysis of a fraction enriched with the characteristic globoid cells contained a relatively large amount of galactosylceramide.[32] Globoid cells experimentally generated by intracerebral injection or leptomeningeal application of galactosylceramide[31,34,495] appear morphologically identical to those seen in patients with Krabbe's disease.[14,647] Biochemical abnormalities are limited to the nervous system, at least in man.

Molecular genetics

The human galactosylceramidase (galactocerebrosidase) gene is localized on chromosome 14q31 and the cDNA and the gene have been cloned.[96,572] More than 40 disease-causing mutations, both nonsense and missense mutations, have been identified.[57,134,195,199,352,413,684,753,757] A frequent abnormality apparently originating in the Nordic countries and thus common among Swedes and Norwegians (but not in the Danish) and their descendants, is characterized by a major deletion in the gene.

Neuroimaging

In GLD, CT may show increased density in the thalami and other regions such as white-matter tracts the cerebral cortex, the cerebellum and the optic radiations. There may be abnormal-appearing white matter, which is hypodense on CT, and hyperintense on T_2-weighted MRI (Fig. 11.50a, b). These abnormalities are less pronounced than in other white-matter disorders. The subcortical U-fibres are spared. By MRI, the white matter abnormalities may have a 'linear' intrinsic pattern. With time, cerebral atrophy ensues. The atrophy also involves the deep grey-matter nuclei. In rare instances, enhancement of the subcortical white matter has been noted after administration of intravenous contrast media. Occasionally, the optic nerves and the chiasm may appear thick and enlarged (Fig. 11.50c). This may be the initial imaging manifestation of the disease. The nerve roots of the cauda equina may also be thick but may also show enhancement after contrast. In late-onset GLD, imaging studies show preferential involvement of the occipital white matter and the splenium of the corpus callosum.

Pathology

Pathology is limited to the nervous system. In the most common infantile type, the brain is atrophic with firm rubbery gliotic white matter. Loss of myelin is nearly complete with the possible exception of subcortical intergyral arcuate U-fibres. Microscopically, marked paucity of myelin with some axonal degeneration is seen throughout the brain. Extensive fibrillary gliosis and infiltration of numerous macrophages (Figs 11.50, 11.51), some multinucleated (epithelioid and globoid cells), are unique characteristic features. The globoid cells are abundant in the region of active demyelination and often clustered around blood vessels (Figs 11.50, 11.51). Oligodendrocytes are markedly reduced.[126,359,662] Correlative MRI and neuropathological studies have shown that the areas of marked hyperintensity on T_2-weighted MRI correspond to the areas of demyelination with globoid cell infiltration.[521] Globoid cells contain PAS-positive storage materials. At the ultrastructural level, the globoid cells contain polygonal or slender tubular structures (Fig. 11.52a, b) that are structurally identical to chemically pure galactosylceramide (galactocerebroside).[792,793] In long surviving cases, the white matter may be totally gliotic and devoid of macrophages.[158,437] Williams *et al.* reported well-preserved dendritic processes of cortical pyramidal neurons

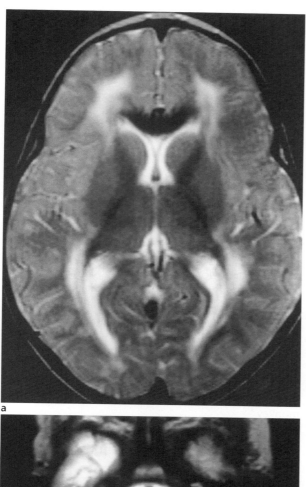

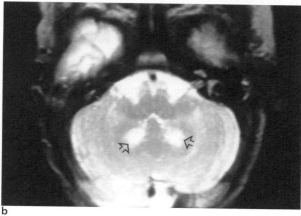

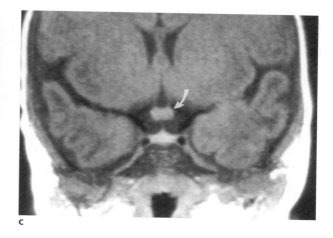

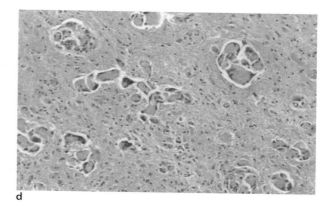

Figure 11.50 *Globoid cell leukodystrophy. (a) Krabbe's disease. Axial MR T₂-weighted image shows increased and abnormal signal intensity in the white matter of the frontal and occipital lobes, particularly in a periventricular distribution. (b) The same patient as in (a): there is abnormally increased signal intensity in the deep cerebellar white matter corresponding to the dentate nuclei (arrows). (c) Coronal T₁-weighted image showing enlarged optic chiasm (arrow), which was the first imaging abnormality in this patient. (d) Demyelinating cerebral white matter with many clustered globoid macrophages. (H&E.)*

in Golgi preparations.[767] However, neuronal loss is conspicuous in the thalamus, cerebellar Purkinje cells and neurons of the dentate nucleus, pons and brainstem in cases examined post-mortem.[126,158,437,521] Giant lamellar inclusions have been reported in denervated Purkinje cells.[286] The optic nerves are usually atrophic but, in some cases, they are markedly enlarged with extensive gliosis (Fig. 11.53). The peripheral nerves may be grossly enlarged and firm.[630] Marked endoneurial fibrosis, and features of segmental demyelination and remyelination with onion bulb formation are often present.[65,379,585,651] Quantitative analysis demonstrated a severe loss of large myelinated fibres but the numbers of unmyelinated fibres were not diminished.[585] Endoneurial macrophages and Schwann cells contain tubular inclusions similar to those in the globoid cells in the

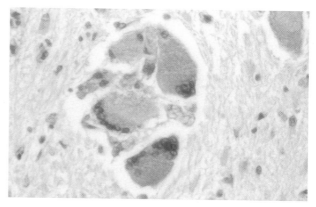

Figure 11.51 *Globoid cell leukodystrophy. Clustered multinucleated globoid cells containing PAS-positive material. (PAS.)*

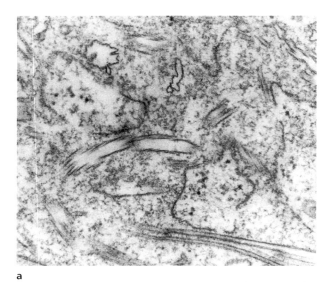

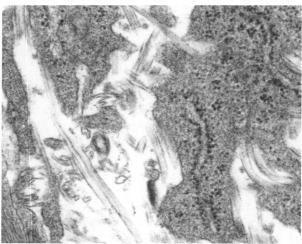

b

Figure 11.52 *Globoid cell leukodystrophy. (a) Tubular inclusions in a macrophage are polygonal on cross-section. (Electron micrograph.) (b) Slender tubular inclusions within electron-lucent spaces in a globoid cell. (Electron micrograph.)*

cerebral white matter.[65,651] MRI study of the late onset GLD shows high-intensity lesions in the white matter suggestive of demyelination.[361,413] Neuropathological reports of late-onset cases, however, are limited. Choi *et al.* described the neuropathology of adult-onset GLD in 18-year-old twins.[98] Their clinical symptoms developed 12 and 7 months before their death, respectively. Both died of severe graft-versus-host disease 2 months after allogeneic bone-marrow transplantation. The brains showed degeneration of the optic radiation and frontoparietal white matter with corticospinal tract degeneration. Multiple necrotic foci with calcium deposits were found within the lesion. Globoid cell infiltration was noted in actively degenerating white matter. In the peripheral nerves of adult GLD, loss of myelinated fibres, disproportionately thin myelin sheaths and inclusions in Schwann cells have been described.[122,276,435,693]

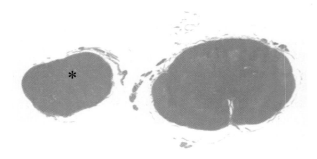

Figure 11.53 *Globoid cell leukodystrophy. Cross-section of a markedly enlarged optic nerve (*), in comparison with the spinal cord. (H&E.)*

Animal models

Genetic galactosylceramidase deficiency (Krabbe's disease) occurs naturally in the mouse (twitcher), in sheep, in dogs (West Highland white terriers and Cairn terriers; blue-tick hound and beagles) and in rhesus monkeys. Clinical and pathological features of these models are closely similar to those of the human disease.[46,359,662] Galactosylceramidase cDNA was cloned and disease-causing mutations have been identified in the mouse,[573] West Highland and Cairn terriers,[724] and the rhesus monkey.[412]

Sphingolipid activator protein (SAP) deficiencies

History, biochemistry and molecular genetics

Several lysosomal hydrolases need the assistance of small non-enzymic glycoprotein cofactors to degrade their substrate sphingolipids. These glycoproteins, also localized within the lysosome, are referred to as activator proteins. If the activator protein for a certain enzyme is genetically defective, the normal function of the enzyme is perturbed, thus resulting in diseases similar to the deficiency of the enzyme itself. The first 'sphingolipid activator protein', the sulfatide activator, now known as saposin B or sap B, was discovered by Mehr and Jatzkewitz.[440] Two genes code for all established and putative sphingolipid activator proteins. One encodes the GM2 activator and is located on human chromosome 5. The other is on chromosome 10, consisting of 15 exons and 14 introns. It codes for the sap precursor protein (prosaposin), which is post-translationally processed to four homologous activator proteins, sap-A (or saposin A, etc.), sap-B, sap-C and sap-D.[576] Deficiency of GM2 activator causes the AB variant of GM2 gangliosidosis[111] (see GM2 gangliosidosis above). Deficiencies of saposin B and C result in metachromatic leukodystrophy-like[638,752] and Gaucher-like[99,100] phenotypes, respectively. Saposin B has been called sulfatide/GM1 activator or SAP-1 and saposin C as SAP-2, respectively, in the past.

No human disease caused by deficiency of saposin A or D is known. However, two siblings with deficiency of all four saposins due to a mutation in the initiation codon of the precursor have been reported.[77,268,590] The parents of these sibs are fourth cousins, both carrying the same mutant allele.[590] An adult patient with neurovisceral lipid storage disease, originally reported as Niemann–Pick disease type C, was later found to be an adult case of total saposin deficiency.[169]

Pathology

Deficiency of GM2 activator protein causes the AB variant of GM2 gangliosidosis. The clinical phenotype and neuropathological findings are very similar to GM2 gangliosidosis caused by the deficiency of β-hexosaminidase A[132,228] (see Gangliosidosis).

The pathology of saposin-B deficiency is similar to that of MLD caused by the deficiency of arylsulfatase A. In the sural nerve biopsy of a 21-year-old patient, Hahn and co-workers reported reduction of myelinated fibres, hypomyelination and onion bulb formation, indicative of chronic recurring demyelination and accumulation of metachromatic and orthochromic globules in Schwann cells and macrophages. These globules showed a hexagonal array or membrane-bound 'tuff stone' appearance, typical ultrastructural features of storage materials in MLD.[253] In addition to the storage of metachromatic materials in macrophages and glial cells in the white matter, scattered cortical neurons with swollen perikarya are present in the brain.[752] Such additional pathology is expected because saposin B has activator functions for degradation of other sphingolipids, such as TCH. Brown metachromasia was demonstrated in the storage macrophages in a rectal biopsy of a 7-year-old child with saposin B deficiency, but submucosal neurons demonstrated non-metachromatic and PAS-positive storage materials with ultrastructural features of membranous cytoplasmic bodies.[587]

In a juvenile patient with saposin C deficiency,[99] there was a striking increase in glucosylceramide and massive neuronal lipid storage in the brain.[506] In the neuropathological report of an 8-year-old boy with saposin C deficiency, the most striking neuronal storage was found in the anterior horn neurons of the spinal cord. There were loss of neurons and neuronophagia similar to type II Gaucher's disease. However, the neuronal storage materials were not the tubular inclusions of glucocerebroside but consisted of lipofuscin as well as concentrically arranged membranous structures at the ultrastructural level. Moderately enlarged neurons were found in the cerebral cortex, thalamus, reticular formation and pons. Perivascular Gaucher cells were absent.[506] Thus, the neuropathological features of saposin-C deficiency are quite different from those of Gaucher's disease, despite the clinical similarity.

One of the two infants with prosaposin deficiency (the other was aborted during pregnancy), who died at 16 weeks, had massive hepatosplenomegaly, and the storage cells in the bone marrow resembled Gaucher cells. However, ultrastructural studies of the liver, nerve and skin revealed more complex inclusions and only a few structures reminiscent of Gaucher's disease. Neuroimaging prior to death indicated an atrophic brain with hydrocephalus. Post-mortem examination was not conducted and thus no information on brain pathology is available.[268] In an adult case of prosaposin deficiency reported by Elleder in 1983 (see above) neurovisceral storage was closely similar to Niemann–Pick disease type C.[169]

Animal model

With targeted disruption of the mouse sphingolipid activator protein (prosaposin) gene, a murine model of total deficiency of sphingolipid activator proteins was generated.[196] In this model, widespread neurovisceral lipid storage and leukodystrophy with extensive axonal dystrophic changes were observed.[500] As already indicated in the section on GM2 gangliosidosis, a mouse model of GM2 gangliosidosis AB variant has been generated by targeted disruption of the GM2 activator protein gene (see above).

MUCOPOLYSACCHARIDOSES

MPS are a genetically heterogeneous group of inborn errors of lysosomal glycosaminoglycan (GAG) metabolism. Each disorder results from the deficiency of the enzyme required at each step of the GAG degradation pathway, and partially degraded GAG accumulate in excessive amounts in virtually all tissues (Table 11.3). There are clinical similarities among different enzyme deficiencies and, conversely, a wide spectrum of clinical severity exists within each enzyme deficiency. All of the MPS share many clinical features, such as a chronic and progressive course, multisystem involvement, organomegaly, dysostosis multiplex, abnormal facies, hearing loss, corneal clouding, and cardiovascular and joint movement sign (and symptom). The pattern of the most prominent storage materials depends on the nature of the enzymic defects. Accumulation of dermatan sulfate in Hurler, Hunter, Maroteaux–Lamy and Sly syndromes is associated with severe skeletal abnormalities, while accumulation of heparan sulfate in Hurler, Hunter and Sanfilippo syndromes is associated with mental retardation resulting from neuronal storage (Table 11.3). However, the major neuronal storage materials in MPS are gangliosides rather than glycosaminoglycans.[274,323] The cellular pathology of affected tissues is generally similar in all MPS cases.[468,759]

Table 11.3 *Mucopolysaccharidoses*

Clinical diagnosis	Affected glycosaminoglycan	Enzyme defect
Hurler's disease (MPS I H) Hurler–Scheie (MPS I H-S) Scheie's disease (MPS I S)	Dermatan sulfate Heparan sulfate	α-L-Iduronidase
Hunter's disease (MPS II)	Dermatan sulfate Heparan sulfate	α-Iduronate-2-sulfatase
Sanfilippo, type A (MPS IIIA) Sanfilippo, type B (MPS IIIB)	Heparan sulfate Heparan sulfate	Heparan N-sulfatase α-N-acetyl-glucosaminidase
Sanfilippo, type C (MPS IIIC)	Heparan sulfate	Acetyl-coenzyme A-α-glucosaminide-N-acetyltransferase
Sanfilippo, type D (MPS IIID)	Heparan sulfate	N-Acetylglucosamine 6-sulfatase
Morquio, type A (MPS IVA)	Keratan sulfate	Galactosamine-6-sulfatase
Morquio, type B (MPS IVB)	Keratan sulfate	β-Galactosidase
Maroteau–Lamy (MPS VI)	Dermatan sulfate	N-Acetyl-galactosamine-4-sulfatase
Sly (MPS VII)	Dermatan sulfate Heparan sulfate Chondroitin sulfate	β-Glucuronidase

Mucopolysaccharidosis I (MPS I, Hurler–Scheie)

History and clinical course

MPS I is usually classified to three phenotypes; Hurler (MPS IH), Hurler–Scheie (MPS IH-S) and Scheie (MPS IS) syndromes. MPS IH is often cited as the prototype of MPS disease. MPS IH was first reported by Gertrude Hurler.[297] It is the most severe form of MPS I and the patient has a coarse face, hepatosplenomegaly, corneal clouding, severe skeletal abnormalities and mental retardation. Clinically, these features are recognized typically between the ages of 9 and 18 months and affected children usually die before the age of 10 years. Acute cardiomyopathy may be a presenting symptom in some infants. MPS IS is at the mildest end of the spectrum in the MPS I phenotype, with normal intellect.[583] The coarse facial features, corneal clouding and joint stiffness are usually recognized after the age of 5 years. Patients may have a normal lifespan. MPS IS was previously classified as MPS V but this term is no longer used and thus there is no MPS V. Patients with MPS IH-S show varying phenotypes intermediate between MPS IH and IS. Survival to adulthood is common. In both MPS IH-S and MPS IS, compression of the cervical spinal cord by thickened dura mater may occur.

Biochemistry

The cause of MPS I is a deficiency of α-L-iduronidase,[40,433] resulting in tissue accumulation and excessive urinary excretion of dermatan and heparan sulfate (Table 11.3; Scheme 11.1A, B). Thus, analysis of urinary glycosaminoglycan was the earliest biochemical procedure for the diagnosis of MPS. In the nervous system, there is a relative accumulation of the normally negligible gangliosides GM2 and GM3 within the neuronal perikarya. The degree of the accumulation is similar to that seen in Niemann–Pick type A, Niemann–Pick type C, MLD, several MPS and many other neurodegenerative diseases. The exact mechanism leading to the secondary ganglioside accumulation in MPS is not completely understood, although inhibition of acid β-galactosidase activity by the accumulated acidic mucopolysaccharides may be an important factor.[346]

Molecular genetics

The gene encoding α-L-iduronidase has been localized to chromosome 4p16. MPS IH, MPS IS and MPS IH-S are allelic owing to mutations in the α-L-iduronidase gene.[456]

Neuroimaging

Patients with MPS IH and MPS II may have a dolicocephalic skull. The frontal bones may also be slightly 'pointed' in the midline. There are no distinguishing imaging findings among the different types of mucopolysaccharidoses. The white matter is abnormal and myelination may be delayed. Multiple cystic areas corresponding to enlarged perivascular spaces are noted particularly in the deep white matter and corpus callosum (Fig. 11.54a). They follow the course of the deep medullary veins. They may also be seen in the basal ganglia. The brain is atrophic with enlarged ventricles (Fig. 11.54b). There is no evidence of periventricular oedema. The subarachnoid spaces are prominent (Fig. 11.54b) and occasionally arachnoid cysts are seen. The skull is thick. In the spine, the vertebrae are malformed and show central beaking (Fig. 11.54c). The most common site for compression of the spinal cord is at C_1-C_2 (Fig 11.54d). Deposition of mucopolysaccharides around the dens leads to laxity of the transverse ligament and subluxations. With time, this ligament thickens. In addition, the foramen magnum may be narrowed. The spinal cord may be compressed and on T_2 weighted MRI it may show increased signal intensity which correlates with the presence of myelomalacia. The dura may also become thickened at other levels and lead to spinal canal stenosis.

Pathology

Widespread accumulation of GAGs results in structural abnormalities in many organs. Hepatosplenomegaly, bony abnormalities (dysostosis multiplex) and hydrocephalus (Fig. 11.54e) are the most pronounced gross pathological features in MPS IH patients. In routine histological examination of paraffin-embedded material, cells distended with large clear vacuoles ('clear cells') (Fig. 11.55) are seen throughout mesodermal tissues such as cartilage, fascia, periostium, blood vessels, heart valves (Fig. 11.55), cornea, choroid plexus (Fig. 11.56) and cerebral leptomeninges. These vacuoles are the sequelae of GAG extraction during the tissue processing and often appear empty or filled with only scanty amorphous or granular material at the ultrastructural level.[552,759] These 'clear cells' are often associated with extensive fibrosis in various visceral organs. The leptomeninges often show extensive fibrosis and obstructive hydrocephalus is common. An association with arachnoid cysts has been reported.[759] Dilatation of the perivascular space with loosely packed fibrous tissues is conspicuous within the cerebral white matter (Figs 11.57–11.59).[137,138,314,648] The basic cellular pathology of the CNS is that of the neuronal storage disease throughout the brain (Fig. 11.60). However, a wide variation can be observed in the extent of the intracytoplasmic storage. A considerable degree of neuronal loss and gliosis is common, resulting in cytoarchitectural derangements. Structural analysis of neurons using Golgi preparations reveals mega-neurites[536] with ectopic neurites in man as well as in feline models.[675,741] The neuronal storage materials stain positively with PAS and are often metachromatic. Alcian blue stain is positive in neuronal perikarya as well as in the dilated perivascular regions. In the cerebellum, Purkinje cells are decreased in number. The remaining Purkinje cells show marked distension of the perikarya (Fig. 11.60) with peculiar fusiform expansion of their dendrites.[181,648] The neuronal storage is also present in the peripheral ganglia. Vacuolation of the Schwann cell cytoplasm has also been documented. In their electron-microscopic study of the cerebral cortical biopsy from a patient with 'gargoylism', which is probably MPS IH in the current classification, Aleu et al.[7] described unique inclusions in storage neurons that were morphologically distinct from MCBs of gangliosidoses[690] and named them 'zebra bodies' (Fig. 11.61). Reports of the neuropathology of the milder forms are very limited. Jellinger et al.[314] reported a 42-year-old woman with a clinical presentation mimicking Friedreich's ataxia. The neuronal storage in that case was limited to the thalamus, hypothalamus, hippocampus, brainstem nuclei, spinal motor neurons and Purkinje cell dendrites. Neurons contained abundant 'ceroid' in their perikarya.[314] Conductive and sensorineural deafness is a common complication of MPS I. Degeneration of the organ of Corti and the neurons of the spiral ganglion with infiltration of vacuolated storage cells in the inner ear has been well documented.[192]

Animal models

Naturally occurring feline and canine models are known. Their clinical phenotype and pathology are closely similar to human MPS I.[613,614,741] These models have been used for investigation of cellular pathogenesis[741] as well as therapeutic manipulation.[613] Recently, a murine MPS I has been generated by targeted disruption of the murine α-L-iduronidase gene.[101,567]

Mucopolysaccharidosis II (MPS II, Hunter)

History and clinical features

MPS II or Hunter syndrome is an X-linked recessive disorder, first described in two brothers by Charles Hunter in 1917.[296] Prominent clinical features are stiff joints, a severe short stature, hepatosplenomegaly, mental retardation and progressive deafness and coarse face. Corneal clouding, however, is not a usual feature. In the majority of cases, clinical diagnosis can be made before the age of 3 years. The affected children usually die before reaching their early teens. A rare mild form exists. Patients with the mild form may develop symptoms later and survive longer into adulthood with minimal or no neurological involvement.[788–790] As noted in the original cases reported by Hunter, nodules or papules over the scapula are frequently observed in MPS II.[184]

Biochemistry

MPS II is caused by a deficiency of iduronate-2-sulfate sulfatase.[39,620] Dermatan sulfate and heparan sulfate accumulate in the tissues and are excreted in the urine (Table 11.3; Scheme 11.1A, B).

Molecular genetics

MPS II is the only X-linked MPS. The gene is mapped to Xq27-28. Many missense and nonsense mutations have been identified. Rarely, female carriers of disease-causing mutations are symptomatic, as often is the case in X-linked recessive disorders.[769]

Pathology

Pathology of visceral organs as well as the brain in the severe form of MPS II is similar to that of MPS IH. Patho-

logical details of the eye[436] and neurovisceral organs examined post-mortem have been reported in the severe form.[375,486] No information on the neuropathology of the mild form is available.

Animal models

Naturally occurring MPS II has been reported in labrador retriever dogs. Deficiency in the activity of induronate-2-sulfate sulfatase has been demonstrated in the cultured fibroblasts of affected dogs. The clinical phenotype and pathological features are closely similar to those of human MPS II.[762] Recently, a mouse model of human MPS II has been generated by gene targeting.[457]

Scheme 11.1 *(A) Stepwise degradation of dermatan sulfate. The deficiency diseases corresponding to the numbered reactions are: 1, MPSII, Hunter syndrome; 2, MPS I, Hurler, Hurler–Scheie and Scheie syndromes; 3, MPSVI, Maroteaux–Lamy syndrome; 4, Sandhoff disease for β-hexosaminidase A and B; 5, MPS VII, Sly syndrome. This schematic drawing depicts all structures known to occur within dermatan sulfate, and does not imply that they occur in equal proportion. (Reproduced from Fig. 136-2 in Ref. 468 by permission of the copyright holder, McGraw Hill.) (Opposite) (B) Stepwise degradation of heparan sulfate. The deficiency diseases corresponding to the numbered reactions are: 1, MPS II, Hunter syndrome; 2, MPS I, Hurler, Hurler–Scheie and Scheie syndromes; 3, MPS IIIA, Sanfilippo syndrome type A; 4, MPS IIIC, Sanfilippo syndrome type C; 5, MPS IIIB, Sanfilippo syndrome type B; 6, no deficiency disease yet known; 7, MPS VII, Sly syndrome; 8, MPS IIID, Sanfilippo syndrome type D. The schematic drawing depicts all structures known to occur within heparan sulfate, and does not imply that they occur stoichiometrically. (Reproduced from Fig. 136-3 in Ref. 468 by permission of the copyright holder, McGraw Hill.) (C) Stepwise degradation of keratan sulfate. The deficiency diseases corresponding to the numbered reactions are: 1, MPS IVA, Morquio syndrome type A; 2, MPS IV B, Morquio syndrome type B; 3, MPS III D, Sanfilippo syndrome type D; 4, Sandhoff disease; and 5, Tay–Sachs and Sandhoff diseases. The alternative pathway releases intact N-acetylglucosamine 6-sulfate, a departure from the usual stepwise cleavage of sulfate and sugar residues. (Reproduced from Fig. 136-4 in Ref. 468 by permission of the copyright holder, McGraw Hill.) (D) Endoglycosidase degradation of chondroitin sulfate and hyaluronan. Arrows show potential sites for hyaluronidase cleavage of chondroitin 4-sulfate (top), chondroitin 6-sulfate (middle) and hyaluronian (bottom) into oligosaccharide fragments. The oligosaccharides are hydrolysed further by stepwise action of N-acetylgalactosamine 4-sulfatase or 6-sulfatase (for oligosaccharides derived from chondroitin 4- or 6-sulfate), β-hexosaminidase A or B, and β-glucuronidase. (Reproduced from Fig. 136-5 in Ref. 468 by permission of the copyright holder, McGraw Hill.)*

(A)

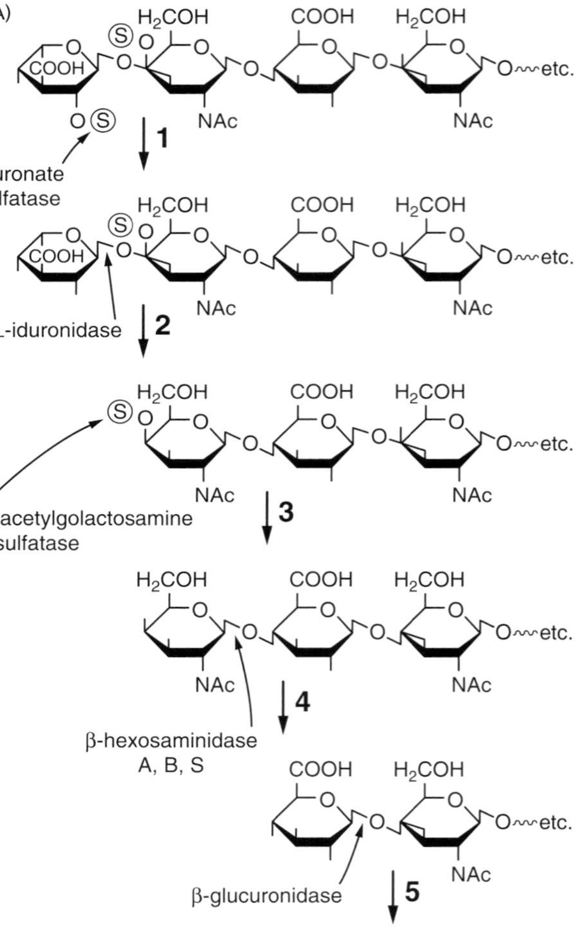

iduronate sulfatase | 1

α-L-iduronidase | 2

N-acetylgolactosamine 4-sulfatase | 3

β-hexosaminidase A, B, S | 4

β-glucuronidase | 5

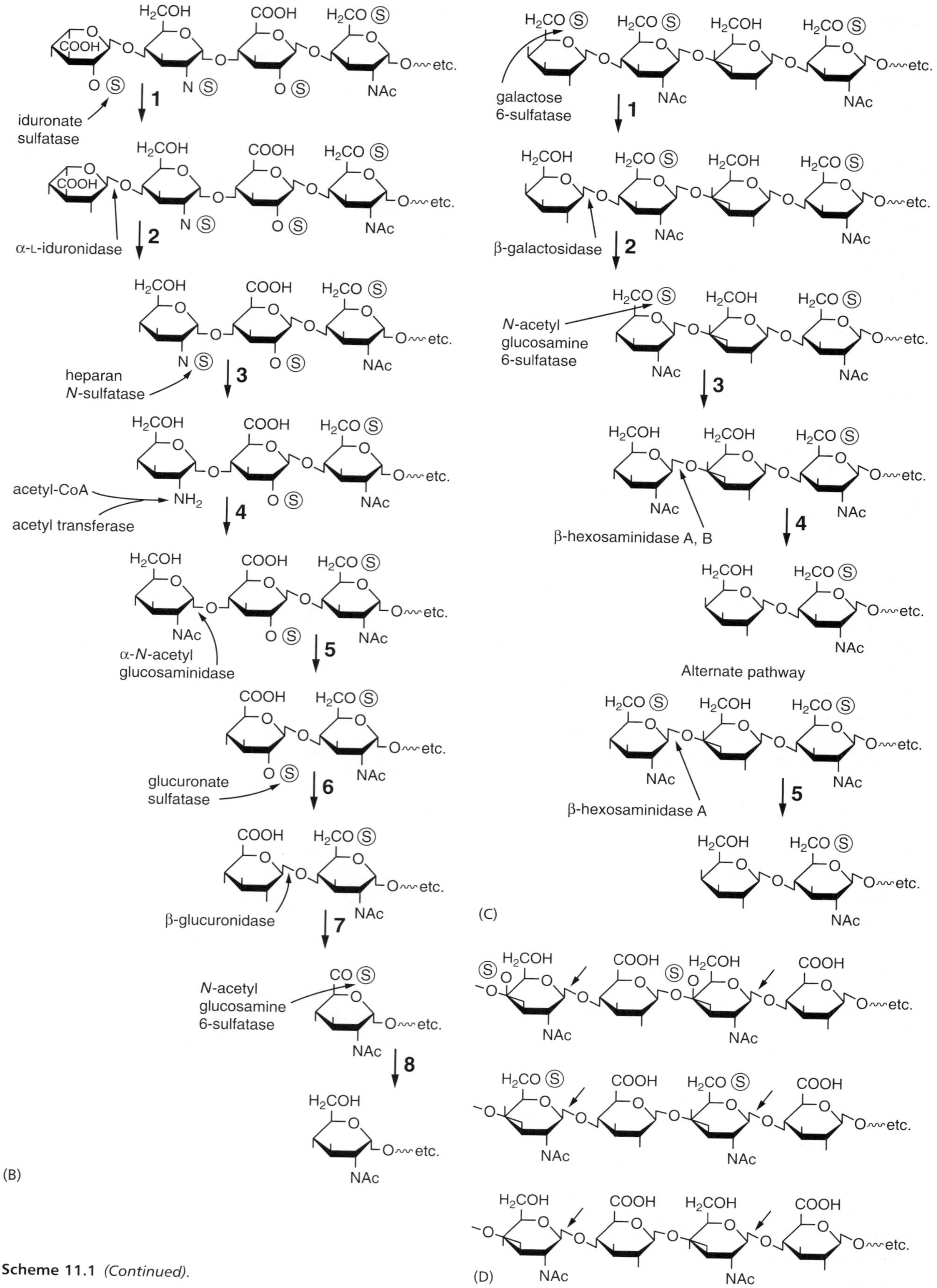

(B)

(C)

(D)

Scheme 11.1 *(Continued)*.

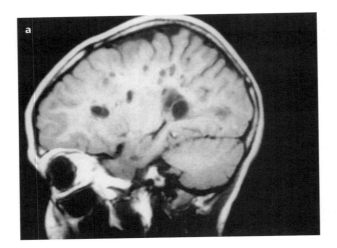

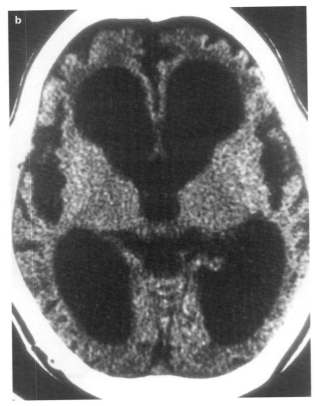

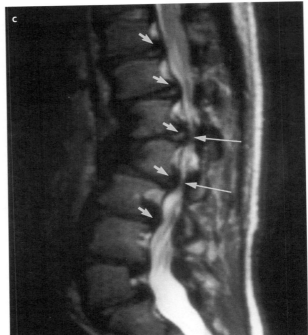

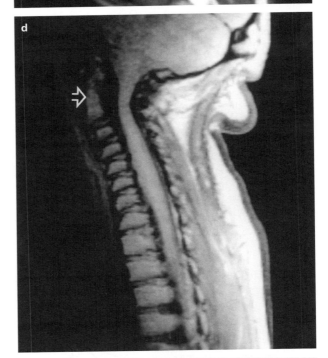

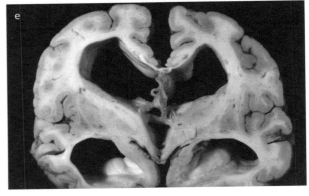

Figure 11.54 *Mucopolysaccharidosis IH (Hurler).* **(a)** *Mucopolysaccharidosis. Parasagittal T₁-weighted MRI in a patient with Hunter's disease showing cyst-like dilated perivascular spaces in the cerebral white matter. (b) Mucopolysaccharidosis. Axial CT image of a patient with Hunter's disease showing cerebral atrophy, markedly enlarged ventricles and prominent subarachnoid spaces. (c) Mucopolysaccharidosis. Midsagittal T₂-weighted MRI in a patient with Hunter's disease showing deformed vertebrae, bulged discs (short arrows) and multilevel stenosis of the spinal canal (long arrows). (d) Hurler's disease. Midsagittal proton density image in a patient with Hurler's disease showing thick dura in the spinal canal and a deformed dens. At the C₁–C₂ level (arrow) the spinal cord is compressed. (e) Coronal section of the brain showing marked hydrocephalus.*

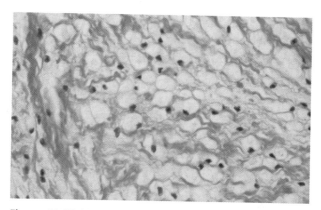

Figure 11.55 *Mucopolysaccharidosis IH (Hurler). Heart valve showing numerous clear cells. (H&E.)*

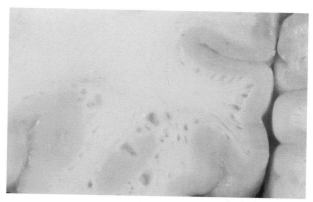

Figure 11.57 *Mucopolysaccharidosis IS (Scheie). Section of cerebrum showing many holes representing dilated perivascular spaces.*

Mucopolysaccharidosis III (MPS III, Sanfilippo)

History and clinical course

In 1963, Sanfilippo and colleagues[578] described a group of eight patients who had severe and progressive intellectual retardation with somatic features that resembled, but was less severe than, MPSIH (Hurler) disease. These patients excreted 'acid mucopolysaccharide' consisting primarily of heparan sulfate.[577] Several years later Rampini reported eight additional patients with similar clinical manifestations and made an extensive literature review.[541] This group of the diseases is now called Sanfilippo syndrome or MPS III. Further biochemical investigations revealed that MPS III includes four distinct genetic diseases caused by deficiencies of four different enzymes (Table 11.3). However, they cannot be differentiated from each other clinically or pathologically. There is great variability in the clinical expression within this syndrome both among the different types and within each type. The onset of clinical

signs, such as speech or behavioural problems, is usually between 2 and 6 years of age in hitherto normal children. Intractable behavioural problems are frequent clinical manifestations. Progressive cognitive and intellectual deteriorations follow.[274] Death occurs usually in the second decade of life.[103,708]

Biochemistry

Heparan sulfate is degraded by the sequential action of several lysosomal enzymes. Deficiency of any one of the enzymes necessary for this degradation pathway results in

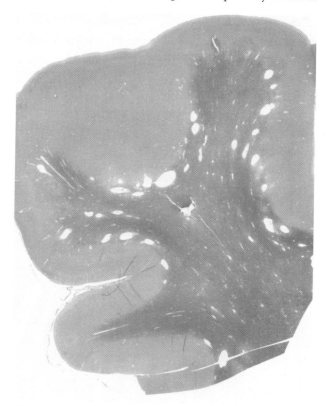

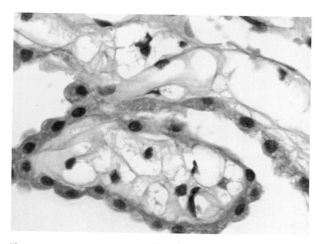

Figure 11.56 *Mucopolysaccharidosis IH (Hurler). Many clear vacuolated cells are seen in the stroma of the choroid plexus. (H&E.)*

Figure 11.58 *Mucopolysaccharidosis IS (Scheie). Section of frontal lobe showing dilatation of perivascular spaces, most pronounced at the corticomedullary junction. (Solochrome and eosin.)*

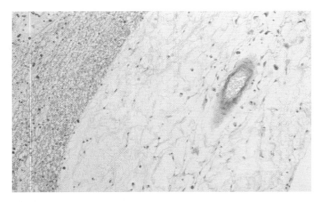

Figure 11.59 *Mucopolysaccharidosis IS (Scheie). Dilated perivascular space containing a loose mesh of fibrous tissue. (LFB and PAS.)*

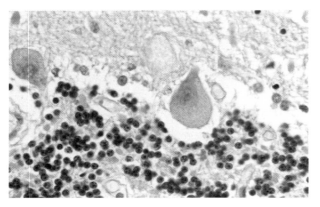

Figure 11.60 *Mucopolysaccharidosis IH (Hurler). Swollen Purkinje cells with storage material. (H&E.)*

the same clinicopathological phenotype. Therefore, the four biochemical types, MPS III A, B, C and D, caused by defects in the four different enzymes (Table 11.3; Scheme 11.1B) cannot be distinguished clinically. Heparan sulfate accounts for most of the GAG accumulated in the tissue and excreted in the urine. In the brain, gangliosides GM2, GM3 and GD2 are elevated owing to the secondary metabolic perturbation induced by the accumulation of heparan sulfate.[273,323] The mechanism causing secondary accumulation of ganglioside is not well understood (see MPS I, above).

Molecular genetics

The genes for the deficient enzyme in type A (heparan *N*-sulfatase) and type D (*N*-acetylglucosamine-6-sulfatase), have been cloned, and many disease-causing mutations have been identified. They are located on chromosome 17q25[597] and 12q14,[557] respectively. The enzyme deficient in MPS III type B (α-*N*-acetylglucosaminidase) has also been cloned recently and several disease-causing mutations have been identified.[798]

Pathology

The pathology of MPS III is similar regardless of the deficient enzymes.[209,247,323,371,427] Clear, vacuolated cells are seen throughout visceral organs but to a far lesser extent than those seen in MPS I or II.[87] Neuronal storage is seen throughout the cerebrum and cerebellum. The extent and the distribution of storage materials vary among different neurons.[608,677] The storage materials are strongly positive with PAS and various stains for lipofuscin and

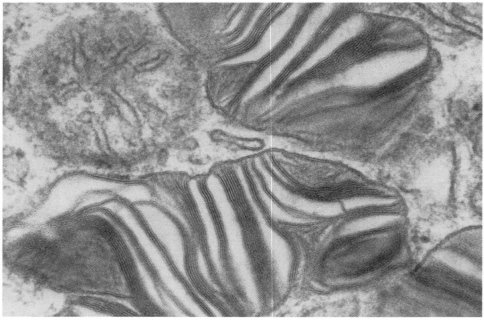

Figure 11.61 *Mucopolysaccharidosis IH (Hurler). Electron micrograph of neuronal inclusion (zebra bodies). (Courtesy of Dr Robert D Terry, University of California, San Diego, California, USA.)*

possess intense autofluorescence under ultra-violet (UV) light.[153,677,772] Ultrastructural features of neuronal storage materials include zebra bodies, membranous cytoplasmic bodies and membrano-granulo-vacuolar inclusions.[247,273,371,427,494] In one type C patient who became symptomatic at the age of 2 years and died at 39 years, marked neuronal loss and gliosis were reported in the cerebral cortex.[376] The extensive storage process also involves virtually every ocular tissue.[139,388]

Animal models

Caprine MPS IIID and canine MPS IIIA are known. Similar to human disease, both animal models show predominantly neurological phenotypes.[185,322] A severe form of caprine model, however, shows corneal clouding and bony and cartilaginous abnormalities. With targeted disruption of the gene, mouse models of MPS IIIA and MPS IIIB have been generated recently.[60,398] The clinical phenotype of these knockout mice is milder than the human disease. Cytoplasmic vacuolation indicative of GAG storage is present in macrophages, hepatocytes, and renal tubular and glomerular epithelium. Electron-dense inclusions are detected in certain neurons. Smilar to the human disease, there are relative increases in GM2 and GM3 gangliosides in the brain.

Mucopolysaccharidosis IVA (MPS IVA, Morquio A)

History and clinical course

The clinical features of patients with MPS IVA are short-trunk dwarfism, a unique form of skeletal dysplasia and

fine corneal opacification. The connective tissue of the cornea, airways and heart valves are also affected, and patients may present with nocturnal dyspnoea and obstructive sleep apnoea, cardiac dysfunction and ophthalmological problems.[479] As in most MPS patients, patients are normal at birth. Clinical signs of kyphosis, growth retardation and genu valgus become apparent by the age of 3.5 years. Odontoid hypoplasia is a universal bony abnormality and cervical myelopathy develops as a grave consequence of the instability of the hypoplastic odontoid processes.[554] Intelligence is usually not affected. The genetically distinct disease, Morquio B disease, due to acid β-galactosidase deficiency and thus allelic to GM1 gangliosidosis, has already been discussed in the section on GM1 gangliosidosis.

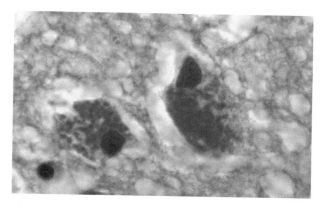

Figure 11.63 *Mucopolysaccharidosis IVA (Morquio A). Storage neurons in hippocampus contain strongly PAS-positive globular inclusions. (PAS.)*

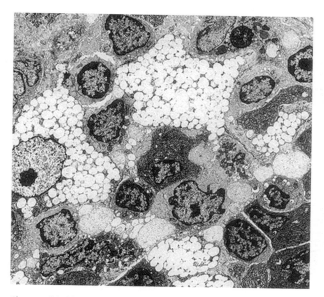

Figure 11.62 *Mucopolysaccharidosis IV (Morquio). Electron micrograph of a tonsil showing histiocytes filled with empty membrane-bound vacuoles. Similar appearances are seen in fibroblasts and histiocytes in other mucopolysaccharidoses.*

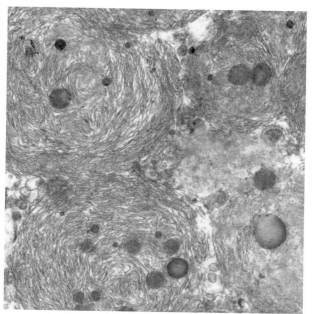

Figure 11.64 *Mucopolysaccharidosis IVA (Morquio A). Neuronal inclusions consist of straight or wavy thin electron-dense membranes and spherical, moderately electron-dense lipid droplets. (Electron micrograph.)*

Biochemistry

MPS IVA is caused by defective degradation of keratan sulfate due to a genetic, deficiency of N-acetylgalactosamine 6-sulfatase (galactose 6-sulfatase) (Scheme 11.1C). A large quantity of keratan sulfate-derived oligosaccharide fragments is excreted in the urine.

Molecular genetics

The gene encoding N-acetylgalactosamine 6-sulfatase has been localized on chromosome 16q24[42] and mutation analysis has already defined a number of different mutations.

Pathology

Similarly to other types of MPS, clear vacuolated cells are seen in many organs in MPS IV (Fig. 11.62). However, MPS IVA is primarily a disease of the skeletal system. Cervical myelopathy resulting from the hypoplastic/dysplastic odontoid process is the most common and serious pathology associated with MPS IVA.[479] Intelligence is usually normal or only slightly abnormal in MPS IVA patients. However, localized neuronal storage in the cerebral cortex, thalamus, hypothalamus, basal ganglia and hippocampus (Fig. 11.63) has been reported.[215,366] The storage materials are PAS positive (Fig. 11.63) and consist of stacked, straight or tangled, loosely packed wavy membranes of various sizes (Fig. 11.64) at the ultrastructural level.[366] The activity of N-acetyl galactosamine-6-sulfate sulfatase was deficient in the liver and brain in the case reported by Koto et al.[366] and, thus, the patient definitely had MPS IVA. However, caution is required because cases reported in the literature often do not have enzymic information and thus are unclear as to whether they are MPS IVA or B.

Animal models

No animal models of MPS IVA are known.

Mucopolysaccharidosis VI (MPS VI, Maroteaux–Lamy)

History and clinical course

MPS VI was first recognized in 1963 by Maroteaux and co-workers as a Hurler-like syndrome with preservation of intelligence and urinary excretion of predominantly dermatan sulfate.[425] Clinically, it is characterized by an extreme short stature, corneal opacities, dysostosis multiplex and progressive cardiopulmonary disease. Growth retardation is usually recognized by 2–3 years of age. Hepatosplenomegaly is often present. The patients usually have normal intelligence without clinical evidence of neurological dysfunction. However, hydrocephalus and nerve entrapment may occur. Carpal tunnel syndrome and generalized restriction of articular movements are often associated with MPS VI. Spastic paraparesis from atlanto-axial subluxation consequent to hypoplasia of the odontoid processes and progressive thickening of the dura have been documented.[339,678,791] Most patients die of heart failure in the second or third decade.

Biochemistry

The MPS VI is caused by genetic deficiency in the activity of N-acetylgalactosamine-4-sulfatase (arylsulfatase B) (Scheme 11.1A).

Molecular genetics

The gene is localized to 5q11-13.[402] The full-length cDNA has been cloned and several disease-causing mutations have been identified.[304,732]

Pathology

Detailed descriptions of the pathology of MPS VI are very limited. Keller et al.[339] reported the pathology of a 27-year-old patient with a severe form of MPS VI. In addition to compressive cervical myelopathy and defective enchondral ossification, the patient had thickened heart valves with endocardial fibrosis and 'increased amounts of GAGs in neurons in the CNS'.[339] Thickening of the sclera and the optic nerve sheaths and atrophy of the optic nerve have also been described.[642] Light- and electron-microscopic studies of the thickened dura showed an extensive accumulation of GAGs in ballooned cells.[791]

Animal models

Feline models of MPS VI are known. The clinical phenotype and pathological lesions closely resemble those described in the man.[148,271]

Mucopolysaccharidosis VII (MPS VII, Sly)

History and clinical course

MPS VII is a very rare form of MPS, first described by Sly et al.[624] in a child with physical features closely similar to Hurler's disease (MPS IH) but with deficiency of lysosomal β-glucuronidase. Short stature, hepatosplenomegaly, dysostosis multiplex and intellectual impairment are the main clinical manifestations, but the spectrum of these symptoms is quite variable in individual cases.[759] Granulocytes often show striking coarse metachromatic granules. Neonatal, infantile and juvenile forms are known. The juvenile form is the mildest, with only limited kyphosis or scoliosis.

Biochemistry

MPS VII is caused by the deficiency of the lysosomal β-glucuronidase, resulting in an accumulation of GAGs containing terminal β-linked glucuronic acid residues: dermatan sulfate, heparan sulfate and chondroitin sulfate (Scheme 11.1A, B, D). The enzyme deficiency has been detected in leukocytes and fibroblasts and in the brain.[728]

Molecular genetics

The β-glucuronidase gene has been cloned and more than two dozen disease-causing mutations have been identified.[197,778,779] The original patient reported by Sly et al.[624] was found to be a compound heterozygote, and a small amount of β-glucuronidase activity was detected in that patient.[610]

Pathology

Reports of the pathology on MPS VII are sparse. Only one detailed post-mortem study of the patient originally described by Sly et al.[624] is reported in the literature.[728] Grossly, dysostosis multiplex, arterial stenosis and fibrous thickening of the cardiac valves with calcification were found. A microscopic feature is that of the typical MPS, and lysosomal storage was found throughout visceral organs as well as in the CNS. Unlike MPS I, II or III, however, the extent of the neuronal storage in the CNS was variable, with the most severe storage being in the hippocampus (h2 and h3, subiculum), presubiculum, substantia nigra, inferior olive, and spinal anterior horn and intermediolateral neurons. The storage materials were autofluorescent, colloidal iron- and PAS positive, and weakly alcian blue positive. The storage was also noted occasionally in glial cells and foamy macrophages in the leptomeninges. Ultrastructurally, membrane-bound lysosomal inclusions consisting of whorls of membranous materials were admixed with a small amount of lipid droplets. The neurons in the Meissner and Auerbach plexuses were distended with cytoplasmic vacuoles containing GAG. Vacuolation was also noted in the non-pigmented ciliary epithelium, corneal fibrocytes and lens epithelium in the eye. The neonatal form of MPS VII causes non-immune hydrops fetalis and many foamy vacuolated cells are present in many visceral organs and also in the Hofbauer cells of the placenta.[69,303,449,467]

Animal models

Canine, feline and murine models of MPS VII are known. These models show a severe clinical phenotype with marked skeletal abnormalities.[64,201,216,272] These models have been extensively used for the investigation of the disease pathogenesis and of therapeutic manipulations with enzyme or somatic cell gene replacement.[63,270,727] Feline β-glucuronidase deficiency has also been reported by two groups of investigators.[201,216]

GLYCOPROTEIN DISORDERS

A series of lysosomal disorders affects primarily degradation of carbohydrate chains of glycoproteins due to genetically defective lysosomal hydrolases.[691] The classification is to some extent arbitrary (Table 11.4). For example, the acid β-galactosidase deficiency already discussed under GM1 gangliosidosis/Morquio B can also be considered a glycoprotein disorder, since degradation of glycoprotein sugar chains with a terminal β-galactose residue is also impaired in this disorder.

Sialidase (neuraminidase) deficiency (sialidosis, mucolipidosis I)

History and clinical course

There are two distinct clinical phenotypes of sialidosis. Type I is characterized by macular cherry-red spots and myoclonus without dysmorphic features or mental retardation.[544] Type II is characterized by dysmorphic features, dysostosis multiplex, cherry-red spots, organomegaly and mental retardation.[340,341,463] In the past, some of the type II patients were classified as mucolipidosis I (ML-I) due to the clinical similarity to ML-II and III.[634] In addition, many of the patients who were originally classified as having the late-onset type II sialidosis (juvenile type II) were later found to have galactosialidosis (see below). Thus, one should be aware of the confusing status of earlier reports on this group of diseases.[202] A 13-year-old girl reported by Gonatas et al. as 'juvenile lipidosis' is the first clinicopathological report of a type I patient.[230] As noted in that patient, intractable myoclonus and decreased visual acuity with a cherry-red spot are usual presenting symptoms between 8 and 25 years of age.[410,544] Type II patients are usually recognized at or shortly after birth by their dysmorphic features and hepatosplenomegaly.[340,463,781] Hydrops fetalis has also been reported as a congenital variant of type II.[48,589]

Biochemistry

Lysosomal α-neuraminidase (sialidase) activity is deficient in both types but the deficiency is more marked in type II than in type I.[484] The extent of the tissue accumulation and urinary excretion of sialyloligosaccharides and sialylglycopeptides appears to be correlated with clinical severity. It is important to note that the sialidase deficiency in sialidosis does not result in a massive accumulation of brain gangliosides,[230] a clear indication that this sialidase is not the primary enzyme to remove sialic acid from higher gangliosides or GM3 ganglioside. Otherwise, there would have been as massive an accumulation of gangliosides in the brain as that seen in genetic gangliosidoses.

Molecular biology

The gene for lysosomal α-neuraminidase, located on chromosome 10,[455] has recently been cloned independently in three laboratories and several disease-causing mutations have been identified.[70,299,532] The mouse gene has also been cloned.[194]

Table 11.4 *Glycoprotein storage disorders*

Clinical diagnosis	Affected compounds	Enzyme defects
Sialidosis (mucolipidosis I)	Sialyloligosaccharides	α-Neuraminidase (sialidase)
α-Mannosidosis	Oligosaccharides with terminal α-mannose	α-Mannosidase
β-Mannosidosis	β-Mannosyl-glcNac, heparan sulfate?	β-Mannosidase heparan-sulfamidase
α-Fucosidosis	Fucose-containing oligosaccharides and glycolipids	α-Fucosidase
Aspartylglycosaminuria	Aspartylglucosamine and glycoasparagines	Glycosylasparaginase
Schindler's disease	α-*N*-Acetyl-galactosamine	α-*N*-Acetyl-galactosaminidase
Galactosialidosis (combined sialidase-β-galactosidase deficiency)	'Protective protein' (see text)	Carboxypeptidase (see text)

Pathology

The most conspicuous pathological feature is the presence of cytoplasmic vacuolation in neurons, oligodendrocytes, vascular endothelial cells and many cells in the visceral organs, in particular hepatocytes, Kupffer cells and histiocytes in the spleen and bone marrow (Fig. 11.65).[9,545,781] These pathological changes are very similar in both type I and II patients. At the ultrastructural level, these vacuoles are membrane bound and usually contain floccular material. They stain variably with PAS and alcian blue. Vacuolation of renal tubular epithelial cells is also conspicuous in some cases. Vacuoles containing short stacked lamellae or small concentric myelin figures have been noted in the spinal neurons as well as in neurons in the myenteric plexus[781] and in Schwann cells.[637] In a 22-year-old patient, Allegranza *et al.*[9] described fine cytoplasmic vacuolation of several neurons of the cortex and of perineuronal and interfascicular oligodendrocytes in the corpus callosum and thalamus. They also observed unique large vacuoles that balloon the perikaryon of some motor neurons of the brainstem and of the anterior horns of the spinal cord. Similar vacuolar changes involve neurons in the dorsal root ganglia, autonomic ganglia and ganglion cells in the myenteric plexus. In addition, they found a neuronal intracytoplasmic storage of lipofuscin-like pigment throughout the brain, which was particularly conspicuous in the thalamus, the pulvinar and in the periventricular and supraoptic nuclei. Lipofuscin-like bodies have been reported in the neurons and hepatocytes in other type I patients.[230,545] Neuronal loss has been reported in the lateral geniculate bodies, substantia nigra, and nuclei of Goll and Burdach. In the cerebellum, loss of Purkinje cells accompanied by Bergmann glia proliferation has been described.[9]

Animal models

A spontaneous mouse mutant, SM/J, appears to be due to a genetic defect in the lysosomal sialidase.[565] A mouse model of lysosomal sialidase deficiency has also been generated by targeted disruption of the gene.[135]

α-Mannosidosis and β-mannosidosis

History and clinical course

α-Mannosidosis was first described by Öckerman as a disease entity.[485] It is classified into the more severe type I and the milder type II. Type I is characterized by severe progressive psychomotor retardation, coarse facies, dysostosis multiplex, hepatosplenomegaly and deafness starting in early childhood. These clinical signs and symptoms can be confused with those of mucopolysaccharidoses. The milder type II patients typically present themselves with speech and hearing disorders, tremor, muscle flaccidity and ataxia in early adolescence. Mental retardation in type II patients is mild to moderate. However, there is a broad clinical spectrum with considerable phenotypic variations and thus, some cases are difficult to classify.[36,129,320,725] Characteristically, α-mannosidosis patients are immunologically compromised and are susceptible to infection. Gingival hyperplasia due to an accumulation of storage in histiocytes is a unique and conspicuous feature in some patients and the diagnosis can be made by gingival biopsy.[147,347]

β-Mannosidosis is an extremely rare disease in man.[756] Facial deformities and mental retardation are usual common features, but other heterogeneous clinical manifestations have been reported.[112,351,395] This is a rare example of a human lysosomal disease that was discovered several years after an equivalent disease was identified in a nonhuman mammalian species (see below).

Biochemistry

In α-mannosidosis, activity of the lysosomal enzyme, acid α-mannosidase, is deficient and a range of undegraded mannose-containing oligosaccharides accumulates in

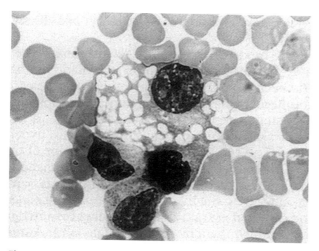

Figure 11.65 *Mannosidosis. Bone marrow film. Many of the plasma cells contain large bold vacuoles. (May–Grunwald–Giemsa.) (From 6th edn, Fig. 11.70.) Similar vacuolated cells are also found in Sialidosis.*

lysosomes. In β-mannosidosis, β-mannosidase activity is markedly deficient in various tissues, serum, leukocytes and cultured fibroblasts. An excess of mannosyl $(1 \rightarrow 4)$-N-acetylglucosamine disaccharide accumulates in the tissue and is excreted in the urine.[112] Heparan sulfate was also detected in the patient reported by Wenger *et al.*[756]

Molecular biology

Both α- and β-mannosidosis are autosomal recessive diseases. The gene for lysosomal α-mannosidosis is localized on chromosome 19q. Many disease-causing mutations have been identified.[52] The gene for β-mannosidosis is localized on chromosome 4q22-25 and the first identification of a mutation associated with human β-mannosidosis has been reported.[8]

Pathology

The pathology of both α- and β-mannosidosis has been well investigated in animal models.[317,318,320,324,408,409,510,740] However, pathological studies in man are very limited. The cardinal pathological feature of human α-mannosidosis is the presence of vacuoles, some of which contain coarse granules, within the cytoplasm of many types of cells, including neutrophils and lymphocytes in peripheral blood and in the bone marrow (Fig. 11.65). These vacuolated cells, however, are not specific and have been recognized in mucopolysaccharidoses, mucolipidoses, sialidosis, galactosialidosis and other lysosomal glycoprotein disorders. Metachromasia as noted in mucopolysaccharidoses is not present. These storage vacuoles show various degrees of diastase-resistant PAS positivity and a positive periodic acid–silver methanamine reaction. They are membrane bound and contain various amounts of reticular or floccular and slight to moderate-ly electron-dense materials at the ultrastructural level. Some vacuoles may appear totally electron lucent and empty.[36,147]

The examination of the brain of α-mannosidosis patients is very limited.[349,646] In a 4.5-year-old child, Kjellman *et al.* observed ballooning of nerve cells with empty cytoplasm throughout the cerebral cortex, brainstem and spinal cord. The neuronal storage was inconspicuous or absent in the basal ganglia. In addition, they observed widespread neuronal loss in the cerebral cortex, and loss of myelin and gliosis in the white matter. In the cerebellum, loss of Purkinje and granular cells was widespread.[349] Histopathological changes of neuronal storage in a 3.5-year-old girl reported by Sung *et al.*[646] are very similar to those in the previous report. However, the extent of neuronal storage was not uniform. The neuronal storage was seen throughout the nervous system, including neurons in the brainstem, spinal cord, and paravertebral sympathetic, trigeminal and dorsal spinal root ganglia. Cytoplasmic ballooning appeared more striking in the larger neurons of the cerebral cortex and striatum. Neurons in the hypothalamus and subthalamic nuclei were severely affected but neuronal storage was variable in different thalamic nuclei. The Purkinje cells in the cerebellum showed focal ballooning of their dendrites but the perikaryal storage was not extensive. Scattered macrophages containing PAS-positive material and astrogliosis were also noted. The affected neurons were ballooned to varying degrees and appeared finely vacuolated on paraffin-embedded tissues. Unlike the case reported by Kjellman *et al.*, Sung *et al.* observed neither neuronal loss in the cerebral cortex nor demyelination in the cerebral white matter.[646] At the ultrastructural level, the perikarya of the affected neurons were filled with storage vacuoles of varying sizes between 1 and 2 μm in diameter, which were bound by a single

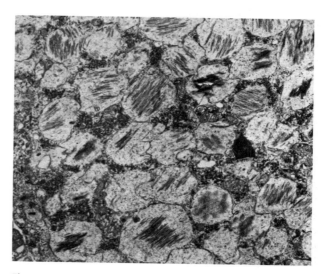

Figure 11.66 *Mannosidosis. Electron micrograph of ventral horn cell of lumbar spinal cord. Storage vacuoles, interdigitating with one another, contain varying amount of fine fibrils in stacks. (From Ref. 646 with permission.)*

membrane and contained loosely dispersed, fine, reticulogranular material (Fig. 11.66). Vacuoles were also observed in astrocytes, endothelial cells and pericytes, but not in oligodendrocytes. On rare occasions, storage vacuoles comprising stacks of fibrils were encountered.[646] The ultrastructural features of these storage vacuoles are similar to those described in bovine and feline α-mannosidosis.[317,740] However, neuroaxonal dystrophy as noted in these animal models has not been documented in man. Detailed pathological reports on the caprine model of β-mannosidosis are available in the literature.[324,408,409,419,510] Basic pathological features are the presence of storage vacuoles in various types of cells including neurons and extensive hypomyelination of the white matter. No reports on the pathology of β-mannosidosis in man are available.

Animal models

Bovine, feline and guinea-pig α-mannosidosis and caprine and bovine β-mannosidosis are known. These models have been extensively used for the investigation of the basic pathological processes as well as for therapeutic strategy.[319,324,408,409,510] With gene-targeting techniques, a mouse model of α-mannosidosis has been generated recently.[639] Biochemical as well as morphological features of this murine model are closely similar to those of the human disease.

Fucosidosis

History and clinical course

Fucosidosis is a rare autosomal recessive lysosomal storage disease first described in Italian siblings as cases of 'new mucopolysaccharide-lipid-storage disease', with progressive mental retardation and neurological deterioration, resulting in death before the age of 5 years.[159] Later, Van Hoof and Hers, who identified α-L-fucosidase deficiency in another similar case, confirmed the deficiency of the enzyme in the earlier cases reported by Durand et al.[711,712] Because of its resemblance to mucopolysaccharidoses, α-fucosidosis was called mucopolysaccharidosis F in some early publications.[406] Although the original siblings reported by Durand et al. died before the age of 5 after rapid deterioration, the clinical course of the majority of patients with α-fucosidosis is slower with survival well into the second and third decades.[300,508] The clinical manifestations include progressive neurological deterioration with mental retardation, seizures, dysostosis multiplex, visceromegaly, angiokeratoma, telangiectasia, ocular abnormalities, hearing loss and recurrent infections. Because of considerable clinical variations among patients, this disease is often classified into two major groups: type I as the severe form as noted in the originally reported patients and type II as the more

common, less severe form. However, as more patients were described, a clinically intermediate type has been recognized. These two types probably represent a continuous clinical spectrum of the disease.[763]

Biochemistry

The basic biochemical defect is a deficiency in activity of lysosomal α-L-fucosidase. L-Fucose is a common constituent of a great variety of biological molecules and, thus, large numbers of glycolipids and glycoproteins (fucoglycolipids and fucoglycoproteins) accumulate in the tissues and also are excreted in urine. The large accumulation of glycoproteins compared with that of oligosaccharides is considered by some as unique to fucosidoses, as no significant accumulation of glycoproteins is noted in mannosidosis.[763]

Molecular biology

α-Fucosidosis is an autosomal recessive disease. Original patients were described in Italy and apparently the incidence is higher in Italy and among those of Italian descent. However, the disease has been reported from many different countries.[763] A large number of mutations suggests genetic heterogeneity.[116] As of January 1999, 22 different mutations had been reported. However, no genotype–phenotype correlation can be made, suggesting that phenotypic differences may be due to secondary unknown factors.[764]

Neuroimaging

Imaging studies show the white matter to have an abnormal appearance. There is diffuse brain atrophy with enlargement of the ventricles and the subarachnoid space. The subcortical U-fibres may be partially preserved. On T_2-weighted MRI, the medial globus pallidus and the thalamus may show increased signal intensity. The putamen may show paradoxical low T_2-weighted intensity, although the basis for this finding is not certain.

Pathology

Pathological studies of fucosidosis are very limited. Only sketchy information is available from a few autopsy reports.[702] The cardinal pathological feature is a varying degree of cytoplasmic vacuolation in many types of cells in the liver, spleen, lymph nodes, endocrine glands, peripheral nerve, brain, conjunctiva and cultured fibroblasts. These vacuoles are very similar to those seen in α-mannosidosis. However, the ultrastructural features of storage vacuoles in α-fucosidosis are more complex. These vacuoles are single-membrane bound and often contain two different components, moderately electron-dense reticular materials and lamellar inclusions with alternating electron-dense and electron-lucent lamellae. These lamellar structures are arranged concentrically or seen as bundles of flat lamellae. These types of inclusion are well described in vacuolated hepatocytes,[190] vascular endothelial cells, macrophages and Schwann cells.[300] In the rectal biopsy specimens from an adult patient α-L-fucose residue was clearly demonstrated in macrophages and vascular endothelial cells by lectin Ulex europeus agglutinin-1 (UEA-1) histochemistry.[300] Grossly, the brain may be atrophic[127] or megalencephalic.[160] Storage vacuoles are conspicuous in both neurons and glial cells throughout the brain. Loss of neurons in the thalamus, dentate nucleus and Purkinje cells in the cerebellum is well documented. Remaining neurons show marked enlargement of their perikarya with membrane-bound vacuoles, containing moderately electron-dense reticular material. Exceptionally, membrane-bound vacuoles with bundles of parallel lamellae are observed. Electron-lucent vacuoles containing reticular material and electron-dense inclusions, displaying either an irregular reticulum or lamellar inclusions are found in astrocytes. White matter shows marked demyelination and gliosis.[84] Notably, numerous Rosenthal fibres (Fig. 11.67a) may be very conspicuous.[206,387] Only clear inclusions are found in oligodendrocytes. Macrophages and vascular endothelial cells contain clear or/and dense inclusions similar to those seen in astrocytes.[406,702] Vacuolar and lamellar inclusions are also described in biopsy specimens of angiokeratoma from fucosidosis patients. Endothelial cells, pericytes, fibroblasts and dark cells of the sweat glands contain almost exclusively vacuolar inclusions, while lamellar inclusions are in Schwann cells, and myoepithelial cells in eccrine sweat glands.[364]

Animal models

α-Fucosidosis has been reported in springer spaniels from Australia,[275,343] the UK[193,403] and the USA.[621,625]

Aspartylglycosaminuria (aspartylglucosaminuria)

History and clinical course

Aspartylglycosaminuria (AGU) is a hereditary metabolic disorder with slowly progressive psychomotor deterioration from infancy with skeletal abnormalities, coarse facies and susceptibility to infection.[23] This disorder is considered to be the most common lysosomal storage disorder of glycoprotein degradation but its occurrence is largely restricted to Finland.[450] It is characterized by urinary excretion and a massive accumulation of aspartylglucosamine (GlucNAc-Asn) and other glycoasparagines in body fluids and tissues.[450] AGU was discovered during a survey of urinary amino acid chromatograms from Finnish patients with mental retardation.[505]

Biochemistry

The basic biochemical defect in AGU is a profound deficiency of glycosylasparaginase (AGA) activity. This enzyme hydrolyzes the N-glycosidic linkage between N-acetylglucosamine and L-asparagine during the lysosomal degradation of asparagine-linked sugar chains of glycoprotein.[20] As the consequence of lacking glycosylasparaginase activity, aspartylglucosamine and other glycoasparagines accumulate in tissues, leukocytes and plasma.[451]

Molecular biology

Human AGA cDNA and genomic DNA have been cloned and at least 15 different disease-causing mutations have been identified.[301,306,308,515]

Pathology

Only limited descriptions of the pathology are available in the literature.[22,258] Macroscopically, the brain is atrophic. The basic pathology is neurovisceral storage. The storage cells are characterized histologically by the presence of numerous vacuoles in the cytoplasm. In the liver, hepatocytes contain large empty vacuoles, in which finely granular or reticular materials dispersed with scattered small opaque 'lipid' droplets were identified at the ultrastructural level (Fig. 11.67b, c). In the brain, neuronal storage, regional loss of neurons and gliosis have been described. The perikarya of storage neurons in the cerebral cortex are distended with poorly defined vacuoles (Fig. 11.67d). These vacuoles are smaller and more numerous than those in the hepatocytes. Some neurons contain lipofuscin-like granules in the perikaryal region. Ultrastructurally, membrane-bound electron-lucent vacuoles and electron-dense residual bodies, consisting of membrane-bound granular material, are noted (Fig. 11.67e).[22,257] Electron-dense and electron-lucent inclusions are also found in macrophages. Pericytes contain many vacuoles but vacuolation is less conspicuous in neuroglial cells and endothelial cells.

Animal models

With targeted disruption of the glycosylasparaginase gene, murine models of AGU have been generated by two groups of investigators. These mice show many of the biochemical as well as pathological features found in human AGU.[231,309,326,327,689]

Schindler's disease (α-N-acetylgalactosaminidase deficiency)

History and clinical course

Lysosomal α-N-acetylgalactosaminidase deficiency was first demonstrated in two German brothers who presented

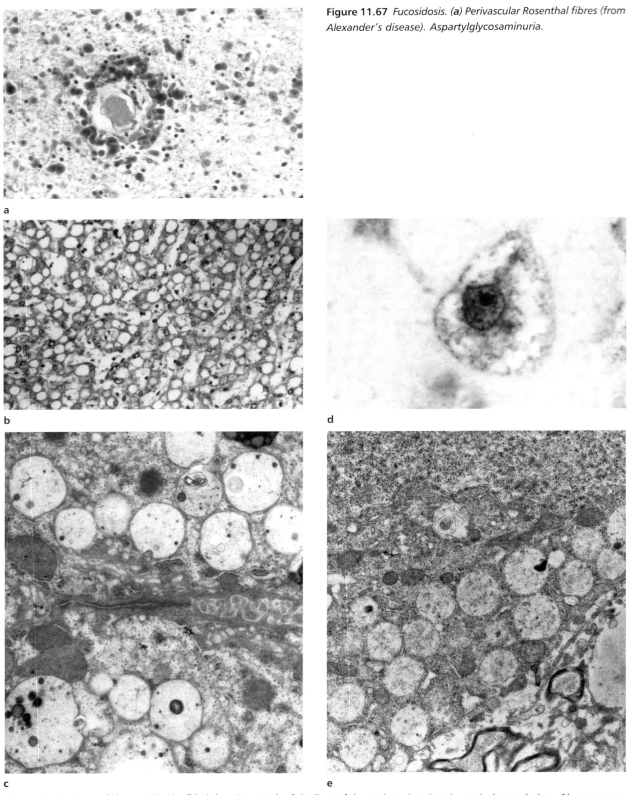

Figure 11.67 *Fucosidosis. (a) Perivascular Rosenthal fibres (from Alexander's disease). Aspartylglycosaminuria.*

a

b

d

c

e

Figure 11.67 *Aspartylglycosaminuria. (b) Light micrograph of the liver of the patient showing the typical vacuolation of hepatocytes, resembling an extreme degree of fatty metamorphosis. (H&E.) (c) Two hepatocytes with numerous membrane-bound electron-lucent storage vesicles and some electron-dense bodies both within and outside the vesicles. (Electron micrograph.) (d) Light micrograph of a swollen cerebral cortical neuron with indistinct vacuolation, a characteristic feature even though it looks like an artefactual 'watery change'. (Luxol fast blue–Cresyl violet.) (e) Electron-lucent storage vesicles in the cytoplasm of a cerebral cortical nerve cell from the brain biopsy. (Electron micrograph.) ((b)–(e) Courtesy of Dr Matti Haltia, University of Helsinki, Helsinki, Finland.)*

with progressive psychomotor deterioration in infancy, bilateral pyramidal tract signs with marked muscular hypotonia, nystagmus, myoclonus and seizures.[584] The light- and electron-microscopic examination of the brain biopsy from one of the patients showed typical axonal pathology as seen in infantile neuroaxonal dystrophy (INAD). However, normal activity of the enzyme in other patients with INAD indicates that the disease in these two brothers characterized by the deficiency of α-N-acetylgalactosaminidase differed from the usual type of INAD despite the pathological similarities.[584] A milder form was found in a 46-year old Japanese woman with angiokeratoma corporis diffusum and glycoproteinuria.[333,334] This patient had slight dysmorphic features and a low intelligence quotient (IQ). The infantile-onset cases have been called type I and the milder adult form type II or Kanzaki's disease. This disease is extremely rare and only a few cases have been reported in the literature.[94,136,345,710] In the cases reported by Chabas et al.,[94] tortuous retinal as well as conjunctival vessels were noted.

Biochemistry

The basic defect is the deficiency of α-N-acetylgalactosaminidase. As a consequence, urinary excretion of glycopeptides with terminal and internal α-N-acetylgalactosamininyl residues have been identified.[142] Excessive intralysosomal storage of α-N-acetylgalactosamine-containing material was demonstrated in cultured fibroblasts using a lectin from Helix pomatia, which is specific for terminal α-N-acetylgalactosamine residues.[710]

Molecular genetics

This is an autosomal recessive disease. The full-length cDNA encording α-N-acetylgalactosaminidase has been isolated and characterized.[748] The gene has remarkable similarities and is probably homologous to human α-galactosidase A, the enzyme deficient in Fabry's disease.[746] Disease-causing mutations have been identified in some patients.[345,748]

Pathology

The light- and electron-microscope features of the biopsy from the frontal lobe from one of the original type I patients described by Schindler et al.[584] showed characteristic pathological features of infantile neuroaxonal dystrophy.[277] At the light-microscopic level, abundant spheroid formation with characteristic straight or curved clear clefts was seen in the cerebral cortex (Fig. 11.68). Tubulovesicular and lamelliform membranous arrays, electron-lucent clefts and electron-dense axoplasmic matrices are the characteristic contents of these spheroids at the ultrastructural level.[774] Similar axonal changes were also present in the peripheral autonomic nerve fibres.[774,775] However, there was no evidence of storage in neurons or other cell types. Remarkably, visceral pathology was absent. Light- and electron-microscopic studies of peripheral blood cells, aspirated and biopsied bone marrow, conjunctiva, jejunal mucosa, muscle, liver and the sural nerve from the type I probands were all essentially normal.[143] In type II patients, whose clinical course was much milder, small clear cytoplasmic vacuoles were noted in granulocytes, monocytes and lymphocytes. Similar cytoplasmic vacuoles were reported in several cell types, including endothelial cells, pericytes, fibroblasts, adipose tissues, Schwann cells, axons of the peripheral nerve, arrector muscles and eccrine sweat gland cells. The localized angiokeratomata in the skin described in the type II patient consisted of hyperkeratosis and dilated, thin-walled vessels.[333,334] The CNS pathology of the type II patient has not been reported.

Animal model

With targeted gene disruption, a murine model of the disease has been generated.[749] No clinicopathological details have been reported.

Galactosialidosis

History and clinical course

An observation by Wenger, that some of the patients who had been thought to have genetic deficiency of lysosomal α-neuraminidase (sialidosis) were simultaneously also deficient in the activity of acid β-galactosidase, leads to the recognition of galactosialidosis as a distinct genetic disorder.[758] Galactosialidosis is characterized clinically by dysmorphic features, psychomotor retardation, macular cherry-red spots and myoclonus. It is usually classified to three types: I, early (severe) infantile; II, late (mild)

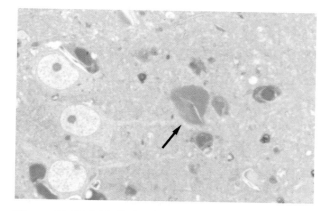

Figure 11.68 Schindler's disease. Brain biopsy from the frontal lobe showing abundant discrete deposits or axonal spheroids (arrow) throughout the cortical neuropil. (Toluidine-blue stained semithin plastic section.) (Courtesy of Dr David Wolf, Mount Sinai School of Medicine New York, USA.)

infantile; and III, juvenile or adult types. The clinical signs and symptoms of the severe infantile type are very similar to those of type II sialidosis. Coarse facies, hepatosplenomegaly, dysostosis multiplex and telangiectasia are common clinical features and affected infants usually cannot survive beyond 1 year of age.[237,350,493,674] Hydrops fetalis has been described.[589] The late (mild) infantile type exhibits coarse facies, hepatosplenomegaly, dysostosis multiplex and corneal clouding, resembling a mucopolysaccharidosis. Macular cherry-red spots are present but seizures are rare. The patient may have mild mental retardation but neurological manifestations appear only in the later years of life.[641] While all known late-infantile patients are Caucasian, a large majority of juvenile type patients reported is Japanese.[446,664–666,674] Patients usually exhibit a mild degree of coarse facies and bony abnormalities. Macular cherry-red spots and angiokeratoma are common but hepatosplenomegaly is rare. Typical neurological features are myoclonus, cerebellar ataxia, seizures and slowly progressive mental retardation.

Biochemistry

Galactosialidosis is caused by mutations in the gene encoding a 32/20-kDa dimeric protective protein, which has cathepsin A-like activity (protective protein/cathepsin A, PPCA). This protein forms a complex with the two lysosomal enzymes, acid β-galactosidase and sialidase, and somehow stabilizes them. Thus, the deficiency of PPCA secondarily causes a combined deficiency of both acid β-galactosidase and sialidase (α-neuraminidase). The deficiency of the protective protein leads to intralysosomal proteolysis of these enzymes and an accumulation of sialyloligosaccharides in the lysosomes and excessive sialyloligosaccharides in urine.[131,758] In the sympathetic ganglia, where many membranous cytoplasmic bodies are detected in neurons, a many-fold increase in gangliosides, in particular GM2 and GM3 gangliosides, has been reported. While a slight increase in gangliosides has also been recorded also in the spinal ganglia and spinal grey matter, it is more important to note that generally gangliosides in most regions of the brain are either normal or slightly decreased, despite the low activity of acid β-galactosidase.[787]

Molecular biology

Galactosialidosis is a rare autosomal recessive disorder caused by mutations in the gene for the galactosialidosis protective protein. The gene has been mapped to chromosome 20q12-q13.1. Several mutations have been identified.

Pathology

The basic pathology is the cytoplasmic vacuolation in many types of cells indicating storage of water-soluble material, such as oligosaccharides. In the severe infantile form, numerous clear cytoplasmic vacuoles are conspicuous features in hepatocytes, Kupffer cells, Schwann cells, fibroblasts, endothelial cells, lymphocytes and plasma cells. These vacuoles are membrane bound and similar to those seen in sialidosis. The glomerular epithelial cells and renal tubular epithelial cells are also finely vacuolated. The neurons in the autonomic ganglion contain numerous membranous cytoplasmic bodies and pleomorphic dense bodies.[784] Similar changes have also been reported in the late infantile/juvenile and adult types.[355,446] Neuropathological investigations have been carried out only in a limited number of patients. In the CNS of a late-infantile patient, gross atrophy of the optic nerves, the thalamus, globus pallidus and the lateral geniculate bodies, the brainstem and the cerebellum have been reported. Histologically, there was marked neuronal loss and fibrillary gliosis in these grossly atrophied structures. Neuronal storage is found only in certain neurons: the Betz cells in the motor cortex, neurons in the basal forebrain, the cranial nerve nuclei, the spinal anterior horn, and in the trigeminal and spinal ganglia.[501] The distribution of the storage neurons is similar, although the extent of neuronal loss may differ in individual patients.[11] Electron-microscopic features of the neuronal storage materials are variable; they are described as membranous cytoplasmic bodies, parallel, wavy–lamellar or tortuous tubular structures, lipofuscin-like irregular shaped pleomorphic bodies, and cytoplasmic vacuoles with fine granules and lamellar materials.[501]

Animal models

A sheep model reported as ovine GM1 gangliosidosis shows deficiency of both β-galactosidase and neuraminidase, and is homologous to human galactosialidase.[531] A mouse model of galactosialidosis has been generated by gene-targeting techniques.[799] Similar to the disease in man, the mice show coarse facies, bony abnormalities and hepatosplenomegaly. Many vacuolated cells and neuronal storage are also present.

NEURONAL CEROID LIPOFUSCINOSIS (NCL, BATTEN'S DISEASE)

The terms neuronal ceroid lipofuscinosis (NCL) and Batten's disease, have often been used interchangeably to describe a clinically and genetically heterogeneous group of diseases, which are pathologically characterized by an accumulation of autofluorescent ceroid lipofuscin materials (inclusions) in the cytoplasm of neurons and other cell types.[796] They are all inherited as autosomal recessive diseases. For many years, NCL has been subclassified into four major groups, infantile (INCL), late-infantile (LINCL), juvenile (JNCL) and adult (ANCL) types, by their clinical presentation and ultrastructural morphology of the abnormal inclusions.[73,224] More recently, at least

Table 11.5 *Neuronal ceroid lipofuscinosis*

	Infantile NCL CLN1	Late infantile NCL				Juvenile NCL CLN3	Adult NCL CLN4	Northern epilepsy CLN8
		CLN2	CLN5	CLN6	CLN7			
Age of onset (years)	0–2	2–4	4–7	4–5	4–7	4–9	11–50	5–10
Morphology EM inclusions	GROD	CV	CV/FP	CV/FP	CV/FP	FP	FP/GROD	CV/GROD
Chromosomal location	1p32	11p15	13q22	15q21-23	Unknown	16p12	Unknown	8p22
Gene product	Palmitoyl-protein thioesterase	Peptatin-insensitive peptidase	Membrane protein	Unknown	Unknown	Lysosomal membrane protein	Unknown	Unknown
Storage material	SAPs A, D fatty acid thioesters	Subunit c	Subunit c	Subunit c	Subunit c	Subunit c	Subunit c	Subunit c SAPs A, D

EM, electron microscopic; GROD, granular osmiophilic deposits; CV, curvilinear bodies; FP, deposits with fingerprint profiles; SAP, sphingolipid activator protein; Subunit c, mitochondrial ATP synthase subunit c.
Adapted from Bennett and Hofmann (1999).[50]

eight genetically distinct gene loci, which are responsible for various types of NCL when mutated, have been identified and gene symbols have been assigned as CLN1–8. CLN1, CLN2, CLN3 and CLN4 correspond to the traditional four major clinical subtypes. As of autumn 1999, four genes (*CLN1, CLN2, CLN3* and *CLN5*) had been identified and their gene products characterized. CLN1 is a lysosomal palmitoyl-protein thioesterase (PPT) and CLN2 is a lysosomal pepstatin-insensitive peptidase. CLN3 and CNL5 are proteins of still unknown physiological functions with multiple membrane-spanning regions. The CNL3 protein is physically associated with lysosomal membranes. Therefore, there is ample evidence that the neuronal ceroid-lipofuscinoses represent a new class of lysosomal disorders.[50,448] Table 11.5 lists the established human forms of neuronal ceroid-lipofuscinosis.[50] Ultrastructural details of neuronal storage bodies in the various types of NCL have been well documented.[224]

Considering animal models of NCL in general, many generic models of NCL have been documented in mammalian species, including cattle, sheep, goats, cats, dogs and mice. Accumulation of saposins and/or subunit c of mitochondrial ATP synthase have been documented in some. However, since most of them were found before the remarkable developments in the biochemical and molecular characterization of NCL during the 1990s, their classification has been for the most part by clinical and pathological phenotypes for the lack of specific analytical, enzymic, or molecular diagnostic criteria.[399] Undoubtedly, many of them will be characterized by genetics and molecular pathology, to be assigned to specific individual forms of NCLs. However, reflecting the

current status of animal models of NCL in general, animal model sections will be included in the description of the individual NCLs only when identified naturally occurring model or mouse knockout models are known.

Infantile neuronal ceroid lipofuscinosis (INCL, Haltia–Santavuori disease)

History and clinical course

INCL is an autosomal recessive disease, which occurs predominantly in Finland. INCL cases have been reported from outside Finland, but with lower incidence. The disease was first described by Hagberg *et al.*[251] It is characterized by psychomotor retardation starting around 10–18 months of age. However, muscular hypotonia, clumsiness in fine motor control and retarded head growth may be detected earlier. MRI can detect hypointensity in the T_2-weighted images as an early sign. By the age of 2 years, the majority of patients shows severe visual deterioration with sluggish papillary reaction, progressive optic atrophy and retinal hypopigmentation. Hyperexcitability with poor sleep resulting from thalamic degeneration and seizures with frequent myoclonic jerks become apparent in the later stage.[581] Most characteristically, the electroencephalogram (ECG) becomes essentially flat in later stages of the disease owing to a nearly complete loss of cortical neurons. The recent identification of the primary defect in INCL has led to the discovery of the existence of late infantile and juvenile forms of the disease.[444] Thus, INCL is not always infantile.

Biochemistry

INCL patients have deficient activity of the lysosomal enzyme PPT.[278,723] PPT is a housekeeping enzyme present in many tissues, and is particularly abundant in the spleen, brain and testis. The storage material includes sphingolipid activator proteins (saposins) A and D. Recently, prenatal and postnatal enzyme analysis for the identification of INCL has been established.[145,709] The mechanism whereby the PPT deficiency leads to accumulation of SAPs and eventual neurodegeneration is not known. Recently, some patients with the clinical phenotypes of LINCL or JNCL have been found to have PPT deficiency.[444,771]

Molecular biology

INCL is caused by a genetic defect in the *CLN1* gene, which encodes palmitoyl protein thioesterase and is located on chromosome 1p32. Over 20 different gene mutations have been reported in patients with the infantile clinical phenotype with an accumulation of granular osmiophilic deposits (GROD).[128,723] All cases of INCL in Finland carry a common missense mutation, $Arg_{122}Trp$.[278]

Pathology

The most significant gross pathology is limited to the brain and its coverings. The head circumference is slightly reduced and the calvaria are abnormally thick. A thick layer of gelatinous tissue covers the inner aspect of the cerebral dura mater. The brain is extremely atrophic, weighing only 250–450 g at the terminal stage. There is marked narrowing of the gyri and widening of the sulci throughout. Optic nerves are atrophic. Atrophy is also noted in the cerebellum and brainstem, while the spinal cord is well preserved. On sectioning the brain, the cerebral cortex and cerebellar folia are markedly thinned and white matter is shrunken and firm in consistency. The histopathology of the brain has been described in three stages.[257,259,260,580] Stage I (up to about 2.5 years of age) is characterized by neuronal storage of colourless or slightly yellowish granules and pronounced astrocytic hyperplasia. At stage II (2.5–4 years of age) the cerebral cortex shows an extensive loss of neurons in association with astrocytic hyperplasia and macrophage infiltration. In stage III (after the age of 4 years) cerebral cortical neurons are almost completely lost (Fig. 11.69) and marked secondary white matter degeneration is present. Interestingly, however, giant cells of Betz in the precentral gyrus (Fig. 11.69) and pyramidal neurons of the CA1 and CA4 sectors of the hippocampus and spinal anterior horn neurons are partially preserved. In the retina, the photoreceptor cells, the bipolar cells and the ganglion cells have completely disappeared and been replaced by reactive gliosis. Accumulation of the storage materials is noted in neurons in the spinal ganglia and autonomic ganglia, many

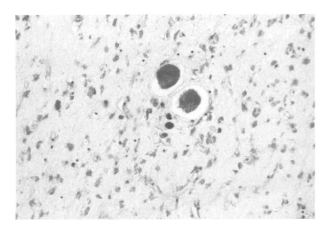

Figure 11.69 *Infantile neuronal ceroid lipofuscinosis. Almost complete loss of cerebral cortical neurons associated with intense glial reaction. (PAS.) (Courtesy of Dr Matti Haltia, University of Helsinki, Helsinki, Finland.)*

epithelial cells including those of eccrine sweat glands, thyroid follicles and testes, skeletal, cardiac, and smooth-muscle cells, endothelial cells and macrophages.[257,259,260] The storage granules show strong yellowish autofluorescence under UV light and are strongly positive for acid phosphatase activity, by PAS and Luxol fast blue. They are immunostained with antibodies against saposins A and D and amyloid β-peptide but not with antibody against subunit c of mitochondrial ATP synthase.[261,704] The ultrastructural features of cytosomes of INCL are membrane-bound cytoplasmic inclusions, 1–3 μm in diameter, often called GROD (Figs 11.70, 11.71).[259,260] Detection of GROD in the neurons of the myenteric and submucosal plexuses and also in some non-neural cells including muscle cells, endothelial cells and chorionic villi was essential for the diagnosis of INCL before the identification of PPT deficiency. Unlike classical LINCL and JNCL, no vacuolated lymphocytes are present in the peripheral blood, but GROD can be detected in their cytoplasm by electron-microscopic investigation.

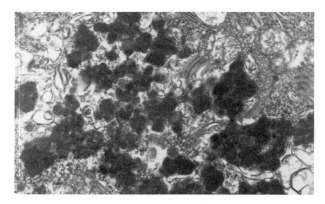

Figure 11.70 *Late infantile neuronal ceroid lipofuscinosis. Granular osmiophilic deposits within a neuron. (Electron micrograph.)*

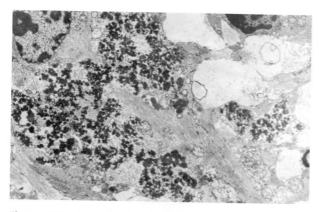

Figure 11.71 *Late infantile neuronal ceroid lipofuscinosis. Granular osmiophilic deposits in an astrocyte. (Electron micrograph.)*

Late infantile neuronal ceroid lipofuscinosis (LINCL, Jansky–Bielschowsky disease)

History and clinical course

Classical LINCL occurs world-wide in many different ethnic groups. However, clusters of cases have been reported in Newfoundland, Costa Rica and western Finland. The early symptoms, such as speech delay, hypotonia, ataxia and grand mal seizures, appear usually between the ages of 2 and 4 years. Motor and cognitive functions deteriorate rapidly, and by the age of 5 years, affected children are completely bed-ridden, mute and cachectic. Visual acuity gradually declines to blindness.[73] The EEG shows an occipital photosensitive response and persists until an advanced state of the illness. The electroretinogram (ERG) is diminished at presentation and soon becomes extinguished, while visual evoked potentials (VEPs) are grossly enhanced, in keeping with the photosensitive EEG response. The pattern of these combined results is very characteristic of late infantile NCL. VEPs persist until very late into the illness, but eventually become diminished when the child reaches a preterminal stage. CT and MRI show varying degree of cerebral and cerebellar atrophy (Figs 11.72, 11.73a, b) depending on the stages of the disease process and may show hyperintensity of bilateral periventricular white matter in proton density and T_2-weighted images.[766]

Biochemistry

The mature form of subunit c of mitochondrial ATP synthase comprises up to 85% of the protein content of the storage material in the brain of patients with classical LINCL.[502,503] Small amounts of sphingolipid activator proteins (saposins) and dolichol are also present as components of the storage material.[470,705] LINCL is caused by deficiency in activity of lysosomal pepstatin-insensitive protease. Recently, an assay for the pepstatin-insensitive protease activity has been developed for enzymic diagnosis.[325,627]

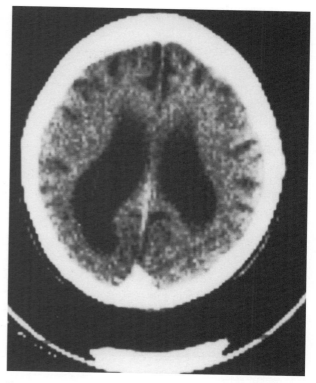

Figure 11.72 *Late infantile neuronal ceroid lipofuscinosis. CT showing marked cerebral atrophy with enlarged ventricles.*

Molecular genetics

The gene responsible for almost all classic LINCL patients (*CLN2*) is mapped to chromosome 11p15 and encodes a pepstatin-insensitive lysosomal peptidase.[623] Immunodepletion of the CLN2 gene product from normal fibroblast extracts caused loss of degradative capacity of subunit c, suggesting that the absence of the gene product provokes the lysosomal accumulation of subunit c.[176] However, a direct substrate–enzyme relationship between subunit c and the pepstatin-insensitive lysosomal peptidase has not yet been demonstrated.

Neuroimaging

In LINCL, MRI studies show diffuse atrophy involving the cerebral hemispheres, the cerebellum and the brainstem (Fig. 11.73a, b). The white matter is abnormally hypodense and its volume appears reduced, particularly in advanced stages of the disease. The cortex is thin but the volume of the deep grey structures is relatively preserved. The calvaria becomes progressively thicker. Similar findings are noted by MRI; however, the basal ganglia may be hypointense in the late stage of the disease.

Pathology

The brain shows severe atrophy (Fig. 11.73c), with a weight of 500–700 g being common at the terminal stage. The cerebral cortex as well as cerebellar folia are thinned. Ventricular dilatation (hydrocephalus *ex vacuo*) with

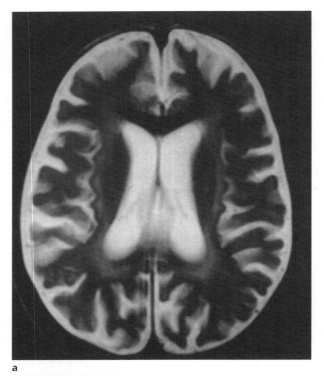

a

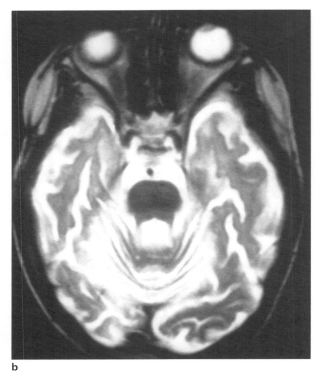

b

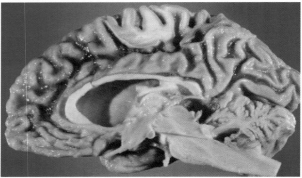

c

Figure 11.73 *Late infantile neuronal ceroid lipofuscinosis. (a) Axial T₂-weighted MRI showing diffuse cerebral cortical atrophy and a greatly enlarged lateral ventricles. (b) T₂-weighted MRI of the same patient as in (a) showing atrophy of the temporal and occipital lobes and significant atrophy of the cerebellum and the brainstem.(Courtesy of Dr Mauricio Castillo, University of North Carolina, Chapel Hill, North Carolina, USA.) (c) Late infantile neuronal ceroid lipofuscinosis. Marked atrophy of cerebrum and cerebellum.*

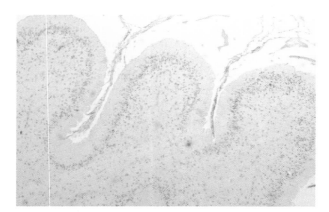

Figure 11.74 *Late infantile neuronal ceroid lipofuscinosis. Extensive loss of neurons is evident in the cerebellum. (H&E.)*

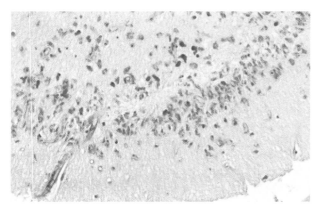

Figure 11.75 *Late infantile neuronal ceroid lipofuscinosis. Extensive gliosis without any identifiable Purkinje or granule cells. (PAS.)*

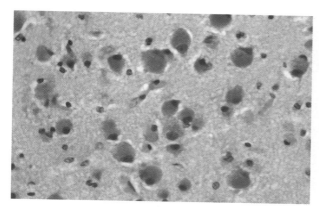

Figure 11.76 *Late infantile neuronal ceroid lipofuscinosis. Ballooned neurons in the cerebral cortex. (H&E.)*

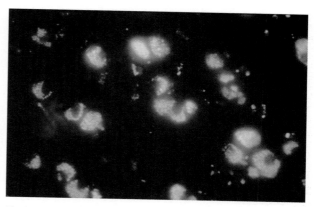

Figure 11.78 *Late infantile neuronal ceroid lipofuscinosis. Storage material in neurons emits strong autofluorescence.*

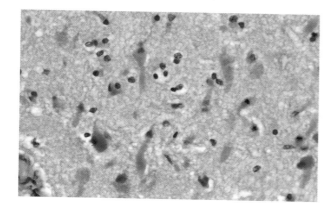

Figure 11.77 *Late infantile neuronal ceroid lipofuscinosis. Affected neurons in the cerebral cortex demonstrate many slender meganeurites. (H&E.)*

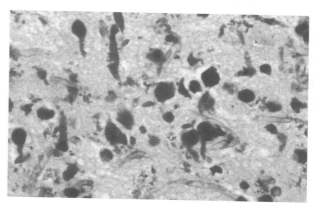

Figure 11.79 *Late infantile neuronal ceroid lipofuscinosis. Storage material in neurons and in glial cells stain strongly positive with PAS stain. (PAS.)*

thinning of the corpus callosum and firm atrophic white matter reflect the severity of the degenerative changes in the brain of LINCL patients. Similarly to INCL, the most pronounced changes noted in the post-mortem brains are severe depletion of neurons and associated astrocytic gliosis and activation of microglia. Increased immunocytochemical staining by BCL-2 and TUNEL suggests that many neurons disappear by apoptosis.[385,533] In the cerebellum, both the granular and Purkinje cells are lost (Figs 11.74, 11.75). The perikarya of remaining neurons are distended with granular storage material (Figs 11.76, 11.77). Meganeurites are conspicuous in some cortical neurons (Fig. 11.77). However, unlike those seen in gangliosidoses and Niemann–Pick type C disease, ectopic neurite formation has not been detected in meganeurites in NCL.[738] A high incidence of neuronal perikaryal spheroids has been reported.[172] Similarly to the storage material in INCL, the neuronal storage material in LINCL emits autofluorescence under UV light (Fig. 11. 78) and stains strongly positive with PAS (Fig. 11.79), Sudan black and Luxol fast blue. Immunoreactivity for subunit c of mitochondrial ATP synthase (SCMAS) (Fig. 11.80) has been demonstrated in the neuronal storage material.[221,380] At the

ultrastructural level, the storage material consists of curvilinear inclusion bodies (Figs 11.81, 11.82), enclosed by a single-unit membrane and associated with SCMAS and acid phosphatase activity. A variable degree of retinal

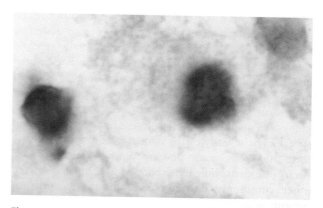

Figure 11.80 *Late infantile neuronal ceroid lipofuscinosis. Neuronal storage material is strongly immunoreactive with an antibody to mitochondria ATP synthase subunit c. (Courtesy of Dr Rosemary Boustany, Duke University Medical Center, North Carolina, USA.)*

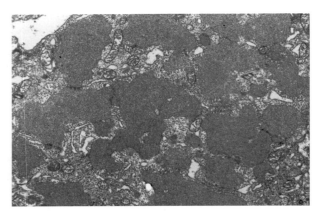

Figure 11.81 *Late infantile neuronal ceroid lipofuscinosis. Low magnification of curvilinear neuronal inclusions. (Electron micrograph.)*

degeneration with loss of neurons and gliosis has been reported. Accumulation of sudanophilic, autofluorescent material with a curvilinear profile has also been well documented in the extracerebral tissues. Thus, rectal or skin biopsies are useful for the diagnosis of LINCL.[217] In an electron-microscopic study of a skin biopsy, curvilinear inclusion bodies were found in sweat gland, peripheral nerve, smooth-muscle and endothelial cells. Peripheral lymphocytes may show clear cytoplasmic vacuoles that contain curvilinear bodies.

Juvenile neuronal ceroid lipofuscinosis (JNCL, Spielmeyer–Vogt–Sjögren–Batten disease)

History and clinical course

JNCL has been reported world-wide but appears to occur with a much higher incidence in populations with Scandinavian or northern European ancestry than in the African–American or Jewish population. The eponym, Batten's disease, was originally coined specifically for this disease, although it is now commonly used to designate all types of NCL. The visual problem is usually an early symptom starting at the age of 4–9 years owing to progressive retinitis pigmentosa. A few years later, gradual and progressive cognitive decline develops. Speech difficulty and seizures follow. By their mid-teens to the age of 20, many patients almost completely lose light perception and speech. The severity of the epilepsy is quite variable. By their mid-teens, many develop signs of parkinsonism. Angry outbursts, violent behaviour and hallucinations are other commonly encountered clinical symptoms of patients with JNCL.[288]

Biochemistry

The major component of the storage material is a protein with the sequence of subunit c of the mitochondrial

ATP synthase, which account for about 85% of the protein in the storage material. Increased levels of phosphorylated dolichols are also found in the storage material. However, the significance of the storage of subunit c and dolichol phosphate in the pathogenesis of JNLC is not clearly understood, as they are also found in other types of NCL and in chronic forms of other lysosomal diseases.[171]

Molecular genetics

The *CLN3* gene was isolated by positional cloning. It is localized in the region of 16p11, 2-12.1. *CLN3* is highly conserved and mammalian homologues have been described in the mouse, rabbit, dog and sheep. However, the physiological function of any of these homologous proteins is not known. Many disease-causing mutations have been reported.[288]

Neuroimaging

The imaging abnormalities in patients with JNCL are similar to those seen in patients with INCL and LINCL. In JNCL, imaging abnormalities appear late in the course of the disease and initial studies may be normal. The cerebellum is profoundly atrophic in patients with JNCL.

Pathology

The most notable laboratory finding is the presence of vacuolated lymphocytes on routine blood smear. Inclusions with a characteristic 'fingerprint' profile are observed in these lymphocytes as well as storage neurons in the brain (Figs 11.83–11.85) by electron-microscopic examination.

Grossly, the brain shows moderate to severe atrophy, in proportion to the length of the disease process. Microscopically, a variable degree of neuronal loss is present in

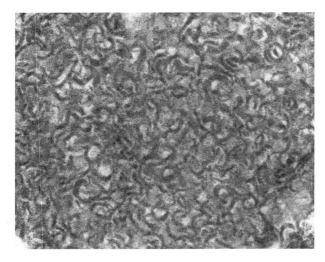

Figure 11.82 *Late infantile neuronal ceroid lipofuscinosis. Higher magnification of inclusions shown in Fig. 11.81. Curvilinear profiles of the inclusion are clearly identified. (Electron micrograph.)*

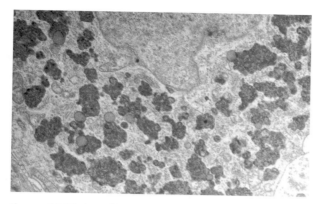

Figure 11.83 *Juvenile neuronal ceroid lipofuscinosis. Low magnification of neuronal inclusions with fingerprint profiles. (Electron micrograph.)*

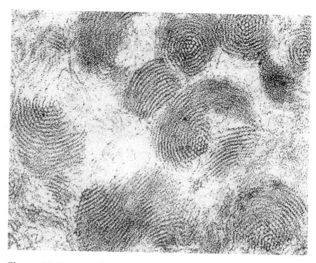

Figure 11.85 *Juvenile neuronal ceroid lipofuscinosis. Fingerprint bodies present in a neuron from the gastrointestinal tract. (Electron micrograph.)*

the cerebrum and cerebellum. With pigmentoarchitectonic analysis, selective loss of neurons in layers II and V of the cerebral cortex and in the striatum and amygdaloid nucleus has been demonstrated.[75] The perikarya of remaining neurons are distended with granular storage material that stains pale yellow on H&E, and strongly positive with PAS, Sudan black and Luxol fast blue. The neuronal storage material is strongly autofluorescent under UV light and immunoreactive for SCMAS (Fig. 11.80). At the ultrastructural level, the storage material consists of inclusions with fingerprint profiles (Figs 11.83, 11.84). Excitotoxicity following dysfunction of GABAergic neurons and of mitochondria has been suggested to be the mechanism of neuronal depletion.[738,742] Extensive neuronal loss occurs in the retina. Death by apoptosis of photoreceptor cells has been demonstrated in a mouse model.[529] Granular storage material is also found in many cell types throughout the visceral organs. The staining characteristics and ultrastructural features of the storage material in the visceral tissue may slightly differ from those in neurons (for more details refer to Hofmann *et al.*[288]). In contrast to classic LINCL, there is no immunohistochemical evidence of SCMAS in the liver, adrenal or endocrine pancreas.[171]

Animal models

There are no naturally occurring animal models of JNCL. However, by targeted disruption of the mouse gene *Cln3*, murine models of JNCL have been generated by two groups of investigators.[238,337] The autofluorescent storage material was demonstrated in both models. Subtle behavioural abnormalities have been noted in older mice.[337]

Adult neuronal ceroid lipofuscinosis (ANCL, Kufs' disease)

History and clinical course

This is a rather heterogeneous group of rare and poorly defined NCL. Some cases reported as Kufs' disease may in fact be adult-onset neuronal lipid storage diseases.[430] The patient originally described by Kufs had a slowly progressive dementing illness beginning at the age of 30 years. However, onset during adolescence has been reported. Presenting clinical features are behavioural changes, seizures, ataxia, cerebellar signs and pyramidal/extrapyramidal movement disorders, followed by dementia. Unlike other NCLs, ANCL patients show no ophthalmological symptoms. Some ANCL cases with visual failure and pigmentary retinal degeneration are most likely to be cases of protracted JNCL. Clinically, ANCL can be subclassified into two subtypes, phenotype A with progressive myoclonus epilepsy and phenotype B with pronounced behavioural changes and dementia.[54,73,430]

Biochemistry and molecular genetics

Sporadic cases of Kufs' disease have been reported.[54] The majority of cases is autosomal recessive inheritance but a

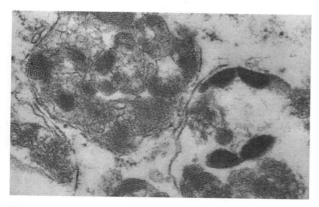

Figure 11.84 *Juvenile neuronal ceroid lipofuscinosis. Cytoplasmic inclusions with fingerprint-like profiles in cerebral cortical neurons. (Electron micrograph.)*

few examples of autosomal dominant inheritance have been described.[67,150,163,392,696] To date, no specific gene has been identified. The putative ACLN gene has been designated as *NCL4*.

Pathology

The brain weight is reduced, with atrophy of the cerebrum, particularly prominent in the frontal and frontoparietal region of the cerebral cortex. The cerebellum may also be atrophic. Microscopically, neuronal storage and variable degrees of neuronal loss are present.[430] With the pigmentoarchitectonic technique, there appears to be selective neuronal storage in the neocortex and subcortical nuclei, as also noted in JNCL.[75,219] Secondary degeneration of white matter associated with astrogliosis and microglial activation has been observed. Staining characteristics of the neuronal storage material are similar to those of other types of NCL. Immunocytochemically, SCMAS and saposins A and D have been demonstrated in the storage material.[171,256,705] At the ultrastructural level, the storage material consists of membrane-bound inclusions containing various combinations of osmiophilic granules, curvilinear, rectilinear and fingerprint profiles, and lipid droplets.[219]

In the majority of cases, no storage material is detected in biopsies from conjunctiva, skin or peripheral nerves. However, in some cases, fingerprint profiles have been found in eccrine sweat gland epithelium, and curvilinear and rectilinear profiles have been noted in skeletal muscles.[426] Osmiophilic inclusions with or without fingerprint profiles have been noted in skin, muscle and rectal biopsies in some cases.[208] Thus, unlike the childhood forms of NCL, storage in the extracerebral tissues is inconsistent and the ultrastructural features of the storage material are quite heterogeneous in ANCL.

Other variant types of NCL

Variant types of NCL include the Finnish variant late infantile NCL, a variant late infantile/early juvenile NCL, the Turkish variant late infantile NCL, and northern epilepsy. They have been separated from the classical forms of CLN by genetic complementation studies. Gene symbols *CLN5*, *CLN6*, *CLN7* and *CLN8* have been assigned to these variants (Table 11.5). Thus, it is important to note that these are not clinical or pathological variants but are distinct genetically from each other and from the classical forms of NCL. The Finnish variant LINCL and northern epilepsy[281a] are almost exclusively found in Finland. These variants are clearly different in their clinical presentations and genetic defects. However, basic neuropathological features are closely similar to the classical form of LINCL/JNCL.[224] Among this group, only the *CLN5* gene has been cloned.[582]

MISCELLANEOUS LYSOSOMAL DISORDERS

I-Cell disease and pseudo-Hurler polydystrophy (mucolipidosis II and III)

I-Cell disease (ICD; mucolipidosis II, ML II) and pseudo-Hurler polydystrophy (PHP; mucolipidosis III, ML III) were originally thought to be a different diseases but now it is established that they are allelic forms of the same disease, caused by the defects in post-translational phosphorylation of many lysosomal enzymes. Clinically, ML II is more severe than ML III.[393]

History and clinical course

The term mucolipidosis was introduced to describe a group of lysosomal storage diseases with clinical features of both the mucopolysaccharidoses and the sphingolipidoses.[636] The mucolipidoses were classified into four clinical phenotypes, types I, II, III and IV. Subsequently, type I became defined as 'sialidoses' (see above),[161,634,635] and type II (I-cell disease) and type III (pseudo-Hurler polydystrophy) were later shown to be allelic variants of the same disorder.[549] Infants with ICD are usually smaller than normal at birth, indicating expression of the disorder *in utero*. The major clinical manifestations include thick, swollen skin, particularly around the ears, congenital hernia and orthopaedic abnormalities, such as clubfoot, dislocation of the hip, kyphosis and other spine abnormalities, growth retardation of the skeletal system, progressive impairment of motion in all joints, hypotonia and mild to severe psychomotor retardation. Facial abnormalities similar to MPS IH are present, but hepatosplenomegaly or corneal clouding is usually not apparent. The ICD phenotype is quite variable but the majority of patients will express clinical symptoms at or shortly after birth, with fatal outcome most often in early childhood. Clinical manifestations of PHP are similar to ICD, but milder and with a protracted course. The onset of clinical symptoms is usually around 3 years of age.[342] Some PHP patients may survive well into adulthood.[706] In both ICD and PHP patients, excessive sialyloligosaccharides are excreted in the urine.[602]

Biochemistry

Lysosomal enzymes are post-translationally modified and acquire the mannose 6-phosphate recognition marker, which is required for proper intracellular routing of newly synthesized lysosomal enzymes to the lysosome. Defective synthesis of the mannose 6-phosphate recognition marker in these disorders results in impairment in the proper targeting of the lysosomal enzymes to the lysosome, their physiological site of function and in leakage of newly synthesized enzymes out of the cells. This recognition marker is generated in the Golgi complex by two-step reactions. The first step is the addition of *N*-acetylglucosamine phosphate to the mannose residue of the sugar chain of the enzymes by the action of UDP-*N*-acetylglucosamine:lysosomal enzyme *N*-acetyl-glucosamine-1-phosphotransferase. The second step is removal of the *N*-acetylglucosamine, which then exposes the terminal mannose 6-phosphate. The first phosphorylation step is defective in all known cases of ICD,[733] but a distinct possibility exists of another genetic form of ICD due to defective removal of *N*-acetyl-glucosamine. The consequence of this defect is that newly synthesized lysosomal enzymes do not reach the lysosome and instead are excreted out of the cell. Thus, the activities of many lysosomal enzymes in solid tissues are defective but they are abnormally elevated in body fluids, including serum.[760,761] Cultured fibroblasts from these patients show defective activities of a large number of lysosomal acid hydrolases. However, in the culture media, the activity of these enzymes is greatly increased and these enzymes are not phosphorylated.[269]

Molecular genetics

ICD and PHP are both inherited as autosomal recessive traits. Genetic defects in three separate genes can cause ICD and PHP. UDP-*N*-acetylglucosamine:lysosomal enzyme *N*-acetylglucosamine-1-phosphotransferase consists of three subunits, α, β and γ. Subunits α and β are generated from a single polypeptide encoded by a single gene, and subunit γ is encoded by its own gene, and the enzyme that removes the glucosamine residue is encoded by the third distinct gene. All three genes have recently been cloned and characterized.[89] Thus, three genetically distinct forms of ICD that are mutually complementary can exist with the same clinical and pathological phenotype. Disease-causing mutations have been identified in the gene coding for the α/β-subunit of the phosphotransferase and in the phosphodiesterase gene.

Pathology

The name 'I-cell' disease is originated from the observation in phase-contrast microscopy of large numbers of granular inclusions in the cultured skin fibroblasts from a patient with the disease. These fibroblasts were called 'inclusion cells' or 'I-cells' and the disorder was named I-cell disease (ICD).[394] Similar I-cell phenomena also occur in PHP fibroblasts in culture.[55,692] The pathological hallmark of ICD is intracytoplasmic membrane-bound vacuoles in lymphocytes and fibroblasts in various tissues, such as skin, conjunctiva, lymph nodes, spleen, gingiva, heart valves and bone in the regions of enchondral and membranous bone formation. Vacuoles have also been reported in Schwann cells, perineural cells, endothelial cells and pericytes,[213,348,431,432] in hepatocytes, myocardial fibres, epithelial cells of renal glomeruli and tubules.[330] These vacuoles showed positive staining for colloidal iron,

PAS, Alcian blue and Sudan III and IV.[348,358] Neuronal and glial changes are minimal. There is no massive neuronal storage. Only a mild accumulation of haematoxyphilic granules is present in the pontomedullary reticular formations and in neurons in the spinal anterior horn. At the ultrastructural level, neurons in the spinal anterior horn were found to contain zebra bodies and membranous cytoplasmic bodies. A few membrane-bound vacuoles with fibrillogranular contents and some lamellar profiles or small lipofuscin granules were described in other neurons. Electron-lucent vacuoles are found in astrocytes, oligodendrocytes and the mesenchymal cells around blood vessels, as well as in endothelial cells.[432] Sympathetic and parasympathetic neurons contain a few lipofuscin granules. Lamellar inclusions similar to MCBs have been described in spinal ganglioa.[461] To the authors' knowledge, no autopsy studies of PHP patients have been reported.

Animal models

A domestic short-haired cat with a deficiency of the enzyme *N*-acetylglucosamine-1-phosphotransferase has been reported.[72,293] Clinically and pathologically, this feline model closely resembles ICD in man. Mannose 6-phosphate receptor-deficient mice have been generated by crossing three mutant mice, carrying null alleles for Igf2, and the 300 kDa and 46 kDa mannose 6-phosphate receptors, Mpr 300 and Mpr 46. The triple-deficient mice phenotypically resemble ICD in man.[149]

Mucolipidosis IV (ML IV)

History and clinical course

In 1974, Berman *et al.*[56] reported a male infant with congenital corneal opacity but with no obvious skeletal or neurological abnormalities. Bone-marrow aspirates, however, showed numerous histiocytes with cytoplasm distended with sudanophilic material. Hepatocytes and conjunctival epithelial cells contained MCBs similar to those of gangliosidoses. Cytoplasmic vacuoles containing finely granular material or lamellated structures were also noted in Kupffer cells in the hepatic sinusoids and some conjunctival epithelial cells.[56] Subsequent reports indicated marked heterogeneity in the clinical symptoms, but major characteristics of this disorder appear to be psychomotor retardation and ophthalmological abnormalities including corneal opacity, retinal degeneration and strabismus. No organomegaly or skeletal abnormalities are present.[97] The clinical course may be protracted.[12,548]

Biochemistry

Abnormalities in the composition of gangliosides, phospholipids and mucopolysaccharides have often been reported in the literature but none appears to reflect directly the primary metabolic defect underlying ML IV.[38,41,118] The lysosomal hydrolases participating in the catabolism of these stored substances are normal. Chen et al.[95] demonstrated abnormalities in the membrane sorting and/or in late steps of endocytosis in fibroblasts from ML IV patients, suggesting a defect in intracellular lysosomal transport.

Molecular genetics

ML IV is an autosomal recessive disorder. Motulsky investigated the genetic and ethnic background of over 70 families with ML IV world-wide, and found that over 90% of patients are Ashkenazi Jews, thus classifying ML IV as one of the genetic disorders occurring with a relatively high frequency in this population.[454] This finding has been further elaborated recently.[538] After many years of false starts, the gene responsible for ML IV has been localized to chromosome 19p13.2-13.3 by linkage analysis.[622] The gene has been identified recently.[45a]

Pathology

The tissue most often examined for diagnosis of ML IV is the epithelium of the conjunctiva. As reported in the original paper by Berman et al.[56] conjunctival biopsies reveal two types of characteristic inclusions: (1) single membrane-bound cytoplasmic vacuoles containing fibrinogranular

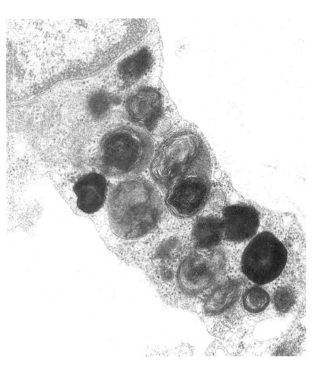

Figure 11.87 *Mucolipidosis IV. Concentric lamellar inclusions in fibroblasts. (Electron micrograph.)*

and small membranous structures, and (2) concentric lamellar structures similar to MCBs of gangliosidoses. The presence of these two types of inclusions in the conjunctival epithelium in a mentally retarded patient is almost the diagnostic feature of ML IV (Figs 11.86, 11.87).[442,553] Vacuoles and/or MCBs have been reported in many other tissues, including muscles, leukocytes, liver and skin fibroblasts.[222] There is a single autopsy report on a 23-year-old ML IV patient, who had mild corneal clouding, severe kyphoscoliosis, multiple joint contractures and bilateral short fourth metatarsals. Vacuolation was noted in the hepatic bile ductal and pancreatic ductal epithelium, Kupffer cells, macrophages in the lung, spleen, and lymph nodes, ganglion cells of the myenteric plexus, parasympathetic and sympathetic ganglia, and in vascular endothelial cells. The brain was atrophic and the corpus callosum was very thin. Histologically, the cortical cytoarchitecture was retained but the parietal and inferior frontal gyri revealed a more columnar (early fetal) organization and widespread neuronal loss and gliosis in the thalamus, hippocampus (CA3), substantia nigra, basis pontis, inferior olivary nucleus, spinal anterior horn and cerebellar Purkinje cell layer. Neurons and microglial cells and possibly astrocytes contained pigmented cytoplasmic granules. These granules were brown on H&E, turquoise–green on LFB, and intensely positive with PAS and Sudan black. White matter and brainstem fibre tracts were weakly stained with LFB. The storage granules in cortical neurons were osmiophilic, amorphous, granular material with a few lamellar membranes at the ultrastructural level. They differed from the lamellar or vacuolar inclusions noted in other cell types.[186] The neuronal

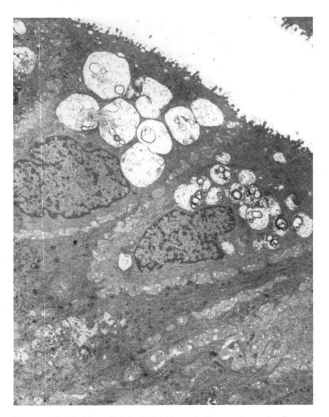

Figure 11.86 *Mucolipidosis IV. Vacuolation and myelin figures in conjunctival epithelial cells. (Electron micrograph.)*

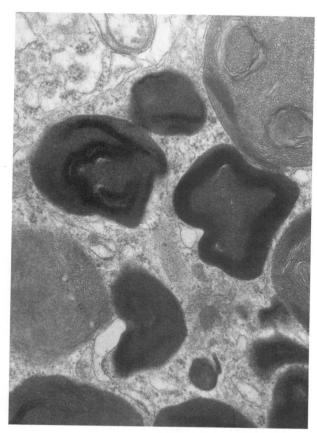

Figure 11.88 *Mucolipidosis IV. Neuronal inclusions consisting of densely packed concentrically arranged membranes or more complex crystalloid pattern. (Electron micrograph.)*

inclusions with additional features, such as a compound body with lamellar and granular components, a dense, strongly osmiophilic inclusion with tightly packed lamellar structures, bodies resembling MCBs and curvilinear bodies, have been reported in the brain biopsy study of a 24-month-old child with ML IV (Fig. 11.88).[688] A recent MRI study detected hypoplastic and dysgenic abnormalities in the corpus callosum and white matter, and cerebral and cerebellar atrophy, particularly in older patients.[189]

Animal models

No animal models of ML IV are known.

Disorders of lysosomal transporters

Two genetic disorders are known that are caused by a genetic defect in transporter proteins across the lysosomal membrane, free sialic acid storage disease and cystinosis.

FREE SIALIC ACID STORAGE DISORDER (SALLA AND INFANTILE SIALIC ACID STORAGE DISEASE)

A genetic defect in the sialic acid transporter results in increased lysosomal accumulation of free sialic acid. Two distinct phenotypes are associated with the disease, the adult type or Salla disease (SD)[28] and the infantile sialic acid storage disease (ISSD).[263,699]

History and clinical course

SD is known almost exclusively among the Finnish population. The eponym 'Salla' refers to the name of a small area in the north-eastern part of Finnish Lappland where the first patients were discovered and where the prevalence of the disease is very high.[28,550] The clinical signs of hypotonia and ocular nystagmus develop at around the age of 3–6 months, and subsequent developmental milestones are delayed. Ataxia, dysarthria and difficulty in walking become gradually apparent. SD patients are severely mentally retarded and IQ levels below 20 are not uncommon. Physical growth is also retarded but without any significant dysmorphic features. There is no hepatosplenomegaly. Their lifespan is not seriously affected. Unlike SD, the allelic infantile form of the disease (ISSD) occurs in many ethnic groups. Infants with ISSD show a more fulminant course with severe psychomotor retardation, dysmorphic features, hepatosplenomegaly, nephrotic syndrome and ascites, and usually die within the first year of life. Cardiomegaly may be present, but corneal opacity or dysostosis multiplex is not present.[391,423] Significant numbers of patients present as hydrops fetalis. Several intermediate types have also been reported.[773]

Biochemistry

The basic metabolic defect is an impairment of an active proton-driven and substrate-specific transport system of free sialic acid across the lysosomal membrane,[421,422,695] resulting in an accumulation of free sialic acid within the lysosome. Thus, tissues and cultured fibroblasts from SD and ISSD patients contain a large amount of free sialic acid.[263,551] Urinary excretion of free sialic acid is also increased. The diagnosis is made by detecting an increased amount of free sialic acid in urine and tissues. Detection of increased intracellular free sialic acid in amniotic fluid cells and chorionic villi has been used for prenatal diagnosis.[381]

Molecular genetics

SD and ISSD are autosomal recessive diseases. ISSD has been found to be allelic to SD.[586] The locus of SD has been assigned to the long arm of chromosome 6, 6q14-q15, by linkage analysis[246] and the gene has recently been cloned.[722] Five Finnish patients with SD were homoallelic for a mutation (R39C), and six different mutations were found in six ISSD patients of different ethnic origins.

Pathology

The cardinal pathology is cytoplasmic storage of colloidal iron- and Alcian blue-positive materials in various types of cells. On routine paraffin sections, the storage materials are dissolved during processing and thus the cytoplasm of the storage cells appears vacuolated.[773] The vacuoles are membrane bound and often contain reticulogranular and occasional laminated material at the ultrastructural level.[699] Notable vacuolated cells include lymphocytes, the proximal renal tubular epithelium, hepatocytes, Kupffer cells, macrophages, eccrine glandular and tubular epithelium, Schwann cells and endothelial cells.[28] In the brain, neurons and glial cells show similar cytoplasmic storage. White matter degeneration of varying degrees is present, with loss of axons and extensive gliosis. Axonal spheroids and microcalcification may be detected.[37,391] Defective patterns of myelination have been observed in a MRI study.[245,629] In two SD patients who died at the age of 41 years, loss of Purkinje cells and abnormal amounts of lipofuscin and neurofibrillary tangles were found in the neocortex, presubiculum, nucleus basalis of Meynert and locus coeruleus.[37]

Animal models

There are no known animal models of SD or ISSD.

CYSTINOSIS
History and clinical course

Cystinosis is a rare lysosomal disorder resulting from defective transport of an amino acid, cystine, across the lysosomal membrane. The transport protein is termed cystinosin. There are two basic phenotypes, nephropathic and non-nephropathic. The majority of the nephropathic form occurs in infancy, although some late-onset cases are known. The first documented case was a 21.5-month-old boy who died of inanition. He had curious white crystal depositions in the liver on post-mortem examination. Biochemical analysis of the visceral organs revealed an abnormal accumulation of cystine.[1] Affected individuals are normal at birth. Gradually, at around the age of 6–18 months, various clinical manifestations including failure to thrive, the renal Fanconi's syndrome characterized by polyuria and dehydration, glucosuria, hypokalaemia and hypophosphataemic rickets become apparent. Growth retardation is one of the most conspicuous clinical features,[203,204] and an average patient has a height around the third percentile at 1 year of age. By 10 years of age, affected children lose virtually all renal function and require dialysis or renal transplantation. Those who survive longer develop further damage including to the thyroid, eye, CNS, pancreas and muscle.[83,321,329,396,726] CT or MRI studies often reveal cerebral cortical atrophy. Impaired cognitive function has been reported in these patients.[182,471] Patients with the non-nephropathic or benign form of cystinosis have crystalline deposits in their bone marrow and leukocytes, but never develop renal disease and their life expectancy is normal. This group of cystinosis is usually discovered serendipitously when an ophthalmologic examination reveals crystalline opacity in the cornea and conjunctiva.

Biochemistry

In affected individuals, free cystine accumulates to between ten and 1000 times the normal level and forms crystals within lysosomes. The rate of cystine accumulation is variable among different tissues. Increased cystine levels in the brain have been noted only in those who survived the longest. Pure cystine crystals can be rectangular or hexagonal. Since the cystine accumulation is intracellular, plasma and urine cystine concentrations are usually not elevated, an important biochemical distinction from cystinuria, in which the urinary cystine level is abnormally high. Elevated cystine content in polymorphonuclear leukocytes and fibroblasts has been used as the diagnostic marker.[203] The underlying cause of the cystine accumulation is a genetic defect in transport of cystine across the lysosomal membrane.

Molecular genetics

Cystinosis displays autosomal recessive patterns of inheritance. The cystinosin gene (*CTNS*) has been cloned and many disease-causing mutations have been identified.[15,26,611,701]

Neuroimaging

Subcortical atrophy may also be seen. The basal ganglia and the periventricular white matter may show calcifications (see Pathology).

Pathology

The kidney is the most severely affected organ (Fig. 11.89). Pathologically, the cystinotic kidney shows different stages of destruction, with giant-cell transformation of the glomerular epithelium, hyperplasia and hypertrophy of the juxtaglomerular apparatus, and occasional dark cells and cytoplasmic inclusions. Ultrastructurally, cystine crystals as well-defined angular or rectagular electron-lucent spaces can be demonstrated (Fig. 11.90). Ultimately, the affected kidney shows the classical

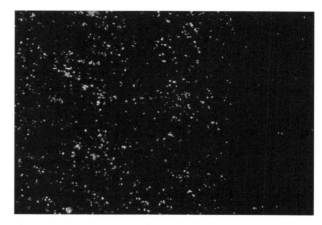

Figure 11.89 *Cystinosis. Reflectile cystine deposits in the kidney. (Dark-field microscopy.)*

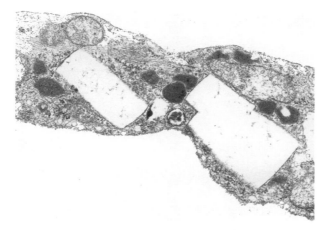

Figure 11.90 *Cystinosis. Rectangular or polygonal profile of cystine crystals in macrophages. (Electron micrograph.)*

pathology of an end-stage renal disease with scarring and fibrosis, chronic interstitial nephritis and tubular degeneration.[203,591,631] Degeneration of the retinal pigment epithelium and accumulation of cystine crystals in the retina, cornea and conjunctiva comprise the well-documented ophthalmic pathology of cystinosis. Cystine storage in the CNS is very limited in young patients. However, deposition of cystine crystals has been demonstrated in longer surviving patients.[321,396,726] Vogel *et al.* examined the brain of a 28-year-old male who received a kidney transplant 18 years before his death.[726] The patient had gait difficulty, intention tremor and progressive dementia. Diffuse ventriculomegaly with cerebral cortical atrophy was detected on CT and MRI. Calcification of the basal ganglia was also found on CT at the age of 20 years. On post-mortem examination cystine crystals were present in moderate quantities in various organs. However, no cystine crystals were seen in the donor kidney. The cerebral cortex was atrophic and the shrunken white matter contained 'yellowish white flecks of gritty material'. Cystic necrosis was present in the globus pallidus and cystine crystals were found in the frontal cortex and substantia nigra, mostly around capillaries when frozen section preparations were examined under polarized light. Numerous angular, needle-shaped and hexagonal crystalline spaces were identified in the cytoplasm of pericytes and possible oligodendrocytes at the ultrastructural level. Necrotic foci and calcium deposits were also described in a 19-year-old patient.[396] In that case cystine crystals were present only in the macrophages in the choroid plexus. Cystine crystals were reported in a brain biopsy sample of the arachnoid and cerebral cortex from a child, who developed non-absorptive hydrocephalus.[563]

Animal models

There are no naturally occurring or transgenically generated models of cystinosis.

Sialuria

This is a very rare disease caused by a defective feedback mechanism of the intracellular synthesis of sialic acid, resulting in overproduction of sialic acid.[187,751] The primary genetic defect has been identified as a mutation in the gene of UDP-*N*-acetylglucosamine-2-epimerase, a key step in sialic acid synthesis.[601] The pathogenetic mechanism is unusual in that the mutation occurs in such a way that it does not affect the catalytic activity of the enzyme but abolishes the ability of the gene to be normally regulated. The unregulated expression of the gene results in overproduction of sialic acid. The excessive sialic acid is stored in the cytoplasm rather than in the lysosome. Since neither the enzyme nor the abnormal accumulaton of the substrate is localized in the lysosome, it is not a lysosomal disorder as defined originally by Hers and later expanded. It is mentioned here because it causes occasional confusion with the free sialic acid storage disease owing to deficiency of the sialic acid transporter across the lysosomal membrane (see above). Clinically, excessive urinary excretion of sialic acid, variable developmental delay and hepatosplenomegaly are present.

Glycogen storage disease type II: acid α-glucosidase (acid maltase) deficiency (Pompe's disease)

History and clinical course

Acid α-glucosidase deficiency (Pompe's disease) was the disease first used by Hers to define the concept of the lysosomal disease based on the discovery of glycogen storage as a result of deficient lysosomal enzyme activity. Pompe's disease is the most severe form of glycogen storage disease. Two major clinical types are known. The first is a generalized, rapid, fatal disorder affecting young infants. The clinical presentations are massive cardiomegaly, macroglossia, hepatomegaly, progressive muscle weakness and hypotonia ('floppy baby'), with death before 1 year of age. In some infants, predominantly muscular symptoms without cardiomegaly have been noted. The second type is characterized by a slowly progressive proximal muscle weakness. The onset is usually in childhood, but some adult-onset cases have also been described. Intermediate types are also known.[287]

Biochemistry

Serum creatinine kinase is elevated in both types but the infantile onset type shows a much higher increase. Responses to adrenaline and glucagon are normal, indicating normal glucose metabolism. Glycogen content in the muscle is increased as much as ten-fold. In cultured fibroblasts and many other tissues, activity of acid α-glucosidase is virtually absent in infantile-onset type and markedly reduced in patients with the late-onset, slowly progressive type.

Molecular genetics

Pompe's disease is an autosomal recessive disorder, caused by mutations in the structural gene for acid α-glucosidase. The gene is localized on chromosome 17q23. In Western nations, it accounts for approximately 15 % of glycogen storage diseases.

Pathology

The most conspicuous pathology in infantile-onset patients is a massive accumulation of glycogen in the liver, heart and skeletal muscles (Fig. 11.91). Grossly, the entire heart is greatly enlarged with thickened ventricular walls as a result of the glycogen accumulation. The glycogen accumulation is predominantly intralysosomal, largely as β-particles, but it is also found in the cytoplasm. Glycogen accumulation is also present in neurons and glia (Fig. 11.92) in the CNS. The accumulation is most marked in the brainstem and spinal cord neurons. Accumulation is also detected in Schwann cells, neurons in the dorsal spinal ganglia and myenteric plexus.[205,223,428,429] In late-onset cases, skeletal muscle is usually the only tissue affected by increased glycogen. Aneurysms and vacuolar degeneration of cerebral arteries have been reported in late-onset acid maltase deficiency.[370]

Animal models

There are several naturally occurring animal models of Pompe's disease.[734] The Lapland dog model appears to be the most analogous to the infantile-onset disease in man.[735] More recently, mouse models of Pompe's disease have been generated in two laboratories by gene targeting.[62,539]

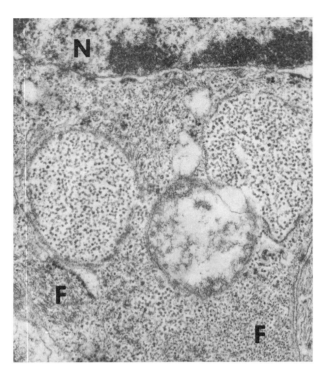

Figure 11.92 *Pompe's disease (infantile glycogenosis type II). Two vacuoles with glycogen accumulation are evident within this astrocyte (F = filaments; N = nucleus). (Electron micrograph.) (From Ref. 205 with permission.)*

Acid lipase deficiency (Wolman's disease, cholesteryl ester storage disease)

History and clinical course

Wolman's disease is an infantile disorder characterized by hepatosplenomegaly, abdominal distension, steatorrhoea, and other gastrointestinal signs and symptoms. The affected infants almost always die before reaching the age of 1 year. Specific symptoms related to the CNS are uncommon. However, affected infants may develop progressive mental deterioration. Radiological demonstration of calcified adrenal gland together with the above symptoms is almost pathognomonic.[4] The clinical phenotype of Wolman's disease is remarkably uniform. A milder form, known as cholesteryl ester storage disease (CESD), is also known. Clinical presentation of this milder form is relatively heterogeneous.[497] Patients have hepatosplenomegaly and widespread lipid deposits in many organs. Hyperlipoproteinaemia is common and patients develop premature atherosclerosis.

Biochemistry and molecular genetics

Cholesteryl esters and triglycerides accumulate in many organs including the liver, adrenal gland and spleen. The activity of a lysosomal acid hydrolase catalysing hydrolysis of cholesteryl esters and triglycerides (acid lipase) is

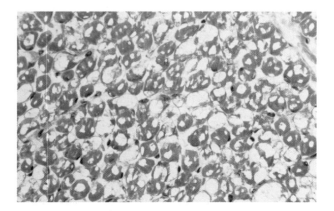

Figure 11.91 *Pompe's disease (infantile glycogenosis type II). Skeletal muscle showing marked vacuolation within the myofibres due to loss of accumulated glycogen during processing. (H&E.)*

severely deficient in all tissues including the liver, spleen, lymph nodes, aorta, peripheral blood leukocytes and cultured skin fibroblasts. Wolman's disease and CESD are allelic and inherited as autosomal recessive traits, involving the structural gene for acid lipase, located on chromosome 10q24-q29.[25]

Pathology

The pathological manifestations of Wolman's disease and CESD are quite similar. The liver, spleen and adrenals are always grossly enlarged with diffuse or focal yellow or orange discoloration. Lipid droplets are found in hepatic parenchymal cells, adrenal cortical cells, Kupffer cells and macrophages (Fig. 11.93). The adrenals often contain flecks of gritty calcified tissue (Fig. 11.94). Sudanophilic lipid droplets are prominent in the muscular layer as well as in the vascular endothelium on frozen sections. Pathological examination of the nervous system is very limited. Swollen neurons in the medulla and retina, foamy cells in the leptomeninges and choroid plexus, accumulation of sudanophilic materials in microglia and perivascular histiocytes, and diffuse fibrillary gliosis

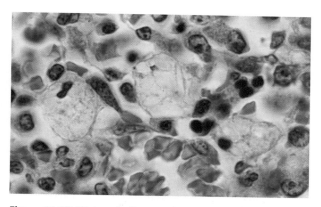

Figure 11.93 *Wolman's disease. Lipid-containing macrophages in bone-marrow smear. (Giemsa.) (Courtesy of Dr James Powers, University of Rochester, New York, USA.)*

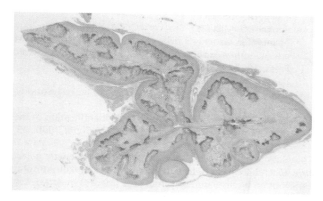

Figure 11.94 *Wolman's disease. Calcium deposition in the adrenal cortex. (H&E.) (Courtesy of Dr James Powers, University of Rochester, New York, USA.)*

have been described in some patients.[243] Storage of sudanophilic granules has also been reported in the ganglion cells of the myenteric plexus.[332] In an ultrastructural study, lipid droplets were reported in Schwann cells, oligodendrocytes, astrocytes and endothelial cell but not in the neurons of the CNS.[86]

Animal models

Naturally occurring autosomal recessive lysosomal acid lipase deficiency is known in Donryu rats. Similar to Wolman's disease in man, this model shows hepatosplenomegaly with many foamy lipid-containing macrophages. Biochemical analysis showed a massive accumulation of cholesteryl esters and triglycerides, and deficiency of acid lipase activity.[377,786] More recently, with targeted disruption of the mouse lysosomal acid lipase gene, a mouse model of acid lipase deficiency has been generated. This model is clinically similar to the milder form (CESD), but mimics Wolman disease biochemically and histopathologically.[155]

Acknowledgements

The authors wish to thank Dr Brian Lake for permission to use figures that have been published in the 6th edition (Figs 11.27, 11.39, 11.62, 11.65, 11.85). They are also grateful for the generosity of Drs Matti Haltia, Robert D. Terry, David Wolf, Rosemary Boustany, James Powers and Mauricio Castillo for allowing us to use their light and electron micrographs and neuroimages for illustrations in this chapter. Dr Robert Bagnell, Department of Pathology and Laboratory Medicine, provided invaluable technical help in the preparation of the photographic work. The secretarial assistance of Ms Carol Troutner is greatly appreciated.

REFERENCES

1 Abderhalden E. Familiare cystindiathese. *Z Physiol Chem* 1903; **38**: 557–61.

2 Abenoza P, Sibley RK. Farber's disease: a fine structural study. *Ultrastruct Pathol* 1987; **11**: 397–403.

3 Abraham K, Lampert P. Intraneuronal lipid deposits in metachromatic leukodystrophy. *Neurology* 1963; **13**: 686–92.

4 Abramov A, Schorr S, Wolman M. Generalized xanthomatosis with calcified adrenals. *J Dis Child* 1956; **91**: 282–6.

5 Adachi M, Wallace BJ, Schneck L, Volk BW. Fine structure of central nervous system in early infantile Gaucher's disease. *Arch Pathol* 1967; **83**: 513–26.

6 Aghion H. La maladie de Gaucher dans l'enfance (forme cardio-renale). Theses pour le doctorat en medecine. Paris: Persan-Beaumont, 1934.

7 Aleu FP, Terry RD, Zellwegar H. Electron microscopy of two cerebral biopsies in gargoylism. *J Neuropathol Exp Neurol* 1965; **24**: 304–17.

8 Alkhayat AH, Kraemer SA, Leipprandt JR *et al.* Human beta-mannosidase cDNA characterization and first identification of a mutation associated with human beta-mannosidosis. *Hum Mol Genet* 1998; **7**: 75–83.

9 Allegranza A, Tredici G, Marmiroli P *et al.* Sialidosis type I. Pathological study in an adult. *Clin Neuropathol* 1989; **8**: 266–71.

10 Alroy J, Orgad U, DeGaspert R *et al.* Canine GM1-gangliosidosis. *Am J Pathol* 1992; **140**: 675–89.

11 Amano N, Yokoi S, Akagi M *et al.* Neuropathological findings of an autopsy case of adult β-galactosidase and neuraminidase deficiency. *Acta Neuropathol (Berl)* 1983; **61**: 283–90.

12 Amir N, Zlotogora J, Bach G. Mucolipidosis type IV: clinical spectrum and natural history. *Pediatrics* 1987; **79**: 953–59.

13 Anderson W. A case of angiokeratoma. *Br J Dermatol* 1898; **10**: 113–17.

14 Andrews JM, Menkes JH. Ultrastructure of experimentally produced globoid cells in the rat. *Exp Neurol* 1970; **29**: 483–93.

15 Anikster Y, Shotelersuk V, Gahl WA. CTNS mutations in patients with cystinosis. *Hum Mutat* 1999; **14**: 454–58.

16 Anzil AP, Blinzinger K, Martinius J. Ultrastructure of storage materials in metachromatic leucodystrophy peripheral neuropathy and in rabbit tissue after sulfatide application with special reference to pleated lamellar systems. *J Microsc* 1973; **18**: 173–86.

17 Anzil AP, Blinzinger K, Mehraen P, Dozic S. Niemann–Pick disease type C: case report with ultrastructural findings. *Neuropediatrics* 1973; **4**: 207–25.

18 Arbisser AL, Donnelly KA, Scott CI Jr *et al.* Morquio-like syndrome with beta-galactosidase deficiency and normal hexosamine sulfatase activity: mucopolysaccharidosis IVB. *Am J Med Genet* 1977; **12**: 195–205.

19 Argov Z, Navon R. Clinical and genetic variations in the syndrome of adult GM2 gangliosidosis resulting from hexosaminidase A deficiency. *Ann Neurol* 1984; **16**: 14–20.

20 Aronson NN Jr. Asparagine-linked glycoproteins and their degradation. In: Mononen I, Aronson NN Jr eds. *Lysosomal storage disease: aspartylglycosaminuria.* Austin, TX: R.G. Landes/Heidelberg: Springer, 1997: 55–75.

21 Arsenio-Nunes ML, Goutieres F. Morphological diagnosis of Niemann–Pick disease type C by skin and conjunctival biopsies. *Acta Neuropathol Suppl* 1981; **7**: 204–7.

22 Arstila AU, Palo J, Haltia M *et al.* Aspartylglucosaminuria. I. Fine structural studies of liver, kidney and brain. *Acta Neuropathol* 1972; **20**: 207–16.

23 Arvio M, Autio S, Mononen T. Clinical manifestations of aspartylglycosaminuria. In: Mononen I, Aronson NN Jr eds. *Lysosomal storage disease: aspartylglycosaminuria.* Austin, TX: R.G. Landes/Heidelberg: Springer, 1997: 19–31.

24 Ashkenazi A, Zaizov R, Matoth Y. Effect of splenectomy on destructive bone changes in children with chronic (type 1) Gaucher disease. *Eur J Pediatr* 1986; **145**: 138–41.

25 Assmann G, Seedorf U. Acid lipase deficiency: Wolman disease and cholesteryl ester storage disease. In: Scriver CR, Beaudet AL, Sly WS, Valle D. eds. *The metabolic and molecular basis of inherited disease.* New York: McGraw Hill, 1995: 2563–87.

26 Attard M, Jean G, Forestier L *et al.* Severity of phenotype in cystinosis varies with mutations in the CTNS gene: predicted effect on the model of cystinosin. *Hum Mol Genet* 1999; **8**: 2507–14.

27 Auer IA, Schmidt ML, Lee VM *et al.* Paired helical filament tau (PHFtau) in Niemann–Pick type C disease is similar to PHFtau in Alzheimer's disease. *Acta Neuropathol* 1995; **90**: 547–51.

28 Aula P, Autio S, Ravio KO *et al.* 'Salla disease'; a new lysosomal storage disorder. *Arch Neurol* 1979; **36**: 88–94.

29 Austin J. Metachromatic sulfatides in cerebral white matter and kidney. *Pro Soc Exp Biol Med* 1959; **100**: 361–70.

30 Austin J, Armstrong D, Fouch H *et al.* Metachromatic leukodystrophy: VII MLD in adults: diagnosis and pathogenesis. *Arch Neurol* 1968; **18**: 225–40.

31 Austin J, Lehfeldt D, Maxwell W. Experimental 'globoid bodies' in white matter and chemical analysis in Krabbe's disease. *J Neuropathol Exp Neurol* 1961; **20**: 284–5.

32 Austin JH. Studies in globoid (Krabbe) leukodystrophy. II. Controlled thin-layer chromatographic studies of globoid body fractions in seven patients. *J Neurochem* 1963; **10**: 921–30.

33 Austin JH. Studies in metachromatic leukodystrophy XII multiple sulfatase deficiency. *Arch Neurol* 1973; **28**: 258–64.

34 Austin JH, Balasubramanian AS, Pattabiraman TN *et al.* A controlled study of enzymatic activities in three human disorders of glycolipid metabolism. *J Neurochem* 1963; **10**: 805–16.

35 Austin JH, Lehfeldt D. Studies in globoid (Krabbe) leucodystrophy. III Significance of experimentally produced globoid-like elements in rat white matter and spleen. *J Neuropathol Exp Neurol* 1965; **24**: 265–89.

36 Autio S, Norden NE, Ockerman P *et al.* Mannosidosis: Clinical, fine-structural and biochemical findings in three cases. *Acta Paediatr* 1973; **62**: 555–65.

37 Autio-Harmainen H, Oldfors A, Sourander P *et al.* Neuropathology of Salla disease. *Acta Neuropathol (Berl)* 1988; **75**: 481–90.

38 Bach G, Cohen MM, Kohn G. Abnormal ganglioside accumulation in cultured fibroblasts from patients with mucolipidosis IV. *Biochem Biophys Res Commun* 1975; **66**: 1483–90.

39 Bach G, Eisenberg F Jr, Cantz M, Neufeld EF. The defect in the Hunter syndrome: deficiency of sulfoiduronate sulfatase. *Proc Nat Acad Sci USA* 1973; **70**: 2134–8.

40 Bach G, Friedman R, Weissmann B, Neufeld EF. The defect in the Hurler and Scheie syndromes: deficiency of α-L-iduronidase. *Proc Nat Acad Sci USA* 1972; **69**: 2048–51.

41 Bach G, Zeigler M, Kohn G *et al.* Mucopolysaccharide accumulation in cultured skin fibroblasts derived from patients with mucopolysaccharidosis IV. *Am J Hum Genet* 1977; **29**: 610–18.

42 Baker E, Guo XH, Orsborn AM *et al.* The Morquio A syndrome (mucopolysaccharidosis IVA) gene maps to 16q24.3. *Am J Hum Genet* 1993; **52**: 96–8.

43 Balicki D, Beutler E. Gaucher disease. *Medicine (Baltimore)* 1995; **74**: 305–23.

44 Banker BQ, Miller JQ, Crocker AC. The cerebral pathology of infantile Gaucher's disease. In: Aronson SM, Volk BM eds. *Cerebral sphingolipidoses.* New York: Academic Press, 1962: 73–99.

45 Bardosi A, Friede R, Ropte S, Goebel HH. A morphometric study on sural nerves in metachromatic leukodystrophy. *Brain* 1987; **110**: 683–94.

45a Bargal R, Avidan N, Ben-Asher E *et al.* Identification of the gene causing mucolipidosis type iV. *Nat Genet* 2000; **23**: 514–16.

46 Baskin GB, Ratterree M, Davison BB *et al.* Genetic galactocerebrosidase deficiency (globoid cell leukodystrophy, Krabbe disease) in rhesus monkeys (*Macaca mulatta*). *Lab Anim Sci* 1998; **48**: 476–82.

47 Baumann N, Masson M, Carreau V *et al.* Adult forms of metachromatic leukodystrophy: Clinical and biochemical approach. *Dev Neurosci* 1991; **13**: 211–15.

48 Beck M, Bendrer SW, Retter H-L et al. Neuraminidase deficiency presenting as non-immune hydrops fetalis. Eur J Pediatr 1984; 143: 135–9.

49 Becker H, Aubock L, Haidvogl M, Bernheimer H. Disseminierte Lipogranulomatose (Farber)-Kasuistischer Bericht des 16. Falles einer Ceramidose. Verh Dtsch Ges Pathol 1976; 60: 254–8.

50 Bennett M.J, Hofmann SL. The neuronal ceroid-lipofuscinoses (Batten disease): a new class of lysosomal storage disease. J Inherit Metab Dis 1999; 22: 535–44.

51 Benninger C, Ullrich-Butt B, Zhan S-S, Schmitt HP. GM2 gangliosidosis B1 variant in a boy of German/Hungarian descent. Clin Neuropathol 1993; 12: 196–200.

52 Berg T, Riise HM, Hansen GM et al. Spectrum of mutations in alpha-mannosidosis. Am J Hum Genet 1999; 64: 77–88.

53 Berger J, Loschl B, Bernheimer H et al. Occurrence, distribution, and phenotype of arylsulfatase A mutations in patients with metachromatic leukodystrophy. Am J Med Genet 1997; 69: 335–40.

54 Berkovic S, Carpenter S, Andermann F et al. Kufs' disease: a critical reappraisal. Brain 1988; 111: 27–62.

55 Berman ER, Kohn G, Yatziv S, Stein H. Acid hydrolase deficiencies and abnormal glycoproteins in mucolipidosis III. Clin Chim Acta 1974; 52: 115–24.

56 Berman ER, Livni N, Shapira E et al. Congenital corneal clouding with abnormal systemic storage bodies: a new variant of mucolipidosis. J Pediatr 1974; 84: 519–26.

57 Bernardini GL, Herrera DG, Carson D et al. Adult-onset Krabbe's disease in siblings with novel mutations in the galactocerebrosidase gene. Ann Neurol 1997; 41: 111–14.

58 Bernheimer H, Karbe E. Morphologische und neurochemische Untersuchungen von zwei Formen der amaurotischen Idiotie des Hundes. Nachweis einer GM2-gangliosidose. Acta Neuropathol 1970; 16: 243–61.

59 Beutler E, Grabowski GA. Gaucher Disease. In: Scriver CR, Beaudet AL, Sly WS, Valle D eds. The metabolic and molecular basis of inherited disease. New York: McGraw-Hill, 1995: 2641–70.

60 Bhaumik M, Muller VJ, Rozaklis T et al. A mouse model for mucopolysaccharidosis type III A (Sanfilippo syndrome). Glycobiology 1999; 9: 1389–96.

61 Bieber FR, Mortimer G, Kolodny E et al. Pathologic findings in fetal GM1 gangliosidosis. Arch Neurol 1986; 43: 736–8.

62 Bijvoet AG, van de Kamp EH, Kroos M et al. Generalized glycogen storage and cardiomegaly in a knockout mouse model of Pompe disease. Hum Mol Genet 1998; 7: 53–62.

63 Birkenmeier EH, Barker JE, Vogler CA et al. Increased life span and correction of metabolic defects in murine mucopolysaccharidosis type VII after syngeneic bone marrow transplantation. Blood 1991; 78: 3081–92.

64 Birkenmeier EH, Davisson MT, Beamer WG et al. Murine mucopolysaccharidosis type VII. Characterization of a mouse with β-glucuronidase deficiency. J Clin Invest 1989; 83: 1258–66.

65 Bischoff A, Ulrich J. Peripheral neuropathy in globoid cell leukodystrophy (Krabbe's disease): ultrastructural and histochemical findings. Brain 1969; 92: 861–70.

66 Bishop DF, Grabowski GA, Desnick RJ. Fabry disease: an asymptomatic hemizygote with significant residual α-galactosidase A activity. Am J Hum Genet 1981; 33: 71A.

67 Boehme DH, Cottrell IC, Leonberg SC, Zeman W. A dominant form of neuronal ceroid lipofuscinosis. Brain 1971; 94: 745–60.

68 Bolhuis PA, Oonk JGW, Kamp PE et al. Ganglioside storage, hexosaminidase lability, and urinary oligosaccharides in adult Sandhof's disease. Neurology 1987; 37: 75–81.

69 Bonduelle M, Lissens W, Goossens A et al. Lysosomal storage disease presenting as transient or persistent hydrops fetalis. Genet Counsel 1991; 2: 227–32.

70 Bonten E, Van der Spoel A, Fornerod M et al. Characterization of human lysosomal neuraminidase defines the molecular basis of the metabolic storage disorder sialidosis. Genes Dev 1996; 10: 3156–69.

71 Bosch EP, Hart MN. Late adult-onset metachromatic leukodystrophy: Dementia and polyneuropathy in a 63-year-old man. Arch Neurol 1978; 35: 475–7.

72 Bosshard NU, Hubler M, Arnold S et al. Spontaneous mucolipidosis in a cat: an animal model of human I-cell disease. Vet Pathol 1996; 33: 1–13.

73 Boustany RM. Batten disease or neuronal ceroid lipofuscinosis. In: Moser HW ed. Handbook of Clinical Neurology Vol. 22 (66): Neurodystrophies and neurolipidoses. Amsterdam: Elsevier Science, 1996: 671–700.

74 Boustany RM, Kaye E, Alroy J. Ultrastructural findings in skin from patients with Niemann–Pick disease type C. Pediatr Neurol 1990; 6: 177–83.

75 Braak H, Braak E. Pathoarchitectonic pattern of iso- and allocortical lesions in juvenile and adult neuronal ceroid-lipofuscinosis. J Inherit Metab Dis 1993; 16: 259–62.

76 Braak H, Braak E, Goebel HH. Isocortical pathology in type C Niemann–Pick disease. A combined Golgi–pigmentoarchitectonic study. J Neuropathol Exp Neurol 1983; 42: 871–87.

77 Bradova V, Smid F, Ulrich-Bott B et al. Prosaposin deficiency: further characterization of the sphingolipid activator protein-deficient sibs. Multiple glycolipid elevations (including lactosylceramidosis), partial enzyme deficiencies and ultrastructure of the skin in this generalized sphingolipid storage disease. Hum Genet 1993; 92: 143–52.

78 Brady RO. Inherited metabolic diseases and pathogenesis of mental retardation. Ann Biol Clin (Paris) 1978; 36: 113–19.

79 Brady RO. Gaucher disease. In: Moser HW ed. Handbook of clinical neurology Vol. 22 (66). Neurodystrophies and Neurolipidoses. Amsterdam: Elsevier, 1996: 123–32.

80 Brady RO, Gal AE, Bradley RM et al. Enzyme defect in Fabry's disease: ceramide trihexosidase deficiency. N Engl J Med 1967; 276: 1163–7.

81 Brady RO, Kanfer JN, Mock MB, Fredrickson DS. The metabolism of sphingomyelin. II. Evidence of an enzymatic deficiency in Niemann–Pick disease. Proc Nat Acad Sci USA 1966; 55: 366–9.

82 Brady RO, Kanfer JN, Shapiro D. Metabolism of glucocerebrosides. II. Evidence of an enzymatic deficiency in Gaucher's disease. Biochem Biophys Res Commun 1965; 18: 221–5.

83 Broyer M, Tete MJ, Guest G et al. Clinical polymorphism of cystinosis encephalopathy. Results of treatment with cysteamine. J Inherit Metab Dis 1996; 19: 65–75.

84 Bugiani O, Borrone C. Fucosidosis: a neuropathological study. Riv Patol Nerv Ment 1976; 97: 133–41.

85 Bundza A, Lowden JA, Charlton KM. Niemann–Pick disease in a poodle dog. Vet Pathol 1979; 16: 530–8.

86 Byrd JC, Powers JM. Wolman's disease: ultrastructural evidence of lipid accumulation in central and peripheral nervous system. Acta Neuropathol (Berl) 1979; 45: 37–42.

87 Cain H, Egner E, Kresse H. Mucopolysaccharidosis IIIA (Sanfilippo disease type A). Histochemical, electron microscopical and biochemical findings. Beitr Pathol 1977; 160: 58–72.

88 Callahan JW. Molecular basis of GM1 gangliosidosis and Morquio disease, type B. Structure–function studies of lysosomal β-galactosidase and the non-lysosomal β-galactosidase-like protein. Biochim Biophys Acta 1999; 1455: 89–103.

89 Canfield WM. Molecular characterization of the mannose 6-phosphate lysosomal enzyme targeting pathway (abstract). *Glycoconj J* 1999; **16**: S41.

90 Carstea ED, Morris JA, Coleman KG *et al*. Niemann–Pick C1 disease gene homology to mediators of cholesterol homeostasis. *Science* 1997; **277**: 228–31.

91 Carstea ED, Polymeropoulos MH, Parker CC *et al*. Linkage of Niemann–Pick disease type C to human chromosome 18. *Proc Nat Acad Sci USA* 1993; **90**: 2002–4.

92 Cashman NR, Antel JP, Hancock LW *et al*. *N*-Acetyl-β-hexosaminidase β locus defect and juvenile motor neuron disease: a case study. *Ann Neurol* 1986; **19**: 568–72.

93 Ceuterick-de Groote C, Martin J-J. Extracerebral biopsy in lysosomal and peroxisomal disorders. Ultrastructural findings, *Brain Pathol* 1998; **8**: 121–32.

94 Chabas A, Coll MJ, Aparicio M, Rodoriguez Diaz E. Mild phenotypic expression of α-*N*-acetylgalactosaminidase deficiency in two adult siblings. *J Inherit Metab Dis* 1994; **17**: 724–31.

95 Chen CS, Bach G, Pagano RE. Abnormal transport along the lysosomal pathway in mucolipidosis type IV disease. *Proc Nat Acad Sci USA* 1998; **95**: 6373–8.

96 Chen YQ, Rafi G, Degala G, Wenger DA. Cloning and expression of DNA encoding human galactocerebrosidase, the enzyme deficient in globoid cell leukodystrophy. *Hum Mol Genet* 1993; **2**: 1841–5.

97 Chitayat D, Meunier CM, Hadgkinson KA *et al*. Mucolipidosis IV: clinical manifestations and natural history. *Am J Med Genet* 1991; **41**: 313–18.

98 Choi KG, Sung JH, Clark HB, Krivit W. Pathology of adult-onset globoid cell leukodystrophy (GLD) (Abstract). *J Neuropathol Exp Neurol* 1991; **50**: 336.

99 Christomanou H, Aignesberger A, Linke RP. Immunochemical characterization of two activator proteins stimulating enzymatic sphingomyelin degradation *in vitro*. Absence of one of them in a human Gaucher disease variant. *Biol Chem Hoppe Seyler* 1986; **367**: 879–90.

100 Christomanou H, Chabas A, Pampols T, Guardiola A. Activator protein deficient Gaucher's disease. A second patient with the newly identified lipid storage disorder. *Klinische Wochenschrift* 1989; **67**: 999–1003.

101 Clark LA, Russel CS, Pownall S *et al*. Murine mucopolysaccharidosis type I: targeted disruption of the murine α-L-iduronidase gene. *Hum Mol Genet* 1997; **6**: 503–11.

102 Clarke JTR, Knaack J, Crawhall JC, Wolf LS. Ceramide trihexosidosis (Fabry's disease) without skin lesions. *N Engl J Med* 1971; **284**: 233–5.

103 Cleary MA, Wraith JE. Management of mucopolysaccharidosis type III (Review). *Arch Dis Child* 1993; **69**: 403–6.

104 Cogan DG, Kuwabara T, Moser H, Hazard GW. Retinopathy in a case of Farber's lipogranulomatosis. *Arch Ophthalmol* 1966; **75**: 752–7.

105 Cohen-Tannoudji M, Marchand P, Akli S *et al*. Disruption of murine HEXA gene leads to enzymatic deficiency and to neuronal lysosomal storage, similar to that observed in Tay–Sachs disease. *Mamm Genome* 1995; **6**: 844–9.

106 Collier J, Greenfield JG. The encephalitis periaxialis of Schilder: a clinical and pathological study with an account of two cases, one of which was diagnosed during life. *Brain* 1924; **47**: 489–519.

107 Colucci WS, Lorell BH, Schoen FJ *et al*. Hypertrophic obstructive cardiomyopathy due to Fabry's disease. *N Engl J Med* 1982; **307**: 926–8.

108 Conradi N, Kyllerman M, Mansson J-E *et al*. Late-infantile Gaucher disease in a child with myoclonus and bulbar signs: neuropathological and neurochemical findings. *Acta Neuropathol* 1991; **82**: 152–7.

109 Conradi NG, Kalimo H, Sourander P. Reaction of vessel walls and brain parenchyma to the accumulation of Gaucher cells in the Norrbottnian type (type III) of Gaucher disease. *Acta Neuropathol (Berlin)* 1988; **75**: 385–90.

110 Conradi NG, Sourander P, Nilsson O *et al*. Neuropathology of the Norbottnian type of Gaucher disease: morphological and biochemical studies. *Acta Neuropathol (Berlin)* 1984; **55**: 99–109.

111 Conzelmann E, Sandhoff K. Deficiency of a factor necessary for stimulation of hexosaminidase A catalyzed degradation of ganglioside GM2 and glycolipid GA2. *Proc Nat Acad Sci USA* 1978; **75**: 3979–83.

112 Cooper AC, Hatton M, Thornley M, Sardharwalla LB. Human β-mannosidase deficiency: biochemical findings in plasma, fibroblasts, white cells, and urine. *J Inherit Metab Dis* 1988; **11**: 17–29.

113 Cork LC, Munnell JF, Lorenz MD. The pathology of feline GM2 gangliosidosis. *Am J Pathol* 1979; **90**: 723–34.

114 Cork LC, Munnell JF, Lorenz MD *et al*. GM2 ganglioside lysosomal storage disease in cats with β-hexosaminidase deficiency. *Science* 1977; **196**: 1014–17.

115 Couce ME, Parisi JE, Schochet SS. Adult onset Niemann–Pick disease type C – Report of two cases. (abstract) *J Neuropathol Exp Neurol* 1997; **56**: 622.

116 Cragg H, Williamson M, Young E *et al*. Fucosidosis: genetic and biochemical analysis of eight cases. *J Med Genet* 1997; **34**: 105–10.

117 Craig JM, Clark JT, Banker BQ. Metabolic neurovisceral disorder with accumulation of unidentified substance: variant of Hurler's syndrome? (abstract) *J Dis Child* 1959; **98**: 577.

118 Crandall BF, Philippart M, Brown WJ *et al*. Mucolipidosis IV. *Am J Med Genet* 1982; **12**: 301–8.

119 Crocker AC. The cerebral defect in Tay–Sachs disease and Niemann–Pick disease. *J Neurochem* 1961; **7**: 68–80.

120 Crocker AC, Cohen J, Farber S. The 'lipogranulomatosis' syndrome; review, with report of patient showing milder involvement. In: Aronson SM, Volk BW. eds. *Inborn disorders of sphingolipid metabolism*. Oxford: Pergamon Press, 1967: 485–503.

121 Crocker AC, Farber S. Niemann–Pick disease: a review of eighteen patients. *Medicine* 1958; **37**: 1–98.

122 Crome I, Hanefeld F, Patrick D, Wilson J. Late onset globoid cell leukodystrophy. *Brain* 1973; **96**: 841–8.

123 Crutchfield KE, Patronas NJ, Dambrosia JM *et al*. Quantitative analysis of cerebral vasculopathy in patients with Fabry disease. *Neurology* 1998; **50**: 1746–9.

124 Cruz-Sanchez EF, Martos JA, Rives A *et al*. Adult type of leukodystrophy. Krabbe disease? *Clin Neurol Neurosurg* 1991; **93**: 217–22.

125 Cummings JF, Wood PA, Walkley SU *et al*. GM2 gangliosidosis in a Japanese spaniel. *Acta Neuropathol* 1985; **67**: 247–53.

126 D'Agostino AN, Sayer GP, Hayles AB. Krabbe disease. Globoid cell type of leukodystrophy. *Arch Neurol* 1963; **8**: 82–96.

127 Dahms BB, Davis RL, Neustein HB, Landing BH. Fucosidosis. Light, histochemical and ultrastructural findings. *Lab Invest* 1979; **40**: 302–3.

128 Das AK, Becerra CH, Yi W *et al*. Molecular genetics of palmitoyl-protein thioesterase deficiency in the US. *J Clin Invest* 1998; **102**: 361–70.

129 Dawson G. The oligosaccharidoses: mannosidosis, fucosidosis and aspartylglucosaminuria. In: Moser HW ed. *Handbook of clinical neurology* Vol. 22 (66): *Neurodystrophies and neurolipidoses*. Amsterdam: Elsevier, 1996: 329–38.

130 Dawson G, Matalon R, Stein AO. Lactosylceramidosis: lactosylceramide galactosylhydrolase deficiency and accumulation of lactosylceramide in cultured skin fibroblasts. *J Pediatr* 1971; **79**: 423–9.

131 d'Azzo A, Andrea G, Strisciuglio P, Galjaard H. Galactosialidosis. In: Scriver CR, Beaudet AL, Sly WS, Valle D eds. *The metabolic basis of inherited diseases*, 7th edn. New York: McGraw-Hill, 1995: 2825–38.

132 de Baecque CM, Suzuki K, Rapin I *et al.* GM2-gangliosidosis AB variant: clinicopathological study of a case. *Acta Neuropathol* 1975; **33**: 207–26.

133 de Duve C, Pressman BC, Gianetto R *et al.* Tissue fractionation studies. VI. Intracellular distribution patterns of enzymes in rat-liver tissue. *Biochem J* 1955; **60**: 604–17.

134 De Gasperi R, Gama Sosa MA, Sartorato EL *et al.* Molecular heterogeneity of late-onset forms of globoid-cell leukodystrophy. *Am J Hum Genet* 1996; **59**: 1233–42.

135 DeGeest L, Mann J, DeSousa-Hitzler C *et al.* Lysosomal neuraminidase deficiency in mice: a model for sialidosis (abstract). *Am J Hum Genet* 1999; **65** (Suppl): A26.

136 De Jong J, Van Den Berg C, Wijburg H *et al.* Alpha-*N*-acetyl-galactosaminidase deficiency with mild clinical manifestations and difficult biochemical diagnosis. *J Pediatr* 1994; **125**: 385–91.

137 Dekaban AS, Constantopoulos G. Mucopolysaccharidosis type I, II, IIIA and V. Pathological and biochemical abnormalities in the neural and mesenchymal elements of the brain. *Acta Neuropathol (Berl)* 1977; **39**: 1–7.

138 Dekaban AS, Constantopoulos G, Herman MM, Steusing JK. Mucopolysaccharidosis type V (Scheie syndrome). *Arch Pathol* 1976; **100**: 237–45.

139 Del Monte MA, Maumenee IH, Green WR, Kenyon KR. Histopathology of Sanfilippo's syndrome. *Arch Ophthalmol* 1983; **101**: 1255–62.

140 Derry DM, Fawcett JS, Andermann F, Wolfe LS. Late infantile systemic lipidosis. Major monosialo-gangliosidosis. Delineation of two types. *Neurology* 1968; **18**: 340–8.

141 Desnick RJ, Bleiden LD, Sharp HL, Moller JH. Cardiac valvular anomalies in Fabry's disease: clinical morphologic and biochemical studies. *Circulation* 1976; **54**: 818–25.

142 Desnick RJ, Wang AM. Schindler disease: an inherited neuroaxonal dystrophy due to alpha-*N*-acetylgalactosaminidase deficiency. *J Inherit Metab Dis* 1990; **13**: 549–62.

143 Desnick RJ, Wang AM. α-*N*-acetylgalactosaminidase deficiency: Schindler disease. In: Scriber CR, Beaudet AL, Sly WS and Valle D eds. *The metabolic and molecular basis of inherited disease*. New York: McGraw-Hill, 1995: 2509–28.

144 de Veber GA, Schwarting GA, Kolodny EH, Kowall NW. Fabry disease: immunochemical characterization of neuronal involvement. *Ann Neurol* 1992; **31**: 409–15.

145 De Vries BBA, Kleijer WJ, Keulemans JLM *et al.* First-trimester diagnosis of infantile neuronal ceroid lipofuscinosis (INCL) using PPT enzyme assay and *CLN1* mutation analysis. *Prenat Diagn* 1999; **19**: 559–62.

146 D'Hooge R, Hartmann D, Manil J *et al.* Neuromotor alterations and cerebellar deficits in aged arylsulfatase A-deficient transgenic mice. *Neurosci Lett* 1999; **273**: 93–6.

147 Dickersin GR, Lott IT, Kolodny EH, Dvorak AM. A light and electron microscopic study of mannosidosis. *Hum Pathol* 1980; **11**: 246–56.

148 Di Natale P, Annella T, Daniele A *et al.* Animal models for lysosomal storage diseases: a new case of feline mucopolysaccharidosis VI. *J Inherit Metab Dis* 1992; **15**: 17–24.

149 Dittmer F, Hafner A, Ulbrich EJ *et al.* I-cell disease-like phenotype in mice deficient in mannose 6-phosphate receptors. *Transgenic Res* 1998; **7**: 473–83.

150 Dom R. Brucher JM, Ceuterrick H *et al.* Adult ceroid lipofuscinosis (Kufs disease) in two brothers: retinal and visceral storage in one; diagnostic muscle biopsy in the other. *Acta Neuropathol* 1979; **45**: 67–72.

151 Donnelly WJC, Sheahan BJ. GM1-gangliosiodosis type II. *Am J Pathol* 1975; **81**: 255–8.

152 Dos Santos MR, Tanaka A, Sa Miranda MC *et al.* GM2-Gangliosidosis B1 variant: analysis of β-hexosaminidase α gene mutations in 11 patients from a defined region in Portugal. *Am J Hum Genet* 1991; **49**: 886–90.

153 Dowspon JH, Wilton-Cox H, Oldfors A, Sourander P. Autofluorescence emission spectra of neuronal lipopigment in mucopolysaccharidosis (Sanfilippo's syndrome). *Acta Neuropathol (Berl)* 1989; **77**: 426–9.

154 Dreborg S, Erikson A, Hagberg B. Gaucher disease – Norrbottnian type. *Eur J Pediatr* 1980; **133**: 107–18.

155 Du H, Duanmu M, Witte D, Grabowski GA. Targeted disruption of the mouse lysosomal acid lipase gene: long-term survival with massive cholesteryl ester and triglyceride storage. *Hum Mol Genet* 1998; **7**: 1347–54.

156 Dubois G, Mussini JM, Auclair M *et al.* Adult sphingomyelinase deficiency: report of 2 patients who initially presented with psychiatric disorders. *Neurology* 1990; **40**: 132–6.

157 Dumontel C, Girod C, Dijoud F *et al.* Fetal Niemann–Pick disease type C: ultrastructural and lipid findings in liver and spleen. *Virchows Arch A Pathol Anat* 1993; **422**: 253–9.

158 Dunn HG, Dolman CL, Farrell DF *et al.* Krabbe leukodystrophy without globoid cells. *Neurology* 1976; **26**: 1035–41.

159 Durand P, Borrone C, Della Cella G. A new mucopolysaccharide lipid-storage disease? *Lancet* 1966; **ii**: 1313–14.

160 Durand P, Borrone C, Della Cella G. Fucosidosis. *J Pediatr* 1969; **75**: 665–74.

161 Durand P, Gatti R, Cavalieri S *et al.* Sialidosis (mucolipidosis I). *Helv Paediatr Acta* 1977; **32**: 391–400.

162 Dustin P, Tondeur M, Jonniaux G *et al.* La maladie de Farber. Etude anatomo-clinique et ultrastructurale. *Bull Acad R Med Belg* 1973; **128**: 733–62.

163 Dyken P, Wisniewski K. Classification of the neuronal ceroid-lipofuscinosis: expansion of the atypical forms. *Am J Med Genet* 1995; **57**: 150–4.

164 Elfenbein IB. Distonic juvenile idiocy without amaurosis, A new syndrome. Light and electron microscopic observation of cerebrum. *Johns Hopkins Med J* 1968; **123**: 205–21.

165 Elleder M, Bradova V, Smid F *et al.* Cardiocyte storage and hypertrophy as a sole manifestation of Fabry's disease. *Virchows Arch A Pathol Anat Histopathol* 1990; **417**: 449–55.

166 Elleder M, Christomanou H, Kustermann-Kuhn B, Harzer K. Leptomeningeal lipid storage patterns in Fabry disease. *Acta Neuropathol (Berl)* 1994; **88**: 579–82.

167 Elleder M, Cihula J. Niemann–Pick disease (variation in the sphingomyelinase deficient group). Neurovisceral phenotype (A) with an abnormally protracted clinical course and variable expression of neurological symptomatology in three siblings. *Eur J Pediatr* 1983; **140**: 323–8.

168 Elleder M, Jirasek A, Smid F *et al.* Niemann–Pick disease type C. Study on the nature of the cerebral storage process. *Acta Neuropathol* 1985; **66**: 325–36.

169 Elleder M, Jirasek A, Vlk J. Adult neurovisceral lipidosis compatible with Niemann–Pick disease type C. *Virchows Arch A Pathol* 1983; **401**: 35–43.

170 Elleder M, Nevoral J, Spicakova V et al. A new variant of sphingomyelinase deficiency (Niemann–Pick): visceromegaly, minimal neurological lesions and low in vivo degradation rate of sphingomyelin. J Inherit Metab Dis 1986; 9: 357–66.

171 Elleder M, Sokola J, Hebiek M. Follow-up study of subunit c of mitochndrial ATP synthase (SCMAS) in Batten disease and in unrelated lysosomal disorders. Acta Neuropathol (Berl) 1997; 93: 379–90.

172 Elleder M, Tyynela J. Incidence of neuronal perikaryal spheroids in neuronal ceroid lipofuscinoses (Batten disease). Clin Neuropathol 1998; 17: 184–9.

173 Emery JM, Green WR, Wyllie RG, Howell RR. GM1-gangliosidosis. Ocular and pathological manifestations. Arch Ophthalmol 1971; 85: 177–87.

174 Erikson A. Gaucher disease. Norrbottnian type (III). Neuropediatric and neurobiological aspects of clinical patterns and treatment. Acta Paediatr Scand Suppl 1986; 326: 1–42.

175 Eto Y, Meier C, Herschkowitz NN. Chemical compositions of brain and myelin in two patients with multiple sulfatase deficiency (a variant form of metachromatic leukodystrophy). J Neurochem 1976; 27: 1071–6.

176 Ezaki J, Tanida I, Kanehagi N, Kominami E. A lysosomal proteinase, the late infantile neuronal ceroid lipofuscinosis gene (CLN2) product, is essential for degradation of a hydrophobic protein, the subunit c of ATP synthase. J Neurochem 1999; 72: 2573–82.

177 Fabry J. Ein Beitrag zur Kenntnis der Purpura haemorrhagica nodularis (Purpura papulosa hemorrhagica Hebrae). Arch Dermatol Forsch Syphilol 1898; 43: 187–200.

178 Farber S. A lipid metabolic disorder disseminated lipogranulomatosis. A syndrome with similarity to, and important difference from Niemann–Pick and Hand–Schuller Christian disease (abstract). Am J Dis Child 1952; 84: 499–500.

179 Farber S, Cohen J, Uzman LL. Lipogranulomatosis. A new lipo-glyco-protein 'storage' disease. J Mt Sinai Hosp 1957; 24: 816–37.

180 Feigin I. Diffuse cerebral sclerosis (metachromatic leukoencephalopathy). Am J Pathol 1954; 30: 715–37.

181 Ferrer I, Cusi V, Pineda M et al. Focal dendritic swelling in Purkinje cells in mucopolysaccharidoses types I, II and III. A Golgi and ultrastructural study. Neuropathol Appl Neurobiol 1988; 14: 315–23.

182 Fink JK, Brouwers P, Barton N et al. Neurologic complications in long-standing nephropathic cystinosis. Arch Neurol 1989; 46: 543–8.

183 Fink JK, Filling-Katz MR, Sokol J et al. Clinical spectrum of Niemann–Pick disease type C. Neurology 1989; 39: 1040–9.

184 Finlayson LA. Hunter syndrome (mucopolysaccharidosis II). Pediatr Dermatol 1990; 7: 150–2.

185 Fischer A. Carmichael KP, Munnell JF et al. Sulfamidase deficiency in a family of Dachshundsanine model of mucopolysaccharidosis IIIA (Sanfilippo A). Pediatr Res 1998; 44: 74–82.

186 Folkerth RD, Alroy J, Lomakina I et al. Mucolipidosis IV: morphology and histochemistry of an autopsy case. J Neuropathol Exp Neurol 1995; 54: 154–64.

187 Fontaine G, Biserte G, Montreuil J et al. La sialurie: un trouble metabolique original. Helv Paediatr Acta 1968; 23 (Suppl 17): 1–32.

188 Fox J, Li Y-T, Dawson G et al. Naturally occurring GM2 gangliosidosis in two muntjak deer with pathological and biochemical features of human classical Tay–Sachs disease (type B GM2 gangliosidosis). Acta Neuropathol 1999; 97: 57–62.

189 Frei KP, Patronas NJ, Crutchfield KE et al. Mucolipidosis type IV: characteristic MRI findings. Neurology 1998; 51: 565–9.

190 Freitag F, Kuchemann K, Blumcke S. Hepatic ultrastructure in fucosidosis. Virchows Arch Abtilung B Zellpathol 1971; 7: 99–113.

191 Fressinaud C, Vallat JM, Mason M et al. Adult-onset metachromatic leukodystrophy presenting as isolated peripheral neuropathy. Neurology 1992; 42: 1396–8.

192 Friedmann I, Spellacy E, Crow J, Watts RW. Histopathological studies of the temporal bones in Hurler's disease [mucopolysaccharidosis (MPS) IH]. J Laryngol Otol 1985; 99: 29–41.

193 Friend SC, Barr SC, Embury D. Fucosidosis in an English springer spaniel presenting as a malabsorption syndrome. Aust Vet J 1985; 62: 415–20.

194 Fronda CL, Zeng GC, Gao LY, Yu RK. Molecular cloning and expression of mouse brain sialidase. Biochem Biophy Res Commun 1999; 258: 727–31.

195 Fu L, Inui K, Nishigaki T et al. Molecular heterogeneity of Krabbe disease. J Inherit Metab Dis 1999; 22: 155–62.

196 Fujita N, Suzuki K, Vanier MT et al. Targeted disruption of the mouse sphingolipid activator protein gene: a complex phenotype, including severe leukodystrophy and widespread storage of multiple sphingolipids. Hum Mol Genet 1996; 5: 711–23.

197 Fukuda S, Tomatsu S, Sukegawa K et al. Molecular analysis of mucopolysaccharidosis type VII. J Inherit Metab Dis 1991; 14: 800–4.

198 Fukuhara N, Suzuki M, Fujita N, Tubaki T. Fabry's disease: on mechanism of the peripheral nerve involvement. Acta Neuropathol (Berl) 1975; 33: 9–21.

199 Furuya H, Kukita Y, Nagano S et al. Adult onset globoid cell leukodystrophy (Krabbe disease): analysis of galactosylceramidase cDNA from four Japanese patients. Hum Genet 1997; 199: 450–6.

200 Fusch C, Huenges R, Moser HW et al. A case of combined Farber and Sandhoff disease. Eur J Pediatr 1989; 148: 558–62.

201 Fyfe JC, Kurzhals RL, Lassaline ME et al. Molecular basis of feline β-glucuronidase deficiency: an animal model of mucopolysaccharidosis VII. Genomics 1999; 58: 121–8.

202 Gahl WA, Krasnewich DM, Williams JC. Sialidoses. In: Moser HW ed. Handbook of clinical neurology Vol. 22 (66). Neurodystrophies and neurolipidoses. Amsterdam: Elsevier, 1996: 353–75.

203 Gahl WA, Reed GF, Thoene JG et al. Cysteamine therapy for children with nephropathic cystinosis. N Engl J Med 1987; 316: 971–7.

204 Gahl WA, Schneider JA, Aula PP. Lysosomal transport disorders: cystinosis and sialic acid storage disorders. In: Scriver CR, Beaud AL, Sly WS, Valle D eds. The metabolic and molecular basis of inherited disease. New York: McGraw-Hill, 1995: 3763–97.

205 Gambetti P, DiMauro S, Baker L. Nervous system in Pompe's disease: ultrastructure and biochemistry. J Neuropathol Exp Neurol 1971; 30: 412–30.

206 Garcia CP, McGarry PA, Duncan CM. Fucosidosis and Alexander's leukodystrophy (abstract). J Neuropathol Exp Neurol 1980; 39: 353.

207 Gaucher P. 1882. De l'epithelioma primitif de la rate. These de Paris.

208 Gelot A, Aurage CA, Rodriguez D et al. In vivo diagnosis of Kuf's disease by extracerebral biopsies. Acta Neuropathol 1998; 96: 102–8.

209 Ghatak NR, Fleming F, Hinman A. Neuropathology of Sanfilippo syndrome. Ann Neurol 1976; 2: 161–6.

210 Gieselmann V, Matzner U, Hess B et al. Metachromatic leukodystrophy: molecular genetics and an animal model. J Inherit Metab Dis 1998; 21: 564–74.

211 Gieselmann V, Polten A, Kreysing J et al. Molecular genetics of metachromatic leukodystrophy. Dev Neurosci 1991; 13: 222–7.

212 Gilbert EF, Callahan J, Viseskul C, Opitz JM. Niemann–Pick disease type C. Pathological, histochemical ultrastructural and biochemical studies. Eur J Pediatr 1981; 136: 263–74.

213 Gilbert EF, Dawson G, Zu Rhein G et al. I-Cell disease. Mucolipidosis II: pathological, histochemical, ultrastructural and biochemical observations in four cases. Z Kinder 1973; 114: 259–92.

214 Gilbert EF, Varakis J, Opitz JM et al. Generalized gangliosidosis type II (juvenile GM1 gangliosidosis). Z Kinderher 1975; 120: 151–80.

215 Gilles FH, Deuel RK. Neuronal cytoplasmic globules in the brain in Morquio's syndrome. Arch Neurol 1971; 25: 393–403.

216 Gitzelmann R, Bosshard NU, Superti-Furga A et al. Feline mucopolysaccharidosis VII due to β-glucuronidase deficiency. Vet Pathol 1994; 31: 435–43.

217 Goebel HH. Neurodegenerative diseases: biopsy diagnosis in children. In: Galcia JH ed. Neuropathology; the diagnostic approach. St Louis, MO: Mosby, 1997: 581–635.

218 Goebel HH, Argyrakis A, Shimokawa K et al. Adult metachromatic leukodystrophy IV ultrastructural studies on the central and peripheral nervous system. Eur Neurol 1980; 19: 294–307.

219 Goebel HH, Braak H. Review article: adult neuronal ceroid-lipofuscinosis. Clin Neuropathol 1989; 8: 109–19.

220 Goebel HH, Busch H. Abnormal lipopigments and lysosomal residual bodies in metachromatic leukodystrophy. Adv Exp Med Biol 1989; 266: 299–309.

221 Goebel HH. Gerhard L, Kominami E, Haltia M. Neuronal ceroid-lipofuscinosis – late infantile or Jansky–Bielschowsky type – revisited. Brain Pathol 1996; 6: 225–8.

222 Goebel HH, Kohlschutter A, Lenard HG. Morphologic and chemical biopsy findings in mucolipidosis IV. Clin Neuropathol 1982; 1: 73–82.

223 Goebel HH, Lenard HG, Kohlschutter, A, Pilz H. The ultrastructure of the sural nerve in Pompe's disease. Ann Neurol 1977; 2: 111–15.

224 Goebel HH, Mole SE, Lake BD eds. The neuronal ceroid lipofuscinoses (Batten disease). Amsterdam: IOS Press, 1999.

225 Goebel HH, Stolte G, Kustermann-Kuhn B, Harzer K. B1 variant of GM2 gangliosidosis in a 12-year-old patient. Pediatr Res 1989; 25: 89–93.

226 Goldblatt J, Sacks S, Beibhton P. The orthopedic aspects of Gaucher disease. Clin Orthopaed 1978; 137: 208–14.

227 Goldman JE, Katz D, Rapin I et al. Chronic GM1 gangliosidosis presenting as dystonia: I Clinical and pathological features. Ann Neurol 1981; 9: 465–75.

228 Goldman JE, Yamanaka T, Rapin I et al. The AB variant of GM2-gangliosidosis. Acta Neuropathol 1980; 52: 189–202.

229 Gonatas K, Gonatas J. Ultrastructural and biochemical observations on a case of systemic late infantile lipidosis and its relationship to Tay–Sachs disease and gargoylism. J Neuropathol Exp Neurol 1965; 24: 318–40.

230 Gonatas NK, Terry RD, Winkler R et al. A case of juvenile lipidosis: The significance of electron microscopic and biochemical observations of a cerebral biopsy. J Neuropathol Exp Neurol 1963; 22: 557–80.

231 Gonzalez-Gomez I, Mononen I, Heisterkamp N et al. Progressive neurodegeneration in aspartylglucosaminuria mice. Am J Pathol 1998; 155: 1293–300.

232 Goodman LA, Livingstone PO, Walkley SU. Proliferation of ectopic dendrites on cortical pyramidal neurons is associated with accumulation of GM2 ganglioside in nonganglioside storage disease. Proc Nat Acad Sci USA 1991; 88: 11330–4.

233 Gordon N. The insidious presentation of juvenile form of metachromatic leukodystrophy. Postgrad Med J 1978; 54: 335–7.

234 Grafe M, Thomas C, Schneider J et al. Infantile Gaucher's disease. A case with neuronal storage. Ann Neurol 1988; 23: 300–3.

235 Gravel RA, Clarke JTR, Kaback D et al. The GM2 gangliosidosis. In: Scriver CR, Beaudet AL, Sly WS, Valle D. eds. The metabolic and molecular basis of inherited disease, 7th edn. New York: McGraw-Hill, 1995: 2639–79.

236 Gravel RA, Clarke JTR, Kaback D et al. The GM2 gangliosidosis. In: Scriver CR, Beaudet AL, Valle D, Sly WS eds. The metabolic and molecular basis of inherited disease, 8th edn. New York: McGraw-Hill, 2001; 3827–76.

237 Gravel RA, Lowden JA, Callahan JW et al. Infantile sialidosis: a phenocopy of type 1 GM1 gangliosidosis distinguished by genetic complementation and urinary oligosaccharides. Am J Hum Genet 1979; 31: 669–79.

238 Greene NDE, Bernard DL, Taschner PEM et al. A murine model for juvenile NCL: gene targeting of mouse Cln3. Mol Genet Metab 1999; 66: 309–13.

239 Greenfield JG. A form of progressive cerebral sclerosis in infants associated with primary degeneration of interfascicular glia. J Neurol Psychopathol 1932–33; 13: 289–302.

240 Gregoire A. Ultrastructure des inclusions metachromatiques dans un cas de leucodystrophie. J Microsc 1964; 3: 343–6.

241 Gregoire A, Perier O, Dustin P. Metachromatic leukodystrophy. An electron microscopic study. J Neuropathol Exp Neurol 1966; 25: 617–36.

242 Guazzi GC, D'Amore I, Van Hoof F et al. Type 3 (chronic) GM1 gangliosidosis presenting as infanto-choreoathetotic dementia, without epilepsy in three sisters. Neurology 1988; 38: 1124–7.

243 Guazzi GC, Martin JJ, Philippart M et al. Wolman's disease. Eur Neurol 1968; 1: 334–62.

244 Guerra WF, Verity MA, Fluharty AL et al. Multiple sulfatase deficiency: clinical, neuropathological, ultrastructural and biochemical studies. J Neuropathol Exp Neurol 1990; 49: 406–23.

245 Haataja L, Parkkola R, Sonninen P et al. Phenotypic variation and magnetic resonance imaging (MRI) in Salla disease, a free sialic acid storage disorder. Neuropediatrics 1994; 25: 238–44.

246 Haataja L, Schleutker J, Laine A-P et al. The genetic locus for free sialic acid storage disease maps to the long arm of chromosome 6. Am J Hum Genet 1994; 54: 1042–9.

247 Hadfield MG, Ghatak NR, Nakoneczna I et al. Pathologic findings in mucopolysaccharidosis type IIIB (Sanfilippo's syndrome B). Arch Neurol 1980; 37: 645–50.

248 Hadfield MG, Mamunes P, David RB. The pathology of Sandhoff's disease. J Pathol 1977; 23: 137–44.

249 Hadley RN, Hagstrom WC. Cardiac lesions in a patient with familial neurovisceral lipidosis (generalized gangliosidosis). Mol Pathol 1971; 55: 237–40.

250 Hagberg B, Sourander P, Svennerholm L. Sulphatide lipidosis in childhood. Am J Dis Child 1962; 104: 644–56.

251 Hagberg B, Sourander P, Svennerholm L. Late infantile progressive encephalopathy with disturbed polyunsaturated fat metabolism. Acta Paediatr 1968; 57: 495–9.

252 Hahn AE, Gilbert JJ, Kwarciak C et al. Nerve biopsy findings in Niemann–Pick type II (NPC). Acta Neuropathol 1994; 87: 149–54.

253 Hahn AF, Gordon BA, Feleki V et al. A variant form of metachromatic leukodystrophy without arylsulfatase deficiency. Ann Neurol 1982; 12: 33–6.

254 Hahn AF, Gordon BA, Gilbert JJ, Hinton GG. The AB-variant of metachromatic leukodystrophy (postulated activator protein deficiency). Light and electron microscopic findings in sural nerve biopsy. Acta Neuropathol (Berl) 1981; 55: 281–7.

255 Hahn CN, del Pilar Martin M, Schroder M et al. Generalized CNS disease and massive GM1 ganglioside accumulation in mice defective in lysosomal acid β-galactosidase. Hum Mol Genet 1997; 6: 205–11.

256 Hall NA, Lake BD, Patrick AD. Recent biochemical and genetic advances in our understanding of Batten disease (ceroid lipofuscinosis). Dev Neurosci 1991; 13: 339–44.

257 Haltia M. Infantile neuronal ceroid-lipofuscinosis: neuropathological aspects. In: Armstrong D, Koppang N, Rider JA eds. Ceroid-lipofuscinosis (Batten's disease). Amsterdam: Elsevier Biomedical Press, 1982: 105–15.

258 Haltia M, Palo J, Autio S. Aspartylglucosaminuria: a generalized storage disease. Acta Neuropathol 1975; 31: 243–55.

259 Haltia M, Rapola J, Santavuori P. Infantile type of so-called neuronal ceroid-lipofuscinosis. Histological and electron microscopical studies. Acta Neuropathol (Berl) 1973; 26: 157–70.

260 Haltia M, Rapola J, Santavuori P, Kernen A. Infantile type of so-called neuronal ceroid-lipofuscinosis. Part 2. Morphological and biochemical studies. J Neurol Sci 1973; 18: 269–85.

261 Haltia M, Tyynela J, Baumann M et al. Immunological studies on sphingolipid activator proteins in the neuronal ceroid lipofuscinosis. Gerontology 1995; 41 (Suppl 2): 239–48.

262 Hammersen G, Oppermann HC, Harms K et al. Oculoneural involvement in an enzymatically proven case of Niemann–Pick disease type B. Eur J Pediatr 1979; 132: 77–84.

263 Hancock LW, Thaler MM, Horwitthz AL, Dawson G. Generalized N-acetylneuraminic acid storage disease: Quantitation and identification of the monosaccharide accumulating in brain and other tissues. J Neurochem 1982; 38: 803–9.

264 Hannun YA, Bell RM. Lysosphingolipids inhibit protein kinase C. Implications for sphingolipidoses. Science 1987; 235: 670–4.

265 Hannun YA, Bell RM. Functions of sphingolipid breakdown products in cellular regulation. Science 1989; 243: 500–7.

266 Hardie RJ, Young EP, Morgan-Hughes JA. Hexosaminidase A deficiency presenting as juvenile progressive dystonia. J Neurol Neurosurg Psychiatry 1988; 51: 446–59.

267 Hartley WJ, Farrow RRH. In: Capen CC, Jones TC, Hackel DB, Migaki G eds. Handbook: animal models of human disease. Fasc II Model No. 241: Registry of Comparative Pathology. Washington, DC: Armed Forces Institute of Pathology, 1982.

268 Harzer K, Paton BC, Poulos A et al. Sphingolipid activator protein (SAP) deficiency in a 16 week-old atypical Gaucher disease patient and his fetal siblings: biochemical signs of combined sphingolipidoses. Eur J Pediatr 1989; 149: 31–9.

269 Hasilik A, Neufeld EF. Biosynthesis of lysosomal enzymes in fibroblasts. J Biol Chem 1980; 255: 4937–45.

270 Haskins M. Bone marrow transplantation therapy for metabolic disease: Animal models as predictors of success and in utero approaches. Bone Marrow Transplant 1996; 18: S25–7.

271 Haskins ME, Aguirre GD, Jezyk PF, Patterson DF. The pathology of the feline model of mucopolysaccharidosis VI. Am J Pathol 1980; 101: 657–74.

272 Haskins ME, Desnick RJ, DiFerrante N et al. β-Glucuronidase deficiency in a dog. A model of human mucopolysaccharidosis VII. Pediatr Res 1984; 18: 980–4.

273 Haust MD, Gordon BA. Ultrastructural and biochemical aspects of the Sanfilippo syndrome, type III genetic mucopolysaccharidosis. Connect Tissue Res 1986; 15: 57–64.

274 Haust MD, Gordon BA, Hong R et al. Clinicopathological conference: an adolescent girl with severe mental impairment and mucopolysacchariduria. Am J Med Genet 1985; 22: 1–27.

275 Healy PJ, Farrow BRH, Nicholas FW et al. Canine fucosidosis: a biochemical and genetic investigation. Vet Sci 1984; 36: 354–9.

276 Hedley-Whyte ET, Boustany RM, Riskind P et al. Peripheral neuropathy due to galactosylceramide-β galactosidase deficiency (Krabbe's disease) in a 73 year old woman. Neuropathol Appl Neurobiol 1988; 14: 515–16.

277 Hedley-Whyte ET, Gilles FH, Uzman BG. Infantile neuroaxonal dystrophy: a disease characterized by altered terminal axons and synaptic endings. Neurology 1968; 18: 891–906.

278 Hellsten E, Vesa J, Olkkonen VM et al. Human palmitoyl-protein thioesterase: evidence for lysosomal targeting of the enzyme and disturbed cellular processing in infantile neuronal ceroid-lipofuscinosis. EMBO J 1996; 15: 5340–5.

279 Hers HG. α-Glucosidase deficiency in generalized glycogen-storage disease (Pompe's disease). Biochem J 1963; 86: 11–16.

280 Hers HG. Inborn lysosomal diseases. Gastroenterology 1965; 48: 625–33.

281 Hess B, Saftig P, Hartmann D et al. Phenotype of arylsulfatase A-deficient mice: relationship to human metachromatic leukodystrophy. Proc Nat Acad Sci USA 1996; 93: 14821–6.

281a Herva R, Tyynela J, Hirvasnieml A, Syrjäkallio-Ylitalo M, Hartia M. Northern Epilepsy: A novel form of neuronal ceriod-lipofuscinosis. Brain Pathology 2000; 10: 215–22.

282 Higashi Y, Murayama S, Pentchev PG, Suzuki K. Cerebellar degeneration in the Niemann–Pick type C mouse. Acta Neuropathol 1993; 85: 175–84.

283 Higashi Y, Murayama S, Pentchev PG, Suzuki K. Peripheral nerve pathology in Niemann–Pick type C mouse. Acta Neuropathol 1995; 90: 158–63.

284 Higashi Y, Pentchev PG, Murayama S, Suzuki K. Pathology of Niemann–Pick type C: studies of murine mutant. In: Ikuta F ed. Neuropathology in brain research. Amsterdam: Elsevier, 1991: 85–102.

285 Hillborg PO. Morbus Gaucher in Norrbotten. Nord Med 1959; 61: 303–13.

286 Hirato J, Nakazato Y, Sasaki A et al. Krabbe's disease with giant lamellar bodies in Purkinje cells. Acta Neuropathol 1994; 88: 78–94.

287 Hirschhorn R. Glycogen storage disease type II: acid α-glucosidase (acid maltase) deficiency. In: Scriver CR, Beaudet AL, Sly WS, Valle D eds. The metabolic and molecular basis of inherited diseases. New York: McGraw-Hill, 1995: 2443–64.

288 Hofmann I, Kohlschutter A, Santavuori P et al. CLN3; juvenile NCL. In: Goebel HH, Mole SE, Lake BD eds. The neuronal ceroid lipofuscinoses (Batten disease). Amsterdam: IOS Press, 1999: 55–76.

289 Horinouchi K, Erlich S, Perl DP et al. Acid sphingomyelinase deficient mice: a model of types A and B Niemann–Pick disease. Nat Genet 1995; 10: 288–93.

290 Horoupian DS, Yang SS. Paired helical filaments in neurovisceral lipidosis (juvenile dystonic lipidosis). Ann Neurol 1978; 4: 404–11.

291 Hozumi I, Nishizawa M, Ariga T et al. Accumulation of gly-cosphingolipids in spinal and sympathetic ganglia of a symptomatic heterozygote of Fabry's disease. J Neurol Sci 1989; 90: 271–80.

292 Huang JQ, Trasler JM, Igdoura S et al. Apoptotic cell death in mouse models of GM2 gangliosidosis and observations on human Tay–Sachs and Sandhoff diseases. Hum Mol Genet 1997; 6: 1879–85.

293 Hubler M, Haskins ME, Arnold S et al. Mucolipidosis type II in a domestic shorthair cat. J Small Anim Pract 1996; 37: 435–41.

294 Hulette CM, Earl NL, Anthony DC, Crain BJ. Adult onset Nie-mann–Pick disease type C presenting with dementia and absent organomegaly. Clin Neuropathol 1992; 11: 293–7.

295 Hund E, Grau A, Fogel W et al. Progressive cerebellar atax-ia, proximal neurogenic weakness and ocular motor dis-turbances: hexosaminidase A deficiency with late clinical onset in four siblings. J Neurol Sci 1997; 145: 25–31.

296 Hunter C. A rare disease in two brothers: evaluation of scapula, limitation of movement of joints and other abnor-malities. Proc R Soc Med 1917; 10: 104–16.

297 Hurler G. Ueber einen Typ multipler Abartungen, vor-wiegend am Skelettsystewm. Z Kinder 1919; 24: 220–34.

298 Ida H, Rennert OM, Kato S et al. Severe skeletal complica-tions in Japanese patients with type 1 Gaucher disease. J Inherit Metab Dis 1999; 22: 63–73.

299 Igdoura SA, Gafuik C, Mertineit C et al. Cloning of the cDNA and gene encoding mouse lysosomal sialidase and cor-rection of sialidase deficiency in human sialidosis and mouse SM/J fibroblasts. Hum Mol Genet 1998; 7: 115–20.

300 Ikeda S, Kondo K, Oguchi K et al. Adult fucosidosis: histo-chemical and ultrastructural studies of rectal mucosa biop-sy. Neurology 1984; 34: 451–6.

301 Ikonen E, Aula P, Gron K et al. Spectrum of mutations in aspartylglucosaminuria. Proc Nat Acad Sci USA 1991; 88: 11222–6.

302 Inzelberg R, Korczyn AD. Parkinsonism in adult-onset GM2 gangliosidosis (Letter). Mov Disord 1994; 9: 375–7.

303 Irani D, Kim HS, El-Hibri H et al. Postmortem observations on β-glucuronidase deficiency presenting as hydrops fetalis. Ann Neurol 1983; 14: 486–90.

304 Isbrandt D, Arlt G, Brooks DA et al. Mucopolysaccharido-sis VI (Maroteaux–Lamy syndrome): six unique arylsulfatase B gene alleles causing variable disease phenotypes. Am J Hum Genet 1994; 54: 454–63.

305 Ishii S, Kase R, Sakuraba H et al. α-Galactosidase transgenic mouse: heterogeneous gene expression and post-transla-tional glycosylation in tissues. Glycoconj J 1998; 15: 591–4.

306 Isoniemi A, Hietala M, Aula P et al. Identification of a novel mutation causing aspartylglucosaminuria reveals a muta-tion hotspot region in the aspartylglucosaminuria gene. Hum Mutat 1995; 5: 318–26.

307 Jaeken J, Proesmans W, Eggermont E et al. Niemann–Pick type C disease and early cholestasis in three brothers. Acta Paediatr (Belg) 1980; 33: 43–6.

308 Jalanko A, Manninen T, Peltonen L. Deletion of the C-ter-minal end of aspartylglucosaminidase resulting in a lysoso-mal accumulation disease: evidence for a unique genomic rearrangement. Hum Mol Genet 1995; 4: 435–41.

309 Jalanko A, Tenhunen K, McKinney CE et al. Mice with an aspartylglucosaminuria mutation similar to humans repli-cate the pathophysiology in patients. Hum Mol Genet 1998; 7: 265–72.

310 Jatzkewitz H. Zwei Typen von Cerebrosid-schwelfel-saureestern als Sog. 'Pralipoide' und Speichersubstanzen bei der Leukodystrophie, Typ Scholz (metachromatische Form der diffusen Sklerose). Z Physiol Chem 1958; 311: 279–82.

311 Jatzkewitz H, Mehl E. Cerebroside-sulphatase and arylsul-fatase A deficiency in metachromatic leukodystrophy (ML). J Neurochem 1969; 16: 19–28.

312 Jatzkewitz H, Sandhoff K. On a biochemically special form of infantile amaurotic idiocy. Biochim Biophys Acta 1963; 70: 354–6.

313 Jellinger K, Anzil AP, Seemann D, Bernheimer H. Adult GM2 gangliosidosis masquerading as slowly progressive mus-cular atrophy: motor neuron disease phenotype. Clin Neu-ropathol 1982; 1: 31–44.

314 Jellinger K, Paulus W, Grisold W, Paschke E. New pheno-type of adult alpha-L-iduronidase deficiency (muco-polysaccharidosis I) masquerading as Friedreich's ataxia with cardiopathy. Clin Neuropathol 1990; 9: 163–9.

315 Johnson WG. Motor neuron diseases resulting from hexosaminidase deficiency. Semin Neurol 1993; 13: 369–74.

316 Johnson WG, Wigger HJ, Karp HR et al. Juvenile spinal mus-cular atrophy: a new hexosaminidase deficiency phenotype. Ann Neurol 1982; 11: 11–16.

317 Jolly RD. The pathology of the central nervous system in pseudolipidosis of angus calves. J Pathol 1971; 103: 113–21.

318 Jolly RD, Thompson KG. The pathology of bovine man-nosidosis. Vet Pathol 1978, 15: 141–52.

319 Jolly RD, Thompson KG, Murphy CE et al. Enzyme replace-ment therapy – an experiment of nature in a chimeric man-nosidosis calf. Pediatr Res 1976; 10: 219–24.

320 Jolly RD, Winchester B, Gehler J et al. Mannosidosis. A com-parative review of biochemical and related clinicopatho-logical aspects of three forms of the disease. J Appl Biochem 1981; 3: 273–91.

321 Jonas AJ, Conley SB, Marshall R et al. Nephropathic cysti-nosis with central nervous system involvement. Am J Med 1987; 83: 966–70.

322 Jones MZ, Alroy J, Boyer PJ et al. Caprine mucopolysac-charidosis – IIID: clinical, biochemical, morphological and immunohistochemical characteristics. J Neuropathol Exp Neurol 1998; 57: 148–57.

323 Jones MZ, Alroy J, Ruledge JC et al. Human mucopolysac-charidosis III D; clinical, biochemical, morphological and immunohistochemical characteristics. J Neuropathol Exp Neurol 1997; 56: 1158–67.

324 Jones MZ, Cunningham JG, Dade AW. Caprine β-mannosi-dosis: Clinical and pathological features. J Neuropathol Exp Neurol 1983; 42: 268–85.

325 Junaid MA, Brooks SS, Wisniewski KE, Pullarkat RK. A novel assay for lysosomal pepstatin-insensitive proteinase and its application for the diagnosis of late-infantile neuronal ceroid lipofuscinosis. Clin Chim Acta 1999; 281: 169–76.

326 Kaartinen V, Mononen I, Gonzales-Gomez I et al. Pheno-typic characterization of mice with targeted disruption of glycosylasparaginase gene: a mouse model for aspartyl-glycosaminuria. J Inherit Metab Dis 1998; 21: 207–9.

327 Kaartinen V, Mononen I, Voncken JW et al. A mouse model for the human lysosomal disease aspartylglycosaminuria. Nat Med 1996; 2: 1375–8.

328 Kaback M, Lim-Steele J, Dabholkar D et al. Tay–Sachs dis-ease-carrier screening, prenatal diagnosis, and the molec-ular era: an international perspective. JAMA 1993; 270: 2307–15.

329 Kaiser-Kupfer MI, Caruso RC, Minkler DS, Gahl WA. Long-term ocular manifestations in nephropathic cystinosis. Arch Opthamol 1986; 104: 706–11.

330 Kamiya M, Tada T, Kuhara H et al. I-Cell disease. A case report and review of the literature. Acta Pathol Jpn 1986; 36: 1679–92.

331 Kamoshita S, Aaron AM, Suzuki K, Suzuki K. Infantile Niemann–Pick disease: a chemical study with isolation and characterization of membranous cytoplasmic bodies and myelin. *Am J Dis Child* 1969; **117**: 379–94.

332 Kamoshita S, Landing BH. Distribution of lesions in myenteric plexus and gastrointestinal mucosa in lipidoses and other neurological disorders of children. *Am J Clin Pathol* 1968; **49**: 312–18.

333 Kanzaki T, Wang AM, Desnick RJ. Lysosomal α-N-acetylgalactosaminidase deficiency, the enzymatic defect in angiokeratoma corporis diffusum with glycopeptiduria. *J Clin Invest* 1991; **88**: 707–11.

334 Kanzaki T, Yokota M, Mizuno N et al. Novel lysosomal glycoaminoacid storage disease with angiokeratoma corporis diffusum. *Lancet* 1989; **i**: 875–7.

335 Kappler J, Von Figura K, Gieselmann V. Late-onset metachromatic leukodystrophy: molecular pathology in two siblings. *Ann Neurol* 1992; **31**: 256–61.

336 Kappler J, Watts RWE, Conzelmann E et al. Low arylsulfatase A activity and choreoathetotic syndrome in three sibblings: differentiation of pseudodeficiency from metachromatic leukodystrophy. *Eur J Pediatr* 1991; **150**: 287–90.

337 Katz ML, Shibuya H, Lin P-C et al. A mouse gene knockout model for juvenile ceroid-lipofuscinosis (Batten disease). *J Neurosci Res* 1999; **57**: 551–6.

338 Kaye EM, Ullman MD, Wilson ER, Barranger JA. Type 2 and type 3 Gaucher disease: a morphological and biochemical study. *Ann Neurol* 1986; **20**: 223–30.

339 Keller C, Briner J, Schneider J et al. Mukopolysaccharidose Typ VI-A (Morbus Maroteaux–Lamy): Korrelation der klinischen und pathologisch-anatomischen Befunde bei einem 27 jahringen Patienten. *Helv Paediatr Acta* 1987; **42**: 317–33.

340 Kelly TE, Bartoshesky L, Harris D et al. Mucolipidosis I (acid neuraminidase deficiency). *Am J Dis Child* 1981; **135**: 703–8.

341 Kelly TE, Graetz G. Isolated acid neuraminidase deficiency: a distinct lysosomal storage disease. *Am J Med Genet* 1977; **1**: 31–46.

342 Kelly TE, Thomas GH, Taylor HA et al. Mucolipidosis III (pseudo-Hurler polydystrophy); clinical and laboratory studies in a series of 12 patients. *Johns Hopkins Med J* 1975; **137**: 156–75.

343 Kelly WR, Clague AE, Barns RJ et al. Canine alpha-L-fucosidosis: a storage disease of springer spaniels. *Acta Neuropathol (Berl)* 1983; **60**: 9–13.

344 Kepes JJ, Berry A III, Zacharias DL. Multiple sulfatase deficiency: bridge between neuronal storage diseases and leukodystrophies. *Pathology* 1988; **20**: 285–91.

345 Keulemann JIM, Reuser AJJ, Kroos MA et al. Human α-N-acetylgalactosaminidase (α-NAGA) deficiency: new mutation and the paradox between genotype and phenotype. *J Med Genet* 1996; **33**: 458–64.

346 Kint JA, Dacremont G, Carton D et al. Mucopolysaccharidoses: secondary induced abnormal distribution of lysosomal isoenzymes. *Science* 1973; **181**: 352–54.

347 Kistler JP, Lott IT, Kolodny EH et al. Mannosidosis: new clinical presentation, enzyme studies, and carbohydrate analysis. *Arch Neurol* 1977; **34**: 45–51.

348 Kitagawa H, Toki J, Morimoto T et al. An autopsy case of I-cell disease. Ultrastructural and biochemical analyses. *Am J Clin Pathol* 1991; **96**: 262–6.

349 Kjellman B, Gamstrop I, Brun A et al. Mannosidosis: a clinical and histopathologic study. *J Pediatr* 1969; **75**: 366–73.

350 Kleijer WJ, Hoogeveen A, Verheuen FW et al. Prenatal diagnosis of sialidosis with combined neuraminidase and β-galactosidase deficiency. *Clin Genet* 1979; **16**: 60–1.

351 Kleijer WJ, Hu P, Thoomes R et al. Beta-mannosidase deficiency: hetergeneous manifestation in the first female patient and her brother. *J Inherit Metab Dis* 1990; **13**: 867–72.

352 Kleijer WJ, Keulemans JL, van der Kraan M et al. Prevalent mutations in the GALC gene of patients with Krabbe disease of Dutch and other European origin. *J Inherit Metab Dis* 1997; **29**: 587–94.

353 Kobayashi T, Furuya H, Furuyama H et al. Adult type Krabbe's disease: clinical, radiological and molecular analyses of four patients (abstract). *Ann Neurol* 1995; **38**: 349.

354 Kobayashi T, Kira J, Shinnoh N et al. Fabry's disease with partially deficient hydrolysis of ceramide trihexoside. *J Neurol Sci* 1985; **67**: 179–85.

355 Kobayashi T, Ohta M, Goto I et al. Adult type mucolipidosis with β-galactosidase and sialidase deficiency. *J Neurosci* 1979; **221**: 137–49.

356 Kobayashi T, Suzuki K. Chronic GM1 gangliosidosis presenting as dystonia: II. Biochemical studies. *Ann Neurol* 1981; **9**: 476–83.

357 Koch J, Gartner S, Li CM et al. Molecular cloning and characterization of a full-length complementary DNA encoding human acid ceramidase – identification of the first molecular lesion causing Farber disease. *J Biol Chem* 1996; **271**: 33110–115.

358 Koga M, Ishihara T, Hoshii Y et al. Histochemical and ultrastructural studies of inclusion bodies found in tissues from three siblings with I-cell disease. *Pathol Int* 1994; **44**: 223–9.

359 Kolodny EH. Globoid cell leukodystrophy. In: Moser HW ed. *Handbook of clinical neurology* Vol. 22 (66): *Neurodystrophies and neurolipidosis*. Amsterdam: Elsevier, 1996: 187–210.

360 Kolodny EH, Fluharty AL. Metachromatic leukodystrophy and multiple sulfatase deficiency: sulfatide lipidosis. In: Scriver CR, Beaudet AL, Sly WS, Valle D eds. *The metabolic and molecular basis of inherited disease*, 7th edn. New York: McGraw Hill, 1995: 2693–739.

361 Kolodny EH, Raghavan S, Krivit W. Late onset Krabbe disease (globoid cell leukodystrophy): clinical and biochemical features of 15 cases. *Dev Neurosci* 1991; **13**: 232–9.

362 Kolodny EH, Ulman MD, Mankin HJ et al. Phenotypic manifestations of Gaucher disease: clinical features in 48 biochemically verified type I patients and comment on type II patients. In: Desnick RJ, Gatt S, Grabowski GA eds. *Gaucher disease: a century of delineation and research*. New York: Alan R. Liss, 1982: 33–65.

363 Kornfeld M. Late onset GM2 gangliosidosis (abstract). *J Neuropathol Exp Neurol* 1999; **58**: 561.

364 Kornfeld M, Snider RD, Wenger DA. Fucosidosis with angiokeratoma: electron microscopic changes in the skin. *Arch Pathol Lab Med* 1977; **101**: 478–85.

365 Kosanke SD, Pierce KR, Read WK. Morphogenesis of light and electron microscopic lesions in porcine GM2-gangliosidosis. *Vet Pathol* 1979; **16**: 6–17.

366 Koto A, Horwitz AL, Suzuki K et al. The Morquio syndrome: Neuropathology and biochemistry. *Ann Neurol* 1978; **4**: 26–36.

367 Kovesi TA, Lee J, Shuckett B et al. Pulmonary infiltration in Niemann–Pick disease type C. *J Inherit Metab Dis* 1996; **19**: 792–3.

368 Krabbe K. A new familial, infantile form of diffuse brain sclerosis. *Brain* 1916; **39**: 74–114.

369 Kraus EJ. Zur Kenntnis der Splenomegalie Gaucher, insbensondere der Histogenese der grobzellen Wucherung. *Z Angewandte Anat* 1920; **7**: 186.

370 Kretzschmar HA, Wagner H, Hubner G et al. Aneurysms and vacuolar degeneration of cerebral arteries in late-onset acid maltase deficiency. J Neurol Sci 1990; **98**: 169–83.

371 Kriel RL, Hauser A, Sung JH, Posalaky Z. Neuroanatomical and electroencephalographic correlations in Sanfilippo syndrome, type A. Arch Neurol 1978; **35**: 838–43.

372 Kruth HS, Comly ME, Butler JD et al. Type C Niemann–Pick disease. Abnormal metabolism of low density lipoprotein in homozygous and heterozygous fibroblasts. J Biol Chem 1986; **261**: 16769–74.

373 Kuemmel TA, Schroeder R, Stoffel W. Light and electron microscopic analysis of the central and peripheral nervous system of acid sphingomyelinase-deficient mice resulting from gene targeting. J Neuropathol Exp Neurol 1997; **56**: 171–9.

374 Kuemmel TA, Thiele J, Schroeder R, Stoffel W. Pathology of visceral organs and bone marrow in an acid sphingomyelinase deficient knock-out mouse line, mimicking human Niemann–Pick disease type A. A light and electron microscopic study. Pathol Res Pract 1997; **193**: 663–71.

375 Kurihara M, Kumagai K, Goto K et al. Severe type Hunter's syndrome. Polysomnographic and neuropathological study. Neuropediatrics 1992; **23**: 248–56.

376 Kurihara M, Kumagai K, Yagishita S. Sanfilippo syndrome type C: a clinicopathological autopsy study of a long-term survivor. Pediatr Neurol 1996; **14**: 317–21.

377 Kuriwaki K, Yoshida H. Morphological characteristics of lipid accumulation in liver constituting cells of acid lipase deficiency rats (Wolman's disease model rats). Pathol Int 1999; **49**: 291–7.

378 Kytzia H-J, Hinrichs U, Maire I et al. Variant of GM2 gangliosidosis with hexosaminidase A having a severely changed substrate specificity. EMBO J 1983; **2**: 1201–5.

379 Lake BD. Segmental demyelination of peripheral nerves in Krabbe's disease. Nature 1968; **217**: 171–2.

380 Lake BD, Hall NA. Immunolocalization studies of subunit c in late-infantile and juvenile Batten disease. J Inherit Metab Dis 1993; **16**: 263–66.

381 Lake BD, Young EP, Nicolaides K. Prenatal diagnosis of infantile sialic acid storage disease in a twin pregnancy. J Inherit Metab Dis 1989; **12**: 152–6.

382 Lake BD, Young EP, Winchester BG. Prenatal diagnosis of lysosomal storage diseases. Brain Pathol 1998; **8**: 132–49.

383 Landing BH, Silverman FN, Craig JM et al. Familial neurovisceral lipidosis. Am J Dis Child 1964; **108**: 503–22.

384 Landrieu P, Said G. Peripheral neuropathy in type A Niemann–Pick disease. A morphological study. Acta Neuropathol 1984; **63**: 66–71.

385 Lane SC, Jolly RD, Schmechel DE et al. Apoptosis as the mechanism of neurodegeneration in Batten's disease. J Neurochem 1996; **67**: 677–83.

386 Lao LM, Kumakiri M, Mima H et al. The ultrastructural characteristics of eccrine sweat glands in a Fabry disease patient with hypohidrosis. J Dermatol Sci 1998; **18**: 109–17.

387 Larbrisseau A, Brochu P, Jasmine G. Fucosidose de type I. Etude anatomique. Arch Franc Pediatr 1979; **36**: 1013–25.

388 Lavery MA, Green WR, Jabs EW et al. Ocular histopathology and ultrastructure of Sanfilippo's syndrome, type III-B. Arch Ophthalmol 1983; **101**: 1263–74.

389 Lee RE. The pathology of Gaucher disease. In: Desnick RJ, Gatt S, Grabowski GA eds. Gaucher disease: a century of delineation and research. New York: Alan R. Liss, 1982: 177–217.

390 Leinekugel P, Michel S, Conzelmann E, Sandhoff K. Quantitative correlation between the residual activity of β-hexosaminidase A and arylsulfatase A and the severity of the resulting lysosomal storage disease. Hum Genet 1992; **88**: 513–23.

391 Lemyre E, Russo P, Melancon SB et al. Clinical spectrum of infantile free sialic acid storage disease. Am J Med Genet 1999; **82**: 385–91.

392 Leonberg SC Jr. A century of Kuf's disease in an American family. In: Armstrong D, Koppang N, Rider JA eds. Ceroid-lipofuscinosis (Batten's disease). Amsterdam: Elsevier Biomedical Press, 1982: 87–93.

393 Leroy JG. The mucolipidoses (including I-cell disease). In: Moser HW ed. Handbook of clinical neurology, Vol. 22 (66): Neurodystrophies and neurolipidoses. Amsterdam: Elsevier, 1996: 377–87.

394 Leroy LG, DeMars RI. Mutant enzymatic and cytological phenotypes in cultured human fibroblasts. Science 1967; **157**: 805–6.

395 Levade T, Graber D, Flurin D et al. Beta-mannosidase deficiency associated with a peripheral neuropathy. Ann Neurol 1994; **35**: 116–19.

396 Levine S, Paparo G. Brain lesions in a case of cystinosis. Acta Neuropathol 1982; **57**: 217–20.

397 Li C, Hong SB, Kopal G et al. Cloning and characterization of the full-length cDNA and genomic sequences encoding murine acid ceramidase. Genomics 1998; **50**: 267–74.

398 Li H-H, Yu W-H, Rozengurt N et al. Mouse model of Sanfilippo syndrome type B produced by targeted disruption of the gene encoding alpha-N-acetylglucosaminidase. Proc Nat Acad Sci USA 1999; **96**: 14505–10.

399 Lingaas F, Mitchison HM, Mole N et al. Animal models of NCL. In: Gobel HH, Mole SE, Lake BD eds. The neuronal ceroid lipofuscinoses (Batten disease). Amsterdam: IOS Press, 1999: 152–67.

400 Lipson AH, Rogers M, Berry A. Collodion babies with Gaucher disease. A further case. Arch Dis Child 1991; **66**: 667.

401 Lipson MH, O'Donnell J, Callahan JW et al. Ocular involvement in Niemann–Pick disease type B. J Pediatr 1986; **108**: 582–4.

402 Littjens T, Baker EG, Beckmann KR et al. Chromosomal localization of ARSB, the gene for human N-acetylgalactosamine-4-sulphatase. Hum Genet 1989; **82**: 67–8.

403 Littlewood JD, Herrtage ME, Palmer AC. Neuronal storage disease in English springer spaniels. Vet Rec 1983; **112**: 86–7.

404 Liu Y, Hoffmann A, Grinberg A et al. Mouse model of GM2 activator deficiency manifests cerebellar pathology and motor impairment. Proc Nat Acad Sci USA 1997; **94**: 8138–43.

405 Liu Y, Suzuki K, Reed JD et al. Mice with type 2 and 3 Gaucher disease point mutations generated by a single insertion mutagenesis procedure (SIMP). Proc Nat Acad Sci USA 1998; **95**: 2503–8.

406 Loeb H, Tondeur M, Jonniaux G et al. Biochemical and ultrastructural studies in a case of mucopolysaccharidosis 'F' (Fucosidosis). Helv Paediatr Acta 1969; **24**: 519–37.

407 Love S, Bridges LR, Case CP. Neurofibrillary tangles in Niemann–Pick disease type C. Brain 1995; **118**: 119–29.

408 Lovell KL, Jones MZ. Distribution of central nervous system lesions in beta-mannosidosis. Acta Neuropathol (Berl) 1983; **62**: 121–6.

409 Lovell KL, Jones MZ. Axonal and myelin lesions in β-mannosidosis: ultrastructural characteristics. Acta Neuropathol (Berl) 1985; **65**: 293–9.

410 Lowden JA, O'Brien JS. Sialidosis: A review of human neuraminidase deficiency. Am J Hum Genet 1979; **31**: 1–18.

411 Lowenthal AC, Cummings JF, Wenger DA et al. Feline sphingolipidosis resembling Niemann–Pick disease type C. Acta Neuropathol 1990; **81**: 189–97.

412 Luzi P, Rafi MA, Victoria T et al. Characterization of the rhesus monkey galactocerebrosidase (GALC) cDNA and gene and identification of the mutation causing globoid cell leukodystrophy (Krabbe disease) in this primate. Genomics 1997; **42**: 319–24.

413 Luzi P, Rafi MA, Wenger DA. Multiple mutations in the GALC gene in a patient with adult-onset Krabbe disease. Ann Neurol 1996; **40**: 116–19.

414 Lyon G, Hagberg B, Evrard PH et al. Symptomatology of late onset Krabbe's leukodystrophy: the European experience. Dev Neurosci 1991; **13**: 240–4.

415 Macaulay RJB, Lowry NJ, Casey RE. Pathologic findings of multiple sulfatase deficiency reflect the pattern of enzyme deficiencies. Pediatr Neurol 1998; **19**: 372–6.

416 Maclaren NK, Max SR, Cornblath M et al. GM3 gangliosidosis: a novel human sphingolipodystrophy. Pediatrics 1976; **57**: 106–10.

417 Maconochie JK, Chong S, Mieli Vergane G et al. Fetal ascites: an unusual presentation of Niemann–Pick disease type C. Arch Dis Child 1989; **64**: 1391–3.

418 Maia M, Alves D, Ribeiro G et al. Juvenile GM2 gangliosidosis variant B: clinical and biochemical study in seven patients. Neuropediatrics 1990; **21**: 18–23.

419 Malachowski JA, Jones MZ. β-Mannosidosis: lesions of the distal peripheral nervous system. Acta Neuropathol (Berl) 1983; **61**: 95–100.

420 Manabe T, Yamane T, Higashi Y et al. Ultrastructural changes in the lung in Niemann–Pick type C mouse. Virchows Arch 1995; **427**: 77–83.

421 Mancini GMS, Beerens CEMT, Aula PP, Verheijen FW. Sialic acid storage disease: a multiple lysosomal transport defect for acidic monosaccharides. J Clin Invest 1991; **87**: 1329–35.

422 Mancini GMS, de Jonge HR, Galjaard H, Verheijen FW. Characterization of a proton-driven carrier for sialic acid in the lysosomal membrane. J Biol Chem 1989; **264**: 15247–54.

423 Mancini GMS, Verheijen FW, Beerens CEMT et al. Sialic acid storage disorders: observations on clinical and biochemical variation. Dev Neurosci 1991; **13**: 327–30.

424 March PA, Thrall MA, Brown DF et al. GABAergic neuroaxonal dystrophy and other cytopathological alterations in feline Niemann–Pick disease type C. Acta Neuropathol 1997; **94**: 164–72.

425 Maroteaux P, Leveque B, Marie J, Lamy M. Une nouvelle dysostose avec elimination urinaire de chondroitin-sulfate B. Presse Med 1963; **71**: 1849–53.

426 Martin JJ, Ceuterick C. Adult neuronal ceroid-lipofuscinosis: personal observations. Acta Neurol Belg 1997; **97**: 85–92.

427 Martin JJ, Ceuterick C, Van Dessel G et al. Two cases of mucopolysaccharidosis type III (Sanfilippo). An anatomopathological study. Acta Neuropathol (Berl) 1979; **46**: 185–90.

428 Martin JJ, de Barsy Th, de Schrijver F et al. Acid maltase deficiency (type II glycogenosis). J Neurol Sci 1976; **30**: 155–66.

429 Martin JJ, de Barsy Th, Van Hoof F, Palladini G. Pompe's disease: an inborn lysosomal disorder with storage of glycogen. A study of brain and striated muscle. Acta Neuropathol (Berl) 1973; **23**: 229–44.

430 Martin JJ, Gottlob I, Goebel HH, Mole SE. CLN4; adult NCL. In: Goebel HH, Mole SE, Lake BD eds. The neuronal ceroid lipofuscinoses (Batten disease). Amsterdam: IOS Press, 1999: 77–90.

431 Martin JJ, Leroy JG, Farriaux J-P et al. I-cell disease (mucolipidosis II). A report on its pathology. Acta Neuropathol (Berl) 1975; **33**: 285–305.

432 Martin JJ, Leroy JG, Vaneygen M, Ceuterick C. I-cell disease: a further report on its pathology. Acta Neuropathol (Berl) 1984; **64**: 234–42.

433 Matalon R, Dorfman A. Hurler's syndrome, an L-iduronidase deficiency. Biochem Biophys Res Commun 1972; **47**: 959–64.

434 Matsuda J, Suzuki O, Oshima A et al. β-Galactosidase-deficient mouse as an animal model for GM1-gangliosidosis. Glycoconj J 1997; **14**: 729–36.

435 Matsumoto R, Oka N, Nagashima Y et al. Peripheral neuropathy in late-onset Krabbe's disease: histochemical and ultrastructural findings. Acta Neuropathol 1996; **92**: 635–9.

436 McDonnell JM, Green WR, Maumenee IH. Ocular histopathology of systemic mucopolysaccharidosis, type II-A (Hunter syndrome, severe). Ophthalmology 1985; **92**: 1772–9.

437 McKelvie P, Vine P, Hopkins I, Poulos A. A case of Krabbe's leukodystrophy without globoid cells. Pathology 1990; **22**: 235–8.

438 McKeran RO, Bradbury P, Taylor D, Stern G. Neurological involvement in type 1 (adult) Gaucher's disease. J Neurol Neurosurg Psychiatry 1985; **48**: 172–5.

439 Meek D, Wolfe LS, Andermann F. Juvenile progressive dystonia: a new phenotype of GM2 gangliosidosis. Ann Neurol 1984; **15**: 348–52.

440 Mehl E, Jatzkewitz H. Eine cerebrosidsulfatase aus Schweineniere. Hoppe Seyler Z Physiol Chem 1964; **339**: 260–75.

441 Mehl E, Jatzkewitz H. Evidence for the genetic block in metachromatic leukodystrophy (ML). Biochem Biophys Res Commun 1965; **19**: 407–11.

442 Merin S, Livni N, Berman ER, Yatziv S. Mucolipidosis IV: Ocular, systemic, and ultrastructural findings. Invest Ophthamol Vis Sci 1975; **14**: 437–48.

443 Miranda SR, Erlich S, Friedrich VL et al. Biochemical, pathological, and clinical response to transplantation of normal bone marrow cells into acid sphingomyelinase-deficient mice. Transplantation 1998; **65**: 884–92.

444 Mitchison HM. Hofmann SL, Becerra CH et al. Mutations in the palmitoyl-protein thioesterase gene (PPT;CLN1) causing juvenile neuronal ceroid lipofuscinosis with granular osmiophilic deposits. Hum Mol Genet 1998; **7**: 291–7.

445 Mitsumoto H, Sliman RJ, Schafer IA et al. Motor neuron disease and adult hexosaminidase A deficiency in two families: evidence for multisystem degeneration. Ann Neurol 1985; **17**: 378–85.

446 Miyatake T, Atsumi T, Obayashi T et al. Adult type neuronal storage disease with neuraminidase deficiency. Ann Neurol 1979; **6**: 232–44.

447 Miyatake T, Suzuki K. Globoid cell leukodystrophy: additional deficiency of psychosine galactosidase. Biochem Biophys Res Commun 1972; **48**: 538–43.

448 Mole S, Gardiner M. Molecular genetics of the neuronal ceroid lipofuscinoses. Epilepsia 1999; **40** (Suppl 3): 29–32.

449 Molyneux AJ, Blair E, Coleman N, Daish P. Mucopolysaccharidosis type VII associated with hydrops fetalis: histopathological and ultrastructural features with genetic implications. J Clin Pathol 1997; **50**: 252–4.

450 Mononen I, Fisher KJ, Kaartinen V, Aronson NN Jr. Aspartylglycosaminuria: protein chemistry and molecular biology of the most common lysosomal storage disorder of glycoprotein degradation. FASEB J 1993; **7**: 1247–56.

451 Mononen T, Mononen I. Biochemistry and biochemical diagrams of aspartylglycosaminuria. In: Mononen I, Aronson NN Jr eds. Lysosomal storage disease: aspartylglycosaminuria. Austin, TX: R.G. Landes/Heidelberg: Springer, 1997: 41–9.

452 Moser HW. Ceramidase deficiency: Farber lipogranulo-matosis. In: Scriver CR, Beaudet AL, Sly WS, Valle D eds. *The metabolic and molecular basis of inherited disease*, 7th edn. New York: McGraw-Hill, 1995: 2589–600.

453 Moser HW, Prensky AL, Wolfe HJ, Rosman NF. Farber's lipogranulomatosis. Report of a case and demonstration of an excess of free ceramide and ganglioside. *Am J Med* 1969; **47**: 869–90.

454 Motulsky AG. Jewish diseases and origin. *Nat Genet* 1995; **9**: 99–101.

455 Mueller OT, Henry WM, Haley LI et al. Sialidosis and galac-tosialidosis: Chromosomal assignment of two genes asso-ciated with neuraminidase-deficiency disorders. *Proc Nat Acad Sci USA* 1986; **83**: 1817–21.

456 Mueller OT, Shows TB, Opitz JM. Apparent allelism of the Hurler, Scheie and Hurler/Scheie syndrome. *Am J Med Genet* 1984; **18**: 547–56.

457 Muenzer J, Fu H. Targeted disruption of the mouse iduronate sulfatase gene (abstract). *Am J Hum Genet* 1999; **65**: A427.

458 Muldoon LL, Neuwelt EA, Pagel MA, Weiss DL. Character-ization of the molecular defect in a feline model for type II GM2-gangliosidosis (Sandhoff disease). *Am J Pathol* 1994; **144**: 1109–18.

459 Murphy JV, Wolf HJ, Balazs EA, Moser HW. A patient with deficiency of arylsulfatases A B, C and steroid sulfatase, associated with storage of sulfatide, cholesterol sulfate and glycosaminoglycans. In: Bersohn J, Grossman HJ eds. *Lipid storage disease, enzymatic defects and clinical implications*. New York: Academic Press, 1971: 67–110.

460 Nagao Y, Nakashima H, Fukuhara Y et al. Hypertrophic car-diomyopathy in late-onset variant of Fabry disease with high residual activity of α-galactosidase A. *Clin Genet* 1991; **39**: 233–7.

461 Nagashima K, Sakakibara K, Endo H et al. I-Cell disease (Mucolipidosis II). Pathological and biochemical studies of an autopsy case. *Acta Pathol Jpn* 1977; **27**: 251–64.

462 Nakamura T, Kaneko H, Nishino I. Angiokeratoma corporis diffusum (Fabry disease): ultrastructural studies of the skin. *Acta Derm Venereol* 1981; **61**: 37–41.

463 Nakano C, Hirabayashi Y, Ohno K et al. A Japanese case of infantile sialic acid storage disease. *Clin Genet* 1996; **18**: 153–6.

464 Nakano T, Ikeda S, Kondo K et al. Adult GM1-gangliosi-dosis. *Neurology* 1985; **35**: 875–80.

464a Naureckiene S, Sleat DE, Lackland H et al. Identification of HE1 as the second gene of Niemann-Pick C disease. *Science* 2000; **290**: 2298–301.

465 Navon R, Argov Z, Brand N, Sandbank U. Adult GM2 gan-gliosidosis in association with Tay–Sachs disease: a new phenotype. *Neurology* 1981; **31**: 1397–401.

466 Navon R, Argov Z, Frisch A. Hexosaminidase A deficiency in adults. *Am J Med Genet* 1986; **24**: 179–96.

467 Nelson J, Kenny B, O'Hara D et al. Foamy changes of pla-cental cells in probable beta glucuronidase deficiency associated with hydrops fetalis. *J Clin Pathol* 1993; **46**: 370–1.

468 Neufeld EF, Muenzer J. The mucopolysaccharidoses. In: Scriver CR, Beaudet AL, Sly WS, Valle D eds. *The metabol-ic and molecular basis of inherited disease*. New York: McGraw-Hill, 1995: 2465–94.

469 Neuwelt EA, Johnson WG, Blank NK et al. Characterization of a new model of GM2-gangliosidosis (Sandhoff's disease) in Korat cats. *J Clin Invest* 1985; **76**: 482–90.

470 Ng Yg, Kin NM, Palo J, Haltia M, Wolfe LS. High levels of brain dolichols in ceroid-lipofuscinosis and senescence. *J Neurochem* 1983; **40**: 1465–73.

471 Nichols SL, Press GA, Schneider JA, Trauner DA. Cortical atrophy and cognitive performance in infantile nephro-pathic cystinosis. *Pediatr Neurol* 1990; **6**: 379–81.

472 Niemann A. Ein unbekanntes Krankheitsbild. *Jahrbuch Kinderheilkunde* 1914; **79**: 1–10.

473 Nilsson O, Grabowski GA, Ludman MD et al. Glyco-sphingolipid studies of visceral tissues and brain from type 1 Gaucher disease variants. *Clin Genet* 1985; **27**: 443–50.

474 Nilsson O, Mansson JE, Hakansson G, Svennerholm L. The occurrence of psychosine and other glycolipid in spleen and liver from the three major types of Gaucher's disease. *Biochim Biophys Acta* 1982; **712**: 453–63.

475 Nilsson O, Svennerholm L. Accumulation of glucosylce-ramide and glucosylsphingosine (psychosine) in cerebrum and cerebellum in infantile and juvenile Gaucher disease, *J Neurochem* 1982; **39**: 709–18.

476 Nordocci N, Bertagnolio B, Rumi V, Angelini L. Progressive dystonia symptomatic of juvenile GM2 gangliosidosis. *Mov Disord* 1992; **7**: 64–7.

477 Norman RM, Urich H, Lloyd OC. The neuropathology of infantile Gaucher's disease. *J Pathol Bacteriol* 1956; **72**: 121–31.

478 Norman RM, Urich H, Tingey AM, Goodbody RA. Tay–Sachs' disease with visceral involvement and its rela-tionship to Niemann–Pick disease. *J Pathol Bacteriol* 1959; **78**: 409–21.

479 Northover H, Cowie RA, Wrait JE. Mucopolysaccharidosis type IVA: a clinical review. *J Inherit Metab Dis* 1996; **19**: 357–65.

480 Norton WR, Poduslo SE. Biochemical studies of metachro-matic leukodystrophy in three siblings. *Acta Neuropathol (Berl)* 1982; **57**: 188–96.

481 Oak S, Rao S, Karmarkar S et al. Papillomatosis of the gall-bladder in metachromatic leukodystrophy. *Pathol Int* 1997; **12**: 424–5.

482 O'Brien JS, Ho MW, Veath ML et al. Juvenile GM1 gan-gliosidosis: clinical, pathological, chemical and enzymatic studies. *Clin Genet* 1972; **3**: 411–34.

483 O'Brien JS, Stern MB, Landing BH et al. Generalized gan-gliosidosis. Another inborn error of ganglioside metabo-lism? *Am J Dis Child* 1965; **109**: 338–46.

484 O'Brien JS, Warner TG. Sialidosis: delineation of subtypes by neuraminidase assay. *Clin Genet* 1980; **17**: 35–8.

485 Ockerman PM. Mannosidosis. *J Pediatr* 1969, **75**: 360–5.

486 Oda H, Sasaki Y, Nakatani Y et al. Hunter's syndrome. An ultrastructural study of an autopsy case. *Acta Pathol Jpn* 1988; **38**: 1175–90.

487 Ogawa K, Sugamata K, Funamoto N et al. Restricted accumulation of globotriaosylceramide in the heart of atyp-ical cases of Fabry's disease. *Hum Pathol* 1990; **21**: 1067–73.

488 Ohnishi A, Dyck PJ. Loss of small peripheral sensory neu-rons in Fabry disease. Histologic and morphometric eval-uation of cutaneous nerves, spinal ganglia, and posterior columns. *Arch Neurol* 1974; **31**:120–7.

489 Ohshima T, Murray GJ, Swaim WD et al. α-galactosidase A deficient mice: a model of Fabry disease. *Proc Nat Acad Sci USA* 1997; **94**: 2540–4.

490 Ohshima T, Schiffmann R, Murray GJ et al. Aging accen-tuates and bone marrow transplantation ameliorates meta-bolic defects in Fabry disease mice. *Proc Nat Acad Sci USA* 1999; **96**: 6423–7.

491 Okada S, O'Brien JS. Generalized gangliosidosis: beta-galac-tosidase deficiency. *Science* 1968; **160**: 1002–4.

492 Okada S, O'Brien JS. Tay–Sachs disease: generalized absence of a β-d-N-acetylhexosaminidase component. *Science* 1969; **165**: 698–700.

493 Okada S, Yutaka T, Kato T et al. A case of neuramidase deficiency associated with a partial β-galactosidase defect. Clinical, biochemical and radiological studies. *Eur J Pediatr* 1979; **130**: 239–49.

494 Oldfors A, Sourander P. Storage of lipofuscin in neurons in mucopolysaccharidosis. Report on a case of Sanfilippo's syndrome with histochemical and electron microscopic findings. *Acta Neuropathol (Berl)* 1981; **54**: 287–92.

495 Olsson R, Sourander P, Svennerholm L. Experimental studies on the pathogenesis of leucodystrophies. I. The effect of intracerebrally injected sphingolipids in the rat brain. *Acta Neuropathol (Berl)* 1966; **6**: 153–63.

496 Opitz JM, Stiles FC, Wise D et al. The genetics of angiokeratoma corporis diffusum (Fabry's disease), and its linkage with Xg (a) locus. *Am J Hum Genet* 1965; **17**: 325–42.

497 Orme RLE. Wolman's disease: an unusual presentation. *Proc R Soc Med* 1970; **63**: 489–90.

498 Oshima A, Yoshida K, Shimmoto M et al. Human β-galactosidase gene mutation in Morquio B disease. *Am J Hum Genet* 1991; **49**: 1091–3

499 Otterbach B, Stoffel W. Acid sphingomyelinase-deficient mice mimic the neurovisceral form of human lysosomal storage disease (Niemann–Pick disease). *Cell* 1995; **81**: 1053–61.

500 Oya Y, Nakayasu H, Fujita N et al. Pathological study of mice with total deficiency of sphingolipid activator proteins (SAP knockout mice). *Acta Neuropathol* 1998; **96**: 29–40.

501 Oyanagi K, Ohama E, Miyashita K et al. Galactosialidosis: neuropathological findings in a case of the late-infantile type. *Acta Neuropathol* 1991; **82**: 331–9.

502 Palmer DN, Fearnley IM, Medd SM et al. Lysosomal storage of the DCCD reactive proteolipid subunit of mitochondrial ATP synthase in human and ovine ceroid-lipofuscinoses (Batten's disease). *Adv Exp Med Biol* 1990; **266**: 211–3.

503 Palmer DN, Fearnley IM, Walker JE et al. Mitochondrial ATP synthase subunit c storage in the ceroid lipofuscinosis (Batten disease). *Am J Med Genet* 1992; **42**: 561–7.

504 Palmer M, Green WR, Maumenee IH et al. Niemann–Pick disease-type C. Ocular histopathologic and electron microscopic studies. *Arch Ophthalmol* 1985; **193**: 817–22.

505 Palo J. Prevalence of phenylketonuria and some other metabolic disorders among mentally retarded patients in Finland. *Acta Neurol Scand* 1967; **43**: 573–9.

506 Pampols T, Pineda M, Giros ML et al. Neuronopathic juvenile glucosylceramidosis due to sap-C deficiency: clinical course, neuropathology and brain lipid composition in this Gaucher disease variant. *Acta Neuropathol* 1999; **97**: 91–7.

507 Parnes S, Karpati G, Carpenter S et al. Hexosaminidase-A deficiency presenting as atypical juvenile-onset spinal muscular atrophy. *Arch Neurol* 1985; **42**: 1176–80.

508 Patel V, Watanabe I, Zeman W. Deficiency of α-l-Fucosidase. *Science* 1972; **176**: 426–7.

509 Patrick AD. A deficiency of glucocerebrosidase in Gaucher's disease. *Biochem J* 1965; **97**: 17C.

510 Patterson JS, Jones MZ, Lovell KL, Abbitt B. Neuropathology of bovine beta-mannosidosis. *J Neuropathol Exp Neurol* 1991; **50**: 538–46.

511 Patterson MC, Vanier MT, Suzuki K et al. Niemann–Pick disease type C: A lipid trafficking disorder. In: Scriver CR, Beaudet AL, Sly WS, Valle D eds. *The metabolic and molecular basis of inherited disease*, 8th edn. New York: McGraw Hill, 2001; 3611–34.

512 Pavone L, Moser HW, Mollica F et al. Farber's lipogranulomatosis: ceramide deficiency and prolonged survival in three relatives. *Johns Hopkins Med J* 1980; **147**: 193–6.

513 Pellissier JF, Berard-Badier M, Pinsard N. Farber's disease in two siblings, sural nerve and subcutaneous biopsies by light and electron microscopy. *Acta Neuropathol (Berl)* 1986; **72**: 178–88.

514 Pellissier JF, Hassoun J, Gambarelli D et al. Niemann–Pick disease (Crocker's type C): ultrastructural study of a case. *Acta Neuropathol (Berl)* 1976; **34**: 65–76.

515 Peltola M, Tikkanen R, Peltonen L, Jalanko A. Ser72Pro active site disease mutation in human lysosomal aspartylglucosaminidase: abnormal intracellular processing and evidence for extracellular activation. *Hum Mol Genet* 1996; **5**: 737–43.

516 Peng L, Suzuki K. Ultrastructural study of neurons in metachromatic leukodystrophy. *Clin Neuropathol* 1987; **6**: 224–30.

517 Pentchev PG, Comly ME, Kruth HS et al. A defect in cholesterol esterification in Niemann–Pick disease (type C) patients. *Proc Nat Acad Sci USA* 1985; **82**: 8247–51.

518 Pentchev PC, Comly ME, Kruth HS et al. Group C Niemann–Pick disease: faulty regulation of low-density lipoprotein uptake and cholesterol storage in cultured fibroblasts. *FASEB J* 1987; **1**: 40–5.

519 Pentchev PG, Kruth HS, Comly ME et al. Type C Niemann–Pick disease. A parallel loss of regulatory responses in both the uptake and esterification of low density lipoprotein-derived cholesterol in cultured fibroblasts. *J Biol Chem* 1986; **261**: 16775–80.

520 Pentchev P, Vanier MT, Suzuki K, Patterson MC. Niemann–Pick disease type C: a cellular cholesterol lipidosis. In: Scriver CR, Beaudet AL, Sly WS, Valle D eds. *The metabolic and molecular basis of inherited disease*, 7th edn. New York: McGraw-Hill, 1995: 2625–39.

521 Percy AK, Odrezin GT, Knowles PD et al. Globoid cell leukodystrophy: comparison of neuropathology with magnetic resonance imaging. *Acta Neuropathol (Berl)* 1994; **88**: 26–32.

522 Petrelli M, Blair JD. The liver in GM1 gangliosidosis types 1 and 2. *Arch Pathol* 1975; **99**: 111–16.

523 Peiffer J. Uber die metachromatischen Leukodystrophien (Type Scholz). *Arch Psychiatrie Z Gesamte Neurol* 1959; **199**: 386–416.

524 Phaneuf D, Wakamatsu N, Huang J-Q et al. Dramatically different phenotypes in mouse models of human Tay–Sachs and Sandhoff diseases. *Hum Mol Genet* 1996; **5**: 1–14.

525 Phelps M, Aicardi J, Vanier MT. Late onset Krabbe's leukodystrophy: a report of four cases. *J Neurol Neurosurg Psychiatry* 1991; **54**: 293–6.

526 Pierce KR, Kosanke SD, Bay WW, Brides CH. Animal model: Porcine cerebrospinal lipodystrophy (GM2 gangliosidosis). *Am J Pathol* 1976; **83**: 419–22.

527 Pin I, Pradines S, Pincemaille O et al. A fatal respiratory form of type C Niemann–Pick disease. *Arch Franc Pediatrie* 1990; **47**: 373–5.

528 Polten A, Fluharty AL, Fluharty CB et al. Molecular basis of different forms of metachromatic leukodystrophy. *N Engl J Med* 1991; **324**: 18–22.

529 Portera-Cailliau C et al. Apoptotic photoreceptor cell death in mouse models of retinitis pigmentosa. *Proc Nat Acad Sci USA* 1994; **91**: 974–8.

530 Prensky A, Ferreira G, Carr S, Moser HW. Ceramide and ganglioside accumulation in Farber's lipogranulomatosis. *Proc Soc Exp Biol Med* 1987; **126**: 725–8.

531 Prieur DJ, Ahern-Rindell AJ, Murnane RD. Animal model of human disease. *Am J Pathol* 1991; **139**: 1511–13.

532 Pshezhetsky AV, Richard C, Michaud L *et al*. Cloning, expression and chromosomal mapping of human lysosomal sialidase and characterization of mutations in sialidosis. *Nat Genet* 1997; **15**: 316–20.

533 Puranam K, Qian WH, Nikbakht K *et al*. Upregulation of Bcl–2 and elevation of ceramide in Batten disease. *Neuropediatrics* 1997; **28**: 37–41.

534 Purpura DP. Ectopic dendritic growth in mature pyramidal neurons in human ganglioside storage disease. *Nature* 1978; **276**: 520–1.

535 Purpura DP, Pappas GD, Baker HJ. Fine structure of meganeurites and secondary growth processes in feline GM1-gangliosidosis. *Brain Res* 1978; **143**: 1–12.

536 Purpura DP, Suzuki K. Distortion of neuronal geometry and formation of aberrant synapses in neuronal storage disease. *Brain Res* 1976; **116**: 1–21.

537 Qu Y, Shapira E, Desnick RJ. Metachromatic leukodystrophy: subtype genotype/phenotype correlations and identification of novel missense mutations (P1481L and P191T) causing the juvenile-onset disease. *Mol Genet Metab* 1999; **67**: 206–12.

538 Raas-Rothschild A, Bargal R, DellaPergola S *et al*. Mucolipidosis type IV: the origin of the disease in the Ashkenazi Jewish populatiomn. *Euro J Human Genet* 1999; **7**: 496–8.

539 Raben N, Nagaraju K, Lee E *et al*. Targeted disruption of the acid alpha-glucosidase gene in mice causes an illness with critical features of both infantile and adult human glycogen storage disease type II. *J Biol Chem* 1998; **273**: 19086–92.

540 Rahman AN, Lindenberg R. The neuropathology of hereditary dystopic lipidosis. *Arch Neurol* 1963; **9**: 373–85.

541 Rampini S. Das Sanfilippo syndrome (polydystrophie oligophrenie, HS-Mukopolysaccharidose). Bericht uber 8 Fallen und Literaturubersicht. *Helv Paediatr Acta* 1969; **24**: 55–91.

542 Rampini S, Clausen J. Farbersche Krankheit (disseminierte Lipogranulomatose). *Helv Paediatr Acta* 1967; **22**: 500–15.

543 Rampini S, Isler W, Baerlocher K *et al*. Die Kombination von Metachromatische Leukodystrophie als selbstandiges Krankheitsbild (Mukosulfatidose). *Helv Paediatr Acta* 1970; **25**: 436–61.

544 Rapin I. Myoclonus in neuronal storage and Lafora diseases. *Adv Neurol* 1986; **43**: 65–85.

545 Rapin I, Goldfisher S, Katzman R *et al*. The cherry-red spot-myoclonus syndrome. *Ann Neurol* 1978; **3**: 234–42.

546 Rapin I, Suzuki K, Suzuki K, Valsamis MP. Adult (chronic) GM2 gangliosidosis. *Arch Neurol* 1976; **33**: 120–30.

547 Raynaud E-J, Escourolle R, Baumann N *et al*. Metachromatic leukodystrophy. Ultrastructural enzymatic study of a case of variant O form. *Arch Neurol* 1975; **32**: 834–6.

548 Reiss S, Sheffer R, Merin S *et al*. Mucolipidosis type IV: a late onset and mild form. *Am J Med Genet* 1993; **47**: 392–4.

549 Reitman ML, Varki A, Kornfeld S. Fibroblasts from patients with I-cell disease and pseudo-Hurler polydystrophy are deficient in uridine 5'-diphosphate *N*-acetylglucosamine:glycoprotein *N*-acetylglucosaminylphosphotransferase activity. *J Clin Invest* 1981; **67**: 1574–9.

550 Renlund M, Aula P, Raivio KO *et al*. Salla disease: a new lysosomal storage disorder with disturbed sialic acid metabolism. *Neurology* 1983; **33**: 57–66.

551 Renlund M. Chester AM, Lundblad A *et al*. Free *N*-acetyl-neuraminic acid in tissues in Salla disease and the enzyme involved in its metabolism. *Eur J Biochem* 1983; **130**: 39–45.

552 Resnick JM, Whitley CB, Leonard S *et al*. Light and electron microscopic features of the liver in mucopolysaccharidosis. *Hum Pathol* 1994; **25**: 276–86.

553 Riedel KG, Zwaan J, Kenyon KR *et al*. Ocular abnormalities in mucolipidosis IV. *Am J Ophthalmol* 1985; **99**: 125–36.

554 Rigante D, Antuzzi D, Ricci R, Segni G. Cervical myelopathy in mucopolysaccharidosis type IV. *Clin Neuropathol* 1999; **18**: 84–6.

555 Rivel J, Vital C, Battin J *et al*. La lipogranulomatose disseminee de Fraber: etudes anatomo-clinique et ultrastructurale de deux observations familiales. *Acta Anat Cytol Pathol* 1977; **25**: 37–42.

556 Robb RM, Kuwabara T. The ocular pathology of type A Niemann–Pick disease. A light and electron microscopic study. *Invest Ophthalmol* 1973; **12**: 366–77.

557 Robertson DA, Callen DF, Baker EG *et al*. Chromosomal localization of the gene for human glucosamine-6-sulphatase to 12q14. *Hum Genet* 1988; **79**: 175–8.

558 Rodriguez M, O'Brien JS, Garrett RS, Powell HC. Canine GM1 gangliosidosis. *J Neuropathol Exp Neurol* 1982; **41**: 618–29.

559 Rodriguez-Lafrasse C, Vanier MT. Sphingosylphosphorylcholine in Niemann–Pick disease brain: accumulation in type A but not type B. *Neurochem Res* 1999; **24**: 199–205.

560 Roels H, Quatacker J, Kint A *et al*. Generalized gangliosidosis-GM1 (Landing disease). II. Morphological study. *Eur Neurol* 1970; **3**: 129–60.

561 Romeo G, Urso M, Piszcane A *et al*. Residual activity of α-galactosidase A in Fabry's disease. *Biochem Genet* 1975; **13**: 615–28.

562 Rose JS, Grabowski GA, Barnett SH, Desnick RJ. Accelerated skeletal deterioration after splenectomy in Gaucher type 1 disease. *Am J Roentgenol* 1982; **139**: 1202–4.

563 Ross DL, Strife CF, Towbin R, Bove KE. Nonabsorptive hydrocephalus associated with nephropathic cystinosis. *Neurology* 1982; **32**: 1330–4.

564 Rottach KG, von Maydel RD, Das VE *et al*. Evidence for independent feedback control of horizontal and vertical saccardes from Niemann–Pick type C disease. *Vision Res* 1997; **37**: 3627–38.

565 Rottier RJ, Bonten E, d'Azzo A. A point mutation in the neu-1 locus causes the neuraminidase defect in the SM/J mouse. *Hum Mol Genet* 1998; **7**: 313–21.

566 Rubin M, Karpati G, Wolf LS *et al*. Adult onset motor neuropathy in the juvenile type of hexosaminidase A and B deficiency. *J Neurol Sci* 1988; **87**: 103–19.

567 Russell C, Hendson G, Jevon G *et al*. Murine MPS I: insights into the pathogenesis of Hurler syndrome. *Clin Genet* 1998; **53**: 349–61.

568 Rutledge JC. Progressive neonatal liver failure due to type C Niemann–Pick disease. *Pediatr Pathol* 1989; **9**: 779–84.

569 Rutsaert J, Menu R, Resibois A. Ultrastructure of sulfatide storage in normal and sulfatide-deficient fibroblasts *in vitro*. *Lab Invest* 1973; **29**: 527–35.

570 Sachs B. On arrested cerebral development, with special reference to its cortical pathology. *J Nerv Ment Dis* 1887; **14**: 541–53.

571 Sacrez R, Juif JG, Gionnet JM, Gruner JE. La maladie de Landing, ou idiote amaurotique infantile précoce avec gangliosidose généralisée. *Pediatrie* 1967; **22**: 143–62.

572 Sakai N, Inui K, Fujii N *et al*. Krabbe disease. Isolation and characterization of a full-length cDNA for human galactocerebrosidase. *Biochem Biophys Res Commun* 1994; **198**: 485–91.

573 Sakai N, Inui K, Tatsumi N *et al*. Molecular cloning and expression of cDNA for murine galactocerebrosidase and mutation analysis of the twitcher mouse, a model of Krabbe's disease. *J Neurochem* 1996; **66**: 1118–24.

574 Samuelsson K, Zetterstrom R. Ceramide in a patient with lipogranulomatosis (Farber's disease) with chronic course. *Scand J Clin Lab Invest* 1971; **27**: 393–405.

575 Sandhoff K. Variation of β-acetylhexosaminidase pattern in Tay–Sachs disease. *FEBS Lett* 1969; **4**: 351–4.

576 Sandhoff K, Harzer K, Furst W. Sphingolipid activator proteins, In: Scriver CR, Beaudet AL, Sly WS, Valle D eds. *The metabolic and molecular basis of inherited disease*. New York: McGraw-Hill, 1995: 2427–41.

577 Sanfilippo S, Good R. A laboratory study of the Hurler syndrome. *Am J Dis Child* 1964; **192**: 140–5.

578 Sanfilippo SJ, Podosin R, Langer L, Good, RA. Mental retardation associated with acid mucopolysacchariduria (heparitin sulfate type). *J Pediatr* 1963; **63**: 837–8.

579 Sango K, Yamanaka S, Hoffmann A *et al.* Mouse models of Tay–Sachs and Sandhoff diseases differ in neurologic phenotype and ganglioside metabolism. *Nat Genet* 1995; **11**: 170–6.

580 Santavuori P, Halfia M, Rapola J *et al.* Infantile type of so-called neuronal ceroid-lipofuscinosis. *Dev Med Child Neurol* 1974; **16**: 644–53.

581 Santavuori P, Gottlob I, Haltia M *et al.* CLN1. Infantile and other types of NCL with GROD. In: Goebel HH, Mole SE, Lake BD eds. *The neuronal ceroid lipofuscinosis (Batten disease)*. Amsterdam: IOS Press, 1999: 16–36.

582 Savukoski M, Klockars T, Holmberg J *et al.* CLN5, a novel gene encoding a putative transmembrane protein mutated in Finish variant late infantile neuronal ceroid lipofuscinosis. *Nat Genet* 1998; **19**: 286–8.

583 Scheie HG, Hambrick GW Jr, Barness LA. A newly recognized forme fruste of Hurler's disease (gargoylism). *Am J Ophthalmol* 1962; **53**: 753–69.

584 Schindler D, Bishop DF, Wolf DE *et al.* Neuroaxonal dystrophy due to lysosomal α-N-acetylgalactosaminidase deficiency. *N Engl J Med* 1989; **320**: 1735–40.

585 Schlaepfer WW, Prensky AL. Quantitative and qualitative study of sural nerve biopsies in Krabbe disease. *Acta Neuropathol (Berl)* 1976; **20**: 55–66.

586 Schleutker J, Leppanen P, Mansson J-E *et al.* Lysosomal free sialic acid storage disorders with different phenotypic presentations – infantile form sialic acid storage disease and Salla disease – represent allelic disorders on 6q14–15. *Am J Hum Genet* 1995; **57**: 893–901.

587 Schlote W, Harzer K, Christomanou H *et al.* Sphingolipid activator protein 1 deficiency in metachromatic leucodystrophy with normal arylsulphatase A activity. A clinical, morphological, biochemical and immunological study. *Eur J Pediatr* 1991; **150**: 584–91.

588 Schmidt B, Selmer T, Ingendoh A, von Figura K. A novel amino acid modification in sulfatases that is defective in multiple sulfatase deficiency. *Cell* 1995; **82**: 271–8.

589 Schmidt M, Fahnenstich H, Haverkamp F *et al.* Sialidose und Galaktosialidose als Ursache des nicht-immunologischen Hydrops fetalis. *Z Geburtshilfe Neonatol* 1997; **201**: 177–80.

590 Schnabel D, Schroder M, Frust W *et al.* Simultaneous deficiency of sphingolipid activator proteins 1 and 2 is caused by a mutation in the initiation cordon of their common gene. *J Biol Chem* 1992; **287**: 3312–15.

591 Schneider JA, Schulman JD. Cystinosis. In: Stanbury JB, Wyngaarden JB, Fredrickson DS *et al.* eds. *The metabolic basis of inherited disease*, 5th edn. New York: McGraw-Hill, 1983: 1844–67.

592 Schneider PB, Kennedy EP. Sphingomyelinase in normal human spleens and in spleens from subjects with Niemann–Pick disease. *J Lipid Res* 1967; **8**: 202–9.

593 Schnorf H, Bosshard NU, Gitzelmann R *et al.* Adult Form der GM2-Gangliosidose: drei Geschwister mit Hex-

osaminidase-A-und-B-Mangel (Morbus Sandhoff) und Literaturubersicht. *Schweiz Med Wochenschr* 1996; **126**: 757–64.

594 Schofer O, Mischo B, Puschel W *et al.* Early-lethal pulmonary form of Niemann–Pick disease type C disease belonging to a second, rare genetic complementation group. *Eur J Pediatr* 1998; **157**: 45–9.

595 Scholtz W. Klinische, pathologisch-anatomische und erbbiologische Untersuchungen bei familiarer, diffuser Hirnsklerose im Kindesalter. *Z Gestamte Neural Psychiatrie* 1925; **99**: 651–717.

596 Schuchman EH, Desnick RJ. Niemann–Pick disease types A and B: acid sphingomyelinase deficiencies. In: Scriver CR, Beaudet AL, Sly WS, Valle D eds. *The metabolic and molecular basis of inherited disease*. New York: McGraw Hill, 1995: 2601–24.

597 Scott HS, Blanch L, Guo XH *et al.* Cloning of the sulphamidase gene and identification of mutations in Sanfilippo A syndrome. *Nat Genet* 1995; **11**: 465–7.

598 Scriver CR, Beaudet AI, Sly W, Valle D eds. *The metabolic and molecular basis of inherited disease*, 7th edn. New York: McGraw-Hill, 1995.

599 Scriver CR, Beaudet AI, Valle D, Sly WS eds. *The metabolic and molecular basis of inherited disease*, 8th edn. New York: McGraw-Hill, 2001.

600 Semeraro LA, Riely CA, Kolodny EH *et al.* Niemann–Pick variant lipidosis presenting as 'neonatal hepatitis'. *J Pediatr Gastroenterol Nutr* 1986; **5**: 492–500.

601 Seppala R, Lehto VP, Gahl WA. Mutations in the human UDP-N-acetylglucosamine 2-epimerase gene define the disease sialuria and the allosteric site of the enzyme. *Am J Hum Genet* 1999; **64**: 1563–9.

602 Sewell AC. Urinary oligosaccharide excretion in disorders of glycolipid, glycoprotein and glycogen metabolism. *Eur J Pediatr* 1980; **134**: 183–94.

603 Shapiro LJ, Aleck KA, Kaback MM *et al.* Metachromatic leukodystrophy without arylsulfatase A deficiency. *Pediatr Res* 1979; **13**: 1179–83.

604 Sheahan NJ, Donnelly WJC, Grimes TD. Ocular pathology of bovine GM1 gangliosidosis. *Acta Neuropathol* 1978; **41**: 91–5.

605 Sherer DM, Metlay LA, Sinkin RA *et al.* Congenital ichthyosis with restrictive dermopathy and Gaucher's disease: a new syndrome with associated prenatal diagnosis and pathology findings. *Obstet Gynecol* 1993; **81**: 842–4.

606 Sherriff FE, Bridges LR, De Souza DSM. Non-Alzheimer neurofibrillary tangles show β-amyloid-like immunoreactivity. *NeuroReport* 1994; **5**: 1897–900.

607 Sheth KJ, Swick HM. Peripheral nerve conduction in Fabry's disease. *Ann Neurol* 1980; **7**: 319–23.

608 Shimamura K, Hakozaki H, Takahashi K *et al.* Sanfilippo B syndrome. A case report. *Acta Pathol Jpn* 1976; **26**: 739–64.

609 Shimmoto M, Kase R, Itoh K *et al.* Generation and characterization of transgenic mice expressing a human mutant α-galactosidase with R301Q substitution causing a variant form of Fabry disease. *FEBS Lett* 1997; **417**: 89–91.

610 Shipley JM, Klinkenberg M, Wu BM *et al.* Mutational analysis of a patient with mucopolysaccharidosis type VII, and identification of pseudogenes. *Am J Hum Genet* 1993; **52**: 517–26.

611 Shotelersuk V, Larson D, Anisker Y *et al.* CTNS mutations in an American-based population of cystinosis patients. *Am J Hum Genet* 1998; **63**: 1352–62.

612 Shows TB, Scrafford-Wolff LR, Brown JA, Meisler M. GM1-gangliosidosis: Chromosome 3 assignment of a β-galactosidase A gene (β-GalA). *Somat Cell Mol Genet* 1979; **5**: 147–58.

613 Shull RM, Hastings NE, Selcer RR et al. Bone marrow transplantation in canine mucopolysaccharidosis I. Effects within the central nervous system. J Clin Invest 1987; 79: 435–43.

614 Shull RM, Helman RG, Spellacy E et al. Morphologic and biochemical studies of canine mucopolysaccharidosis I. Am J Pathol 1984; 114: 487–95.

615 Shulman LM, David NJ, Weiner WJ. Psychosis as the initial manifestation of adult onset Niemann–Pick disease type C. Neurology 1995; 45: 1739–43.

616 Sidransky E, Sherer DM, Ginns EI. Gaucher disease in the neonate: a distinct Gaucher phenotype is analogous to a mouse model created by targeted disruption of the glucocerebrosidase gene. Pediatr Res 1992; 32: 494–8.

617 Sidransky E, Tayebi N, Stubblefield BK et al. The clinical, molecular and pathological characterization of a family with two cases of lethal perinatal type 2 Gaucher disease. J Med Genet 1996; 33: 132–4.

618 Siegel DA, Walkley SU. Growth of ectopic dendrites on cortical pyramidal neurons in neuronal storage diseases correlates with abnormal accumulation of GM2 ganglioside. J Neurochem 1994; 62: 1852–62.

619 Sima AA, Robertson DM. Involvement of peripheral nerve and muscle in Fabry's disease. Arch Neurol 1978; 35: 291–301.

620 Sjoberg I, Fransson LA, Matalon R, Dorfman A. Hunter's syndrome: a deficiency of L-idurono-sulfate-sulfatase. Biochem Biophys Res Commun 1973; 54: 1125–32.

621 Skelly BJ, Sargan DR, Winchester BG et al. Genomic screening for fucosidosis in english springer spaniels. Am J Vet Res 1999; 60: 726–9.

622 Slaugenhaupt SA, Acierno JS Jr, Helbling LA et al. Mapping of the mucolipidosis type IV gene to chromosome 19p and definition of founder haplotypes. Am J Hum Genet 1999; 65: 773–8.

623 Sleat DE. Donnelly R, Lackland H et al. Association of mutations in a lysosomal protein with classical late infantile neuronal ceroid lipofuscinosis. Science 1997; 277: 1802–5.

624 Sly WS, Quinton BA, McAlister WH, Rimoin DL. Beta glucuronidase deficiency: report of clinical, radiologic and biochemical features of a new mucopolysaccharidosis. J Pediatr 1973; 82: 249–57.

625 Smith MO, Wenger DA, Hill SL, Matthews J. Fucosidosis in a family of American-bred English springer spaniels. J Am Vet Med Assoc 1996; 209: 2088–90.

626 Soffer D, Yamanaka T, Wenger DA et al. Central nervous system involvement in adult-onset Gaucher's disease. Acta Neuropathol (Berl) 1980; 49: 1–6.

627 Sohar I, Sleat DE, Jadot M, Lobel P. Biochemical characterization of a lysosomal protease deficient in classical late infantile neuronal ceroid lipofuscinosis (LINCL) and development of an enzyme-based assay for diagnosis and exclusion of LINCL in human specimens and animal models. J Neurochem 1999; 73: 700–11.

628 Sokol J, Blanchette-Mackie J, Kruth GS et al. Type C Niemann–Pick disease. Lysosomal accumulation and defective intracellular mobilization of low density lipoprotein cholesterol. J Biol Chem 1988; 263: 3411–17.

629 Sonninen P, Autti T, Varho T et al. Brain involvement in Salla disease. Am J Neuroradiol 1999; 20: 433–43.

630 Sourander P, Olsson Y. Peripheral neuropathy in globoid cell leukodystrophy (Morbus Krabbe). Acta Neuropathol (Berl) 1968; 11: 69–81.

631 Spear GS. Pathology of the kidney in cystinosis. Pathol Ann 1974; 9: 81–92.

632 Specola N, Vanier MT, Goutieres F et al. The juvenile and chronic forms of GM2 gangliosidosis: clinical and enzymatic heterogeneity. Neurology 1990; 40: 145–50.

633 Sperl W, Bart G, Vanier MT et al. A family with visceral course of Niemann–Pick disease, macular halo syndrome and low sphingomyelin degradation rate. J Inherit Metab Dis 1994; 17: 93–103.

634 Spranger J, Cantz M. Mucolipidosis I, the cherry-red spot-myoclonus syndrome and neuraminidase deficiency. Birth Defects Orig Article Ser 1978; XIV (6B), 105–12.

635 Spranger J, Gehler J, Cantz M. Mucolipidosis I-a sialidosis. Am J Med Genet 1977; 1: 21–9.

636 Spranger JW, Wiedemann HR. The genetic mucolipidoses. Humangenetik 1970; 9: 113–39.

637 Steinman L, Tharp BR, Dorfman LJ et al. Peripheral neuropathy in the cherry-red spot-myoclonus syndrome (Sialidosis type I). Ann Neurol 1980; 7: 450–6.

638 Stevens RL, Fluharty AL, Kihara H et al. Cerebroside sulfatase activator deficiency induced metachromatic leukodystrophy. Am J Hum Genet 1981; 33: 900–6.

639 Stinchi S, Lullmann-Rauch R, Hartmann D et al. Targeted disruption of the lysosomal alpha-mannosidase gene results in mice resembling a mild form of human alpha-mannosidosis. Hum Mol Genet 1999; 8: 1365–72.

640 Stone DL, van Diggelen OP, de Klerk JB et al. Is the perinatal lethal form of Gaucher disease more common than classic type 2 Gaucher disease? Eur J Hum Genet 1999; 7: 505–9.

641 Strisciuglio P, Sly WS, Dodson WE et al. Combined deficiency of β-galactosidase and neuraminidase: natural history of the disease in the first 18 years of an American patient with late infantile onset form. Am J Med Genet 1990; 37: 573–7.

642 Sturmer J. Mukopolysaccharidose Typ VI-A (Morbus Maroteaux–Lamy). Klinisch-Pathologischer Fallbericht. Klin Monatsbl Augenheilk 1989; 194: 273–81.

643 Sugita M, Dulaney JT, Moser HW. Ceramidase deficiency in Farber's disease (lipogranulomatosis). Science 1972; 178: 1100–2.

644 Sun CC, Panny S, Comb J, Gutberlett R. Hydrops fetalis associated with Gaucher disease. Pathol Res Pract 1984; 179: 101–4.

645 Sung JH. Autonomic neurons affected by lipid storage in the spinal cord of Fabry's disease: distribution of autonomic neurons in the sacral cord. J Neuropathol Exp Neurol 1979; 38: 87–98.

646 Sung JH, Hayano M, Desnick RJ. Mannosidosis: pathology of the nervous system. J Neuropathol Exp Neurol 1977; 36: 807–20.

647 Suzuki K. Ultrastructural study of experimental globoid cells. Lab Invest 1970; 23: 612–19.

648 Suzuki K. Neuronal storage disease: a review. In: Zimmerman HM ed. Progress in neuropathology Vol. III. New York: Grune and Stratton, 1976: 173–202.

649 Suzuki K. Metabolic disease. In: Johannessen JV ed. Electron microscopy in human medicine. Vol. 6: Nervous system, sensory organs and respiratory tract. London: McGraw-Hill, 1979: 3–53.

650 Suzuki K. Neuropathology of late onset gangliosidoses. Dev Neurosci 1991; 13: 205–10.

651 Suzuki K, Grover WD. Krabbe's leukodystrophy (globoid cell leukodystrophy). An ultrastructural study. Arch Neurol 1970; 22: 385–96.

652 Suzuki K, Parker CC, Pentchev PG et al. Neurofibrillary tangles in Niemann–Pick disease type C. Acta Neuropathol 1995; 89: 227–38.

653 Suzuki K, Parker CC, Pentchev PG. Niemann–Pick disease type C: neuropathology revisited. Dev Brain Dysfunc 1997; 10: 306–20.

654 Suzuki K, Proia RL, Suzuki K. Mouse models of human lysosomal diseases. Brain Pathol 1998; 8: 195–215.

655 Suzuki K, Suzuki K. The gangliosidoses. In: Moser H ed. *Neurodystropies and neurolipidosis* Revised Series 22. Amsterdam: Elsevier, 1996: 247–80.

656 Suzuki K, Suzuki Y. Globoid cell leucodystrophy (Krabbe's disease): deficiency of galactocerebroside β-galactosidase. *Proc Nat Acad Sci USA* 1970; **66**: 302–9.

657 Suzuki K, Suzuki K, Chen G. Metachromatic Leucodystrophy: isolation and chemical analysis of metachromatic granules. *Science* 1966; **151**: 1231–3.

658 Suzuki K, Suzuki K, Chen GC. Isolation and chemical characterization of metachromatic granules from a brain with metachromatic leukodystrophy. *J Neuropathol Exp Neurol* 1967; **26**: 537–50

659 Suzuki K, Suzuki K, Chen GC. Morphological, histochemical and biochemical studies on a case of systemic late infantile lipidosis (generalized gangliosidosis). *J Neuropathol Exp Neurol* 1968; **27**: 15–28.

660 Suzuki K, Suzuki K, Kamoshita S. Chemical pathology of GM1-gangliosidosis (generalized gangliosidosis). *J Neuropathol Exp Neurol* 1969; **28**: 25–73.

661 Suzuki K, Suzuki K, Rapin I et al. Juvenile GM2-gangliosidosis. *Neurology* 1970; **20**: 190–204.

662 Suzuki K, Suzuki Y, Suzuki K. Galactosylceramide lipidosis: Globopid -cell leukodystrophy (Krabbe disease). In: Scriver CR, Beaudet AL, Sly W, Valle D eds. *The metabolic and molecular basis of inherited disease*, 7th edn. New York: Mc-Graw-Hill, Inc. 1995: 2671–92.

663 Suzuki Y, Jacob JC, Suzuki K et al. GM2 gangliosidosis with total hexosaminidase deficiency. *Neurology* 1971; **21**: 313–28.

664 Suzuki Y, Nakamura N, Shimada Y et al. Macular cherry-red spots and beta-galactosidase deficiency in an adult: an autopsy case with progressive cerebellar ataxia, myoclonus, thrombocytopathy, and accumulation of polysaccharide in liver. *Arch Neurol* 1977; **34**: 157–61.

665 Suzuki Y, Nakamura N, Fukuoka K et al. β-Galactosidase deficiency in juvenile and adult patients. *Hum Genet* 1977; **36**: 219–29.

666 Suzuki Y, Namba E, Tsuji A et al. Clinical heterogeneity in galactosialidosis. *Dev Brain Dysfunc* 1988; **1**: 285–93.

667 Suzuki Y, Sakuraba H, Oshima A. β-Galactosidase deficiency (β-galactosidosis): GM1 gangliosidosis and Morquio B disease. In: Scriver CR, Beaudet Al, Sly WS, Valle D eds. *The metabolic and molecular basis of inherited diseases*. New York: McGraw-Hill, 1995: 2785–823.

668 Svennerholm L. Some aspects of the biochemical changes in leucodystrophy. In: Folchi-pi J, Bauer H eds. *Brain lipids and lipoproteins, and the leucodystrophies*. Amsterdam: Elsevier, 1963: 104–19.

669 Svennerholm L, Vanier M-T, Mansson J-E. Krabbe disease: a galactosylsphingosine (psychosine) lipidosis. *J Lipid Res* 1980; **21**: 53–64.

670 Sweeley CC, Klinosky B. Fabry's disease: classification as a sphingolipidosis and partial characterization of a novel glycolipid. *J Biol Chem* 1963; **238**: 3148–50.

671 Tabira T, Goto I, Kuroiwa Y. Neuropathological and biochemical studies in Fabry's disease. *Acta Neuropathol (Berl)*. 1974; **30**: 345–54.

672 Tagliavini F, Pietrini V, Pilleri G et al. Adult metachromatic leukodystrophy: clinicopathological report of two familial cases with slow course. *Neuropathol Appl Neurobiol* 1979; **5**: 233–43.

673 Takada G, Satoh K, Komatsu K et al. Transitory type of sphingomyelinase deficient Niemann–Pick disease: clinical and morphological studies and follow-up of two sisters. *Tohoku J Exp Med* 1987; **153**: 27–36.

674 Takano T, Shimmoto M, Fukuhara Y et al. Galactosialidosis: clinical and molecular analysis of 19 Japanese patients. *Brain Dysfunc* 1991; **4**: 271–80.

675 Takashima S, Becker LE, Chan FW, Augustin R. Golgi and computer morphometric analysis of cortical dendrites in metabolic storage disease. *Exp Neurol* 1985; **88**: 652–72.

676 Takebayashi S, Bassewitz H, Themann H. Feinstructurelle Veranderungen der Niere bei generalisierter Gangliosidose GM1. *Virchow Arch Abtilung B Zellpathol* 1970; **5**: 301–13.

677 Tamagawa K, Morimatsu Y, Fujisawa K et al. Neuropathological study and chemico-pathological correlation in sibling cases of Sanfilippo syndrome type B. *Brain Dev* 1985; **7**: 599–609.

678 Tamaki N, Kojima N, Tanimoto M et al. Myelopathy due to diffuse thickening of the cervical dura mater in Maroteaux–Lamy syndrome: report of a case. *Neurosurgery* 1987; **21**: 416–19.

679 Tanaka A, Ohno K, Suzuki K. GM2 ganglioside B1 variant. A wide geographic and ethnic distribution of the specific β-hexosaminidase α-chain mutation originally identified in a Puerto Rican patient. *Biochem Biophys Res Commun* 1988; **156**: 1015–19.

680 Tanaka A, Sakazaki H, Murakami H et al. Molecular genetics of Tay–Sachs disease in Japan. *J Inherit Metab Dis* 1994; **17**: 593–600.

681 Tanaka J, Garcia JH, Max SR et al. Cerebral sponginess and GM3 gangliosidosis: ultrastructure and probable pathogenesis. *J Neuropathol Exp Neurol* 1975; **34**: 249–62.

682 Tanaka J. Nakamura H, Miyawaki S. Cerebellar involvement in murine sphingomyelinosis: A new model of Niemann–Pick disease. *J Neuropathol Exp Neurol* 1988; **47**: 291–300.

683 Taniike M, Yamanaka S, Proia RL et al. Neuropathology of mice with targeted disruption of Hexa gene, a model of Tay–Sachs disease. *Acta Neuropathol* 1995; **89**: 296–304.

684 Tatsumi N, Inui K, Sakai N et al. Molecular defects in Krabbe disease. *Hum Mol Genet* 1995; **4**: 1865–8.

685 Tay W. Symmetrical changes in the region of the yellow spot in each eye of an infant. *Trans Ophthalmol Soc UK* 1881; **1**: 155–7.

686 Tayebi N, Cushner SR, Kleijer W et al. Prenatal lethality of a homozygous null mutation in the human glucocerebrosidase gene. *Am J Med Genet* 1997; **73**: 41–7.

687 Tedeschi G, Bonavita S, Banerjee TK et al. Diffuse central neuronal involvement in Fabry disease: a proton MRS imaging study. *Neurology* 1999; **52**: 1663–7.

688 Tellez-Nagel I, Rapin I, Iwamoto T et al. Mucolipidosis IV. Clinical, ultrastructural, histochemical, and chemical studies of a case, including a brain biopsy. *Arch Neurol* 1976; **33**: 828–35.

689 Tenhunen K, Uusitalo A, Autti T et al. Monitoring the CNS pathology in aspartylglucosaminuria mice. *J Neuropathol Exp Neurol* 1998; **57**: 1154–63.

690 Terry RD, Weiss M. Studies in Tay–Sachs disease II. Ultrastructure of the cerebrum. *J Neuropathol Exp Neurol* 1963; **22**: 18–55.

691 Thomas GH, Beaudet AL. Disorders of glycoprotein degradation and structure: α-mannosidosis, β-mannosidosis, fucosidosis, sialidosis, aspartylglucosaminuria and carbohydrate-deficient glycoprotein syndrome. In: Scriver CR, Beaudet A, Sly WS, Valle D eds. *The metabolic and molecular basis of inherited disease*. New York: McGraw-Hill, 1995: 2529–61.

692 Thomas GH, Taylor HA, Reynolds LW, Miller CS. Mucolipidosis III (pseudo Hurler polydystrophy). Multiple lysosomal enzyme abnormalities in serum and cultured fibroblast cells. *Pediatr Res* 1973; **7**: 751–6.

693 Thomas PK, Halpern J-P, King RHM, Patrick D. Galactosyl-ceramide lipidosis: novel presentation as slowly progressive spinocerebellar degeneration. *Ann Neurol* 1984; **16**: 618–20.

694 Thomas PK, King RHM, Kocen RS, Brett EM. Comparative ultrastructural observations on peripheral nerve abnormalities in the late infantile, juvenile and late onset forms of metachromatic leukodystrophy. *Acta Neuropathol (Berl)* 1977; **39**: 237–45.

695 Tietze F, Seppala R, Renlund M *et al*. Defective lysosomal egress of free sialic acid in fibroblasts of patients with infantile free sialic acid storage disease. *J Biol Chem* 1989; **264**: 15316–22.

696 Tobo M, Mitsuyama Y, Ikari K, Itoi K. Familial occurrence of adult-type neuronal ceroid lipofuscinosis. *Arch Neurol* 1984; **41**: 1091–4.

697 Tome FMS, Fardeau M, Lenoir G. Ultrastructure of muscle and sensory nerve in Fabry's disease. *Acta Neuropathol (Berl)* 1977; **38**: 187–94.

698 Tondeur M, Resibois A. Fabry's disease in children. *Virchow Arch Abteilung B Zellpathol* 1969; **2**: 239–54.

699 Tondeu M, Libert J, Vamos E *et al*. Infantile form of sialic acid storage disorder: clinical, ultrastructural, and biochemical studies in two siblings. *Eur J Pediatr* 1982; **139**: 142–47.

700 Toppet M, Vamos-Hurwitz E, Jonniaux G *et al*. Farber's disease as a ceramidosis: clinical, radiological and biochemical aspects. *Acta Paediatr* 1978; **67**: 113–19.

701 Town M, Jean G, Cherqui S *et al*. A novel gene encoding an integral membrane protein is mutated in nephropathic cystinosis. *Nat Genet* 1998; **18**: 319–24.

702 Troost J, Straks W, Willemse J. Fucosidosis II. Ultrastructure. *Neuropaediatrie* 1977; **8**: 163–71.

703 Tybulewicz VLJ, Tremblay ML, LaMarca ME *et al*. Aninal model of Gaucher's disease from targeted disruption of the mouse glucocerebrosidase gene. *Nature* 1992; **357**: 407–10.

704 Tyynela J, Baumann M, Henseler M *et al*. Sphingolipid activator proteins in the neuronal ceroid-lipofuscinosis: an immunological study. *Acta Neuropathol (Berl)* 1995; **89**: 391–8.

705 Tyynela J, Suopanki J, Baumann M, Haltia M. Sphingolipid activator proteins (SAPs) in neuronal ceroid lipofuscinosis (NCL). *Neuropediatrics* 1997; **28**: 49–52.

706 Umehara F, Matsumoto W, Kuriyama M *et al*. Mucolipidosis III (pseudo-Hurler polydystrophy); clinical studies in aged patients in one family. *J Neurol Sci* 1997; **146**: 167–72.

707 Ushiyama M, Ikeda S, Nakayama J *et al*. Type III (chronic) GM1-gangliosidosis. Histochemical and ultrastructural studies of rectal biopsy. *J Neurol Sci* 1985; **71**: 209–23.

708 Van de Kamp J, Niermeijer MF, von Figura K, Giesberts MA. Genetic heterogeneity and clinical variability in the Sanfilippo syndrome (types A B, and C). *Clin Genet* 1981; **20**: 152–60.

709 Van Diggelen OP, Keulemans JLM, Winchester B *et al*. A rapid fluorogenic palmitoyl-protein thioesterase assay for pre- and postnatal diagnosis of INCL. *Mol Genet Metab* 1999; **66**: 240–4.

710 Van Diggelen OP, Schindler D, Willemsen R *et al*. Alpha-*N*-acetylgalactosaminidase deficiency, a new lysosomal storage disorder. *J Inherit Metab Dis* 1988; **11**: 349–57.

711 Van Hoof F, Hers HG. Mucopolysaccharidoses by absence of alpha-fucosidase. *Lancet* 1968; **i**: 1198.

712 Van Hoof F, Hers HG. The abnormalities of lysosomal enzymes in mucopolysaccharidoses. *Eur J Biochem* 1968; **7**: 34–44.

713 Vanier M, Svennerholm L. Chemical pathology of Krabbe disease: the occurrence of psychosine and other neutral sphingoglycolipids. In: Volk BW, Schneck L eds. *Current trends in sphingolipidoses and allied disorders* Vol. 68. New York: Plenum Press, 1976: 115–26.

714 Vanier MT. Lipid changes in Niemann–Pick disease type C brain: personal experience and review of the literature. *Neurochem Res* 1999; **24**: 481–9.

715 Vanier MT, Rousson RM, Mandon G *et al*. Diagnosis of Niemann–Pick disease type C on chorionic villus cells. *Lancet* 1989; **i**: 1014–15.

716 Vanier M T, Suzuki K. Niemann–Pick diseases. In: Moser HW ed. *Handbook of clinical neurology*, Vol. 22 (66): *Neurodystrophies and neurolipidoses*, Amsterdam: Elsevier, 1996: 133–62.

717 Vanier MT, Suzuki K. Recent advances in elucidating Niemann–Pick C disease. *Brain Pathol* 1998; **8**: 163–74.

718 Vanier MT, Svennerholm L. Chemical pathology of Krabbe's disease, II. Fatty acid composition of cerebrosides, sulfatides and sphingomyelins in brain. *Acta Paediatr Scand* 1974; **63**: 501–6.

719 Vanier MT, Svennerholm L. Chemical pathology of Krabbe's disease, III. Ceramide hexosides and gangliosides of brain. *Acta Paediatr Scand* 1975; **64**: 641–8.

720 Vanier MT, Wenger DA, Comly ME *et al*. Niemann–Pick disease group C: clinical variability and diagnosis based on defective cholesterol esterification. A collaborative study on 70 patients. *Clin Genet* 1988; **33**: 331–48.

721 Verdru P, Lammens M, Dom R *et al*. Globoid cell leukodystrophy: a family with both late -infantile and adult type. *Neurology* 1991; **41**: 1382–4.

722 Verheijen FW, Verbeek E, Aula N *et al*. A new gene, encoding an anion transporter, is mutated in sialic acid storage diseases. *Nat Genet* 1999; **23**: 462–5.

723 Vesa J, Hellsten E, Verkruyse LA *et al*. Mutations in the palmitoyl-protein thioesterase gene causing infantile neuronal ceroid lipofuscinosis. *Nature* 1995; **376**: 584–7.

724 Victoria T, Rafi MA, Wenger DA. Cloning of the canine GALC cDNA and identification of the mutation causing globoid cell leukodystrophy in West Highland White and Cairn terriers. *Genomics* 1996; **33**: 457–62.

725 Vidgoff J, Lovrien EW, Beals R K, Buist NRM. Mannosidosis in three brothers – a review of the literature. *Medicine* 1977; **56**: 335–48.

726 Vogel DG, Malekzadeh MH, Cornford ME *et al*. Central nervous system involvement in nephropathic cystinosis. *J Neuropathol Exp Neurol* 1990; **49**: 591–9.

727 Vogler C, Levy B, Galvin NJ *et al*. Enzyme replacement in murine mucopolysaccharidosis type VII: Neuronal and glial response to β-glucuronidase requires early initiation of enzyme replacement therapy. *Pediatr Res* 1999; **45**: 838–44.

728 Vogler C, Levy B, Kyle JW *et al*. Mucopolysaccharidosis VII: postmortem biochemical and pathological findings in a young adult with beta-glucuronidase deficiency. *Modern Pathol* 1994; **7**: 132–7.

729 Volk BW, Schneck L, Adachi M. The clinic, pathology and biochemistry of Tay–Sachs disease. In: Vinken PJ, Bruyn GW eds. *Handbook of clinical neurology*. Amsterdam: North-Holland, 1970: 385–426.

730 Von Hirsch TH, Peiffer J. Uber histologische Methoden in der Differentialdiagnose von Leukodystrophien und Lipoidosen. *Arch Psychiatrie Z Neurol* 1955; **194**: 88–104.

731 Von Scheidt W, Eng CM, Fitzmaurice TF *et al*. An atypical variant of Fabry's disease confined to the heart. *N Engl J Med* 1991; **324**: 395–9.

732 Voskovoeva E, Isrrandi K, Von Figura K et al. Four novel mutant alleles of the arylsulfatase B gene in two patients with intermediate form of mucopolysaccharidosis VI (Maroteaux–Lamy syndrome). Hum Genet 1994; 93: 259–64.

733 Waheed AB, Pohlman R, Hasilik A et al. Deficiency of UDP-N-acetylglucosamine: lysosomal enzyme N-acetylglucosamine-1-phosphotransferase in organs of I-cell patients. Biochem Biophys Res Commun 1982; 105: 1052–8.

734 Walvoot HC. Glycogen storage diseases in animals and their potential value as models of human disease. J Inherit Metab Dis 1983; 6: 3–16.

735 Walvoort HC, Dormans JAMA, van den Ingh TSGAM. Comparative pathology of the canine model of glycogen storage type II (Pompe's disease). J Inherit Metab Dis 1985; 8: 38–46.

736 Walkley SU. Further studies on ectopic dendrite growth and other geometrical distortions of neurons in feline GM1 gangliosidosis. Neuroscience 1987; 21: 313–31.

737 Walkley SU. Pyramidal neurons with ectopic dendrites in storage diseases contain elevated levels of GM2 ganglioside. Neuroscience 1995; 68: 1027–35.

738 Walkley SU. Cellular pathology of lysosomal storage disorders. Brain Pathol 1998; 8: 175–93.

739 Walkley SU, Baker HJ. Sphingomyelin lipidosis in a cat: Golgi studies. Acta Neuropathol 1984; 65: 138–44.

740 Walkley SU, Blakemore WF, Purpura DP. Alterations in neuron morphology in feline mannosidosis. A Golgi study. Acta Neuropathol (Berl) 1981; 53: 75–9.

741 Walkley SU, Haskins ME, Shull RM. Alterations in neuron morphology in mucopolysaccharidosis type I. A Golgi study. Acta Neuropathol (Berl) 1988; 75: 611–20.

742 Walkley SU, March PA, Schroeder CE et al. Pathogenesis of brain dysfunction in Batten disease. Am J Med Genet 1995; 57: 196–203.

743 Walkley SU, Pierok AL. Ferric ion-ferrocyanide staining in ganglioside storage disease establishes that meganeurites are of axon hillock origin and distinct from axonal spheroids. Brain Res 1986; 382: 379–86.

744 Walkley SU, Siegel DA, Dobrenis K. GM2 ganglioside and pyramidal neuron dendritogenesis. Neurochem Res 1995; 20: 1287–99.

745 Walkley SU, Wurzelmann S, Rattazzi MC, Baker HJ. Distribution of ectopic neurite growth and other geometrical distortion of CNS neurons in feline GM2 gangliosidosis. Brain Res 1990; 510: 63–73.

746 Wang AM, Desnick RJ. Structural organization and complete sequence of the human α-N-acetylgalactosaminidase gene: homology with the α-galactosidase A gene provides evidence for evolution from a common ancestral gene. Genomics 1991; 10: 133–42.

747 Wang AM, Ioannou YA, Zeidner KM et al. Fabry disease: generation of a mouse model with α-galactosidase A deficiency (abstract). Am J Hum Genet 1996; 59 Suppl: A208.

748 Wang AM, Schindler D, Desnick R. Schindler disease: the molecular lesion in the alpha-N-acetylgalactosaminidase gene that causes an infantile neuroaxonal dystrophy. J Clin Invest 1990; 86: 1752–6.

749 Wang AM, Stewart CL, Desnick RJ. α-N-Acetylgalactosaminidase: characterization of the murine cDNA and genomic sequences and generation of the mice by targeted gene disruption (abstract). Am J Hum Genet 1993; 53: A99.

750 Weintraub H, Abramovici A, Sandbank U et al. Neurological mutation characterized by dysmyelination in NCTR-Balb/C mouse with lysosomal lipid storage disease. J Neurochem 1985; 45: 665–72.

751 Weiss P, Teitze F, Gahl WA et al. Identification of the metabolic defect in sialuria. J Biol Chem 1989; 264: 17635–6.

752 Wenger DA, DeGala G, Williams C et al. Clinical, pathological, and biochemical studies on an infantile case of sulfatide/GM1 activator protein deficiency. Am J Med Genet 1989; 33: 255–65.

753 Wenger DA, Rafi MA, Luzi P. Molecular genetics of Krabbe disease (globoid cell leukodystrophy): diagnostic and clinical implications. Hum Mutat 1997; 19: 268–79.

754 Wenger DA, Sattler M, Kudoh T et al. Niemann–Pick disease: a genetic model in Siamese cats. Science 1980; 208: 1471–3.

755 Wenger DA, Sattler M, Mueller OT et al. Adult GM1 gangliosidosis: clinical and biochemical studies on two patients and comparison to other patients called variant or adult GM1 gangliosidosis. Clin Genet 1980; 17: 323–34.

756 Wenger DA, Sujansky E, Fennessey PV, Thompson JN. Human β-mannosidase deficiency. N Engl J Med 1986; 315: 1201–5.

757 Wenger DA, Suzuki K, Suzuki Y, Suzuki K. Galactosylceramide lipidosis: globoid cell leukodystrophy (Krabbe disease). In: Scriver CR, Beaudet AL, Sly WS, Valle D eds. The metabolic and molecular basis of inherited disease, 8th edn. New York: McGraw-Hill, 2001: 3669–94.

758 Wenger DA, Tarby TJ, Wharton C. Macular cherry-red spots and myoclonus with dementia. Coexistent neuraminidase and β-galactosidase deficiencies. Biochem Biophys Res Commun 1978; 82: 589–95.

759 Whitley CB. The mucopolysaccharidoses. In: Moser HW ed. Handbook of Clinical Neurology Vol. 22 (66): Neurodystrophies and neurolipidosis. Amsterdam: Elsevier, 1996: 281–327.

760 Wiesmann UN, Lightbody J, Vassella F, Herschkowitz NN. Multiple lysosomal enzyme deficiency due to enzyme leakage? N Engl J Med 1971; 284: 109–10.

761 Wiesmann UN, Vassella F, Herschkowitz NN. I-Cell disease: leakage of lysosomal enzymes into extracellular fluids. N Engl J Med 1971; 285: 1090–1.

762 Wilkerson MJ, Lewis DC, Marks SL, Prieur DJ. Clinical and morphological features of mucopolysaccharidosis type II in a dog: naturally occurring model of Hunter syndrome. Vet Pathol 1998; 35: 230–3.

763 Willems PJ, Gatti R, Darby JK et al. Fucosidosis revisited: a review of 77 patients. Am J Med Genet 1991; 38: 111–31.

764 Willems PJ, Seo H-C, Coucke P et al. Spectrum of mutations in fucosidosis. Eur J Hum Genet 1999; 7: 60–67.

765 Willemsen R, Tybulewicz E, Sidransky E et al. A biochemical and ultrastructural evaluation of the type 2 Gaucher mouse. Mol Chem Neuropathol 1995; 24: 179–92.

766 Williams RE, Gottlob I, Lake BD et al. Classic late infantile NCL. In: Gobel HH, Mole SE, Lake BD eds. The neuronal ceroid lipofuscinoses (Batten disease). Amsterdam: IOS Press, 1999: 37–54.

767 Williams RS, Ferrante RJ, Caviness VS. The isolated human cortex. A Golgi analysis of Krabbe's disease. Arch Neurol 1979; 36: 134–9.

768 Willner JP, Grabowski GA, Gordon RE et al. Chronic GM2 gangliosidosis masquerading as atypical Friedreich ataxia: clinical, morphologic, and biochemical studies of nine cases. Neurology 1981; 31: 787–98.

769 Winchester B, Young E, Geddes S et al. Female twin with Hunter disease due to non-random inactivation of the X-chromosome: a consequence of twinning. Am J Med Genet 1992; 44: 834–8.

770 Winkelman MD, Banker G, Victor M, Moser HW. Non-infantile neuronopathic Gaucher's disease: a clinicopathologic study. Neurology 1983; 33: 994–1008.

771 Wisniewski KE, Commell F, Kaczmanski W et al. Palmitoyl-protein thioesterase deficiency in a novel granular variant of LINCL. Pediatr Neurol 1998; 18: 119–23.

772 Wisniewski K, Rudelli R, Laure-Kamionowska M et al. Sanfilippo disease, type A with some features of ceroid lipofuscinosis. Neuropediatrics 1985; 16: 98–105.

773 Wolburg-Buchholz K, Schlote W, Baumkotter J et al. Familial lysosomal storage disease with generalized vacuolation and sialic aciduria. Sporadic Salla disease. Neuropediatrics 1985; 16: 67–75.

774 Wolf D. Infantile neuroaxonal dystrophy associated with α-acetylgalactosaminidase deficiency: on relating axonal spheroids to a lysosomal enzyme deficiency. In: Asbury AK, Budka H, Sluga E eds. Sensory neuropathies. Vienna: Springer-Verlag, 1995: 197–207.

775 Wolf D. Neuroaxonal dystrophy in infantile alpha-N-acetylgalactosaminidase deficiency. J Neurol Sci 1995; 132: 44–56.

776 Wolf HJ, Pietra GG. The visceral lesions of metachromatic leukodystrophy. Am J Pathol 1964; 44: 921–30.

777 Wolf LS, Callahan J, Fawcett JSD et al. GM1-gangliosidosis without chondrodystrophy or visceromegaly. Neurology 1970; 20: 23–44.

778 Wu RM, Sly WS. Mutational studies in a patient with the hydrops fetalis form of mucopolysaccharodosis type VII. Hum Mutat 1993; 2: 446–57.

779 Yamada S, Tomatsu S, Sly WS et al. Four novel mutations in mucopolysaccharidosis type VII including a unique base substitution in exon 10 of the beta glucuronidase gene that creates a novel 5'-splice site. Hum Mol Genet 1995; 4: 651–5.

780 Yamanaka S, Johnson MD, Grinberg A et al. Targeted disruption of the Hexa gene results in mice with biochemical and pathologic features of Tay–Sachs disease. Proc Nat Acad Sci USA 1994; 91: 9975–79.

781 Yamano T, Shimada M, Matsuzaki K et al. Pathological study on a severe sialidosis (α-neuraminidase deficiency). Acta Neuropathol (Berl) 1986; 71: 278–84.

782 Yamano T, Shimada M, Okada S et al. Ultrastructural study of biopsy specimens of rectal mucosa. Arch Pathol Lab Med 1982; 106: 673–7.

783 Yamano T, Shimada M, Okada S et al. Ultrastructural study on nervous system of fetus with GM1-gangliosidosis type 1. Acta Neuropathol 1983; 64: 15–20.

784 Yamano T, Shimada M, Sugino H et al. Ultrastructural study on a severe infantile sialidosis (beta-galactosidase-alpha-neuraminidase deficiency). Neuropediatrics 1985; 16: 109–12.

785 Yoshida K, Ikeda S, Kawaguchi K, Yanagisawa N. Adult GM1 gangliosidosis. Neurology 1994; 44: 2376–82.

786 Yoshida H, Kuriyama M. Genetic lipid storage disease with lysosomal acid lipase deficiency in rats. Lab Anim Sci 1990; 40: 486–9.

787 Yoshino H, Miyashita K, Miyatani N et al. Abnormal glycosphingolipid metabolism in the nervous system of galactosialidosis. J Neurol Sci 1990; 97: 53–65.

788 Young ID, Harper PS. Mild form of Hunter's syndrome: clinical delineation based on 31 cases. Arch Dis Child 1982; 57: 828–36

789 Young ID, Harper PS. The natural history of the severe form of Hunter's syndrome: a study based on 52 cases. Dev Med Child Neurol 1983; 25: 481–9.

790 Young ID, Harper PS, Newcombe RG, Archer IM. A clinical and genetic study of Hunter's syndrome. 2. Differences between the mild and severe forms. J Med Genet 1982; 19: 408–11.

791 Young R, Kleinman G, Ojemann RG et al. Compressive myelopathy in Maroteaux-Lamy syndrome: clinical and pathological findings. Ann Neurol 1980; 8: 336–40.

792 Yunis EJ, Lee RE. The ultrastructure of globoid (Krabbe) leukodystrophy. Lab Invest 1969; 21: 415–19.

793 Yunis EJ, Lee RE. Tubules of globoid leukodystrophy: a right handed helix. Science 1970; 169: 64–6.

794 Zappatini-Tommasi L, Dumontel C, Guibaud P, Girod C. Farber disease: an ultrastructural study. Virchows Arch A Pathol Anat 1992; 420: 281–90.

795 Zarbin MA, Green WR, Moser HW, Morton SJ. Farber's disease: light and electron microscopic study of the eye. Arch Ophthalmol 1985; 103: 73–80.

796 Zeman W, Dyken P. Neuronal ceroid lipofuscinosis (Batten's disease): relationship to amaurotic family idiocy? Pediatrics 1969; 44: 570–83.

797 Zevin S, Abrahamov A, Hadas-Halpern I et al. Adult type Gaucher disease in children: genetic, clinical features and enzyme replacement therapy. Q J Med 1993; 86: 565–73.

798 Zhao HG, Li HH, Bach G et al. The molecular basis of Sanfilippo syndrome type B. Proc Nat Acad Sci USA 1996; 93: 6101–5.

499 Zhou XY, Morreau H, Rottier R et al. Mouse model for the lysosomal disorder galactosialidosis and correction of the phenotype with overexpressing erythroid precursor cells. Genes Dev 1995; 9: 2623–34.

800 Ziegler RJ, Yew NS, Li C et al. Correction of enzymatic and lysosomal storage defects in Fabry mice by adenovirus-mediated gene transfer. Hum Gene Ther 1999; 10: 1667–82.

801 Zimran A, Kay A, Saven A et al. Gaucher disease: clinical, laboratory, radiologic and genetic features in 53 patients. Medicine (Baltimore) 1992; 71: 337–53.

12

Peroxisomal and mitochondrial disorders

JAMES M. POWERS AND DARRYL C. DE VIVO

INTRODUCTION

Peroxisomal and mitochondrial disorders have been estimated to be responsible for approximately 30% of human metabolic diseases, with mitochondrial being about twice as common as peroxisomal disorders.[10] Although most of their metabolic functions are divergent, both peroxisomes and mitochondria are involved in the β-oxidation of fatty acids and the oxidation of phytanic acid.[392] Long-chain fatty acids are oxidized in mitochondria, whereas very long-chain fatty acids (> C22, VLCFA) and branched-chain fatty acids are initially oxidized in peroxisomes and then transferred to mitochondria for completion of the process.[395] In yeast, where β-oxidation of fatty acids is confined to peroxisomes, the acetyl-coenzyme A (CoA) produced there must be transported by carnitine into mitochondria to be degraded to CO_2 and H_2O.[384] Peroxisomes are abundant in cells characterized by a 'vigorous mitochondrial population'.[72] Both peroxisomes and mitochondria have been highly conserved throughout evolution; both are believed to have evolved to their present state because these organelles bestowed a selective advantage on the host cells. Mammalian peroxisomes may have evolved from a primitive respiratory system that developed in order to deal with the hydrogen peroxide generated by aerobic living, such as the glycosomes of protozoa that are parasitic to man. Mitochondria are believed to be prokaryotic structures: perhaps bacteria, that colonized or parasitized the cytoplasm of eukaryotic cells long ago.[6]

The diseases induced by abnormalities in these organelles provide additional connections. Firstly, disorders of both peroxisomes and mitochondria produce systemic, multiorgan (multisystemic) lesions. In disorders of peroxisomes, the central nervous system (CNS), eyes, skeleton, liver and adrenal are most severely involved,[273] while in mitochondrial disorders the CNS, skeletal muscle, eyes, heart, liver and kidney bear the brunt of the defect.[88] Both types of disorders involve grey and white matter. Both are associated with optic atrophy, atypical pigmentary retinopathy and sensorineural deafness. Both may display hepatic lesions ranging from portal fibrosis to cirrhosis. Secondly, both have shown marked phenotypic heterogeneity and poor genotype–phenotype correlations, suggesting a role for modifier genes or epigenetic factors. The correlations, however, are improving with the insights provided by molecular data. For example, the nature of the affected gene mutation with the consequent residual activity of its gene product and mosaicism are beginning to explain some phenotypic differences in the peroxisome biogenesis disorders (PBDs). Similarly, the phenotypic severity in some of the mitochondrial disorders seems to correlate directly with the percentage of mutant mitochondrial DNA (mtDNA) in affected individuals, even though the biochemical correlations are still imprecise. Thirdly, several peroxisomal disorders exhibit mitochondrial abnormalities, including Zellweger's syndrome (ZS), the first peroxisomal disease recognized in man.[126,128,149,156] Fourthly, fatty/organic acids appear to play pivotal pathogenic roles in both types of disorders.

In spite of these points of similarity there are even greater differences. Neurological deficits in peroxisomal disorders tend to reflect involvement of either grey matter, particularly neuronal migration abnormalities, or white matter, particularly dysmyelination and demyelination. Neuronal loss, spongy myelinopathy and striated muscle involvement are typical of mitochondrial disorders. Angulate lysosomes in hepatic macrophages typify some peroxisomal disorders, while neutral lipid droplets in hepatocytes (steatosis) are seen in some disorders of mitochondria. Perhaps the most important difference is that mitochondria possess their own DNA, while

Table 12.1 *Disorders of peroxisomes and mitochondria*

	Peroxisomes	Mitochondria
Major localization	CNS	CNS
	WM > GM	GM > WM
Histopathological lesions	Demyelination/dysmyelination	Dead neurons
	Misguided neurons	Spongy myelin
Spongy change		●
Vascularity		●
Mineralization		●
Inflammation	●	
Oligodendroglial loss	●	
Astrocytosis	●	●
Microgliosis	●	●
Ultrastructural lesions	Abnormal peroxisomes,	Abnormal mitochondria with paracrystalloids
	Spicules in angulate lysosomes (PBD);	
	Lamellae (ALD/AMN)	
Biochemical defect	Fatty acids (VLCFA)	Organic acids (lactic acid)
Molecular defect	Importation	Multiple for nDNA
		Heteroplasmy for mtDNA
Systemic involvement	●	●
Adrenal	●	
Ears	●	●
Eyes	●	●
Gastrointestinal		●
Heart		●
Kidney	●	●
Liver	● (Angulate lysosomes)	● (Steatosis)
Skeletal muscle		●
Skeleton	●	

WM, white matter; GM, grey matter.

peroxisomes do not. This leads to a bewildering array of inheritance patterns and even more heterogeneity than is seen in peroxisomal diseases.

PEROXISOMES AND PEROXISOMAL DISORDERS (Table 12.1)

Peroxisomes, originally called a 'microbody' under the electron microscope,[299] are found in all nucleated cells of plants (glyoxysomes) and mammals. Human peroxisomes are characterized ultrastructurally by a granular, electron-dense matrix surrounded by a unit membrane; a shape that varies from primarily spherical, with diameters of approximately 0.1–1.0 μm, to elongated tubular (reticulum); and the presence of catalase within the matrix as demonstrated by enhanced electron density after diaminobenzidine staining. The latter technique can also identify peroxisomes at the light-microscopic level, but specific antibodies to peroxisomal matrix and membrane proteins[171,314] have become another popular and informative method. Membrane-bound or particulate catalase activity, versus cytosolic or soluble, has been the traditional biochemical marker. Catalase appears to be the least efficiently imported matrix pro-

tein; hence, its absence in particulate form does not indicate that peroxisomes must lack all matrix proteins.[130a] Much of our understanding of mammalian peroxisomes has been derived through studies of hepatic and renal tubular peroxisomes; the investigation of yeast peroxisomes, which are highly homologous to those of mammals, has recently led to rapid and dramatic insights into peroxisomal biogenesis and diseases.[36,190,130a] The peroxisomes in the CNS are smaller (microperoxisomes) than those of liver and kidney,[152] and probably possess slightly different biochemical properties.[375] In the mature mammalian CNS peroxisomes appear to be largely restricted to oligodendrocytes, while in the developing CNS they are present in neuroblasts, immature neurons and oligodendrocytes.[152] In human fetuses, catalase-positive neurons are observed in the basal ganglia, thalamus and cerebellum at 27–28 weeks and in the frontal cortex at 35 weeks of gestation. As in other mammals their neuronal prominence decreases with postnatal age. Catalase-positive glia are identified in deep white matter at 31–32 weeks of gestation, and throughout the remainder of gestation they appear to shift from deep to superficial white matter.[153]

The peroxisome is named for its peroxide-based respiration in which a variety of oxidases (e.g. D- and L-amino

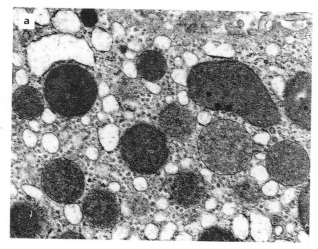

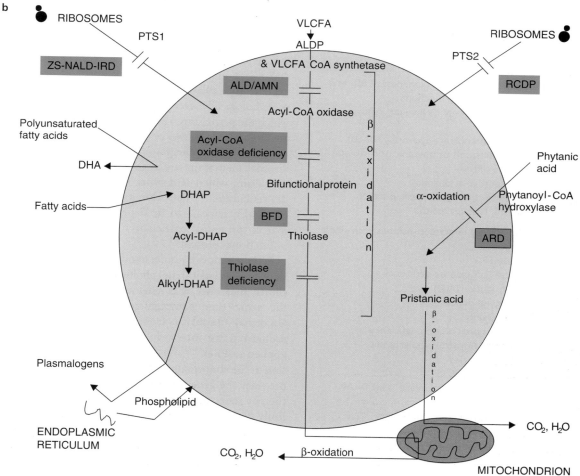

Figure 12.1 *(a) Normal peroxisomes and mitochondria. Peroxisomes with limiting single membranes and a homogeneous granular matrix admixed with mitochondria displaying internal cristae, electron-dense granules and limiting double membranes in an hepatocyte. (Electron microscopy of a biopsy.) (b) Metabolic pathways of neuroperoxisomal disorders. DHA, docosahexaenoic acid. PTS, peroxisomal targeting signal; for other abbreviations see Tables 12.2. and 12.4.*

acid) generate hydrogen peroxide that is decomposed by catalase or peroxidatically to yield O_2 and H_2O, or H_2O, respectively[72,190] (Fig. 12.1b). The relevance of peroxisomes in normal mammalian cells only came to be appreciated

fully after morphological and biochemical abnormalities of this organelle were noted in a few rare human diseases. Peroxisomal (and mitochondrial) abnormalities were recognized first in the cerebrohepatorenal syndrome of

Zellweger (ZS),[128] which is the prototype of PBDs.[191,130a] These diseases display biochemical defects in most or all of the known functions of peroxisomes in man: β-oxidation of long chain and VLCFA, pristanic acid and cholestanoic acids; α-oxidation of phytanic acid; pipecolic acid degradation; glyoxylate detoxification; glutaryl-Co A metabolism; and the biosynthesis of ether-phospholipids (plasmalogens), docosahexaenoic acid (DHA), cholesterol and dolichol.[392a] There are over 50 matrix enzymes in peroxisomes to execute these functions.[36,190,339,392] Additional and more current information is available on a website created and maintained by Dr Stephen Gould (http://www.peroxisome.org/).

Peroxisomal disorders have been classified in several ways, none of which is entirely satisfactory. This chapter uses a classification scheme that is based on peroxisomal morphology and clinical presentation (Table 12.2).

Table 12.2 *Classification of peroxisomal disorders*

Group I.	Disorders of peroxisome biogenesis (PBD) and multiple peroxisomal functions
	Cerebrohepatorenal (Zellweger) syndrome (ZS)
	Neonatal adrenoleukodystrophy (NALD)
	Infantile Refsum's or phytanic acid storage disease (IRD)
	Hyperpipecolic acidaemia
	Rhizomelic chondrodysplasia punctata (RCDP), type I, classical
Group II.	Morphologically intact peroxisomes with single enzymopathy
	A. Pseudo-PBD
	1. Acyl-CoA oxidase deficiency (pseudo-NALD)
	2. Thiolase deficiency (pseudo-ZS)
	3. Bifunctional protein deficiency
	4. Di- and trihydroxycholestanoic deficiencies
	5. RCDP types II, III (DHAP acyltransferase, alkyl DHAP synthase deficiencies)
	6. Mevalonate kinase deficiency
	7. Zellweger-like syndrome
	B. Adrenoleukodystrophy (ALD) and adrenomyeloneuropathy (AMN)
	C. Refsum's disease, classical, adult (ARD) and atypical Refsum's disease
	D. Miscellaneous
	1. Glutaric aciduria, type III (glutaryl-CoA oxidase deficiency)
	2. Hyperoxaluria type I (alanine glyoxylate aminotransferase deficiency)
	3. Acatalasaemia
Group III.	Others

DHAP, dihydroxyacetone phosphate.

In PBDs, previously referred to as general or generalized peroxisomal diseases,[232,328] morphologically identifiable or biochemically particulate peroxisomes are absent or severely deficient owing to a fundamental defect in their assembly. Both membrane and matrix proteins are synthesized on polysomes and are post-translationally imported into pre-existing peroxisomes through the interaction of specific targeting signals on the proteins and their receptors.[190,392] Two major peroxisomal targeting signals (PTSs), PTS1 and 2, have been identified. Most mammalian matrix proteins contain a carboxy-terminal serine–lysine–leucine (SKL) sequence characteristic of PTS1, while thiolase, alkyl-dihydroxyacetone phosphate (DHAP) synthase and phytanoyl-CoA hydroxylase display PTS2 amino-terminal sequences, which are proteolytically cleaved after import into the peroxisome. The PTS motifs needed to direct membrane proteins (e.g. ALDP/ABCD1 and PMP 70/ABCD3)[84a] to the peroxisome are yet unknown, but are distinct from PTS1 or 2 and do not require adenosine triphosphate (ATP). The ATP-dependent import of matrix proteins and lipid uptake expand the alkaline peroxisomal compartment to a morphologically recognizable and critical size, after which the peroxisomes proliferate through PEX 11-mediated fission (see below) or budding from the peroxisomal reticulum. The phospholipids destined for the peroxisomal membrane are synthesized in the endoplasmic reticulum, which is distinct from the peroxisome and its reticulum.[190] The abundance of peroxisomes in a cell also appears to be dependent on the import of matrix proteins, particularly acyl-CoA oxidase and bifunctional protein.[54]

Early attempts to understand the pathogenesis of PBD were largely classical morphological studies,[105,385] followed shortly thereafter by biochemical approaches.[393] At about the same time complementation analysis, in which abnormal fibroblasts from two different patients are induced to fuse into a multinucleated heterokaryon, was applied to PBD.[41,234,302,334] As with other diseases, correction of the abnormalities occurs only if one abnormal cell provides the gene product that is deficient in the other, thereby reflecting distinct genotypes. Thus far, 12 genetically distinct complementation groups (CG) have been identified in PBD;[130a,234] all display an impairment of matrix protein import.[392] The chromosomal localization for some of these genes has been established: 7q21-22(CG1), 12p13.3(CG2), 6p21.1(CG4), 8q21.1(CG7) and 6q22-24(CG11).[231] More recently, 24 genes involved in peroxisome biogenesis or assembly (PEX genes) have been cloned; their gene products have been designated 'peroxins' or PEX #p,[94] some of which have human homologues and correlate with specific complementation groups and characteristic phenotypes[131,231,392] (Table 12.3). All known peroxins, with the exception of 3, 11, 16, and 19, are involved in matrix protein import. PEX 3, 16, and particularly 19 are critical for peroxisomal membrane protein import.

Table 12.3 *Human PEX-genes and peroxins*

PEX gene	Peroxin	Complementation group	Phenotype
PEX 1	143 kDa; AAA-ATPase; cytosolic and vesicle associated	1 (E)	ZS, NALD, IRD
PEX 2	35 kDa; integral peroxisomal membrane protein (PMP)	10 (F)	ZS, IRD
PEX 3	42 kDa; PMP	12	ZS
PEX 5	67 kDa; PTS1-receptor; cytosolic and peroxisomal	2	NALD, ZS, IRD
PEX 6	104 kDa; AAA-ATPase; cytosolic and vesicle associated	4 (C)	ZS, NALD
PEX 7	36 kDa; PTS2-receptor; cytosolic and peroxisomal	11	RCDP
PEX 10	37 kDa; PMP	7 & 5 (B)	ZS, NALD
PEX 12	40 kDa; PMP	3	ZS, NALD, IRD
PEX 13	44 kDa; PMP	13 (H)	ZS, NALD
PEX 16	39 kDa; PMP peroxisomal membrane	9 (D)	ZS
PEX 19	33 kDa; binds multiples PMPs; cytosolic and peroxisomal	14 (A)	ZS

Numerical complementation groups from Kennedy-Krieger Institute.[229]
Lettered complementation groups from Japan.[334]

Genotype–phenotype correlations have been poor, because defects in the same gene can produce different phenotypes and defects in different genes can produce the same phenotype.[36,231,279,392] For example, the ZS phenotype can be due to mutations in PEX 1, 2, 3, 5, 6, 10, 12, 13, 16 or 19. The most common complementation group is group 1, due to a defect in PEX 1, in which the ZS, neonatal adrenoleukodystrophy (NALD), and infantile Refsum's disease (IRD) phenotypes (referred to as the Zellweger spectrum) are seen in decreasing order of prevalence and severity.[298] PEX 1p stabilizes PEX 5p, the PTS1 receptor, and PEX 1p and PEX 6p interact with each other to facilitate PTS1- and 2-mediated matrix protein import.[392] A defect in either gene, particularly the missense mutation G843D in PEX 1, is responsible for about 80% of ZS–NALD–IRD phenotypes, which currently are viewed as a continuum.[118] The reason for the phenotypic variability with the same genotype appears to be due to the specific nature of the gene defect and the resultant deficiency of mRNA/protein, leading to a variable import defect of matrix proteins. For example, the G843D mutation has approximately 15% residual matrix protein import activity and correlates with the mildest IRD phenotype, while the C.2097inST mutation has no import activity and is associated with the most severe ZS phenotype. A comparable situation has been found with PEX 5, 6, 7, 10 and 12.[131a,231] The temperature sensitivity of peroxisomal permeability may also play a role.[161] It has become apparent that most Zellweger spectrum patients, with an incidence of one per 25 000–50 000 births, suffer from a defect in PTS1-matrix protein import. By contrast Rhizomelic Chondrodysplasia Punctata (RCDP), which is the only PBD associated with PEX 7, displays a selective defect in PTS2-matrix protein import.

Two knockout mouse models of ZS, one targeting PEX 2[109] and the other PEX 5,[18] have demonstrated an impairment in neocortical neuronal migration, as well as other PBD abnormalities. Dietary supplementation with DHA did not alter the neuronal migration defect in the PEX 5 knockout.[166]

Diagnosis

The diagnosis of peroxisomal disorders is based initially on clinical symptomatology, followed by confirmatory laboratory studies.[329,392a] All of the peroxisomal disorders, except for ALD/AMN which is X-linked, are transmitted by an autosomal-recessive pattern. Dysmorphic facies or rhizomelia (shortening of forelimbs), particularly when accompanied by hypotonia and seizures, in the neonatal period; or signs of central white matter disease (e.g. spasticity, ataxia or aphasia), myelopathy and neuropathy in male children or adults should alert the clinician to the possibility of a peroxisomal disorder. Plasma VLCFA levels, particularly C_{26}, are elevated in virtually all peroxisomal disorders and therefore are an excellent laboratory screening test. It would be ideal, but some technical aspects of the assay are difficult. If VLCFA levels are abnormal and the patient is suspected of having a peroxisomal disorder other than ALD/AMN, plasma levels of di- and trihydroxycholestanoic (THCA), pristanic, phytanic and pipecolic acids and DHA should be measured. It also might be necessary to assess *de novo* plasmalogen biosynthesis, fatty acid β-oxidation, phytanic acid α-oxidation and immunostaining for peroxisomal matrix/membrane proteins in fibroblast cultures.[329] In atypical cases, when the preceding tests are ambiguous and a peroxisomal aetiology is still deemed likely, a liver biopsy to ascertain the presence and morphology of peroxisomes by catalase histochemistry, immunohistochemistry and electron microscopy[301] may be useful. Prenatal diagnosis can be performed in at-risk families through the analysis of VLCFA; the suspected defective enzyme (activity measurements) or protein (immunoblotting) is available for most peroxisomal disorders and tests are highly reliable. Adrenoleukodystrophy (ALD) is the most difficult, especially if the ALD-protein (ALDP) is expressed in the index patient. DNA analysis is necessary in such cases. The identification of mutant PEX genes allows the identification of heterozygotes or carrier status and may become the definitive test.[329]

If the diagnosis is not made ante-mortem and a peroxisomal disorder is suspected, samples of plasma, brain, liver and adrenal should be frozen at post-mortem examination for biochemical analyses. Sections of brain, liver and adrenal are fixed for light and electron microscopy and immunohistochemistry. Small samples of skeletal muscle and spleen are snap-frozen for molecular studies, and a section of skin should be removed for fibroblast cultures. Even if such measures are not taken, such as in retrospective archival investigations, VLCFA and phytanic acids determinations can be made on formalin-fixed wet tissue samples of brain and adrenal[224] because of their post-mortem stability and insolubility in aqueous solutions.

General pathology and neuropathological overview of peroxisomal disorders

The major organ systems that are involved in peroxisomal disorders are the CNS, peripheral nervous system (PNS), skeleton, eyes, liver, adrenal and kidney.[273] In the PBDs and those single enzyme deficiencies that simulate them clinically (pseudo-PBDs) various extraneural lesions are usually seen: dysmorphic facies and stippled calcifications to shortened proximal long bones; portal fibrosis to micronodular cirrhosis and steatosis; periodic acid–Schiff (PAS)-positive macrophages with angulate lysosomes containing trilaminar spicules; striated adrenocortical cells containing lamellae and lamellar-lipid profiles to adrenal atrophy; and renal cortical microcysts to macrocysts.[92,273,301] The eyes typically display cataracts, atypical pigmentary retinopathy, degeneration of photoreceptor cells, ganglion cell loss and optic atrophy; angulate lysosomes with spicular inclusions (Fig. 12.2; see below) in retinal macrophages and electron-opaque membranous cytoplasmic bodies in ganglion cells are observed ultrastructurally.[65,66] Of the PBDs, ZS is the most severe clinically and in general manifests the most severe lesions. However, skeletal involvement is most impressive in RCDP and its phenocopies, hepatic macrophages in IRD and lymphoid/thymus macrophages in NALD.[272] The characteristic ultrastructural inclusion in PBDs is the membrane-bound angulate lysosome containing rigid-appearing trilaminar spicules consisting of two electron-dense leaflets of 3–5 nm, separated by a regular electron-lucent space of 6–12 nm. These structures also are seen in brain, adrenal, retina and rarely

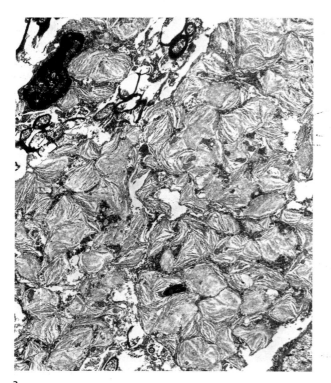

a

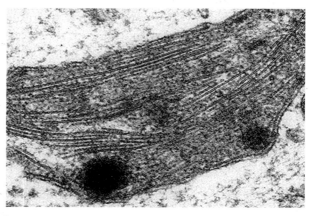

b

Figure 12.2 *(a) Adrenoleukodystrophy. Angulate lysosomes containing trilaminar straight spicules in a CNS macrophage from a symptomatic ALD heterozygote. (Electron microscopy of autopsy material.) (b) Infantile Refsum's disease. Angulate lysosome containing trilaminar inclusions in hepatocyte of IRD. (Electron microscopy of a biopsy.)*

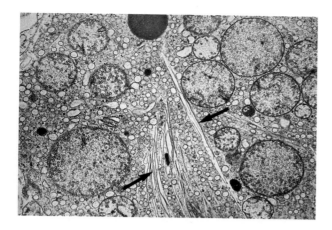

Figure 12.3 *Adrenoleukodystrophy. Electron micrograph of lamellae and lamellar-lipid profiles (arrows) among dilated smooth endoplasmic reticulum and variably sized mitochondria in a 22-week fetal zone adrenocortical cell of ALD. (Autopsy.)*

other macrophages of ALD/adrenomyeloneuropathy (AMN).[65,121,282] In spite of their prominence in peroxisomal disorders, especially PBDs, they are non-specific;[93] for example, they have been reported in skin biopsies of other degenerative metabolic diseases, particularly in late infantile and juvenile neuronal ceroid-lipofuscinoses[99] (see also Chapter 11, this Volume). Hence, their identification in macrophages of the CNS or an affected visceral organ is of paramount diagnostic importance. They contrast morphologically with the most characteristic inclusions of ALD/AMN, which are linear to gently curved, lamellae and lamellar-lipid profiles lying free in the cytoplasm of adrenocortical, Leydig and Schwann cells[284,285] and brain macrophages[270,319] (Fig 12.3). Lamellae are not membrane bound and fundamentally consist of two 2.5-nm electron-dense leaflets separated by a variable electron-lucent space of 1–7 nm. They often lie within or at the edge of large clear spaces (lamellar-lipid profiles). Cells that possess spicules or lamellae/lamellar-lipid profiles are birefringent and retain their birefringence after acetone extraction.[168,301] The lamellae/lamellar-lipid profiles, apparently in contrast to the spicules,[301] can be extracted with xylene or *n*-hexane. This non-polar lipid has been identified as abnormal cholesterol esters containing saturated VLCFA.[157] Additional details about their morphology, composition and formation are available.[274,282,288,301] In view of the known facts, that the only biochemical defect in ALD is the accumulation of saturated VLCFA and that VLCFA are increased in all PBDs and pseudo-PBDs, angulate lysosomes with spicules in peroxisomal disorders most probably contain lysosomally modified VLCFA. Peroxisomes vary greatly in their morphology: virtually undetectable, atrophic or hypertrophic in PBDs, malformed to normal in pseudo-PBDs, and normal in most other single enzymopathies.

Neuropathological lesions in peroxisomal disorders are of three major types: (1) abnormalities in neuronal migration or differentiation, which are characteristic of PBDs and pseudo-PBDs, particularly ZS; (2) defects in the formation or maintenance of central white matter, the former typically seen in PBD and the latter in ALD/AMN and NALD; and (3) postdevelopmental neuronal degenerations, which are most frequent in AMN, PBDs and Refsum's disease.[279] Pathological data on most of the peroxisomal disorders are scant, except for ZS, NALD and ALD/AMN, and should be considered to be provisional.[273] The prototypes of the PBD group, ZS, and of the single enzymopathy group, ALD/AMN, will be emphasized. Abnormal white matter is prominent in ZS and predominant in NALD and ALD; consequently, an overview of primary diseases of myelin[271] can provide a perspective for the white matter lesions described below and later in the mitochondrial section.

LEUKODYSTROPHIES AND OTHER DEFECTS IN MYELINATION

The term 'leukodystrophy' is generally used to describe genetic (inherited) and progressive disorders that primarily and directly affect CNS myelin. The classical leukodystrophies have been historically classified as 'dysmyelinative' primary diseases of myelin. Other diseases displaying a comparable confluent loss of myelin, but lacking the genetic, progressive or primary myelin involvement have been referred to as 'leukoencephalopathies'. The genetic defect in the leukodystrophies may result in the synthesis of biochemically abnormal myelin or in a molecular abnormality in myelin-forming cells, usually oligodendrocytes, which has an adverse impact on myelin in other ways. Irrespective of the biochemical/molecular abnormality, the end result is typically a confluent destruction, or failed development, of central white matter. In the latter and much less common 'hypomyelinative' leukodystrophies, such as Pelizaeus–Merzbacher disease (PMD), a molecular defect in oligodendrocytes impedes the formation of myelin. There are also several neonatal–infantile diseases, including PBDs, in which it is difficult to decide whether there is hypomyelination and, if so, whether it represents a delay in CNS myelin formation or an arrest of myelination. Both of these situations are hypomyelinative at autopsy and, at least theoretically, could be considered as hypomyelinative leukodystrophies. However, the former is usually not progressive and, hence, it may be more prudent to consider such delays in myelination as leukoencephalopathies. It takes considerable experience with numerous controls and a sound knowledge of the timing of regional myelinogenesis in the CNS[39,179,405] to make these determinations neuropathologically. Computed tomography (CT) has not improved our diagnostic sensitivity of white matter disorders; but magnetic resonance imaging (MRI) has, particularly on T2-weighted images in which the same patterns of classical gross neuropathological lesions can be more easily appreciated.[176,381] Longitudinal studies using MRI, especially with recent modifications including magnetization transfer and diffusion anisotropy, promise to provide powerful pathogenetic insights.

Most leukodystrophies fall into the dysmyelinative category, where myelin is initially formed to a variable extent but subsequently breaks down. The myelin may break down because it is biochemically abnormal, such as in metachromatic leukodystrophy (MLD) and ALD; because an oligodendroglial toxin accumulates owing to the molecular defect in the oligodendrocyte, such as has been proposed in globoid cell leukodystrophy (GLD, Krabbe disease); or for unknown reasons, such as in sudanophilic (orthochromatic) leukodystrophies (SLDs). When myelin is catabolized, its protein and lipid constituents, particularly galactolipids (cerebroside and sulfatide) and cholesterol, are liberated and can be appreciated with traditional carbohydrate (e.g. PAS) and lipid (e.g. oil red O) stains. Galactolipids are PAS positive; sulfatide, which contains anionic sulfate groups, is also metachromatic. When biochemically normal myelin is degraded by cells with normal catabolic enzymes, these staining reactions are ephemeral. However, if galactocerebrosidase or arylsulfatase activity is absent or markedly diminished, these staining qualities persist. Consequently, in GLD lacking galactocerebrosidase the myelin debris that accumulates is PAS positive, while in MLD it is PAS positive and metachromatic. The liberated cholesterol is esterified primarily by macrophages and usually persists for much longer as cytoplasmic vacuoles (lipophages, gitter cells, compound granular corpuscles). Therefore, if the myelin is biochemically 'normal' and the host possesses normal catabolic enzymes, the myelin debris should consist primarily of cholesterol esters. Normal cholesterol esters, the 'floating fraction' of neurochemists, are stained convincingly with neutral lipid or sudanophilic dyes, hence the term 'sudanophilic'. Because cholesterol esters are not metachromatic, they are also 'orthochromatic'.[271,283]

Histological examination reveals a concurrent dynamic process with various cells participating at specific times. In general, the affected myelin sheaths display morphological changes of vacuolation, blebbing, fragmentation and loss of stainability with traditional myelin stains which is accompanied by cellular reactions characteristic of each disease. Most commonly, in the dysmyelinative leukodystrophies, axons lacking sheaths are admixed with numerous macrophages containing myelin debris, which is often diagnostically distinctive, and hypertrophic or reactive astrocytes. Later, the macrophages migrate to venules either to die there by apoptosis or to exit the brain; the reactive astrocytes involute and produce a chronic astroglial scar, which may be anisomorphic or isomorphic. In the 'hypomyelinative' leukodystrophies, there is little need for a macrophage response but reactive astrocytosis is usually prominent.

The classical dysmyelinative leukodystrophies (ALD, MLD, GLD and probably some SLDs) involve defects in myelin lipids that are qualitatively similar in the CNS and PNS; hence, involvement of both CNS and PNS myelin is commonly observed. If the defect involves myelin proteins that are largely restricted to one compartment (e.g. the CNS proteolipid protein), then the myelin lesions are likewise restricted (e.g. to CNS in PMD). All leukodystrophies mentioned above display similar gross CNS features: reduced brain weight, optic atrophy, bilaterally symmetrical diffuse to confluent loss or lack of deep cerebral and cerebellar white matter that is replaced by firm tan to grey astrocytic tissue (sclerosis), relative sparing of subcortical arcuate fibres, atrophy of the corpus callosum and compensatory hydrocephalus.

Light and electron microscopy, however, show each leukodystrophy to have its own characteristic and usually diagnostic lesions, in addition to the common features of reduced myelin staining, loss of oligodendrocytes, relative sparing of axons, macrophages containing myelin debris and reactive astrocytosis to fibrillary astrogliosis. Axonal loss is greater and inflammatory cells, other than macrophages, are conspicuously absent in the leukodystrophies compared with the prototypic demyelinative diseases, multiple sclerosis (MS) and acute disseminated (allergic) encephalomyelitis (ADEM). ALD is the exception, because it is markedly inflammatory and mimics MS.[270,274,319] It differs from MS, however, by the typical localization of lymphocytes just within (rather than at) the demyelinative edge, by the relative paucity of B-lymphocytes and plasma cells[278] and by the T-helper cell–cytokine pattern.[203] In MS and ADEM (discussed in Chapter 8, Volume II), lymphocytic or lymphocytic/plasmacytic reactions, more axonal sparing, lesion asymmetry when bilateral, random involvement of subcortical fibres, sudanophilic myelin debris, and restriction of lesions to the CNS reflect the immune destruction of biochemically normal central myelin in which myelin proteins appear to be a major target.

An additional group of primary diseases of myelin, sometimes referred to as myelinolytic or spongy myelinopathies, shares the common histopathological feature of spongy or vacuolated myelin due to intramyelinic oedema. The splits in myelin usually occur at the intraperiod (extracellular face) line. They typically elicit little to no macrophage or reactive astrocytic response. In spite of this common histopathological lesion, their aetiologies are diverse and usually toxic–metabolic, and include vitamin B_{12} deficiency, aminoacidurias and mitochondrial disorders.[271] Canavan's disease, which is described more fully in Chapter 8, this Volume, bridges this classification scheme by exhibiting a spongiform myelinopathy (i.e. myelinolytic) and a confluent, progressive and genetically determined myelin lesion (i.e. a leukodystrophy). Peroxisomal disorders are not characterized by spongy myelin, except in one family with atypical Refsum's disease in which a mitochondrial defect was not completely excluded.[368]

Table 12.4 *Overview of peroxisomal disorders*

	ZS	NALD	RCDP	BFD	ALD	AMN
Major localization	Cer GM	Cer WM	CNS	Cer GM	Cer WM	SC
Histopathology	Dysgenesis	Demyelination	Microencephaly	Dysgenesis	Demyelination	Axonopathy
Misguided neurons	+++	+	0?	++	0	0
Cer/Cbl myelination	Hypo	De	Hypo	Hypo/De	De	Dys/De
Oligodendroglial loss	+/–	++	+/–	+/–	+++	++
Astrocytosis	++	++	+/–	+	+++	++
Microgliosis	+/–	++	+/–	+	+++	+
Inflammation	0	++	0	+	+++	+/–
Adrenal lamellae	+	+	0	+	+++	+++
Angulate lysosomes	+	++	0	+	+	+
Biochemical defect	Multiple	Multiple	↓Plasmalogens	↑VLCFA ↑Cholestanoic acids	↑VLCFA	
Molecular defect	PEX 1 import	PEX 1 import	PEX 7 import	D-BFP activity or import	ALDP import	

0, negative; +/–, rare; +, mild; ++, moderate; +++, severe.
ALD, adrenoleukodystrophy; ALDP, ALD protein; AMN, adrenomyeloneuropathy; BFD, bifunctional protein deficiency; Cbl, cerebellar; Cer, cerebral; CNS, central nervous system; D-BFP, dextro isomer of bifunctional protein; De, demyelination; Dys, dysmyelination; GM, grey matter; Hypo, hypomyelination; NALD, neonatal adrenoleukodystrophy; PEX, peroxin; RCDP, rhizomelic chondrodysplasia punctata; SC, spinal cord; VLCFA, very long-chain fatty acid; WM, white matter; ZS, Zellweger's syndrome.

An overview of peroxisomal disorders is presented in Table 12.4.

GROUP I: DISORDERS OF PEROXISOME BIOGENESIS

'Classical' Zellweger's syndrome

These infants usually present at birth with characteristic dysmorphic facies, seizures, severe hypotonia and profound psychomotor retardation; they usually die by 6 months of age. Additional clinical and radiological findings include cataracts, pigmentary retinopathy, optic atrophy, sensorineural hearing deficits, equinovarus deformity, hepatomegaly, and stippled calcifications of the patellae, femora and humeri. Systemic pathological findings may also include biliary dysgenesis, ventriculoseptal defects, islet cell hyperplasia, and hypoplasia of the thymus and lung. Renal microcysts, predominantly cortical and varying from 0.1 to 0.5 cm, arise from both tubules and glomeruli.[35,253,258,408] The adrenal cortex displays scattered and infrequent adrenocortical striated cells with lamellar-lipid profiles and PAS-positive macrophages with spicules.[129] Many of these lesions have been documented in affected fetuses.[280] Hepatic peroxisomes originally had been reported as absent;[128] subsequently, immunofluorescent studies identified peroxisomal membrane proteins in the form of malformed peroxisomal 'ghosts' lacking matrix proteins.[314] As a result, elevations in VLCFA,

phytanic, pristanic, pipecolic, di- and trihydroxycholestanoic acids, with decreases in plasmalogens and DHA, are seen. Phytanic acid is derived exclusively from dietary sources, while pristanic acid comes from phytanic acid breakdown and dietary sources; hence, the presence and prevalence of both may vary with age, diet and catabolic enzyme activity.[392,394]

Neuropathology of Zellweger's syndrome

The major lesions are seen in the CNS where abnormal neuronal migrations dominate.[105,385] These infants classically show a unique combination of centrosylvian or parasylvian pachygyria (medial) and polymicrogyria (lateral and extending into the lateral frontal lobe and the lateral parieto-temporo-occipital region) (Fig. 12.4); this localization for the major neocortical malformation is consistent, but may be associated with other areas of polymicrogyria and pachygyria. There may also be an abnormal vertical tilt to the sylvian fissure. The limbic areas of the brain are typically spared. Coronal sections of the cerebrum exhibit a thickened cortex with either excessive superficial plications or obvious subcortical heterotopias. The micropolygyric cortex usually reveals fusion of the molecular layers and better preservation of the supragranular cortex (Fig. 12.5). The outer cortex is typically occupied by medium to large pyramidal cells

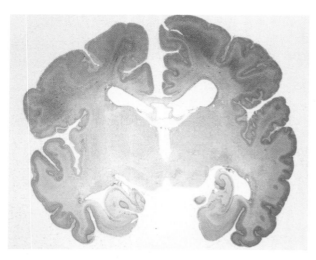

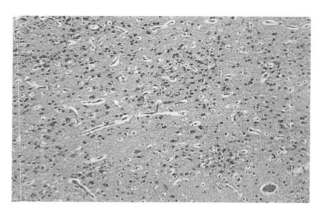

Figure 12.6 *Zellweger's syndrome. Pachygyric heterotopia in ZS consisting of many pyramidal neurons. (H&E.)*

Figure 12.4 *Zellweger's syndrome. Coronal section of a 4-week-old, PEX-1 ZS male demonstrating bilateral parasylvian medial pachygyria with prominent subcortical heterotopia and asymmetric lateral polymicrogyria, particularly of insular cortex. (Nissl.)*

destined for deep cortex, while the usually superficial neuronal populations are detained in deep cortex and subcortical white matter. The pachygyric cortex has a similar alteration, but more severe; the subcortical heterotopias are likewise more prominent (Fig. 12.6). These cortical abnormalities differ from those of classical four-layered polymicrogyria or lissencephaly–pachygyria in that all neuronal classes seem to be affected, with those destined for the outer layers tending to be more impeded. The cerebellum is grossly unremarkable, but it is common to find heterotopic Purkinje cells (often poly-dendritic) or combinations of Purkinje cells and granule cells in the white matter, especially in the nodulus. Dysplastic claustra are accompanied by dysplastic medullary olives, and often dysplasia of the dentate nuclei. These dysplasias appear to reflect a problem with neuronal differ-

entiation or the terminal stages of migration and are not true heterotopias, i.e. the neurons reach their expected destinations but are not properly organized.[273,279] For example, the olives and dentate nuclei may lack their normal serpiginous configuration or consist of discontinuous islands of neurons; the olives may also simply display a peripheral palisading of neurons (Fig. 12.7). Striated and globose PAS-positive macrophages, containing abnormal lipid cytosomes, have been identified in grey and white matter of cerebrum and cerebellum (Fig. 12.8).[4,74,401] Morphological evidence for a restricted neuronal lipidosis is seen in the form of striated neuronal perikarya and dystrophic spheroids containing lamellar-lipid profiles in Clarke's and lateral cuneate nuclei[290b] (Figs 12.9–12.11). Ventricular enlargement is common, as are periventricular cysts and ependymal abnormalities.[315]

Brains from fetuses at risk of developing ZS disclose neocortical migratory defects as early as postmenstrual estimated gestational age (EGA) 14 weeks in the form of micropolygyric ripples and subtle subcortical heterotopias. Thin abnormal cortical plates with more obvious sub-

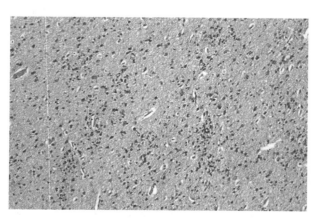

Figure 12.5 *Zellweger's syndrome. Micropolygyric heterotopia in ZS with fewer pyramidal and more granular neurons than its pachygyric counterpart. (H&E.)*

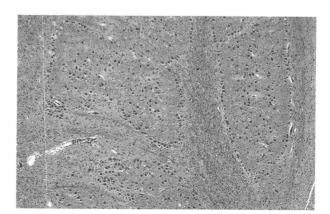

Figure 12.7 *Zellweger's syndrome. Discontinuous and simplified inferior olive with peripheral palisading of neurons in a 4-week-old, PEX-1 ZS male. (H&E.)*

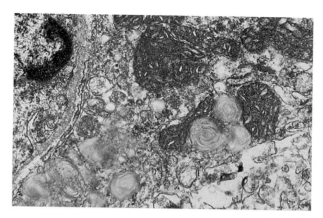

Figure 12.8 *Zellweger's syndrome. Electron-opaque membranous cytoplasmic bodies, typical of ZS, in an astrocyte of occipital cortex in a 13-week-old ZS male. (Autopsy.)*

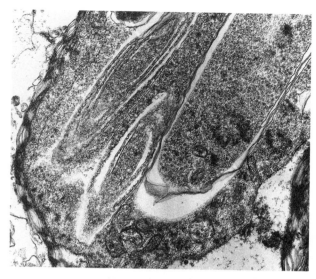

Figure 12.11 *Zellweger's syndrome. Electron micrograph of lamellae and lamellar-lipid profiles in axonal swelling within DNC of the same ZS patient as in Figure 12.10. (Autopsy.)*

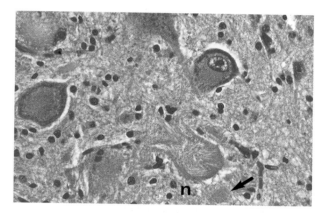

Figure 12.9 *Zellweger's syndrome. Striated neuron (n) of DNC with spheroid (arrow) in the same ZS patient as in Fig. 12.8. (H&E.)*

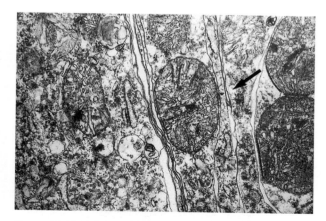

Figure 12.10 *Zellweger's syndrome. Lamellae and lamellar-lipid profiles (arrow) between mitochondria in DNC perikaryon of a 12-week-old ZS male. (Electron microscopy of autopsy material.)*

cortical heterotopias occur at EGA 22–24 weeks (Fig. 12.12). Astrocytes, neuroblasts, immature neurons, radial glia and PAS-positive macrophages contain abnormal pleomorphic cytosomes; these include electron-opaque membranous cytoplasmic bodies, perhaps representing gangliosides containing saturated VLCFA. Some neurites also exhibit lamellar-lipid profiles. Dysplastic alterations of the inferior olivary and dentate nuclei are present, as well as renal cortical microcysts, fetal zone adrenocortical striated cells and patellar mineralization.[289] These fetal lesions confirm the prediction that the insult (presumably metabolic) causing the neocortical migration defect is operating throughout the entire neocortical neuronal migratory period.[105] Deficiencies of the cell adhesion molecule L1[372a] and doublecortin[295a] have been noted in foetal Zellweger brains.

The CNS white matter in ZS is commonly abnormal (Fig. 12.13), but does not contain classical inflammatory cells (lymphocytes or plasma cells). While some have referred to it as a leukodystrophy,[258] most would not and the nature of the defect is still unclear.[4,273] It appears to be dysmyelinative, and primarily hypomyelinative, in that there usually is little sudanophilic lipid accumulation in macrophages. Reactive astrocytosis may be relatively inconspicuous in immature white matter or severe, particularly in areas with heterotopias (Fig. 12.14); it can even extend throughout the white matter of the neuraxis. Many abnormal lipid cytosomes are seen in astrocytes and oligodendrocytes,[401] some of which might be VLCFA gangliosides, and its well-established plasmalogen deficiency could interfere with normal myelination.[273,279] However, a decrease in the normal complement of myelinated axons due to severe pachygyria–polymicrogyria and superimposed hypoxic–ischaemic damage due to seizures and

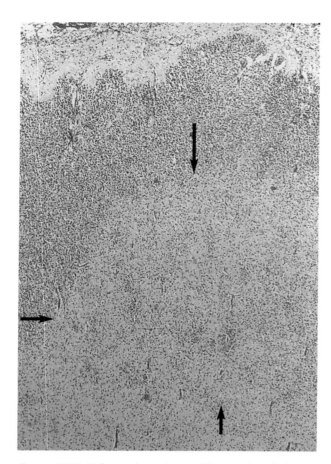

Figure 12.12 *Zellweger's syndrome. Abnormal cortical plate with subcortical heterotopia (arrows) in incipient pachygyric superior parietal gyrus of a 22-week ZS male fetus. (H&E.)*

chronic debilitation are probable complicating factors. It is important to emphasize that, irrespective of the precise pathogenesis of the white matter lesion in ZS, it is not inflammatory and differs morphologically from that of ALD.

Neonatal adrenoleukodystrophy (NALD)

This less severe, and highly variable, PBD has features in common with both ZS and ALD.[27,137,164,211,374] Clinically, these infants resemble ZS, but they usually die around 36 months of age and wide variations even with survival into adolescence are reported.[17,175] Despite its name, NALD is transmitted as an autosomal-recessive trait, and the coexistence of NALD and ALD in the same kindred has never been reported. Hepatic lesions are common. Peroxisomes in the liver have been reported as missing, decreased in size or enlarged, with consequent biochemical abnormalities in all peroxisomal functions. Adrenocortical atrophy with striated adrenocortical cells mimics the adrenal lesion of ALD. The diffuse distribution of PAS-positive macrophages with angulate lysosomes containing spicules in the liver, thymus, spleen, lymph node, lung, gastrointestinal tract and adrenal contrasts with their

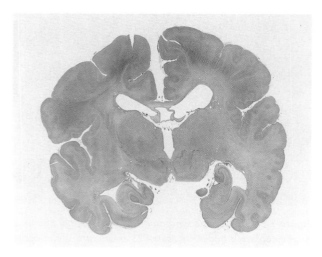

Figure 12.13 *Zellweger's syndrome. Coronal section of a 4-week-old, PEX-1 ZS male demonstrating an asymmetric paucity of myelin most notably in the posterior limbs. (LFB–PAS.)*

hepatic predominance in IRD. The PNS has been unremarkable or has shown evidence of demyelination and thin myelin sheaths, and lamellar-lipid profiles (see ALD) have been visualized in Schwann cells.[222] One case of NALD demonstrated severe atrophy of the auditory sensory epithelium and tectorial membrane.[158]

The CNS in NALD, in contrast to ZS, shows greater involvement of white matter than neuronal migrations. Both ZS and NALD are associated with a slight increase in brain weight and are often macrocephalic. Heterotopic Purkinje cells are observed. Neuronal loss has been reported in the olives, dentate nuclei and thalami of two patients with NALD. PAS-positive macrophages are present in the cortex of the cerebrum and particularly the cerebellum, similar to ZS, as are rare swollen neurons in the arcuate nucleus and perhaps in the pons.[374] Polymicrogyria may be diffuse, focal or multifocal and associated with subcortical heterotopias; pachygyria and dysplastic olives have not been reported. Diffuse dysmyelination/demyelination

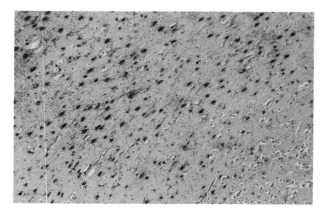

Figure 12.14 *Zellweger's syndrome. Subcortical cerebral white matter of a ZS patient with reactive astrocytosis. (GFAP.)*

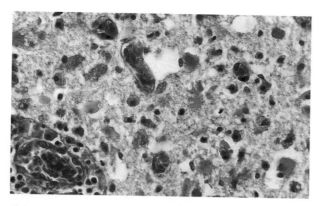

Figure 12.15 *Neonatal adrenoleukodystrophy. Inflammatory demyelinative lesion in occipital white matter of a 14-year-old NALD male. (LFB–PAS.)*

of cerebral and cerebellar white matter, often with a prominent perivascular lymphocytic reaction, is another distinguishing CNS feature and resembles ALD (Fig. 12.15). PAS-positive macrophages containing both spicules and lamellae are present, and variable degrees of reactive astrocytosis to chronic fibrillary astrogliosis are seen. Sparing of the arcuate fibres has been reported and sudanophilic macrophages are commonly observed within white matter lesions. In summary, NALD displays adrenal atrophy, systemic PAS-positive macrophages, inflammatory demyelinative CNS lesions and increases in saturated VLCFA; ZS exhibits chondrodysplasia, renal microcysts, pachygyria–polymicrogyria with dysplastic claustra, dentate nuclei and olives, and the accumulation of both saturated and monounsaturated VLCFA.[175]

Infantile Refsum's or phytanic acid storage disease

Patients with IRD display mental retardation, dysmorphic facies of a minor degree, retinitis pigmentosa, sensorineural hearing deficits, failure to thrive, and hypocholesterolaemia.[267] All biochemical peroxisomal parameters are abnormal and peroxisomes are either deficient or reduced in number. The presentation usually occurs after the neonatal period, the clinical course is much milder, and patients typically survive at least to their early teens. Some patients, who are phenotypically IRD, develop clinical and radiological evidence of a leukoencephalopathy. At the present time, these patients are arbitrarily reclassified as NALD. The most conspicuous pathological alteration is the prominence of PAS-positive macrophages containing angulate lysosomes in the liver; subsequently, spicular structures accumulate in hepatocytes.[330] Hepatomegaly with micronodular cirrhosis was reported at autopsy in a 12-year-old boy.[366] The adrenals were interpreted as hypoplastic, because they were small and lacked striated cells. It appears more likely that this represents atrophy, because a few scattered striated cells could be overlooked. CNS migration defects were not

observed, but the cerebellar cortex was diffusely small; granule cells were preferentially reduced in number and Purkinje cells were abnormally situated in the molecular layer. This was also interpreted as hypoplasia, but MRI studies[381] and a similar neuropathological lesion in chronic RCDP are more consistent with an atrophic process.[277] The cerebral white matter demonstrated focal decreases in the number of myelinated axons, particularly in the periventricular region, corpus callosum, corticospinal tracts and optic nerves; MRI studies have shown more widespread cerebral involvement, including the posterior limb and pyramidal fibres in the brainstem.[176,381] Inflammatory cells were not seen, but there were numerous perivascular collections of non-sudanophilic and PAS-negative macrophages with dense gliosis. Occasional perivascular macrophages were also noted in the white matter of the brainstem and cerebellum. Ultrastructurally, brain macrophages contained lamellae, but lacked angulate lysosomes. Astrocytes also displayed lamellar inclusions. Two 'atypical' IRD siblings, who died at 3.5 years and 8 months, have also been reported. Marked adrenal atrophy with striated cells (not illustrated) and sparse PAS-positive macrophages were associated with displaced Purkinje cells in the molecular layer, peripheral palisading of neurons in the olive and cirrhosis with PAS-positive macrophages.[58]

With respect to the sensorineural hearing deficit, which is also seen in ZS, NALD, ARD, RCDP, and acyl-CoA oxidase deficiency, one IRD patient exhibited good preservation of ganglion cells and nerve fibres in the organ of Corti, but severe atrophy of the sensory epithelium and stria vascularis.[366]

Hyperpipecolic acidaemia

Only four cases have been reported.[191] Their nosological definition had been uncertain, but now is assigned to the PBD.[131a] Minor dysmorphic features, hepatomegaly, developmental delay, hypotonia, pigmentary retinopathy and progressive neurological dysfunction are reported. Two cases, who died at or before 27 months of age, have come to post-mortem examination.[53,117] Micronodular cirrhosis and hepatocytic glycolipid inclusions were seen, in addition to dilatations of renal tubules. The neuropathological findings were discordant. In neither case were abnormal neuronal migrations noted; the brain was either normal or slightly increased in weight. In one case, the white matter of brain showed multiple areas of demyelination and astrocytosis, which were most prominent in the internal capsule, pons, medulla and cerebellum. Abnormal, often striated, material was observed in both macrophages and astrocytes. Macrophages also contained sudanophilic spherical droplets, and the striated macrophages were PAS positive and contained angulate lysosomes with spicules. Myelin was interpreted as degenerate ultrastructurally, but post-mortem autolysis may have complicated this interpretation.[117] In the other case, the cerebral white matter was hypoplastic (similar to the RCDP case of Agamanolis and Novak[3] described below) and showed a moderate decrease in myelin staining without myelin breakdown. The putamina were pale and gliotic. The other noteworthy neuropathological alteration was an accumulation of 1–1.5 µm PAS-positive, diastase-resistant, alcian blue-negative, non-sudanophilic, non-fluorescent granules in astrocytes, satellite cells and perivascular foot processes. This material seemed to correlate ultrastructurally with irregular membranovesicular profiles within the cytoplasm of astrocytes.[53] The adrenal glands in both cases were reported to be within normal limits, but rare PAS-positive, striated macrophages were found within the adrenal cortex of the Gatfield case[117] (personal observation, slide courtesy of Dr Daria Haust).

Rhizomelic chondrodysplasia punctata, type I, classical

Classical RCDP presents at birth with severe shortening and stippled calcifications of the humerus and femur, vertebral defects, joint contractures, dysmorphic facies, psychomotor and growth retardation, cataracts and optic atrophy, sensorineural hearing deficits and microcephaly. Most also have icthyosis. Death usually supervenes by the end of the first year, but some milder variants with the same biochemical defect survive into the juvenile period.[269] The rhizomelic form is the only form of chondrodysplasia punctata[345] that appears to be associated with a peroxisomal defect. Plasmalogen deficiency is even more severe than that seen in ZS, and the phytanic acid oxidation defect approximates that of adult Refsum's disease and ZS. Acyl-CoA:dihydroxyacetone phosphate acyltransferase (DHAPAT) and alkyl DHAP synthase activities are also deficient.[393,394] In some hepatocytes peroxisomes cannot be identified, while in others they are irregularly shaped and enlarged.[191] Catalase is in the particulate fraction of cultured skin fibroblasts. VLCFA are normal. Post-mortem examinations of the infantile cases have been limited.[122,269] Although most of these infants are microencephalic, no satisfactory morphological correlation for their severe psychomotor retardation is found. Microscopic examination of the CNS in those who have died at about 1 year of age is essentially unremarkable. However, in one of the brains stated to be microscopically normal, the inferior olives showed focal discontinuities and were considered to be a mild form of the defect seen in ZS.[269] The white matter of a 3-year-old girl with RCDP was diffusely reduced in size but appeared to be normally myelinated, except in the occipital lobe; diffuse cerebellar degeneration and a corresponding neuronal loss in the olives were observed.[3] The present authors confirmed the microencephaly in two chronic RCDP patients and focal dysplasia of the olive in one; they both displayed severe cerebellar atrophy due to losses of Purkinje and granule cells (Figs 12.16, 12.17). Neuronal loss in the olives

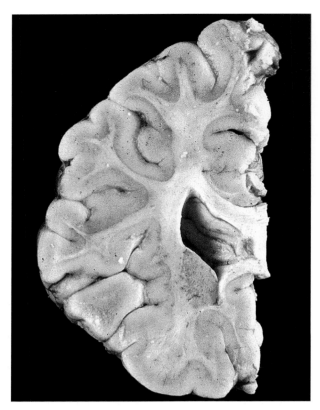

Figure 12.16 *Rhizomelic chondrodysplasia. Microencephalic brain of an 11-year-old RCDP boy with reduced volume of frontal white matter.*

and a variable pallor of myelin with corresponding reactive astrocytosis were also noted. Thus, a postdevelopmental cerebellar atrophy occurs in RCDP patients with prolonged survivals, and phytanic acid has been implicated in its pathogenesis.[277] Neocortical migration defects are generally considered to be absent, supporting the hypothesis that the migration defects in PBD and pseudo-PBD are due to elevated VLCFA.[191,289] However,

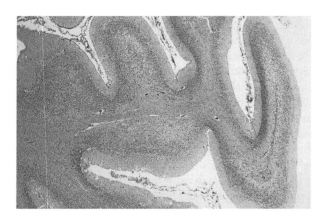

Figure 12.17 *Rhizomelic chondrodysplasia. Loss of granule neurons and Purkinje cells, worse distally, in atrophic cerebellum of a 9-year-old RCDP girl.*

one patient with short humeri and femora, widespread stippled calcifications, collecting tubule and glomerular cysts, and cataracts displayed pachygyria of the posterior frontal and pararolandic region and focal microgyria of the frontal pole.[279,404] This case preceded the era of biochemical or genetic confirmatory tests, so it is uncertain whether this is a case of peroxisomal RCDP. Additional MRI or post-mortem brain examinations are needed.

GROUP II: INTACT PEROXISOMES WITH SINGLE ENZYMOPATHY

Pseudo-PBD

Acyl-CoA oxidase deficiency (pseudo-NALD)

Only eight cases have been reported.[266,392a] While dysmorphic features were not observed in some, mild anomalous facial features were noted in others. All displayed moderate to severe neonatal hypotonia, seizures and psychomotor retardation. Sensorineural hearing deficits and abnormal electroretinograms were reported. The only biochemical abnormality was elevated VLCFA; hepatic peroxisomes were heterogeneous in size, many of them were enlarged and angulated, and they were increased in number. Macrophages with angulate lysosomes were not identified. Neuropathological data are still unavailable, but neuroradiological studies indicate an absence of migration defects, diffuse and progressive (in one out of three patients) CT hypodensities in cerebral white matter, a thin corpus callosum (in one out of three patients) and cerebellar hypoplasia (in one out of three patients). The white matter abnormality of the progressive case demonstrated abnormal contrast enhancement, suggesting an inflammatory component, such as in NALD and ALD. With MRI the white matter abnormality was seen as an abnormally high signal intensity on T2-weighted images, but contrast material was not administered.[188] A knockout mouse model has been developed, but neuropathological data were not provided.[106]

Thiolase deficiency (3-oxoacyl-CoA thiolase deficiency; pseudo-ZS)

Only one patient (of consanguineous parents) who died at the age of 11 months has been reported; increased VLCFA and bile acid intermediates were present.[127,325] She resembled classical ZS in that she had dysmorphic facies, profound hypotonia, renal cortical microcysts, striated adrenocortical cells (but also adrenal atrophy), ventriculoseptal defect, hepatomegaly with hepatic fibrosis and hepatocytic lamellae with lipid droplets. However, inflammatory demyelination and astrocytosis of cerebellar white matter, heterotopic subcortical Purkinje cells, focal polymicrogyria,[273] and adrenal atrophy with striated cells are more reminiscent of NALD. The specific nosological placement of this patient is uncertain.[392a]

Bifunctional protein deficiency (2-enoyl-CoA hydratase/D-3 hydroxacyl-CoA dehydrogenase)

This deficiency has the following distinguishing features. Firstly, this is by far the most common of the pseudo-PBD single enzymopathies.[398] Secondly, the deficient enzyme is D-, not L-, bifunctional protein (also referred to as multifunctional protein 2, multifunctional enzyme II and multifunctional β-oxidation protein 2) as originally reported.[383,397] Thirdly, this is a more severe clinical phenotype than acyl-CoA oxidase deficiency.[398] Biochemically, these patients demonstrate elevations in VLCFA, bile acid intermediates and perhaps phytanic and pristanic acids.[392,398] One patient with the clinical features of NALD has been reported; he died at 5½ months of age. However, peroxisomes were present and catalase was particulate. Autopsy findings consisted of mild portal fibrosis, glomerular microcysts and adrenal atrophy with 'lipid-containing balloon cell'; striated cells were not reported. The CNS revealed polymicrogyria, focal heterotopias, 'demyelination' of cerebral white matter and periventricular cysts. A few perivascular foamy macrophages were also present.[397] In another case, previously classified as atypical acyl-CoA oxidase deficiency, there was dysmyelination and inflammatory demyelination of the CNS white matter (occipital lobes and cerebellum), resembling that of NALD and ALD. There were also some mild cerebral and cerebellar heterotopias and focal dysplasia of olivary and Clarke's nuclei. Microgyria were observed, but not pachygyria or polymicrogyria. PAS-positive macrophages with angulate lysosomes were found in the liver, thymus, adrenals and lymph nodes. Adrenocortical atrophy with striated cortical cells was present.[241] A third patient displayed centrosylvian pachygyria–polymicrogyria, reminiscent of, but milder than, ZS, diffuse hemispheric hypomyelination with subcortical heterotopic neurons, Purkinje cell heterotopias and simplified convolutions of the dentate nucleus and inferior olive[172] (Fig. 12.18). Two other PBD patients of the same complementation group, aged 6 and 14 months at death, exhibited myelin pallor with reactive astrocytosis in both, but with mild chronic lymphocytic perivasculitis and macrophages in the older patient; one also displayed simplified olives with peripheral palisades of neurons.[279] In summary, focal polymicrogyria and an inflammatory leukoencephalopathy, more consistent with NALD, as well as centrosylvian pachygyria–polymicrogyria, a non-inflammatory leukoencephalopathy and olivary dysplasia, more consistent with ZS, have been reported in PBD.

The remaining diseases in the pseudo-PBD category, Zellweger-like syndrome[352] in which multiple peroxisomal enzymes were deficient, di- and trihydroxycholestanoic acidaemia,[59] and RCDP type III,[76] are rare and lack neuropathological data.[392] MRI of hypotonic and ataxic infants with mevalonate kinase deficiency revealed severe cerebellar atrophy; one post-mortem case was reported to have

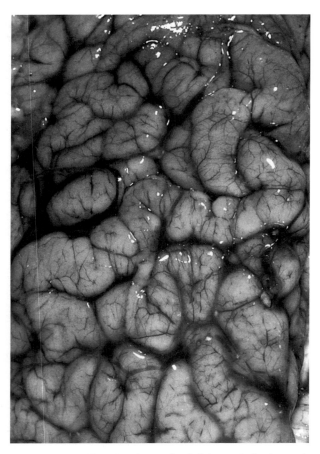

Figure 12.18 *Bifunctional protein deficiency. Polymicrogyric pattern in an 11.5-month-old BPD male.*

vermal agenesis, granule cell necrosis of the cerebellum and pseudolaminar necrosis with gliosis of the cerebral cortex.[183] A 12-day-old patient with RCDP type II (DHAPAT deficiency) is reported to have had some heterotopias, but the description 'multiple heterotopic foci of immature neurons in the vicinity of the third ventricle' suggests normal findings in an infant. The olive was also reported to be 'broadened'.[140]

Adrenoleukodystrophy (ALD) and adrenomyeloneuropathy (AMN)

ALD has two major phenotypes: X-linked juvenile (childhood cerebral) ALD and its adult variant, AMN.[230] Much less frequent (< 15%) types are adolescent and adult cerebral, which differ from childhood only in the age of onset; adrenal insufficiency-only (Addisonian); asymptomatic; and rare olivopontocerebellar[186,250] and spinocerebellar[212] types with prominent cerebellar and brainstem inflammatory demyelination. Approximately 30% of hemizygote (female) carriers demonstrate the AMN phenotype, usually mild.[16,230,233]

The molecular genetics of ALD has been a field of intense activity in the past decade, but genotype–phenotype correlations are still poor. The same genetic defect is

associated with juvenile ALD, AMN and even Addisonianonly ALD.[98,234,279,341,356] This has generated the hypothesis that a modifier gene and/or environmental factors are responsible for the phenotypic variation.[230] It is also unclear how the genetic defect is related to the major biochemical abnormality identified in ALD: decreased activity of VLCF acyl-CoA synthetase (lignoceroyl-CoA ligase) with a consequent elevation of VLCFAs. VLCFAs have been identified in many myelin components, but especially in cholesterol esters,[157] gangliosides,[159] phosphatidylcholine[363] and proteolipid protein.[31]

The ALD gene is localized to the Xq 28 region, occupies 21–26 kilobases (kb) of genomic DNA, contains 10 exons, and encodes a mRNA of 3.7–4.3 kb to translate a protein of 745–750 amino acids. This ALD protein (ALDP), instead of being the deficient synthetase, was found to be an integral membrane protein of peroxisomes with the properties of an ATP binding cassette (ABC) halftransporter.[235] A 3.7 kb ALDP transcript is present in all tissues, but is highest in the adrenal glands, intermediate in brain and almost undetectable in liver. ALDP is markedly expressed in microglia, astrocytes and endothelial cells; oligodendrocytes have little to no ALDP, except for those in the corpus callosum and internal capsule. ALDP is not detectable in the fibroblasts of about two-thirds of ALD patients. A large number of mutations have been identified: approximately 54% are missense, 25% are frameshift, 10% are nonsense and 7% are large deletions. A mutational hotspot is noted in exon 5. All mutations examined, except about one-third of the missense, do not express detectable ALDP in fibroblasts, while all have ALDP mRNA.[16,98,341]

The X-linked juvenile form usually presents between 6 and 9 years of age with behavioural, auditory, visual and gait abnormalities or adrenocortical insufficiency (Addison's disease). The disease is rapidly progressive, typically leading to death within 3 years.[319] CT and MRI confirm the gross neuropathological lesions previously described,

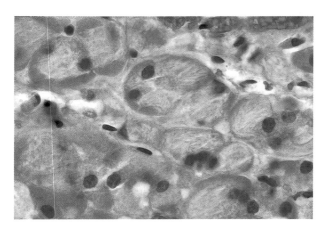

Figure 12.19 *Adrenoleukodystrophy/adrenomyeloneuropathy. Ballooned adrenocortical cells of ALD/AMN with diagnostic striations. (H&E.)*

as well as the usual progression of the lesions from the parieto-occipital to frontal lobes. Enhancement at the advancing edge of the demyelinative lesion is highly characteristic.[233] The adrenal cortex and testis are the only two non-neural organs that show significant lesions.[273,274,284]

Adrenocortical cells, particularly those of the inner fasciculata-reticularis, become ballooned and, of diagnostic import, striated due to accumulations of lamellae, lamellar-lipid profiles and fine lipid clefts[285] (Figs 12.19–12.21). The striated material, consisting of the same abnormal cholesterol esters as in CNS striated lipophages,[168] appears to lead to cell dysfunction, atrophy and apoptotic death.[286,288] Histoenzymic decreases in mitochondrial α-glycerophosphate dehydrogenase, 3β-hydroxysteroid dehydrogenase and reduced triphosphopyridine nucleotide (TPNH) diaphorase have been reported, and they show excessive peripheral cytolysis under the electron microscope. Moreover, the striated cells appear to adapt poorly to a tissue culture environment.[288] Ultimately, primary atrophy of the adrenal cortex ensues. Inflammatory cells are rarely observed and are probably an epiphenomenon: antiadrenal antibodies are not detected. The adrenal cortex in AMN displays the same qualitative changes as, but tends to be more atrophic than, most

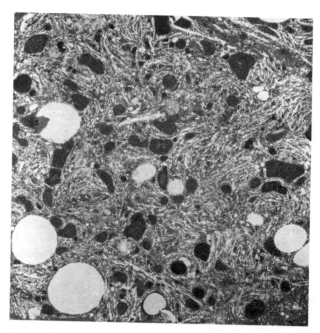

Figure 12.21 *Juvenile adrenoleukodystrophy. Predominantly fine, clear lipid clefts in an adrenocortical cell of a juvenile ALD patient. (Biopsy.)*

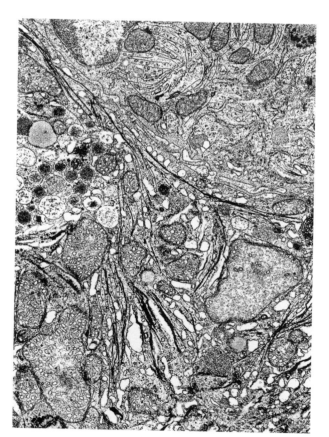

Figure 12.20 *Juvenile adrenoleukodystrophy. Lamellae and lamellar-lipid profiles in adrenocortical cells of juvenile ALD; medullary cell granules on left. (Biopsy.)*

adrenals of ALD patients; this is related to the longer duration of hypoadrenalism and consequent corticosteroid replacement therapy in AMN.[274] The same striated adrenocortical cells have been identified in ALD heterozygotes, both symptomatic and asymptomatic, but they are limited to small, multifocal clusters.[281] This resembles ZS but is in striking contrast to ALD/AMN and to the fetal adrenal zone in affected fetuses, where this lesion is diffuse.[281a]

Testicular lesions in prepubertal ALD males are usually present only at the ultrastructural level and consist of lamellae and lamellar-lipid profiles in the interstitial cells of Leydig and their precursors. The testis in AMN and adult cerebral ALD demonstrates the same Leydig cell alterations as noted already in childhood ALD, but there is also Leydig cell loss. No inflammatory cells have been seen, except in a single case of adult ALD. Degenerative changes in the seminiferous tubules in AMN appear indistinguishable from those of adult cerebral ALD and vary from a maturation arrest of spermatocytes to a Sertoli cell-only phenotype in which all germ cells are depleted. Ultrastructurally, vacuolation of the Sertoli cell's endoplasmic reticulum followed by widened intercellular spaces appears to be the initial lesion of the seminiferous tubules.[287]

Neuropathology of ALD

In addition to the gross and microscopic features common to most leukodystrophies, ALD has its own distinguishing characteristics.[274,319] Mild to moderate premature ath-

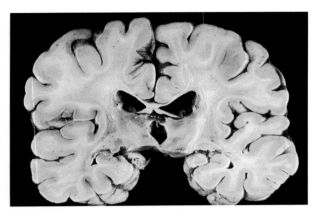

Figure 12.22 *Adrenomyeloneuropathy/adrenoleukodystrophy. Bilaterally symmetrical, confluent demyelination of parietal white matter, particularly of the posterior limb of the internal capsule, with sparing of subcortical myelin in AMN/ALD.*

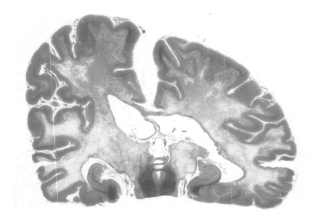

Figure 12.23 *Juvenile adrenoleukodystrophy. More severe loss of myelin, including most arcuate fibres, in juvenile ALD. (LFB–H&E.)*

erosclerosis can be seen in adult patients. The loss of myelin is almost always most prominent in the parieto-occipital region (Fig. 12.22). The advancing edges, usually frontal, are more asymmetrical and may display a white to pink 'softening' that blends imperceptibly into normal white matter. Cavitation and calcification of white matter may be seen in severe cases. Arcuate fibres are relatively spared, but the posterior cingulum, corpus callosum, fornix, hippocampal commissure, posterior limb of the internal capsule and optic system are typically involved (Fig. 12.23). The cerebellar white matter usually exhibits a similar, but milder, confluent loss of myelin and sclerosis. Secondary corticospinal tract degeneration extending down through the peduncles, basis pontis, medullary pyramids and spinal cord is characteristic (Fig. 12.24). The brainstem may also display primary demyelinative foci, especially in the basis pontis. The spinal cord is spared, except for the descending tract degeneration. Cerebral and cerebellar grey matter may be intact, or atrophic if there is severe (e.g. cavitary) damage to the centrum semiovale or cerebellar white matter.

Histopathologically, there are marked losses of myelinated axons (myelin > axons) and oligodendrocytes; apoptotic nuclear changes have not been seen in oligodendrocytes with traditional stains, but some appear pyknotic. Random preservation of individual myelinated axons in foci of myelin loss is common, but these myelin sheaths may be thin or irregular. The advancing edges of myelin loss are sites of intense perivascular inflammation, particularly lymphocytes, lipophage accumulation and reactive astrocytosis (Figs 12.25, 12.26). The predominant lipophage has granular to vacuolated cytoplasm, which is intensely sudanophilic and PAS positive. The second type stains less intensely and usually demonstrates striated cytoplasm due to the presence of clear clefts. The number of striations generally correlates inversely with sudanophilia and PAS positivity. Striated macrophages retain birefringence after acetone extraction, while granular macrophages generally do not.[168] This non-polar lipid

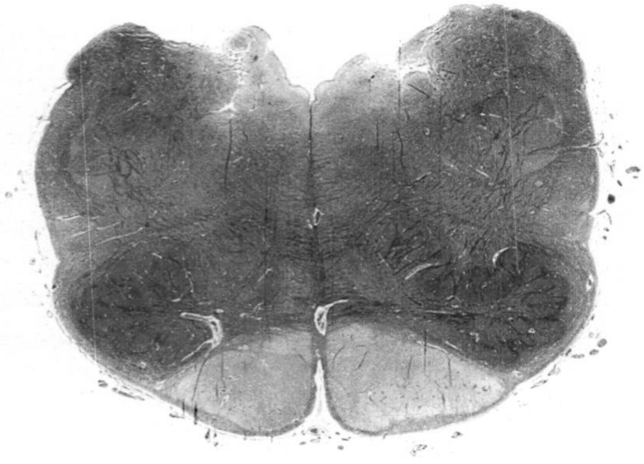

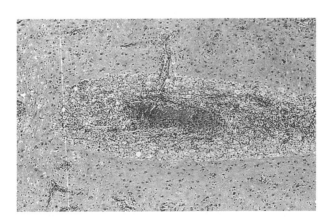

Figure 12.24 *Juvenile adrenoleukodystrophy. Loss of myelinated fibres in asymmetrical medullary pyramids of the same ALD patient as in Fig. 12.23. (LFB–H&E.)*

Figure 12.25 *Juvenile adrenoleukodystrophy. Subacute inflammatory demyelinating lesion of juvenile ALD. (H&E.)*

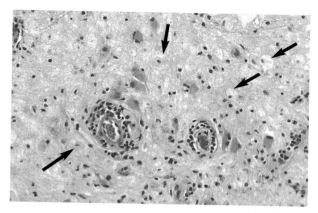

Figure 12.26 *Adrenoleukodystrophy. Inflammatory demyelinating lesion of ALD: perivascular lymphocytes and lipophages, interstitial lipophages (arrows) and reactive astrocytes in demyelinated white matter displaying a reduction in oligodendrocytes. (H&E.)*

is cholesterol esterified with saturated VLCFA[157] and it does not accumulate until after the phase of myelin breakdown.[274,363] Small numbers of perivascular lymphocytes, hypertrophic astrocytes and lipophages are noted even in sclerotic lesions.

The lymphocytes display both T-cell, including CD4, and B-cell phenotypes,[132] with the T-cell predominant in one study.[278] Plasma cells are much less frequent. Immunoglobulins identified in ALD lesions were elutable at neutral pH, implying that they are not bound to a tissue component and are probably due to a disruption of the blood–brain barrier (BBB).[30] Inflammatory foci are usually most intense immediately within the advancing edge where myelin and oligodendrocytes have already been lost, axons are relatively spared and many interstitial lipophages are present. It was primarily this finding that prompted a two-stage pathogenetic theory:[273,274,284,319] firstly, a biochemical defect in the myelin membrane leads to its breakdown (dysmyelination) and, secondly, an inflammatory immune response directed at a CNS antigen exposed during this dysmyelination causes additional and a more extensive destruction of myelin (demyelination). CD8 cytotoxic lymphocytes (CTLs) appear to be intimately associated with interfascicular oligodendrocytes of normal white matter, which suggests a prominent pathogenic role for CTLs in the early myelin lesion of ALD/AMN.[163a] Hypertrophy, and perhaps hyperplasia, of glial fibrillary acidic protein (GFAP)-positive astrocytes and macrophage infiltration are also seen just outside the advancing edge, where some splitting of myelin sheaths and oedema are observed. These astrocytes and macrophages outside of and at the edge show both tumour necrosis factor-α (TNF-α) and interleukin-1 (IL-1) immunoreactivity. Adhesion molecule (ICAM) and class I and II upregulation also are noted. These data generated the additional hypotheses that cytokines, par-

ticularly TNF-α, initiate the secondary phase of inflammatory demyelination in which macrophages and T-lymphocytes are the main effector cells.[278] Subsequent studies demonstrated an upregulation of TNF receptor II mRNA, but surprisingly not TNF-α mRNA, in acute ALD lesions.[203] The absence of the cell-mediated immunosuppressive cytokine, IL-4, and the presence of γ-interferon align the T-helper cell response in ALD closer to the Th1 subtype. More recently, an excess of inducible nitric oxide synthase has been identified in ALD brains;[125] as well as CDIb, c and d, which raises the possibility of lipid antigen presentation. Abnormal myelin lipids and proteins, particularly gangliosides and proteolipid protein, containing saturated VLCFA have been proposed as the cytokine trigger/immunologic target.[230,273,274,279]

The Wallerian-like degeneration of the corticospinal tracts exhibits equivalent losses of axons and myelin, mild hypertrophy of astrocytes and a few lipophages. In contrast to non-ALD secondary tract degeneration, ALD tract degeneration often contains foci of perivascular lymphocytes and striated lipophages.[274,319]

Ultrastructural examination of old, sclerotic lesions usually reveals little more than astrocytic processes filled with dense cytofilaments. Crystals, consistent with hydroxyapatite, are rarely seen within myelinated axons and in the extracellular space. Active lesions contain demyelinated intact axons, demyelinated degenerate

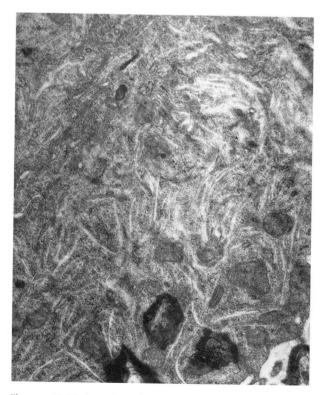

Figure 12.27 *Juvenile adrenoleukodystrophy. CNS macrophage in juvenile ALD containing predominantly fine, clear lipid clefts. (Autopsy.)*

axons, thinly myelinated axons, a variety of inflammatory cells, and two populations of macrophages. The predominant macrophage contains myelin debris and opaque lipid droplets (cholesterol esters), while the other contains lipid droplets, lamellae, lamellar-lipid profiles and angulate lysosomes containing spicules[274] (Fig. 12.27). The latter macrophages are those that retain birefringence after acetone extraction. Beyond this active edge of demyelination, the extracellular space is enlarged; splitting and fragmentation of myelin sheaths is observed.[319,351] Convincing evidence of lamellar inclusions in oligodendrocytes is rare.[43,357] The extent and intensity of CNS white-matter lesions in ALD do not correlate with clinical or pathological involvement of the adrenal cortex. A possible role for testosterone in triggering the onset of ALD or the AMN/ALD transition has been suggested.[274]

Neuropathology of AMN

Typically, AMN patients present with stiffness or clumsiness of the legs in the third or fourth decade, which progresses slowly but inexorably over the next few decades to severe spastic paraparesis.[133] The patients have been divided into 'pure' and 'cerebral', the latter indicating the presence of brain lesions.[16,230,233]

In AMN patients the spinal cord bears the brunt of the disease, as well as in symptomatic female heterozygotes[44,273,274,276,279,320] (Fig. 12.28). Loss of myelinated axons

and a milder loss of oligodendrocytes is observed in the long ascending and descending tracts of spinal cord, especially in the fasciculus gracilis and lateral corticospinal tracts (Fig. 12.29). The pattern of fibre loss is consistent with a distal axonopathy, in that the greatest losses are observed in the lumbar corticospinal and cervical gracile and dorsal spinocerebellar tracts. Axonal loss is usually commensurate with or greater than myelin loss. Gangliosides containing VLCFAs, present in AMN axonal membranes, are postulated to be the major pathogenic element,[273,274,276,279] perhaps by interfering with neurotrophic factor–receptor interactions. Sudanophilia and inflammation are minimal or absent. Astrogliosis, usually isomorphic, is moderate, but the predominant reactive cells are activated microglia. Some sparing of individual myelinated fibres is noted, even in severely affected tracts. Perivascular accumulations of striated and granular PAS-positive lipophages are present, particularly in relatively preserved tracts. Spinal grey matter is unremarkable. In semithin and thin sections, the affected tracts may show segmental demyelination, myelin corrugation, axonal ovoids, axons with thin myelin sheaths and probably axonal atrophy[276,293] (Fig. 12.30). Macrophages with pleomorphic cytoplasmic inclusions, mainly spicules, have been visualized. The severity of the myelopathy does not appear to correlate with the duration of neurological symptoms, presence or duration of endocrine abnormalities, or extent of supraspinal neuropathological lesions. Atrophy of neurons in the dorsal root ganglia, predominantly involving the largest and usually without appreciable neuronal loss, and lipidic mitochondrial inclusions have been demonstrated.[271a,275] Thus, this slowly progressive myelopathy with a late onset and perikaryal preservation even at autopsy should be amenable to therapeutic intervention.

The involvement of cerebral and cerebellar white matter in AMN is variable, but usually minimal compared with ALD.[274,276,279,320] In some there may be no lesions of white matter; but most, if not all, probably contain at least microscopic dysmyelinative foci, measuring millimetres in

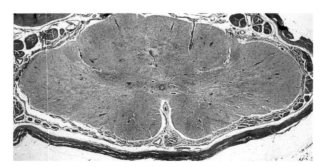

Figure 12.28 *Adrenomyeloneuropathy. Severe loss of myelinated fibres in long tracts of AMN spinal cord with sparing of the propriospinal fibres. (LFB–PAS.)*

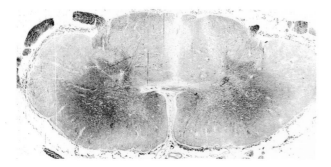

Figure 12.29 *Adrenomyeloneuropathy. More localized loss of myelinated fibres in both the gracile tracts and the posterolateral columns in a AMN patient. (Modified Bielschowsky.)*

Figure 12.30 *Adrenomyeloneuropathy. Loss of myelinated fibres and myelin ovoids in the gracile tract of AMN; semithin longitudinal section. (Toluidine blue.)*

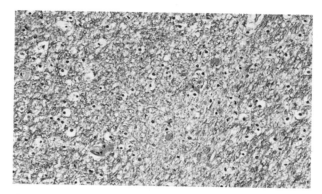

Figure 12.31 *Adrenomyeloneuropathy. Dysmyelinative lesion of the cerebral white matter displaying myelin pallor and PAS-positive macrophages in AMN. (LFB–PAS.)*

diameter, of myelin pallor with relative to total axonal and oligodendrocytic sparing, activation of microglia and the development of PAS-positive, striated macrophages (Fig. 12.31). Reactive astrocytosis and lymphocytes are absent or minimal. These lesions probably explain some neuropsychological deficiencies observed in 'pure' AMN.[101] Other patients with AMN demonstrate confluent losses of myelin staining in the cerebrum and, to a lesser extent, the cerebellum without significant inflammation and with sparing of arcuate fibres.[320] Still others display inflammatory demyelinative lesions with axonal loss, qualitatively similar to ALD but much more localized. Mixtures of these lesions may coexist in the same patient. Involvement of the posterior limbs can result in secondary corticospinal tract degeneration in the midbrain, pons, medulla and spinal cord, accompanied by mild reactive astrocytosis and a few lymphocytes. The concurrence of primary inflammatory demyelinative lesions in basis pontis can further complicate the interpretation of pyramidal tract degeneration. In AMN, however, the pyramidal tracts more commonly seem to undergo a dying-back axonopathy, and pyramidal signs appear early in AMN, even in 'pure' AMN. Thus, the corticospinal tracts in some 'cerebral' AMN patients may undergo both anterograde and retrograde axonal degeneration, whereas 'pure' AMN appears to develop only a retrograde, dying-back axonopathy. Finally, about 25% of patients with AMN (AMN/ALD) experience the myeloneuropathy for several decades before they develop confluent cerebral inflammatory demyelination qualitatively and usually quantitatively similar to childhood cerebral ALD; they usually die within a few years of this transition. In addition to these primary dysmyelinative and inflammatory demyelinative lesions, patients with AMN demonstrate non-inflammatory, bilateral, fairly symmetrical supraspinal lesions displaying comparable losses of axons and myelin (i.e. system degenerations); these involve the medial and lateral lemnisci, brachium conjunctivum, middle and inferior cerebellar peduncles, optic system, and particularly the geniculo-calcarine tracts.[274,320]

Refsum's disease, classical or adult (ARD) and atypical Refsum's disease

Peroxisomal phytanoyl-co A hydroxylase (phytanic acid α-hydroxylase) is the enzyme that is deficient in ARD.[165,339] The initial α-oxidation of phytanic acid, the elevation of which is the only biochemical abnormality in classical ARD, occurs in the peroxisome; the subsequent β-oxidation of its degradative product, pristanic acid, in man may be completed in the peroxisome[339] or in mitochondria.[395] Phytanic acid is a 20-carbon, branched-chain fatty acid, which is completely of dietary origin. Hence, dietary restriction can be an effective treatment, particularly for the peripheral neuropathy. The typical ARD patient presents before 20 years of age with decreased visual acuity due to pigmentary retinopathy, peripheral neuropathy, cerebellar ataxia, sensorineural hearing deficits, cardiac problems and dry skin to ichthyosis.[347] Many of these features are typical of PBD. Chronic RCDP has comparably elevated phytanic acid levels and icthyosis, but demonstrates low plasmalogens and cerebellar atrophy,[277] while ARD has normal plasmalogens and lacks cerebellar atrophy.

In view of the fact that dietary therapy is so successful and prevalent, neuropathological studies are essentially restricted to those performed decades ago.[45] Neuropathological lesions are most prominent in peripheral nerves where onion bulbs predominate. Osmiophilic granular, granulomembranous and crystalloid bodies are seen in Schwann cell cytoplasm.[107] The relationship of any of these structures to the increased phytanic acid found in peripheral nerve in this disease is unclear. Oil red O positive-lipid droplets, presumably phytanic acid,[45] in CNS have been noted in the leptomeninges, subpial glia, ependymal cells and choroid plexus epithelium. Excessive lipid is also detected in pallidum and around cerebral and retinal blood vessels.[367] There is an apparent increase in lipofuscin in CNS neurons. Other CNS lesions include system degenerations with marked loss of myelin (presumably myelinated fibres) in olivary and dentate nuclei and olivocerebellar fibres; and loss of myelin (presumably myelinated fibres) with gliosis in superior and middle cerebellar peduncles, pyramidal tracts and medial lemnisci. Neuronal loss is noted in the inferior olivary, dentate, cochlear, vestibular, gracile and cuneate nuclei. Thus, the CNS lesions of ARD seem to resemble those of AMN and MERRF (see below), in that they are mainly tract degenerations, but with superimposed lipid accumulations. Cerebral cortical neurons, Purkinje cells and spinal ganglion cells are also reduced in number. Degeneration and loss of anterior horn cells and ascending tract degeneration have been interpreted as being secondary to the peripheral neuropathy. Neuropathological studies do not record diffuse white-matter changes, but a CT report illustrates this alteration in cerebrum and cerebellum.[176] The reason why myelin is the major site of disease in the PNS, but not in the CNS, is probably due to the fact that phytanic acid concentrations in the PNS of ARD are much greater[201] and PNS myelin has a higher turnover rate.

Miscellaneous

Most of the few remaining conditions listed in Table 12.2 are rare; the patients have biochemical evidence of peroxisomal dysfunction, but lack either neuropathological data or noteworthy neurological features. Neuroradiological abnormalities in CNS myelination have been found in RCDP type II due to isolated DHAPAT deficiency,[392a] and cerebellar atrophy seems characteristic of mevalonic aciduria.[147a]

GROUP III: OTHERS

An archival case of orthochromatic leukodystrophy with epithelioid cells of Norman-Gullotta[136] had elevated VLCFA and equivocally elevated phytanic acid, as well as 'typical lamellar inclusions'.[224] One patient demonstrated ataxia and increased concentrations of pristanic acid, phytanic acid and C_{27} bile acids.[64] Two other patients had a peripheral neuropathy, one of whom was also ataxic; they demonstrated panperoxisomal dysfunction.[202] Another patient with a neuromuscular disorder resembling Werdnig–Hoffmann disease also had a panperoxisomal defect.[24] Three patients with a sensorimotor neuropathy and elevated levels of pristanic acid and C_{27}-bile acid intermediates were found to have a deficiency of α-methylacyl-CoA racemase, which is responsible for the conversion of pristanoyl-CoA and the C_{27}-bile acyl-CoAs to their (S)-stereoisomers.[111] Finally, patients with the typical, but milder, biochemical abnormalities of ZS may present with only pigmentary degeneration of retina and sensorineural hearing loss.[131a]

SPECIFIC TREATMENT OF PEROXISOMAL DISORDERS

Docosahexaenoic acid (DHA) has been used in the treatment of PBD with some success.[213,215] Glucocorticoid replacement therapy is needed by ALD/AMN patients who are Addisonian. Bone-marrow transplantation in ALD patients with mild neurological symptomatology has been the most effective therapy thus far.[16,230] Treatment of neurologically symptomatic ALD with corticosteroids and β-interferon to suppress the inflammatory response, as well as with thalidomide to block the postulated pathogenic role of TNF-α apparently has not been successful. Dietary restriction and treatment with glyceryl trierucate/glyceryl trioleate (Lorenzo's oil), in spite of the publicity and its ability to reduce promptly plasma VLCFA, have not had a statistically significant effect on the progression of AMN or ALD.[382] Lovastatin, a cholesterol-lowering agent, also reduces VLCFA plasma levels and gains entry into the CNS;[346] the latter has been a limiting factor for erucic acid. Riboflavin appeared to have a favourable biochemical effect on the first patient reported with glutaric aciduria, type III.[28] Dietary restriction has had a profound impact on ARD. Phytanic acid restriction has also had a positive clinical effect on an ataxic patient

with di- and trihydroxycholestanaemia[59] and another ataxic patient[64] with increased plasma levels of phytanic, pristanic and C_{27} bile acids.

CONSIDERATIONS ON THE CELLULAR PATHOGENESIS OF PEROXISOMAL DISORDERS

Much has been learned about the morphological, biochemical, cellular and molecular intricacies of peroxisomes and their disorders. However, much more needs to be discovered about how the recently identified molecular defects translate into biochemical and cellular abnormalities, and how they produce the characteristic tissue lesions. At present, VLCFAs are believed to play a central role in the pathogenesis of ALD/AMN. The relative insolubility of VLCFAs at normal body temperatures and their incorporation into membrane and myelin constituents, perhaps in particular phosphatidylcholine, gangliosides and the CNS-restricted proteolipid protein, have an adverse impact on the fluidity of these membranes by increasing their viscosity.[146,288] This is thought to lead to myelin instability and dysmyelination. Their incorporation into axonal membranes, particularly as gangliosides, may interfere with normal receptor–neurotrophic factor interactions, resulting in perikaryal and axonal atrophy with axonal loss. Their incorporation into plasma membranes of growth cones and radial glia may impair neuronal migrations in ZS and other dysmorphogenetic types.

A similar mechanism has been proposed for phytanic acid in the PNS myelin of ARD. This branched-chain fatty acid, with a 'thorny' configuration, may take the place of normal straight-chain fatty acids and also cause a membrane (myelin) instability, but in this case the melting point of the membrane would be lower than normal because of the presence of phytanate.[201,347] In the cerebellar atrophy of chronic RCDP, and perhaps IRD, the tissue plasmalogen deficiency is viewed as a possible contributing factor. Finally, the importance of DHA to retinal photoreceptor cells suggests a pathogenic role for its deficiency in the atypical pigmentary retinopathy of PBD.

Thus, it appears plausible to propose that abnormal fatty acids, particularly VLCFAs and phytanic acid, accumulate in peroxisomal disorders, are incorporated into cell membranes (including myelin and axons) and perturb their microenvironments. This would lead to dysmyelination and dysfunction, atrophy and death of vulnerable cells. Tissue plasmalogens and DHA may contribute to their vulnerability.

MITOCHONDRIA AND MITOCHONDRIAL DISORDERS

Mitochondria, originally called bioblasts by Altmann[6] and renamed mitochondria by Benda,[26] are cytoplasmic constituents of all aerobic nucleated cells. Although there is considerable variation in the size and shape of mitochondria, the basic morphology is much the same in that all share the ultrastructural characteristics of double unit membranes, outer and inner, an intermembranous space and the innermost matrix; the latter is subdivided by infoldings of the inner mitochondrial membrane (cristae) and frequently contains electron-dense granules containing minerals (e.g. calcium and phosphate) and lipid. The majority are larger than peroxisomes, particularly when elongated, and the round forms in man usually vary between 0.5 and 1.0 μm in diameter. Specialized morphological techniques are not needed to recognize mitochondria under the electron microscope because of their characteristic ultrastructure. They can be identified with acid fuchsin staining at the light-microscopic level (Altmann's stain), but they need to be fixed or postfixed in potassium dichromate-containing solutions, such as Zenker's or Regaud's. Commercial antibodies to mitochondrial proteins are available, such as to cytochrome *c* oxidase (COX, not to be confused with the more recently discovered cyclo-oxygenase that is also abbreviated COX), and can identify mitochondria immunohistochemically.

The principal functions of mitochondria are the oxidation of pyruvate, ketone bodies, fatty acids and amino acids, and the synthesis of adenosine triphosphate (ATP). They also play a role in calcium sequestration and the detoxification of ammonia in the urea cycle. By the middle of the twentieth century it was obvious that mitochondria represented the intracellular domain of intermediary metabolism and acetyl-CoA was the centre point. The cytochrome system was described in 1925;[174] oxidation–reduction processes were described in 1929;[396] and the elucidation of the Krebs cycle, ATP and oxidative phosphorylation followed.[184] The chemiosmotic theory was proposed to explain the proton-motive force that facilitated the synthesis of ATP.[221] In 1962 the first patient with a mitochondrial disorder, which included ultrastructural abnormalities, was identified by Luft *et al.*;[200] only one other patient with this disorder has been reported and the molecular defect is still unknown. Two important morphological observations took place in 1963: the recognition that intramitochondrial fibres had the characteristics of DNA,[243] and the description of ragged-red fibres (RRFs) in biopsied skeletal muscle.[104] Following the ultrastructural characterization of mitochondria,[254] subsequent studies demonstrated that the inner mitochondrial membrane was largely impermeable to molecules of all sizes and special adaptive mechanisms were necessary for the translocation of metabolites and proteins from the intermembranous space into the matrix. The protein importation process was found to be energy dependent and required the macromolecules to be unfolded before traversing mitochondrial membranes and then refolded after entering the mitochondrial matrix.[318] Chaperone proteins, such as 'heat shock' or 'stress' proteins, play important roles in this process. The leader sequence, consisting of 20–80 positively charged and non-polar amino

acid residues, guides the protein to the matrix and is cleaved by a mitochondrial specific protease. All but 13 of mitochondrial proteins are imported by this process. In striking contrast to the peroxisomal disorders, only a few mitochondrial diseases have been attributed to defects of protein importation. Fatty acids with chain lengths exceeding 8 or 10 carbon atoms require carnitine to enter mitochondria. There are several diseases related to abnormalities in the carnitine pathway (see Chapter 10, Volume II).

Mitochondria contain their own DNA, which is distinct from nuclear DNA in several ways.[80] All mtDNA is derived from the fertilized ovum.[113] Therefore, mtDNA characteristics are inherited exclusively from the mother, and the terms mitochondrial, maternal and cytoplasmic inheritance[124] are interchangeable. Each mitochondrion contains two to ten copies of the mtDNA genome. It is estimated that cells have hundreds to thousands of mitochondria and, therefore, more than 10 000 copies of mtDNA may exist in each cell. The mtDNA genome is a small, double-stranded circular molecule containing 16 569 base pairs (bp);[7] it contains one heavy and one light strand, and each strand contains its own origin of replication. The mitochondrial genome does not contain introns, and the only non-coding region in mtDNA is the displacement loop (D-loop). The D-loop contains 1000 bp and is the site of origin for replication of the heavy strand and the promoter regions for light and heavy strand transcription. The mitochondrial genome requires its own transcription and translation factors for synthesis of mitochondrial proteins and contains 37 genes, of which 13 code for structural proteins in the respiratory chain. The mitochondrial genome also contains 24 genes for protein synthesis, including two ribosomal RNAs and 22 transfer RNAs. There are equivalent genes in yeast.[409] The number of nuclear-encoded genes that directly or indirectly influence mitochondrial function is far greater. For example, the genes that code for the respiratory chain (oxidative phosphorylation) consist of 13 of mitochondrial origin and 70 or more of nuclear origin. In addition, an increasing number of nuclear genes are responsible for the importation of proteins and the assembly of respiratory chain complexes.[79] The proximity of mtDNA in the matrix to the respiratory chain embedded in the inner mitochondrial membrane, which is the major source of free radicals in a cell, is one factor that predisposes mtDNA to spontaneous mutations. The limited ability of mitochondria to repair mtDNA mutations is another.

The mitochondrial genotype may be homoplasmic or heteroplasmic. If homoplasmic, the thousands of mtDNA genomes per cell are identical; it is heteroplasmic when the genomes represent a mixture of wild-type (normal) and mutated (abnormal) types. The cellular phenotype is determined by the proportion of wild-type to mutated genomes. The severity of a mitochondrial disease is often directly proportional to the percentage of mutant mtDNA genomes, but conflicting data exist.[56a] It is believed that once the proportion of wild-type to mutated genomes exceeds a threshold, the biological behaviour of the cell changes (threshold effect) due to an impaired energy state. This concept may be an oversimplification of the biological state existing in the cell.[56,348] In chronic progressive external ophthalmoplegia (PEO) it is estimated that the threshold may vary from 60 to 70%, while in the syndromes of mitochondrial encephalomyopathy with lactic acidosis and stroke-like episodes (MELAS) and myoclonus epilepsy and ragged red fibres (MERRF) it varies from 90 to 95%.[246] The theoretical threshold is influenced by several factors, including the age of the patient and the energy demands of the tissue or organ. The latter is somewhat analogous to the mosaicism of peroxisomal disorders. Brain and muscle cells have a high energy demand, as do the tissues of a developing child, so in these situations the threshold for phenotypic transformation is lower. In addition to the threshold effect, an important concept needed to understand mitochondrial diseases is the principle of mitotic (replicative) segregation, which refers to the stochastic or random redistribution of mtDNA genomes during mitochondrial and cell divisions. Threshold effects and mitotic (replicative) segregation influence the oxidative capability of the cellular progeny and help to explain the phenotypic heterogeneity of maternally transmitted human diseases.

RRFs (illustrated and described more fully in the mitochondrial myopathies, Chapter 10, Volume II) are morphological reflections of large-scale rearrangements of mtDNA or pathogenic point mutations that affect the transfer (t) RNA genes. Both lesions interfere with intramitochondrial protein synthesis. In addition, nuclear mutations can produce multiple mitochondrial mtDNA deletions or can cause a reduction in the number of mtDNA copies, and these too may display RRFs. In contrast, point mutations affecting structural genes are not usually associated with RRF, although exceptions are being described with increasing frequency. Acquired injury to the mitochondrial genome, such as in zidovudine treatment, also causes RRF.[13] The emerging rule appears to be that RRFs are the morphological signature of mtDNA lesions that affect intramitochondrial protein synthesis, which may be the result of a primary molecular defect involving either the mitochondrial or nuclear genome. It is clear that RRFs do not exist in the many other mitochondrial diseases that affect other mitochondrial metabolic pathways and processes.

While ultrastructural abnormalities in mitochondria are easily identified in RRFs they have been less commonly recognized in the CNS, even in areas typically involved in the pathological process.[9,115,198,387] This may be due, in part, to the paucity of brain biopsies with the opportunity to preserve adequately mitochondrial structure and the vulnerability of mitochondria to agonal changes and post-mortem autolysis. It may also reflect the apoptotic removal of neurons that accumulate mutant mtDNA.[220] A monoclonal antibody to an inner mitochondrial membrane protein, MI168, that effectively labels RRF,[259] has been used immunohistochemically to demonstrate abnormal mitochondria in vascular smooth-muscle cells, choroid plexus epithelium, ependyma, astrocytes and specific neurons: neocortical, cerebellar cortex (Purkinje and granule cells) and inferior medullary olive in Leigh's syndrome (LS).[260] Oncocytic transformation of choroidal epithelium due to a proliferation of mitochondria has also been reported in LS[177] and MELAS.[247] Reviews of abnormal mitochondria in several diseases, including mitochondrial, should be consulted for further details.[120,390]

The classification of mitochondrial disorders has been even more problematic than that of the peroxisome. Previous attempts to classify them by clinical profile, such as mitochondrial myopathy and encephalopathy, or by morphological criteria proved unsatisfactory because of the clinical and histopathological heterogeneity of mitochondrial diseases. Biochemical classifications preceded the important discoveries of primary mutations in the mitochondrial genome.[150,389] Currently, mitochondrial disorders are characterized according to the genomic site of the molecular lesion, but correlation with the biochemical abnormalities is often problematic (Table 12.5).

From the clinical perspective three major categories emerge: defects of fatty acid oxidation, pyruvate meta-

Table 12.5 *Biomolecular classification of mitochondrial disorders*

Inherited conditions

  Nuclear DNA defects

    Substrate transport (e.g. carnitine deficiency)

    Substrate utilization (e.g. pyruvate dehydrogenase or carboxylase deficiency; Leigh's syndrome)

    Krebs cycle (e.g. fumarase deficiency)

    Oxidation–phosphorylation coupling (e.g. Luft's disease)

    Respiratory chain (e.g. Leigh's syndrome)

    Protein importation (e.g. ornithine transcarbamoylase deficiency)

    Intergenomic signalling (e.g. MNGIE, mtDNA depletion syndrome)

  Mitochondrial DNA defects

    Sporadic large-scale rearrangements (e.g. Kearns–Sayre syndrome)

    Transmitted large-scale rearrangements (e.g. a diabetes mellitus–deafness syndrome)

    Point mutations affecting structural genes (e.g. Leber's hereditary optic neuropathy)

    Point mutations affecting synthetic genes (e.g. MELAS, MERRF, Leigh's syndrome)

Acquired conditions

  Infections (e.g. Reye's syndrome)

  Toxic (e.g. MPTP)

  Drugs (e.g. zidovudine)

  Ageing (e.g. hypoxia-induced oxidative stress)

---

bolism, and the respiratory chain. Patients with defects of fatty acid oxidation typically experience metabolic decompensation during fasting and are discussed in Chapter 10, this Volume. Clinically, these patients have cardiac and skeletal muscle symptoms. Liver and kidney are less commonly involved, and brain is only secondarily affected by hypoketotic hypoglycaemia or cerebral oedema. This category encompasses defects of carnitine; defects of the inner mitochondrial membrane system, including very long-chain acyl-CoA (VLCAD) and long-chain 3-hydroxyacyl-CoA (LCHAD) dehydrogenase deficiencies; and defects in the mitochondrial matrix or β-oxidation system, including short-chain (SCAD),

medium-chain (MCAD), and long-chain (LCAD) acyl-CoA dehydrogenase deficiencies. Their clinical picture is often indistinguishable from Reye's syndrome. Elevated serum free fatty acids, hypoketonaemia, primary or secondary carnitine deficiency, hypoglycaemia and dicarboxylic aciduria are commonly associated with defects of fatty acid oxidation (Fig. 12.32a).

Lactic acidosis (acidaemia) is the laboratory signature of defects involving pyruvate metabolism and the respiratory chain. The lactate/pyruvate ratio may be normal when the oxidation–reduction potential is preserved, or elevated when the primary defect involves

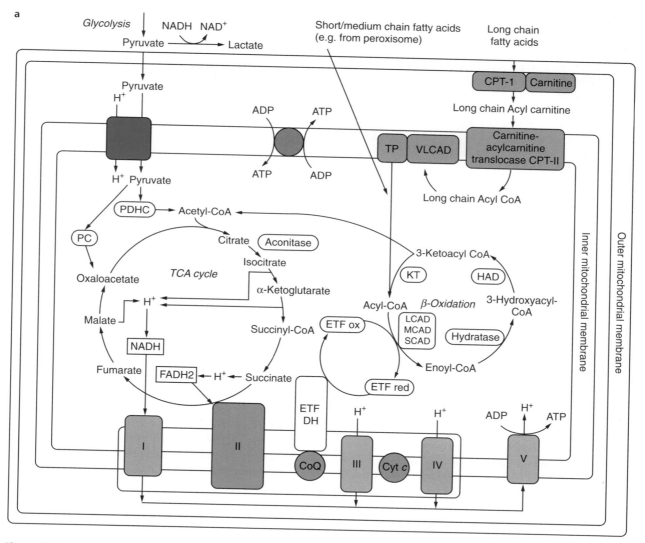

Figure 12.32 *(a) Schematic representation of mitochondrial metabolism. Respiratory chain components or complexes encoded exclusively by the nuclear DNA are brown; complexes containing some subunits encoded by the nuclear genome and others encoded by the mitochondrial genome are light blue. PC, pyruvate carboxylase; PDHC, pyruvate dehydrogenase complex; CPT, carnitine palmitoyltransferase; VLCAD, very long-chain acyl-CoA dehydrogenase; TP, trifunctional protein; LCAD, long-chain acyl-CoA dehydrogenase; MCAD, medium-chain acyl-CoA dehydrogenase; SCAD, short-chain acyl-CoA dehydrogenase; HAD, 3-hydroxyacyl-CoA dehydrogenase; KT, 3-ketothiolase; ETFox, oxidized form of electron-transfer flavoprotein; ETFred, reduced form of electron-transfer flavoprotein; ETF-DH, ETF-coenzyme Q oxidoreductase; I, II, III, IV, V, respiratory chain complexes I, II, III, IV and V; CoQ, coenzyme Q10; Cyt c, cytochrome c. (b) and (c) Continued over page.*

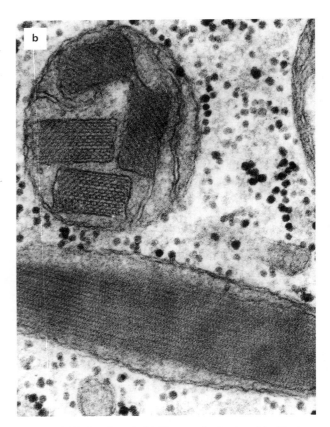

Figure 12.32 Continued. *(b) Abnormal mitochondria. Electron micrograph of abnormal mitochondria with paracrystalline inclusions. (Biopsy.) (c) continued over.*

the respiratory chain. The spectrum of defects in pyruvate metabolism ranges from life-threatening congenital lactic acidosis to a benign clinical syndrome of intermittent weakness or ataxia.[378] Such defects are associated with elevated serum and tissue concentrations of pyruvate, lactate and alanine. The lactate:pyruvate ratio is relatively preserved with these defects, because the oxidation–reduction potential is maintained. Defects of the respiratory chain (oxidative phosphorylation defects) show wide-ranging phenotypes, which include the well-characterized neuropathological entities of LS, MELAS, MERRF and Leber's hereditary optic neuropathy (LHON). The clinical presentation of respiratory chain defects is due to the involvement of organs that have a high oxidative metabolic demand, such as brain and muscle; hence, these diseases have been referred to as mitochondrial encephalomyopathies.[332] Biochemical defects of the respiratory chain are associated with lactic acidosis; however, unlike defects of pyruvate metabolism, respiratory chain defects are associated with elevated lactate:pyruvate ratios, usually higher than 20.

Leigh's syndrome, originally Leigh's disease or subacute necrotizing encephalomyelopathy, may be the result of nuclear DNA abnormalities involving substrate utilization or the respiratory chain, or may result from mtDNA abnormalities, such as point mutations. After a more thorough investigation, the genotypic–phenotypic correlation in LS is even weaker.[87] In addition to rare examples of mtDNA deletion (sporadic), depletion or point mutations, LS may be caused by COX deficiency (autosomal recessive transmission), pyruvate dehydrogenase E1α deficiency (X-linked), complex I deficiency (autosomal recessive) and ATPase 6 gene deficiencies (maternal).

Yeast genetics are becoming increasingly useful in the elucidation of mitochondrial disorders. The yeast *SHY1* gene was instrumental in the resolution of studies on COX-LS[79] and expanded the understanding of intergenomic processes. The *SCO1* and *SCO2* assembly genes facilitated the discovery of the human *SCO2* mutation.[257] Several mouse models have been informative, such as ant1 deficient and Tfam deficient.[388] These models also provide an opportunity to study the molecular and cellular consequences of impaired energy production, generation of reactive oxygen species and the activation of apoptotic mechanisms leading to the death of neurons. Two websites provide updates on mitochondria (http://www.umdf.org/ and http://www.hnrc.cpmc.columbia.edu/melas.htm/).

Inheritance patterns

The unique interplay of nuclear and mtDNA genomes on the respiratory chain results in numerous disparate patterns of inheritance. A biochemical defect involving the respiratory chain may be transmitted in either mendelian or non-mendelian patterns. The strictly maternal inheritance of mitochondria determines the pattern of vertical transmission of mtDNA mutations. Clinical conditions related to mtDNA mutations are transmitted from the mother to all her male and female progeny, but only daughters can pass the condition to succeeding generations. This is reminiscent of mendelian inheritance including autosomal dominant and X-linked patterns, but both genders are equally affected and there is no father-to-son transmission. Expression of the maternally inherited genetic defect is determined by replicative segregation and by the threshold effect, as has been demonstrated in several diseases with heteroplasmic mtDNA mutations: LHON, MERRF, MELAS, the syndrome of neuropathy, ataxia and retinitis pigmentosa (NARP syndrome) and a syndrome of diabetes mellitus–deafness–optic atrophy (Wolfram's syndrome). Deletions of mtDNA generally occur sporadically, as is the case with Kearns–Sayre syndrome (KSS) and PEO.

However, classical mendelian inheritance patterns exist in most mitochondrial diseases. The autosomal-recessive pattern of inheritance is the most common and includes all the known defects of fatty acid oxidation, pyruvate carboxylase deficiency, defects of the Krebs cycle, mtDNA depletion syndrome and several defects involving the respiratory chain. The syndrome of mitochondrial myopathy (almost invariably PEO) due to multiple mtDNA deletions is usually inherited as an autosomal-

c

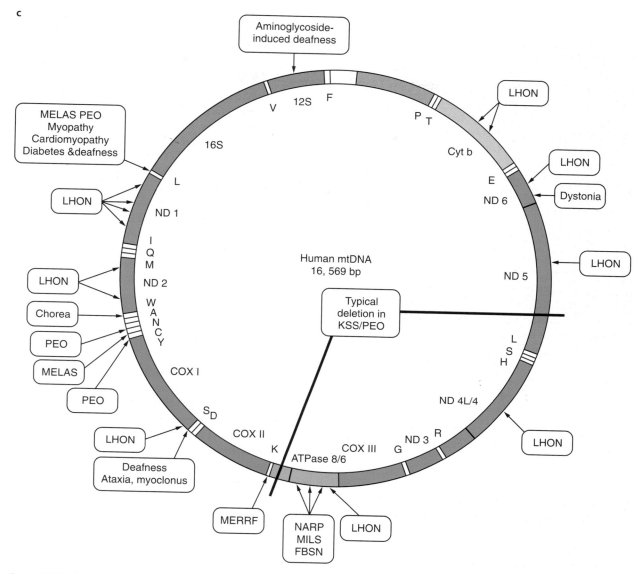

Figure 12.32 Continued. *(c) Morbidity map of human mitochondrial DNA diseases of the CNS. Differently coloured areas of the 16 569-bp mitochondrial DNA represent the structural genes for the seven subunits of complex I (NADH–CoQ oxidoreductase, ND), the three subunits of cytochrome c oxidase (COX), cytochrome b, the two subunits of ATP synthetase (ATPase 6 and 8), the 12S and 16S rRNAs, and the 22 tRNAs identified by one-letter codes for the corresponding amino acids. mtDNA, mitochondrial DNA; NADH-CoQ, nicotinamide–adenine dinucleotide coenzyme Q; rRNA, ribosomal ribonucleic acid; tRNA, transfer ribonucleic acid; FBSN, familial bilateral striatal necrosis; KSS, Kearns–Sayre syndrome; MELAS, mitochondrial encephalomyopathy, lactic acidosis, and stroke-like episodes; MERRF, myoclonus epilepsy with ragged-red fibres; MILS, maternally inherited Leigh's syndrome; NARP, neuropathy, ataxia, and retinitis pigmentosa; PEO, progressive external ophthalmoplegia. (a, c) Modified by permission from DiMauro et al.[87]*

dominant trait,[67] or more rarely autosomal-recessive.[33] The X-linked pattern of inheritance is seen in ornithine transcarbamoylase deficiency and most examples of pyruvate dehydrogenase complex deficiency (PDHC).

Diagnosis

The diagnosis of mitochondrial disorders is based initially on the clinical presentation followed by confirmatory lab-oratory data.[85,87] The clinical manifestations of mitochondrial diseases, particularly those that involve the CNS, are protean and result from dysfunction of organ systems that are highly dependent on aerobic metabolism, which include the brain, ears, eyes, skeletal and cardiac muscle, liver and kidney. Impairments of vision and sensorineural hearing loss are common. Convulsions and myoclonus, as well as lethargy and coma, may occur. Peripheral neuropathy may also be present and has been described with defects of long-chain fatty acid metabolism, generalized COX deficiency and the NARP mutation. The respiratory pattern may be affected, causing central hypoventilation or apnoea. Incoordination, ataxia, hypotonia, and extrapyramidal or pyramidal signs are common. Eye findings may include optic atrophy, retinal pigmentary degeneration, ptosis, ophthalmoparesis and ophthalmoplegia, strabismus and nystagmus. Limb weakness is common and muscular atrophy frequently occurs. Cardiomyopathy develops in many patients with mitochondrial diseases, and conduction defects may result in dysrhythmias or complete heart block. Kidney involvement produces tubular dysfunction with a generalized aminoaciduria, hyperphosphaturia and acidosis. This multisystemic involvement may be associated with short stature and poor weight gain. Presentations in neonates and infants cause a delay in psychomotor development, sucking and swallowing difficulties, failure to thrive and the acquisition of microcephaly, because the rate of brain growth is compromised. Endocrinopathies are being increasingly noted in patients with mitochondrial diseases, such as diabetes mellitus,[380,413] hypothyroidism,[95] hypoparathyroidism, isolated growth hormone deficiency,[139,295] and adrenal insufficiency.[42]

The blood lactate levels reflect the energy state of the tissues and are important indicators of respiratory chain defects. Excess pyruvate may be converted to lactate or alanine. The lactate/pyruvate ratio can be preserved or elevated, depending on the tissue oxidation–reduction potential. It is important to note that normal levels of blood lactate and pyruvate, however, do not exclude a respiratory chain defect, such as maternally inherited LS. The cerebrospinal fluid (CSF) lactate and pyruvate levels are more informative, but even these may rarely be normal. Cerebral ventricular lactate is elevated (cerebral lactic acidosis) in disorders of pyruvate metabolism and the respiratory chain, which can be documented by MR spectroscopy.[97] Serum creatine kinase is usually close to normal, with the exception of the myopathy associated with mtDNA depletion. CSF protein is often mildly elevated. Many other biochemical changes and profiles can help to establish a specific diagnosis.[80]

Imaging data are also often of great value.[87,176,381] Bilateral hypodense (CT) and hyperintense (MRI) signals in the putamen, caudate nucleus and globus pallidus are typical of LS, whereas infarct-like lesions, particularly in the posterior cerebral hemispheres and outside the distribution of major blood vessels, with basal ganglia calcifications are typical of MELAS. A diffuse hyperintense signal abnormality on T2-weighted images of cerebral and cerebellar white matter is characteristic of KSS and chronic PEO,[60,403] as is mineralization of the basal ganglia. Proton MR spectroscopy can demonstrate elevated lactate levels in the involved parenchyma[22] and in CSF in PDHC, LS, MELAS[134] and MERRF. In addition to these classical neuroradiological patterns, many patients display variations and non-specific findings.[377]

RRFs in fresh-frozen, cryostat sections of skeletal muscle are typically demonstrated with Gomori's one-step trichrome stain or even more effectively with a modified succinic dehydrogenase (SDH) reaction; in the latter they are seen as hyperintense 'ragged blue fibres'. Mitochondrial proliferation in affected blood vessels is best demonstrated with SDH and is most characteristic of MELAS. Scattered COX-negative fibres suggest impaired mitochondrial protein synthesis and are typically seen in mtDNA deletions and in mutations of tRNA genes of mtDNA. COX-positive RRFs are typical of MELAS or patients with mutations in structural mitochondrial genes (other than COX genes),[87] but they also may be COX negative.[55] Diffuse and less severely decreased COX staining, also involving smooth muscle and muscle spindles, is suggestive of LS. Most recently, immunohistochemistry using antibodies directed against mtDNA- or nuclear DNA-encoded proteins has proved useful. For example, in an atypical mitochondrial encephalomyopathy with a tRNA[Ile] (nt4269) A to G mutation, the immunohistochemical reactivity of antibodies to mtDNA-encoded COX II was compared with the immunoreactivity of antibodies against nuclear encoded-COX IV. In addition to establishing a mtDNA defect because of a selective loss of COX II, it apparently also demonstrated heteroplasmy/threshold effect in CNS neurons by a mosaic staining pattern.[169] Polymerase chain reaction (PCR) techniques also can be performed, even on single fibres dissected out of thick sections. Electron microscopy no longer shares its historical value, but it can reveal abnormal mitochondria when the enzyme histochemical results are equivocal.

Lymphocytes, cultured skin fibroblasts or muscle biopsies can be analysed biochemically for the activities of respiratory chain enzymes. Fresh muscle is preferable, but the activities of individual respiratory chain complexes I and IV, as well as the combined activities of complexes I plus III or II plus III can be measured in frozen muscle specimens. Isolated defects of complex I, III or IV can be due to either mutations in nuclear genes, especially if transmitted by autosomal recessive inheritance, or mutations in mtDNA protein-encoding genes in sporadic patients or those with maternal inheritance. In contrast, combined defects of complexes I, III and IV suggest mtDNA involvement, either primary or secondary.

A molecular assay, however, is needed to define precisely the pathogenic mutation and is usually achieved by first screening for the most common mutations associated with a particular clinical-laboratory phenotype, e.g. the A3243G mutation in MELAS that accounts for about 80% of typical cases (reviewed in Refs 86, 349). Blood is usually adequate for MELAS, MERRF, some LHON, KSS and Pearson's syndrome; but muscle DNA is preferable, particularly when investigating mtDNA large-scale deletions. Prenatal testing for nuclear DNA defects and mtDNA point mutations affecting structural genes is available. Prenatal testing for mtDNA point mutations affecting synthetic genes is unreliable, because of the unpredictability of replicative segregation and the consequent heteroplasmy.

When the diagnosis is not made ante-mortem and a mitochondrial disorder is still suspected, samples of skeletal muscle may be taken at autopsy for light and electron microscopy and immunohistochemistry. Small samples of skeletal muscle should be snap-frozen in liquid nitrogen for enzyme histochemistry, enzyme biochemical assays and molecular studies. Biochemical studies of blood, brain, liver or skeletal muscle taken at autopsy are severely compromised by autolysis and are essentially fruitless. Even when all else fails, it is still possible to extract DNA from formalin-fixed tissues[240] or from paraffin sections[313] to identify at least the common mutations.

General pathology and neuropathological overview of mitochondrial disorders

The major organ systems that are involved in mitochondrial disorders are the CNS, eyes, skeletal muscle, heart, liver and kidneys. The PNS can also be affected and may demonstrate axonal degeneration, demyelination or both. The general pathological correlates of the systemic signs and symptoms mentioned above include RRFs and other myopathic features in skeletal muscle, lipid accumulations in skeletal and cardiac muscle, hypertrophic cardiomyopathy, hepatic steatosis and portal fibrosis. Mitochondria show abnormal variations in size (megaconial) and shape (pleoconial), and often contain intramitochondrial protein paracrystalloids (Fig. 12.32b).

Mitochondrial disorders, just as hypoxia, can affect both neurons and oligodendrocytes; hence, both grey and white matter are typically involved in most mitochondrial encephalomyopathies. Grey matter involvement varies from rarefaction and spongy change, through neuronal loss and astrogliosis, to areas of ischaemic-like necrosis. White matter involvement usually varies from myelin pallor, through a spongy myelinopathy due to the accumulation of intramyelinic oedema, to cystic necrosis. Involvement of the CNS can be divided into three major neuropathological patterns: the first is widespread damage to brain tissue resulting in microencephaly and ventriculomegaly; this is usually associated with congenital lactic acidosis, urea cycle defects and some diseases of fatty acid oxidation. The localization may be primarily that of a poliodystrophy or polioencephalopathy (grey matter), a leukoencephalopathy (white matter) or combined grey and white matter lesions. The second pattern is more limited to grey matter and is best typified by LS, in which there is symmetrical subcortical damage particularly affecting the brainstem, cerebellar roof nuclei, basal ganglia and thalamus; histologically, there is rarefaction of the

neuropil to neuronal loss with a corresponding decrease of myelin, reactive astrocytosis, and proliferation or swelling of cerebral microvessels. In some disorders, particularly in MELAS, multifocal ischaemic-like necrosis develops and often favours the posterior cerebrum. In others, such as MERRF, more selective neuronal loss and tract degeneration predominate. The third pattern is one of a spongy myelinopathy (a leukoencephalopathy); this is commonly seen in KSS.[343] MRI may reflect this latter pattern with a hyperintense signal of CNS white matter in T2-weighted images. A few mitochondrial diseases also demonstrate developmental anomalies, such as agenesis of the corpus callosum and heterotopic olivary nuclei (e.g. PDHC), and neocortical neuronal migration abnormalities (e.g. glutaric aciduria type II).

The neuropathological features of LS, KSS, LHON, MELAS, MERRF and, to some extent, congenital lactic acidosis, are fairly consistent (see below). Numerous biochemical, genetic and molecular defects can produce the same clinical phenotype and, hence, the neuropathological features of these major mitochondrial diseases will be described after reviewing their places in the molecular classification.

An overview of mitochondrial disorders is presented in Table 12.6 and Fig. 12.32c.

INHERITED CONDITIONS ASSOCIATED WITH NUCLEAR DNA DEFECTS

Defects of substrate transport

These involve various defects in carnitine metabolism and are discussed in Chapter 10, Volume II, as are the substrate utilization defects involving fatty acid oxidation.

Defects of substrate utilization

The clinical spectrum of defects in pyruvate metabolism ranges from rapidly fatal congenital lactic acidosis to a benign clinical syndrome manifested by intermittent weakness or ataxia.[378]

Classical pyruvate carboxylase deficiency

This autosomal-recessive condition is life-threatening and is reflected by hypotonia, psychomotor retardation, failure to thrive and metabolic acidosis.[81] Thirty-five patients have been reported,[378] 16 of whom had the severe French phenotype with absence of enzyme protein and 18 had a less severe but equally fatal North American phenotype in which a mutated protein is present in tissues with some residual activity. Biotin deficiency affects pyruvate carboxylase, as well as three other biotin-dependent carboxylase reactions. Neuropathological data are scant,[15,308] and in some (the French phenotype) the lesions are those of congenital (fatal, cerebral) lactic acidosis[316,402] (see below). One child with pyruvate carboxylase

Table 12.6 *Overview of mitochondrial disorders*

	CLA	LS	KSS	MELAS	MERRF
Major localization	Cer WM	Subcort GM	CNS WM	Cer GM	Dentate and olivary nuclei
Histopathology	Cell death	Cell death (prolonged)	Spongy myelin	Cell death (rapid)	Neuronal loss with tract degeneration
RRF	0	0 to +/–	+	+	+
Spongy GM	+/–	+++	+/–	+	+/–
Spongy WM	+	+	+++	+/–	+/–
Neuronal loss	+/–	++	+	+++	+++
Astrocytosis	+/–	++	+/–	++	++
Oligodendroglial loss	+++	+/–	+	++	+
Microgliosis	+/–	++	+/–	+++	+
Vascularity	+/–	+++	+/–	++	+/–
Mineralization	0	0	++	+++	+/–
Biochemical defect	PC, PDHC, respiratory chain	Complex IV or I, PDHC	Respiratory chain	Respiratory chain	Respiratory chain
Molecular defect	Multiple nDNA	Multiple nDNA	4977 bp deletion mtDNA	A3243G tRNA[Leu] mtDNA	A8344G tRNA[Lys] mtDNA

0, negative; +/–, rare; +, mild; ++, moderate; +++, severe.
A, adenine; bp, base pairs; Cer, cerebral; CLA, congenital lactic acidosis; CNS, central nervous system; G, guanine; GM, grey matter; KSS, Kearns–Sayre syndrome; leu, leucine; LS, Leigh's syndrome; lys, lysine; MELAS, mitochondrial encephalomyopathy, lactic acidosis, stroke-like episodes; MERRF, myoclonus epilepsy with ragged red fibres; mtDNA, mitochondrial deoxyribonucleic acid; nDNA, nuclear deoxyribonucleic acid; PC, pyruvate carboxylase; PDHC, pyruvate dehydrogenase complex; RRF, ragged red fibres; Subcort, subcortical; tRNA, transfer ribonucleic acid; WM, white matter.

deficiency displayed mild hepatic steatosis, hypoplasia or atrophy of hypomyelinated cerebral white matter with perivascular macrophages and numerous ectopic neurons, severe neocortical neuronal loss, and ectopic glia in the subarachnoid space.[15] In respect to the biotin-related multiple carboxylase deficiency, an intermittently ataxic 3.5-year-old child demonstrated anterior vermal atrophy, a multifocal, subacute necrotizing myelopathy involving all funiculi and diffuse lymphocytic meningoencephalitis with microgliosis restricted to the grey matter.[308]

Pyruvate dehydrogenase complex (PDHC) deficiency

Approximately 200 patients with PDHC deficiency have been reported. Defects in most patients involve the E1α-subunit; a male predominance is expected because the gene is located on the X chromosome. However, phenotype–genotype correlations are complex in PDHC deficiency.[77,82,83] There are two major presentations: neonatal and infantile. In the neonatal presentation hypotonia, episodic apnoea, convulsions, weak suck, dysmorphic facies simulating the fetal alcohol syndrome, lethargy, low birth weight, failure to thrive and coma are seen.[5,57,219]

About 70 patients have been noted with the infantile form. They usually present between 3 and 6 months of age with psychomotor retardation, hypotonia, convulsions, episodic apnoea, ataxia, pyramidal and extrapyramidal signs, lethargy, dysmorphic features, deceleration of head and somatic growth, ophthalmoplegia, optic atrophy, peripheral neuropathy, ptosis, dysphagia and cranial nerve palsies. A brain biopsy of an infantile case displayed a cortical focus of neuronal loss with glial and vascular proliferation, and hypomyelination of subcortical white matter.[292] Of the 70 infantile cases, 21 came to autopsy and LS was found in 81% of them.[21] Hypoplasia to agenesis of the corpus callosum and ectopic medullary olives are highly characteristic of PDHC deficiency, particularly the neonatal group[57,80,300b,333] (Fig. 12.33). Both malformations develop early in fetal life (6–12 weeks), when glycolysis is the primary source of energy production in the brain. Oxidative phosphorylation assumes a prominent role in the last few fetal months and the postnatal period.[336] Seven children had a benign phenotype with fluctuating ataxia, postexercise fatigue, transient paraparesis and thiamine responsiveness. These children had normal mental and motor development between episodes.[84] Two sisters with familial intermittent lactic acidosis due to lipoate acetyl-

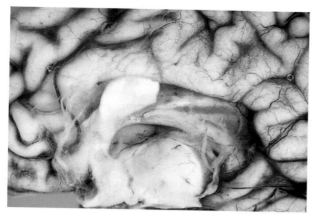

Figure 12.33 *Pyruvate dehydrogenase complex deficiency. Partial agenesis (posterior) of the corpus callosum in PDHC deficiency.*

transferase deficiency died of spontaneous lactic acidosis at around 3 and 7 years of age. They both showed decreased myelin staining of CNS white matter without a cellular reaction.[51]

Defects of the Krebs cycle

Krebs cycle defects are rare, but clinical reports of partial deficiencies in dihydrolipoyl (lipoamide) dehydrogenase, α-ketoglutarate dehydrogenase and succinate dehydrogenase have been described.[83] Some had episodic infantile diseases, but others had seizures, dystonic movements and imaging abnormalities of the basal ganglia that were consistent with LS. The postmortem examination of a 7-month-old male with combined dihydrolipoyl and alpha-ketoglutarate dehydrogenese activities revealed LS-like lesions: 'myelin loss and cavitation were found in discrete areas of the basal ganglia, thalami and brainstem. The cerebral cortices appeared to be free of pathology'.[300c] Sudden death was a common event in both dihydrolipoyl dehydrogenase and α-ketoglutarate dehydrogenase deficiencies.

Fumarase deficiency

Approximately nine infants and children have been described since the original report.[412] They usually exhibited delayed development, hypotonia, microcephaly and failure to thrive. Other findings consisted of polyhydramnios, dysmorphic facies, hepatomegaly, infantile spasms, intermittent vomiting, dystonia, amaurosis, repeated infections and neutropenia. The neuropathological features are said to approximate those of females deficient in PDHC, who have extreme cerebral atrophy and microencephaly due to frameshift mutations that completely abolish E1α protein synthesis.[40] At autopsy the brain of one patient showed microencephaly, hypomyelination and 'islets of cell' heterotopias in the cere-

bellum and parieto-occipital areas.[119] The fumarase gene has been assigned to chromosome 1 and is transmitted as an autosomal-recessive trait, with consanguinity noted in several families.

Defects of oxidation–phosphorylation coupling

Luft's disease (non-thyroidal hypermetabolism)

Only two sporadic patients have been described; abundant RRFs were found unassociated with neurological symptomatology. The biochemical defect is still unknown.

Defects of the respiratory chain (oxidative phosphorylation)

The respiratory chain consists of five enzyme complexes that are embedded in the inner mitochondrial membrane. Electrons are collected from numerous sources by complexes I and II, transfer to complex III via coenzyme Q_{10} (ubiquinone), sequentially move through cytochrome C and complex IV, and then react with oxygen. At the same time, protons are pumped across the inner mitochondrial membrane at complexes I, III and IV, resulting in a proton gradient. The potential energy in this proton gradient is used by complex V to condense adenosine diphosphate (ADP) and inorganic phosphate into ATP, which is transferred across the inner mitochondrial membrane by adenine nucleotide translocase.

The respiratory chain complexes are uniquely influenced by both nuclear and mitochondrial genes, except for complex II which is completely controlled by the nuclear genome. Many previously reported cases designated as respiratory chain or oxidative phosphorylation (OXPHOS) disorders were studied prior to our understanding of mitochondrial genetics, so it is difficult to classify them at the present time. This is complicated by the great diversity of clinical presentations, some of which occur without neurological or neuromuscular symptoms.[11] Defects in complex I or IV are relatively common and are the most frequent causes of LS.[2,91,227,296] It is noteworthy, however, that relatively few to no mutations in the complex I mitochondrial and complex IV mitochondrial or nuclear structural genes could be identified. In the case of COX, loss-of-function mutations (e.g. frameshift, stop, splice-site) have been identified in the nuclear *SURF 1* gene, the human homologue of *SHY1*, located on chromosome 9q34. That gene and another nuclear gene, *SCO2* gene, located on chromosome 22q13 encode mitochondrial proteins that are involved in the assembly and maintenance of COX activity and mitochondrial respiration.[257,364,365,411] A few pontocerebellar[73] and cerebellar hypoplasias, as well as olivopontocerebellar atrophy,[336] have been associated with abnormalities of the respiratory chain. Alpers disease (see Chapter 8, Volume I) has been linked biochemically to several respiratory chain defects, most notably the mtDNA depletion syndrome.[80,336] Also

Navajo neurohepatopathy, an autosomal recessive condition of full-blooded Navajo children manifested by severe peripheral neuropathy and cirrhosis, has been linked to mtDNA depletion syndrome.[386a] Currently, Friedreich's ataxia and at least one form of Hereditary Spastic Paraplegia (SPG7) are considered OXPHOS diseases, because their gene products (frataxin and paraplegin, respectively) have a mitochondrial localization and their mutated forms induce abnormalities in the respiratory chain.[335a]

Complex I (reduced nicotinamide–adenine dinucleotide phosphate–coenzyme Q reductase) is the largest complex and consists of over 40 polypeptides, seven of which are of mtDNA origin. More than 60 patients can be subclassified into myopathic or multisystemic types. The myopathy usually presents in children or young adults as exercise intolerance and limb weakness. The multisystemic or encephalomyopathic type can present in three forms: fatal congenital lactic acidosis, a milder encephalomyopathy in children or adults, and LS.[227,296,369] The prognosis is influenced by the age at presentation (congenital worst) and the extent of organ involvement (muscle-only best). Atypical presentations, such as adults with ataxia, dementia, parkinsonism and dystonia due to olivopontocerebello- and striatonigral-like lesions,[370] are not uncommon. One female infant with a point mutation in the *NDUFV1* flavoprotein gene displayed a fatal leukodystrophy with myoclonic epilepsy.[327]

Deficiencies of complex II (succinate–coenzyme Q reductase), which consists of only four nuclear-encoded polypeptides, are rare and usually present as multisystemic encephalomyopathies[80] and LS.[34] Complex III (coenzyme Q–cytochrome C oxidoreductase) consists of 11 polypeptide subunits, of which only one is encoded by mtDNA. Clinical presentations include: fatal congenital or child/adult multisystemic disease, pure myopathy in children and adolescents, pure (histiocytoid) cardiomyopathy in infants[256] and exercise intolerance.[8] A functional deficiency of complex III due to a primary deficiency in muscle coenzyme Q_{10} has been found in some patients with familial cerebellar ataxia and atrophy, pyramidal signs, seizures and mental retardation.[239a]

Complex IV (cytochrome *c* oxidase; COX) contains 13 polypeptide units, three of which are encoded by mtDNA. Its deficiencies can also be divided into myopathic (fatal and benign infantile) and multisystemic.[379] The infantile forms are indistinguishable and both have severe lactic acidosis; however, the benign form spontaneously improves over several months and normalizes by 1–3 years. The multisystemic form usually manifests as autosomal-recessive LS, which is commonly due to a partial generalized defect in COX.[227,296,379] The COX deficiency is secondary to a primary mutation in an assembly gene, such as *SURF 1* or *SCO2*.[349] COX-LS can be distinguished from PDHC-LS by the latter's neonatal to early infantile presentation (versus late infantile), death by 1 year (versus 4–5 years), seizures, recurrent apnoea, relative preservation of the lactate:pyruvate ratio and brain malformations. Atypical presentations, such as a pseudo-leukodystrophic pattern on neuroimaging,[75,407] have been reported.

Complex V (mitochondrial ATP synthase) contains 14 polypeptides, two of which are encoded by mtDNA, and has two major domains: the hydrophilic F_1 in the matrix and the hydrophobic F_0 embedded in the inner membrane. Single cases of a slowly progressive congenital myopathy with RRF[324] and a multisystemic form that developed in a 17-year-old male who originally presented with a carnitine-deficient lipid storage myopathy[61] are reported. The most noteworthy member of this group is NARP (neuropathy, ataxia and retinitis pigmentosa), which usually presents in adolescents or young adults with a slowly progressive course; its phenotype is highly variable and may resemble Usher's syndrome or adult Refsum's disease;[376] but it also may include developmental delay, dementia, seizures, proximal weakness, an axonal sensory neuropathy, and even KSS or MELAS phenotypes.[312,376] Lactic acidosis is inconsistent, and neurogenic atrophy without RRF is seen. The major molecular defect is a heteroplasmic T to G mutation in the ATPase 6 gene at nucleotide 8993 (T8993G).[311,335,376] ATPase 6, or subunit a, is a mtDNA-encoded subunit that catalyses ATP synthesis and translocates protons into the matrix. Patients with NARP/T8993G usually do not have severe CNS clinical problems, except for ataxia and rarely recurrent intractable seizures. Post-mortem examinations of NARP appear to be lacking. Neuroimaging data, however, have revealed mild cerebral and cerebellar atrophy,[151] areas of abnormal signals in periventricular white matter with oligoclonal bands in CSF,[376] bilateral necrosis of lenticular nuclei 'compatible with old lacunar infarcts' (but probably not) with subsequent diffuse oedema of the left hemisphere,[312] and olivopontocerebellar atrophy.[336] Some maternal relatives may develop LS (maternally inherited), if the proportion of mutated mtDNA (T8993G) reaches a level of 90–95%. This maternally inherited LS (MILS) usually presents with a neonatal, rapidly progressive form of LS, but milder phenotypes also are seen. Lactic acidosis is usually present, but RRF are still lacking. The atypical pigmentary retinopathy, present in approximately 40% of (T8993G) maternally inherited LS, distinguishes this LS from LS associated with COX or PDHC deficiencies, and even from LS due to T8993C which has a milder[310] and perhaps more ataxic[114] phenotype. Seizures occur in two-thirds of MILS, one-half of PDHC-LS and less than one-tenth of COX-LS. With both 8993 mutations the phenotypic severity correlates directly with the percentage of mutated mtDNA; both cause a single amino acid substitution in the F_0 domain: the T to G transversion changes leucine to arginine, while the T to C substitutes proline. Coincidentally, subunit c of ATP synthase has been localized in lysosomal inclusions that accumulate in late infantile and juvenile ceroid-lipofuscinoses.[255]

Defects of protein importation

Protein targeting deficiencies or errors have rarely been reported, but are anticipated to be an important subgroup in the future. Defects of major importation factors may be incompatible with life, thus explaining the scarcity of such diseases.[110] Defects in the leader sequences of methylmalonyl-CoA mutase[193] and PDHC,[355] resulting in one form of methylmalonic aciduria and PDHC-LS, respectively, have been published. A mutated but catalytically active alanine glyoxylate aminotransferase, the peroxisomal matrix protein deficient in primary hyperoxaluria type I, was detected in the mitochondrial matrix;[294] this misdirectional error attests to the similarities between peroxisomes and mitochondria. The human deafness-dystonia syndrome may be due to a defect in protein import.[182]

Defects of intergenomic signalling

At least two mtDNA associated clinical syndromes have been described that result from a primary molecular defect involving the nuclear genome, in addition to the intergenomic cross-talk mentioned above in COX-LS. More are expected in the future.[145a] The first is multiple deletions of mtDNA, which is characterized by PEO or PEO and multisystemic disease. As a rule, the autosomal-dominant PEO form has disease limited to the musculature,[409] while autosomal-recessive PEO is multisystemic.[47,68] The former presents in the third decade with PEO, progressive limb weakness, bilateral cataracts, depression and premature death. Linkage analysis has revealed genetic heterogeneity in a Finnish family mapped to chromosome 10 and an Italian family to chromosome 3. One form of the autosomal-recessive PEO has a childhood onset and is accompanied by a severe cardiomyopathy. Another form is the mitochondrial neurogastrointestinal encephalopathy syndrome (MNGIE),[145,245] which previously has been referred to as myoneurogastrointestinal encephalopathy (MNGIE),[21] POLIP (polyneuropathy, ophthalmoplegia, leukoencephalopathy and intestinal pseudo-obstruction),[338] oculogastrointestinal muscular dystrophy,[162] MEPOP (mitochondrial encephalomyopathy with sensorimotor polyneuropathy, ophthalmoplegia and pseudo-obstruction),[306] and CIPO (chronic intestinal pseudo-obstruction with myopathy and ophthalmoplegia).[195] In addition to mtDNA deletions, there is a depletion of mtDNA in MNGIE. The disease has been mapped to 22q 13.32-qter, and the gene encodes thymidine phosphorylase.[245] Gastrointestinal dysfunction, cirrhosis, peripheral neuropathy, ophthalmoplegia and MRI evidence of a leukoencephalopathy are prominent.[21,145,338] The severely atrophic gastropathy–enteropathy seen in MNGIE patients is of debatable aetiology; some see it as neurogenic[338] and others as myogenic.[162,198] Neuropathological data have been somewhat discordant. A mixed axonal and demyelinative sensorimotor peripheral neuropathy, leptomeningeal and adventitial fibrosis of PNS blood vessels;[21] or widespread endoneurial fibrosis, an axonal neuropathy and central optic neuropathy, and pallor of CNS white matter with sparing of the corpus callosum due in part to a loss of myelinated fibres without gliosis[338] have been reported at autopsy. A focus of spongy myelinopathy of the medial posterior columns, most marked at lumbar levels and without vascular changes, was also noted in one patient.[162] RRFs are characteristic of both autosomal-dominant and recessive forms, including 80% of MNGIE patients. An additional patient with multiple mtDNA deletions exhibited marked cerebellar ataxia, a parkinsonian extrapyramidal movement disorder, PEO, dysphagia and severe peripheral neuropathy. At autopsy, the cerebellum and brainstem were atrophic owing to a marked and diffuse loss of hemispheric Purkinje, nigral and olivary neurons; a moderate loss of dentate neurons with gliosis and myelin pallor, and microgliosis of the dentate nucleus, substantia nigra, red nucleus, inferior colliculus and superior cerebellar peduncle. The cerebral white matter displayed diffuse myelin pallor with gliosis, while there was astrogliosis of the superficial occipital cortex and diffuse microvacuolation of the molecular layer. Severe hippocampal (CA1–4) neuronal loss was evident, despite the lack of seizures until his terminal admission for respiratory insufficiency. Myelin pallor (probably with axonal loss) throughout the posterior columns and neuronal loss in DRG were noted. A mosaic pattern of COX-deficient/succinic dehydrogenase-positive neurons was noted.[68] Thus, many of the neuropathological features of this patient simulate those of MERRF (see below).

A second defect in intergenomic signalling is the autosomal-recessive mtDNA depletion syndrome with variable tissue expression,[226] in which a nuclear gene defect is associated with a quantitative reduction in mtDNA copy number. The mechanism(s) for depletions of mtDNA is (are) still unknown. Two main phenotypes have emerged: a fatal congenital or infantile myopathic form with limb weakness and hypotonia, and a fatal hepatopathy.[300] Lactic acidosis is characteristic of the congenital myopathy and hepatopathy, and RRFs are noted in the congenital myopathy. The severity of the phenotype correlates directly with the deficiency of mtDNA: congenital 83–98% and infantile 66–83%. Others present with CNS or PNS involvement,[386] including LS,[228] and spinal muscular atrophy.[268] It may be of interest to note that some patients with milder childhood forms of chromosome 5p-spinal muscular atrophy have demonstrated abnormalities in fatty acid metabolism comparable to patients with primary defects in mitochondrial fatty acid β-oxidation.[68a] Hepatic involvement varies from mild microvesicular and macrovesicular steatosis with portal fibrosis, through cirrhosis with macrovesicular steatosis and cholestasis, to massive hepatic necrosis. Either RRFs[386] or pseudo-RRFs[228] are present. Abnormal mitochondria and decreased COX histochemical activity are seen in the liver. Imaging studies have revealed partial agenesis of the corpus callosum, cortical atrophy and abnormal CNS white matter.[386] In another study a 5-month-old girl with massive hepatic necrosis and a normal head CT scan was reported to lack CNS lesions at autopsy. Another patient with LS, clinically and radiologically (MRI), exhibited rarefaction and gliosis with microcavitary foci containing macrophages in putamen (particularly lateral) and caudate nucleus, gliosis of the external pallidum and substantia nigra; hyperplastic and prominent capillaries were present in the medial putamen and substantia nigra; and Alzheimer type II astrocytes were numerous in cerebral cortex, basal ganglia, dentate nucleus and brainstem.[228] Two other interesting findings in this LS case were: (1) diffuse, patchy and subcortical myelin pallor associated with scant, perivascular, LFB-negative foamy macrophages and mild chronic astrogliosis; and (2) a bilateral decrease in myelinated fibres of medial fasciculus gracilis in a section of lower thoracic cord. Other cases of mtDNA depletion syndrome, in which a neuropathological post-mortem examination was performed,[112,386] were reported to show no abnormalities of the brain. Those who lack CNS pathology may have sufficient wild-type mtDNA in the brain,[386] but this issue needs further study. Finally, one patient demonstrated a spongy myelinopathy of cerebral and cerebellar white matter,[145a] and two other patients have the clinical features of Navajo neurohepatopathy.[386a]

Neuropathology of congenital lactic acidosis

Deficiencies of pyruvate carboxylase, PDHC or the respiratory chain, particularly of complexes I or IV, may result in a rapidly progressive and fatal neonatal phenotype consisting primarily of hypotonia, psychomotor retardation, failure to thrive and coma. Affected neonates usually die before 8 months of age. Some cases have shown only 'hypoxic' lesions, such as bilateral loss of neurons in Sommer's sector.[90] However, that same patient was reported to have 'focal infarcts in the basal ganglia', which raises the possibility of an atypical LS. Others seem to constitute a neuropathological subset in which lesions of white matter predominate. Brain size varies from microencephalic to macrocephalic, but ventriculomegaly due to compensatory hydrocephalus rarely occurs. The cardinal neuropathological feature of congenital (fatal, cerebral) lactic acidosis consists of focal to diffuse degeneration to cystic necrosis of cerebral and cerebellar white matter. Cystic degeneration of the white matter is usually bilateral and symmetrical, but varies from case to case in respect to its primary lobar involvement; cases with frontal predominance and others with parieto-occipital involvement are reported. The deep cerebellar white matter near the dentate nucleus is preferentially affected in some cases.[108,196] Two out of three patients confirmed to be PDHC deficient,[5,57,219] as well as those mentioned above with unconfirmed biochemical defects, revealed that either subcortical or periventricular white matter may be preferentially involved by the necrotizing process (Figs

12.34–12.36); the latter results in periventricular (paraventricular, subependymal, germinal matrix) cysts. The other patient demonstrated profound hypoplasia or atrophy of the centrum semiovale with absent medullary pyramids.[219] The microscopic appearance of the destructive lesions in white matter is not described well in most reports, but they may display a loss of oligodendrocytes and axons, microcystic spaces and usually a feeble astrocytic response.[108,196] They may also contain lipophages, if the lesions develop close to the time of death. At least some of those lacking a macrophage response develop *in utero*.[5,219] The grey matter is comparatively spared, but variable neuronal loss may be observed in the cerebral cortex, basal ganglia, brainstem and cerebellum in these patients. They lack the other associated changes of LS (see below). The 'vascular proliferation' illustrated in one PDHC-deficient patient[219] seems more likely to be dilated blood vessels. Two cases with the most dramatic neuropathological findings lack enzyme confirmation.[108,196] Agenesis to hypoplasia of the corpus callosum and medullary pyramids, heterotopic medullary olives, neuroglial heterotopia in the meninges, subependymal neuronal

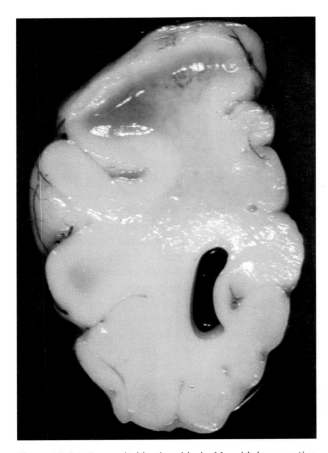

Figure 12.34 *Congenital lactic acidosis. Mucoid degeneration of the subcortical white matter in a 16-day-old female with unclassified congenital (cerebral, fatal) lactic acidosis (blood lactate in mmoles/litre: 11.9, CSF 8.6; normal values <2.2, <2.5, respectively).*

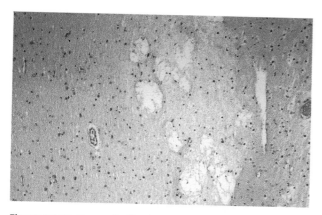

Figure 12.35 *Congenital lactic acidosis. Microcystic change and reduced oligodendrocytes of subcortical white matter in the same CLA infant as in Fig. 12.34. (H&E.)*

heterotopia, dysplasia of the dentate nucleus, a spongy myelinopathy of white matter near the cysts with fibrillary astrogliosis and probable hypomyelination[5,57,108,196,219] are also reported. The patients with congenital lactic acidosis confirmed to be pyruvate carboxylase deficient[15,316,402] exhibited lesions similar to those of PDHC, except for the malformations.

Hypoxia–ischaemia was believed to play the major pathogenic role in the cavitated infarcts and gliosis of the cerebral white matter of one patient, rather than lactic acid,[402] perhaps because this infant also had bilateral germinal matrix haemorrhages. In the other cases of congenital lactic acidosis, due to either pyruvate carboxylase or PDHC deficiency, no such vascular lesions were noted. Hence, while superimposed hypoxia cannot be excluded as a contributing factor, these destructive lesions of white matter are more likely to be caused by other factors. It might be worthwhile to recall that cavitary lesions of cerebral white matter are characteristic of swayback in lambs, which classically occurs in areas with copper-deficient soil. In this disease, a deficiency of the copper-dependent COX is believed to be pathogenic.[49] No studies were found that have determined brain lactic acid levels in swayback; but we found markedly elevated brain lactate in Menkes' disease, which is considered to be a genetic human counterpart of swayback.

Neuropathological overlap cases are reported in LS (see below), and this includes congenital lactic acidosis with its prominent leukoencephalopathy.[331]

Neuropathology of Leigh's syndrome

Most of the key neuropathological and clinical features of LS were described in the original report of 'subacute necrotizing encephalomyelopathy in an infant'.[194] This entity, however, has had an interesting evolution and is now more accurately designated a syndrome.[78] LS has been shown to be due primarily to deficiencies in the respiratory chain (COX or complex IV and complex I) and PDHC in those LS cases for whom a specific aetiology has been identified, 80% of classical and 41% of a 'Leigh-like' group.[227,296,369] As such, it is the prototype of nuclear-encoded mitochondrial encephalomyopathies and usually lacks RRFs, but mtDNA mutations can also produce LS (e.g. point mutations in the ATPase 6 gene and mtDNA synthetic genes) and RRFs may be seen in LS (see discussion on RRFs above). The classical clinical presentation is infantile (below 2 years) and consists predominantly of hypotonia, nystagmus, failure to thrive, respiratory difficulties, ataxia and psychomotor retardation; rarely, LS infants may demonstrate central hypertension, presumably from involvement of the nucleus tractus solitarius.[242] The mode of inheritance historically was autosomal recessive, and that transmission pattern is probably responsible for about 50% of LS, but sporadic, X-linked and maternal modes of transmission also occur.[89] Neonates to adults, and perhaps even animals,[37] also may be affected. Males are more commonly reported (3:2). Some clinical clues may suggest a specific biochemical or molecular causation in an LS patient. Pigmentary retinopathy, particularly with 'bony spicules', is indicative of the T8993G mutation of the ATPase gene in maternally inherited LS. COX-LS differs from PDHC-LS by the neonatal to early infantile onset, more rapidly progressive course of seizures and recurrent apnoea with death at 1 year, and normal lactate:pyruvate ratios in the latter. COX-LS tends to have a late infantile presentation with death at 4–5 years and an elevated lactate:pyruvate ratio of over 20. Most classical neuropathological reviews of LS preceded our molecular and even biochemical understanding of LS.[50,71,167,225] Consequently, neuropathological correlates for these more clinically distinctive forms of LS are unknown,[40] but PDHC-LS is associated with CNS malformations. Imaging data suggest that involvement of the dorsal pons may be characteristic of COX-LS,[22,317] perhaps reflecting its relative chronicity; this lesion has also been observed

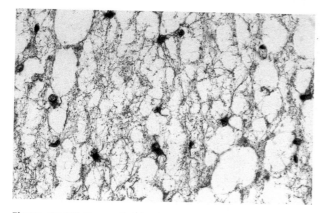

Figure 12.36 *Congenital lactic acidosis. Mild astrocytosis of microcystic white matter in the same CLA infant as in Fig. 12.34. (PTAH.)*

in complex I-LS (see below). Lactic acidosis in plasma usually is present, but it may be restricted to CSF or absent from both.[50,87,227,399] Hepatic lesions (usually steatosis) and hypertrophic cardiomyopathy are seen in a minority of cases, and RRFs have been reported in two patients with COX-LS.[14,223] RRFs were also seen in one unclassified patient reported as Leigh's disease, who had LS-like midbrain lesions, Purkinje cell dendritic abnormalities, cardiomyopathy and pigmentary retinopathy.[69] Others consider this case to be KSS. Infrequently, focal demyelination or axonal degeneration without inflammation has been reported in the PNS and dorsal root ganglia (DRG) without ganglion cell loss.[167] An unpublished 18-year-old LS patient did not demonstrate significant lesions in the PNS, except for increased numbers of Nageotte's nodules, focal accumulations of lymphocytes and microcalcifications in atrophic DRG. This was associated with a bilaterally symmetrical lenticular loss of myelin staining in the dorsomedial gracile tracts (anterior root zone) of cervical cord, at which level bilaterally asymmetrical neuronal loss of the anterior horns was also noted. The gracile lesion demonstrated an equal to near-equal loss of axons and vascular dilatation. Most preterminal pathological findings are essentially restricted to the CNS, and include the presence of abnormal mitochondria.[391]

The neuropathological heterogeneity of LS has been commented on previously. The neuraxis is commonly involved from the optic nerves to the spinal cord. Some optic nerves are atrophied and demonstrate a central pattern of degeneration. The external examination of the brain is usually unremarkable, but focal grey–brown and cystic lesions can be readily appreciated in slices of brainstem tegmentum and basal ganglia–thalamus. There are two cardinal diagnostic features of LS: the topographic distribution of lesions and their histopathological characteristics. Both grey and white matter are involved; the lesions typically are bilaterally symmetrical and subcortical (Figs 12.37–12.41). The most frequent sites of neuropathological involvement in decreasing order are: substantia nigra, inferior colliculi and periaqueductal grey matter, medullary tegmentum, spinal cord, cerebellar roof nuclei and adjacent white matter, pontine tegmentum, corpus striatum (putamen more than caudate), the inferior medullary olives, subthalamic nuclei and thalami.[40,50,167] The rapidly progressive infantile cases of LS with death before 1 year tend to have lesions restricted to the midbrain at autopsy, while older LS children also display lesions in the medulla, cerebellum, basal ganglia and spinal cord. While the topographical–temporal relationship is fairly consistent, the severity of the lesions does not necessarily follow this pattern. For example, acute CNS lesions were more severe in basal ganglia than in the periaqueductal grey matter of a 5-year-old with a 2-month fatal course[102] (Figs 12.42, 12.43). MRI consistently demonstrates T2 hyperintense lesions in the putamen, particularly the anterior portion, while the midbrain lesions are less commonly appreciated.[22,217,377] This

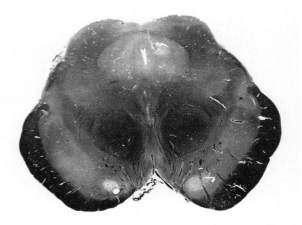

Figure 12.37 *Leigh's syndrome. Midbrain of a 5-year-old male with unclassified LS displaying bilaterally symmetrical necrotizing lesions in the medial substantia nigra and moderately severe lesions of periaqueductal grey and remaining substantia nigra. (LFB–PAS.)*

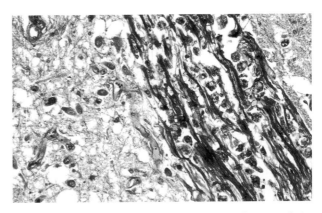

Figure 12.38 *Leigh's syndrome. Higher magnification of Fig. 12.37 showing rarefaction and neuronal sparing of the medial substantia nigra with subacute necrosis of III nerve fibres. (LFB–PAS.)*

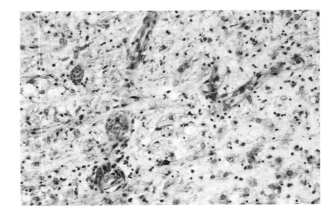

Figure 12.39 *Myoclonus epilepsy with ragged red fibres (MERRF)/Leigh's syndrome. Marked rarefaction to liquefaction of the medullary tegmentum in an 18-year-old, A8344G MERRF–LS overlap male. (LFB–Nissl.)*

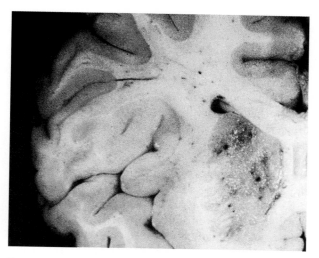

Figure 12.40 *Leigh's syndrome. Hyperaemia and 'softening' of the caudate nucleus in the same unclassified LS patient as in Fig. 12.37.*

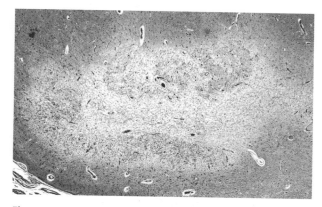

Figure 12.41 *Leigh's syndrome. Marked pallor and vacuolation of the inferior olive in a 4-year-old, complex I–LS male. (H&E.)*

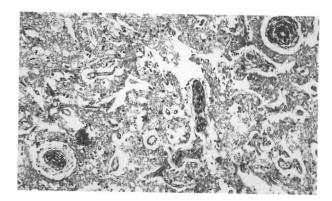

Figure 12.42 *Leigh's syndrome. Marked rarefaction and loosening of neuropil with increased vascularity in the putamen of the same unclassified LS patient as in Fig. 12.37. (H&E.)*

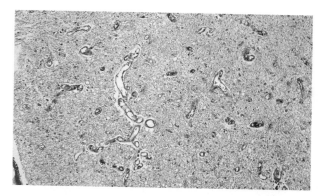

Figure 12.43 *Leigh's syndrome. Mild rarefaction of the periaqueductal grey with vascular dilatation in the same unclassified LS patient as in Fig. 12.37. (LFB–PAS.)*

apparent discrepancy could be explained if the putaminal lesions were caused by transient changes, e.g. cytotoxic oedema. Spinal cord lesions seem preferentially to involve the posterior columns and anterior horns of the cervical cord (Fig. 12.44). They vary from the focal lenticular lesion described above to a lesion that can involve almost the entire posterior columns. These lesions also tend to be necrotizing and may have some spongy myelin around their periphery. Other necrotizing lesions seem to be centred on spinal grey matter, particularly the anterior horns, and spill over into the adjacent white matter producing a butterfly pattern that is bilateral and symmetrical[50,167,225] (Fig. 12.45). The cerebral cortex is rarely involved,[387] as confirmed by functional neuroimaging;[22] but, when present, the lesions may extend to the pial surface. Lesions of the centrum semiovale that vary from myelin pallor to spongy or vacuolated myelin to cystic necrosis are common.[50] The same study reported frequent Purkinje cell loss, torpedoes and staghorn dendrites, particularly in long-term survivors with severe neuronal loss in the medullary olives, who lacked a history of seizures.

The histopathological features of rarefaction to spongy change to vacuolar change to cavitary necrosis of neuropil and adjacent white matter, with vascular prominence and glial reactivity, are equally distinctive. The

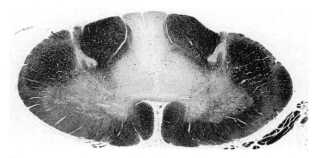

Figure 12.44 *Leigh's syndrome. Bilaterally symmetrical loss of myelin staining in the cervical posterior column of a 7-year-old female with unclassified LS. (Spielmeyer.)*

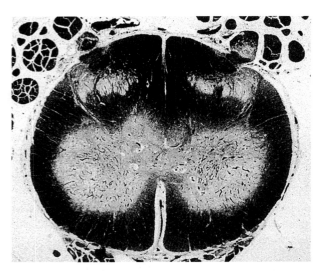

Figure 12.45 *Leigh's syndrome. Bilaterally symmetrical loss of myelin staining in the lumbar anterior horns and adjacent white matter of the same unclassified LS female as in Fig. 12.44. (Spielmeyer.)*

affected neuropil reveals pallor and fine spongy change, probably reflecting cytotoxic oedema due to increased fluid in swollen astrocytes[387] and dendrites; this process seems to progress to a more severe vacuolation, due in part to intramyelinic oedema,[9,178] and then to liquefaction, microglial proliferation, and astrocytic hypertrophy and hyperplasia (Fig. 12.46); followed by microcystic to grossly visible cystic or cavitary necrosis with lipophages, chronic fibrillary astrogliosis and loss of oligodendrocytes. Neurons and their axons are also lost or may show non-specific signs of injury: chromatolysis, eosinophilia, atrophy, axonal destruction and axonal spheroids;[9] however, some neurons are characteristically well-preserved, even in the necrotizing stage, which helps to distinguish these lesions from those of hypoxia–ischaemia. The vascularity of affected areas is clearly increased, particularly around destructive lesions, but most of this vascularity appears to represent dilatation of capillary lumina,

swelling of endothelial cells and a concentration of blood vessels due to tissue atrophy, rather than true proliferation. Evidence for proliferation is largely subjective, but most agree that there is some; more objective evidence[216] suggests that increased vascularity precedes the rarefaction and spongiform change. A thorough immunohistochemical evaluation of these lesions with proliferation antibodies, such as Ki-67, appears to be lacking. In most lesions inflammatory cells of neutrophilic or lymphocytic origin are absent or inconspicuous; however, neutrophils in association with pools of eosinophilic proteinaceous fluid, indicative of vasogenic oedema, and hypercellular endothelial cells with prominent nucleoli may be seen in necrotizing brainstem lesions. In a 4-year-old LS patient lymphocytes were prevalent in and around some lesions[369] (Fig. 12.47). This same patient also demonstrated astrocytes with cytologically atypical nuclei in his lesions, as well as encephalitic-like infiltrates of microglia and lymphocytes in the medulla and pons; he also had a MELAS-like lesion of the posterior frontoparietal region (Fig. 12.48). Comparable clinicoradiological–neuropathological overlaps with MELAS, lacking its characteristic mtDNA mutation, have been reported;[376] this was probably case 3 of Kalimo *et al.*[170] Neuropathological overlap with MERFF[353] and Pearson's syndrome (see below) also occurs.

The histopathological and topographical features of LS are almost identical or similar to those of acute Wernicke's disease.[50,167,225] Histologically, the absence of acute haemorrhage or haemosiderin and the involvement of CNS myelin in LS, and topographically, the involvement of the substantia nigra with preservation of the mamillary bodies in LS are the features that distinguish LS from Wernicke's disease.

Juvenile and adult cases of LS are uncommon. There is some confusion in the literature as to whether the reported patients survived to those time periods following a

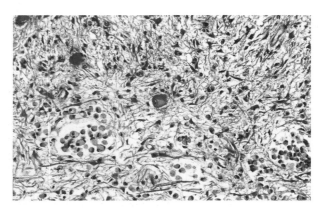

Figure 12.46 *Leigh's syndrome. Higher magnification of Fig. 12.41 displaying chronic fibrillary astrogliosis, lipophages and rare surviving neurons in a complex I–LS male. (H&E.)*

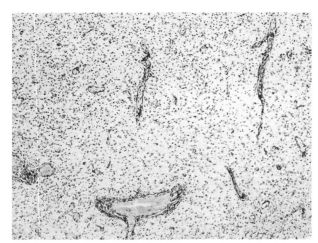

Figure 12.47 *MERRF/Leigh's syndrome. Lower magnification of Fig. 12.39 with increased vascularity and perivascular cuffing in MERRF–LS overlap. (LFB–Nissl.)*

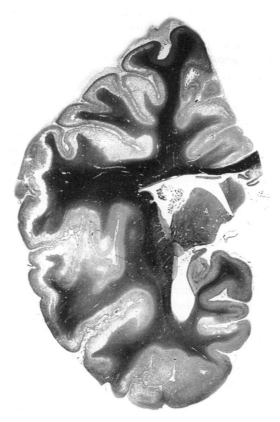

Figure 12.48 *Leigh's syndrome with MELAS-like features. MELAS-like posterior cerebral necrotic lesion in a complex I–LS male. (LFB–PAS.)*

childhood presentation or had the onset of disease after childhood.[240] This is an area where almost all case reports lack biochemical or molecular characterization and were pre-MRI; a mitochondrial aetiology was largely defined from clinicopathological correlations. For example, one patient[340] died at the age of 32 years, but her disease started when she was 5 years of age. She had the same distribution of lesions as infantile LS, but with a predilection for brainstem. Another patient with a childhood onset and death in the third decade displayed the classical widespread distribution of lesions.[177] A multifocal pattern with prominent midbrain and medial thalamic lesions was seen in a true adult-onset LS,[131] and the lesions were more restricted to the brainstem and medial thalamus in another.[373] Two other patients, as well as a diabetic patient with the NARP-MILS T8993G mutation in ATPase 6, had adult onsets (approximately 55 years, 49 years and 43 years).[141,147,240] Lesions in the patient of Ho *et al.*[147] were primarily localized to periaqueductal grey matter, the medullary tegmentum, and lower thoracic–upper lumbar cord, and those of Hegedüs and Németh[141] to the periaqueductal grey matter, left inferior colliculus and left dentate nucleus. The T8993G patient of Nagashima *et al.*[240] developed the clinical signs of LS and had lesions essentially restricted to medial thal-

ami and superior colliculi by MRI and at autopsy. Thus, in a small number of non-alcoholic, adult-onset LS (many reviewed by Nagashima *et al.*[240]), the lesions tend to be preferentially localized to the brainstem, particularly the midbrain, and medial thalamus. The rapid clinical course (a few months) of most adult LS is comparable to those infants with LS who die before 1 year of age. Clinicopathological correlations in both groups support the notion that the midbrain is generally the first area affected.[40,50] In addition, the periaqueductal lesions in one patient[141] were thought to cause aqueductal stenosis with consequent obstructive hydrocephalus. Optic atrophy may be more common in adults. The prominent and concomitant early involvement of medial thalami seems to be characteristic of adult-onset LS, but further studies are needed.

One family lacking biochemical or imaging studies had juvenile onsets at 13, 15 and 22 years of age with prolonged survival times.[170] Most of their neuropathological lesions were those of LS, but case 3 also displayed infarcts in the cerebrum and cerebellum more consistent with MELAS. A 37-year-old male patient reported as 'juvenile LS', again without biochemical or molecular confirmation, presented at the age of 7 years with deafness and shortly thereafter developed optic atrophy and a protracted course of chronic sensorimotor neuropathy, ataxia, deafness and retinitis pigmentosa.[209] From 30 to 37 years of age a global encephalopathy ensued, culminating in episodes of respiratory distress. MRI at approximately 28 years of age only showed mild cerebral atrophy. Sural nerve biopsy revealed evidence of chronic demyelination and onion bulbs; the published illustration also appears to show chronic axonal degeneration in the form of clusters of thinly myelinated regenerating axons. Serum phytanic acid was normal. CNS findings are problematic and atypical for LS. Small, bilaterally symmetrical lesions reported to consist of 'neuronal loss, spongiosis, vascular hypertrophy, numerous macrophages and reactive astrocytes' were observed in the ventral tegmentum of an asymmetrical lower midbrain–upper pons section. Bilaterally symmetrical lesions with a myelin stain were also present in the superior cerebellar peduncles in the upper pons. In addition, bilateral and almost symmetrical lesions in the dentate nuclei and adjacent white matter were illustrated, while two symmetrical lesions in the inferior olives with some perivasculitis were described. Loss of Purkinje cells, many torpedoes and occasional ectopic Purkinje cells in the granular layer with moderate pallor of the posterior columns were noted. The substantia nigra, colliculi, periaqueductal grey matter, brachium conjunctivum, basal ganglia and thalami were apparently unremarkable. The clinical findings in this patient are more suggestive of NARP, the neuropathological features of which have not been described; but the neuropathology in this patient seems most consistent with an atypical LS.

Out of the neuropathological quagmire of LS, several facts seem to emerge: (1) there is marked heterogeneity in the neuropathology, which does not appear to correlate with any biochemical or molecular abnormality, but bilateral symmetry and hypervascularity are highly characteristic; (2) the lesions are ultimately necrotizing and involve both grey and white matter; (3) the lesions are of varying ages and polymorphous, implying a dynamic process due to episodic insults; (4) lesions in the grey matter of the midbrain are the earliest and most constant neuropathological lesion, in both paediatric and most adult patients, whereas the most frequent and earliest neuroradiological changes develop in the putamina; and (5) primary and non-necrotizing lesions of myelin, as well as Purkinje cell abnormalities in long-term survivors often associated with necrotizing lesions of the medullary olives, are more common than was once appreciated.

INHERITED CONDITIONS ASSOCIATED WITH MTDNA DEFECTS

Sporadic large-scale rearrangements and deletions

Kearns–Sayre syndrome

KSS is the prototype and is defined by the following triad: disease onset before 20 years of age, PEO and pigmentary retinopathy. This triad must be accompanied by either cardiac conduction block, a cerebellar syndrome or a CSF protein greater than 100 mg/dl. Dominant clinical features include progressive eye signs, such as ptosis, pigmentary retinopathy and ophthalmoparesis to ophthalmoplegia; cerebellar ataxia, mental retardation, episodic coma, sensorineural hearing loss; short stature; cardiac conduction defects; and endocrinopathies, such as diabetes mellitus, hypoparathyroidism (with seizures and mineralization of basal ganglia) and isolated growth hormone deficiency.[139,295] Overlap occurs with other clinically distinct syndromes, such as MELAS,[413] in the absence of a MELAS point mutation. KSS/MELAS overlaps have also been reported with the A3243G MELAS point mutation.[400] Pseudo-KSS/MELAS overlap can result from the coincidence of embolic infarcts in patients with KSS.[52] KSS may rarely be due to a mtDNA duplication, but the most common molecular defect is a single 4977-bp deletion, termed the 'common deletion', which obliterates both structural and several tRNA genes and impairs protein synthesis.[323] KSS is heteroplasmic, but there has been a poor correlation between the size (approximately 9–50% of mtDNA) or site of the deletion and the severity of the clinical phenotype. This statement may not be as true for skeletal muscle with the advent of improved biochemical methods.[326]

The skeletal muscle changes consist largely of RRFs (see Chapter 10, Volume II). The rarely described but apparently consistent cardiac abnormalities are those of a hypertrophic cardiomyopathy with abnormal mitochondria and myocardial fibrosis, often without lesions in the conduction system; one patient, however, exhibited abnormal mitochondria in cells of the conduction system[155] and another demonstrated COX-deficient conduction fibres bearing the common deletion.[239]

The ocular pathology is variable.[262] The original study of Kearns and Sayre[173] stated that it was typical of pigmentary retinopathy: loss of the outer nuclear, rod/cone layers and pigment epithelium (PE) in association with a normal optic nerve. There were also areas of gliosis, fibrosis and clumps of melanin along blood vessels. Subsequent studies have usually confirmed these observations, but have demonstrated the variability of all pigmentary retinopathies and more severe retinal lesions with a thinning of the inner nuclear layer, loss of ganglion cells and optic atrophy.[25,100,135,204] Most ophthalmological pathologists refer to it as an atypical pigmentary retinopathy, similar to the pigmentary retinopathy of peroxisomal disorders. It is considered histopathologically distinctive by some, resulting from a primary defect in the PE.[100] The 'salt and pepper' pattern and the rarity of 'bone spicule' pigmentation are characteristic of KSS. Suspicious mitochondria[100] to definitely abnormal mitochondria without paracrystalline inclusions[204] have been identified in the PE of KSS.

The ophthalmoplegia of KSS may be relevant to other mitochondrial disorders that display a problem with eye movements. KSS was once included in the 'ophthalmoplegia plus' group of diseases.[96] Extraocular muscles (EOMs) are richly endowed with mitochondria;[213] hence, at least theoretically, one would expect the ophthalmoplegia of KSS and other mitochondrial diseases to reflect a fundamental mitochondrial dysfunction in EOMs. Indeed, abnormal mitochondria have been identified in EOMs of KSS or ophthalmoplegia plus, as well as other myopathic features.[1,135,173,322] However, abnormalities in neurons and myelinated fibres of the appropriate brainstem nuclei have also been observed.[70,135] Most of the limited data is consistent with a primary mitochondrial myopathy of EOM in KSS.[135]

The pathological lesion responsible for the sensorineural hearing loss of KSS has not been extensively investigated. One patient demonstrated a severe loss of myelinated fibres in the VIIIth cranial nerves, most obvious in the cochlear divisions, without changes in their nuclei.[135] Another patient displayed a 60–70% loss of neurons in spiral ganglia.[197]

Sporadic PEO

Patients with RRFs display a slowly progressive course of chronic PEO, ptosis, and pharyngeal and proximal limb weakness with its onset in adolescence or young adulthood. The common 4977-bp deletion of KSS is typical. COX-negative RRFs and excessive lactic acidosis after exercise are characteristic. There are two similar, but genetically transmitted, syndromes: autosomal-dominant multiple mtDNA deletions (see above) and maternally inherited mtDNA point mutations, usually the MELAS A3243G (see below).

Pearson's syndrome

This is a non-neurological disorder of infants, who exhibit pancytopenia, recurrent infections, disturbed pancreatic exocrine function, chronic diarrhoea, failure to gain weight and liver abnormalities.[263,304,406] The pathogenic deletions in mtDNA are identical to those reported in KSS.[303] Bone-marrow biopsy reveals vacuolated cells of the erythroid and myeloid series with sideroblasts. At autopsy, these changes may be replaced by a generalized hyperplasia. In the pancreas acinar cells are atrophic to necrotic with fibrosis and haemosiderosis; some lymphocytes, neutrophils and xanthoma cells with fat necrosis may occur. The islets are preserved. Sudanophilic lipid droplets have been observed in hepatocytes and in renal tubular epithelium. The survivors of this infantile condition develop KSS[32,189,206] or LS[309,406] as young children.

Neuropathology of Kearns–Sayre syndrome

The histopathological features of the CNS in the traditional mitochondrial encephalomyopathies due to inherited mtDNA defects, the RRF diseases (KSS, MELAS, and MERRF) have been reviewed.[262,343] They include varying degrees of spongy change, neuronal loss, infarct-like necrosis, mineral deposits, gliosis and tract degeneration. In contrast to LS, neuropathological reports of KSS are few and less controversial, except for a recent report of an atypical KSS (allegedly a *forme fruste* of Pearson's syndrome) with an unique 2905-bp deletion that challenges the presence of iron in the mineral deposits of the basal ganglia.[25]

On external examination the brain and optic nerves are often unremarkable,[173] but atrophy of the optic nerves, cerebrum and cerebellum has been reported.[25,135] Neuroimaging studies, however, in both KSS and PEO consistently report diffuse cerebral and cerebellar atrophy; the former does not correlate with neurological deficits, while the latter does.[22,381,403] Diffuse to confluent grey–tan discolorations and translucent softenings in the white matter, as well as discolorations and atrophy of basal ganglia, are seen in coronal slices.[251,406] The white-matter change may spare the corpus callosum, internal capsules and arcuate fibres[48,103] (Fig. 12.49). Neuroimaging of white-matter lesions reveals bilaterally symmetrical T2 hyperintense MRI lesions (hypodense on CT) in cerebral and cerebellar white matter, globus pallidus, substantia nigra, dorsal midbrain and thalami. The cerebral and cerebellar white matter abnormality is more diffuse than generally appreciated neuropathologically; there is a peripheral, or subcortical, predilection and a relative sparing of periventricular, callosal and capsular white matter.

The histopathological hallmark of KSS is a spongy to vacuolar leukoencephalopathy (myelinopathy) (Fig. 12.50). The spongy myelin may be restricted to the brainstem and involve the medial longitudinal fasciculi, medi-

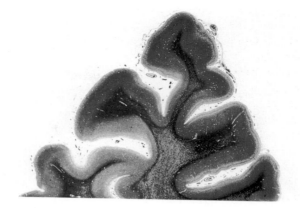

Figure 12.49 *Kearns–Sayre syndrome. Decreased argyrophilia of frontal white matter with sparing of arcuate fibres due to severe intramyelinic edema in a 41-year-old KSS male carrying the common 4977 mtDNA deletion. (Glees.)*

al leminisci and spinothalamic tracts,[135] but generally is more widespread. Spongy myelin is noted in the following sites in decreasing order of frequency: white matter of cerebrum (~84%), midbrain tegmentum (~80%), pontine and medullary tegmentum (~76%), white matter of cerebellum (~56%), cervical spinal cord (~50%), thalamus/hypothalamus (~45%) and basal ganglia, particularly globus pallidus (~30%).[343] Involvement of the subcortical U or arcuate fibres varies greatly, even from one area to another in the same patient; but generally they are involved (Figs 12.51–12.53). The histopathological nature of the myelin lesion also varies from myelin pallor to mild spongy myelinopathy to coarse vacuolation. Even in the most severe vacuolation, astrocytosis, macrophage response and vascular dilatation are usually inconspicuous with routine stains; immunostaining with anti-GFAP and antimacrophage antibodies can reveal considerable numbers of astrocytes and macrophages in the most severely vacuolated areas. Axons and oligodendrocytes are

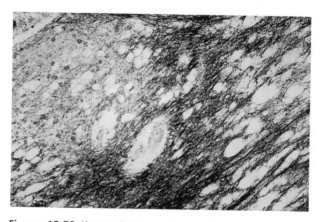

Figure 12.50 *Kearns–Sayre syndrome. Spongy change and vacuolation of myelinated fibres in the nucleus and tract of the lateral lemniscus with neuronal sparing in a 19-year-old KSS female carrying an 8 kb mtDNA duplication. (LFB–Nissl.)*

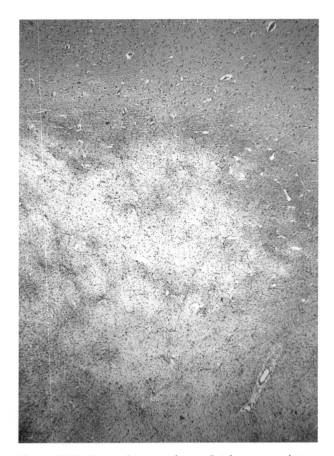

Figure 12.51 *Kearns–Sayre syndrome. Patchy spongy change of subcortical white matter, including the arcuate fibres, in an unclassified KSS patient. (H&E.)*

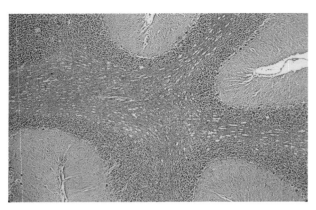

Figure 12.53 *Kearns–Sayre syndrome. Spongy myelin in cerebellar white matter of an unclassified KSS patient. (H&E.)*

relatively well preserved, even ultrastructurally,[251] but a moderate to severe loss of both can occur in the subcortical white matter (Fig. 12.54). Although the callosum and internal capsules are said to be spared grossly and on neuroimaging, a mild spongy myelinopathy can be observed in both sites with the light microscope. Ultrastructurally, the spongy alteration in myelin corresponds to splits at the intraperiod line or extracellular face.[251] Abnormal mitochondria have been seen in Purkinje cells of KSS by some,[343] but not by others.[251] As expected, the cerebral and cerebellar cortices are spared from the spongy myelinopathy, except in some cases when the vacuolation of arcuate fibres extends into the deep cerebral cortex which is richly endowed with myelinated fibres.[205] Alzheimer type 2 or reactive, hypertrophic astrocytes may be associated with these cortical excursions. Neuronal loss in the brainstem, particularly the substantia nigra, cranial nerve nuclei and red nucleus, has been reported in some KSS patients. Purkinje cell loss is common and dendrit-

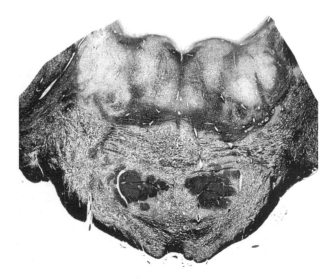

Figure 12.52 *Kearns–Sayre syndrome. Lower magnification of Fig. 12.50 showing vacuolated myelin in pontine tegmentum of KSS. (LFB–Nissl.)*

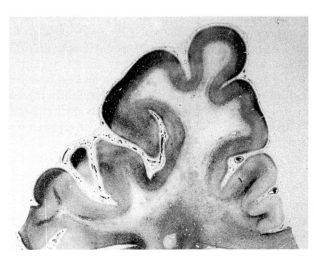

Figure 12.54 *Kearns–Sayre syndrome. Loss of axons in frontal white matter of the same KSS female illustrated in Figs 12.50 and 12.52. (Glees.)*

ic cacti are reported,[360] but the dentate neurons are usually spared. However, antisynaptophysin antibodies have shown disruption of the axonal connections of Purkinje cells with dentate neurons in one patient.[360] Moreover, dentate neurons, not Purkinje cells, in KSS have revealed a selective loss of a mtDNA-encoded subunit of COX (COX II).[361] Loss of spinal grey neurons, including the DNC, is also commonly reported when the cord is examined.

Mild vascular dilatation and congestion in spongy foci or increased vascularity due to atrophy of affected parenchyma[251] can be seen in KSS. There also are cases that demonstrate some neuropathological overlap with LS, in which increased vascularity is more prominent, such as a 19-year-old female with an 8-kb mtDNA duplication[38] (Fig. 12.55). However, unequivocal vascular proliferation in uncomplicated (non-overlap) cases of sporadic KSS seems to be rare, if it occurs at all.

Mineralization of the basal ganglia[173] and thalamus is common in KSS,[343] but is also seen in a few other subcortical sites, just as in MELAS. As pointed out in the original report,[173] and confirmed by many others,[251] there are iron encrustations (siderosis) of vascular walls in the globus pallidus, together with a golden brown to brown pigment in parenchymal astrocytes and microglia in the globus pallidus and caudate nucleus. Both changes are noted in the ageing brain (see Chapter 4, Volume II). There is no evidence that mineralization of the basal ganglia in mitochondrial disorders differs qualitatively from that of ageing. In KSS, and MELAS, this appears to represent a premature and quantitatively exaggerated lesion, but some have raised the unlikely possibility that it may be related to hypoparathyroidism in KSS.[264] The 'golden brown pigment' in ageing is histologically, histochemically and ultrastructurally typical of lipofuscin; some lipofuscins, even brown ones such as neuromelanin, contain histochemically demonstrable iron. It has been known at least since

1922 that most mineralizations in the CNS, including the iron-encrusted blood vessels of the globus pallidus, usually react with both iron and calcium stains. This substance was referred to as 'pseudocalcium' by Spatz.[321] Therefore, the term siderocalcinosis or simply mineralization is more appropriate than either siderosis or calcification. At least some of the pigment in the caudate nucleus in KSS, presumably the golden brown, has the ultrastructural appearance of lipofuscin.[251] As demonstrated in MELAS[291] and in ageing, however, some parenchymal mineralizations of the basal ganglia stain only for calcium and some also stain for iron (Prussian blue). It is to be expected, therefore, that some basal ganglia mineralization in KSS (and MELAS) should lack iron when analysed by microprobe analysis.[25]

Transmitted large-scale rearrangements

A familial diabetes mellitus–deafness syndrome with cardiomyopathy has been associated with a 10.4-kb mtDNA deletion.[19] The same phenotype can be caused by a mtDNA point mutation (A3243G) in the tRNA leucine gene (the common MELAS mutation).

Point mutations affecting structural genes

In addition to NARP (see above under complex V of respiratory chain defects), the other major mtDNA disease in this category is the maternally transmitted Leber's hereditary optic neuropathy (LHON).[192] In LHON lactic acidosis is absent, while it is inconsistent in NARP. In LHON RRFs are absent, just as they are in NARP. The typical presentation of LHON is that of an acute to subacute, painless, bilateral blurring or clouding of vision with a central scotoma in a young adult;[389] but unilateral blindness followed by visual loss in the other eye within weeks or months and early onset at 5 years of age are also seen. Preservation of the pupillary reflex is characteristic. Disc oedema and circumpapillary telangiectatic microangiopathy reflect a retrobulbar problem. The condition is relatively static after the initial visual loss. Patients with the most common mutation, G11778A, usually have uncomplicated optic atrophy, but atypical presentations also occur. Neurological and psychiatric signs and symptoms include Babinski's sign, incoordination, dystonia, tremor, ataxia, peripheral neuropathy and cardiac conduction abnormalities. Clinical and radiological abnormalities, typical of multiple sclerosis and including elevated CSF immunoglobulin G (IgG) production with oligoclonal bands, are documented. LHON has also been associated with multiple system degenerations involving the posterior columns and pyramidal tracts, a MELAS-like syndrome and bilateral striatal necrosis with putaminal lesions on neuroimaging (LS-like). At least 11 different missense mutations have been associated with LHON.[336] The G11778A point mutation in the ND4 gene of complex I is usually homoplasmic. There is a striking male predominance (4:1), implying some X-linked

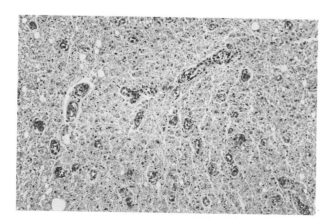

Figure 12.55 *Kearns–Sayre syndrome. Subacute necrotic lesion in the thoracic posterior column with capillary dilatation, reminiscent of LS, in the same KSS female as in Fig. 12.54. (H&E.)*

influence on the mitochondrial defect. The neuropathology of uncomplicated LHON is relatively straightforward, but a paucity of data together with the intrinsic limitations of post-mortem evaluations of dynamic ante-mortem lesions are recognized.[154] Ganglion cell atrophy and loss, and nerve fibre atrophy in the retina are combined with a central (maculopapillary bundle) to complete cross-sectional optic neuropathy, which mimics tobacco–alcohol amblyopia. The inner nuclear layer and photoreceptor cells may be involved; the optic radiations may demonstrate tract degeneration with anterograde degeneration of the lateral geniculate nucleus. If complicated or atypical, CNS sites beyond the optic system and the PNS show additional lesions. For example, posterior column degeneration with gliosis and peripheral neuropathy have been reported.[187] Clinical heterogeneity of the G11778A mutation recently has been broadened due to presentations of parkinsonism[337a] or an acute periaqueductal syndrome,[300a] without optic atrophy.

While LHON and Wolfram's syndrome (diabetes insipidus, diabetes mellitus, optic atrophy and deafness; DIDMOAD) share clinical and molecular features, they have distinct mtDNA haplotypes. Wolfram's syndrome may represent another primary nuclear genome defect with multiple mtDNA deletions.[23,148]

Point mutations affecting synthetic genes

More than 50 pathogenic point mutations and at least four distinct clinical conditions are associated with mtDNA point mutations affecting tRNA genes: MELAS, MERRF, a maternally inherited myopathy/cardiomyopathy and a maternally inherited syndrome of diabetes mellitus and deafness (A3243G). Lactic acidosis and RRFs commonly accompany these four syndromes. MELAS and MERRF will be discussed below.

MELAS, first described in 1984,[261] is relatively common in that approximately 110 MELAS patients were reported within a decade.[143] Patients are usually symptomatic before 40 years of age, and almost all have normal development followed by the onset of exercise intolerance, stroke-like episodes, seizures and dementia in the first decade. Recurrent migraine-like headaches, hearing loss, short stature, learning difficulties, seizures, hemiparesis, hemianopia and limb weakness are common. Lactic acidosis and RRFs are nearly universal. The CSF is normal in about one-half of the patients; the other half has the expected mild elevation in protein. Over one-third have basal ganglia mineralizations on neuroimaging, and 10% have PEO. Most angiographic and functional imaging data show differences between these lesions and those of documented ischaemic stroke.[143,252] The heteroplasmic A3243G mutation in the tRNA leucine gene[130] is present in about 80% of MELAS patients. This mutation appears to affect the activities of at least both complex I and IV of the respiratory chain.[154] Overlap syndromes with LS,

KSS and MERRF occur;[115,144,348] the coincidence of bilateral striatal necrosis (see Chapter 6, Volume II) and MELAS associated with a T3308C mutation in the mitochondrial ND1 gene are also reported.[46]

General autopsy findings include hypertrophic cardiomyopathy, hepatic steatosis, glomerulosclerosis and hyaline degeneration of the islets.[20] There is a generalized mitochondrial microangiopathy without paracrystalline aggregates,[238] and gastrointestinal smooth-muscle cells display numerous abnormal mitochondria without paracrystalline aggregates.[198,244]

Neuropathology of MELAS

Those cases autopsied prior to 1993 have been reviewed.[143,145] Recently, a series of seven patients, of whom five were confirmed to have the A3243G mutation, were reported.[359] The predominant gross findings are diffuse cerebral and cerebellar atrophy with the hallmark infarct-like lesions of the cortex and subcortical white matter (Fig. 12.56). These hallmark lesions are multifocal and asymmetrical, favour the posterior cerebrum and do not usually fall within the vascular territory of a major cerebral artery or border zones; they rarely involve the brainstem.[244] The appearance of the infarct-like lesions, both neuroradiologically and neuropathologically, resembles true infarcts by showing some gross swelling due to oedema in the acute stage and cystic or cavitating change in the chronic stage. Microscopically, the acute to subacute stage displays neuronal eosinophilia, astrocytic nuclear swelling to protoplasmic astrocytosis to reactive hyper-

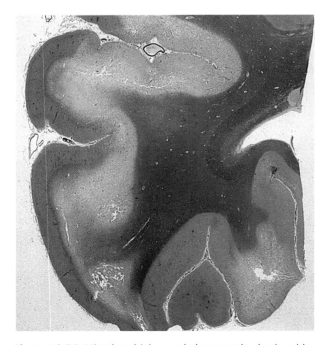

Figure 12.56 *Mitochondrial encephalomyopathy, lactic acidosis, stroke-like episodes (MELAS). Acute to subacute infarct-like necrosis of the posterior temporal cortex and subcortical white matter in a 10-year-old MELAS female. (LFB–PAS.)*

trophy and lipophages, with cytotoxic and vasogenic oedema (Figs 12.57, 12.58), or it may exhibit coagulative necrosis of almost all elements. Both are most commonly distributed in pseudolaminar, pancortical, deep cortical–subcortical white matter, and pancortical–subcortical white-matter patterns. In most cases the crests of gyri are preferentially involved. MELAS lesions may also be seen

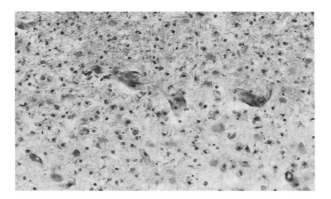

Figure 12.57 *MELAS. Reactive astrocytes, weakly PAS-positive lipophages and swollen endothelia of deep cortex in the same MELAS patient as in Fig. 12.56. (LFB–PAS.)*

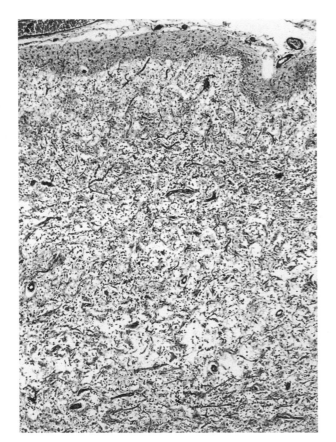

Figure 12.58 *Leigh's syndrome and MELAS overlap. Higher magnification of Fig. 12.48 showing cortical necrosis with reactive astrocytosis of the preserved molecular layer in complex I–LS–MELAS overlap. (LFB–PAS.)*

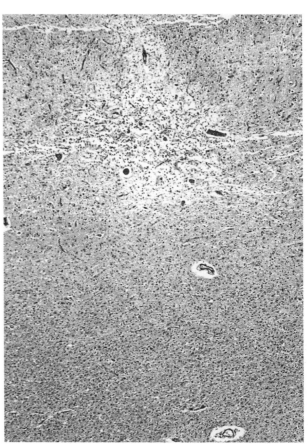

Figure 12.59 *Leigh's syndrome and MELAS overlap. Focal cortical necrosis in the same complex I–LS–MELAS overlap patient as in Fig. 12.58. (LFB–PAS.)*

as small foci of cortical necrosis[359,372] (Fig. 12.59). Reactive, hypertrophic astrocytosis is often most prominent when there is a pseudolaminar pattern, where swollen eosinophilic astrocytes in the molecular layer and in the preserved deep cortical layers border the necrotic lesions (Fig. 12.60). The deep cortex also tends to be a major site of increased vascularity. As in LS, dilated small blood vessels with swollen to proliferative endothelia are most conspicuous within and at the edge of lesions, but increased vascularity can also occur in viable cortex near the lesions. The vessel lumina are open and, to the authors' knowledge, have not been reported to be occluded;[248] the neighbouring leptomeningeal arteries and arterioles are also patent. By contrast, myocytes and rarely the endothelium of surface arterioles and small arteries have shown increased numbers of mitochondria. Abnormalities in their size and shape, but without paracrystalline inclusions, and degenerative changes in myocytes were also noted.[248] The same study did not identify these changes in intraparenchymal blood vessels, except for a rare capillary endothelial cell, or in neurons and glia. The authors postulated that this mitochondrial vasculopathy was responsible for the infarct-like lesion of MELAS. The bulk of the available data does not support this

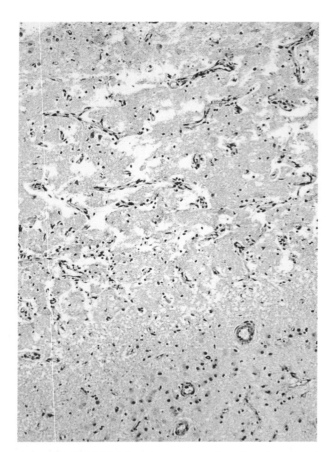

Figure 12.60 *MELAS. Reactive astrocytosis at the edge of, and prominent vascularity within, coagulative necrosis of deep cortex in the same MELAS patient as in Fig. 12.56. (H&E.)*

hypothesis; it still is conceivable, however, that abnormal mitochondria in leptomeningeal arterioles, a major site of CNS vascular autoregulation, may contribute synergistically to the formation of MELAS lesions. An *in situ* hybridization study using a probe to mitochondrial ribosomal RNA has demonstrated a close similarity between parenchymal vascular changes in thrombotic infarcts and MELAS; these data suggest that, in both, the microvascular changes are the consequence rather than the cause of brain necrosis.[198] Abnormal mitochondria were also observed in the epithelium of the choroid plexus and its blood vessels[247,359] and, most recently, as well as in the staghorn or cactus deformities of Purkinje cell dendrites.[359,372] The same dendritic deformities are highly characteristic of Menkes' kinky hair disease[142,218] and have been observed in LS[50] and KSS,[360] as well as the LD patient described above.[69]

The chronic infarct-like lesions, as expected, show loss of affected parenchyma, atrophy, microcystic and cystic spaces, isolated neuronal sparing and chronic fibrillary astrogliosis (Figs 12.61, 12.62). In addition to the Purkinje cell abnormalities described above, there is loss of Purkinje cells,[359] granule cells[372] and occasionally dentate neurons,[160] generalized atrophy of cerebral cortex and fib-

rillary astrogliosis of atrophic cerebral and cerebellar white matter without loss of myelin staining.[359,372] Spongy change of the cerebral white matter, similar to that seen in LS, has been reported occasionally in MELAS.[160] The possibility that such cases represent overlap syndromes cannot be eliminated. Almost all of those documented to have the A3243G defect do not report a spongy myelinopathy of cerebral or cerebellar white matter.[145,244,359,372] However, the case of Nicoll *et al.*[244] did demonstrate mild, multifocal areas of spongy myelin in cerebral subcortical and cerebellar white matter.

The basal ganglia rarely display infarct-like lesions.[377] However, the other hallmark lesion of MELAS is mineralization of the basal ganglia, predominantly of the globus pallidus and caudate nucleus[343] (Fig. 12.63); but it can also be more disseminated and involve the internal capsule, lateral thalamus and dentate nucleus.[185] It is detected in about 43% of MELAS patients by CT,[143] and histopathologically in at least 65%.

The optic nerves rarely may be mildly gliotic and demonstrate a mild spongy myelinopathy.[62] The spinal cord may display neuronal loss, secondary degeneration

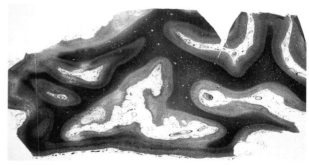

Figure 12.61 *MELAS. Infarct-like lesion of occipital lobe with cystic atrophy of cortex in the same MELAS female as in Fig. 12.60. (LFB–PAS.)*

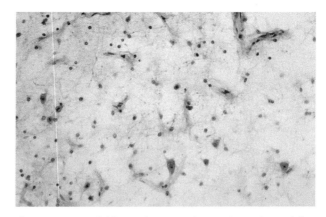

Figure 12.62 *Leigh's syndrome and MELAS overlap. Higher magnification of Fig. 12.58 showing rarefied cortex with persistent cortical microvessels and a few preserved neurons in the same complex I–LS–MELAS overlap as in Fig. 12.58. (LFB–PAS.)*

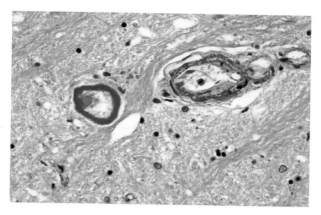

Figure 12.63 *MELAS. Early mineralization of pallidal blood vessels in the same MELAS female as in Fig. 12.56. (H&E.)*

of the corticospinal tracts, and a mild spongy myelinopathy in the lateral and posterior columns.[249] The peripheral nerves have shown a loss of myelinated fibres and fibrosis.[143]

The terms status spongiosus(-is) and spongiform change as they relate to mitochondrial diseases, in particular to MELAS, have caused some confusion in the literature.[40,343] Historically, status spongiosus has been a non-specific term that referred to vesicular/vacuolar lesions of either grey or white matter, whereas spongiform change has usually been restricted to grey matter lesions, particularly in prion diseases (see Chapter 5, Volume II). Status spongiosus has also been used to describe burned-out or end-stage grey-matter lesions in a number of metabolic diseases, including LS and MELAS. The microscopic feature common to both is a spongy change, which may reflect an early, acute, or a late, chronic process. Mitochondrial disorders, as a group, are characterized by 'spongy' changes, both in grey and in white matter. In the white matter, 'sponginess' is usually caused by intramyelinic oedema, a form of cytotoxic or intracellular oedema. However, in most conditions that demonstrate intramyelinic oedema, the split in the myelin occurs at the intraperiod line, the fusion of the extracellular faces of the myelin-forming cells' plasma membranes; this is continuous, at least potentially, with the extracellular space. A spongy or vacuolar myelinopathy is most conspicuous in KSS, particularly in the cerebral and cerebellar white matter and in tracts of myelinated fibres; but it also occurs in brainstem nuclei where myelinated fibres are intimately admixed with neuronal perikarya. The latter pattern is also true for LS, and one can uncommonly observe a true spongy myelinopathy of cerebral and cerebellar white matter.[9,50,167] An enlarged extracellular space due to oedema or axonal loss[9] and intra-astrocytic accumulations of fluid[387] may complicate the interpretation of this white-matter spongy lesion. However, LS mainly displays spongy changes in the grey matter. This change appears to be due to astrocytic, and probably to some dendritic swelling; this is a more appropriate example of cytotoxic

oedema. LS is further complicated by having a subacute to chronic necrotizing element to its lesions and, hence, some of the spongy appearance may reflect: (1) vasogenic oedema and vacuolated lipophages; or (2) liquefaction and microcystic residual lesions with fibrillary gliosis. MELAS, like LS, is necrotizing, but the process is more acute, and also affects preferentially the grey matter. Its infarct-like lesions in the acute stage display cytotoxic oedema like infarcts do. Most of the cases of uncomplicated MELAS reported to have 'status spongiosus' or 'spongy' lesions referred to the cerebral cortex, not to the white matter, and appeared to describe old necrotic lesions with microcystic change.[138,180,248] Two other reports of 'spongy alterations' or 'spongy degeneration' in the cerebral cortex are likely to represent acute foci of cytotoxic oedema.[62,237] In view of the heterogeneity of mitochondrial diseases and well-documented overlapping cases, admixtures of these spongy lesions in a single patient are to be expected and do occasionally occur. The imprecise and confusing terminology demands caution when considering the histopathological nature and significance of 'spongy' lesions in mitochondrial disorders. The superimposition of preterminal hypoxia-induced cytotoxic oedema in the grey matter further complicates the interpretation and prevalence of such spongy change. In summary, a spongy or vacuolar myelinopathy is frequent in KSS, infrequent in LS and rare in MELAS, while spongy change of the grey matter (devoid of significant numbers of myelinated fibres) is frequent in LS, infrequent in MELAS and rare in KSS.

Abnormal mitochondria have been reported rarely in non-vascular or non-choroidal cells of the brain, such as neurons, in MELAS.[123,160] There is also some controversy regarding the prevalence of mutant mtDNA in the MELAS brain. One study reports relatively low levels in histologically unaffected brain regions, such as the temporal lobe, virtually undetectable levels in affected occipital lobes, and high levels in unaffected liver and kidney.[199] The authors conclude that their data are inconsistent with the hypothesis that defective mitochondria are responsible for the infarct-like lesions. By contrast, two other studies report high levels of mutant DNA in MELAS brain: 82%[123] and over 90%.[350]

The second major disease due to a point mutation in a synthetic gene is MERRF. First described in 1980,[116] it is less common than MELAS but equally heterogeneous. The major clinical features of this maternally inherited disease are cerebellar ataxia, generalized seizures, myoclonus, dementia, hearing loss, impaired deep sensation, optic atrophy, short stature and lipomas. Pigmentary retinopathy apparently has not been described in MERRF, while diabetes mellitus and chronic PEO are uncommon.[154] Age of onset usually varies from childhood to the fifth decade; the clinical course varies from slow progression to rapid deterioration. Lactic acidosis is less striking than in MELAS, and RRFs are consistent. A heteroplasmic point mutation in the tRNA lysine gene

(A8344G) is the major cause of MERRF. Overlap with LS is reported.[29]

General autopsy findings have included muscular wasting, hepatic steatosis, myocardial fibrosis and abnormal mitochondria in cardiac myocytes.[358]

Neuropathology of MERRF

The neuropathological lesions of MERRF have been reviewed.[115,343] Neuroimaging reveals diffuse cerebral and cerebellar atrophy and patchy T2 hyperintense MRI lesions in white matter.[22,176] The hallmark lesion of MERRF is a neuronal system degeneration, particularly involving the dentatorubral fibres to produce a Ramsay–Hunt syndrome. Gross findings are usually lacking, but may consist of a brown discoloration of the dentate nuclei.[103] Neuronal loss and astrocytosis in the dentate nucleus is usually severe (Fig. 12.64), and grumous degeneration[12] may be seen. The inferior medullary olives are devastated to the same degree, while the red nuclei and substantia nigra are somewhat less severely affected. In the spinal cord the gracile, cuneate and Clarke's nuclei show a significant reduction of neurons; the DRGs show neuronal loss and Nageotte's nodules.[358] A moderate loss of pallidal neurons, particularly of the outer segment, rarely associated with mineralization,[22,103] is typical. Losses of Purkinje cells and cerebral cortical neurons are mild, except in the anterior vermis where they can be moderate. In spite of mild neuronal loss in the cerebral cortex, positron emission tomographic (PET) studies have shown decreased cortical metabolism with normal cortical blood flow and cerebral pH.[29] The superior cerebellar peduncles show a marked loss of myelinated fibres and gliosis. A 'dying-back' pattern, to the authors' knowledge, has not been detected; but it would be imprudent at present to assume that this is simply centrifugal tract degeneration secondary to dentate neuronal loss. Comparable degeneration of the olivocerebellar tracts, dorsal spinocerebellar tracts and posterior columns is seen.

Although this issue is not discussed by Takeda *et al.*, their illustrations suggest a greater loss of gracile fibres in the lower, as opposed to upper, spinal cord.[358] This might indicate that centrifugal, rather than centripetal (dying-back), degeneration is taking place. Nevertheless, MERRF lesions resemble some of those seen in Joseph–Machado disease, dentatorubropallidoluysial atrophy[115] and Friedreich's ataxia,[358] as well as in adult Refsum's disease and AMN. Mitochondria provide energy needed for axonal transport and may play a crucial role in the pathogenesis of these tract degeneration: defective axonal transport can produce an axonopathy, often a dying-back or distal axonopathy (see Chapter 6, Volume II). For example, Friedreich's ataxia, a nuclear DNA trinucleotide (GAA) repeat disorder, also displays severe neuronal loss in dentate nucleus, Clarke's nucleus and DRG, with the neuropathological pattern of a distal or dying-back axonopathy in spinal cord[307] (see Chapter 6, Volume II); its gene product, frataxin, plays a role in mitochondrial iron metabolism.[181]

Abnormally large mitochondria with vesicular cristae and mitochondria with equivocal paracrystalline inclusions have been identified in cerebellar cortex and dentate nucleus, respectively.[115] Biochemical deficits in complexes I, III, IV and combined I/IV have been reported in MERRF (reviewed in Ref. 344). In that same study, a selective and severe immunohistochemical deficiency in the mtDNA-encoded subunit II of complex IV (COX II) was demonstrated not only in the remaining neurons of the dentate nucleus and medullary olives, but also in the Purkinje cells and in scattered neurons within the medullary nuclei and cerebral cortex (Fig. 12.65). A microdissection-PCR study of mutant mtDNA in MERRF revealed that the percentage of mutant mtDNA in Purkinje cells was approximately 97% and in dentate neurons approximately 95%; however, the degree of cell loss was 45% for dentate neurons and only 7% for Purkinje cells. Thus, additional factors seem to contribute to cell death.[410]

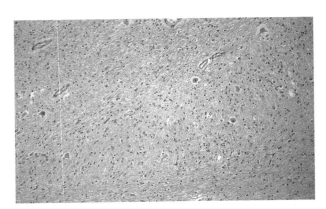

Figure 12.64 *MERRF. Loss of neurons and mild chronic astrogliosis of the dentate nucleus in a 20-year-old patient with unclassified MERRF. (H&E.)*

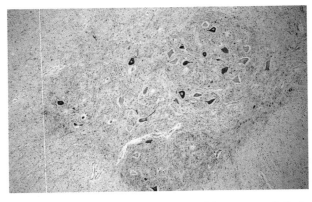

Figure 12.65 *MERRF. Mosaic pattern of immunoreactivity in anterior horn neurons of an unclassified MERRF patient. (Anti-COX II.)*

ACQUIRED CONDITIONS

There are numerous clinical situations in which mitochondria are secondarily involved. These entities are more appropriately discussed in sections that deal with the primary clinical disease: Reye's syndrome (Chapter 10, this Volume), MPTP toxicity (see Chapter 13, this Volume), zidovudine toxicity (see Chapter 1, Volume II), ageing and oxidative stress (see Chapter 4, Volume II).

SPECIFIC TREATMENT OF MITOCHONDRIAL DISEASES

Gastrointestinal disturbances are common in the mitochondrial disorders and are particularly prominent in MNGIE. Early placement of a gastrostomy tube and fundoplication ensure adequate intake of calories, medications, vitamins and other dietary cofactors. Selective organ failure may be managed by transplantation. Heart transplants have been performed in a few patients with KSS and other mitochondrial diseases that severely affect cardiac function.[305] Convulsions are a prominent clinical feature in defects of pyruvate metabolism and the respiratory chain, but can be treated with antiepileptic drugs. Seizures occur in approximately 31% of patients with LS and 95–100% of patients with MELAS and MERRF; they are uncommon in KSS, and when present are often associated with hypoparathyroidism.

The ketogenic diet is effective in controlling seizures in patients with PDHC deficiency. A high-fat diet also provides an alternative fuel (ketone bodies) for brain metabolism, effectively bypassing the PDHC enzyme defect. Ketone bodies are metabolized in the mitochondrion to acetyl-CoA, avoiding the block associated with the conversion of pyruvate to acetyl-CoA. Occasional patients are cofactor dependent and benefit from high doses of vitamins such as thiamine and α-lipoic acid (cofactors for PDHC) and biotin (an essential cofactor for the four carboxylases, including pyruvate carboxylase). Rarely, patients may have a defect in coenzyme Q_{10} biosynthesis, which is responsive to coenzyme Q_{10} supplementation.

Coenzyme Q_{10} is localized primarily in the inner mitochondrial membrane and serves as a membrane protectant. Oxidative stress is increasingly recognized as a fundamental mechanism for tissue injury and cell death. The use of high-dose antioxidants as treatment for patients with mitochondrial diseases has gained clinical acceptance; these include L-carnitine, coenzyme Q_{10}, vitamins E and C, α-lipoic acid and selenium. Patients with KSS have been shown to have relative CNS folate deficiency and treatment with folinic acid has been attempted. Vitamins K and C may be effective in bridging the gap in the electron shuttle associated with complex III deficiency. Lactic acid is a metabolic signature of mitochondrial disease. Chronic cerebral lactic acidosis occurs in deficiencies of PDHC, pyruvate carboxylase and the respiratory chain; it has been speculated that chronic cerebral lactic acidosis contributes to the pathophysiology of mitochondrial diseases, particularly MELAS. Sodium bicarbonate is ineffective in managing the cerebral acidosis. Dichloroacetate is an experimental agent that crosses the BBB and effectively lowers brain lactic acid concentrations. Its value in mitigating cerebral lactic acidosis in mitochondrial diseases is currently under investigation.

There have been early attempts at gene therapy for mitochondrial diseases. *In vitro* studies have demonstrated selective inhibition of mutant human mtDNA replication by peptide nucleic acids.[362] The mtDNA defect has been reversed in human skeletal muscle[63] and complete restoration of a wild-type mtDNA genotype has been seen in the regenerating muscle fibres of a patient with a tRNA point mutation and mitochondrial encephalomyopathy.[337] A novel therapy for mitochondrial myopathy has also been proposed by producing a gene shifting paradigm with graded physical exercise.[354] This response to exercise occurs with somatic mutations affecting mtDNA and sparing the muscle satellite cells that are involved in muscle regeneration after tissue injury. Another novel treatment strategy has been developed in cultured cells containing the NARP mutation (T8993G) using oligomycin.[210] Oligomycin specifically interferes with ATP synthesis in the mutant cells, allowing clonal expansion of wild-type cells. The goal of treatment in patients harbouring mtDNA point mutations is to alter favourably the balance between wild-type and mutated mitochondrial genomes. Upregulation of the wild-type genomes theoretically would reduce the proportion of the mutated genomes below the cellular threshold, restoring the biological integrity of the cell. These successful *in vitro* and *in vivo* experiments will guide the future direction of gene therapy in mitochondrial disease associated with mtDNA mutations.[268a]

CONSIDERATIONS ON THE CELLULAR PATHOGENESIS OF MITOCHONDRIAL DISORDERS

Mitochondria provide essential functions for the cell, including the production of energy, and energy is necessary to carry out cellular activities. Within the nervous system, cellular work is primarily related to the generation and propagation of action potentials. The functional activation of energy metabolism is localized to the neuropil which contains neuronal processes and astrocytic elements. Axonal terminals, dendrites and synapses account for approximately 90% of the cerebral glucose metabolism in the mature brain.[342] It is estimated that astrocytes contribute to the increased energy metabolism during functional activation, and these cellular elements are essential in the reuptake of glutamate from the synaptic cleft and the metabolism of glucose to lactate. Current evidence suggests that lactate produced by astrocytes is taken up by neurons for oxidation to water and CO_2.[207,208,371]

Mitochondrial disorders differentially affect oxidative metabolism, causing an overproduction of lactate by accelerated glycolysis. Metabolically, this results in the accumulation of tissue lactate and hydrogen ion, decreased cellular ATP, loss of functional activation of cellular elements within the neuropil and the accumulation of extracellular glutamate. An excess of glutamate promotes an influx of calcium through N-methyl-D-aspartate (NMDA) receptors and leads to the accumulation of intracellular calcium. Mitochondrial dysfunction impairs sequestration of cytoplasmic calcium in the mitochondrial matrix, which results in the activation of calcium-dependent mechanisms that promote cell death.[236] Release of cytochrome c from damaged mitochondria may activate apoptotic mechanisms and lead to cell death,[220] but others are unable to detect apoptosis in mitochondrial encephalomyopathies.[329a] Accumulation of tissue free radicals also promotes damage to cellular structural elements and accelerates DNA damage.

These biochemical mechanisms associated with energy failure produce cellular death and spongy change of the neuropil. Spongy change of the brain is the neuropathological hallmark of LS and KSS, and occurs to some extent in MELAS; this appears to be due to cytotoxic (including intramyelinic) oedema caused by the failure of energy-dependent ionic pumps in glia and neurons. The spongy myelinopathy of KSS may also be related, in part, to CNS folic acid deficiency. Seizures impose an added metabolic burden on the brain region involved in the epileptogenic focus. Regional energy failure in the presence of a focal seizure enhances tissue injury. Focal seizure activity, which is particularly prominent in MELAS, may contribute to the regional brain necrosis that characterizes this clinical syndrome.

The role of chronic tissue lactic acidosis in mitochondrial disorders and in the genesis of spongy change is unclear, but its presence is probably responsible for microvascular alterations that are particularly prominent in the clinical syndromes associated with cerebral lactic acidosis (LS and MELAS). In contrast, microvascular alterations and spongy change are rarely seen in MERRF, and cerebral lactic acidosis is minimal in this condition. Vascular dilatation and proliferation mainly appear to be responses to the necrotic lesions of LS and MELAS, rather than the cause, and have been likened to the penumbra around ischaemic lesions. This protective response to ischaemic lesions may be a double-edged sword. While it does provide seemingly beneficial increases in blood to ischaemic tissues, at the same time it may contribute to tissue damage by delivering a persistent supply of glucose to the area and by promoting glycolysis with a deleterious acute rise in local lactate levels.[265,297] A release of excitotoxins and the generation of free radicals may contribute to the necrotizing process.[49] In contrast to infarcts caused by ischaemia, the CNS in LS and MELAS appears to have increased vascular perfusion, but it suffers from a tissue failure of oxidative phosphorylation due to an inherent mitochondrial dysfunction, which leads to inadequate oxygen utilization and cell death. Researchers are beginning to discover some of the molecular mechanisms involved in the selective vulnerability of hemispheric oligodendrocytes in CLA, brainstem neuropil in LS, cerebral cortex in MELAS, myelin in KSS and specific neuronal populations in MERRF. The developmental stage of the patient and nature of the metabolic insult, the density of neurotransmitter receptors (e.g. glutamate) and synaptic activity of specific neuronal populations, the percentage of mutant mtDNA and the threshold of the affected cells may all play a major role in the pathogenesis of mitochondrial disorders. The cellular threshold is determined by the percentage of mutant mtDNA and the cell's demand for oxidative metabolism. This threshold varies from one cell to another, as determined by its biological function and by its metabolic activity during development.

Acknowledgements

The authors wish to express their great appreciation, particularly to Mrs Tina Blazey, and to Mrs Linda Crandall and Ms Grace Holloway, for their outstanding performance in preparing this manuscript for publication; we also thank Ms Christine Kerwin and Ms Frances Vito for their help and Nancy Dimmick for her outstanding skill in processing the illustrations. Dr JM Powers is most grateful for the hospitality and generosity of the following colleagues, who permitted him to examine and photograph case material used in this chapter: Professor Seth Love, Frenchay Hospital, Bristol; Professor Francesco Scaravilli, National Hospital, Queen Square, London; and Professors Peter Barth, Derek Troost and Ronald Wanders, Academic Medical Centre of the University of Amsterdam.

REFERENCES

1 Adachi M, Torii J, Volk BW et al. Electron microscopic and enzyme histochemical studies of cerebellum, ocular and skeletal muscles in chronic progressive ophthalmoplegia with cerebellar ataxia. Acta Neuropathol 1973; 23: 300–12.

2 Adams PL, Lightowlers RN, Turnbull DM. Molecular analysis of cytochrome c oxidase deficiency in Leigh's syndrome. Ann Neurol 1997; 41: 268–70.

3 Agamanolis DP, Novak RW. Rhizomelic chondrodysplasia punctata: report of a case with review of the literature and correlation with other peroxisomal disorders. Paediatr Pathol Lab Med 1995; 15: 503–13.

4 Agamanolis DP, Robinson HB Jr, Timmons GD. Cerebro-hepato-renal syndrome. Report of a case with histochemical and ultrastructural observations. J Neuropath Exp Neurol 1976; 35: 226–46.

5 Aleck KA, Kaplan AM, Sherwood G, Robinson BH. In utero central nervous system damage in pyruvate dehydrogenase deficiency. Arch Neurol 1988; 45: 987–9.

6 Altmann R. Die Elementarorganismen und ihre Beziehungen zu den Zellen. Leipzig: Veit, 1890.

7   Anderson S, Bankier AT, Barrell BG et al. Sequence and organisation of the human mitochondrial genome. Nature 1981; 290: 457–65.

8   Andreu AL, Hanna MG, Reichmann H et al. Exercise intolerance due to mutations in the cytochrome b gene of mitochondrial DNA. N Engl J Med 1999; 341: 1037–44.

9   Anzil AP, Weindl A, Struppler A. Ultrastructure of a cerebral white matter lesion in a 41-year-old man with Leigh's encephalomyelopathy (LEM). Acta Neuropathol 1981; 7 (Suppl): 233–8.

10 Applegarth DA, Dimmick JE, Hall JG. eds. Organelle diseases. Clinical features, diagnosis, pathogenesis and management. London: Chapman & Hall Medical, 1997.

11 Aprille JR. Mitochondrial cytopathies and mitochondrial DNA mutations. Curr Opin Paediatr 1991; 3: 1045–53.

12 Arai N. Grumose degeneration of the dentate nucleus. A light and electron microscopic study in progressive supranuclear palsy and denatorubro-pallidoluysian atrophy. J Neurol 1989; 90: 131–45.

13 Arnaudo E, Dalakas M, Shanske S et al. Depletion of muscle mitochondrial DNA in AIDS patients with zido-vudine-induced myopathy. Lancet 1991; 337: 508–10.

14 Arts WF, Scholte HR, Loonen MC et al. Cytochrome c oxidase deficiency in subacute necrotising encephalomyelopathy. J Neurol Sci 1987; 77: 103–15.

15 Atkin BM, Buist NRM, Utter MF et al. Pyruvate carboxylase deficiency and lactic acidosis in a retarded child without Leigh's disease. Paediatr Res 1979; 13: 109–16.

16 Aubourg P. X-linked adrenoleukodystrophy. In: Moser H ed. Handbook of clinical neurology Vol. 66. Amsterdam: Elsevier, 1996: 447–83.

17 Aubourg P, Scotto J, Rocchiccioli F et al. Neonatal adrenoleukodystrophy. J Neurol Neurosurg Psychiatry 1986; 49: 77–86.

18 Baes M, Gressens P, Baumgart E et al. A mouse model for Zellweger syndrome. Nat Genet 1997; 17: 49–57.

19 Ballinger SW, Shoffner JM, Trounce I et al. Maternally transmitted diabetes and deafness associated with a 10.4 kb mitochondrial DNA deletion. Nat Genet 1992; 1: 11–15.

20 Ban S, Mori N, Saito K et al. An autopsy case of mitochondrial encephalomyopathy (MELAS) with special reference to extra-neuromuscular abnormalities. Acta Pathol Jpn 1992; 42: 818–25.

21 Bardosi A, Creutzfeldt W, DiMauro S et al. Myo-, neuro-gastrointestinal encephalopathy (MNGIE syndrome) due to partial deficiency of cytochrome-c-oxidase. A new mitochondrial multisystem disorder. Acta Neuropathol 1987; 74: 248–58.

22 Barkovich AJ, Good WV, Koch TK, Berg BO. Mitochondrial disorders: analysis of their clinical and imaging characteristics. Am J Neuroradiol 1993; 14: 1119–37.

23 Barrientos A, Volpini V, Casademont J et al. A nuclear defect in the 4p16 region predisposes to multiple mitochondrial DNA deletions in families with Wolfram syndrome. J Clin Invest 1996; 97: 1570–6.

24 Baumgartner MR, Verhoeven NM, Jakobs C et al. Defective peroxisome biogenesis with a neuromuscular disorder resembling Werdnig–Hoffmann disease. Neurology 1998; 51: 1427–32.

25 Becher MW, Wills ML, Noll WW et al. Kearns–Sayre syndrome with features of Pearson's marrow-pancreas syndrome and a novel 2905-base pair mitochondrial DNA deletion. Hum Pathol 1999; 30: 577–81.

26 Benda C. Weitere Mitteilungen über die Mitochondria. Arch Physio 1899; 4: 376–83.

27 Benke PJ, Reyes PF, Parker JC Jr. New form of adrenoleukodystrophy. Hum Genet 1981; 58: 204–8.

28 Bennett MJ, Pollitt RJ, Goodman SI et al. Atypical riboflavin-responsive glutaric aciduria, and deficient peroxisomal glutaryl-CoA oxidase activity: a new peroxisomal disorder. J Inherit Metab Dis 1991; 14: 165–73.

29 Berkovic SF, Carpenter S, Evans A et al. Myoclonus epilepsy and ragged-red fibres (MERRF). Brain 1989; 112: 1231–60.

30 Bernheimer H, Budka H, Müller P. Brain tissue immunoglobulins in adrenoleukodystrophy: a comparison with multiple sclerosis and systemic lupus erythematosus. Acta Neuropathol 1983; 59: 95–102.

31 Bizzozero OA, Zuniga G, Lees MB. Fatty acid composition of human proteolipid protein in peroxisomal disorders. J Neurochem 1991; 56: 872–8.

32 Blaw ME, Mize CE. Juvenile Pearson syndrome. J Child Neurol 1990; 5: 187–90.

33 Bohlega S, Tanji K, Santorelli FM et al. Multiple mitochondrial DNA deletions associated with autosomal recessive ophthalmoplegia and severe cardiomyopathy. Neurology 1996; 46: 1329–34.

34 Bourgeron T, Rustin P, Chretien D et al. Mutation of a nuclear succinate dehydrogenase gene results in mitochondrial respiratory chain deficiency. Nat Genet 1995; 11: 144–9.

35 Bowen P, Lee CSN, Zellweger H, Lindenberg R. A familial syndrome of multiple congenital defects. Bull Johns Hopkins Hosp 1964; 114: 402–14.

36 Braverman N, Dodt G, Gould SJ, Valle D. Disorders of peroxisome biogenesis. Hum Mol Genet 1995; 4: 1791–8.

37 Brenner O, Wakshlag JJ, Summers BA, de Lahunta A. Alaskan husky encephalopathy – a canine neurodegenerative disorder resembling subacute necrotizing encephalomyelopathy (Leigh syndrome). Acta Neuropathol 2000; 100: 50–62.

38 Brockington M, Alsanjari N, Sweeney MG et al. Kearns–Sayre syndrome associated with mitochondrial DNA deletion or duplication: a molecular genetic and pathological study. J Neurol Sci 1995; 131: 78–87.

39 Brody BA, Kinney HC, Kloman A, Gilles FH. Sequence of central nervous system myelination in human infancy. I. An autopsy study of myelination. J Neuropathol Exp Neurol 1987; 46: 283–30.

40 Brown GK, Squier MV. Neuropathology and pathogenesis of mitochondrial diseases. J Inherit Metab Dis 1996; 19: 553–72.

41 Brul S, Westerveld A, Strijland A et al. Genetic heterogeneity in the cerebrohepatorenal (Zellweger) syndrome and other inherited disorders with a generalised impairment of peroxisomal functions. A study using complementation analysis. J Clin Invest 1988; 81: 1710–15.

42 Bruno C, Minetti C, Tang Y et al. Primary adrenal insufficiency in a child with a mitochondrial DNA deletion. J Inherit Metab Dis 1998; 21: 155–61.

43 Budka H, Molzer B, Bernheimer H et al. Clinical, morphological and neurochemical findings in adrenoleukodystrophy and its variants. In: Yonezawa T ed. International symposium on the leucodystrophy and allied diseases. Kyoto: Japanese Society of Neuropathology, 1981: 209–24.

44 Budka H, Sluga E, Heiss WD. Spastic paraplegia associated with Addison's disease: adult variant of adrenoleukodystrophy. J Neurol 1976; 213: 237–50.

45 Cammermeyer J. Refsum's disease. In: Vinken PJ, Bruyn GW eds. Handbook of clinical neurology Vol. 21. Amsterdam: North-Holland, 1975: 231–61.

46   Campos Y, Martín MA, Rubio JC et al. Bilateral striatal necrosis and MELAS associated with a new T3308C mutation in the mitochondrial ND1 gene. Biochem Biophys Res Commun 1997; 238: 323–5.

47   Carrozzo R, Hirano M, Fromenty B et al. Multiple mtDNA deletion features in autosomal dominant and recessive diseases suggest distinct pathogeneses. Neurology 1998; 50: 99–106.

48   Castaigne P, Lhermitte F, Escourolle R et al. Étude anatomo-clinique d'une observation d' 'ophtalmoplegia plus' avec analyse des lésions musculaires, nerveuses centrales, oculaires, myocardiques et thyroïdiennes. Rev Neurol 1977; 133: 369–86.

49   Cavanagh JB. Selective vulnerability in acute energy depression syndromes. Neuropathol Appl Neurobiol 1993; 19: 461–70

50   Cavanagh JB, Harding BN. Pathogenic factors underlying the lesions in Leigh's disease. Tissue responses to cellular energy deprivation and their clinico-pathological consequences. Brain 1994; 117: 1357–76.

51   Cederbaum SD, Blass JP, Minkoff N et al. Sensitivity to carbohydrate in a patient with familial intermittent lactic acidosis and pyruvate dehydrogenase deficiency. Paediatr Res 1976; 10: 713–20.

52   Chabrol B, Paquis V. Cerebral infarction associated with Kearns–Sayre syndrome. Neurology 1997; 49: 308.

53   Challa VR, Geisinger KR, Burton BK. Pathologic alterations in the brain and liver in hyperpipecolic acidemia. J Neuropathol Exp Neurol 1983; 42: 627–38.

54   Chang C-C, South S, Warren D et al. Metabolic control of peroxisome abundance. J Cell Sci 1999; 112: 1579–90.

55   Chinnery PF, Elliott C, Green GR et al. The spectrum of hearing loss due to mitochondrial DNA defects. Brain 2000; 123: 82–92.

56   Chinnery PF, Taylor DJ, Brown DT et al. Very low levels of the mtDNA A3243G mutation associated with mitochondrial dysfunction in vivo. Ann Neurol 2000; 47: 381–4.

56a   Chinnery PF, Taylor DJ, Manners D et al. No correlation between muscle A3243G mutation load and mitochondrial function in vivo. Neurology 2001; 56, 1101–4.

57   Chow CW, Anderson RMcD, Kenny GCT. Neuropathology in cerebral lactic acidosis. Acta Neuropathol 1987; 74: 393–6.

58   Chow CW, Poulos A, Fellenberg AJ et al. Autopsy findings in two siblings with infantile Refsum disease. Acta Neuropathol 1992; 83: 190–5.

59   Christensen E, Van Eldere J, Brandt NJ et al. A new peroxisomal disorder: di- and trihydroxycholestanaemia due to a presumed trihydroxycholestanoyl-CoA oxidase deficiency. J Inherit Metab Dis 1990; 13: 363–6.

60   Chu BC, Terae S, Takahashi C et al. MRI of the brain in the Kearns–Sayre syndrome: report of four cases and a review. Neuroradiology 1999; 41: 759–64.

61   Clark JB, Hayes DJ, Byrne E, Morgan-Hughes JA. Mitochondrial myopathies: defects in mitochondrial metabolism in human skeletal muscle. Biochem Soc Trans 1983; 11: 626–7.

62   Clark JM, Marks MP, Adalsteinsson E et al. MELAS: clinical and pathologic correlations with MRI, xenon/CT, and MR spectroscopy. Neurology 1996; 46: 223–7.

63   Clark KM, Bindoff LA, Lightowlers RN et al. Reversal of a mitochondrial DNA defect in human skeletal muscle (Letter). Nat Genet 1997; 16: 222–4.

64   Clayton PT, Johnson AW, Mills KA et al. Ataxia associated with increased plasma concentrations of pristanic acid, phytanic acid, and C_{27} bile acids but normal fibrob-

last branched-chain fatty acid oxidation. J Inherit Metab Dis 1996; 19: 761–8.

65   Cohen SMZ, Brown FR, Martyn L et al. Ocular histopathologic and biochemical studies of the cerebrohepatorenal syndrome (Zellweger's syndrome) and its relationship to neonatal adrenoleukodystrophy. Am J Ophthalmol 1983; 96: 488–501.

66   Cohen SMZ, Green WR, de la Cruz ZC et al. Ocular histopathologic studies of neonatal and childhood adrenoleukodystrophy. Am J Ophthalmol 1983; 95: 82–96.

67   Cormier V, Rotig A, Tardieu M et al. Autosomal dominant deletions of the mitochondrial genome in a case of progressive encephalomyopathy. Am J Hum Genet 1991; 48: 643–8.

68   Cottrell DA, Ince PG, Blakely EL et al. Neuropathological and histochemical changes in a multiple mitochondrial DNA deletion disorder. J Neuropathol Exp Neurol 2000; 59: 621–7.

68a   Crawford TO, Sladky JT, Hurko O et al. Abnormal fatty acid metabolism in childhood spinal muscular atrophy. Ann Neurol 1999; 45: 337–43.

69   Crosby TW, Chou SM. 'Ragged-red' fibres in Leigh's disease. Neurology 1974; 24: 49–54.

70   Daroff RB, Solitare GB, Pincus JH, Glaser GH. Spongiform encephalopathy with chronic progressive external ophthalmoplegia. Neurology 1966; 16: 161–9.

71   Dayan AD, Ockenden BG, Crome L. Necrotising encephalomyelopathy of Leigh. Neuropathological findings in 8 cases. Arch Dis Child 1970; 45: 39–48.

72   de Duve C, Baudhuin P. Peroxisomes (microbodies and related particles). Physiol Rev 1966; 46: 323–57.

73   de Koning TJ, de Vries LS, Groenendaal F et al. Pontocerebellar hypoplasia associated with respiratory-chain defects. Neuropediatrics 1999; 30: 93–5.

74   de Leon GA, Grover WD, Huff DS et al. Globoid cells, glial nodules, and peculiar fibrillary changes in the cerebrohepato-renal syndrome of Zellweger. Ann Neurol 1977; 2: 473–84.

75   de Lonlay-Debeney P, von Kleist-Retzow J-C, Hertz-Pannier L et al. Cerebral white matter disease in children may be caused by mitochondrial respiratory chain deficiency. J Paediatr 2000; 136: 209–14.

76   de Vet ECJM, Ijlst L, Oostheim W et al. Alkyl-dihydroxyacetonephosphate synthase: fate in peroxisome biogenesis disorders and identification of the point mutation underlying a single enzyme deficiency. J Biol Chem 1998; 273: 10296–301.

77   De Vivo DC. Complexities of the pyruvate dehydrogenase complex. Neurology 1998; 51: 1247–9.

78   De Vivo DC. Leigh syndrome: historical perspective and clinical variations. BioFactors 1998; 7: 269–71.

79   De Vivo, DC. Solving the COX puzzle. Ann Neurol 1999; 46: 142–3.

80   De Vivo DC, DiMauro S. Mitochondrial diseases. In: Swaiman KF, Ashwal S eds. Paediatric neurology principles and practice. London: Mosby, 1999: 494–509.

81   De Vivo DC, Haymond MW, Leckie MP et al. The clinical and biochemical implications of pyruvate carboxylase deficiency. J Clin Endocrinol Metab 1977; 45: 1281–96.

82   De Vivo DC, Haymond MW, Obert KA. Defective activation of the pyruvate dehydrogenase complex in subacute necrotising encephalomyelopathy (Leigh disease). Ann Neurol 1979; 6: 483–94.

83   De Vivo DC, Hirano M, DiMauro S. Mitochondrial disorders. In: Moser HW ed. Handbook of clinical neurology Vol. 66. Amsterdam: Elsevier 1996: 389–431.

84   De Vivo DC, Van Coster RN. Leigh syndrome: clinical and biochemical correlates. In: Fukuyama Y, Kamoshita S, Oht-

suka C, Suzuki Y eds. *Modern perspectives of child neurology*. Tokyo: Asahi Daily News Co., 1991: 27–37.

84a Dean M, Rzhetsky A, Allikmets R. The human ATP-binding cassette (ABC) transporter superfamily. *Genome Res* 2001; **11**: 1156–66.

85 DiMauro S. Mitochondrial encephalomyopathies. In: Rosenberg RN, Prusiner SB, DiMauro S et al. eds. *The molecular and genetic basis of neurological disease*. Boston, MA: Butterworth-Heinemann, 1993: 665–94.

86 DiMauro S, Andreu AL. Mutations in mtDNA: are we scraping the bottom of the barrel? *Brain Pathol* 2000; **10**: 431–41.

87 DiMauro S, Bonilla E, De Vivo DC. Does the patient have a mitochondrial encephalomyopathy? *J Child Neurol* 1999; **14**: S23–35.

88 DiMauro S, Bonilla E, Lombes A et al. Mitochondrial encephalomyopathies. *Paediatr Neurol* 1990; **8**: 483–506.

89 DiMauro S, De Vivo DC. Genetic heterogeneity in Leigh syndrome. *Ann Neurol* 1996; **40**: 5–7.

90 DiMauro S, Mendell JR, Sahenk Z et al. Fatal infantile mitochondrial myopathy and renal dysfunction due to cytochrome-c-oxidase deficiency. *Neurology* 1980; **30**: 795–804.

91 DiMauro S, Servidei S, Zeviani M et al. Cytochrome c oxidase deficiency in Leigh syndrome. *Ann Neurol* 1987; **22**: 498–506.

92 Dimmick JE, Applegarth DA. Pathology of peroxisomal disorders. *Perspect Paediatr Pathol* 1993; **17**: 45–98.

93 Dingemans KP, Mooi WJ, van den Bergh Weerman MA. Angulate lysosomes. *Ultrastruct Pathol* 1983; **5**: 113–22.

94 Distel B, Erdmann R, Gould SJ et al. A unified nomenclature for peroxisome biogenesis factors. *J Cell Biol* 1996; **135**: 1–3.

95 Doriguzzi C, Palmucci L, Mongini T et al. Endocrine involvement in mitochondrial encephalomyopathy with partial cytochrome c oxidase deficiency. *J Neurol Neurosurg Psychiat* 1989; **52**: 122–5.

96 Drachman DA. Ophthalmoplegia plus. The neurodegenerative disorders associated with progressive external ophthalmoplegia. *Arch Neurol* 1968; **18**: 654–74.

97 Dubeau F, De Stefano N, Zifkin BG et al. Oxidative phosphorylation defect in the brains of carriers of the tRNA$^{leu(UUR)}$ A3243G mutation in a MELAS pedigree. *Ann Neurol* 2000; **47**: 179–85.

98 Dubois-Dalcq M, Feigenbaum V, Aubourg P. The neurobiology of X-linked adrenoleukodystrophy, a demyelinating peroxisomal disorder. *Trends Neurosci* 1999; **22**: 4–12.

99 Dumontel C, Rousselle C, Guigard M-P, Trouillas J. Angulate lysosomes in skin biopsies of patients with degenerative neurological disorders: high frequency in neuronal ceroid lipofuscinosis. *Acta Neuropathol* 1999; **98**: 91–6.

100 Eagle RC, Hedges TR, Yanoff M. The atypical pigmentary retinopathy of Kearns–Sayre syndrome. A light and electron microscopic study. *Ophthalmology* 1982; **89**: 1433–40.

101 Edwin D, Speedie LJ, Kohler W et al. Cognitive and brain magnetic resonance imaging findings in adrenomyeloneuropathy. *Ann Neurol* 1996; **40**: 675–8.

102 Eisengart MA, Powers JM, Rose AL. Subacute necrotising encephalomyelopathy. *Am J Dis Child* 1974; **127**: 730–2.

103 Ellison D, Love S. Mitochondrial encephalopathies. In: Ellison D, Love S eds. *Neuropathology. A reference text of CNS pathology*. London: Mosby, 1997: 24.1–24.9.

104 Engel WK, Cunningham CG. Rapid examination of muscle tissue: an improved trichrome stain method for fresh-frozen biopsy sections. *Neurology* 1963; **13**: 919–23.

105 Evrard P, Caviness VS, Prats-Vinas J, Lyon G. The mechanism of arrest of neuronal migration in the Zellweger malformation: an hypothesis based upon cytoarchitectonic analysis. *Acta Neuropathol* 1978; **41**: 109–17.

106 Fan C-Y, Pan J, Chu R et al. Hepatocellular and hepatic peroxisomal alterations in mice with a disrupted peroxisomal fatty acyl-coenzyme A oxidase gene. *J Biol Chem* 1996; **271**: 24698–710.

107 Fardeau M, Engel WK. Ultrastructural study of a peripheral nerve biopsy in Refsum's disease. *J Neuropathol Exp Neurol* 1969; **28**: 278–94.

108 Farkas-Bargeton E, Goutières F, Richardet JM et al. Leucoencéphalopathie familiale associée à une acidose lactique congénitale. *Acta Neuropathol* 1971; **17**: 156–68.

109 Faust PL, Hatten ME. Targeted deletion of the PEX2 peroxisome assembly gene in mice provides a model for Zellweger syndrome, a human neuronal migration disorder. *J Cell Biol* 1997; **139**: 1293–305.

110 Fenton WA. Mitochondrial protein transport – a system in search of mutations. *Am J Hum Genet* 1995; **57**: 235–8.

111 Ferdinandusse S, Denis S, Clayton PT et al. Mutations in the gene encoding peroxisomal α-methylacyl-CoA racemase cause adult-onset sensory motor neuropathy. *Nat Genet* 2000; **24**: 188–91.

112 Figarella-Branger D, Pellissier JF, Scheiner C et al. Defects of the mitochondrial respiratory chain complexes in three paediatric cases with hypotonia and cardiac involvement. *J Neurol Sci* 1992; **108**: 105–13.

113 Fine PE. Mitochondrial inheritance and disease. *Lancet* 1978; **ii**: 659–62.

114 Fujii T, Hattori H, Higuchi Y et al. Phenotypic differences between T→C and T→G mutations at nt 8993 of mitochondrial DNA in Leigh syndrome. *Pediatr Neurol* 1998; **18**: 275–7.

115 Fukuhara N. MERRF: a clinicopathological study. Relationships between myoclonus epilepsies and mitochondrial myopathies. *Rev Neurol* 1991; **147**: 476–9.

116 Fukuhara N, Tokiguchi S, Shirakawa K, Tsubaki T. Myoclonus epilepsy associated with ragged-red fibres (mitochondrial abnormalities): disease entity or a syndrome? Light- and electron-microscopic studies of two cases and review of literature. *J Neurol Sci* 1980; **47**: 117–33.

117 Gatfield PD, Taller E, Hinton GG et al. Hyperpipecolatemia: a new metabolic disorder associated with neuropathy and hepatomegaly: a case study. *Can Med Assoc J* 1968; **99**: 1215–33.

118 Geisbrecht BV, Collins CS, Reuber BE, Gould SJ. Disruption of a PEX1–PEX6 interaction is the most common cause of the neurologic disorders Zellweger syndrome, neonatal adrenoleukodystrophy, and infantile Refsum disease. *Proc Nat Acad Sci USA* 1998; **95**: 8630–5.

119 Gellera C, Uziel G, Rimoldi M et al. Fumarase deficiency is an autosomal recessive encephalopathy affecting both the mitochondrial and the cytosolic enzymes. *Neurology* 1990; **40**: 495–9.

120 Ghadially FN. Mitochondria. In: Ghadially FN ed. *Ultrastructural pathology of the cell and matrix*. Boston, MA: Butterwoth-Heinemann, 1997: 195–342.

121 Ghatak NR, Nochlin D, Peris M, Myer EC. Morphology and distribution of cytoplasmic inclusions in adrenoleukodystrophy. *J Neurol Sci* 1981; **50**: 391–8.

122 Gilbert EF, Opitz JM, Spranger JW et al. Chondrodysplasia punctata: rhizomelic form. Pathologic and radiologic studies of three infants. *Eur J Paediatr* 1976; **123**: 89–109.

123 Gilchrist JM, Sikirica M, Stopa E, Shanske S. Adult-onset MELAS. Evidence for involvement of neurons as well as cerebral vasculature in strokelike episodes. *Stroke* 1996; **27**: 1420–3.

124 Giles RE, Blanc H, Cann HM, Wallace DC. Maternal inheritance of human mitochondrial DNA. *Proc Nat Acad Sci USA* 1980; **77**: 6715–19.

125 Gilg AG, Pahan K, Singh K, Singh I. Inducible nitric oxide synthase in the central nervous system of patients with X-linked adrenoleukodystrophy. *J Neuropathol Exp Neurol* 2000; **59**: 1063–9.

126 Goldfischer S. Pathogenesis of Zellweger's cerebro-hepato-renal syndrome and related peroxisome deficiency diseases. In: Fahimi HD, Sies H eds. *Peroxisomes in biology and medicine.* Berlin: Springer, 1987: 323–34.

127 Goldfischer S, Collins J, Rapin I et al. Pseudo-Zellweger syndrome: deficiencies in several peroxisomal oxidative activities. *J Paediatr* 1986; **108**: 25–32.

128 Goldfischer S, Moore CL, Johnson AB et al. Peroxisomal and mitochondrial defects in the cerebro-hepato-renal syndrome. *Science* 1973; **182**: 62–4.

129 Goldfischer S, Powers JM, Johnson AB et al. Striated adrenocortical cells in cerebro-hepato-renal (Zellweger) syndrome. *Virchows Arch A Pathol Anat Histopathol* 1983; **401**: 355–61.

130 Goto Y, Nonaka I, Horai S. A mutation in the tRNA^Leu(UUR) gene associated with the MELAS subgroup of mitochondrial encephalomyopathies. *Nature* 1990; **348**: 651–3.

130a Gould SJ, Raymond GV, Valle D. The peroxisome biogenesis disorders. In Scriver CR, Beaudet AL, Sly WS and Valle D. (eds.), *The metabolic & molecular bases of inherited disease,* eighth edition. New York NY: McGraw-Hill Book Company, 2001; 3181–218.

131 Gray F, Louarn F, Gherardi R et al. Adult form of Leigh's disease: a clinicopathological case with CT scan examination. *J Neurol Neurosurg Psychiatry* 1984; **47**: 1211–15.

132 Griffin DE, Moser HW, Mendoza Q et al. Identification of the inflammatory cells in the central nervous system of patients with adrenoleukodystrophy. *Ann Neurol* 1985; **18**: 660–4.

133 Griffin JW, Goren E, Schaumburg H et al. Adreno-myeloneuropathy: a probable variant of adrenoleukodystrophy. I. Clinical and endocrinologic aspects. *Neurology* 1977; **27**: 1107–13.

134 Grodd W, Krageloh-Mann I, Klose U, Sauter R. Metabolic and destructive brain disorders in children: findings with localised proton MR spectroscopy. *Radiology* 1991; **181**: 173–81.

135 Groothuis DR, Schulman S, Wollman R et al. Demyelinating radiculopathy in the Kearns–Sayre syndrome: a clinicopathological study. *Ann Neurol* 1980; **8**: 373–80.

136 Gullotta F, Heyer R, Tropitzsch G et al. Ungewöhnliche orthochromatische Leukodystrophie bei drei geschwistern. *Neuropädiatrie* 1970; **2**: 173–86.

137 Haas JE, Johnson ES, Farrell DL. Neonatal-onset adrenoleukodystrophy in a girl. *Ann Neurol* 1982; **12**: 449–57.

138 Hart ZH, Chang C, Perrin EVD et al. Familial poliodystrophy, mitochondrial myopathy, and lactate acidemia. *Arch Neurol* 1977; **34**: 180–5.

139 Harvy JN, Barnett D. Endocrine dysfunction in Kearns–Sayre syndrome. *Clin Endocrinol* 1992; **37**: 97–104.

140 Hebestreit H, Wanders RJA, Schutgens RBH et al. Isolated dihydroxyacetonephosphate-acyl-transferase deficiency in rhizomelic chondrodysplasia punctata: clinical presentation, metabolic and histological findings. *Eur J Paediatr* 1996; **155**: 1035–9.

141 Hegedüs K, Németh G. The adult form of subacute necrotising encephalopathy. *Surg Neurol* 1984; **21**: 572–6.

142 Hirano A, Llena JF, French JH, Ghatak NR. Fine structure of the cerebellar cortex in Menkes kinky-hair disease. X-chromosome-linked copper malabsorption. *Arch Neurol* 1977; **34**: 52–6.

143 Hirano M, Pavlakis SG. Mitochondrial myopathy, encephalopathy, lactic acidosis, and strokelike episodes (MELAS): Current concepts. *J Child Neurol* 1994; **9**: 4–13.

144 Hirano M, Ricci E, Koenigsberger MR et al. MELAS: an original case and clinical criteria for diagnosis. *Neuromusc Disord* 1992; **2**: 125–35.

145 Hirano M, Silvestri G, Blake DM et al. Mitochondrial neurogastrointestinal encephalomyopathy (MNGIE): clinical, biochemical, and genetic features of an autosomal recessive mitochondrial disorder. *Neurology* 1994; **44**: 721–7.

145a Hirano M and Vu TH. Defects of intergenomic communication: Where do we stand? *Brain Pathology* 2000; **10**: 451–61.

146 Ho JK, Moser H, Kishimoto Y, Hamilton JA. Interactions of a very long chain fatty acid with model membranes and serum albumin. Implications for the pathogenesis of adrenoleukodystrophy. *J Clin Invest* 1995; **96**: 1455–63.

147 Ho K-L, Piligian JT, Chason JL. Adult form of subacute necrotising encephalomyelopathy. *Arch Pathol Lab Med* 1979; **103**: 344–7.

147a Hoffmann GF, Charpentier C, Mayatepek E. et al. Clinical and biochemical phenotype in 11 patients with mevalonic aciduria. *Pediatrics* 1993; **91**: 915–21.

148 Hofmann S, Bezold R, Jaksch M et al. Wolfram (DIDMOAD) syndrome and Leber hereditary optic neuropathy (LHON) are associated with distinct mitochondrial DNA haplotypes. *Genomics* 1997; **39**: 8–18.

149 Holmes RD, Moore KH, Ofenstein JP et al. Lactic acidosis and mitochondrial dysfunction in two children with peroxisomal disorders. *J Inherit Metab Dis* 1993; **16**: 368–80.

150 Holt IJ, Harding AE, Morgan-Hughes JA. Deletions of muscle mitochondrial DNA in patients with mitochondrial myopathies. *Nature* 1988; **331**: 717–19.

151 Holt IJ, Harding AE, Petty RKH, Morgan-Hughes JA. A new mitochondrial disease associated with mitochondrial DNA heteroplasmy. *Am J Hum Genet* 1990; **46**: 428–33.

152 Holtzman E. Peroxisomes in nervous tissue. *Ann N Y Acad Sci* 1982; **386**: 523–5.

153 Houdou S, Kuruta H, Hasegawa M. Developmental immunohistochemistry of catalase in the human brain. *Brain Res* 1991; **556**: 267–70.

154 Howell N. Human mitochondrial diseases: answering questions and questioning answers. *Int Rev Cytol* 1999; **186**: 49–116.

155 Hübner G, Gokel JM, Pontgratz D et al. Fatal mitochondrial cardiomyopathy in Kearns–Sayre syndrome. *Virchows Arch Pathol Anat Histopathol* 1986; **408**: 611–21.

156 Hughes JL, Poulos A, Robertson E et al. Pathology of hepatic peroxisomes and mitochondria in patients with peroxisomal disorders. *Virchows Arch A Pathol Anat Histopathol* 1990; **416**: 255–64.

157 Igarashi M, Belchis D, Suzuki K. Brain gangliosides in adrenoleukodystrophy. *J Neurochem* 1976; **27**: 327–8.

158 Igarashi M, Neely JG, Anthony PF, Alford BR. Cochlear nerve degeneration coincident with adrenocerebroleukodystrophy. *Arch Otolaryngol* 1976; **102**: 722–6.

159 Igarashi M, Schaumburg HH, Powers J et al. Fatty acid abnormality in adrenoleukodystrophy. *J Neurochem* 1976; **26**: 851–60.

160   Ihara Y, Namba R, Kuroda R et al. Mitochondrial encephalomyopathy (MELAS): pathological study and successful therapy with coenzyme Q10 and idebenone. J Neurol Sci 1989; 90: 263–71.

161   Imamura A, Tsukamoto T, Shimozawa N et al. Temperature-sensitive phenotypes of peroxisome-assembly processes represent the milder forms of human peroxisome-biogenesis disorders. Am J Hum Genet 1998; 62: 1539–43.

162   Ionasescu V. Oculogastrointestinal muscular dystrophy. Am J Med Genet 1983; 15: 103–12.

163   Ito M, Mock DJ, Goodman AD, Powers JM. An immuno-histochemical/in situ PCR study of potential environmental–host proinflammatory factors in ALD. J Neuropathol Exp Neurol 2000; 59: 453.

163a   Ito M, Blumberg BM, Mock DJ et al. Potential Environmental and Host Participants in the Early White Matter Lesion of Adreno-Leukodystrophy: Morphologic Evidence for CD8 Cytotoxic T Cells, Cytolysis of Oligodendrocytes and CD1-Mediated Lipid Antigen Presentation. J Neuropathol Exp Neurol 2001; 60: 1004–90.

164   Jaffe R, Crumrine P, Hashida Y, Moser HW. Neonatal adrenoleukodystrophy. Clinical, pathologic, and biochemical delineation of a syndrome affecting both males and females. Am J Pathol 1982; 108: 100–11.

165   Jansen GA, Wanders RJA, Watkins PA, Mihalik SJ. Phytanoyl-coenzyme A hydroxylase deficiency – the enzyme defection in Refsum's disease. N Engl J Med 1997; 337: 133–4.

166   Janssen A, Baes M, Gressens P et al. Docosahexaenoic acid deficit is not a major pathogenic factor in peroxisome-deficient mice. Lab Invest 2000; 80: 31–5.

167   Jellinger K, Seitelberger F. Subacute necrotising encephalomyelopathy (LEIGH). Ergebnisse Inneren Medizin Kinderheilkunde 1970; 29: 155–219.

168   Johnson AB, Schaumburg HH, Powers JM. Histochemical characteristics of the striated inclusions of adrenoleukodystrophy. J Histochem Cytochem 1976; 24: 725–30.

169   Kaido M, Fujimura H, Taniike M et al. Focal cytochrome c oxidase deficiency in the brain and dorsal root ganglia in a case with mitochondrial encephalomyopathy (tRNA^Ile 4269 mutation): histochemical, immunohisto-chemical, and ultrastructural study. J Neurol Sci 1995; 131: 170–6.

170   Kalimo H, Lundberg PO, Olsson Y. Familial subacute necrotising encephalomyelopathy of the adult form (adult Leigh syndrome). Ann Neurol 1979; 6: 200–6.

171   Kamei A, Houdou S, Takashima S et al. Peroxisomal disorders in children: immunohistochemistry and neuropathology. J Paediatr 1993; 122: 573–9.

172   Kaufmann WE, Theda C, Naidu TC et al. Neuronal migration abnormality in peroxisomal bifunctional enzyme defect. Ann Neurol 1996; 39: 268–71.

173   Kearns TP, Sayre GP. Retinitis pigmentosa, external ophthalmoplegia, and complete heart block. Unusual syndrome with histologic study in one of two cases. Arch Ophthalmol 1958; 60: 280–9.

174   Keilin D. Cytochrome, a respiratory pigment common to animals, yeast and higher plants. Proc R Soc Lond B Biol Sci 1925; 98: 312–39.

175   Kelley RI, Datta NS, Dobyns WB et al. Neonatal adrenoleukodystrophy: new cases, biochemical studies and differentiation from Zellweger and related peroxisomal polydystrophy syndromes. Am J Med Genet 1986; 23: 869–901.

176   Kendall BE. Disorders of lysosomes, peroxisomes and mitochondria. Am J Neuroradiol 1992; 13: 621–53.

177   Kepes JJ. Oncocytic transformation of choroid plexus epithelium. Acta Neuropathol 1983; 62: 145–8.

178   Kimura S, Kobayashi T, Amemiya F. Myelin splitting in the spongy lesion in Leigh encephalopathy. Paediatr Neurol 1991; 7: 56–8.

179   Kinney HC, Brody BA, Kloman A, Gilles FH. Sequence of central system myelination in human infancy. II. Patterns of myelination in autopsied infants. J Neuropathol Exp Neurol 1988; 47: 217–34.

180   Kishi M, Yamamura Y, Kurihara T et al. An autopsy case of mitochondrial encephalomyopathy: biochemical and electron microscopic studies of the brain. J Neurol Sci 1988; 86: 31–40.

181   Knight SAB, Kim R, Pain D, Dancis A. Insights from model systems: the yeast connection to Friedreich ataxia. Am J Hum Genet 1999; 64: 365–71.

182   Koehler CM, Leuenberger D, Merchant S et al. Human deafness dystonia syndrome is a mitochondrial disease. Proc Natl Acad Sci USA 1999; 96: 2141–6.

183   Kozich V, Gibson KM, Zeman J et al. Case report. Mevalonic aciduria. J Inherit Metab Dis 1991; 41: 265–6.

184   Krebs HA, Kornberg HL. A survey of the energy transformations in living matter. Ergeb Physiol 1957; 49: 212–98.

185   Kuriyama M, Umezaki H, Fukuda Y et al. Mitochondrial encephalomyopathy with lactate-pyruvate elevation and brain infarctions. Neurology 1984; 34: 72–7.

186   Kuroda S, Hirano A, Yuasa S. Adrenoleukodystrophy: cerebello-brain stem dominant case. Acta Neuropathol 1983; 60: 149–52.

187   Kwittken J, Barest HD. The neuropathology of hereditary optic atrophy (Leber's disease); the first complete anatomic study. Am J Pathol 1958; 34: 185–207.

188   Kyllerman M, Blomstrand S, Mansson JE et al. Central nervous system malformations and white matter changes in pseudo-neonatal adrenoleukodystrophy. Neuropediatrics 1990; 21: 199–201.

189   Larsson NG, Holme E, Kristiansson B et al. Progressive increase of the mutated mitochondrial DNA fraction in Kearns–Sayre syndrome. Paediatr Res 1990; 28: 131–6.

190   Lazarow PB. Peroxisome structure, function, and biogenesis – human patients and yeast mutants show strikingly similar defects in peroxisome biogenesis. J Neuropathol Exp Neurol 1995; 54: 720–5.

191   Lazarow PB, Moser HW. Disorders of peroxisome biogenesis. In: Scriver CR, Beaudet AL, Sly WS, Valle D eds. The metabolic and molecular bases of inherited disease Vol. II. New York: McGraw-Hill, 1995: 2287–324.

192   Leber T. Uber hereditare und congenital-angelegte Sehnervenleiden. Graefes Arch Ophthalmol 1871; 17: 249–91.

193   Ledley FD, Jansen R, Nhaum SU et al. Mutation eliminating mitochondrial leader sequence of methylmalonyl. CoA mutase causes methylmalonic acidemia. Proc Natl Acad Sci USA 1990; 87: 3147–50.

194   Leigh D. Subacute necrotising encephalomyelopathy in an infant. J Neurol Neurosurg Psychiatry 1951; 14: 216–21.

195   Li V, Hostein J, Romero NB et al. Chronic intestinal pseudoobstruction with myopathy and ophthalmoplegia. A muscular biochemical study of a mitochondrial disorder. Dig Dis Sci 1992; 37: 456–63.

196   Lie SO, Löken AC, Strömme JH, Aagenaes Ö. Fatal congenital lactic acidosis in two siblings. I. Clinical and pathological findings. Acta Paediatr Scand 1971; 60: 129–37.

197   Lindsay JR, Hinojosa R. Histopathologic features of the inner ear associated with Kearns–Sayre syndrome. *Arch Otolaryngol* 1976; **102**: 747–52.

198   Love S, Hilton DA. Assessment of the distribution of mitochondrial ribosomal RNA in MELAS and in thrombotic cerebral infarcts by *in situ* hybridisation. *J Pathol* 1996; **178**: 182–9.

199   Love S, Nicoll JAR, Kinrade E. Sequencing and quantitative assessment of mutant and wild-type mitochondrial DNA in paraffin sections from cases of MELAS. *J Pathol* 1993; **170**: 9–14.

200   Luft R, Ikkos D, Palmieri G et al. A case of severe hypermetabolism of nonthyroid origin with a defect in the maintenance of mitochondrial respiratory control: a correlated clinical, biochemical, and morphological study. *J Clin Invest* 1962; **41**: 1776–804.

201   MacBrinn MC, O'Brien JS. Lipid composition of the nervous system in Refsum's disease. *J Lipid Res* 1968; **9**: 552–61.

202   MacCollin M, DeVivo DC, Moser AB, Beard M. Ataxia and peripheral neuropathy: a benign variant of peroxisome dysgenesis. *Ann Neurol* 1990; **28**: 833–6.

203   McGuinness MC, Powers JM, Bias WB et al. Human leukocyte antigens and cytokine expression in cerebral inflammatory demyelinative lesions of X-linked adrenoleukodystrophy and multiple sclerosis. *J Neuroimmunol* 1997; **75**: 174–82.

204   McKechnie NM, King M, Lee WR. Retinal pathology in the Kearns–Sayre syndrome. *Br J Ophthalmol* 1985; **69**: 63–75.

205   McKelvie PA, Morley JB, Byrne E, Marzuki S. Mitochondrial encephalomyopathies: a correlation between neuropathological findings and defects in mitochondrial DNA. *J Neurol Sci* 1991; **102**: 51–60.

206   McShane MA, Hammans SR, Sweeney M et al. Pearson syndrome and mitochondrial encephalomyopathy in a patient with a deletion of mtDNA. *Am J Hum Genet* 1991; **48**: 39–42.

207   Magistretti PJ, Pellerin L. Cellular bases of brain energy metabolism and their relevance to functional brain imaging: evidence for a prominent role of astrocytes. *Cerebral Cortex* 1996; **6**: 50–61.

208   Magistretti PJ, Pellerin L, Rothman DL, Shulman RG. Energy on demand. *Science* 1999; **283**: 496–7.

209   Malandrini A, Palmeri S, Fabrizi GM et al. Juvenile Leigh syndrome with protracted course presenting as chronic sensory motor neuropathy, ataxia, deafness and retinitis pigmentosa: a clinicopathological report. *J Neurol Sci* 1998; **155**: 218–21.

210   Manfredi G, Gupta N, Vazquez-Memije ME et al. Oligomycin induces a decrease in the cellular content of a pathogenic mutation in the human mitochondrial ATPase 6 gene. *J Biol Chem* 1999; **274**: 9386–91.

211   Manz HJ, Schuelein M, McCullough DC et al. New phenotypic variant of adrenoleukodystrophy. *J Neurol Sci* 1980; **45**: 245–60.

212   Marsden CD, Obeso JA, Lang AE. Adrenoleukomyeloneuropathy presenting as spinocerebellar degeneration. *Neurology* 1982; **32**: 1031–2.

213   Martinez AJ, Hay S, McNeer KW. Extraocular muscles. Light microscopy and ultrastructural features. *Acta Neuropathol* 1976; **34**: 237–53.

214   Martinez M, Pineda M, Vidal R, Martin B. Docosahexaenoic acid: a new therapeutic approach to peroxisomal patients. Experience with two cases. *Neurology* 1993; **43**: 1389–97.

215   Martinez M, Vazquez E. MRI evidence that docosahexaenoic acid ethyl ester improves myelination in generalised peroxisomal disorders. *Neurology* 1998; **51**; 26–32.

216   Matthews PM, Nagy Z, Brown GK et al. Isolated capillary proliferation in Leigh's syndrome. *Clin Neuropathol* 1994; **13**: 139–41.

217   Medina L, Chi TL, De Vivo DC, Hilal SK. MR findings in patients with subacute necrotising encephalomyelopathy (Leigh syndrome): correlation with biochemical defect. *Am J Roentgenol* 1990; **154**: 1269–74.

218   Menkes JH, Alter M, Steigleder GK et al. A sex-linked recessive disorder with retardation of growth, peculiar hair, and focal cerebral and cerebellar degeneration. *Paediatrics* 1962; **29**; 764–79.

219   Michotte A, De Meirleir L, Lissens W et al. Neuropathological findings of a patient with pyruvate dehydrogenase E1α deficiency presenting as a cerebral lactic acidosis. *Acta Neuropathol* 1993; **85**: 674–8.

220   Mirabella M, Di Giovanni S, Silvestri G et al. Apoptosis in mitochondrial encephalomyopathies with mitochondrial DNA mutations: a potential pathogenic mechanism. *Brain* 2000; **123**: 93–104.

221   Mitchell P. Coupling of phosphorylation to electron and hydrogen transfer by a chemiosmotic type of mechanism. *Nature* 1961; **191**: 144–8.

222   Mito T, Takada K, Akaboshi S et al. A pathological study of a peripheral nerve in a case of neonatal adrenoleukodystrophy. *Acta Neuropathol* 1989; **77**: 437–40.

223   Miyabayashi S, Narisawa K, Iinuma K et al. Cytochrome c oxidase deficiency in two siblings with Leigh encephalomyelopathy. *Brain Dev* 1984; **6**: 362–72.

224   Molzer B, Gullotta F, Harzer K et al. Unusual orthochromatic leukodystrophy with epitheloid cells (Norman–Gullotta): increase of very long chain fatty acids in brain discloses a peroxisomal disorder. *Acta Neuropathol* 1993; **86**: 187–9.

225   Montpetit VJA, Andermann F, Carpenter S et al. Subacute necrotising encephalomyelopathy. A review and a study of two families. *Brain* 1971; **94**: 1–30.

226   Moraes CT, Shanske S, Tritschler HJ et al. mtDNA depletion with variable tissue expression: a novel genetic abnormality in mitochondrial diseases. *Am J Hum Genet* 1991; **48**: 492–501.

227   Morris AAM, Leonard JV, Brown GK et al. Deficiency of respiratory chain complex I is a common cause of Leigh disease. *Ann Neurol* 1996; **40**: 25–30.

228   Morris AAM, Taanman J-W, Blake J et al. Liver failure associated with mitochondrial DNA depletion. *J Hepatol* 1998; **28**: 556–63.

229   Moser AB, Rasmussen M, Naidu S et al. Phenotype of patients with peroxisomal disorders subdivided into sixteen complementation groups. *J Paediatr* 1995; **127**: 13–22.

230   Moser HW. Adrenoleukodystrophy: phenotype, genetics, pathogenesis, and therapy. *Brain* 1997; **120**: 1485–508.

231   Moser HW. Minireview. Genotype–phenotype correlations in disorders of peroxisome biogenesis. *Mol Genet Metab* 1999; **68**: 316–27.

232   Moser HW. New approaches in peroxisomal disorders. *Dev Neurosci* 1987; **9**: 1–18.

233   Moser HW, Naidu S, Kumar AJ, Rosenbaum AE. The adrenoleukodystrophies. *CRC Crit Rev Neurobiol* 1987; **3**: 29–88.

234   Moser HW, Powers JM, Smith KD. Adrenoleukodystrophy: molecular genetics, pathology, and Lorenzo's oil. *Brain Pathol* 1995; **5**: 259–66.

235   Mosser J, Lutz Y, Stoeckel ME et al. The gene responsible for adrenoleukodystrophy encodes a peroxisomal membrane protein. *Hum Molec Genet* 1994; **3**: 265–71.

236   Moudy AM, Handran SD, Goldberg MP *et al.* Abnormal calcium homeostasis and mitochondrial polarisation in a human encephalomyopathy. *Proc Natl Acad Sci USA* 1995; **92**: 729–33.

237   Mukoyama M, Kazui H, Sunohara N *et al.* Mitochondrial myopathy, encephalopathy, lactic acidosis, and stroke-like episodes with acanthocytosis: a clinicopathological study of a unique case. *J Neurol* 1986; **233**: 228–32.

238   Müller-Höcker J, Hübner G, Bise K *et al.* Generalised mitochondrial microangiopathy and vascular cytochrome *c* oxidase deficiency. Occurrence in a case of MELAS syndrome with mitochondrial cardiomyopathy – myopathy and combined complex I/IV deficiency. *Arch Pathol Lab Med* 1993; **117**: 202–10.

239   Müller-Höcker J, Jacob U, Seibel P. The common 4977 base pair deletion of mitochondrial DNA preferentially accumulates in the cardiac conduction system of patients with Kearns–Sayre syndrome. *Mod Pathol* 1998; **11**: 295–301.

239a   Musumeci O, Naini A, Slonim AE *et al.* Familial cerebellar ataxia with muscle coenzyme Q10 deficiency. *Neurology* 2001; **56**: 849–55.

240   Nagashima T, Mori M, Katayama K *et al.* Adult Leigh syndrome with mitochondrial DNA mutation at 8993. *Acta Neuropathol* 1999; **97**: 416–22.

241   Naidu S, Hoefler G, Watkins PA *et al.* Neonatal seizures and retardation in a girl with biochemical features of X-linked adrenoleukodystrophy: a possible new peroxisomal disease entity. *Neurology* 1988; **38**: 1100–7.

242   Narita T, Yamano T, Ohno M *et al.* Hypertension in Leigh syndrome – a case report. *Neuropediatrics* 1998; **29**: 265–7.

243   Nass S, Nass MM. Intramitochondrial fibres with DNA characteristics. *J Cell Biol* 1963; **19**: 593–629.

244   Nicoll JAR, Moss TH, Love S *et al.* Clinical and autopsy findings in two cases of MELAS presenting with stroke-like episodes but without clinical myopathy. *Clin Neuropathol* 1993; **12**: 38–43.

245   Nishino I, Spinazzola A, Hirano M. Thymidine phosphorylase gene mutations in MNGIE, a human mitochondrial disorder. *Science* 1999; **283**: 689–92.

246   Nonaki I. Mitochondrial diseases. *Curr Opin Neurol Neurosurg* 1992; **5**: 622–32.

247   Ohama E, Ikuta F. Involvement of choroid plexus in mitochondrial encephalomyopathy (MELAS). *Acta Neuropathol* 1987; **75**: 1–7.

248   Ohama E, Ohara S, Ikuta F *et al.* Mitochondrial angiopathy in cerebral blood vessels of mitochondrial encephalomyopathy. *Acta Neuropathol* 1987; **74**: 226–33.

249   Ohara S, Ohama E, Takahashi H *et al.* Alterations of oligodendrocytes and demyelination in the spinal cord of patients with mitochondrial encephalomyopathy. *J Neurol Sci* 1988; **86**: 19–29.

250   Ohno T, Tsuchida H, Fukuhara N *et al.* Adrenoleukodystrophy: a clinical variant presenting as olivopontocerebellar atrophy. *J Neurol* 1984; **231**: 167–9.

251   Oldfors A, Fyhr I-M, Holme E *et al.* Neuropathology in Kearns–Sayre syndrome. *Acta Neuropathol* 1990; **80**: 541–6.

252   Ooiwa Y, Uematsu Y, Terada T *et al.* Cerebral blood flow in mitochondrial myopathy, encephalopathy, lactic acidosis, and strokelike episodes. *Stroke* 1993; **24**: 304–9.

253   Opitz JM, ZuRhein GM, Vitale L *et al.* The Zellweger syndrome (cerebro-hepato-renal syndrome). *Birth Defects* 1969; **5**: 144–66.

254   Palade GE. An electron microscope study of the mitochondrial structure. *J Histochem Cytochem* 1953; **1**: 188–203.

255   Palmer DN, Fearnley IM, Medd SM *et al.* Lysosomal storage of the DCCD reactive proteolipid subunit of mitochondrial ATP synthase in human and ovine ceroid lipofuscinoses. *Adv Exp Med Biol* 1989; **266**: 211–22.

256   Papadimitriou A, Neustein HB, DiMauro S *et al.* Histiocytoid cardiomyopathy of infancy: deficiency of reducible cytochrome b in heart mitochondria. *Paediatr Res* 1984; **18**: 1023–8.

257   Papadopoulou LC, Sue CM, Davidson MM *et al.* Fatal infantile cardioencephalomyopathy with COX deficiency and mutations in SCO2, a COX assembly gene. *Nat Genet* 1999; **23**: 333–7.

258   Passarge E, McAdams AJ. Cerebro-hepato-renal syndrome: a newly recognised hereditary disorder of multiple congenital defects, including sudanophilic leukodystrophy, cirrhosis of the liver, and polycystic kidneys. *J Paediatr* 1967; **71**: 691–702.

259   Paulus W, Lehr A, Peiffer J *et al.* Immunohistochemical demonstration of mitochondria in routinely processed tissue using a monoclonal antibody. *J Pathol* 1990; **160**: 321–8.

260   Paulus W, Peiffer J. Intracerebral distribution of mitochondrial abnormalities in 21 cases of infantile spongy dystrophy. *J Neurol Sci* 1990; **95**: 49–62.

261   Pavlakis SG, Phillips PC, DiMauro S *et al.* Mitochondrial myopathy, encephalopathy, lactic acidosis, and strokelike episodes: a distinctive clinical syndrome. *Ann Neurol* 1984; **16**: 481–8.

262   Pavlakis SG, Rowland LP, De Vivo DC *et al.* Mitochondrial myopathies and encephalomyopathies. In: Plum F ed. *Advances in contemporary neurology*. Philadelphia, PA: FA Davis Co., 1988: 95–133.

263   Pearson HA, Lobel JS, Kocoshis SA *et al.* A new syndrome of refractory sideroblastic anaemia with vacuolisation of marrow precursors and exocrine pancreatic dysfunction. *J Paediatr* 1979; **95**: 976–84.

264   Pellock J, Behrens M, Lewis L *et al.* Kearns–Sayre syndrome and hypoparathyroidism. *Ann Neurol* 1978; **3**: 455–8.

265   Plum F. What causes infarction in ischemic brain? The Robert Wartenberg lecture. *Neurology* 1983; **33**: 222–33.

266   Poll-Thé BT, Roels F, Ogier H *et al.* A new peroxisomal disorder with enlarged peroxisomes and a specific deficiency of acyl-CoA oxidase (pseudo-neonatal adrenoleukodystrophy). *Am J Hum Genet* 1988; **42**: 422–34.

267   Poll-Thé BT, Saudubray JM, Ogier HAM *et al.* Infantile Refsum disease: an inherited peroxisomal disorder. Comparison with Zellweger syndrome and neonatal adrenoleukodystrophy. *Eur J Paediatr* 1987; **146**: 477–83.

268   Pons R, Andreetta F, Wang CH *et al.* Mitochondrial myopathy simulating spinal muscular atrophy. *Paediatr Neurol* 1996; **15**: 153–8.

268a   Pons R, De Vivo DC. Mitochondrial disease. *Current Treatment Options in Neurology* 2001; **3**: 271–88.

269   Poulos A, Sheffield L, Sharp P *et al.* Rhizomelic chondrodysplasia punctata: clinical, pathologic and biochemical findings in two patients. *J Paediatr* 1988; **113**: 685–90.

270   Powell H, Tindall R, Schultz P *et al.* Adrenoleukodystrophy. Electron microscopic findings. *Arch Neurol* 1975; **32**: 250–60.

271   Powers JM. A neuropathologic overview of the neurodystrophies and neurolipidoses. In: Moser H ed. *Handbook of clinical neurology* Vol. 66. Amsterdam: Elsevier, 1996: 1–32.

271a   Powers JM, DeCiero D, Cox C *et al.* The dorsal root ganglia in adrenomyeloneuropathy: Neuronal atrophy and abnormal mitochondria. *J Neuropathol Exp Neurol* 2001; **60**: 493–501.

272 Powers JM. Peroxisomal diseases. In: Duckett S ed. *Paediatric neuropathology*. Philadelphia, PA: Williams & Wilkins, 1995: 630–9.

273 Powers JM. Presidential address: the pathology of peroxisomal disorders with pathogenetic considerations. *J Neuropathol Exp Neurol* 1995; **54**: 710–19.

274 Powers JM. Review article. Adreno-leukodystrophy (adreno-testiculo-leuko-myelo-neuropathic-complex). *Clin Neuropathol* 1985; **4**: 181–99.

275 Powers JM, DeCiero D, Cox C *et al*. The dorsal root ganglia in adrenomyeloneuropathy (AMN). *J Neuropathol Exp Neurol* 1999; **58**: 559.

276 Powers JM, DeCiero DP, Ito M *et al*. Adrenomyeloneuropathy: a neuropathologic review featuring its noninflammatory myelopathy. *J Neuropathol Exp Neurol* 2000; **59**: 89–102.

277 Powers JM, Kenjarski TP, Moser AB, Moser HW. Cerebellar atrophy in chronic rhizomelic chondrodysplasia punctata: A potential role for phytanic acid and calcium in the death of its Purkinje cells. *Acta Neuropathologica* 1999; **98**: 129–34.

278 Powers JM, Liu Y, Moser A, Moser H. The inflammatory myelinopathy of adreno-leukodystrophy. *J Neuropathol Exp Neurol* 1992; **51**: 630–43.

279 Powers JM, Moser HW. Peroxisomal disorders: genotype, phenotype, major neuropathologic lesions, and pathogenesis. *Brain Pathol* 1998; **8**: 101–20.

280 Powers JM, Moser HW, Moser AB *et al*. Foetal cerebrohepatorenal (Zellweger) syndrome: dysmorphic, radiologic, biochemical, and pathologic findings in four affected foetuses. *Hum Pathol* 1985; **16**: 610–20.

281 Powers JM, Moser HW, Moser AB *et al*. Pathologic findings in adrenoleukodystrophy heterozygotes. *Arch Pathol Lab Med* 1987; **111**: 151–3.

282 Powers JM, Moser HW, Moser AB, Schaumburg HH. Foetal adrenoleukodystrophy: the significance of pathologic lesions in adrenal gland and testis. *Hum Pathol* 1982; **13**: 1013–19.

283 Powers JM, Rubio A. Selected leukodystrophies. *Semin Paediatr Neurol* 1995; **2**: 200–10.

284 Powers JM, Schaumburg HH. Adreno-leukodystrophy (sex-linked Schilder's disease). *Am J Pathol* 1974; **76**: 481–500.

285 Powers JM, Schaumburg HH. Adreno-leukodystrophy. Similar ultrastructural changes in adrenal cortical and Schwann cells. *Arch Neurol* 1974; **30**: 406–8.

286 Powers JM, Schaumburg HH. The adrenal cortex in adrenoleukodystrophy. *Arch Pathol* 1973; **96**: 305–10.

287 Powers JM, Schaumburg HH. The testis in adrenoleukodystrophy. *Am J Pathol* 1981; **102**: 90–8.

288 Powers JM, Schaumburg HH, Johnson AB, Raine CS. A correlative study of the adrenal cortex in adrenoleukodystrophy-evidence for a fatal intoxication with very long chain saturated fatty acids. *Invest Cell Pathol* 1980; **3**: 353–76.

289 Powers JM, Tummons RC, Caviness VS Jr *et al*. Structural and chemical alterations in the cerebral maldevelopment of foetal cerebro-hepato-renal (Zellweger) syndrome. *J Neuropathol Exp Neurol* 1989; **48**: 270–89.

290 Powers JM, Tummons RC, Moser AB *et al*. Neuronal lipidosis and neuroaxonal dystrophy in cerebro-hepato-renal (Zellweger) syndrome. *Acta Neuropathol* 1987; **73**: 333–43.

291 Prayson RA, Wang N. Mitochondrial myopathy, encephalopathy, lactic acidosis, and strokelike episodes (MELAS) syndrome. An autopsy report. *Arch Pathol Lab Med* 1998; **122**: 978–81.

292 Prick M, Gabreëls F, Renier W *et al*. Pyruvate dehydrogenase deficiency restricted to brain. *Neurology* 1981; **31**: 398–404.

293 Probst A, Ulrich J, Heitz PhU, Herschkowitz N. Adrenomyeloneuropathy. A protracted, pseudosystematic variant of adrenoleukodystrophy. *Acta Neuropathol* 1980; **49**: 105–15.

294 Purdue PE, Takada Y, Danpure CJ. Identification of mutations associated with peroxisome-to-mitochondrion mistargeting of alanine/glyoxylate aminotransferase in primary hyperoxaluria type 1. *J Cell Biol* 1990; **111**: 2341–51.

295 Quade A, Zierz S, Klingmuller D. Endocrine abnormalities in mitochondrial myopathy with external ophthalmoplegia. *Clin Invest* 1992; **70**: 396–402.

295a Qin J, Mizuguchi M, Itoh M, Takashima S. A novel migration-related gene product, doublecortin, in neuronal migration disorder of fetuses and infants with Zellweger syndrome. *Acta Neuropathologica* 2000; **100**: 168–73.

296 Rahman S, Blok RB, Dahl H-HM *et al*. Leigh syndrome: clinical features and biochemical and DNA abnormalities. *Ann Neurol* 1996; **39**: 343–51.

297 Rehncrona S, Rosen I, Siesjo BK. Excessive cellular acidosis: an important mechanism of neuronal damage in the brain? *Acta Physiol Scand* 1980; **110**: 435–7.

298 Reuber BE, Collins CS, Germain-Lee E *et al*. Mutations in PEX 1 are the most common cause of peroxisome biogenesis disorders. *Nat Genet* 1997; **17**: 445–8.

299 Rhodin J. Correlation of ultrastructural organisation and function in normal and experimentally changed proximal convoluted cells of the mouse kidney. PhD Thesis, Karolinska Institutet, Stockholm, 1954.

300 Ricci E, Moraes CT, Servidei S *et al*. Disorders associated with depletion of mitochondrial DNA. *Brain Pathol* 1992; **2**: 141–7.

300a Riggs JE, Ellis BD, Hogg JP *et al*. Acute periaqueductal syndrome associated with the G11778A mitochondrial DNA mutation. *Neurology* 2001; **56**: 570–1.

300b Robinson BH. Lactic acidemia: Disorders of pyruvate carboxylase and pyruvate dehydrogenase. In Scriver CR, Beaudet AL, Sly WS and Valle D (eds.), *The metabolic & molecular bases of inherited disease,* 8th edition. New York, NY: McGraw-Hill Book Company, 2001; 2275–95.

300c Robinson BH, Taylor J, Sherwood WG. Deficiency of dihydrolipoyl dehydrogenase (a component of the pyruvate and a-ketoglutarate dehydrogenase complexes): A cause of congenital chronic lactic acidosis in infancy. *Pediatr Res* 1977; **11**: 1198–202.

301 Roels F, Especl M, Poggi F *et al*. Human liver pathology in peroxisomal disorders: a review including novel data. *Biochimie* 1993; **75**: 281–92.

302 Roscher AA, Hoefler S, Hoefler G *et al*. Genetic and phenotypic heterogeneity in disorders of peroxisome biogenesis – a complementation study involving cell lines from 19 patients. *Paediatr Res* 1989; **26**: 67–72.

303 Rötig A, Bourgeron T, Chretien D *et al*. Spectrum of mitochondrial DNA rearrangements in the Pearson marrow-pancreas syndrome. *Hum Mol Genet* 1995; **4**: 1327–30.

304 Rötig A, Cormier V, Blanche S *et al*. Pearson's marrow-pancreas syndrome. A multisystem mitochondrial disorder in infancy. *J Clin Invest* 1990; **86**: 1601–8.

305 Rowland LP. Myopathies, cardiomyopathies, and heart transplantation: a tribute to Giovanni Salviati. *Ital J Neurol Sci* 1999; **20**: 381–5.

306 Rowland LP. Progressive external ophthalmoplegia and ocular myopathies. In: Vinkens PJ, Bruyn GW, Klawans HL eds. *Handbook of clinical neurology*. Amsterdam: Elsevier, 1992: 287–329.

307 Said G, Marion M-H, Selva J, Jamet C. Hypotrophic and dying-back nerve fibres in Friedreich's ataxia. *Neurology* 1986; **36**: 1292–9.

308 Sander JE, Malamud N, Cowan MJ et al. Intermittent ataxia and immunodeficiency with multiple carboxylase deficiencies: a biotin-responsive disorder. *Ann Neurol* 1980; **8**: 544–7.

309 Santorelli FM, Barmada MA, Pons R et al. Leigh-type neuropathology in Pearson syndrome associated with impaired ATP production and a novel mtDNA deletion. *Neurology* 1996; **47**: 1320–3.

310 Santorelli FM, Mak S-C, Vazquez-Memije ME et al. Clinical heterogeneity associated with the mitochondrial DNA T8993C point mutation. *Paediatr Res* 1996; **39**: 914–17.

311 Santorelli FM, Shanske S, Macaya A et al. The mutation at nt 8993 of mitochondrial DNA is a common cause of Leigh's syndrome. *Ann Neurol* 1993; **34**: 827–34.

312 Santorelli FM, Tanji K, Shanske S, DiMauro S. Heterogeneous clinical presentation of the mtDNA NARP/T8993G mutation. *Neurology* 1997; **49**: 270–3.

313 Santorelli FM, Tanji K, Shanske S et al. The mitochondrial DNA A8344G mutation in Leigh syndrome revealed by analysis in paraffin-embedded sections: revisiting the past. *Ann Neurol* 1998; **44**: 962–4.

314 Santos MJ, Imanaka T, Shio H et al. Peroxisomal membrane ghosts in Zellweger syndrome – aberrant organelle assembly. *Science* 1988; **239**: 1536–8.

315 Sarnat HB, Trevenen CL, Darwish HZ. Ependymal abnormalities in cerebro-hepato-renal disease of Zellweger. *Brain Dev* 1993; **15**: 270–7.

316 Saudubray JM, Marsac C, Charpentier C et al. Neonatal congenital lactic acidosis with pyruvate carboxylase deficiency in two siblings. *Acta Paediatr Scand* 1976; **65**: 717–24.

317 Savoiardo M, Uziel G, Strada L et al. MRI findings in Leigh's disease with cytochrome-C-oxidase deficiency. *Neuroradiology* 1991; **33** (Suppl): 507–8.

318 Schatz G. The protein import machinery of mitochondria. *Prot Sci* 1993; **2**: 141–6.

319 Schaumburg HH, Powers JM, Raine CS et al. Adrenoleukodystrophy. A clinical and pathological study of 17 cases. *Arch Neurol* 1975; **33**: 577–91.

320 Schaumburg HH, Powers JM, Raine CS et al. Adrenomyeloneuropathy: a probable variant of adrenoleukodystrophy. II. General pathologic, neuropathological, and biochemical aspects. *Neurology* 1977; **27**: 1114–19.

321 Schiffer D. Calcification in nervous tissue. In: Minckler J ed. *Pathology of the nervous system* Vol. 2. New York: McGraw-Hill, 1971: 1342–60.

322 Schneck L, Adachi M, Briet P et al. Ophthalmoplegia plus with morphological and chemical studies of cerebellar and muscle tissue. *J Neurol Sci* 1973; **19**: 37–44.

323 Schon EA, Rizzuto R, Moraes CT et al. A direct repeat is a hotspot for large-scale deletion of human mitochondrial DNA. *Science* 1989; **244**: 346–9.

324 Schotland DL, DiMauro S, Bonilla E et al. Neuromuscular disorder associated with a defect in mitochondrial energy supply. *Arch Neurol* 1976; **33**: 475–9.

325 Schram AW, Goldfischer S, van Roermund CWT et al. Human peroxisomal 3-oxoacyl-coenzyme A thiolase deficiency. *Proc Natl Acad Sci USA* 1987; **84**: 2494–6.

326 Schröder R, Vielhaber S, Wiedemann FR et al. New insights into the metabolic consequences of large-scale mtDNA deletions: a quantitative analysis of biochemical, morphological, and genetic findings in human skeletal muscle. *J Neuropathol Exp Neurol* 2000; **59**: 353–60.

327 Schuelke M, Smeitink J, Mariman E et al. Mutant NDUFV1 subunit of mitochondrial complex I causes leukodystrophy and myoclonic epilepsy. *Nat Genet* 1999; **21**: 260–1.

328 Schutgens RBH, Heymans HSA, Wanders RJA. Review. Peroxisomal disorders: a newly recognised group of genetic diseases. *Eur J Paediatr* 1986; **144**: 430–40.

329 Schutgens RBH, Wanders RJA. Laboratory diagnosis of peroxisomal disorders. In: Applegarth DA, Dimmick JE, Hall JG eds. *Organelle diseases. Clinical features, diagnosis, pathogenesis and management.* London: Chapman & Hall Medical, 1997: 193–209.

329a Sciacco M, Fagiolari G, Lamperti C et al. Lack of apoptosis in mitochondrial encephalomyopathies. *Neurology* 2001; **56**: 1070–4.

330 Scotto JM, Hadchouel M, Odievre M et al. Infantile phytanic acid storage disease, a possible variant of Refsum's disease: three cases, including ultrastructural studies of the liver. *J Inherit Metab Dis* 1982; **5**: 83–90.

331 Seitz RJ, Langes K, Frenzel H et al. Congenital Leigh's disease: panencephalomyelopathy and peripheral neuropathy. *Acta Neuropathol* 1984; **64**: 167–71.

332 Shapira Y, Harel S, Russel A. Mitochondrial encephalomyopathies. A group of neuromuscular disorders with defects in oxidative metabolism. *Israel J Med Sci* 1977; **13**: 161–4.

333 Shevell MI, Matthews PM, Scriver CR et al. Cerebral dysgenesis and lactic acidemia: an MRI/MRS phenotype associated with pyruvate dehydrogenase deficiency. *Paediatr Neurol* 1994; **11**: 224–9.

334 Shimozawa N, Suzuki Y, Orii T et al. Standardisation of complementation grouping of peroxisome-deficient disorders and the second Zellweger patient with peroxisomal assembly factor-1 (PAF-1) defect (Letter). *Am J Hum Genet* 1993; **52**: 843–4.

335 Shoffner JM, Fernhoff PM, Krawiecki NS et al. Subacute necrotising encephalopathy: oxidative phosphorylation defects and the ATPase 6 point mutation. *Neurology* 1992; **42**: 2168–74.

335a Shoffner JM. Oxidative phosphorylation diseases. In Scriver CR, Beaudet AL, Sly WS, Valle D eds., *The metabolic and molecular bases of inherited disease*, 8th edition. New York: McGraw-Hill Book Company, 2001: 2367–423.

336 Shoffner JM, Wallace DC. Oxidative phosphorylation diseases. In: Scriver CR, Beaudet AL, Sly WS, Valle D eds. *The metabolic and molecular bases of inherited disease* Vol. I. New York: McGraw-Hill Book Company, 1995: 1535–609.

337 Shoubridge EA, Johns T, Karpati G. Complete restoration of a wild-type mtDNA genotype in regenerating muscle fibres in a patient with a tRNA point mutation and mitochondrial encephalomyopathy. *Hum Mol Genet* 1997; **6**: 2239–42.

337a Simon DK, Pulst SM, Sutton JP et al. Familial multisystem degeneration with parkinsonism associated with the 11778 mitochondrial DNA mutation. *Neurology* 1999; **53**: 1787–93.

338 Simon LT, Horoupian DS, Dorfman LJ et al. Polyneuropathy, ophthalmoplegia, leukoencephalopathy, and intestinal pseudo-obstruction: POLIP syndrome. *Ann Neurol* 1990; **28**: 349–60.

339 Singh I. Review article. Biochemistry of peroxisomes in health and disease. *Mol Cell Biochem* 1997; **167**: 1–29.

340 Sipe JC. Leigh's syndrome: The adult form of subacute necrotising encephalomyelopathy with predilection for the brain stem. *Neurology* 1973; **23**: 1030–8.

341 Smith KD, Kemp S, Braiterman LT et al. X-linked adrenoleukodystrophy: genes, mutations, and phenotypes. Neurochem Res 1999; 24: 521–35.

342 Sokoloff L. Energetics of functional activation in neural tissues. Neurochem Res 1999; 24: 321–9.

343 Sparaco M, Bonilla E, DiMauro S, Powers JM. Neuropathology of mitochondrial encephalomyopathies due to mitochondrial DNA defects. J Neuropathol Exp Neurol 1993; 52: 1–10.

344 Sparaco M, Schon EA, DiMauro S, Bonilla E. Myoclonic epilepsy with ragged-red fibres (MERRF): an immunohistochemical study of the brain. Brain Pathol 1995; 5, 125–33.

345 Spranger JW, Opitz JM, Bidder U. Heterogeneity of chondrodysplasia punctata. Humangenetik 1971; 11: 190–212.

346 Stanislaus R, Pahan K, Singh AK, Singh I. Amelioration of experimental allergic encephalomyelitis in Lewis rats by lovastatin. Neurosci Lett 1999; 269: 71–4.

347 Steinberg D. Refsum disease. In: Scriver CR, Beaudet AL, Sly WS, Valle D eds. The metabolic and molecular bases of inherited disease Vol. II. New York: McGraw-Hill, 1995: 2351–69.

348 Sue CM, Bruno C, Andreu AL et al. Infantile encephalopathy associated with the MELAS A3243G mutation. J Paediatr 1999; 134: 696–700.

349 Sue CM, Schon EA. Mitochondrial respiratory chain diseases and mutations in nuclear DNA: a promising start? Brain Pathol 2000; 10: 442–50.

350 Suomalainen A, Majander A, Pihko H et al. Quantification of tRNA Leu 3243 point mutation of mitochondrial DNA in MELAS patients and its effects on mitochondrial transcription. Hum Mol Genet 1993; 2: 525–34.

351 Suzuki K, Grover WD. Ultrastructural and biochemical studies of Schilder's disease. I. Ultrastructure. J Neuropathol Exp Neurol 1970; 29: 392–404.

352 Suzuki Y, Shimozawa N, Orii T et al. Zellweger-like syndrome with detectable hepatic peroxisomes: a variant form of peroxisomal disorder. J Paediatr 1988; 113: 841–5.

353 Sweeney MG, Hammans SR, Duchen LW et al. Mitochondrial DNA mutation underlying Leigh's syndrome: clinical, pathological, biochemical, and genetic studies of a patient presenting with progressive myoclonic epilepsy. J Neurol Sci 1994; 121: 57–65.

354 Taivassalo T, Fu K, Johns T et al. Gene shifting: a novel therapy for mitochondrial myopathy. Hum Mol Genet 1999; 8: 1047–52.

355 Takakubo F, Cartwright P, Hoogenraad N et al. An amino acid substitution in the pyruvate dehydrogense Ela gene, affecting mitochondrial import of the precursors protein. Am J Hum Genet 1995; 57: 772–80.

356 Takano H, Koike R, Onodera O et al. Mutational analysis and genotype–phenotype correlation of 29 unrelated Japanese patients with X-linked adrenoleukodystrophy. Arch Neurol 1999; 56: 295–300.

357 Takeda S, Ohama E, Ikuta F. Adrenoleukodystrophy – early ultrastructural changes in the brain. Acta Neuropathol 1989; 78: 124–30.

358 Takeda S, Wakabayashi K, Ohama E, Ikuta F. Neuropathology of myoclonus epilepsy associated with ragged-red fibres (Fukuhara's disease). Acta Neuropathol 1988; 75: 433–40.

359 Tanahashi C, Nakayama A, Yoshida M et al. MELAS with the mitochondrial DNA 3243 point mutation: a neuropathological study. Acta Neuropathol 2000; 99: 31–8.

360 Tanji K, DiMauro S, Bonilla E. Disconnection of cerebellar Purkinje cells in Kearns–Sayre syndrome. J Neurol Sci 1999; 166: 64–70.

361 Tanji K, Vu TH, Schon EA et al. Kearns–Sayre syndrome: unusual pattern of expression of subunits of the respiratory chain in the cerebellar system. Ann Neurol 1999; 45: 377–83.

362 Taylor RW, Chinnery PF, Turnbull DM, Lightowlers RN. Selective inhibition of mutant human mitochondrial DNA replication in vitro by peptide nucleic acids. Nat Genet 1997; 15: 212–15.

363 Theda C, Moser AB, Powers JM, Moser HW. Phospholipids in X-linked adreno-leukodystrophy white matter-fatty acid abnormalities before the onset of demyelination. J Neurol Sci 1992; 110: 195–204.

364 Tiranti V, Hoertnagel K, Carrozzo R et al. Mutations of SURF-1 in Leigh disease associated with cytochrome c oxidase deficiency. Am J Hum Genet 1998; 63: 1609–21.

365 Tiranti V, Jaksch ME, Hofmann SE et al. Loss-of-function mutations of SURF-1 are specifically associated with Leigh syndrome with cytochrome c oxidase deficiency. Ann Neurol 1999; 46: 161–6.

366 Torvik A, Torp S, Kase BF et al. Infantile Refsum's disease: a generalised peroxisomal disorder. Case report with postmortem examination. J Neurol Sci 1988; 85: 39–53.

367 Toussaint D, Danis P. An ocular pathologic study of Refsum's syndrome. Am J Ophthalmol 1971; 72: 342–7.

368 Tranchant C, Aubourg P, Mohr M et al. A new peroxisomal disease with phytanic and pipecolic acid oxidation. Neurology 1993; 43: 2044–8.

369 Triepels RH, van den Heuvel LP, Loeffen JL et al. Leigh syndrome associated with a mutation in the NDUFS7 (PSST) nuclear encoded subunit of complex I. Ann Neurol 1999; 45: 787–90.

370 Truong DD, Harding AE, Scaravilli F et al. Movement disorders in mitochondrial myopathies. Mov Disord 1990; 5: 109–17.

371 Tsacopoulos M, Magistretti PJ. Metabolic coupling between glia and neurons. J Neurosci 1996; 16: 877–85.

372 Tsuchiya K, Miyazaki H, Akabane H et al. MELAS with prominent white matter gliosis and atrophy of the cerebellar granular layer: a clinical, genetic, and pathological study. Acta Neuropathol 1999; 97: 520–4.

372a Tsuru A, Mizuguchi M, Uyemura K, Takashima S. Abnormal expression of cell adhesion molecule L1 in migration disorders: A developmental immunohistochemical study. Clin Neuropathol 1997; 16: 122–6.

373 Ulrich J, Fankhauser-Mauri C. Subacute necrotising encephalopathy (Leigh) in an adult. Eur J Neurol 1978; 17: 241–6.

374 Ulrich J, Herschkowitz N, Hertz Ph et al. Adrenoleukodystrophy. Preliminary report of a connatal case. Light and electron microscopical, immunohistochemical and biochemical findings. Acta Neuropathol 1978; 43: 77–83.

375 Usuda N, Kuwabara T, Ichikawa R et al. Immunoelectron microscopic evidence for organ differences in the composition of peroxisome-specific membrane polypeptides among three rat organs: liver, kidney, and small intestine. J Histochem Cytochem 1991; 39: 1357–66.

376 Uziel G, Moroni I, Lamantea E et al. Mitochondrial disease associated with the T8993G mutation of the mitochondrial ATPase 6 gene: a clinical, biochemical, and molecular study in six families. J Neurol Neurosurg Psychiatry 1997; 63: 16–22.

377 Valanne L, Ketonen L, Majander A et al. Neuroradiologic findings in children with mitochondrial disorders. Am J Neuroradiol 1998; 19: 369–77.

378 Van Coster RN, Fernhoff PM, De Vivo DC. Pyruvate carboxylase deficiency: a benign variant with normal development. Paediatr Res 1991; 30: 1–4.

379 Van Coster R, Lombes A, De Vivo DC *et al*. Cytochrome *c* oxidase-associated Leigh syndrome: phenotypic features and pathogenetic speculations. *J Neurol Sci* 1991; **104**: 97–111.

380 van den Ouweland JM, Lemkes HH, Trembath RC *et al*. Maternally inherited diabetes and deafness is a distinct subtype of diabetes and associates with a single point mutation in the mitochondrial tRNA (Leu(UUR)) gene. *Diabetes* 1994; **43**: 746–51.

381 van der Knapp MS, Valk J eds. *Magnetic resonance of myelin, myelination, and myelin disorders*. Berlin: Springer, 1995.

382 van Geel BM, Assies J, Haverkort EB *et al*. Progression of abnormalities in adrenomyeloneuropathy and neurologically asymptomatic X-linked adrenoleukodystrophy despite treatment with 'Lorenzo's oil'. *J Neurol Neurosurg Psychiatry* 1999; **67**: 290–9.

383 van Grunsven EG, van Berkel E, Mooijer PAW *et al*. Peroxisomal bifunctional protein deficiency revisited: resolution of its true enzymatic and molecular basis. *Am J Hum Genet* 1999; **64**: 99–107.

384 van Roermund CWT, Hettema EH, van den Berg M *et al*. Molecular characterisation of carnitine-dependent transport of acetyl-CoA from peroxisomes to mitochondria in *Saccharomyces cerevisiae* and identification of a plasma membrane carnitine transporter, Agp2p. *Eur Mol Biol Org J* 1999; **18**: 5843–52.

385 Volpe JJ, Adams RD. Cerebro-hepato-renal syndrome of Zellweger. An inherited disorder of neuronal migration. *Acta Neuropathol* 1972; **20**: 175–98.

386 Vu TH, Sciacco M, Tanji K *et al*. Clinical manifestations of mitochondrial DNA depletion. *Neurology* 1998; **50**: 1783–90.

386a Vu TH, Tanji K, Holve SA *et al*. Navajo neurohepatopathy: A mitochondrial DNA depletion syndrome? *Hepatology* 2001; **34**: 116–20.

387 Vuia O. The cortical form of subacute necrotising encephalopathy of the Leigh type. A light- and electron-microscopic study. *J Neurol Sci* 1975; **26**: 295–304.

388 Wallace DC. Mitochondrial disease in man and mouse. *Science* 1999; **283**: 1482–8.

388a Wallace DC, Lott MT, Brown MD, Kerstann K. Mitochondria and neuro-ophthalmologic diseases. In Scriver CR, Beaudet AL, Sly WS, Valle D (eds), *The metabolic & molecular bases of inherited disease*, 8th edn. New York, NY: McGraw-Hill Book Company, 2001: 2425–509.

389 Wallace DC, Singh G, Lott MT *et al*. Mitochondrial DNA mutation associated with Leber's hereditary optic neuropathy. *Science* 1988; **242**: 1427–30.

390 Walter GF. Myoencephalopathies with abnormal mitochondria: a review. *Clin Neuropathol* 1983; **2**: 101–13.

391 Walter GF, Brucher JM, Martin JJ *et al*. Leigh's disease – several nosological entities with an identical histopathological complex? *Neuropathol Appl Neurobiol* 1986; **12**: 95–107.

392 Wanders RJA. Peroxisomal disorders: Clinical, biochemical, and molecular aspects. *Neurochem Res* 1999; **24**: 565–80.

392a Wanders RJA, Barth PG, Heymans HSA. Single peroxisomal enzyme deficiencies. In Scriver CR, Beaudet AL, Sly WS, Valle D (eds.), *The metabolic & molecular bases of inherited disease*, 8th edn. New York, NY: McGraw-Hill Book Company, 2001: 3219–48.

393 Wanders RJA, Heymans HSA, Schutgens RBH *et al*. Review article. Peroxisomal disorders in neurology. *J Neurol Sci* 1988; **88**: 1–39.

394 Wanders RJA, Schutgens RBH, Barth PG. Peroxisomal disorders: a review. *J Neuropathol Exp Neurol* 1995; **54**: 726–39.

395 Wanders RJA, Tager JM. Lipid metabolism in peroxisomes in relation to human disease. *Mol Aspects Med* 1998; **19**: 71–154.

396 Warburg O, Negelein E. Uber das Absorptions Spektrum des atmungsferent. *Biochemische Z* 1929; **214**: 64–100.

397 Watkins PA, Chen WW, Harris CJ *et al*. Peroxisomal bifunctional enzyme deficiency. *J Clin Invest* 1989; **83**: 771–7.

398 Watkins PA, McGuinness MC, Raymond GV *et al*. Distinction between peroxisomal bifunctional enzyme and acyl-CoA oxidase deficiencies. *Ann Neurol* 1995; **38**: 472–7.

399 Wijburg FA, Wanders RJA, van Lie Peters EM *et al*. NADH:Q_1 oxidoreductase deficiency without lactic acidosis in a patient with Leigh syndrome: implications for the diagnosis of inborn errors of the respiratory chain. *J Inherit Metab Dis* 1991; **14**: 297–300.

400 Wilichowski E, Korenke GC, Ruitenbeek W *et al*. Pyruvate dehydrogenase complex deficiency and altered respiratory chain function in a patient with Kearns–Sayre/MELAS overlap syndrome and A3243G mtDNA mutation. *J Neurol Sci* 1998; **157**: 206–13.

401 Wisniewski T, Powers J, Moser A, Moser H. Ultrastructural evidence for a gliopathy in cerebro-hepato-renal (Zellweger) syndrome. *J Neuropathol Exp Neurol* 1989; **48**: 366.

402 Wong LTK, Davidson GF, Applegarth DA *et al*. Biochemical and histologic pathology in an infant with cross-reacting material (negative) pyruvate carboxylase deficiency. *Paediatr Res* 1986; **20**: 274–9.

403 Wray SH, Provenzale JM, Johns DR, Thulborn KR. MR of the brain in mitochondrial myopathy. *Am J Neuroradiol* 1995; **16**: 1167–73.

404 Yakovac WC. Calcareous chondropathies in the newborn infant. *Arch Pathol* 1954; **57**: 62–77.

405 Yakovlev PI, Lecours AR. The myelogenetic cycles of regional maturation of the brain. In: Minkowski A ed. *Regional development of the brain in early life*. Oxford: Blackwell, 1967: 3–70.

406 Yamadori I, Kurose A, Kobayashi S *et al*. Brain lesions of the Leigh-type distribution associated with a mitochondriopathy of Pearson's syndrome: light and electron microscopic study. *Acta Neuropathol* 1992; **84**: 337–41.

407 Zafeiriou DI, Koletzko B, Mueller-Felber W *et al*. Deficiency in complex IV (cytochrome *c* oxidase) of the respiratory chain, presenting as a leukodystrophy in two siblings with Leigh syndrome. *Brain Dev* 1995; **17**: 117–21.

408 Zellweger H. The cerebro-hepato-renal (Zellweger) syndrome and other peroxisomal disorders. *Dev Med Child Neurol* 1987; **29**: 821–9.

409 Zeviani M, Antozzi C. Defects of mitochondrial DNA. *Brain Pathol* 1992; **2**: 121–32.

410 Zhou L, Chomyn A, Attardi G, Miller CA. Myoclonic epilepsy and ragged red fibres (MERRF) syndrome: selective vulnerability of CNS neurons does not correlate with the level of mitochondrial tRNA[lys] mutation in individual neuronal isolates. *J Neurosci* 1997; **17**: 7746–53.

411 Zhu Z, Yao J, Johns T *et al*. SURF1, encoding a factor involved in the biogenesis of cytochrome *c* oxidase, is mutated in Leigh syndrome. *Nat Genet* 1998; **20**: 337–43.

412 Zinn AB, Kerr DS, Hoppel CL. Fumarase deficiency: a new cause of mitochondrial encephalomyopathy. *N Engl J Med* 1986; **315**: 469–75.

413 Zupanc ML, Moraes CT, Shanske S *et al*. Deletion of mitochondrial DNA in patients with combined features of Kearn–Sayre and MELAS syndrome. *Ann Neurol* 1991; **29**: 680–3.

13

Neurotoxicology

DOYLE GRAHAM AND THOMAS J. MONTINE

INTRODUCTION

Neurotoxicology has significance that reaches far beyond the identification of xenobiotics (neurotoxicants) or endogenous agents (neurotoxins) that are deleterious to the nervous system. Although considered separate fields of study, neurotoxicology, neurodegeneration, stroke, trauma and metabolic diseases of the nervous system provide complementary information about the mechanisms of neuronal dysfunction and death, as well as response to injury in the nervous system. Indeed, there are several examples of compounds first identified as neurotoxicants that subsequently came into use as models of neurodegenerative disease in man, perhaps the most striking being 1-methyl-4-phenyl-1,2,3,6-tetrahydropyridine (MPTP). Moreover, many compounds initially identified as neurotoxicants have become fundamental tools used by neuroscientists, e.g. tetrodotoxin, curare, kainic acid and 6-hydroxydopamine. Conversely, progress in other fields of neuroscience continually advances our understanding of the mechanisms of neurotoxicants.

Pathologists' experience with neurological illness caused by xenobiotics typically is limited. However, it should not be misinterpreted that these diseases are rare. The recent history of neurotoxicology is replete with occupational and environmental accidents that have yielded a tremendous quantity of preventable disease and death. Examples include tri-o-cresyl-phosphate (TOCP) in the USA, Europe and South Africa in the 1930s, mercury contamination of the Minamata Bay region in Japan in the 1950s, hexachlorophene, hexane, methyl n-butylketone, chlordecone and repeated large-scale mercury neurotoxicity in the 1970s, and parkinsonism secondary to MPTP injection and dementia secondary to domoic acid intoxication in the 1980s. It would be incorrect to conclude that xenobiotic-induced neurological disease in humans is of historical interest only or limited to isolated contaminations; exposure to environmental and occupational neurotoxicants continues to this day. In addition, epidemiological studies are linking low-level chronic exposure to some xenobiotics with an increased risk of cerebrovascular and neurodegenerative diseases.

In addition to the xenobiotics that damage the nervous system, a large field of research examines the excess generation or abnormal metabolism of endogenous neurotoxins and their role in both ageing and diseases such as trauma, stroke, epilepsy and neurodegeneration. Examples of endogenous neurotoxins include free radicals, excitatory amino acids, trace elements, lipid peroxidation products, catechol derivatives and advanced glycation endproducts (AGEs). Just as the separation between neurotoxicology and other fields that investigate neuron dysfunction and death is arbitrary, so is the separation between exogenous neurotoxicants and endogenous neurotoxins. Indeed, it is likely that many neurotoxicants act, at least in part, via neurotoxins.

NEUROTOXICANTS

Oedema is the most striking macroscopic finding in acute toxic encephalopathies (Fig. 13.1). The brain is heavy and swollen, even after fixation, with broadened cortical gyri and obliterated sulci. In severe cases, transtentorial and cerebellar tonsillar herniae may occur. Cerebral oedema secondary to vascular damage, as in lead encephalopathy, or direct damage to central nervous system (CNS) myelin, as in triethyltin encephalopathy, is largely confined

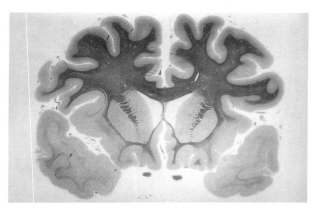

Figure 13.1 *Acute encephalopathy. Exposure to a mixture of toxicants. Coronal section of brain from a patient who died from acute encephalopathy following exposure to a mixture of toxicants. (H&E/LFB-CV.)*

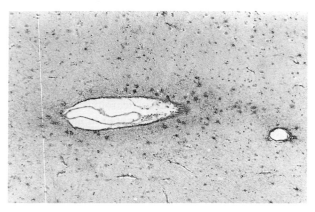

Figure 13.2 *Acute encephalopathy. Intoxication with inorganic lead. Photomicrograph of basal ganglia from patient who died from acute encephalopathy following intoxication with inorganic lead. (Immunohistochemistry for GFAP for astrocytes.)*

to the white matter. In contrast, oedema resulting from diffuse cytotoxic damage, as in thallium intoxication, affects both grey and white matter and has been observed to impart a 'motheaten' appearance to the cortical ribbon. The histological manifestations of cerebral oedema can be slight. Myelin pallor and mild gliosis may be observed by standard histochemical stains, while antibodies to glial fibrillary acidic protein (GFAP) may highlight reactive gliosis (Fig. 13.2).

Neuronal degeneration after exposure to toxicants may be diffuse, e.g. thallium intoxication, or associated with damage to specific structures, e.g. methylmercury- or dimethylmercury-induced degeneration of the calcarine and cerebellar cortices. Whether the primary lesion is focal or generalized, secondary degeneration of fibre pathways may be observed. Intraneuronal inclusions are uncommon in neurotoxicant-induced disease of the CNS, but have been reported in neurons after intoxication with heavy metals.[24]

Glial response to injury includes astrocyte hypertrophy with the development of prominent eosinophilic cell bodies that are strongly immunoreactive for GFAP. In many instances of systemic exposure to toxicants, GFAP immunoreactivity is most prominent around blood vessels (Fig. 13.2). As astrocytic reaction to injury enters a chronic phase, the morphological features are less pronounced. These morphological changes have been quantified by immunoblotting studies that showed early but transient elevation in GFAP immunoreactivity after exposure to neurotoxicants.[204,205] Another response to injury by astrocytes is the formation of Alzheimer type II astrocytes that is associated with encephalopathy from hyperammonaemic states. Microglia are inconspicuous elements of the uninjured CNS, but can assume prominence after tissue damage. Diffuse prominence of microglia, has been reported after neurotoxicant exposure. Histopathological changes in CNS myelin usually begin with the observation of myelin pallor. After neurotoxicant exposure, myelin pallor is more commonly due to a combination of oedema and gliosis, although examples of demyelination exist, e.g. glue sniffer encephalopathy.[143] Intramyelinic oedema follows hexachlorophene or triethyltin intoxication.

Axonal degeneration is a common finding in toxicant-induced peripheral neuropathies. An optimal technique for viewing axons along several internodes is teased fibre preparations showing linear collections of phagocytic cells that are digesting myelin and axonal debris, an appearance generally referred to as 'dying-back' axonopathy. As originally proposed, this process describes a specific sequence, namely toxic injury to the neuronal soma that results in dying back of the distal axon. Others have suggested an alternative pathogenesis of multifocal 'chemical transection' of the axon followed by Wallerian-type degeneration of the distal segment. Segmental demyelination is another common pathological lesion in the peripheral nervous system (PNS) after toxicant exposure. Inappropriately thin myelin sheaths, shortening of internodal distances and variation in myelin thickness among internodal segments of the same axon are observed during the remyelination that follows demyelination. Recurrent episodes of demyelination with remyelination may lead to Schwann cell hyperplasia. Some neurotoxicant-induced diseases are characterized by giant axonal swellings (Fig. 13.3). These large eosinophilic collections within axons are composed mostly of massive accumulations of neurofilaments. Similar neurofilament-filled axonal swellings are seen also in a rare familial neuropathy termed giant axonal neuropathy. This is in distinction to the morphologically similar axonal spheroids that contain tubulovesicular material and that have been observed in characteristic locations in older individuals as well as in patients with neuraxonal dystrophies.

Catalogue of human neurotoxicants

Knowledge of a neurotoxicant typically begins when a cluster of neurological symptoms that appears in a group

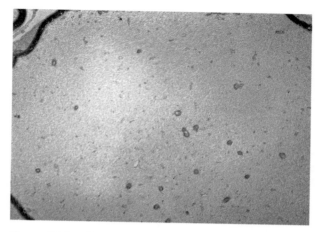

Figure 13.3 n-Hexane, 3,4-dimethyl-2,5-hexanedione intoxication. Electron photomicrograph of an anterior root axon from a rat injected i.p. with an analogue of n-hexane, 3,4-dimethyl-2,5-hexanedione, at a dose of 0.25 mmoles/kg/per day for 14 days. The massively enlarged axon is surrounded by a thin layer of myelin. The axoplasm contains large numbers of disorganized neurofilaments.

of patients that share some activity. Unfortunately, man is often the sentinel species for neurotoxicants. The suspect neurotoxicants are removed then from the environment, physicians follow the patients and laboratory scientists investigate the mechanisms of action. A compilation of pathological data for neurotoxicant-induced disease obtained from such case series is shown in Table 13.1.

NEUROTOXINS

In many instances, neurotoxicant exposure is the aetiology of a disease but the pathogenesis involves the generation or release of endogenous neurotoxins. In addition to neurotoxicant-induced diseases, the pathogenesis of other neurological diseases is thought to receive significant contributions from endogenous neurotoxins. Examples include stroke, hypoglycaemia, trauma, epilepsy, encephalitis, and some metabolic diseases and neurodegenerative diseases. An overview of the major neurotoxins thought to contribute to disease in man is given below.

Free radicals

Free radicals are atoms or molecules with one or more unpaired electron(s) in the outer valence shell. A growing body of research indicates that free-radical production under controlled conditions is a component of second messenger signalling in cells. However, excess or uncontrolled free-radical production is detrimental to cells by either direct damage to macromolecules or liberation of neurotoxic byproducts.[103,104]

Several sites for free-radical generation exist in the nervous system; however, the major source appears to be oxidative phosphorylation in mitochondria. Considering the relatively high oxygen consumption of the brain compared with other organs and the limited ability of neurons to regenerate, slight inefficiencies in oxidative phosphorylation present a huge burden of free-radical generation over a lifetime. Other sources of free radicals may become significant during pathological states. These include excessive stimulation of excitatory amino acid receptors (EAARs), enzymes such as cyclo-oxygenases, lipoxygenases, myeloperoxidase, xanthine oxidase and monoamine oxidase, auto-oxidation of catechols such as dopamine, and aggregated $A\beta$ peptides.

There are many types of free radicals; however, research in biological systems has focused on oxygen-, nitrogen- and carbon-centred free radicals, with oxygen-centred free radicals being the most extensively studied. During the sequential four-electron reduction of molecular oxygen to water (Reaction 13.1), two free radicals, superoxide anion (O_2^-) and hydroxyl radical ($\cdot OH$), are produced along with hydrogen peroxide (H_2O_2); these three molecules are collectively referred to as reactive oxygen species (ROS). Hydroxyl radical is the most reactive ROS and is capable of oxidizing lipids, carbohydrates, protein and nucleic acids. Hydroxyl radical is formed from O_2^- and H_2O_2 by the Haber–Weiss reaction (Reaction 13.2) or from H_2O_2 and ferrous iron by Fenton chemistry (Reaction 13.3).

$$O_2 \rightarrow O_2^- \rightarrow H_2O_2 \rightarrow \cdot OH \rightarrow H_2O \quad (13.1)$$

$$\begin{array}{ccccc} \text{Molecular} & \text{Superoxide} & \text{Hydrogen} & \text{Hydroxyl} & \text{Water} \\ \text{oxygen} & \text{anion} & \text{peroxide} & \text{radical} & \end{array}$$

$$O_2^- + H_2O_2 \rightarrow O_2 + OH^- + \cdot OH \quad (13.2)$$

$$Fe^{2+} + H_2O_2 \rightarrow Fe^{3+} + OH^- + \cdot OH \quad (13.3)$$

Nitric oxide ($NO\cdot$) is a free-radical product of nitric oxide synthase-catalysed oxidation of L-arginine to citrulline. $NO\cdot$ has several physiological functions including vasodilatory and neuromodulatory, but is produced also during pathological states such as excitotoxicity, inflammation and ischaemia–reperfusion.[14] $NO\cdot$ reacts with O_2^- to produce peroxynitrite ($ONOO^-$), a powerful oxidant that can directly modify cellular macromolecules, e.g. proteins to form nitrotyrosine.[15] In addition, upon protonation $ONOO^-$ can form hydroxyl radical and nitrogen dioxide radical ($NO_2\cdot$). Carbon-centred free radicals are generated during the metabolism of some molecules and are also produced on fatty acyl chains during lipid peroxidation.

Excitatory amino acids

Excitatory amino acids (EAAs), primarily L-glutamate, and their cell-surface receptors (EAARs) have been proposed to participate in a wide array of neurological dis-

Table 13.1 *Human neurotoxicants*

Neurotoxicant	Neurological findings	Neuropathological and imaging findings
Acrylamide	Encephalopathy[a] Truncal ataxia[b] SMPN[c]	Not documented Not documented Axonal degeneration that predominantly affects large myelinated axons[82,122]
Aluminium	Dementia, myoclonus, epilepsy and focal neurological signs have been observed in patients undergoing chronic renal dialysis[1] Encephalopathy[a]	Spongiosis in cerebral midcortical layers, mild reactive astrocytosis, and increased prominence of microglia have been observed[30,230] Only diffuse brain oedema was observed at autopsy[170]
Amiodarone and chloroquine	SMPN	Sural nerve biopsies show demyelinating neuropathy with variable loss of unmyelinated axons Ultrastructural analyses show cytoplasmic lamellar inclusions in Schwann cell cytoplasm[66,124,172] Skeletal muscle biopsies show changes of denervation and vacuolar change
Amphetamine and methamphetamine	Cerebral infarction and intracerebral haemorrhage[a,55,134,217] Neuropsychiatric disturbances[c]	Two studies, one post-mortem and one MRI, both show bilateral infarcts of the globus pallidus[265,270] Post-mortem and MRS studies in chronic abusers indicate neurotransmitter abnormalities in the dopaminergic, serotonergic and cholinergic systems, but not extensive neuron loss[37,140,290]
Arsenic (inorganic)	SMPN, often painful[a,c,d,59]	Nerve biopsies show axonal degeneration with regeneration after acute exposure and demyelination with chronic exposure[46,90,130,207]
Arsenic (organic)	Encephalopathy[a]	Petechial haemorrhages with perivascular demyelination and haemorrhagic necrosis of the cerebral white matter and the brainstem[125]
Bismuth	Encephalopathy[a]	Degeneration of pyramidal neurons in cerebellum and hippocampus with microglial reaction is characteristic[157]
Cadmium	Neurobehavioural deficits in children (often with coincident exposure to other metals)[106] SMPN,[c] olfactory disorders[c] and parkinsonism[a, d] in adults[208,243]	Not documented
Carbon disulfide	Encephalopathy,[b] neuropsychiatric symptoms[c] and parkinsonism[d] (mixed with CCl$_4$)[220]	Diffuse oedema of brain with swollen endothelial cells and perivascular haemorrhages, neuronal loss in the cerebral cortex, hippocampus, striatum and cerebellum, and scattered white matter damage characterized by myelin loss and gliosis are observed[3] Cerebral cortical atrophy and basal ganglia infarcts are seen by neuroimaging[117]

(Continued.)

Table 13.1 *(Continued)*

Neurotoxicant	Neurological findings	Neuropathological and imaging findings
	Distal SMPN[c]	Axonopathy is characteristic; one instance showed neurofilament accumulation[19,180,181,203]
Carbon monoxide	Encephalopathy[a] and parkinsonism[d]	Generalized oedema is observed
		Hypoxic/ischaemic damage to cerebrum, bilateral necrosis of globus pallidus and perivascular demyelination have been reported in survivors of acute poisonings[42,88,89,141,223,229,258]
		Not documented
	Impaired cognitive function after low-level exposure[5]	
Chlordecone (Kepone)	Tremor, opsoclonus and encephalopathy[b]	Sural nerve biopsies show decreased number of unmyelinated fibres and endoneurial fibrosis[168]
Cocaine	Increased risk of cerebrovascular disease, cerebral perfusion defects and cerebral atrophy[74,80,133]	Autopsies show brain infarcts and haemorrhages[291]
	Decreased head circumference[e,304]	Imaging studies show increased cerebrovascular resistance in cocaine abusers[109]
	Movement and psychiatric abnormalities, especially during withdrawal or in response to some medications[c]	Evidence for brain structural damage in newborns exposed to cocaine is mixed[16]
		Alteration in striatal dopamine neurotransmission in cocaine abusers is reported[161,162,291]
Colchicine	Proximal weakness	Skeletal muscle biopsy shows vacuolar myopathy
	SMPN	Sural nerve biopsy shows axonal degeneration of large myelinated fibres[149,231]
Cyanide and methylcyanide (acetonitrile)	Encephalopathy[a] and parkinsonism[d]	Generalized oedema was reported after fatal acute exposure
		Delayed changes of global hypoxic/ischaemic damage have been observed: bilateral necrosis of the globus pallidus and striatum, laminar necrosis of the cerebral cortex and loss of cerebellar Purkinje cells[68,98,192,237,280,283]
Dimethyaminopropionitrile	Flaccid neurogenic bladder, male sexual dysfunction, sensory loss in sacral dermatomes and distal SMPN[b]	Sural nerve biopsy from a severely intoxicated patient showed mildly decreased density of myelinated and unmyelinated axons with axonal swellings containing neurofilaments[219]
Disulfiram	SMPN	Sural nerve biopsies show axonal degeneration, segmental demyelination and sometimes neurofilamentous swellings[113, 285]
Domoic acid	Headache, seizures, hemiparesis, ophthalmoplegia and coma[a]	Neuronal loss is seen primarily in the hippocampus and amygdala[218,275]
	Anterograde memory deficits and SMPN[d]	
Ethanol[f]	Fetal alcohol syndrome[b]	Abnormalities of brain development that most commonly include microcephaly, neuroglial heterotopias, brainstem and cerebellum malformations with hydrocephalus, and agenesis of the corpus callosum[47,214,293]

(Continued over page.)

Table 13.1 (Continued)

Neurotoxicant	Neurological findings	Neuropathological and imaging findings
	Dementia[c]	Degeneration of cerebral grey matter and white matter, especially frontal lobes, is reported[105,148]
	Wernicke–Korsakoff syndrome[c]	Petechial haemorrhages, neuronal loss, gliosis and capillary proliferation are present in the mammillary bodies and periventricular grey matter of the midbrain and hindbrain
		Older lesions may cavitate[125]
	Slowly progressive truncal ataxia[c]	Atrophy of superior cerebellar vermis and cerebellar hemispheres is characteristic[125]
	Distal SMPN[c]	Nerve biopsies show primarily distal axonal degeneration[125]
	Marchifava–Bignami disease[c]	Partial demyelination and necrosis of the corpus callosum have been observed[125]
	Increased risk from cerebrovascular accidents[c]	Non-specific[74,80,87]
Ethylene glycol	Encephalopathy[a]	Generalized oedema with scattered petechial haemorrhages throughout the brain and meningitis have been observed
		Oxalate crystal deposition in the meninges and brain is characteristic[18,81,234,260]
Ethylene oxide	Acute encephalopathy[102]	Not documented
	Cognitive impairment[c,49]	Diffuse cerebral atrophy is observed by MRI[25]
	SMPN[b]	Axonal degeneration with regeneration is observed[102,151,248]
Hexane and 2-hexanone (methyl n-butylketone)	Euphoria, narcosis[a]	Not documented
	Distal SMPN[b,c]	Axonal swelling with thinned myelin sheaths and axonal degeneration is present in the distal portion of long axons of the spinal cord and PNS
		Axonal regeneration is observed in the PNS[2,4,21,64,110,131,144,232 267,269,279,296]
		Autopsy of a patient with a 12-year history of glue sniffing showed diffuse cerebral and cerebellar atrophy[64]
Isonicotinic acid hydrazide (INH)	SMPN	Peripheral nerve biopsies show loss of myelinated and unmyelinated fibres[206,211]
	'Slow acetylators' are more vulnerable to developing neuropathy	
Lead (inorganic)	Encephalopathy[a,b] (more common in children)	Generalized oedema with scattered petechial haemorrhages occurs; however, herniation is unusual
		Microscopically, a protein-rich perivascular exudate, endothelial necrosis and thrombosis are observed throughout the neuraxis
		Microglial nodules have been reported
		Focal degeneration of cerebellar Purkinje and internal granule cells with reactive gliosis have been demonstrated[111,147]

(Continued.)

Table 13.1 (Continued)

Neurotoxicant	Neurological findings	Neuropathological and imaging findings
	Neurobehavioural deficits or delays[9,75,249]	Not documented
	Motor neuropathy, primarily of upper extremities[b,c] (more common in adults)	Axonal degeneration with regeneration has been reported[111,147]
	Asymptomatic adults may be at increased risk from cerebrovascular accidents[c,249]	Non-specific
Lead (organic)	Encephalopathy[a]	Atrophy of cerebellar vermis and adjacent hemispheres is observed.[132,284] Microscopic sections show Purkinje cell loss, internal granular cell atrophy, and Bergmann gliosis. One report documented other changes that suggest global hypoxia as a contributing factor[284]
	Adults may be at increased risk from cerebrovascular accidents[c]	Non-specific
Leptophos	Rigidity, spasticity, and other central and peripheral nervous system findings[245]	Not documented
Lithium	Ataxia, often in combination with other medications	Cerebellar atrophy with degeneration of internal granule cells and Purkinje cells[163,241]
	Superior sagittal sinus thrombosis[289]	
Manganese	Extrapyramidal movement disorder[c,d] and psychiatric disturbances[b,114]	Bilateral neuron loss in the pallidum and subthalamic nucleus, with or without involvement of the putamen, gliosis and sometimes pigment deposition have been observed[10,11,44,274,295]
		PET shows preservation of presynaptic and postsynaptic nigrostriatal dopaminergic function[213]
Mercury (inorganic)	Dementia and emotional lability	Degeneration of cerebellar granule cells and deposition of mercury granules in the inferior olive, dentate nucleus and choroid plexus have been reported[54]
		Persistence of mercury in the brain has been shown in man for up to 17 years after exposure[209]
	SMPN[c]	Axonal degeneration and demyelination are observed in sural nerve biopsies[43]
Mercury (organic)	Gait ataxia Concentric visual field deficits	Degeneration of the calcarine and cerebellar cortices, particularly in the depths of sulci, is characteristic
		Less severely affected structures include the precentral, postcentral and temporal cortices
		Brain degeneration is more severe in children exposed in utero
		The atrophic cerebral cortex shows neuronal degeneration and reactive astrocytosis

(Continued over page.)

Table 13.1 (Continued)

Neurotoxicant	Neurological findings	Neuropathological and imaging findings
		The cerebellum shows selective loss of the internal granular cells. Secondary, symmetrical degeneration of the pyramidal tracts has been noted[38,201,255]
	Perioral and extremity paresthaesias	Findings in the PNS have been variable, ranging from no abnormality to degeneration of dorsal root ganglion cells and posterior columns[38,255]
Methanol	Blindness[a,b]	Retinal ganglion cell degeneration with delayed optic nerve atrophy has been reported [17,116]
	Parkinsonism[d]	Bilateral putaminal necrosis with or without haemorrhage and widespread hypoxic/ischaemic damage are characteristic[116,150,171,221]
Methotrexate (intraventricular or intrathecal)	Confusion, seizures and ataxia (combined with craniospinal irradiation)	Disseminated necrotizing leukoencephalopathy, often periventricular, with minimal inflammation has been reported[227,242,250]
Methyl bromide	Encephalopathy with seizures[a] SMPN, weakness, co-ordination defects, extrapyramidal movement disorders, and psychosis[b,c,190,300]	Cerebral oedema with petechial and subarachnoid haemorrhages is reported[190, 226] One patient who was maintained artificially for 30 days after acute exposure had, at autopsy, symmetrical lesions in the mammillary bodies and inferior colliculi that resembled the changes of Wernicke's encephalopathy[270]
Mevacor	Myopathy that may be severe (often in combination with cyclosporine)	Myofibre necrosis and regeneration with lymphocytic infiltrate that may mimic myositis are reported[45,264]
MPTP	Parkinsonism	Post-mortem examination years after exposure shows reduction in pigmented neurons of the substantia nigra without Lewy bodies[152] Clinical and neuroimaging studies in man localize the lesion to the nigrostriatal dopaminergic system[9,292] PET studies years after exposure show a faster rate of dopaminergic neurodegeneration in those patients exposed to MPTP than in controls[288]
Nucleoside analogue reverse transcriptase inhibitors, e.g. zidovudine	Sensory neuropathy and weakness in patients with HIV infection[135, 191] Multiple neurological abnormalities in HIV-negative children treated prophylactically in utero and after birth have been observed[22]	There are several patterns of neuropathy, probably from increased susceptibility to drug toxicity in patients with HIV infection[101] Fibre atrophy and necrosis, vacuole formation and mitochondrial abnormalities characterize the myopathy[177] Some HIV-negative children treated prophylactically have brain white matter lesions and necrosis on MRI[22]
Platinum (cis-diamminedichloro-platinum II)	Tinnitus, high-frequency hearing loss and sensory neuropathy	Myelinated and unmyelinated fibre loss in sural nerve biopsies is reported[212,277] A post-mortem study indicated neuronopathy rather than axonopathy[145]

(Continued.)

Table 13.1 (Continued)

Neurotoxicant	Neurological findings	Neuropathological and imaging findings
Polychlorinated biphenyls and polychlorodibenzofurans	Sensory neuropathy[39,276] Neurobehavioural deficits or delays[9,40,126,138,278]	Not documented
Thallium	Encephalopathy[a]	Generalized oedema of both grey and white matter with focal haemorrhages, chromatolysis of ganglion cells in the brain and spinal cord, and formation of microglia with minimal astrogliosis have been reported[228]
		Highest brain levels of thallium were in the grey matter[53]
	SMPN, primarily with features of axonopathy[60]	Axonal degeneration with secondary myelin loss is observed[53,136,158]
	Autonomic neuropathy[d]	Not documented
Triethyltin and hexachlorophene[g]	Encephalopathy[a,b] Seizures and persistent cognitive deficits[d,69]	Generalized oedema of the white matter characterized by intramyelinic vacuoles has been reported[166,167,194,256,257]
Trimethyltin	Limbic–cerebellar syndrome[a,20,239]	Central chromatolysis, membrane-bound neuronal cytoplasmic inclusions, neuronophagia and widespread neuron loss are most concentrated in limbic structures[20,146]
Tri-o-cresyl phosphate and other organophosphorous compounds	Cholinergic crisis[a] Distal SMPN[d]	None reported Axonal degeneration of central and peripheral long axons with axonal regeneration in the PNS is characteristic
Trichloroethylene	Sensorimotor neuropathy primarily restricted to cranial nerve V	Symmetrical demyelination and axonal degeneration of cranial nerve V as well as associated ganglion cell degeneration were observed[31,71] possibly related to reactivation of herpes simplex virus[36]
	Dementia[c]	A single report describes subcortical gliosis and intraneuronal argentophilic bodies throughout the cerebral cortex[254]
Toluene	Euphoria[a] Amnesia, dementia, cerebellar ataxia, pyramidal tract and oculomotor dysfunction, tremor and deafness[b,23,73,93,176,236]	Not documented Damage is primarily to white matter with brain atrophy PAS-positive macrophages with cytoplasmic membrane-bound trilaminar inclusions are characteristic White matter has increased levels of very long-chain fatty acid cholesteryl esters[143,238]
Vincristine	SMPN	Sural nerves show axonal degeneration with regeneration[246]

[a]Acute (< 1 month); [b]subacute (< 1 year); [c]chronic (> 1 year); [d]delayed; [e]prenatal exposure; [f]in combination with nutritional deficiencies; [g]infants and children.

HIV, human immunodeficiency virus; MRI, magnetic resonance imaging; MRS, magnetic resonance spectroscopy; PAS, periodic acid–Schiff; PET, positron emission tomography; SMPN, sensorimotor peripheral neuropathy.

eases.[160,173,174] A large number of experiments and trials has provided indirect or pharmacological support for a role of EAARs in neurological diseases. In addition, exposure to high doses of EAAR agonists and the subsequent development neurological disease in man have underscored the importance of EAAs in disease. Perhaps the most striking example is the domoic acid intoxications that occurred in the Maritime Provinces of Canada in late 1987.[218,275] A total of 107 patients were identified who experienced an acute illness that most commonly presented as gastrointestinal disturbance, severe headache and short-term memory loss within 24–48 h after ingesting mussels. A subset of the more severely afflicted patients were subsequently shown to have chronic memory deficits, motor neuropathy and decreased medial temporal lobe glucose metabolism by positron emission tomography (PET). Neuropathological investigation of patients who died within 4 months of intoxication disclosed neuronal loss with reactive gliosis that was most prominent in the hippocampus and amygdala, but also affected regions of the thalamus and cerebral cortex. The responsible agent was identified as domoic acid, a potent structural analogue of glutamate that had been concentrated in cultivated mussels.

Experimental studies have outlined a cascade of events through which EAAR stimulation may lead to neurodegeneration. Initially, the synaptic concentration of EAAs is increased by either increased release from neurotransmitter pools, decreased reuptake, or both. Rapid neurodegeneration is mediated by a depolarization-dependent increase in sodium and chloride permeability that is followed by osmotic swelling and neuronal lysis. Delayed toxicity, which develops after the agonist has been removed, appears to operate through disruption of intraneuronal calcium levels with subsequent inappropriate activation of calcium-dependent enzymes, mitochondrial damage and increased generation of free radicals.[35,48,240]

Some investigators have proposed that neurodegenerative diseases, such as amyotrophic lateral sclerosis (ALS), Huntington's disease (HD), Parkinson's disease (PD), and Alzheimer's disease (AD) also may derive in part from excitotoxicity.[12–14] Under these chronic conditions, it is proposed that excitotoxicity is linked to impaired energy metabolism. Indeed, it has been demonstrated that impairment of energy metabolism in tissue culture facilitates the transition of glutamate from neurotransmitter to excitotoxin, and that delayed excitotoxicity follows exposure to inhibitors of cellular respiration.[13,100,202] These experimental findings have been synthesized into a hypothesis that defective mitochondrial respiration reduces energy charge, increases ROS production and enhances the sensitivity of neurons to physiological concentrations of endogenous EAAs, thereby contributing to chronic neurodegeneration.

Trace elements

Iron (Fe) and copper (Cu) are both present in grey matter and subserve many physiological functions. Both elements can exist as free ions or bound to proteins; free ions and some bound ions can participate in oxidation–reduction (redox) reactions. Accumulation of redox active iron or copper is central to many neurotoxic hypotheses because they act as catalysts for Fenton chemistry and catechol autoxidation, and can participate in redox chemistry with Aβ peptides.[120,182] Brain iron and copper levels are relatively stable during adult life.[165] Bulk iron, but not copper, levels are significantly increased in diseased regions of brain in patients with AD or PD, and some data indicate that the increased iron in tissue may be redox active.[112,128,129,165,262]

Like iron and copper, manganese (Mn) ions are also paramagnetic and capable of redox reactions; however, manganese does not catalyse the Fenton reaction. In addition to its role in normal physiology, most notably Mn-superoxide dismutase, occupational and iatrogenic exposure to manganese is associated clinically with dystonia and parkinsonism, and pathologically with a pallidoluysian degeneration.[127] Manganese intoxication is discussed at greater length in a later section, Biochemical mechanisms of selected neurotoxicants.

Similarly to iron, copper and manganese, zinc (Zn) is central to many important biochemical reactions. Unlike these other elements, zinc does not directly participate in free-radical generation in biological systems. Nevertheless, excess zinc can be neurotoxic.[51] The mechanisms of neurotoxicity associated with excess zinc are not fully understood but may be related to a pool of zinc that is released from a subset of glutaminergic neurons upon depolarization. In this capacity, zinc has been proposed to contribute to brain damage after hypoxia/ischaemia, trauma, epilepsy and neurodegeneration.[41] In the specific case of AD, some research has suggested that zinc levels are elevated in diseased regions of the AD brain and that zinc may alter the regulation of amyloid precursor protein gene transcription and the proteolytic processing of amyloid precursor protein and Aβ peptides.[50] Since perturbation of amyloid precursor protein metabolism appears to be central to neurodegeneration in at least some forms of AD, these findings suggest that zinc may indirectly influence the neurotoxicity of these peptides.

Lipid peroxidation products

Free-radical-mediated damage to polyunsaturated fatty acids, termed lipid peroxidation, differs from other forms of free-radical damage to macromolecules because it is a self-propagating process that generates neurotoxic byproducts. Thus, there are two deleterious outcomes to lipid peroxidation, i.e. structural damage to membranes and generation of bioactive secondary products.

Membrane damage derives from the generation of fragmented fatty acyl chains, lipid–lipid cross-links and lipid–protein cross-links.[67] In addition, lipid hydroperoxyl radicals can undergo endocyclization to produce novel fatty acid esters that may disrupt membranes.[189,233] Fragmentation of lipid hydroperoxides, in addition to producing abnormal fatty acid esters, liberates a number of diffusible products, some of which are potent electrophiles.[65,224] The most abundant diffusible products of lipid peroxidation are chemically reactive aldehydes such as malondialdehyde (MDA), acrolein, and 4-hydroxy-2-nonenal (HNE).[65] Alternatively, enzymatic hydrolysis of abnormal fatty acyl groups generated by lipid peroxidation can liberate abnormal products from damaged lipid.

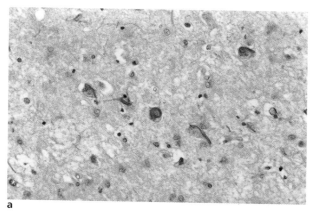

MDA   Acrolein   HNE

Some products of lipid peroxidation are thought to contribute significantly to its deleterious effects in tissue. Reactive aldehydes produced from lipid peroxidation react with a number of cellular nucleophiles, including protein, nucleic acids and some lipids.[65] Indeed, many of the cytotoxic effects of lipid peroxidation can be reproduced directly by electrophilic lipid peroxidation products such as acrolein and HNE.[67] These include depletion of glutathione, dysfunction of structural proteins, reduction in enzyme and transporter activities, and induction of cell death. A large body of experimental data now exists that points to reactive aldehyde products of lipid peroxidation as potent neurotoxins. Studies of human brain and cerebrospinal fluid (CSF) post-mortem and animal models of AD, PD, ALS and HD have all detected elevated levels of neurotoxic lipid peroxidation products or their protein adducts in disease tissue compared with control[32,72,183–185,215,299] (Fig. 13.4). In addition, two studies of living patients have shown that lipid peroxidation products in CSF obtained from the lumbar cistern are increased early in the course of probable AD, HD and sporadic ALS.[186,215]

In addition to chemically reactive lipid peroxidation products, chemically stable products of lipid peroxidation may also contribute to disease through receptor-mediated signalling. For example, peroxidation and fragmentation of polyunsaturated fatty acyl groups in phosphatidylcholines can generate platelet-activating factor (PAF) analogues that stimulate the PAF receptor, thereby stimulating inflammatory responses.[169] In addition, one isomer of the isoprostanes, which are products of arachidonic acid peroxidation, has been shown to be a potent vasoconstrictor both peripherally and in the cerebral vasculature, probably through a receptor-mediated mechanism.[115,189]

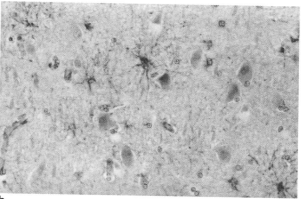

Figure 13.4 *Alzheimer's disease. Photomicrographs of (**a**) entorhinal cortex or (**b**) temporal cortex from a patient with AD. Tissue sections were stained with antiserum specific for (**a**) 2-pentylpyrrole or (**b**) Michael-type protein adducts from 4-hydroxy-2-nonenal and then developed with diaminobenzidine as chromogen substrate (brown) and hematoxylin as counterstain. The temporal cortex (**b**) was also immunohistochemically stained for GFAP antiserum (red chromogen substrate).*

Advanced glycation endproducts

Analogous to protein adduction by lipid peroxidation products, non-enzyme-catalysed post-translational modification of protein by reducing sugars, a process termed glycation, is also associated with some forms of neurodegeneration. Subsequent irreversible rearrangements, fragmentations, dehydrations and condensations yield a complex mixture of protein-bound products termed AGEs.[261] AGEs have been studied most extensively from the perspective of diabetes mellitus and its complications, where their accumulation is correlated with the degree of hyperglycaemia. However, accumulation of AGEs in tissue is also associated with advancing age and with some diseases not characterized by hyperglycaemia but associated with oxidative stress, e.g. uraemia and AD. Moreover, molecules other than reducing sugars can lead to AGE formation under conditions of increased oxidative stress, such as other carbohydrates and even ascorbate.[61,62,99]

AGEs can damage structural proteins and enzymes, thus rendering them dysfunctional.[7] AGEs can also be redox active and may themselves generate oxidative stress and induce neuronal apoptosis.[137,297] In addition to these deleterious biochemical reactions, AGE-modified proteins may bind to an AGE receptor (RAGE) that exists on several cell types, including neurons and glia. One role of RAGE is thought to be incorporation of AGE-modified proteins for degradation. However, binding of ligands, including Aβ peptides, to RAGE on neurons in culture stimulates production of ROS, and binding to RAGE on microglia in culture leads to cellular activation.[298]

AGE formation in human neurological disease has been investigated most extensively in AD. These studies have focused on immunohistochemical localization of AGEs in the brain. Antibodies to AGEs are consistently immunoreactive with senile plaques and neurofibrillary tangles (NFTs) in the hippocampus of AD patients, but have also been observed in vessel walls, granulovacuolar degeneration and Hirano bodies.[57,139,195,244,263,272] AGE immunoreactivity has been reported in the substantia nigra and locus coeruleus of patients with PD, and in the frontal and temporal cortex, but not the hippocampus, of patients with dementia with Lewy bodies.[34] AGEs have also been detected on intraneuronal hyaline inclusions of spinal cord from patients with ALS linked to mutations in *SOD1* and in mice that express mutant human *SOD1*,[253] and on NFTs from patients with progressive supranuclear palsy, Guamanian parkinsonism–dementia complex and Guamanian ALS.[244]

Catechol metabolites

Catechols such as dopamine and noradrenaline are vulnerable to oxidations, rearrangements and condensations under physiological conditions. Within synaptic vesicles high concentrations of antioxidants and metal ion chelators stabilize catechols. However, conditions in the extracellular fluid and cytosol are favourable for chemical transformation of the catechol nucleus. Several products from catechols have been proposed to participate in dopaminergic neurodegeneration. The evidence for some is stronger than others; however, as yet none of these molecules has been shown to contribute significantly to the progression of PD.

Oxidation of the catechol nucleus is one mechanism for generating biologically active catechol products.[95,97] These reactions begin with trace metal-catalysed single-electron oxidations of the catechol to the semiquinone and quinone which, in biological systems, are accompanied by the formation of superoxide anion. The quinoid species may be reduced and potentially can enter a redox cycle with generation of ROS at the expense of cellular reductants. This quinone may react also with intramolecular or extramolecular nucleophiles, such as those on protein, and contribute to toxicity.[97,107,154] Alternatively, oxidized cate-

chols react quickly with intracellular thiolates, such as glutathione and cysteine, to yield catechol thioethers. Glutathionyl- and cysteinyl-dopamine have been proposed as biomarkers of dopamine oxidation *in vivo*.[77–79,266] Other products from this pathway include benzothiazine derivatives and mercapturyl conjugates, both of which have been proposed to contribute to dopaminergic neurotoxicity.[155,222,251,252,302]

A second class of reactions that can alter catecholamines is condensation with carbohydrates to form isoquinolines. This is the same mechanism for generating fluorophores in catacholaminergic tissue. The most extensively studied group of isoquinolines is salsolinol.[197] The (R)-enantiomers of salsolinols have been detected in dopaminergic regions of the brain as well as in CSF in man.[193,199] Moreover, (R)-N-methylsalsolinol has been reported to be a dopaminergic neurotoxin in rats.[198,199]

A third mechanism for the modification of catechols is direct attack by free radicals, typically hydroxyl radical, although the same chemistry can occur with nitrogen-based radicals. Hydroxyl radical attack on dopamine can generate 6-hydroxydopamine, a well-known selective dopaminergic neurotoxin that has been used extensively in experimental lesioning studies on the dopaminergic system.[303] The dopaminergic selectivity of 6-hydroxydopamine results from it being a substrate for the dopamine transporter. The cytotoxicity of 6-hydroxydopamine derives from its facile oxidation. If formed to significant amounts, 6-hydroxydopamine clearly could contribute to dopaminergic neurodegeneration. Indeed, some animal studies have suggested that 6-hydroxydopamine formation is a component of amphetamine-induced dopaminergic neurotoxicity.

BIOCHEMICAL MECHANISMS OF SELECTED NEUROTOXICANTS

This section distinguishes between two classes of agent. The first group, including carbon monoxide (CO), cyanide (CN) and methanol, produces CNS damage as a delayed consequence of acute, life-threatening exposure. These agents produce histotoxic lesions in several sites of the CNS, probably as the result of global hypoxic/ischaemic injury. With the exception of methanol, this group of toxicants exerts little direct toxicity in the CNS.

The second group of compounds discussed in this section is neuron cytotoxicants and axonotoxicants. MPTP, manganese, n-hexane and carbon disulfide (CS_2) are the examples belonging to this class. In this instance, exposure yields little systemic toxicity and tissue damage is largely restricted to loss of vulnerable neurons or axons with sparing of other tissue elements. Both classes of neurotoxicants derive significant contributions from the generation of endogenous neurotoxins.

Histotoxicants

CO, CN and methanol comprise the histotoxic neurotoxicants. It must be stressed that all three agents are systemic toxicants with profound effects on the cardio-respiratory system. Patients who survive acute intoxication often develop delayed neurological sequelae. In these cases, pathological examination reveals lesions in the basal ganglia and hippocampus, as well as other sites of the CNS, which follow the typical temporal, topographical and morphological patterns of global hypoxic/ischaemic injury.[89,223]

CARBON MONOXIDE (CO)

Delayed encephalopathy from acute CO exposure is relatively common in intoxicated patients requiring hospitalization.[42,88] The clinical picture in encephalopathic patients is often broad, including motor, cognitive and psychiatric dysfunction in addition to parkinsonism. The older medical literature contains several reports of post-mortem examination of patients who survived the initial intoxication but later succumbed. In summary, grey matter lesions consist of bilateral cystic necrosis of the globus pallidus that frequently extends into the adjacent internal capsule, laminar necrosis of the cerebral cortex, neuronal loss in the cornu ammonis of the hippocampus, granular atrophy of the arterial border zones and focal necrosis of the cerebellum. Several patterns of white matter necrosis also have been identified as sequelae of acute CO intoxication in man. The central importance of pallidal lesions to parkinsonian symptoms was underscored by a case report that described bilateral lucencies of the globus pallidus by computed tomography (CT) in a survivor of CO intoxication who had a pure parkinsonian syndrome.[141] Other reports describing patients with more complex neurological dysfunction have also demonstrated lesions in the basal ganglia by CT or MRI.[42,229,258] A more recent study has associated mild cognitive impairments with low-level CO exposure; however, pathological examination was not performed in these cases.[5] Data from carefully controlled studies on rats, cats and monkeys have generally indicated that systemic hypotension is the best predictor of CNS damage after CO intoxication, although direct cytotoxic action of CO may contribute to the leukoencephalopathy.[216] One laboratory demonstrated that, at least in part, neurodegeneration induced by systemic CO exposure could be impeded by EAAR antagonists.[123]

CYANIDE (CN)

Three autopsy studies document the pathological changes in the brains of patients who died more than 24 h after acute CN intoxication.[108,280] In one case, the patient remained comatose for 36 h before death, and although the globus pallidus bilaterally was reported grossly as 'soft' no histological examination was made. The second patient survived for 16 days after intoxication, but did not demonstrate an extrapyramidal movement disorder. Pathological changes were limited to laminar necrosis of the cerebral cortex and marked cerebellar Purkinje cell degradation. The most recent case concerned a man who survived for 19 months after attempting suicide with KCN. Within 4 months he had developed generalized rigidity, bradykinesia and resting tremor of the arms. At autopsy, the putamen and the globus pallidus were shrunken and 'spongy', the subthalamic nucleus showed neuronal loss and gliosis, the occipital lobes contained laminar necrosis in the arterial border zone, there was neuronal loss in the zona compacta of the substantia nigra and marked loss of Purkinje cells was seen in the cerebellar hemispheres. The hippocampi were noted specifically to be unremarkable.[280] These autopsies have been corroborated by more recent neuroimaging studies.[68,98,237,283] Elegant experiments in rats and monkeys led to the conclusion that hypoxic/ischaemic damage, rather than direct histotoxicity, is the major cause of delayed CNS damage after CN exposure.[26,27]

Chronic exposure to CN has been linked to cassavism, a spastic paraparesis of the lower extremities that has been observed in indigent populations around the globe that consume large amounts of cassava roots in their diets.[268] While some investigators have proposed that hydrolysis of cyanogenic glucosides with release of CN is the mechanism of toxicity, others have proposed that alternative agents, also contained within these roots, may play a central role in the development of this disease.[210] Chronic occupational exposure to CN has been associated with a variety of non-specific neurological signs and symptoms; however, these examples are complicated by exposure to multiple agents and pathological data are not available.

METHANOL (CH$_3$OH)

Methanol-induced damage to the basal ganglia, in contrast to CO, is directed principally at the putamen, rather than the globus pallidus. Patients surviving methanol intoxication have been observed to develop cystic necrosis of the putamen that commonly involves adjacent structures, ischaemic cell change in the hippocampus, laminar necrosis of the cerebral cortex and cystic necrosis of cerebral white matter.[171,221] While retinal ganglion cell degeneration appears to be mediated through formate, a metabolite of methanol, it is not clear what direct role methanol or its metabolites play in other CNS lesions. The striking similarity between the pathological changes produced by methanol, CO or CN exposure promotes the hypothesis that all share similar pathogenic mechanisms. However, there are examples of methanol-intoxicated patients who lacked clinical evidence of marked hypoxia or hypotension but who latter developed CNS lesions. Furthermore, there is clearly preferential involvement of the putamen after methanol exposure, while other causes of global hypoxia/ischaemia tend to involve the globus pallidus. It seems likely that methanol and its metabolites, in addition to global hypoxia/ischaemia, contribute directly to the development of CNS lesions other than retinal degeneration.

Neuronal cytotoxicants

MPTP

The history of MPTP-induced parkinsonism in young adults who inadvertently injected themselves with this compound is well known. MPTP has been shown to act as a protoxicant that, after entering the brain, is metabolized by glial monoamine oxidase-B (MAO-B) to the toxic metabolite 1-methyl-4-phenylpyridinium (MPP^+), which is then selectively transported into nigral neurons via the mesencephalic dopamine transporter. Once inside these neurons, MPP^+ is thought to act primarily as a mitochondrial toxin by inhibiting complex I activity in the mitochondrial electron transport chain, thereby reducing ATP production and increasing ROS generation.[153] MPTP-induced dopaminergic neurodegeneration can be diminished by free-radical scavengers, inhibitors of the inducible form of nitric oxide synthase, and by EAAR antagonists. In addition, mice lacking both alleles of the Cu/Zn-superoxide dismutase gene (sod1) or the glutathione peroxidase gene (gpx1) are significantly more vulnerable to MPTP-induced dopaminergic neurodegeneration than are littermate controls.[142,301]

The search for xenobiotics that may act similarly to MPTP and so be environmental toxicants that promote PD has not been fruitful. The one exception may be pyridinium metabolites of haloperidol that have the potential to damage dopaminergic neurons.[281] The search for endogenous neurotoxins that may act like MPTP has generated several intriguing candidates, including N-methylsalsolinol 1-tricholoromethyl-1,2,3,4-tetrahydro-β-carboline and some of the catechol oxidation products discussed above; however, none has been shown to contribute significantly to PD progression.[28,155,187,197,222]

MANGANESE

There have been many case series and individual reports world-wide concerning occupational exposure to manganese, as well as a few accounts of apparent iatrogenic exposure to manganese.[63,70,91,179,200,259] In one of the larger studies, a cohort of 13 symptomatic patients employed as manganese miners was identified.[175] The duration of exposure to manganese dust ranged from 8 months to 20 years. Consistently observed signs and symptoms were psychomotor disturbances or locura manganica (manganic madness) in the early phases of disease that were followed by generalized muscle weakness, gait abnormalities and impaired speech. Other commonly reported features were clumsiness, tremor, impotence, memory dysfunction and sleep disturbances. Some years later, a separate group of investigators re-examined most of these patients and concluded that bradykinesia and dystonia were the major clinical findings.[10,11]

A separate cohort of six workers from a ferromanganese factory displayed bradykinesia, rigidity clumsiness and gait abnormalities, but not neuropsychiatric disturbances, as the most common signs and symptoms.[118] All six had been exposed to elevated manganese concentrations for over 2 years and had elevated blood and hair manganese levels. Repeat neurological examination 4 years later demonstrated slow progression of symptoms, despite cessation of manganese exposure, and limited response to levodopa therapy.[119] This same group of investigators performed PET studies on four patients with early parkinsonism secondary to chronic manganese exposure.[294] Their results suggested that the early effects of manganism are directed at cerebral structures that are postsynaptic to the nigrostriatal system, including the striatum and the pallidum. Subsequent PET studies showed preservation of presynaptic and postsynaptic nigrostriatal dopaminergic function in patients exposed to manganese.[213] Furthermore, diffusely decreased cerebral glucose metabolism was observed in patients who demonstrated extrapyramidal movement disorders but who did not manifest neuropsychiatric impairment.

Only a few autopsy studies of patients who suffered from manganism have been performed.[10,11,295] Consistent pathological findings are atrophy of the basal ganglia, characterized by neuronal loss and mild gliosis. The lesion tends to focus in the pallidoluysian system, but the striatum and even the thalamus may be equally affected.[33] Involvement of the substantia nigra and the red nucleus has been reported in some cases. Lewy bodies were identified in the substantia nigra of one case; however, it is unclear whether or not this patient had PD.[44] More recent neuroimaging studies of symptomatic patients have shown prominent involvement of the globus pallidus but with sparing of the dopaminergic system.[44]

Many experiments directed at understanding the mechanisms of manganese-induced neurotoxicity have been performed in experimental animals and in vitro. Results have varied depending upon the system used, the method of administration, and the age of the animal. Existing evidence supports the following possible mechanisms: (i) Mn^{3+}-accelerated catechol auto-oxidation with generation of cytotoxic quinones and partially reduced oxygen species[8,58,94,178,188,286] that may be augmented by increased dopamine turnover;[10] (ii) inhibition of cellular protective mechanisms by manganese;[156,287] (iii) enhancement of mitochondrial P-450 activity;[156] and (iv) disruption of mitochondrial calcium levels and inhibition of oxidative phophorylation.[83–85] This last mechanism is particularly interesting in light of the observation that neurodegeneration after direct injection of manganese into rat striatum could be partially blocked by an EAAR antagonist or interruption of the corticostriatal glutaminergic pathway.[29] These investigators also observed a reduction in tissue ATP levels, and they propose that manganese-induced neurodegeneration is mediated by EAAR stimulation secondary to impaired cellular respiration.

Axonotoxicants

Distal sensorimotor polyneuropathy is probably the most common clinical manifestation of neurotoxicant exposure in man. A variety of toxicants, including hexane, methyl n-butylketone (2-hexanone), CS_2, acrylamide and organophosphorus esters, results in degeneration of the distal portions of the longest, largest myelinated axons in the PNS and CNS, an observation encapsulated in the term central–peripheral distal axonopathy. A morphologically striking subset of the central–peripheral distal axonopathies comprises those characterized by neurofilamentous axonal swellings. Investigations have detailed the biochemical steps through which two chemically dissimilar compounds, CS_2 and n-hexane, may produce clinically and morphologically identical lesions.[96]

Cases of neuropathy from exposure to hexane date to the 1960s and have been reported from around the world.[110,296] Inhalant abuse of hexane-containing mixtures has also been an important source of exposure and is responsible for some of the most severe cases of hexane-induced neuropathy.[4] Toxicity from CS_2 exposure was recognized in the late nineteenth century in Europe.[52] Today, CS_2 is still used widely as a chemical solvent and as a reactant in the production of cellophane and rayon from cellulose. The acute toxicity of CS_2 resulting from high-level exposure is manifested as narcosis and psychosis. Reduction of ambient levels of CS_2 in the workplace has diminished the occurrence of these overt, acute signs, but also provided an appropriate environment for chronic low-level exposure.

Despite the very different chemical structures, chronic exposure to either hexane or CS_2 can produce identical pathological changes in nerves. The characteristic lesion produced by both hexane and CS_2 develops in the distal axon of the longest and largest sensory and motor nerves of the central and peripheral tracts. Initially, multifocal fusiform axonal swellings develop at the proximal side of nodes of Ranvier at distal but preterminal sites (Fig. 13.5a). Ultrastructural changes at the swellings

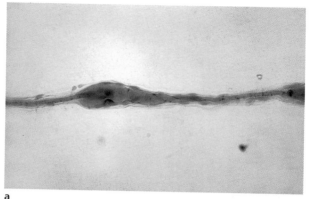

a

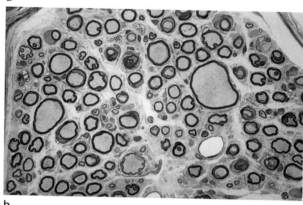

b

Figure 13.5 *Carbon disulfide intoxication. Muscular branch of posterior tibial nerve from a rat exposed to CS_2 at 800 ppm, 6 h/day, 5 days/week for 13 weeks in an inhalation chamber. (a) Teased fibre preparation illustrating a large paranodal axonal swelling. (b) Epon-embedded cross-section containing massively enlarged myelinated axons, some of which are surrounded by inappropriately thin myelin.*

include massive accumulations of disorganized 10-nm neurofilaments, decreased numbers of microtubules, thin myelin, and segregation of axoplasmic organelles and cytoskeletal components. As axonal swellings enlarge, thinning and retraction of myelin become increasingly apparent (Fig. 13.5b). Demyelination may occur partially through mechanical retraction at associated swellings, but evidence suggests that a direct action upon Schwann cells is also possible.[225] Schwann cells develop increased cytoplasmic contents and proliferate around swollen and demyelinated axons with intrusion of their cell processes into the axoplasm. Distal to the swellings, axons may become shrunken and then degenerate. With continued exposure, more proximal swellings occur with subsequent degeneration. Investigations of hexane and CS_2 have detailed their fate within biological systems and provided insight into their mechanisms of action. The key to their shared clinical and pathological profiles appears to be the ability of each compound to generate protein-bound electrophilic species that can covalently cross-link proteins.

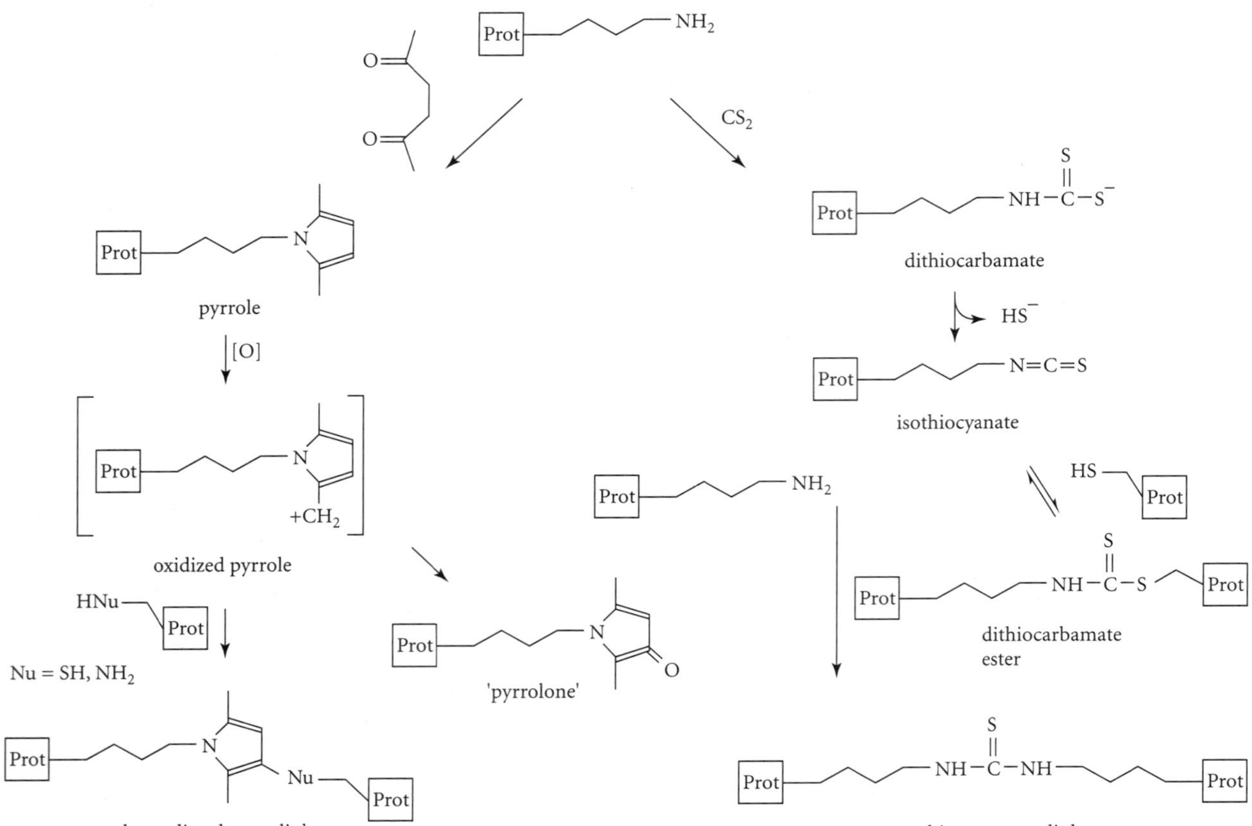

pyrrole

oxidized pyrrole

Nu = SH, NH₂

pyrrole-mediated cross-link

'pyrrolone'

dithiocarbamate

isothiocyanate

dithiocarbamate ester

thiourea cross-link

Hexane is successively metabolized by hepatic ω-1 oxidation to its toxic metabolite 2,5-hexanedione.[56] Intermediates in this oxidative pathway are also potentially neurotoxic and one, methyl *n*-butyl ketone (2-hexanone), has also been associated with distal axonopathies in humans.[2,21] Neurotoxicity requires irreversible binding of the diketone to protein amino functions to form pyrrole adducts.[86] While pyrrole formation is necessary for neurotoxicity, it is not sufficient. The pyrrole adduct must be oxidized to an electrophile that can yield protein cross-linking.[6,235,271] Neurofilament proteins are thought to be among the critical targets of hexane-mediated protein cross-linking because γ-diketones that do not result in neurofilamentous swellings, such as 3-acetyl-2,5-hexanedione, also do not result in degeneration of the axon. However, other targets exist because axons without neurofilaments are also vulnerable to γ-diketone-induced degeneration.

The ability of CS₂ to cross-link covalently neurofilament proteins has also been demonstrated and probably explains how these chemically dissimilar compounds produce identical changes in the axon.[96,282] The cross-linking sequence starts with CS₂ adding to a protein amine group, forming a monoalkyl dithiocarbamate. The next step requires generation of isothiocyanate through either loss of sulfhydryl ion from dithiocarbamate or oxidation of dithiocarbamate disulfide to isothiocyanate. Once formed, isothiocyanate protein adducts can react with sulfhydryl or amine groups to produce dithiocarbamate

ester or thiourea cross-linking structures, respectively. Because dithiocarbamate esters form reversibly under physiological conditions they too may serve as a source of isothiocyante. The relative stability of thiourea and the greater abundance of amine groups in biological systems suggest that thiourea may be the more biologically relevant cross-linking structure.

TOXICANTS AS RISK FACTORS FOR NEUROLOGICAL DISEASE

Several epidemiological studies suggest that PD may be significantly influenced by exposure to environmental toxicants. Although not in full agreement, epidemiological studies have converged on the potentially overlapping risk factors of rural living, consumption of well water and agrochemical exposure.[92,121,159,164,247,273,274] Experience with MPTP provides sufficient clinical, pathological and experimental data to conclude that parkinsonism that very closely mimics PD can result from toxicant exposure. Moreover, PET studies have made the extremely important observation that transient exposure to MPTP may result in long-term acceleration of dopaminergic neurodegeneration.[288] However, the identity of specific toxicants that increase the risk of PD and their relative effects on different subsets of parkinsonian patients remain to be elucidated.

Debate over the role of aluminium in AD has a contentious history that has evolved in three phases. First, aluminium was proposed to be aetiologically related to AD. Exposure of rabbits to high levels of aluminium produces a cerebral neurodegenerative disease that is characterized by structures that superficially resemble NFTs. Accidental exposure of adults to high levels of aluminium can yield a dementing illness; however, it is not characterized by the pathological hallmarks of AD, i.e. senile plaques and NFTs. In the second phase, aluminium levels were proposed to be increased in brains of AD patients and to contribute to disease pathogenesis. However, most studies have failed to show that bulk levels of aluminium in the brains of AD patients are increased compared with age-matched controls. Using localizing techniques, some groups have observed increased aluminium in NFTs, in the nucleus of tangle-bearing neurons, and in senile plaques; however, these results have not been confirmed by others.[165] The current phase in the debate over aluminium in AD is epidemiological, and seeks to determine whether exposure to aluminium is a risk factor for developing AD. Most data, but not all, do not favour this hypothesis. Interested readers should examine the arguments presented by others.[76,196]

REFERENCES

1 Alfrey AC, LeGendre GR, Kaehny WD. The dialysis encephalopathy syndrome. *N Engl J Med* 1976; **294**: 184–8.

2 Allen N, Mendell JR, Billmaier DJ et al. Toxic polyneuropathy due to methyl *n*-butyl ketone. An industrial outbreak. *Arch Neurol* 1975; **32**: 209–18.

3 Alpers BJ, Lewy FH. Changes in the nervous system following carbon disulfide poisoning in animals and in man. *Arch Neurol Psychiat* 1940; **44**: 725–39.

4 Altenkirch H, Mager J, Stoltenburg G, Helmbrecht J. Toxic polyneuropathies after sniffing a glue thinner. *J Neurol* 1977; **214**: 137–52.

5 Amitai Y, Zlotogorski Z, Golan-Katzav V et al. Neuropsychological impairment from acute low-level exposure to carbon monoxide. *Arch Neurol* 1998; **55**: 845–8.

6 Anthony DC, Boekelheide K, Graham DG. The effect of 3,4 dimethyl substitution on the neurotoxicity of 2,5-hexanedione. I. Accelerated clinical neuropathy is accompanied by more proximal swellings. *Toxicol Appl Pharmacol* 1983; **71**: 362–71.

7 Arai K, Maguchi S, Fujii S et al. Glycation and inactivation of human Cu-Zn-superoxide dismutase. *J Biol Chem* 1987; **262**: 16969–72.

8 Archibald FS, Tyree C. Manganese poisoning and the attack of trivalent manganese upon catecholamines. *Arch Biochem Biophys* 1987; **256**: 638–50.

9 Ballard PA, Tetrud JW, Langston JW. Permanent human parkinsonism due to 1-methyl-4-phenyl-1,2,3,6-tetrahydropyridine (MPTP): seven cases. *Neurology* 1985; **35**: 949–56.

10 Barbeau A. Manganese and extrapyramidal disorders. A critical review and tribute to Dr. George C. Cotzias. *Neurotoxicology* 1984; **5**: 13–36.

11 Barbeau A, Inoue N, Cloutier T. Role of manganese in dystonia. *Adv Neurol* 1976; **14**: 339–51.

12 Beal MF. Aging, energy, and oxidative stress in neurodegenerative diseases. *Ann Neurol* 1995; **38**: 357–66.

13 Beal MF. Does impairment of energy metabolism result in excitotoxic neuronal death in neurodegenerative illnesses? *Ann Neurol* 1992; **31**: 119–30.

14 Beal MF. Excitotoxicity and nitric oxide in Parkinson's disease pathogenesis. *Ann Neurol* 1998; **44**: S110–14.

15 Beal MF, Ferrante RJ, Browne SE et al. Increased 3-nitrotyrosine in both sporadic and familial amyotrophic lateral sclerosis. *Ann Neurol* 1997; **42**: 644–54.

16 Behnke M, Eyler F, Conlon M et al. Incidence and description of structural brain abnormalities in newborns exposed to cocaine. *J Pediatr* 1998; **132**: 291–4.

17 Benton CD Jr, Calhoun FP Jr. The ocular effects of methyl alcohol poisoning. Report of a catastrophe involving 320 persons. *Am J Ophthalmol* 1952; **36**: 1677–85.

18 Berger JR, Ayyar R. Neurological complications of ethylene glycol intoxication. Report of a case. *Arch Neurol* 1981; **38**: 724–6.

19 Bergouignan FX, Vital C, Henry P, Eschapasse P. Disulfiram neuropathy. *J Neurol* 1988; **235**: 382–3.

20 Besser R, Kramer G, Thumler R et al. Acute trimethyltin limbic-cerebellar syndrome. *Neurology* 1987; **37**: 945–50.

21 Billmaier D, Allen N, Craft B et al. Peripheral neuropathy in a coated fabrics plant. *J Occup Med* 1974; **16**: 665–71.

22 Blanche S, Tardieu M, Rustin P et al. Persistent mitochondrial dysfunction and perinatal exposure to antiretroviral nucleoside analogues. *Lancet* 1999; **354**: 1084–9.

23 Boor JW, Hurtig HI. Persistent cerebellar ataxia after exposure to toluene. *Ann Neurol* 1977; **2**: 440–2.

24 Bouldin TW, Goines ND, Bagnell CR, Krigman MR. Pathogenesis of trimethyltin neuronal toxicity. Ultrastructural and cytochemical observations. *Am J Pathol* 1981; **104**: 237–49.

25 Brashear A, Unverzagt F, Farber M et al. Ethylene oxide neurotoxicity: a cluster of 12 nurses with peripheral and central nervous system toxicity. *Neurology* 1996; **46**: 992–8.

26 Brierley JB, Brown AW, Calverley J. Cyanide intoxication in the rat–physiological and neuropathological aspects. *J Neurol Neurosurg Psychiat* 1976; **39**: 129–40.

27 Brierley JB, Prior PF, Calverley J, Brown AW. Cyanide intoxication in *Macaca mulatta*. *J Neurol Sci* 1977; **31**: 133–57.

28 Bringmann G, God R, Feineis D et al. The TaClo concept: 1-trichloromethyl-1,2,3,4-tetrahydro-beta-carboline (TaClo), a new toxin for dopaminergic neurons. *J Neural Trans Suppl* 1995; **46**: 235–44.

29 Brouillet EP, Shinobu L, McGarvey U et al. Manganese injection into the rat striatum produces excitotoxic lesions by impairing energy metabolism. *Exp Neurol* 1993; **120**: 889–94.

30 Burks JS, Alfrey AC, Huddlestone J et al. A fatal encephalopathy in chronic haemodialysis patients. *Lancet* 1976; **i**: 764–8.

31 Buxton PH, Hayward M. Polyneuritis cranialis associated with industrial trichloroethylene poisoning. *Neurol Neurosurg Psychiat* 1967; **30**: 511–17.

32 Calingasan NY, Uchida K, Gibson GE. Protein-bound acrolein: a novel marker of oxidative stress in Alzheimer's disease. *J Neurochem* 1999; **72**: 751–6.

33 Canavan MM, Cobb S, Drinker CK. Chronic manganese poisoning. Report of a case, with autopsy. *Arch Neurol Psychiat* 1934; **32**: 501–13.

34 Castellani R, Smith MA, Richey PL, Perry G. Glycoxidation and oxidative stress in Parkinson disease and diffuse Lewy body disease. *Brain Res* 1996; **737**: 195–200.

35 Castilho RF, Ward MW, Nicholls DG. Oxidative stress, mitochondrial function, and acute glutamate excitotoxicity in

cultures cerebellar granule cells. *J Neurochem* 1999; **72**: 1394–401.

36 Cavanagh J, Buxton P. Trichloroethylene cranial neuropathy: is it really a toxic neuropathy or does it activate latent herpes virus? *J Neurol Neurosurg Psychiat* 1989; **52**: 297–303.

37 Chang L, Ernst T, Grob C, Poland R. Cerebral (1)H MRS alterations in recreational 3,4-methylenedioxymethamphetamine (MDMA, 'ecstasy') users. *J Mag Reson Imag* 1999; **10**: 521–6.

38 Chang LW. Mercury. In: Spencer PS, Schaumburg HH, eds. *Experimental and clinical neurotoxicology*. Baltimore, MD: Williams and Wilkins, 1980: 508–26.

39 Chen R, Tang S, Miyata H *et al*. Polychlorinated biphenyl poisoning: correlation of sensory and motor nerve conduction, neurologic symptoms, and blood levels of polychlorinated biphenyls, quaterphenyls, and dibenzofurans. *Environ Res* 1985; **37**: 340–8.

40 Chen YCJ, Guo YL, Hsu CC, Rogan WJ. Cognitive development of Yu-Cheng ('oil disease') children prenatally exposed to heat-degraded PCBs. *JAMA* 1992; **268**: 3213–18.

41 Choi DW, Koh JY. Zinc and brain injury. *Annu Rev Neurosci* 1998; **21**: 347–75.

42 Choi IS. Delayed neurologic sequellae in carbon monoxide intoxication. *Arch Neurol* 1983; **40**: 433–5.

43 Chu C, Huang C, Ryu S, Wu T. Chronic inorganic mercury induced peripheral neuropathy. *Acta Neurol Scand* 1998; **98**: 461–5.

44 Chu NS, Hochberg FH, Calne DB, Olanow CW. Neurotoxicology of manganese. In: Chang LW, Dyer R eds. *Handbook of neurotoxicology*. New York: Marcel Dekker, 1995: 91–104.

45 Chucrallah A, deGirolami U, Freeman R, Federman M. Lovastatin/gemfibrozil myopathy: a clinical, histochemical and ultrastructural study. *Eur Neurol* 1992; **32**: 293–6.

46 Chuttani PN, Chopra JS. Arsenic poisoning. In: Vinken PJ, Bruyn GW eds. *Handbook of clinical neurology* Vol 36. Amsterdam: Elsevier, 1979: 199–216.

47 Clarren SK, Alvord EC Jr, Sumi SM *et al*. Brain malformations related to prenatal exposure to ethanol. *J Pediatr* 1978; **92**: 64–7.

48 Coyle JT, Puttfarcken P. Oxidative stress, glutamate, and neurodegenerative disorders. *Science* 1993; **262**: 689–95.

49 Crystal HA, Schaumburg HH, Grober E *et al*. Cognitive impairment and sensory loss associated with chronic low-level ethylene oxide exposure. *Neurology* 1988; **38**: 567–9.

50 Cuajungco M, Lees G. Zinc and Alzheimer's disease: is there a direct link? *Brain Res – Brain Res Rev* 1997; **23**: 219–36.

51 Cuajungco M, Lees G. Zinc metabolism in the brain: relevance to human neurodegenerative disorders. *Neurobiol Dis* 1997;**4**: 137–69.

52 Davidson M, Feinlab M. Carbon disulfide poisoning: a review. *Am Heart J* 1972; **83**: 100–14.

53 Davis LE, Standefer JC, Kornfeld M *et al*. Acute thallium poisoning: toxicological and morphological studies of the nervous system. *Ann Neurol* 1981; **10**: 38–44.

54 Davis LE, Wands JR, Weiss SA *et al*. Central nervous system intoxication from mercurous chloride laxatives. *Arch Neurol* 1974; **30**: 428–31.

55 Delaney P, Estes M. Intracranial hemorrhage with amphetamine abuse. *Neurology* 1980; **30**: 1125–8.

56 Di Vincenzo GD, Kaplan CJ, Dedinas J. Characterization of the metabolites of methyl *n*-butyl ketone, methyl iso-butyl ketone, and methyl ethyl ketone in guinea pig serum and their clearance. *Toxicol Appl Pharmacol* 1976; **36**: 311–17.

57 Dickson DW, Sinicropi S, Yen SH *et al*. Glycation and microglial reaction in lesions of Alzheimer's disease. *Neurobiol Aging* 1996; **17**: 733–43.

58 Donaldson J, McGregor D, Labella F. Manganese neurotoxicity: a model for free radical mediated neurodegeneration? *Can J Physiol Pharmacol* 1982; **60**: 1398–405.

59 Donofrio PD, Wilbourn AJ, Albers JW *et al*. Acute arsenic intoxication presenting as Guillain–Barré-like syndrome. *Muscle Nerve* 1987; **10**: 114–20.

60 Dumitru D, Kalantri A. Electrophysiologic investigation of thallium poisoning. *Muscle Nerve* 1990; **13**: 433–7.

61 Dunn JA, Ahmed MU, Murtiashaw MH *et al*. Reaction of ascorbate with lysine and protein under autoxidizing conditions: formation of *N*-(carboxymethyl)lysine by reaction between lysine and products of autoxidation of ascorbate. *Biochemistry* 1990; **29**: 10964–70.

62 Dyer DG, Blackledge JA, Thorpe SR, Baynes JW. Formation of pentosidine during nonenzymatic browning of proteins by glucose. *J Biol Chem* 1991; **266**: 11654–60.

63 Ejima A, Imamura T, Nakamura S *et al*. Manganese intoxication during total parenteral nutrition. *Lancet* 1992; **339**: 426.

64 Escobar A, Aruffo C. Chronic thinner intoxication: clinicopathologic report of a human case. *J Neurol Neurosurg Psychiat* 1980; **43**: 986–94.

65 Esterbauer H, Schaur RJ, Zollner H. Chemistry and biochemistry of 4-hydroxynonenal, malondialdehyde and related aldehydes. *Free Radic Biol Med* 1991; **11**: 81–128.

66 Estes M, Ewing-Wilson D, Chou S *et al*. Chloroquine neuromyotoxicity. Clinical and pathologic prospective. *Am J Med* 1987; **82**: 447–55.

67 Farber JL. Mechanisms of cell injury. In: Craighead JE ed. *Pathology of environmental and occupational disease*. St Louis, MO: Mosby-Year Book, 1995: 287–302.

68 Feldman JM, Feldman MD. Sequellae of attempted suicide by cyanide ingestion: a case report. *Int J Psychiat Med* 1990; **20**: 173–9.

69 Feldman R, White R, Eriator I. Trimethyltin encephalopathy. *Arch Neurol* 1993; **50**: 1320–4.

70 Feldman RG. Manganese as possible ecoetiologic factor in Parkinson's disease. In: Langston JW, Young A eds. *Neurotoxins and neurodegenerative disease* Vol. 648. New York: New York Academy of Sciences, 1992: 266–7.

71 Feldman RG. Trichlorethylene. In: Vinken PJ, Bruyn GW eds. *Handbook of clinical neurology* Vol. 36. Amsterdam: Elsevier, 1979: 457–64.

72 Ferrante RJ, Browne SE, Shinobu LA *et al*. Evidence of increased oxidative damage in both sporadic and familial amyotrophic lateral sclerosis. *J Neurochem* 1997; **69**: 2064–74.

73 Filley CM, Heaton RK, Rosenberg NL. White matter dementia in chronic toluene abuse. *Neurology* 1990; **40**: 532–4.

74 Filley CM, Kelly JP. Alcohol- and drug-related neurotoxicity. *Curr Opin Neurol Neurosurg* 1993; **6**: 443–7.

75 Finkelstein Y, Markowitz M, Rosen J. Low-level lead-induced neurotoxicity in children: an update on central nervous system effects. *Brain Res Rev* 1998; **27**: 168–76.

76 Forbes W, Hill G. Is exposure to aluminum a risk factor for the development of Alzheimer disease? – Yes. *Arch Neurol* 1998; **55**: 740–1.

77 Fornstedt B, Pileblad E, Carlsson A. *In vivo* autoxidation of dopamine in guinea pig striatum increases with age. *J Neurochem* 1990; **55**: 655–9.

78 Fornstedt B, Rosengren E, Carlsson A. The apparent autoxidation rate of catechols in dopamine-rich regions of human brains increases with degree of depigmentation of substantia nigra. *J Neural Transm* 1989; **1**: 279–95.

79 Fornstedt B, Rosengren E, Carlsson A. Occurrence and distribution of 5-S-cysteinyl derivatives of dopamine, dopa, and dopac in the brains of eight mammalian species. *Neuropharmacology* 1986; **25**: 451–4.

80 Freilich RJ, Byrne E. Alcohol and drug abuse. *Curr Opin Neurol Neurosurg* 1992; **5**: 391–5.

81 Friedman EA, Greenberg JB, Merrill JP, Dammin GJ. Consequences of ethylene glycol poisoning. *Am J Med* 1962; **32**: 891–902.

82 Fullerton PM. Electrophysiological and histological observations on peripheral nerves in acrylamide poisoning in man. *J Neurol Neurosurg Psychiat* 1969; **32**: 186–92.

83 Gavin C, Gunter K, Gunter T. Manganese and calcium transport in mitochondria: implications for manganese toxicity. *Neurotoxicology* 1999; **20**: 445–53.

84 Gavin CE, Gunter KK, Gunter TE. Manganese and calcium efflux kinetics in brain mitochondria. Relevance to manganese toxicity. *Biochem J* 1990; **266**: 329–34.

85 Gavin CE, Gunter KK, Gunter TE. Mn^{2+} sequestration by mitochondria and inhibition of oxidative phosphorylation. *Toxicol Appl Pharmacol* 1992; **115**: 1–5.

86 Genter MB, Szakal-Quin G, Anderson CW *et al*. Evidence that pyrrole formation is a pathogenetic step in γ-diketone neuropathy. *Toxicol Appl Pharmacol* 1987; **87**: 351–62.

87 Gill JS, Hornby RS, Hitchcock ER, Beevers DG. Alcohol consumption – a risk factor for hemorrhagic and non-hemorrhagic stroke. *Am J Med* 1991; **90**: 489–96.

88 Ginsberg MD. Carbon monoxide. In: Spencer PS, Schaumburg HH eds. *Experimental and clinical neurotoxicology*. Baltimore, MD: Williams and Wilkins, 1980: 374–94.

89 Ginsberg MD, Hedley-Whyte ET, Richardson EP Jr. Hypoxic–ischemic leukoencephalopathy in man. *Arch Neurol* 1976; **33**: 5–14.

90 Goebel HH, Schmidt PF, Bohl J *et al*. Polyneuropathy due to acute arsenic intoxication: biopsy studies. *J Neuropathol Exp Neurol* 1990; **49**: 137–49.

91 Gorell J, Johnson C, Rybicki B *et al*. Occupational exposure to manganese, copper, lead, iron, mercury and zinc and the risk of Parkinson's disease. *Neurotoxicology* 1999; **20**: 239–47.

92 Gorell JM, Johnson CC, Rybicki BA *et al*. The risk of Parkinson's disease with exposure to pesticides, farming, well water, and rural living. *Neurology* 1998; **50**: 1346–50.

93 Grabski DA. Toluene sniffing producing cerebellar degeneration. *Am J Psychiat* 1961; **118**: 461–2.

94 Graham DG. Catecholamine toxicity: a proposal for the molecular pathogenesis of manganese neurotoxicity and Parkinson's disease. *Neurotoxicology* 1984; **5**: 83–96.

95 Graham DG. Oxidative pathways for catecholamines in the genesis of neuromelanin and cytotoxic quinones. *Mol Pharmacol* 1978; **14**: 633–43.

96 Graham DG, Amarnath V, Valentine WM *et al*. Pathogenetic studies of hexane and carbon disulfide neurotoxicity. *Crit Rev Toxicol* 1995; **25**: 91–112.

97 Graham DG, Tiffany SM, Bell WR Jr Gutknecht WF. Autoxidation versus covalent binding of quinones as the mechanism of toxicity of dopamine, 6-hydroxydopamine, and related compounds toward C1300 neuroblastoma cells *in vitro*. *Mol Pharmacol* 1978; **14**: 644–53.

98 Grandas F, Artieda J, Obeso JA. Clinical and CT scan findings in a case of cyanide intoxication. *Mov Dis* 1989; **4**: 188–93.

99 Grandhee SK, Monnier VM. Mechanism of formation of the Maillard protein cross-link pentosidine. *J Biol Chem* 1991; **266**: 11649–53.

100 Greene JG, Porter HP, Eller RV, Greenamyre JT. Inhibition of succinate dehydrogenase by malonic acid produces an exci-totoxic lesion in rat striatum. *J Neurochem* 1993; **61**: 1151–54.

101 Griffin GW, Wesselingh SL, Griffin DE *et al*. Peripheral nerve disorders in HIV infection. In: Price RW, Perry SW eds. *HIV, AIDS, and the brain*. New York: Raven Press, 1994: 159–82.

102 Gross JA, Haas ML, Swift TR. Ethylene oxide neurotoxicity: report of four cases and review of the literature. *Neurology* 1979; **29**: 978–83.

103 Gutteridge JMC, Westermarck T, Halliwell B. Oxygen radical damage in biological systems. In: Johnson JE, Walford R, Harman D, Miquel J eds. *Free radicals, aging, and degenerative diseases*. New York: Alan R. Liss, 1986: 99–139.

104 Halliwell B. Reactive oxygen species and the central nervous system. *J Neurochem* 1992; **59**: 1609–23.

105 Harper C. The neuropathology of alcohol-specific brain damage, or does alcohol damage the brain? *J Neuropathol Exp Neurol* 1998; **57**: 101–10.

106 Hastings L. Neurotoxicity of cadmium. In: Chang LW, Dyer RS eds. *Handbook of neurotoxicology*. New York: Marcel Dekker, 1995: 171–212.

107 Hastings TG, Lewis DA, Zigmond MJ. Role of oxidation in the neurotoxic effects of intrastriatal dopamine injections. *Proc Natl Acad Sci USA* 1996; **93**: 1956–61.

108 Haymaker W, Ginzler AM, Ferguson RL. Residual neuropathological effects of cyanide poisoning. A study of the central nervous system of 23 dogs exposed to cyanide compounds. *Military Surgeon* 1952; **111**: 231–45.

109 Herning R, King D, Better W, Cadet J. Neurovascular deficits in cocaine abusers. *Neuropsychopharmacology* 1999; **21**: 110–18.

110 Herskowitz A, Ishii N, Schamburg H. *n*-Hexane neuropathy: a syndrome occurring as a result of industrial exposure. *N Engl J Med* 1971; **285**: 82–5.

111 Hirano A, Iwata M. Neuropathology of lead intoxication. In: Vinken PJ, Bruym GW eds. *Handbook of clinical neurology* Vol. 36. Amsterdam: Elsevier, 1979: 35–64.

112 Hirsch EC, Brandel J-P, Galle P *et al*. Iron and aluminum increase in the substantia nigra of patients with Parkinson's disease: an x-ray microanalysis. *J Neurochem* 1991; **56**: 446–51.

113 Hirschberg M, Ludolph A, Groemeyer K, Gullotta F. Development of a subacute tetraparesis after disulfiram intoxication. Case report. *Eur Neurol* 1987; **26**: 222–8.

114 Hochberg F, Miller G, Valenzuela R *et al*. Late motor deficits of Chilean manganese miners: a blinded control study. *Neurology* 1996; **47**: 788–95.

115 Hoffman SW, Moore S, Ellis EF. Isoprostanes: free radical-generated prostaglandins with constrictor effects on cerebral arterioles. *Stroke* 1997; **28**: 844–9.

116 Hsu H, Chen C, Chen F *et al*. Optic atrophy and cerebral infarcts caused by methanol intoxication: MRI. *Neuroradiology* 1997; **39**: 192–4.

117 Huang C, Chu C, Chen R *et al*. Chronic carbon disulfide encephalopathy. *Eur Neurol* 1996; **36**: 364–8.

118 Huang C-C, Chu N-S, Lu C-S *et al*. Chronic manganese intoxication. *Arch Neurol* 1989; **46**: 1104–6.

119 Huang C-C, Lu C-S, Chu N-S *et al*. Progression after chronic manganese exposure. *Neurology* 1993; **43**: 1479–83.

120 Huang X, Atwood C, Hartshorn M *et al*. The A beta peptide of Alzheimer's disease directly produces hydrogen peroxide through metal ion reduction. *Biochemistry* 1999; **38**: 7609–16.

121 Hubble JP, Kurth JH, Glatt SL *et al*. Gene-toxin interaction as a putative risk factor for Parkinson's disease with dementia. *Neuroepidemiology* 1998; **17**: 96–104.

122 Igisu H, Goto I, Kawamura *et al*. Acrylamide encephaloneuropathy due to well water pollution. *J Neurol Neurosurg Psychiat* 1975; **38**: 581–4.

123 Ishimaru H, Katoh A, Suzuki H et al. Effects of N-methyl-D-aspartate receptor antagonists on carbon monoxide-induced brain damage in mice. J Pharmacol Exp Ther 1992; **261**: 349–52.

124 Jacobs J, Costa-Jussa' F. The pathology of amiodarone neurotoxicity. II. Peripheral neuropathy in man. Brain 1985; **108**: 753–69.

125 Jacobs JM, Le Quesne PM. Toxic disorders. In: Adams JH, Duchen LW eds. Greenfield's neuropathology 5th edn. New York: Oxford University Press, 1992: 881–987.

126 Jacobson J, Jacobson S. Evidence for PCBs as neurodevelopmental toxicants in humans. Neurotoxicology 1997; **18**: 415–24.

127 Jellinger K. Exogenous lesions of the pallidum. In: Vinken PJ, Bruyn GW, Klawans HL eds. Handbook of clinical neurology. Amsterdam: Elsevier, 1986: 465–91.

128 Jellinger K, Kienzl E, Rumpelmair G et al. Iron–melanin complex in substantia nigra of parkinsonian brains: an x-ray microanalysis. J Neurochem 1992; **59**: 1168–71.

129 Jellinger K, Paulus W, Grundke-Iqbal I et al. Brain iron and ferritin in Parkinson's and Alzheimer's diseases. J Neural Transm 1990; **2**: 327–40.

130 Jenkins RB. Inorganic arsenic and the nervous system. Brain 1966; **89**: 479–97.

131 Joong S, Kim JM. Giant axonal swelling in 'Huffer's' neuropathy. Arch Neurol 1976; **33**: 583–6.

132 Kaelan C, Harper C, Vieira BI. Acute encephalopathy and death due to petrol sniffing: neuropathological findings. Aust NZ J Med 1986; **16**: 804–7.

133 Kaku DA, Lowenstein DH. Emergence of recreational drug abuse as a major risk factor for stroke in young adults. Ann Intern Med 1990; **113**: 821–7.

134 Karch S, Stephens B, Ho C. Methamphetamine-related deaths in San Francisco: demographic, pathologic, and toxicologic profiles. J Forensic Sci 1999; **44**: 359–68.

135 Kelleher T, Cross A, Dunkle L. Relation of peripheral neuropathy to HIV treatment in four randomized clinical trials including didanosine. Clin Ther 1999; **21**: 1182–92.

136 Kennedy P, Cavanagh J. Spinal changes in the neuropathy of thallium poisoning. A case with neuropathological studies. J Neurol Sci 1976; **29**: 295–301.

137 Kikuchi S, Shinpo K, Moriwaka F et al. Neurotoxicity of methylglyoxal and 3-deoxyglucosone on cultured cortical neurons: synergism between glycation and oxidative stress, possibly involved in neurodegenerative diseases. J Neurosci Res 1999; **57**: 280–9.

138 Kimbrough RD. Human health effects of polychlorinated biphenyls (PCBs) and polybrominated biphenyls (PBBs). Annu Rev Pharmacol Toxicol 1987; **27**: 87–111.

139 Kimura T, Takamatsu J, Ikeda K et al. Accumulation of advanced glycation end products of the Maillard reaction with age in human hippocampal neurons. Neurosci Lett 1996; **208**: 210–11.

140 Kish S, Kalasinsky K, Furukawa Y et al. Brain choline acetyltransferase activity in chronic, human users of cocaine, methamphetamine, and heroin. Mol Psychiatry 1999; **4**: 26–32.

141 Klawans HL, Stein RW, Tanner CM, Goetz CG. A pure parkinsonian syndrome following acute carbon monoxide intoxication. Arch Neurol 1982; **39**: 302–4.

142 Klivenyi P, Andreassen OA, Ferrante RJ et al. Mice deficient in cellular glutathione peroxidase show increased vulnerability to malonate, 3-nitropropionic acid, and 1-methyl-4-phenyl-1,2,5,6-tetrahydropyridine. J Neurosci 2000; **20**: 1–7.

143 Kornfeld M, Moser A, Moser H et al. Solvent vapor abuse leukoencephalopathy. Comparison to adrenoleukodystrophy. J Neuropathol Exp Neurol 1994; **53**: 389–98.

144 Korobkin R, Asbury AK, Sumner AJ, Nielsen SL. Glue-sniffing neuropathy. Arch Neurol 1975; **32**: 158–62.

145 Krarup-Hansen A, Rietz B, Krarup C et al. Histology and platinum content of sensory ganglia and sural nerves in patients treated with cisplatin and carboplatin: an autopsy study. Neuropathol Appl Neurobiol 1999; **25**: 29–40.

146 Kreyberg S, Torvik A, Bjorneboe A et al. Trimethyltin poisoning: report of a case with postmortem examination. Clin Neuropathol 1992; **11**: 256–9.

147 Krigman MR, Bouldin TW, Mushak P. Lead. In: Spencer PS, Schaumburg HH eds. Experimental and clinical neurotoxicology. Baltimore, MD: Williams and Wilkins, 1980: 490–507.

148 Kril J, Halliday G, Svoboda M, Cartwright H. The cerebral cortex is damaged in chronic alcoholics. Neuroscience 1997; **79**: 983–98.

149 Kuncl R, Duncan G, Watson D et al. Colchicine myopathy and neuropathy. N Engl J Med 1987; **316**: 1562–8.

150 Kuteifan K, Oesterle H, Tajahmady T et al. Necrosis and hemorrhage of the putamen in methanol poisoning shown on MRI. Neuroradiology 1998; **40**: 158–60.

151 Kuzuhara S, Kanazawa I, Nakanishi T, Egashira T. Ethylene oxide polyneuropathy. Neurology 1983; **33**: 377–80.

152 Langston JW, Forno LS, Tetrud J et al. Evidence of active nerve cell degeneration in the substantia nigra of humans years after 1-methyl-4-phenyl-1,2,3,6-tetrahydropyridine exposure. Ann Neurol 1999; **46**: 598–605.

153 Langston JW. Organic neurotoxicants. In: Calne DB ed. Neurodegenerative diseases. Philadelphia, PA: WB Saunders, 1994: 225–40.

154 LaVoie M, Hastings T. Dopamine quinone formation and protein modification associated with the striatal neurotoxicity of methamphetamine: evidence against a role for extracellular dopamine. J Neurosci 1999; **19**: 1484–91.

155 Li H, Dryhurst G. Irreversible inhibition of mitochondrial complex I by 7-(2-aminoethyl)-3,4-dihydro-5-hydroxy-2H-1,4-benzothiazine-3-carboxylic acid (DHBT-1): a putative nigral endotoxin of relevance to Parkinson's disease. J Neurochem 1997; **69**: 1530–41.

156 Liccione JJ, Maines MD. Selective vulnerability of glutathione metabolism and cellular defense mechanisms in rat striatum to manganese. J Pharmacol Exp Ther 1988; **247**: 156–61.

157 Liessens J, Monstrui J, Vanden E et al. Bismuth encephalopathy. A clinical and anatomicropathological report of one case. Acta Neurol 1978; **78**: 301–9.

158 Limos LC, Ohnishi A, Suzuki N et al. Axonal degeneration and focal muscle fiber necrosis in human thallotoxicosis: histopathological studies of nerve and muscle. Muscle Nerve 1982; **5**: 698–706.

159 Liou HH, Tsai MC, Chen CJ et al. Environmental risk factors and Parkinson's disease: a case–control study in Taiwan. Neurology 1997; **48**: 1583–8.

160 Lipton SA, Rosenberg PA. Excitatory amino acids as a final common pathway for neurological disorders. N Engl J Med 1994; **330**: 613–22.

161 Little K, McLaughlin D, Zhang L et al. Brain dopamine transporter messenger RNA and binding sites in cocaine users: a postmortem study. Arch Gen Psych 1998; **55**: 793–9.

162 Little K, Zhang L, Desmond T et al. Striatal dopaminergic abnormalities in human cocaine users. Am J Psych 1999; **156**: 238–45.

163 Mangano W, Montine T, Hulette C. Pathologic assessment of cerebellar atrophy following acute lithium intoxication. Clin Neuropathol 1997; **16**: 30–3.

164 Marder K, Logroscino G, Alfaro B et al. Environmental risk factors for Parkinson's disease in an urban multiethnic community. Neurology 1998; **50**: 279–81.

165 Markesbery W, Ehmann W. Brain trace elements in Alzheimer disease. In: Katzman R, Bick KL eds. *Alzheimer's disease*. New York: Raven Press, 1994: 353–64.

166 Martin-Bouyer G, Lebreton R, Toga M *et al*. Outbreak of accidental hexachlorophene poisoning in France. *Lancet* 1982; i: 91–5.

167 Martinez AJ, Boehm R, Hadfield MG. Acute hexachlorophene encephalopathy: clinico-neuropathological correlation. *Acta Neuropathol (Berl)* 1974; **28**: 93–103.

168 Martinez AJ, Taylor JR, Dyck PJ *et al*. Chlordecone intoxication in man. II. Ultrastructure of peripheral nerves and skeletal muscle. *Neurology* 1978; **28**: 631–5.

169 McIntyre TM, Zimmerman GA, Prescott SM. Biologically active oxidized phospholipids. *J Biol Chem* 1999; **274**: 25189–92.

170 McLaughlin AIG, Kazantzis G, King E *et al*. Pulmonary fibrosis and encephalopathy associated with the inhalation of aluminium dust. *Br J Ind Med* 1962; **19**: 253–63.

171 McLean DR, Jacobs H, Mielke BW. Methanol poisoning: a clinical and pathological study. *Ann Neurol* 1980; **8**: 161–7.

172 Meier C, Kauer B, Muller U, Ludin H. Neuromyopathy during chronic amiodarone treatment. *J Neurol* 1979; **220**: 231–9.

173 Meldrum B, Garthwaite J. Excitatory amino acid neurotoxicity and neurodegenerative disease. *Trends Pharmac Sci* 1990; **11**: 379–87.

174 Meldrum BS. Excitatory amino acid receptors and disease. *Curr Opin Neurol Neurosurg* 1992; **5**: 508–13.

175 Mena I, Marin O, Fuenzalida S, Cotzias GC. Chronic manganese poisoning. Clinical picture and manganese turnover. *Neurology* 1967; **17**: 128–36.

176 Meulenbelt J, de Groot G, Savelkoul TJF. Two cases of acute toluene intoxication. *Br J Indt Med* 1990; **47**: 417–20.

177 Mhiri C, Baudrimont M, Bonne G, *et al*. Zidovudine myopathy: a distinctive disorder associated with mitochondrial dysfunction. *Ann Neurol* 1991; **29**: 606–14.

178 Migheli R, Godani C, Sciola L *et al*. Enhancing effect of manganese on L-DOPA-induced apoptosis in PC12 cells: role of oxidative stress. *J Neurochem* 1999; **73**: 1155–63.

179 Mirowitz SA, Westrich TJ, Hirsch JD. Hyperintense basal ganglia on T1-weighted MR images in patients receiving parenteral nutrition. *Radiology* 1991; **181**: 117–20.

180 Moddel G, Bilbao JM, Payne D, Ashby P. Disulfiram neuropathy. *Arch Neurol* 1978; **35**: 658–60.

181 Mokri B, Ohnishi A, Dyck PJ. Disulfiram neuropathy. *Neurology* 1981; **31**: 730–5.

182 Monks TJ, Hanzlik RP, Cohen GM *et al*. Quinone chemistry and toxicology. *Toxicol Appl Pharmacol* 1992; **112**: 2–16.

183 Montine K, Reich E, Olson SJ *et al*. Distribution of reducible 4-hydroxynonenal adduct immunoreactivity in Alzheimer's disease is associated with APOE genotype. *J Neuropathol Exp Neurol* 1998; **57**: 415–25.

184 Montine KS, Kim PJ, Olson SJ *et al*. 4-Hydroxy-2-nonenal pyrrole adducts in human neurodegenerative disease. *J Neuropathol Exp Neurol* 1997; **56**: 866–71.

185 Montine KS, Olson SJ, Amarnath V *et al*. Immunochemical detection of 4-hydroxynonenal adducts in Alzheimer's disease is associated with APOE4. *Am J Pathol* 1997; **150**: 437–43.

186 Montine TJ, Beal MF, Cudkowicz ME *et al*. Increased cerebrospinal fluid F$_2$-isoprostane concentration in probable Alzheimer's disease. *Neurology* 1999; **52**: 562–5.

187 Montine TJ, Picklo MJ, Amarnath V *et al*. Neurotoxicity of endogenous cysteinylcatechols. *Exp Neurol* 1997; **148**: 26–33.

188 Montine TJ, Underhill TM, Linney E, Graham DG. Fibroblasts that express aromatic amino acid decarboxylase have increased sensitivity to the synergistic cytotoxicity of L-dopa and manganese. *Toxicol Appl Pharmacol* 1994; **128**: 116–22.

189 Morrow JD, Roberts LJ. The isoprostanes: unique bioactive products of lipid peroxidation. *Prog Lipid Res* 1997; **36**: 1–21.

190 Moses H, Klawans HL. Bromide intoxication. In: Vinken PJ, Bruyn GW eds. *Handbook of clinical neurology* Vol. 36. Amsterdam: Elsevier, 1979: 291–318.

191 Moyle G, Sadler M. Peripheral neuropathy with nucleoside antiretrovirals: risk factors, incidence and management. *Drug Safety* 1998; **19**: 481–94.

192 Mueller M, Borland C. Delayed cyanide poisoning following acetonitrile ingestion. *Postgrad Med J* 1997; **73**: 299–300.

193 Muller T, Przuntek H, Kuhn W *et al*. No increase of synthesis of (R) salsolinol in Parkinson's disease. *Mov Disord* 1999; **14**: 514–5.

194 Mullick FG. Hexachlorophene toxicity – human experience at the Armed Forces Institute of Pathology. *Pediatrics* 1973; **51**: 395–9.

195 Munch G, Cunningham AM, Riederer P, Braak E. Advanced glycation end products are associated with Hirano bodies in Alzheimer's disease. *Brain Res* 1998; **796**: 307–10.

196 Munoz D. Is exposure to aluminum a risk factor for the development of Alzheimer disease? – No. *Arch Neurol* 1998; **55**: 737–9.

197 Nagatsu T. Isoquinoline neurotoxins in the brain and Parkinson's disease. *Neurosci Res* 1997; **29**: 99–111.

198 Naoi M, Maruyama W. *N*-methyl(*R*)salsolinol, a dopamine neurotoxin, in Parkinson's disease. *Adv Neurol* 1999; **80**: 259–64.

199 Naoi M, Maruyama W, Dostert P, Hashizume Y. *N*-methyl-(*R*) salsolinol as a dopaminergic neurotoxin: from an animal model to an early marker of Parkinson's disease. *J Neural Transm Suppl* 1997; **50**: 89–105.

200 Nelson K, Golnick J, Korn T, Angle C. Manganese encephalopathy: utility of early magnetic resonance imaging. *Br J Ind Med* 1993; **50**: 510–13.

201 Nierenberg D, Nordgren R, Chang M *et al*. Delayed cerebellar disease and death after accidental exposure to dimethylmercury. *N Engl J Med* 1998; **338**: 1672–6.

202 Novelli A, Reilly JA, Lysko PG, Henneberry RC. Glutamate becomes neurotoxic via the *N*-methyl-D-aspartate receptor when intracellular energy levels are reduced. *Brain Res* 1988; **451**: 205–12.

203 Nukada H, Pollock M. Disulfiram neuropathy. A morphometric study of sural nerve. *J Neurol Sci* 1981; **51**: 51–67.

204 O'Callaghan JP. Assessment of neurotoxicity using assays of neuron- and glial-localized proteins: chronology and critique. In: Tilson H, Mitchell C eds. *Neurotoxicology*. New York: Raven Press, 1992: 83–100.

205 O'Callaghan JP. Quantitative features of reactive gliosis following toxicant-induced damage of the CNS. *Ann NY Acad Sci* 1992; **679**: 195–211.

206 Ochoa J. Isoniazid neuropathy in man: quantitative electron microscopic study. *Brain* 1970; **93**: 831–50.

207 Ohta M. Ultrastructure of sural nerve in a case of arsenical neuropathy. *Acta Neuropathol (Berl)* 1970; **16**: 233–42.

208 Okuda B, Iwamoto Y, Tachibana H, Sugita M. Parkinsonism after acute cadmium poisoning. *Clin Neurol Neurosurg* 1997; **99**: 263–5.

209 Opitz H, Schweinsberg F, Grossmann T *et al*. Demonstration of mercury in the human brain and other organs 17 years after metallic mercury exposure. *Clin Neuropathol* 1996; **15**: 139–44.

210 Osuntokun BO. An ataxic neuropathy in Nigeria. A clinical, biochemical and electrophysiological study. *Brain* 1968; **91**: 215–47.

211 Ott T, Rabinowicz T, Moran D. Étude clinique et histopathologique d'un cas de polynerite survenue au cours du traitement par l'isoniazide. *Revue Neurology* 1959; **100**: 103–17.

212 Pages M, Pages A, Bories-Azeau L. Severe sensorimotor neuropathy after cisplatin therapy. *J Neurol Neurosurg Psych* 1986; **49**: 333–4.

213 Pal P, Samii A, Calne D. Manganese neurotoxicity: a review of clinical features, imaging and pathology. *Neurotoxicology* 1999; **20**: 227–38.

214 Peiffer J, Majewski F, Fischbach H et al. Alcohol embryo- and fetopathy. *J Neurol Sci* 1979; **41**: 125–37.

215 Pendersen WA, Fu W, Keller JN et al. Protein modification by the lipid peroxidation product 4-hydroxynonenal in the spinal cords of amyotrophic lateral sclerosis patients. *Ann Neurol* 1998; **44**: 819–24.

216 Penney DG. Acute carbon monoxide poisoning: animal models: a review. *Toxicology* 1990; **62**: 123–60.

217 Perez JJ, Arsura E, Strategos S. Methamphetamine-related stroke: four cases. *J Emerg Med* 1999; **17**: 469–71.

218 Perl TM, Bedard L, Kosatsky T et al. An outbreak of toxic encephalopathy caused by eating mussels contaminated with domoic acid. *N Engl J Med* 1990; **322**: 1775–80.

219 Pestronk A, Keogh JP, Griffin JW. Dimethylaminopropionitrile. In: Spencer PS, Schaumburg HH eds. *Experimental and clinical neurotoxicology*. Baltimore, MD: Williams and Wilkins, 1980: 422–9.

220 Peters HA, Levine RL, Matthews CG, Chapman LJ. Extrapyramidal and other neurologic manifestations associated with carbon disulfide fumigant exposure. *Arch Neurol* 1988; **45**: 537–40.

221 Phang PT, Passerini L, Mielke B et al. Brain hemorrhage associated with methanol poisoning. *Crit Care Med* 1988; **16**: 137–40.

222 Picklo MJ, Amaranth V, Graham DG, Montine TJ. Endogenous catechol thioethers may be pro-oxidant or anti-oxidant. *Free Rad Biol Med* 1999; **27**: 271–7.

223 Plum F, Posner JB, Hain RF. Delayed neurological deterioration after anoxia. *Arch Intern Med* 1962; **110**: 56–63.

224 Porter NA, Caldwell SE, Mills KA. Mechanisms of free radical oxidation of unsaturated lipids. *Lipids* 1995; **30**: 277–90.

225 Powell HC, Koch T, Garrett R, Lampert PW. Schwann cell abnormalities in 2,5-hexanedione neuropathy. *J Neurocytol* 1978; **7**: 517–28.

226 Prain JH, Smith GH. A clinical–pathological report of eight cases of methyl bromide poisoning. *Br J Ind Med* 1952; **9**: 44–9.

227 Price R, Jamieson P. The central nervous system in childhood leukemia. II. Subacute leukoencephalopathy. *Cancer* 1975; **35**: 306–18.

228 Prick JJG. Thallium poisoning. In: Vinken PJ, Bruyn GW eds. *Handbook of clinical neurology* Vol. 36. Amsterdam: Elsevier, 1979: 239–78.

229 Pulst S-M, Walshe TM, Romero JA. Carbon monoxide poisoning with features of Gilles de la Tourette's syndrome. *Arch Neurol* 1983; **40**: 443–4.

230 Reusche E, Seydel U. Dialysis-associated encephalopathy: light and electron microscopic morphology and topography with evidence of aluminum by laser microprobe mass analysis. *Acta Neuropathol* 1992; **86**: 249–58.

231 Riggs J, Schochet S, Gutmann L et al. Chronic human colchicine neuropathy and myopathy. *Arch Neurol* 1986; **43**: 521–3.

232 Rizzuto N, Terzian H, Galiazzo-Rizzuto S. Toxic polyneuropathies in Italy due to leather cement poisoning in shoe industries. *J Neurol Sci* 1977; **31**: 343–54.

233 Roberts LJ, Montine TJ, Markesbery WR et al. Formation of isoprostane-like compounds (neuroprostanes) *in vivo* from docosahexaenoic acid. *J Biol Chem* 1998; **273**: 13605–12.

234 Roscher AA. A new histochemical method for the demonstration of calcium oxalate in tissues following ethylene glycol poisoning. *Am J Clin Pathol* 1971; **55**: 99–104.

235 Rosenberg CK, Anthony DC, Szakal-Quin G et al. Hyperbaric oxygen accelerates the neurotoxicity of 2,5-henanedione. *Toxicol Appl Pharmacol* 1987; **87**: 374–9.

236 Rosenberg NL, Kleinschmidt-DeMasters BK, Davis KA et al. Toluene abuse causes diffuse central nervous system white matter changes. *Ann Neurol* 1988; **23**: 611–14.

237 Rosenberg NL, Myers JA, Martin WR. Cyanide-induced parkinsonism: clinical, MRI, and 6-fluorodopa PET studies. *Neurology* 1989; **39**: 142–4.

238 Rosenberg NL, Spitz MC, Filley CM et al. Central nervous system effects of chronic toluene abuse–clinical, brainstem evoked response and magnetic resonance imaging studies. *Neurotoxicol Teratol* 1988; **10**: 489–95.

239 Ross WD, Emmett EA, Steiner J, Tureen R. Neurotoxic effects of occupational exposure to organotins. *Am J Psychiat* 1981; **138**: 1092–5.

240 Rothman SM, Olney JW. Glutamate and the pathophysiology of hypoxic–ischemic brain damage. *Ann Neurol (Paris)* 1986; **19**: 105–11.

241 Roy M, Stip E, Black D et al. Cerebellar degeneration following acute lithium intoxication. *Rev Neurol (Paris)* 1998; **154**: 546–8.

242 Rubinstein L, Herman M, Long T, Wilbur J. Disseminated necrotizing leukoencephalopathy: a complication of treated central nervous system leukemia and lymphoma. *Cancer* 1975; **35**: 291–305.

243 Rydzewski B, Sulkowski W, Miarzynska M. Olfactory disorders induced by cadmium exposure: a clinical study. *Int J Occup Med Environ Health* 1998; **11**: 235–45.

244 Sasaki N, Fukatsu R, Tsuzuki K et al. Advanced glycation end products in Alzheimer's disease and other neurodegenerative diseases. *Am J Pathol* 1998; **153**: 1149–55.

245 Schaumburg HH, Spencer PS. Selected outbreaks of neurotoxic disease. In: Spencer PS, Schaumburg HH eds. *Experimental and clinical neurotoxicology*. Baltimore, MD: Williams and Wilkins, 1980: 883–9.

246 Schochet SS, Lampert PW, Earle KM. Neuronal changes induced by intrathecal vincristine sulfate. *J Neuropathol Exp Neurol* 1968; **27**: 645–7.

247 Schoenberg BS. Environmental risk factors for Parkinson's disease: the epidemiologic evidence. *Can J Neurol Sci* 1987; **14**: 407–13.

248 Schroder JM, Hoheneck M, Weis J, Deist H. Ethylene oxide polyneuropathy: clinical follow-up study with morphometric and electron microscopic findings in a sural nerve biopsy. *Neurology* 1985; **232**: 83–90.

249 Services US Department of Health and Human Services. *Toxicological profile for lead*. Washington, DC: US Department of Health & Human Services, 1993.

250 Shapiro W, Chernik N, Posner J. Necrotizing encephalopathy following intraventricular installation of methotrexate. *Arch Neurol* 1973; **28**: 96–102.

251 Shen XM, Dryhurst G. Further insights into the influence of L-cysteine on the oxidation chemistry of dopamine: reaction pathways of potential relevance to Parkinson's disease. *Chem Res Toxicol* 1996; **9**: 751–63.

252 Shen XM, Xia B, Wrona MZ, Dryhurst G. Synthesis, redox properties, *in vivo* formation, and neurobehavioral effects of *N*-acetylcysteinyl conjugates of dopamine: possible metabolites of relevance to Parkinson's disease. *Chem Res Toxicol* 1996; **9**: 1117–26.

253 Shibata N, Hirano A, Kato S et al. Advanced glycation end-

products are deposited in neuronal hyaline inclusions: a study of familial amyotrophic lateral sclerosis with superoxide dismutase-1 mutation. *Acta Neuropathol* 1999; **97**: 240–6.

254 Shibayama H, Kitoh J, Marui Y *et al*. An unusual case of Pick's disease. *Acta Neuropathol* 1983; **59**: 79–87.

255 Shiraki H. Neuropatholigic aspects of organic mercury intoxication, including Minamata disease. In: Vinken PJ, Bruyn GW eds. *Handbook of clinical neurology* Vol. 36. Amsterdam: Elsevier, 1979: 83–145.

256 Shuman RM, Leech RW, Alvord EC Jr. Neurotoxicity of hexachlorophene in the human: I. A clinicopathologic study of 248 children. *Pediatrics* 1974; **54**: 689–95.

257 Shuman RM, Leech RW, Alvord EC Jr. Neurotoxicity of hexachlorophene in humans. II. A clinicopathological study of 46 premature infants. *Arch Neurol* 1975; **32**: 320–5.

258 Silverman CS, Brenner J, Murtagh FR. Hemorrhagic necrosis and vascular injury in carbon monoxide poisoning: MR demonstration. *Am J Neuroradiol* 1993; **14**: 168–70.

259 Sjogren B, Iregren A, Frech W *et al*. Effects on the nervous system among welders exposed to aluminum and manganese. *Occup Environ Med* 1996; **53**: 32–40.

260 Smith DE. Morphological lesions due to acute and subacute poisoning with antifreeze (ethylene glycol). *Arch Pathol* 1951; **51**: 423–33.

261 Smith M, Sayre L, Monnier V, Perry G. Radical ageing in Alzheimer's disease. *Trends Neurosci* 1995; **18**: 172–6.

262 Smith MA, Harris PLR, Sayre LM, Perry G. Iron accumulation in Alzheimer's disease is a source of redox-generated free radicals. *Proc Natl Acad Sci USA* 1997; **94**: 9866–8.

263 Smith MA, Taneda S, Richey PL *et al*. Advanced Maillard reaction end products are associated with Alzheimer disease pathology. *Proc Natl Acad Sci USA* 1994; **91**: 5710–14.

264 Spach D, Bauwens J, Clark C, Burke W. Rhabdomyolysis associated with lovastatin and erythromycin use. *West J Med* 1991; **154**: 213–15.

265 Spatt J, Glawar B, Mamoli B. A pure amnestic syndrome after MDMA ('ecstasy') ingestion. *Neurol Neurosurg Psych* 1997; **62**: 418–19.

266 Spencer JPE, Jenner P, Daniel SE *et al*. Conjugates of catecholamines with cysteine and GSH in Parkinson's disease: possible mechanisms of formation involving reactive oxygen species. *J Neurochem* 1998; **71**: 2112–22.

267 Spencer PS, Couri D, Schaumburg HH. *n*-Hexane and methyl *n*-butyl ketone. In: Spencer PS, Schaumburg HH eds. *Experimental and clinical neurotoxicology*. Baltimore, MD: Williams and Wilkins, 1980: 456–75.

268 Spencer PS, Ludolph AC, Kisby GE. Are human neurodegenerative disorders linked to environmental chemicals with excitotoxic properties? In: Langston JW, Young A eds. *Neurotoxins and neurodegenerative disease*. New York: New York Academy of Sciences, 1992: 154–60.

269 Spencer PS, Schaumburg HH, Raleigh RL, Terhaar CJ. Nervous system degeneration produced by the industrial solvent methyl *n*-butyl ketone. *Arch Neurol* 1975; **32** 219–22.

270 Squier MV, Thompson J, Rajgopalan B. Case report: neuropathology of methyl bromide intoxication. *Neuropathol Appl Neurobiol* 1992; **18**: 579–84.

271 St. Clair MBG, Amarnath V, Moody MA *et al*. Pyrrole oxidation and protein cross-linking as necessary steps in the development of γ-diketone neuropathy. *Chem Res Toxicol* 1988; **1**: 179–85.

272 Takedo A, Yasuda T, Miyata T *et al*. Immunohistochemical study of advanced glycation end products in ageing and Alzheimer's disease brain. *Neurosci Lett* 1996; **221**: 17–20.

273 Tanner C. Epidemiology of Parkinson's disease. *Neurol Clin* 1992; **10**: 317–29.

274 Tanner CM, Langston JW. Do environmental toxins cause Parkinson's disease? A critical review. *Neurology* 1990; **3**: 17–30.

275 Teitelbaum JS, Zatorre RJ, Carpenter S *et al*. Neurologic sequellae of domoic acid intoxication due to the ingestion of contaminated mussels. *N Engl J Med* 1990; **322**: 1781–7.

276 Thomke F, Jung D, Besser R *et al*. Increased risk of sensory neuropathy in workers with chloracne after exposure to 2,3,7,8-polychlorinated dioxins and furans. *Acta Neurol Scand* 1999; **100**: 1–5.

277 Thompson S, Davis L, Kornfeld M *et al*. Cisplatin neuropathy. Clinical, electrophysiologic, morphologic and toxicologic studies. *J Cancer* 1984; **54**: 1269–75.

278 Tilson H, Jacobson J, Rogan W. Polychlorinated biphenyls and the developing nervous system: cross-species comparisons. *Neurotoxicol Teratol* 1990; **12**: 239–48.

279 Towfighi J, Gonatas NK, Pleasure D *et al*. Glue sniffer's neuropathy. *Neurology* 1976; **26**: 238–43.

280 Uitti RJ, Rajput AH, Ashenhurst EM, Rozdilsky B. Cyanide-induced parkinsonism: a clinicopathologic report. *Neurology* 1985; **35**: 921–5.

281 Usuki E, Pearce R, Parkinson A, Castagnol NJ. Studies on the conversion of haloperidol and its tetrahydropyridine dehydration product to potentially neurotoxic pyridinium metabolites by human liver microsomes. *Chem Res Toxicol* 1996; **9**: 800–6.

282 Valentine WM, Amarnath V, Graham DG, Anthony DC. Covalent cross-linking of proteins by carbon disulfide. *Chem Res Toxicol* 1992; **5**: 254–62.

283 Valenzuela R, Court J, Godoy J. Delayed cyanide induced dystonia. *J Neurol Neurosurg Psychiat* 1992; **55**: 198–9.

284 Valpey R, Sumi SM, Copass MK, Goble GJ. Acute and chronic progressive encephalopathy due to gasoline sniffing. *Neurology* 1978; **28**: 507–10.

285 van Rossum F, Ross R, Bouts G. Disulfiram polyneuropathy. *Clin Neurol Neurosurg* 1984; **86**: 81–7.

286 Vescovi A, Facheris L, Zaffaroni A *et al*. Dopamine metabolism alterations in a manganese-treated pheochromocytoma cell line (PC12). *Toxicology* 1991; **67**: 129–42.

287 Vescovi A, Gebbia M, Cappelletti G *et al*. Interactions of manganese with human brain glutathione-*S*-transferase. *Toxicology* 1989; **57**: 183–91.

288 Vingerhoets F, Snow B, Tetrud J *et al*. Positron emission tomographic evidence of progression of human MPTP-included dopaminergic lesions. *Ann Neurol* 1994; **36**: 765–70.

289 Wasay M, Bakshi R, Kojan S *et al*. Superior sagittal sinus thrombosis due to lithium: local urokinase thrombolysis treatment. *Neurology* 2000; **54**: 532–3.

290 Wilson J, Kalasinsky K, Levey A *et al*. Striatal dopamine nerve terminal markers in human, chronic methamphetamine users. *Nat Med* 1996; **2**: 699–703.

291 Wilson J, Levey A, Bergeron C *et al*. Striatal dopamine, dopamine transporter, and vesicular monoamine transporter in chronic cocaine users. *Ann Neurol* 1996; **40**: 428–39.

292 Winder H, Tetrud J, Rehncrona S *et al*. Bilateral fetal mesencephalic grafting in two patients with parkinsonism induced by 1-methyl-4-phenyl-1,2,3,6-tetrahydropyridine (MPTP). *N Engl J Med* 1992; **327**: 1556–63.

293 Wisniewski K, Dambska M, Sher JH, Qazi Q. A clinical neuropathological study of the fetal alcohol syndrome. *Neuropediatrics* 1983; **14**: 197–201.

294 Wolters EC, Huang C-C, Clark C *et al*. Positron emission tomography in manganese intoxication. *Ann Neurol* 1989; **26**: 647–51.

295 Yamada M, Ohno S, Okayasu I *et al*. Chronic manganese poisoning: a neuropathological study with determination of manganese distribution in the brain. *Acta Neuropathol* 1986; **70**: 273–8.

296 Yamada S. An occurrence of polyneuritis by *n*-hexane in the polyethylene laminating plants. *Jpn J Ind Health* 1964; **6**: 192–6.

297 Yan SD, Chen X, Schmidt AM *et al*. Glycated tau protein in Alzheimer disease: a mechanism for induction of oxidant stress. *Proc Natl Acad Sci USA* 1994; **91**: 7787–91.

298 Yan SD, Zhu H, Fu J *et al*. Amyloid-beta peptide-receptor for advanced glycation endproduct interaction elicits neuronal expression of macrophage-colony stimulating factor: a proinflammatory pathway in Alzheimer disease. *Proc Natl Acad Sci USA* 1997; **94**: 5296–301.

299 Yoritaka A, Hattori N, Uchida K *et al*. Immunohistochemical detection of 4-hydroxynonenal protein adducts in Parkinson disease. *Proc Natl Acad Sci USA* 1995; **93**: 2696–701.

300 Zatuchni J, Hong K. Methyl bromide poisoning seen initially as psychosis. *Arch Neurol* 1981; **38**: 529–30.

301 Zhang J, Graham DG, Montine TJ, Ho YS. Enhanced *N*-methyl-4-phenyl-1,2,3,6-tetrahydropyridine toxicity in mice deficient in Cu/Zn-superoxide dismutase or glutathione peroxidase. *J Neuropathol Exp Neurol* 2000; **59**: 53–61.

302 Zhang J, Price JO, Graham DG, Montine TJ. Secondary excitotoxicity contributes to dopamine-induced apoptosis of dopaminergic neuronal cultures. *Biochem Biophys Res Commun* 1998; **248**: 812–16.

303 Zigmond M, Hastings T, Abercrombie E. Neurochemical responses to 6-hydroxydopamine and L-DOPA therapy: implications for Parkinson's disease. *Ann NY Acad Sci* 1992; **648**: 71–82.

304 Zuckerman B, Frank DA, Hingson R *et al*. Effects of maternal marijuana and cocaine use on fetal growth. *N Engl J Med* 1989; **320**: 762–8.

14

Trauma

DAVID I. GRAHAM, TOM A. GENNARELLI AND TRACY K. McINTOSH

INTRODUCTION

Brain damage resulting from a head injury, often referred to as traumatic brain injury (TBI), is complex. The different causes, mechanisms, types and distributions of brain injury will be reviewed in this chapter.

Head injury, 'a silent epidemic', remains an important problem in modern society: deaths from head injury comprise 1–2% of all deaths from all causes, and between one-third and one-half of all deaths due to trauma result from head injury.[206] In a study that analysed 174 160 injured patients, those with head injury comprised 34% of all the cases, but resulted in 62% of all the deaths,[186] there being a three times higher mortality in patients with a head injury than in those without a head injury. Of the survivors, those with a head injury were substantially more impaired than those without a head injury; the latter, therefore, also being an important cause of morbidity.[185]

The nature and distribution of TBI are diverse and there are many influences on the outcome from head injury. The process of head injury can be separated into four phases: the primary injury, the delayed consequences of the primary injury, secondary or additional injury, and recovery and functional outcome, each of which may be modulated by numerous factors (Fig. 14.1). The precise type, location and extent (size) of primary injury are determined by the proximate cause, that is, whether the injury is produced by a road traffic accident, a fall, an assault or by a gunshot. Furthermore, the primary injury is influenced by host factors such as age, pre-existing disease, psychosocial status and whether the nutritional status is optimal prior to injury. Certainly the influence of sedative, psychoactive or other exogenous drugs, and particularly alcohol, influence the primary injury.[628,651] Most recently recognized has been the role of the genetic make-up of the individual in the response and outcome from TBI.[163,513,583]

The delayed consequences of the primary injury have only recently begun to be understood. These are various events that have been triggered by the primary injury and include neurobiological processes involving cellular dysfunction such as free radical formation, receptor-mediated mechanisms, and calcium- and inflammation-mediated damage. In various combinations and degrees of severity, the resultant cellular dysfunction defines the nature and extent of the primary injury, the outcome of which may not become apparent for several days or even weeks after the injury.

Additional or secondary injury can be produced by many factors including ischaemia, raised intracranial pressure, seizures, infection, brain swelling or the influences from extracranial injury. Eventually, the recovery and functional outcome are the products of the primary injury and its delayed consequences, the secondary injury, and

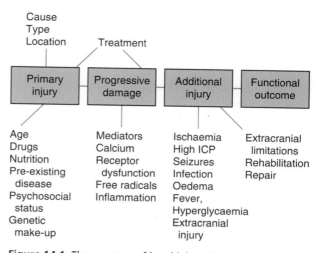

Figure 14.1 *The progress of head injury. Head injury is shown as a process that has many influences as it proceeds from primary injury to functional outcome.*

the repair and rehabilitation that are achieved. The influence of extracranial complications, such as heterotopic ossification or joint contractures, will also limit the functional outcome.

Blunt (non-missile) injury and penetrating head injury are the two main types of head injury.

BLUNT HEAD INJURY

Brain damage resulting from a blunt head injury is particularly distressing as many of the patients are adolescent or in early adult life, remain severely or moderately disabled,[283] and require care in institutions or from their families for many years.[286,386,428] Even if physical disability is not severe, the cognitive and behavioural problems or changes in personality may become a great strain on family and friends.[81] Intentional injuries due to homicides, assaults and suicides or unintentional injuries due to falls or road traffic accidents are the leading causes of death under the age of 45 years in industrialized nations, and head injuries account for between 25 and 33% of all deaths from trauma.[327] Each year in the UK there are some nine deaths from head injury per 100 000 population and they account for 1% of all deaths and 25% of deaths from trauma. Death rates from head injuries are even higher in the USA and in Australia.[327] A survey of head injuries by the European Brain Injury Consortium found that 3% of patients with head injury remained vegetative and 16% were severely disabled, 20% moderately disabled and 31% had made a good recovery 6 months after their injury.[427] The accumulating population of disabled survivors from head injury results in an estimated prevalence in the USA of 24 per 100 000 population per year with major persisting impairment, i.e. about 64 600 individuals.[327] This estimate is much less than that derived earlier because of the 25% decline in hospital admission rates seen in recent years. There is, however, hope that some causes of head injury are becoming less common. Head injuries due to road traffic accidents seem to be effectively mitigated by modern protective devices such as the combination of seatbelts and airbags. These are substantially reducing the number of severe brain injuries.[475]

It is difficult to overemphasize the importance of blunt head injury. Attempts at prevention must clearly continue but so also must the identification of at least potentially avoidable factors such as the delayed recognition of intracranial haematoma[111,528] and the appropriate medical treatment of the processes that may be triggered by the injury.[364,365,590]

The genesis of blunt head injuries

The types of mechanical loading to the head are numerous and complex[187] and include static loading and the various types of dynamic loading (Fig. 14.2). Static loading occurs when forces are applied to the head gradually and is usually a slow process. Although this mechanism is uncommon, it does occur in situations such as earthquakes and landslides in which the head is squeezed slowly or is crushed, usually taking more than 200 ms to develop. Sufficient force results in multiple, comminuted or 'eggshell' fractures of the vault or base of the skull. However, coma and severe neurological signs, except from damaged cranial nerves, are characteristically not seen until the skull deformation is so severe that the brain becomes compressed and distorted, at which time serious or fatal brain laceration occurs.

The most common mechanical input to the head is dynamic loading. In this instance the forces causing injury act in less than 200 ms, and in most cases in less than 20 ms. The duration of the loading is a critical factor in determining the type of head injury produced. Dynamic loading can be of two types: impulsive or impact. Impulsive loading occurs when the head is set into motion or when the moving head is stopped without its being either struck or arrested by impact. These conditions are not infrequent since a blow to the thorax or face can often set the head into violent motion without direct impact to the skull. In these circumstances, there is no impact to the cranium and thus contact does not occur. The resulting head injuries are caused solely by the inertia produced by the manner in which the head has moved. Although there is no doubt that facial impact can cause sufficient forces in the brain to result in any of the inertial injuries, recent evidence has raised the question of whether this is true for situations not involving impact to the face. It is not certain that in real-world accidents sufficiently high levels of inertial forces develop to produce serious inertial injuries if impact to the head or face does not occur.[407] Thus, when the head is stopped or set into motion by indirect impact to the chest or thorax, it is not clear whether situations occur in which the head moves in the appropriate manner to generate the high-intensity strains necessary to cause the full spectrum of inertial injuries.

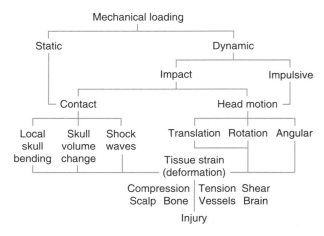

Figure 14.2 *Mechanical events that contribute to primary head injury.*

Impact loading occurs when a blunt object strikes the head and is the most common type of dynamic loading. It usually results in a combination of contact and inertia, i.e. sudden deceleration of the head when the cranium hits the ground, e.g. the drunk, against a windscreen, wall, etc., or as a result of a car crash. The response of the head to impact is dependent on the blunt object that strikes the head or on the object that the head strikes. For example, inertia can be minimal in certain impact conditions, especially if the head is prevented from moving when it is struck. The result is that most of the impact energy is delivered to the head as contact and results in a complex set of effects collectively known as contact phenomena. These contact phenomena are a group of mechanical events that occur both near to and distant from the point of impact. The magnitude and importance of these events vary with the size of the impacting object and with the magnitude of the force delivered to the contact point. The latter is determined by the mass, surface area, velocity and hardness of the impacting object. These factors determine the manner in which energy is transferred to the head. For objects larger than 5.0 cm^2, localized skull deformation occurs with in-bending of the skull immediately beneath the point of impact and out-bending of the skull peripheral to the impact site. If the degree of local skull deformation exceeds the tolerance of the skull, fracture occurs. Penetration, perforation or localized depressed fracture of the skull is more likely if the object has a surface area less than 5.0 cm^2. In addition, shock waves that travel at the speed of sound propagate throughout the skull from the point of impact, as well as directly through the brain. The shock waves cause local changes in tissue pressure. If these changes cause sufficient brain distortion, then small localized intraparenchymal petechial haemorrhages result.

Strain or brain deformation is the proximate cause of tissue injury, whether induced by inertia or by contact. There are three types of strain: compression, tension and shear. The injury that results in a given circumstance is determined by the type and location of the induced strains and by the ability of the tissue to withstand those particular strains. Strain is best understood as the amount of deformation that the tissue undergoes as a result of a mechanical force (the stress) being applied. Tensile strain, for example, is the amount of elongation that occurs when a material is stretched. If a column of rubber 10 cm in length becomes 11 cm when stretched by hanging a 100-g weight from it, it undergoes a 10% tensile strain (stretched length minus original length divided by original length). In contrast, a glass column under the same stress or load (100 g) may become only 10.1 cm long, i.e. a 1% strain. The inherent properties of these two materials are different, not only in how much strain occurs under identical loading conditions but also with regard to how much strain is necessary to cause failure (breakage) of the material. Thus, the rubber column may tolerate a 20% strain before it breaks, whereas the glass column

may break with a 0.5% strain. In this example, the glass rod would have broken but the rubber column would not, even though the rubber underwent greater strain. This example demonstrates static strain, in which the duration of applied force is very long. Dynamic strain occurs in situations in which the load is applied briefly and is a more complicated mechanism because of a property of biological tissues called viscoelasticity. A viscoelastic material is one in which tolerance to strain changes with the rate at which the material is loaded. Characteristically, biological tissues withstand strain better if they are deformed slowly rather than quickly, i.e. they become more brittle and will break at lower strain levels under rapidly applied loads. The three principal tissues affected in head injury – bone, blood vessels and brain – vary considerably in their tolerance to deformation. Bone, for example, is considerably stronger than vascular or brain tissue and more force is therefore required to induce injurious levels of strain. The amount of strain that bone can tolerate is less than that needed to injure the brain, i.e. bone breaks at a strain of 1–2%, whereas brain and vascular tissue may not tear unless a 10–20% strain is applied. It does, however, take considerable force to cause a 1–2% strain in bone. Bone shares with vascular tissue and brain the property of being able to withstand compressive strain better than shear or tensile strain. There is proportionately less difference between the three strain tolerances for bone, whereas there is a considerable difference in the ability of brain tissue to withstand compression and shear.

Since the brain is virtually incompressible *in vivo* and since it has a very low tolerance to tensile and shear strain, the latter two types of strain are the usual causes of brain damage. The same is true for vascular tissue. Whether damage to vascular tissue or brain occurs depends on the exact properties of these two tissues. Vascular tissue tends to fail under more rapidly applied loads than does the brain and, depending on the type of input to the head, conditions exist that can cause relatively pure injury to the vascular tissues or to the tissues of the brain within the skull.

Experimental models of human blunt TBI

Two reciprocal hypotheses are implicit in experimental models that produce injury to the brain: namely that human TBI can be duplicated in non-humans, and that non-human TBI replicates human injury. Associated with these hypotheses are assumptions including the view that the mechanism of production of the TBI is not important, and that species differences can be ignored. It may be argued that, if the desired type of brain injury can be produced, the mechanism by which the injury is produced is irrelevant. However, the knowledge of the precise mechanism has important implications for the prevention, mitigation and development of safety measures in 'real-life' injury. That species differences can be ignored is less easy to accept, because anatomical, physiological and, perhaps, receptor, neurotransmitter and genomic differences between species are quite profound. Thus, an injury model may have a substantially different response to the same input because, for example, an injury may occur in a different neurochemical pathway.

Although the earliest recorded experimental head injuries were performed by Galen on piglets,[169] the geneology of modern models of experimental brain injury stems from the work of Denny-Brown and Russell.[122] In a series of elegant studies, they divided experimental brain injury into two principal categories which were named acceleration concussion and percussion concussion. They were able to reproduce the clinical state of concussion by delivering controlled blows to the freely movable head by a calibrated pendulum, a situation similar to the common clinical one of an impact to a head that is free to move. Denny-Brown and Russell[122] also established that acceleration of the head was a vital factor in the production of concussion since it was much more difficult to produce if the head was fixed. These two general categories are still recognized today and it remains useful to continue to classify current models of head injury into these two categories. Models using fluid percussion and rigid indentation are essentially the modern versions of Denny-Brown and Russell's percussion concussion and both can be produced by percussion to the dura centrally, or laterally with contralateral dural opening. In fluid percussion, a small volume of fluid is injected into the extradural space, most commonly by an impacted fluid column or, more recently, by rapid pump infusion.[596] Models using a solid indenter that is rapidly applied to the dura at varying velocities and depths of indentation are the modern versions of rigid percussion. Inertial injury models and impact acceleration models are the modern versions of Denny-Brown and Russell's acceleration concussion. Models of inertial injury apply an acceleration to the head without impact or, more properly in most cases, by distributing loading widely to minimize the effects of impact. Impact acceleration models provide impact through an impactor, a piston or a weight dropped either directly onto the skull or onto a steel plate attached to the skull that serves to minimize localized skull loading and fracture. Special types of models of TBI have also been developed. Injection models inject fluid or blood into the extradural, subdural or intracerebral compartments, while local tensile models provide an underpressure or a suction injury to the intact or opened dura.[391,460]

FLUID PERCUSSION MODELS

The similarities outnumber the differences between fluid and rigid percussion models. However, central and lateral input sites differ. Both central and lateral fluid percussion models are characterized by brief behavioural unresponsiveness (e.g. coma) and metabolic alterations as well as changes in cerebral blood flow and blood–brain barrier (BBB) permeability. Motor as well as memory deficits have been characterized in both models, but few direct comparisons between the two models have been made.[384,523]

Central fluid percussion

Central fluid percussion tends to cause variable and relatively small contusions in the vicinity of the fluid pulse than does lateral fluid percussion. In addition, in the cat and rat there is scattered axonal damage mainly in the brainstem.[538] Direct axial movement of the lower brainstem has been implicated as the cause for these changes.[585]

Lateral fluid percussion

This widely used model is also characterized by variable contusions which tend to be ipsilateral to the percussion site, although a small amount of histological change has been seen in the contralateral hemisphere.[368] There is unilateral axonal damage scattered throughout the white matter of the ipsilateral cerebral hemisphere, as well as an occasional tissue tear at the junction between deep grey and white matter.[55,222] Hippocampal damage, principally unilateral, is more characteristic of this model than of the central fluid percussion model,[550] but in contrast, there is less brainstem abnormality with lateral than with central percussion. Lateral fluid percussion with contralateral craniotomy and dural opening has been attempted to parallel similar models using rigid indentation, but this model has little to offer at the moment.

RIGID PERCUSSION MODELS

Central rigid percussion

As described in the ferret[348] and more recently in the rat,[128] central rigid percussion can produce a variable-sized contusion in the parasagittal cortex beneath the impact, and coma of variable duration. Axonal damage has been described in the ventral halves of the cerebral hemispheres, but not scattered widely through the convexities as in human diffuse traumatic axonal injury (DAI).

Lateral rigid percussion

Relatively brief coma is produced by this model, which is consistent with the small amount of axonal damage seen scattered throughout the hemispheres. There is, however, axonal damage at the periphery of the indentation and in the hemisphere beneath the indentation there is a variable-sized contusion.

Lateral rigid percussion with contralateral dural opening

This model also produces brief coma, but the amount of contusional damage can be altered to be more on the coup side (ipsilateral to impact) than on the contrecoup side (contralateral to impact), depending on the input conditions. Hemispheric axonal damage occurs in both locations around and lateral to the contusional injuries, but there is relatively little widespread hemispheric or brainstem axonal damage.

ACCELERATION MODELS

Inertial acceleration models

These, depending on the acceleration conditions, can produce relatively pure acute subdural haematoma,[190] brief disturbances of consciousness or prolonged coma and DAI.[191,549] The latter is associated with haemorrhagic tissue tears in the central white matter, as well as at the parasagittal grey–white junction (so-called gliding contusions). These models tend to be characterized by a variable period of coma, and widespread axonal damage throughout the white matter of the cerebral hemispheres, the upper brainstem and the cerebellum.[28,86,363,546,549,552]

Impact acceleration models

Although the first impact acceleration models were characterized principally by variable-sized contusions which, to some degree, could be altered depending on the impact characteristics,[156,541,595] prolonged coma has been produced in a more recent model with widespread axonal damage.[383] These models continue to be characterized by variable and somewhat uncontrolled skull fractures.[346]

INJECTION MODELS

The injection of blood and other fluids intracranially has been used to study various types of haematoma. The injection of blood into the subdural space mimics acute subdural haematoma,[69,138,414] and there are characteristically large areas of necrosis underlying the subdural haematoma of the type not infrequently seen in man. Injection into the extradural space has been used in the past principally to study intracranial pressure (ICP) dynamics. Similarly, the injection of blood in the brain to create an intracerebral haematoma to determine the relationship between regional blood flow and metabolism, and ICP has been studied.[277]

LOCAL TENSILE LOADING MODELS

Application of local tensile loading, or suction, to the intact or open dura has been proposed as a localized model of coup contusion by several groups. Whether the application is by suction through a syringe or applied through a specially modified fluid percussion device, the models are characterized by the absence of generalized cerebral phenomena or coma, and by a discrete, well-localized coup contusion that is confined to the area of suction.

IN VITRO MODELS

The mechanical-loading conditions leading to traumatic axonal injury have been studied using tissue in culture.[170,358,420,425,554,621] These have shown that the causes of cellular damage are complex and involve multiple pathways that may end in dysfunction or death. These pathways include ionic derangements, excitotoxicity, free radical generation, lipid damage and disruption of the cytoskeleton.

The important models

Cerebral concussion is common in man after a head injury,[182] and both acceleration and percussion concussion appear to have been achieved experimentally, at least in short-term behavioural changes. Diffuse brain injury is, however, more important with regard to patients who die or remain vegetative or impaired.[15,16,282,374] Models using acceleration concussion appear to duplicate this better than percussion concussion, but the degree of replication to man is less than that seen with concussion. The exception may be the severe end of diffuse brain injury, where widespread diffuse traumatic axonal injury occurs. This condition appears to be quite faithfully replicated by an angular acceleration model.[191,549]

Contusion is another common clinical phenomenon and appears to be reproduced by suction and local tensile models more closely and without distant or global effects compared with other models. Percussion models produce contusion as well, but have associated concussive events. The only other common model of injury is that of acute subdural haematoma, which is frequent in human head injury, and is associated with a poor outcome.[188] This condition remains poorly modelled in general, but some phenomena are replicated well by injection and acceleration. Skull fracture, brain swelling and extradural haematoma are currently not well duplicated routinely and consistently by any of the existing models. Intracerebral haematoma, which occurs in a small but important number of patients, is perhaps best modelled by injection, but there are too few recent studies to judge its ability to mimic the clinical condition.

It is possible to summarize the specific attributes of each model in terms of its ability to reproduce abnormalities known to occur in human head injury.[181,486] Cerebral concussion can be produced by all varieties of fluid percussion and rigid indentation. Inertial injury and impact acceleration also adequately reproduce concussive events, whereas injection and suction models do not. Axonal injury can be produced in a limited manner by central and lateral fluid percussion and by central and lateral rigid indentation. A larger amount of axonal damage can be produced by impact acceleration and by rigid indentation with contralateral dural opening.[309] Models using inertial acceleration are perhaps the best to replicate the pattern of axonal damage seen in man. Injection and suction models are not useful for axonal injury. Contusional injury can be produced by many models, perhaps the best and most specific being local tensile models. Models based on impact acceleration, inertial acceleration, and fluid and rigid percussion can also mimic contusion, but are often compounded by other pathological changes. Subdural haematoma is best replicated by injection and by inertial acceleration. Again, there are not any good models that produce brain swelling, intracerebral haematoma or skull fracture.

The plethora of models designed to study brain injury stresses the fact that brain injury is complex. Therefore, matching injury models to man must always allow for this complexity. For example, it must be remembered that human head injury is rarely ever as pure as in experimental models. From a clinical series, solitary lesions in humans occur in 26% of cases while two, three or more than three lesions occur in 26%, 21% and 27%, respectively.[182] As injury severity worsens, the multiplicity of lesions increases and, perhaps except for very acute deaths, the incidence of single lesions in an autopsy series of head-injured patients will be almost zero.

It is likely that after the adaptation of the controlled cortical impact model[240,553] and the fluid percussion injury model[82] to the mouse there will be an increasing use of transgenic animals.[426,429,561,618,639] Thus, since the total complexity of human injury may not be adequately addressed in the purer and simplified animal models, there exists the concern that some models may be studying traumatic phenomena rather than traumatic disease.[183]

Current concepts of the pathophysiology of traumatic brain injury

It has been recognized since Neolithic times that injury to the head, and particularly to the brain, triggers a complex set of events (Fig. 14.3). That brain injury is complex is not a new concept, since it has long been recognized that it has different causes, and there are different mechanisms of damage that result in different types of clinical injury. These tend to be recognized as having a different pathophysiology and therefore requiring different treatments.[75]

PRINCIPLES OF HEAD INJURY CARE

The current care of the head-injured patient emphasizes four principles: evacuation of mass lesions, detection and treatment of increased ICP, prevention and treatment of cerebral ischaemia, and treatment of systemic (extracranial) complications. Although these principles have been recognized for some time, their achievement remains difficult in daily clinical practice. For example, the incidence of avoidable cerebral ischaemic events remains disproportionately high. In achieving these current principles in

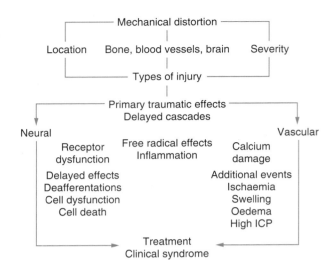

Figure 14.3 *Mechanisms of brain injury. A complex set of events is triggered by mechanical loading of the brain: some are immediate, others are delayed.*

management, control of intracranial hypertension remains of foremost clinical importance. The management of ICP in general includes the following possible regimens: the correct positioning of the head, sedation, paralysis, hyperventilation, the administration of mannitol or other hyperosmotic agents, drainage of cerebrospinal fluid (CSF), barbiturates, hypothermia, hyperintense hyperosmolality and radical decompressive craniotomy. Clinical research continues to try to clarify the order of priority of these types of treatment, and perhaps in the future there will be agreement as to their best sequence. The prevention and management of cerebral ischaemia have played an important role in the care of the head-injured patient because it has become well recognized that superimposed ischaemia results in a substantially worse outcome. The general concept is to match cerebral blood flow to the particular metabolic needs of the brain after injury. In order to do so, hypotension must be avoided and the patient can be better managed in a normovolaemic than in a hypovolaemic state. Preservation of cerebral perfusion pressure, i.e. the difference between the mean arterial and intracranial pressures, requires that it remains above 9.3 kPa (70 mmHg) in order to avoid deleteriously low cerebral oxygenation. Cerebral oxygenation should be optimized to ensure that the delivery and utilization of oxygen are appropriate to the metabolic needs of the brain; one way of achieving this is to ensure that the jugulovenous oxygen saturation is greater than 55%. Minimizing secondary insults caused by hyperthermia or hyperglycaemia requires that body temperature be kept at less than 38°C and that the serum glucose does not exceed 200 mg/dl.[75,95]

Using these principles, head injuries are treated according to the type of injury. A clinical distinction between focal and diffuse brain damage is important because of the potential need for surgical evacuation of mass lesions. Therefore, it has been held that focal brain injuries are fundamentally different from diffuse brain injuries. Certainly the potential cascade of events that can follow the localized damage in focal injury is different from the more global changes that may result when the brain damage is diffuse. However, the pathophysiology of the two share many common events, and these will now be discussed.

Brain injury can be viewed as a clinical syndrome, a phenotype resulting from a combination of principally neural and/or vascular events brought about by mechanical distortion of the head. The primary traumatic events appear to be mediated by four basic mechanisms, the consequences of which are not instantaneous. Thus, brain injury involves processes that are set in motion at the time of head injury, but may require hours or days to achieve completion. These four mechanisms of cellular abnormality are receptor dysfunction, free radical oxidative effects, calcium-mediated damage and inflammatory events, and can therefore have the potential for causing delayed cell damage or delayed cell death. These events, depending on whether they primarily affect neural or vascular tissue, may produce additional events or epiphenomena, such as brain swelling, cerebral oedema and increased ICP. This sequence of events may be similar in focal and diffuse brain injuries, but appears to be different because of varying degrees of involvement of neural and vascular tissues, and because of combinations of the types of cellular dysfunction.

The initial traumatic events

Comparing research into the pathophysiology of TBI to that of cerebral ischaemia discloses many similarities between the two; indeed it is difficult to distinguish brain injury due to trauma from that due to ischaemia. One difference, however, is that the initial events of trauma involve mechanical distortion of the brain. Primary mechanical disruption of axons and instantaneous cell death are relatively uncommon in TBI. Rather, a possible initial abnormality in TBI is mechanoporation.[192] Mechanoporation is the creation of a traumatic defect in the cell membrane that occurs as the lipid bilayer is transiently separated from the stiffer protein inclusions such as receptors or channels. This event provides the opportunity for considerable ionic fluxes, whereby ions of many species rapidly move either into or out of the cell according to their preinjury concentration gradients. Thus, there would be initial movement of potassium to the outside and sodium, chloride and calcium to the inside of the cell.

It is likely that the traumatic membrane defect is present for only a relatively brief period and that within minutes, or perhaps at most a few hours, this defect closes, either by simple flow of the lipid bilayer or by an active process due to calcium-activated phospholipase A_2 (PLA_2) generation of lysolecithin patching, fusion of the membrane[635] or other mechanisms.[157] The persistence of traumatic membrane defects by achieving a metastable state of the micropore is less likely. However, the magnitude of the traumatic membrane defects will parallel the amount of tissue deformation which, in turn, can be measured by the amount of immediate traumatic ionic flux. For example, when changes in intracellular calcium in isolated axons or in nerve cells in tissue culture subjected to deformation are measured, there are transient rises in intracellular calcium that parallel the amount of injury delivered to the system.[167] In mild cases, intracellular calcium levels become normal after seconds to minutes, but in more severe cases, even without tissue disruption, intracellular calcium can rise to such high levels that it becomes injurious to the cell and can result in delayed events.[183,366]

There is increasing evidence that mechanically induced depolarization and other changes are likely to result in aberrant cell signalling pathways which will be subsequently reflected in an acute genomic response.[535] Using well-characterized experimental models of TBI, the temporal and regional patterns of induction of various classes of genes such as the immediate-early gene and heat shock proteins have been studied. The immediate-early genes c-fos, c-Jun and jun B are transcription factors that regulate the expression of a variety of target genes that include growth factors, cytoskeletal proteins and metabolic enzymes, and it has been suggested that the classic stress proteins – the heat shock proteins – might have a neuroprotective role in vivo. A wide range of disorders including TBI induces the immediate-early genes. After TBI there is a very rapid rise and then a fall in the immediate-early genes, but the relationship between this response and subsequent structural changes and any post-traumatic memory deficit is not known. However, the pattern of immediate-early gene induction after fluid percussion brain injury is similar to that observed in models of seizures, focal and global ischaemia and hypoxia–ischaemia. The protein Fos forms a heterodimer with Jun and regulates the expression of certain target genes including nerve growth factor, amyloid precursor protein and opioid precursor proteins, all of which have been shown to be upregulated after TBI. In addition, the expression of fos and jun has been associated with synaptic plasticity and programmed cell death (apoptosis), an event that has been recently described in TBI.

After ischaemia, seizures and trauma there is an induction of the 72 heat shock protein (HSP72). Immunoreactivity is seen in neurons, glia and endothelial cells, particularly around the site of maximal injury. These responses are in contrast to the glucose-regulated proteins grp78 and grp94, which share sequence homology with HSP72 but are only mildly affected following fluid percussion brain injury. The precise role of heat shock protein induction in response to central nervous system (CNS) disease has still not been defined and may simply serve as a marker of a generalized stress response injury.

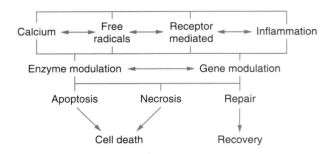

Figure 14.4 *Cellular damage after head injury.*

It appears that after the initial events of TBI, delayed cellular dysfunction may occur by numerous mechanisms. The most studied of these cascades of events include inflammation, receptor-mediated dysfunction, free radical and oxidative damage and calcium- or other ion-mediated damage (Fig. 14.4). The sum of the results of these processes will modulate gene expression or protein regulation and ultimately lead to cell death or repair by mechanisms still under investigation (see below). However, the phenotype of TBI may be largely determined by the combination and severity of these processes (Fig. 14.5). Here, the potential interactions between these four major mechanisms of delayed cellular damage are depicted. In differing types of TBI, one or several of these mechanisms may be predominant and some may be unimportant for that specific type of TBI. This hypothetical mechanism is illustrated in Fig. 14.6, where the brain damage associated with subdural haematoma, contusion and DAI is shown for illustrative purpose. DAI is proposed to have relatively little damage associated with inflammation, whereas inflammation is shown as the predominant mechanism for brain damage in contusion. Recent evidence suggests that widespread neuronal loss is progressive and continuous for many months or years postinjury.[54,129,470,548] The mechanisms underlying delayed cell death may be due to the release or activation of endogenous 'autodestructive' pathways. This new information has underpinned the development of novel ther-

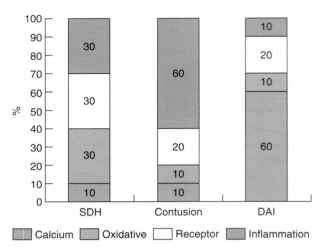

Figure 14.6 *Phenotypes of traumatic brain injury and cellular cascades.*

apeutic agents designed to modify gene expression, the synthesis and release of substances, receptor or functional activity with subsequent modulation of cellular damage and improvement in the neurological and behavioural outcomes.[67,134]

Cellular and molecular consequences of TBI

BRAIN INJURY AND NEURODEGENERATIVE DISEASES

Head injury has been convincingly implicated as a risk factor for Alzheimer's disease (AD) in several epidemiological studies[29,57,104,234,251,404,422] (Fig. 14.7). Brain damage associated with dementia pugilistica (punch-drunk syndrome) and its associated neurobehavioural picture of memory loss and Parkinson-like symptoms include diffuse beta-amyloid (Aβ) deposits and neurofibrillary tangles,[179,591] both of which have also been identified and associated with brain trauma (see below). Most experimental brain injury studies in rodents, however, have been unable to find evidence for diffuse or neuritic Aβ plaques. However, in experimental models of TBI, upregulation of β-amyloid precursor protein (β-APP) has been reported to occur in the acute post-traumatic period (within hours) and is associated with axonal damage. This increased expression of β-APP has been observed after weight-drop brain injury[344,345] and lateral fluid percussion brain injury in rats.[426,471] Recent studies using transgenic mice which overexpress human β-APP twofold failed to note any evidence of Aβ plaques or a worse behavioural outcome after controlled cortical impact brain injury.[129] However, a subsequent study using a strain of transgenic mice that overexpressed mutant human Aβ tenfold showed increased neuronal cell loss in vulnerable hippocampal regions, significantly impaired cognitive scores and increased regional concentrations of Aβ 1–42 without evidence of amyloid plaque formation.[551]

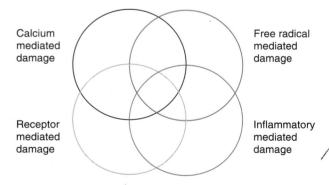

Figure 14.5 *Mechanisms of delayed cellular damage. Interactions of mechanisms of delayed cellular damage can affect vascular, neural or glial elements.*

In contrast to the experimental literature, increased numbers of diffuse Aβ plaques have been reported in head-injured patients who died 6–18 days after head injury.[498] Subsequent studies by these authors using larger series of patients demonstrated in 152 head-injured patients, with survival times between 4 h and 2.5 years, that 30% of cases showed Aβ deposits. A correlation was not observed between Aβ deposits and cerebral contusions, intracranial haematoma, ischaemic brain damage, brain swelling or the pathology of raised ICP, suggesting that the deposition of this peptide may represent a consequence of the acute phase response of neurons to stress in susceptible individuals.[217,497] Another study, however, was unable to detect any significant increase in Aβ deposits after human head injury.[23]

Cytokines such as interleukin-1β (IL-1β), which are known to be upregulated directly within injured CNS or by peripheral immune cells after trauma (see above), are known to induce β-APP expression and synthesis.[205] Griffin and colleagues[229] showed that activated microglia containing IL-1β immunoreactivity were increased three-fold in the acute period after human head injury, which correlated with a seven-fold increase in the number of neurons expressing β-APP.

Based on the recognition that the ε4 allele of the apolipoprotein E (ApoE) gene is a major genetic risk factor for sporadic AD, the relation of the ApoE gene polymorphism to the β-APP deposits in fatal head injury has been explored.[218,444] Patients with ApoE ε4 who died from head injury have been shown to be more that four times as likely to cortical Aβ deposits than patients lacking ApoE ε4. These data have been interpreted to indicate that head injury can act as a trigger for Aβ deposition. Moreover, several studies have now shown that patients with ApoE ε4 have a worse outcome after traumatic brain injury than those who do not have the ε4 allele. A higher frequency of ApoE ε4 among patients with prolonged post-traumatic brain injury was observed in those who did not recover consciousness than in those who did. In a prospectively recruited series of patients, 57% of patients with ApoE ε4 had an unfavourable outcome [dead, vegetative state, or severe disability according to the Glasgow Outcome Scale (GOS)] 6 months after injury, compared with 27% of the patients without ApoE ε4.[583] This remained significant when controlled for age, the severity of the initial injury as assessed by the Glasgow Coma Score (GCS), and initial computed tomographic (CT) scan findings. A subsequent study reported that ApoE ε4 is strongly associated with more than 7 days of post-traumatic unconsciousness and suggested that patients with ApoE ε4 are unlikely to have a good functional outcome.[163,558] Moreover, a study of 30 professional boxers (aged 23–76 years) showed that those with 12 professional bouts or more and who had ApoE ε4 had significantly greater scores on the clinical scale of chronic TBI.[292] Studies exploring the influence of ApoE ε4 genotype on the longer-term outcome after trauma, and particularly whether ApoE ε4 predisposes to a late neurodegenerative decline, are needed. However, of note is the evidence that there is a synergistic interaction between a history of head injury and possession of the ApoE ε4 allele as risk factors for AD.[403]

CYTOSKELETON-RELATED NEURODEGENERATIVE PATHOLOGY

In addition to amyloid plaques, Alzheimer's disease is characterized by neurofibrillary tangles, which consist of abnormally phosphorylated tau protein[232] (Fig. 14.7). Neurofibrillary tangles in brains from ex-boxers have also been shown to be immunopositive for the tau protein, suggesting that tau pathology may be a feature of dementia pugilistica-associated neurodegeneration.[591] In brain-injured humans, cleaved forms of tau proteins are markedly elevated in the CSF.[644] Although relatively little is known about alterations in tau in the traumatically injured brain, there is some indication that phosphorylated tau may accumulate in injured axons and cell bodies after experimental TBI.[258,547] In addition, increased tau immunoreactivity has been observed in oligodendrocytes in the acute post-traumatic period after TBI in man.[269]

Several neurodegenerative diseases are associated with disorganization of the neurofilamentous cytoskeleton (see Chapters 4 and 6, Volume II).[293,522] Intriguingly, many aspects of the neurofilamentous alterations, which accompany neurodegenerative diseases, are also present in the pathology of TBI. Increased neurofilamentous immunoreactivity in axonal swellings, indicative of neurofilamentous protein accumulation, is a well-established consequence of traumatic axonal injury.[401] This disruption of the neurofilamentous cytoskeleton and loss of neurofilamentous proteins occurs in regions of grey and white matter after TBI.[489,508] Abnormal phosphorylation of neurofilamentous proteins in neuronal cell bodies and dephosphorylation of neurofilamentous proteins in axons[92,140,502,626] have been reported after experimental TBI. Recently, in a model of traumatic axonal injury, neurofilamentous-rich inclusions were observed in brain-injured pigs also exhibiting β-APP-immunopositive plaque-like profiles.[547] While it is not well understood how disturbances in the neurofilament cytoskeleton contribute to the morbidity or mortality of TBI, abnormal neurofilamentous organization may be related to worsened outcome after experimental brain injury. Transgenic mice expressing a neurofilamentous fusion protein and exhibiting perikaryal neurofilamentous accumulation had greater initial neuromotor dysfunction, slower recovery of function and larger cortical lesions than their wild-type littermates after TBI.[432] Together, these data suggest that the study of neurodegenerative disease may provide great insight into the mechanisms and treatment of cytoskeletal pathology associated with TBI.

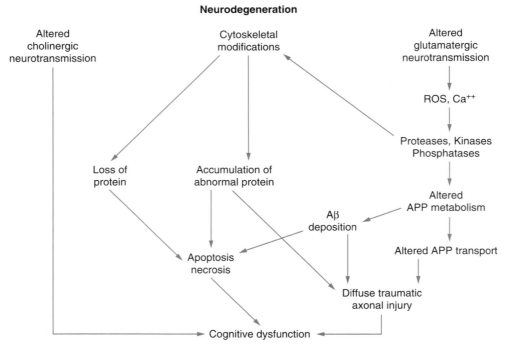

Figure 14.7 *Traumatic brain injury: neurodegeneration. ROS, reactive oxygen species; APP, amyloid precursor protein; Aβ, amyloid β peptide.*

BRAIN INJURY, CALCIUM AND THE CYTOSKELETON

Alterations in brain calcium homoeostasis[365,366,400] and receptors/channels associated with calcium entry [voltage-sensitive channels or ionophore-associated glutamate receptors such as *N*-methyl-D-aspartate (NMDA) receptors] have been related to the development of regional cerebral oedema, vasospasm and delayed cell death. Traumatic, ischaemic or anoxic injury to neurons is associated with widespread neuronal depolarization (including the induction of cortical spreading depression) and release of excitatory amino acid neurotransmitters such as glutamate,[204,447,461,476,652] leading to the opening of NMDA receptor-associated ion channels and influx of calcium. Post-traumatic increases in global calcium flux have been documented using ^{45}Ca autoradiography[158] and indirectly via cytochemical evidence for redistribution of membrane pump calcium ATPase and ecto calcium ATPase activity, and calcium influx in myelinated nerve fibres of the guinea-pig optic nerve after stretch[400] and the analysis of calcium-mediated gene expression.[365] Both calcium channel blockers and competitive and non-competitive NMDA receptor antagonists have been shown to be efficacious in the treatment of experimental TBI (see Ref. 364 for a review), but to date have been disappointing in human studies.[134]

Post-traumatic increases in intracellular calcium can precipitate an attack on the cellular membrane via the activation of calcium-dependent phospholipases. Trauma-induced activation of PLA$_2$ and phospholipase C (PLC) may participate in the release of free fatty acids (FFAs) and diacylglycerol (DAGs), which can directly affect membrane permeability.[35,36,540,615] Brain injury-induced DAG

formation has also been associated with post-traumatic cerebral oedema.[123,124] Controlled cortical impact brain injury in rats induces sustained and time-dependent (delayed) activation of phospholipase-mediated signalling pathways (including increases in FFA and DAG), leading to membrane phospholipid degradation.[257]

Increased intracellular calcium can also stimulate the release of reactive oxygen species (ROS) from mitochondria or via cytoplasmic generation[238,239,317–319,445,598] (Fig. 14.8). These highly reactive molecules cause peroxidative destruction of the cell membrane, oxidize cellular proteins and nucleic acids, and attack the cerebral vasculature. Other endogenous sources of ROS include excitatory amino acid neurotransmitters, cyclo-oxygenase or nitric oxide synthase, from inflammatory cells such as macrophages and neutrophils.[136] Expression of the immediate-early genes *c-fos* and *c-jun* is induced by ROS,[30] while oxidative damage can disrupt calmodulin-regulated gene transcription and intracellular transduction cascades.[634] Free reactive iron, a catalyst for the formation of ROS, may also act in trauma-induced peroxidative tissue damage. The formation of ROS has been documented directly in a weight-drop model of brain injury[556] and indirectly by measuring the production of low molecular weight antioxidants by the injured brain.[38,539]

Calcium can also irreversibly activate the non-lysosomal cysteine protease calpain, which can proteolyse a wide range of cytoskeletal proteins. In many cases, calpain-mediated proteolysis yields characteristic protein fragments. Cytoskeletal protein substrates for calpain include spectrin, tubulin, the microtubule-associated proteins (MAP-2, MAP-1B) and the neurofilament pro-

Oncogenesis

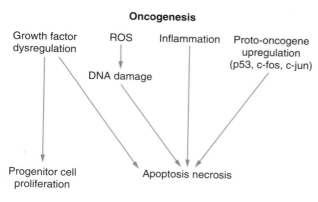

Figure 14.8 *Traumatic brain injury: oncogenesis. ROS, reactive oxygen species.*

teins.[44,289,294,521,543] Calpain is also known to be involved in the degradation of other enzymes (kinases, phosphatases) and membrane-associated proteins, including ion channels and transporters, glutamate receptors, neurotrophin receptors and adhesion molecules.[574] The activation of calpain, when prolonged and unregulated, produces irreversible structural and functional alterations to the cytoskeleton that have been implicated in neuronal toxicity.[34,613]

Calpain activation after brain injury can be determined by the detection of autolysed calpain directly, or indirectly by the identification of calpain-specific proteolytic fragments. Kampfl *et al.*[295] reported that calpain activation occurs as early as 15–30 min postinjury and continues for at least 24 h in regions that sustain neuronal loss and axonal injury after lateral controlled cortical impact brain injury in rats. This increase in calpain activity may be associated with a redistribution of calpain from the cytosol to the cell membrane.[507,647] Calpain-mediated degradation of the membrane-associated cytoskeletal protein spectrin has been demonstrated in the acute post-traumatic period, continuing for a prolonged period (days) after TBI in rats.[441,507] In addition to spectrin, marked loss of MAP-2 has been reported to be both an acute and a persistent post-traumatic event in several models of brain injury in rats.[252,345,478,479] Experimental controlled cortical impact trauma in the rodent also results at 3 h postinjury in reduced levels of 68- and 200-kDa neurofilament proteins,[489] together with disturbances in the spatial orientation of dendritic neurofilaments within injured brain regions.[480] The axonal cytoskeleton also appears to be vulnerable after TBI. In several species, traumatic injury has been shown to produce structural disruptions, altered distribution and even degradation of neurofilaments and microtubules.[272,395,401,611]

Therapeutic strategies to block or antagonize the proteolytic effects of calpain on the cytoarchitecture of the cell have met with some success in the laboratory. Saatman *et al.*[507] showed in rats that administration of the selective calpain antagonist AK295 will significantly attenuate both post-traumatic motor and cognitive

deficits after lateral fluid percussion brain injury. Moreover, calpain inhibitor-2 treatment has been reported to attenuate loss of spectrin and neurofilament proteins after brain injury in rats.[479,480] While pretreatment with the NMDA receptor antagonist dizocilpine maleate (MK-801) did not affect alterations in MAP-2 produced by weight-drop brain injury in the rat,[345] postinjury administration of the broad-spectrum glutamate antagonist kynurenate significantly attenuated proteolysis of MAP-2 initiated by lateral fluid percussion brain injury in the rat.[252]

Postinjury inflammation also mediates delayed neuronal damage after TBI (Fig. 14.9). Alterations in bloodborne immunocompetent cells have been described after trauma, and since the BBB is opened for hours to days during the acute post-traumatic period, entry into the brain of these cells may directly influence neuronal death and/or survival. Infiltration and accumulation of polymorphonuclear leukocytes (PMNs) into brain parenchyma has been documented in experimental TBI in rats[367] and in the first 3 days after human TBI.[255] The entry of PMNs into injured brain and activation of microglia/macrophages is believed to be pathogenic (in mediating the local inflammatory response), and conversely, to play a role in repair and/or regeneration. Marked increases in regional concentrations of the cytokines IL-1B, IL-6 and tumour necrosis factor (TNF) have been observed after experimental and human TBI.[153,154,360,458,579,622] Although recent studies documenting the beneficial effects of pharmacological blockade of the complement cascade and the cytokines IL-1B[622] and TNF[125] suggest that the release and/or upregulation of these pathways may be indeed pathogenic, studies using mice genetically engineered to be deficient in either TNF (TNF−/−) or interleukin 6 (IL-6) and in wild-type litter mates subjected to experimental closed TBI has shown that in spite of an increased post-traumatic morbidity in TNF/leukotriene-α-deficient mice in the acute post-traumatic period, there is a neuroprotective effect of these cytokines.[561] The results suggest that these cytokines may play a role in facilitating long-term behavioural recovery, thereby underscoring the

Inflammation

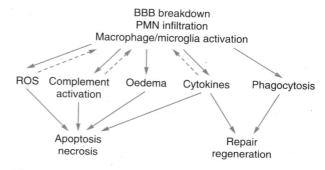

Figure 14.9 *Traumatic brain injury: inflammation. BBB, blood-brain barrier; ROS, reactive oxygen species.*

potential for postinjury cellular and molecular changes to be either pathological or protective, depending on when they are expressed during the postinjury cascade.

Future studies using novel inhibitors of cytokine function and inflammatory mediators and other transgenic strains of experimental animals should begin to address the importance of these immunological factors in mediating specific regional cellular damage after brain injury.

TBI AND APOPTOTIC/NECROTIC CELL DEATH

Apoptosis is considered to be the morphological hallmark of programmed cell death, and has normally been associated with the formation of the normal CNS during development[456] (see also Chapter 3, this Volume). Apoptotic cell death is associated with internucleosomal chromatin cleavage, which can be enzymatically identified *in situ* using the terminal deoxynucleotidyl transferase-mediated dUTP nick-end labelling (TUNEL) technique.[173] TUNEL immunohistochemistry has been used since the early 1990s to establish that neural cell apoptosis is a component of the pathology of neurodegenerative diseases such as Alzheimer's, Parkinson's and Huntington's diseases.[419,477,545] Rink *et al.*[495] were the first to report that between 12 h and 3 days after lateral fluid percussion brain injury in the rat, a small but significant number of injured neurons in the cortex and hippocampus exhibited TUNEL reactivity. Two types of TUNEL(+) cells were identified: type I which were neuron-like, with diffuse TUNEL reactivity throughout the cell, and type II which were compact, spherical and intensely TUNEL(+). Using electron microscopy, these authors reported that while type I cells were vacuolated and necrotic, type II cells exhibited signs of classical apoptosis.[495] Conti and co-workers[109] extended the initial observations by demonstrating that there was a biphasic increase at 24 h and 1 week postinjury in the number of apoptotic cells in the cortex. In addition, apoptotic neurons were present in the injured thalamus, but did not appear until 1 week postinjury, suggesting a delayed pattern of apoptosis. These initial observations have been confirmed by a number of investigators using the controlled cortical impact model of TBI in rats and mice.[102,106,160,305,442] A bis-benzamide dye has also been used to demonstrate post-traumatic apoptotic nuclear condensation in neurons in injured brain regions.[102,160,442] In contrast to lateral fluid percussion brain injury, neuronal apoptosis after controlled cortical impact brain injury in rats remains restricted to the injured cortex, and is maximal at 24 h postinjury.[102,442] At more severe levels of impact, neuronal apoptosis has been observed in the hippocampus.[106,305] In addition to neurons, oligodendrocytes (in the white matter) and astrocytes appear to undergo apoptosis after experimental TBI.[109,442] The presence of apoptotic cell death has been recently suggested by the presence of TUNEL(+) neurons and oligodendrocytes in human head-injured tissue.[442,536,555,620] Although TUNEL has been widely used to visualize apoptotic cells in tissue sections, these results must be cautiously interpreted because DNA degradation leading to the formation of free 3′-hydroxyl groups can occur in the late phases of necrosis. Identification of apoptotic cells has been based on light microscopy to evaluate the presence of chromatin margination, and nuclear and cytoplasmic condensation within TUNEL(+) cells.[89,109]

Based on the observations that morphological features of both necrosis and apoptosis appear in the same neural cell, and that apoptotic neural cells exhibit only some of the characteristics of developmental apoptosis, it has been argued that a continuum between apoptosis and necrosis exists[77,446] (Fig. 14.10). However, it is equally likely that the nature and/or intensity of the insult may regulate whether a complex cell such as a neuron undergoes apoptosis or necrosis. Moderate levels of experimental TBI result in both necrosis and apoptosis, with necrosis contributing more than apoptosis to the total number of dying cells.[109,442] The presence of a continuum suggests that intracellular pathways leading to apoptosis and necrosis may not be mutually exclusive. For example, although it has been proposed that the calcium-activated neutral proteases (calpains) may mediate necrosis, and that caspase-3 is only activated in apoptotic cells,[612] calpain activation may also lead to apoptosis.[560]

Moreover, as long as adenine triphosphate (ATP) is present within the injured cell, apoptotic pathways may be able to be initiated, and once ATP is depleted (as a result of damage to the mitochondria), the injured cell may shift towards necrotic pathways. This hypothesis may, in part, explain why neurons dying as a result of a pathological stimulus may exhibit features of both apoptosis and necrosis (i.e. the apoptotic features may represent the temporal extent to which apoptotic pathways were active). Mitochondrial dysfunction associated with decreases in ATP has been documented after experimental TBI,[571,605,625] although more recent data from the lateral fluid percussion brain injury model suggest that TBI-induced decreases in ATP levels may not be sufficient to inhibit apoptosis.[347] Reversal of trauma-induced mitochondrial damage by cyclosporin A treatment inhibits traumatic cortical cell loss[520] and axonal injury.[65,455]

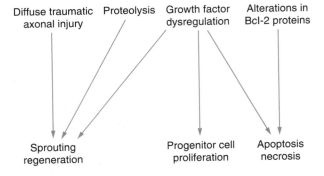

Figure 14.10 *Traumatic brain injury: neurodevelopment.*

The current literature suggests that a complex mechanism, involving altered anti- and pro-cell death signalling pathways, is likely to play a major role in mediating post-traumatic apoptotic cell death. Under normal circumstances, the death-inducing activity of members of the Bcl-2 family (*Bax, Bad, Bid, Bcl-x$_S$*) appears to be in a dynamic equilibrium with their survival-promoting cognates (*Bcl-2, Bcl-x$_L$*).[411] The Bcl-2 family of genes may also participate in pathological apoptotic and necrotic cell death.[56] Neurotoxin- or ischaemia-mediated apoptotic death is preceded by increased Bax messenger RNA (mRNA) and protein, and decreased expression of *Bcl-2* in cells that are destined to die,[200,201] while an increase in *Bcl-2* immunoreactivity has been observed in neurons, glia and endothelial cells that survived focal ischaemic injury.[90] Similarly, increased expression of *Bcl-2* has been observed in neurons that survive the traumatic insult both in the rat and in brain-injured man,[100,102] while Bax has been reported to be translocated to the nucleus of apoptotic cells after experimental brain injury.[305] A role for Bcl-2 in neuronal cell death after TBI has been further supported by recent observations that transgenic mice overexpressing the human Bcl-2 protein exhibited significantly less neuronal loss in the injured cortex and hippocampus after experimental TBI.[431,490] Bcl-2 family members may control cell death by regulating the release of cytochrome *c* from the mitochondria.[633] Once in the cytosol, cytochrome *c* aids in the activation of the caspases, apoptosis-promoting cysteine family of proteases.

One consequence of shifts in intracellular levels of Bcl-2 family proteins is the activation of the death-inducing cysteine proteases and caspase.[588] Activation of caspases has been associated with neuronal and oligodendroglial cell death resulting from multiple kinds of stimuli such as growth factor deprivation, hypoxia, free radical generation, ionizing radiation and ischaemia.[233,433,438,463] Currently, 14 members of the mammalian caspase family have been identified and separated into two categories: the 'activator' caspases such as caspase-8 and -9, and, the 'executioner' caspases such as caspase-2, -3, -6 and -7.[588] Activation of caspase-9, which has been demonstrated *in vivo* after experimental cerebral ischaemia[325] and traumatic spinal cord injury,[90] has been suggested to occur before and to mediate the activation of caspase-3.[588] Activation of caspase-3 has been reported in injured cerebral cortex in the acute period after experimental[472] and human[100] brain injury, and in the chronic period after traumatic spinal cord injury.[144,559] A role for caspases in the pathobiology of TBI was found in studies by Faden and co-workers.[141] More recently, Clark and co-workers reported that while post-traumatic administration of the caspase inhibitor z-DEVD-fmk attenuated neuronal apoptosis and reduced the extent of cortical injury after experimental brain trauma, brain-injured, z-DEVD-fmk-treated rats were as impaired in motor function as their vehicle-treated counterparts.[101]

The current hypothesis regarding the mechanism(s) of caspase-mediated cell death proposes that caspases cleave multiple protein substrates, resulting in cell death.[588] Caspases may cleave antiapoptotic regulators such as the inhibitor of the nuclease responsible for DNA fragmentation, as well as cytoskeletal proteins, e.g. spectrin and actin, resulting in the disassembly of the dying cell.[355] The characteristic internucleosomal DNA fragmentation that is observed in apoptotic human cells has been suggested to be mediated via a specific endonuclease, the 40-kDa DNA fragmentation factor (DFF40).[355] DFF40 is present in the cytosol as a heterodimer with a 45-kDa subunit, DFF45, and upon cleavage of DFF45 by activated caspase-3, translocates to the nucleus as the active nuclease.[355] Homologues of the human proteins DFF40 and DFF45 in rodents are the caspase-activated DNAse (CAD) and inhibitor of CAD (ICAD) proteins, respectively.[145] Cleavage of rat DFF45 homologue and subsequent translocation of DFF40-like protein to the nucleus has been demonstrated in the cortex and hippocampus of rats after TBI.[646] Moreover, the post-traumatic cleavage of the DFF45-like protein was attenuated in brain-injured animals treated with the caspase-3 inhibitor, z-DEVD-fmk.[101]

Disruption of the balance between mitogen activated protein kinase (MAPK)-mediated intracellular signalling pathways may also control the fate of the cell, since activation of c-Jun N-terminal kinase (JNK) or p38MAPK may lead to cell death while extracellular signal-regulated kinase (ERK1/2) and Akt kinase are critical regulators of cell survival.[624] *In vivo*, systemic administration of kainic acid leads to an acute and sustained decrease in phospho-ERK1/2 levels, and a concomitant increase in phospho-JNK in apoptotic neurons within the cortex and the hippocampus.[412] Delayed neuronal death after global cerebral ischaemia has been reported to be associated with a sustained increase in activated JNK,[459] while increased ERK1/2 signalling is associated with neuroprotection in a model of ischaemic preconditioning.[533] Activated JNK has been observed in both apoptotic neurons as well as in apoptotic oligodendrocytes after compressive spinal cord injury.[430] Inhibition of JNK directly or blocking its upstream activators attenuates apoptotic cell death *in vitro*[624] and *in vivo*.[515] Recently, gene-targeted disruption of the brain isoform of JNK, JNK3, resulted in mice that are resistant to excitotoxic-induced hippocampal cell death and exhibit reduced seizure activity and mortality.[632] To date, there is very little information regarding the role of JNK/ERK signalling pathways in mediating cell death after TBI.

Although controlled DNA fragmentation, i.e. breakage of both DNA strands, is a biochemical hallmark of apoptosis, both single and double DNA strand breaks may precede or induce apoptotic cell death.[532,601] Activation of endonucleases can result in double-strand DNA breaks in DNA associated with oxidative damage[354] and has been replicated in the induction of neural apoptosis.[50,227]

Oxygen free radicals, or ROS such as superoxide anion, the hydroxyl radical or singlet oxygen, are generated as a consequence of reduction of oxygen to water, or as a byproduct of certain enzymic reactions. Both ischaemic and traumatic brain injury reported to result in single- or double-stranded DNA breaks in neuronal and glial DNA[100,109,288,354,357,532,536] have been associated with an increase in ROS, suggesting that oxidative stress could be one pathway of secondary injury.[88,98,265] In addition to causing DNA strand breaks, ROS can mediate the formation of DNA–protein adducts and/or oxidative adducts of the nitrogen bases.[107] While increased species of oxidized nitrogenous bases have been detected in cortical DNA after focal cerebral ischaemia,[354] it is unclear whether the increase in free radical production observed after TBI leads to oxidative DNA damage.

DNA damage is known to activate intracellular pathways that lead to either growth arrest, apoptosis or repair and elimination of damaged DNA,[151] depending on the cell type, extent of damage and/or environment. One major component of the DNA damage response is the induction and upregulation of the tumour suppresser gene, p53, also termed the 'guardian of the genome'.[88] Induction of p53 mRNA has been associated with neuronal damage after excitotoxic and ischaemic brain injuries.[98,107,151,263,265,511] After both lateral fluid percussion and controlled cortical impact brain injury, increased mRNA and p53 protein were observed in regions that exhibited neuronal apoptosis and in neurons that were TUNEL(+).[305,435] Increased p53 mRNA was also observed in the pyramidal CA1 neurons of the hippocampus, in a region where cell death does not occur after lateral fluid percussion brain trauma.[435] Further evidence for a pathological role for p53 in CNS injury is provided by reports that p53-deficient mice are resistant to excitotoxic, ischaemic and traumatic injuries.[118,421,592] Because wild-type p53 is a transcription factor for genes such as wild-type p53 activated fragment (WAF1/p21),[33] the pro-apoptotic factor, Bax,[418] and the growth arrest and DNA damage-inducible gene, GADD45,[645] the consequences of p53 induction may be multiple. While WAF1 and GADD45 can cause cell cycle arrest and facilitate DNA repair and eventual cell survival,[645] Bax can induce cell death (see above).

Base-excision and nucleotide-excision repair are two primary mechanisms that are responsible for repairing damaged DNA.[514] The base-excision repair (BER) pathway is believed to repair oxidative DNA damage and recent reports suggest that BER occurs in response to the DNA damage that develops after ischaemic brain injury.[265,304,355,357,532] Indirect evidence for the activation of DNA repair after ischaemia arises from the observations of increased activity of poly (ADP-ribose) polymerase (PARP).[146,532] While the exact role of PARP activation in DNA repair has yet to be determined, the ability of PARP to bind to damaged DNA suggests that it may serve a role in targeting the repair enzymes to the lesioned area on the DNA molecule.[518] TBI in rats induced PARP activation as early as 30 min postinjury.[331] Because PARP uses nicotinamide adenine dinucleotide as its substrate and thereby depletes cellular stores of energy, PARP activation after CNS injury may be detrimental.[142,618]

Since one of the hallmarks of apoptotic cell death is a minimal activation of the immune system as a result of cell loss, it remains possible that neuronal apoptosis after an ischaemic or traumatic insult may represent a protective response by the brain, i.e. a mechanism by which the brain is able to remove injured and damaged cells with only minimal effect on the remaining brain tissue. In this regard, induction of apoptosis using staurosporine resulted in a larger cortical lesion in rats subjected to focal cerebral ischaemia.[97] More recently, Clark and co-workers[101] demonstrated that although caspase-3 inhibition reduced the number of apoptotic neurons in the cortex after experimental TBI, the motor function of caspase inhibitor-treated animals was as impaired as the controls. Similarly, the cortical and hippocampal damage after TBI in transgenic mice overexpressing the antiapoptotic protein Bcl-2 was significantly reduced compared with the wild-type mice, but motor and cognitive deficits in brain-injured Bcl-2 transgenic mice were not alleviated.[490]

Despite almost three decades of basic preclinical research, the pathological mechanisms underlying cell death and behavioural dysfunction after TBI are not fully understood. However, unconventional 'outside-the-box' strategies and approaches to evaluating TBI may lead to the identification of novel therapeutic targets, particularly to attenuate the chronic consequences in patients who survive the initial traumatic insult.[134,364,385]

Investigation of head-injured patients

Modern techniques include imaging, and physiological and biochemical methods.

IMAGING

Although skull radiographs remain the standard for the diagnosis of skull fracture, CT scans or magnetic resonance imaging (MRI) are much more precise for the diagnosis of brain injury. Both are sensitive to blood products and thus are useful for the diagnosis of extradural, subdural and intraparenchymal haemorrhage as well as contusional damage. MRI is the more sensitive and can detect small tissue tear haemorrhages associated with traumatic axonal injury as well as non-haemorrhagic axonal damage. Not unexpectedly, some of these findings are seen in the less severe injuries of concussion.[4,24,164,172,308,417,531,546]

PHYSIOLOGICAL MONITORING

This includes radionucleotide imaging, functional MRI (fMRI) and positron emission scanning (PET).

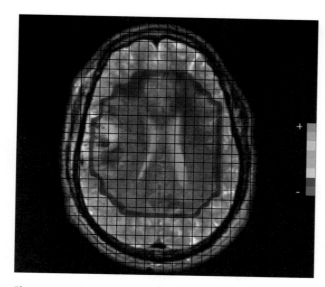

Figure 14.11 *Glutamate map. Derived from [¹H]MR spectroscopy superimposed on T2-weighted MRI showing right temporal contusion associated with a high glutamate level.*

Although invasive monitoring can measure virtually any compound in brain or CSF, non-invasive monitoring can now assess many neurochemical compounds. Magnetic resonance spectroscopy, for example, can measure intracellular pH, ATP, creatinine, phosphorous and magnesium, as well as a host of metabolites such as lactate, N-acetylaspartate, choline, aspartate and glutamate (Fig. 14.11). The spatial resolution of these measures continues to improve.[39,43,108,171,378,491,494,604]

BIOCHEMICAL MARKERS

Recognition of brain injury is usually clinically or pathologically obvious but biochemical markers in the CSF or serum have been shown to be useful in cases where the diagnosis cannot be confidently made on clinical grounds. Although innumerable compounds have been measured after TBI, the identification of neuron-specific enolase and the S-100 protein offers new promise in the biochemical detection of TBI because of their specificity. Neuron-specific enolase is only known to be produced within neurons and S-100 within Schwann cells or oligodendroglia, and thus their presence in the CSF or serum is indicative of neuronal or glial damage.[250,253,267,268,369,453,503,504,599,614,631]

Pathology of head injury

The classification of brain damage has to take into account two extremes: the patient who remains unconscious from the moment of injury until death; and the patient who is apparently normal after the initial injury but who, as a result of a complication, lapses into fatal coma. Even an apparently trivial head injury may set in motion a series of events leading to a fatal outcome unless their onset is recognized early and, where feasible, appropriate treatment instituted. Emphasis in the past has therefore tended to be placed on primary or immediate brain damage, and secondary damage or complications of the original injury.[215]

However, it is now usual for clinicians and pathologists to classify brain damage as focal or diffuse.[216] Focal damage includes contusions on the surface of the brain, intracranial haematomas and the various types of secondary brain damage, including haemorrhage and infarction in the brainstem, that can be produced by intracranial expanding lesions, as well as abscess formation and other less commonly encountered lesions such as pontomedullary tears and avulsion of the pituitary stalk and cranial nerves.

Diffuse brain damage is fundamentally different and exists in four principal forms. Three of these are encountered in patients who survive long enough to reach hospital: DAI, hypoxic brain damage and diffuse brain swelling; the fourth, diffuse vascular injury, however, appears to be virtually restricted to patients who die within 24 h and often much sooner and consists of multiple small haemorrhages throughout the brain. These types of brain damage, when sufficiently severe, cause coma not by compression of the brainstem but by diffuse injury to the cerebral hemispheres and/or the brainstem. In an unconscious patient without any evidence of intracranial haematoma – a situation that occurs in almost 50% of patients who have sustained a blunt head injury – it is usually concluded that the patient has sustained diffuse brain damage but even with improved imaging its precise type may not be identifiable during life. It may also be difficult to define post-mortem unless the brain is properly fixed before dissection and appropriate histological studies are undertaken.

The frequency and types of pathology encountered between 1968 and 1982 and 1987 and 1990 after blunt head injury are given in Table 14.1. Differences in the two cohorts reflect changes in admission policy to the neurosurgical unit and changes in medical practice. Each case underwent post-mortem examination in which the brain was suspended in 10% formol saline for 3–4 weeks before being dissected. The cerebral hemispheres were sliced in the coronal plane, the cerebellum at right angles to the folia and the brainstem horizontally, and comprehensive histological studies were undertaken. Males contributed 78% and females 22%; the age range was 9 weeks to 89 years and the duration of survival from 1 to 14 years 3 months. The majority of the injuries were attributable to road traffic accidents (53%) or to falls (35%). There was a fracture of the skull in 75% of the cases. The clinical records were assessed with particular reference to any deterioration in the level of consciousness after a lucid interval. The lucid interval was defined as being total if the patient had been able to talk rationally after injury, and partial if talking had been confused and disorientated:[492] 32% of the cases had 'talked' at some time after their injury. Patients who had talked had clearly not sustained

Table 14.1 *Data from a consecutive series of 635 fatal blunt head injuries between 1968 and 1982 and 163 between 1987 and 1990 (autopsies undertaken in the Institute of Neurological Sciences, Glasgow, UK)*

	1968–1982 (*n* = 635)	1987–1990 (*n* = 163)
Sex		
Male	497 (78%)	116 (71%)
Female	138 (22%)	47 (29%)
Type of injury		
Road traffic accident	335 (53%)	77 (47%)
Falls	222 (35%)	68 (42%)
Assaults	31 (5%)	8 (5%)
Other	47 (7%)	10 (6%)
Skull fracture	120 (79%)	125 (77%)
Focal		
Surface contusions		
Absent	7 (5%)	21 (12%)
Mild	13 (9%)	27 (17%)
Moderate	116 (76%)	104 (64%)
Severe	15 (10%)	11 (7%)
Intracranial haematoma	381 (87%)	103 (63%)
Raised intracranial pressure	131 (87%)	116 (71%)
Diffuse		
Diffuse axonal injury	184 (29%)	102 (63%)
Hypoxic damage		
Absent/mild	68 (45%)	104 (64%)
Moderate	50 (33%)	37 (23%)
Severe	33 (22%)	22 (13%)
Brain swelling		
Total	60 (40%)	86 (53%)
Bilateral	22 (15%)	5 (3%)
Meningitis	4 (3%)	3 (2%)

severe brain damage at the moment of injury, although the outcome was not always good.[262] The principal types of brain damage will now be described.

LESIONS OF THE SCALP

The scalp is often lacerated or bruised at the time of head injury and such lesions are the best indication of the site of impact. The other important features of lacerations are that they may bleed copiously and be a potential route for the entry of infection.

FRACTURE OF THE SKULL

The presence of a fracture of the skull indicates that the impact has had considerable force but many patients with

a fracture may not have evidence of TBI and make a smooth and uneventful recovery. However, patients with a fracture of the skull have a much higher incidence of intracranial haematoma[207,529] than those who do not have a fracture.[74,409] If there is radiological evidence of a fracture of the skull and some impairment of consciousness, one patient in four in an accident and emergency department will develop an intracranial haematoma. With a skull fracture and preserved orientation the risk is 1 in 6000. Impact against a flat surface will produce fissure fractures which often extend into the base of the skull, while impact against a smaller or irregular object will produce a more localized fracture which is often depressed, i.e. the fragments of the inner table of the skull are depressed by at least the thickness of the skull. A depressed fracture is said to be compound if there is an associated laceration of the scalp, and penetrating or open if there is also a tear in the dura. Fractures of the base of the skull are evidence of severe impact and they often pass through the middle ear or the anterior cranial fossa, producing, in some cases, a CSF otorrhoea or rhinorrhoea or damage to local cranial nerves (especially facial, acoustic, optic and olfactory). In addition, they may allow air and/or bacteria to enter the head, producing pneumocephalus or possibly infection, respectively. When the impact has been particularly severe there may be a 'hinge or ring' fracture extending across the base of the skull, usually in the region of the posterior part of the pituitary fossa or in the rostral part of the clivus, and the adjacent squamous parts of the temporal bones.

Contrecoup fracture

This term is used to describe fractures that are located at a distance from the point of injury and that are not direct extensions of a fracture originating at the point of injury. They occur principally in the roofs of the orbits and the ethmoid plates in association with a fall on the occiput. Growing fractures occur in infancy; the dura is so firmly attached to the skull in this age group that it is readily torn in association with a fracture, resulting in the interposition of soft tissue and meninges between the edges of the fracture. Brain tissue protruding into the fracture may prevent it from healing and indeed enlarge it. As a result there may, some months after the injury, be a protruding swelling consisting mainly of brain tissue at the site of the fracture.

The occurrence of a fracture of the skull depends on the material properties of the skull, the magnitude and direction of the impact, the size of the impacted area, and the thickness and strength of the skull in various areas. The local inbending that occurs when an object strikes the skull produces a compression strain on the outer table and a tensile strain on the inner table. Since bone is weaker during tension than during compression, sufficient inbending causes a fracture to originate in the inner table. It will then propagate along the lines of least resistance from the impact site. The length, direction and width of the fracture depend on the amount of energy absorbed by the skull and its thickness at the impact site. A sufficiently small object will focus the impact energy at the site of contact and is most likely to cause a depressed fracture or skull perforation. A larger object distributes the impact force over a wider area and is less likely to cause a fracture.

Contact with the skull base can occur directly or indirectly, and thus some fractures of the base of the skull are due to local contact effects. Direct impacts occur to the occiput or mastoid, whereas indirect impacts to the face allow energy to funnel through the facial bones or the mandible to produce a fracture of the base of the skull.[362] Distortion and shock waves both contribute to fractures of the vault that occur away from the impact site, to skull base fractures and to contrecoup contusions. Remote fracture of the vault can develop if the impact occurs over a thick portion of the skull or if the striking object is relatively broad. Local in-bending has little effect, but the skull bends outward around the impact zone. This causes the opposite effects of the more common situation, in that the outer table undergoes tensile loading and the inner table experiences a compressive strain. If the area of out-bending occurs in a thin area of the skull, a fracture begins in the outer table some distance from the point of impact. The fracture will still propagate along the lines of least resistance, usually, but not always, toward the impact site. Often the area of the least resistance is not over the vault, and the various characteristic types of skull base fracture occur.

Impact to the skull does not always cause simple in-bending or out-bending near the site of the impact. Occasionally, the circumstances are such that global changes occur in the shape of the skull. This type of deformation results in increases or decreases in intracranial volume. These changes are brief, especially if a fracture does not occur, because the elasticity of the skull soon returns it to its normal shape. However, the rapid changes in volume can be sufficient to produce levels of negative pressure at points where the skull has pulled away from the brain; the resulting tensile loading of the surface of the brain at these locations can then cause contrecoup contusions. This mechanism has also been impugned as a cause of small paraventricular petechiae, presumably as they expand in response to a brief negative ICP. Although global skull deformation occurs, the frequency with which trauma attributed to this mechanism takes place is still debated, and these injuries are probably most commonly due to inertia.

Linear fracture

Linear fractures occur solely because of the contact effects due to impact. Head motion, acceleration and inertia do not play a role. A linear fracture is caused by an impacting object that is hard, so that most of the impact energy is not utilized to set the head into motion and enough energy is available for local deformation of the skull. The object must also be of intermediate size. It has to be sufficiently large (greater than 5 cm^2) that skull penetration does not readily occur and sufficiently small that the contact phenomena are not distributed widely over the surface of the head. Acceleration injuries may be superimposed if substantial head motion occurs after impact.

Depressed fracture

Depressed fractures are similar to linear fractures except that there are more contact forces, usually because of a smaller impact surface. The contact phenomena are more focused or more intense, and exceed the elasticity of the skull, thus allowing skull perforation.

Basal fracture

These are due either to direct impact to the area of the skull base (occiput, mastoid) or to energy transmitted to the skull base from the face. In the latter case, stress waves that propagate from the point of impact cause sufficient changes in the shape of the skull to cause a fracture. A special circumstance exists with many ring fractures of the base of the skull. These can be caused by several mechanisms: impact to the chin (that usually results in mandibular fracture), force transmitted up the temporal mandibular joints, or a 'head whip'. The latter occurs, usually in frontal car crashes, when the torso is well restrained (usually from a restraint system) and the head is free to move violently forward. In any of these cases, an abrupt hyperextension of the head occurs and because of the tenacious attachment of the neck muscles to the base of the skull a ring avulsion fracture occurs where the muscles remain attached, but the base undergoes fracture resulting in pontomedullary vascular stretch or rent.[315,316,326,362,377,526,610]

FOCAL BRAIN DAMAGE IN BLUNT HEAD INJURY

Contusions and lacerations of the brain

These are common and are characteristic of blunt head injury. Nevertheless, patients, particularly those with diffuse brain damage, may die as a result of a head injury with minimal or even without contusions. However, the appearance of contusions is so characteristic that it can often be stated categorically that a patient has sustained a head injury recently or some time in the past. A distinction is sometimes made between contusions and lacerations: in the former the pia–arachnoid is not breached but with lacerations the pia–arachnoid and the underlying brain are torn.

Contusions characteristically occur at the crests of gyri but not all contusions are immediately apparent on external examination of the brain because they may be restricted to the deeper layers of the cortex, with or without involvement of the adjacent white matter (Figs 14.12,

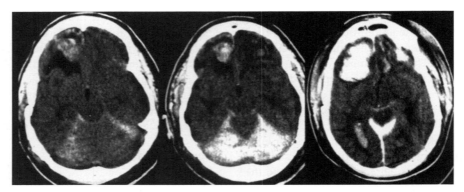

Figure 14.12 *Cerebral contusions. Evolution of bifrontal contusions 1, 4 and 8 h after road traffic accident. Subdural blood is also present layered upon the tentorium posteriorly.*

14.13). In the early stages they are characterized by groups of punctate haemorrhages or streaks of haemorrhage at right angles to the cortical surface. That they can develop very rapidly is shown by the fact that contusions of this type may be very obvious in patients who have died almost instantaneously (Fig. 14.14). Thereafter the haemorrhage becomes more extensive and the blood often permeates into the adjacent white matter (Fig. 14.15a, b). With the passage of time these acute contusions located at the crests of gyri become shrunken and are often brown (Fig. 14.16) because of the persistence of haemosiderin. They can be distinguished from foci of old ischaemic damage which are almost invariably more severe and lie within the depths of sulci. Contusions present similar features in all age groups apart from early infancy; blunt head injury in this age group produces tears, which are often apparent macroscopically, in the subcortical white matter and in the inner layers of the cerebral cortex, particularly in the frontal and temporal lobes.[79,175,352]

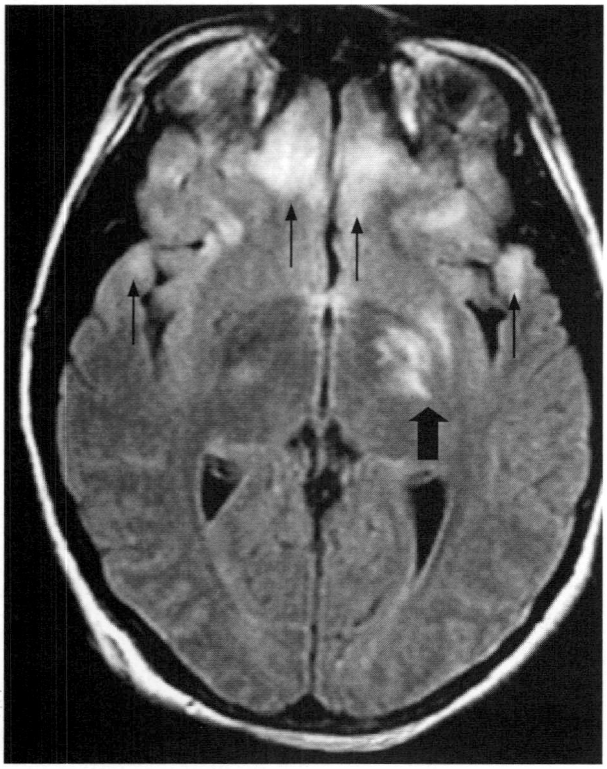

Contusions have a characteristic distribution whatever the site of the original injury. Thus, they affect particularly the frontal poles, the orbital surfaces of the frontal lobes (Fig. 14.17), the temporal poles, the lateral and inferior surfaces of the temporal lobes, and the cortex above and below the sylvian fissures (Fig. 14.14). The last of these, although common, are not identifiable before the brain is sliced. Contusions of the parietal and occipital lobes and of the cerebellum are uncommon unless they are directly related to a fracture of the skull (Fig. 14.18). In the acute stage there is frequently some swelling of brain tissue adjacent to contusions (see Fig. 14.55). Contusions and swelling may influence the early clinical state,[492] but because they are essentially a focal type of brain damage

Figure 14.13 *Cerebral contusions. T1-weighted MRI shows typical bifrontal contusions in the orbital gyri and contusions of both temporal tips (thin arrows). Also present are basal ganglionic lesions (thick arrow) associated with diffuse traumatic axonal injury.*

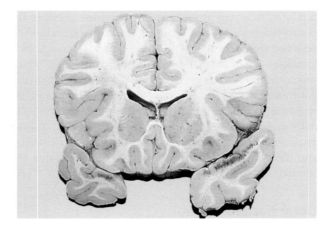

Figure 14.14 *Cerebral contusions. Early contusions take the form of linear perivascular haemorrhages in the cortex and related structures. The patient died within minutes of a road traffic accident. Reproduced by permission from Ref. 216.*

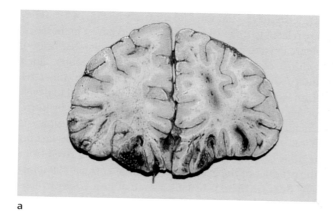

a

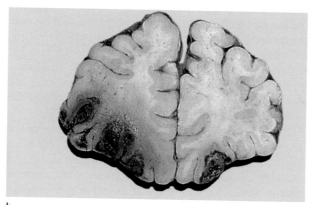

b

Figure 14.15 *Cerebral contusions. Contusions on the orbital surface of the frontal lobes extending into the adjacent white matter: (a) in a patient who survived for 44 h; (b) in a patient who survived for 12 days. Reproduced by permission from Ref. 216.*

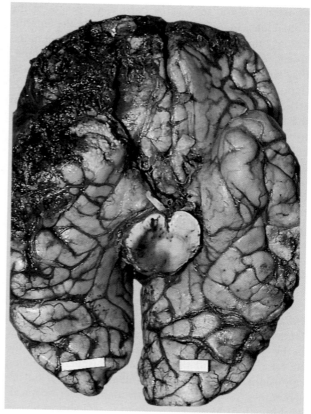

Figure 14.17 *Cerebral contusions. Recent contusions in the frontal and temporal lobes. There was a right-sided acute subdural haematoma and the patient died 32 h after injury from secondary damage in the brainstem. Reproduced by permission from Ref. 216.*

in regions relatively unimportant to immediate survival, patients with quite severe contusions may make a smooth and uneventful recovery if other types of brain damage, or complications such as intracranial haematoma are not present. Healed contusions have been

reported as an incidental finding in 2.5% of 2000 consecutive necropsies in a general hospital.[617]

Contusions have been the subject of detailed and comprehensive studies,[21,349,350,353] and numerous subdivisions have been defined. Fracture contusions occur at the site

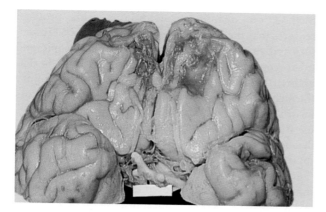

Figure 14.16 *Cerebral contusions. Old contusions in the frontal lobe and over the lateral aspect of the left temporal lobe; incidental findings post-mortem. Reproduced by permission from Ref. 216.*

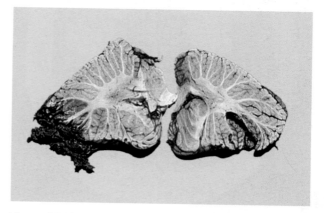

Figure 14.18 *Cerebral contusions. Recent contusions on the under aspects of each cerebellar hemisphere. There was a fracture of the occipital bone. Reproduced by permission from Ref. 216.*

of a fracture and tend to be particularly severe in the frontal lobes in association with fractures in the anterior fossa. Coup contusions occur at the site of impact in the absence of a fracture. Although there are many exceptions, they tend to be more severe in relation to a blow to the stationary head than when the moving head is suddenly arrested.[349] Their size depends on the size of the area of the skull between the striking object and the skull. Contrecoup contusions occur in the brain away from the point of impact and, although not exclusively, they occur more in relation to sudden deceleration of the head than to a blow. The classic example is a fall on the occiput resulting in severe contusions in and adjacent to the frontal and temporal poles. Herniation contusions occur where the parahippocampal gyri and the cerebellar tonsils make contact against the edge of the tentorium and the foramen magnum, respectively, at the time of injury. They are most frequently observed in association with missile injuries[162] but they may also occur with blunt injuries.

Contusions on the surface of the brain must be differentiated from gliding contusions, a term introduced by Lindenberg and Freytag[350] to describe focal haemorrhage in the cerebral cortex and subjacent white matter at the superior margins of the cerebral hemispheres. Gliding contusions are usually bilateral but asymmetrical and are sometimes restricted to the white matter macroscopically, although histological examination will almost always show some involvement of the cortex. A more appropri-

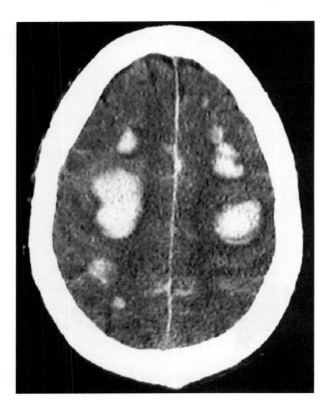

Figure 14.19 *Gliding contusions. Large 'gliding' contusions in the parasagittal white matter are associated with traumatic axonal injury.*

ate term may be parasagittal contusions (Fig. 14.19). They are related to diffuse brain damage and have a higher incidence in patients with traumatic axonal injury (see below).

Most of the literature on cerebral contusions, albeit instructive and informative, has been based on subjective impressions. Adams *et al.*[11,21] therefore attempted to develop a quantitative approach to cerebral contusions by introducing the concept of a contusion index. This index is based on the extent and depth of contusions in various regions of the brain, and for each region is derived from the product of the extent and depth of contusional damage. Because there is usually a zone of non-haemorrhagic necrosis that cannot be identified macroscopically deep to the haemorrhagic part of a contusion, the regional indices had to be based on microscopic studies because the related necrosis was considered to be part of the contusion (Fig. 14.20a, b). Using this technique it is possible to derive a total contusion index for an individual brain, mean contusion indices for specific anatomical sites and mean total contusion indices for a series of cases or for subsets.

The index has confirmed that whatever the site of the injury, contusions on the surface of the brain are most severe in the frontal and temporal lobes, and above and below the sylvian fissures. Contusions are more severe in patients with a fracture of the skull and in patients who do not experience a lucid interval. The analysis also sheds doubt on the interpretation of contrecoup contusions because irrespective of whether the injury was frontal or occipital, contusions were most severe in the frontal lobes (see below). Thus, while contusions can be most severe diametrically opposite to the point of injury, particularly in relation to falls on the occiput, it does not follow that because the most severe contusions are in a particular region of the brain, the injury occurred in the diametrically opposite part of the skull. It has also been established that patients can die as a result of a head injury without there being any contusions on the surface of the brain and that surface contusions are less severe in patients with DAI.

More recently, Ryan *et al.*[506] developed a sector scoring method for quantifying contusions. This protocol requires that the brain is divided into a total of 116 sectors and the presence and extent of macroscopic and microscopic brain damage in each are recorded in diagrams that summarize the distribution of injury throughout the brain. By counting the number of sectors in which damage is present an injury sector score ranging from 0 to 116 is obtained. The sector score provides detailed information about the anatomical distribution of injury that is needed for biomechanical correlations.[49]

In patients who die almost immediately after a head injury a contusion is composed essentially of perivascular haemorrhage, hence the linear disposition of the haemorrhage that is often apparent macroscopically. Blood extends into the adjacent cortex, where neurons in the affected region undergo necrosis as shown by the presence of ischaemic cell change. Haemorrhage may also extend

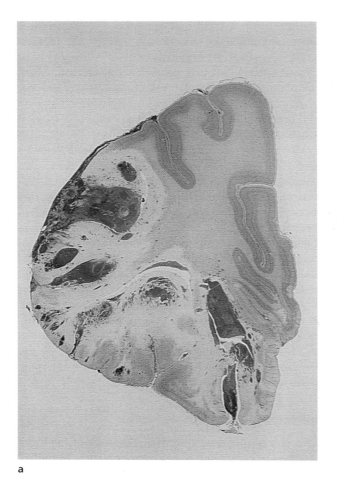

a

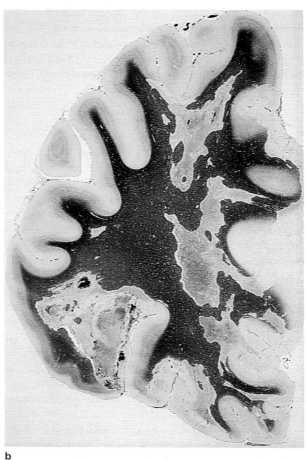

b

Figure 14.20 *Contusion index. This takes into account the depth and extent of the contusion. Note the amount of associated necrosis. (a) Left frontal lobe on its lateral and inferior aspects. (b) Left frontal lobe on its inferior and medial aspects. (a, b, celloidin; a, H&E; b, myelin.) Reproduced by permission from Ref. 216.*

into the white matter. The dynamics of the inflammatory response to contusional injury has been studied[87,451,452] with the increasing recognition that there are different components to the response, each with a different time course. For example, examination of contused brain from 12 patients undergoing neurosurgery between 3 h and 5 days after trauma, showed that the inflammatory response was limited to vascular margination of PMNs in patients undergoing surgery within 24 h of trauma, whereas in material obtained within 3–5 days after trauma the cellular response was a mixture comprising polymorphs, reactive microglia, monocytes/macrophages and both CD4- and CD8-positive T-lymphocytes.[264] There were essentially similar findings in a quantitative immunohistochemical study of contusions from 104 patients aged between 6 and 81 years with closed head injury who survived between a few minutes and 30 weeks. Immunoreactivity for macrophage-related protein-8 (MRP-8) and MRP-14, only expressed on macrophages or activated microglia, could only be detected in contused brain tissue with a survival longer than 72 h.[147] Immunohistochemistry for various inflammatory cells[244] and for astrocytes[245] has provided useful information about their

time course. Although the results of these various studies show intraindividual and interindividual variability, the immunohistochemical findings in the appropriate context may be a valuable contribution towards estimating the age of human contusions. With increasing survival, there is proliferation of capillaries, astrocytes and microglia. The dead tissue is removed, resulting in a shrunken, gliotic, fenestrated scar often containing residual haemosiderin-filled macrophages. An old contusion tends to be triangular in shape, its broad base being at the crest of a gyrus and its apex in the digitate white matter.

Ultrastructural studies have provided evidence of microvascular collapse, swelling of endothelium and perivascular oedema.[71,603]

Coup contusions

Contusions beneath the site of impact are due to local tissue strains arising from local bending of the skull that exceed the tolerances of the local pial, vascular and cortical brain tissue. In order for such localized effects to occur, the impacting object must be relatively small and hard and the area of the skull that is struck must remain elastic. Rupture of pial blood vessels usually occurs because of high tensile strains, such as suction, that are produced when the focally depressed elastic skull rapidly returns to its normal configuration. If skull elasticity is exceeded by the force of the blow, direct compressive injury to the cortical surface may occur.

Contrecoup contusions

Superficial focal areas of vascular disruption and cortical damage remote from the site of impact occur principally because of head motion (inertia) and can result from either translational or angular movements of the head. Movement of the brain towards the site of impact causes tensile strains in the area opposite to that of the impact. If the tensile strains that result are greater than the vascular tolerance, contusion results. However, unlike coup contusions, impact is not necessary for contrecoup contusions to occur. The term coup is therefore a misnomer, since the critical mechanism is most often acceleration rather than impact. In situations in which the head undergoes impulsive loading, contrecoup contusions occur solely because of the effects of acceleration. If an impact causes considerable global deformation of the skull, tensile strains can also occur remote from the site of impact and cause contusional damage, but the predominant mechanism for contrecoup contusions is acceleration of the head.

It is important to recognize that predicting the mechanism of an injury by drawing a straight line from an area of contrecoup contusion to a localized lesion on the scalp is fraught with error. Because of the complexity of head motions that occur in any clinical accident and because of the anatomical irregularities of the inner surface of the skull, contrecoup contusions are often not exactly opposite the point of impact. Thus, the frequently occurring contusions of the temporal and frontal poles are contrecoup in almost every instance, irrespective of the site of impact. In fact, it is perhaps correct to define a contrecoup contusion as one that is not immediately below the site of impact, irrespective of its exact location.

The relative proportion of coup versus contrecoup contusions depends on the response of the head to impact, i.e. on how much of the impact energy is converted into head motion. A small, hard impact object, e.g. a hammer, tends to produce focal deformation of the skull leading to an underlying coup contusion, but since much of the energy is dissipated at the site of impact there is little head acceleration and consequently slight or very limited contrecoup contusion. In contrast, a softer or larger impact object results in less local injury beneath the point of impact as more of the energy is used in setting the head into motion. In this case a large contrecoup lesion occurs, the coup contusion being smaller or non-existent.

Coup lesions predominate if the head is accelerated and contrecoup contusions predominate if the head is decelerated. This is a clinical rule of limited usefulness and is true only to the extent that many acceleration injuries to the head are from small, hard impactors, e.g. weapons used in assaults, and many deceleration injuries occur against broad surfaces, e.g. pavements or floors during falls, or against softer surfaces, e.g. padded motor vehicle interiors. Thus, most 'acceleration' injuries have a greater proportion of contact phenomena and less head acceleration than do 'deceleration' injuries, in which the proportion is usually reversed.

Contusions are mainly impact-related phenomena and it is therefore not surprising, as indicated above, that they are significantly more severe in patients with a fracture of the skull than in those who do not have a fracture. In early experiments on acceleration injury in non-human primates, impact phenomena occurred at short-duration, high acceleration levels that were sufficient to cause fracture of the skull and contusions of the brain.[13] As in man, the contusions occurred particularly at the frontal and temporal poles and their depth and surface extent increased as the mechanical input to the head increased. It appeared that the extent of the contusions was primarily determined by the immediate traumatic event but that the depth of a contusion could increase with time. As the mechanical input increased, contusions at the frontal pole occurred before contusions at the temporal pole.

Intracranial haemorrhage

This is a common complication especially of the more severe varieties of blunt head injury, being present in 55% of the cases in the Glasgow database, although the great majority had been surgically evacuated. It is the most common cause of clinical deterioration and death in patients who have experienced a lucid interval after their injury.[74,111,492,501] In a series of patients in whom it was judged that death might have been prevented by more effective management,[119,284] almost two-thirds were found to have an intracranial haematoma. Although there is not a consistent relationship between fracture of the skull and the occurrence of a haematoma, the majority of patients who develop intracranial haematoma have a fracture of the skull.[409] Frequently the fracture is contralateral to the haematoma.

In the past it has been assumed that the main effects of an intracranial haematoma are delayed until it is large enough to cause distortion and herniation of the brain and a raised ICP. Routine imaging of head-injured patients has, however, shown that intracranial haematomas are often apparent before they produce clinical deterioration and may even be present in a patient who would not previously have been suspected of having this complication.[74,111] This raises the possibility that progressive swelling of the underlying hemisphere (see below) may contribute materially to the failure of spatial compensation (see Chapter 4, this Volume) to accommodate the expanding lesion. Haemorrhage usually begins at the time of injury, i.e. it is a primary event, but the clinical presentation is usually that of a complication because of the interval between the onset of haemorrhage and the appearance of the clinical features of an intracranial expanding lesion.[60,387,416,563,564,581,597]

In traumatic intracranial haemorrhage, there may be bleeding into the extradural, subdural or subarachnoid spaces, into the brain or into the ventricles. Some degree of subarachnoid haemorrhage is common in association with contusions and intraventricular haemorrhage is a frequent occurrence in patients with traumatic axonal injury (see below), but extradural, subdural and intracerebral haematomas are the usual causes of expanding intracranial lesions in head injury. Because of the frequency with which intracerebral and subdural haematomas occur together (a 'burst' lobe), perhaps the most useful classification is to consider the haematomas as being extradural or intradural. Even this simple classification presents certain problems since in many clinical series the various haematomas occur in combination rather than singly (Table 14.2).

Extradural (epidural) haematoma

This occurs in approximately 2% of all types of head injury.[273,349,469] In fatal head injuries extradural haematoma (EDH) is found in between 5%[112] and 15%[161] of cases, and was present in 8% of the cases in the Glasgow database. In most series the peak incidence is in the second and third decades after a fall or traffic accident. An EDH is most unusual in the first 2 years of life.[83] A fracture of the skull is present in the great majority of patients[273] but an EDH can occur in the absence of a fracture, especially in children. However, a proportion of children thought not to have a fracture radiologically have been found to have one at operation.[405]

This type of haemorrhage usually takes place from meningeal blood vessels, and as the haematoma enlarges it gradually strips the dura from the skull to form a circumscribed ovoid mass (Fig. 14.21a–c) that progressively indents and flattens the adjacent brain. The dura is normally firmly attached to the skull[373] and extradural haematomas have therefore been referred to as 'fracture haematomas', since they occur both as a consequence of a fracture and stripping of the endosteum at the time of the fracture. Since the initial injury may be apparently trivial and the patient experiences a lucid interval, there is frequently little or only minimal evidence of other types of brain damage. By contrast, extradural haematoma may occur also in patients with other types of brain damage and for this reason some patients may have been unconscious from the time of the original injury.[58,110,273]

Classically, the haematoma occurs as a result of tearing of a middle meningeal artery (about 50% of cases) in the region of the squamous part of the temporal bone where the bone is thin and easily fractured, but in some 20–30% of cases the haematoma occurs elsewhere,[111] e.g. in the frontal and parietal regions or in the posterior fossa. Supratentorial EDH may also occur after injury to the middle meningeal veins (about 30%), diploic veins (about 10%) or the dural sinuses, and after laceration of the carotid artery before it enters the intracranial dura.[111] As acute EDH is more likely to be due to bleeding from an artery than from a venous source, it is likely to reach its ultimate volume within minutes of the injury occurring.[373] Occasionally, patients with EDH may present with a subacute or chronic course: 13% in a series of 116 patients in one study[578] and 14.3% in a series of 292 in another.[608] In between 40 and 50% of cases with EDH neuroimaging shows subdural haematoma (SDH) and cerebral contusions, thereby contradicting the commonly held view that patients with an EDH do not have any significant intradural pathology,[469] and this will therefore influence the clinical outcome.[110,469] EDH is occasionally bilateral.

In a few patients EDH may be managed without operation.[72] A series of patients with small to moderate sized EDHs thought not to require neurosurgical intervention was followed by serial imaging.[42,74,530] These studies have shown that the size of the EDH may increase by up to 50% until about 10–14 days after injury. After the second week the haematomas become smaller and in the majority of patients have completely resolved by 4–6 weeks after injury. However, non-operative management is not without controversy as in a prospective study of 22 patients with small asymptomatic EDHs, 32% eventually required surgery.[313]

In fire-related deaths where the head has been exposed to intense heat, there may be fissure fractures of the skull and heat haematomas in the extradural space. These haematomas have a pink, spongy appearance which is said to be characteristic of thermal injury and is different from the dark red appearance of the blood in the conventional EDH; they also follow closely the distribution of the charring on the outer surface of the skull. The pathogenesis of this type of haematoma is not known, although it has been presumed that the victim must have been alive in order for it to develop. The combination of EDH and fracture of the skull in fire victims may therefore pose difficulties in interpretation for the forensic pathologist.

An EDH can be considered as a complication of a skull fracture in which the dural blood vessels are torn. The rupture of these blood vessels can occur as the fracture propagates across them, or the blood vessel may be injured without fracture if skull deformation and bending are sufficient to tear it. EDH, like skull fracture, is not related to head motion or acceleration. Vascular disruption of dural or of skull blood vessels occurs because of contact-related skull fracture or contact-related skull deformation.

Intradural haematoma

This takes three forms: 'pure' SDH, usually brought about by rupture of the veins that bridge the subdural space where they connect the vertex of the cerebral hemispheres to the sagittal sinus, 'pure' intracerebral haematoma that is presumably brought about by the rupture of intrinsic cerebral blood vessels at the time of head injury, and a combination of these, i.e. blood in the subdural space,

Table 14.2 *Incidence and type of acute intracranial haematoma after head injury*

Reference	Population studied	n	Overall haematoma incidence (%)	Type of haematoma (%)				
				Extradural only	Extradural and intradural	Subdural only	Subdural and intracerebral	Intracerebral only
Strang et al.[564]	Emergency room attenders (Scotland)	3568	0.2					
Miller and Jones[416]	Admission to a neurosurgical unit providing primary care (Edinburgh, UK)	1919	4	22 (combined)		34	44	
Brocklehurst et al.[60]	Admission to a neurosurgical unit providing primary care (Hull, UK)	4011	2	29 (combined)		53 (combined)		18
Teasdale et al.[581]	Transfers to neurosurgery (Glasgow, UK)	Pre-CT 223 / Post-CT 492	34 / 26	27	8	25	26	13
Stone et al.[563]	Patients in a neurosurgical centre (Chicago, USA)	486		8	5	70 (combined)		17
Turazzi et al.[597]	Patients in a coma in a neurosurgical centre (Italy)	Pre-CT 1000 / Post-CT 385	35 / 33	25 (combined)		41	34	
Marshall et al.[387]	Patients in four neurosurgical centres (USA)	746	40	12		60		28 (including contusions)

Reproduced by permission from Ref. 70.

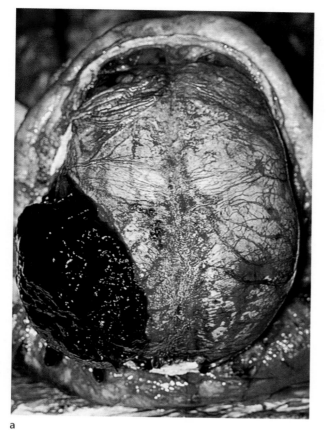

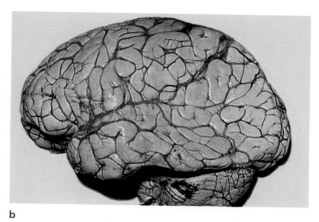

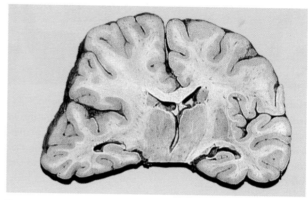

Figure 14.21 *Extradural haematoma. (a) Ovoid circumscribed clot of blood on the outer aspect of the dura mater overlying the left temporoparietal region. (b) Same case as above. Note the distortion of the brain produced by the haematoma. (c) There is an absence of associated damage to the brain. Reproduced by permission from Ref. 216.*

contusions on the surface of the brain and an adjacent intracerebral haematoma, this frequently being referred to as a 'burst' lobe.

Acute SDH

Since 'pure' SDH, which was found in 13% of the cases in the Glasgow database, is usually brought about by rupture of the bridging veins, there may be very little evidence of other brain damage. Some SDHs are arterial in origin, the haemorrhage arising from a cortical artery.[111,638] The principal causes are falls, car accidents and assaults, or they may be caused by a whiplash injury when there is no injury to the head. The haematoma may develop very rapidly or over a period of several hours. Because the blood can spread freely throughout the subdural space, it tends to cover the entire hemisphere (Fig. 14.22a, b),

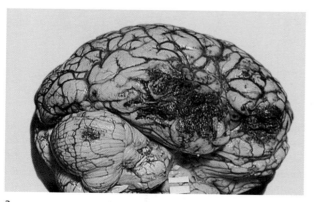

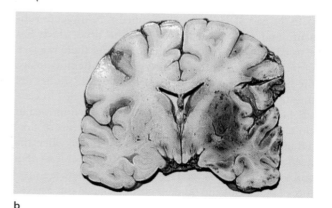

Figure 14.22 *Acute subdural haematoma. (a) There is contusional injury over the lateral aspect of the right cerebral hemisphere; compare with Fig. 14.21b. (b) Same case as (a). There is extensive damage to the right cerebral hemisphere. Reproduced by permission from Ref. 216.*

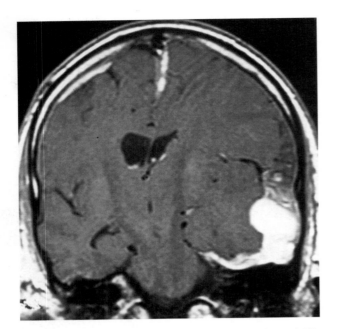

Figure 14.23 *Subacute subdural haematoma. Coronal T1-weighted MRI of subacute haematoma showing large mixed intensity left temporofrontal blood and marked left to right midline shift. Small amounts of subdural blood are also present over the right convexity and in the interhemispheric fissure to the left of the falx.*

resulting in an SDH which is more extensive than an EDH. Occasionally a SDH can extend between an occipital lobe and the tentorium cerebelli or between a temporal lobe and the base of the skull. Rarely they may be located between the medial surface of a cerebral hemisphere and the falx.[259] There is an association between an SDH between the cerebral hemispheres after minor injury and anticoagulation therapy[392] and in patients who have haemophilia,[527] although it may also result from rupture of a saccular aneurysm.[493] About 40% of patients have a complicated SDH with a mortality rate of over 50%, indicating that outcome is influenced, in part, by the associated parenchymal damage. A large proportion of survivors is disabled.[528]

In the past SDHs have been defined as being acute, subacute and chronic depending on the time which has elapsed between injury and diagnosis, but there is a lack of uniformity of nomenclature,[70,290] and attempts to age the haematoma on the basis of histological studies are unsatisfactory. The neurosurgical opinion tends to classify SDHs as acute when the haematoma is composed of clotted blood, as subacute when there is a mixture of clotted and fluid blood (Fig. 14.23), and chronic when the haematoma is fluid. The blood is clotted for at least 48 h and sometimes for several days; thereafter, there is a mixture of blood clot and fluid blood; and after about 3 weeks clot is no longer present. However, with increasing use of CT scanning early after injury such approaches have become less relevant. An acute clotted SDH has high CT density compared with brain for about 7–10 days, after

which liquefaction progressively occurs, with a change to isodensity and later hypodensity. Isodense and hypodense collections are now generally termed chronic subdurals: more usually haematomas (black, tarry liquid; 'old engine oil'), but sometimes hygromas (clear yellow; proteinaceous fluid). Despite the presence of the intracranial expanding lesion and distortion of the brain, the gyral and sulcal pattern on the side of the haematoma is preserved, and convolutional flattening is not a feature, unlike in the contralateral hemisphere. This is because the subdural blood is in contact with both gyri and sulci and therefore exerts uniform compression on the subjacent brain, thus preventing flattening of the surface of the brain.[121] As will be described below, there is a significant correlation between acute SDH and swelling of the subjacent cerebral hemisphere.

A review of the biomechanics of 'pure' acute SDH identified patients with acute SDH where rupture of the bridging veins was judged to be the primary pathological process; in 72% of these cases the head injury had been produced by a fall or an assault, whereas in only 24% the cause had been a road traffic accident.[189,190] These figures are in marked contrast to patients without mass lesions who had been unconscious for more than 24 h, i.e. patients with diffuse brain damage, of whom 89% had been in road traffic accidents and only 10% had experienced falls and assaults.

Experimental studies on acceleration of the head in non-human primates have helped to clarify the situation (Fig. 14.24). In animals subjected to acceleration at high strain rates, there was an admixture of concussion and acute SDH. Increasing the magnitude of acceleration and maintaining a constant duration of the acceleration led to increasingly severe injury up to acute and rapidly fatal

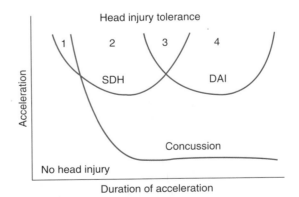

Figure 14.24 *Clinicopathological correlations with amount and duration of angular acceleration. The complex relation between the amount of angular acceleration (y-axis) and the duration for which it occurs (x-axis) is shown for concussion, subdural haematoma (SDH) and diffuse traumatic axonal injury (DAI). Above each tolerance line the injury occurs so that in region 1 SDH occurs without concussion, in region 2 SDH occurs with concussion, in region 3 both SDH and DAI occur, and in region 4 only DAI occurs. Reproduced by permission from Ref. 216.*

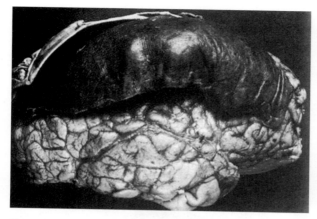

Figure 14.25 *Chronic subdural haematoma. The haematoma is encapsulated and not attached to the dura mater or the arachnoid. Reproduced by permission from Ref. 216.*

SDH. However, acute SDH did not occur where the duration of acceleration was increased. This indicates that bridging veins are more liable to tear when the acceleration (or deceleration) is applied rapidly than when the acceleration occurs more slowly. This accords with the finding of a high incidence of acute SDH in individuals who sustain falls or are assaulted, since these types of injury are associated with very high rates of acceleration or deceleration. In contrast, in road traffic accidents the deceleration rate is usually much slower.

Chronic SDH

This may present weeks or months after a head injury that may have seemed at the time to have been trivial, especially in the elderly. However, a history of head injury is absent in between 25 and 50% of cases.[159,388] Associated factors include epilepsy, shunting procedures and coagulation disturbances, and in about 50% there is alcohol abuse.[570] The precise pathogenesis of chronic SDH is not clear, because it is now known from imaging that most acute SDHs normally resolve spontaneously and do not progress to a chronic SDH.[133] However, the haematoma may become encapsulated in a membrane (Fig. 14.25) and slowly increase in size, possibly as a result of repeated small haemorrhages into it[381] rather than as an osmotic effect. Support for this hypothesis has been provided by ultrastructural studies of the small blood vessels located within the capsule of the haematoma,[575,629,630] from which it was concluded that there had been repeated bleeding from capillaries with wide lumina, attenuated endothelium and wide endothelial gap junctions. Because chronic SDH is most common in the older age groups (75% of patients are over the age of 50 years) and in whom there may be some cerebral atrophy, and since the haematoma expands fairly slowly, the period of spatial compensation (see Chapter 4, this Volume) may be so long that the cerebral hemispheres may be severely distorted (Fig. 14.26a, b) before there is any significant increase in ICP. In untreated cases, however, death is usually attributable to

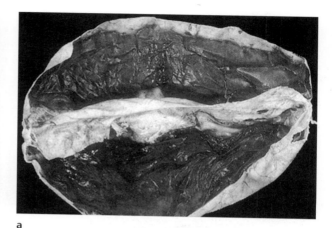

a

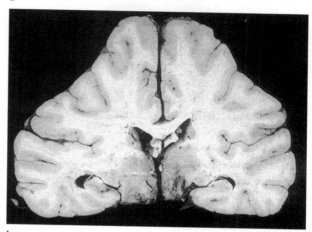

b

Figure 14.26 *Chronic subdural haematoma. (a) Bilateral encapsulated haematomas. (b) Distortion of the brain and secondary haemorrhagic infarction in the brainstem and thalamus, produced by the haematomas. Reproduced by permission from Ref. 216.*

brain damage secondary to increased ICP and compression of the brainstem, although apparently incidental chronic SDHs may occasionally be encountered postmortem in elderly individuals. Chronic SDH is not infrequently bilateral. Most large series report a mortality rate of about 10%.[408]

Subdural hygroma

This is a collection of clear, xanthochromic or bloodstained fluid within the subdural space. It is generally accepted to be due to a valve-like tear in the arachnoid which allows the escape of CSF into the subdural space. The hygroma enlarges because CSF becomes trapped in the subdural space. However, membrane formation surrounding the hygroma is unusual. Hygromas have been reported in between 7 and 12% of all intracranial mass lesions.[562] Fluid can also collect in the subdural space as brain shrinkage occurs for whatever reason. In simple hygromas associated injuries are absent or minor, whereas in complex hygromas there is associated extracerebral haematoma or intraparenchymal injury.[562]

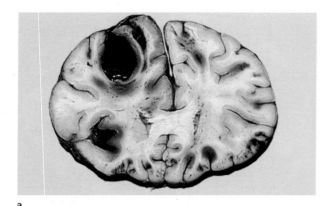

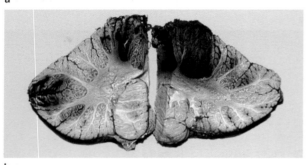

b

Figure 14.27 *Traumatic haematomas. (a) In addition to contusions there is a number of intracerebral haematomas in the frontal lobes of this patient who died 24 h after a road traffic accident. (b) They may also occur in the cerebellum. Reproduced by permission from Ref. 216.*

'Pure' intracerebral haematomas

Present in 15% of the cases in the Glasgow database, these are haematomas that are not in contact with the surface of the brain. They are often multiple and although between 80 and 90% are found in the frontal and temporal regions (Fig. 14.27a) they may occur deep within the hemispheres and in the cerebellum (Fig. 14.27b). Their precise pathogenesis is not clear but it seems likely that

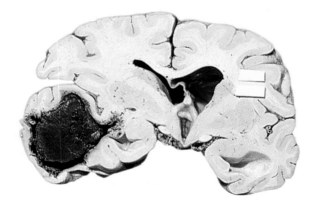

Figure 14.28 *Delayed post-traumatic intracranial haematoma. Following evacuation of an acute extradural haematoma, an intracerebral haematoma developed in the temporal lobe 10 days later. Reproduced by permission from Ref. 216.*

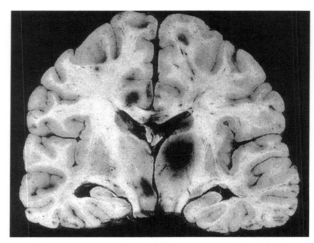

Figure 14.29 *Traumatic basal ganglia haematomas. There are two small haematomas in the deep grey matter. There is also haemorrhage in the corpus callosum. Reproduced by permission from Ref. 216.*

they are caused by the direct rupture of intrinsic cerebral blood vessels at the time of injury. It may be difficult to differentiate clearly a post-traumatic intracerebral haematoma from a "burst lobe" or severe focal contusion.

Traumatic intracerebral haematomas are sometimes delayed and develop in between 1.5 and 7% of patients with severe head injuries.[448] This definition used to be based on the time from the injury to presentation, but since the advent of imaging a delayed haematoma is now defined as 'a lesion of increased attenuation (as seen on CT scan) developing after admission to hospital, in a part of the brain which the admission CT scan had suggested was normal'.[196] They develop in the same general location as contusions and about 80% will become apparent within 48 h of injury, rarely they may be delayed for 1 week or longer after injury.[434] The pathogenesis of these delayed haematomas is not known (Fig. 14.28).[143]

As a result of imaging the occurrence of relatively small haematomas deeply seated in the brain (Fig. 14.29) that tend to be referred to as 'basal ganglia' haematomas[557] is well known. In patients with this type of haematoma there is a reduced incidence of a lucid interval and an increased incidence of gliding contusions and DAI.[7] This suggests that patients found to have a basal ganglia haematoma shortly after a head injury are likely to have sustained diffuse brain damage at the time of injury.

Tissue tear haemorrhages associated with diffuse traumatic axonal injury

Tissue tear haemorrhages are multiple areas of intracerebral damage to blood vessels and axons occurring in association with DAI. They are mentioned here to distinguish them from other types of intracerebral haematomas, but are actually a part of the pathological picture of the severe form of DAI. Tissue tear haemorrhages are distinguished by their multiplicity, their small size (usually varying from petechial to 1.0 cm), and their parasagittal location in the central (not polar) portion of the brain.

They are caused only by high levels of shear and tensile strains as a result of head acceleration and are not related to stress wave concentration due to contact forces. Tissue tear haemorrhages appear to be small areas where the tolerance of the brain to shear and tension forces has been exceeded, allowing the tissue to separate sufficiently to tear both axons and small blood vessels. Their locations are characteristically in the superomedial and frontoparietal white matter, the corpus callosum, the centrum semiovale, the periventricular white and grey matter, the internal capsule and the basal ganglia. In the brainstem, they occur in the dorsal area of the midbrain and the upper pons. Tissue tear haemorrhages represent areas of maximum acceleration-induced brain damage.

A fall may be precipitated by spontaneous intracranial haemorrhage, and may be severe enough to produce a fracture of the skull, cerebral contusions and intracranial haemorrhage. The interpretation of the findings postmortem can be difficult or even impossible and much depends in medicolegal cases on the statements of witnesses and on the site of the haematoma, particularly if it is solitary, when the possibility of a ruptured saccular aneurysm or pre-existing hypertension has to be borne in mind. Even when all the possibilities have been taken into consideration, it may be difficult to reach a final conclusion as to the pathogenesis of the haematoma. If the haematoma is in the subfrontal or temporal region, it is more likely to be traumatic than spontaneous.

'Burst lobe'

This is a convenient term to describe the coexistence of cerebral contusions, SDH from superficial cortical blood vessels, and a haematoma in the white matter deep to the contusions. Since contusions tend to be most severe in the

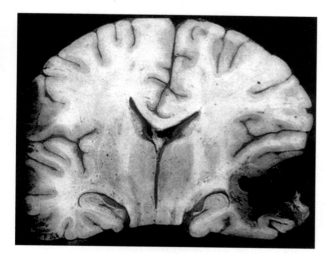

Figure 14.30 'Burst lobe'. The haematoma in the right temporal lobe was in continuity with an acute subdural haematoma. Contusions in the left cerebral hemisphere are restricted to the crests of gyri. Reproduced by permission from Ref. 216.

frontal and temporal poles, these are also the usual sites for a 'burst' lobe (Fig. 14.30). They occurred in 26% of the cases in the Glasgow database.

Intraventricular haemorrhage

The reported incidence varies between 1 and 7% of patients with severe head injuries.[165,274,517] The source of the haemorrhage in the majority of patients is the extension of midline haemorrhages into the ventricles. In many of these patients there are also lesions in the corpus callosum and interventricular septum, a pattern that is often in keeping with DAI (see below). In some cases the haemorrhage appears to be due to tears of subependymal veins or of blood vessels within the choroid plexus. Intraventricular haemorrhage may be a cause of hydrocephalus, which is otherwise uncommon. The outcome is variable, depending on the frequency of associated injuries, particularly those related to DAI.

Trauma is the most common cause of subarachnoid haemorrhage, although a ruptured saccular aneurysm must be considered in some cases.[166,225] In patients with traumatic SDH, the findings on CT scan at admission can predict outcome.[225,226] Fibrous scarring of the meninges secondary to resorption of large amounts of subarachnoid haemorrhage or SAH (haemosiderosis) has been linked to the late complication of 'normal pressure hydrocephalus'.

Mass lesions in the posterior cranial fossa

These are uncommon after trauma. For example, extradural haematoma has an incidence of between about 3 and 7% of all EDHs,[256,440] and subdural haematoma is even less common, representing less than 1% of the total number of acute SDHs.[623,637]

An infratentorial EDH occurs after a blow to the occiput. In the majority of patients haemorrhage results from a tear of the outer wall of a transverse or sigmoid sinus, rather than directly under the site of a fracture. Occasionally bleeding from the diploe may give rise to a posterior fossa EDH.

In most instances SDH in the posterior fossa also occurs after injury to the occipital area. A fracture of the occiput is present in between 20 and 80% of cases, being less common than with posterior fossa EDH. The pathogenesis of the bleeding is attributed to tearing of bridging veins, injury to the venous sinuses or a tear of the tentorium.

The inferior surface of the cerebellum is particularly vulnerable to contusion and haematoma formation. Associated features are separation of the suture lines or occipital fractures.[623]

Brain damage secondary to raised ICP

This subject has been dealt with in Chapter 4 of this Volume where various factors have been emphasized, including the importance of measurement of ICP and the criterion of pressure necrosis in one or both parahippocampal gyri as evidence of high ICP due to a supratentorial expanding lesion.[12] A high ICP with associated distortion, shift and herniation of the brain is common in head injury, and there was evidence that the ICP had been high in 75% of the patients in the Glasgow database.[220] The usual causes were intracranial haematoma or brain swelling. In these cases there was a high incidence of secondary haemorrhage or infarction in the brainstem (68%) with a contralateral peduncular lesion in the midbrain (17%) and of infarction in the territories supplied by the posterior cerebral arteries (36%), the anterior cerebral arteries (12%) and the superior cerebellar arteries (6%).

Some types of brain damage conventionally attributable to a high ICP can, however, occur in the absence of pressure necrosis in one or both hippocampal gyri.[219] This apparent anomaly was found infrequently and only in 16 of 324 cases, eight of whom survived for less than 20 h after their injury. When ICP increases rapidly for any reason, death often supervenes before there is sufficient time for internal herniation to appear. In such cases, pressure necrosis in the parahippocampal gyri is absent. Other explanations were surgical evacuation of mass lesions, the development of bilateral hemispheric swelling in association with diffuse hypoxic brain damage, the swelling under these circumstances rarely being sufficient to cause infarction in the territories supplied by the posterior cerebral arteries or secondary damage in the brainstem, and rarely a large external cerebral hernia occurring after craniotomy. In the 71 cases in the Glasgow database without evidence of a high ICP the most common causes of death were traumatic axonal injury in 29, hypoxic brain damage in 25, brain swelling in 13 and infection in nine.[219] The recognition and mapping of the vascular complications of brain swelling and raised ICP have become particularly important in differentiating between traumatic and non-traumatic axonal damage (see below).

Infection

In a small number of head injuries a brain abscess may develop. Most commonly this is due to a penetrating head injury when infected material may be carried directly into the cranial cavity (see Fig. 14.62) from a compound depressed fracture of the skull, when bone or missile fragments are left *in situ* in patients with intracranial gunshot wounds, and after operation for removal of contused brain or intracranial haematoma.

Subdural empyema may develop after penetrating wounds of the skull, the insertion of ICP monitoring devices, craniofacial injuries or infection of an SDH. Subdural empyema is usually found over the convexities of the cerebral hemispheres or in the parasagittal regions. It is rarely seen in the basal areas of the skull, but it may spread over the tentorium cerebelli. Cranial osteomyelitis may develop, but it is usually a complication of craniotomy and less often contamination of or inadequate débridement of an open skull wound.

Meningitis is a well-recognized complication of a blunt head injury and is usually due to the spread of micro-organisms through an open fracture of the calvaria or through a sometimes unrecognized fracture of the base of the skull bringing the subarachnoid space into continuity with major air sinuses. The latter is often associated with a CSF rhinorrhoea or otorrhoea, or an aerocele. If there is a small defect in the dura at the base of the skull, meningitis may be delayed for many months or even years: a small traumatic fistula may also be a cause of recurrent episodes of meningitis. In a small number of cases (less than 3%) infection may complicate the insertion of an ICP monitoring device. Shunt-associated infections may present in various ways. Infected ventriculoatrial shunts may present as shunt nephritis and ventriculoperitoneal shunt infections may present as meningitis, ventriculitis or abdominal sepsis.

Other types of focal brain damage

These include a number of disorders.

In accidents causing hyperextension of the head on the neck, traumatic separation of the pons and medulla is a well-recognized cause of death.[351,544] Such cases usually fall within the domain of medicolegal medicine and in many there is an associated ring fracture at the base of the skull or dislocation and/or fracture of the first or second cervical vertebra.[334] While complete tears are immediately fatal, patients with smaller or incomplete tears at the pontomedullary junction may survive for some time after injury (Fig. 14.31)[47,59,473,474] and such lesions may be recognized by appropriate imaging.[641]

Almost any of the cranial nerves may be damaged at the time of injury. For example, trauma is the most common

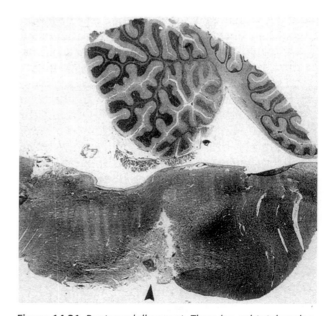

Figure 14.31 *Pontomedullary rent. There is a subtotal wedge-shaped rent (arrow) between the pons and the medulla. This patient survived for 26 days after a head injury, and there were established reactive changes in the walls of the rent. (Luxol fast blue–cresyl violet.) Reproduced by permission from Ref. 216.*

cause of loss of the sense of smell and is encountered in about 7% of all head injuries.[572] This is not surprising in view of the relative severity of contusions affecting the undersurfaces of the frontal lobes and the frequency of fractures in the anterior cranial fossae. Injury to the optic nerve and chiasm occurs in 0.3–5.2% of patients with head injuries. The most vulnerable part of the optic nerve is that portion which lies within the optic canal.[202] If there is severe trauma to the apex of the orbit there may also be disruption of the sphenoidal fissure and damage to the IIIrd, IVth and VIth cranial nerves and the ophthalmic branch of the Vth nerve. The IIIrd, IVth and Vth cranial nerves may be injured directly, but also secondarily as a result of tentorial herniation, thrombosis of the cavernous sinus or the development of a traumatic caroticocavernous fistula. Injuries to the supraorbital and infraorbital nerves are said to be the most common form of injury to the Vth nerve after head injury. Damage to the Gasserian ganglion is uncommon but has been described either in association with fractures involving the base of the middle fossa or as a result of a backward and medial rotation of the petrous tip of the temporal bone, the fragment damaging the foramen lacerum exposing the carotid artery and injuring the trigeminal root ganglion. The facial nerve may be damaged anywhere along its course, although injury within the temporal bone is the most common site: an associated fracture is usual. Hearing and labyrinthine function may be impaired after a head injury from damage to the VIIIth cranial nerves and their end organs, or there may be trauma to the middle ear. Injuries to the VIIIth cranial nerve are commonly associated with a fracture of the petrous temporal bone. Injury to the lower cranial nerves and the internal jugular vein are uncommon in closed head injury, being described most often as a consequence of gunshot wounds. The frequency with which injury to the cranial nerves occurs has been underestimated, MRI now providing a much more sensitive means of identifying damage than was previously possible with CT.[174]

The types of damage that can occur in the hypothalamus and pituitary gland are reviewed in Chapter 17 of this Volume. Furthermore, the pituitary stalk may occasionally be torn at the time of head injury, leading to infarction in the anterior lobe of the pituitary gland. In a review of 100 fatal cases of blunt head injury, infarction was found in the anterior lobe of the pituitary gland in 38.[242] Several potential mechanisms have been put forward to explain the type of damage, including a basal skull fracture that extends into the sella turcica, elevation of the ICP leading to distortion and compression of the pituitary stalk and the hypophyseal arteries, and hypotensive shock, analogous to the situation occurring in postpartum necrosis of the pituitary. The identification of injury to the hypothalamus and the pituitary stalk has been greatly facilitated *in vivo* with the advent of MRI. These studies and those carried out in the laboratory have shown that the singular vascular supply to the pituitary gland deter-

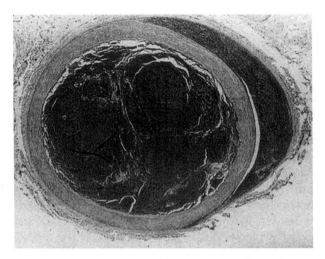

Figure 14.32 *Traumatic thrombosis of an internal carotid artery. Note the dissection in the wall of the artery. Reproduced by permission from Ref. 216.*

mines the pattern of vascular damage in the anterior lobe of the pituitary depending on whether the patient has experienced a high or low transection of the pituitary stalk.

Damage to blood vessels may occur. Angiography is complementary to imaging and is used primarily for the study of injuries to blood vessels, particularly those in the neck after penetrating injuries. It is now possible to identify various vascular lesions, including dissection or occlusion of the internal carotid (Fig. 14.32) or vertebral arteries, traumatic pseudoaneurysm, traumatic arteriovenous fistula, venous thrombosis and an assessment of vasospasm.

The frequency and distribution of cerebral infarction consequent upon these various vascular abnormalities are reviewed later (see below).

The wide use of imaging techniques after head injury has shown that in many patients there are small haemorrhagic and non-haemorrhagic lesions in the brain. This is particularly true of MRI in the detection of lesions attributable to shearing injury, the principal neuropathological correlates of which are lesions in lobar white matter, in the corpus callosum and in the dorsolateral sector of the rostral brainstem adjacent to the superior cerebellar peduncle(s). These areas have since become known as the 'shearing injury triad'. However, such lesions are not restricted to these areas, being found also in periventricular structures, the hippocampal formation, the internal capsule and occasionally deep within the cerebellar hemispheres.

Petechial haemorrhages are not uncommonly found post-mortem in patients dying from severe head injury. While many of these may indeed have histological evidence of traumatic axonal injury there are others including diffuse vascular injury (see below) in which the haemorrhages can be ascribed to a number of causes that include ischaemic damage in the territory supplied by the pericallosal arteries, usually secondary to a supracallosal hernia, fat embolism and a host of vascular and haematological abnormalities that constitute some of the medical complications of head injuries.[329]

Another complication of head injury is traumatic subarachnoid haemorrhage. Death may be rapid and the cases fall within the provenance of legal medicine. In most such cases a large amount of fresh blood is present within the basal cisterns, and around the brainstem and the cranial nerve roots.[312,333] If there is a history of assault, the possibility of trauma to the vertebral artery should always be borne in mind, particularly if there is an external bruise to the side or back of the neck, either behind or just below the ear.[223,241] Whatever the circumstances, the vertebral artery can be damaged in the canal within the first cervical vertebra whether or not the transverse process is fractured, just below the axis in the space between the transverse processes of the axis and the atlas as it emerges from the canal and penetrates the spinal dura just below the foramen magnum, or within the subarchnoid space within or above the foraman magnum.[312] The autopsy demonstration of damage to the vertebral artery usually requires the use of CT scanning or post-mortem angiography. These are followed by painstaking dissection to determine whether or not the bleeding was due to rupture of a saccular aneurysm. If such a bleeding point is not found then the upper cervical region is dissected and processed using a number of specialized techniques that may require the removal of the specimen or block and its subsequent dissection, possibly after decalcification.

DIFFUSE (MULTIFOCAL) BRAIN DAMAGE

The concept of diffuse brain damage in patients who have sustained a blunt head injury is not new. Thus, its importance has been emphasized as being the cause not only of 'instantaneous loss of cerebral function so frequently observed after head injury' but also of many of the long-continued disturbances of consciousness often followed by residual symptoms in patients who were rendered unconscious at the moment of injury. Diffuse brain damage was also the dominant theme in the early experimental work[122] and, more recently, a comprehensive clinical study has emphasized that immediate prolonged unconsciousness unaccompanied by an intracranial mass lesion occurs in almost half of severely head-injured patients and is associated with 35% of all head-injury deaths.[188] Furthermore, there is some evidence that in patients who have sustained a minor head injury there may be persisting, if mild, diffuse damage in the brain for up to 99 days after TBI.

Diffuse brain damage is more difficult to define and delineate than the more obvious focal types of damage because macroscopic abnormalities may be minimal or even trivial, while much of it can only be recognized microscopically even when the brain has been properly fixed before dissection. There are four principal types of diffuse brain damage: of these three are seen frequently in patients who survive their injury long enough to be admitted to hospital, namely diffuse traumatic axonal injury, ischaemic brain damage and brain swelling; the fourth, diffuse vascular injury, seems to be restricted to patients who die very soon after their head injury.[594]

Traumatic axonal injury

Strich[566] was the first to define clearly the occurrence of 'diffuse degeneration of the cerebral white matter' in a series of patients with severe post-traumatic dementia. This type of brain damage resulting from head injury is now widely recognized, although it has been referred to by other authors under different names, i.e. shearing injury,[464,568,569] diffuse damage to white matter of immediate impact type[20] diffuse white matter shearing injury,[650] inner cerebral trauma,[224] and now, for the most severe forms, by the internationally recognized term of DAI.[17,191] Strich has always taken the view that diffuse damage to white matter is brought about by the shearing of nerve fibres at the moment of injury, but others have contended that it is secondary to hypoxic or ischaemic brain damage, cerebral oedema or secondary damage to the brainstem resulting from an intracranial expanding lesion.[275,276,466]

When the term DAI was first introduced in the early 1980s,[17,191] it provided an appealing description for the structural changes that occurred in the types of diffuse TBI in which few or no macroscopically visible changes were present. Subsequent to the initial description, axonal change was found to be present in human minor head injury[48] and was hypothesized to be the structural basis of concussion.[192] At that time, clinicians tended towards the view that DAI was the main cause of diffuse brain injury (coma lasting longer than 6 h, without mass lesions to explain it). Pathological studies using silver impregnation techniques demonstrated axonal change in 34% of all cases of fatal head injury, and in 53% of deaths that occurred after 12-h survival.[473] It was also found that DAI was a major factor in patients who had been vegetative or severely disabled after their injury.[374]

As the concepts of axonal change and diffuse brain injury were developed, the overriding hypothesis was that of a clinical spectrum, all due to a common axonal pathology, but differing in amount, location and severity. Thus, it was postulated that, as physiological disturbances of function became more severe, there was a progressively larger amount of axonal damage.[184,192] It therefore became possible to conceive of a spectrum of events that began with concussive syndromes and ended in the more severe forms of brain impairment, which included immediate coma associated with decerebrate posturing, prolonged coma and incomplete recovery (Fig. 14.33).

This concept, also supported by neuropathological studies of human and experimental head injuries, has resulted in the definition of three grades of DAI. In grade I DAI there was widespread axonal damage in the corpus

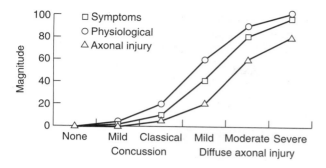

Figure 14.33 *The continuum of diffuse brain injury.*

callosum as well as in the white matter of the cerebral hemispheres and in the brainstem. In grade II DAI there are, in addition, focal abnormalities in the corpus callosum, often associated with small haemorrhages called tissue tear haemorrhages. In grade III DAI, the most severe form, there are, in addition to the findings of grade II, axonal abnormalities and commonly abnormalities in the rostral brainstem resulting from tissue tear haemorrhages.

These concepts were widely accepted, particularly in neuropathology and experimental neurotrauma. However, it soon became evident axonal damage could be identified in patients who did not conform to the clinical concept of DAI. Thus, tissue tear haemorrhages had been seen on CT scans in conditions other than those associated with immediate, prolonged coma after a head injury. It was further recognized that grade I DAI can be found without there being immediate coma and the term DAI was incorrectly used by some investigators to describe morphologically abnormal axons in the absence of trauma. Often this is focal axonal damage as occurs in normal ageing or adjacent to focal lesions in the CNS such as haematomas, infarcts, abscesses and tumours where axons are disrupted.[192] Focal axonal change must therefore be clearly separated from DAI, although there appears to be a sequence of descriptive alterations that is common to many, if not all, types of axonal damage, similar to that first described by Cajal.[78,567]

Clinicopathological studies on DAI[9,17,20] have helped to define the time course of the structural abnormalities in white matter, but have not provided direct evidence of axonal shearing (see below). Similar structural abnormalities have been produced in non-human primates without there being any increase in ICP or an episode of hypoxia.[17,191]

There are three distinctive features of the pathology of DAI in its most severe form: (1) diffuse damage to axons; (2) a focal lesion in the corpus callosum; and (3) focal lesions in the dorsolateral sector(s) of the rostral brainstem adjacent to the superior cerebellar peduncles. Since the last two can often be identified macroscopically, it may be easy to make the presumptive diagnosis of grade III DAI post-mortem on the basis of the macroscopic examination of the brain, but the diffuse damage to axons can

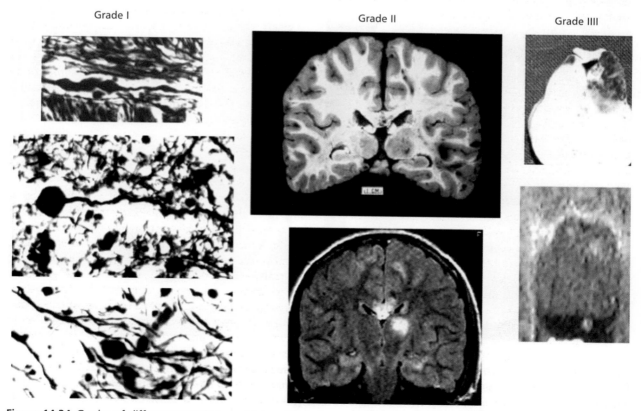

Figure 14.34 *Grades of diffuse traumatic axonal injury. Grade I axonal damage only; grade II lesions in the corpus callosum; grade III lesions in the dorsolateral sector(s) of the brainstem.*

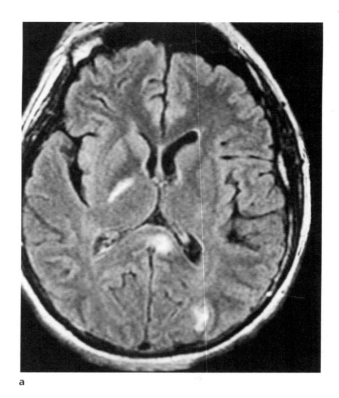

a

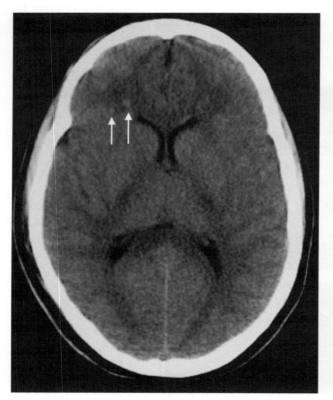

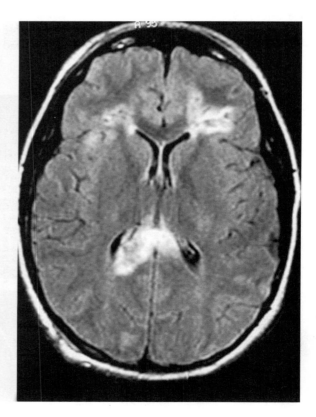

b

Figure 14.35 *Diffuse axonal injury: tissue tear haemorrhages. (a) Diffuse traumatic axonal injury with tissue tear haemorrhage in the splenium of the corpus callosum, right thalamus and the occipital white matter. (b) CT (left) and T1-weighted MRI (right) show-ing greater sensitivity of MRI in detecting lesions associated with diffuse traumatic axonal injury. On CT only two small tissue tear haemorrhages (arrows) are seen, while large MRI intensities are seen in the frontal white matter at Steinert's angle and the splenium of the corpus callosum. (c) and (d) Continued.*

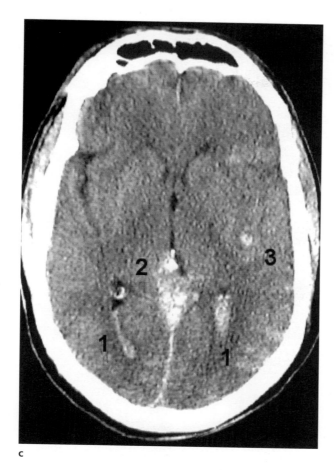

c

only be seen by light or electron microscopy. This may also be the case with the focal lesions in the corpus callosum and in the brainstem. In patients who sustain milder forms of DAI, however, there may be no macroscopic abnormalities in the brain[48] (Fig. 14.34).

The appearances of the individual lesions depend on the length of survival after injury. In the early stages after injury (hours to days) the focal lesion in the corpus callosum is typically haemorrhagic (Fig. 14.35a–d). Although often not measuring more than 3–5 mm across, the lesions usually extend over an anteroposterior distance of several centimetres. They generally occur in the inferior part of the corpus callosum and on one or other side of the midline (Fig. 14.36a); they may, however, extend to the midline (Fig. 14.36b, c) to involve the interventricular septum (which is often ruptured and may therefore be the cause of the not infrequently associated intraventricular haemorrhage) and the fornix (Fig. 14.36c). Haemorrhagic lesions are sometimes restricted to the splenium where they are frequently bilateral, particularly affecting its lateral margins (Fig. 14.36d). After several days the lesion becomes granular and less easy to identify macroscopically (Fig. 14.36e), and with the passage of time comes ultimately to be represented by a shrunken and sometimes cystic area (Fig. 14.36f).

Histological studies have established that the haemorrhage is first perivascular and then extends into the adjacent tissue. Silver impregnation reveals numerous axonal swellings adjacent to the focal lesions 15–18 h after injury, followed by the usual reactive changes in microglia, astrocytes and capillary endothelium, the appearance of lipid-containing macrophages and the progressive removal of the damaged tissue. The end-stage is a rarefied lesion traversed by astrocytic fibres among which there are haemosiderin-containing macrophages. The use of antibodies to β-APP, the microglial-associated antigen CD68 (PG-M1) and to astrocytes [glial fibrillary acidic protein (GFAP)] has greatly enhanced our knowledge of various cellular responses, and the time course that has proved of importance in Forensic practice.[176]

The lesions in the dorsolateral sector(s) of the rostral brainstem follow an essentially similar course (Fig. 14.37). In patients of short survival they are usually haemorrhagic, when they can be readily identified macroscopically in the dorsolateral part of the midbrain and the rostral pons, almost always involving the superior cerebellar peduncle (Fig. 14.38a–e). When bilateral, one lesion is usually larger than the other. As with lesions in the corpus callosum, with the passage of time these focal lesions become brown and often granular and are ultimately represented by shrunken, sometimes cystic, scars (Fig. 14.38f). The sequence of histological changes is similar to that described above for the corpus callosum but on occasion, particularly if the lesion is small, it is represented in the early stages by a rarefied and coarsely vacuolated focus, a traumatic tissue tear in which haemorrhage is absent or minimal (Fig. 14.39) that can only be identified microscopically.

d

Figure 14.35 Continued. (**c**) CT lesions associated with diffuse traumatic axonal injury: intraventricular haemorrhage (1), tissue tear haemorrhage in the corpus callosum and periventricular region (2), and tissue tear haemorrhage in hemispheric white matter (3). (**d**) T1-weighted coronal MRI image of diffuse traumatic axonal injury lesions in the corpus callosum and the fornix, and a gliding contusion in the left frontal parasagittal white matter.

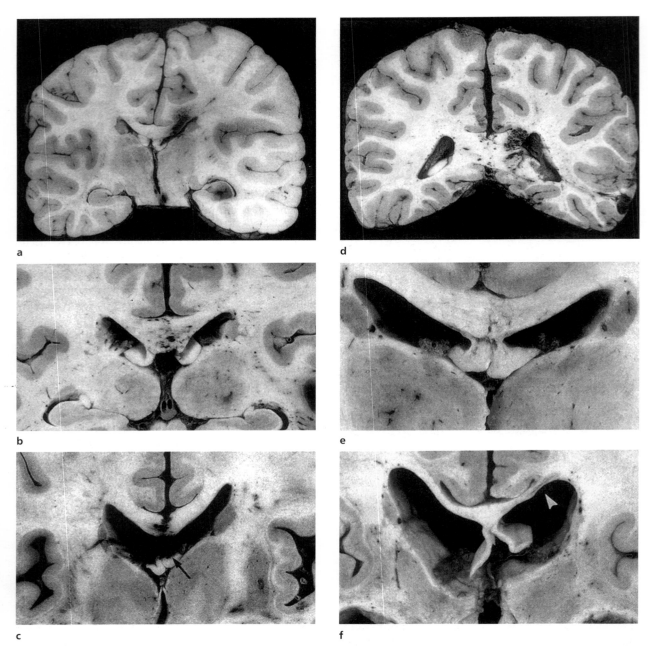

Figure 14.36 *Diffuse axonal injury: lesions in the corpus callosum. (a) There is an acute haemorrhagic lesion to the right of the midline. There is also a small haematoma in the right hippocampus (6 days' survival). (b) Multiple small haemorrhagic foci in and adjacent to the midline (5 days' survival). (c) In addition to a haemorrhagic lesion in the corpus callosum, the interventricular septum is ruptured and there are small foci of haemorrhage in the fornix (arrow) (10 days' survival). (d) Haemorrhagic lesion accentuated in the lateral part of the splenium (5 days' survival). (e) Disintegrating non-haemorrhagic lesion (12 weeks' survival). (f) Shrunken cystic lesion (arrowhead) (21 months' survival). Reproduced by permission from Ref. 216.*

Because the lesions in the corpus callosum and in the dorsolateral sector(s) of the rostral brainstem are often small, it is not surprising that pathologists may think that they are of little significance. When both are present, however, the patient has sustained severe DAI.

In patients of short (days) survival damage to axons is shown by the presence of large numbers of eosinophilic (Fig. 14.40a) and argyrophilic bulbs on nerve fibres (Fig. 14.40b) – the 'retraction' balls of Cajal[78] – in the white

matter of the cerebral hemispheres, the cerebellum and the brainstem. Their distribution is not uniform or symmetrical but they occur particularly in the subcortical parasagittal white matter (Fig. 14.40c), in the corpus callosum, particularly posteriorly, remote from the focal lesions referred to above (Fig. 14.40d), in the fornix, in the internal capsule and in the deep grey matter (Fig. 14.40e), in the white matter adjacent to the outer limits of the caudate nucleus and in cerebellar folia

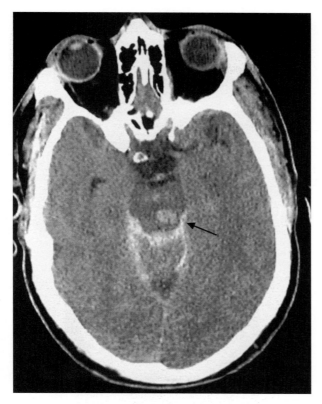

Figure 14.37 *Diffuse axonal injury: lesions in the brainstem. Unenhanced CT image of tissue tear haemorrhage in the dorsolateral sector of the midbrain in diffuse traumatic axonal injury. Traumatic subarachnoid haemorrhage is seen in the perimesencephalic cistern.*

dorsal to the dentate nuclei. Various tracts in the brainstem are involved but as has been emphasized there is often particularly severe but asymmetrical involvement of the corticospinal tracts, the medial lemnisci, the medial longitudinal bundles and the central tegmental tracts[566] (Fig. 14.40f). It is quite common to find large numbers of axonal swellings in nerve fibres running in one direction, and none in an immediately adjacent tract running in a different direction (Fig. 14.40b). In addition to typical bulbs, axons may be varicose and swollen (Fig. 14.40g).

After a few weeks the most striking abnormality is the presence of large numbers of small clusters of microglia throughout the white matter of the cerebral hemispheres, the cerebellum and the brainstem: the clusters of microglia are well seen in 20-μm-thick celloidin sections stained by cresyl violet (Fig. 14.41), or by immunocytochemistry. By this stage the damaged axons have become fragmented and the myelin sheaths broken up, with the result that axonal swellings are rarely identifiable. After 2–3 months wallerian-type degeneration (Fig. 14.42) becomes easy to detect, particularly with the Marchi method.[567] This is often particularly conspicuous in the medial lemnisci and in the pyramidal tracts throughout the brainstem and the spinal cord, but it can also be iden-

tified in the white matter of the cerebral hemispheres including subcortical white matter and the internal capsules.[566,568] By this time there is usually some reduced bulk and increased consistency of the white matter of the cerebral hemispheres, thinning of the corpus callosum (Fig. 14.43) and compensatory enlargement of the ventricular system (Fig. 14.44).

Any other type of brain damage due to blunt head injury may occur in association with DAI, but in an analysis of the cases of DAI in the Glasgow database there was a statistically significant lower incidence of cerebral contusions, intracranial haematoma and evidence of a high ICP compared with patients who did not have DAI. In the patients with DAI there was also a statistically significant lower incidence of lucid interval, fracture of the skull and injury due to a fall, and a higher incidence of head injury due to road traffic accidents. Although contusions tend to be less in patients with DAI, 'gliding' contusions[9] are often prominent, as are small haematomas deep in the cerebral hemispheres[7] and in the Ammon's horns. However, it has to be emphasized that the presence of an intracranial haematoma does not preclude coexisting DAI.[111,302,510]

Grading of diffuse traumatic axonal injury in man

Oppenheimer[457] was the first to show that occasional clusters of microglia can be found in patients dying from some unrelated cause within 15 h but more easily between 24 and 48 h after a minor head injury; Clark[99] also drew attention to the frequent occurrence of such clusters in the white matter in patients dying as a result of a head injury. Further, Pilz[473] described the frequent occurrence of axonal swellings in fatal head injuries in man and Adams et al.[10] detailed nine cases of what has been referred to as microscopic DAI. More recently immunostaining with an antibody to β-APP showed multifocal axonal injury in five cases of mild head injury (GCS of 14–15) with a recorded loss of consciousness for as little as 60 s and with a survival from intercurrent disease up to 99 days after the initial head injury,[48] thereby extending earlier observations by the same group.[49] In these cases macroscopic focal lesions in the corpus callosum or in the brainstem were not seen but on histological examination there were the typical structural features of multiple axonal swellings diffusely scattered throughout the brain.

In a review of 122 cases of traumatic axonal injury in the Glasgow database using the same criteria as defined for the subhuman primates (see below) it was possible to identify ten cases of grade I DAI.[6] There were 29 cases with grade II DAI, i.e. there was a focal lesion in the corpus callosum in addition to diffuse axonal damage; the focal lesions were identified only microscopically in 11 of these cases. The majority of the cases (83) had sustained grade III DAI because there were focal lesions both in the corpus callosum and in the dorsolateral

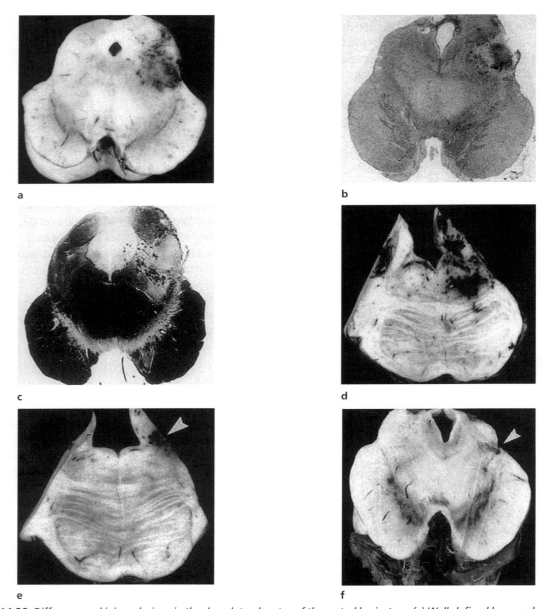

Figure 14.38 *Diffuse axonal injury: lesions in the dorsolateral sector of the rostral brainstem. (a) Well-defined haemorrhagic lesion in the midbrain (12 days' survival). (b) Same lesion as (a). (Cresyl violet.) (c) Same lesion as (a). (Heidenhain.) (d) Large haemorrhagic lesion in the rostral pons (5 days' survival). (e) Small haemorrhagic lesion (arrow) centred on a superior cerebellar peduncle (2 days' survival). (f) Old shrunken lesion (arrow) in the midbrain (9 months' survival). Reproduced by permission from Ref. 216.*

sector(s) of the rostral brainstem; in only 49 of these cases were both the focal lesions apparent macroscopically, even in a properly fixed and dissected brain. Thus, of the 122 cases, the severity of DAI could be defined only by histological assessment in 24, while its presence in 31 cases would have been missed unless appropriate histological studies had been undertaken. Grades II and III can be said to be severe if the focal lesions are apparent macroscopically. In a study of 34 cases of severe DAI,[46] an increased incidence of gliding contusions and basal ganglia haematomas in patients with DAI was found.[9] It has also been shown that if DAI was caused by a fall it was usually from a considerable height,[8] although doubt has been

raised about this.[3] Further experience has established[212] that DAI can also occur after an assault.[266] Most of the patients were involved in a brawl that resulted in an exchange of punches, but in some there were also additional blows to the head by kicking or heavy objects. In some instances, as a result of punching, the victim had an accelerated fall, striking his head on the ground, kerb or pavement. The lack of full information about the assault leaves open the possibility that the victims sustained injuries other than those simply due to punching. This study therefore did not determine whether DAI was produced by the assault itself, by the ensuing fall to the ground, the subsequent deceleration, or by a combination

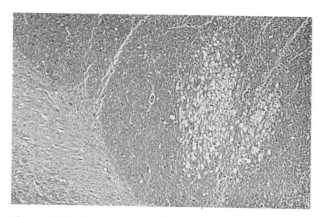

Figure 14.39 *Traumatic tissue tear: diffuse axonal injury. There is a rarefied lesion in a superior cerebellar peduncle (3 days' survival). Reproduced by permission from Ref. 216.*

of these. It was initially thought that the combination of head motions did not include the acceleration/deceleration conditions that are necessary to produce DAI,[194,379] but increasing experience with witnessed accounts would suggest otherwise. It is worth noting at this stage that DAI has not been reported as a sequela of boxing.[115,178]

In the early studies on traumatic axonal injury it was stressed that none of the cases had 'talked' immediately after their injury.[20] In a more recent study 17 (14%) of 122 cases with DAI experienced a complete or partial lucid interval.[6] The two with a complete lucid interval had grade I injury, while the remaining 15 had grade II. Thus, none of the patients who talked had the most severe type, i.e. grade III, of DAI. Furthermore, all of the patients who talked died as a result of some other type of pathology: raised ICP brought about by oedema related to contusions, diffuse brain swelling or intracranial haematoma in 15, fat embolism in one and massive gastrointestinal haemorrhage in one.

Histological identification of axonal injury in man

By the conventional histological techniques of haematoxylin and eosin (H&E) and silver impregnation it is not possible to identify with certainty axonal bulbs until about 15 h after injury. Thus, a diagnosis of DAI could not, until the advent of immunohistochemistry, be made in patients who survived for only a short time after their injury. However, the diagnosis in cases with a shorter survival can now be made and has been greatly facilitated by the use of immunocytochemistry on either freshly frozen brain tissue[208] or paraffin-embedded material.[198]

Various axonally transported proteins have been suggested as possible markers for axonal damage. For example, anti-ubiquitin[235] and anti-68-, 170- and 200-kDa neurofilament protein[208,443] immunostaining have been tried with some success. However, in an extensive comparative study using antibodies to nine different antigens, immunostaining for β-APP produced the most sensitive and reliable staining of axonal damage.[537] There is an increased expression of β-APP throughout grey matter in

head-injured patients, but particularly in populations of neurons closely associated with axonal damage.[198] However, the accumulation of β-APP is not restricted to head-injured patients and has been reported in the dystrophic myelinated axons of elderly subjects, in association with cerebral infarction and haematomas, and in human immunodeficiency virus (HIV) encephalitis (Fig. 14.45). It is therefore not a marker for head injury but rather it is an indicator of local anatomical or more generalized metabolic change within the brain. Thus, all types of focal axonal injury will immunostain for β-APP in formalin-fixed paraffin-embedded sections.

Axonal β-APP immunoreactivity was present in all cases who survived for 2–3 h or more, thereby demonstrating the usefulness of β-APP immunostaining as an early marker for axonal injury. The reliability of β-APP immunostaining for detecting axonal injury has been confirmed in a number of studies, indicating that the frequency of axonal injury has probably been grossly underestimated and that it may be an almost universal consequence of fatal head injury.

Distribution and time course of axonal injury in man

In the original descriptions of severe DAI[17,20,224] using classic silver methods, emphasis was placed on the concentration of axonal damage in and around midline structures, namely the corpus callosum, the parasagittal white matter and in the rostral pons. This pattern of axonal injury has been confirmed and extended using immunostaining for β-APP and it is now suggested that blocks be taken from a wider sample of tissue.[180] The recommended set of blocks include the corpus callosum and parasagittal posterior frontal white matter, the splenium of the corpus callosum, the deep grey matter (to include the posterior limb of the internal capsule), the cerebellar hemispheres, the midbrain (to include the decussation of the superior cerebellar peduncles) and the pons (to include the superior or middle cerebellar peduncles), with suggested additional samples from the corpus callosum and parasagittal anterior frontal white matter, and the temporal lobe (to include the hippocampi). However, increasing experience suggests that the pattern of axonal injury is likely to be different in different patients depending upon the loading conditions and that quantitative studies will be required to improve clinicopathological correlations. It is therefore recommended that the brain be sampled widely to establish the presence and distribution of any axonal damage.

β-APP immunostaining has been demonstrated in axonal swellings 1.75 h after head injury[49] and with antigen retrieval techniques β-APP positivity has been noted within 60–90 h postinjury. A study of 25 further cases of blunt head injury by immunostaining for β-APP suggested that the amount of axonal damage increased up to 24 h postinjury and levelled off thereafter.[199] Using axonal bulb formation as incontrovertible evidence of axonal damage,

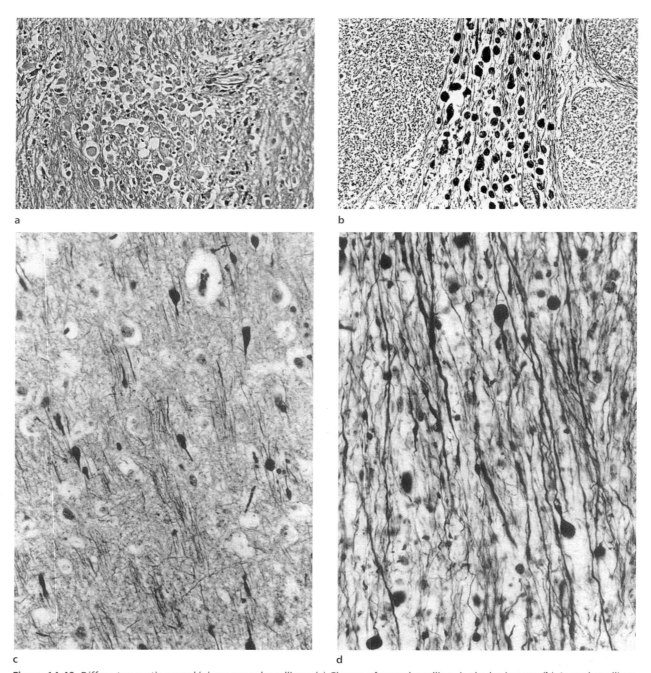

Figure 14.40 *Diffuse traumatic axonal injury: axonal swellings. (a) Clumps of axonal swellings in the brainstem. (b) Axonal swellings in the tegmentum of the midbrain, all on axons running in the same direction. (c) Axonal swellings in the parasagittal white matter. (d) Axonal swellings in the corpus callosum. (e) Axonal swellings in the thalamus. (f) Axonal swellings in the central tegmental tract. (g) Irregularly beaded axon in the corpus callosum. (a, H&E; b–e, Palmgren.) Reproduced by permission from Ref. 216.*

it was confirmed that damage increased only during the first 12–24 h after injury, suggesting that not all the immediate postinjury changes were irreversible.[487] With longer survival, axonal bulbs diminish in number but can still be identified at 4 weeks[46] and for about 3 months after injury.[48,374] However, between 10 and 14 days not all bulbs are β-APP positive, although axons may remain so for about 2 weeks: the occasional granular deposit can be seen for up to 6 months postinjury.[176] The relationship between

the size of axonal swellings with survival time has been explored in post-mortem brain tissue.[619] In 66 cases of head injury with known post-traumatic survival using an image analysis system on β-APP-immunostained axons, a strong positive and significant relationship between the mean size of axonal swelling and survival time which plateaued at around 85 h postinjury was found. It was concluded that in the forensic setting such observations might contribute evidence about trauma and postinjury survival,

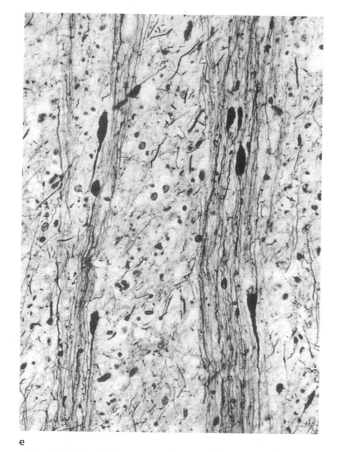

e

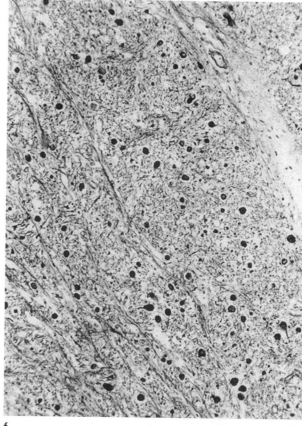

f

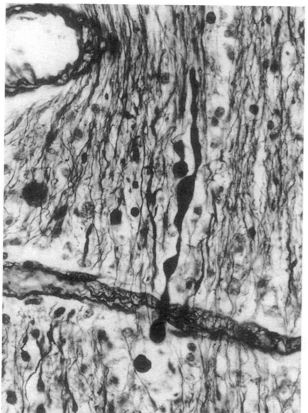

g

but should always be assessed with other evidence. As the number of bulbs decreases so changes in microglia, macrophages and astrocytes become more marked.[176]

Diffuse axonal damage is an important pathological substrate of prolonged traumatic coma that is not due to a mass lesion and, like cerebral concussion, is caused only by inertial and not by contact phenomena.[191,406] Similar to concussion, which is a milder form of the same type of damage, DAI occurs only from angular or rotational acceleration. The amount and location of axonal damage in all

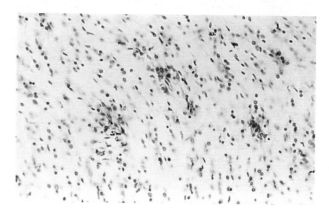

Figure 14.41 *Diffuse traumatic axonal injury: clusters of microglia in the white matter. (Cresyl violet.) Reproduced by permission from Ref. 216.*

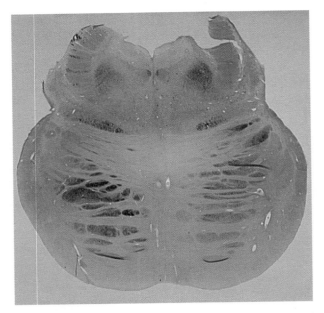

Figure 14.42 *Diffuse traumatic axonal injury: degeneration of long tracts. Degeneration in ascending and descending tracts in a patient who survived in a vegetative state for 9 months after a head injury. (Marchi preparation.) Reproduced by permission from Ref. 216.*

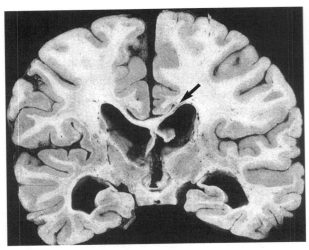

Figure 14.44 *Diffuse traumatic axonal injury. Enlargement of the ventricular system in a patient who survived in a vegetative state for 21 months after a head injury. Arrow indicates the corpus callosum. Reproduced by permission from Ref. 216.*

likelihood determine the severity of injury and the quality of recovery. Critical factors in the amount of axonal damage are the magnitude, duration and rate of onset of the angular acceleration, as well as the direction of head motion. DAI is produced by long acceleration loading (20–25 ms), while loading with shorter onset (5–10 ms) produces acute SDH. Thus, DAI is most likely to occur when the head is impulsively loaded or when impact is against a relatively soft, broad object (e.g. motor vehicle interiors). The former is uncommon clinically, but the latter is the most frequent circumstance producing DAI. In fact, although the mechanisms causing SDH and DAI are closely related, there is a marked difference in the type of accident that produces each condition. Almost all cases of DAI, especially its severe form, arise from road traffic accidents, e.g. impact to padded dashboards, resilient windshields, deformable hoods and energy-absorbing steering columns, in which acceleration is long. Conversely, most SDHs occur because of falls or assaults in which the impact duration is short and the angular acceleration is abrupt.

The direction in which the head moves plays an important role in the amount and distribution of axonal damage in a given situation. For equivalent levels of angular acceleration, the brain is most vulnerable if it is moved laterally. The brain tolerates sagittal movement best, and head motions in the horizontal plane are somewhere in between lateral and sagittal movements. Although some degree of axonal damage can occur in any direction, the full-blown picture of widely scattered damage to the cerebral hemispheres and brainstem, along with tissue tear haemorrhages, occurs most

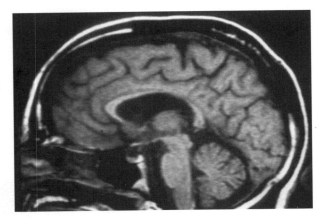

Figure 14.43 *Diffuse traumatic axonal injury: long survival. T1-weighted MRI image 11 years after severe diffuse traumatic axonal injury showing marked atrophy in the posterior one-third of the corpus callosum.*

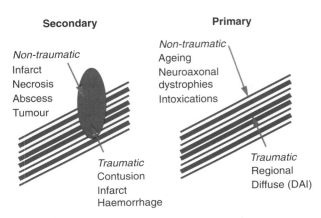

Figure 14.45 *Types of axonal damage.*

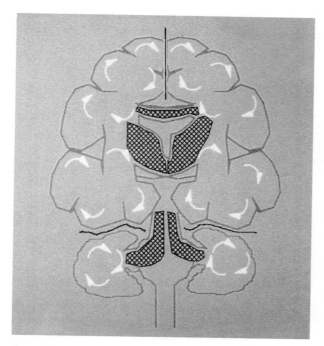

Figure 14.46 *Movement of head undergoing rotation acceleration. A schematic coronal view of the brain is shown to illustrate the movement that occurs when the entire head undergoes rotational acceleration. The arrows depict the local movement of the brain. Note that in certain locations in the central brain and brainstem, portions of the brain move in opposite directions, thus generating shear and tensile strains shown in cross-hatched areas. It is these regions that show the greatest and most consistent amounts of axonal injury. Reproduced by permission from Ref. 216.*

probably owing to geometrical changes in the strain pattern induced by the falx and tentorium during lateral motions (Fig. 14.46). Newer imaging techniques are increasingly capable of identifying white-matter damage (Fig. 14.47).

Patients who sustain severe DAI are unconscious from the moment of injury, do not experience a lucid interval, and remain unconscious, vegetative or at least severely disabled until death.[15,282] Their clinical state has been referred to in the past as primary brainstem injury, but although there is damage to the brainstem in DAI, it is always accompanied by evidence of diffuse brain damage.

Recent literature has suggested that the amount and distribution of β-APP immunoreactivity after hypoxia may mimic DAI.[301] While by definition this cannot be the case (absence of definite history of TBI), it raises the possibility that in a forensic setting there may be instances in which β-APP immunoreactivity may be sufficiently widespread to raise the possibility of trauma. Dolinak *et al.*,[131,132] in follow-up studies, concluded that if the minimum number of brain blocks is taken from the recommended areas[176] then global hypoxia per se is an unusual cause of axonal injury,[131] whereas hypoglycaemia may be a cause of widespread axonal injury.[132] In both cir-

cumstances particular attention has to be paid to the vascular consequences of brain swelling and raised ICP (Fig. 14.48a, b).

DAI in experimental models

In the earlier series of experiments undertaken by Gennarelli and his group in Philadelphia, USA, all of the focal types of brain damage encountered in non-missile head injury in man were produced experimentally in non-human primates.[14] Prolonged traumatic unconsciousness in the absence of an intracranial expanding lesion was, however, not produced. When the model was modified to allow acceleration of the head in the oblique and lateral planes as well as sagittal, and when the duration of the acceleration was increased, prolonged traumatic coma was produced in the absence of an intracranial expanding lesion[17,191] (Fig. 14.49a, b). The structural abnormalities in these brains were identical to those seen in DAI in man: these consisted of focal lesions in the corpus callosum and in the dorsolateral sector(s) of the rostral brainstem, and microscopic evidence of diffuse damage to axons.

In this experimental situation using classic silver impregnation it was possible to define three grades of DAI[191] which were used later to develop the grading system in man (see above). As in man, axonal damage was particularly conspicuous in the parasagittal white matter of the cerebral hemispheres, in the corpus callosum, in the superior cerebellar peduncles, in the medial lemnisci, in the medial longitudinal bundles, in the central tegmental tracts and in the corticospinal tracts in the brainstem. So far, non-human primates have not been kept alive long enough to allow the demonstration of wallerian degeneration.

In these experiments there were occasional mild surface contusions at conventional sites and small amounts of blood in the subarachnoid and subdural spaces. Gliding contusions were conspicuous and there were frequently haematomas deep in the cerebral hemispheres similar to those seen in man. The progression from sagittal through oblique to lateral angular acceleration was associated with increased duration of coma, more severe post-traumatic disability and more severe DAI.[194] Furthermore, as the degree of traumatic coma increased from transient to severe, both the incidence and severity of DAI increased, the latter in proportion to the duration of the coma. There was also a close correlation between outcome and the presence and severity of DAI: when the animal made a good recovery there was no evidence of DAI; animals that remained moderately disabled usually had grade I or grade II DAI; while in the great majority of animals that remained severely disabled or in persistent coma until death the structural abnormalities were those of grade III. DAI was most readily produced by lateral acceleration of the head and this correlated highly with the production of severe traumatic coma, poor neurological recovery, and the occurrence and severity of DAI.

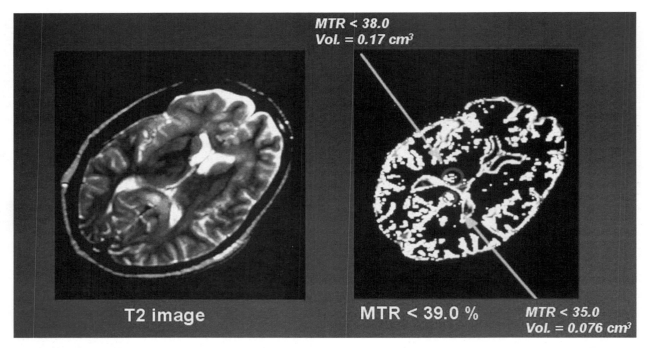

Figure 14.47 *Diffuse traumatic axonal injury: neuroimaging. T2 (left) and magnetic transfer (right) MRI images demonstrating greater sensitivity to white-matter abnormalities in diffuse traumatic axonal injury.*

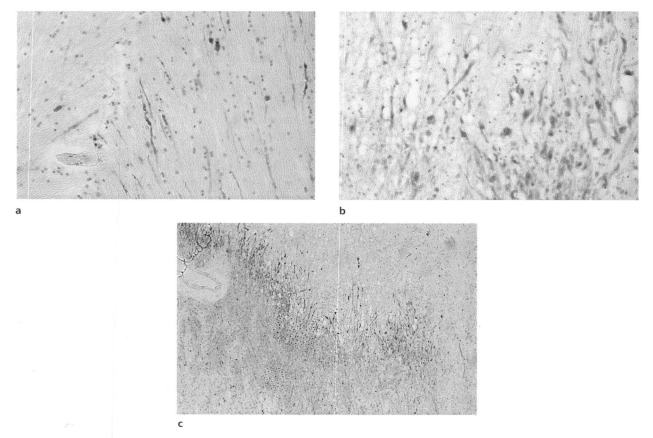

Figure 14.48 *Diffuse traumatic axonal injury. (a) Scattered immunoreactive axons. (b) Larger number of scattered immunoreactive axons. (c) Compare with the pattern of immunoreactive axons in a and b. In this instance the immunoreactivity is Z-shaped and defines the margin of a cerebral infarct. (a–c, ICC βAPP.)*

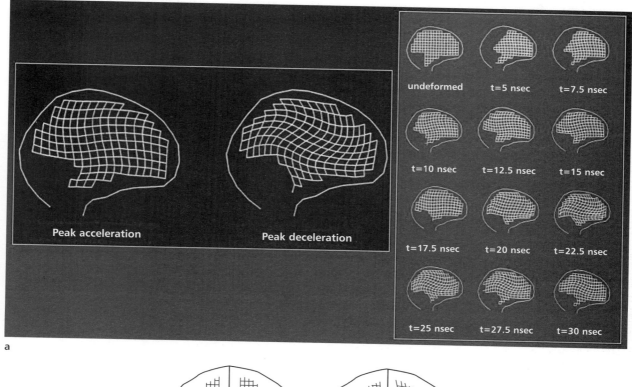

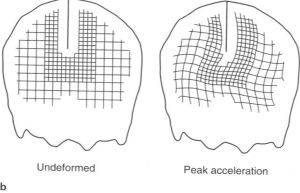

Figure 14.49 *Head motions of the brain. (a) Sagittal head motion. The maximum deformation is at the surface of the brain which predisposes to rupture of the bridging veins and bleeding into the subdural space. (b) Oblique head motion. In contrast to (a) the maximum deformation is in midline structures determined in part by the compartmentalization of the intracranial cavity. It is in the central white-matter tracts that axonal injury is therefore maximal.*

This accords well with the clinicopathological findings in man:[17] if the acceleration/deceleration is short as occurs in falls, the principal findings are SDH and contusions; if it is of longer duration as occurs in road traffic accidents, DAI is more likely to be produced. Because traumatic coma occurred instantaneously in the non-human primates,[191] and since none of the 45 human cases of severe DAI experienced a lucid interval, in contrast to the 42% of patients found not to have DAI who did experience a lucid interval,[17] there is now no doubt that a cascade of pathological events in axons occurs at the moment of injury and that it is related to shear and tensile strains. The fact that the lesions in the corpus callosum and in the dorsolateral sector(s) in the rostral brainstem are often haemorrhagic suggests that these strains can also produce rupture of small blood vessels. It further seems likely that axonal damage is the most important single factor contributing to the severity of brain damage and to the outcome in any patient who sustains a blunt head injury because it occurs at the moment of injury.

Fluid percussion induced traumatic brain injury is the most commonly used model of human head injury. Originally developed for the rabbit and cat, it has been modified for use in a range of species including mouse, rat, doe and pig.[181,549] In addition to contusions, lateral fluid percussion induces axonal damage including tissue tears.[55,222,368] Prolonged survival, albeit in the absence of coma, is associated with brain atrophy,[54,129,470,548] which has been attributed in large measure to degenerative changes in white matter.

As the brain size decreases the rotational acceleration required to replicate events in human head injury increases exponentially. For example, it has been calculated that in the original experiments 20 000 kg of thrust was just enough to generate sufficient non-impact rotational acceleration to induce DAI in a 50–75-g non-human primate brain.[549] Adaptation of the same injury apparatus allowed the development of rotational acceleration brain injury in miniature swine; this model now having been the basis of multiple studies including characterization of axonal pathology[502,552] and degenerative hippocampal cell loss[547,549] and their correlation with various imaging modalities.[308,546]

Structural changes and time course of axonal injury

The classic view that in man the axons are torn at the time of injury, i.e. primary axotomy (immediate axonal disruption), no longer appears to be true in most cases, although it undoubtedly occurs in man in instances of pontomedullary rent. Primary axotomy is uncommon, although it has been identified by electron microscopy in a population of small-diameter fibres in a non-human primate model of acceleration–deceleration injury (Fig. 14.50).[402] Perhaps this is not unexpected given the severity of the injury and the obvious physical disruption of tissue that can occur under conditions of high mechanical loading. Under conditions of mild to moderate TBI it is now apparent that there is a process of delayed axotomy in which the actual disruption of some axons does not occur until some time after the original injury. Initial studies in mild TBI using anterograde tracers[484] demonstrated focal impairment of axoplasmic transport at about 60 min postinjury and that with survival further changes occurred in the affected segment which became swollen and lobulated, axotomy only becoming apparent between 6 and 12 h after injury. Thereafter, the proximal segment continued to expand becoming maximal between 24 and 72 h, whereas the distal segment underwent rapid degeneration. Ultrastructural studies showed the accumulation of various membranous organelles to be greatest at the paranode. While these alterations were occurring there was a notable absence of abnormalities in the axolemma,[484] although earlier studies using freeze-fracture had demonstrated changes in the glial–axonal junction between 1 and 6 h after injury.[394] Later, altered permeability of the axolemma was demonstrated after the extracellular infusion of horseradish peroxidase (HRP) in a cat model of fluid percussion.[468] After moderate but not mild injury localized collections of HRP could be identified in axons and were associated over a 3-h time course with disassembly of neurofilaments. These features progressed with the further passage of organelles into bulbous dilations of axons, the core of which contained disorganized neurofilaments. Eventually disruption or secondary axotomy took place. Additional studies showed that the axonal changes developed in the apparent absence of any marked alterations in either nerve

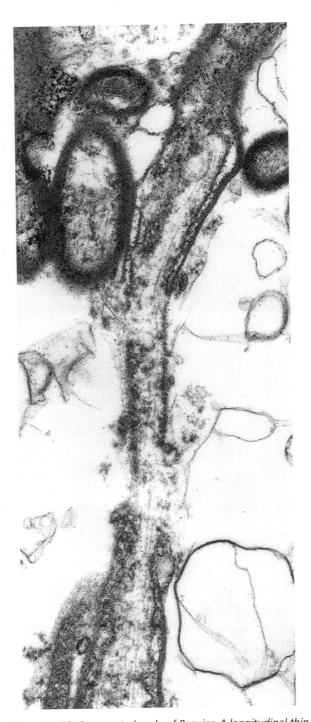

Figure 14.50 *Fragmented node of Ranvier. A longitudinal thin section of a node of Ranvier from a non-human primate 35 min after lateral head acceleration. The paranodal regions related to this node can be seen at the top and bottom of the figure. The nodal axolemma retains the electron dense undercoating. There is fragmentation of the axolemma between the node and upper paranode. The axoplasm has a flocculent ultrastructure which is suggestive of autolysis. Courtesy of Dr WL Maxwell, University of Glasgow, UK.*

cells[247,481] or blood vessels. Furthermore, recent studies using scanning and transmission electron microscopy have shown a considerable microvascular response[397,399] and that the axonal changes are not model specific.[193,402] Comparative studies now suggest that the time course of secondary axotomy is influenced by the species, the injury model and the intensity of the injury.[401,485] In general, the time taken for secondary axotomy to occur in cats and pigs is longer than in the rat and is longest in man.[482,485] However, there is considerable heterogeneity of response and it is not clear whether all axons showing the changes necessarily proceed to actual axotomy. However, it does appear that local factors, at least in part, determine the distribution of the axonal change insofar as fibres that decussate, change anatomical direction or pass around blood vessels appear particularly prone to injury.[481] Furthermore, it was initially thought that changes occurred particularly in large-calibre axons,[14,93] although in certain models it is small-calibre nerve fibres that are particularly at risk.[398]

Ultrastructural analysis of the axonal response within 10–15 min after stretch injury in the optic nerves of the guinea-pig indicates that the earliest morphological changes is the development of a membrane-bound nodal bleb containing a small quantity of axoplasm protruding from a damaged node of Ranvier[398] (Fig. 14.51a, b). Ballooning of the axolemma occurs in damaged nodes and this is correlated with loss of subaxolemma density.[398] Axotomy in the formation of typical axonal swellings occurs between 24 and 72 h after injury. After fluid percussion many axons have undergone degeneration by 2 weeks.[483] However, in a proportion of the fibres there is an attempt at regeneration as shown by the outgrowth of sprouts and growth cones features that have been seen up to 3 months postinjury.[488]

A well-recognized feature of axonal injury is that of wallerian degeneration, but it was not until recently that the importance of deafferentation of various target sites was recognized,[150] one consequence of which would be a phase of excitation that contributes to the ensuing morbidity.[246,248] Such changes may well enhance the process of plasticity and indeed Erb and Povlishock[150] found that focal deafferented sites in the dorsal lateral vestibular nucleus of the cat were reinnervated by the same neurotransmitter system that was initially lost, thereby providing a possible explanation, not only for the immediate morbidity but for subsequent adaptive plasticity and associated recovery. The exact subcellular events and their time course in injured axons is not clear, although pathological rises in intracellular calcium after TBI can precipitate damage to the lipid bilayer of the cell membrane by the activation of calcium-dependent phospholipases and production of ROS.[365,367] Physical stretch at the time of injury results in damage to the axolemma and related axoplasm at the injured node of Ranvier (mechanoporation),[192] but there is now doubt about this concept.[554,621] Irrespective of the mode of induction this change in mem-

brane structure disrupts the capability of the axon to maintain physiological ionic gradients and results in changes in concentrations of calcium, potassium and sodium and chloride within the axoplasm. These changes in ion concentration in certain fibres may activate neutral proteases which in turn disrupt the axonal cytoarchitecture, including spectrin,[66] tubulin, MAPs and neurofilaments.[508,626] The activation of calpain and regional calpain-induced cytoskeletal protolysis have been documented in laboratory animals[295,296,507,509] and in man.[361] However, this hypothesis has not been universally

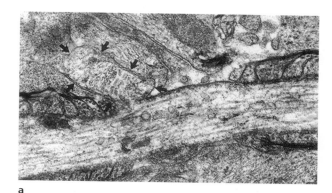

a

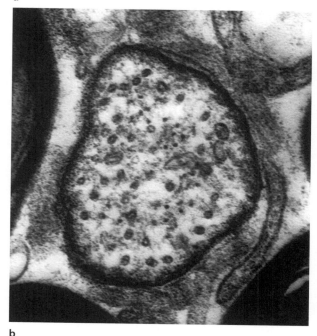

b

Figure 14.51 *Experimental stretch injury. (a) Axonal damage in the optic nerve of the guinea-pig. A membrane-bound nodal bleb (arrows) containing a small amount of axoplasm extends from a damaged node of Ranvier. (b) Node of Ranvier. A transverse, thin section of a node of Ranvier from the optic nerve of an adult guinea-pig. Note the smooth profile, the dense undercoating characteristic of the nodal axolemma, and the relatively high number of microtubules and low number of neurofilaments. The node is intimately related to astrocyte processes. Courtesy of Dr WL Maxwell, University of Glasgow, UK.*

accepted as the ultrastructural studies have revealed neither a progressive degradation of neurofilaments nor the classic granular disorganization associated with calcium-mediated abnormalities.[482] An alternative hypothesis was put forward by Povlishock and his group that TBI can either mechanically or functionally disturb the neurofilament subunits, thereby impairing axoplasmic transport.[626] Although changes in all three neurofilament subunits were identified it was found that antibodies to the 68-kDa subunit were particularly useful, in that within 60 min of TBI there was a highly localized accumulation of the intraaxonal 68-kDa subunit. Moreover, with increasing survival 68-kDa-immunoreactive neurofilaments became increasingly disorganized and were internalized to the core of the axon as organelles began to accumulate in the periphery of axonal swellings.

These ultrastructural observations were considered to be inconsistent with the calcium hypothesis and more in keeping with changes that could be attributed to a direct mechanical effect upon the cytoskeleton.[482] Further work has suggested that a number of mechanisms may be operating in axons after TBI and that any influx of calcium need not always cause direct cytoskeletal dissolution but may alter the side-arms of neurofilaments, causing them to collapse and become compacted.[482] Evidence in support of the latter comes from quantitative studies using computer-generated images showing an early loss of highly phosphorylated epitopes from the side-arms of the neurofilaments,[487] a view that also appears to be supported by recent biochemical and light and confocal microscopy data.[480]

Changes in axons are heterogeneous, thereby raising the distinct possibility that the hypotheses discussed above are not mutually exclusive and that depending on many factors a number of changes may be initiated that reflect a particular mechanism that has been activated. Thus, in a proportion of fibres using the oxalate/pyroantimonate technique for the identification of calcium and the lead citrate technique for cytochemical localization of membrane pump calcium ATPase and ecto-ATPase activity, a series of changes occurred between 15 min and 6 h after stretch. This was interpreted as providing support for the hypothesis that a post-traumatic influx of calcium is a mechanism by which changes in axoplasmic transport take place[400] (Fig. 14.52a, b). Further support was obtained by morphometric identification of rapid loss of microtubules in the same model.[396] What is increasingly apparent is that the changes are complex, that there are both direct and indirect consequences of mechanical loading, and that ensuing functional impairment is a product of many factors which may not include morphological abnormality.[593]

Ischaemic brain damage

Full understanding of the frequency and distribution of hypoxic brain damage in blunt head injury was not reached until the late 1970s.[209] In the first comprehensive study hypoxic brain damage was identified in 138 of 151 (91%) of a group of fatal head injuries: the damage was classified as severe in 27%, moderately severe in 43% and mild in 30%. It was noted to be more frequent in the hippocampus (81%) and in the basal ganglia (79%) than in the cerebral cortex (46%) and in the cerebellum (44%). Clinicopathological correlations indicated the importance of episodes of hypoxaemia, raised ICP and transient failures of cerebral perfusion pressure due to a reduction in cerebral blood flow (CBF), while in some of the patients there were known episodes of cardiac arrest or status epilepticus. This study led to an increased recognition and treatment of hypoxia and hypotension at the scene of the accident, during interhospital transfer and in critical care units, and to the detection and relief of cerebral compression in traumatic intracranial haematoma. These avoidable factors required that the management and organization of patient care be altered, but an audit of the amount and distribution of ischaemic damage in a second cohort of 112 cases found ischaemic brain damage in 88% of the cases: it was concluded that this type of brain damage is still common after severe head injury and it seemed likely that it remained an important cause of mortality and morbidity (Fig. 14.53a–e).[214] Even today, with improved resuscitation techniques irreversible hypoxic brain damage in patients with fatal head injury remains high, much of it being attributable to the effects of shift, distortion and the sequelae of raised ICP.

The hippocampus is selectively vulnerable to a variety of hypoxic events, including cardiac arrest, status epilepticus and hypoglycaemia (see Chapter 5, this Volume). Confirmation of the frequency and distribution of hippocampal damage in fatal blunt head injury was established in a series of 122 cases in which damage was found in 94 (84%): the lesions always involved the CA1 subfield and were bilateral in 70 cases (Fig. 14.54).[324] Although hypoxia and a high ICP were likely to have contributed to these abnormalities, more recent work has demonstrated that such changes may occur in their absence at all ages[322,323] and in experimental models.[321,549,550] The basis of this vulnerability remains unclear as ^{31}P and ^{1}H magnetic resonance spectroscopy between 20 min and 4 h after diffuse injury in pigs has not demonstrated any changes in ATP, pH, PCr/P or lactate concentration.[549] Pathological neuronal excitation has been proposed as a possible mechanism for this pattern of selective vulnerability and the excitatory amino acid neurotransmitter glutamate has been found to be increased in the extracellular fluid of the hippocampus in the rat after fluid percussion brain injury[152,299,300] and after experimentally induced SDH.[69] In both models treatment with glutamate antagonists has been shown to attenuate the increase in extracellular neurotransmitter, as well as its metabolic and pathological effects.[465,642] Thus, mechanisms such as excitotoxicity are likely to play a role in the genesis of ischaemic brain damage in TBI[447,476] especially as blood flow is well above ischaemic thresholds in some of the models.[454,627]

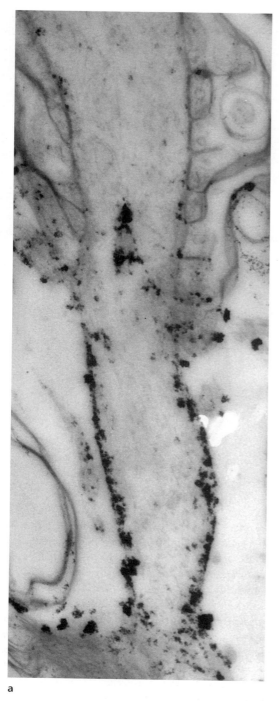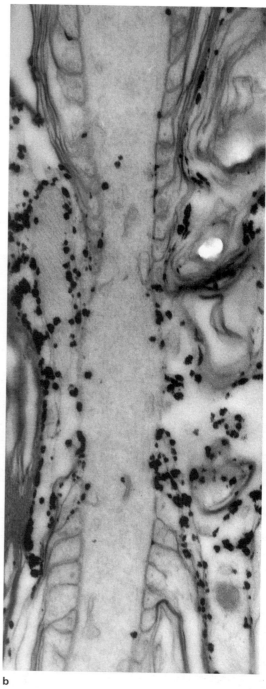

a   b

Figure 14.52 *Experimental stretch injury. ATPase staining of node. Longitudinal sections of control and experimental nodes of Ranvier from the optic nerve of adult guinea-pigs. Sections were incubated in 0.5 mM CaCl₂ for the demonstration of membrane pump calcium ATPase activity. In the control node (**a**) reactive product occurs on the axoplasmic face of the nodal axolemma. In the experimental node (**b**) 4 h after stretch injury there is no reaction product on the axoplasmic face. Courtesy of Dr WL Maxwell, University of Glasgow, UK.*

There is now considerable clinical evidence that the outcome after TBI may be made worse by secondary insults such as hypoxia or hypotension.[94,291,413] However, earlier clinical studies of acute head injury had failed to demonstrate evidence of cerebral ischaemia. Given that CBF studies in head-injured patients are not usually conducted until some hours or days after injury, it is perhaps not too surprising that cerebral ischaemia if present may have occurred in the first few hours after clinical brain injury and may not have been detected at the time of the first CBF study, although a reduction of CBF had occurred in the early hours after injury. That this indeed can be the

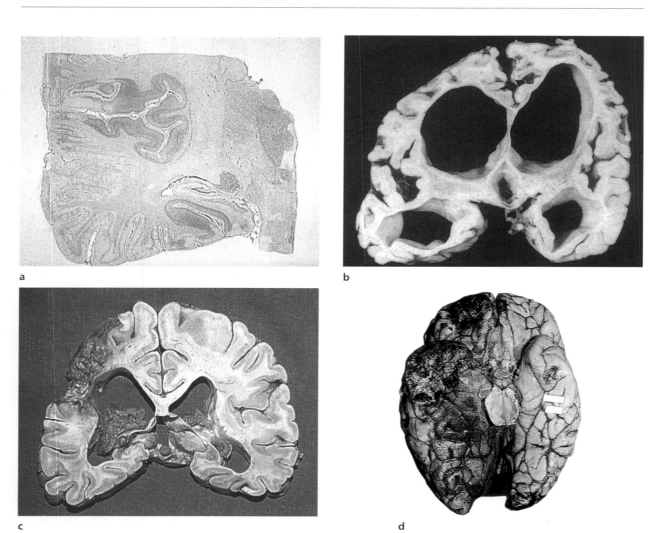

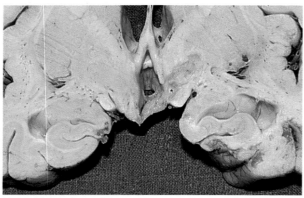

Figure 14.53 *Ischaemic brain damage: cerebral hemispheres. (a) Multiple foci of necrosis in the grey matter of the left temporal lobe of a 3-year-old patient who died 80 h after a head injury. (Celloidin, cresyl violet.) The necrosis was not apparent macroscopically. (b) Longstanding ischaemic damage in a patient who survived in a vegetative state for 4 years after a head injury. (c) Old infarction in a patient who survived severely disabled for 2.5 years after a head injury. Note the infarct in the distribution of the left middle cerebral artery. (d) Recent vascular complications of internal herniation in a patient who survived for 4 days after a head injury. (e) Longstanding vascular complication of internal herniation in patient who survived for 2 months after a head injury. Reproduced by permission from Ref. 216.*

case has been reported with low CBF during the first 6 h after injury and at levels below the threshold for infarction (<18 ml/100 g per minute) were present in one-third of cases.[51,524,525] Thus, there was confirmation that an acute period of ischaemia does occur in a subset of severely head-injured patients. CBF as measured by xenon CT carried out during the first 4 h after injury has shown that in patients without an intracranial mass lesion there is a trend towards low initial flows with subsequent increases in CBF for 24 h and that low CBF in the first 24 h postinjury is significantly correlated with a low initial GCS.[306,380,500] The changes are likely to be heterogeneous, particularly as it has now been shown that in addition to any global ischaemia there are likely to be further decreases in regional CBF in relation to focal lesions.[524] Therefore, it is difficult to escape the conclusion that either a regional or global reduction in CBF and subsequent ischaemia may occur within the first few hours

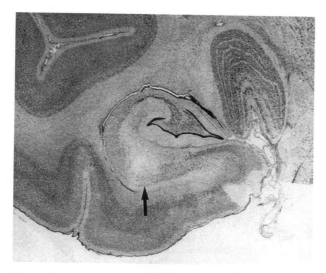

Figure 14.54 *Ischaemic brain damage: hippocampus. Focus of neuronal necrosis (arrow) in the hippocampus. (Cresyl violet.) Reproduced by permission from Ref. 216.*

of severe TBI and that a decreased cerebral perfusion has important effects on brain viability and subsequent neurological outcome.

Multimodality monitoring in severely head-injured patients has identified the particular value of brain oxygen monitoring with the recognition that periods of desaturation of the cerebrovenous blood occur that in turn affect cerebral oxygen consumption and metabolic needs and adversely influence outcome.[127,307,602,643] Since the initial studies of Jenkins *et al.*[278,279] who showed in a 'double insult' model the additive influence of trauma and global ischaemia, there has been ample laboratory evidence in support of the adverse influence of hypoxia on the cellular, molecular and behavioural sequelae of trauma.[91,103,120,270,279]

Recent experimental studies have been particularly concerned with the concept of injury-induced vulnerability in which, after TBI, the brain may be at risk of even minor changes in CBF, increases in ICP and apnoea. This is true for head-injured patients[127,130,291,307,413,643] and in experimental models of head injury.[53,91,103,120,127,270,278,279,307,602,643] The key neurochemical event that appears to trigger a cascade of metabolic dysfunction is the increased extracellular concentration of glutamate after TBI[152,299] which in turn causes a massive flux of potassium.[300] Ionic fluxes, particularly those associated with potassium, result in an increase in glycolysis, an accumulation of lactic acid[302,636] and an activation of ATP-dependent–sodium potassium pumps. The acute increase in glycolytic energy demand after fluid percussion in rats may last for some 30–60 min during which time nerve cells are exposed to increased levels of lactic acid,[303] the effects of which can be attenuated either by blocking the excitatory amino acid receptors or by restricting the activity of the sodium potassium pump. CBF has been shown to be reduced during the first

60 min after experimental TBI,[627,640] but not always in circumstances in which oxidative metabolism is compromised.[261,609] These studies therefore show that post-traumatic ischaemia is not necessarily required to induce significant ionic and metabolic changes after TBI. Furthermore, this mismatch between glucose and CBF can be seen after mild, moderate and severe TBI.[260,299] Although critical levels of blood flow have not been determined, it is known that during these periods of relative cerebral ischaemia there is an accumulation of intracellular calcium.[116,158] After an initial acute increase in injury-induced hyperglycolysis[587] the brain undergoes metabolic depression demonstrated by a reduction in both glucose and oxidative metabolism and both a decrease in and impaired autoregulation of CBF.[148] These laboratory studies have indicated that the neurochemical, ionic and metabolic cascades after experimental TBI are multifactorial, each element having a different time course with important implications for therapy.

The correlation between the cerebral metabolic rate of glucose (CMRglc) and the level of consciousness within the first 30 days of 43 patients with TBI has been studied using [^{18}F]fluorodeoxyglucose positron emission tomography (FDG-PET). In 88% of the studies there was a regional reduction in cerebral glucose utilization (CMRglc $\leq$ 4.9 mg/100 g per minute) and in 80% of severely head-injured patients compared with 67% of the mild to moderately head-injured patients there were greater global reductions, although there was considerable variation according to the severity of injury, the GCS correlating poorly with the global cortical CMRglc value.[39] The interpretation of these findings is uncertain, with some investigations having assumed that metabolism as a whole is depressed and therefore glucose utilization will be low: such a hypometabolic state reflects a reduced oxidative metabolism secondary to coma-induced neuronal damage. However, this hypothesis is difficult to reconcile with the finding that there was hyperglycolysis in over 50% of patients studied within 7 days of TBI.[40]

Reference has been made already to the importance of relative ischaemia after TBI and several factors need to be considered that include the stretching and distortion of blood vessels secondary to mass lesions and the development of internal herniae (see Chapter 4, this Volume), arterial hypotension associated with multiple injuries, post-traumatic changes in the cerebral microvasculature[116,126,376,397,399] and vasospasm. Using transcranial Doppler ultrasonography it has been possible to demonstrate vasospasm in a number of severely head-injured patients, this being one factor that may contribute to the development of post-traumatic hypoperfusion.[332,389] In 24 of 75 patients with TBI transcranial Doppler and CT angiography revealed cerebral vasospasm. In three patients who died, the cerebral blood vessels had the histological features of post-traumatic vasospasm similar to those seen in cerebral vasospasm after postaneurysmal subarachnoid haemorrhage.[653]

Brain swelling

Brain swelling occurs frequently after head injury and may be a major factor contributing to an increase in ICP, but its pathogenesis and the extent to which it is due to cerebral vasodilation, i.e. congestive brain swelling, or to cerebral oedema, i.e. an increase in tissue water content, is not yet clear. Brain swelling and oedema are discussed in detail in Chapter 4 of this Volume, but three main types of brain swelling are encountered in patients who have sustained a TBI: swelling adjacent to contusions and intracerebral haemorrhages, diffuse swelling of one cerebral hemisphere, and diffuse swelling of both cerebral hemispheres.

Swelling of white matter adjacent to contusions

This is common (Fig. 14.55). Adjacent to the physically disrupted and necrotic tissue there is a zone of damaged blood vessels where there is increased permeability at capillary level and loss of normal physiological regulation at the arteriolar level.[126,415] The water content of the brain tissue around cerebral contusions is increased and this type of oedema corresponds to that referred to as vasogenic.[73,382] A similar sequence of events may occur around an intracerebral haematoma. Hypoxia increases the regional breakdown of the BBB to circulating proteins.[576,577]

Diffuse swelling of one cerebral hemisphere is most often seen in association with an ipsilateral acute SDH.[18] When the haematoma is evacuated the brain simply expands to fill the space so created (Fig. 14.56), a situation similar to that which has been created in experimental studies and attributed to engorgement of a non-reactive vascular bed secondary to cerebral ischaemia produced by a high ICP.[330] The extent to which ischaemia contributes to this vasomotor paralysis remains in some doubt but this type of brain swelling can occur very soon after the occurrence of SDH in man[356] and experimentally.[182] If a craniectomy is undertaken to evacuate the haematoma with the

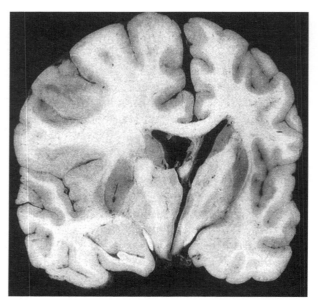

Figure 14.56 *Brain swelling: unilateral. There is diffuse swelling of the left cerebral hemisphere on the same side as an acute subdural haematoma that had been evacuated. Reproduced by permission from Ref. 216.*

aim of reducing ICP, the brain tissue simply herniates through the craniectomy. Because it is difficult to conceive of cerebral oedema occurring so rapidly, it is likely that this type of swelling is due in the first instance to vasodilation with or without significant pre-existing ischaemia. If this state persists, however, a subsequent breakdown of the BBB may lead to cerebral oedema. Indeed, it has been suggested that, in patients in whom SDH does not become clinically manifest until 2–3 days after the injury, progressive development of brain swelling is more likely to be the cause of clinical deterioration and an increase in ICP than enlargement of the haematoma itself.[415]

Diffuse brain swelling is more difficult to account for. The crucial evidence that it is due to cerebral oedema is lacking, despite the fact that extravasation of HRP into extracellular spaces in the brain has been demonstrated shortly after experimental TBI.[116,126]

Diffuse swelling of the entire brain (Fig. 14.57) occurs mainly in children and adolescents.[213] Its presence is indicated during life by the demonstration of small symmetrical ventricles and occlusion of the basal cisterns on CT.[580] This problem has been studied in considerable detail.[62,650] Some of the children with diffuse brain swelling had experienced a lucid interval while others had not, and the available evidence suggests that the diffuse swelling is brought about by an increase in cerebral blood volume. If this persists, it seems again possible that true cerebral oedema will subsequently occur. Bruce *et al.*[62] and Zimmerman *et al.*[650] suggested that hyperaemia was a major factor contributing to diffuse brain swelling in children and adolescents. More recent studies have

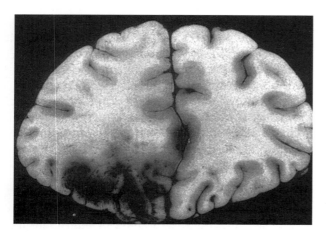

Figure 14.55 *Brain swelling in relation to contusions. Reproduced by permission from Ref. 216.*

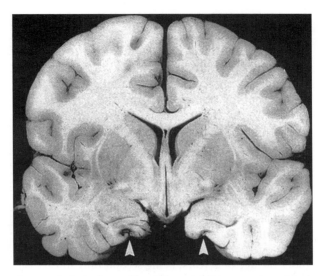

Figure 14.57 *Brain swelling: bilateral. Diffuse swelling of both cerebral hemispheres in a 5 year old who survived for 30 h after a head injury. Note the absence of contusions and the presence of bilateral tentorial herniae (arrows). Reproduced by permission from Ref. 216.*

indicated that although hyperaemia does occur in this age group it is not severe enough to account for the brain swelling.[424]

One of the problems facing pathologists in assessing the presence of diffuse brain swelling post-mortem on the basis of convolutional flattening, obliteration of sulci and small symmetrical ventricles is that brain swelling occurs in association with the onset of brainstem death and is a feature at autopsy. Although the brain may swell post-mortem,[516] it seems likely in the context of TBI that any swelling identified at autopsy was the cause of clinical brainstem failure rather than a consequence of it.

Some brain swelling occurs in almost every patient with severe TBI and in 5–10% of patients with moderate degrees of injury.[382] There is still a widespread misconception that the increase in brain volume after TBI is due to vasogenic oedema.[71,73] This is in spite of numerous clinical trials that have failed to show efficacy supporting the use of corticosteroids, and laboratory studies have clearly demonstrated that the extracellular fluid volume may increase for less than 30 min postinjury,[68] possibly because of the hypertensive surge associated with injury. It is more likely that there is a net shift of small ions together with obligated water from the intravascular to the extracellular compartment: within about 60 min of the injury the extracellular volume decreases as water and ions become intracellular.[389] At the most severe end of the spectrum, the injured brain is unable to restore ionic homoeostasis, ICP rises, cerebral perfusion pressure is compromised and death may ensue. The CT scan appearances are those of 'loss of grey–white definition' or the 'ground glass appearance', but such changes do not occur in all patients with diffuse injuries.[271] Vasogenic oede-

ma probably becomes important around focal contusions on the second through the 10th–15th day postinjury. MRI- and CT-based techniques have shown that cerebral blood volume is uniformly reduced initially after acute brain injury, although many patients will demonstrate a phase of hyperaemic CBF from the second to the seventh day post-injury especially after the removal of an intracranial haematoma.[271] When the microcirculation is competent and CBF remains above about 20 ml per 100 g per minute, recovery of brain swelling will be more rapid than if blood flow in the microcirculation is below threshold levels.[271]

Diffuse vascular injury

Multiple small haemorrhages are frequently seen in the brains of patients who die very soon after a head injury. Indeed, it is remarkable how conspicuous they can be in patients who appeared to have died instantaneously (Fig. 14.58); it has been suggested that when present in the brainstem they are indicative of damage of a type and distribution that is incompatible with life.[594] In the experience of the authors, however, there is a spectrum of change: multiple haemorrhages, particularly in the cerebral hemispheres, are compatible with survival for up to several hours. Many of these haemorrhages can be identified macroscopically, while others can be seen microscopically as haemorrhages around small blood vessels. They can occur in any part of the brain but they tend to be particularly conspicuous in the white matter of the anterior parts of the frontal and temporal lobes, and in and adjacent to midline structures including the periventricular white matter, the thalamus and the brainstem. In the brainstem they are particularly numerous beneath the ependyma around the aqueduct and in the floor of the fourth ventricle; they occur rarely in the caudal pons or medulla.[594] They have been referred to as primary brainstem haemorrhages,[594] but in the authors' opinion they are more appropriately considered as a primary type of diffuse brain damage in view of their wide distribution.

Similar haemorrhages may be seen in the corpus callosum and in the dorsolateral sector(s) of the rostral brainstem but, unlike typical examples of DAI, they are neither restricted to nor particularly severe in these sites. The mechanism of their occurrence has not been established; it may, however, be further evidence that various structures in the brain, such as the subdural bridging veins and axons, have different responses to acceleration and deceleration (see above).

Fat embolism

Some patients who sustain a head injury also have multiple injuries, including limb and other fractures. They are therefore at risk of developing systemic fat embolism. Indeed, fulminating fat embolism is a well-recognized, if uncommon, cause of rapid progressive neurological deterioration in such a patient without an acute intracranial expanding lesion. The subject of fat embolism is dealt with in Chapter 6 of this Volume, but it is important for pathologists to appreciate that classic petechial haemorrhages may be absent despite the presence of extensive fat embolism. In patients with multiple injuries, therefore, the brain should be screened routinely for fat embolism.

Other causes of small haemorrhages

There are many causes of multiple petechial haemorrhage in the brains of patients who survive for some time after TBI. These range from various haematological complications associated with thrombocytopenia to small blood vessel disease due to sepsis, or an adverse reaction to drug therapy. The interpretation of these haemorrhages requires careful correlation with the circumstances under which a presumed head injury has occurred, the clinical findings and any associated structural damage, including signs of asphyxia. In patients who are pregnant, amniotic fluid embolism should be considered.

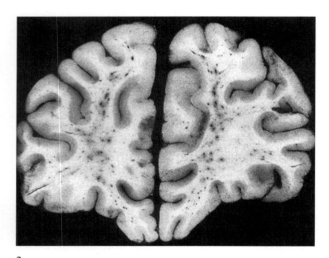

a

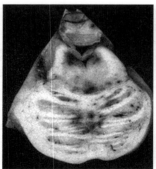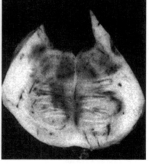

b

Figure 14.58 *Diffuse vascular injury. There are multiple small haemorrhages: (a) in the white matter of the frontal lobes (30 min survival); (b) in the brainstem (less than 10 min survival). Reproduced by permission from Ref. 216.*

Head injury in infancy and childhood

Trauma to the brain and spinal cord during birth is described in Chapter 9 of this Volume. Head injuries are common in the paediatric age group and most are minor and of little consequence. However, head injury is the single most common cause of death and new disabilities in childhood[359] and the third leading cause of death in children aged less than 12 months.[22,137,616] Fracture of the skull occurs in between 23 and 39% of cases and a surgical lesion in between 8 and 9% of children admitted to hospital after TBI, with an overall mortality in cases with a GCS of less than 8 of between 9 and 52%.[616]

According to Duhaime *et al.*,[137] child abuse accounts for almost one-quarter of all children admitted to hospital under the age of 2 years, being second only to car accidents as the cause of death.[45] Between the ages of 2 and 4 years, falls are the most common cause of TBI and in older children bicycling and car accidents are the most common causes of injury.

Fracture of the skull in infancy (during the first year of life) is not uncommon as the skull is relatively thin and breaks easily after impact. An overriding mechanism of injury from impact involves the extensive deformation of skull and brain that occurs when the unfused infant skull is impacted. Most skull fractures are linear and are not associated with underlying brain damage, although intracranial bleeding may result. In many instances simple depressed skull fractures are managed without operation, although for cosmetic reasons some require surgical elevation. Fracture of the skull in infancy can be associated with two particular complications. The first is the development of a subepicranial hygroma, when a fracture is associated with a dural tear and allows CSF to dissect beneath the periosteum,[149] and most of these pseudomeningoceles resolve spontaneously. Histologically there are reactive changes in the brain and meninges that extend from the ventricle to the skull fracture.[505] A second complication, unique to infants, is a growing skull fracture which results from the herniation of contused and swollen brain through the torn dura mater, thereby separating the bones along the line of the fracture. The fracture tends to "grow" during the period of rapid growth of the brain. Dense scarring at the junction between the brain and dura mater prevents secondary closure of the dura, thereby perpetuating the growing fracture.[519] Surgical repair is required.

EDH in infancy rarely results from injury to the middle meningeal artery: venous bleeding from the bone is the usual cause. Chronic SDHs occur most commonly at 6 months of age and are rare after 1 year of age.[616]

Child abuse is a major cause of head injury in infants but its true incidence is unknown. The first child abuse syndrome to be widely recognized was that of the 'battered child'. The term 'the shaken baby syndrome' was used in infants with acute SDH and subarachnoid haemorrhage, retinal haemorrhages and periosteal new bone formation at epiphyseal regions of long bones, and was attributed to the to-and-fro shaking of a child's body producing a whiplash motion of the child's head on the neck.[76] The term 'shaken baby' has been questioned as inertial forces generated by shaking alone were insignificant compared with those caused by impact.[138,139] These and related studies gave origin to the 'shaking impact syndrome' in which the injuries are attributed to both inertial and impact forces. Current debate revolves around the question of whether shaking alone is sufficient to cause injuries observed in infants with the shaking impact syndrome. The consensus view is that head-injured infants undergo shaking followed by sudden inertial injury from impact. There is some evidence that between the ages of 2 and 5 years the still maturing brain responds differently to head injury than in an older child. For example, there is said to be a smaller risk of developing a traumatic intracranial haematoma in children less than 5 years old than in adults.[25,582] EDH occurs in between 1–2%[249] and 6.5%[61] of head-injured children and acute SDH occurs in only 25% as frequently as in adults.[648]

The findings in an autopsy series of 87 children[213] were compared with data derived from the CT findings in 262 children with acute head injury.[649] The impression that contusions of the brain are less common in head-injured children than in adults is not correct since they were present in 90% of the autopsied cases. This would suggest that the figure of 16% in the CT studies underestimates quite considerably the true incidence of contusions.[649] Further, CT evidence of diffuse brain damage 'shearing injury' is less common in children (4%) than in adults (7%), most of the children having been passengers in high-speed road traffic accidents.[649] However, comparisons of the different types of brain damage in fatal blunt head injury in relation to age and type of injury[5,648] would suggest that the presence of DAI is dependent on the cause of the accident, but not on age. The incidence of ischaemic brain damage was also found to be high in children and its pathogenesis was similar to that in adults, and morphological evidence of the ICP having been high in life was not that dissimilar in the two groups. The one exception was diffuse cerebral swelling, which was found by CT scanning in over 40% of comatose children after head injury.[62] The principal CT findings were small ventricles and compression of the basal cisterns, while the principal pathological features were the enlargement of the cerebral hemispheres and obliteration of the CSF spaces. Where ICP monitoring had been carried out pressures in excess of 2.7 kPa (20 mmHg) were recorded in over 80% of the cases.[64] The bilateral hemispheric swelling has been attributed to cerebral hyperaemia[63] with an increase in cerebral blood volume.[328] However, more recent studies have failed to demonstrate hyperaemia in all cases,[328] although it was present in 28 of 32 severely head-injured children at some point after admission to hospital.[423,424] In a post-mortem series of 87 children, swelling of the brain was found in 61

cases, in 45 of which it was bilateral.[213] In 27 of the 45 cases the swelling was attributable to ischaemic damage, contusions or intracranial haematomas, or to a combination of these factors: in the remaining 18 an underlying cause could not be found. There are also examples of unilateral hemispheric swelling attributable to infarction, contusions and intracranial haematoma.

Children with haematological disorders, especially haemophilia, are at particular risk for developing intracranial haemorrhage after a trivial head injury. Another special at-risk group of children comprises those who have been shunted for hydrocephalus.

There have been continuing uncertainties about the nature, the distribution and the pathology in accidental and non-accidental injury in infants and children. Recent clinicopathological studies by Geddes et al.[175,177] on 53 cases of non-accidental paediatric head injury, of which 37 were infants aged 20 days to 9 months and 16 were children aged between 13 months and 2 years 6 months, showed that traumatic axonal injury of the type seen in DAI of adults (see above) was only seen in children older than 12 months: in infants less than 12 months hypoxia/ischaemia was the principal finding and any axonal pathology was invariably limited to the craniocervical junction. Therefore, contrary to some literature,[203,237,534] DAI is not a feature of non-accidental head injury in infants in whom structural damage that results from hypoxia/ischaemia is thought to be consequent upon respiratory distress and/or apnoea due to axonal injury at the craniocervical junction.

Outcome after blunt head injury

It has long been recognized in survivors of severe head injury that changes in cognition and behaviour contribute more to disability than any physical disability such as a hemiparesis.[285] Prospective studies have identified neurobehavioural abnormalities for up to 3 months postinjury.[81,195,341] More recently, in a prospective hospital-based cohort study of 2962 patients aged 14 years or more with head injury and a 1-year follow-up, the principal finding was a higher than expected disability in both young and old people admitted to hospital with an apparently mild head injury.[589]

Predictors of neurobehavioural outcome in adults include age (greater than 50 years is a poor prognostic factor), the acute GCS (as a predictor of duration of coma), abnormal brainstem reflexes, ventricular enlargement (correlated with length of coma), neurological deficit and the duration of post-traumatic amnesia.[81] The relationship between these predictors of outcome and structural (CT, MRI) and functional imaging [single-photon emission computed tomography (SPECT), PET] has also been examined.[336] Apparently, although of considerable diagnostic value in acute treatment, CT is only a modest predictor of neurobehavioural outcome after severe head injury,[339] whereas CT evidence of presumed DAI (midline haemorrhages or multiple haemorrhages at the grey/white matter interface) predicted a poorer GOS at 6 months compared with CT findings of diffuse swelling or focal lesions.[600] Levin *et al.*[339] did not find a relationship between CT features of diffuse swelling, mass effect, etc., and cognition at 1 year, possibly because MRI will detect 80–85% more intracranial lesions than CT.[337,343] These studies concluded that the correlations between the site of lesions seen on MRI and specific neuropsychological domains were again only modest, although strikingly good correlations were seen in some cases,[337,340,343] and at the severe end of the GOS MRI could predict recovery from the vegetative state.[297] Multivariant models have been used to predict outcome of severe head injury, a combination of age, GCS motor score and pupillary response providing a high prediction of subsequent GOS category.[52,96]

The neurobehavioural outcome of head injury in children is similar to that in adults, with lesions frequently seen in the orbitofrontal and dorsolateral frontal lobes and in the temporal poles.[41,338,342,410] Uncomplicated mild head injury does not have clinically significant long-term effects on the child's cognitive, academic or psychosocial functioning,[155] although this has been questioned.[22] Predictors of outcome in children include age (plasticity of the developing brain often permits good recovery), acute GCS scores, post-traumatic amnesia (poorer if longer than 1 week) and imaging studies (anatomical location of lesions, especially if deep in the cerebral hemispheres).[81] Outcome in paediatric head injury correlates with the admission and 6-h modified GCS score – children's Coma Scale.[237]

SEVERE DISABILITY AND THE VEGETATIVE STATE

A survey of head injuries by the European Brain Injury Consortium provided data on outcome for 94% of the cases assessed by these centres 6 months after injury:[427] 31% died, 3% were vegetative, 16% severely disabled, 20% moderately disabled and 31% had made a good recovery. Neuropathological studies have provided the structural basis of the GOS after head injury.

The structural basis of severe disability after head injury has been comprehensively studied.[224,275,276,466] Emphasis has been placed on the frequency of abnormalities in the rostral brainstem, intracranial haematoma, brain swelling, and respiratory and circulatory distress, in the belief that post-traumatic encephalopathy is on the whole dominated by the complications of trauma and their sequelae.[275,276] In one series of 80 cases of prolonged unconsciousness after head injury, by far the most common findings were either secondary damage to the brainstem[275] or transtentorial herniation.[466] These conclusions are at variance with those of Strich,[569] who has always placed particular emphasis on the presence of diffuse brain damage in patients who remain vegetative after head injury and on her failure to identify any cases of prolonged post-traumatic coma where damage was confined to the brainstem.

Reviews[15,282] showed that of 35 cases of the vegetative state and 30 severely disabled cases surviving for at least 1 month after head injury, severely disabled cases were older, had a higher incidence of fracture of the skull and of evacuated intracranial haematoma, and had more cortical contusions. DAI was less common in the severely disabled cases, particularly its most severe grade. Structural changes in the thalamus was much less common in severely disabled cases. Half of the severely disabled patients had neither grade II nor III DAI nor thalamic damage, and ten of these 15 cases did not have ischaemic brain damage either. These combinations did not occur in a single vegetative case. It was concluded that half of the severely disabled cases had only focal brain damage, a feature not found in any vegetative case. In the severely disabled patients with lesions similar to those of the vegetative state it is likely that more damage occurred in the vegetative cases.[19] However, any TBI may be complicated by hypoxia/ischaemia, which is also capable of being causative in the vegetative state.[105,135,310]

This therefore remains a somewhat controversial field, not only because there are problems of nomenclature but also in the interpretation of the pathogenesis of lesions in the brainstem. There seems to be increasing evidence from clinicopathological studies that the most common causes of the vegetative state and severe disability after blunt head injury, at least in patients who survive their injury for more than 4 weeks, are DAI and diffuse ischaemic brain damage, of which the more important is DAI.

MODERATE DISABILITY

The macroscopic and microscopic features of the brains of 20 moderately disabled patients who had survived for between 1 and 47 years after TBI have been described.[16] Most of the deaths had been sudden and attributed to sudden unexpected death in epilepsy (SUDEP),[311,436,586] post-traumatic epilepsy being a feature in 15 of the cases. An intracranial haematoma had been evacuated in 15 and 11 of these also had epilepsy. DAI was found in six cases: five grade I and one grade II. There was not a case of diffuse thalamic damage, nor a case with severe ischaemic brain damage. The conclusions were that the dominant lesion was focal damage from an evacuated intracranial haematoma, with DAI and thalamic damage being only mild in only one case.[16]

POST-TRAUMATIC EPILEPSY

The definition, mechanisms and pathology of epilepsy are dealt with in Chapter 15 of this Volume. In the case of post-traumatic epilepsy a clear distinction has been made between early epilepsy (occurring within 7 days of injury) and late epilepsy (occurring after 7 days).[280,287] Almost 50% of all post-traumatic seizures occur within 24 h after head injury and children are at greater risk than adults during the first 24 h after head injury; also, patients with superficial contusions or haematomas are likely to develop seizures between 1 and 7 days post-injury. Of patients who develop late seizures, about 20% are observed within 4 weeks and 50% occur within 12 months of head injury. Patients who experience three or more seizures in the first 12 months after head injury are twice as likely to experience persistent seizures.[335]

The severity of head injury is the most important predictor of both early and late post-traumatic seizures. Seizures are more frequent in patients with more severe injuries and are uncommon in mild head injury.[32] The risk of early post-traumatic seizures is increased with prolonged unconsciousness, fracture of the skull, intracerebral haematomas or contusions, SDHs and neurological deficits.[31,281,314] In civilian populations late-onset post-traumatic seizures are associated with intracranial haematomas, depressed fracture of the skull, loss of consciousness greater than 24 h, age greater than 65 years and early seizures.[31,32]

Post-traumatic seizures are associated with various complications. For example, early post-traumatic seizures can cause further or secondary insults through increased metabolic demands, raised ICP and excess release of neurotransmitters.[606] Moreover, early seizures may be associated with aspiration pneumonia or status epilepticus. Late post-traumatic seizures are associated with important cognitive, psychosocial and emotional effects, and have a major impact on employment, social and domestic life.[437,449]

The incidence of late epilepsy is much higher after missile head injuries than after blunt head injuries (about 40% compared with 5%), and the incidence has remained the same despite marked improvement over decades in patient transport, surgical techniques, medical management and the prophylactic use of anticonvulsants.[85] Continuous electroencephalographic (EEG) monitoring has now established that during the first week after moderate to severe TBI 20% of patients develop seizures.[607] There is a highly significant relationship between the degree of focal brain destruction and the liability of epilepsy. This close relationship suggests that focal brain damage is the most important cause of post-traumatic epilepsy in many types of head injury.

MEDICAL COMPLICATIONS AFTER BLUNT HEAD INJURY

The importance of these is being increasingly recognized as the complex interactions between the injured brain and other organs are better understood. As a result of the optimization of care that encompasses the skills of the neurosurgeon and those who work in critical care units, treatment strategies are specifically designed for the multiple injured patient who in addition may have a head injury.[590] Given the increased risk of the already injured brain to additional insults, considerable attention is given to maintaining adequate pulmonary and cardiovascular support. Additional considerations are attention

to fluid and electrolyte balance, including the syndrome of inappropriate antidiuretic hormone and cerebral salt wasting, the recognition and treatment of venous thrombosis, pulmonary embolism and disseminated intravascular coagulation and, more recently, to providing adequate nutrition and metabolic support. Overly rapid correction of hyponatraemia may be associated with central pontine myelinolysis (see Chapter 10, this Volume).

The medical complications after blunt head injury are therefore many and in those who die it is usually possible for the pathologist to identify one or more factors that have contributed to the death. Usually, patients who die within 7 days of injury do so from intracranial damage; thereafter, medical complications become increasingly important. In many instances the outcome is a product of both intracranial and extracranial events.

PROGRESSIVE NEUROLOGICAL DISEASE

Despite the occasional striking association between a head injury and the onset of neurological disease, many of the cases reported have been found to be unconvincing.[565,569] Diseases in which a possible connection with head injury has been reported include Pick's disease,[231] Parkinson's disease,[231] motor neuron disease and Creutzfeldt–Jakob disease.[37] It must, however, be accepted that in most instances a direct correlation between any of these diseases and a previous head injury has not yet been established.

Large numbers of concussive or subconcussive blows, such as may be incurred by various sportsmen and in particular by boxers, sometimes induce the development of neurological signs and progressive dementia.[113,117,390,393] This condition, known as dementia pugilistica or the punch-drunk syndrome, may develop years after the last injury, affects amateur[372] as well as professional boxers, and is most likely to develop in boxers with long careers who have been dazed if not knocked out on many occasions. In detailed studies of the brains of 15 ex-boxers there was a characteristic pattern of damage, the principal features of which were abnormalities in the septum pellucidum with enlargement of the cavum, and fenestration of its leaves (Fig. 14.59).[115] In some cases there was thinning of the adjacent fornices and corpus callosum, scarring and neuronal loss in the cerebellum, degeneration of the substantia nigra as shown by loss of neurons and pigment, and the presence of numerous neurofibrillary tangles (Fig. 14.60) diffusely throughout the cerebral cortex and the brainstem, and Aβ-containing plaques.[496] These tangles broadly conformed to the topographic pattern found in AD, but more recently the neuropathological findings in a 23-year-old boxer were described, in which the distribution and features suggest that the mechanism of tangle formation induced by repetitive head injury may be different from that in head injury. In contrast to the

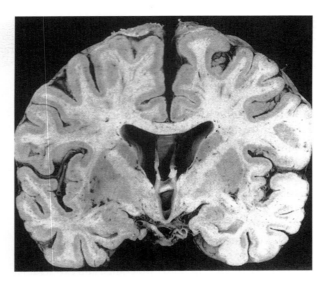

Figure 14.59 *Dementia pugilistica. Professional boxer who died aged 83 years. There is cerebral atrophy, enlargement of the ventricular system and a wide cavum with torn walls in the interventricular septum. Reproduced by permission from Ref. 216.*

numerous tangles, there was a remarkably sparse occurrence or, in most cases, a total absence of classic senile plaques[178,179,591] (see Chapter 4, Volume II).

Of the various environmental (non-genetic) risk factors for AD there is increasing awareness of the importance of a history of previous head injury.[114,254,375,403,404,422,439] Support for this hypothesis has been obtained from patients

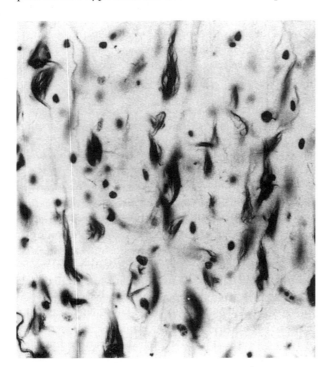

Figure 14.60 *Dementia pugilistica. Professional boxer. There are abundant neurofibrillary tangles in the cortex of the temporal lobe. (Modified Bielschowsky.) Reproduced by permission from Ref. 216.*

subjected to domestic violence[499] and the demonstration of large numbers of diffuse, i.e. non-neuritic, plaques composed of Aβ in the brains of boxers with dementia pugilistica.[104] These diffuse plaques are not identifiable with Congo red or standard silver stains. Such data suggest that there are similarities between the molecular neuropathology of dementia pugilistica and AD. Further studies established that the plaques were widely and symmetrically distributed and were not associated with the various pathologies of TBI,[217] and there was an increased number of APP-immunoreactive neurons,[497] especially in the medial temporal lobe,[370,371] indicating that the upregulation of β-APP can trigger the deposition of Aβ, in keeping with the amyloid hypothesis of AD. Sustained or repeated upregulation may trigger a sequence of events culminating in AD by the overproduction or sustained production of β-APP, and a subsequent increase in Aβ and its deposition as diffuse plaques, perhaps mediated through glial cytokines.[228–230,548]

After the recognition that possession of the ε4 allele of the *ApoE* gene is a major genetic risk factor for sporadic AD, the relation of the *ApoE* gene polymorphism to the Aβ deposits in fatal head injury was explored[218,444] (see above). Subsequent studies have now shown that patients with *ApoE* ε4 have a worse outcome after TBI,[558] and that patients with *ApoE* ε4 are unlikely to have a good functional outcome.[163] *ApoE* genotype influences outcome after TBI associated boxers.[292] Thus, there is increasing evidence of a synergistic interaction between a history of a head injury and possession of the *ApoE* ε4 allele as risk factors for AD.[221,403]

Subarachnoid haemorrhage occurs almost always in all types of head injury. The consequent obliteration of the subarachnoid space as the blood is organized is a recognized cause of normal pressure hydrocephalus, and this may lead to dementia (see Chapter 4, this Volume). There are, however, other causes of enlargement of the ventricles in patients who survive for some time after a severe head injury, such as a reduction in the mass of the brain as a consequence of DAI or diffuse ischaemic brain damage. Quantitative MRI studies of trauma-related changes in which preinjury and postinjury images are compared should provide useful information about grey–white-matter alterations in relation to outcome.[168,584]

MISSILE HEAD INJURY

These have been much less common than blunt head injuries in a civilian population. However, in certain regions, particularly in the USA, the number of missile wounds has been increasing alarmingly. If the current trend continues, with fewer severe road traffic-related brain injuries and more missile injuries, then the latter will assume much more importance in the future. Although missiles can include knives and cross-bow bolts, the most severe craniocerebral injuries are caused by guns.[243] In Phoenix, USA, 10% of all admissions to the trauma clinic are from gunshot wounds, with a mortality of 60%.[467]

There are considerable differences between missile head injuries in civilian and military practice. For example, the amount of damage caused by penetration of the head by a bullet from a rifle with a high muzzle velocity of 731–975 m/s is such that death is instantaneous. In contrast, civilians injured by handguns with low muzzle velocities of less than 305 m/s are more likely to reach hospital for treatment. However, although this difference has been emphasized in the past, the availability of high-velocity weapons in civilian life has blurred the distinction.[243]

The amount of damage depends on factors such as the mass, shape and velocity of the missile(s), and it will increase the greater the amount of energy released by the missile during its passage through the head. Therefore, more damage is associated with a missile that 'yaws' rather than 'tumbles', one that is hollow-point than one that does not shatter, and a shotgun. Other factors include the properties of the scalp and skull of the victim, and whether the missile deforms on impact.

The injury may be classified as depressed, penetrating or perforating.[349] In depressed injuries the missile does not enter the cranial cavity but produces a depressed fracture of the skull and subjacent fracture contusions. Brain damage is therefore focal and consciousness is frequently lost only briefly or not at all. Clinical examination may be misleading because the scalp laceration may not lie directly over the fracture, or an apparently intact outer table may conceal a depression of the inner table of the skull.

In penetrating injuries the object enters the cranial cavity but does not pass through it. If the object is small and sharp, such as a nail, there may be very little direct injury to the skull or the brain; this damage may escape clinical detection if the missile is no longer embedded in the skull. Brain damage is again focal and loss of consciousness is unusual. Not frequently, patients injured by a penetrating missile such as a screwdriver are admitted to a neurosurgical unit with the missile still in position and the patient fully conscious. Occasionally, however, the missile

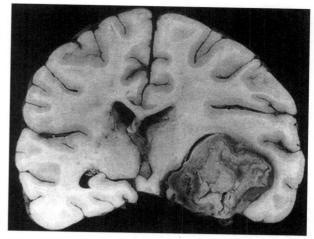

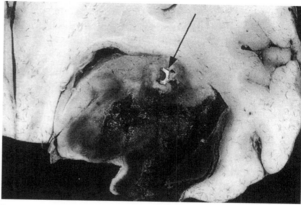

b

Figure 14.62 *Missile head injury. (a) Abscess in the right temporal lobe. (b) Airgun pellet (arrow) in the wall of the abscess. The abscess presented 21 months after the original injury. Reproduced by permission from Ref. 216.*

may penetrate deeply enough to damage some vital structure (Fig. 14.61). With penetrating head injuries there is an 11% risk of intracranial infections, 60% of which develop within 6 weeks after injury (Fig. 14.62a, b).[573]

In a perforating injury the missile, usually a bullet, traverses the cranial cavity and leaves through an exit wound. Brain damage is often severe but a high-velocity bullet may on occasion pass through the head without knocking the victim down or causing impairment of consciousness.[565] The exit wound in the skull is characteristically larger than the entry wound. Bullets of low velocity cause more damage at the site of entry and rarely pass completely through the skull; the bullet, however, may ricochet from the skull and traverse the brain in various directions.[162] Injuries from low-velocity missiles tend to be complicated by fragments of bone, scalp and, sometimes, clothing driven into the brain,[542] all of which increase the risk of intracranial infection.

There are three fairly distinct zones in a cross-section of the wound canal produced by a missile entering the

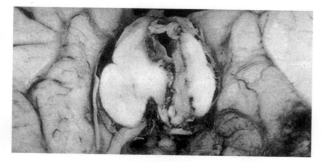

Figure 14.61 *Missile head injury. In this case the tip of a toy sword had penetrated directly into the midbrain. Reproduced by permission from Ref. 216.*

brain.[349] This cavity is permanent and in general either equals or is slightly larger than the diameter of the missile (Fig. 14.63) and is filled with blood. Enveloping the central cavity is an intermediate band of haemorrhagic tissue necrosis which in turn is surrounded by a marginal layer of pinkish-grey discoloured tissue, both of which follow the creation of a temporary cavity which collapses rapidly after formation around the permanent missile tract. The temporary cavity may be up to 30 times the diameter of the missile and is largely dependent on the velocity of the missile. The temporary cavity is smaller in low- than high-velocity missile injuries. Radial displacement forces from the missile track frequently cause remote contusions affecting the frontal and temporal poles and the undersurface of the cerebellum; bleeding into the basal ganglia, hypothalamus and upper brainstem is also common and large subdural haematomas may develop. Contrecoup fractures may also occur in the orbital plates.[80] Post-mortem MRI has identified many of the lesions,[298] especially when correlated with histology.

The cellular changes in the brain after gunshot wounding have allowed its degree, distribution and time course to be identified. For example, in a study of 14 patients who survived for between 1.5 and 86 h, immunohistochemistry for β-APP revealed widely distributed axonal damage throughout the cerebral hemispheres and in the brainstem.[320] Axonal and neuronal changes in 20 cases with survival of less than 90 min have also been identified, with the recognition that changes extended about 18 mm radially from the centre of the wound, tapering gradually along the track from entry point to exit point.[450] Injuries to the dural venous sinuses may occur, as a result of which the haemorrhage can be profuse and difficult to control. Gunshot wounds may also result in direct damage to blood vessels, resulting in massive haemorrhage or traumatic (false) aneurysms.[1,2,236] Between 0.4 and 0.7% of all aneurysms are said to be traumatic in origin. There is also a high frequency (32–51%) of epilepsy.[512] In studies on experimental missile injuries there was extensive subarachnoid, intraventricular and subependymal haemorrhage.[26,27] There were also perivascular ring haemorrhages, oedema and blood vessels surrounded by zones of decreased or increased staining intensity both close to and away from the missile track, as well as selective swelling of astrocytes that was more evident in the grey than in the white matter. Adjacent neurons, oligodendrocytes, pericytes and endothelial cells appeared normal. Some of these changes have been attributed to a marked rise in ICP,[84] the exact cause of which is not clear as it is out of proportion to the size of the intracranial haemorrhage.

REFERENCES

1 Aarabi B. Traumatic aneurysms of the brain due to high velocity missile wounds. *Neurosurgery* 1988; **22**: 1056–63.
2 Aarabi B, Taghipour M, Kamgarpour A, Alibail E. Traumatic intracranial aneurysms due to craniocerebral missile wounds. In: Aarabi B, Kaufman HH eds. *Missile wounds of the head and neck* Vol II. AANS Publications Committee, 1999: 293–314.
3 Abou-hamden A, Blumbergs PC, Scott G *et al.* Axonal injury in falls. *J Neurotrauma* 1997; **14**: 699–713.
4 Abu-Judeh HH, Parker R, Singh M *et al.* SPET brain perfusion imaging in mild traumatic brain injury without loss of consciousness and normal computed tomography. *Nucl Med Commun* 1999; **20**: 505–10.
5 Adams JH, Doyle D, Ford I *et al.* Brain damage in fatal non-missile head injury in relation to age and type of injury. *Scott Med J* 1989; **34**: 399–401.
6 Adams JH, Doyle D, Ford I *et al.* Diffuse axonal injury in head injury: definition, diagnosis and grading. *Histopathology* 1989; **15**: 49–59.
7 Adams JH, Doyle D, Graham DI *et al.* Deep intracerebral (basal ganglia) haematomas in fatal non-missile head injury in man. *J Neurol Neurosurg Psychiatry* 1986; **49**: 1039–43.
8 Adams JH, Doyle D, Graham DI *et al.* Diffuse axonal injury in head injuries caused by a fall. *Lancet* 1984; **ii**: 1420–1.
9 Adams JH, Doyle D, Graham DI *et al.* Gliding contusions in non-missile head injury in humans. *Arch Pathol Lab Med* 1986; **110**: 485–8.
10 Adams JH, Doyle D, Graham DI *et al.* Microscopic diffuse axonal injury in cases of head injury. *Med Sci Law* 1985; **25**: 265–9.
11 Adams JH, Doyle D, Graham DI *et al.* The contusion index; a reappraisal in man and experimental non-missile head injury. *Neuropathol Appl Neurobiol* 1985; **11**: 299–308.
12 Adams JH, Graham DI. The relationship between ventricular fluid pressure and the neuropathology of raised intracranial pressure. *Neuropath Appl Neurobiol* 1976; **2**: 323–32.
13 Adams JH, Graham DI, Gennarelli TA. Contemporary neuropathological considerations regarding brain damage in head injury. In: Becker DP, Povlishock JT editors. *Central nervous system trauma status report*. Washington DC: National Institute of Neurological Communicative Disorders and Stroke, 1985: 65–77.
14 Adams JH, Graham DI, Gennarelli TA. Neuropathology of acceleration-induced head injury in the subhuman primate. In: Grossman RG, Gildenberg PL eds. *Head injury: basic and clinical aspects*. New York: Raven Press, 1982: 141–50.

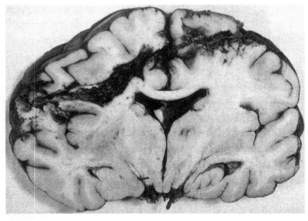

Figure 14.63 *Missile head injury. Track of a bullet wound through the brain. Reproduced by permission from Ref. 216.*

15 Adams JH, Graham DI, Jennett B. The neuropathology of the vegetative state after acute brain insults. *Brain* 2000; **123**: 1327–38.

16 Adams JH, Graham DI, Jennett B. The structural basis of moderate disability following traumatic brain damage. *J Neurol Neuropathol Psychiatry* in press.

17 Adams JH, Graham DI, Murray LS, Scott G. Diffuse axonal injury due to non-missile injury in humans: an analysis of 45 cases. *Ann Neurol* 1982; **12**: 557–63.

18 Adams JH, Graham, DI, Scott G et al. Brain damage in non-missile head injury. *J Clin Pathol* 1980; **33**: 1132–45.

19 Adams JH, Jennett B, McLellan DR et al. The neuropathology of the vegetative state after head injury. *J Clin Pathol* 1999; **52**: 804–6.

20 Adams JH, Mitchell DE, Graham DI, Doyle D. Diffuse brain damage of immediate impact type. *Brain* 1967; **100**: 489–502.

21 Adams JH, Scott G, Parker LS et al. The contusion index: a quantitative approach to cerebral contusions in head injury. *Neuropathol Appl Neurobiol* 1980; **6**: 319–24.

22 Adelson PD, Kochanek PM. Head injury in children. *J Child Neurol* 1998; **13**: 2–15.

23 Adle-Biassette H, Duyckaerts C, Wasowicz M et al. β-AP deposition and head trauma. *Neurobiol Aging* 1996; **17**: 415–19.

24 Alavi A, Mirot A, Newberg A et al. Fluorine-18-FDG evaluation of crossed cerebellar diaschisis in head injury. *J Nucl Med* 1997; **38**: 1717–20.

25 Alberico AM, Ward JD, Choi SC et al. Outcome after severe head injury. Relationship to mass lesions, diffuse injury, and ICP course in pediatric and adult patients. *J Neurosurg* 1987; **67**: 648–56.

26 Allen IV, Kirk J, Maynard RL et al. An ultrastructural study of experimental high velocity penetrating head injury. *Acta Neuropathol (Berl)* 1983; **59**: 277–82.

27 Allen IV, Scott R, Tanner JA. Experimental high velocity missile head injury. *Injury* 1982; **14**: 183–93.

28 Alsop DC, Murai H, Detre JA et al. Detection of acute pathologic changes following experimental traumatic brain injury using diffusion-weighted magnetic resonance imaging. *J Neurotrauma* 1996; **13**: 515–21.

29 Amaducci LA, Fratiglioni L, Rocca WA et al. Risk factors for clinically diagnosed Alzheimer's disease: a case-control study of an Italian population. *Neurology* 1986; **36**: 922–31.

30 Amstad PA, Krupitza G, Cerutti PA. Mechanism of c-fos induction by active oxygen. *Cancer Res* 1992; **52**: 3952–60.

31 Annegers JF, Grabow JD, Groover RV et al. Seizures after head trauma: a population study. *Neurology* 1980; **30**: 683–9.

32 Annegers JF, Hauser WA, Coan SP et al. A population-based study of seizures after traumatic brain injuries. *N Engl J Med* 1998; **338**: 20–4.

33 Artuso M, Esteve A, Bresil H et al. The role of the ataxia telangiectasia gene in the p53, WAF1/CIP1(p21)- and GADD45-mediated response to DNA damage produced by ionizing radiation. *Oncogene* 1995; **11**: 1427–35.

34 Bartus RT. The calpain hypothesis of neurodegeneration: evidence for a common cytotoxic pathway. *Neuroscientist* 1997; **3**: 314–27.

35 Bazan NG, Allan G, Rodriguez de Turco EB. Role of phospholipase A_2 and membrane derived lipid second messengers in membrane function and transcriptional activation of genes: implications in cerebral ischemia and neuronal excitability. *Prog Brain Res* 1993; **96**: 247–57.

36 Bazan NG, Rodriguez de Turco EB, Allan G. Mediators of injury in neurotrauma: intracellular signal transduction and gene expression. *J Neurotrauma* 1995; **12**: 791–814.

37 Behrman S, Mandybur T, McMenemey WH. Un cas de maladie Creutzfeld–Jakob à la suite d'un traumatisme cerebrale. *Rev Neurol* 1962; **107**: 453–9.

38 Beit-Yannai E, Kohen R, Horowitz M et al. Changes of biological reducing activity in rat brain following closed head injury: a cyclic voltammetry study in normal and heat-acclimated rats. *J Cereb Blood Flow Metab* 1997; **17**: 273–9.

39 Bergsneider M, Hovda DA, Lee SM et al. Dissociation of cerebral glucose metabolism and level of consciousness during the period of metabolic depression following human traumatic brain injury. *J Neurotrauma* 2000; **17**: 389–401.

40 Bergsneider M, Hovda DA, Shalmon E et al. Cerebral hyperglycolysis following severe traumatic brain injury in humans: a positron emission tomography study. *J Neurosurg* 1997; **86**: 241–51.

41 Berryhill P, Lilly MA, Levin HS et al. Frontal lobe changes after severe closed head injury in children: a volumetric study of magnetic resonance imaging. *Neurosurgery* 1995; **37**: 392–9.

42 Bezircioglu H, Ersahin Y, Demircivi F et al. Nonoperative treatment of acute extradural hematomas: analysis of 80 cases. *J Trauma* 1996; **41**: 696–8.

43 Bigler ED. Neuroimaging in pediatric traumatic head injury: diagnostic considerations and relationships to neurobehavioral outcome. *J Head Trauma Rehabil* 1999; **14**: 406–23.

44 Billger M, Wallin M, Karlsson JO. Proteolysis of tubulin and microtubule-associated proteins 1 and 2 by calpain I and II. Difference in sensitivity of assembled and disassembled microtubules. *Cell Calcium* 1988; **9**: 33–44.

45 Billmire ME, Myers PA. Serious head injury in infants: accident or abuse? *Pediatrics* 1985; **75**: 340–2.

46 Blumbergs PC, Jones NR, North JB. Diffuse axonal injury in head trauma. *J Neurol Neurosurg Psychiatry* 1989; **52**: 838–41.

47 Blumbergs PC, Oatey PE, Sandhu A et al. Pontomedullary tear in a speedboat accident, report of a case with MRI diagnosis. *Zentral bl Neurochir* 1991; **52**: 89–93.

48 Blumbergs PC, Scott G, Manavis J et al. Staining of amyloid precursor protein to study axonal damage in mild head injury. *Lancet* 1994; **344**: 1055–6.

49 Blumbergs PC, Scott G, Manavis J et al. Topography of axonal injury as defined by amyloid precursor protein and the sector scoring method in mild and severe closed head injury. *J Neurotrauma* 1995; **12**: 565–72.

50 Boobis AR, Fawthrop DJ, Davies DS. Mechanisms of cell death. *Trends Pharmac Sci* 1989; **10**: 275–80.

51 Bouma GJ, Muizelaar JP, Stringer WA et al. Ultra-early evaluation of regional cerebral blood flow in severely head-injured patients using xenon-enhanced computerized tomography. *J Neurosurg* 1992; **77**: 360–8.

52 Braakman R, Gelpke GJ, Habbema JDF et al. Systematic selection of prognostic features in patients with severe head injury. *Neurosurgery* 1980; **6**: 362–70.

53 Bramlett HM, Dietrich WD, Green EJ. Secondary hypoxia following moderate fluid percussion brain injury in rats exacerbated sensorimotor and cognitive deficits. *J Neurotrauma* 1999; **16**: 1035–47.

54 Bramlett HM, Dietrich WD, Green EJ, Busto R. Chronic histopathological consequences of fluid-percussion brain injury in rats: effects of post-traumatic hypothermia. *Acta Neuropathol* 1997; **93**: 190–9.

55 Bramlett HM, Kraydieh S, Green EJ, Dietrich WD. Temporal and regional patterns of axonal damage following traumatic brain injury: a beta-amyloid precursor protein immunocytochemical study in rats. *J Neuropathol Exp Neurol* 1997; **56**: 1132–41.

56 Bredesen DE. Neural apoptosis. *Ann Neurol* 1995; **38**: 839–51.

57 Bretler MMB, Claus JJ, Van Duijn CM *et al*. Epidemiology of Alzheimer's disease. *Epidemiol Rev* 1992; **14**: 59–82.

58 Bricolo A, Pasut LM. Extradural haematoma: toward zero mortality. A prospective study. *Neurosurgery* 1984; **14**: 8–12.

59 Britt RH, Herrick MK, Mason RT, Dorfman LJ. Traumatic lesions of the pontomedullary junction. *Neurosurgery* 1980; **6**: 623–31.

60 Brocklehurst G, Gooding M, James G. Comprehensive care of patients with head-injuries. *BMJ* 1987; **294**: 345–7.

61 Bruce D, Schut L, Bruno L *et al*. Outcome following severe head injuries in children. *J Neurosurg* 1978; **48**: 679–88.

62 Bruce DA, Alavi A, Bilaniuk L *et al*. Diffuse cerebral swelling following head injuries in children: the syndrome of 'malignant brain edema'. *J Neurosurg* 1981; **54**: 170–8.

63 Bruce DA, Langfitt TW, Miller JD *et al*. Regional cerebral blood flow, intracranial pressure, and brain metabolism in comatose patients. *J Neurosurg* 1973; **38**: 131–44.

64 Bruce DA, Raphaely RC, Goldberg AI. The pathophysiology, treatment and outcome following severe head injury in children. *Childs Brain* 1979; **5**: 174–91.

65 Buki A, Okonkwo DO, Povlishock JT. Postinjury cyclosporin A administration limits axonal damage and disconnection in traumatic brain injury. *J Neurotrauma* 1999; **16**: 511–21.

66 Buki A, Siman R, Trojanowski JQ, Povlishock JT. The role of calpain-mediated spectrum proteolysis in traumatically induced axonal injury. *J Neuropathol Exp Neurol* 1999; **58**: 365–75.

67 Bullock MR, Lyeth BG, Muizelaar JP. Current status of neuroprotection trials for traumatic brain injury: lessons from animal models and clinical studies. *Neurosurgery* 1999; **45**: 207–17.

68 Bullock R. Injury and cell function. In: Reilly P, Bullock R eds. *Head injury: pathophysiology and management of severe closed injury*. London: Chapman and Hall Medical, 1997: 121–41.

69 Bullock R, Butcher SP, Chen M-H *et al*. Correlation of the extracellular glutamate concentration with extent of blood flow reduction after subdural hematoma in the rat. *J Neurosurg* 1991; **74**: 794–802.

70 Bullock R, Graham DI. Non-penetrating injuries of the head. In: Cooper GJ, Dudley HAF, Gann DS *et al* eds. *Scientific foundation of trauma: non-penetrating blunt injury*. Oxford: Butterworth Heinemann, 1997: 101–26.

71 Bullock R, Maxwell WL, Graham DI *et al*. Glial swelling following human cerebral contusion: an ultrastructural study. *J Neurol Neurosurg Psychiatry* 1991; **54**: 427–34.

72 Bullock R, Smith RM, Dellen JR van. Nonoperative management of extradural hematoma. *Neurosurgery* 1985; **16**: 602–6.

73 Bullock R, Statham P, Patterson J *et al*. The time course of vasogenic edema after focal human head injury – evidence from SPECT mapping of blood brain barrier deficit. *Acta Neurochir* 1990; **51** (Suppl): 286–8.

74 Bullock R, Teasdale G. Surgical management of traumatic intracranial haematomas. In: Braakman R ed. *Head injury. Handbook of clinical neurology* Vol. 15 No. 57. Amsterdam: Elsevier, 1990: 244–98.

75 Bullock RM, Chesnut RM, Clifton GL *et al*. Guidelines for the management of severe traumatic brain injury. Part 1. *J Neurotrauma* 2000; **17**: 453–553.

76 Caffey J. The whiplash shaken infant syndrome – manual shaking by the extremeties with whiplash-induced intracranial and intraocular bleedings, linked with residual permanent brain damage and mental retardation. *Pediatrics* 1974; **54**: 396–403.

77 Cailliau CP, Price DL, Martin LJ. Non-NMDA and NMDA receptor-mediated excitotoxic neuronal deaths in adult brain are morphologically distinct: further evidence for an apoptosis–necrosis continuum. *J Compl Neurol* 1997; **378**: 88–104.

78 Cajal S, Ramon Y. *Degeneration and regeneration of the nervous system* Vol. 2. May RM transl and ed. New York: Hafner, 1959.

79 Calder IM, Hill I, Scholtz CL. Primary brain trauma in non-accidental injury. *J Clin Pathol* 1984; **37**: 1095–100.

80 Campbell GA. The pathology of penetrating wounds of the brain and its enclosures. In: Aarabi B, Kaufman HH eds. *Missile wounds of the head and neck* Vol. I. AANS Publications Committee, 1999: 73–89.

81 Capruso DX, Levin HS. Neurobehavioral sequelae of head injury. In: Cooper PR, Golfinos JG, eds. *Head injury* 4th edn. New York: McGraw-Hill, 2000: 525–53.

82 Carbonell WS, Maris DO, McCall T, Grady MS. Adaptation of the fluid percussion injury model to the mouse. *J Neurotrauma* 1998; **15**: 217–29.

83 Carcassone M, Choux M, Grisoli F. Extradural hematomas in infants. *J Pediatr Surg* 1977; **12**: 69–73.

84 Carey ME, Sarna GS, Farrell B *et al*. Experimental missile wound to the brain. *J Neurosurg* 1989; **71**: 754–64.

85 Caveness WF, Meirowsky AM, Rish BL *et al*. The nature of post-traumatic epilepsy. *J Neurosurg* 1979; **50**: 545–53.

86 Cecil KM, Lenkinski RE, Meaney DF *et al*. High-field proton magnetic resonance spectroscopy of a swine model for axonal injury. *J Neurochem* 1998; **70**: 2038–44.

87 Cervos-Navarro J, Lafuente JV. Traumatic brain injuries: structural changes. *J Neurol Sci* 1991; **103**: 3–14.

88 Chan PH. Role of oxidants in ischemic brain damage. *Stroke* 1996; **27**: 1124–9.

89 Charriaut-Marlangue C, Ben-Ari Y. A cautionary note in the use of TUNEL stain to determine apoptosis. *Neuroreport* 1995; **7**: 61–4.

90 Chen J, Graham SH, Chan PH *et al*. Bcl-2 is expressed in neurons that survive focal ischemia in the rat. *Neuroreport* 1995; **6**: 394–8.

91 Chen M, Clark RSB, Kochanek PM *et al*. 72-kDA heat shock protein and mRNA expression after controlled cortical impact injury with hypoxemia in rats. *J Neurotrauma* 1998; **15**: 171–81.

92 Chen X-H, Meaney DF, Xu B-N *et al*. Evolution of neurofilament subtype accumulation in axons following diffuse brain injury in the pig. *J Neuropathol Exp Neurol* 1999; **58**: 588–96.

93 Cheng CLY, Povlishock JT. The effect of traumatic brain injury on the visual system: a morphologic characterization of reactive axonal change. *J Neurotrauma* 1988; **5**: 47–60.

94 Chesnut RM. Secondary brain insults after head injury: clinical perspectives. *New Horiz* 1995; **3**: 366–75.

95 Chesnut RM, Ghajar J, Maas AIR *et al*. Early indicators of prognosis in severe traumatic brain injury. Part 2. *J Neurotrauma* 2000; **17**: 559–627.

96 Choi SC, Narayan RK, Anderson RL *et al*. Enhanced specificity of prognosis in severe head injury. *J Neurosurg* 1988; **69**: 381–5.

97 Chopp M, Li Y, Jiang N. Increase in apoptosis and concomitant reduction of ischemic lesion volume and evidence for synaptogenesis after transient focal cerebral ischemia in rat treated with staurosporine. *Brain Res* 1999; **828**: 197–201.

98 Chopp M, Li Y, Zhang ZG, Freytag SO. p53 expression in brain after middle cerebral artery occlusion in the rat. *Biochem Biophys Res Commun* 1992; **182**: 1201–7.

99 Clark JM. Distribution of microglial clusters in the brain after head injury. *J Neurol Neurosurg Psychiatry* 1974; **37**: 463–74.

100 Clark RS, Kochanek PM, Chen M *et al*. Increases in BCL-2 and cleavage of caspase-1 and caspase-3 in human brain after head injury. *FASEB J* 1999; **13**: 813–21.

101 Clark RS, Kochanek PM, Watkins SC *et al*. Caspase-3 mediated neuronal death after traumatic brain injury in rats. *J Neurochem* 2000; **74**: 740–53.

102 Clark RSB, Chen J, Watkins SC *et al*. Apoptosis-suppressor gene *bcl-2* expression after traumatic brain injury in rats. *J Neurosci* 1997; **17**: 9172–82.

103 Clark RSB, Kochanek PM, Dixon CE *et al*. Early neuropathologic effects of mild or moderate hypoxemia after controlled cortical impact injury in rats. *J Neurotrauma* 1997; **14**: 179–89.

104 Clinton J, Ambler MV, Roberts GW. Post-traumatic Alzheimer's disease: preponderance of a single plaque type. *Neuropath Appl Neurobiol* 1991; **17**: 69–74.

105 Cole G, Cowie VA. Long survival after cardiac arrest: case report and neuropathological findings. *Clin Neuropathol* 1987; **6**: 104–9.

106 Colicos MA, Dash PK. Apoptotic morphology of dentate gyrus granule cells following experimental cortical impact injury in rats: possible role in spatial memory deficits. *Brain Res* 1996; **739**: 120–31.

107 Collins AR, Dusinska M, Gedik CM, Stetina R. Oxidative damage to DNA: do we have a reliable biomarker? *Environ Health Persp* 1996; **104** (Suppl 3): 465–9.

108 Condon B, Oluoch-Olunya D, Hadley D *et al*. Early ¹H magnetic resonance spectroscopy of acute head injury: four cases. *J Neurotrauma* 1998; **15**: 563–71.

109 Conti AC, Raghupathi R, Trojanowski JQ, McIntosh TK. Experimental brain injury induces regionally distinct apoptosis during the acute and delayed post-traumatic period. *J Neurosci* 1998; **18**: 5663–72.

110 Cook RJ, Dorsch NWC, Fearnside MR *et al*. Outcome prediction in extradural haematomas. *Acta Neurochir (Wien)* 1988; **95**: 90–4.

111 Cooper PR. Post-traumatic intracranial mass lesions. In: Cooper PR, Golfinos JG eds. *Head injury* 4th edn. New York: McGraw-Hill, 293–348.

112 Cordobes F, Labato RD, Rivas JJ *et al*. Observations on 82 patients with extradural hematoma. Comparison of results before and after advent of computerized tomography. *J Neurosurg* 1981; **54**: 179–86.

113 Corsellis JAN. Boxing and the brain. *BMJ* 1989; **298**: 105–9.

114 Corsellis JAN, Brierley JB. Observations on the pathology of insidious dementia following head injury. *J Ment Sci* 1959; **105**: 714–20.

115 Corsellis JAN, Bruton CJ, Freeman-Browne D. The aftermath of boxing. *Psychol Med* 1973; **3**: 270–303.

116 Cortez SC, McIntosh TK, Noble LJ. Experimental fluid percussion brain injury: vascular disruption and neuronal and glial alterations. *Brain Res* 1989; **482**: 271–82.

117 Critchley M. Medical aspects of boxing particularly from a neurological standpoint. *BMJ* 1957; **I**: 357–66.

118 Crumrine RC, Thomas AL, Morgan PF. Attenuation of p53 expression protects against focal ischemic damage in transgenic mice. *J Cereb Blood Flow Metab* 1994; **14**: 887–91.

119 Dacey RG, Alves WN, Rimel RW *et al*. Neurosurgical complications after apparently minor head injury. *J Neurosurg* 1986; **65**: 203–10.

120 Dave JR, Bauman RA, Long JB. Hypoxia potentials traumatic brain injury – induced expression of C-fos in rats. *Neuroreport* 1997; **8**: 395–8.

121 Dawson SL, Hirsch CS, Lucas FV, Sebek BA. The contrecoup phenomenon: reappraisal of a classic problem. *Hum Pathol* 1980; **II**: 155–66.

122 Denny-Brown JP, Russell WR. Experimental cerebral concussion. *Brain* 1941; **64**: 93–164.

123 Dhillon HS, Carbary T, Dose J *et al*. Activation of phosphatidylinositol bisphosphate signal transduction pathway after experimental brain injury: a lipid study. *Brain Res* 1995; **698**: 100–6.

124 Dhillon HS, Donaldson D, Dempsey RJ, Prasad MR. Regional levels of free fatty acids and evans blue extravasation after experimental brain injury. *J Neurotrauma* 1994; **11**: 405–15.

125 Dietrich WD, Alonso O, Busto R, Finklestein SP. Posttreatment with intravenous basic fibroblast growth factor reduces histopathological damage following fluid-percussion brain injury in rats. *J Neurotrauma* 1996; **13**: 309–16.

126 Dietrich WD, Alonso O, Halley M. Early microvascular and neuronal consequences to traumatic brain injury: a light and electron microscopic study in rats. *J Neurotrauma* 1994; **11**: 289–301.

127 Dings J, Meixensberger J, Amschler J *et al*. Brain tissue PO₂ in relation to cerebral perfusion pressure, TCD findings and TCD CO₂ reactivity after severe head injury. *Acta Neurochir* 1996; **138**: 425–34.

128 Dixon CE, Clifton GL, Lighthall JW *et al*. A controlled cortical impact model of traumatic brain injury in the rat. *J Neurosci Meth* 1991; **39**: 253–62.

129 Dixon CE, Kochanek PM, Yan HQ *et al*. One-year study of spatial memory performance, brain morphology and cholinergic markers after controlled cortical impact in rats. *J Neurotrauma* 1999; **16**: 109–22.

130 Doberstein CE, Hovda DA, Becker DP. Clinical considerations in the reduction of secondary brain injury. *Ann Emerg Med* 1993; **22**: 933–7.

131 Dolinak D, Smith C, Graham DI. Global hypoxia *per se* is an unusual cause of axonal injury. *Acta Neuropathol* 2000; **100**: 553–60.

132 Dolinak D, Smith C, Graham DI. Hypoglycaemia is a cause of axonal injury. *Neuropathol Appl Neurobiol* 2000; **26**: 448–53.

133 Dolinskas CS, Zimmerman RA, Bilaniuk LT, Gennarelli TA. Computed tomography of post-traumatic extracerebral hematomas. *J Trauma* 1979; **19**: 163–9.

134 Doppenberg EMR, Bullock R. Clinical neuro-protection trials in severe traumatic brain injury: lessons from previous studies. *J Neurotrauma* 1997; **14**: 71–80.

135 Dougherty JH, Rawlinson DG, Levy DE *et al*. Hypoxic–ischemic brain injury and the vegetative state: clinical and neuropathologic correlation. *Neurology* 1981; **31**: 991–7.

136 Dugan LL, Choi DW. Excitotoxicity, free radicals, and cell membrane changes. *Ann Neurol* 1994; **35**: S17–21.

137 Duhaime A, Alario AJ, Lewander WJ *et al*. Head injury in very young children: mechanisms, injury types, and ophthalmologic findings in 100 hospitalized patients younger than 2 years of age. *Paediatrics* 1992; **90**: 179–85.

138 Duhaime AC, Christian CW, Rorke LB, Zimmerman RA. Non-accidental head injury in infants in the 'shaken-baby' syndrome. *N Engl J Med* 1998; **338**: 1822–9.

139 Duhaime AC, Gennarelli TA, Thibault LE *et al*. A clinical, pathological and biochemical study. *J Neurosurg* 1987; **66**: 409–15.

140 Dunn-Meynell AA, Levin BE. Histological markers of neuronal, axonal and astrocytic changes after lateral rigid impact traumatic brain injury. *Brain Res* 1997; **761**: 25–41.

141 Eldadah BA, Faden AI. Caspase pathways, neuronal apoptosis, and CNS injury. *J Neurotrauma* 2000; **17**: 811–29.

142 Eliasson MJ, Sampei K, Mandir AS et al. Poly(ADP-ribose) polymerase gene disruption renders mice resistant to cerebral ischemia. Nat Med 1997; 3: 1089–95.

143 Elsner H, Rigamonti D, Corradino G et al. Delayed traumatic intracerebral hematomas. J Neurosurg 1990; 72: 813–15.

144 Emery E, Aldana P, Bunge R et al. Apoptosis after traumatic spinal cord injury. J Neurosurg 1998; 89: 911–20.

145 Enari M, Sakahira H et al. A caspase-activated DNase that degrades DNA during apoptosis, and its inhibitor ICAD. Nature 1998; 391: 43–50.

146 Endres M, Wang ZQ, Namura S et al. Ischemic brain injury is mediated by the activation of poly(ADP-ribose)polymerase. J Cereb Blood Flow Metab 1997; 17: 1143–51.

147 Engel S, Schluesener H, Mittelbronn M, Seid K et al. Dynamics of microglial activation after human traumatic brain injury are revealed by delayed expression of macrophage-related proteins MRP8 and MRP14. Acta Neuropathol 2000; 100: 313–22.

148 Engelborghs K, Haseldonckx M, Van Reempts J et al. Impaired autoregulation of cerebral blood flow in an experimental model of traumatic brain injury. J Neurotrauma 2000; 17: 667–77.

149 Epstein JA, Epstein BS, Small M. Subepicranial hygroma. A complication of head injuries in infants and children. J Pediatr 1961; 59: 562–6.

150 Erb DE, Povlishock JT. Neuroplasticity following traumatic brain injury: a study of GABAergic terminal loss and recovery in the cat dorsal lateral vestibular nucleus. Exp Brain Res 1991; 83: 253–67.

151 Evan G, Littlewood TD. A matter of life and death. Science 1998; 281: 1317–22.

152 Faden AI, Demediuk P, Panter SS, Vink R. The role of excitatory amino acids and NMDA receptors in traumatic brain injury. Science 1989; 244: 798–800.

153 Fan L, Young PR, Barone FC et al. Experimental brain injury induces expression of interleukin-1β mRNA in the rat brain. Mol Brain Res 1995; 30: 125–30.

154 Fan L, Young PR, Barone FC et al. Experimental brain injury induces differential expression of tumor necrosis factor-α mRNA in the CNS. Mol Brain Res 1996; 36: 287–91.

155 Fay GC, Jaffe KM, Polissar NL et al. Mild pediatric traumatic brain injury: a cohort study. Arch Phys Med Rehabil 1993; 74: 895–901.

156 Feeney DM, Boyeson MG, Linn RT et al. Responses to cortical injury. I. Methodology and local effects of contusions in the rat. Brain Res 1981; 211: 67–77.

157 Fern R. Axon resealing: filling in the holes. Neuroscientist 1995; 1: 253–54.

158 Fineman I, Hovda DA, Smith M et al. Concussive brain injury is associated with a prolonged accumulation of calcium: a ^{45}Ca autoradiographic study. Brain Res 1993; 624: 94–102.

159 Fogelholm R, Waltimo O. Epidemiology of chronic subdural haematoma. Acta Neurochir 1975; 32: 247–50.

160 Fox GB, Fan L, Levasseur RA, Faden AI. Sustained sensory/motor and cognitive deficits with neuronal apoptosis following controlled cortical impact brain injury in the mouse. J Neurotrauma 1998; 15: 599–614.

161 Freytag E. Autopsy findings in head injuries from blunt forces. Arch Pathol 1963; 75: 402–13.

162 Freytag E. Autopsy findings in head injuries from firearms. Arch Pathol 1963; 76: 215–25.

163 Friedman G, Froom P, Sazbon L I et al. Apolipoprotein E-epsilon 4 genotype predicts a poor outcome in survivors of traumatic brain injury. Neurology 1999; 52: 244–48.

164 Friedman SD, Brooks WM, Jung RE et al. Proton MR spectroscopic findings correspond to neuropsychological function in traumatic brain injury. Am J Neuroradiol 1998; 19: 1879–85.

165 Fujitsu K, Kuwabara M, Hirata K et al. Traumatic intraventricular hemorrhage: report of twenty-six cases and consideration of the pathogenetic mechanism. Neurosurgery 1988; 23: 423–30.

166 Gaetani P, Tancioni F, Tartara F et al. Prognostic value of the amount of post-traumatic subarachnoid haemorrhage in a six month follow up period. J Neurol Neurosurg Psychiatry 1995; 59: 635–7.

167 Galbraith JA, Thibault LE, Matteson RA. Mechanical and electrical responses of the squid giant axon to simple elongation. J Biomech Eng 1993; 115: 13–22.

168 Gale SD, Johnson SC, Bigler ED, Blatter DD. Nonspecific white matter degeneration following traumatic brain injury. J Int Neuropsychol Soc 1995; 1: 17–28.

169 Galen on anatomical procedures, the later books. Duckworth WLH Transl. Cambridge: Cambridge University Press, 1962.

170 Gallant PE, Galbraith JA. Axonal structure and function after axolemmal leakage in the squid giant axon. J Neurotrauma 1997; 14: 811–22.

171 Garada B, Klufas RA, Schwartz RB. Neuroimaging in closed head injury. Semin Clin Neuropsychiatry 1997; 2: 188–95.

172 Gass A, Filippi M, Grossman RI. The contribution of MRI in the differential diagnosis of posterior fossa damage. J Neurol Sci 2000; 172: S43–9.

173 Gavrieli Y, Sherman Y, Ben-Sasson SA. Identification of programmed cell death in situ via specific labeling of nuclear DNA fragmentation. J Cell Biol 1992; 119: 493–501.

174 Gean AD. Imaging of head trauma. New York: Raven Press 1994: 497–556.

175 Geddes JF, Hackshaw AK, Vowles GH et al. Neuropathology of inflicted head injury in children. I: Patterns of brain damage. Brain 2001; 124: 1290–8.

176 Geddes JF, Vowles GH, Bler TW, Ellison DW. The diagnosis of diffuse axonal injury: implications for forensic practice. Neuropathol Appl Neurobiol 1997; 23: 339–47.

177 Geddes JF, Vowles GH, Hackshaw AK et al. Neuropathology of inflicted head injury in children II: microscopic brain injury in infants. Brain 2001; 124: 1299–306.

178 Geddes JF, Vowles GH, Nicoll JAR, Revesz T. Neuronal cytoskeletal changes are an early consequence of repetitive head injury. Acta Neuropathol 1999; 98: 171–8.

179 Geddes JF, Vowles.GH, Robinson SFD, Sutcliff JC. Neurofibrillary tangles, but not Alzheimer-type pathology, in a young boxer. Neuropath Appl Neurobiol 1996; 22: 12–16.

180 Geddes JF, Whitwell HL, Graham DI. Traumatic axonal injury: practical issues for diagnosis in medico-legal cases. Neuropathol Appl Neurobiol 2000; 26: 105–16.

181 Gennarelli TA. Animate models of human head injury. J Neurotrauma 1994; 11: 357–68.

182 Gennarelli TA. Head Injury in man and experimental animals: clinical aspects. Acta Neurochir 1983; 32 (Suppl): 1–13.

183 Gennarelli TA. The pathobiology of traumatic brain injury. Neuroscientist 1997; 3: 73–81.

184 Gennarelli TA. The spectrum of traumatic axonal injury. Neuropathol Appl Neurobiol 1996; 22: 509–13.

185 Gennarelli TA, Champion HC, Copes WS, Sacco WJ. Comparison of mortality, morbidity and severity of 59,713 head injured patients with 114,447 patients with extracranial injuries. J Trauma 1994; 37: 962–8.

186 Gennarelli TA, Champion HC, Sacco WJ et al. Mortality of patients with head injury and extracranial injury treated in trauma centers. J Trauma 1989; 29: 1193–202.

187 Gennarelli TA, Meaney DF. Mechanisms of primary head injury. In: Wilkins RH, Rengachary SS eds. Neurosurgery 2nd edn. New York: McGraw-Hill, 1996: 2611–22.

188 Gennarelli TA, Spielman GM, Langfitt TW et al. The influence of the type of intracranial lesion on outcome from severe head injury, a multicenter study using a new classification system. J Neurosurg 1982; 56: 26–32.

189 Gennarelli TA, Thibault LE. Biological models of head injury. In: Becker DP, Povlishock JT eds. Central nervous system trauma status report. Bethesda, MD: National Institute of Neurological and Communicative Disorders and Stroke, National Institutes of Health, 1985: 391–404.

190 Gennarelli TA, Thibault LE. Biomechanics of acute subdural hematoma. J Trauma 1982; 22: 680–6.

191 Gennarelli TA, Thibault LE, Adams JH et al. Diffuse axonal injury and traumatic coma in the primate. Ann Neurol 1982; 12: 564–74.

192 Gennarelli TA, Thibault LE, Graham DI. Diffuse axonal injury: an important form of traumatic brain injury. Neuroscientist 1998; 4: 202–15.

193 Gennarelli TA, Thibault LE, Tipperman R et al. Axonal injury in the optic nerve: a model simulating diffuse axonal injury in the brain. J Neurosurg 1989; 71: 244–53.

194 Gennarelli TA, Thibault LE, Tomei G et al. Directional dependence of axonal brain injury due to centroidal and non-centroidal acceleration. In: Proceedings of the 33rd Stapp Car Crash Conference. New York: Society of Automotive Engineers, 1987: 35–53.

195 Gentilini M, Nichelli P, Schoenhuber R et al. Neuropsychological evaluation of mild head injury. J Neurol Neurosurg Psychiatry 1985; 48: 137–40.

196 Gentleman D, North F, MacPherson P. Diagnosis and management of delayed traumatic haematomas. Br J Neurosurg 1989; 3: 367–72.

197 Gentleman SM, Greenberg BD, Savage MJ et al. Aβ42 is the predominant form of amyloid β protein in the brain of short term survivors of head injury. Neuroreport 1997; 8: 1519–22.

198 Gentleman SM, Hush MJ, Sweeting CJ et al. β-Amyloid precursor protein (β-APP) as a marker for axonal injury after head injury. Neurosci Lett 1993; 160: 139–44.

199 Gentleman SM, Roberts GW, Gennarelli TA et al. Axonal injury: a universal consequence of fatal closed head injury? Acta Neuropathol 1995; 89: 537–43.

200 Gillardon F, Lenz C, Waschke KF et al. Altered expression Bcl-2, Bcl-x, Bax, and c-Fos colocalizes with DNA fragmentation and ischemic cell damage following middle cerebral artery occlusion in rats. Mol Brain Res 1996; 40: 254–60.

201 Gillardon F, Wickert H, Zimmermann M. Up-regulation of Bax and down-regulation of Bcl-2 is associated with kainate-induced apoptosis in mouse brain. Neurosci Lett 1995; 192: 85–8.

202 Gjerris F. Traumatic lesions of the visual pathways. In: Vinken PJ, Bruyn GW eds. Handbook of neurology. New York: Elsevier, 1976: 27–57.

203 Gleckman AM, Bell MD, Evans RJ, Smith TW. Diffuse axonal injury in infants with non-accidental craniocerebral trauma: enhanced detection by beta-amyloid precursor protein immunohistochemical staining. Arch Pathol Lab Med 1999; 123: 146–51.

204 Globus M, Busto R, Dietrich W et al. Effect of ischemia on the in vivo release of striatal dopamine, glutamate, and gamma aminobutyric acid studied by intracerebral microdialysis. J Neurochem 1988; 51: 1455–64.

205 Goldgaber D, Harris HW, Hla T et al. Interleukin 1 regulates synthesis of amyloid beta-protein precursor mRNA in human endothelial cells. Proc Natl Acad Sci USA 1989; 86: 7606–10.

206 Goldstein M. Traumatic Brain Injury: a silent epidemic. Ann Neurol 1990; 27: 327.

207 Golfinos JG, Cooper PR. Skull fracture and post-traumatic cerebrospinal fluid fistulae. In: Cooper PR, Golfinos JG eds. Head injury 4th edn. New York: McGraw-Hill, 2000: 155–74.

208 Grady MS, McLaughlin MR, Christman CW et al. The use of antibodies targeted against the neurofilament subunits for the detection of diffuse axonal injury in humans. J Neuropathol Exp Neurol 1993; 31: 299–306.

209 Graham DI, Adams JH, Doyle D. Ischaemic brain damage in fatal non-missile head injuries. J Neurol Sci 1978; 39: 213–34.

210 Graham DI, Adams JH, Nicoll JAR et al. The nature, distribution and causes of traumatic brain injury. Brain Pathol 1995; 5: 397–406.

211 Graham DI, Bell JE, Ironside JW. Colour atlas and text of neuropathology. London: Mosby-Wolfe, 1995.

212 Graham DI, Clark JC, Adams JH, Gennarelli TA. Diffuse axonal injury caused by assault. J Clin Pathol 1992; 45: 840–1.

213 Graham DI, Ford I, Adams JH et al. Fatal head injury in children. J Clin Pathol 1989; 42: 18–22.

214 Graham DI, Ford I, Adams JH et al. Ischaemic brain damage is still common in fatal non-missile head injury. J Neurol Neurosurg Psychiatry 1989; 52: 346–50.

215 Graham DI, Gennarelli TA. Pathology of brain damage after head injury. In: Cooper PR, Golfinos JG eds. Head Injury 4th edn. New York: McGraw-Hill, 2000: 133–53.

216 Graham DI, Gennarelli TA. Trauma. In: Graham DI, Lantos PL eds. Greenfield's neuropathology 6th edn. London: Arnold, 1997: 197–262.

217 Graham DI, Gentleman SM, Lynch A, Roberts GW. Distribution of β-amyloid protein in the brain following severe head injury. Neuropathol Appl Neurobiol 1995; 21: 27–34.

218 Graham DI, Gentleman SM, Nicoll JAR et al. Is there a genetic basis for the deposition of beta-amyloid after fatal head injury? Cell Mol Neurobiol 1999; 19: 19–30.

219 Graham DI, Lawrence AE, Adams JH et al. Brain damage in fatal non-missile head injury without high ICP. J Clin Pathol 1988; 41: 34–7.

220 Graham DI, Lawrence AE, Adams JH et al. Brain damage in non-missile head injury secondary to a high ICP. Neuropathol Appl Neurobiol 1987; 13: 209–317.

221 Graham DI, McIntosh TK, Maxwell WL et al. Recent advances in neurotrauma. J Neuropathol Exp Neurol 2000; 59: 641–51.

222 Graham DI, Raghupathi R, Saatman KE et al. Tissue tears in the white matter after lateral fluid percussion brain injury in the rat: relevance to human brain injury. Acta Neuropathol 2000; 99: 117–24.

223 Gray JT, Puetz SM, Jackson SZ, Green MA. Traumatic subarachnoid haemorrhage: a 10 year case study and review. Forensic Sci Int 1999; 105: 13–23.

224 Grcevic N. Neuropathological correlates of supratentorial lesions in traumatic and nontraumatic apallic syndrome. In: Ore GD, Gerstenbrand F, Lucking CH et al. eds. The apallic syndrome. Berlin: Springer, 1977: 109–13.

225 Greene KA, Jacobowitz R, Marciano FF et al. Impact of traumatic subarachnoid hemorrhage on outcome in non penetrating head injury. Part II: Relationship to clinical course and outcome variables during acute hospitalization. J Trauma 1996; 41: 964–71.

226 Greene KA, Marciano FF, Johnson BA et al. Impact of traumatic subarachnoid hemorrhage on outcome in non penetrating head injury. Part I: A proposed computerized tomography grading scale. J Neurosurg 1995; 83: 445–52.

227 Greenlund LJ, Deckwerth TL, Johnson EM Jr. Superoxide dismutase delays neuronal apoptosis: a role for reactive oxygen species in programmed neuronal death. *Neuron* 1995; **14**: 303–15.

228 Griffin WS, Sheng JG, Royston MC *et al*. Glial–neuronal interactions in Alzheimer's disease: the potential role of a 'cytokine cycle' in disease progression. *Brain Pathol* 1998; **149**: 32–40.

229 Griffin WST, Sheng JG, Gentleman SM *et al*. Microglial interleukin-1β expression in human head injury: correlations with neuronal and neuritic β-amyloid precursor protein expression. *Neurosci Lett* 1994; **176**: 133–6.

230 Griffin WST, Sheng JG, Roberts GW, Mrak RE. Interleukin-1 expression in different plaques in Alzheimer's disease: significance in plaque evolution. *J Neuropathol Exp Neurol* 1995; **54**: 276–81.

231 Grimberg L. Paralysis agitans and trauma. *J Nerv Ment Dis* 1934; **79**: 14–42.

232 Grundke-Iqbal I, Iqbal K, Tung YC *et al*. Abnormal phosphorylation of the microtubule-associated protein tau in Alzheimer cytoskeletal pathology. *Proc Natl Acad Sci USA* 1986; **83**: 4913–17.

233 Gu C, Casaccia-Bonnefil P, Srinivasan A, Chao MV. Oligodendrocyte apoptosis mediated by caspase activation. *J Neurosci* 1999; **19**: 3043–9.

234 Gualtieri T, Cox DR. The delayed neurobehavioral sequelae of traumatic brain injury. *Brain Injury* 1991; **5**: 219–32.

235 Gultekin SH, Smith TW. Diffuse axonal injury in craniocerebral trauma. A comparative histological and immunohistochemical study. *Arch Pathol Lab Med* 1994; **118**: 168–71.

236 Haddad FS, Haddad GF, Taha J. Traumatic aneurysms caused by missiles: their presentation and management. *Neurosurgery* 1991; **28**: 1–7.

237 Hahn Y, Chyung C, Barthel MJ *et al*. Head injuries in children under 36 months of age: demography and outcome. *Childs Nerv Syst* 1988; **4**: 34–40.

238 Hall E, Wolf DL, Braughler J. Leukotrienes, antioxidants, and free radical scavengers. In: Gilad GM, Gorio A, Kreutzberg GW eds. *Process of recovery from neural trauma*. Germany: Springer, 1986: 63–73.

239 Hall ED, Yonkers PA, Andrus PK *et al*. Biochemistry and pharmacology of lipid antioxidants in acute brain and spinal cord injury. *J Neurotrauma* 1992; **9**: S425–42.

240 Hannay HJ, Feldman Z, Phan P *et al*. Validation of a controlled cortical impact model of head injury in mice. *J Neurotrauma* 1999; **16**: 1103–14.

241 Harland WA, Pitts JF, Watson AA. Subarachnoid haemorrhage due to upper cervical trauma. *J Clin Pathol* 1983; **36**: 1335–41.

242 Harper CG, Doyle D, Adams JH, Graham DI. Analysis of abnormalities in pituitary gland in non-missile head injury: study of 100 consecutive cases. *J Clin Pathol* 1986; **39**: 769–73.

243 Harrington T, Apostolides P. Penetrating brain injury. In: Cooper PR, Golfinos JG eds. *Head injury* 4th edn. New York: McGraw-Hill, 2000: 349–59.

244 Hausmann R, Kaiser A, Lang C *et al* A quantitative immunohistochemical study on the time-dependent course of acute inflammation cellular response to human brain injury. *Int J Legal Med* 1999; **112**: 227–32.

245 Hausmann R, Ries R, Fieguth A. Immunohistochemical investigations on the course of astroglial GAP expression following human brain injury. *Int J Legal Med* 2000; **113**: 70–5.

246 Hayes RL, Jenkins LW, Lyeth BG. Neuropharmacological mechanisms of traumatic brain injury: acetylcholine and excitatory amino acids. *J Neurotrauma* 1991; **8**: S173–87.

247 Hayes RL, Katayama Y, Jenkins LW *et al*. Regional rates in glucose utilization in the cat following concussive head injury. *J Neurotrauma* 1988; **5**: 121–7.

248 Hayes RL, Lyeth BG, Jenkins LW. Neurochemical mechanisms of mild and moderate head injury: implications for treatment. In: Levin HS, Eisenberg HM, Benton AL eds. *Mild head injury*. New York: Oxford University Press, 1989: 54–79.

249 Hendricks E, Harwood-Nash D, Hudson A. Head injuries in children: a survey of 4465 consecutive cases of the Hospital for Sick Children, Toronto, Canada. *Clin Neurosurg* 1964; **11**: 46–65.

250 Herrmann M, Jost S, Kutz S *et al*. Temporal profile of release of neurobiochemical markers of brain damage after traumatic brain injury is associated with intracranial pathology as demonstrated in cranial computerized tomography. *J Neurotrauma* 2000; **17**: 113–22.

251 Heyman A, Wilkinson WE, Stafford JA *et al*. Alzheimer's disease: a study of epidemiological aspects. *Ann Neurol* 1984; **15**: 335–41.

252 Hicks RR, Smith DH, McIntosh TK. Temporal response and effects of excitatory amino acid antagonism on microtubule-associated protein 2 immunoreactivity following experimental brain injury in rats. *Brain Res* 1995; **678**: 151–60.

253 Hinkle DA, Baldwin SA, Scheff SW, Wise PM. GFAP and S100beta expression in the cortex and hippocampus in response to mild cortical contusion. *J Neurotrauma* 1997; **14**: 729–38.

254 Hollander D, Strich SJ. Atypical Alzheimer's disease with congophilic angiopathy presenting with dementia of acute onset. In: Wolstenholme GEW, O'Connor M eds. *Alzheimer's disease and related conditions*. Ciba Foundation Symposium. London: Churchill, 1970: 105–24.

255 Holmin S, Biberfeld P, Mathiesen T. Intracerebral inflammation after human brain contusion. *Neurosurgery* 1998; **42**: 291–9.

256 Holzschuh M, Schuknecht B. Traumatic epidural haematomas of the posterior fossa: 20 new cases and a review of the literature since 1961. *Br J Neurosurg* 1989; **3**: 171–80.

257 Homayoun P, Rodriguez de Turco EB, Parkins NE *et al*. Delayed phospholipid degradation in rat brain after traumatic brain injury. *J Neurochem* 1997; **69**: 199–205.

258 Hoshino S, Tamaoka A, Takahashi M *et al*. Emergence of immunoreactivities for phosphorylated tau and amyloid-beta protein in chronic stage of fluid percussion in rat brain. *Neuroreport* 1998; **9**: 1879–83.

259 Houtteville J-P, Toumi K, Theron J *et al*. Interhemispheric subdural haematomas: seven cases and review of the literature. *Br J Neurosurg* 1988; **2**: 357–68.

260 Hovda DA, Lee SM, Smith ML *et al*. The neurochemical and metabolic cascade following brain injury: moving from animals models to man. *J Neurotrauma* 1995; **12**: 903–6.

261 Hovda DA, Yoshino A, Kawamata T *et al*. Diffuse prolonged depression of cerebral oxidative metabolism following concussive brain injury in the rat: a cytochrome oxidase histochemistry study. *Brain Res* 1991; **567**: 1–10.

262 Hsiang JNK, Yeung T, Yu ALM *et al*. High-risk mild head injury. *J Neurosurg* 1999; **87**: 234–8.

263 Hughes PE, Alexi T, Yoshida T *et al*. Excitotoxic lesion of rat brain with quinolinic acid induces expression of p53 mRNA and protein and p53-inducibile genes Bax and Gadd45 in brain areas showing DNA fragmentation. *Neuroscience* 1996; **74**: 1143–60.

264 Hulmin S, Soderlund J, Biberfeld P, Mathiesen T. Intracerebral inflammation after brain contusion. *Neurosurgery* 1998; **42**: 291–8.

265 Ikeda Y, Long DM. The molecular basis of brain injury and brain edema: the role of oxygen free radicals. *Neurosurgery* 1990; **27**: 1–11.

266 Imajo T, Challener RC, Roessman U. Diffuse axonal injury by assault. *Am J For Med Pathol* 1987; **8**: 217–19.

267 Ingebrigsten T, Romner B. Serial S-100 protein serum measurements related to early magnetic resonance imaging after minor head injury. Case report. *J Neurosurg* 1996; **85**: 945–8.

268 Ingebrigsten T, Waterloo K, Jacobsen EA et al. Traumatic brain damage in minor head injury: relation of serum S-100 protein measurements to magnetic resonance imaging and neurobehavioral outcome. *Neurosurgery* 1999; **45**: 468–75; Discussion 475–6.

269 Irving EA, Nicoll J, Graham DI, Dewar D. Increased tau immunoreactivity in oligodendrocytes following human stroke and head injury. *Neurosci Lett* 1996; **213**: 189–92.

270 Ishige N, Pitts LH, Hashimoto T et al. Effect of hypoxia on traumatic brain injury in rats: Part 1. Changes in neurological function, electroencephalograms and histopathology. *Neurosurgery* 1987; **21**: 848–53.

271 Ito J, Marmarou A, Barzo P et al. Characterization of edema by diffusion weighted imaging in experimental traumatic brain injury. *J Neurosurg* 1996; **84**: 97–103.

272 Jafari SS, Nielson M, Graham DI, Maxwell WL. Axonal cytoskeletal changes after nondisruptive axonal injury. II. Intermediate sized axons. *J Neurotrauma* 1998; **15**: 955–66.

273 Jamieson KG, Yelland JDN. Extradural hematoma: report of 167 cases. *J Neurosurg* 1968; **29**: 13–23.

274 Jayakumar PN, Kolluri VRS, Basavakumar DG et al. Prognosis in traumatic intraventricular haemorrhage. *Acta Neurochir (Wien)* 1990; **106**: 48–51.

275 Jellinger K. Pathology and pathogenesis of apallic syndromes following closed head injuries. In: Ore GD, Gerstenbrand F, Lucking CH et al. eds. *The apallic syndrome*. Berlin: Springer, 1977: 88–103.

276 Jellinger K, Seitelberger F. Protracted post-traumatic encephalopathy: pathology, pathogenesis and clinical implications. *J Neurol Sci* 1970; **10**: 51–94.

277 Jenkins A, Maxwell WL, Graham DI. Experimental intracerebral haematoma in the rat: sequential light microscopical changes. *Neuropathol Appl Neurobiol* 1989; **15**: 477–86.

278 Jenkins LW, Lyeth BG, Lewelt W et al. Combined pretrauma scopolamine and phencyclidine attenuate posttraumatic increased sensitivity to delayed secondary ischemia. *J Neurotrauma* 1988; **5**: 275–82.

279 Jenkins LW, Monzynski K, Lyeth BG et al. Increased vulnerability of the mildly traumatized brain to cerebral ischemia: the use of controlled secondary ischemia as a research tool to identify common or different mechanisms contributing to mechanical and ischemic brain injury. *Brain Res* 1989; **477**: 212–24.

280 Jennett B. Early traumatic epilepsy. *Arch Neurol* 1974; **30**: 394–8.

281 Jennett B. *Epilepsy after non-missile head injuries*. Chicago, IL: William Heinnemann, 1975.

282 Jennett B, Adams JH, Murray LS, Graham DI. Neuropathology in vegetative and severely disabled patients after head injury. *Neurology* 2001; **56**: 486–90.

283 Jennett B, Bond M. Assessment of outcome after severe brain damage: a practical scale. *Lancet* 1975; **1**: 480–4.

284 Jennett B, Carlin J. Preventable mortality and morbidity after head injury. *Injury* 1978; **10**: 31–9.

285 Jennett B, Snoek J, Bond MR et al. Disability after severe head injury: observation on the use of the Glasgow Outcome Scale. *J Neurol Neurosurg Psychiatry* 1981; **44**: 285–93.

286 Jennett B, Teasdale G, Galbraith S et al. Severe head injuries in three countries. *J Neurol Neurosurg Psychiatry* 1977; **40**: 291–8.

287 Jennett B, Teather D, Bennie S. Epilepsy after head injury. *Lancet* 1973; **ii**: 652–3.

288 Jin K, Chen J, Nagayama T et al. *In situ* detection of neuronal DNA strand breaks using the Klenow fragment of DNA polymerase I reveals different mechanisms of neuron death after global cerebral ischemia. *J Neurochem* 1999; **72**: 1204–14.

289 Johnson GVW, Litersky JM, Jope RS. Degradation of microtubule-associated protein 2 and brain spectrin by calpain: a comparative study. *J Neurochem* 1991; **56**: 1630–8.

290 Jones NR, Blumbergs PC, North JB. Acute subdural haematomas: aetiology, pathology and outcome. *Aust N Z J Surg* 1986; **56**: 907–13.

291 Jones PA, Andrews PJD, Midgley S et al. Measuring the burden of secondary insults in head-injured patients during intensive care. *J Neurosurg Anesthesiol* 1994; **6**: 4–14.

292 Jordan BD, Relkin NR, Ravdin LD et al. Apolipoprotein E epsilon4 associated with chronic traumatic brain injury in boxing. *JAMA* 1997; **278**: 136–40.

293 Julien JP, Mushynski WE. Neurofilaments in health and disease. *Prog Nucl Acid Res Mol Biol* 1998; **61**: 1–23.

294 Kamakura K, Ishiura S, Suzuki K et al. Calcium-activated neutral protease in the peripheral nerve, which requires mM order Ca^{2+}, and its effect on the neurofilament triplet. *J Neurosci Res* 1985; **13**: 391–403.

295 Kampfl A, Posmantur R, Nixon R et al. Mu-calpain activation and calpain mediated cytoskeletal proteolysis following traumatic brain injury. *J Neurochem* 1996; **67**: 1575–83.

296 Kampfl A, Postmantur RM, Zhao X et al. Mechanisms of calpain proteolysis following traumatic brain injury: implications for pathology and therapy: a review and update. *J Neurotrauma* 1997; **14**: 121–34.

297 Kampfl A, Schmutzhard E, Fran ZG et al. Predication of recovery from post-traumatic vegetative state with cerebral magnetic resonance imaging. *Lancet* 1998; **13**: 1763–7.

298 Karger B, Puskas Z, Rewald B et al. Morphological findings in the brain after experimental gunshots using radiology, pathology and histology. *Int J Legal Med* 1998; **111**: 314–19.

299 Katayama Y, Becker DP, Tamura T, Hovda DA. Massive increases in extracellular potassium and the indiscriminate release of glutamate following concussive brain injury. *J Neurosurg* 1990; **73**: 889–900.

300 Katayama Y, Maeda T, Koshinaga M et al. Role of excitatory amino-acid mediated ionic fluxes in traumatic brain injury. *Brain Pathol* 1995; **5**: 427–35.

301 Kaur B, Rutty GN, Timperley WR. The possible role of hypoxia in the formation of axonal bulbs. *J Clin Pathol* 1999; **52**: 203–9.

302 Kawamata T, Katayama Y, Hovda DA et al. Administration of excitatory amino acid antagonists via microdialysis attenuates the increase in glucose utlization seen following concussive brain injury. *J Cereb Blood Flow Metab* 1992; **12**: 12–24.

303 Kawamata T, Katayama Y, Hovda DA et al. Lactate accumulation following concussive brain injury: the role of ionic fluxes induced by excitatory amino acids. *Brain Res* 1995; **674**: 196–204.

304 Kawase M, Fujimura M, Morita-Fujimura Y, Chan PH. Reduction of apurinic/apyrimidinic endonuclease expression after transient global cerebral ischemia in rats: implication of the failure of DNA repair in neuronal apoptosis. *Stroke* 1999; **30**: 441–8.

305 Kaya SS, Mahmood A, Li Y et al. Apoptosis and expression of p53 response proteins and cyclin D1 after cortical impact in rat brain. Brain Res 1999; 818: 23–33.

306 Kelly DF, Martin NA, Kordestani R et al. Cerebral blood flow as a predictor of outcome following traumatic brain injury. J Neurosurg 1997; 86: 633–41.

307 Kiening KL, Unterberg AW, Bardt TF et al. Monitoring of cerebral oxygenation in patients with severe head injuries: brain tissue PO₂ versus jugular vein oxygen saturation. J Neurosurg 1996; 85: 751–7.

308 Kimura H, Meaney DF, McGowan JC et al. Magnetization transfer imaging of diffuse axonal injury following experimental brain injury in the pig: characterization of magnetization transfer ratio with histopathologic correlation. J Comput Assist Tomogr 1996; 20: 540–6.

309 King AI, Ruan JS, Zhou C et al. Recent advances in biomechanics of brain injury research: a review. J Neurotrauma 1995; 12: 651–8.

310 Kinney HC, Samuels MA. Neuropathology of the persistent vegetative state. A review. J Neuropathol Exp Neurol 1994; 53: 548–58.

311 Kloster R, Engelskjon T. Sudden unexpected death in epilepsy (SUDEP): a clinical perspective and a search for risk factors. J Neurol Neurosurg Psychiatry 1999; 67: 439–44.

312 Knight B. Forensic pathology. London: Arnold, 1991: 176–84.

313 Knuckey HW, Gelbard S, Eastein MH. The management of 'asymptomatic' epidural haematomas: a prospective study. J Neurosurg 1989; 70: 392–6.

314 Kollevold T. Immediate and early cerebral seizures after head injuries. Part 1. J Oslo City Hosp 1976; 26: 99–114.

315 Kondo T, Saito K, Nishigami J, Ohshima T. Fatal injuries of the brain stem and/or upper cervical spinal cord in traffic accidents: nine autopsy cases. Sci Justice 1995; 35: 197–201.

316 Konrad CJ, Fieber TS, Schuepfer GK, Gerber HR. Are fractures of the base of the skull influenced by the mass of the protective helmet? A retrospective study in fatally injured motorcyclists. J Trauma 1996; 41: 854–8.

317 Kontos H, Povlishock JT. Oxygen radicals in brain injury. Cent Nerv Syst Trauma 1986; 3: 257–63.

318 Kontos HA. Oxygen radicals in central nervous system damage. Chem Biol Interact 1989; 72: 229–55.

319 Kontos HA. Oxygen radicals in cerebral vascular injury. Circ Res 1985; 57: 508–16.

320 Koszyca B, Blumbergs PC, Manavis J et al. Widespread axonal injury in gunshot wounds to the head using amyloid precursor protein as a marker. J Neurotrauma 1998; 15: 674–83.

321 Kotapka MJ, Gennarelli TA, Graham DI et al. Selective vulnerability of hippocampal neurons in acceleration-induced experimental head injury. J Neurotrauma 1991; 8: 247–58.

322 Kotapka MJ, Graham DI, Adams JH et al. Hippocampal damage in fatal paediatric head injury. Neuropathol Appl Neurobiol 1993; 19: 128–33.

323 Kotapka MJ, Graham DI, Adams JH, Gennarelli TA. Hippocampal pathology in fatal human head injury without high intracranial pressure. J Neurotrauma 1994; 11: 317–24.

324 Kotapka MJ, Graham DI, Adams JH, Gennarelli TA. Hippocampal pathology in fatal non-missile human head injury. Acta Neuropathol 1992; 83: 530–4.

325 Krajewski S, Krajewska M, Ellerby LM. Release of caspase-9 from mitochondria during neuronal apoptosis and cerebral ischemia. Proc Natl Acad Sci USA 1999; 96: 5752–7.

326 Krantz KP. Head and neck injuries to motorcycle and moped riders – with special regard to the effect of protective helmets. Injury 1985; 16: 253–8.

327 Kraus JF, McArthur DL. Epidemiology of head injury. In: Cooper PR, Golfinos JF eds. Head injury 4th edn. New York: McGraw-Hill, 2000: 1–26.

328 Kuhl DE, Alavi A, Hoffman EJ et al. Local cerebral blood volume in head-injured patients. Determination by emission computed tomography of ⁹⁹ᵐTc-labelled red cells. J Neurosurg 1980; 52: 309–20.

329 Lafuente JV, Cervos-Navarro J. Craniocerebral trauma induces hemorheological disturbances. J Neurotrauma 1999; 16: 425–30.

330 Langfitt TW, Weinstein JD, Kassell NF. Cerebral vasomotor paralysis produced by intracranial hypertension. Neurology 1965; 15: 662–41.

331 LaPlaca MC, Raghupathi R, Verma A et al. Temporal patterns of poly(ADP-ribose) polymerase activation in the cortex following experimental brain injury in the rat. J Neurochem 1999; 73: 205–13.

332 Lee JH, Martin NA, Alsina G et al. Haemodynamically significant cerebral vasospasm and outcome after head injury: a prospective study. J Neurosurg 1997; 87: 221–3.

333 Leestma JE. Forensic neuropathology. New York: Raven Press 1988, pp. 197–8.

334 Leestma JE, Kalelkar MB, Teas S. Pontomedullary avulsion associated with cervical hyperextension. Acta Neurochir 1983; 32 (Suppl): 69–73.

335 Le Roux PD. Prevention and management of seizures in the head-injured patient. In: Cooper PR, Golfinos JG eds. Head injury 4th edn. New York: McGraw-Hill, 2000: 499–516.

336 Levin HS. Prediction of recovery from traumatic brain injury. J Neurotrauma 1995; 12: 913–22.

337 Levin HS, Amparo E, Eisenberg HM et al. Magnetic resonance imaging and computerized tomography in relation to the neurobehavioural sequelae of mild and moderate head injuries. J Neurosurg 1987; 66: 706–13.

338 Levin HS, Culhane KA, Medelsohn D et al. Cognition in relation to magnetic resonance imaging in head-injured children and adolescents. Arch Neurol 1993; 50: 897–905.

339 Levin HS, Gary HE, Eisenberg HM et al. Neurobehavioural outcome 1 year after severe head injury: experience of the Traumatic Coma Data Bank. J Neurosurg 1990; 73: 699–709.

340 Levin HS, Handel SF, Goldman AM et al. Magnetic resonance imaging after 'diffuse' non-missile injury. Arch Neurol 1985; 42: 963–8.

341 Levin HS, Mattis S, Ruff RM et al. Neurobehavioral outcome following minor head injury: a three center study. J Neurosurg 1987; 66: 234–43.

342 Levin HS, Mendelsohn D, Lilly MA et al. Magnetic resonance imaging in relation to functional outcome of pediatric closed head injury: a test of the Ommaya–Gennarelli model. Neurosurgery 1997; 40: 432–40.

343 Levin HS, Williams DH, Eisenberg HM et al. Serial MRI and neurobehavioural findings after mild to moderate closed head injury. J Neurol Neurosurg Psychiatry 1992; 55: 255–62.

344 Lewen A, Li GL, Nilsson P et al. Traumatic brain injury in rat produces changes of β-amyloid precursor protein immunoreactivity. Neuroreport 1995; 6: 357–60.

345 Lewen A, Li GL, Olsson Y, Hillered L. Changes in microtubule-associated protein 2 and amyloid precursor protein immunoreactivity following traumatic brain injury in rat: influence of MK-801 treatment. Brain Res 1996; 719: 161–71.

346 Lewis SB, Finnie JW, Blumbergs PC et al. A head impact model of early axonal injury in the sheep. J Neurotrauma 1996; 13: 505–14.

347 Lifshitz J, Raghupathi R, Welsh FA, McIntosh TK. Mitochondrial respiratory function and ATP concentration

defits in cortical and hippocampal regions following lateral fluid-percussion brain injury in the rat. *J Neurotrauma* 1999; **16**: 990.

348 Lighthall JW. Controlled cortical impact: a new experimental brain injury model. *J Neurotrauma* 1988; **5**: 1–15.

349 Lindenberg R. Trauma of meninges and brain. In: Minckler J ed. *Pathology of the nervous system* Vol. 2. New York: McGraw Hill, 1971: 1705–65.

350 Lindenberg R, Freytag E. A mechanism of cerebral contusions: a pathologic–anatomic study. *Arch Pathol* 1960; **69**: 440–69.

351 Lindenberg R, Freytag E. Brainstem lesions of traumatic hypertension of the head. *Arch Pathol* 1970; **90**: 509–15.

352 Lindenberg R, Freytag E. Morphology of brain lesions from blunt trauma in infancy. *Arch Pathol* 1969; **87**: 298–305.

353 Lindenberg R, Freytag E. Morphology of cerebral contusions. *Arch Pathol* 1957; **63**: 23–42.

354 Liu PK, Hsu CY, Dizdaroglu M et al. Damage, repair, and mutagenesis in nuclear genes after mouse forebrain ischemia-reperfusion. *J Neurosci* 1996; **16**: 6795–806.

355 Liu X, Zou H, Slaughter C, Wang X. DFF. A heterodimeric protein that functions downstream of capase-3 to trigger DNA fragmentation during apoptosis. *Cell* 1997; **89**: 175–84.

356 Lobato RD, Sarabia R, Cordobes F et al. Posttraumatic cerebral hemispheric swelling. *J Neurosurg* 1988; **68**: 417–423.

357 Love S, Barber R, Wilcock GK. Apoptosis and expression of DNA repair proteins in ischaemic brain injury in man. *Neuroreport* 1998; **9**: 955–9.

358 Lucas JH, Emery DG, Rosenberg LJ. Physical injury of neurons: important roles for sodium and chloride ions. *Neuroscientist* 1997; **3**: 85–101.

359 Luerssen T. Head injuries in children. *Neurosurg Clin North Am* 1991; **2**: 399–410.

360 McClain C, Cohen D, Phillips R et al. Increased plasma and ventricular fluid interleukin-6 levels in patients with head injury. *J Lab Clin Med* 1991; **118**: 225–31.

361 McCracken E, Hunter AJ, Patel S et al. Calpain activation and cytoskeletal protein breakdown in the corpus callosum in head-injured patients. *J Neurotrauma* 1999; **16**: 749–61.

362 McElhaney JH, Hopper RH, Nightingale RW, Myers BS. Mechanisms of basilar skull fracture. *J Neurotrauma* 1995; **12**: 669–78.

363 McGowan JC, McCormack TM, Grossman RI et al. Diffuse axonal pathology detected with magnetization transfer imaging following brain injury in the pig. *Magn Reson Med* 1999; **41**: 727–33.

364 McIntosh TK, Juhler M, Wieloch T. Novel pharmacological strategies in the treatment of experimental traumatic brain injury. *J Neurotrama* 1998; **15**: 731–69.

365 McIntosh TK, Saatman KE, Raghupathi R. Calcium and pathogenesis of traumatic CNS injury: cellular and molecular mechanisms. *Neuroscientist* 1997; **3**: 169–75.

366 McIntosh TK, Saatman KE, Raghupathi R et al. The molecular and cellular sequelae of experimental traumatic brain injury: pathogenetic mechanisms. *Neuropathol Appl Neurobiol* 1998; **24**: 251–67.

367 McIntosh TK, Smith DH, Meaney DF et al. Neuropathological sequelae of experimental brain injury: relationship to neurochemical and biomechanical mechanisms. *Lab Invest* 1996; **74**: 315–42.

368 McIntosh TK, Vink R, Noble L et al. Traumatic brain injury in the rat: characterization of a lateral fluid percussion model. *Neuroscience* 1989; **28**: 233–44.

369 McKeating EG, Andrews PJ, Mascia L. Relationship of neuron specific enolase and protein S-100 concentrations in systemic and jugular venous serum to injury severity and outcome after traumatic brain injury. *Acta Neurochir Suppl (Wien)* 1998; **71**: 117–19.

370 McKenzie JE, Gentleman SM, Roberts GW et al. Increased numbers of β-APP-immunoactive neurons in the entorhinal cortex after head injury. *Neuroreport* 1994; **6**: 161–4.

371 McKenzie JE, Gentleman SM, Roberts GW et al. Quantification of β-APP immunoreactive pre-α cells in the entorhinal cortex using image analysis. *Neurodegeneration* 1995; **4**: 299–306.

372 McLatchie G, Brooks N, Galbraith S et al. Clinical neurological examination and computed tomographic head scanning in active amateur boxers. *J Neurol Neurosurg Psychiatry* 1987; **50**: 96–9.

373 McLaurin Rl, Ford LE. Extradural hematoma. Statistical survey of 47 cases. *J Neurosurg* 1965; **23**: 296–304.

374 McLellan DR, Adams JH, Graham DI et al. Structural basis of the vegetative state and prolonged coma after nonmissile head injury. In: Papo I, Cohadon F, Massarotti M eds. *Le coma traumatique*. Padova: Liviana Editrice, 1986: 165–85.

375 McMenemey WH, Grant HC, Behrman S. Two examples of 'presenile dementia' (Pick's disease and Stern–Garcin syndrome) with a history of trauma. *Arch Psychiatrie Nervenkrank* 1965; **208**: 162–76.

376 MacPherson P, Graham DI. Correlation between angiographic findings and the ischaemia of head injury. *J Neurol Neurosurg Psychiatry* 1978; **41**: 122–7.

377 Maeda H, Higuchi T, Imura M et al Ring fracture of the base of the skull and atlanto-occipital avulsion due to anteroflexion on motorcycle riders in a head-on collision accident. *Med Sci Law* 1993; **33**: 266–9.

378 Mamelak M. The motor vehicle collision injury syndrome. *Neuropsychiatry Neuropscyhol Behav Neurol* 2000; **13**: 125–35.

379 Margulies SS, Thibault LE, Gennarelli TA. Physical model simulations of brain injury in the primate. *J Biomech* 1989; **23**: 823–36.

380 Marion DW, Darby J, Yonas H. Acute regional cerebral blood flow changes caused by severe head injuries. *J Neurosurg* 1992; **74**: 407–14.

381 Markwalder T-M. Chronic subdural hematomas: a review. *J Neurosurg* 1981; **54**: 637–45.

382 Marmarou A. Traumatic brain edema: an overview. *Acta Neurochir* 1994; **60** (Suppl): 421–4.

383 Marmarou A, Foda MAA-E, Brink W van den et al. A new model of diffuse brain injury in rats. *J Neurosurg* 1994; **80**: 291–300.

384 Marmarou A, Shima K. Comparative studies of edema produced by fluid percussion injury with lateral and central modes of injury in cats. *Adv Neurol* 1990; **52**: 233–6.

385 Marshall LF. Head injury: recent, past, and future. *Neurosurgery* 2000; **47**: 546–61.

386 Marshall LF, Becker DP, Bowers SA et al. The National Traumatic Coma Data Bank. Part 1: Design, purpose, goals, and results. *J Neurosurg* 1983; **59**: 276–84.

387 Marshall LF, Kauber MR et al. Traumatic Coma Data Bank Study Group. Outcome after severe head injury. *J Neurosurg* 1991; **75** (Suppl): 528–36.

388 Marshall LF, Toole BM, Bowers SA. The National Traumatic Coma Data Bank. Part 2: Patients who talk and deteriorate: implications for treatment. *J Neurosurg* 1983; **59**: 285–8.

389 Martin NA, Patwardhan RV, Alexander MJ et al. Characterization of cerebral haemodynamic phases following severe head trauma: hypoperfusion, hyperemia and vasospasm. *J Neurosurg* 1997; **87**: 9–19.

390 Martland HS. Punch drunk. *JAMA* 1928; **91**: 1103–7.

391 Mathew P, Bullock R, Graham DI *et al* A new experimental model of contusion in the rat: histopathological analysis and temporal patterns of cerebral blood flow disturbances. *J Neurosurg* 1996; **85**: 860–70.

392 Mattle H, Kohler S, Huber P *et al*. Anticoagulation-related intracranial extracerebral haemorrhage. *J Neurol Neurosurg Psychiatry* 1989; **52**: 829–37.

393 Mawdsley C, Ferguson FR. Neurological disease in boxers. *Lancet* 1963; **ii**: 795–801.

394 Maxwell W, Kansagra AM, Graham DI *et al*. Freeze-fracture studies of reactive myelinated nerve fibres after diffuse axonal injury. *Acta Neuropathol* 1988; **76**: 395–406.

395 Maxwell WL. Histopathological changes at central nodes of Ranvier after stretch injury. *Micro Res Technique* 1996; **34**: 522–35.

396 Maxwell WL, Graham DI. Loss of axonal microtubules and neurofilaments after stretch-injury to guinea pig optic nerve fibers. *J Neurotrauma* 1997; **14**: 603–14.

397 Maxwell WL, Irvine A, Adams JH *et al*. Response of cerebral microvasculature to brain injury. *J Pathol* 1988; **155**: 327–35.

398 Maxwell WL, Irvine A, Graham DI *et al*. Focal axonal injury: axon response to stretch. *J Neurocytol* 1991; **20**: 157–64.

399 Maxwell WL, Irvine A, Watt C *et al*. The microvascular response to stretch injury in the adult guinea pig visual system. *J Neurotrauma* 1991; **8**: 271–9.

400 Maxwell WL, McCreath BJ, Graham DI, Gennarelli TA. Cytochemical evidence for redistribution of membrane pump calcium-APPase and ecto-Ca-ATPase activity, and calcium influx in myelinated nerve fibers of the optic nerve after stretch injury. *J Neurocytol* 1995; **24**: 925–42.

401 Maxwell WL, Povlishock JT, Graham DI. A mechanistic analysis of nondisruptive axonal injury: a review. *J Neurotrauma* 1997; **14**: 419–40.

402 Maxwell WL, Watts C, Graham DI, Gennarelli TA. Ultrastructural evidence of axonal shearing as a result of lateral acceleration of the head in non-human primates. *Acta Neuropathol* 1993; **86**: 136–44.

403 Mayeux R, Ottman R, Maestre G *et al*. Synergistic effects of traumatic head injury and apolipoprotein-ε4 in patients with Alzheimer's disease. *Neurology* 1995; **45**: 555–7.

404 Mayeux R, Ottman R, Tang M-X *et al*. Genetic susceptibility and head injury as risk factors for Alzheimer's disease among community-dwelling elderly persons and their first-degree relatives. *Ann Neurol* 1993; **33**: 494–501.

405 Mazza C, Pasqualin A, Ferriotti G, Pian R da. Traumatic extradural haematoma in children. *Acta Neurochir* 1982; **65**: 67–80.

406 Meaney DF, Smith DH, Shreiber DI *et al*. Biomechanical analysis of experimental diffuse axonal injury. *J Neurotrauma* 1994; **12**: 689–94.

407 Meaney DF, Thibault LE, Gennarelli TA. Rotational brain injury tolerance criteria as a function of vehicle crash parameters. In: *Proceedings of International Research Council on the Biokinetics of Impact (IRCOBI)*, Bron, France, 1994: 234–9.

408 Mellergard P, Wisten O. Operations and re-operations for chronic subdural haematomas during a 25-year period in a well defined population. *Acta Neurochir (Wien)* 1996; **138**: 708–13.

409 Mendelow AD, Teasdale G, Jennett B *et al*. Risks of intracranial haematoma in head injured adults. *BMJ* 1983; **287**: 1173–6.

410 Mendelsohn D, Levin HS, Bruce D *et al*. Late MRI after head injury in children: relationship to clinical features and outcome. *Childs Nerv Syst* 1992; **8**: 445–52.

411 Merry DE, Veis DJ, Hickey WF, Korsmeyer SJ. Bcl-2 protein expression is widespread in the developing nervous system

and retained in the adult PNS. *Development* 1994; **120**: 301–11.

412 Mielke K, Brecht S, Dorst A, Herdegen T. Activity and expression of JNK1, p38, and ERK kinases, c-jun N-terminal phosphorylation, and c-jun promoter binding in the adult rat brain following kainate-induced seizures. *Neuroscience* 1999; **91**: 471–83.

413 Miller JD. Head injury. *J Neurol Neurosurg Psychiatry* 1993; **56**: 440–7.

414 Miller JD, Bullock R, Graham DI *et al*. Ischemic brain damage in a model of acute subdural hematoma. *Neurosurgery* 1990; **27**: 433–9.

415 Miller JD, Corales RL. Brain edema as a result of head injury: fact or fallacy. In: Vlieger M, Lange SA de, Becks JWS eds. *Brain edema*. New York: John Wiley: 99–115.

416 Miller JD, Jones PR. The work of a regional head injury service. *Lancet* 1985; **i**: 1141–4.

417 Mittl RL, Grossman RI, Hiehl JF *et al*. Prevalence of MR evidence of diffuse axonal injury in patients with mild head injury and normal head CT findings. *Am J Neuroradiol* 1994; **15**: 1583–9.

418 Miyashita M, Reed JC. Tumor suppressor, p53 is a direct transcriptional activator of the human bax gene. *Cell* 1995; **80**: 293–9.

419 Mochizuki H, Goto K, Mori H, Mizuno Y. Histochemical detection of apoptosis in Parkinson's disease. *J Neurol Sci* 1996; **137**: 120–3.

420 Morrison B, Saatman KE, Meaney DF, McIntosh TK. *In vitro* central nervous system models of mechanically induced trauma: a review. *J Neurotrauma* 1998; **15**: 911–28.

421 Morrison RS, Wenzel HJ, Kinoshita Y *et al*. Loss of the p53 tumor suppressor gene protects neurons from kainate-induced cell death. *J Neurosci* 1996; **16**: 1337–45.

422 Mortimer JA, Van Duijn CM, Chandra L *et al*. Head trauma as a risk factor for Alzheimer's disease: a collaborative re-analysis of case–control studies. *Int J Epidemiol* 1991; **20**: S28–35.

423 Muizelaar J, Ward J, Marmarou A *et al*. Cerebral blood flow and metabolism in severely head-injured children. Part 2: Autoregulation. *J Neurosurg* 1989; **71**: 72–6.

424 Muizelaar JP, Marmarou A, Salles AAF de *et al*. Cerebral blood flow and metabolism in severely head-injured children. *J Neurosurg* 1989; **71**: 63–71.

425 Mukin AG, Inanova SA, Knoblach SM, Faden AI. New *in vitro* model of traumatic neuronal injury: evaluation of secondary injury and glutamate receptor-mediated neurotoxicity. *J Neurotrauma* 1997; **14**: 651–63.

426 Murai H, Pierce JE, Raghupathi R *et al*. Twofold overexpression of human beta-amyloid precursor proteins in transgenic mice does not affect the neuromotor, cognitive, or neurodegenerative sequelae following experimental brain injury. *J Comp Neurol* 1998; **392**: 428–38.

427 Murray GD, Teasdale GM, Braakman R *et al*. The European Brain Injury Consortium survey of head injuries. *Acta Neurochir (Wien)* 1999; **141**: 223–36.

428 Murray LS, Teasdale GM, Murray GD *et al*. Does prediction of outcome alter patient management? *Lancet* 1993; **341**: 1487–91.

429 Nakagawa Y, Nakamura M, McIntosh TK *et al*. Traumatic brain injury in young, amyloid-beta peptide overexpressing transgenic mice induces marked ipsilateral hippocampal atrophy and diminished Abeta deposition during aging. *J Comp Neurol* 1999; **411**: 390–8.

430 Nakahara S, Yone K, Sakou T *et al*. Induction of apoptosis signal regulating kinase 1(ASK1) after spinal cord injury in rats: possible involvement of ASK1-JNK and p38 pathways in neuronal apoptosis. *J Pharmacol Exp Ther* 1999; **58**: 442–50.

431 Nakamura M, Raghupathi R, Merry DE et al. Overexpression of Bcl-2 is neuroprotective following experimental brain injury in the adult rat. J Comp Neurol 1999; 412: 681–92.

432 Nakamura M, Saatman KE, Galvin JE et al. Increased vulnerability of NFH-LacZ transgenic mouse to traumatic brain injury-induced behavioral deficits and cell loss. J Cereb Blood Flow Metab 1999; 19: 762–70.

433 Namura S, Zhu J, Fink K et al. Activation and cleavage of caspase-3 in apoptosis induced by experimental cerebral ischemia. J Neurosci 1998; 18: 3659–68.

434 Nanassis K, Frowein RA, Karimi A. Delayed post-traumatic intracerebral bleeding. Neurosurg Rev 1989; 12 (Suppl 1): 243–51.

435 Napieralski JA, Raghupathi R, McIntosh TK. The tumor-suppressor gene, p53, is induced in injured brain regions following experimental traumatic brain injury. Mol Brain Res 1999; 71: 78–86.

436 Nashef L. Sudden unexpected death in epilepsy: terminology and definitions. Epilepsia 1997; 38 (Suppl 11): 56–8.

437 Nashef L, Garner S, Sander JW et al. Circumstances of death in sudden death in epilepsy: interviews of bereaved relatives. J Neurol Neurosurg Psychiatry 1998; 64: 345–52.

438 Nath R, Probert A, McGinnis KM, Wang KKW. Evidence for activation of caspase-3-like protease in excitotoxin- and hypoxia/hypoglycemia-injured neurons. J Neurochem 1998; 71: 186–95.

439 Nemetz PN, Leibson C, Naessens JM et al. Traumatic brain injury and time to onset of Alzheimer's disease: a population-based study. Am J Epidemiol 1999; 149: 32–40.

440 Neubauer UJ. Extradural hematoma of the posterior fossa. Twelve years experience with CT-scan. Acta Neurochir (Wien) 1987; 87: 105–11.

441 Newcomb JK, Kampfl A, Posmantur RM et al. Immunohistochemical study of calpain-mediated breakdown products to α-spectrin following controlled cortical impact injury in the rat. J Neurotrauma 1997; 14: 369–83.

442 Newcomb JK, Zhao X, Pike BR, Hayes RL. Temporal profile of apoptotic-like changes in neurons and astrocytes following controlled cortical impact injury in the rat. Exp Neurol 1999; 158: 76–88.

443 Ng HK, Mahaliyana RD, Poon WS. The pathological spectrum of diffuse axonal injury in blunt head trauma: assessment with axon and myelin stains. Clin Neurol Neurosurg 1994; 96: 24–31.

444 Nicoll JAR, Roberts GW, Graham DI. Apolipoprotein E ε4 allele is associated with deposition of amyloid β-protein following head injury. Nat Med 1995; i: 135–7.

445 Nicotera P, Bellomo G, Orrenius S. Calcium-mediated mechanisms in chemically induced cell death. Annu Rev Pharmacol Toxicol 1992; 32: 449–70.

446 Nicotera P, Leist M, Manzo L. Neuronal cell death: a demise with different shapes. Trends Pharmacol Sci 1999; 20: 46–51.

447 Nilsson P, Hillered L, Ponten U, Urgerstedt V. Changes in cortical extracellular levels of energy-related metabolites and amino acids following concussive brain injury in rats. J Cereb Blood Flow Metab 1990; 10: 631–7.

448 Ninchoji T, Uemura K, Shimayama I et al. Traumatic intracerebral haematomas of delayed onset. Acta Neurochir (Wien) 1984; 71: 69–90.

449 O'Donaghue MF, Duncan JS, Sander JW. The subjective handicap of epilepsy: a new approach to measuring treatment outcome. Brain 1998; 121: 317–43.

450 Oehmichen M, Meissner C, Konig HG. Brain injury after gunshot wounding: morphometric analysis of cell destruction caused by temporary cavitation. J Neurotrauma 2000; 17: 155–62.

451 Oehmichen M, Raff G. Timing of cortical contusion. Correlation between histomorphological alterations and post-traumatic interval. Z Rechtsmed 1980; 84: 79–94.

452 Oehmichen W, Eisenmenger W, Raff G, Berhaus G. Brain macrophages in human cortical contusions as indicator of survival period. Forensic Sci Int 1986; 30: 281–301.

453 Ogata M, Tsuganezawa O. Neuron-specific enolase as an effective immunohistochemical marker for injured axons after fatal brain injury. Int J Legal Med 1999; 113: 19–25.

454 Okiyama K, Rosenkrantz TS, Smith DH et al. (S)-Emopamil attenuates regional cerebral blood flow reduction following experimental brain injury. J Neurotrauma 1994; 11: 83–95.

455 Okonkwo DO, Buki A, Siman R, Povlishock JT. Cyclosporin A limits calcium-induced axonal damage following traumatic brain injury. Neuroreport 1999; 10: 353–8.

456 Oppenheim RW. Cell death during development of the nervous system. Annu Rev Neurosci 1991; 14: 453–501.

457 Oppenheimer DR. Microscopic lesions in the brain following head injury. J Neurol Neurosurg Psychiatry 1968; 31: 299–306.

458 Ott L, McClain CJ, Gillespie M, Young B. Cytokines and metabolic dysfunction after severe head injury. J Neurotrauma 1994; 11: 447–72.

459 Ozawa H, Shioda S, Dohi K et al. Delayed neuronal cell death in the rat hippocampus is mediated by the mitogen-activated protein kinase signal transduction pathway. Neurosci Lett 1999; 262: 57–60.

460 Ozawa Y, Nakamura T, Sunami K et al. Study of regional cerebral blood flow in experimental head injury: changes following cerebral contusion and during spreading depression. Neurol Med Chir (Tokyo) 1991; 31: 685–90.

461 Palmer AM, Burns MA. Preservation of redox, polyamine, and glucine modulatory domains of the N-methyl-D-aspartate receptor in Alzheimer's disease. J Neurochem 1994; 62: 187–96.

462 Palmer AM, Marion DW, Botscheller ML et al. Traumatic brain injury-induced excitotoxicity assessed in a controlled cortical impact model. J Neurochem 1993; 61: 2015–24.

463 Park DS, Morris EJ, Stefanis L et al. Multiple pathways of neuronal death indiced by DNA-damaging agents, NGF deprivation, and oxidative stress. J Neurosci 1998; 18: 830–40.

464 Peerless SJ, Rewcastle NB. Shear injuries of the brain. Can Med Assoc J 1967; 96: 577–82.

465 Pellerin L, Magistretti PJ. Glutamate uptake into astrocytes stimulates aerobic glycolysis: a mechanism coupling neuronal activity to glucoutilization. Proc Natl Acad Sci USA 1994; 91: 106225–9.

466 Peters G, Rothemund E. Neuropathology of the traumatic apallic syndrome. In: Ore GD, Gerstenbrand F, Lucking CH et al. eds. The apallic syndrome. Berlin: Springer, 1977; 78–87.

467 Petersen S, Bowlby KJ. Trauma report. Phoenix, AR: St. Joseph's Hospital and Medical Center, 1997.

468 Pettus EH, Christman CW, Giebel ML, Povlishock JT. Traumatically induced altered membrane permeability: its relationship to traumatically induced reactive axonal change. J Neurotrauma 1994; 11: 507–22.

469 Phonprasert C, Suwanwela C, Hongsaprabhas C et al. Extradural hematoma: analysis of 138 cases. J Trauma 1980; 20: 679–83.

470 Pierce JES, Smith DH, Trojanowski JQ, McIntosh TK. Enduring cognitive, neurobehavioral and histopathological changes persist for up to one year following severe experimental brain injury in rats. Neuroscience 1998; 87: 359–69.

471 Pierce JES, Trojanowski JQ, Graham DI *et al.* Immunohistochemical characterization of alterations in the distribution of amyloid percursor proteins and amyloid β peptide following experimental brain injury in the rat. *J Neurosci* 1996; **16**: 1083–90.

472 Pike BR, Zhao X, Newcomb JK *et al.* Regional calpain and caspase-3 proteolysis of α-spectrin after traumatic brain injury. *Neuroreport* 1998; **9**: 2437–42.

473 Pilz P. Axonal injury in head injury. *Acta Neurochir* 1983; **32** (Suppl): 119–23.

474 Pilz P, Strohecker J, Grobovschek M. Survival after pontomedullary tear. *J Neurol Neurosurg Psychiatry* 1982; **45**: 422–7.

475 Pintar FA, Yoganandan N, Gennarelli TA. Airbag effectiveness on brain trauma in frontal crashes. *J Assoc Advance Automot Med* 2000: 167–74.

476 Pohl D, Bittigau P, Ishimaru MJ *et al.* N-Methyl-D-aspartate antagonists and apoptotic cell death triggered by head trauma in developing rat brain. *Proc Natl Acad Sci USA* 1999; **96**: 2508–13.

477 Portera CP, Hedreen JC, Price DD, Koliatsos VE. Evidence for apoptotic cell death in Huntigton disease and excitotoxic animal models. *J Neurosci* 1995; **15**: 3775–87.

478 Postmantur R, Hayes RL, Dixon CE, Taft WC. Neurofilament 68 and neurofilament 200 protein levels decrease after traumatic brain injury. *J Neurotrauma* 1994; **11**: 533–45.

479 Posmantur R, Kampfl A, Taft WC *et al.* Diminished microtubule associated protein 2 immunoreactivity following cortical impact injury. *J Neurotrauma* 1996; **13**: 125–37.

480 Posmantur RM, Kampfl A, Liu SJ *et al.* Cytoskeletal derangements of cortical neuronal processes three hours after traumatic brain injury in rats: an immunofluorescence study. *J Neuropathol Exp Neurol* 1996; **55**: 68–90.

481 Povlishock JT. Traumatically induced axonal damage without concomitant change in focally related neuronal somata and dendrites. *Acta Neuropathol* 1986; **70**: 53–79.

482 Povlishock JT. Traumatically induced axonal injury: pathogenesis and pathobiological implications. *Brain Pathol* 1992; **2**: 1–12.

483 Povlishock JT, Becker DP. Fate of reactive axonal swellings induced by head injury. *Lab Invest* 1985; **42**: 540–52.

484 Povlishock JT, Becker DP, Cheng DLY, Vaughan GW. Axonal change in minor head injury. *J Neuropathol Exp Neurol* 1983; **42**: 225–42.

485 Povlishock JT, Christman CW. The pathobiology of traumatically-induced axonal injury in animals and humans: a review of current thoughts. *J Neurotrauma* 1995; **12**: 555–64.

486 Povlishock JT, Hayes RL, Michel ME, McIntosh TK eds. Workshop on animal models of traumatic brain injury. *J Neurotrauma* 1994; **11**: 723–32.

487 Povlishock JT, Jenkins LW. Are the pathobiological changes evoked by traumatic brain injury immediate and irreversible? *Brain Pathol* 1995; **5**: 415–26.

488 Povlishock JT, Kontos HA. Continuing axonal and vascular change following experimental brain trauma. *Cent Nerv Syst Trauma* 1985; **2**: 285–97.

489 Povlishock JT, Marmarou A, McIntosh TK *et al.* Impact acceleration injury in the rat: evidence for focal axolemmal change and related neurofilament sidearm alteration. *J Neuropathol Exp Neurol* 1997; **56**: 347–59.

490 Raghupathi R, Fernandez SC, Murai H *et al.* Bcl-2 overexpression attenuates cortical cell loss following traumatic brain injury in transgenic mice. *J Cereb Blood Flow Metab* 1998; **18**: 1259–69.

491 Rango M, Lenkinski RE, Alves WM *et al.* Brain pH in head injury: an image-guided 31P magnetic resonance spectroscopy study. *Ann Neurol* 1990; **28**: 661–7.

492 Reilly PL, Graham DI, Adams JH, Jennett B. Patients with head injury who talk and die. *Lancet* 1974; **ii**: 375–7.

493 Rengachary S, Szymanski DC. Subdural hematomas of arterial origin. *Neurosurgery* 1981; **8**: 166–72.

494 Ricker JH, Zafonte RD. Functional neuroimaging and quantitative electroencephalography in adult traumatic head injury: clinical applications and interpretive cautions. *J Head Trauma Rehabil* 2000; **15**: 859–68.

495 Rink A, Fung K-M, Trojanowski JQ *et al.* Evidence of apoptotic cell death after experimental traumatic brain injury in the rat. *Am J Pathol* 1995; **147**: 1575–83.

496 Roberts GW, Allsop D, Bruton CJ. The occult aftermath of boxing. *J Neurol Neurosurg Psychiatry* 1990; **53**: 373–8.

497 Roberts GW, Gentleman SM, Lynch A *et al.* β-Amyloid protein deposition in the brain after severe head injury: implications for the pathogenesis of Alzheimer's disease. *J Neurol Neurosurg Psychiatry* 1994; **57**: 419–25.

498 Roberts GW, Gentleman SM, Lynch A, Graham DI. βA4 amyloid protein deposition in brain after head trauma. *Lancet* 1991; **338**: 1422–3.

499 Roberts GW, Whitwell HL, Acland PR, Bruton CJ. Dementia in a punch-drunk wife. *Lancet* 1990; **335**: 918–19.

500 Robertson CS, Contant CF, Gokaslan ZL *et al.* Cerebral blood flow, arteriovenous oxygen difference, and outcome in head injured patients. *J Neurol Neurosurg Psychiatry* 1992; **55**: 594–603.

501 Rockswold GI, Leonard PM, Nagib MG. Analysis of management in 33 closed head injury patients who talked and deteriorated. *Neurosurgery* 1987; **21**: 51–5.

502 Ross DT, Meaney DF, Sabol M *et al.* Distribution of forebrain diffuse axonal injury following inertial closed head injury in miniature swine. *Exp Neurol* 1994; **126**: 291–9.

503 Ross SA, Cunningham RT, Johnston CF, Rowlands BJ. Neuron-specific enolase as an aid to outcome prediction in head injury. *Br J Neurosurg* 1996; **10**: 471–6.

504 Rothoerl RD, Woertgen C, Holzschuh M *et al.* S-100 serum levels after minor and major head injury. *J Trauma* 1998; **45**: 765–7.

505 Roy S, Sarkar C, Tandon P *et al.* Craniocerebral erosion (growing fractures of the skull in children). Part 1. Pathology. *Acta Neurochir* 1987; **87**: 112–18.

506 Ryan GA, McLean AJ, Vilenius ATS. Brain injury patterns in fatally injured pedestrians. *J Trauma* 1994; **36**: 469–76.

507 Saatman KE, Bozyczko-Coyne D, Marcy VR *et al.* Prolonged calpain-mediated spectrin breakdown occurs regionally following experimental brain injury in the rat. *J Neuropathol Exp Neurol* 1996; **55**: 850–60.

508 Saatman KE, Graham DI, McIntosh TK. The neuronal cytoskeleton is at risk after mild and moderate brain injury. *J Neurotrauma* 1998; **15**: 1047–58.

509 Saatman KE, Murai H, Bartus RT *et al.* Calpain inhibitor AK295 attenuates motor and cognitive deficits following experimental brain injury in the rat. *Proc Natl Acad Sci USA* 1996; **93**: 3428–33.

510 Sahuquillo-Baris J, Lamarca-Ciura J, Vilalta-Castan J *et al.* Acute subdural haematoma and diffuse axonal injury after severe head trauma. *J Neurosurg* 1988; **68**: 894–900.

511 Sakhi S, Bruce A, Sun N *et al.* p53 induction is associated with neuronal damage in the CNS. *Proc Natl Acad Sci USA* 1994; **91**: 7525–9.

512 Salazar AM, Aarabi B, Levi L, Feinsod M. Post traumatic epilepsy following craniocerebral missile wounds following cradiocerebral missile wounds in recent armed conflicts. In: Aarabi B, Kaufman HH eds. *Missile wounds of head and neck* Vol. II. AANS Publications Committee, 1999: 281–92.

513 Samatovicz RA. Genetics and brain injury: apolipoprotein E. *J Head Trauma Rehabil* 2000; **15**: 869–74.

514 Sancar A. Excision repair in mammalian cells. *J Biol Chem* 1995; **270**: 15915–18.

515 Saporito MS, Brown EM, Miller MS, Carswell S. CEP-1347/KT-7515, an inhibitor of c-jun N-terminal kinase activation, attenuated the 1-methyl-4-phenyl tetrahydropyridine-mediated loss of nigrostriatal dopaminergic neurons *in vivo*. *J Pharmacol Exp Ther* 1999; **288**: 421–7.

516 Sarwar M, McCormick WF. Decrease in ventricular and sulcal size after death. *Radiology* 1978; **127**: 409–11.

517 Sato M, Tanaka S, Kohama A, Fujii C. Traumatic intraventricular haemorrhage. *Acta Neurochir (Wien)* 1987; **88**: 95–103.

518 Satoh MS, Lindahl T. Role of poly(ADP-ribose) formation in DNA repair. *Nature* 1992; **356**: 356–8.

519 Scarfo GB, Mariottini A, Tamaccini D, Palma L. Growing skull fractures: progressive evolution of brain damage and effectiveness of surgical treatment. *Childs Nerv Syst* 1989; **173**: 653–7.

520 Scheff SW, Sullivan PG. Cyclosporin A significantly ameliorates cortical damage following experimental traumatic brain injury in rodents. *J Neurotrauma* 1999; **16**: 783–92.

521 Schlaepfer WW, Zimmerman U-JP. The degradation of neurofilaments by calpains. In: Mellgren RL, Murachi T eds. *Intracellular calcium-dependent proteolysis*. Boca Raton, FL: CRC Press, 1990: 241–9.

522 Schmidt ML, Carden MJ, Lee VMY, Trojanowski JQ. Phosphate-dependent and independent neurofilament epitopes in the axonal swellings of patients with motor neuron disease and controls. *Lab Invest* 1987; **56**: 282–94.

523 Schmidt RH, Grady MS. Regional patterns of blood–brain barrier breakdown following central and lateral fluid percussion injury in rodents. *J Neurotrauma* 1993; **10**: 415–30.

524 Schroeder ML, Muizelaar JP, Bullock R *et al*. Focal ischemia due to traumatic contusion, documented by stable, xenon CT and ultrastructural studies. *J Neurosurg* 1994; **82**: 966–71.

525 Schroeder ML, Muizelaar JP, Kuta AJ. Documented reversal of global ischaemia immediately after removal of an acute subdural hematoma. *J Neurosurg* 1994; **80**: 324–7.

526 Schulz E, Jahn R. Ring fractures of the base of the skull. *Z Rechtsmed* 1983; **90**: 137–45.

527 Seeler RA, Imana RB. Intracranial hemorrhage in patients with hemophilia. *J Neurosurg* 1973; **39**: 181–5.

528 Servadei F. Prognostic factors in severely head injured adult patients with acute subdural haematomas. *Acta Neurochir (Wein)* 1997; **139**: 279–85.

529 Servadei F, Ciucci G, Pagano F *et al*. Skull fracture as a risk factor of intracranial complications in minor head injuries. *J Neurol Neurosurg Psychiatry* 1988; **51**: 526–8.

530 Servadei F, Faccani G, Roccella P *et al*. Asymptomatic extradural haematomas. Results of a multicenter study of 158 cases in minor head injury. *Acta Neurochir (Wien)* 1989; **96**: 39–45.

531 Servadei P, Vergoni G, Pasini A *et al*. Diffuse axonal injury with brainstem localisation: report of a case in a mild head injured patient. *J Neurosurg Sci* 1994; **38**: 129–30.

532 Shaikh AY, Ezekiel UR, Liu PK, Hsu CY. Ischemic neuronal apoptosis: a view based on free radical-induced DNA damage and repair. *Neuroscientist* 1998; **4**: 88–95.

533 Shamloo M, Rytter A, Wieloch T. Activation of the extracellular signal-regulated protein kinase cascade in the hippocampal CA1 region in a rat model of global cerebral ischemic preconditioning. *Neuroscience* 1999; **93**: 81–8.

534 Shannon P, Smith CR, Deck J *et al*. Axonal injury and the neuropathology of shaken baby syndrome. *Acta Neuropathol* 1998; **95**: 625–31.

535 Sharp FR, Lu A, Tang Y, Millhorn DE. Multiple molecular penumbras after cerebral ischemia. *J Cereb Blood Flow Metab* 2000; **20**: 1011–32.

536 Shaw K, MacKinnon M-A, Raghupathi R *et al*. TUNEL-positive staining in white and grey matter after head injury in Man. *Clin Neuropathol* 2001; **20**: 106–12.

537 Sherriff FE, Bridges LR, Gentleman SM *et al*. Markers of axonal injury in post mortem human brain. *Acta Neuropathol* 1994; **88**: 433–9.

538 Shima K, Marmarou A. Evaluation of brain-stem dysfunction following severe fluid percussion head injury to the cat. *J Neurosurg* 1991; **74**: 270–7.

539 Shohami E, Beit-Yannai E, Horowitz M, Kohen R. Oxidative stress in closed-head injury: brain antioxidant capacity as an indicator of functional outcome. *J Cereb Blood Flow Metab* 1997; **17**: 1007–19.

540 Shohami E, Shapira Y, Yadid G *et al*. Brain phospholipase A_2 is activated after experimental closed head injury. *J Neurochem* 1989; **53**: 1541–6.

541 Shreiber DI, Bain AC, Ross DT *et al*. Experimental investigation of cerebral contusion: histopathological and immunohistochemical evaluation of dynamic cortical deformation. *J Neuropathol Exp Neurol* 1999; **58**: 153–64.

542 Sights WP. Ballistic analysis of shot gun injuries to the central nervous system. *J Neurosurg* 1969; **31**: 25–33.

543 Siman R, Baudry M, Lynch G. Brain fodrin: substitute for calpain I, an endogenous calcium-activated protease. *Proc Natl Acad Sci USA* 1984; **81**: 3572–6.

544 Simpson DA, Blumbergs PC, Cooter RD *et al*. Pontomedullary tears and other gross brainstem injuries after vehicular accidents. *J Trauma* 1989; **29**: 1519–25.

545 Smale G, Nichols NR, Brady DR *et al*. Evidence for apoptotic cell death in Alzheimer's disease. *Exp Neurol* 1995; **133**: 225–30.

546 Smith DH, Cecil KM, Meaney DF *et al*. Magnetic resonance spectroscopy of diffuse brain trauma in the pig. *J Neurotrauma* 1998; **15**: 665–74.

547 Smith DH, Chen X-H, Nonaka M *et al*. Accumulation of amyloid β and tau and the formation of neurofilament inclusions following diffuse brain injury in the pig. *J Neuropathol Exp Neurol* 1999; **58**: 982–92.

548 Smith DH, Chen X-H, Pierce JES *et al*. Progressive atrophy and neuron death for one year following brain trauma in the rat. *J Neurotrauma* 1997; **14**: 715–27.

549 Smith DH, Chen XH, Xu BN *et al* Characterization of diffuse axonal pathology and selective hippocampal damage following inertial brain trauma in the pig. *J Neuropathol Exp Neurol* 1997; **56**: 822–34.

550 Smith DH, Lowenstein DH, Gennarelli TA, McIntosh TK. Persistent memory dysfunction is associated with bilateral hippocampal damage following experimental brain injury. *Neurosci Lett* 1994; **168**: 151–4.

551 Smith DH, Nakamura M, McIntosh TK *et al*. Brain trauma induces massive hippocampal neuron death linked to a surge in β-amyloid levels in mice overexpressing mutant amyloid precursor protein. *Am J Pathol* 1998; **153**: 1005–110.

552 Smith DH, Nonaka M, Miller R *et al*. Immediate coma following inertial brain injury dependent on axonal damage in the brainstem. *J Neurosurg* 2000; **93**: 315–22.

553 Smith DH, Soares HD, Pierce JS *et al*. A model of parasagittal controlled cortical impact model in the mouse: cognitive and histopathologic effects. *J Neurotrauma* 1995; **12**: 169–78.

554 Smith DH, Wolf JA, Lusardi TA *et al*. High tolerance and delayed elastic response of cultured axon dynamic stretch injury. *J Neurosci* 1999; **19**: 4203–9.

555 Smith FM, Raghupathi R, MacKinnon M-A et al. TUNEL positive staining of surface contusions after fatal head injury in man. Acta Neuropathol 2000; 100: 537–45.

556 Smith SL, Hall ED. Mild pre- and posttraumatic hypothermia attenuates blood–brain barrier damage following controlled cortical impact injury in the rat. J Neurotrauma 1996; 13: 1–9.

557 Soloniuk D, Pitts LH, Lovelly M et al. Traumatic intracerebral haematomas: timing of appearance and indications for operative removal. J Trauma 1986; 26: 787–94.

558 Sorbi S, Nacmias N, Piacentini S et al. ApoE as a prognostic factor for post-traumatic coma. Nat Med 1995; i: 852.

559 Springer JE, Azbill RD, Knapp PE. Activation of caspase-3 apoptotic cascade in traumatic spinal cord injury. Nat Med 1999; 5: 943–6.

560 Squier MKT, Miller ACK, Malkinson AM, Cohen JJ. Calpain activation in apoptosis. J Cell Physiol 1994; 159: 229–37.

561 Stahel PF, Shohami E, Younis FM et al. Experimental closed head injury: analysis of neurological outcome, blood–brain barrier dysfunction, intracranial neutrophil infiltration, and neuronal cell death in mice deficient in genes for pro-inflammatory cytokines. J Cereb Blood Flow Metab 2000; 20: 369–80.

562 Stone JL, Lang RGR, Sugar O, Moody RA. Traumatic subdural hygroma. Neurosurgery 1981; 8: 542–50.

563 Stone JL, Rifai MHS, Sugar O et al. Subdural hematomas. I. Acute subdural hematoma: progress in definition, clinical pathology, and therapy. Surg Neurol 1983; 19: 216–31.

564 Strang L, MacMillan R, Jennett B. Head injury in accident and emergency departments in Scottish hospitals. Injury 1978; 10: 154–9.

565 Strich SJ. Cerebral trauma. In: Blackwood W, Corsellis JAN eds. Greenfield's neuropathology 3rd edn. London: Arnold, 1076: 327–60.

566 Strich SJ. Diffuse degeneration of the cerebral white matter in severe dementia following head injury. J Neurol Neurosurg Psychiatry 1956; 19: 163–85.

567 Strich SJ. Notes on Marchi method for staining degenerating myelin in the peripheral and central nervous system. J Neurol Neurosurg Psychiatry 1968; 31: 110–14.

568 Strich SJ. Shearing of nerve fibres as a cause of brain damage due to head injury. Lancet 1961; ii: 443–8.

569 Strich SJ. The pathology of brain damage due to blunt head injuries. In: Walker AE, Caveness WF, Critchley M eds. The late effects of head injury. Springfield, IL: Charles C Thomas, 1969: 501–24.

570 Stroobandt G, Fransen P, Thauvoy C, Menard E. Pathogenetic factors in chronic subdural haematoma and causes of recurrence after drainage. Acta Neurochir (Wien) 1995; 137: 6–14.

571 Sullivan PG, Keller JN, Mattson MP, Scheff SW. Traumatic brain injury alters synaptic homeostasis: implications for impaired mitochondrial and transport function. J Neurotrauma 1998; 15: 789–98.

572 Sumner D. Post-traumatic anosmia. Brain 1964; 87: 107–20.

573 Taha JM, Haddad FS. Central nervous system infections after craniocerebral missile wounds. In: Aarabi B, Kaufman HH eds. Missile wounds of the head and neck Vol. II. AANS Publications Committee, 1999: 271–80.

574 Takahashi K. Calpain substrate specificity. In: Mellgren RL, Murachi T eds. Intracellular calcium-dependent proteolysis. Boca Raton, FL: CRC Press, 1990: 55–74.

575 Tanaka T, Kaimori K, Sako K et al. Histological study of operated cases of chronic subdural haematoma in adults: relationship between dura mater and outer membrane. No Shinkei Geka 1997; 25: 701–5.

576 Tanno H, Nockels RP, Pitts LH, Noble LJ. Breakdown of the blood–brain barrier after fluid percussive brain injury in the rat: Part 1: Distribution and time course of protein extravasation. J Neurotrauma 1992; 9: 21–32.

577 Tanno H, Nockels RP, Pitts LH, Noble LJ. Breakdown of the blood–brain barrier after fluid percussive brain injury in the rat: Part 2: Effects of hypoxia on permeability to plasma proteins. J Neurotrauma 1992; 9: 335–47.

578 Tatagiba M, Sepehrnia A, El Axm M et al. Chronic epidural hematoma – report of eight cases and review of the literature. Surg Neurol 1989; 32: 453–8.

579 Taupin V, Toulmond S, Serrano A et al. Increase in IL-6, IL-1 and TNF levels in rat brain following traumatic lesion. Influence of pre- and post-traumatic treatment with Ro54864, a peripheral-type (p site) benzodiazepine ligand. J Neuroimmunol 1993; 42: 177–86.

580 Teasdale E, Cardoso E, Galbraith S, Teasdale G. CT scan in severe diffuse head injury: physiological and clinical correlations. J Neurol Neurosurg Psychiatry 1984; 47: 600–603.

581 Teasdale G, Galbraith S, Murray L et al. Management of traumatic intracranial haematoma. BMJ 1982; 285: 1695–7.

582 Teasdale GM, Murray G, Anderson E et al. Risks of acute traumatic intracranial haematoma in children and adults: implications for managing head injuries. BMJ 1990; 300: 363–7.

583 Teasdale GM, Nicoll JA, Murray G, Fiddes M. Association of apolipoprotein E polymorphism with outcome after head injury. Lancet 1997; 350: 1069–71.

584 Thatcher RW, Chamacho M, Salazar A et al. Quantitative MRI of the gray–white matter distribution in traumatic brain injury. J Neurotrauma 1997; 14: 1–14.

585 Thibault L, Meaney DF, Marmarou A, Andersen B. Biomechanical aspects of the fluid percussion model of brain injury. J Neurotrauma 1993; 9: 311–22.

586 Thom M. Neuropathologic findings in post-mortem studies of sudden death in epilepsy. Epilepsia 1997; 38 (Suppl 11): 532–4.

587 Thomas S, Prins ML, Samil M, Hovda DA. Cerebral metabolic response to traumatic brain injury sustained early in development: a 2-deoxy-D-glucose autoradiographic study. J Neurotrauma 2000; 17: 649–65.

588 Thornberry NA, Lazebnik YA. Caspases: enemies within. Science 1998; 281: 1312–16.

589 Thornhill S, Teasdale GM, Murray GD et al. Disability in young people and adults one year after head injury: prospective cohort study. BMJ 2000; 320: 1631–5.

590 Tien R, Chesnut RM. Medical management of the traumatic brain-injured patient. In: Cooper PR, Golfinos JG eds. Head injury 4th edn. New York: McGraw-Hill, 457–82.

591 Tokuda T, Ikeda S, Yanagisawa N et al. Re-examination of ex-boxers' brains using immunohistochemistry with antibodies to amyloid β-protein and tau protein. Acta Neuropathol 1991; 82: 281–5.

592 Tomasevic G, Raghupathi R, Oga M et al. Experimental TBI in mice lacking the tumor suppressor p53 gene. J Neurotrauma 1998; 16: 999.

593 Tomei G, Spagnoli D, Ducati A et al. Morphology and neurophysiology of focal axonal injury experimentally induced in the guinea pig optic nerve. Acta Neuropathol 1990; 80: 506–13.

594 Tomlinson BE. Brain-stem lesions after head injury. In: Sevitt S, Stoner HB eds. The pathology of trauma. London: Royal College of Pathologists. J Clin Pathol 1970; 23 (Suppl 4): 154–65.

595 Tornheim PA, Linwnicz BH, Hirsch CS et al. Acute responses to blunt head trauma. Experimental model and gross pathology. J Neurosurg 1983; 59: 431–8.

596 Toulmond S, Duval D, Serrano A et al. Biochemical and histological alterations induced by fluid percussion brain injury in the rat. Brain Res 1993; 620: 24–31.

597 Turazzi S, Bricolo A, Pastut ML et al. Changes produced by CT scanning in the outlook of severe head injury. Acta Neurochir (Wien) 1987; 85: 87–95.

598 Tymianski M, Tator CH. Normal and abnormal calcium homeostasis in neurons: a basis for the pathophysiology of traumatic and ischemic central nervous system injury. Neurosurgery 1996; 38: 1176–95.

599 Uzan M, Hanci M, Guzel O et al. The significance of neuron specific enolase levels in cerebrospinal fluid and serum after experimental traumatic brain damage. Acta Neurochir (Wien) 1995; 135: 141–3.

600 Uzzell BP, Dolinskas CA, Wiser RF et al. Influence of lesions detected by computed tomography on outcome and neuropyschological recovery after severe head injury. Neurosurgery 1987; 20: 396–402.

601 Vamvakas S, Vock EH, Lutz WK. On the role of DNA double-strand breaks in toxicity and carcinogenesis. Crit Rev Toxicol 1997; 27: 155–74.

602 Van Den Brink WA, Van Santbrink H, Steyerberg EW et al. Brain oxygen tension in severe head injury. Neurosurgery 2000; 46: 868–76.

603 Vaz R, Sarmento A, Borges N et al. Ultrastructural study of brain microvessels in patients with traumatic cerebral contusions. Acta Neurochir (Wien) 1997; 139: 215–20.

604 Velakoulis D, Lloyd JH. The role of SPECT scanning in a neuropsychiatry unit. Aust N Z J Psychiatry 1998; 32: 511–22.

605 Verweij BH, Muizelaar JP, Vinas FC et al. Mitochondrial dysfunction after experimental and human brain injury and its possible reversal with a selective N-type calcium channel antagonist (SNX111). Neurol Res 1997; 19: 334–9.

606 Vespa P, Prins M, Ronne-Engstrom E et al. Increase in extracellular glutamate caused by reduced cerebral perfusion pressure and seizures after human traumatic brain injury: a microdialysis study. J Neurosurg 1998; 89: 971–82.

607 Vespa PM, Nuwer MR, Nenov V et al. Increased incidence and impact of nonconvulsive and convulsive seizures after traumatic brain injury as detected by continuous electroencephalographic monitoring. J Neurosurg 1999; 91: 750–60.

608 Viljoen JJ, Wessels LS. Subacute and chronic extradural haematomas. S Afr J Surg 1990; 28: 133–7.

609 Vink R, Faden AI, McIntosh TK. Changes in cellular bionergetic state following graded traumatic brain injury in rats: determination by phosphorus 31 magnetic resonance spectroscopy. J Neurotrauma 1988; 5: 315–30.

610 Voigt GE, Skold G. Ring fractures of the base of the skull. J Trauma 1974; 14: 494–505.

611 Vowles GH, Scholtz CL, Cameron JM. Diffuse axonal injury in early infancy. J Clin Pathol 1987; 40: 185–9.

612 Wang KKW. Calapin and caspase: can you tell the difference? Trends Neurosci 2000; 23: 20–6.

613 Wang KKW, Yuen P-W. Calpain inhibition: an overview of its therapeutic potential. Trends Pharmacol Sci 1994; 15: 412–19.

614 Waterloo K, Ingebrigtsen T, Romner B. Neuropsychological functions in patients with increased serum levels of protein S-100 after minor head injury. Acta Neurochir (Wien) 1997; 139: 26–31; Discussion 31–2.

615 Wei EP, Lamb RG, Kontos HA. Increased phospholipase C activity after experimental brain injury. J Neurosurg 1982; 56: 695–8.

616 Weiner HL, Weinberg JS. Head injury in the pediatric age group. In: Cooper PR, Golfinos JG eds. Head injury 4th edn. New York: McGraw-Hill, 2000: 419–56.

617 Welte E. Uber die Zusammenhange zwishen anatomischem Befund und Klinishcem Bild bei Rindenprellungsherden nach stumpfen Schadeltrauma. Arch Psychiatrie Nervenkrank 1948; 179: 243–315.

618 Whalen MJ, Carlos TM, Dixon CE et al. Effect of traumatic brain injury in mice deficient in intracellular adhesion molecule-1: assessment of histopathologic and functional outcome. J Neurotrauma 1999; 16: 299–309.

619 Wilkinson AE, Bridges LR, Sivaloganathan S, Correlation of survival time with size of axonal swellings in diffuse axonal injury. Acta Neuropathol 1999; 98: 197–202.

620 Williams S, Raghupathi R, MacKinnon M-A et al. In-situ DNA fragmentation occurs in white matter up to 12 months after head injury in man. Acta Neuropathol in press.

621 Wolf JA, Stys PK, Lusardi T et al. Traumatic axonal injury induces calcium influx modulated by tetrotoxin-sensitive sodium changes. J Neurosci 2001; 21: 1923–30.

622 Woodroofe MN, Sarna GS, Wadhwa M et al. Detection of interleukin-1 and interleukin-6 in adult rat brain, following mechanical injury, by in vivo microdialysis: evidence of a role for microglia in cytokine production. J Neuroimmunol 1991; 33: 227–36.

623 Wright RL. Traumatic hematomas of the posterior cranial fossa. J Neurosurg 1966; 25: 402–9.

624 Xia Z, Dickens M, Raingeaud J et al. Opposing effects of ERK and JNK-p38 MAP kinases on apoptosis. Science 1995; 270: 1326–31.

625 Xiong Y, Peterson PL, Muizelaar JP, Lee CP. Mitochondrial dysfunction and calcium perturbation induced by traumatic brain injury. J Neurotrauma 1997; 14: 23–34.

626 Yaghmai A, Povlishock JT. Traumatically induced reactive change as visualized through the use of monoclonal antibodies targeted to the neurofilament subunits. J Neuropathol Exp Neurol 1992; 51: 158–76.

627 Yamakami I, McIntosh TK. Alterations in regional cerebral blood flow following brain injury in the rat. J Cereb Blood Flow Metab 1991; 11: 655–60.

628 Yamaki I, Vink R, Faden AI et al. Effects of acute ethanol intoxication on experimental brain injury in the rat: neurobehavioural and phosphorous-31 nuclear magnetic resonance spectroscopy studies. J Neurosurg 1995; 82: 813–21.

629 Yamashima T, Yamamoto S. How do vessels proliferate in the capsule of a chronic subdural hematoma? Neurosurgery 1984; 15: 672–8.

630 Yamashima T, Yamamoto S, Friede RL. The role of endothelial gap junctions in the enlargement of chronic subdural hematoma. J Neurosurg 1983; 59: 298–303.

631 Yamazaki Y, Yada K, Morii S et al. Diagnostic significance of serum neuron-specific enolase and myelin basic protein assay in patients with acute head injury. Surg Neurol 1995; 43: 267–70; discussion 270–1.

632 Yang DD, Kuan CY, Whitmarsh AJ et al. Absence of excitotoxicity-induced apoptosis in the hippocampus of mice lacking the Jnk3 gene. Nature 1997; 389: 865–70.

633 Yang JY, Liu X, Bhalla K et al. Prevention of apoptosis by Bcl-2: release of cytochrome c from mitochondria blocked. Science 1997; 275: 1129–32.

634 Yao Y, Yin D, Jas GS et al. Oxidative modification of a carboxylterminal vicinal methionine in calmodulin by hydrogen peroxide inhibits calmodulin-dependent activation of the plasma membrane CaATPase. Biochemistry 1996; 35: 2767–87.

635 Yawo H, Kuno M. How a nerve fiber repairs its cut end: involvement of phospholipase A$_2$. Science 1983; 222: 1351–2.

636 Yoshino A, Hovda DA, Kawamata T *et al*. Dynamic changes in local cerebral glucose utilization following cerebral concussion in rats: evidence of a hyper- and subsequent hypometabolic state. *Brain Res* 1991; **561**: 106–19.

637 Young Ha, Schimidek HH. Complications accompanying occipital skull fracture. *J Trauma* 1982; **22**: 914–20.

638 Young-Su P, Ishikawa J. Wide craniotomy–small dural incisions and intentionally delayed removal of intracerebral contusional hemorrhage for acute subdural hematoma. *No Shinkei Geka* 1997; **25**: 1081–9.

639 Yranheikki J, Koistinaho J, Copin JC, Crespigny A de *et al*. Spreading depression-induced expression of c-fos and cyclooxygenase-2 in transgenic mice that overexpress human copper/zinc-superoxide dismutase. *J Neurotrauma* 2000; **17**: 713–18.

640 Yuan X, Prough DS, Smith TL *et al*. The effects of traumatic brain injury on regional cerebral blood flow in rats. *J Neurotrauma* 1988; **5**: 289–301.

641 Zampella EJ, Duvall ER, Langford KH. Computed tomography and magnetic resonance imaging in traumatic locked-in syndrome. *Neurosurgery* 1988; **22**: 591–3.

642 Zauner A, Bullock R. The role of excitatory amino acids in severe brain trauma: opportunities for therapy. A review. *J Neurotrauma* 1995; **12**: 547–54.

643 Zauner A, Doppenberg EMR, Woodward JJ *et al*. Continuous monitoring of substrate delivery and clearance: initial experience in 24 patients with severe acute brain injuries. *Neurosurgery* 1997; **41**: 1082–93.

644 Zemlan FP, Rosenberg WS, Luebbe PA *et al*. Quantification of axonal damage in traumatic brain injury: affinity purification and characterization of cerebrospinal fluid tau proteins. *J Neurochem* 1999; **72**: 741–50.

645 Zhan Q, Chen I-T, Antinore MJ, Fornace AJ. Tumor suppressor p53 can participate in transcriptional induction of the GADD45 promoter in the absence of direct DNA binding. *Mol Cell Biol* 1998; **18**: 2768–78.

646 Zhang C, Raghupathi R, Saatman KE *et al*. Regional and temporal alterations in DNA fragmentation factor (DFF)-like proteins following experimental brain trauma in the rat. *J Neurochem* 1999; **73**: 1650–9.

647 Zhao X, Posmantur R, Kampfl A *et al*. Subcellular localization and duration of mu-calpain and m-calpain activity after traumatic brain injury in the rat: a casein zymography study. *J Cereb Blood Flow Metab* 1998; **18**: 161–7.

648 Zimmerman R, Bilaniuk L. Computed tomography in pediatric head trauma. *J Neuroradiol* 1981; **8**: 257–71.

649 Zimmerman RA, Bilaniuk LT, Bruce DA *et al*. Computed tomography of craniocerebral injury in the abused child. *Radiology* 1979; **130**: 687–90.

650 Zimmerman RA, Larissa T, Bilaniuk LT, Gennarelli TA. Computed tomography of shearing injuries of the cerebral white matter. *Radiology* 1978; **127**: 393–6.

651 Zink BJ, Walsh RF, Feustel PJ. Effects of alcohol in traumatic brain injury. *J Neurotrauma* 1993; **10**: 275–86.

652 Zipfel GJ, Babcock DJ, Lee JM, Choi DW. Neuronal apoptosis after CNS injury: the roles of glutamate and calcium. *J Neurotrauma* 2000; **17**: 857–69.

653 Zubkov AY, Pilkington AS, Bernanke DH *et al*. Post traumatic cerebral vasospasm: clinical and morphological presentations. *J Neurotrauma* 1999; **16**: 763–70.

15

Epilepsy

MRINALINI HONAVAR AND BRIAN S. MELDRUM

INTRODUCTION

Epilepsy is most effectively defined by its pathophysiology as 'an episodic disorder of the nervous system arising from the excessively synchronous and sustained discharge of a group of nerve cells', as initially proposed by Hughlings Jackson in 1873.[178] An isolated seizure does not constitute epilepsy, nor do multiple seizures secondary to fever, syncope, hypoglycaemia or other intermittent metabolic disorders. Seizures occurring in the context of inborn errors of metabolism, which have a sustained primary effect on the nervous system, are, however, regarded as epilepsy.

CLASSIFICATION

The classification of epilepsy is based on two frameworks, aetiology with a traditional dichotomy of 'idiopathic' or 'primary' versus 'symptomatic' or 'secondary' and semeiology with a traditional dichotomy of 'petit mal' (absence attacks with momentary arrest of movement and impairment of consciousness) and 'grand mal' (tonic–clonic seizures with violent motor activity alternating flexion and extension of limbs and trunk). The Commission on Classification in 1981[66] produced a scheme dependent only on the clinical features of the seizures with a primary dichotomy of 'generalized' versus 'focal' seizures. Generalized seizures are subdivided into absence (typical or atypical), myoclonic, clonic, tonic, tonic–clonic and atonic seizures. Partial or focal seizures are subdivided into simple partial, complex partial and partial evolving to secondarily generalized seizures. Patients may, however, have attacks of several types, either at different stages of the illness or mingled at one period, as in some patients with juvenile myoclonic epilepsy who may have, in addition to the myoclonic seizures, absences and tonic clonic seizures.

A more recent official classification from the International League against Epilepsy[65] is a hybrid, first dividing seizures into 'localization related' and 'generalized', and then subdividing into 'idiopathic', 'symptomatic' and 'cryptogenic'. Idiopathic epilepsies or syndromes are disorders not preceded or occasioned by another; they are defined by their age-related onset and clinical and electroencephalographic (EEG) features and are presumed to have a primarily genetic origin. Symptomatic epilepsies and syndromes are the consequence of a disorder of the central nervous system (CNS). Cryptogenic is now used to describe disorders that do not conform to an identified idiopathic syndrome and are presumed to be symptomatic (see Table 15.1).

In symptomatic or secondary epilepsy there is a primary pathology independent of epilepsy such as a malformation or developmental abnormality, post-traumatic scar, tumour, abscess or parasitic lesion that is presumed to have caused a local reduction in seizure threshold. These pathologies explain the epilepsy to a very limited extent in that they are commonly found in the brain in the absence of seizures and the causal relationship between the primary pathology and epileptogenesis is poorly understood. In addition, the morphological abnormalities seen in brains of epileptic subjects may be a consequence of the seizures, effects of antiepileptic therapy or simply incidental findings unrelated to the seizures. The lesion of 'hippocampal' or 'mesial temporal' sclerosis found in complex partial seizures is a special case in that

Table 15.1 *Classification of epileptic syndromes*

Localization related (focal or partial)	Cryptogenic or symptomatic
Idiopathic (age-related onset)	West's syndrome (infantile spasms, Blitz–Nick–Salaam
Benign childhood epilepsy with centrotemporal spikes	Krämpfe)
Childhood epilepsy with occipital paroxysms	Lennox–Gastaut syndrome
Frontal lobe seizures (sleep related)	Epilepsy with myoclonic astatic seizures
Primary reading epilepsy	Epilepsy with myoclonic absences
Symptomatic	Symptomatic
Chronic progressive epilepsia partialis continua	Non-specific aetiology
(Koshevnikoff's syndrome): includes Rasmussen's	Early myoclonic encephalopathy
syndrome	Early infantile encephalopathy with suppression burst
Developmental malformations	Specific syndromes
Tuberous sclerosis	Malformations
Lissencephaly–pachgyria	Aicardi's syndrome
Sturge–Weber syndrome	Lissencephaly–pachgyria
Syndromes characterized by seizures with specific modes	Tuberous sclerosis
of precipitation (reflex epilepsies and others)	Inborn errors of metabolism
Temporal lobe epilepsies	Non-ketotic hyperglycinaemia
(can be subdivided aetiologically or anatomically:	Phenylketonuria
mesiobasal limbic versus lateral temporal)	Tay–Sachs disease
Frontal lobe: includes supplementary motor, cingulate,	Pyridoxine dependency
anterior frontopolar, orbitofrontal, dorsolateral, opercular	Early and late infantile ceroid–lipofuscinosis
and motor cortex epilepsies	(Santavuori–Haltia–Hagberg disease and
Parietal lobe	Jansky–Bielschowski disease)
Occipital lobe	Infantile Huntington's disease
Cryptogenic (presumed to be symptomatic but aetiology	Juvenile Gaucher's disease
unknown)	Juvenile ceroid–lipofuscinosis
	(Spielmeyer–Vogt–Sjögren disease)
Generalized epilepsies	Lafora disease
Idiopathic (with age-related onset)	Progressive myoclonic epilepsy
Benign neonatal familial convulsions	Dyssynergia cerebellaris myoclonia with epilepsy
Benign neonatal convulsions	(Ramsay–Hunt syndrome)
Benign myoclonic epilepsy in infancy	Cherry red spot myoclonus (sialidosis with deficit in
Childhood absence epilepsy (pyknolepsy)	neuraminidase)
Juvenile absence epilepsy	Adult ceroid–lipofuscinosis (Kufs' disease)
Juvenile myoclonic epilepsy	
Epilepsy with grand mal (GTCS) on awakening	

the lesion may be both secondary to seizures and a focal cause of seizures. An important feature of localization-related seizures is that they may be amenable to surgical treatment; this may require not only identification and delineation of the primary pathology, but also functional delineation of the epileptic focus.

EPIDEMIOLOGY

Epilepsy is found in all ethnic groups that have been investigated. Epidemiological studies around the world show prevalence figures ranging from 1.5 per 1000 in Japan[347] to 19.5 per 1000 in Colombia,[133] although most studies have found the prevalence of epilepsy to lie between 4 and 10 per 1000.[344] Most reports give rates of incidence of 20–70 per 100 000 per annum, but there are studies in which there is much greater variation.[344] The incidence of seizures is highest in the first year of life, especially in the first month.[108,153] It falls in each successive age group and

rises again after the age of 60 years. In all populations there is a slightly higher prevalence of epilepsy amongst males. Differences in methodology account for some of the variation between studies.[153,344] Different methods of case collection, definition, diagnosis and classification of epilepsy make it difficult to draw comparisons. In studies that have looked only at children, the prevalence of epilepsy varied from 4.7 per 1000 in Kiel, Germany,[91] and 8.2 per 1000 in Tokyo,[388] to 31 per 1000 in Melipilla, Chile.[58] The first study looked at medical records and registers, while the account by Tsuboi[388] is based on clinical and EEG examination of a cohort of 17 044 children aged 3 years followed up for 6 years. Chiofalo *et al.*[58] investigated 2085 children, 9 years of age, using a questionnaire and subjecting a proportion to clinical and EEG examination. In Rochester, Minnesota, USA, Hauser and Kurland[153] demonstrated that the incidence of seizures was 120 per 100 000 if recurrent, febrile and single convulsions were included, but was 54 per 100 000 if only recurrent seizures were considered.

There are, however, genuine differences in the prevalence and incidence of epilepsy in different regions, owing to variations in geographical, environmental and socio-economic factors. Aetiological factors vary in their relative importance. The distribution of types of seizures varies and the prognosis is different owing to differences in the availability of treatment. Partial seizures are the most common type of seizures seen in many of the populations studied.[34,131,185,189,195] In contrast, Li et al.[225] classified 81% of the cases surveyed as 'generalized epilepsy' in a population of 63 195 in urban areas in the People's Republic of China.

The high prevalence of epilepsy in developing countries is attributed to intracranial infections (particularly those due to parasitosis), perinatal brain damage, head injury and toxic agents.[356] In Nigeria, for instance, the very high incidence of partial epilepsy compared with that in more developed countries was thought to be the consequence of the increased incidence of febrile illnesses (such as malaria) leading to febrile convulsions, birth injury and CNS infections.[78]

It is difficult to determine the aetiology of the seizures, particularly when carrying out large population-based epidemiological studies. In most instances the cause is presumed. In the recent past no aetiology has been found in between 65 and 79% of cases.[71,122,153,189,225] The introduction of magnetic resonance imaging (MRI) has undoubtedly changed this (see below). Forsgren[122] reviewed a series of reports in different populations that estimated the proportions of cases of epilepsy in which an aetiology was postulated. There is great variation in the proportions between studies, but world-wide head injury, birth trauma, cerebrovascular disease and infections are the most common causes of symptomatic epilepsy.

Prenatal and perinatal factors that are associated with an increased risk of subsequently developing epilepsy have been reviewed.[402] Intrauterine infections and cerebrovascular insufficiency, and congenital malformations may result in seizures after birth. Intrapartum events that are associated with a high risk of seizures later are use of midcavity forceps, evidence of fetal distress including low fetal heart rate, prolonged second stage of labour and emergency Caesarean section.[268,279] Hypoxic–ischaemic encephalopathy or cerebrovascular insufficiency due to intrapartum and postnatal events, in many instances in babies who have had potentially traumatic births, is considered an important risk factor.[402] In a prospective clinical study, infants with perinatal hypoxia, defined as those with Apgar scores of 5 or less after 1 h, were found to have a five-fold increased risk of epilepsy compared with controls.[31] Risk factors for different types of seizures have been investigated, and there appears to be some difference.[334–336] A history of maternal seizures, febrile convulsions and head injury increases the risk of developing generalized tonic–clonic seizures and partial complex seizures. Risk of the latter is also enhanced with neonatal seizures, viral encephalitis and cerebral palsy. Febrile convulsions were the only risk factor identified for absence of seizures.

At least one additional handicapping medical condition may accompany epilepsy in up to 65% of patients.[71,206,406] The most common are mental retardation, seen in up to 28% of patients, motor handicap, and hearing and visual impairment. Epilepsy starting in the first few years of life is more likely to be associated with mental subnormality, and tends more frequently to manifest as generalized seizures.[366] Neurological deficit is associated more commonly with focal epilepsy.

The prognosis is generally better if the onset of epilepsy is before the age of 10 years,[12] but is poor in patients with neurological deficit present at birth, and in those with mental retardation.

DEATH IN EPILEPSY

There is an overall increased risk of premature death in patients with epilepsy.[13,64] The risk is even higher in patients with symptomatic epilepsy, which is attributed to the underlying aetiology rather than to the epilepsy itself. The most common causes are pneumonia, cancer and stroke. There is a significant excess of deaths due to accidents, and drowning appears to be the most frequent cause of death due to seizure-related accidents.[370] Sudden unexpected death in epilepsy (SUDEP) occurs in about 10% of patients, and is the major form of death in patients in the 20–40 year age group.[103,218] It has been defined as sudden, unexpected, witnessed or unwitnessed, non-traumatic and non-drowning death in patients with epilepsy, with or without evidence for a seizure and excluding documented status epilepticus, in which post-mortem examination does not reveal a toxicological or an anatomical cause for death.[278] It has been postulated that death results from cardiac arrhythmia or respiratory failure during or immediately after a seizure.[103,159] However, ventricular arrhythmias have not been found to be more common in patients with epilepsy than in the general population, although occasional cases of near fatal cardiac arrhythmia have been documented in epileptic patients.[193,226,312] The risk of SUDEP is higher in young patients, males, and those with generalized seizures, severe or frequent seizures, on multiple antiepileptic drugs, or with poor compliance with medication, head injury and alcohol abuse.[102,283,383,401]

Post-mortem studies have revealed pulmonary oedema and generalized visceral congestion, with an increase in organ weights, in the majority of cases of SUDEP in some series,[103,218,384] while others have shown no significant abnormality.[159,385] In up to 70% of brains examined, morphological lesions were found that could be attributed to the cause of epilepsy, or result from the epilepsy, such as malformations, hippocampal sclerosis, tumours, old infarcts, scars and old contusions. In approximately one-third of cases cerebral oedema was noted without any internal herniation, and in rare cases histological examination showed acute hypoxic changes in neocortical and brainstem neurons, suggesting a short interval between the fatal event and death.

An experimental model of epilepsy in sheep, in which pulmonary oedema and sudden death were generated, showed that cardiac arrhythmia occurred in all the animals, but did not account for death in any.[188] There was no evidence of pulmonary venous constriction, and the pulmonary oedema found was considered to be neurogenic in origin, due to markedly elevated pulmonary vascular pressures, resulting from a combination of pulmonary vascular hypertension, occurring as a consequence of seizures, and hypoxia.[187] The oedema was not considered to have been of sufficient magnitude to impair alveolar gas exchange. However, there was marked hypoventilation with a precipitous drop in arterial oxygen tension after the induction of seizures in the animals dying suddenly, supporting the role of centrally induced respiratory failure in this model of sudden death in epilepsy.

GENETICS

Since the early 1990s there have been great advances in the understanding of the genetic basis of epilepsy, and with the information about the genetics has come an understanding of the cellular mechanisms of the disorders.[19,130,317,332] Some primary generalized forms of epilepsy have a clear genetic basis: in several syndromes mendelian patterns of inheritance can be demonstrated; in some others inheritance is complex, associated with chromosome deletions or assumed to be polygenic (Table 15.2). The chromosomal locus of the defect has been definitively or tentatively determined in some syndromes, and mutations have been identified in genes for factors such as ion channels, elements of excitatory and inhibitory neurotransmitter receptors, neuromodulators and protein kinases, which result in a predisposition to hyperexcitability.

Benign familial neonatal convulsions are remarkable in that a very precisely defined phenotype, including onset at the age of 2–7 days, has apparent genetic heterogeneity. Linkage studies in families with autosomal dominant inheritance have shown a locus on chromosome 20q in some families and chromosome 8q in others. Both loci correspond to genes encoding voltage-sensitive potassium channels in the KQT group (KCNQ2/KCNQ3) that jointly generate the M current. Different families have shown missense, frameshift and splice-site variant mutations.[341] The mutated potassium ion channels probably produce the seizures by directly altering the excitability in the cell populations in which they are expressed.[222]

Juvenile myoclonic epilepsy (JME) is the most frequent form of primary generalized epilepsy with tonic–clonic seizures, and has complex non-mendelian inheritance. Linkage analysis indicates a gene locus in chromosome 6p in one family.[227] Another gene locus on chromosome 15 that encodes the α_7-subunit of the neuronal nicotinic acetylcholine receptor is currently being investigated in a large group of families with JME. Juvenile absence epilepsy shows an allelic association with a polymorphism in the receptor gene GRIK1, which codes for the GluR5 subunit of the kainate receptor.[345]

There is a clear genetic predisposition to febrile convulsions.[317] It is presumed to be polygenic as a definite pattern of inheritance has not been identified; there is an enhanced risk of epilepsy in the relatives of probands, and a much higher risk in monozygotic than in dizygotic twins. Comparison of polymorphisms in patients with temporal lobe epilepsy with and without hippocampal sclerosis shows that a polymorphism relating to the gene for a proinflammatory cytokine, interleukin-1β (IL-1β), is associated with the cases with hippocampal sclerosis,[190] suggesting that a genetically determined enhanced inflammatory response might favour the occurrence of hippocampal sclerosis in response to an early life stress. First described in a large Tasmanian family, generalized epilepsy with febrile seizures plus (GEFS+), an autosomal dominant condition in which febrile seizures persist beyond the usual age of resolution of 5–6 years, has shown linkage to chromosome 19q.[332] A strong candidate locus present within the target interval for GEFS+ is a gene that encodes a sodium ion channel β₁-subunit, and a missense mutation was revealed in affected individuals of the family. A new locus on chromosome 2 has also been found in a French kindred with GEFS+. There is also a genetic basis for a variety of photosensitive epileptiform phenomena, including paroxysmal EEG discharges induced by intermittent photic stimulation in children without epilepsy.[282]

Table 15.2 includes two idiopathic syndromes of partial epilepsy that are genetic in origin. Benign childhood epilepsy with centrotemporal spikes has complex or autosomal dominant inheritance with age-dependent penetrance. Twenty-two families have been linked to chromosome 15q, in the region of the α_7-subunit of the nicotinic acetylcholine receptor.[280] A rare syndrome with onset in childhood in which frontal lobe seizures are manifest as clusters of brief motor attacks during sleep, autosomal dominant nocturnal frontal lobe epilepsy (ADNFLE),[349] has a gene locus on 20q that maps to the same region as the neuronal nicotinic acetylcholine receptor α_4-subunit. A missense mutation in the second transmembrane domain of this receptor subunit is present in all affected members of a large Australian kindred.[374] The functional role of this α_4-nicotinic receptor may be to control the synaptic release of glutamate. It is interesting that ADNFLE and one of the forms of benign familial neonatal convulsions are mapped to the same region of chromosome 20, but are caused by mutations in distinct genes separated by just 30 kb.[130] Linkage

Table 15.2 *Genetic characteristics of some epileptic syndromes*

Syndrome (age of onset)	Inheritance	Chromosome (year of description of linkage)	Gene/protein
Benign familial neonatal convulsions (EBN1, EBN2) (2–7 days; remission at 3 months)	Autosomal dominant Autosomal dominant	20q (1989) 8q (1993)	KCNQ2/VS K⁺ channel KCNQ3/(M-current)
Benign familial infantile convulsions (4–6 months)	Autosomal dominant	19q (1997)	
Generalized epilepsy with febrile seizures plus (median 1 year; remission by 11 years)	Autosomal dominant	19q (1998) 2q (1999)	β_1-subunit/Na⁺ channel α-subunit/Na⁺ channel
Autosomal dominant nocturnal frontal lobe epilepsy, ADNFLE (median 8 years)	Autosomal dominant	20q (1995) 15q (1998)	α4-subunit/nicotinic ACh receptor
Benign childhood epilepsy with rolandic spikes (3–13 years)	Complex	15q (1998)	
Childhood absence epilepsy (3–13 years)	Complex	(?) 8q (1998)	
Juvenile myoclonic epilepsy, JME (12–18 years)	Complex	(?) 6p (1988) 15q (1997)	
Northern epilepsy syndrome (epilepsy with mental retardation, EPMR) (5–10 years)	Autosmal recessive	8p (1994)	(?) Cathepsin B
Progressive myoclonus epilepsy, Unverricht–Lundborg type (6–15 years)	Autosomal recessive	21q (1991)	Cyastatin B (protease inhibitor)
Myoclonus epilepsy of Lafora, Lafora body disease (10–16 years)	Autosomal recessive	6q (1995)	Laforin (protein phosphatase)
Miller–Dieker lissencephaly	*De novo* deletion (or balanced chromosome rearrangement)	17p (1983)	LIS-1/platelet-activating factor hydrolase
Angelman syndrome	Complex: 4 different genotypes, including maternally inherited deletions	15q (1991)	UBE3A/ubiquitin ligase 3ᴬ GABRB3/GABA_A receptor β_3-subunit

has also been reported to a second ADNFLE locus at 15q close to a cluster of acetylcholine receptors, α_3, α_5 and β_4.[311]

A familial form of temporal lobe epilepsy is described, with mild seizures of mesial or lateral origin, in which the typical hippocampal pathology of temporal lobe epilepsy is not seen. In one family in which auditory disturbances are also a feature, the epilepsy susceptibility gene has been mapped to chromosome 10q, where candidate genes include those for two adrenergic receptors, glutamate dehydrogenase and a subunit of calcium-calmodulin protein kinase.[296]

Angelman syndrome, with profound mental retardation, atypical absences and myoclonic epilepsy,[10,407] is most commonly (70% of cases) due to a large maternally inherited deletion in chromosome 15q11–13, which usually

includes the *UBE3A* gene (coding for ubiquitin ligase 3A) and three genes for subunits of the γ-aminobutyric acid-A (GABA_A) receptor. A mutation in the *UBE3A* gene causes a form of Angelman syndrome (class IV) in which the epilepsy is less severe than in the form associated with a maternally inherited deletion (class I).[266] A role for loss of GABA_A receptor subunits is suggested by studies with GABA_A β_3-subunit knockout mice, which show some behavioural features seen in Angelman syndrome including the seizure syndrome.[85]

Studies of single gene mutations in mice have identified five recessively inherited syndromes that manifest absence-like attacks with behavioural arrest and bilateral spike-and-wave discharges all of which involve subunits of the voltage-gated calcium channels in the brain.[30] Thus, the *tottering* mouse has a point mutation and the *leaner* mouse a frame shift in the gene for the α_{1A}-subunit. In *lethargic* mice the mutation produces protein truncation in the β_4-subunit; in *stargazer* mice it is the γ-subunit and in *ducky* mice the $\alpha_2\delta$-subunit that is affected. These mouse syndromes all have other neurological signs, most commonly ataxia, and various developmental abnormalities in the brain, but they clearly signal Ca^{2+} channel defects as potential causes of generalized epilepsies.

There is a group of about 150 genetic disorders[144,234] with a metabolic or developmental defect involving the brain in which epileptic seizures occur. McKusick[234] lists about 25 autosomal dominant syndromes, which include acute intermittent porphyria, neurofibromatosis and tuberous sclerosis. There are about 100 autosomal recessive syndromes including phenylketonuria and other disorders of amino acid metabolism; a wide range of disorders of lipid metabolism including Batten's disease, Krabbe's disease and Tay–Sachs disease; and many disorders associated with cerebral malformations such as the lissencephaly syndromes I and II. McKusick's third group, X-linked phenotypes, includes Aicardi's syndrome, which is characterized by infantile spasms, chorioretinal lacunae, agenesis of the corpus callosum and mental retardation.[5] Post-mortem studies in a small number of cases show a consistent occurrence of sulcogyral abnormalities (Fig. 15.1). These genetic syndromes are considered to be 'secondary epilepsy', because a gross pathological process involving the nervous system usually precedes seizure onset. The distinction between secondary epilepsy in genetic disorders and primary genetic forms of epilepsy is not, however, absolute. In some of these disorders epilepsy may be the presenting symptom, such as pyridoxine dependency and progressive myoclonus epilepsies. In northern epilepsy syndrome, a progressive epilepsy with mental retardation, the seizure onset precedes the period of mental decline;[377] however, the neuropathology of the syndrome has not been described. The locus for the disorder appears to be in the telomeric region of chromosome 8, in the region of the gene of a protease cathepsin B. Cathepsin has no known role in the control of neuronal excitability, and it is postulated that the defective protease may lead to the accumulation of a neurotoxic product, resulting in cell degeneration and subsequent seizures.

The genetic classification of the mitochondrial disorders, many of which are associated with seizures, divides them into two main groups, those caused by mutations in nuclear DNA of the thousands of proteins needed to regulate mitochondrial function and which are transmitted by mendelian inheritance, and those caused by mutations in mitochondrial DNA (mtDNA).[89] There are two categories of mutations of mtDNA, major rearrangements such as deletions and duplications, which are sporadic events, and point mutations which are maternally inherited. The most common mitochondrial syndromes, myoclonus epilepsy with ragged-red fibres (MERRF), mitochondrial encephalopathy, lactic acidosis and stroke episodes (MELAS) and maternally inherited Leigh syndrome (MILS), are associated with different point mutations, while Kearns–Sayres syndrome is characterized by a mtDNA deletion (see also Chapter 12, this Volume).

Some further genetic epilepsy syndromes are discussed below under 'Cortical dysplasia' and 'Myoclonus epilepsy'.

SYMPTOMATIC EPILEPSY

Cerebral malformations

Chronic seizures are a clinical feature of numerous and varied developmental disorders of the brain. They may be seen with malformations such as agenesis of the corpus callosum[5] and disturbances in growth, both micrencephaly and megalencephaly.[126] Seizures are also common in a group of abnormalities characterized by disordered cortical architecture and aberrant neuronal arrangement. They are an early and frequent feature of lissencephaly or argyria and pachygyria,[87] and hemimegalencephaly,[200] and are also often associated with less severe defects such as laminar and nodular heterotopia, polymicrogyria and schizencephaly. Most of these malformations of cortical development are associated with mental retardation and motor dysfunction (see Chapter 7, this Volume).

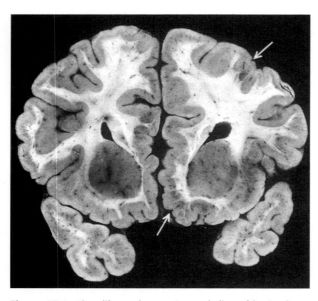

Figure 15.1 *Aicardi's syndrome. Coronal slice of brain showing gyral malformation (arrowed) and an absent corpus callosum from a 10-year-old blind, subnormal girl, whose EEG was typical of that seen in Aicardi's syndrome. The patient's younger sister had Down's syndrome. Personal communication from Professor Colin Binnie, King's College Hospital, London, UK.*

Cortical dysplasia

The term cortical dysplasia describes a malformative lesion predominantly affecting cerebral neocortex, resulting in disorganized brain cytoarchitecture. In general, normal cortical lamination is disturbed and neurons are abnormally located. Adjacent white matter is often involved.

The role of microdysgenesis, mild cortical dysplasia or other subtle developmental abnormalities in cytoarchitecture of the brain, as a cause of primary epilepsy has been the subject of speculation since the beginning of the twentieth century.[6] Veith and Wicke[393] suggested that the microdysgenesis observed in 34% of brains with epilepsy was of pathological significance. The changes seen in seven out of eight cases of primary generalized seizures by Meencke and Janz[256] consisted of the presence of unipolar and bipolar neurons immediately beneath the pia, and protrusion of neural tissue, sometimes containing neurons, into the leptomeninges (Fig. 15.2a). There was an increased density of Retzius–Cajal cells and large pyramidal neurons in the molecular layer, blurred demarcation between layers I and II of the neocortex, and inappropriate columnar arrangement of neurons.

Increased numbers of nerve cells were seen in the white matter (Fig. 15.2b). There were increased numbers of large nerve cells in the stratum radiatum of the hippocampus, and in the cerebellum, ectopic Purkinje cells were found in the molecular and granule cell layers and in the white matter. In a further study of the brains of children, which included morphometrical analysis of neuronal density, Meencke[255] reported a high incidence of microdysgenesis in West's syndrome (9/24), Lennox–Gastaut syndrome (7/12), childhood absence epilepsy (11/12) and juvenile myoclonic epilepsy (2/3). Some of these were associated with perinatal and postnatal ischaemic lesions. However, doubts have been expressed about the significance of such findings, as many of these appearances may be seen in the brains of normal individuals.[192,231]

A wide range of histological abnormalities has been included under the heading of 'microdysgenesis', without macroscopic abnormality, and with morphologically normal neurons and glia within the lesions. In addition to the features above, indistinct cortical lamination, pronounced vertical lamination, small grey-matter heterotopia, increased neuronal satellitosis, rows of perivascular glia, and dentate gyrus granule cell dispersion or duplication are described.[16,40,287] Tiny microdysgenetic nodules or

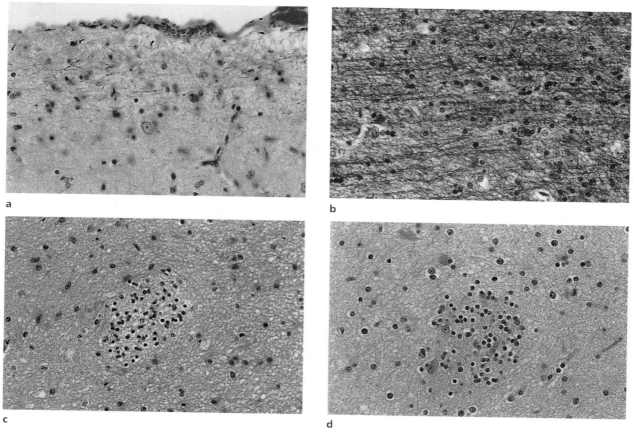

a

b

c

d

Figure 15.2 *Microdysgenesis. This was seen as an additional finding in temporal lobe resection specimens with mesial temporal sclerosis (a, b) and a dysembryoplastic neuroepithelial tumour (c, d). (a) Subpial neuron in temporal neocortex. (b) Neurons in temporal white matter. (c) Microdysgenetic nodule in white matter composed of oligodendroglia-like cells, astrocytes and occasional neurons. (d) Microdysgenetic nodule in neocortex. (a, b: Luxol fast blue/cresyl violet; c, d: H&E.)*

glioneuronal hamartia which consist of minute, multifocal, circumscribed aggregates in the cortex of randomly orientated neurons with glial cells, predominantly astrocytes, may also be seen (Fig. 15.2c, d).[413,414,417] Small clusters of oligodendroglia-like cells are frequently included within the lesion. These glioneuronal aggregates show normal or only slightly increased cellularity compared with normal cortex.

These changes have also been described in temporal and frontal cortical resections from patients with partial seizures[16,40,191,287] in some instances associated with a tumour or porencephaly. As with primary generalized epilepsy, the role of microdysgenesis as a substrate of epilepsy in localized seizures has been questioned. Counts of nerve cell density by Hardiman *et al.*[146] showed neuronal ectopia in 96% of 49 temporal neocortical resections and in 72% of controls, although severe ectopia, defined by them as more than eight neurons per mm[2] white matter, was found in 43% of the epileptic material but not in any of the controls. Microdysgenetic changes such as neuronal clustering and areas devoid of neurons in the temporal neocortex were described in association with the severe neuronal ectopia. In contrast, Babb *et al.*[22] compared the volumetric cell density of cortical neurons in the inferior and middle temporal gyri from 45 resected temporal lobes and in four normal controls and did not find a difference. More recent studies have also confirmed the presence of microdysgenetic features in both temporal lobe resections and autopsy controls, but neuronal clustering in cortical layers II–IV, perivascular oligodendroglial clusters, glioneuronal hamartia and increased numbers of white-matter neurons were significantly increased in patients with temporal lobe epilepsy.[109,191] Whether all these changes are truly of developmental origin or a secondary consequence of the seizure activity, related to the pathogenesis of the epilepsy or simply epiphenomena, remains unanswered.

A morphologically distinct form of cortical dysplasia is focal cortical dysplasia (cortical dysplasia with neuronal cytomegaly),[381] seen in specimens resected from patients with partial epilepsy. The abnormal area usually appears normal externally, but may on occasion be represented by a wider than normal gyrus or a zone of partial lissencephaly,[180] while the cut surface shows blurred grey-and white-matter demarcation (Fig. 15.3a). The lamination of the cortex is disturbed, and large, bizarre neurons with prominent dendritic arborization are present throughout the cortex and in the white matter, accompanied by large balloon cells with pleomorphic nuclei and glassy eosinophilic cytoplasm of uncertain histogenesis (Fig. 15.3b, c). The orientation of the large neurons is not clear and some show axons pointing in inappropriate directions while others are more correctly positioned. Occasional abnormal cells may be found in the brain adjacent to the main lesion. The abnormal large neurons are strongly immunoreactive for high and medium molecular weight

neurofilament epitopes.[99] The balloon cells express glial fibrillary acidic protein erratically, and some cells express both glial and neuronal markers.[399,400] The large neurons have been shown to express increased levels of markers of neuronal immaturity, microtubule-associated proteins

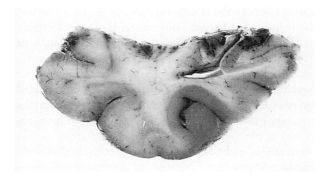

a

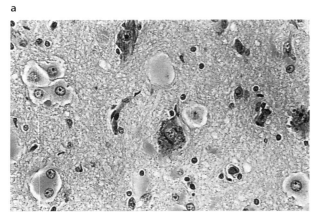

b

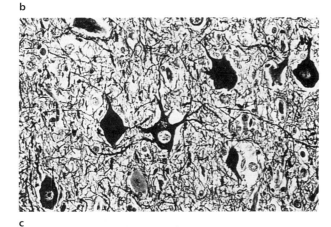

c

Figure 15.3 *Focal cortical dysplasia. (a) Slice of a temporal lobectomy of a 16-year-old girl with partial complex seizures. The abnormality was seen on external examination. The lesion in the inferior and middle temporal gyri shows a wide cortex with blurred demarcation between the grey and white matter. The abnormality extended along the whole length of the specimen. There was no mesial temporal sclerosis. (b) Disordered cortex containing large neurons and balloon cells. The abnormal cells are frequently seen in the underlying white matter as well. (c) Bizarre neuron with prominent coarse dendritic arborization. (b: H&E; c: Glees and Marsland silver impregnation.)*

2c and 1b and nestin.[73,422,423] Abnormal patterns of expression and levels of distribution of several proteins involved in the Wnt signalling pathway have been found in the abnormal large neurons and balloon cells of focal cortical dysplasia.[70] The Wnt pathway transduces signals from the extracellullar space to the nucleus to determine gene transcription, and participates in the determination of neuronal fate in neurodevelopment; the abnormalities found indicate a failure of these cells to differentiate and commit to cell fate.

There is increasing evidence that the morphological abnormalities are associated with alterations in the neuronal circuitry, which may be responsible for the epileptogenicity of focal cortical dysplasia. Using antibodies to parvalbumin, calbindin D_{28k} and calretinin, calcium binding proteins that identify GABAergic interneurons in the cerebral cortex, a reduction in inhibitory neurons immunoreactive for the proteins has been demonstrated in the affected cortex, compared with the surrounding normal cortex.[120,371] Some of the large abnormal neurons also stained positively and had morphological features resembling different types of interneurons.[120] An increased intensity of immunostaining for the excitatory glutamate receptors, GluR-2/3 α-amino-3-hydroxy-5-methyl-4-isoxazolepropionic acid (AMPA) and N-methyl-D-aspartate receptor-1 (NMDAR-1) subunits, has been reported in the dysplastic cortex, with the large abnormal neurons preferentially expressing both subunits, which has been interpreted as an enhancement of excitatory circuitry.[371] In addition, enhanced immunolabelling for GluR-1 and GluR-2/3 and a highly specific increase in NMDAR-2 have been linked to 'developmental immaturity' and to altered excitability.[196,246] By studying the relative abundance of messenger RNA (mRNA) transcripts in single cells, Crino et al.[72] identified changes that are specific to dysplastic neurons. Thus, increases in mRNA for GluR-4, and NMDA receptors NR-2B and NR-2C are seen in dysplastic but not in heterotopic neurons in dysplastic cortex. Decreases in GABAα$_1$, GABAα$_2$, GABAβ$_2$ and GluR-1 were seen in both dysplastic and heterotopic neurons.

Preoperative diagnosis of focal cortical dysplasia is difficult, as it is infrequently demonstrable by computed tomographic (CT) scanning, and not always visualized on MRI.[158,180] Improved resolution of MRI is leading to identification of more focal cortical dysplasias.[210,323] The results of surgery are not consistently favourable, and seizures either fail to improve or worsen in approximately one-third of patients. EEG findings in some suggest that the lesions may extend further than is appreciated by current methods of imaging. Quantitative MRI measuring regional distribution of grey and white matter supports the view that the structural disorganization is much more widespread than suggested by visual inspection for cortical dysgenesis.[359]

The relationship of this lesion to one form of hemimegalencephaly, which also presents with intractable seizures and in which similar large neurons and astrocytes are seen,[331] is unclear. In other cases of hemimegalencephaly the affected hemisphere shows a wide variety of cortical abnormalities. The lesions of focal cortical dysplasia also bear some resemblance to those of a forme fruste of tuberous sclerosis. The cytoarchitectural abnormalities in tuberous sclerosis are, however, much more extensive and a characteristic feature of the cortical tubers is the presence of subpial clusters of giant astrocytes and sheaves of astrocytic processes.[299,308] The diagnosis of forme fruste of tuberous sclerosis is made in cortical lesions with the histological picture of classic tuberous sclerosis (see Chapter 7, this Volume), but without any other lesions in the brain or the visceral and cutaneous stigmata of the disorder. Epilepsy is also a feature of classic tuberous sclerosis. It is seen in 82–90% of patients with the disease, and is the most frequent presenting symptom.[134] Macrogyria, a focal form of cortical dysplasia, is composed of diffusely thick cortex with indistinct cortical lamination, and includes the condition of bilateral central macrogyria.[239] Abnormalities of neuroglial morphology are not generally seen.

The term glioneuronal hamartoma is probably best retained for a tumour-like malformation that presents as a mass. It is composed of mature but disorganised neuronal and glial elements, which may be accompanied by a vascular and a connective tissue component. The hypothalamic neuronal hamartoma that presents with gelastic seizures is a well-defined mass of grey matter with mature neurons, resembling those of the principal hypothalamic nuclei, and with myelinated and unmyelinated fibres coursing through.[339]

It has been suggested that the various forms of cortical dysplasia constitute a spectrum of change, composed of distinct and specific microscopic abnormalities, resulting from disruptions in the process of neocortical development occurring at different times.[269] Type I lissencephaly, as in the Miller–Dieker syndrome, arises from arrest of neuronal migration around 10–14 weeks of development and may be associated with facial dysmorphism.[90] The Miller–Dieker syndrome is most commonly the result of a de novo deletion in chromosome 17, involving a platelet-activating factor hydrolase that appears to be developmentally significant.[151] In general, focal cortical dysplasia, with neuronal cytomegaly and balloon cells, is regarded as an early developmental disruption, occurring around the time of the last mitotic division when neuronal phenotypes are being specified. Neuronal heterotopia and polymicrogyria result from events in an intermediate period, between 10 and 24 weeks of gestation, when active neuroblast migration occurs. The lesions of cortical microdysgenesis – cortical laminar disturbance, marginal glioneuronal heterotopia, persistence of the subpial granular cell layer, neurons in the molecular layer and single heterotopic neurons in the white matter – are seen as abnormalities of late cortical development. There is some correlation between the frequency of seizures and the three groups of lesions. This concept has some support from animal models for specific malformations that have been developed to study the underlying mechanisms of epileptogenesis, reviewed recently by Jacobs *et al.*[179] Lesions similar to cortical dysplasia and lissencephaly are produced by giving teratogens, such as methylazoxymethanol acetate (MAM) and ionizing radiation, early, during the time of cortical neuroblast generation and migration, resulting in death of the dividing cells and injury to migrating cells. These animals do not have spontaneous seizures but have an increased propensity to seizures and a lowered threshold to proconvulsant substances. In the MAM-treated animal there are increased numbers of CA1 and neocortical neurons that respond to an intracellular depolarizing current pulse with a high-frequency burst of action potentials, and this type of neuron is thought to participate in epileptogenesis. The local application of an insult, a freezing probe or an injection of ibotenic acid, during the late stages of cortical development leads to a focal region of cortical neuronal death without injury to migrating cells and has been used to produce models of four-layered polymicrogyria and nodular heterotopia. Slice preparations from these animals are hyperexcitable. Some studies show that there is an increase in postsynaptic glutamate receptors and a decrease in $GABA_A$ receptors in the microgyric cortex, and others that the affected area lacks thalamic sensory afferents, which project instead to the adjacent cortex, which increases the excitatory connectivity in this area. The area surrounding the microgyrus is epileptogenic while the malformation itself is not.

Vascular malformations

The other group of developmental abnormalities in which epilepsy is a common clinical manifestation are vascular malformations of the brain. Seizures are often the sole clinical feature and occasionally the diagnosis is made only after surgery for epilepsy.[104,207] Epilepsy is more common with supratentorial lesions than with lesions elsewhere in the brain. Venous and capillary malformations occur more frequently, but are rarely associated with seizures, compared with arteriovenous malformations and cavernous angiomas. The mechanism of seizure production in vascular malformations is not completely understood, but mass effect, haemorrhage, gliosis and neuronal loss are factors that are implicated. There is progressive gliosis within and around arteriovenous malformations, with neuronal loss in the adjacent cortex. Much of this is considered to be ischaemic in origin, due to the steal phenomenon, and may contribute to the epileptogenesis. Haemorrhage leading to deposition of haemosiderin and subsequent iron-induced free radical generation and lipid peroxidation probably also plays a role in epileptogenesis.

Sturge–Weber syndrome is a congenital malformation of cephalic vasculature, characterized by a telangiectatic

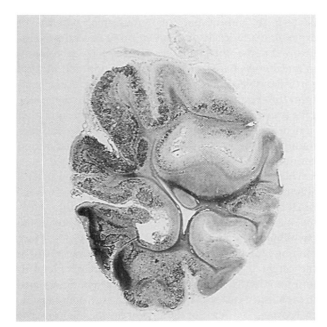

a

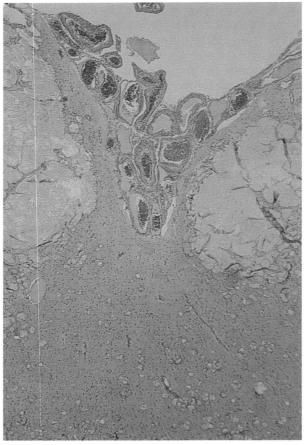

b

Figure 15.4 *Sturge–Weber syndrome. (a) Coronal slice through the occipital lobe of a total hemispherectomy showing calcific deposits. (b) Leptomeningeal angiomatosis overlying the calcified cortex. (a: H&E; b: H Van Gieson.)*

venous angioma of the leptomeninges over the parieto-occipital region or all of one cerebral hemisphere, and ipsilateral facial angiomatous naevus (Fig. 15.4). Calcified deposits may be visible on the skull X-ray.[135] Up to 90% of patients have seizures, which may be partial or generalized, and commonly commence in infancy.

Infections

Seizures may occur during or as a sequel to any inflammatory disorder of the brain. Epilepsy may result from meningitis, encephalitis in the acute stage and the resultant scarring in the brain, cerebral abscess and granulomatous inflammation. Annegers *et al.*[11] examined the records of 714 survivors of encephalitis and meningitis between 1935 and 1981 to evaluate the risk of seizures after infections of the CNS. Nineteen per cent of patients had seizures during the acute phase of the infection. The 20-year risk of developing seizures after viral encephalitis ranged from 10% in those who had not experienced seizures in the acute illness to 22% in those who had. The risk was 2.4% without early seizures and 13% with early seizures in patients after bacterial meningitis. Aseptic meningitis does not increase the risk of developing epilepsy. The presence of permanent neurological deficit after bacterial meningitis identifies those at high risk of developing epilepsy.[315] Most patients develop partial seizures with secondary generalization, and while postmeningitic seizures are commonly associated with medial temporal sclerosis, most postencephalitic epilepsy results from neocortical foci.[242,315] The occurrence of bacterial meningitis in young children and the susceptibility of the hippocampus to early insult may explain this difference.

The incidence of seizures is high in patients with cerebral abscesses, affecting 25% of patients at presentation.[238] In patients who survive, long-term follow-up shows an incidence of epilepsy of up to 72%, with children faring worse than adults.[44,219,274] This appears not to be influenced by the method of treatment. Patients with tuberculous meningitis may develop seizures as an early feature or as a late complication of the infection.[429] Seizures are a common symptom in patients with intracerebral tuberculomas, occurring even with cerebellar lesions.[79]

Parasitic infections

Epilepsy is a well-recognized complication of a variety of parasitic infestations, and these constitute an important cause of epilepsy in parts of the world where such diseases are common. In an extensive review of the relationship of parasitosis to epilepsy, Bittencourt *et al.*[35] examined the major parasitic infestations of the CNS. The seizures are usually partial and may become generalized, with the exception of cerebral malaria in which seizures are more often generalized from the outset. Epilepsy is seen in up to 60% of cases of neurocysticercosis, and is frequently the presenting feature. Cysticercosis is an important cause of epilepsy in Mexico,[110] it is the most common cause of adult-onset epilepsy in Portugal[273] and was found to be the aetiology in 5% of adults evaluated for recent-onset epilepsy in India.[3] Seizures are commonly seen in toxoplasmosis, in the acquired immunodeficiency syndrome (AIDS) and in babies with congenital infections, in African trypanosomiasis; and in hydatid disease, when it affects the brain.[35,95]

Rasmussen's syndrome

Rasmussen's syndrome or encephalitis is an unusual seizure disorder refractory to anticonvulsant therapy, characterized by progressive unilateral neurological deficit, and the morphological changes of a chronic inflammatory process restricted to one cerebral hemisphere.[322] Seizures begin abruptly, usually in childhood, and consist of focal seizures, partial complex seizures and generalized seizures, followed by hemiplegia, hemianopsia and intellectual deterioration. Progressive cerebral atrophy, which may be localized to part or may involve the whole hemisphere, is demonstrated radiologically. Surgery is the treatment of choice. The pathological changes vary in severity. Atrophy of gyri may be seen macroscopically (Fig. 15.5a) and is patchy in the hemispherectomy specimens. The change can be subtle in those cases coming to surgery 1–2 years after the onset of the seizures, with slight discoloration and granularity accompanying focal thinning of the cortex. In more chronic cases, there is more widespread hemiatrophy with ventricular dilatation.

The microscopic changes are widespread and are also seen in macroscopically normal areas. There may be leptomeningeal thickening with collections of lymphocytes and macrophages. Perivascular inflammatory cell cuffs consisting mainly of lymphocytes and macrophages and aggregates of cells composed of microglial cells and lymphocytes, the 'microglial nodules', are seen in the cortex, in the white matter and less often in the basal ganglia (Fig. 15.5b–d). Neuronophagia is a consistent finding. In longstanding cases, the thinned cortex is spongy and gliotic and there is virtually complete loss of neurons. Capillary proliferation may be prominent. The inflammation is sparse in the scarred, shrunken cortex, but more active inflammation is usually found elsewhere in the specimen.[167,321] Post-mortem studies confirm the essentially unilateral nature of the disorder; the contralateral hemisphere, the brainstem and the cerebellum are free of inflammatory pathology.[136,333] In rare instances there has been clinical and radiological evidence of bilateral hemispheric involvement, confirmed at autopsy in one case.[57,88]

There is some resemblance to Kozhevnikov's epilepsy, a chronic tick-borne viral encephalitis with intractable epilepsy, rarely seen outside Russia.[294,425] Rasmussen's

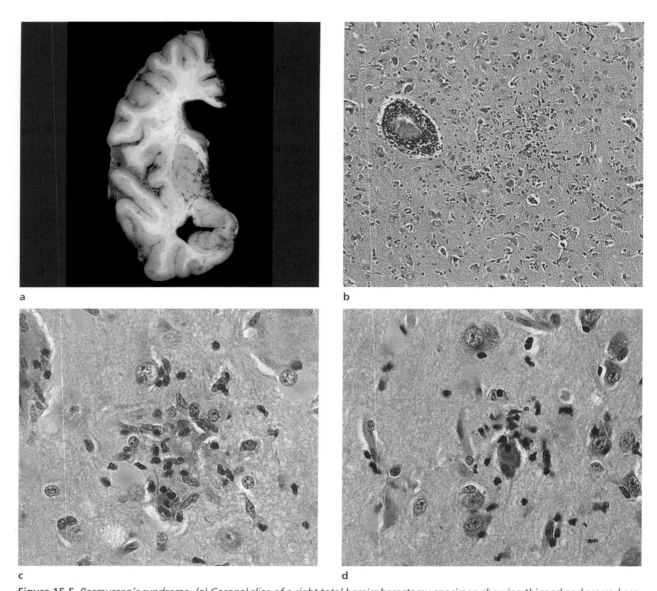

a

b

c

d

Figure 15.5 *Rasmussen's syndrome. (a) Coronal slice of a right total hemispherectomy specimen showing thinned and scarred cortex in the parasagittal and perisylvian regions. The putamen and globus pallidus are mildly discoloured. (b) Perivascular lymphocytic cuff with inflammatory cells infiltrating the adjacent parenchyma. (c) Cellular aggregates composed of lymphocytes, microglial cells and astrocytes. (d) Neuronophagia. These inflammatory changes and striking astrogliosis are widespread in the cortex, white matter and deep grey nuclei, extending well beyond macroscopically abnormal areas. (b–d: H&E.)*

syndrome, however, lacks the clinical profile of an encephalitic illness, and although the histological appearances are strongly suggestive of a viral infection, no aetiological agent has yet been isolated. *In situ* hybridization and polymerase chain reaction studies have implicated Epstein–Barr virus[403] and cytomegalovirus,[316] although other studies using similar techniques have failed to demonstrate the presence of viral genomic material.[118,167] Reports of patients developing ipsilateral uveitis and choroiditis before or shortly after the onset of seizures have added to the speculation of a viral aetiology.[127,136,149] It has also been suggested that immune complex deposition and vasculitis may be responsible for the disorder.[9] Immunofluorescence staining showed granular accumulation of

immunoglobulin G (IgG), IgM, IgA, C3 and C1q within blood-vessel walls, and there was ultrastructural evidence of vascular injury in a hemispherectomy specimen from a young child with the clinical and pathological features of the syndrome. More recently, Rogers *et al.*[337] postulated that an autoimmune process underlies the condition. Two rabbits used to raise antibodies to GluR-3 receptor proteins developed seizures and had pathological features similar to those of Rasmussen's encephalitis. Further, on examining the sera of four children with pathologically proven Rasmussen's syndrome, immunoreactivity to GluR-3 was demonstrated in three, all of whom had progressive disease or ongoing seizures. There appears to be a correlation between GluR-3 immunoreactivity and disease activity. The fourth patient, who did not have antibodies to GluR-3, had been free from seizures for 2 years after a hemispherectomy. Plasmapheresis leading to a reduction in plasma GluR-3 antibodies is associated with clinical improvement. The antibodies to GluR-3 modulate neuronal excitability by acting as agonists at the glutamate receptor.[390] The finding of additional cerebral pathology in resection specimens of Rasmussen's syndrome, such as cortical dysplasia, tuberous sclerosis, forme fruste of tuberous sclerosis, cavernous angioma and tumour, has led to the suggestion that these lesions induce seizures causing alterations in the blood–brain barrier, that subsequently permit a viral or autoimmune disorder to develop.[148,298,421] The latter hypothesis is supported by the presence of antibodies to GluR-3 receptor in a patient with concomitant Rasmussen's syndrome and cortical dysplasia.[298]

Trauma

Epilepsy has long been established as a late consequence of head injury. The risk of developing post-traumatic epilepsy is related to the severity and type of injury. In a study of 356 casualties of the Korean campaign between 1951 and 1954, it was shown that patients with severe cortical injury producing neurological deficits, but with an intact dura mater, have a 7–39% incidence of epilepsy, while in those where the dura mater has been penetrated, the incidence rises to 20–57%.[51] Similar results were reported in an assessment of the records of servicemen in World War I who sustained gunshot wounds to the head.[18] The incidence of post-traumatic epilepsy in a study of 500 soldiers from World War II who had experienced non-missile, closed head injury was 6%[310] and rose to 43% in a series evaluating the progress of 820 men after gunshot wounds with dural penetration.[340] Depressed skull fractures, dural penetration, cortical laceration, loss of brain tissue, intracerebral haematoma and retained foreign material are factors that contribute to the increased risk of post-traumatic epilepsy.[182,184,343] Seizures early after the head injury are also predictive of an increased risk of late epilepsy. The incidence of post-traumatic epilepsy is lower as a result of civilian injuries,[74,183] presumably reflecting the higher proportion of closed head injuries in this group. Russell and Whitty[340] stressed the importance of the site of injury. The incidence of epilepsy was highest when the injury was to the parietal lobe and the motor area.

It is likely that epileptogenesis results from a combination of factors. The presence of a gliotic scar has been considered a factor in the development of not only post-traumatic epilepsy, but also that caused by healed abscesses and ischaemic lesions, and it is hypothesized that seizures result from disordered neuroglial function.[304,306,314] Using an animal model of post-traumatic epilepsy, Hoeppner and Morrell[163] demonstrated that the collagenous component of the scar, rather than the glial, was more significant in epileptogenesis. Strategies to reduce epileptiform activity favoured reduced collagenous scar formation. The increased risk of developing seizures following the occurrence of traumatic haematoma, spontaneous haematoma and haemorrhagic infarction led Willmore[409] to postulate that the presence of blood in the neuropil is a critical aetiological factor, and that iron liberated from haemoglobin and transferrin may be important in epileptogenesis. Cortical ferrous or ferric chloride injections into rat and cat sensorimotor cortex induced recurrent focal epileptiform discharges.[410] Tissue obtained from the injection site shortly after the injection showed increased levels of superoxide radicals. These are thought to contribute to the tissue damage that is responsible for epileptogenesis through lipid peroxidation, and pretreatment with antioxidants prevents the severe tissue necrosis and astrogliosis, and the development of seizures that follows the cortical injection of ferric chloride in rats.[409]

It is suggested that post-traumatic temporal lobe epilepsy differs from that not related to trauma. The patients are older, there is less Ammon's horn neuronal loss in the temporal lobectomy specimens, and they have better seizure outcomes after temporal lobe surgery.[245] Old cortical or white-matter scars are found in half of the specimens from patients with post-traumatic epilepsy.

Tumours

Intracranial tumours are a common cause of seizures. Brain tumours, along with cerebral infarcts, were the most common causes identified in a study of late-onset epilepsy carried out on 221 patients over the age of 25 years.[77] The mean incidence of epilepsy in the presence of cerebral neoplasms is 35%.[216] Tumours in the supratentorial compartment, particularly those involving cerebral cortex, compared with those in the white matter or the deep cerebral nuclei, are much more frequently associated with seizures.[197,216,354] The incidence of epilepsy appears to correlate inversely with the rate of tumour growth; low-grade glioma is more than twice as likely to present with seizures than is glioblastoma. This is reflected in the prognosis; in a retrospective study of 560 patients with primary intracerebral tumours, the median survival was 37 months in the 164 patients presenting with epilepsy, compared with 6 months in those who presented with other symptoms.[365] The occurrence of epilepsy in different histological types of tumours of the CNS was averaged from reports of several large series, and showed that seizures were seen in 70.9% of oligodendrogliomas, 58.5% of astrocytomas, 36.9% of meningiomas and 28.9% of glioblastoma.[197] Seizures were also seen in about one-third of a variety of other tumours. In a report of a series of children operated for low-grade astrocytoma and oligodendroglioma, epilepsy was the presenting feature in 76% and the only clinical sign in 62%; there was a significant reduction to 19% in the incidence of seizures after surgery.[160]

Data obtained from accounts of the surgical management of chronic epilepsy show that tumours presenting with seizures and without clinical evidence of space occupation are predominantly low-grade intrinsic neoplasms, with astrocytoma, oligodendroglioma, ganglioglioma and dysembryoplastic neuroepithelial tumour being most frequently seen.[38,41,165,251,418] The mixed neuronal–glial tumours, ganglioglioma and dysembryoplastic neuroepithelial tumour are rare, and present almost invariably with epilepsy; epilepsy is the most common presenting feature in up to 90% of gangliogliomas and in virtually all dysembryoplastic neuroepithelial tumours.[80,165,319,324,415] Irrespective of the histological type and grade, glial tumours associated with chronic intractable seizures appear to constitute a distinct clinicopathological group, with a long history and indolent behaviour.[25,125] The long–term outcome has been shown to be better than that expected of patients with similar tumours who do not have chronic epilepsy. Certainly, results of surgery for dysembryoplastic neuroepithelial tumour in terms of both control of epilepsy and tumour recurrence are very good, even when the removal of the tumour was thought to be incomplete.[80,154,201]

Disorganization of cortical laminar architecture, neuronal clustering, ectopic neurons and neuronocytomegaly are among the dysplastic changes seen in the cortex adjacent to some tumours associated with chronic epilepsy. A defining feature of dysembryoplastic neuroepithelial tumour, cortical dysplasia has also been found with gangliogliomas and low-grade astrocytomas from patients with epilepsy.[80,165,318,319,415] There is evidence to suggest that the epileptogenicity of the mixed neuronal–glial tumours may result from the neuronal component; a variety of neurotransmitter producing enzymes, neurotransmitter receptors, neuropeptides and calcium-binding proteins have been demonstrated in dysembryoplastic neuroepithelial tumour and gangliogliomas.[413,417] Hyperexcitability of the cortex surrounding tumours associated with seizures has been suggested by a study demonstrating decreased GABA and somatostatin neurons in the cortex adjacent to low-grade astrocytomas compared with controls.[140] An ultrastructural study has shown that loss of the inhibitory synapses on the body and initial segment of the axon of pyramidal cells, and the presence of numerous excitatory synapses on dendrites, in peritumoral cortex from a patient with epilepsy, account for the hyperexcitable state.[240]

CHANGES SECONDARY TO EPILEPSY

Neuropathological changes secondary to epilepsy can be classified under four aetiological headings.

- Acute neuronal damage secondary to status epilepticus provides the most definitively identifiable pathology; relevant clinical and experimental data are discussed in the following section.

- There is tentative evidence from post-mortem studies that chronic seizures result in the loss of neurons and reactive gliosis (that is not necessarily secondary to nerve cell loss).
- Seizures may result in traumatic injury to the brain through falls.
- There is the possibility of iatrogenic damage relating to surgical or medical treatment.

That seizures of limited duration cause cell loss and gliosis is an inference from quantitative studies showing reduced neuronal counts in material from patients with epilepsy compared with age-matched, seizure-free patients[75,76] and from studies of temporal lobectomy specimens where seizures are secondary to a tumour or other mass lesion.[124,224] Neuronal loss seems to involve the same neuronal groups that are vulnerable to status epilepticus. There is loss of pyramidal cells in the hippocampus similar to but less severe than that after status epilepticus. There may also be neocortical cell loss.

Superficial erosions and contusions may be found in the brains of chronic epileptics, as a result of frequent falls and head injury. The reported incidence of such findings at autopsy varies from 11 to 36%,[241,346] but is now seen much less frequently. The lesions are usually seen on the orbital surface of the frontal lobes, the frontal and temporal poles and the inferior surface of the temporal lobes.

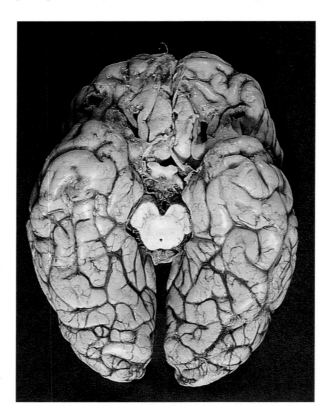

Figure 15.6 *Previous traumatic injury. Multiple old contusions on the orbital surfaces of both frontal lobes in the brain of an elderly man with longstanding epilepsy, resulting from falls during seizures.*

Multiple lesions with different chronology may be found (Fig. 15.6). Contrecoup lesions of the temporal pole are not accompanied by hippocampal sclerosis.[241]

Epileptic brain damage

Bouchet and Cazauvieilh[39] in 1825 first described a pattern of damage that is characteristically found in patients with epilepsy who were thought to require institutional care. They described a predominantly unilateral atrophic hardening of Ammon's horn (Fig. 15.7), a (lobular) atrophy of the cerebellum (Fig. 15.8) and diffuse cortical atrophy. Subsequent landmarks in the description of epileptic brain damage include the contributions of Sommer,[367] Pfleger,[309] Spielmeyer,[369] Scholz[351,352] and Margerison and Corsellis.[241]

Sommer's contribution was notable for the precision of his description of the cell loss in the hippocampus, in terms of both the cell types involved and their topographical distribution (pyramidal cell loss in the 'Sommer sector', roughly corresponding to the CA1 subfield of Lorente de No[228]). The pyramidal cell layer of the Ammon's horn is divided into zones CA1–CA4 (Fig. 15.9). In addition to severe neuronal loss in the highly vulnerable CA1 area, neurons are lost from the endfolium in CA4 and CA3 areas. The CA2 area or 'resistant zone' is relatively well preserved. The small neurons of the dentate fascia may also be depleted. The cell loss is accompanied by fibrillary gliosis. The changes are usually seen along the full length of the hippocampus. Pfleger[309] described what appeared to be haemorrhagic lesions in the amygdala and hippocampus of patients dying shortly after status epilepticus and concluded that local vascular events associated with the seizures were causing focal lesions. Spielmeyer was impressed by the similarity, in terms of acute cellular changes ('ischaemic cell change') and the selective pattern of cell loss, to the effects of cerebral ischaemia. The common features included the laminar pattern in the cortex with diffuse loss initially in lamina

III and then lamina II, with the more severe cases often showing preservation of lamina V and VI, and the lobular pattern of cerebellar damage with Purkinje cells showing the highest vulnerability followed by granule cells. He proposed that vasospasm associated with the seizure onset was responsible for the pathology. Penfield's direct intraoperative observations and the subsequent quantitative studies by others[55] revealed that seizure activity is associated with local vasodilatation and enhanced cerebral blood flow rather than ischaemia. There is, however, a marked increase in oxygen and glucose utilization.[55] Scholz and others developed the concept of 'consumptive hypoxia'. That the enhanced metabolic activity associated with seizure activity contributes to pathological outcome continues to be part of the thinking about mechanisms; it plays a role in the modified excitotoxic theory presented in the following section.

Postmortem studies of chronic epileptic brain damage culminated in those of Stauder[373] Sano and Malamud[346] and Margerison and Corsellis,[241] all of which emphasized the correlation between clinical and EEG signs of temporal lobe epilepsy and the occurrence of hippocampal sclerosis. In the 55 brains studied by Margerison and Corsellis damage was most frequently found in the hippocampus (55%), compared with the cerebellum (45%), the amygdaloid nucleus (27%), the thalamus (25%) and the cortex (22%) (Fig. 15.9). Cerebellar damage occurred as an isolated lesion in some patients, but thalamic or amygdalar damage was always accompanied by hippocampal damage. More than one-third of the patients with hippocampal sclerosis did not show damage in the Sommer sector or CA1 but showed bilateral or unilateral endfolium sclerosis. The overall pattern of 'hypoxic' brain damage in the institutionalized patients is very similar to the overall pattern of acute hypoxic/ischaemic brain damage found in adults or children dying shortly after severe status epilepticus (see below). It raises the question of whether such damage is the result of an early severe seizure or the cumulative effect of minor degrees of damage associated with less prolonged seizures, or both phenomena. Similar patterns of damage can be seen after cardiac arrest or other hypoxic/ischaemic episodes, but such episodes do not figure in the history of most epileptic patients. Birth injury or asphyxia gives rise to a different pattern of pathology with a predominant emphasis on the basal ganglia, and if hippocampal damage is present it does not show the CA1 and CA4 selectivity characteristic of epileptic brain damage. These issues are discussed further below (see section on Mesial temporal sclerosis and complex partial seizures, below).

Subpial gliosis or Chaslin's gliosis[56] is seen in longstanding epilepsy (Fig. 15.10). A dense band of glial fibres expands the normally fine glia limitans. The gliosis varies from area to area, often extending deeper into the cortex. It is not restricted to any particular region of the brain or to any particular type of epilepsy. It was considered by Chaslin to be a primary lesion in its own right, the

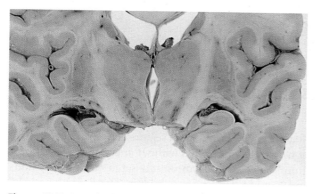

Figure 15.7 *Atrophic hippocampus. Markedly shrunken left hippocampus from the brain of a chronic epileptic subject. The adjacent parahippocampal gyrus is also atrophic. The right side is normal.*

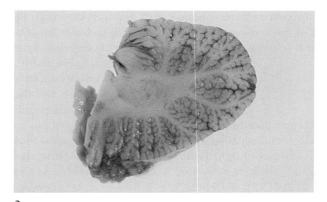

a

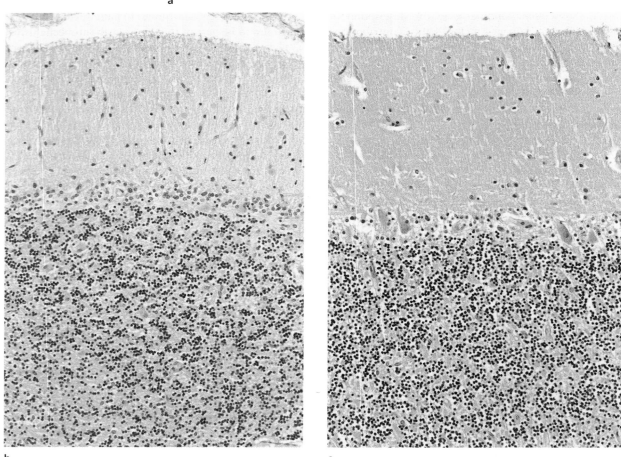

b   c

Figure 15.8 *Cerebellar atrophy. (a) This may be seen in some patients with chronic epilepsy. (b) Histological examination shows loss of Purkinje cells, proliferation of Bergmann glia and a sparse granule cell layer compared with (c) normal cerebellar cortex. (b, c: H&E.)*

proliferation of glial fibres causing the seizures. Subsequently it was recognized to be a secondary change. Corsellis and Meyer[69] reported seeing it in patients with grand mal seizures, and in those who had undergone chemical or electric convulsive therapy. Similar gliosis may also be present in the periventricular subependymal areas and around blood vessels in the white matter. It may be secondary to acute changes in the composition of extracellular fluid (unknown but potentially involving ionic composition at one extreme and trophic factors at the other).

Status epilepticus

Status epilepticus refers to seizure activity that is continuous, or intermittent but without intervening recovery, for a prolonged period, commonly set at 60 min for adults and 30 min for infants and children. This definition is relevant to the pathological literature but it has recently been proposed that for therapeutic purposes the operational definition of status epilepticus should be 'continuous seizures lasting at least 5 minutes or two or more discrete seizures between which there is incomplete recovery of consciousness'.[230] Generalized status epilepticus is a medical emergency that continues to have a high morbidity and mortality in spite of the general introduction into emergency treatment of rapid intervention with pharmacological and general measures.[358] It occurs in

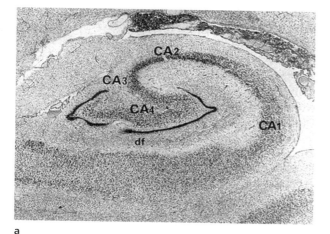

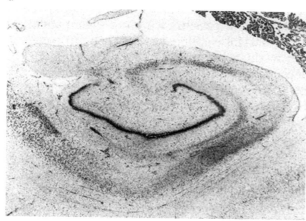

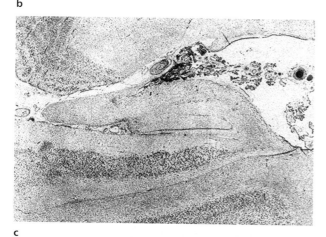

Figure 15.9 *Normal hippocampus. (a) The pyramidal cell layer is divided into zones CA1–CA4 (see text). (b) Acute selective necrosis of the hippocampus after status epilepticus. Relative preservation of CA2 can be seen. (c) The classic Ammon's horn of hippocampal sclerosis. (a–c: Cresyl violet.)*

patients who were previously seizure free and in patients with known epilepsy. In the latter group non-compliance with antiepileptic medication is the most common cause of status epilepticus.[8] In patients without a history of epilepsy the most common causes are cerebrovascular disease and drug overdose, but tumour, trauma, cardiac arrest and alcohol withdrawal are also significant. Unfavourable outcomes (neurological morbidity or mortality) are associated with particular precipitating circumstances (cardiac arrest, head injury), hyperpyrexia (which may be secondary to the seizure) and seizure duration longer than 2 h.[8]

In 1904 Clark and Prout[60] described 38 cases of status epilepticus, seven of whom died during or after the status and came to post-mortem. The predominant finding in the cerebral cortex was chromatolysis in pyramidal neurons of laminae II and III, often associated with lymphocytic infiltration. Subsequently, reports on adults dying shortly after status epilepticus are scarce; since Scholz's 1951 review[351] there have been two case reports[264,285] and a summary[68] describing 12 adult cases, only five of whom showed acute neuronal damage. These studies report little gross abnormality and little acute swelling (except sometimes in the hippocampus), while occasionally there is congestion or discoloration. Cell loss or ischaemic cell change is seen in the hippocampus, sometimes with an acute glial reaction (Fig. 15.9b). Laminar neuronal loss occurs usually in a patchy fashion in the neocortex (Fig. 15.11); in the cerebellum there is Purkinje cell loss and, when damage is severe, granule cell loss. The thalamus and other cerebral deep grey matter are more exceptionally involved.

Hospital-based studies of infants and children have indicated a particularly unfavourable outcome of prolonged febrile convulsions and status epilepticus. Aicardi and Chevrie[4] in a study of 239 infants and children, found mental or neurological residua in 57% of their patients. Population-based studies give a much more optimistic prognosis for febrile convulsions and status epilepticus.[253,254,395] Post-mortem studies in children present a more consistent picture of damage than studies in adults and suggest a higher degree of vulnerability in

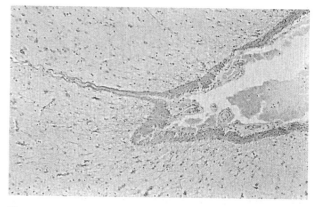

Figure 15.10 *Chaslin's subpial gliosis. Lobectomy specimen that showed mesial temporal sclerosis. (GFAP immunocytochemistry.)*

infants and children up to 3 years of age.[68,123,289,428] Loss of pyramidal neurons in the Sommer sector is often almost total. In the cerebellum, loss of Purkinje cells may be severe and associated with cell loss in the granular layer. There is nerve cell loss in cortical laminae II and III. The thalamus may show severe focal damage, whereas striatal damage is less common. There is no definitive difference in the pattern of damage in young children compared with adults; the difference is the greater chance of finding damage in children and its greater severity.

Domoic acid poisoning, resulting from consumption of blue mussels that have fed on *Chondria armata* or *Pseudonitzschia pungens*, produces an acute clinical picture with confusion and signs of limbic seizures. Chronically there is commonly anterograde amnesia, particularly for visuospatial material.[382] Four elderly men came to post-mortem 7 days to 3 months after the acute intoxication and showed consistent patterns of neuronal loss and astrocytosis. The hippocampus and amygdala showed the most severe lesions with the characteristic pattern of pyramidal cell loss in hippocampal subfields (H2 being relatively preserved). Loss of dentate granule cells was seen in three of the four patients. All four had lesions in the claustrum, secondary olfactory areas, septal area and nucleus accumbens, three had damage in lamina VI of the insular and subfrontal cortex and two had thalamic damage, particularly the dorsomedial nucleus. The pattern of cortical damage is clearly different from that seen after generalized status epilepticus. It might be thought to reflect the excitotoxic action of domoic acid, as kainate receptors have a high density in laminae V and VI; a similar pattern of damage is, however, seen in rodents receiving intrahippocampal kainate[181] and the cortical damage can be prevented by administration of an NMDA receptor antagonist, implying that the local pattern of enhanced excitatory activity is responsible for the cortical pathology. A further elderly male developed temporal lobe epilepsy 1 year after exposure to domoic acid that had resulted in exceptionally prolonged initial limbic status epilepticus. This pattern of limbic system damage is closely similar to that seen in rodents or non-human primates in which limbic seizures are induced either by kainate or domoate or by pilocarpine.[52] The seizures were controlled with phenytoin but the patient had severe amnesia. At death 3 years after the initial exposure the brain showed severe bilateral hippocampal atrophy and patchy neuronal loss in medial and basal amygdala. Neuronal loss and gliosis was also seen in the mesial temporal cortex, dorsal and ventral septal nuclei. This is perhaps the best documented case in which mesial temporal sclerosis acquired late in life was, after a latent interval, associated with the onset of temporal lobe epilepsy.

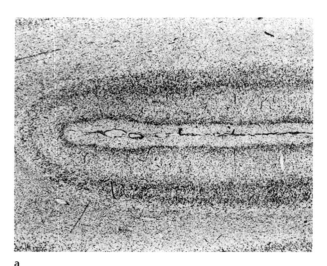

a

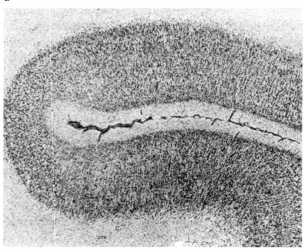

b

Figure 15.11 *Status epilepticus. (a) Cerebral cortex of an infant dying shortly after an episode of status epilepticus. Extensive neuronal necrosis has destroyed the middle layers, and particularly the third. The resulting pallor is seen when compared with the normal cortex (b). (Cresyl violet.)*

The assumption that the acute brain damage seen in children dying after status epilepticus was hypoxic/ischaemic damage secondary to events occurring during or after the seizures dominated thinking until 1973.[302,351,427] A role for systemic factors was supported by the clinical observation that most children succumbing after status epilepticus had periods of cardiorespiratory failure during or after the status epilepticus. Meldrum and Brierley[259] used prolonged seizures induced by bicuculline in physiologically monitored baboons to examine these issues. They showed that status lasting for longer than 90 min was associated with the acute appearance of ischaemic cell change in the hippocampus, neocortex and cerebellum, and that its incidence and severity correlated with the duration of cortical seizure activity, severity of hyperthermia and delayed arterial hypotension. When secondary systemic changes were minimized by motor paralysis and artificial respiration, damage to the cerebellum was diminished but the pattern of hippocampal damage was unaltered.[261] Meldrum[257,258] concluded that the local enhancement of excitatory activity and metabolic rate was contributing critically to the hippocampal damage. These observations in baboons were subsequently confirmed by a wide range of studies in rodents, using the same or related models of either generalized or limbic system seizures.[29,360,363,389] Acute hippocampal pathology could occur after bicuculline-induced seizures in the absence of any local ischaemia or hypoxia.[281] The role of systemic changes in cortical and cerebellar damage was complex. Hyperpyrexia clearly exacerbates damage, especially in the cerebellum, but mild or moderate degrees of hypoxia or arterial hypotension could be protective,[36] possibly because they limited seizure activity or because 'oxidative damage' was reduced following the metabolic or excitotoxic stress. An increase in superoxide generation has been demonstrated in bicuculline-induced seizures in newborn pigs.[15]

The importance of local neuronal or metabolic activity related to the seizure is emphasized by the pathology observed clinically and experimentally with focal seizures. Predominantly limbic seizures can be induced in rodents and non-human primates by the systemic or intracerebral injection of kainate (or domoate) and by the systemic administration of pilocarpine, with or without lithium. These models produce damage predominantly within the limbic circuit, involving the hippocampus, the amygdala, the claustrum, some thalamic nuclei, the pyriform and olfactory cortex, the thalamic nuclei and the pars reticularis of the substantia nigra.[29,176,263,386,389]

Within the hippocampus the pattern of damage is similar to that seen with other models except that CA3 damage is often most prominent in kainate seizures. The pyriform cortex damage is commonly very severe in kainate or pilocarpine seizures. Nigral damage is also seen in some rodent models of generalized epilepsy, e.g. flurothyl seizures,[176,281] but has not been described for limbic or generalized status in children or adults or in non-human primates. Focal motor seizures also clearly show regional damage that correlates with anatomical pathways of spread of enhanced neuronal activity. Thus, in severe unilateral seizures cerebellar damage is found in the hemisphere contralateral to the seizures and the neocortical and thalamic degeneration. In an experimental model of focal cortical epilepsy neurodegeneration is observed in the thalamus. The most definitive experimental demonstration of the role of neuronal activity is provided by the model in the rat, employing perforant path stimulation.[293,360,361] This can induce cell loss restricted to the end-folium.

The most important factor linking seizure activity to selective neuronal death appears to be the entry of sodium and more particularly calcium into neurons.[257,258,404] Overloading the mechanisms for intracellular sequestration of calcium and outward transport of calcium is associated with marked increases in the intracellular concentration of calcium that activates a wide range of enzymes with diverse secondary consequences. The use of the oxalate/pyroantimonate method to visualize free calcium in the rat brain after 30–90 min of seizure activity showed that in the hippocampal neuropil focal swellings on dendrites contained free calcium and grossly swollen mitochondria heavily laden with calcium[111,137] and pyramidal cell bodies also showed distended mitochondria with heavy calcium loading (Fig. 15.12). The nucleus also showed enhanced calcium content. Among the enzymes activated by the rise in intracellular $[Ca^{2+}]$ are various proteases including calpain with the effect of damaging the cytoskeleton and forming xanthine oxidase.[260] A large number of kinases are activated, including calmodulin kinase. Activation of phospholipase A_2 leads to the formation of free fatty acids including arachidonic acid initiating a cascade involving cyclooxygenase and lipoxygenase. Calcium also activates (through calmodulin) nitric oxide synthase, converting arginine to nitric oxide which may be cytotoxic. Within the nucleus there is activation of endonucleases. What determines irreversibility in this process is not clear; mitochondrial swelling and calcium loading can be quite severe but if seizure activity is blocked with diazepam morphological recovery can occur in 30–60 min.[112,138]

When the insult is severe the pattern of morphological change is that of ischaemic cell change, ending with necrotic fragments undergoing neuronophagia. It appears that seizures can also trigger apoptotic cell death, which does not entrain a glial response.

Activation of NMDA receptors during the course of the epileptic discharges clearly plays a crucial role in the enhanced calcium entry and subsequent cell death. Thus, compounds that act as antagonists at the NMDA receptor can prevent most of the limbic pathology induced by systemic kainate even when they do not reduce the duration of status epilepticus.[61,117,223] They can also protect against thalamic damage in focal cortical status.[62] NMDA receptor activation depends on the pattern of synaptic activation, rather than on a sustained increase in extracellular glutamate concentration, so that in this respect epileptic brain damage does not match the paradigms of excitotoxic damage (periventricular lesions in neonatal rodents, and in vitro nerve cell death due to glutamate or NMDA exposure).

In vivo and in vitro the neuronal toxicity of NMDA can be enhanced by mitochondrial poisons. In status epilepticus the mitochondria are being poisoned by calcium overload; in this circumstance there is evidence that superoxide is generated; this can be toxic to the cell generally but it can also damage mtDNA in a cumulative fashion. Such damage also occurs with ageing and may facilitate selective nerve cell loss in a variety of conditions.[27] This is a possible mechanism whereby repeated seizures, none of which was severe enough to produce acute neuronal degeneration, might facilitate cell loss.

Experimental evidence for such a process is limited but includes (1) data in electrically kindled rats which experience only brief limbic seizures but develop evidence of hilar cell loss[48,50] and (2) experiments with silver stains showing occasional isolated degenerating neurons after

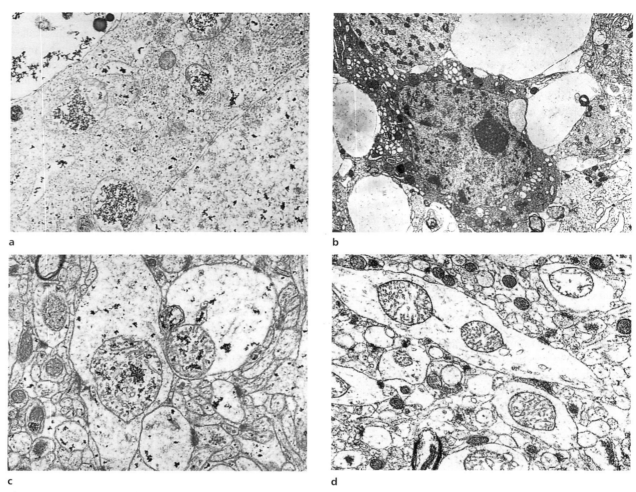

Figure 15.12 *Experimental seizures. (a) Rat hippocampal pyramidal neuron (oxalate-pyroantimonate/osmium) showing free calcium in a swollen mitochondrion, endoplasmic reticulum and nucleus after 90 min of seizure activity. In the upper left corner a swollen astrocytic process is visible. (b) Necrotic hippocampal pyramidal neuron showing cytoplasmic condensation and vacuolation surrounded by dilated astrocytic processes following bicuculline-induced status epilepticus in the rat. (c) Focal dendritic swellings containing dilated mitochondria loaded with calcium in the hippocampus following 90 min of seizure activity (oxalate and pyroantimonate/osmium method). (d) Focal dendritic swellings containing grossly swollen mitochondria in the rat hippocampus following 90 min of seizure activity. Note the presence of normal mitochondria. Photographs by T Griffiths, deceased.*

single seizures or after-discharges.[169] The stronger evidence comes from hippocampal cell density studies in lobectomy specimens where there is a mass lesion that is the presumed primary cause of the focal seizures and there is no history of an early prolonged seizure, trauma, etc. Such studies consistently show cell densities lower than those in control patients but of lesser severity than those with Ammon's horn sclerosis.[20,124,198,224] Levesque *et al.*[224] found no correlation with the total number of seizures but a correlation with the type of mass lesion, gliomas being associated with a lesser degree of cell loss (less than 30%), whereas neuronal heterotopia was associated with loss equivalent in severity to mesial temporal sclerosis. Hamartomas were associated with an intermediate level of cell loss. In a smaller series Fried *et al.*[124] found a correlation between cell loss and location of the mass lesion; mesial temporal lesions being associated with lower cell counts. Dam[75,76] in her post-mortem study found a 20% neuronal loss in all hippocampal subfields with age over 65 years in normals and a loss in epilepsy in all hippocampal fields and in granule cells that increased with the duration in years of the epilepsy.

Febrile convulsions

Febrile convulsions are usually manifest as generalized seizures occurring in children under the age of 5 years during the course of a febrile illness. In clinical practice it may be difficult to differentiate true febrile convulsions in which the infective agent does not directly involve the brain from seizures secondary to meningitis or encephalitis.

Febrile convulsions have an incidence significantly greater than that of epilepsy. A national cohort study in the UK found that 398 children out of 14 676 (2.7%) had one or more febrile convulsions.[394,395] Similar figures (2.4% and 2.9%) have been reported in population studies from Minnesota, USA[152] and six temperate climate populations.[221] The incidence is higher in tropical countries.[105,141] Simple febrile convulsions are brief and without detectable consequence. There is an increased incidence of afebrile seizures. Annegers et al.[12,14] found that the 1% risk of recurrent seizures before the age of 20 years in the general population was increased to 3% for those showing brief febrile convulsions and to 8% with febrile status. These increases may largely reflect common genetic and acquired underlying factors. However, when the duration exceeds a threshold somewhere between 15 and 30 min, or convulsions are repeated two or more critically three or more times in 24 h, or sustained focal features are seen, the likelihood of subsequent neurological or behavioural impairment, or the occurrence of complex partial seizures (but not primary generalized seizures) is enhanced.[14] There is an excess of both primary generalized, tonic–clonic seizures and complex partial seizures. The primary generalized seizures occur predominantly in children with neurological abnormalities prior to the complex febrile convulsion, suggesting that both have common acquired antecedents.[14,395] Recurrent afebrile seizures are more common after a prolonged afebrile status epilepticus than after lengthy febrile convulsions.

Mesial temporal sclerosis and complex partial seizures

A link between mesial temporal sclerosis found in temporal lobectomy specimens and a history of a prolonged first convulsion in early childhood (commonly febrile) first arose from study of material from Murray Falconer,[47] who found initial status in 11 out of 17 cases with Ammon's horn sclerosis (64%) and 0 out of nine cases without Ammon's horn sclerosis. This observation has been confirmed in many subsequent studies.[41,97,115,198,235,297] Sagar and Oxbury[342] showed a clear correlation between the severity of Ammon's horn sclerosis (assessed by cell density counts in Sommer sector, endfolium and dentate granule cell layer) and a prolonged seizure before the age of 3 years. A recent well-documented study of temporal lobectomy specimens further analysed this correlation.[248] All 18 of 20 patients with non-mass lesions that showed hippocampal sclerosis reported an initial precipitating injury (before the age of 5 years in all but two). The five children who had 'non-seizure' precipitating injuries (which included trauma with coma) had long latencies to onset of chronic temporal lobe epilepsy (mean 17 years) and relatively poor outcome. Of those with prolonged seizures four had meningitis or encephalitis and three had hemiconvulsions, hemiplegia and epilepsy. Four had only brief seizures recurring in the first 2–5 years of life, starting with a difficult delivery in two cases. Thus,

11 out of 18 had either a prolonged initial seizure or recurrent febrile convulsions. This study and a larger retrospective study (120 temporal lobectomies) from the same epilepsy centre[245] confirms that the patients with initial prolonged seizures had a shorter latent interval before the onset of complex partial seizures and more severe CA1 neuronal loss than patients with either birth injury or cerebral trauma as their initial precipitating injury. The birth injury and trauma patients had temporal pathologies other than hippocampal neuron loss in 50% or more of the cases. In Cavanagh and Meyer's study[47] the group with Ammon's horn sclerosis did not have a higher incidence of possible birth trauma than the group without Ammon's horn sclerosis. Birth trauma enhances the risk of subsequent epilepsy but is now thought to play a limited role in causing mesial temporal sclerosis. The poor outcome of surgical treatment in the group with birth trauma suggests that epileptic foci may be extrahippocampal or extratemporal in accordance with the more widespread brain damage in this group.[245]

The feature of temporal lobectomy specimens with Ammon's horn sclerosis on which Cavanagh and Meyer[47] placed most emphasis was the occurrence of a laminar necrosis involving layers II and III diffusely in the mesial cortex, i.e. middle, inferior, fusiform and hippocampal (equivalent to the entorhinal gyrus in lower mammals) gyri. This was almost always severe and widespread when the Ammon's horn sclerosis was severe, it could be severe when the Ammon's horn sclerosis was mild and could be present when Ammon's horn sclerosis was absent. Amygdaloid sclerosis was less consistently observed than cortical necrosis. This observation led to the widespread adoption of the term mesial temporal sclerosis, rather than hippocampal or Ammon's horn sclerosis for this pathology. Babb et al.[22] performed cell density measurements and failed to find cell loss in the entorhinal cortex. More recently, a laminar pattern (layer III) of cell loss has been described in the entorhinal cortex in four patients with temporal lobe epilepsy in the absence of similar damage in temporal neocortex.[94] Similar patterns of laminar cortical damage are reported in several experimental models of generalized or limbic epilepsy.[48,93] A more restricted lesion involving patchy loss of immunostaining for AMPA and kainate receptors and for GABAergic neurons has been described in the temporal cortex.[84] Changes in the entorhinal cortex are of interest in that in combined slice preparations (entorhinal cortex plus hippocampus) the entorhinal cortex sometimes has the lower threshold for initiating epileptic discharges.[372,426]

A further morphological change characteristically observed in association with mesial temporal sclerosis is dispersion of the dentate granule cell layer.[171] The normal compact narrow lamina of granule cells is broadened with diffuse margins, with cells extending into the molecular layer, sometimes in a radial array (Fig. 15.13). This feature is associated with severe hippocampal cell loss and a widespread pattern of dentate mossy fibre sprouting.[106] It

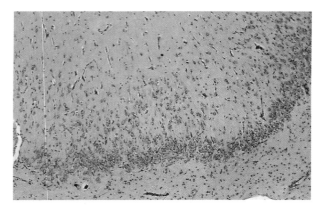

Figure 15.13 *Dentate granule cell dispersion. Section taken from a temporal lobectomy specimen with mesial temporal sclerosis. The normal well–demarcated outline of the granular cell layer is blurred by cells extending out into the molecular layer. (Luxol fast blue/cresyl violet.)*

has been suggested that the ectopic granule cell may result either from alterations in cell migration or from structural plasticity induced by an insult in early life when granule cell development continues.[171,291] Dentate granule cell progenitor division has been found to be enhanced by initial limbic seizures in rat models of epileptogenesis;[276] prolonged seizures and pyramidal neuronal degeneration were not necessary for the upregulation. Similar appearances have been reported in rodents after status epilepticus induced by pilocarpine.[262,301]

Attempts to quantify nerve cell loss in the amygdala have focused on the lateral nucleus because it is commonly included in anterior temporal or amygdalohippocampal resections and is readily identified histologically.[173,412] A mean neuronal loss of 67 or 59% is reported to occur without any close correlation with the severity or pattern of hippocampal damage, suggesting that damage to the amygdala and to the hippocampus involves distinct processes.

Astrogliosis is a prominent histological feature of medial temporal sclerosis, although its role in the pathogenesis of seizures has received little attention. Glial Na/K-ATPase activation has been found to be defective in the temporal neocortex in patients with hippocampal–amygdalar epilepsy.[139] While recent quantitation studies do not agree about astrocytosis in temporal white matter, astrocytic nuclear hypertrophy has been demonstrated consistently.[194,208,270]

Epileptic focus studied by immunocytochemistry and molecular probes

Improved understanding of the molecular biology of the systems that control neuronal function has permitted study of the expression of specific peptides or proteins that form enzymes, receptor units, transporters, ion channels, etc. (reviewed by de Lanerolle *et al.*[213]). Changes in the

regional or cellular expression of many proteins can be studied by immunocytochemistry using monoclonal or polyclonal antibodies to particular isoforms of a receptor, enzyme or transporter.

The most venerable description of morphological changes in neurons associated with epilepsy is that of DeMoor,[86] who used the Golgi technique to study neuronal morphology in the cortex of patients with dementia and epilepsy, and observed moniliform changes with a loss of dendrites and appearance of nodular deformations on apical dendrites. Scheibel *et al.*[350] examined the dentate fascia in temporal lobe epilepsy and also found a loss of dendritic spines and nodular deformities. Similar changes have been described in models of chronic focal cortical epilepsy.[325]

Focal seizures may be explicable in terms of a local impairment of GABA-mediated inhibitory processes, and hence numerous studies have concerned markers of GABAergic activity.[329,330] Using immunocytochemistry of glutamic acid decarboxylase, the enzyme synthesizing GABA, as a marker for GABAergic neurons and synaptic boutons, Babb *et al.*[24] found a relative preservation of GABAergic neurons in the human epileptic hippocampus. de Lanerolle *et al.*,[211] using an anti-GABA antibody, came to a similar conclusion.

The GABA$_A$ benzodiazepine receptor has been studied both by quantitative autoradiography[145,186] and with a monoclonal antibody to the α_1-subunit.[416] Severe losses in GABA$_A$ receptor density are found in the hippocampus of patients with mesial temporal sclerosis but they correlate rather closely with the loss of pyramidal and granule cells, with the possible exception of CA1 region where the reduction in flumazenil binding is greater than the loss of pyramidal neurons.[145]

Hilar neurons can be differentiated into numerous categories according to their Golgi morphology[7] or their immunocytochemistry. Polymorphic hilar neurons that are positive for somatostatin, neuropeptide Y and substance P are selectively lost,[214] whereas the basket cells that are strongly GAD positive and lie closer to or within the granule cell layer are preserved. Interneurons positive for somatostatin, neuropeptide Y and substance P found in relation to the CA1–CA3 pyramidal fields are not lost.

Autoradiographic studies of glutamate receptors in temporal lobectomy specimens have yielded rather mixed results, possibly because of variability in opposing effects of loss of receptor density through neuronal loss and upregulation of receptors. De Lanerolle *et al.*[215] described enhanced kainic acid binding in the dentate gyrus, as did Represa *et al.*[328] in a post-mortem study of children with a variety of epileptic syndromes. Geddes *et al.*[132] reported a decrease in NMDA receptor density in the hippocampus but an increase in density and laminar distribution in the parahippocampal gyrus. McDonald *et al.*[232] reported the binding properties of the NMDA receptor to be altered in the hippocampus. Hosford *et al.*[170] described a reduction in NMDA receptor density in the dendritic fields of CA3 (after correction for cell loss). AMPA binding was enhanced in the molecular layer of the dentate gyrus. Studies of mRNA levels for glutamate ionotropic receptor subunits using *in situ* hybridization in temporal lobectomy and post-mortem hippocampi[249,250] indicate an increase in kainate receptor subunit (KA2, GluR5) mRNA levels per granule cell in hippocampal sclerosis, probably in association with dentate mossy fibre sprouting. Some regionally selective increases in mRNA levels for AMPA and NMDA receptor subunits were observed in temporal lobectomy specimens with or without hippocampal sclerosis (corrected for neuronal loss). Immunohistochemistry has shown an altered cellular pattern of expression of AMPA receptor subunits in the epileptogenic hippocampus, with increased GluR-1 immunoreactivity on dendrites of hilar and CA3 neurons and Glu-R2/3 immunoreactivity on dentate granule cell dendrites.[212]

The hippocampal localization of various calcium binding proteins has been studied by immunocytochemistry in both human epileptic foci and experimental models. In the non-epileptic human hippocampus parvalbumin is found in interneurons but not principal cells, whereas calbindin D_{28k} is found in dentate granule cells, CA2 pyramidal neurons and interneurons.[361] Little abnormality is found in patients with a mass lesion in the temporal lobe, but patients with ammon's horn sclerosis show an apparent preferential survival of cells that are calbindin or parvalbumin positive.[364] Cajal–Retzius-like cells that are immunoreactive for calretinin and calbindin D_{28k} are prominent in the hippocampal molecular layer (dentate fascia and CA1) in Ammon's horn sclerosis.[37] They are particularly

associated with early seizure onset. A study of the morphology and connectivity of calbindin, calretinin- and substance P-positive interneurons in control and epileptic dentate gyrus showed marked changes associated with epilepsy.[236] That synaptic reorganization is an important process in the epileptic hippocampus is also supported by evidence that immunoreactivity for the highly polysialylated neural cell adhesion molecule is markedly enhanced; expression of this molecule is associated with synaptic plasticity, remodelling and neuronal migration.[265]

Seizures induced electrically or chemically in rodents commonly lead to the expression of immediate-early genes in susceptible sites. Limbic seizures rapidly induce an increase in the mRNA for nerve growth factor in dentate granule cells.[129]

The mossy fibre system that is the excitatory axonal output of the dentate granule cells terminating on hilar interneurones and pyramidal cells of the CA3 subfield can be readily visualized by the Timm histochemical method (staining zinc) and by dynorphin immunoreactivity. Using these methods in temporal lobectomy specimens reveals that in specimens with Ammon's horn sclerosis there is extensive sprouting of the mossy fibre system such that novel terminals are found in the inner molecular layer of the dentate and in the CA1 region[23,172,375] (Fig. 15.14). Similar appearances are found in rodent models of temporal lobe epilepsy such as amygdala-kindled rats[49,81,327,376] and kainate-lesioned rats.[247,326] The sprouting also involves the formation of novel connections to CA1. Although it has been suggested that the sprouting is a response to hilar cell loss, it may not

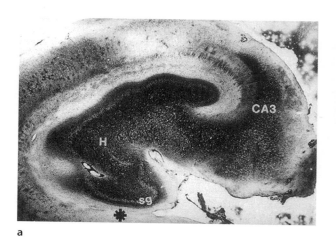
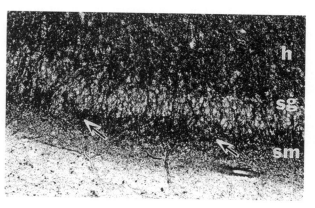

a

b

Figure 15.14 *Synaptic reorganization and axon sprouting in temporal lobe epilepsy. (a) Transverse section of dentate gyrus and hippocampus stained with the Timm method. The specimen was obtained from a patient who underwent temporal lobectomy for treatment of temporal lobe epilepsy. The terminal projections of the mossy fibre pathway are darkly stained, and include the hilus (H) of the dentate gyrus and the CA3 region of the hippocampus: sg, stratum granulosum. The region indicated by the asterisk is shown at higher power in (b). (b) Higher power of the same section demonstrating granule cells in the stratum granulosum (sg) and densely packed dark granules in the hilus (h) that correspond to the synaptic terminals of mossy fibre axons of granule cells. In association with epilepsy in humans and animal models, dark staining granules corresponding to mossy fibre terminals are observed along the border of the stratum granulosum and stratum moleculare (sm), where they are not normally found (arrows). The development of mossy fibre synaptic terminals in this region is an indication of axon sprouting and reorganization of the pattern of synaptic connections of the mossy fibre pathway. Photographs courtesy of T Sutula, University of Wisconsin, Maddison, USA.*

require significant cell loss but may be a response to release of neurotrophins during seizure activity.[42,391] In the pilocarpine/status epilepticus model it appears not to be dependent on granule cell neurogenesis as irradiation does not block mossy fibre sprouting.[300]

Although the process of sprouting has been most thoroughly documented in respect of the mossy fibre system in the dentate gyrus, it very probably involves many other systems in the hippocampus and cortex, including neuropeptide Y fibres in the inner molecular layer.[213]

Pathogenesis and physiology of epilepsy

The pathogenesis of epilepsy is poorly understood. A wide variety of molecular and cellular changes involving neurons and glia have been postulated as critical determinants of the tendency to spontaneous seizures. In studying pathogenesis it is necessary to identify the critical processes that link an initial genetic defect or an insult to the brain to the subsequently manifest susceptibility to spontaneous seizures. These critical processes commonly occupy 1–20 years in man, but in a widely studied animal model of epileptogenesis, electrical kindling in the rat, occur over a period of 2 weeks. It is also necessary to understand the permanent changes in neuronal function and molecular properties. It must be remembered that any morphological or functional change of neurons and glia found in association with any epilepsy syndrome may be a critical change contributing to spontaneous seizures, or to some early stage in the process of epileptogenesis, an adaptive response tending to decrease seizures or a coincidental effect of the primary insult that initiated epileptogenesis. Studying the time course of any such change may provide vital information about its significance. Thus, hilar cell loss after status epilepticus might be indirectly but cannot be directly responsible for epileptic discharges because it precedes epilepsy by many years.

Changes in extracellular fluid volume or ionic composition undoubtedly play a key role in sustained abnormal neuronal discharges *in vivo* and *in vitro*. They may contribute to neuronal synchronization independently of any effects on synaptic function. Thus, astrocytic and neuronal transport and fluxes of chloride, hydroxyl ions, protons, sodium, potassium, calcium and magnesium all play a part in epileptic discharges. Agents acting on sodium, potassium and calcium channels all modify epileptic discharges. Furosemide, a chloride cotransport inhibitor, blocks changes in extracellular space and prevents synchronized discharges in many seizure models without decreasing excitatory synaptic responses.[162]

Astrocytes derived from a seizure focus have been shown to differ from normal astrocytes in many functional respects, including an enhanced capacity to regulate extracellular [K^+] and evidence of abnormal properties of excitability and calcium fluxes.[67]

Attempts to demonstrate altered GABAergic inhibitory function in human epileptic foci have given very mixed results, variously showing enhancement, impairment or no change. An ingenious attempt to reconcile some apparently discordant observations is the 'dormant basket cell' hypothesis which suggests that the hilar cell loss associated with status epilepticus or prolonged perforant path stimulation deprives well-preserved GABAergic basket cells of their excitatory input and thereby disrupts a critical inhibitory feedback loop.[28,361,362] There is also the possibility that critical GABAergic neurons such as the chandelier cells are particularly vulnerable to ischaemia or status epilepticus.[84] Experiments with bilateral microdialysis probes chronically implanted in the hippocampi of patients with intractable temporal lobe epilepsy have led to the suggestion that there is a decrease in GABA transporters that leads to a decreased non-synaptic release of GABA.[100]

An enhanced functional efficacy of NMDA receptors at various points within the hippocampus of fully kindled rats has been described in considerable detail.[202,203] Studies of cortical slices from patients with focal epilepsy undergoing cortical resection also show augmented NMDA receptor function, as judged by changes in extracellular calcium concentration induced by NMDA iontophoresis.[229] Cells from kindled animals also show changes in the properties of some voltage-operated calcium channels.[271,272]

MYOCLONUS EPILEPSY

Myoclonus is defined as sudden brief shock-like involuntary movements caused by muscle contractions or muscle inhibitions arising from the CNS.[113] A single muscle or groups of muscles can be involved, and the jerks may be single or multiple and repetitive. Myoclonus occurs in a wide variety of conditions and can be found with almost all types of epilepsy. It may occur as a result of lesions at any level of the CNS: cortical, subcortical, brainstem or spinal cord.[243] Electrophysiological studies demonstrate that myoclonus of cerebral cortical origin is mediated via the pyramidal tract. Other forms consist of abnormalities in the extrapyramidal system, the brainstem or in the spinal cord without abnormalities demonstrated in the EEG.[142]

Myoclonic seizures are frequently seen in the epilepsies of childhood, such as Lennox–Gastaut syndrome, and primary generalized epilepsy. Berkovic and Andermann[32] reviewed the progressive myoclonus epilepsies, a large group of disorders characterized by severe myoclonus, seizures and progressive neurological deterioration. The diseases are heterogeneous and are uncommon. Two broad groups emerge, the first consisting of disorders where myoclonus is a presenting and major clinical feature, with neurological deficit appearing later, and the second group in which myoclonic seizures are a part of a progressive encephalopathy, and may be overshadowed by other neurological features. The latter includes, amongst many other conditions, inborn errors of metabolism such as GM2 and GM1 gangliosidoses, Neimann–Pick disease and Krabbe's disease, and acquired disorders such as subacute sclerosing panencephalitis. Creutzfeldt–Jakob disease, Alzheimer's disease and post-hypoxic encephalopathy, where myoclonus may be part of the clinical picture, are included in this group. The group of progressive myoclonic epilepsies in which myoclonus predominates also consists of a large number of varied conditions, many of them rare congenital metabolic disorders. The most common of these are Lafora body disease and Unverricht–Lundborg disease, two conditions that have long been confused with each other but are now distinguished clearly on clinical, pathological and genetic grounds.

Lafora body disease is recognized as an abnormality of carbohydrate metabolism, resulting in the accumulation of glucose polymer, polyglucosan, in various cells in the body.[424] It is an autosomal recessive disorder, with a gene locus recently mapped to chromosome 6q.[357] The responsible gene encodes laforin, a protein tyrosine phosphatase that regulates intracellular concentrations of phosphotyrosine.[267] Phosphatases are involved in glycogen metabolism, regulation of ion channels and synaptic transmission, but it is uncertain as to how laforin deficit leads to epilepsy.[317] The disease presents between the ages of 10 and 18 years with generalized seizures followed by myoclonus. Seizures with visual symptoms are common, and vision usually deteriorates. Cerebellar signs develop. Intellectual deterioration occurs early and progresses to dementia. The brain shows mild diffuse cortical atrophy on histological examination, and more appreciable neuronal loss in the globus pallidus and the dorsal medial nucleus of the thalamus. The hallmark of the condition is the characteristic intracytoplasmic neuronal inclusion, the Lafora body. Lafora bodies vary in size from 1 to 30 μm in diameter, and one or multiple inclusions may be present in each cell. They may be found in nerve cell processes and apparently free in the neuropil. They have a concentric–lamellar target-like appearance, with a basophilic core surrounded by a pale amphophilic zone (Fig. 15.15). The pale outer zone may show dark radial stria. The centre of the inclusion stains intensely with periodic acid–Schiff (PAS) and Alcian blue, resisting predigestion with diastase and hyaluronidase, while the periphery stains less intensely.[147,355] The core often contains a protein granule that is stained by the ninhydrin–Schiff or alloxan–Schiff procedures.[147,420] Lafora bodies show metachromatic staining with methyl violet and toluidine blue. Another form of the inclusion has also been described, with a homogeneous core and a surrounding clear halo.[83] Electron microscopy shows that the inclusion is not membrane bound and is composed of glycogen-like granules interspersed with fine filaments and fine granular material.[45] The inclusions are distributed throughout the cerebral cortex and are most numerous in the central region and the prefrontal motor cortex.[355] They are readily found in the globus pallidus, thalamus and substantia nigra. Fewer inclusions are present in the caudate nucleus and the putamen. The rest of the cerebral deep grey matter and brainstem nuclei are less severely affected. Numerous Lafora bodies are found in the cerebellum. There is modest loss of Purkinje cells and of the granule cells with a glial reaction, while the dentate nucleus is severely affected and shows nerve cell loss and large numbers of inclusions. Only the occasional inclusion is found in the spinal cord. Lafora bodies may also be found in glial cells and in capillary endothelial cells in the brain, in the retina, the peripheral nerves, the skeletal and cardiac muscle, the liver and the cells of the sweat ducts in skin.[1,45,46,353,392] The diagnosis can be confirmed in life by demonstrating Lafora bodies in a liver or skin biopsy, particularly axillary skin, although the absence of inclusions does not rule it out.[26,43,45,92,284]

Unverricht–Lundborg disease, Baltic myoclonus or progressive myoclonus epilepsy without Lafora bodies, is an autosomal recessive disorder, resulting from mutations in a gene localized to the distal long arm of chromosome 21, which is highly prevalent in Finland, Sweden and Estonia.[107,205,220,288] The affected gene codes for a cysteine proteinase inhibitor called cystatin B, a fairly ubiquitous protein, which is thought to protect against intracellular degradation by proteinases that leak from lysosomes.[357] The mechanism for the neurological features of the disease and the epilepsy remain unexplained, as cystatin B has no known direct functional relationship to excitability. Mediterranean myoclonus, described first in subjects from northern Africa, has many similar clinical features, but was thought to be a separate condition. Linkage studies have, however, shown that the genetic locus for the two disorders is identical.[237] It presents in childhood with myoclonus provoked by light, touch and other stimuli, and tonic–clonic seizures. Other neurological abnormalities, such as ataxia, intention tremor, dysarthria, emotional lability and intellectual decline (which is usually mild), set

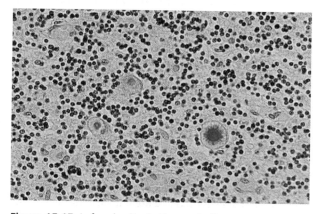

Figure 15.15 *Lafora bodies in the cerebellar cortex. The intracytoplasmic inclusion has a dense basophilic core and a pale periphery. (H&E.) Courtesy of Professor F Scaravilli, Institute of Neurology, London, UK.*

in late and very gradually. Phenytoin has an adverse effect and is associated with rapid progression of the disorder.[107] The most consistent biochemical abnormality detected, originally observed by Unverricht, is the increased urinary excretion of indican.[204]

Pathological studies were carried out in 32 of the 93 cases reported by Koskiniemi et al.[205] Sural nerve, muscle, liver and rectal biopsies from 26 cases showed no significant changes. Post-mortem examination of the brain in six cases showed severe diffuse loss of Purkinje cells, accompanied by moderate proliferation of Bergman glia. Surviving Purkinje cells were swollen or vacuolated. The internal granule cell layer and dentate nucleus were preserved. Neuronal degeneration was also seen in the medial thalamic nucleus. These findings have been confirmed by others. Detailed examination of the CNS has in addition demonstrated mild to moderate cerebral cortical atrophy and neuronal degeneration in the striatum, the anterior and lateral thalamus, the mamillary body, the brainstem nuclei and the spinal anterior horn cells.[143] No Lafora bodies were found, although corpora amylacea were found in abundance in some areas. It has been speculated that the extensive Purkinje cell loss is a result of the effect of phenytoin on these patients. Cochius et al.[63] described membrane-bound vacuoles on electron microscopy in sweat gland secretory cells in five out of seven patients, which may assist in confirming the diagnosis.

A form of progressive myoclonus epilepsy has been described in two North American families so far, characterized by onset of generalised seizures, myoclonus and progressive epilepsy in the third decade, in which a mutation in the Neuroserpin gene, mapped to chromosome 3q26, has been demonstrated.[378] Neuroserpin is a serine protease inhibitor, a regulator of extracellular proteolytic reactions, and the mutation, which causes an arginine for serine substitution S52R, is associated with widespread accumulation of the abnormal protein as eosinophilic intracytoplasmic inclusions in the cell bodies and processes of neurons throughout the CNS.

One clinical form of the wide spectrum of disorders of the nervous system resulting from disordered mitochondrial function is that of myoclonus epilepsy and the mitochondrial myopathy with ragged-red fibres (MERRF) in the skeletal muscle in sections stained with Gomori's trichrome.[128,338,387] The disease begins in the second decade, usually with myoclonus and ataxia. Tonic–clonic seizures are invariably present and dementia is frequently seen. Other features include hearing loss, optic atrophy and neuropathy, while muscle weakness is mild or absent. MERRF may be sporadic or familial. The inheritance is heterogenous, and while in some cases it is autosomal, the majority show a point mutation of mtDNA.[89] In addition to the mitochondrial abnormalities found in muscle biopsies from these patients, autopsy studies show neurodegenerative lesions in the CNS. A post-mortem study of two cases showed dentatorubral and palli-doluysian degeneration with changes in the spinal cord resembling those of Friedreich's ataxia. Degeneration was also noted in the cerebellar cortex, the substantia nigra, the locus coeruleus, the inferior olivary, gracile and cuneate nuclei and in the pontine tegmentum.[379] A report of three members of one family with MERRF showed nerve cell loss in the dentate and inferior olivary nuclei with striking gliosis of the white matter of the cerebellum and of the brainstem. There was mild neuronal loss in the red nuclei and a reduction in the number of cerebellar Purkinje cells. The spinal cord showed pallor of the posterior columns.[33] The biochemical abnormalities are also heterogeneous.

The combination of progressive cerebellar ataxia and myoclonus with or without seizures, referred to as the Ramsay Hunt syndrome, was thought to result from degeneration primarily of the dentate nucleus. Hunt's original report in 1921[174] described six patients with cerebellar ataxia, intention tremor and myoclonus, and included the pathological findings of one case showing atrophy of the dentate nucleus and rarefaction of the superior cerebellar peduncle. It is now clear that the Ramsay Hunt syndrome is not a disease entity and consists of a variety of clinically biochemical and genetically defined conditions. Most cases of this clinical syndrome are examples of mitochondrial encephalopathy and Unverricht–Lundborg disease.[33,244]

NEUROSURGERY AND NEUROSURGICAL PATHOLOGY

The first documented craniotomy successfully carried out for the treatment of seizures was by Sir Victor Horsley in 1886 for post-traumatic epilepsy caused by an indriven fragment of bone.[168] The basis of modern surgery for epilepsy, rests, however, on the pioneering work on the resection of epileptogenic foci by Penfield and co-workers.[121,303,307] Since then there has been increasing interest in the use of surgery such that neurosurgical treatment is now an established option in the management of chronic drug-resistant epilepsy. Two categories of procedures are carried out, namely functional surgery and resective surgery. Functional surgery is less frequently performed, and aims to control the seizures rather than to cure them. Procedures such as section of the corpus callosum, temporal lobotomy and multiple subpial transection attempt to disconnect neuronal circuitry and to prevent the propagation of the seizures. Rarely, stereotactic lesions are made to ablate deep epileptic foci or to control the seizures when there are multiple foci.

Section of the corpus callosum is carried out with the expectation that division of the main interhemispheric connection will prevent seizures from generalizing from one hemisphere to the other. In a large number, the generalized seizures abate, while the partial seizures remain. In some the latter increase in severity. Multiple subpial transection was devised as a method of controlling partial seizures that arise in cortical regions, such as the speech or primary motor areas, that cannot be resected without the patient developing unacceptable neurological deficit.[275] Horizontal intracortical fibres are severed by a series of cuts in the molecular layer to limit the spread of epileptic activity without adverse effects on cortical function. Neuropathological examination of biopsies or small resections that were obtained from 17 patients undergoing multiple subpial transection showed six cases of cortical dysplasia, six of Rasmussen's syndrome, four with non-specific astrogliosis and one dysembryoplastic neuroepithelial tumour.[164] Seizures were controlled in ten patients. There was no difference between the diagnoses in the seven patients whose seizures failed to improve, and the rest who did. Success of surgery relates more to the extent of the abnormality than to the pathology of the underlying lesion.

The aim of resective surgery is primarily to remove the epileptic focus. It also serves to disconnect the rest of the brain from the focus if removal is incomplete, and may reduce the total number of abnormally excitable neurons. Surgery was originally performed in cases where an epileptogenic focus could be localized well by EEG. As neuroimaging techniques improved, more patients were considered candidates for surgery. Procedures carried out consist of temporal lobe resection, resections from other lobes and hemispherectomy. Table 15.3 shows the range of abnormalities seen in surgical resections from chronic epilepsy. The sections that follow detail the findings in the various types of resection carried out.

Temporal lobectomy

Temporal lobectomy is carried out for the relief of drug-resistant temporal lobe epilepsy. Temporal lobe resections may be excision of the neocortex only, and with evidence pointing to the importance of the hippocampal complex in the generation of partial complex seizures,[116,241] removal of the medial temporal structures only or, what is more commonly performed, an anterior temporal lobectomy in which neocortex and deep medial temporal structures are removed. Penfield described a technique for resecting the anterior temporal lobe including the amygdala and hippocampus, removing tissue piecemeal using suction.[305] Falconer introduced the *en bloc* anterior temporal lobectomy, which provides better material for pathological study.[114] A portion of tissue approximately 30 g in weight when taken from the dominant hemisphere and 40 g when non-dominant, consisting of 4–6 cm of the temporal lobe from the temporal pole back, is usually available for examination (Figs 15.16, 15.17). Part of the superior temporal gyrus is included along the superolateral cut border, and the uncus and parahippocampal gyrus in its medial cut border. A 1.5–3-cm length of the hippocampus is obtained, and

Table 15.3 *Lesions seen in surgical resections*

Ammon's horn sclerosis (mesial temporal sclerosis)	
Malformations	Malformations of cortical development
	Microdysgenesis
	Nodular heterotopia
	Focal cortical dysplasia
	Tuberous sclerosis
	Glioneuronal hamartomas
	Hemimegalencephaly
	Polymicrogyria
	Vascular malformations
	Arteriovenous malformation
	Cavernous angioma
	Sturge–Weber syndrome
	Arachnoid cyst
Scars	Traumatic
	Inflammatory
	Postinfectious
	Abscess
	Rasmussen's syndrome
	Hypoxic–ischaemic
	Intrauterine
	Perinatal
	Later
Neoplasms	Neuroglial
	Ganglioglioma
	Dysembryoplastic neuroepithelial tumour
	Glial
	Astrocytoma
	Oligodendroglioma
	Oligoastrocytoma
	Others
Non-specific changes	
No abnormality	

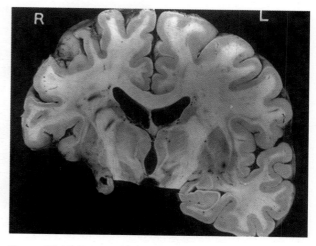

Figure 15.16 *Temporal lobectomy. Coronal slice of the brain showing the defect of an en-bloc anterior temporal lobe resection performed some years earlier.*

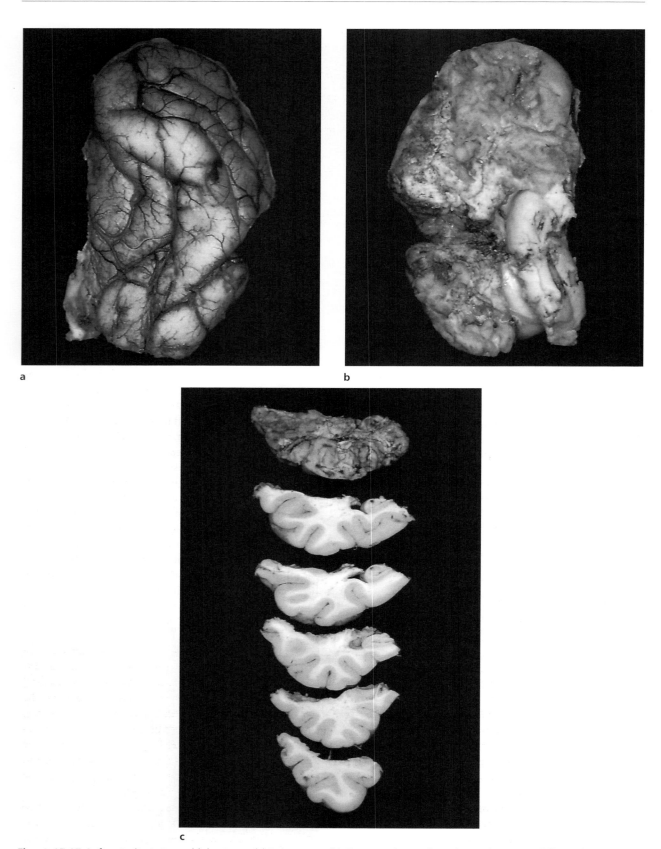

a

b

c

Figure 15.17 *Left anterior temporal lobectomy. (a) Lobectomy. (b) The resection surface shows the exposed floor of the tempo-ral horn of the lateral ventricle with approximately the anterior two-thirds of the hippocampus, along the medial margin. (c) Coronal slices arranged with the temporal pole below to show part of the amygdala in slice 2 and the hippocampus in slices 3–5. The hippocampus is shrunken and the temporal horn of the lateral ventricle appears spacious.*

Table 15.4 *Neuropathological findings in temporal lobe epilepsy*

Pathology	Mathieson[251]	Babb and Brown[21]	Bruton[41]	Wolf et al.[414]	Honavar et al.[166]
Mesial temporal sclerosis	140	79	107	51[a]	122
Glioneuronal malformations	18	15	10	42	11
Vascular malformations	19	6	4	13	6
Scars	54	4	10	1	9
Tumours	115	18	37	75[a]	58
Others	171	7	15	10	1
Non-specific	167	–	25	Not specified	33
No pathology	173	–	41	Not specified	–
Total	857	129	249	216	241

[a]Include cases with dual pathology.

usually a portion of the amygdala, 2–5 mm thick. Methods for handling and examining the resected specimens have been detailed.[41,166,418]

The most frequently seen pathological abnormality in temporal lobectomy specimens is mesial temporal or hippocampal sclerosis, reported in up to 63% of cases.[21,41,101,166,251,414] The terms mesial temporal sclerosis, hippocampal sclerosis and Ammon's horn sclerosis are used synonymously in this section. Neuropathological findings from some of the larger series are listed in Table 15.4. The variation between studies arises in part from differing methods of reporting results. Babb and Brown,[21] Mathieson[251] and Honavar et al.[166] restrict the diagnosis of mesial temporal sclerosis to cases where it is the only principal abnormality, whereas Bruton[41] and Wolf et al.[414] include those with double pathology, a focal lesion and mesial temporal sclerosis. Restrictions are also placed by the absence of adequate representation of the hippocampal formation in the surgical specimen to allow proper assessment. Wolf et al.[414] showed an incidence of 71.8% when they considered only cases in which the hippocampus was intact and was available for examination. This also reflects the number of cases in which no significant abnormality or only minor non-specific changes are seen.

Histologically, three patterns of cell loss are described in the hippocampus:[41,241] Classical Ammon's horn sclerosis in which the neuronal loss is most severe in the Sommer sector and endfolium, less in the dentate fascia and least in the resistant zone; total Ammon's horn sclerosis characterized by severe neuronal loss in all the hippocampal subzones and endfolium sclerosis, a mild lesion where the loss of neurons is; restricted to the endfolium. These patterns appear to have no clinical significance and do not correlate with the severity of the seizures on the outcome of surgery. The neuronal loss is accompanied by fibrillary gliosis leading to atrophy of the hippocampus. Gliosis may affect the amygdala, the uncus and the parahippocampal gyrus to complete the picture of medial temporal sclerosis.

Focal lesions that are found in these resections include most of the conditions listed in Table 15.3. Tumours constitute the second largest group. Dual pathology, in most instances represented by a focal lesion and hippocampal sclerosis, is reported in up to 30% of temporal lobectomies.[41,224,414] Neuronal counts show milder degrees of cell loss when associated with a tumour, compared with those where hippocampal sclerosis is the primary abnormality.

Marked reduction or complete control of seizures is achieved when a definite pathological abnormality is demonstrated in the specimen.[115,116] This is as valid for medial temporal sclerosis as for focal lesion. Bruton[41] showed significant reduction or abolition of seizures in 80% of patients with medial temporal sclerosis followed up for an average of 8 years after temporal lobectomy. Nakasato et al.[277] demonstrated that while all cases of temporal lobe epilepsy showed some neuronal loss, worthwhile seizure control after temporal lobectomy was seen in 90% of those with severe cell loss and in only 65% of those with mild cell loss. A subgroup has been identified with neuronal loss predominantly in the anterior hippocampus in whom the benefits of surgery are greater than those in the anterior and posterior hippocampus. The latter group of patients with medial temporal sclerosis may not be relieved of epilepsy after temporal lobectomy.[22]

Selective amygdalohippocampectomy consists of removal of the anterior hippocampus and the anterior parahippocampal gyrus and the amygdala, and at least partial interruption of the anterior commissure and the uncinate fasiculus.[405] Material available for pathological study consists of small pieces of hippocampus, on average 1–2 g in weight, and small fragments of the amygdala. Recognition and orientation of structures may be difficult, although usually enough of the hippocampal pyramidal cell layer can be identified (Fig. 15.18).

Table 15.5 shows the histopathological findings of two groups, one in Zurich and the other at the Maudsley Hospital, London, UK. Mesial temporal sclerosis accounts for 22% of cases in one[313] and 67% in the other.[166] Patients selected for this type of surgery vary; nearly all the rest of the cases reported by Plate et al. are focal lesions, mainly neoplasms, restricted to the medial temporal region.

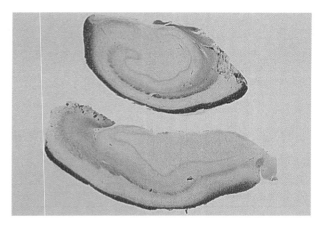

Figure 15.18 *Amygdalohippocampectomy. Proper orientation of fragments of the hippocampus assists in diagnosing Ammon's horn sclerosis with certainty. (Luxol fast blue/cresyl violet.)*

Table 15.5 *Neuropathological findings in amygdalohippocampectomy*

Pathology	Plate et al.[313] (224 cases)	Honavar et al.[166] (44 cases)
Mesial temporal sclerosis	49	30
Glioneuronal malformation	16	1
Vascular malformations	20	–
Tumours	126	3
Others	13	10

Cortical resection

The location of the epileptogenic focus dictates the site of the cortical resection. The lesions are similar to the focal abnormalities found in temporal lobectomies, although much higher proportions of focal cortical dysplasia and Rasmussen's syndrome are seen.[166,419]

The most radical of resective procedures employed, hemispherectomy or removal of a large part of one cerebral hemisphere, was first used in the management of intractable seizures by McKenzie.[233] Krynauw[209] published a series of 12 patients with infantile hemiplegia and epilepsy treated by hemispherectomy and demonstrated seizure relief. The method is indicated in patients with intractable unilateral partial seizures as their predominant seizure type, arising from multiple epileptic foci within one hemisphere, associated with significant contralateral motor deficit. Surgical techniques currently being carried out range from total hemispherectomy, in which virtually all of the hemisphere is removed, preserving only the deep grey nuclei, to functional hemispherectomy, where portions of cerebral tissue are removed, functionally disconnecting the remainder. Persistent subdural bleeding in the cavity resulting from a total hemispherectomy led to procedures being devised where parts of the hemisphere, such as frontal and occipital lobes, remained, although disconnected from the rest of the brain, or the dura was firmly tethered following removal of the whole hemisphere, to avoid the complication. Superficial cerebral haemosiderosis developed as a result of the persistent bleeding, a late fatal complication of hemispherectomy, characterized by gradual neurological deterioration.[295] Postmortem examination in three cases who died many years after hemispherectomy for seizure control showed a haemorrhagic subdural membrane lining the hemispherectomy cavity. The membrane also covered the basal ganglia and extended into the third ventricle through the dilated foramen of Munro. The rest of the ventricle showed granular ependymitis. There was haemosiderosis of the surface of the cerebellum, brainstem and spinal cord.

The pathological findings in hemispherectomy specimens from some published series are shown in Table 15.6. The main groups of disorders responsible for chronic unilateral epilepsy and hemiplegia that are subjected to this operative procedure are developmental abnormalities, lesions resulting from anoxic–ischaemic damage and Rasmussen's.[119,166,209,397,411,419] Lesions resulting from an anoxic–ischaemic encephalopathy in the prenatal or perinatal period are most frequently seen overall. The changes observed fall into three categories: (1) cystic porencephaly, frequently in the territory of the middle cerebral artery (Fig. 15.19). The main trunk of the middle cerebral artery is reported to show intimal proliferation and disruption of the internal elastic lamina and occasionally a recanalized thrombus;[411] (2) scarring with ulegyria, also localized most often to the middle cerebral artery territory; and (3) diffuse lesions consisting of gyral atrophy and gliosis, sometimes accompanied by small cortical and subcortical cysts.

Table 15.6 *Neuropathological findings in hemispherectomy specimens*

Pathology	Wilson[411]	Farrell et al.[119]	Wolf et al.[419]	Honavar et al.[166]	Total
Malformation	–	15	5	4	24
Anoxic–ischaemic	35	16	5	10	66
Rasmussen's syndrome	–	3	3	15	21
Sturge–Weber syndrome	2	3	1	1	7
Other	–	1	5	–	6
Total	37	38	19	30	124

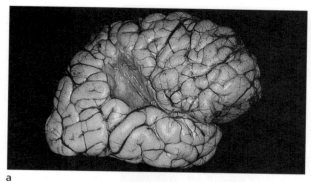

a

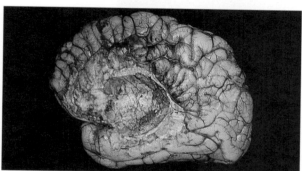

b

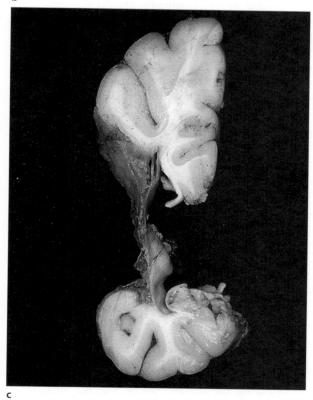

c

Figure 15.19 *Hemispherectomy. (a) Specimen from a boy with infantile hemiplegia and intractable seizures. There is a cystic defect on the lateral aspect of the frontoparietal region. (b) The medial surface of the total hemispherectomy specimen shows the severed corpus callosum. (c) A coronal slice demonstrates the extent of the defect. The thin gliotic wall of the collapsed cyst rests on the ventricular lining. The gyri at the periphery of the cyst are not malformed.*

The control of seizures is good and the morbidity low, such that hemispherectomy is considered the treatment of choice in patients with infantile hemiplegia and seizures, hemimegalencephaly, Sturge–Weber syndrome and Rasmussen's encephalitis.[82,175,200,292,396,398]

Neuroimaging

The newer neuroimaging technologies allow correlation of *in vivo* data with the neuropathology of surgical specimens and autopsy material not only in terms of gross morphology but also in terms of the pattern of cellular change and ligand binding to receptor sites. Techniques such as functional MRI, positron emission tomography (PET) and single photon emission computed tomography (SPECT) allow the study of regional blood flow and metabolism. In addition, magnetic resonance spectroscopy (MRS) allows the study of certain chemical substances in brain regions. Interictal studies with MRS show that the phosphocreatine/inorganic phosphate ratio is decreased on the side of the focus in temporal lobe epilepsy.[320] The *N*-acetyl aspartate signal is commonly reduced around a temporal lobe focus, apparently reflecting neuronal loss.[157]

Studies correlating neuroimages obtained *in vivo* with morphology of surgically resected or post-mortem brain tissue are progressively enhancing the ability to diagnose epileptic pathology and provide appropriate treatment. Thus, the presurgical evaluation of patients with complex partial seizures has been improved by quantitative MRI.[177] Hippocampal sclerosis, found in a high proportion of patients giving a history of a complex febrile convulsion, can be readily identified by MRI as reduction in volume of mesial temporal structures, which may be associated with altered signal intensity (Fig. 15.20).[2,53,54,408] Measurement of absolute hippocampal volume (rather than asymmetry) is necessary to detect cases with bilateral atrophy;[199,217] absolute hippocampal volume has been shown to correlate with pyramidal cell density counts.[217] It is also possible to identify acute changes after status epilepticus (enhanced T2-weighted image at 24 h) and to follow the course of subsequent atrophy.[286] MRI measurements of hippocampal volume also provide direct and indirect evidence for progressive reduction in volume on the side of focal origin of severe seizures with secondary generalization.[290,380]

The non-invasive detection of cortical dysgenesis in patients with otherwise unexplained focal or generalized seizures has been greatly facilitated by high-resolution MRI that allows differentiation of white and grey matter.[210,323] This readily differentiates abnormalities of gyration such as focal microgyria and macrogyria and heterotopias (Fig. 15.21a, b), and indicates the possibility of surgical treatment in cases of generalized or focal epilepsy previously considered 'cryptogenic'. As mentioned above, the anatomical pathology does not define the epileptogenic abnormality. Minor degrees of pathology may be very widespread.[359]

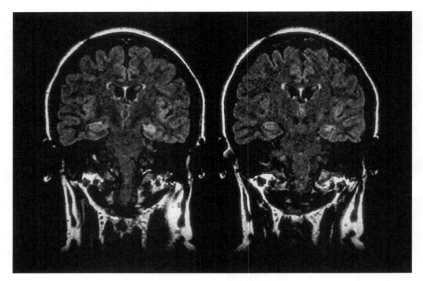

Figure 15.20 *Chronic temporal lobe epilepsy. FLAIR MRI in the coronal plane showing higher signal abnormality in the smaller left hippocampus. Photographs courtesy of Dr CC Penney, King's Health Care NHS Trust, London, UK.*

Interictal, ictal and postictal SPECT, most commonly with the tagged tracer technetium-99m-hexamethyl propylene-amine-oxime, is being used increasingly in the evaluation of epilepsy to diagnose and localize epileptogenic regions, by studying the changes in cerebral perfusion. Epileptogenic areas show ictal hyperperfusion and interictal hypoperfusion. Ictal SPECT in mesial temporal lobe epilepsy shows hyperperfusion of the whole temporal lobe, the mesial temporal cortex

remaining hyperperfused for some time postictally (Fig. 15.22).[98,150,161] The adjacent cortex may show hypoperfusion. Studies with PET using the glucose analogue fluorodeoxyglucose to estimate regional metabolic rate for glucose in patients with a focus in the anterior temporal lobe show that during the interictal period there is a region of hypometabolism in the temporal lobe that is much more extensive than the focus as defined by light-microscopic pathology or by electrophysiology.[156] Ictal PET, not

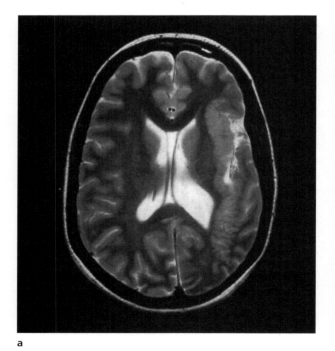

a

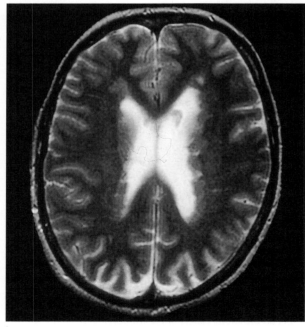

b

Figure 15.21 *(a) Polymicrogyria. T2-weighted axial MRI from a girl with congenital hemiparesis and focal motor seizures demonstrating thickened perisylvian cortex with irregular inner contour and loss of sulcation. (b) Subependymal nodular heterotopia. Bilateral nodules of grey matter in T2-weighted axial MRI from a 35-year-old woman with intractable seizures for 20 years. Photographs courtesy of Dr CC Penney, King's Health Care NHS Trust, London, UK.*

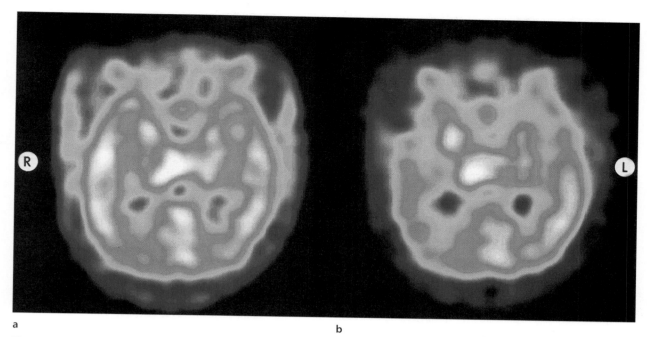

a   b

Figure 15.22 *SPECT images from a 32-year-old man with right temporal lobe epilepsy. (a) Interictal image carried out 24 h after the seizure, showing marginal residual hyperperfusion of the right mesial temporal cortex. (b) Postictal image acquired following injection of HMPAO 30 s after the end of a typical seizure that lasted for 40 s. The typical postictal pattern for a mesial temporal seizure is shown, with hyperperfusion of the mesial temporal cortex on the right and marked hypoperfusion of the lateral temporal cortex on the same side. There is some hypoperfusion of the left temporal lobe. Images courtesy of Dr R Duncan, South Glasgow University Hospital NHS Trust, Glasgow, UK.*

routinely carried out, demonstrates hypermetabolism in the epileptogenic zone with supression of metabolic activity in the surrounding areas.[59] The hypometabolism is greater with hippocampal sclerosis than with focal lesions in the neocortex, and may extend to the ipsilateral frontal lobe and basal ganglia.[96] There is correlation between the degree of hypometabolism and the loss of hippocampal volume on MRI and hippocampal cell loss. A comparison of MRI, SPECT and PET shows that PET is the most sensitive diagnostic method in temporal lobe epilepsy in the interictal period, although overall the highest diagnostic sensitivity and specificity are achieved by ictal SPECT.[368] In extratemporal lobe epilepsies, results with both SPECT and PET are of more limited value; the patterns of change in blood flow and metabolism are less constant owing to greater variation in the underlying pathology.

PET and SPECT have been used to assess receptor binding sites interictally in patients with complex partial seizures. Increases have been described in μ-opiate receptor number or binding affinity (assessed with [^{11}C]carfentanil) in the lateral temporal cortex on the side of the focus.[252] Benzodiazepine binding is decreased in mesial temporal structures on the side of the focus (as evaluated by PET with [^{11}C]flumazenil and by SPECT with [^{123}I]iomazenil).[155] This may not be fully explained by the loss of GABA$_A$ receptors associated with nerve cell loss in hippocampal structures.[416] In a series of 19 patients with partial seizures of limbic or neocortical origin without MRI abnormality the region of reduced benzodiazepine receptor density corresponds to the epileptogenic focus in all patients, with a correlation between seizure frequency and the extent of receptor reduction.[348] In focal cortical dysplasia the seizure onset zone shows reduced flumazenil binding on preoperative PET and reduced postoperative bendzodiazepine-receptor autoradiography.[17]

The combination of *in vivo* neuroimaging with current quantitative neuropathological techniques offers an opportunity to study the natural history of a wide range of epilepsy syndromes, including those that do not normally come to the attention of neuropathologists.

REFERENCES

1 Acharya JN, Satishchandra P, Asha T, Shankar SK. Lafora's disease in south India: a clinical electrophysiologic, and pathologic study. *Epilepsia* 1993; **34**: 476–87.

2 Adam C, Haulac M, Saint-Hilaire J-M *et al*. Value of magnetic resonance imaging-based measurements of hippocampal formations in patients with partial epilepsy. *Arch Neurol* 1994; **51**: 130–8.

3 Ahuja GK, Mohanta A. Late onset epilepsy: a prospective study. *Acta Neurol Scand* 1982; **66**: 216–66.

4 Aicardi J, Chevrie JJ. Convulsive status epilepticus in infants and children. A study of 239 cases. *Epilepsia* 1970; **11**: 187–97.

5 Aicardi J, Lefebvre J, Lerique-Koechlin A. A new syndrome: spasms in flexion, callosal agenesis, ocular abnormalities. *Electro-encephalogr Clin Neurophysiol* 1965; **19**: 609–10.

6 Alzheimer A. Die Gruppierung der Epilepsie. *Allegemeine Z Psychiatrie* 1907; **64**: 418–48.

7 Amaral DG. A golgi study of cell types in the hilar region of the hippocampus in rat. *J Comp Neurol* 1978; **182**: 851–914.

8 Aminoff MJ, Simon RP. Status epilepticus. Causes, clinical features and consequences in 98 patients. *Am J Med* 1980; **69**: 657–66.

9 Andrews JM, Thompson JA, Pysher TJ *et al*. Chronic encephalitis, epilepsy and cerebrovascular immune complex deposits. *Ann Neurol* 1990; **28**: 88–90.

10 Angelman H. 'Puppet' children: a report of three cases. *Dev Med Child Neurol* 1965; **7**: 681–7.

11 Annegers JF, Hauser WA, Beghi E *et al*. The risk of unprovoked seizures after encephalitis and meningitis. *Neurology* 1988; **38**: 1407–10.

12 Annegers JF, Hauser WA, Elveback LR. Remission of seizures and relapse in patients with epilepsy. *Epilepsia* 1979; **20**: 729–37.

13 Annegers JF, Hauser WA, Shirts SB. Heart disease mortality and morbidity in patients with epilepsy. *Epilepsia* 1984; **25**: 699–740.

14 Annegers JF, Hauser WA, Shirts SB, Kurland LT. Factors prognostic of unprovoked seizures after febrile convulsions. *N Engl J Med* 1987; **316**: 493–8.

15 Armstead WM, Mirro R, Leffler CW, Busija DW. Cerebral superoxide anion generation during seizures in newborn pigs. *J Cereb Blood Flow Metab* 1989; **9**: 175–9.

16 Armstrong DD. The neuropathology of temporal lobe epilepsy. *J Neuropathol Exp Neurol* 1993; **52**: 433–43.

17 Arnold S, Berthele A, Drzezga A *et al*. Reduction of benzodiazepine receptor binding is related to the seizure onset zone in extratemporal focal cortical dysplasia. *Epilepsia* 2000; **41**: 818–24.

18 Ashcroft PB. Traumatic epilepsy after gunshot wounds at the head. *BMJ* 1941; **i**: 739–44.

19 Avoli M, Rogawski MA, Avanzini G. Generalized epileptic disorders: an update. *Epilepsia* 2001; **42**: 445–57.

20 Babb TL. Research on the anatomy and pathology of epileptic tissue. In: Luders H ed. *Neurosurgery of epilepsy*. New York: Raven Press, 1991: 719–27.

21 Babb TL, Brown WJ. Pathological findings in epilepsy. In: Engel J ed. *Surgical treatment of the epilepsies*. New York: Raven Press, 1987: 511–40.

22 Babb TL, Brown WJ, Pretorius J *et al*. Temporal lobe volumetric cell densities in temporal lobe epilepsy. *Epilepsia* 1984; **25**: 729–40.

23 Babb TL, Kupfer WR, Pretorius JK *et al*. Synaptic reorganization by mossy fibers in human epileptic fascia dentata. *Neuroscience* 1991; **42**: 351–63.

24 Babb TL, Pretorius JK, Kupfer WR, Crandall PH. Glutamate decarboxylase-immunoreactive neurons are preserved in human epileptic hippocampus. *J Neurosci* 1989; **9**: 2562–74.

25 Bartolomei JC, Christopher S, Vives K *et al*. Low-grade gliomas of chronic epilepsy: A distinct clinical and pathological entity. *J Neuro-oncol* 1997; **34**: 79–84.

26 Baumann RJ, Kocoshis SA, Wilson D. Lafora disease: liver histopathology in presymptomatic children. *Ann Neurol* 1983; **14**: 86–9.

27 Beal MF. Aging, energy, and oxidative stress in neurodegenerative diseases. *Ann Neurol* 1995; **38**: 357–66.

28 Bekenstein JW, Lothman EW. Dormancy of inhibitory interneurons in a model of temporal lobe epilepsy. *Science* 1993; **259**: 97–100.

29 Ben Ari Y, Tremblay E, Ottersen OP, Meldrum BS. The role of epileptic activity in hippocampal and 'remote' cerebral lesions induced by kainic acid. *Brain Res* 1980; **191**: 79–97.

30 Benatar MG. Calcium channelopathies. *Q J Med* 1999; **92**: 133–41.

31 Bergamasco B, Benna P, Ferrero P, Gavinelli R. Neonatal hypoxia and epileptic risk: a clinical prospective study. *Epilepsia* 1984; **25**: 131–6.

32 Berkovic SF, Andermann F. The progressive myoclonus epilepsies. In: Pedley TA, Meldrum BS eds. *Recent advances in epilepsy*. Edinburgh: Churchill Livingstone, 1986; **3**: 157–87.

33 Berkovic SF, Carpenter S, Evans A *et al*. Myoclonus epilepsy and ragged-red fibres (MERRF). *Brain* 1989; **112**: 1231–60.

34 Bharucha NE, Bharucha EP, Bharucha AE *et al*. Prevalence of epilepsy in the Parsi community of Bombay. *Epilepsia* 1988; **29**: 111–15.

35 Bittencourt PRM, Garcia CM, Lorenzana P. Epilepsy and parasitosis of the central nervous system. In: Pedley TA, Meldrum BS eds. *Recent advances in epilepsy*. Edinburgh: Churchill Livingstone, 1988: 123–59.

36 Blennow G, Brierley JB, Meldrum BS, Siesjö BK. Epileptic brain damage. *Brain* 1978; **101**: 687–700.

37 Blümcke I, Beck H, Suter B *et al*. An increase of hippocampal calretinin-immunoreactive neurons correlates with early febrile seizures in temporal lobe epilepsy. *Acta Neuropathol* 1999; **97**: 31–9.

38 Boon PA, Williams PD, Fried I *et al*. Intracranial, intra-axial, space-occupying lesions in patients with intractable partial seizures: an anatomical, neuropsychological and surgical correlation. *Epilepsia* 1991; **32**: 467–76.

39 Bouchet C, Cazauvieilh M. De l'épilepsie considerée dans ses rapports avec l'aliénation mentale. *Arch Gén Med* 1825; **9**: 510–42.

40 Bränström T, Silfvenius H, Olivercrona M. The range of disorders of cortical organization in surgically treated epilepsy patients. In: Guerrini R, Andermann F, Canapicchi R *et al*. eds. *Dysplasias of cerebral cortex and epilepsy*. New York: Raven Press, 1996: 57–64.

41 Bruton CJ. The neuropathology of temporal lobe epilepsy. *Maudsley Monogr* 1988; **31**: 1–158.

42 Bugra K, Pollard H, Charton G *et al*. aFGF, bFGF and flg mRNAs show distinct patterns of induction in the hippocampus following kainate-induced seizures. *Eur J Neurosci* 1994; **6**: 58–66.

43 Busard HLSM, Gabreels-Festen AAWM, Remei WO *et al*. Axilla skin biopsy: a reliable test for the diagnosis of Lafora's disease. *Ann Neurol* 1987; **21**: 599–601.

44 Carey ME, Chou SN, French LA. Long-term neurological residua in patients surviving brain abscess with surgery. *J Neurosurg* 1971; **34**: 652–6.

45 Carpenter S, Karpati G. Sweat gland duct cells in Lafora disease: diagnosis by skin biopsy. *Neurology* 1981; **31**: 1564–8.

46 Carpenter S, Karpati G, Andermann F *et al*. Lafora's disease: peroxisomal storage in skeletal muscle. *Neurology* 1974; **24**: 531–8.

47 Cavanagh JB, Meyer A. Aetiological aspects of Ammon's horn sclerosis associated with temporal lobe epilepsy. *BMJ* 1956; 1403–7.

48 Cavazos JE, Das I, Sutula TP. Neuronal loss induced in limbic pathways by kindling: evidence for induction of hippocampal sclerosis by repeated brief seizures. *J Neurosci* 1994; **14**: 3106–21.

49 Cavazos JE, Golarai G, Sutula TP. Mossy fiber synaptic reorganization induced by kindling: time course of development, progression and permanence. *J Neurosci* 1991; **11**: 2795–803.

50 Cavazos JE, Sutula TP. Progressive neuronal loss induced by kindling: a possible mechanism for mossy fiber synaptic reorganization and hippocampal sclerosis. *Brain Res* 1990; **527**: 1–6.

51 Caveness WF. Epilepsy, a product of trauma in our time. *Epilepsia* 1976; **17**: 207–15.

52 Cendes F, Andermann F, Carpenter S *et al*. Temporal lobe epilepsy caused by domoic acid intoxication: evidence for glutamate receptor-mediated excitotoxicity in humans. *Ann Neurol* 1995; **37**: 123–6.

53 Cendes F, Andermann F, Dubeau F *et al*. Early childhood prolonged febrile convulsions, atrophy and sclerosis of mesial structures, and temporal lobe epilepsy: an MRI volumetric study. *Neurology* 1993; **43**: 1083–7.

54 Cendes F, Andermann F, Gloor P *et al*. MRI volumetric measurement of amygdala and hippocampus in temporal lobe epilepsy. *Neurology* 1993; **43**: 719–25.

55 Chapman AG. Cerebral energy metabolism and seizures. In: Pedley TA, Meldrum BS eds. *Recent advances in epilepsy 2*. Edinburgh: Churchill Livingstone, 1985: 19–63.

56 Chaslin P. Note sur l'anatomie pathologique de l'épilepsie dite essentielle – la sclérose nevroglique. *Comptes Rendus des Séances de la Société de Biologie* 1889; **1**: 169–71.

57 Chinchilla D, Dulac O, Robain O *et al*. Reappraisal of Rasmussen's syndrome with special emphasis on treatment with high doses of steroids. *J Neurol Neurosurg Psychiatry* 1994; **57**: 1325–33.

58 Chiofalo N, Kirschbaum A, Fuentes A *et al*. Prevalence of epilepsy in Melipilla, Chile. *Epilepsia* 1979; **20**: 261–6.

59 Chugani HT, Runthaka PJ, Shewmon DA. Ictal patterns of cerebral glucose utilisation in children with epilepsy. *Epilepsia* 1994; **35**: 813–22.

60 Clark LP, Prout TP. Status epilepticus: A clinical and pathological study in epilepsy. *Am J Insanity* 1903–4; **60**: 291–306, 645–675; **61**: 81–108.

61 Clifford DB, Olney JW, Benz AM *et al*. Ketamine, phencyclidine, and MK-801 protect against kainic acid-induced seizure-related brain damage. *Epilepsia* 1990; **31**: 382–90.

62 Clifford DB, Zorumski CF, Olney JW. Ketamine and MK-801 prevent degeneration of thalamic neurons induced by focal cortical seizures. *Exp Neurol* 1989; **105**: 272–9.

63 Cochius J, Carpenter S, Andermann E *et al*. Sweat gland vacuoles in Unverricht–Lundbord disease: a clue to diagnosis? *Neurology* 1994; **44**: 2372–5.

64 Cockerell OC, Johnson AL Sander JW *et al*. Mortality from epilepsy: results from a prospective population-based study. *Lancet* 1994; **344**: 918–21.

65 Commission on Classification and Terminology of the International League against Epilepsy. Proposal for revised classification of epilepsies and epileptic syndromes. *Epilepsia* 1989; **30**: 389–99.

66 Commission on Classification and Terminology of the International League against Epilepsy. Proposal for revised clinical and electroencephalograph classification of epileptic seizures. *Epilepsia* 1981; **22**: 489–501.

67 Cornell-Bell AH, Williamson A. Hyperexcitability of astrocytes and neurons in epileptic human cortex. In: Federoff S, Juurlink BH, Doucette R eds. *Biology and pathology of astrocyte–neuron interactions*. New York: Plenum, 1993: 51–66.

68 Corsellis JAN, Bruton CJ. Neuropathology of status epilepticus in humans. In: Delgado-Escueta AV, Wasterlain CG, Treiman D, Porter RJ eds. *Status epilepticus: mechanisms of brain damage and treatment*. New York: Raven Press, 1983: 129–39.

69 Corsellis JAN, Meyer A. Histological changes in the brain after uncomplicated electroconvulsant treatment. *J Ment Sci* 1954; **100**: 375–83.

70 Cotter D, Honavar M, Lovestone S *et al*. Disturbance in Notch-1 and WNT signalling proteins in neuroglial balloon cells and abnormal large neurons in focal cortical dysplasia in human cortex. *Acta Neuropathol* 1999; **98**: 465–72.

71 Cowan LD, Bodensteiner JB, Leviton A, Doherty L. Prevalence of the epilepsies in children and adolescents. *Epilepsia* 1989; **30**: 94–106.

72 Crino PB, Duhaime AC, Baltuch G, White R. Differential expression of glutamate and GABA$_A$ receptor subunit mRNA in cortical dysplasia. *Neurology* 2001; **56**: 906–13.

73 Crino PB, Trojanowski JQ, Eberwine J. Internexin, MAP1B, and nestin in cortical dysplasia as markers of developmental maturity. *Acta Neuropathol* 1997; **93**: 619–27.

74 D'Alessandro R, Ferrara R, Benassi G. Computed tomographic scans in post traumatic epilepsy. *Arch Neurol* 1988; **45**: 42–3.

75 Dam AM. Epilepsy and neuron loss in the hippocampus. *Epilepsia* 1980; **21**: 617–29.

76 Dam AM. Hippocampal neuron loss in epilepsy and after experimental seizures. *Acta Neurol Scand* 1982; **66**: 601–42.

77 Dam AM, Fuglsang-Fredriksen A, Svarre-Olsen U, Dam M. Late-onset epilepsy: etiologies, types of seizure, and value of clinical investigation, EEG, and computerized tomography scan. *Epilepsia* 1985; **26**: 227–31.

78 Danesi MA. Classification of the epilepsies: an investigation of 945 patients in a developing country. *Epilepsia* 1985; **2**: 131–6.

79 Dastur HM. Diagnosis and neurosurgical treatment of tuberculous disease of the CNS. *Neurosurgery* 1983; **6**: 111–17.

80 Daumas-Duport C, Scheithauer BW, Chodkiewicz J-P *et al*. Dysembryoplastic neuroepithelial tumour. A surgically curable tumour of young patients with intractable partial seizures. *Neurosurgery* 1988; **23**: 545–56.

81 Davenport CJ, Brown WJ, Babb TL. Sprouting of GABAergic and mossy fiber axons in dentate gyrus following intrahippocampal kainate in the rat. *Exp Neurol* 1990; **109**: 180–90.

82 Davies KG, Maxwell RE, French LA. Hemispherectomy for intractable seizures: long-term results in 17 patients followed for up to 38 years. *J Neurosurg* 1993; **78**: 733–48.

83 Davison C, Keschner M. Myoclonus epilepsy. *Arch Neurol Psychiatry* 1940; **43**: 524–46.

84 DeFelipe J, Huntley GW, del Rio MR *et al*. Microzonal decreases in the immunostaining for non-NMDA ionotropic excitatory amino acid receptor subunits GluR 2/3 and GluR 5/6/7 in the human epileptogenic neocortex. *Brain Res* 1994; **657**: 150–8.

85 DeLorey TM, Handforth A, Homanics GE *et al*. Mice lacking the β3 subunit of the GABA$_A$ receptor have the epilepsy phenotype and many of the behavioural characteristics of Angelman syndrome. *J Neurosci* 1998; **18**: 8505–14.

86 DeMoor J. Le méchanisme et la signification de l'état moniliforme des neurones. *Annales de la Société Royale des Sciences Médicales et Naturelles de Bruxelles* 1898; **7**: 205–50.

87 De Rijk-Van Andel JF, Arts WFM *et al*. Diagnostic features and clinical signs of 21 patients with lissencephaly type I. *Dev Med Child Neurol* 1990; **32**: 707–17.

88 DeToledo JC, Smith DB. Partially successful treatment of Rasmussen's encephalitis with Zidovudine: symptomatic improvement followed by involvement of the contralateral hemisphere. *Epilepsia* 1994; **35**: 352–5.

89 DiMauro S, Kulikova R, Tanji K *et al*. Mitochondrial genes for generalized epilepsies. In: Delgado-Escueta AV, Wilson WA, Olsen RW, Porter RJ eds. *Jasper's Basic mechanisms of the epilepsies* 3rd edn. *Advances in Neurology* 1999; **79**: 411–19.

90 Dobyns WB, Curry CJR, Hoyme HE *et al*. Clinical and molecular diagnosis of Miller–Dieker syndrome. *Am J Hum Genet* 1991; **48**: 584–94.

91 Doose H, Sitepu B. Childhood epilepsy in a German city. *Neuropediatrics* 1983; **14**: 220–4.

92 Drury I, Blaivas M, Abou-Khalil BW, Beydoun A. Biopsy results in a kindred with Lafora disease. *Arch Neurol* 1993; **50**: 102–5.

93 Du F, Schwarcz R. Aminooxyacetic acid causes selective neuronal loss in layer III of the rat medial entorhinal cortex. *Neurosci Lett* 1992; **147**: 185–8.

94 Du F, Whetsell WO Jr, Abou-Khalil B *et al*. Preferential neuronal loss in layer III of the entorhinal cortex in patients with temporal lobe epilepsy. *Epilepsy Res* 1993; **16**: 223–33.

95 Dukes CS, Luft BJ, Durack DT. Toxoplasmosis of the central nervous system. In: Scheld WM, Whitley RJ, Durack DT eds. *Infections of the central nervous system*. Raven Press, 1991: 801–23.

96 Duncan JS. Imaging and epilepsy. *Brain* 1997; **120**: 339–77.

97 Duncan JS, Sagar HJ. Seizure characteristics, pathology, and outcome after temporal lobectomy. *Neurology* 1987; **37**: 405–9.

98 Duncan R, Patterson J, Roberts R *et al*. Ictal/postictal SPECTin the pre-surgical localisation of complex partial seizures. *J Neurol Neurosurg Psychiatry* 1993; **56**: 141–8.

99 Duong T, De Rosa MJ, Poukeus V *et al*. Neuronal cytoskeletal abnormalities in human cerebral cortical dysplasia. *Acta Neuropathol (Berl)* 1994; **87**: 493–503.

100 During MJ, Ryder KM, Spencer DD. Hippocampal GABA transporter function in temporal-lobe epilepsy. *Nature* 1995; **376**: 174–7.

101 Earle KM, Baldwin M, Penfield W. Incisural sclerosis and temporal lobe seizures produced by hippocampal herniation at birth. *Arch Neurol Psychiatry* 1953; **69**: 27–42.

102 Earnest MP, Thomas GE, Eden RA. Sudden unexpected death in epilepsy. *Neurology* 1988; **38** (Suppl 1): 248–9.

103 Earnest MP, Thomas GE, Eden RA, Hossack KF. The sudden unexplained death syndrome in epilepsy: demographic, clinical and postmortem features. *Epilepsia* 1992; **33**: 310–16.

104 Edgar R, Baldwin M. Vascular malformations associated with temporal lobe epilepsy. *J Neurosurg* 1960; **17**: 638–56.

105 Edgell HP, Stanfield JP. Paediatric neurology in Africa: a Ugandan report. *BMJ* 1972; **i**: 548–52.

106 El Bahh B, Lespinet V, Lurton D *et al*. Correlation between granule cell dispersion, mossy fiber sprouting, and hippocampal cell loss in temporal lobe epilepsy. *Epilepsia* 1999; **40**: 1393–401.

107 Eldridge R, Iivanainen M, Stern R *et al*. 'Baltic' myoclonus epilepsy: hereditary disorder of childhood made worse by Phenytoin. *Lancet* 1983; **ii**: 838–42.

108 Ellenberg JH, Hirtz DG, Nelson KB. Age at onset of seizures in young children. *Ann Neurol* 1984; **15**: 127–34.

109 Emery JÁ, Roper SN, Rojiani AM. White matter neuronal heterotopia in temporal lobe epilepsy: a morphometric and immunohistochemical study. *J Neuropathol Exp Neurol* 1997; **56**: 1276–82.

110 Escobedo F, Garcia-Ramos G, Sotelo J. Parasitic disorders and epilepsy. In: Nistico G, Di Perry R, Meinardi H eds. *Epilepsy: an update on research and therapy*. New York: Alan R Liss, 1983: 227–33.

111 Evans M, Griffiths T, Meldrum BS. Early changes in the rat hippocampus following seizures induced by bicuculline or L-allylglycine: a light and electron microscope study. *Neuropathol Appl Neurobiol* 1983; **9**: 39–52.

112 Evans MC, Griffiths T, Meldrum BS. Kainic acid seizures and the reversibility of calcium loading in vulnerable neurons in the hippocampus. *Neuropathol Appl Neurobiol* 1984; **10**: 285–30.

113 Fahn S, Marsden CD, Van Woert MH. Definition and classification of myoclonus. *Adv Neurol* 1986; **43**: 1–5.

114 Falconer MA. Discussion of the surgery of temporal lobe epilepsy; surgical and pathological aspects. *Proc R Soc Med* 1953; **46**: 971–5.

115 Falconer MA. Mesial temporal (Ammon's horn) sclerosis as a common cause of epilepsy. Aetiology, treatment and prevention. *Lancet* 1974; **2**: 767–70.

116 Falconer MA, Serafetinides EA, Corsellis JAN. Etiology and pathogenesis of temporal lobe epilepsy. *Arch Neurol* 1964; **10**: 233–48.

117 Fariello RG, Golden GT, Smith GG, Reyes PF. Potentiation of kainic acid epileptogenicity and sparing from neuronal damage by an NMDA receptor antagonist. *Epilepsy Res* 1989; **3**: 206–13.

118 Farrell MA, Cheng L, Cornford ME *et al*. Cytomegalovirus and Rasmussen's encephalitis. *Lancet* 1991; **337**: 1551–2.

119 Farrell MA, DeRosa MJ, Curran JG *et al*. Neuropathologic findings in cortical resections (including hemispherectomies) performed for the treatment of intractable childhood epilepsy. *Acta Neuropathol* 1992; **83**: 246–59.

120 Ferrer I, Pineda M, Tallada M *et al*. Abnormal local-circuit neurons in epilepsia partialis continua associated with focal cortical dysplasia. *Acta Neuropathol* 1992; **83**: 647–52.

121 Foerster O, Penfield W. The structural basis of traumatic epilepsy and results of radical operation. *Brain* 1930; **53**: 99–119.

122 Forsgren L. Prevalence of epilepsy in adults in northern Sweden. *Epilepsia* 1992; **33**: 450–8.

123 Fowler M. Brain damage after febrile convulsions. *Arch Dis Child* 1957; **32**: 67–76.

124 Fried I, Kim JH, Spencer DD. Hippocampal pathology in patients with intractable seizures and temporal lobe masses. *J Neurosurg* 1992; **76**: 735–40.

125 Fried I, Kim JH, Spencer DD. Limbic and neocortical gliomas associated with intractable seizures: a distinct clinicopathological group. *Neurosurgery* 1994; **34**: 815–23.

126 Friede RL. Disturbances in bulk growth: megalencephaly, minencephaly atelencephaly and others. In: *Developmental neuropathology*. New York: Springer, 1989: 296–308.

127 Fukuda T, Oguni H, Yanagaki S *et al*. Chronic localized encephalitis (Rasmussen's syndrome) preceded by ipsilateral uveitis: a case report. *Epilepsia* 1994; **35**: 1328–31.

128 Fukuhara N, Tokiguchi S, Shirakawa K, Tadao T. Myoclonus epilepsy associated with ragged-red fibres (mitochondrial abnormalities): disease entity or a syndrome? *J Neurol Sci* 1980; **47**:117–37.

129 Gall CM, Isackson PJ. Limbic seizures increase neuronal production of messenger RNA for nerve growth factor. *Science* 1989; **245**: 758–61.

130 Gardiner RM. Genetic basis of the human epilepsies. *Epilepsy Res* 1999; **36**: 91–5.

131 Gastaut H, Gastaut JL, Goncalves E *et al*. Relative frequency of different types of epilepsy: a study employing the classification of the International League against Epilepsy. *Epilepsia* 1975; **11**: 102–13.

132 Geddes JW, Cahan LD, Cooper SM *et al*. Altered distribution of excitatory amino acid receptors in temporal lobe epilepsy. *Exp Neurol* 1990; **108**: 214–20.

133 Gomez JG, Arciniegas E, Torres J. Prevalence of epilepsy in Bogota, Colombia. *Neurology* 1978; **28**: 90–8.

134 Gomez MR. Tuberous sclerosis. In: Gomez MR ed. *Neurocutaneous diseases*. Boston, MA: Butterworths, 1989: 30–52.

135 Gomez MR, Bebin EM. Sturge-Weber syndrome. In: Gomez MR ed. *Neurocutaneous diseases*. Boston, MA: Butterworths, 1987: 356–67.

136 Gray F, Serdaru M, Baron H *et al*. Chronic localised encephalitis (Rasmussen's) in an adult with epilepsia partialis continua. *J Neurol Neurosurg Psychiatry* 1987; **50**: 747–51.

137 Griffiths T, Evans MC, Meldrum BS. Intracellular calcium accumulation in rat hippocampus during seizures induced by bicuculline or ʟ-allylglycine. *Neuroscience* 1983; **10**: 385–95.

138 Griffiths T, Evans MC, Meldrum BS. Status epilepticus: the reversibility of calcium loading and acute neuronal pathological changes in the rat hippocampus. *Neuroscience* 1984; **12**: 557–67.

139 Grisar T, Delgado-Escueta AV. Astroglial contribution in human temporal lobe epilepsy: K⁺ activation of Na⁺, K⁺-ATPase in bulk isolated glial cells and synaptosomes. *Brain Res* 1986; **364**: 1–11.

140 Haglund MM, Berger MS, Kunkel DD *et al*. Changes in gamma-aminobutyric acid and somatostatin in cortex associated with low-grade gliomas. *J Neurosurg* 1992; **77**: 209–16.

141 Hall J. A pattern of convulsions in childhood. *West Indian Med J* 1964; **13**: 244–8.

142 Halliday AM. The electrophysiological study of myoclonus in man. *Brain* 1967; **90**: 241–84.

143 Haltia M, Kristensson K, Sourander P. Neuropathological studies in three Scandinavian cases of progressive myoclonus epilepsy. *Acta Neurol Scand* 1969; **45**: 63–77.

144 Hamosh A, Scott AF, Amberger J *et al*. Online Mendelian inheritance in man (OMIM). *Hum Mutat* 2000; **15**: 57–61.

145 Hand KSP, Baird VH, Van Paesschen W *et al*. Central benzodiazepine receptor autoradiography in hippocampal sclerosis. *Br J Pharmacol* 1997; **122**: 358–64.

146 Hardiman O, Burke T, Phillips J *et al*. Microdysgenesis in resected temporal neocortex. *Neurology* 1988; **38**: 1041–7.

147 Harriman DGF, Millar JHD. Progressive familial myoclonic epilepsy in three families: its clinical features and pathological basis. *Brain* 1955; **78**: 325–49.

148 Hart YM, Andermann F, Robitaille Y *et al*. Double pathology in Rasmussen's syndrome. A window on the etiology? *Neurology* 1998; **50**: 731–5.

149 Harvey AS, Andermann F, Hopkins IJ *et al*. Chronic encephalitis (Rasmussen's syndrome) and ipsilateral uveitis. *Ann Neurol* 1992; **32**: 826–9.

150 Harvey AS, Bowe JM, Hopkins IJ *et al*. Ictal ⁹⁹ᵐTc-HMPAO single photon emission computed tomography in children with temporal lobe epilepsy. *Epilepsia* 1993; **34**: 869–77.

151 Hattori M, Adachi H, Tsujimoto M *et al*. Miller–Dieker lissencephaly gene encodes a subunit of brain platelet-activating factor. *Nature* 1994; **370**: 216–18.

152 Hauser WA, Annegers JF, Anderson VE, Kurland LT. The risk of seizure disorder, among relatives of children with febrile convulsions. *Neurology* 1985; **35**: 1268–73.

153 Hauser WA, Kurland LT. The epidemiology of epilepsy in Rochester, Minnesota, 1935 through 1967. *Epilepsia* 1975; **16**: 1–66.

154 Hennessy MJ, Elwes RDC, Honavar M *et al*. Predictors of outcome and pathological considerations in the surgical treatment of intractable epilepsy associated with temporal lobe lesions. *J Neurol Neurosurg Psychiatry* 2001; **70**: 450–8.

155 Henry TR, Frey KA, Sackellares JC *et al*. In vivo cerebral metabolism and central benzodiazepine-receptor binding in temporal lobe epilepsy. *Neurology* 1993; **43**: 1998–2006.

156 Henry TR, Mazziotta JC, Engel J Jr *et al*. Quantifying interictal metabolic activity in human temporal lobe epilepsy. *J Cereb Blood Flow Metab* 1990; **10**: 748–57.

157 Hetherington H, Kuzniecky R, Pan J *et al*. Proton nuclear magnetic resonance spectroscopic imaging of human temporal lobe epilepsy at 4.1T. *Ann Neurol* 1995; **38**: 396–404.

158 Hirabayashi S, Binnie CD, Janota I, Polkey CE. Surgical treatment of epilepsy due to cortical dysplasia: clinical and EEG findings. *J Neurol Neurosurg Psychiatry* 1993; **56**: 765–70.

159 Hirsch CS, Martin DL. Unexpected death in young epileptics. *Neurology* 1971; **21**: 682–90.

160 Hirsch J-F, Rose CS, Pierre-Kahn A *et al*. Benign astrocytic and oligodendrocytic tumours of the cerebral hemispheres in children. *J Neurosurg* 1989; **70**: 568–72.

161 Ho SS, Newton MR, McIntosh AM *et al*. Perfusion patterns during temporal lobe seizures: relationship to surgical outcome. *Brain* 1997; **120**: 1921–8.

162 Hochman DW, Baraban SC, Owens JWM, Schwartzkroin PA. Dissociation of synchronization and excitability in furosemide blockade of epileptiform activity. *Science* 1995; **270**: 99–102.

163 Hoeppner TJ, Morrell F. Control of scar formation in experimentally induced epilepsy. *Exp Neurol* 1986; **94**: 519–36.

164 Honavar M. Neuropathology of failed multiple subpial transection. *Bol Epilepsia* 1996; **2**: 51–2.

165 Honavar M, Janota I, Polkey CE. Histological heterogeneity of dysembryoplastic neuroepithelial tumour: identification and differential diagnosis in a series of 74 cases. *Histopathology* 1999; **34**: 342–56.

166 Honavar M, Janota I, Polkey CE. Neuropathological findings in surgery for epilepsy. Four hundred and thirty resections for treatment of chronic epilepsy: an 18-year experience. *Bol Epilepsia* 1997; **2**: 14–28.

167 Honavar M, Janota I, Polkey CE. Rasmussen's encephalitis in surgery for epilepsy. *Dev Med Child Neurol* 1992; **34**: 3–14.

168 Horsley V. Brain surgery. *BMJ* 1886; **ii**: 670–5.

169 Horvath Z, Hsu M, Pierre E *et al*. Structural impairment of hippocampal neurons following a single epileptic afterdischarge. *Epilepsy Res* 1996; **12** (Suppl): 325–34.

170 Hosford DA, Crain BJ, Cao Z *et al*. Increased AMPA-sensitive quisqualate receptor binding and reduced NMDA receptor binding in epileptic human hippocampus. *J Neurosci* 1991; **11**: 428–34.

171 Houser CR. Granule cell dispersion in the dentate gyrus of humans with temporal lobe epilepsy. *Brain Res* 1990; **535**: 195–204.

172 Houser CR, Miyashiro J, Swartz BE *et al*. Altered patterns of dynorphin immunoreactivity suggest mossy fiber reorganization in human hippocampal epilepsy. *J Neurosci* 1990; **10**: 267–82.

173 Hudson LP, Munoz DG, Miller L *et al*. Amygdaloid sclerosis in temporal lobe epilepsy. *Ann Neurol* 1993; **33**: 622–31.

174 Hunt JR. Dyssynergia cerebellaris myoclonica – primary atrophy of the dentate system. *Brain* 1921; **44**: 490–538.

175 Ignelzi RJ, Bucy PC. Cerebral decortication in the treatment of infantile cerebral hemiatrophy. *J Nerv Ment Dis* 1968; **147**: 14–30.

176 Inamura K, Smith ML, Hansen AJ, Siesjo BK. Seizure-induced damage to substantia nigra and globus pallidus is accompanied by pronounced intra- and extracellular acidosis. *J Cereb Blood Flow Metab* 1989; **9**: 821–9.

177 Jackson GD, Connelly A, Duncan JS *et al*. Detection of hippocampal pathology in intractable partial epilepsy: Increased sensitivity with quantitative magnetic resonance T2 relaxometry. *Neurology* 1993; **43**: 1793–9.

178 Jackson H. On the anatomical, physiological and pathological investigation of epilepsies. *West Riding Lunatic Asylum medical reports* 1873; **3**: 315. Reprinted in: Taylor J ed. *Selected writings of John Hughlings Jackson*. London: Hodder and Stoughton, 1931; 90–111.

179 Jacobs KM, Kharazia VN, Prince DA. Mechanisms underlying epileptogenesis in cortical malformations. *Epilepsy Res* 1999; **36**: 165–88.

180 Janota I, Polkey CE. Cortical dysplasia in epilepsy. In: Pedley TA, Meldrum BS eds. Recent advances in epilepsy Vol. 5. Edinburgh: Churchill Livingstone, 1992: 37–49.

181 Jarrard LE, Meldrum BS. Selective excitotoxic pathology in the rat hippocampus. Neuropathol Appl Neurobiol 1993; 19: 381–9.

182 Jennett B. Epilepsy and acute traumatic intracranial haematoma. J Neurol Neurosurg Psychiatry 1975; 38: 378–81.

183 Jennett WB, Lewin W. Traumatic epilepsy after closed head injury. J Neurol Neurosurg Psychiatry 1960; 22: 295–301.

184 Jennett WB, Miller JD, Braakman R. Epilepsy after non-missile depressed skull fracture. J Neurosurg 1974; 41: 108–216.

185 Joensen P. Prevalence, incidence, and classification of epilepsy in the Faroes. Acta Neurol Scand 1986; 74: 150–5.

186 Johnson EW, De Lanerolle NC, Kim JH et al. 'Central' and 'peripheral' benzodiazepine receptors: opposite changes in human epileptogenic tissue. Neurology 1992; 42: 811–15.

187 Johnston SC, Darragh TM, Simon RP. Postictal pulmonary edema requires pulmonary vascular pressure increases. Epilepsia 1996; 37: 428–32.

188 Johnston SC, Horn JK, Valente J, Simon RP. The role of hypoventilation in a sheep model of epileptic sudden death. Ann Neurol 1995; 37: 531–7.

189 Joshi V, Katiyar BC, Mohan PK et al. Profile of epilepsy in a developing country: a study of 1,000 patients based on the International Classification. Epilepsia 1977; 18: 549–54.

190 Kanemoto K, Kawasaki J, Miyamoto T et al. Interleukin (IL)-1β, IL-1α, and IL-1 receptor antagonist gene polymorphisms in patients with temporal lobe epilepsy. Ann Neurol 2000; 47: 571–4.

191 Kasper BS, Stefan H, Buchfelder M, Paulus W. Temporal lobe microdysgenesis in epilepsy versus control brains. J Neuropathol Exp Neurol 1999; 58: 22–8.

192 Kaufmann WE, Galaburda AM. Cerebrocortical microdysgenesis in neurologically normal subjects. Neurology 1989; 39: 238–44.

193 Keilson MJ, Hauser WA, Magrill JP, Goldman M. ECG abnormalities in patients with epilepsy. Neurology 1987; 37: 1624–6.

194 Kendal C, Everall I, Polkey C, Al-Sarraj S. Glial cell changes in white matter in temporal lobe epilepsy. Epilepsy Res 1999; 36: 43–51.

195 Keränen T, Sillanpää M, Riekkinen PJ. Distribution of seizure types in an epileptic population. Epilepsia 1988; 29: 1–7.

196 Kerfoot C, Vinters HV, Mathern GW. Cerebral cortical dysplasia: giant neurons show potential for increased excitation and axonal plasticity. Dev Neurosci 1999; 21: 260–70.

197 Ketz E. Brain tumours and epilepsy. In: Vinken PL, Bruyn GW eds. Handbook of clinical neurology Vol. 16. Amsterdam: North-Holland, 1974: 254–69.

198 Kim JH, Guimaraes PO, Shen MY et al. Hippocampal neuronal density in temporal lobe epilepsy with and without gliomas. Acta Neuropathol (Berl) 1990; 80: 41–5.

199 King D, Spencer SS, McCarthy G et al. Bilateral hippocampal atrophy in medial temporal lobe epilepsy. Epilepsia 1995; 36: 905–10.

200 King M, Stephenson JBP, Ziervogel M et al. Hemimegalencephaly – a case for hemispherectomy? Neuropediatrics 1985; 16: 46–55.

201 Kirkpatrick PJ, Honavar M, Janota I, Polkey CE. Control of temporal lobe epilepsy following en-bloc resection of low-grade tumours. J Neurosurg 1993; 78: 19–25.

202 Kohr G, Konick Y, Mody I. Properties of NMDA receptor channels in neurons acutely isolated from epileptic (kindled) rats. J Neurosci 1993; 13: 3612–27.

203 Kohr G, Mody I. Kindling increases N-methyl-D-aspartate potency at single N-methyl-D-aspartate channels in dentate gyrus granule cells. Neuroscience 1994; 62: 975–81.

204 Koskiniemi M. Findings in routine laboratory examination in progressive myoclonus epilepsy. Acta Neurol Scand 1975; 51: 12–20.

205 Koskiniemi M, Donner M, Majuri H et al. Progressive myoclonus epilepsy: a clinical and histopathological study. Acta Neurol Scand 1974; 50: 307–32.

206 Koul R, Razdan S, Motta A. Prevalence and pattern of epilepsy (Lath/Mirgi/Laran) in rural Kashmir, India. Epilepsia 1988; 29: 116–22.

207 Kraemer DL, Awad IA. Vascular malformations and epilepsy: clinical considerations and basic mechanisms. Epilepsia 1994; 35 (Suppl 6): S30–43.

208 Krishnan B, Armstrong DL, Grossman RG et al. Glial cell nuclear hypertrophy in complex partial seizures. J Neuropathol Exp Neurol 1994; 53: 502–7.

209 Krynauw RA. Infantile hemiplegia treated by removing one cerebral hemisphere. J Neurol Neurosurg Psychiatry 1950; 13: 243–67.

210 Kuzniecky RI. Magnetic resonance; imaging in developmental disorders of the cerebral cortex. Epilepsia 1994; 35 (Suppl): S44–56.

211 Lanerolle NC de, Brines M, Williamson A et al. Neurotransmitters and their receptors in human temporal lobe epilepsy. In: Ribak CE, Gall CM, Mody I eds. The dentate gyrus and its role in seizures. Epilepsy Research (Suppl 7). Amsterdam: Elsevier, 1992: 235–50.

212 Lanerolle NC de, Eid T, Campe G von et al. Glutamate receptor subunits GluR1 and GluR2/3 distribution shows reorganization in the human epileptogenic hippocampus. Eur J Neurosci 1998; 10: 1687–703.

213 Lanerolle NC de, Kim JH, Brines ML. Cellular and molecular alterations in partial epilepsy. Clin Neurosci 1994; 2: 64–81.

214 Lanerolle NC de, Kim JH, Robbins RJ, Spencer DD. Hippocampal interneuron loss and plasticity in human temporal lobe epilepsy. Brain Res 1989; 495: 387–95.

215 Lanerolle NC de, Sundaresan S, Brines ML et al. Distribution of NMDA, quisqualic acid and kainic acid receptors in the hippocampus in human temporal lobe epilepsy. Epilepsia 1990; 31: 625.

216 LeBlanc FE, Rasmussen T. The epilepsies. In: Magnus O, Lorentz de Haas AM eds. Handbook of clinical neurology (Series eds: Vinken PJ, Bruyn GW) Vol. 15. Amsterdam: North Holland, 1974.

217 Lee N, Tien RD, Lewis DV et al. Fast spin-echo, magnetic resonance imaging-measured hippocampal volume: correlation with neuronal density in anterior temporal lobectomy patients. Epilepsia 1995; 36: 899–904.

218 Leestma JE, Walczak T, Hughes JR et al. A prospective study on sudden unexpected death in epilepsy. Ann Neurol 1989; 26: 195–203.

219 Legg NJ, Gupta PC, Scott DF. Epilepsy following cerebral abscess. A clinical and EEG study of 70 patients. Brain 1973; 96: 259–68.

220 Lehesjoki AE, Koskiniemi M, Sistonen P et al. Localization of a gene for progressive myoclonus epilepsy to chromosome 21q22. Proc Nat Acad Sci USA 1991; 88: 3696–9.

221 Lennox-Buchthal MA. Febrile convulsions. Amsterdam: Elsevier, 1973.

222 Lerche H, Biervert C, Alekov AK et al. A reduced K+ current due to a novel mutation in KCNQ2 causes neonatal convulsions. Ann Neurol 1999; 46: 305–12.

223 Lerner-Natoli M, Rondouin G, Relaidi M et al. N-(2-Thienyl)cyclohexyl 1-piperidine (TCP) does not block kainic acid-induced status epilepticus but reduces secondary hippocampal damage. Neurosci Lett 1991; 122: 174–8.

224 Levesque MF, Nakasato N, Vinters HV, Babb TL. Surgical treatment of limbic epilepsy associated with extrahippocampal lesions: the problem of dual pathology. *J Neurosurg* 1991; **75**: 364–70.

225 Li S-c, Schoenberg BS, Wang C-c *et al*. Epidemiology of epilepsy in urban areas of the People's Republic of China. *Epilepsia* 1985; **26**: 391–4.

226 Liedholm LJ, Gudjonsson O. Cardiac arrest due to partial epileptic seizures. *Neurology* 1992; **42**: 824–9.

227 Liu AW, Delgado-Escueta AV, Serratosa JM *et al*. Juvenile mycolonic epilepsy locus in chromosome 6p21.2-p11: linkage to convulsions and electroencephalography trait. *Am J Hum Genet* 1995; **57**: 368–81.

228 Lorente de No R. I. Studies on the structure of the cerebral cortex. II. Continuation of the study of the ammonic system. *J Psychol Neurol* 1934; **46**: 143–77.

229 Louvel J, Pumain R. *N*-methyl-D-aspartate-mediated responses in epileptic cortex in man: an *in vitro* study. In: Engel J ed. *Neurotransmitters, seizures and epilepsy* IV. Amsterdam: Elsevier, 1992: 487–95.

230 Lowenstein DW, Alldredge BK. Status epilepticus. *N Engl J Med* 1998; **338**: 970–6.

231 Lyon G, Gastaut H. Considerations on the significance attributed to unusual cerebral histological findings recently described in eight patients with primary generalized epilepsy. *Epilepsia* 1985; **26**: 365–7.

232 McDonald JW, Garofalo EA, Hood T *et al*. Altered excitatory and inhibitory amino acid receptor binding in hippocampus of patients with temporal lobe epilepsy. *Ann Neurol* 1991; **29**: 529–41.

233 McKenzie KG. The present status of a patient who had the right cerebral hemisphere removed. *JAMA* 1938; **111**: 168.

234 McKusick VA. *Mendelian inheritance in man*. Baltimore, MD: Johns Hopkins University Press, 1992.

235 McMillan T, Powell GE, Janota I, Polkey CE. Relationships between neuropathology and cognitive functioning in temporal lobectomy patients. *J Neurol Psychiatry* 1987; **50**: 167–76.

236 Maglóczky ZS, Wittner L, Borhegyi ZS *et al*. Changes in the distribution and connectivity of interneurons in the epileptic human dentate gyrus. *Neuroscience* 2000; **96**: 7–25.

237 Malafosse A, Lehesjoki AE, Genton P *et al*. Identical genetic locus for Baltic and Mediterranean myoclonus. *Lancet* 1992; **339**: 1080–1.

238 Mampalam TJ, Rosenblum ML. Trends in the management of bacterial brain abscesses: a review of 102 cases over 17 years. *Neurosurgery* 1988; **23**: 451–8.

239 Marchal G, Andermann F, Tampieri D *et al*. Generalised cortical dysplasia manifested by diffusely thick cerebral cortex. *Arch Neurol* 1989; **46**: 430–4.

240 Marco P, Sola RG, Ramon y Cajal S, DeFelipe J. Loss of inhibitory synapses on the soma and axon initial segment of pyramidal cells in human epileptic peritumoural neocortex: implications for epilepsy. *Brain Res Bulle* 1997; **44**: 47–66.

241 Margerison JH, Corsellis JAN. Epilepsy and the temporal lobes. *Brain* 1966; **89**: 499–530.

242 Marks DA, Kim J, Spencer D, Spencer SS. Characteristics of intractable seizures following meningitis and encephalitis. *Neurology* 1992; **42**: 1513–18.

243 Marsden CD, Hallett M, Fahn S. The nosology and pathophysiology of myoclonus. In: Marsden CD, Fahn S eds. *Movement disorders*. London: Butterworth Scientific, 1982: 196–248.

244 Marsden CD, Harding AE, Obeso JA. Progressive myoclonic ataxia (the Ramsay Hunt syndrome). *Arch Neurol* 1990; **47**: 1121–5.

245 Mathern GW, Babb TL, Vickrey BG *et al*. Traumatic compared to non-traumatic clinical–pathologic associations in temporal lobe epilepsy. *Epilepsy Res* 1994; **19**: 129–39.

246 Mathern GW, Cepeda C, Hurst RS *et al*. Neurons recorded from pediatric epilepsy surgery patients with cortical dysplasia. *Epilepsia* 2000; **41** (Suppl 6): S162–7.

247 Mathern GW, Cifuentes F, Leite JP *et al*. Hippocampal EEG excitability and chronic spontaneous seizures are associated with aberrant synaptic reorganization in the rat intrahippocampal kainate model. *Electroencephalogr Clin Neurophysiol* 1993; **87**: 326–39.

248 Mathern GW, Pretorius JK, Babb TL. Influence of the type of initial precipitating injury and at what age it occurs on course and outcome in patients with temporal lobe seizures. *J Neurosurg* 1995; **82**: 220–7.

249 Mathern GW, Pretorius JK, Kornblum HI *et al*. Altered hippocampal kainate-receptor mRNA levels in temporal lobe epilepsy patients. *Neurobiol Dis* 1998; **5**: 151–76.

250 Mathern GW, Pretorius JK, Kornblum HI *et al*. Human hippocampal AMPA and NMDA mRNA levels in temporal lobe epilepsy patients. *Brain* 1997; **120**: 1937–59.

251 Mathieson G. Pathology of temporal lobe foci. *Adv Neurol* 1975; **11**: 163–85.

252 Mayberg HS, Sadzot B, Meltzer CD *et al*. Quantification of Mu and non-Mu opiate receptors in temporal lobe epilepsy using positron emission tomography. *Ann Neurol* 1991; **30**: 3–11.

253 Maytal J, Shinnar S. Febrile status epilepticus. *Paediatrics* 1990; **86**: 611–16.

254 Maytal J, Shinnar S, Mosher SI, Alvarez IA. Low morbidity and mortality on status epilepticus in children. *Paediatrics* 1989; **83**: 323–31.

255 Meencke HJ. Pathology of childhood epilepsies. *Cleveland Clin J Med* 1990; **56** (Suppl 1.1): S111–20.

256 Meencke HJ, Janz D. Neuropathological findings in primary generalized epilepsy: a study of eight cases. *Epilepsia* 1984; **25**: 8–21.

257 Meldrum BS. Metabolic effects of prolonged epileptic seizures and the causation of epileptic brain damage. In: Rose FC ed. *Metabolic disorders of the nervous system*. London: Pitman, 1981: 175–87.

258 Meldrum BS. Metabolic factors during prolonged seizures and their relation to nerve cell death. *Adv Neurol* 1983; **34**: 261–75.

259 Meldrum BS, Brierley JB. Prolonged epileptic seizures in primates: ischaemic cell change and its relation to ictal physiological events. *Arch Neurol* 1973; **28**: 10–17.

260 Meldrum BS, Garthwaite J. Excitatory amino acid neurotoxicity and neurodegenerative disease. *Trends Pharmacol Sci* 1990; **11**: 379–87.

261 Meldrum BS, Vigoroux RA, Brierley JB. Systemic factors and epileptic brain damage. Prolonged seizures in paralysed artificially ventilated baboons. *Arch Neurol* 1973; **29**: 82–7.

262 Mello LE, Cavalheiro EA, Tan AM *et al*. Granule cell dispersion in relation to mossy fibre sprouting, hippocampal cell loss, silent period and seizure frequency in the pilocarpine model of epilepsy. *Epilepsy Res* 1992; **9** (Suppl): 51–9.

263 Menini C, Meldrum BS, Riche D *et al*. Sustained limbic seizures induced by intraamygdaloid kainic acid in the baboon: symptomatology and neuropathological consequences. *Ann Neurol* 1980; **8**: 501–9.

264 Meyer A, Beck E, Shepherd M. Unusually severe lesions in the brain following status epilepticus. *J Neurol Psychiatry* 1955; **18**: 24–33.

265 Mikkonen M, Soininen H, Kälviäinen R *et al*. Remodelling of neuronal circuitries in human temporal lobe epilepsy: increased expression of highly polysialylated neural cell

adhesion molecule in the hippocampus and the entorhinal cortex. *Ann Neurol* 1998; **44**: 923–34.

266 Minassian BA, DeLorey TM, Olsen RW *et al*. Angelman syndrome: correlations between epilepsy phenotypes and genotypes. *Ann Neurol* 1998; **43**: 485–93.

267 Minassian BA, Lee JR, Herbrick JA *et al*. Mutations in a gene encoding a novel protein tyrosine phosphatase cause progressive myoclonus epilepsy. *Nat Genet* 1998; **20**: 171–4.

268 Minchom P, Niswander K, Chalmers I *et al*. Antecedents and outcome of very early neonatal seizures in infants born at or near term. *Br J Obstetr Gynaecol* 1987; **94**: 431–9.

269 Mischel PS, Nguyen LP, Vinters HV. Cerebral cortical dysplasia associated with pediatric epilepsy. Review of neuropathologic features and proposal for a grading system. *J Neuropathol Exp Neurol* 1995; **54**: 137–53.

270 Mitchell LA, Jackson GD, Kalnis RM *et al*. Anterior temporal abnormality in temporal lobe epilepsy. A quantitative MRI and histopathologic study. *Neurology* 1999; **52**: 327–36.

271 Mody I. The molecular basis of kindling. *Brain Pathol* 1993; **3**: 395–403.

272 Mody I, Reynolds JN, Salter MW *et al*. Kindling-induced epilepsy alters calcium currents in granule cells of rat hippocampal slices. *Brain Res* 1990; **531**: 88–94.

273 Monteiro L, Nunes B, Mendonca D, Lopes J. Spectrum of epilepsy in neurocysticercosis: a long-term follow-up of 143 patients. *Acta Neurol Scand* 1995; **90**: 1–8.

274 Morgan H, Wood MW, Murphy F. Experiences with 88 consecutive cases of brain abscess. *J Neurosurg* 1973; **38**: 698–704.

275 Morrell F, Walter WW, Bleck TP. Multiple subpial transection: A new approach to the surgical treatment of focal epilepsy. *J Neurosurg* 1989; **70**: 231–9.

276 Nakagawa E, Aimi Y, Yasuhara O *et al*. Enhancement of progenitor cell division in the dentate gyrus triggered by initial limbic seizures in rat models of epilepsy. *Epilepsia* 2000; **41**: 10–18.

277 Nakasato N, Levesque MF, Babb TL. Seizure outcome following standard temporal lobectomy: correlation with hippocampal neuron loss and extrahippocampal pathology. *J Neurosurg* 1992; **77**: 194–200.

278 Nashef L. Sudden unexpected death in epilepsy: terminology and definitions. *Epilepsia*. 1997; **38** (Suppl 11): S6–8.

279 Nelson KB, Ellenberg JH. Antecedents of seizure disorders in childhood. *Am J Dis Child* 1986; **140**: 1053–61.

280 Neubauer BA, Fiedler B, Himmelein B *et al*. Centrotemporal spikes in families with rolandic epilepsy: linkage to chromosome 15q14. *Neurology* 1998; **51**: 1608–12.

281 Nevander G, Ingvar M, Auer RN, Siesjo BK. Status epilepticus in well-oxygenated rats causes neuronal necrosis. *Ann Neurol* 1985; **18**: 281–90.

282 Newmark ME, Penry JK. *Photosensitivity and epilepsy: a review*. New York: Raven Press, 1979: 1–220.

283 Nilsson L, Farahmand BY, Persson P-G *et al*. Risk factors for sudden unexpected death in epilepsy: a case–control study. *Lancet* 1999; **353**: 888–93.

284 Nishimura RN, Ishak KG, Reddick R *et al*. Lafora disease: diagnosis by liver biopsy. *Ann Neurol* 1980; **8**: 409–15.

285 Noël P, Cornil A, Chailly P, Flament-Durand J. Mesial temporal haemorrhage, consequence of status epilepticus. *J Neurol Neurosurg Psychiatry* 1977; **40**: 932–5.

286 Nohria V, Lee N, Tien RD *et al*. Magnetic resonance imaging evidence of hippocampal sclerosis in progression: a case report. *Epilepsia* 1994; **35**: 1332–6.

287 Nordborg C, Sourander P, Silfvenius H *et al*. Mild cortical dysplasia in patients with intractable partial seizures: a histological study. In: Wolf P, Dam M, Janz D, Dreifuss FE eds. *Adv Epileptol* Vol. 16. New York: Raven Press, 1987: 29–33.

288 Norio R, Koskiniemi M. Progressive myoclonus epilepsy: genetic and nosological aspects with special reference to 107 Finnish patients. *Clin Genet* 1979; **15**: 382–98.

289 Norman RM. The neuropathology of status epilepticus. *Med Sci Law* 1964; **4**: 46–51.

290 O'Brien TJ, So EL, Meyert FB *et al*. Progressive hippocampal atrophy in chronic intractable temporal lobe epilepsy. *Ann Neurol* 1999; **45**: 526–9.

291 O'Connor W, Masukawa L, Freese A *et al*. Hippocampal cell distribution in temporal lobe epilepsy: a comparison between patients with and without an early risk factor. *Epilepsia* 1996; **37**: 440–9.

292 Ogunmekan AO, Hwang PA, Hoffman HJ. Sturge–Weber–Dimitri disease: role of hemispherectomy in prognosis. *Can J Neurol Sci* 1989; **16**: 78–80.

293 Olney JW, De Gubareff T, Sloviter RS. 'Epileptic' brain damage in rats induced by sustained electrical stimulation of the perforant path. II. Ultrastructural analysis of acute hippocampal pathology. *Brain Res Bull* 1983; **10**: 699–712.

294 Omorokov LI. Kozhenikov's epilepsy in Siberia. In: Andermann F ed. *Chronic encephalitis and epilepsy: Rasmussen's syndrome*. Oxford: Butterworth-Heinemann, 1991: 263–9.

295 Oppenheimer DR, Griffith HB. Persistent intracranial bleeding as a complication of hemispherectomy. *J Neurol Neurosurg Psychiatry* 1966; **29**: 229–40.

296 Ottman R, Risch N, Hauser WA *et al*. Localization of a gene for partial epilepsy to chromosome 10q. *Nat Genet* 1995; **10**: 56–60.

297 Ounsted C, Lindsay J, Norman R. *Biological factors in temporal lobe epilepsy*. London: W Heinemann Medical Books, 1966: 1–135.

298 Palmer CA, Geyer JD, Keating JM *et al*. Rasmussen's encephalitis with concomitant cortical dysplasia: the role of GluR3. *Epilepsia* 1999; **40**: 242–7.

299 Palmini A, Andermann F, Olivier A *et al*. Focal neuronal migration disorders and intractable partial epilepsy: a study of 30 patients. *Ann Neurol* 1991; **30**: 741–9.

300 Parent JM, Tada E, Fike JR, Lowenstein DH. Inhibition of dentate granule cell neurogenesis does not prevent seizure-induced mossy fibre synaptic reorganization in the rat. *J Neurosci* 1999; **19**: 4508–19.

301 Parent JM, Yu TW, Leibowitz RT *et al*. Dentate granule cell neurogenesis is increased by seizures and contributes to aberrant network reorganization in the adult hippocampus. *J Neurosci* 1997; **17**: 3727–38.

302 Peiffer J. Morphologische aspekte der epilepsien. *Pathogenetische, Pathogisch-Anatomische und Klinische Probleme der Epilepsien* 1963: 1–185.

303 Penfield W. Epilepsy and surgical therapy. *Arch Neurol Psychiatry* 1936; **36**: 449–84.

304 Penfield W. The mechanism of cicatricial contraction in the brain. *Brain* 1927; **50**: 499–517.

305 Penfield W, Baldwin M. Temporal lobe seizures and the technic of subtotal temporal lobectomy. *Ann Surg* 1952; **136**: 625–34.

306 Penfield W, Humphreys S. Epileptogenic lesions of the brain – a histological study. *Arch Neurol Psychiatry* 1940; **43**: 240–61.

307 Penfield W, Jasper H. *Epilepsy and the functional anatomy of the human brain*. London: Churchill, 1954: 1–896.

308 Perot P, Weir B, Rasmussen T. Tuberous sclerosis: surgical therapy for seizures. *Arch Neurol* 1966; **15**: 498–506.

309 Pfleger L. Beobachtungen über Schrumpfung und Sklerose des Ammonshorns bei Epilepsie. *Allgemeine Z Psychiatrie* 1880; **36**: 359–65.

310 Phillips G. Traumatic epilepsy after closed head injury. *J Neurol Neurosurg Psychiatry* 1954; **17**: 1–10.

311 Phillips HA, Scheffer IE, Crossland KM *et al*. Autosomal dominant nocturnal frontal-lobe epilepsy: genetic heterogeneity and evidence for a second focus at 15q24. *Am J Hum Genet* 1998; **63**: 1101–9.

312 Phizackerley PJR, Poole EW, Whitty CWM. Sino-auricular heart block as an epileptic manifestation: a case report. *Epilepsia* 1954; **3**: 89–91.

313 Plate K, Wieser H-G, Yasargil MG, Wiestler OD. Neuropathological findings in 224 patients with temporal lobe epilepsy. *Acta Neuropathol* 1993; **86**: 433–8.

314 Pollen DA, Trachtenberg MC. Neuroglia: gliosis and focal epilepsy. *Science* 1970; **167**: 1252–3.

315 Pomeroy SL, Holmes SJ, Dodge PR, Feigin RD. Seizures and other neurologic sequelae of bacterial meningitis in children. *N Engl J Med* 1990; **323**: 1651–7.

316 Power C, Poland SD, Blume WT *et al*. Cytomegalovirus and Rasmussen's encephalitis. *Lancet* 1990; **ii**: 1282–4.

317 Prasad AN, Prasad C, Stafstrom CE. Recent advances in the genetics of epilepsy: insights from human and animal studies. *Epilepsia* 1999; **40**: 1329–52.

318 Prayson RA, Estes ML, Morris HH. Coexistence of neoplasia and cortical dysplasia in patients presenting with seizures. *Epilepsia* 1993; **34**: 609–15.

319 Prayson RA, Khajavi K, Comair YG. Cortical architectural abnormalities and MIB1 immunoreactivity in ganglio-gliomas: a study of 60 patients with intracranial tumours. *J Neuropathol Exp Neurol* 1995; **54**: 513–20.

320 Pritchard JW. Nuclear magnetic resonance spectroscopy of seizure states. *Epilepsia* 1994; **35**: 514–20.

321 Rasmussen T. Further observations on the syndrome of chronic encephalitis and epilepsy. *Appl Neurophysiol* 1978; **41**: 1–12.

322 Rasmussen T, Olszewski J, Lloyd-Smith D. Focal seizures due to chronic localized encephalitis. *Neurology* 1958; **8**: 435–45.

323 Raymond AA, Fish DR, Sisodiya SM *et al*. Abnormalities of gyration, heterotopias, tuberous sclerosis, focal cortical dysplasia, microdysgenesis, dysembryoplastic neuroepithelial tumour and dysgenesis of the archicortex in epilepsy. Clinical, EEG and neuroimaging features in 100 adult patients. *Brain* 1995; **118**: 629–60.

324 Raymond AA, Halpin SF, Alsanjari N *et al*. Dysembryoplastic neuroepithelial tumour. Features in 16 patients. *Brain* 1994; **117**: 461–75.

325 Reid SA, Sypert GW, Boggs WM, Willmore LJ. Histopathology of the ferric-induced chronic epileptic focus in cat: a Golgi study. *Exp Neurol* 1979; **66**: 205–19.

326 Represa A, Jorwuera I, Le Gall *et al*. Epilepsy induced collateral sprouting of hippocampal mossy fibers: does it induce the development of ectopic synapses with granule cell dendrites. *Hippocampus* 1993; **3**: 257–68.

327 Represa A, Le Gall La Salle G, Ben-Ari Y. Hippocampal plasticity in the kindling model of epilepsy in rats. *Neurosci Lett* 1989; **99**: 345–50.

328 Represa A, Robain O, Tremblay E, Ben-Ari Y. Hippocampal plasticity in childhood epilepsy. *Neurosci Lett* 1989; **99**: 351–5.

329 Ribak CE, Hunt CA, Bakay RAE, Oertel WH. A decrease in the number of GABAergic somata is associated with the preferential loss of GABA-ergic terminals at epileptic foci. *Brain Res* 1986; **363**: 78–90.

330 Ribak CE, Joubran C, Kesslak JP, Bakay RAE. A selective decrease in the number of GABAergic somata occurs in pre-seizing monkeys with alumina gel granuloma. *Epilepsy Res* 1989; **4**: 126–38.

331 Robain O, Chiron C, Dulac O. Electron microscopic and Golgi study in a case of hemimegalencephaly. *Acta Neuropathol* 1989; **77**: 664–6.

332 Robinson R, Gardiner M. Genetics of childhood epilepsy. *Arch Dis Child* 2000; **82**: 121–5.

333 Robitaille Y. Neuropathologic aspects of chronic encephalitis. In: Andermann F ed. *Chronic encephalitis and epilepsy: Rasmussen's syndrome*. London: Butterworth-Heinemann, 1991: 79–110.

334 Rocca WA, Sharbrough LW, Hauser WA *et al*. Risk factors for absent seizures: a population-based case–control study in Rochester, Minnesota. *Neurology* 1987; **37**: 1309–14.

335 Rocca WA, Sharbrough LW, Hauser WA *et al*. Risk factors for complex partial seizures: a population based case–control study. *Ann Neurol* 1987; **21**: 22–31.

336 Rocca WA, Sharbrough LW, Hauser WA *et al*. Risk factors for generalised tonic–classic seizures. A population-based case control study in Rochester Minnesota. *Neurology* 1987; **37**: 1315–22.

337 Rogers SW, Andrews PI, Gahring LC *et al*. Autoantibodies to glutamate receptor GluR3 in Rasmussen's encephalitis. *Science* 1994; **265**: 648–51.

338 Rosing HS, Hopkins LC, Wallace DC *et al*. Maternally inherited mitochondrial myopathy and myoclonic epilepsy. *Ann Neurol* 1985; **17**: 228–37.

339 Russell DS, Rubinstein LJ. Tumours and tumour-like lesions of maldevelopmental origin. In: *Pathology of tumours of the nervous system* 1989: 664–765.

340 Russell WR, Whitty CWM. Studies in traumatic epilepsy. I. Factors influencing the incidence of epilepsy after brain wounds. *J Neurol Neurosurg Psychiatry* 1952; **15**: 93–8.

341 Ryan SG. Ion channels and the genetic contribution to epilepsy. *J Child Neurol* 1999; **14**: 58–66.

342 Sagar HJ, Oxbury JM. Hippocampal neuron loss in temporal lobe epilepsy: Correlation with early childhood convulsions. *Ann Neurol* 1987; **22**: 334–40.

343 Salazar AM, Jabbari B, Vance SC *et al*. Epilepsy after penetrating head injury I. Clinical correlates: a report of the Vietnam Head Injury Study. *Neurology* 1985; **35**: 1406–14.

344 Sander JWA, Shorvon SD. Incidence and prevalence studies in epilepsy and their methodological problems: a review. *J Neurol Neurosurg Psychiatry* 1987; **50**: 829–39.

345 Sander T, Hildman T, Kretz R *et al*. Allelic association of juvenile absence epilepsy with a GluR5 kainate receptor gene (GRIK1) polymorphism. *Am J Med Genet* 1997; **74**: 416–21.

346 Sano K, Malamud N. Clinical significance of sclerosis of the cornu ammonis. *Arch Neurol Psychiatry* 1953; **70**: 40–53.

347 Sato S. An epidemiologic and clinico-statistical study of epilepsy in Niigata City. *Clin Neurol* 1964; **4**: 461–71 (in Japanese).

348 Savic I, Svanborg E, Thorell JO. Cortical benzodiazepine receptor changes are related to frequency of partial seizures: a positron emission tomography study. *Epilepsia* 1996; **37**: 236–44.

349 Scheffer IE, Bhatia KP, Lopes-Cendes I *et al*. Autosomal dominant frontal epilepsy misdiagnosed as sleep disorder. *Lancet* 1994; **343**: 515–17.

350 Scheibel ME, Crandall PH, Scheibel AB. The hippocampal–dentate complex in temporal lobe epilepsy. *Epilepsia* 1974; **15**: 55–80.

351 Scholz W. *Die Krampfschädigungen des Gehirns*. Berlin: Springer, 1951.

352 Scholz W. The contribution of patho-anatomical research to the problem of epilepsy. *Epilepsia* 1959; **1**: 36–55.

353 Schwarz GA, Yanoff M. Lafora's disease. *Arch Neurol* 1965; **12**: 172–88.

354 Scott GM, Gibberd FB. Epilepsy and other factors in the prognosis of gliomas. *Acta Neurol Scand* 1980; **61**: 227–39.

355 Seitelberger F. Myoclonus body disease. In: Minckler J ed. *Pathology of the nervous system* Vol. I. New York: McGraw-Hill, 1968: 1121–34.

356 Senanayake N, Román GC. Epidemiology of epilepsy in developing countries. *Bull World Health Organ* 1993; **71**: 247–58.

357 Serratosa JM, Gardiner RM, Lehesjoki A-E *et al*. The molecular genetic basis of the progressive myoclonus epilepsies. In: Delgado-Escueta AV, Wilson WA, Olsen RW, Porter RJ eds. *Jasper's Basic mechanisms of the epilepsies* 3rd edn. *Advances in Neurology* Vol. 79. New York: Raven Press, 1999: 383–98.

358 Shorvon S. *Status epilepticus*. Cambridge: Cambridge University Press, 1994.

359 Sisodiya SM, Free SL, Stevens JM *et al*. Widespread cerebral structural changes in patients with cortical dysgenesis and epilepsy. *Brain* 1995; **118**: 1039–50.

360 Sloviter RS. 'Epileptic' brain damage in rats induced by sustained electrical stimulation of the perforant path. I. Acute electrophysiological and light microscopic studies. *Brain Res* 1983; **10**: 675–97.

361 Sloviter RS. Permanently altered hippocampal structure, excitability, and inhibition after experimental status epilepticus in the rat: 'dormant basket cell' hypothesis and its possible relevance to temporal lobe epilepsy. *Hippocampus* 1991; **1**: 41–66.

362 Sloviter RS. The functional organization of the hippocampal dentate gyrus and its relevance to the pathogenesis of temporal lobe epilepsy. *Hippocampus* 1994; **35**: 640–54.

363 Sloviter RS, Dean E, Sollas AL, Goodman JH. Apoptosis and necrosis induced in different hippocampal neuron populations by repetitive perforant path stimulation in the rat. *J Comp Neurol* 1996; **366**: 516–33.

364 Sloviter RS, Sollas AL, Barbaro NM, Laxer KD. Calcium-binding protein (Calbindin-D28K) and parvalbumin immunocytochemistry in the normal and epileptic human hippocampus. *J Comp Neurol* 1991; **308**: 381–96.

365 Smith DF, Hutton JL, Sandemann D *et al*. The prognosis of primary intracerebral tumours presenting with epilepsy: the outcome of medical and surgical management. *J Neurol Neurosurg Psychiatry* 1991; **54**: 915–20.

366 Sofijanov NG. Clinical evaluation and prognosis of childhood epilepsies. *Epilepsia* 1982; **23**: 61–9.

367 Sommer W. Erkrankung des Ammonshornes als aetiologisches Moment der Epilepsie. *Arch Psychiatrie Nervenkrankheiten* 1880; **10**: 631–75.

368 Spencer SS, Theodore WH, Berkovic SF. Clinical applications: MRI, SPECT and PET. *Magn Reson Imaging* 1995; **13**: 1119–24.

369 Spielmeyer W. Die Pathogenese des epileptischen Krampfes. *Z Gesamte Neurol Psychiatrie* 1927; **109**: 501–20.

370 Spitz MC. Injuries and death as a consequence of seizures in people with epilepsy. *Epilepsia* 1998; **39**: 904–7.

371 Spreafico R, Battaglia G, Arcelli P *et al*. Cortical dysplasia. An immunocytochemical study of three patients. *Neurology* 1998; **50**: 27–36.

372 Stanton PJ, Jones RSG, Mody I, Heinemann H. Epileptiform activity induced by lowering extracellular [Mg^{2+}] in combined hippocampal–entorhinal cortex slices: modulation by receptors for norepinephrine and N-methyl-D-aspartate. *Epilepsy Res* 1987; **1**: 53–62.

373 Stauder KH. Epilepsie und Schlafenlappen. *Arch Psychiatrie Nervenkrankheiten* 1935; **104**: 181–211.

374 Steinlein OK, Mulley JC, Propping P *et al*. A missense mutation in the neuronal nicotinic acetylcholine receptor α4 subunit is associated with autosomal dominant nocturnal frontal lobe epilepsy. *Nat Genet* 1995; **11**: 1–7.

375 Sutula T, Cascino G, Cavazos J *et al*. Mossy fiber synaptic reorganization in the epileptic human temporal lobe. *Ann Neurol* 1989; **26**: 321–30.

376 Sutula T, Xiad-Xian H, Cavazos J, Scott G. Synaptic reorganization in the hippocampus induced by abnormal functional activity. *Science* 1988; **239**: 1147–50.

377 Tahvanainen E, Ranta S, Hirvasniemi A *et al*. The gene for a recessively inherited human cell childhood progressive epilepsy with mental retardation maps to the distal short arm of chromosome 8. *Proc Nat Acad Sci USA* 1994; **91**: 7267–70.

378 Takao M, Benson MD, Murrell JR *et al*. Neuroserpin mutation S52R causes neuroserpin accumulation in neurons and is associated with progressive myoclonus epilepsy. *J Neuropathol Exp Neurol* 2000; **59**: 1070–86.

379 Takeda S, Wakabayashi K, Ohama E, Ikuta F. Neuropathology of myoclonus epilepsy associated with ragged-red fibres (Fukuhara's disease). *Acta Neuropathol* 1988; **75**: 433–40.

380 Tasch E, Cendes F, Li LM *et al*. Neuroimaging evidence of progressive neuronal loss and dysfunction in temporal lobe epilepsy. *Ann Neurol* 1999; **45**: 568–76.

381 Taylor DC, Falconer MA, Bruton CJ, Corsellis JAN. Focal dysplasia of the cerebral cortex in epilepsy. *J Neurol Neurosurg Psychiatry* 1971; **34**: 369–87.

382 Teitelbaum JS, Zatorre RJ, Carpenter S *et al*. Neurologic sequelae of domoic acid intoxication due to the ingestion of contaminated mussels. *N Engl J Med* 1990; **322**: 1781–7.

383 Tennis P, Cole TB, Annegers JF *et al*. Cohort study of incidence of sudden unexplained death in persons with seizure disorder treated with antiepileptic drugs in Saskatchewan, Canada. *Epilepsia* 1995; **36**: 29–36.

384 Terrence CF, Rao GR, Perper JA. Neurogenic pulmonary edema in unexpected, unexplained death of epileptic patients. *Ann Neurol* 1981; **9**: 4458–64.

385 Thom M. Neuropathologic findings in postmortem studies of sudden death in epilepsy. *Epilepsia* 1997; **38** (Suppl 11): S32–4.

386 Towfighi J, Kofke WA, O'Connell BK *et al*. Substantia nigra lesions in mercaptopropionic acid induced status epilepticus: a light and electron microscopic study. *Acta Neuropathol (Berl)* 1989; **77**: 612–20.

387 Tsairis P, Engel WK, Kark P. Familial myoclonic epilepsy syndrome associated with skeletal muscle mitochondrial abnormalities. *Neurology* 1973; **23**: 408.

388 Tsuboi T. Prevalance and incidence of epilepsy in Tokyo. *Epilepsia* 1988; **29**: 103–10.

389 Turski L, Ikonomidou C, Turski WA *et al*. Review: Cholinergic mechanisms and epileptogenesis. The seizures induced by pilocarpine: a novel experimental model of intractable epilepsy. *Synapse* 1989; **3**: 154–71.

390 Twyman RE, Gahring LC, Spiess J, Rogers SW. Glutamate receptor antibodies activate a subset of receptors and reveal an agonist binding site. *Neuron* 1995; **14**: 755–62.

391 Van der Zee CEEM, Rashid K, Le K *et al*. Intraventricular administration of antibodies to nerve growth factor retards kindling and blocks mossy fiber sprouting in adult rats. *J Neurosci* 1995; **15**: 5316–23.

392 Van Heycop ten Ham MW, Jager H de. Progressive myoclonus epilepsy with Lafora bodies: clinical–pathological features. *Epilepsia* 1963; **4**: 95–119.

393 Veith G, Wicke R. Cerebrale Differenzierungsstorungen bie Epilepsie. In: *Jahrbuch*. Koln-Opalden: Westdeutscher Verlag, 1968: 515–34.

394 Verity CM, Golding J. Risk of epilepsy after febrile convulsions: a national cohort study. *BMJ* 1991; **303**: 1373–6.

395 Verity CM, Ross PM, Golding J. Outcome of childhood status epilepticus and lengthy febrile convulsions: findings of national cohort study. *BMJ* 1993; **307**: 225–8.

396 Vigevano F, Di Rocco C. Effectiveness of hemispherectomy in hemimegalencephaly with intractable seizures. *Neuropediatrics* 1990; **21**: 222–3.

397 Villemure JG, Rasmussen T. Functional hemispherectomy in children. *Neuropediatrics* 1993; **24**: 53–5.

398 Vining EPG, Freeman JM, Brandt J et al. Progressive unilateral encephalopathy of childhood (Rasmussen's syndrome): a reappraisal. *Epilepsia* 1993; **34**: 639–50.

399 Vinters HV, Fisher RS, Cornford ME et al. Morphological substrates of infantile spasms: studies based on surgically resected cerebral tissue. *Childs Nerv Syst* 1992; **8**: 8–17.

400 Vital A, Marchal C, Loiseau H et al. Glial and neuronoglial malformative lesions associated with medically intractable epilepsy. *Acta Neuropathol* 1994; **87**: 196–201.

401 Walczak TS, Leestma JE, Hughes JR et al. Sudden unexpected death in epilepsy: clinical and pathological features in a prospectively identified group. *Ann Neurol* 1988; **24**: 135.

402 Wallace SJ. Prenatal and perinatal risk factors for epilepsy. In: Pedley TA, Meldrum BS eds. *Recent advances in epilepsy* Vol. 5. Edinburgh: Churchill Livingstone, 1992: 91–106.

403 Walter GF, Renella RR. Epstein–Barr virus in brain and Rasmussen's encephalitis. *Lancet* 1989; **i**: 279–80.

404 Wasterlain CG, Fujikawa DG, Penix L, Sankar R. Pathophysiological mechanisms of brain damage from status epilepticus. *Epilepsia* 1993; **34** (Suppl 1): S37–53.

405 Weiser HG. Selective amygdalohippocampectomy: indications and follow up. *Can J Neurol Sci* 1991; **18**: 617–27.

406 Wendt LV, Rantakallio P, Saukkonen A-L, Mäkinin H. Epilepsy and associated handicaps in a 1 year birth cohort in northern Finland. *Eur J Pediatr* 1985; **144**: 149–51.

407 Williams CA, Angelman H, Clayton-Smith J et al. Angelman syndrome: consensus for diagnostic criteria. *Am J Med Genet* 1995; **56**: 237–8.

408 Williamson PD, French JA, Thadani VM et al. Characteristics of medial temporal lobe epilepsy: II. Interictal and ictal scalp electroencephalophalography, neuropsychological testing, neuroimaging, surgical results, and pathology. *Ann Neurol* 1993; **34**: 781–7.

409 Willmore LJ. Post-traumatic epilepsy – mechanisms and prevention. In: Pedley TA, Meldrum BS eds. *Recent advances in Epilepsy*. Edinburgh: Churchill Livingstone, 1992: 107–17.

410 Willmore LJ, Sypert GW, Munson JB. Recurrent seizures induced by cortical iron injection: a model of posttraumatic epilepsy. *Ann Neurol* 1978; **4**: 329–36.

411 Wilson PJE. Cerebral hemispherectomy for infantile hemiplegia – a report of 50 cases. *Brain* 1970; **93**: 147–80.

412 Wolf HK, Aliashkevich AF, Blümke I et al. Neuronal loss and gliosis of the amygdaloid nucleus in temporal lobe epilepsy: a quantitative analysis of 70 surgical specimens. *Acta Neuropathol* 1997; **93**: 606–10.

413 Wolf HK, Birkholz T, Wellmer J et al. Neurochemical profile of glioneuronal lesions from patients with pharmacoresistant focal epilepsies. *J Neuropathol Exp Neurol* 1995; **54**: 689–97.

414 Wolf HK, Campos MG, Zentner J et al. Surgical pathology of temporal lobe epilepsy. Experience with 216 cases. *J Neuropathol Exp Neurol* 1993; **52**: 499–506.

415 Wolf HK, Müller MB, Spänle M et al. Ganglioglioma: a detailed histopathological and immunohistochemical analysis of 61 cases. *Acta Neuropathol* 1994; **88**: 166–73.

416 Wolf HK, Spänle M, Müller MB et al. Hippocampal loss of GABA$_A$ receptor α_1 subunit in patients with chronic pharmacoresistant epilepsies. *Acta Neuropathol* 1994; **88**: 313–19.

417 Wolf HK, Wellmer J, Muller MB et al. Glioneuronal malformative lesions and dysembryoplastic neuroepithelial tumors in patients with chronic pharmacoresistant epilepsies. *J Neuropathol Exp Neurol* 1995; **54**: 245–54.

418 Wolf HK, Wiestler OD. Surgical pathology of chronic epileptic seizure disorders. *Brain Pathol* 1993; **3**: 371–80.

419 Wolf HK, Zentner J, Hufnagel A et al. Surgical pathology of chronic epileptic seizure disorders: experience with 63 specimens from extratemporal corticectomies, lobectomies and functional hemispherectomies. *Acta Neuropathol (Berl)* 1993; **86**: 466–72.

420 Wolman M. Minerals, pigments and inclusion bodies. In: Filipe MI, Lake BD eds. *Histochemistry in pathology* 2nd edn. Edinburgh: Churchill Livingstone, 1990: 419–39.

421 Yacubian EM, Rosemberg S, Marie SKN et al. Double pathology in Rasmussen's encephalitis: etiologic considerations. *Epilepsia* 1996; **37**: 495–500.

422 Yamanouchi H, Jay V, Otsubo H et al. Early forms of microtubule-associated proteins are strongly expressed in cortical dysplasia. *Acta Neuropathol* 1998; **95**: 466–70.

423 Yamanouchi H, Zhang W, Jay V, Becker LE. Enhanced expression of of microtubule-associated protein 2 in large neurons of cortical dysplasia. *Ann Neurol* 1996; **39**: 57–61.

424 Yokoi S, Austin J, Witmer F, Sakai M. Studies in myoclonus epilepsy (Lafora body form). *Arch Neurol* 1968; **19**: 15–33.

425 Zemskaya AG, Yatsuk SL, Samoilov VI. Intractable or partial epilepsy of infectious or inflammatory etiology: recent surgical experience in the USSR. In: Andermann F ed. *Chronic encephalitis and epilepsy: Rasmussen's syndrome*. London: Butterworth-Heinemann, 1991: 271–9.

426 Zhang CI, Glovell T, Heinemann H. Effects of NMDA- and AMPA-receptor antagonists on different forms of epileptiform activity in rat temporal cortex slices. *Epilepsia* 1994; **35** (Suppl 5): S68–73.

427 Zimmerman HM. The basis of convulsive attacks in children – an experimental study. *N Y Pathol Soc* 1959; **35**: 801–10.

428 Zimmerman HM. The histopathology of convulsive disorders in children. *J Pediatr* 1938; **13**: 859–90.

429 Zuger A, Lowry FD. Tuberculosis of the central nervous system. In: Scheld WM, Whitley RJ, Durack DT eds. *Infections of the central nervous system*. New York: Raven Press, 1991: 801–23.

16

Ophthalmic neuropathology

PHILIP J. LUTHERT AND SUSAN LIGHTMAN

INTRODUCTION

There are multiple links between the pathology of the brain and its coverings and the pathology of the eye. The optic nerve and retina are extensions of the cerebral hemispheres and the close physical proximity of the orbit and anterior cranial fossa results in local extension of disease from one compartment to the other. The following account is not intended to provide a substitute for the many excellent texts on ophthalmic pathology. An introduction to the subject is provided that will be of value to neuropathologists with an interest in the eye and orbit finding themselves having to tackle an overlapping problem. The emphasis will be on areas having a particular relevance to neuropathology.

The aim of the following discussion is to consider the eye and orbit as part of the routine examination of the central nervous system (CNS). There are few integrated studies of the eye and brain. For example, very little is known of the cerebral pathology associated with conditions as common as glaucoma and amblyopia, despite the possibility that the former may be associated with cerebral small-vessel disease and the latter has been well described in non-human primate studies. It is becoming increasingly clear that system degenerations involve many sites of the CNS beyond the defining pathways (e.g. corticospinal tracts in motor neuron disease) but often, studies of retinal ganglion cell or photoreceptor cell pathology have not been carried out in these conditions. Many ophthalmic pathology units are based in specialist eye hospitals with no mortuary. Neuropathogists are therefore in an ideal position to advance the histopathological description of many eye diseases that are largely unstudied, but many opportunities are missed. Perhaps part of the difficulty lies with the practicalities of removing the eyes at post-mortem examination. These, and other issues relating to the handling of ocular specimens, are discussed in the next section.

Practical issues

At post-mortem examination the eye can be removed from the front or from behind following deroofing of the orbit.[202] If the latter approach is taken it is possible to remove just the posterior pole, that is the optic nerve with a disc of retina up to approximately 2 cm across. A great deal of information may be obtained from such a specimen, but the improved architecture and extra tissue available for examination offered by removal and fixation of the eye intact make this latter approach the preferred option. Although, in principle, limited removal is cosmetically less problematic, the resulting loss of pressure within the eye requires packing of the orbit to maintain the normal profile of the lids. It therefore involves relatively little extra work to remove the eyes intact and insert a prosthesis. The latter can, however, be problem with infants as small glass eyes may not be available. Nevertheless, the importance of careful examination of the eyes in cases of possible non-accidental injury makes removal of the eyes in these cases mandatory.

There are many views as to how eyes should be fixed. Immersion in a glutaraldehyde-based electron microscopy fixative undoubtedly improves retinal architecture and its adherence to the retinal pigment epithelium (RPE). Fresh glutaraldehyde may, however, not be available and buffered formol saline is often used. Fixation in alcohol firms the globe for slicing but is not essential. Indeed, primary fixation in alcohol is to be avoided as it renders the vitreous opaque and alters the staining properties of other components of the eye.

Like the brain, the eye is a composite organ with many different elements that respond to a given pathological event in a variety of relatively stereotyped ways. One of the challenges of ophthalmic pathology is integrating what may be quite a complex series of observations into a coherent whole. The eye must be examined and dissected in such a way as to optimize information gathering. External examination, including determining whether it is a left or right eye, and a careful search for extraocular tumour in appropriate cases should be supported with photography. In the case of presumed choroidal melanoma, vortex veins arising at the back of the eye should be sampled, as vascular spread is not uncommon. Transillumination is of value in the localization of any intraocular pathology such as a haemorrhage, scar or tumour that might dictate how the eye should be opened. Usually, a block is taken extending from the pupil to the optic nerve (PO block) that is 7–10 mm thick. Ideally, the centre of the pupil should be at the centre of the anterior face of the block and the optic nerve similarly located at the posterior face. In the absence of any focal pathology or evidence of surgery two near-horizontal caps or calottes are removed. A skin-grafting blade or a mounted disposable microtome blade is a useful tool for this. A horizontal block will include the macula. The superior limbus and adjacent cornea are important sites for surgical access to the anterior chamber/trabecular meshwork and intraocular lenses are often orientated vertically. In an operated eye, even when a limbal scar cannot be identified macroscopically, it is appropriate to open the eye vertically. If there is focal pathology, such as a choroidal melanoma, an oblique meridian is taken so that the resulting block includes the centre of the lesion, the pupil and the optic nerve head (Fig. 16.1). Intraocular examination

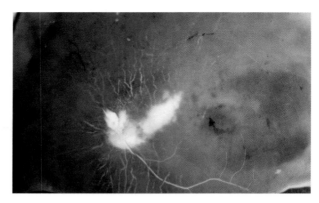

Figure 16.2 *Artefact. There is myelin extrusion into the vitreous and blood vessels in the vicinity of the optic nerve head.*

should be made with adequate illumination and with the assistance of a dissecting microscope. A relatively common artefact is the presence of extruded myelin following compression of the optic nerve (Fig. 16.2). Again, supporting photography is important and can be a vital aid in the subsequent interpretation of histological findings.

The extent of histological examination depends on many factors. The authors' current practice is to examine five levels through the PO block. Most eyes can be processed with other surgical specimens. If there is an expanse of solid tissue, as in a large choroidal melanoma, a more protracted, 3-day protocol is beneficial. As with large CNS blocks, the cutting of histological sections from eyes requires expertise, but any experienced, conscientious histologist should be able to produce high-quality results.

DEVELOPMENTAL ABNORMALITIES

Normal development

Development of the eye and orbit is complex, with participation of ectoderm, neuroectoderm, mesenchyme and neural crest derivatives.[199,232] The presence of the globe drives much of the development and growth of the orbit. Failure to implant an ocular prosthesis in early childhood results in impaired orbital expansion. The optic primordia of the eye form as outpouchings of the developing forebrain at the 2-mm, 18th-day stage of gestation.[165] The primordia expand, giving rise to the optic vesicles that invaginate, while remaining connected to the third ventricle by the optic stalk. The optic vesicle is covered by neural crest tissue, except close to the ectoderm where interaction with the surface ectoderm leads to the formation of the lens and cornea. The expanded optic vesicle gives rise to the optic cup with inner and outer layers separated by a potential space that is, topographically, in continuity with the ventricular cavity of the brain. The outer portion becomes the retinal pigment epithelium and the inner the neural retina.

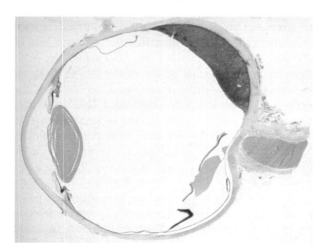

Figure 16.1 *Tissue block for intraocular pathology. A section from a PO block passing through the pupil, the optic nerve and a choroidal melanoma.*

Inferior closure of the optic cup extends posteriorly along the optic stalk, enclosing the hyaloid blood vessels that, within the nerve, become the central retinal vein and artery. In the adult, the central retinal artery gains access to the nerve inferomedially and approximately 10 mm behind the globe. Capillary precursors migrate from the optic disc towards the periphery of the retina following vascular endothelial growth factor (VEGF) which is being released by an advancing wave of astroglia.[264] Disruption of the association between astrocytes and blood vessels in development leads to abnormal patterns of vascularization and haemorrhage.[267] Macrophage marker-positive microglial cells also appear in the retina around this time, although other microglia may be present earlier.[209] Oligodendrocytes normally do not pass beyond the lamina cribrosa. In approximately 1% of individuals, however, myelinated fibres extend from the optic nerve head across the anterior retina.[234]

The genetics of normal ocular development are being increasingly understood, with remarkable parallels becoming established between *Drosophila* and man, despite the wide divergence of organization of the final result. A discussion of the molecular genetics of eye development is beyond the scope of this chapter but details may be found elsewhere.[85,244]

Malformations of the retina

ALBINISM

The fascination of albinism for clinical neuroscientists lies in the associated misrouting of the axons of retinal ganglion cells at the chiasm,[136] and for ophthalmic pathologists in the maldevelopment of the fovea, yet there are few reports of human pathology of the eye or brain in this condition.[87,176] Albinism may be classified by mode of inheritance, by loss or reduction of tyrosinase activity, by clinical extent of depigmentation and by severity of ocular phenotype. Forms with mild or absent retinal abnormalities are sometimes classified as having albinoidism.[101]

Foveal hypoplasia is failure of formation of the foveal pit and is associated with loss of the avascular zone at the centre of the normal macula. Other ocular manifestations include impaired visual acuity, reduction and irregularity of RPE pigmentation, strabismus, nystagmus and an increased susceptibility to photoreceptor degenerations. The foveal maldevelopment and the chiasmal decussation of temporal optic nerve fibres that would normally project to the ipsilateral lateral geniculate body can be explained by mistiming of proliferation of retinal neuroblasts. This, in turn, appears to be due to decreased dopamine levels at a critical point in development, secondary to a reduction in tyrosinase activity.[137]

The albino retina is especially sensitive to light damage[121] and also is more sensitive than normal retina to photoreceptor cell loss due to mutant opsin[186] and to ischaemia/reperfusion injury.[184] Histologically, there is loss of normal-looking melanosomes in the pigmented ocular structures, and macromelanosomes or melanin macroglobules are often described.

ASTROGLIAL HAMARTOMATA

Rarely, hamartomatous astroglial lesions with a predominantly pilocytic pattern have been described, usually but not always in the context of tuberous sclerosis or, less often, neurofibromatosis. They are essentially non-progressive in nature, although secondary retinal detachment or haemorrhage may lead to loss of vision (Fig. 16.3).

CYST FORMATION

Developmental retinal cysts have been described,[101] but more often these are acquired following, for instance, prolonged retinal detachment, cystoid macular oedema or retinitis.[101]

RETINAL DYSPLASIA

This developmental abnormality of the inner retina usually occurs with other ocular abnormalities such as microphthalmia or anterior chamber malformations, including Peter's anomaly.[132] Retinal dysplasia is manifested as interconnecting tubular arrangements of parts of the retina, which in section appear like rosettes (Fig. 16.4). It is important, however, to avoid the relatively common mistake of interpreting acquired retinal folds in a disorganized eye as evidence of dysplasia. Trisomy 13–15 and maternal lysergic acid diethylamide consumption are recognized associations.

COLOBOMA FORMATION

As at other sites, developmental migration and fusion of structures can fail and if the optic fissure is not

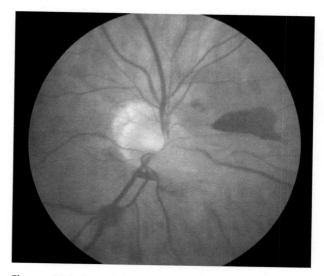

Figure 16.3 *Astroglial hamartoma. Courtesy of Professor A Bird.*

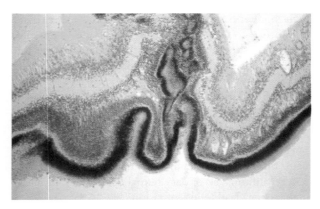

Figure 16.4 *Retinal dysplasia. There is disorganization of the retina.*

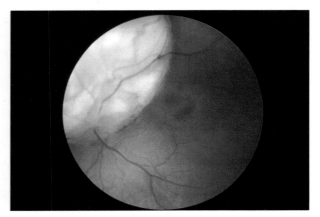

Figure 16.5 *Retinal coloboma. If developmental migration and fusion fail and if the optic fissure is not obliterated the remaining gap is known as a coloboma. Courtesy of Professor A Bird.*

obliterated the remaining gap is known as a coloboma (Fig. 16.5) (derived from the Greek for mutilation). These may be unilateral or bilateral and involve anterior or posterior structures of the eye, or both. The most severe form is associated with microphthalmos, with or without cyst formation. If the retina is involved the RPE is absent and the neuroretina absent or markedly attenuated, usually with an associated choroidal defect. Classically the defect is inferonasal, with its apex at the optic nerve head. Colobomas may be associated with cerebral pathology, as in Aicardi's syndrome[81] and other complex disorders.[111] A mutation in the *Pax 2* gene has been implicated in one family with optic nerve colobomas and renal problems.[223]

Malformations of the optic nerve

OPTIC NERVE HEAD MALFORMATIONS

The optic nerve head adopts a variety of configurations, many representing relatively minor departures from normal anatomy. More obvious abnormalities include pit formation and colobomas (see above), the latter some-

times being associated with choristoma formation. In the morning glory syndrome the optic nerve head adopts a funnel-like configuration with a surrounding rim of chorioretinal tissue. This may be seen in isolation or in association with a variety of other CNS malformations, including agenesis of the corpus callosum and abnormalities of the base of the skull.[71] Defects involving the circumference of the optic nerve head are also seen in Aicardi's syndrome, where there is often circumpapillary depigmentation associated with coloboma formation and patches of retinochoroidal depigmentation elsewhere.

OPTIC NERVE APLASIA AND HYPOPLASIA

True optic nerve aplasia is rare[214] and while bilateral cases associated with widespread CNS malformations including holoprosencephaly have been reported most instances are sporadic and unilateral. These probably arise following catastrophic failure of optic pathway development. Maternal drug consumption and diabetes, other CNS abnormalities, endocrine defects and albinism have all been associated with optic nerve hypoplasia.

Malformations of the orbit

The craniofacial synostoses and dysostoses lead to a variety of orbital malformations.[135] The two most important synostoses are Crouzon's disease and Apert's syndrome and the best-defined dysostosis is Treacher–Collins syndrome. These malformations have a varying impact on the eye. If the lids do not cover the globe, exposure keratopathy arises. Malformation of the optic canal and other distortions can lead to optic atrophy. Similarly, disturbances of lacrimal drainage may be seen. Milder abnormalities of orbital development are seen in neurofibromatosis type 1.[141] Failure of development of the globe can, in turn, lead to maldevelopment of the orbit.

ORBITAL CYSTS

Dermoid cysts of the orbit, as elsewhere, have adnexal elements as well as epidermis in their wall and contain varying amounts of keratin and lipid. They are most commonly superotemporal in position and associated with what on computed tomographic (CT) scan is clearly a longstanding bony defect. They may extend through the sphenoid bone into the temporal fossa. More rarely, intracranial components are present. The wall is often incomplete with a granulomatous reaction to the keratin that, in some cases, extends into the orbital fat, generating a picture resembling fat necrosis if the presence of the cyst is not appreciated. Epidermoid cysts lack adnexal components.

Entrapped embryonic conjunctiva can form conjunctival dermoid cysts lined by simple, goblet cell-bearing cuboidal epithelium, one or two cells thick. Critically, they lack keratinization but may contain sebaceous glands, hair follicles and sweat glands as these structures are present in the caruncle. Conjunctival dermoid cysts must be distinguished from inclusion cysts and from the solid dermoids of the limbus.

Microphthalmia with cyst results from failure of fusion of the optic fissure and is therefore related to colobomata. The cyst may dominate the clinical picture and is usually lined by astroglial tissue. The ocular remnant may be so small as to be inapparent clinically. Microphthalmia may occur in isolation but may also be part of a syndrome.[135] Rarely, enterogenous cysts[154] and cysts lined by respiratory epithelium[192] have been reported in the orbit. The differential diagnosis of congenital cysts includes a number of presumably acquired lesions. These include cholesterol granuloma, aneurysmal bone cysts, giant cell reparative granuloma and haematic cysts.

MENINGOCELES AND ENCEPHALOCELES

Portions of the coverings of the brain, with or without parenchymal components, may become trapped within the orbit during development. Patients usually present with proptosis or as part of a more major malformation. Recently, the diagnosis of one case was made prenatally.[125] Most remain attached by a meningeal stalk that extends between frontal, ethmoidal, lacrimal or maxillary bones in the most common, anterior form of the condition. In the posterior form the connection runs through an orbital fissure or the optic foramen. Even when there is no communication between the intracranial compartment and orbit, embryonic entrapment is the most likely mechanism of formation. Classically, glial elements predominate. Additional variable components include scattered ganglion cells, ependyma and foci of mineralization.

Vascular malformations

ORBITAL VASCULAR MALFORMATIONS

Vascular malformations and related lesions of the eye and orbit are relatively common in clinical practice. Capillary haemangiomas involving the orbit may present in the first few weeks of life but more commonly involve the eyelid with potential adverse effects on the cornea as well as being cosmetically disfiguring. Histologically, the phases described for subcutaneous lesions can be seen. Cavernous haemangiomas (Fig. 16.6) are often found incidentally on neuroimaging. Only if vision is threatened or there is excessive proptosis would surgery normally be considered. They are well-defined lesions composed of dilated, blood-filled channels lined by a simple endothelium and separated by a relatively sparse fibrous stroma. Orbital varices and arteriovenous malformations may present with proptosis and, where there is involvement of the face, may be unsightly. Surgical debulking is often of only limited success. The sluggish flow in true varices leads to thrombosis and phlebolith formation, the latter being of

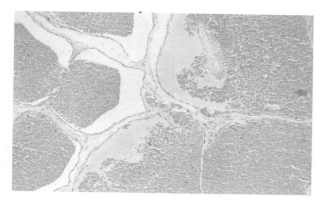

Figure 16.6 *Cavernous haemangioma. Large vascular spaces are lined by a single layer of endothelium and separated by thin fibrous stroma.*

diagnostic importance on imaging. The existence of lymphangiomas of the orbit is debated. Although it is often stated that the orbit does not have lymphatics, this may not be the case. Certainly there is a distinct entity with large ectatic vessels with walls composed only of simple endothelium and separated by broad expanses of fibrous tissue. Lymphoid aggregates, often with well-developed germinal centres, are typically present. The vascular channels often contain red cells, but proponents of the lymphangioma interpretation regard this as a secondary phenomenon. Fuller descriptions of orbital vascular lesions are given elsewhere.[166]

INTRAOCULAR VASCULAR MALFORMATIONS

In von Hippel–Lindau disease, von Hippel's contribution was the description of retinal angiomatosis. This is probably best considered a congenital, hamartomatous lesion, although one *de novo* occurrence has been described.[254] Clinically, the ocular lesions may involve the optic nerve head as well as the retina. Rarely, haemangioblastoma may be seen arising in the optic nerve.[142] Typically, pink nodular lesions are seen (Fig. 16.7) and the blood vessels leak

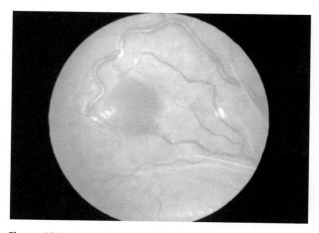

Figure 16.7 *Retinal angioma in von Hippel–Lindau disease. The lesion appears as a pink nodular lesion. Courtesy of Professor A Bird.*

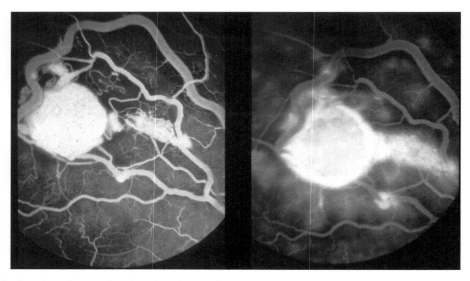

Figure 16.8 *Retinal angioma in von Hippel–Lindau disease. (Fluorescein angiogram.) Courtesy of Professor A Bird.*

fluorescein (Fig. 16.8). Histologically, the appearances are similar to those of Lindau's cerebellar haemangioblastoma, although in the ophthalmic literature these lesions are usually described, perhaps more appropriately, as capillary haemangiomas.[101] The stromal cells are a feature and are considered by some as lipidized astrocytes.[107] Exudation from the lesion is particularly apparent in the eye and such exudate would provide a rich source of lipid.

The molecular basis of these lesions has recently been elucidated. The von Hippel–Lindau tumour suppressor gene (*VHL*) normally binds and inhibits hypoxia-induced transcription factors. In mutant proteins binding is lost and unrestrained angiongenesis can occur.[196]

Sturge–Weber syndrome may be associated with conjunctival and episcleral vascular lesions, but the main ophthalmic interest in this condition lies with diffuse haemangiomas of the choroid.[66,102] Similar, more localized lesions are seen sporadically. In the context of Sturge–Weber syndrome, these lesions usually present under 10 years of age. Secondary pigmentary changes at the periphery of the lesion have led to enucleation to exclude choroidal melanoma. Glaucoma is a common complication.

One of the intriguing differences between the retina and brain is the overrepresentation of disorders of vascularization in the retina. Many of these are acquired and will be discussed below. Congenital conditions include, most importantly, Coats' disease (Fig. 16.9). In this condition, most prevalent in young males, telangectatic retinal vessels lack an adequate blood–retinal barrier and leakage of plasma protein leads to intraretinal and sub-retinal exudates. In eyes removed surgically, the latter typically have led to total retinal detachment with cholesterol crystals and foamy macrophages in the subretinal fluid (Fig. 16.10). In such eyes, it may be difficult to identify the primary vascular pathology and a similar, so-called Coats'-like reaction is seen in other conditions. Other

congenital and acquired retinal telangectatic disorders, including familial exudative vitreoretinopathy have been described.[101]

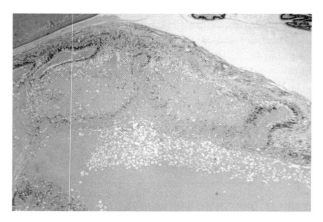

Figure 16.9 *Coats' disease. The retina overlaying lipid-rich sub-retinal fluid is disorganized.*

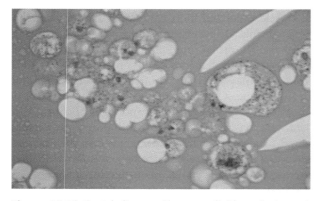

Figure 16.10 *Coats' disease. There are lipid- and pigment-containing macrophages. The pigment is from the retinal pigment epithelium.*

TRAUMA

Ocular trauma is a substantial subject in its own right[175] and the coverage here will be highly selective. From a retinal point of view, the most common problems are those associated with non-accidental injury and these are discussed at length below. Penetrating injury often has disastrous consequences for the retina and the pathologist usually receives end-stage phthisical eyes in which retinal architecture is not infrequently totally lost. Blunt trauma may lead to scleral or choroidal rupture. The retina often detaches and there may be retinal tears. When the latter occur at the junction with the ora serrata the condition is known as retinal dialysis. Finally, the retina may develop a whitish appearance over a period of several hours following the injury, an appearance known as commotio retinae. The pathological correlates of this include oedema, and in a primate model, shearing of photoreceptor outer segments followed by photoreceptor cell loss and some pigment migration into the retina.[226]

An important practical consideration in examining traumatized eyes is to look for evidence of sympathetic ophthalmia in the form of granulomatous choroidal inflammation.[46] The pathogenesis of sympathetic ophthalmia appears to have an autoimmune basis[213] and similar histopathology is seen in the Vogt–Koyanagi–Harada syndrome.[163] Failure to alert clinicians to this admittedly rare complication of ocular trauma (accidental or surgical) may put the remaining eye at risk.

Non-accidental injury

The problem of non-accidental injury of infants has become a social as well as a medical issue. The ophthalmic pathology of fatal cases has become an essential part of the post-mortem examination and it is important that the neuropathology and ophthalmic pathology are considered together. Non-accidental trauma may be direct or indirect. Direct injury may lead to perforation of the globe or other anterior disease. Indirect injury, as in shaking, can result in avulsion of the root of the iris or dislocation of the lens, but the main focus of this section will be retinal haemorrhage.

NATURE OF THE INJURY

The injury in these cases is almost always unwitnessed and neither denials nor confessions of the accused can be totally relied upon. The hypothesis has, however, developed that shaking of infants with lack of support of the head can cause subdural and retinal haemorrhage. The subdural haemorrhage is often mild and the critical cerebral event is most frequently hypoxic damage, with or without perfusion-threatening cerebral oedema. In more severe cases, there may be frank contusion of the brain, sometimes with tears.

Most commentators agree that simple domestic falls, from a bed or a table, even when of sufficient severity to cause a skull fracture, are neurologically benign.[240] This has contributed to the concept of angular forces being critical in shaking injury, but there is much debate as to the minimum severity of shaking required to cause damage, with estimates varying from as mild as vibration from domestic machinery to sustained shaking as hard as possible. Both extremes seem unlikely and the threshold will vary between individuals, with extreme youth probably being an additional risk factor. From a medicolegal point of view, the lack of precision of the minimum force required to generate significant pathology is a cause for concern.

A further area of controversy revolves around whether or not impact is necessary in addition to shaking.[95] Certainly, in experimental studies, shaking followed by impact generates angular forces substantially in excess of those obtainable by shaking alone.[61] The absence of physical evidence of impact does not exclude the possibility, as a soft surface such as a mattress would not inevitably cause bruising.

OPHTHALMIC PATHOLOGICAL FINDINGS IN NON-ACCIDENTAL INJURY

Retinal haemorrhages are generally the main feature of note (Fig. 16.11), although it is important to look for changes at the front of the eye, particularly in relation to the lens and the iris. The retinal pathology is well represented by opening the eye in the coronal plane just anterior to the ora serrata; in this way the retina is less likely to become completely detached. The retina can be photographed in a way that facilitates comparison with clinical photographs or drawings. The anterior and posterior portions of the specimen can be trisected for processing, generating blocks analogous to those taken normally. Many, however, find opening the eye in the conventional way easier.

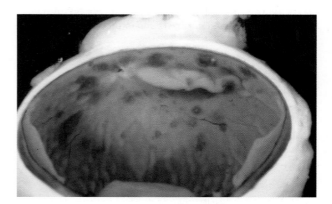

Figure 16.11 *Shaken baby syndrome. There are focal, recent haemorrhages in the retina at the posterior pole. Although the white spots present are said to be characteristic of Purtscher's retinopathy, they may be seen in cases of presumed shaking.*

The typical finding is of retinal haemorrhages that may be present in any retinal layer and are often present in all layers (Fig. 16.12). As in other circumstances, haemorrhages into the nerve fibre layer are flame-shaped and those in outer retinal layers are somewhat constrained by Müller cell processes and so adopt a dot- or blot-like configuration, depending on size. Retinal haemorrhages often extend to the anterior-most retina at the ora serrata, sometimes with equatorial sparing.[100] In severe cases there is near total confluence of haemorrhage over the majority of the extent of the retina and there may be retinal detachment (Fig. 16.13). In general, more severe retinal pathology mirrors more severe intracranial damage.[259] Not infrequently, bleeding extends into the potential space between the retina and the vitreous (subhyaloid haemorrhage) and in more severe instances there is bleeding into the vitreous. Increased severity of injury appears to be related to the presence of retinal detachment with subretinal haemorrhage and the formation of macular folds. It is important to note that retinal folds of artefactual origin are present in most infant eyes. That seen consistently at the ora serrata is known as Lange's fold.

Perineural haemorrhage, that is bleeding around the optic nerve, in the subdural or subarachnoid space, is a common feature (Figs 16.14–16.15). It is usually apparent macroscopically and the cut end of the optic nerve should always be photographed. Both here and in relation

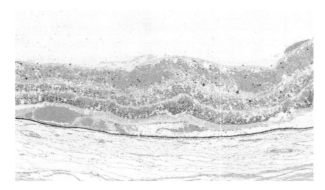

Figure 16.12 *Shaken baby syndrome. There are recent retinal haemorrhages in all retinal layers and in the subretinal space.*

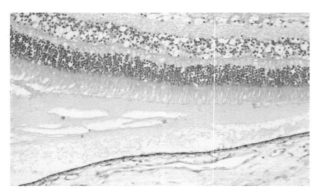

Figure 16.13 *Shaken baby syndrome. There is retinal detachment. Note the layer of subretinal fluid.*

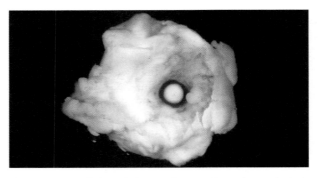

Figure 16.14 *Shaken baby syndrome. There is particularly marked subdural haemorrhage around the optic nerve.*

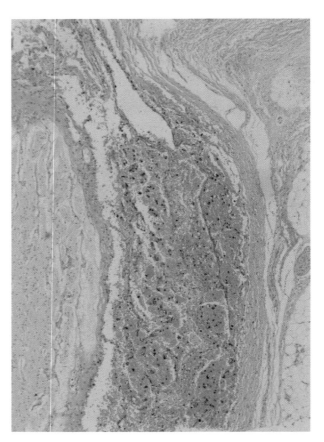

Figure 16.15 *Shaken baby syndrome. There is subdural haemorrhage around the optic nerve.*

to the retina, a search for stainable iron using Perls' method should be undertaken (Fig. 16.16). It takes at least 48 h for this to form and its presence may be evidence of previous trauma. Certainly up to 8 weeks of age, and maybe longer, haemosiderin may reflect trauma of childbirth (Fig. 16.16), retinal haemorrhages being a common finding in the newborn.

Not all infants die acutely from shaking and long-term complications persisting after clearance of the acute haemorrhage include retinal scarring, retinal folds and retinoschisis. Permanent visual disability may be the result of cortical as opposed to ocular damage.[118]

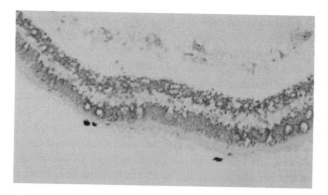

Figure 16.16 *Perinatal retinal haemorrhages. There are Perls'-positive cells in the subretinal space and in the inner retina.*

MECHANISM OF RETINAL HAEMORRHAGE

The precise mechanism of haemorrhage remains unclear. It is believed, however, that one important component is shearing forces between the jelly-like vitreous and the retina, to which it is firmly attached, especially at its anterior margin and around the optic nerve head. Splinting of the chest and raised intracranial pressure (ICP) may conspire to increase pressure in the central retinal vein, making haemorrhage more likely. Certainly, rapid increases in ICP are a well recognized cause of retinal haemorrhage and given the apparent vulnerability of the infant retinal vascular tree to physical stress, venous congestion is likely to be a contributory factor. Similarly, a Valsalva manoeuvre, in isolation, can cause extensive haemorrhage into the retina.[54,59] Exclusion of alternative intracranial pathology, in particular a vascular malformation, that may have bled and caused perineural and retinal haemorrhages is a vital role for the neuropathologist in these cases.[253]

OPTIC NERVE DAMAGE

Survivors of non-accidental injury may have retinal scarring and optic atrophy. The latter may in part be due to damage to the nerve fibre layer, but rarely avulsion of the optic nerve just behind the globe may be seen. Recently, acutely increased β-amyloid precursor protein (APP) expression in the retrolaminar optic nerve has been described.[96] This may arise from shearing forces at this site or from locally disturbed haemodynamics secondary to perineural haemorrhage.

INTEGRATING OPHTHALMIC AND NEUROPATHOLOGICAL FINDINGS

The role of ICP in the pathogenesis of retinal haemorrhage becomes critical when integrating pathology within the eye and within the intracranial compartment. If there is cerebral oedema without significant subdural haemorrhage or other pathology indicative of trauma, can the presence of retinal haemorrhages be interpreted as evidence of trauma? If the haemorrhages are relatively minor then probably not. Can unsupported flexion and extension of the head in vulnerable individuals cause critical medullary–upper cervical cord injury that generates apnoea of sufficient duration to cause fatal cerebral oedema? Could such a sequence of events be associated with a thin film of subdural blood and scattered retinal haemorrhages? In many cases, there is very severe intracranial and retinal pathology and no such dilemmas exist. The way forward is to examine the eyes in a wide range of cases from children dying with non-trauma-related intracranial disease in order to improve knowledge and understanding.

NEOPLASIA

For the purposes of this chapter, only retinoblastoma, tumours of the optic nerve and lymphoma will be discussed. Orbital tumours were well reviewed by McCartney in the previous edition of this text[166] and several other sources may be referred to.[135,258] In clinical practice, uveal melanoma[10] is the most significant problem, but metastases are said to be the most common intraocular malignancy.[27] The reader is referred elsewhere for consideration of intraocular tumours other than retinoblastoma and lymphoma.[102,201]

Retinoblastoma

Retinoblastoma is the most common intraocular neoplasm in children and is reasonably considered a variant of a primitive neuroectodermal tumour. Children most commonly present with leukocoria (white behind the pupil) or strabismus and the clinical differential diagnosis includes Coats' disease, *Toxocara* infestation and persistent hyperplastic primary vitreous. Most children present before the age of 3 years and tumours may be present at birth. Increasingly within the UK, children with proven or suspected retinoblastoma are referred to a specialist centre so the number of cases seen outside these units is dropping.

The understanding of the molecular basis of retinoblastoma was one of the landmark discoveries in oncology. Many patients with retinoblastoma have a germline mutation in the *RB* gene and, in accordance with Knudson's 'two-hit' hypothesis,[147] only require a single additional tissue mutation to develop a tumour. Most germline mutations arise sporadically and are not inherited. Approximately 90% of patients with the germline mutation will develop at least one, and commonly three or four retinoblastomas. These patients tend to differ from those with two acquired mutations. They more often have multiple tumours involving both eyes and may develop similar tumours in the parasellar or pineal region (trilateral retinoblastoma). They often present at a younger age and are more likely to develop non-ocular tumours later in life. Osteogenic sarcomas of the lower limbs are particularly common. The risk of non-ocular tumours is increased by radiotherapy or chemotherapy.[56]

Retinoblastoma arises from the inner or outer nuclear layer of the retina and may grow inwards into the vitreous space, or outwards lifting the retina, or both. More rarely, growth is diffuse within the retina or there may be tumour regression. The mechanism of regression is unknown and it may occur in one eye in the face of continued growth of a separate tumour in the contralateral eye. Macroscopically, the eye usually contains pale necrotic-looking tumour with foci of mineralization. Sometimes tumour seeding is evident, but it may be difficult to distinguish this from genuine multifocal tumours. Tumour spread is classically a long the optic nerve and it can extend into the intracranial compartment either along the nerve or through the subarachnoid space. Spread into the choroid is a poor prognostic sign and extraocular extension is associated with a high mortality. When treated early the prognosis is remarkably good with a cure rate of approximately 95%.

Histologically, sheets of tumour cells are seen, often as viable perivascular cuffs separated by necrosis. Mineralization is often marked. In better-differentiated tumours, Flexner–Wintersteiner rosettes (Fig. 16.17), with well-defined lumina, are regularly seen, while Homer Wright rosettes are less common. Occasionally, particularly well-differentiated structures known as fleurettes, with short runs of photoreceptors with cone-like, eosinophilic inner segments, may be found.[242] Evidence for glial differentiation has come from immunohistochemical studies with glial fibrillary acidic protein (GFAP) and from *in vitro* investigations.

A rare, benign form of retinal tumour has been named retinocytoma or retinoma and spontaneously regressed retinoblastoma is probably the same entity.[169] The malignant transformation of a retinoma into a retinoblastoma has been described[65] and this may explain how adult retinoblastomas occasionally develop.

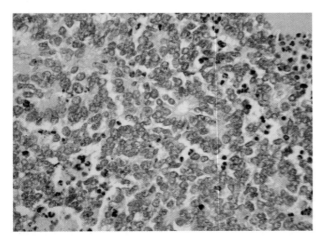

Figure 16.17 *Retinoblastoma. A Flexner–Wintersteiner rosette is present close to the centre of the field.*

Histopathologically, the diagnosis is rarely a problem, although it is important to be alert to the possibility of atypical presentations of other childhood small-cell malignant tumours. The only other primary intraocular tumour that may cause difficulties is the medulloepithelioma. This rare tumour exists in benign and malignant forms and was previously known as a diktyoma. The defining component is primitive neuroepithelium that forms duct-like structures, cysts and interconnecting cords of cells. The cysts contain hyaluronic acid. In the malignant form, there can also be sheets of primitive, malignant-looking cells that may form Homer Wright or Flexner–Wintersteiner rosettes. A more extensive description of retinoblastoma is given by McLean.[169]

Tumours of the optic nerve and nerve sheath

Optic nerve and optic nerve sheath tumours typically present with proptosis, progressive visual failure or both. They are relatively rare, and current neuroimaging is sufficiently accurate to make diagnostic biopsy of certain lesions, in particular optic nerve glioma, inappropriate.

OPTIC NERVE HEAD TUMOURS

Primary tumours of the optic nerve head include a variety of haemangiomas, gliomas and, peculiarly, melanocytomas.[21,40] Secondary involvement is usually by extension from neighbouring tumours, for instance retinoblastoma or meningioma. Primary retinal–cerebral B-cell lymphoma can also extend along the optic nerve.

OPTIC NERVE GLIOMAS

These low-grade, pilocytic astrocytomas most commonly present during the first decade of life, sometimes at birth (see also Chapter 11, Volume II). A comprehensive review is given by Dutton.[62] Neurofibromatosis type 1 (NF-1) is a risk factor and NF1 patients are more likely to have optic nerve as opposed to chiasmal lesions and may present differently.[161] Axial proptosis is a common presenting feature, although older children may first report visual loss. Presumably because of the gradual expansion of the optic nerve with displacement of axons before their destruction, acuity can be relatively well preserved. More posteriorly placed tumours may generate chiasmal field defects or symptoms attributable to pituitary stalk and hypothalamic involvement. In about one-half of cases, tumour growth halts and it is reasonable to consider the lesion a hamartoma. In others, growth over and above what can be explained in terms of microcystic degeneration or haemorrhage takes place and the lesion's behaviour appears genuinely neoplastic. The presence of compound nuclear organizer regions (AgNORs) has been used as evidence to support the hypothesis that these lesions are true neoplasms.[24]

Macroscopically, there is diffuse expansion of the nerve and the dura often remains intact. At low power, it is often possible to see expansion of individual axonal compartments with their intervening fibroglial septae intact. Histologically, the expansion is due to increased numbers of pilocytic astrocytes with varying degrees of microcyst and Rosenthal fibre formation (Fig. 16.18). Mineralization may be seen. There is thickening of the perineural components with meningothelial hyperplasia (Fig. 16.19) and intervening glial processes. The former may mislead if a superficial biopsy is taken, the appearances being suggestive of a meningioma.[42]

Malignant astrocytomas of the optic nerve[116] are usually seen in adults[19] and often represent extension of a chiasmal lesion.

OPTIC NERVE SHEATH MENINGIOMAS

Optic nerve sheath meningiomas, while in many respects similar to their intracranial counterparts, differ in several ways. Orbital meningiomas appear to present at a younger age. In one study of meningiomas in children aged 1–16 years, four out of nine were found in the orbit,[224] and Eggers and Jakobiec found 25% of orbital meningiomas in the first decade of life and the rest in the fifth.[67] It is not clear whether the earlier presentation can be explained solely as a consequence of the tumour arising at a site more likely to be apparent clinically. The facts that younger cases behave more aggressively[230,263] and that the female predominance of adult tumours is not seen in paediatric cases suggest that there may be something fundamentally different between orbital meningiomas in young and old patients. NF-2 is a known risk factor.[47]

Most orbital meningiomas clearly arise from the optic nerve sheath (Fig. 16.20) and grow around the nerve. Unlike optic nerve gliomas, the nerve may often be seen coursing through the tumour on neuroimaging. Meningiomas are more likely to extend outside the nerve sheath. An intraocular meningioma has been reported[171] and intraocular extension is also described.[37] It is also well recognised that meningiomas may arise in the orbit apparently separate from the nerve.[262]

Lymphoma

Lymphoproliferative disease of the conjunctiva and orbit is a common clinicopathological problem[25,43,45] and intraocular lymphoma, while relatively rare, presents a particular challenge to ophthalmolgist and pathologist alike. Recent advances in the understanding and classification of lymphomas,[119] in particular the elucidation of the evolution of extranodal marginal zone lymphoma, combined with the availability of antibodies that work reliably in paraffin-embedded sections, have made the diagnosis of orbital lymphoid lesions much more straightforward. There is now little need for diagnoses such as atypical benign lymphoid hyperplasia or grey-zone lymphoma.

Anteriorly situated lymphomas often present with a 'salmon patch' (Fig. 16.21), a pale pink, fleshy subconjunctival lesion, and they are not infrequently bilateral. More posterior lesions may present with proptosis and, perhaps because they present later, these lesions have a worse prognosis. On imaging, orbital lymphomas usually have relatively well-defined borders within the orbit and cloak the globe with little tendency to compress it. The lacrimal gland may be involved. The majority of these lymphomas are low-grade extranodal marginal zone, B-cell lymphomas and if related to the conjunctiva fall within the class of mucosa-associated lymphoid tissue (MALT) tumours (Fig. 16.22). In common with MALT lymphomas elsewhere, these tumours appear to evolve from a reactive, benign follicular hyperplasia. The prognosis for this group is good.[188] There is presumably some stimulus that drives the reactive process but its nature remains unknown. In the authors' experience, follicle centre cell lymphomas are the next most commonly encountered orbital lymphoma, but almost any category

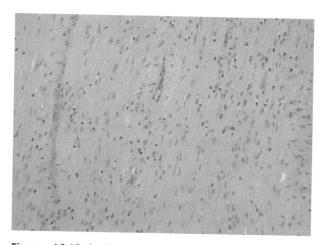

Figure 16.18 *Optic nerve glioma. There are numerous Rosenthal fibres.*

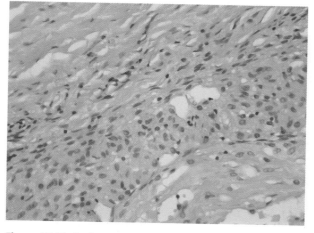

Figure 16.19 *Optic nerve glioma. There is meningothelial hyperplasia in the meninges adjacent to the optic nerve.*

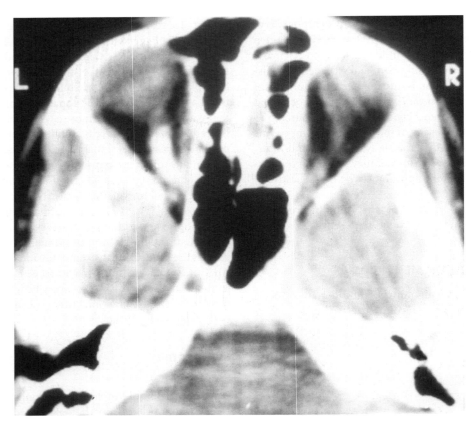

Figure 16.20 *Optic nerve meningioma. (CT scan.) Courtesy of Mr J Kanski.*

of non-Hodgkin's lymphoma may be seen. Increased expression of *bcl-2* in neoplastic follicles is particularly useful for distinguishing follicular lymphoma from benign lymphoid hyperplasia or, more frequently, an extranodal marginal zone B-cell lymphoma in which neoplastic lymphocytes are colonizing coexisting reactive follicles. T-cell lymphomas are rare[44] and Hodgkin's lymphoma appears rarer still. Many orbital lymphomas are localized to the orbits at presentation but a significant percentage eventually develop systemic disease. The orbit may also be involved secondarily.

Within the eye, the retina and choroid may be involved by lymphoma. The overall clinical picture and pathology of disease at these sites differ substantially. The retina behaves very much like an extension of the brain. Patients are usually elderly and present with a refractory inflammatory picture (uveitis) with clusters of cells within the vitreous. Bilateral disease is common. Discrete deposits may become apparent in relation to the retina. Vitreous biopsy, at its simplest a neat sample of vitreous taken into a syringe via a hypodermic needle, may be diagnostic[3] but is often unrewarding. The vitreous is a technically challenging fluid with which to work and as the centre of the eye is relatively hypoxic, degenerate cells may predominate. If they are numerous, however, a neoplastic, rather reactive process is more likely. In some instances only reactive, inflammatory cells can be retrieved, but if the infiltrate is largely composed of B-cells

suspicion for lymphoma is increased. High intravitreal levels of interleukin-10 (IL-10) as opposed to IL-6 and IL-12 might be of value in distinguishing lymphoma from chronic inflammation. The trend is for IL-10 to be relatively raised in lymphoma, but exceptions are not uncommon[4,23] and studies of vitreous cytokine profiles for the moment remain largely in the research realm. A further technique, used effectively in some centres, is to immunophenotype the cells using flow cytometry.[50] If all else fails, retinal biopsy or aspiration of subretinal fluid may be of diagnostic value.[39] Retinal biopsy is especially appropriate where treatment decisions regarding the

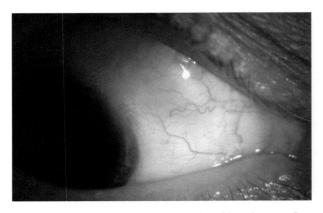

Figure 16.21 *Lymphoma. Anteriorly placed lymphomas often present with a 'salmon patch'.*

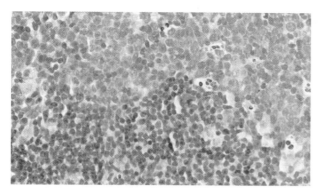

Figure 16.22 *Lymphoma. Extranodal, marginal zone lymphoma (MALT-associated). Regions of larger cells may be seen as in the upper portion of this field.*

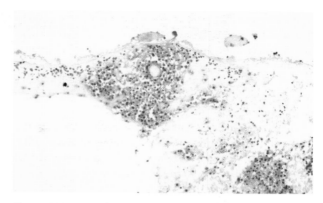

Figure 16.24 *Lymphoma. Necrotic retina in a case of high-grade B-cell lymphoma. (CD20 staining in red.)*

contralateral eye cannot be made without a tissue diagnosis. If possible, a full-thickness retinochoroidal biopsy should be taken. This increases the likelihood of finding lymphoma, which often extends in the plane between the RPE and Bruch's membrane[51] and extends the investigation to include primary choroidal processes. A trans-scleral approach may be of value, especially if it is not possible to obtain a good view from the front.[112] Further confirmation of the presence of lymphoma can be sought by looking for gene rearrangements by polymerase chain reaction (PCR).[257]

Histologically, retinal lymphomas are usually of the high-grade, large B-cell type, of identical appearance to the majority of primary cerebral lymphomas (Figs 16.23, 16.24). Indeed, 20% of patients with primary cerebral lymphoma have involvement of the optic nerve or retina. Conversely, over 50% of patients with retinal lymphoma have cerebral disease.[84] The tumour grows under the RPE and through the retina, often with a perivascular pattern of growth and much associated necrosis. There is variable spillover of cells into the vitreous.

Choroidal involvement by lymphoma (Fig. 16.25) is usually a manifestation of systemic disease. It is interesting how differently two so closely related tissues, one within a blood–tissue barrier and the other outside one, can

behave. The bilaterality of ocular lymphoma along with the apparent multifocal nature of cerebral lymphoma and the isolation of the CNS compartment from the rest of the body raise questions as to how separate foci of tumour are generated. Spread from eye to eye along central visual pathways is possible, but blood-borne spread with precise targeting of metastatic spread is an intriguing alternative.

VASCULAR DISEASE

Retinal ischaemia and neovascularization

Retinal ischaemia occurs in a wide range of clinical contexts and is extremely important. Recent developments in the understanding of the mechanisms of angiogenesis have brought the prospect of a new era of therapeutics in a wide range of conditions resulting in blindness.[216] For instance, blocking α_v-integrin binding with a cyclic peptide has been shown to inhibit new vessel formation in a

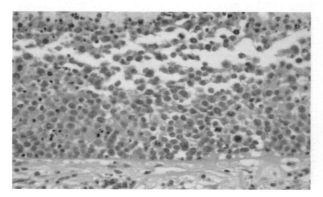

Figure 16.23 *Lymphoma. High-grade B-cell tumour of the retina lying on Bruch's membrane.*

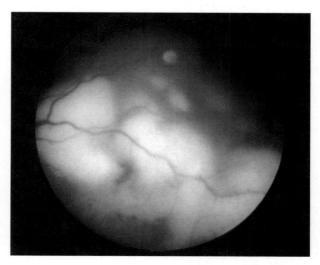

Figure 16.25 *Choroidal lymphoma. This is usually a manifestation of systemic disease.*

murine model of retinopathy of prematurity.[117] As well as the conditions considered in this section, in the newborn, neovascularization complicates retinopathy of prematurity and the most sight-threatening complication of age-related macular disease is new blood-vessel formation. Angiogenesis at the front of the eye causes corneal opacity and neovascular glaucoma.

There are interesting contrasts between ischaemia in the retina and in the brain and it is in many instances difficult to know whether there are specific processes to the retina or whether the ability to visualize retinal vascular pathology so much more readily is responsible for apparent differences.

The inner retina is supplied by two vascular beds from the terminal branch of the ophthalmic artery, the central retinal artery, and is drained by the central retinal vein. The outer retina is supplied by the choriocapillaris that lies immediately under the RPE and Bruch's membrane. It has been estimated that the choroidal circulation contributes approximately two-thirds of the oxygenation to the retina.[6] The choriocapillaris is supplied by the short posterior ciliary arteries, which penetrate the sclera in a ring around the optic nerve. These blood vessels are branches of the medial and lateral long posterior ciliary arteries (themselves branches of the ophthalmic artery), which also supply part of the anterior choriocapillaris. Choroidal blood flow rate is remarkably high, an order of magnitude greater than that of the brain.

'COTTON-WOOL' SPOTS

Arteriolar occlusions in the inner retinal vascular plexus lead to what are clinically recognized as 'cotton-wool' spots (Fig. 16.26) and are histologically evident as small infarcts in the nerve fibre layer. They were classically described in diabetic retinopathy but are found in hypertension, collagen vascular disorders, the acquired immunodeficiency syndrome (AIDS) and many other conditions.[53] They last from 4 to 12 weeks and when resolved a small inner retinal scar that is only discernible

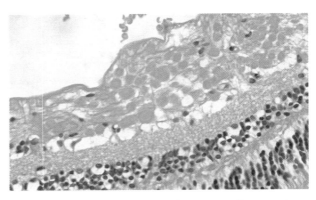

Figure 16.27 *Intraocular trauma. There are swollen axonal profiles in the nerve layer (cotton-wool spot).*

by histology is all that remains. Morphologically, cotton-wool spots are comprised of a cluster of swollen axons, hypoxia having led to a cessation of orthograde and retrograde axonal transport. Morphologically similar structures are seen following direct trauma to the eye (Fig. 16.27). The accumulation of organelles and other material within the centre of each swelling is evident as a dark centre, giving rise to the term cytoid body.

CAPILLARY NON-PERFUSION AND MICROANEURYSM FORMATION

In diabetic retinopathy, retinal vein occlusions, sickle cell disease and related conditions, areas of non-perfusion develop (Figs 16.28, 16.29). These are readily demonstrated clinically by fluorescein angiography, and in retinal whole mounts, by protease digestion to visualize regions of endothelial and pericyte loss or by indian ink injection (Fig. 16.30). Around the edge of such areas, microaneurysms form. They are difficult to see in conventionally prepared sections and may be similar to Charcot–Bouchard aneurysms in the brain. Loss of adventitial support and loss of pericyte-mediated tone have been proposed as possible mechanisms of formation. Whether similar microaneurysms form within the brain

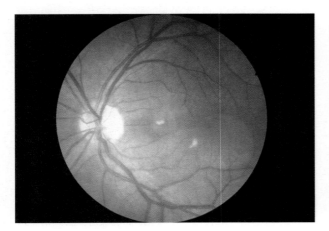

Figure 16.26 *Cotton-wool spots. These are due to occlusion of arterioles in the inner retinal vascular plexus.*

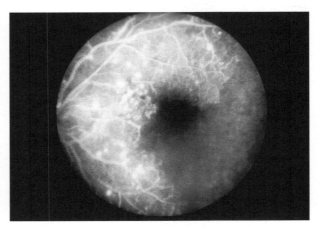

Figure 16.28 *Eales' disease. Fluorescein angiogram showing marked peripheral vascular closure and ischaemia.*

in diabetes is not clear. Similar microvascular pathology, with thickening of blood-vessel walls and vessel occlusion, are seen in radiation retinopathy. This has been described most frequently after radiotherapy for ocular disease, but treatment of intracranial lesions is also a well-recognized cause.[11]

CENTRAL AND BRANCH RETINAL ARTERY OCCLUSION

Branch retinal artery occlusions usually result from emboli from the usual wide range of sources.[217] Central retinal artery occlusion may also be embolic and can also arise from local atherosclerosis, giant cell arteritis and intraocular or orbital surgery. The key pathological findings are of oedema and evolving neuronal cell death acutely with, chronically, astrogliosis and inner retinal atrophy with loss of nerve fibre and ganglion cell layers, as well as the inner two-thirds of the inner nuclear layer (Fig. 16.31).

CENTRAL AND BRANCH RETINAL VEIN OCCLUSION

Retinal vein occlusions cause oedema and haemorrhages in the nerve fibre layer and deeper parts of the retina. In general, there is not a total loss of inner retina and most commonly thinning of the nerve fibre layer and ganglion

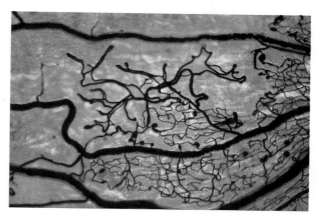

Figure 16.30 *Diabetic retinopathy. Indian ink injection whole mount of retina. Areas of vascular closure (upper field) are bounded by ectatic vessels with microaneurysms.*

cell loss secondary to neovascular angle-closure glaucoma are seen. Any hypercoagulable state will predispose to retinal vein occlusion, but the main aetiological factor is thought to be arterial disease. Venous occlusion occurs especially at the lamina cribrosa and where branch arteries and veins cross. At these locations artery and vein share adventitial coverings: distortion of the vein due to arterial disease may provoke thrombus formation in the adjacent vein.[103] Local disease such as glaucoma, papilloedema or optic nerve drusen are also important risk factors.

RETINAL NEOVASCULARIZATION

Retinal ischaemia that is insufficient to cause total tissue loss often provokes neovascularization. This is best documented in diabetic retinopathy but is also seen in other conditions including sickle cell disease (Fig. 16.29) and retinopathy of prematurity. Initially, new blood vessels form in the nerve fibre layer and intraretinal microvascular abnormalities (IRMAs) result.[133] Later, in the proliferative phase of disease, they extend preretinally, through the inner limiting membrane (Fig. 16.32). These

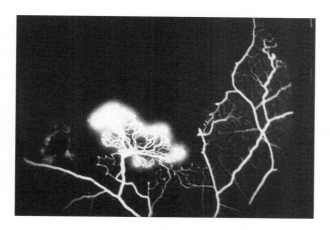

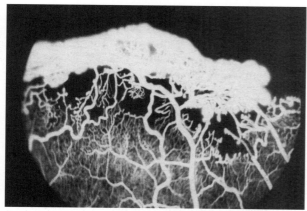

Figure 16.29 *Sickle cell disease. Fluorescein angiogram showing peripheral vascular closure and neovascularization. Courtesy of Professor A Bird.*

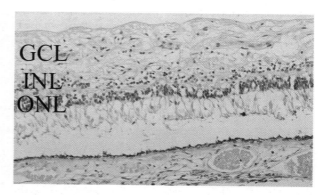

Figure 16.31 *Ischaemic inner retinal atrophy. There is total loss of ganglion cells in the ganglion cell layer (GCL) and substantial loss of the inner portion of the inner nuclear layer (INL) with relative preservation of the outer nuclear layer (ONL).*

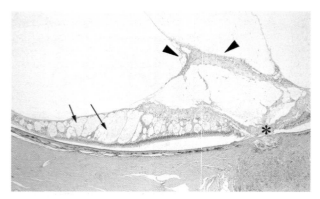

Figure 16.32 *Neovascularization. Neovascularization (arrowheads) arising from the optic nerve head (asterisk). Note the presence of cystoid macular oedema in the retina to the left of the optic nerve head (arrows).*

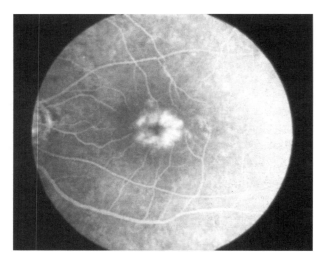

Figure 16.33 *Cystoid macular oedema. Fluorescein angiogram.*

immature vessels may be fenestrated and leak protein. They may bring with them fibroglial tissue which contracts and causes retinal detachment. They are also prone to haemorrhage, often massively, into the vitreous with catastrophic effects on vision.

Release of VEGF by the hypoxic retina is an important component of pathogenesis. It is released following experimental ischaemia[179] and is seen in clinical situations where ischaemia and angiogenesis are taking place.[2] Other factors are likely to be involved. Insulin-like growth factor promotes neovascularization, possibly by increasing VEGF expression, and it has been proposed that $\alpha_v\beta_3$-integrin mediates basic fibroblast growth factor (bFGF)-driven angiogenesis and that $\alpha_v\beta_5$ is involved in VEGF-mediated new blood-vessel formation.[86]

Retinal haemorrhages

Retinal haemorrhages are seen in many situations: following trauma, in microvasculopathies such as diabetes, and sickle cell disease, and in conditions in which venous return or arteriolar autoregulation is impaired. The pattern of haemorrhage is determined by the local environment. Haemorrhages in the nerve fibre layer are flame shaped. Deeper within the retina extravasated blood is confined by radial Müller cell processes into 'dot' and 'blot' patterns.

Cystoid macular oedema

The macula reacts to many pathological stimuli by becoming oedematous. As in the brain, this may be vasogenic, and in its earliest stages vision may be normal but retinal blood vessels are seen to leak on fluorescein angiography. In the eye the integrity of tight junctions between the RPE cells is also of importance in maintaining the blood–retinal barrier, and local RPE–choroidal pathology can also cause cystoid macular oedema (CME).

A remarkably wide range of insults cause macular oedema, perhaps because the macula is relatively undervascularized, given its metabolic requirements. The organization of the fovea may also not resist the accumulation of extracellular fluid as well as elsewhere in the retina, and certainly the radial pattern of photoreceptor axons in Henle's layer contributes to the star-like pattern of oedema sometimes seen (Fig. 16.33). Causes include diabetic retinopathy and other vascular retinopathies, uveitis, retinal degenerations and intraocular tumours. Particularly important from a clinical perspective is macular oedema arising following intraocular surgery, especially cataract extraction (Irvine–Gass syndrome).

The histopathology is of cystic spaces, usually in the inner nuclear and outer plexiform layers (Fig. 16.32). Outer layers are more likely to be involved if the RPE is compromised. The cysts may be filled by watery or more proteinaceous fluid and with time secondary astrogliosis and photoreceptor cell loss develop. There is debate as to the balance between intracellular fluid accumulation in Müller cells and extracellular fluid in various forms of CME.[79,93]

Details of the pathogenesis may vary according to the underlying pathology, but clearly disruption of the blood–retinal barriers is important. The mechanism of oedema formation following cataract extraction is unclear, although vitreous traction and inflammatory mediators have been implicated.

Ischaemic optic neuropathy and papilloedema

ISCHAEMIC OPTIC NEUROPATHY

The vascular supply to the optic nerve head is complex. Its laminar and prelaminar components are supplied by peripapillary choroidal blood vessels organized in an incomplete anastomotic ring (of Zinn–Haller) that are, in

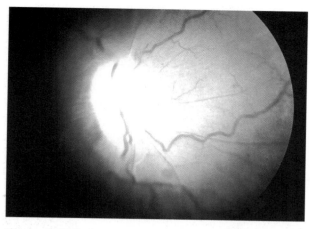

Figure 16.34 *Ischaemic optic neuropathy. There is marked swelling of the disc. Courtesy of Mr J Kanski.*

turn, supplied by the multiple short posterior ciliary vessels that perforate the globe in a ring around the optic nerve. In non-arteritic ischaemic optic neuropathy (ION), it is usually this system of blood vessels that is affected and the term anterior ION is often used in this context. Patients are typically elderly and have an increased likelihood of being hypertensive or diabetic. Symptoms are often noted on wakening and it is supposed that hypoperfusion is an important factor in pathogenesis.[123] The marked swelling of the disc seen clinically (Fig. 16.34) reflects the anterior nature of the disease and with time this evolves into optic atrophy. Arteritic ION is discussed below.

PAPILLOEDEMA

Swelling of the optic nerve head (Fig. 16.35) occurs in many situations, including raised ICP.[221] Macroscopically it is best assessed under the dissecting microscope. His-

tologically, sections should be taken through the centre of the optic nerve head, which may appear full. The lateral displacement of the peripapillary retina is more specific, giving rise to a concertina-like appearance (Fig. 16.36). Necrotic-looking material may be present in the peripapillary subretinal space and swollen axons are often seen. Venous congestion with oedema and hypoxia and physical disruption of axonal transport may all contribute to the pathogenesis of papilloedema.

INFLAMMATORY AND IMMUNE DISEASE

A large number of infectious and non-infectious inflammatory diseases affect the retina and optic nerve. The detailed histopathology of inflammation at these sites has been dealt with in detail elsewhere.[101,214] Similarly, other sources should be consulted for the wide range of pathology associated with intraocular infection in general. The following provides an overview of some of the more commonly encountered conditions affecting primarily the retina or optic nerve. Occasionally, infections relevant to the brain, such as Whipple's disease, may affect other parts of the eye (Fig. 16.37).

Infective retinitis

The retina is vulnerable to many of the viruses that can affect the brain. The ability to visualize the retina, however, provides interesting insights into evolution of disease. As with the rest of the CNS, the advent of AIDS has increased the prevalence of many forms of viral retinitis. However, although human immunodeficiency virus (HIV) can be found in the retina, giant cell retinitis equivalent to that seen in HIV encephalitis has not been

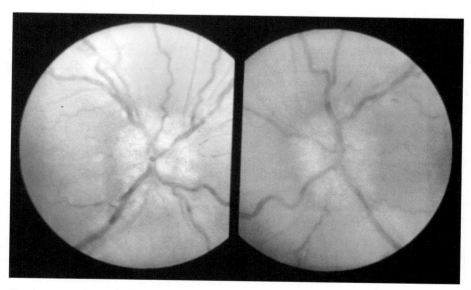

Figure 16.35 *Papilloedema. There are bilateral swollen optic nerves.*

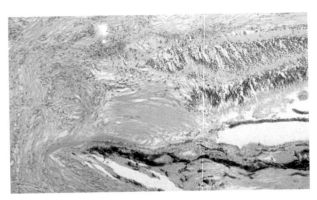

Figure 16.36 *Papilloedema. The retina is displaced laterally from the edge of the optic nerve head. Courtesy of WB Saunders Co.; from Cogan and Luthert.*[40]

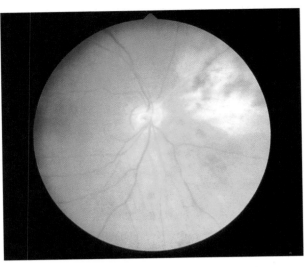

Figure 16.38 *CMV retinitis. Clinically there is haemorrhage, exudate and retinal necrosis in the absence of evident intraocular inflammation.*

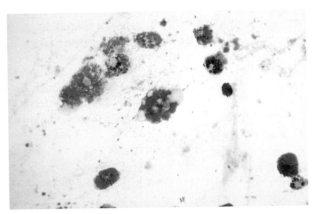

Figure 16.37 *Whipple's disease. PAS-positive staining, swollen macrophages in a vitreous specimen. Courtesy of Professor I Cree.*

described (see also Chapter 1, Volume II). Microinfarcts of the nerve fibre layer (cotton-wool spots) are, however, well recognized.

Cytomegalovirus (CMV) infection is a particular problem in AIDS. Clinically, there is haemorrhage, exudate and retinal necrosis in the absence of evident intraocular inflammation (Fig. 16.38). In patients on highly active antiretroviral therapy (HAART) there may be inflammation. Histopathologically, there is retinal destruction with classical intranuclear inclusions in astroglia and neurons (Fig. 16.39). There may be some secondary choroidal inflammation and there is generally little vitritis. Human herpes virus 6 has been shown to coinfect with CMV in some cases.[78] Herpes simplex type II retinitis has been described in association with neonatal encephalitis.[36] Again, necrotizing retinitis is seen but in this instance usually with more associated inflammation in adjacent tissues. In adults, two clinical patterns of disease, progressive outer retinal necrosis (PORN), now known as varicella-zoster retinitis, and acute retinal necrosis (ARN) (Fig. 16.40), are well recognized. Herpes zoster-varicella (HZV) is an important cause of both, with PORN only occurring in severely immunocompromised cases.[110] ARN, in which

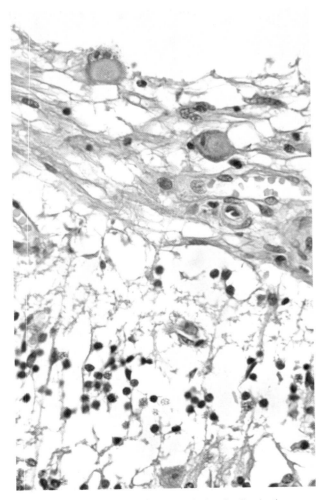

Figure 16.39 *CMV retinitis. Viral inclusion bodies in the nerve fibre layer of the retina.*

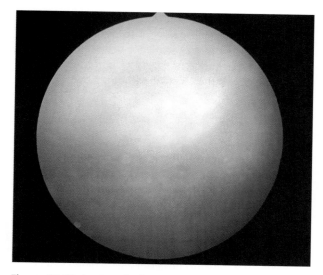

Figure 16.40 *Acute retinal necrosis (HZV).*

there is often an intense vasculitis involving arteries and veins, may also be caused by herpes simplex virus (HSV) types I and II. Cerebrospinal fluid (CSF) antibody production against specific viruses has been used to identify causative viruses in ARN without resorting to retinal biopsy.[68] It is also possible to use vitreous biopsy for PCR diagnosis of CMV, HZV, HSV-I and II and Epstein–Barr virus (EBV). Involvement of the intracranial compartment is also suggested by the possibility that disease may spread from one eye to the other via the optic pathways. The optic nerve may be involved and systemic steroids or rarely surgical decompression may be required. Herpes viruses are also important causes of disease elsewhere in the eye. Finally, measles virus has been shown to cause a maculopathy in the context of subacute sclerosing panencephalitis.[80]

Candida, and less frequently *Cryptococcus neoformans*, which more commonly causes a choroiditis, can cause discrete, fluffy lesions on the retina and infection will often spread into the vitreous and cause endophthalmitis. Other fungal infections such as *Aspergillus* cause endophthalmitis and most of the time fungal infection can be diagnosed clinically. Toxoplasmosis is another cause of retinal necrosis, and retinal biopsy may sometimes be required to distinguish this infection from lymphoma. Typically, cysts are present in the retina and there is a granulomatous inflammatory cell reaction in the choroid (Fig. 16.41). In some instances, it appears as though the retinal pathology develops following an acutely acquired systemic infection, but more often there is reactivation of earlier acquired infection. Cysts can be found at the edge of healed toxoplasma retinochoroidal scars. In immunosuppressed patients, toxoplasma retinitis can be especially destructive and may also be associated with CNS disease.

Sarcoid

The clinical manifestations of ocular sarcoid are protean. There may be anterior or posteior uveitis or both. In the posterior segment, 'snowballs' in the vitreous and waxy retinal deposits described as 'candle-wax drippings' (Fig. 16.42) are classically seen. Retinal periphlebitis is common. Optic nerve involvement is often present (Fig. 16.43). If the risk of sight-threatening complications, including new blood-vessel formation, is to be minimized, rapid, effective immunosuppressive treatment is mandatory. Cerebral involvement is much more common in patients with retinal or optic nerve disease than in those without. Histologically, typical granulomata with only scant lymphocytes are seen.

Behçet's disease

In Behçet's disease, clinically, there is intraocular inflammation with ischaemic vasculitis, retinitis (Fig. 16.44) and optic nerve involvement. The prognosis for vision is poor when ischaemia is extensive.

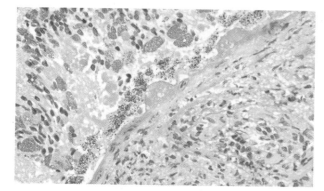

Figure 16.41 *Toxoplasmosis. Cysts are seen in the necrotic-looking retina which is separated from a granulomatous chronic inflammatory cell infiltrate in the choroid by disorganized retinal pigment epithelium.*

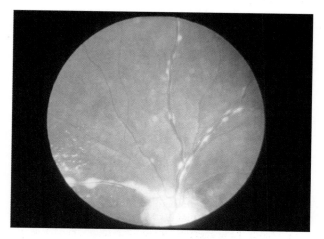

Figure 16.42 *Sarcoidosis. Candle-wax drippings. Courtesy of Mr J Kanski.*

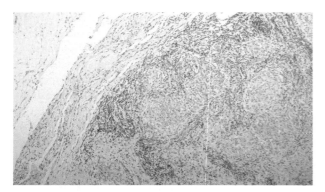

Figure 16.43 *Sarcoidosis. Granulomata in the optic nerve. Courtesy of WB Saunders Co.; from Cogan and Luthert.*[40]

Optic neuritis and demyelination

The clinical definition of optic neuritis stems mainly from the clinical appearances of a swollen disc with, unlike in acute papilloedema, significant reduction in vision. There may also be retrobulbar disease with a normal nerve. The histopathological correlates of this 'neuritis' are poorly characterized and in many instances there may not be any true inflammatory cell infiltrate. Most intraocular infections can cause optic neuritis,[214] with HIV, secondary syphilis, Lyme disease and infection secondary to sinus disease being worthy of specific mention. The most common cause of optic neuritis, however, is the idiopathic form that is often associated with multiple sclerosis (MS) and which, in a significant number of cases of MS, may be the presenting feature.

The pathology of the optic nerve is essentially that of white-matter tracts anywhere in the nervous system, but the frequency of involvement is very high, with 35 of 36 nerves of 18 patients being affected in one study.[243] The retina may also be involved. Clinically, sheathing of retinal veins may be seen and the histopathological correlate of this is perivascular cuffing by lymphocytes that is best demonstrated in retinal digests.[143] Inflammation of the choroid and rarely the ciliary body have also been seen. Deficits in the nerve fibre layer of the retina are also well recognized clinically. The presence of lesions in a non-myelinated tract indicates the importance and possible primary nature of the vascular pathology in MS.

Vasculitis

Ischaemic optic neuropathy is the most common ophthalmic complication of temporal arteritis.[122] There are several clinical features in addition to pain and tenderness that distinguish this form of ischaemic optic neuropathy from the non-arteritic variety. There may be premonitory visual symptoms and bilateral disease at presentation occasionally occurs. Visual loss is usually more severe. Involvement of the short posterior ciliary blood vessels has been reported in cases coming to post-mortem examination[124] and the pathology may be more posterior in the nerve than in typical non-arteritic ischaemic optic neuropathy. Much less often, retinal blood vessels may be primarily involved. To optimize the chances of finding significant pathology in a temporal artery biopsy, the specimen should be as long as possible, cut into short segments and examined at multiple levels. It is important to exclude non-specific age-related changes that not infrequently lead to disruption of the internal elastic lamina. Granulomatous inflammation or transmural scarring indicative of old disease must be seen for the diagnosis to be made.[167]

Paraneoplastic disease

In common with other parts of the CNS, the retina may be a target for autoimmune-mediated damage in patients with cancer [carcinoma-associated retinopathy (CAR)]. Retinal pathology may exist in isolation or coincident with changes in the brain or spinal cord. Typically, but not exclusively, small-cell anaplastic carcinoma of

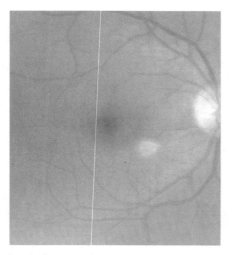
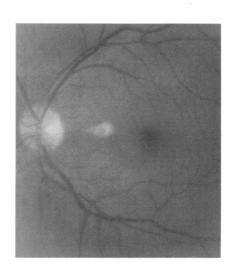

Figure 16.44 *Behçet's disease. Bilateral macular retinitis.*

the bronchus is discovered, sometimes after the presentation of visual symptoms. Patients present with relatively rapid visual loss, night blindness or abnormalities of colour vision, and many have a circulating antibody that recognizes a 23-kDa retinal protein[241] now known to be recoverin, a phototransduction protein expressed in rods and cones.[256] The photoreceptor cells are the most common target but the optic nerve may be involved.[17] Patients with cutaneous melanoma may also develop a retinopathy and present with usually mild visual loss. The target in this condition appears to be retinal bipolar cells; the antigen is as yet uncharacterized.[252]

A curious condition with the descriptive title of bilateral diffuse uveal melanocytic proliferation is also considered to be a paraneoplastic disorder.[92] Carcinoma of the bronchus in men and ovarian cancer in women are the most common associations. In general, the melanocytic proliferation appears benign but this may not invariably be the case.[172] (For other paraneoplastic syndromes see Chapter 11, Volume II.)

DEGENERATIVE DISEASE

Many disease processes are characterized by degeneration of the optic nerve or retina. As elsewhere, the most important of these, glaucoma and age-related macular degeneration, are age related and increasing in importance. There are many interesting parallels with neurodegenerative disease in the brain and it is likely that increasing crossover of therapeutic strategies will be seen. The accessibility of the eye makes it an especially attractive target for new modes of therapy including gene delivery and transplantation.

Two populations of neurons in the retina are of critical clinical importance: the retinal ganglion cells, including their axonal projection through the optic nerve, and the photoreceptors. Damage to the former leads to optic atrophy, there being a wide range of causes. Loss of photoreceptor cells is seen in a wide range of inherited and acquired retinal degenerations.

Glaucoma

A typical patient with glaucoma has reduced visual fields, cupping of the optic disc (Fig. 16.45) and raised intraocular pressure (IOP). The main histopathological feature, other than disc cupping, is loss of retinal ganglion cells and their axons. The condition can therefore be considered an optic neuronopathy. Cases can be differentiated by the presence or absence of clear aetiology (primary or secondary), IOP (normal or raised), the state of the anterior chamber angle, the site of aqueous drainage (open or closed), age of onset and the suddenness of onset (acute or chronic). The most common form of glaucoma is chronic open angle glaucoma of adults.

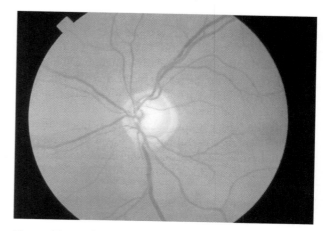

Figure 16.45 *Glaucoma. Glaucomatous cupping of the optic nerve.*

Comprehensive examination of cases with glaucoma can be time-consuming and complex. Many parts of the eye may be involved and the primary pathology may be complicated by repeated surgical and other therapeutic procedures. A full description of the surgical pathology of glaucoma is therefore beyond the scope of this chapter and the emphasis will be on retinal and optic nerve head changes.

RETINAL AND OPTIC NERVE HEAD PATHOLOGY IN GLAUCOMA

Surgical pathology

By the time eyes come to enucleation the glaucomatous changes at the back of the eye are usually readily identifiable. Macroscopically, the optic nerve head is excavated and may appear paler than normal. If, as is often the case because of surgical intervention, the eye is opened vertically, sections must be cut at levels from the temporal face of the block so that the macula can be assessed. Sections through the centre of the optic nerve head are also important (Fig. 16.46). As always, transverse sections of the optic nerve should be taken unless the nerve has been cut flush by the surgeon.

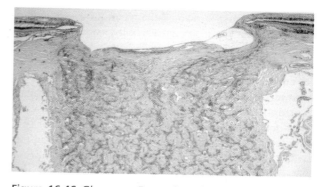

Figure 16.46 *Glaucoma. Excavation of the optic nerve head (cupping). Courtesy of WB Saunders Co.; from Cogan and Luthert.*[40]

Thinning of the nerve fibre layer of the retina may be subtle but in advanced cases is easily assessed, even given the need to take into account its increasing thickness towards the optic nerve. Similarly, ganglion cell loss will be seen, especially in the region of the macula. The outer retina appears relatively normal, although there may be photoreceptor cell loss.[200] The inferior oblique muscle, which is the only extraocular muscle to insert directly into the sclera, is a useful landmark as it lies across the back of the macula. Curiously, the numbers of retinal corpora amylacea, which increase with age, decrease in glaucoma.[148]

An important additional pathology in the retina is evidence of central retinal artery or vein occlusion. This is discussed in the section on vascular disease. The cause of the glaucoma often lies at the front of the eye and treatment often modifies the appearances here, generating quite complex patterns of pathology. Readers are referred to one of the excellent accounts of anterior segment disease in glaucoma.[228]

Experimental pathology in man and animal models of glaucoma

There are interesting parallels between some of the principles underlying the pathogenesis of glaucoma and other neurodegenerative disease. There is great interest in the possibility of selective vulnerability and, as elsewhere, large numbers of cells and their axons have to be lost before patients become symptomatic. One focus of clinical research is to develop screening tests, sensitive enough to detect preclinical disease.

The ganglion cell projection from the retina comprises at least two systems, the magnocellular pathway and the parvocellular pathway, so called because of location of their dominant projection to the lateral geniculate body. The magnocellular pathway arises from parasol ganglion cells and the parvocellular from midget ganglion cells. The two pathways have different functional properties and functional screening tests endeavour to exploit visual stimuli handled particularly by the magnocellular pathway because it is believed that this pathway is affected first. On the grounds of morphometric studies of retinal ganglion cells,[97] optic nerve axon diameters and secondary changes in the lateral geniculate body, as well as experimental radiolabel measurements of axonal transport,[49] it has been concluded that the magnocellular pathway is selectively vulnerable to glaucomatous damage. There is, however, some need for caution in interpreting these data as atrophy without selective cell loss may generate similar shifts in size distributions.[183] The discussion of this important matter continues. In a recent primate study, the earliest pathology was shrinkage of ganglion cell dendritic arbours, with atrophy of cell bodies of both midget and parasol cells occurring later.[250]

The nature of the reactive pathology at the optic nerve head is also of interest. There is astrocytosis and tenasin

expression[203] and nitric oxide synthase (NOS) isoforms are increased,[189] as is cyclo-oxygenase 1.[190] Inhibition of NOS-2 with aminoguanidine has been demonstrated to be protective in a rat model of glaucoma.[191]

MECHANISMS OF OPTIC NERVE HEAD DAMAGE IN GLAUCOMA

The key question in glaucoma pathogenesis is: what are the mechanisms of nerve fibre and ganglion cell loss? Mechanical factors, namely shearing stresses, particularly as axons pass over the edge of the optic nerve head or traverse between the overlapping, perforated plates of collagen in the lamina cribrosa, are likely to play a role. Impaired axonal transport has been demonstrated and axonal swellings can be seen at the optic nerve head. Certainly, raised IOP is a significant risk factor and although, surprisingly, definitive evidence supporting the therapeutic benefit of lowering IOP is lacking, it is widely held to be the case and, indeed, provides the mainstay of therapy. Vascular disease is also a risk factor and impaired perfusion of the optic nerve head may play a role. Optic nerve head blood flow is reduced but establishing a causal link is problematic.[108] As with raised intracranial pressure and reduced cerebral blood flow, raised IOP will reduce perfusion pressure to the optic nerve head and reduce blood flow once the capacity of the vascular bed to autoregulate has been lost. Interestingly, although they are not specific for glaucoma, flame-shaped optic nerve head haemorrhages are seen in glaucoma and these may be a manifestation of loss of autoregulation. The state of the circulation of the optic nerve head may modulate the effects of raised IOP and in some patients, ganglion cell loss progressed despite normal IOP. This may reflect previous damage due to raised pressure continuing in the face of controlled pressure or non-pressure-related pathogenesis in these patients. The notion that factors other then raised IOP are important is strengthened by the observation that some individuals have raised pressure and no apparent optic nerve damage.

It has been proposed that the mechanism of cell death in glaucoma is apoptotic,[89,193,210,225] possibly secondary to excitotoxicity. Many neurons, including retinal ganglion cells, are glutamatergic and retinal ganglion cells express N-methyl-D-aspartate (NMDA) receptors. Indeed, the first, classical experiments demonstrating excitotoxicity were carried out in the retina. In human and experimental glaucoma,[20,58] levels of glutamate in the vitreous are reported as being elevated and glutamate antagonists may be of benefit.[114] Larger ganglion cells, that is those apparently more susceptible to glaucoma, are more vulnerable to glutamate toxicity.[57] It is feasible that hypoxic damage could be responsible for the release of glutamate and, experimentally, optic nerve section also leads to glutamate release. It might not be expected, however, that the rate and duration of release would be sufficient to maintain high levels of glutamate in the vitreous. One possible explanation is that a positive pattern of positive feedback involving NMDA and non-NMDA glutamate receptors is responsible.[235] It is also possible that reversed glutamate transport from Müller cells is of some significance.[170]

Most therapeutic approaches strive to reduce IOP, but there is growing interest in the role of neuroprotection in glaucoma.[106,155]

Non-glaucomatous optic neuropathies

A wide range of insults, alone or in combination, lead to optic neuropathy, often by a final common pathway that involves impairment of mitochondrial oxidative phosphorylation. Axonal transport and ganglion cell perikaryal homoeostasis are likely targets. It is not entirely clear why the optic nerve is so vulnerable, but as with other sites affected in some of these disorders, high metabolic rate, or relatively limited metabolic reserve must be important. A common feature of these conditions is selective loss of the papillomacular bundle. It is tempting to speculate that the high concentration of ganglion cells at the macula, combined with relatively limited retinal circulation, is of some significance.

MITOCHONDRIAL OPTIC NEUROPATHIES

Patients with Leber's hereditary optic neuropathy, a condition not to be confused with Leber's congenital amaurosis, often present with relatively rapid onset of severe blindness, often in one eye followed by the other. It is now known that mutations in mitochondrial DNA play a significant role and to date over ten mutations have been described that confer either relatively high or low risk. The genetics and biochemistry of mitochondrial cytopathies are discussed in detail in Chapter 12 in this Volume. In many individuals, it appears as though an additional mitochondrial stressor is required for blindness to develop. Genetic and environmental factors are likely to be important. Certainly there appears to be an association with smoking and alcoholism.

The most common mutation is at nucleotide 11778 and men are four times more likely to be affected than women. Histologically, the main finding is of loss of ganglion cells and optic atrophy with loss of axons and myelin. Despite their huge requirement for oxidative phosphorylation, photoreceptors are relatively well preserved. They may be able to tolerate mitochondrial dysfunction better than retinal ganglion cells can as, experimentally, they have been shown to resist short periods of mitochondrial poisoning.[261] They also normally metabolize glucose to lactate. Optic atrophy is also seen in MERRF (myoclonic epilepsy and ragged-red fibres).[247]

In Leigh's disease, loss of myelin and sometimes axons has been described[28] in the optic pathways including the optic chiasm.[99]

Other parts of the eye may be affected in mitochondrial disease. For example, in a case of mitochondrial encephalomyopathy lactic acidosis and stroke-like episodes (MELAS) with a mitochondrial DNA (mtDNA) nucleotide 3243 point mutation, there were abnormalities of RPE pigmentation and loss of photoreceptors, particularly at the macula. In addition, there were widespread ultrastructural abnormalities of mitochondria.[219] Retinal degeneration is also seen in NARP (neuropathy, ataxia and retinitis pigmentosa)[128] and in the Kearns–Sayre syndrome (chronic progressive external ophthalmoplegia). Again the macula is most affected and there is the suggestion that there is failure of rod outer segment phagocytosis rather than a primary defect in photoreceptors.[63,134,168]

A further retinal degeneration associated with a mitochondrial abnormality is gyrate atrophy. In this rare autosomal recessive condition there is early-onset visual field loss with in the teens, the development of well-defined patches of atrophy of the choroid and retina.[35] In this instance, the mutation is not in the mtDNA but in the gene for the mitochondrial enzyme ornithine aminotransferase (OAT) on chromosome 10. There may be associated cognitive and muscular abnormalities. Hyperornithinaemia is a feature of diagnostic importance. In a mouse model of OAT deficiency, the primary pathology appeared to be in the RPE.[248] Histopathology of a human case showed a sharp transition between normal and atrophic retina, RPE and choroid and normal-looking tissue. Mitochondrial abnormalities were present in photoreceptors and elsewhere within the eye.[260]

OTHER INHERITED OPTIC NEUROPATHIES

Several inherited optic atrophies have been described with autosomal dominant and autosomal recessive patterns of inheritance. Dominant optic atrophy can present in infancy or in later childhood and while in many cases optic atrophy is the sole manifestation of disease various other sensory and motor neuropathies may be associated. Similarly, recessive optic atrophy may occur in isolation or with other CNS abnormalities or diabetes mellitus. Hearing loss not infrequently occurs with optic atrophy, and important syndromic forms include Charcot–Marie–Tooth disease, Friedreich's ataxia and Wolfram's syndrome. There are few reports of histopathology in these conditions but the features are non-specific with ganglion cell and nerve fibre loss, particularly the maculopapullar bundle in the retina. There is atrophy with fibre loss in the optic nerve.[138,144]

ACQUIRED OPTIC NEUROPATHIES

Nutritional deficiency is a widely accepted cause of both sporadic and epidemic optic neuropathy. Surprisingly, the specific deficiency has yet to be defined and it is probable that a combination of factors, in terms of both nutritional lack and associated toxic influences such as tobacco, is important. It is the presence of cyanide in tobacco smoke that may be critical.[82] A specific role for vitamin B_{12} has been seen in patients with pernicious anaemia and experimental B_{12} deficiency can cause optic nerve demyelination. It is therefore likely to contribute to the condition in dietary malnutrition. Folate deficiency in strict vegetarians is also of importance.

As would be expected from the vulnerability of retinal ganglion cells in general, there are many reports of toxic optic neuropathy; however, clear-cut cause-and-effect relationships are not always seen. Methanol is one well-investigated exception. There are two reports in the literature[187] and the focus of the pathology was in the retrolaminar part of the optic nerve. This area may be vulnerable as it represents a vascular 'watershed'. Ethambutol toxicity is also well characterized, but here the primary pathology may be due to the drug's ability to chelate cations.[153] The reader is referred to other texts for comprehensive lists of potential optic nerve toxins.[166]

SEQUELAE OF OPTIC NERVE DEGENERATION

Optic nerve damage, depending on the site of injury, leads to retrograde or anterograde degeneration, or both. In anterograde (ascending) degeneration the primary pathology is retinal, usually affecting the ganglion cells directly. In longstanding cases the centripetal degeneration leads to neuronal atrophy in the layers 2, 3 and 5 of the ipsilateral lateral geniculate body and 1, 4 and 6 on the opposite side.[31,220] Alterations in activity may be sufficient to cause changes. In amblyopia due to visual deprivation changes in the lateral geniculate body are also seen.[227]

Primary photoreceptor cell degeneration

CLASSIFICATION OF INHERITED PHOTORECEPTOR DEGENERATIONS

Inherited photoreceptor degenerations have traditionally been classified clinically and can be divided into those primarily affecting the rods in the peripheral retina [retinitis pigmentosa (RP)] and those primarily affecting the macula (macular dystrophies). They can also be classified according to mode of inheritance or whether or not the retinal degeneration occurs in isolation or as part of a syndrome. Retinitis pigmentosa may be autosomal dominant, autosomal recessive or sex-linked, or present sporadically. Syndromic forms include abetalipoproteinaemia, Friedreich-like ataxia with retinitis pigmentosa,[265] Refsum's disease, Batten's disease, Usher's syndrome, Kearns–Sayre syndrome and the Laurence–Moon and Bardet–Biedl syndromes.

Over recent years there has been considerable progress in the molecular genetics of outer retinal degenerations.[5,105,207] Although many individual conditions are rare, as a group, inherited photoreceptor degenerations are responsible for about the same level of blind registrations in the working population as diabetes. Parallel disorders

in the dog, where outer retinal degeneration is known as progressive retinal atrophy, also present a major problem.[204] There are currently 36 known or assumed gene loci for retinal degenerations and many identified genes have many different disease-causing mutations. Defects in single genes can lead to multiple phenotypes and single phenotypes may arise as a result of mutations in several different genes.

RETINITIS PIGMENTOSA

Patients with retinitis pigmentosa typically present with progressive loss of night-time vision and a ring-shaped field loss that extends peripherally and centrally.[15] The clinical course may vary markedly, even within single families or with different mutations in a single gene.[38] Cone loss appears to follow the primary rod degeneration and loss of central daytime vision may ultimately occur.

The classical clinical findings of retinitis pigmentosa include irregularity of pigmentation of the RPE with abnormal pigmentation along the course of attenuated blood vessels in a 'bone spicule' configuration (Figs 16.47,

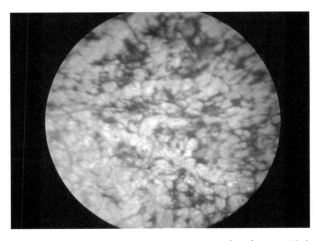

Figure 16.47 *Retinitis pigmentosa. Courtesy of Professor A Bird.*

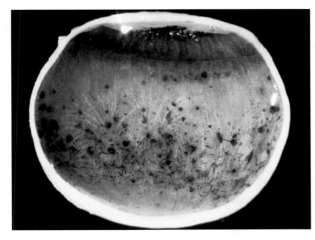

Figure 16.48 *Retinitis pigmentosa. Calotte of an eye from a patient showing characteristic bone-spicule patterning of the migrated pigment epithelium.*

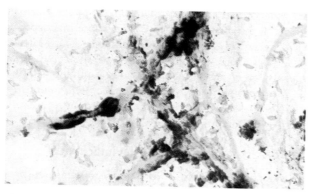

Figure 16.49 *Retinitis pigmentosa. Retinal whole mount that has been protease digested to reveal the vascular architecture with associated retinal pigment epithelium.*

16.48) and pallor of the optic disc. The pigmentation is due to retinal pigment epithelial cells that, following the loss of photoreceptors, have migrated into the retina, often then adhering to connective tissue elements around intraretinal blood vessels (Fig. 16.49). Degenerating photoreceptors often lose their outer segments early, and in part because of this and in some instances because of mutations in rhodopsin itself[237] there is mislocalization of rhodopsin to around the cell body (Fig. 16.50). In type 2 Usher's syndrome there are abnormalities in the cilium connecting the outer and inner segments,[13] and in type 1B Usher's syndrome there is a mutation in myosin VIIa, which localizes to the cilium.[162] Mislocalization of rhodopsin and other phototransduction proteins is therefore a common feature of retinal degenerations.

In chronic degenerations, rods respond by sprouting neurites which can extend substantial distances into the inner retina, apparently following along the surface of Müller cell processes.[32,160,177]

Inner retinal degeneration is also seen[222] and is likely to be trans-synaptic in part,[233] but secondary vascular changes can lead to strangulation of ganglion cell nerve fibres and retrograde ganglion cell loss.[245] Not surprisingly, gliosis is often marked. Blood–retinal barrier breakdown has been demonstrated by the use of immunohisto-chemistry for albumin and in some cases cystoid macu-lar oedema may develop.[246] Macrophages, often with pigment, are present throughout the retina and epireti-nal membranes (see below) may form.[239] A recent com-prehensive review of the histopathology of retinitis pigmentosa is given by Milam *et al.*[178]

MACULAR DEGENERATIONS

Four macular degenerations are of particular current interest as, clinically, they share features with age-related macular disease (see below) and their genetic basis has just been established.[266] Abnormal accumulation of lipofuscin is a recurring feature in these disorders (Fig. 16.51) and electroretinographic (ERG) abnormalities are a feature of non-adult forms of neuronal ceroid lipofuscinosis. The mnd mouse also has features of neuronal ceroid lipofus-cinosis and a retinal degeneration.[29] A recent, exciting clinical development is the ability to image ocular lipofuscin-associated autofluorescence in patients (Fig. 16.51).[218]

Sorsby's fundus dystrophy (SFD)

Sorsby described a retinal degeneration with subretinal deposits and choroidal neovascularization (Fig. 16.52). Histologically, the most striking abnormality is the accumulation of granular material between the RPE and Bruch's membrane (Fig. 16.53),[26,33] and also over the ciliary body. The composition of this material is hetero-

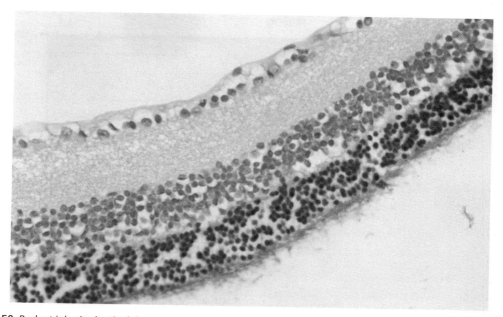

Figure 16.50 *Rodent inherited retinal degeneration. There is mislocalization of opsin (stained red) around outer nuclear layer neurons.*

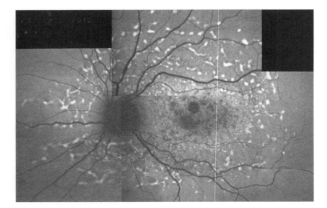

Figure 16.51 *Stargardt's disease.* In vivo *RPE autofluorescence image. Courtesy of Professor A Bird.*

geneous and includes protein, lipid and mineralization. There are breaks in Bruch's membrane with internal extension of choroidal blood vessels (choroidal neovascularization). The retinal changes are relatively non-specific with, in end-stage cases, marked atrophy and gliosis.

The condition displays autosomal dominant inheritance and is due to a mutation in the *tissue inhibitor of metalloproteinase-3* gene (*TIMP-3*).[77] TIMP-3, unlike other TIMPs, is insoluble and binds to connective tissue components. It is produced by the RPE[52,139] and normally binds to Bruch's membrane. In SFD, the subretinal deposit contains TIMP-3[75] and it is possible that the mutation causes its dimerization by the generation of paired cysteines.[149] TIMP-3 is present in thickened Bruch's membrane and drusen in normal ageing.[76,140]

Inherited drusen disorders (Malattia leventinese and Doyne's honeycomb dystrophy)

These conditions are characterized by macular degeneration with abnormalities of the retinal pigment epithelium and drusen formation. Drusen (from the German word for mound or gland) are focal, subretinal deposits that are visible clinically as subretinal spots.[72] Malattia leventinese and Doyne's honeycomb dystrophy have recently been shown to be the result of mutations in the *EGF-containing fibrillin-like extracellular matrix protein 1* (*EFEMP1*) gene.[231] Histologically, the appearances are very similar to those in AMD.

Stargardt's disease/fundus flavimaculatus

This condition, which is now known to be caused by a mutation in the retinal adenosine triphosphate (ATP)-binding cassette protein ABCR,[16] displays autosomal recessive inheritance and patients often present with visual deterioration in childhood. The fundal appearances vary but drusen-like flecks are a characteristic feature (Fig. 16.51). Histological reports are scarce but again increased lipofuscin within the RPE is seen.[64] There is loss of RPE and increased lipofuscin is also present in photoreceptors.

Best's disease

In Best's disease, a yellowish deposit accumulates under the retinal pigment epithelium at the posterior pole in childhood. It is also known as vitelliform macular degeneration type 2. This material, which clinically resembles egg yolk (Fig. 16.54), hence 'vitelliform', increases in volume and ultimately extends through the RPE into the subretinal space. At this stage significant visual impairment will be present and this deteriorates with the development of retinal atrophy or subretinal neovascularization. There are few descriptions of the histopathology, but abnormal accumulation of lipofuscin within the RPE and debris under the RPE are features.[83,195,251] Recently the gene responsible for the condition has been identified[205] and called *bestrophin*. Its function is currently unknown.

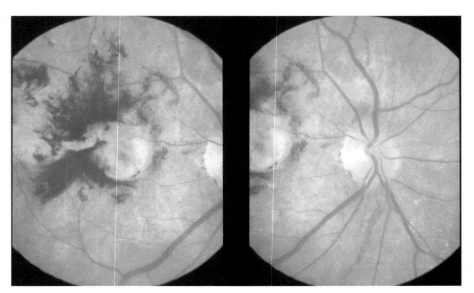

Figure 16.52 *Sorsby's dystrophy. Choroidal neovascular membrane. Courtesy of Professor A Bird.*

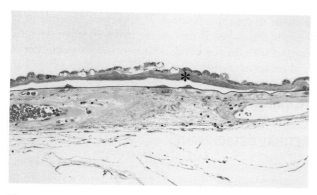

Figure 16.53 *Sorsby's fundus dystrophy. Toluidine blue-stained resin section of the retinal pigment epithelium and subjacent choroid. Note the deposition of material beneath the RPE (asterisk).*

VULNERABILITY OF PHOTORECEPTORS

Photoreceptors are remarkably sensitive to a wide range of pathological insults. Acquired disease will be discussed later and the focus of this section is the array of inherited retinal degenerations in which there is primary photoreceptor cell loss. A remarkable number of mutations in a large number of genes have been implicated in retinal degeneration, probably more so than for any other cell type. More than 40 disease-causing rhodopsin mutations have been described. Broadly speaking, genes concerned with the phototransduction pathway or with structural integrity of the photoreceptor outer segment are involved. The former include controlling transcription factors[238] as well as enzymes. Simply overexpressing opsin is enough to cause degeneration.[198]

This vulnerability may, in part, be a consequence of the heavy metabolic demands placed on photoreceptors. There are substantial ion movements across the outer seg-ment, especially in the dark when the channels are open. The vascular supply to the outer retina is also a little unusual. There are no blood vessels in the outer nuclear layer or between the inner and outer segments. Instead, there is a remarkably rich blood supply externally, under the retinal pigment epithelium, in the form of the choriocapillaris. This highly fenestrated vascular bed has the highest blood flow of any tissue in the body. The integrity of the blood–retinal barrier is maintained by tight junctions between the retinal pigment epithelial cells. There is also a capillary bed within the outer plexiform layer. The inner segments of the photoreceptors, where nearly all of the cells' mitochondria are found, are therefore relatively hypoxic. However, there is evidence that photoreceptors are relatively resistant to hypoxic damage. Another peculiar feature of photoreceptors is that they are illuminated by potentially damaging radiation. Prolonged exposure to intense illumination kills photoreceptors, especially in albino animals, and light damage can exacerbate photoreceptor cell loss in experimental inherited degenerations. Furthermore, some patients with retinitis pigmentosa have an altitudinal field defect with selective degeneration of the inferior retina, possibly due to increased incident light. In nearly every situation investigated, photoreceptors die by apoptosis[208] (Figs 16.55, 16.56).

THERAPEUTIC STRATEGIES

Outer retinal degenerations also present a particularly exciting therapeutic challenge.[164] Unlike many other parts of the CNS, the retina is relatively accessible. Administration of growth factors into the vitreous cavity is proving successful experimentally in a variety of inherited and acquired retinal degenerations[34,74,150,151] and might be used in the clinic. More promising, however, is the growing availability of slow-release implantable devices of the

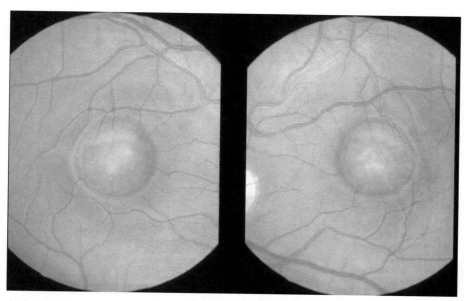

Figure 16.54 *Best's disease. There is a yellowish deposit accumulation under the retinal pigment epithelium. Courtesy of Professor A Bird.*

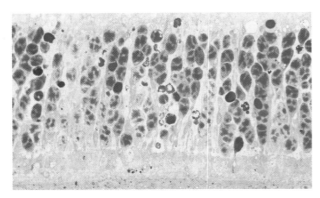

Figure 16.55 *Experimental retinal degeneration. Apoptotic-looking photoreceptor cells.*

type that have been used to deliver ganciclovir in CMV retinitis.[173] An alternative delivery method is the implantation of genetically modified cells. Gene therapy is also showing great promise. Recently, structural and functional abnormalities in the *rds* mouse have been reversed using an adeno-associated virus (AAV) system to deliver the normal gene to the photoreceptors.[6] The *rds* mouse has a mutation in the *rds/peripherin* gene, which is required to maintain disc outer segment morphology. In man, mutations in this gene cause both retinitis pigmentosa and macular dystrophy.[255] A ribozyme approach has also been successful using the AAV system in a rat model of rhodopsin RP.[156] Finally, rather than using transplants of genetically modified cells to deliver specific trophic factors, there is much interest in the use of cells that are naturally supportive of photoreceptors. One strategy is to transplant Schwann cells, which produce a cocktail of trophic molecules.[152] The other is to transplant rod photoreceptors.[181] The rationale here is that in many retinal degenerations the mutant gene is only expressed in the rods yet there is a secondary cone degeneration which is the cause of the major handicap to patients. There are many reasons why this might occur but it is now clear that at least part of the explanation is that rods generate

a factor that supports cones.[180] Therefore, transplanting healthy rods, even if they never make effective synaptic contact with the rest of the neuroretina, may rescue cones and preserve useful vision.

Acquired retinal degenerations

RETINAL DETACHMENT

The retina depends on close physical and functional relationships with the RPE for its continued survival. The best example of functional dependence comes from the RCS rat. In this animal, a spontaneous mutation results in failure of rod outer segment phagocytosis by the RPE, with secondary degeneration of photoreceptor cells. In man, it is more common for the retina to become detached from the RPE, although retinal photoreceptor degenerations secondary to mutations in the RPE are becoming more widely appreciated. Retinal detachment can develop because of a break in the retina (rhegmatogenous detachment), scarring leading to retinal traction, or the accumulation of serous or exudative fluid under the retina.

The resulting pathology has been well characterized in animal models and to a lesser extent in man. As in other retinal degenerations, the photoreceptors lose their outer segments, redistribute opsin to the cell body[158] and progressively die (Fig. 16.57) by apoptosis.[30] In an experimental model in the kitten, the peak of apoptosis is around 3 days post-detachment.[41] In a rabbit study, one-half of the photoreceptors had died by 2 weeks.[14] Red and green cones appear to be most resistant.[194] The pathogenesis of cell death is probably multifactorial. Loss of reciprocal growth factor support, hypoxia due to separation from the choriocapillaris, failure of outer segment phagocytosis and physical disturbance of the retina are all likely to play a part. Recent studies of hyperoxia in detachment have shown improved photoreceptor survival[174] and reduced Müller cell reactive changes, suggesting that hypoxia may be of prime importance.[157] Reattachment minimizes pho-

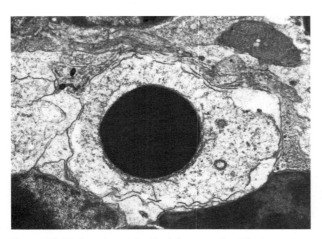

Figure 16.56 *Experimental retinal degeneration. Electron micrograph of an apoptotic photoreceptor cell.*

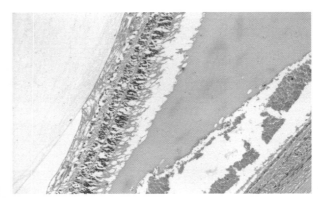

Figure 16.57 *Retinal detachment. Note the accumulation of proteinaceous material between the retina and the retinal pigment epithelium. There is early disorganization of photoreceptor outer and inner segments.*

toreceptor cell loss,[12] especially if rapid but ultrastructural abnormalities are present.[8,109]

There are early reactive changes in the RPE cells, which lose their apical villi, become rounded in appearance, begin to proliferate[9] and can migrate into the subretinal space or, if there is a retinal break, into the vitreous cavity. It is even possible for RPE cells to migrate through the retina onto its anterior surface.[126] Secondary changes also occur in retinal Müller cells and astrocytes. Along with retinal oedema, there is Müller cell hypertrophy with upregulation of GFAP expression,[70] and astrocytes and Müller cells migrate through the inner limiting membrane (Fig. 16.58). Here, with RPE cells if present, an epiretinal membrane may form and if more than a single cell thick, contraction may occur. This process is known as proliferative vitreoretinopathy (PVR) and is the most common cause of surgical failure following retinal detachment surgery.[127] Macrophages or macrophage-like microglia are also seen. The former could come from a resident population of macrophages in the subretinal space analogous to those seen lining the ventricular system of the brain or they may migrate from the choroid. Epiretinal membranes may also form secondary to intraocular inflammation (Fig. 16.59).

Intriguing changes also take place in surviving retinal neurons. Rods show neurite sprouting similar to that seen in retinitis pigmentosa and, in addition, bipolar cells and horizontal cells extend neuritic processes for substantial distances.[159]

LIGHT DAMAGE

Exposure to high levels of incident light, especially at the blue end of the spectrum, leads to photoreceptor cell death. In albino rodents slow, progressive photoreceptor cell death takes place over the lifetime of the animal at exposures as low as those found in many animal facilities. This age-related photoreceptor cell death can confound studies of age-related decline in cognitive tasks requiring visual queues. It also poses interpretational difficulties in long-term toxicology studies. It is advisable to use pigmented animals in any long-term study where retinal structure or function is an issue. Photocoagulation is routinely used in ophthalmology and causes death of photoreceptors and RPE cells (Fig. 16.60), leading to chorioretinal scar formation.

RETINAL TOXICOLOGY

Several classes of drug have been shown to cause retinal pathology. In most cases the effects are dose related. The pathogenesis is, in many instances, poorly understood but high affinity for pigment appears to be of importance in the case of quinolines and phenothiazines.

Prolonged, high-dose chloroquine or hydroxychloroquine treatment can cause a retinopathy that starts with macular pigmentary abnormalities and may evolve into a horizontally elongated bull's-eye pattern of macular depigmentation with associated paracentral field defects. Ganglion cell loss with photoreceptor degeneration and pigment migration have been reported.[212] Other agents, such as tamoxifen and canthaxanthine, may cause a striking fundus appearance with a perimacular ring of inner retinal refractile crystalline material. Phenothiazine therapy may lead to a widespread abnormality with pigment clumping and relatively large areas of atrophy. Although symptoms are reversible if treatment is stopped early, the fundus appearances may continue to progress.

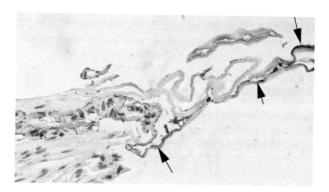

Figure 16.58 *Retinal pigment epithelium. A surgically stripped epiretinal membrane immunohistochemically stained for GFAP. Note the thin, wrinkled inner limiting membrane (arrows).*

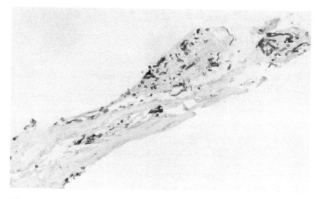

Figure 16.59 *Epiretinal membrane. There are scattered, Grocott-positive yeasts (Candida).*

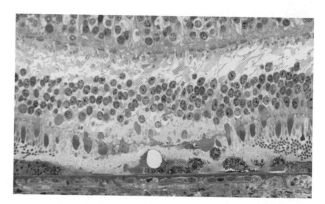

Figure 16.60 *Photocoagulation burn. There is focal destruction of photoreceptors and retinal pigment epithelium 5 days after a photocoagulation burn.*

Age-related macular degeneration

CLINICAL FEATURES AND HISTOPATHOLOGY

Age-related macular degeneration (AMD) is in many ways the Alzheimer's disease of the eye, but without many of the advances that have come about since the central role of APP was identified. It is the most common cause of irreversible blindness in the Western world in patients over the age of 65 years and there is little therapy that offers lasting benefit. As with Alzheimer's disease, the socioeconomic consequences of AMD are enormous.

Many of the clinical and pathological terms used are potentially confusing. The key clinical features of AMD are the formation of focal deposits known as drusen under the retinal pigment epithelium (Fig. 16.61) that may ultimately be associated with loss of RPE (geographical atrophy) or with the formation of a subretinal fibrovascular complex at the macula, known as a disciform scar (Figs 16.61, 16.62). The blood vessels in a disciform scar come from the choroid, through Bruch's membrane, in a process known as choroidal neovascularization. It is this process, in particular, that has devastating consequences for sight. The scar separates the retina from the RPE and sudden visual loss arises when haemorrhagic complications set in.

AMD is reasonably considered an extreme end-point of an ageing process and it seems likely that the primary pathology resides within the RPE cell (Fig. 16.63). Although not strictly postmitotic, these cells have only limited ability to maintain their numbers by replication and yet they are subject to severe metabolic stress throughout the lifetime of the individual. In particular, they phagocytose large numbers of rod outer segments every day. This is associated with the net accumulation of lipofuscin with age.[197,218] *In vitro*, lipofuscin accumulates

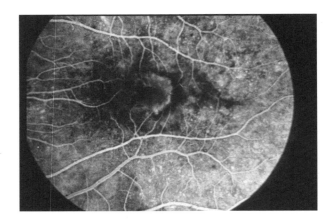

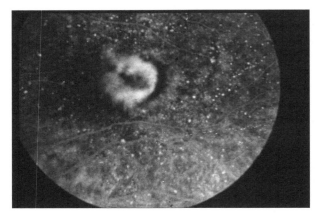

Figure 16.62 *Age-related macular degeneration. Fluorescein angiogram showing neovascular membrane. Courtesy of Professor A Bird.*

more rapidly when RPE cells are fed peroxidized, as opposed to normal, photoreceptor outer segments.[22] Lipofuscin in the RPE is similar to that at other sites, although its chemistry differs in that it contains *N*-retinylidene-*N*-retinylethanolamine (A2-E), a metabolite of vitamin A, which is derived from rod outer segments. Recent studies

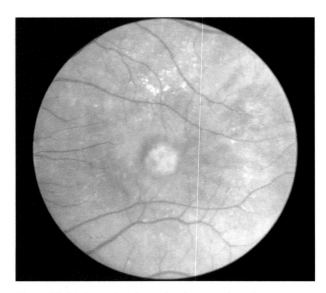

Figure 16.61 *Age-related macular degeneration. There are scattered drusen and a neovascular membrane is present at the macula. Courtesy of Professor A Bird.*

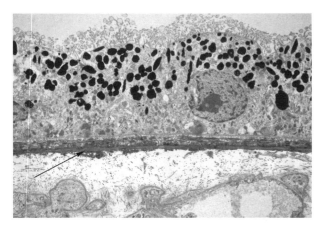

Figure 16.63 *Bruch's membrane. Electron micrograph of retinal pigment epithelium, Bruch's membrane (arrow) and inner choroid.*

have suggested that lipofuscin may be deleterious to RPE cells. It appears to increase the sensitivity of the RPE to phototoxicity from blue light by increasing lysosomal instability,[249] perhaps by promoting the formation of reactive oxygen species.[88] A2-E may also inhibit lysosomal proteolysis[69,130] and inhibit phagocytosis.[236] As in the brain, abnormal accumulation of lipofuscin in ceroid lipofuscinoses is damaging to RPE. This has been well described in the *mnd* mouse. Increased macular RPE lipofuscin is associated with decreased photoreceptor number,[55] but the nature of any potential causal link remains to be defined.

A parallel ageing change is the thickening of Bruch's membrane due to accumulation of lipid[131] and proteinaceous debris.[113,211] This may interfere with nutrient and waste trafficking between the RPE and choriocapillaris.[182]

Focal deposits between the RPE basement membrane and Bruch's membrane are known as drusen and these are seen to accumulate in many individuals with age.[1] Hard drusen are discrete and round (Fig. 16.64). Soft drusen are larger with poorly defined borders and are an important risk factor for geographical atrophy and choroidal neovascularization.[48] Histologically, hard drusen are readily identified as eosinophilic masses under the RPE. They may have a central core, which often contains a major histocompatibility complex (MHC) class II-expressing cell process. Soft drusen material is harder to see but clearly expands the space between the RPE and Bruch's membrane.

A further type of sub-RPE deposit has been described. This forms between the basal plasma membrane of the RPE and its basement membrane (Fig. 16.65), that is, it lies internal to drusen. It is widely known as basal laminar deposit and forms earliest at the far periphery of the retina, where the daily load of rod outer segment to RPE cell is at its highest. The biochemistry of these deposits has been problematic,[146] but by immunohistochemistry they contain TIMP-3 (Fig. 16.66) (see above), vitronectin[115] and apoliproprotein E and other proteins, many which also accumulate in Alzheimer's disease. Part of the protein component appears to be ubiquitinated (Fig. 16.67). They also contain a variety of carbohydrate residues.[145,185] The

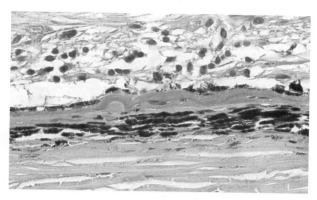

Figure 16.65 *Drusen. A small druse and more diffuse subretinal deposit (basal laminar and basal linear deposits) in a case of age-related macular degeneration.*

ultrastructural features of these various sub-RPE deposits have been studied extensively.[104] They are heterogeneous and include wide-spacing material, presumably a form of collagen, granular material and membranous vesicles.

In geographical atrophy there is RPE attenuation and loss. *In vivo* studies have shown an increase in autofluorescence (presumably from lipofuscin) around the edge of a patch of atrophy.[129]

In choroidal neovascularization, new blood vessels break through Bruch's membrane and a fibrovascular (disciform) scar forms in either the sub-RPE or subretinal space, or both. The presence of large drusen or basal laminar deposits increases the risk of progression to disciform scar formation.[229] Choroidal neovascularization is a feature of many other conditions not discussed here.

PATHOGENESIS

The pathogenesis of AMD is not understood. Genetic factors are important,[98] but are likely to confer risk rather than be strictly causal. The apparent increase in AMD and epidemiological data support the notion of environmental factors associated with the Western lifestyle as being important,[120] but the nature of the factor is unknown. Smoking seems to be a consistent risk factor in several

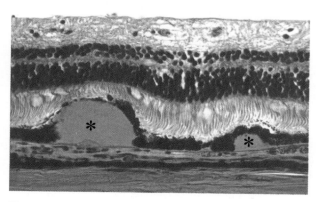

Figure 16.64 *Drusen. There are two eosinophilic bodies (asterisks).*

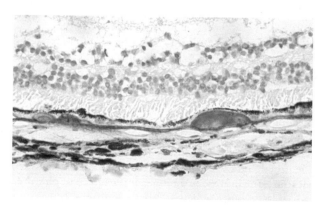

Figure 16.66 *Drusen. Subretinal deposits in a case of age-related macular degeneration. There is immunoreactivity for TIMP-3.*

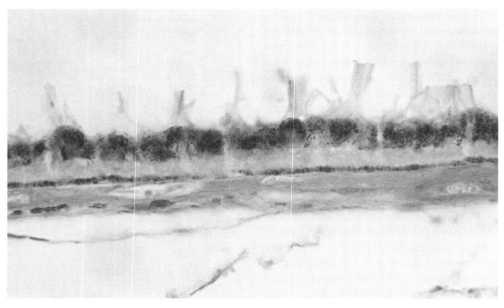

Figure 16.67 *Basal laminar deposit. Ubiquitin immunoreactivity of basal laminar deposit in a case of age-related macular degeneration.*

studies. Perhaps surprisingly, lifetime light exposure is not. There is an urgent need for initiatives to further our understanding of this condition.

The pathogenesis of choroidal neovascularization, which can be considered to be a complication of the primary pathology in AMD, is also not understood. Bruch's membrane offers a barrier to vessel formation, and when breaks in it form in other conditions the risk of new blood-vessel formation is increased. Disturbances in the release or bioavailability of angiogenesis factors are also, almost inevitably, going to be of importance. It is not surprising that the juxtaposition of one of the richest vascular beds in the body, that is the choriocapillaris, with the outer retina, the most avascular neural portion of the CNS, is associated with a high risk of neovascularization.

Miscellaneous retinal and vitreo-retinal degenerations

X-linked recessive retinoschisis usually develops at the macula and consists of splitting of the retina within the nerve fibre layer. The overlying vitreous may be condensed and retinal holes may form in the inner and outer layers. Where both are present retinal detachment results, although vitreous traction as well as hole formation is probably important in the genesis of this complication. The gene for this condition, *XLRS1*, has recently been identified[94] and it appears to be expressed in Müller cells, although the murine orthologue is expressed in photoreceptors.[215] Goldman–Favre disease is similar but shows autosomal recessive inheritance and there is a retinitis pigmentosa-like component to the disease.[206]

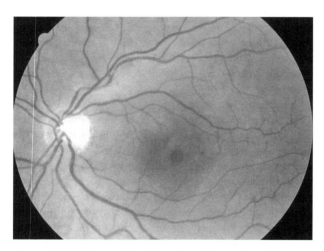

Figure 16.68 *Macular hole. The retina at the centre of the macula is thin and 'macular holes' may form. Courtesy of Mr H Towler.*

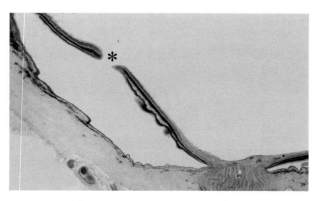

Figure 16.69 *Retinal macula with a macular hole. The macular hole is marked by an asterisk.*

Familial exudative vitreoretinopathy is an autosomal dominant condition characterized by failure of vascularization of the developing peripheral retina with secondary neovascularization, scarring and retinal detachment similar to that seen in retinopathy of prematurity, where there is a clear association with postnatal oxygen supplementation.[18] The differential diagnosis also includes Coats' disease and *Toxocara canis* infection.

The retina at the centre of the macula is thin and macular holes may form (Figs 16.68, 16.69). These may be post-traumatic or arise in association with other pathology but are often idiopathic. Elderly women are especially at risk. The sequence of events leading to macular hole formation, starting with foveolar detachment, progressing through an eccentric hole and ending up with a complete, circular retinal defect, with or without posterior vitreous detachment, has been well described.[91] A preretinal opacity or operculum may be apparent and this may contain vitreous collagen, glial elements or, in some instances, cone photoreceptors.[73] The pathogenesis of idiopathic macular holes remains a matter of debate. Tangential vitreous traction is likely to be of importance and recent attention has been drawn to the possible role of foveal Müller cells.[90] Surgical treatment is directed towards closing the hole or preventing progression to a full-thickness hole. This usually involves removing the vitreous (vitrectomy) and thus one potential source of traction. Various locally applied adjuncts such as autologous human serum and transforming growth factor-β have been used in an attempt to promote hole closure.

Lattice degeneration of the retina is relatively common and reported to be present 10–15% of cases in autopsy series, but it is less apparent clinically. The degeneration is often bilateral and generally present in adolescence. It is seen between the equator and the ora serrata and consists of linear or oval circumferential lesions that may run to several millimetres in length. Histopathologically, the retina is thinned with loss of blood vessels. There is liquefaction of overlying vitreous with dense vitreous adhesions at the edges of the lesion. There may be secondary pigmentary change with RPE cell migration into the retina. The clinical importance of lattice degeneration is that

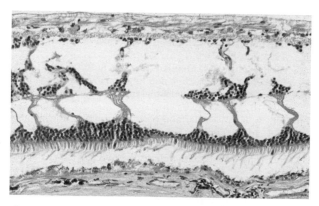

Figure 16.71 *Peripheral microcystoid degeneration. There are spaces throughout much of the thickness of the retina.*

it predisposes to retinal breaks and hence rhegmatogenous retinal detachment. There is a suggestion of a genetic component to lattice degeneration of the retina, but a much clearer pattern of inheritance is seen in two related conditions, Wagner's vitreoretinal degeneration and Stickler's syndrome, both of which show autosomal dominant inheritance. The latter is caused by mutations in type II procollagen and the syndrome includes skeletal abnormalities.

Paving-stone, or cobblestone, degeneration consists of pale retinal patches close to the ora serrata and is a common incidental finding (Fig. 16.70). The pathology consists of outer retinal thinning in the absence of overlying vitreous abnormality. There is atrophy of the choriocapillaris and a vascular pathogenesis seems most likely. Other retinal degenerations include typical peripheral cystoid degeneration where small, multiple and sometimes confluent cystic spaces are present in the outer plexiform layer of the retina immediately posterior to the ora serrata (Fig. 16.71). This condition is extremely common and adverse clinical sequelae are rare. Of more importance is reticular peripheral cystoid degeneration, which is usually seen in conjunction with typical peripheral cystoid degeneration. Here, the cystic spaces are within the nerve fibre layer and there is a risk of evolution to clinically significant retinoschisis.

REFERENCES

1 Abdelsalam A, Del Priore L, Zarbin MA. Drusen in age-related macular degeneration: pathogenesis, natural course, and laser photocoagulation-induced regression. *Surv Ophthalmol* 1999; **44**: 1–29.

2 Aiello LP, Avery RL, Arrigg PG *et al*. Vascular endothelial growth factor in ocular fluid of patients with diabetic retinopathy and other retinal disorders. *N Engl J Med* 1994; **331**: 1480–7.

3 Akpek EK, Ahmed I, Hochberg FH *et al*. Intraocular–central nervous system lymphoma: clinical features, diagnosis, and outcomes. *Ophthalmology* 1999; **106**: 1805–10.

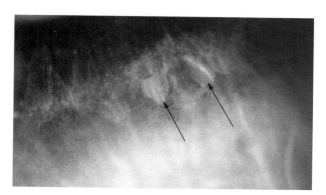

Figure 16.70 *Paving-stone degeneration. The degeneration (arrows) is just posterior to the ora serrata.*

4 Akpek EK, Maca SM, Christen WG, Foster CS. Elevated vitreous interleukin-10 level is not diagnostic of intraocular–central nervous system lymphoma. *Ophthalmology* 1999; **106**: 2291–5.

5 Ali RR, Sarra GM, Stephens C *et al*. Restoration of photoreceptor ultrastructure and function in retinal degeneration slow mice by gene therapy. *Nat Genet* 2000; **25**: 306–10.

6 Alm A, Bill A. Ocular and optic nerve blood flow at normal and increased intraocular pressures in monkeys (*Macaca irus*): a study with radiolabeled microspheres including flow determinations in brain and other tissues. *Exp Eye Res* 1973; **15**: 15–29.

7 al Maghtheh M, Gregory C, Inglehearn C *et al*. Rhodopsin mutations in autosomal dominant retinitis pigmentosa. *Hum Mutat* 1993; **2**: 249–55.

8 Anderson DH, Guerin CJ, Erickson PA *et al*. Morphological recovery in the reattached retina. *Invest Ophthalmol Vis Sci* 1986; **27**: 168–83.

9 Anderson DH, Stern WH, Fisher SK *et al*. Retinal detachment in the cat: the pigment epithelial–photoreceptor interface. *Invest Ophthalmol Vis Sci* 1983; **24**: 906–26.

10 Anon. Histopathologic characteristics of uveal melanomas in eyes enucleated from the Collaborative Ocular Melanoma Study. COMS report no. 6. *Am J Ophthalmol* 1998; **125**: 745–66.

11 Bagan SM, Hollenhurst RW. Radiation retinopath after irradiation of intracranial lesions. *Am J Ophthalmol* 1979; **88**: 694–7.

12 Barr CC. The histopathology of successful retinal reattachment. *Retina* 1990; **10**: 189–94.

13 Barrong SD, Chaitin MH, Fliesler SJ *et al*. Ultrastructure of connecting cilia in different forms of retinitis pigmentosa. *Arch Ophthalmol* 1992; **110**: 706–10.

14 Berglin L, Algvere PV, Seregard S. Photoreceptor decay over time and apoptosis in experimental retinal detachment. *Graefes Arch Clin Exp Ophthalmol* 1997; **235**: 306–12.

15 Bird AC. Retinal photoreceptor dystrophies. Edward Jackson Memorial Lecture. *Am J Ophthalmol* 1995; **119**: 543–62.

16 Birnbach CD, Jarvelainen M, Possin DE, Milam AH. Histopathology and immunocytochemistry of the neurosensory retina in fundus flavimaculatus. *Ophthalmology* 1994; **101**: 1211–19.

17 Boghen DR, Sebag M, Michaud J. Paraneoplastic optic neuritis and encephalomyelitis. *Arch Neurol* 1988; **45**: 353–6.

18 Boldrey EE, Egbert P, Gass JD, Friberg T. The histopathology of familial exudative vitreoretinopathy. A report of two cases. *Arch Ophthalmol* 1985; **103**: 238–41.

19 Brodovsky S, Hove MW ten, Pinkerton RM *et al*. An enhancing optic nerve lesion: malignant glioma of adulthood. *Can J Ophthalmol* 1997; **32**: 409–13.

20 Brooks DE, Garcia GA, Dreyer EB *et al*. Vitreous body glutamate concentration in dogs with glaucoma. *Am J Vet Res* 1997; **58**: 864–7.

21 Brown GC, Shields JA. Tumors of the optic nerve head. *Surv Ophthalmol* 1985; **29**: 239–64.

22 Brunk UT, Wihlmark U, Wrigstad A *et al*. Accumulation of lipofuscin within retinal pigment epithelial cells results in enhanced sensitivity to photo-oxidation. *Gerontology* 1995; **41** (Suppl 2): 201–12.

23 Buggage RR, Velez G, Myers PB *et al*. Primary intraocular lymphoma with a low interleukin 10 to interleukin 6 ratio and heterogeneous IgH gene rearrangement. *Arch Ophthalmol* 1999; **117**: 1239–42.

24 Burnstine MA, Levin LA, Louis DN *et al*. Nucleolar organizer regions in optic gliomas. *Brain* 1993; **116**: 1465–76.

25 Cahill M, Barnes C, Moriarty P *et al*. Ocular adnexal lymphoma – comparison of MALT lymphoma with other histological types. *Br J Ophthalmol* 1999; **83**: 742–47.

26 Capon MR, Marshall J, Krafft JI *et al*. Sorsby's fundus dystrophy. A light and electron microscopic study. *Ophthalmology* 1989; **96**: 1769–77.

27 Castro PA, Albert DM, Wang WJ, Ni C. Tumors metastatic to the eye and adnexa. *Int Ophthalmol Clin* 1982; **22**: 189–223.

28 Cavanagh JB, Harding BN. Pathogenic factors underlying the lesions in Leigh's disease. Tissue responses to cellular energy deprivation and their clinico-pathological consequences. *Brain* 1994; **117**: 1357–76.

29 Chang B, Bronson RT, Hawes NL *et al*. Retinal degeneration in motor neuron degeneration: a mouse model of ceroid lipofuscinosis. *Invest Ophthalmol Vis Sci* 1994; **35**: 1071–76.

30 Chang CJ, Lai WW, Edward DP, Tso MO. Apoptotic photoreceptor cell death after traumatic retinal detachment in humans. *Arch Ophthalmol* 1995; **113**: 880–6.

31 Chaturvedi N, Hedley-Whyte E, Dreyer E. Lateral geniculate nucleus in glaucoma. *Am J Ophthalmol* 1993; **116**: 182–8.

32 Chong NH, Alexander RA, Barnett KC *et al*. An immunohistochemical study of an autosomal dominant feline rod/cone dysplasia (Rdy cats). *Exp Eye Res* 1999; **68**: 51–7.

33 Chong NH, Alexander RA, Gin T *et al*. TIMP-3, collagen, and elastin immunohistochemistry and histopathology of Sorsby's fundus dystrophy. *Invest Ophthalmol Vis Sci* 2000; **41**: 898–902.

34 Chong NH, Alexander RA, Waters L *et al*. Repeated injections of a ciliary neurotrophic factor analogue leading to long-term photoreceptor survival in hereditary retinal degeneration. *Invest Ophthalmol Vis Sci* 1999; **40**: 1298–305.

35 Chong NVD, Downes SM, Freeman GM *et al*. *Medical retina CD-ROM*. London: BMA, 1999.

36 Cibis GW, Fylnn JT, Davis EB. Neonatal herpes simplex retinitis. *Graefes Arch Clin Exp Ophthalmol* 1975; **196**: 39–47.

37 Cibis GW, Whittaker CK, Wood WE. Intraocular extension of optic nerve meningioma in a case of neurofibromatosis. *Arch Ophthalmol* 1985; **103**: 404–6.

38 Cideciyan AV, Hood DC, Huang Y *et al*. Disease sequence from mutant rhodopsin allele to rod and cone photoreceptor degeneration in man. *Proc Natl Acad Sci USA* 1998; **95**: 7103–8.

39 Ciulla TA, Pesavento RD, Yoo S. Subretinal aspiration biopsy of ocular lymphoma. *Am J Ophthalmol* 1997; **123**: 420–2.

40 Cogan DG, Luthert PJ. Pathology of the optic nerve. In: Albert DM, Jakobiec FA eds. *Principles and practice of ophthalmology* 2nd edn. Philadelphia, PA: WB Saunders, 2000: 3874–85.

41 Cook B, Lewis GP, Fisher SK, Adler R. Apoptotic photoreceptor degeneration in experimental retinal detachment. *Invest Ophthalmol Vis Sci* 1995; **36**: 990–6.

42 Cooling RJ, Wright JE. Arachnoid hyperplasia in optic nerve glioma: confusion with orbital meningioma. *Br J Ophthalmol* 1979; **63**: 596–9.

43 Coupland SE, Foss HD, Anagnostopoulos I *et al*. Immunoglobulin VH gene expression among extranodal marginal zone B-cell lymphomas of the ocular adnexa. *Invest Ophthalmol Vis Sci* 1999; **40**: 555–62.

44 Coupland SE, Foss HD, Assaf C *et al*. T-cell and T/natural killer-cell lymphomas involving ocular and ocular adnexal tissues: a clinicopathologic, immunohistochemical, and molecular study of seven cases. *Ophthalmology* 1999; **106**: 2109–20.

45 Coupland SE, Krause L, Delecluse HJ et al. Lymphoprolif-erative lesions of the ocular adnexa. Analysis of 112 cases. Ophthalmology 1998; 105: 1430–41.

46 Croxatto JO, Rao NA, McLean IW, Marak GE. Atypical histopathologic features in sympathetic ophthalmia. A study of a hundred cases. Int Ophthalmol 1982; 4: 129–35.

47 Cunliffe IA, Moffat DA, Hardy DG, Moore AT. Bilateral optic nerve sheath meningiomas in a patient with neurofibro-matosis type 2. Br J Ophthalmol 1992; 76: 310–12.

48 Curcio CA, Millican CL. Basal linear deposit and large drusen are specific for early age-related maculopathy. Arch Oph-thalmol 1999; 117: 329–39.

49 Dandona L, Hendrickson A, Quigley HA. Selective effects of experimental glaucoma on axonal transport by retinal ganglion cells to the dorsal lateral geniculate nucleus. Invest Ophthalmol Vis Sci 1991; 32: 1593–9.

50 Davis JL, Viciana AL, Ruiz P. Diagnosis of intraocular lym-phoma by flow cytometry. Am J Ophthalmol 1997; 124: 362–72.

51 Dean JM, Novak MA, Chan CC, Green WR. Tumor detach-ments of the retinal pigment epithelium in ocular/central nervous system lymphoma. Retina 1996; 16: 47–56.

52 Della NG, Campochiaro PA, Zack DJ. Localization of TIMP-3 mRNA expression to the retinal pigment epithelium. Invest Ophthalmol Vis Sci 1996; 37: 1921–4.

53 Destro M, Gragoudas ES. Arterial occlusions. In: Albert DM, Jakobiec FA eds. Principles and practice of ophthalmology 2nd edn. Philadelphia, PA: WB Saunders, 2000: 1879–900.

54 Dieckert JP. Nonpenetrating posterior segment trauma. In: Albert DM, Jakobiec FA eds. Principles and practice of oph-thalmology 2nd edn. Philadelphia, PA: WB Saunders, 2000: 5227–40.

55 Dorey CK, Wu G, Ebenstein D et al. Cell loss in the aging retina. Relationship to lipofuscin accumulation and mac-ular degeneration. Invest Ophthalmol Vis Sci 1989; 30: 1691–9.

56 Draper GJ, Sanders BM, Kingston JE. Second primary neo-plasms in patients with retinoblastoma. Br J Cancer 1986; 53: 661–71.

57 Dreyer EB, Pan ZH, Storm S, Lipton SA. Greater sensitivity of larger retinal ganglion cells to NMDA-mediated cell death. NeuroReport 1994; 5: 629–31.

58 Dreyer EB, Zurakowski D, Schumer RA et al. Elevated glu-tamate levels in the vitreous body of humans and monkeys with glaucoma. Arch Ophthalmol 1996; 114: 299–305.

59 Duane TD. Valsalva hemorrhagic retinopathy. Trans Am Ophthalmol Soc 1972; 70: 298–313.

60 Duhaime AC, Christian CW, Rorke LB, Zimmerman RA. Non-accidental head injury in infants – the 'shaken-baby syn-drome'. N Engl J Med 1998; 338: 1822–9.

61 Duhaime AC, Gennarelli TA, Thibault LE et al. The shaken baby syndrome. A clinical, pathological, and biomechani-cal study. J Neurosurg 1987; 66: 409–15.

62 Dutton JJ. Gliomas of the anterior visual pathway. Surv Ophthalmol 1994; 38: 427–52.

63 Eagle RC Jr, Hedges TR, Yanoff M. The Kearns–Sayre syn-drome. A light and electron microscopic study. Trans Am Ophthalmol Soc 1982; 80: 218–34.

64 Eagle RC Jr, Lucier AC, Bernadino VB Jr et al. Retinal pig-ment epithelial abnormalities in fundus flavimaculatus: a light and electron microscope study. Ophthalmology 1980; 87: 1189–200.

65 Eagle RC Jr, Shields JA, Donoso L, Milner RS. Malignant transformation of spontaneously regressed retinoblastoma, retinoma/retinocytoma variant. Ophthalmology 1989; 96: 1389–95.

66 Ebert EM, Boger WPI, Albert DM. Phakomatoses. In: Albert D, Jakobiec F eds. Principles and practice of ophthalmology 2nd edn. Philadelphia, PA: WB Saunders, 2000; 5117–46.

67 Eggers H, Jakobiec FA, Jones IS. Tumors of the optic nerve. Doc Ophthalmol 1976; 41: 43–128.

68 el Azazi M, Samuelsson A, Linde A, Forsgren M. Intrathe-cal antibody production against viruses of the herpesvirus family in acute retinal necrosis syndrome. Am J Ophthal-mol 1991; 112: 76–82.

69 Eldred GE. Lipofuscin fluorophore inhibits lysosomal pro-tein degradation and may cause early stages of macular degeneration. Gerontology 1995; 41 (Suppl 2): 15–28.

70 Erickson PA, Feinstein SC, Lewis GP, Fisher SK. Glial fibril-lary acidic protein and its mRNA: ultrastructural detection and determination of changes after CNS injury. J Struct Biol 1992; 108: 148–61.

71 Eustis HS, Sanders MR, Zimmerman T. Morning glory syn-drome in children. Association with endocrine and central nervous system anomalies. Arch Ophthalmol 1994; 112: 204–7.

72 Evans K, Gregory CY, Wijesuriya SD et al. Assessment of the phenotypic range seen in Doyne honeycomb retinal dys-trophy. Arch Ophthalmol 1997; 115: 904–10.

73 Ezra E, Munro PM, Charteris DG et al. Macular hole oper-cula. Ultrastructural features and clinicopathological cor-relation. Arch Ophthalmol 1997; 115: 1381–7.

74 Faktorovich EG, Steinberg RH, Yasumura D et al. Photo-receptor degeneration in inherited retinal dystrophy delay-ed by basic fibroblast growth factor. Nature 1990; 347: 83–6.

75 Fariss RN, Apte SS, Luthert PJ et al. Accumulation of tissue inhibitor of metalloproteinases-3 in human eyes with Sorsby's fundus dystrophy or retinitis pigmentosa. Br J Ophthalmol 1998; 82: 1329–34.

76 Fariss RN, Apte SS, Olsen BR et al. Tissue inhibitor of met-alloproteinases-3 is a component of Bruch's membrane of the eye. Am J Pathol 1997; 150: 323–8.

77 Felbor U, Stohr H, Amann T et al. A second independent Tyr168Cys mutation in the tissue inhibitor of metallopro-teinases-3 (TIMP3) in Sorsby's fundus dystrophy. J Med Genet 1996; 33: 233–6.

78 Fillet AM, Reux I, Joberty C et al. Detection of human her-pes virus 6 in AIDS-associated retinitis by means of in situ hybridization, polymerase chain reaction and immunohis-tochemistry. J Med Virol 1996; 49: 289–95.

79 Fine BS, Bruckner AJ. Macular edema and cystoid macular edema. Am J Ophthalmol 1981; 92: 466–81.

80 Font RL, Jenis EH, Tuck KO. Measles maculopathy associat-ed with subacute sclerosing panencephalitis. Arch Pathol 1973; 96: 168–74.

81 Font RL, Marines HM, Cartwright J, Bauserman SC. Aicar-di syndrome. A clinicopathologic case report including elec-tron microscopic observations. Ophthalmology 1991; 98: 1727–31.

82 Foulds WS, Chisholm IA, Bronte SJ, Wilson TM. Vitamin B 12 absorption in tobacco amblyopia. Br J Ophthalmol 1969; 53: 393–7.

83 Frangieh GT, Green WR, Fine SL et al. A histopatholoic study of Best's vitelliform dystrophy. Arch Ophthalmol 1982; 100: 1115–21.

84 Freeman LN, Schachat AP, Knox DL. Clinical features, lab-oratory investigations, and survival in ocular reticulum cell sarcoma. Ophthalmology 1987; 94: 1631–9.

85 Freund C, Horsford DJ, McInnes RR. Transcription factor genes and the developing eye. Hum Mol Genet 1996; 5: 1471–88.

86 Friedlander M, Theesfeld CL, Sugita M et al. Involvement of integrins alpha v beta 3 and alpha v beta 5 in ocular neo-vascular diseases. Proc Natl Acad Sci USA 1996; 93: 9764–9.

87 Fulton AB, Albert DM, Craft JL. Human albinism: light and electron microscopy study. *Arch Ophthalmol* 1978; **96**: 305–10.

88 Gaillard ER, Atherton SJ, Eldred G, Dillon J. Photophysical studies on human retinal lipofuscin. *Photochem Photobiol* 1995; **61**: 448–53.

89 Garcia VE, Shareef S, Walsh J, Sharma SC. Programmed cell death of retinal ganglion cells during experimental glaucoma. *Exp Eye Res* 1995; **61**: 33–44.

90 Gass JD. Muller cell cone, an overlooked part of the anatomy of the fovea centralis: hypotheses concerning its role in the pathogenesis of macular hole and foveomacular retinoschisis. *Arch Ophthalmol* 1999; **117**: 821–3.

91 Gass JD. Reappraisal of biomicroscopic classification of stages of development of a macular hole. *Am J Ophthalmol* 1995; **119**: 752–9.

92 Gass JD, Gieser RG, Wilkinson CP et al. Bilateral diffuse uveal melanocytic proliferation in patients with occult carcinoma. *Arch Ophthalmol* 1990; **108**: 527–33.

93 Gass JDM, Anderson DR, Davis EB. A clinical, fluorescein angiographic, and electron microscopic correlation of cystoid macular edema. *Am J Ophthalmol* 1985; **100**: 82–6.

94 Gehrig A, White K, Lorenz B et al. Assessment of RS1 in X-linked juvenile retinoschisis and sporadic senile retinoschisis. *Clin Genet* 1999; **55**: 461–5.

95 Gilliland MG, Folberg R. Shaken babies – some have no impact injuries. *J Forensic Sci* 1996; **41**: 114–16.

96 Gleckman AM, Bell MD, Evans RJ, Smith TW. Diffuse axonal injury in infants with nonaccidental craniocerebral trauma: enhanced detection by beta-amyloid precursor protein immunohistochemical staining. *Arch Pathol Lab Med* 1999; **123**: 146–51.

97 Glovinsky Y, Quigley HA, Pease ME. Foveal ganglion cell loss is size dependent in experimental glaucoma. *Invest Ophthalmol Vis Sci* 1993; **34**: 395–400.

98 Gorin MB, Breitner JC, Jong PT de et al. The genetics of age-related macular degeneration. *Mol Vis* 1999 (Nov 3); **5**: 29.

99 Gray F, Louarn F, Gherardi R et al. Adult form of Leigh's disease: a clinicopathological case with CT scan examination. *J Neurol Neurosurg Psychiatry* 1984; **47**: 1211–15.

100 Green MA, Lieberman G, Milroy CM, Parsons MA. Ocular and cerebral trauma in non-accidental injury in infancy: underlying mechanisms and implications for paediatric practice. *Br J Ophthalmol* 1996; **80**: 282–7.

101 Green WR. Retina. In: Spencer WH ed. *Ophthalmic pathology: an atlas and textbook* 4th edn. Philadelphia, PA: WB Saunders, 1996: 667.

102 Green WR. Uveal tract. In: Spencer WH ed. *Ophthalmic pathology: An atlas and textbook* 4th edn. Philadelphia, PA: WB Saunders, 2000: 1439–2120.

103 Green WR, Chan CC, Hutchins GM, Terry JM. Central retinal vein occlusion: a prospective histopathologic study of 29 eyes in 28 cases. *Trans Am Ophthalmol Soc* 1981; **79**: 371–422.

104 Green WR, Enger C. Age-related macular degeneration histopathologic studies. The 1992 Lorenz E. Zimmerman Lecture. *Ophthalmology* 1993; **100**: 1519–35.

105 Gregory EK, Bhattacharya SS. Genetic blindness: current concepts in the pathogenesis of human outer retinal dystrophies. *Trends Genet* 1998; **14**: 103–8.

106 Gross RL, Hensley SH, Gao F, Wu SM. Retinal ganglion cell dysfunction induced by hypoxia and glutamate: potential neuroprotective effects of beta-blockers. *Surv Ophthalmol* 1999; **43** (Suppl 1): S162–70.

107 Grossniklaus HE, Thoma JW, Vigneswaran N et al. Retinal hemangioblastoma. A histologic, immunohistochemical, and ultrastructural evaluation. *Ophthalmology* 1992; **99**: 140–5.

108 Grunwald JE, Piltz J, Hariprasad SM, DuPont J. Optic nerve and choroidal circulation in glaucoma. *Invest Ophthalmol Vis Sci* 1998; **39**: 2329–36.

109 Guerin CJ, Anderson DH, Fariss RN, Fisher SK. Retinal reattachment of the primate macula. Photoreceptor recovery after short-term detachment. *Invest Ophthalmol Vis Sci* 1989; **30**: 1708–25.

110 Guex CY, Rochat C, Herbort CP. Necrotizing herpetic retinopathies. A spectrum of herpes virus-induced diseases determined by the immune state of the host. *Ocul Immunol Inflamm* 1997; **5**: 259–65.

111 Gunduz K, Gunalp I, Saatci I. Septo-optic dysplasia associated with bilateral complex microphthalmos. *Ophthalmic Genet* 1996; **17**: 109–13.

112 Gunduz K, Shields JA, Shields CL et al. Transscleral choroidal biopsy in the diagnosis of choroidal lymphoma. *Surv Ophthalmol* 1999; **43**: 551–5.

113 Guymer R, Luthert P, Bird A. Changes in Bruch's membrane and related structures with age. *Prog Retin Eye Res* 1999; **18**: 59–90.

114 Haefliger IO, Fleischhauer JC, Flammer J. In glaucoma, should enthusiasm about neuroprotection be tempered by the experience obtained in other neurodegenerative disorders? *Eye* 2000; **14**: 464–72.

115 Hageman GS, Mullens RF, Russell SR et al. Vitronectin is a constituent of ocular drusen and the vitronectin gene is expressed in human retinal pigmented epithelial cells. *FASEB J* 1999; **13**: 477–84.

116 Hamilton AM, Garner A, Tripathi RC, Sanders MD. Malignant optic nerve glioma: report of a case with electron microscope study. *Br J Ophthalmol* 1973; **57**: 253–64.

117 Hammes H, Brownlee M, Jonczyk A et al. Subcutaneous injection of a cyclic peptide antagonist of vitronectin receptor-type integrins inhibits retinal neovascularization. *Nat Med* 1996; **2**: 529–33.

118 Han DP, Wilkinson WS. Late ophthalmic manifestations of the shaken baby syndrome. *J Pediatr Ophthalmol Strabismus* 1990; **27**: 299–303.

119 Harris NL, Jaffe ES, Stein H et al. A revised European–American classification of lymphoid neoplasms: a proposal from the International Lymphoma Study Group. *Blood* 1994; **84**: 1361–92.

120 Hawkins BS, Bird A, Klein R, West SK. Epidemiology of age-related macular degeneration. *Mol Vis* 1999 (Nov 3); **5**: 26.

121 Hayes JM, Balkema GW. Visual thresholds in mice: comparison of retinal light damage and hypopigmentation. *Vis Neurosci* 1993; **10**: 931–8.

122 Hayreh SS, Podhajsky PA, Zimmerman B. Ocular manifestations of giant cell arteritis. *Am J Ophthalmol* 1998; **125**: 509–20.

123 Hayreh SS, Zimmerman MB, Podhajsky P, Alward WL. Nocturnal arterial hypotension and its role in optic nerve head and ocular ischemic disorders. *Am J Ophthalmol* 1994; **117**: 603–24.

124 Henkind P, Charles NC, Pearson J. Histopathology of ischemic optic neuropathy. *Am J Ophthalmol* 1970; **69**: 78–90.

125 Hingorani M, Mannor G, Vardy SJ et al. Prenatal diagnosis of orbital heterotopic brain tissue. *J Paediatr Surg* 1998; **32**: 1348–50.

126 Hiscott P, Gray R, Grierson I, Gregor Z. Cytokeratin-containing cells in proliferative diabetic retinopathy membranes. *Br J Ophthalmol* 1994; **78**: 219–22.

127 Hiscott P, Sheridan C, Magee RM, Grierson I. Matrix and the retinal pigment epithelium in proliferative retinal disease. *Prog Retin Eye Res* 1999; **18**: 167–90.

128 Holt IJ, Harding AE, Petty RKH, Morgan-Hughes JA. A new mitochondrial disease associated with mitochondrial DNA heteroplasmy. *Am J Hum Genet* 1990; **46**: 428–33.

129 Holz FG, Bellmann C, Margaritidis M *et al*. Patterns of increased *in vivo* fundus autofluorescence in the junctional zone of geographic atrophy of the retinal pigment epithelium associated with age-related macular degeneration. *Graefes Arch Clin Exp Ophthalmol* 1999; **237**: 145–52.

130 Holz FG, Schutt F, Kopitz J *et al*. Inhibition of lysosomal degradative functions in RPE cells by a retinoid component of lipofuscin. *Invest Ophthalmol Vis Sci* 1999; **40**: 737–43.

131 Holz FG, Sheraidah G, Pauleikhoff D, Bird AC. Analysis of lipid deposits extracted from human macular and peripheral Bruch's membrane. *Arch Ophthalmol* 1994; **112**: 402–6.

132 Hunter WS, Zimmermam LE. Unilateral retinal dysplasia. *Arch Ophthalmol* 1965; **74**: 23–30.

133 Imesch PD, Bindley CD, Wallow IH. Clinicopathologic correlation of intraretinal microvascular abnormalities. *Retina* 1997; **17**: 321–9.

134 Isashiki Y, Nakagawa M, Ohba N *et al*. Retinal manifestations in mitochondrial diseases associated with mitochondrial DNA mutation. *Acta Ophthalmol Scand* 1998; **76**: 6–13.

135 Jakobiec FA, Bilyk JR, Font RL. Orbit. In: Spencer WH ed. *Ophthalmic pathology: an atlas and textbook* 4th edn. Philadelphia, PA: WB Saunders, 1998: 2438–933.

136 Jeffery G. The albino retina: an abnormality that provides insight into normal retinal development. *Trends Neurosci* 1997; **20**: 165–9.

137 Jeffery G, Brem G, Montoliu L. Correction of retinal abnormalities found in albinism by introduction of a functional tyrosinase gene in transgenic mice and rabbits. *Brain Res Dev Brain Res* 1997; **99**: 95–102.

138 Johnston PB, Gaster RN, Smith VC *et al*. A clinicopathologic study of autosomal dominant optic atrophy. *Am J Ophthalmol* 1979; **88**: 868–75.

139 Jomary C, Neal MJ, Iwata K, Jones SE. Localization of tissue inhibitor of metalloproteinases-3 in neurodegenerative retinal disease. *Neuroreport* 1997; **8**: 2169–72.

140 Kamei M, Hollyfield JG. TIMP-3 in Bruch's membrane: changes during aging and in age-related macular degeneration. *Invest Ophthalmol Vis Sci* 1999; **40**: 2367–75.

141 Kaste SC, Pivnick EK. Bony orbital morphology in neurofibromatosis type 1 (NF1). *J Med Genet* 1998; **35**: 628–31.

142 Kerr DJ, Scheithauer BW, Miller GM *et al*. Hemangioblastoma of the optic nerve: case report. *Neurosurgery* 1995; **36**: 573–80.

143 Kerrison JB, Flynn T, Green WR. Retinal pathologic changes in multiple sclerosis. *Retina* 1994; **14**: 445–51.

144 Kjer P, Jensen OA, Klinken L. Histopathology of the eye: optic nerve and brain in a case of dominant optic atrophy. *Acta Ophthalmol Scand* 1983; **61**: 300–12.

145 Kliffen M, Mooy CM, Luider TM, Jong PT de. Analysis of carbohydrate structures in basal laminar deposit in aging human maculae. *Invest Ophthalmol Vis Sci* 1994; **35**: 2901–5.

146 Kliffen M, Schaft TL van der, Mooy CM, Jong PT de. Morphologic changes in age-related maculopathy. *Microsc Res Tech* 1997; **36**: 106–22.

147 Knudson AGJ. Mutation and cancer: a statistical study of retinoblastoma. *Proc Natl Acad Sci USA* 1971; **68**: 820–8.

148 Kubota T, Holbach LM, Naumann GO. Corpora amylacea in glaucomatous and non-glaucomatous optic nerve and retina. *Graefes Arch Clin Exp Ophthalmol* 1993; **231**: 7–11.

149 Langton KP, Barker MD, McKie N. Localization of the functional domains of human tissue inhibitor of metalloproteinases-3 and the effects of a Sorsby's fundus dystrophy mutation. *J Biol Chem* 1998; **273**: 16778–81.

150 LaVail MM, Unoki K, Yasumura D *et al*. Multiple growth factors, cytokines, and neurotrophins rescue photoreceptors from the damaging effects of constant light. *Proc Natl Acad Sci USA* 1992; **89**: 11249–53.

151 LaVail MW, Yasumura D, Matthes MT *et al*. Protection of mouse photoreceptors by survival factors in retinal degenerations. *Invest Ophthalmol Vis Sci* 1998; **39**: 592–602.

152 Lawrence JM, Sauve Y, Keegan DJ *et al*. Schwann cell grafting into the retina of the dystrophic RCS rat limits functional deterioration. *Invest Ophthalmol Vis Sci* 2000; **41**: 518–28.

153 Leopold IH. Zinc deficiency and visual impairment? *Am J Ophthalmol* 1978; **85**: 871–5.

154 Leventer DB, Merriam JC, Defendini R *et al*. Enterogenous cyst of the orbital apex and superior orbital fissure. *Ophthalmology* 1994; **101**: 1614–21.

155 Levin LA. Direct and indirect approaches to neuroprotective therapy of glaucomatous optic neuropathy. *Surv Ophthalmol* 1999; **43** (Suppl 1): S98–101.

156 Lewin AS, Drenser KA, Hauswirth WW *et al*. Ribozyme rescue of photoreceptor cells in a transgenic rat model of autosomal dominant retinitis pigmentosa. *Nat Med* 1998; **4**: 967–71.

157 Lewis G, Mervin K, Valter K *et al*. Limiting the proliferation and reactivity of retinal Muller cells during experimental retinal detachment: the value of oxygen supplementation. *Am J Ophthalmol* 1999; **128**: 165–72.

158 Lewis GP, Erickson PA, Anderson DH, Fisher SK. Opsin distribution and protein incorporation in photoreceptors after experimental retinal detachment. *Exp Eye Res* 1991; **53**: 629–40.

159 Lewis GP, Linberg KA, Fisher SK. Neurite outgrowth from bipolar and horizontal cells after experimental retinal detachment. *Invest Ophthalmol Vis Sci* 1998; **39**: 424–34.

160 Li ZY, Kljavin IJ, Milam AH. Rod photoreceptor neurite sprouting in retinitis pigmentosa. *J Neurosci* 1995; **15**: 5429–38.

161 Listernick R, Darling C, Greenwald M *et al*. Optic pathway tumors in children: the effect of neurofibromatosis type 1 on clinical manifestations and natural history. *J Pediatr* 1995; **127**: 718–22.

162 Liu X, Vansant G, Udovichenko IP *et al*. Myosin VIIa, the product of the Usher 1B syndrome gene, is concentrated in the connecting cilia of photoreceptor cells. *Cell Motil Cytoskeleton* 1997; **37**: 240–52.

163 Lubin JR, Ni C, Albert DM. Clinicopathological study of the Vogt–Koyanagi–Harada syndrome. *Int Ophthalmol Clin* 1982; **22**: 141–56.

164 Luthert PJ, Chong NH. Photoreceptor rescue. *Eye* 1998; **12**: 591–6.

165 McCartney ACE. Embryological development of the eye. In: Garner A, Klintworth GK eds. *Pathobiology of ocular disease: a dynamic approach*. New York: Marcel Dekker, 1994: 1255–84.

166 McCartney ACE. Optic nerve and orbit. In: Graham DI, Lantos PL eds. *Greenfield's neuropathology* 6th edn. London: Arnold, 1997: 973–1006.

167 McDonnell PJ, Moore GW, Miller NR *et al*. Temporal arteritis. A clinicopathologic study. *Ophthalmology* 1986; **93**: 518–30.

168 McKechnie NM, King M, Lee WR. Retinal pathology in the Kearns Sayre syndrome. *Br J Ophthalmol* 1985; **69**: 63–75.

169 McLean IW. Retina: retinoblastomas, retinocytomas, and pseudoretinoblastomas. In: Spencer WH ed. *Ophthalmic pathology: an atlas and textbook* 4th edn. Philadelphia, PA: WB Saunders, 1996: 1332–438.

170 Maguire G, Simko H, Weinreb RN, Ayoub G. Transport-mediated release of endogenous glutamate in the vertebrate retina. *Pflugers Arch* 1998; **436**: 481–4.

171 Mani H, Peyman GA, Leff SI. Intraocular meningothelial meningiomas. *Int Ophthalmol* 1988; **12**: 207–11.

172 Margo CE, Pavan PR, Gendelman D, Gragoudas E. Bilateral melanocytic uveal tumors associated with systemic non-ocular malignancy. Malignant melanomas or benign paraneoplastic syndrome? *Retina* 1987; **7**: 137–41.

173 Marx JL, Kapusta MA, Patel SS et al. Use of the ganciclovir implant in the treatment of recurrent cytomegalovirus retinitis. *Arch Ophthalmol* 1996; **114**: 815–20.

174 Mervin K, Valter K, Maslim J et al. Limiting photoreceptor death and deconstruction during experimental retinal detachment: the value of oxygen supplementation. *Am J Ophthalmol* 1999; **128**: 155–64.

175 Mieler WF. Overview of ocular trauma. In: Albert D, Jakobiec FA eds. *Principles and practice of ophthalmology* 2nd edn. Philadelphia, PA: WB Saunders, 2000: 5179.

176 Mietz H, Green WR, Wolff SM et al. Foveal hypoplasia in complete oculocutaneous albinism. A histopathologic study. *Retina* 1992; **12**: 254–60.

177 Milam AH, Li ZY, Cideciyan AV, Jacobson SG. Clinicopathologic effects of the Q64ter rhodopsin mutation in retinitis pigmentosa. *Invest Ophthalmol Vis Sci* 1996; **37**: 753–65.

178 Milam AH, Li ZY, Fariss RN. Histopathology of the human retina in retinitis pigmentosa. *Prog Retin Eye Res* 1998; **17**: 175–205.

179 Miller JW, Adamis AP, Shima DT et al. Vascular endothelial growth factor/vascular permeability factor is temporally and spatially correlated with ocular angiogenesis in a primate model. *Am J Pathol* 1994; **145**: 574–84.

180 Mohand SS, Deudon CA, Hicks D et al. Normal retina releases a diffusible factor stimulating cone survival in the retinal degeneration mouse. *Proc Natl Acad Sci USA* 1998; **95**: 8357–62.

181 Mohand SS, Hicks D, Simonutti M et al. Photoreceptor transplants increase host cone survival in the retinal degeneration (rd) mouse. *Ophthalmic Res* 1997; **29**: 290–7.

182 Moore DJ, Hussain AA, Marshall J. Age-related variation in the hydraulic conductivity of Bruch's membrane. *Invest Ophthalmol Vis Sci* 1995; **36**: 1290–7.

183 Morgan JE. Selective cell death in glaucoma: does it really occur? *Br J Ophthalmol* 1997; **94**: 875–80.

184 Muller A, Villain M, Favreau B et al. Differential effect of ischemia/reperfusion on pigmented and albino rabbit retina. *J Ocul Pharmacol Ther* 1996; **12**: 337–42.

185 Mullins RF, Russell SR, Anderson GH, Hageman GS. Drusen associated with aging and age-related macular degeneration contain proteins common to extracellular deposits associated with athersclerosis, elastosis, amyloidosis and dense deposit disease. *FASEB J* 2000; **14**: 835–46.

186 Naash MI, Ripps H, Li S et al. Polygenic disease and retinitis pigmentosa: albinism exacerbates photoreceptor degeneration induced by the expression of a mutant opsin in transgenic mice. *J Neurosci* 1996; **16**: 7853–8.

187 Naeser P. Optic nerve involvement in a case of methanol poisoning. *Br J Ophthalmol* 1988; **72**: 778–81.

188 Nakata M, Matsuno Y, Katsumata N et al. Histology according to the Revised European–American Lymphoma Classification significantly predicts the prognosis of ocular adnexal lymphoma. *Leuk Lymphoma* 1999; **32**: 533–43.

189 Neufeld AH, Hernandez MR, Gonzalez M. Nitric oxide synthase in the human glaucomatous optic nerve head. *Arch Ophthalmol* 1997; **115**: 497–503.

190 Neufeld AH, Hernandez MR, Gonzalez M, Geller A. Cyclooxygenase-1 and cyclooxygenase-2 in the human optic nerve head. *Exp Eye Res* 1997; **65**: 739–45.

191 Neufeld AH, Sawada A, Becker B. Inhibition of nitric-oxide synthase 2 by aminoguanidine provides neuroprotection of retinal ganglion cells in a rat model of chronic glaucoma. *Proc Natl Acad Sci USA* 1999; **96**: 9944–8.

192 Newton C, Dutton JJ, Klintworth GK. A respiratory epithelial choristomatous cyst of the orbit. *Ophthalmology* 1985; **92**: 1754–7.

193 Nickells RW. Apoptosis of retinal ganglion cells in glaucoma: an update of the molecular pathways involved in cell death. *Surv Ophthalmol* 1999; **43** (Suppl 1): S151–61.

194 Nork TM, Millecchia LL, Strickland BD et al. Selective loss of blue cones and rods in human retinal detachment. *Arch Ophthalmol* 1995; **113**: 1066–73.

195 O'Gorman S, Flaherty WA, Fishman GA et al. Histopathological findings in Best's vitelliform macular dystrophy. *Arch Ophthalmol* 1988; **106**: 1261–8.

196 Ohh M, Kaelin WGJ. The von Hippel–Lindau tumour suppressor protein: new perspectives. *Mol Med Today* 1999; **5**: 257–63.

197 Okubo A, Rosa RHJ, Bunce CV et al. The relationships of age changes in retinal pigment epithelium and Bruch's membrane. *Invest Ophthalmol Vis Sci* 1999; **40**: 443–9.

198 Olsson JE, Gordon JW, Pawlyk BS et al. Transgenic mice with a rhodopsin mutation (Pro23His): a mouse model of autosomal dominant retinitis pigmentosa. *Neuron* 1992; **9**: 815–30.

199 O'Rahilly R. The prenatal development of the human eye. *Exp Eye Res* 1975; **21**: 93–112.

200 Panda S, Jonas JB. Decreased photoreceptor count in human eyes with secondary angle-closure glaucoma. *Invest Ophthalmol Vis Sci* 1992; **33**: 2532–6.

201 Parsons MA, Sahel JA. Pathology of the uveal tract. In: Albert DM, Jakobiec FA eds. *Principles and practice of ophthalmology* 2th edn. Philadelphia, PA: WB Saunders, 3634–84.

202 Parsons MA, Start RD. Necropsy techniques in ophthalmic pathology. *J Clin Pathol* in press.

203 Pena JD, Varela HJ, Ricard CS, Hernandez MR. Enhanced tenascin expression associated with reactive astrocytes in human optic nerve heads with primary open angle glaucoma. *Exp Eye Res* 1999; **68**: 29–40.

204 Petersen-Jones SM. A review of research to elucidate the causes of the generalized progressive retinal atrophies. *Vet J* 1998; **155**: 5–18.

205 Petrukhin K, Koisti MJ, Bakall B et al. Identification of the gene responsible for Best macular dystrophy. *Nat Genet* 1998; **19**: 241–7.

206 Peyman GA, Fishman GA, Sanders DR, Vichek J. Histopathology of Goldmann–Favre syndrome obtained by a full-thickness eye-wall biopsy. *Ann Ophthalmol* 1977; **9**: 479–84.

207 Phelan JK, Bok D. A brief review of retinitis pigmentosa and the identified retinitis pigmentosa genes. *Mol Vis* 2000; **6**: 116–24.

208 Portera CC, Sung CH, Nathans J, Adler R. Apoptotic photoreceptor cell death in mouse models of retinitis pigmentosa. *Proc Natl Acad Sci USA* 1994; **91**: 974–8.

209 Provis JM, Diaz CM, Penfold PL. Microglia in human retina: a heterogeneous population with distinct ontogenies. *Perspect Dev Neurobiol* 1996; **3**: 213–22.

210 Quigley HA, Nickells RW, Kerrigan LA et al. Retinal ganglion cell death in experimental glaucoma and after axotomy occurs by apoptosis. *Invest Ophthalmol Vis Sci* 1995; **36**: 774–86.

211 Ramrattan RS, Schaft TL van der, Mooy CM et al. Morphometric analysis of Bruch's membrane, the choriocapillaris, and the choroid in aging. *Invest Ophthalmol Vis Sci* 1994; **35**: 2857–64.

212 Ramsey MS, Fine BS. Chloroquine toxicity in the human eye: histopathologic observations by electron microscopy. *Am J Ophthalmol* 1972; **73**: 229–35.

213 Rao NA. Mechanisms of inflammatory response in sympathetic ophthalmia and VKH syndrome. *Eye* 1997; **11**: 213–16.

214 Rao NA, Spencer WH. Optic nerve. In: Spencer WH ed. *Ophthalmic pathology: an atlas and textbook* 4th edn. Philadelphia, PA: WB Saunders, 1998: 513–622.

215 Reid SN, Akhmedov NB, Piriev NI *et al*. The mouse X-linked juvenile retinoschisis cDNA: expression in photoreceptors. *Gene* 1999; **227**: 257–66.

216 Robinson GS, Aiello LP. Angiogenic factors in diabetic ocular disease: mechanisms of today, therapies for tomorrow. *Int Ophthalmol Clin* 1998; **38**: 89–102.

217 Ros MA, Magargal LE, Uram M. Branch retinal artery occlusion: a review of 201 eyes. *Ann Ophthalmol* 1989; **3**: 103–7.

218 Ruckmann A von, Fitzke FW, Bird AC. Fundus autofluorescence in age-related macular disease imaged with a laser scanning ophthalmoscope. *Invest Ophthalmol Vis Sci* 1997; **38**: 478–86.

219 Rummelt V, Folberg R, Ionasescu V *et al*. Ocular pathology of MELAS syndrome with mitochondrial DNA nucleotide 3243 point mutation. *Ophthalmology* 1993; **100**: 1757–66.

220 Sadun AA, Smythe BA, Scaechter JD. Optic neuritis or ophthalmic artery aneurysm? Case presentation with histopathologic documentation utilizing a new staining method. *J Clin Neuroophthalmol* 1984; **4**: 265–73.

221 Sanders MD. The Bowman Lecture. Papilloedema: 'the pendulum of progress'. *Eye* 1997; **11**: 267–94.

222 Santos A, Humayun MS, Juan E de *et al*. Preservation of the inner retina in retinitis pigmentosa. A morphometric analysis. *Arch Ophthalmol* 1997; **115**: 511–15.

223 Sanyanusin P, Schimmenti LA, McNoe LA *et al*. Mutation of the PAX2 gene in a family with optic nerve colobomas, renal anomalies and vesicoureteral reflux. *Nat Genet* 1995; **9**: 358–64.

224 Sheikh BY, Siqueira E, Dayel F. Meningioma in children: a report of nine cases and a review of the literature. *Surg Neurol* 1996; **45**: 328–35.

225 Shorstein NH, Dawson WW, Sherwood MB. Mid-peripheral pattern electrical retinal responses in normals, glaucoma suspects, and glaucoma patients. *Br J Ophthalmol* 1999; **83**: 15–23.

226 Sipperley JO, Quigley HA, Gass DM. Traumatic retinopathy in primates. The explanation of commotio retinae. *Arch Ophthalmol* 1978; **96**: 2267–73.

227 Sloper JJ. Edridge–Green Lecture: Competition and cooperation in visual development. *Eye* 1993; **7**: 319–31.

228 Spencer WH. Glaucoma. In: Spencer WH ed. *Ophthalmic pathology: an atlas and textbook* 2nd edn. Philadelphia, PA: WB Saunders, 1996: 438–512.

229 Spraul CW, Grossniklaus HE. Characteristics of Drusen and Bruch's membrane in postmortem eyes with age-related macular degeneration. *Arch Ophthalmol* 1997; **115**: 267–73.

230 Stafford SL, Perry A, Suman VJ *et al*. Primarily resected meningiomas: outcome and prognostic factors in 581 Mayo Clinic patients, 1978 through 1988. *Mayo Clin Proc* 1998; **73**: 936–42.

231 Stone EM, Lotery AJ, Munier FL *et al*. A single EFEMP1 mutation associated with both Malattia Leventinese and Doyne honeycomb retinal dystrophy. *Nat Genet* 1999; **22**: 199–202.

232 Stone J. The origins of the cells of the vertebrate retina. *Prog Retin Eye Res* 2000; **7**: 1–19.

233 Stone JL, Barlow WE, Humayun MS *et al*. Morphometric analysis of macular photoreceptors and ganglion cells in retinas with retinitis pigmentosa. *Arch Ophthalmol* 1992; **110**: 1634–9.

234 Straatsma BR, Foos RY, Heckenlively J *et al*. Myelinated retinal nerve fibers. *Am J Ophthalmol* 1981; **91**: 25–38.

235 Sucher NJ, Lipton SA, Dreyer EB. Molecular basis of glutamate toxicity in retinal ganglion cells. *Vision Res* 1997; **37**: 3483–93.

236 Sundelin S, Wihlmark U, Nilsson SE, Brunk UT. Lipofuscin accumulation in cultured retinal pigment epithelial cells reduces their phagocytic capacity. *Curr Eye Res* 1998; **17**: 851–7.

237 Sung CH, Makino C, Baylor D, Nathans J. A rhodopsin gene mutation responsible for autosomal dominant retinitis pigmentosa results in a protein that is defective in localization to the photoreceptor outer segment. *J Neurosci* 1994; **14**: 5818–33.

238 Swain PK, Chen S, Wang QL *et al*. Mutations in the cone–rod homeobox gene are associated with the cone–rod dystrophy photoreceptor degeneration. *Neuron* 1997; **19**: 1329–36.

239 Szamier RB. Ultrastructure of the preretinal membrane in retinitis pigmentosa. *Invest Ophthalmol Vis Sci* 1981; **21**: 227–36.

240 Taylor D. Child abuse and the eye. The ophthalmology child abuse working party. *Eye* 1999; **23**: 3–10.

241 Thirkill CE, Keltner JL, Tyler NK, Roth AM. Antibody reactions with retina and cancer-associated antigens in 10 patients with cancer-associated retinopathy. *Arch Ophthalmol* 1993; **111**: 931–7.

242 Ts'o MO, Zimmerman LE, Fine BS. The nature of retinoblastoma. I. Photoreceptor differentiation: a clinical and histopathologic study. *Am J Ophthalmol* 1970; **69**: 339–49.

243 Ulrich J, Groebke-Lorenz W. The optic nerve in multiple sclerosis. A morphological study with retrospective clinico-pathological correlations. *Neuro-ophthalmology* 1983; **3**: 149–59.

244 Van Heyningen V. Developmental eye disease – a genome era paradigm. *Clin Genet* 1998; **54**: 272–82.

245 Villegas-Perez MP, Vidal SM, Lund RD. Mechanism of retinal ganglion cell loss in inherited retinal dystrophy. *NeuroReport* 1996; **7**: 1995–9.

246 Vinores SA, Kuchle M, Derevjanik NL *et al*. Blood–retinal barrier breakdown in retinitis pigmentosa: light and electron microscopic immunolocalization. *Histol Histopathol* 1995; **10**: 913–23.

247 Wallace DC, Zheng X, Lott JM. Familial mitchondrial encephalomyopathy (MERRF): genetic, pathophysiological, and biochemical characterization of a mitochondrial DNA disease. *Cell* 1988; **55**: 601–10.

248 Wang T, Milam AH, Steel G, Valle D. A mouse model of gyrate atrophy of the choroid and retina. Early retinal pigment epithelium damage and progressive retinal degeneration. *J Clin Invest* 1996; **97**: 2753–62.

249 Wassell J, Davies S, Bardsley W, Boulton M. The photoreactivity of the retinal age pigment lipofuscin. *J Biol Chem* 1999; **274**: 23828–32.

250 Weber AJ, Kaufman PL, Hubbard WC. Morphology of single ganglion cells in the glaucomatous primate retina. *Invest Ophthalmol Vis Sci* 1998; **39**: 2304–20.

251 Weingeist TA, Kobrin JL, Watzke RC. Histopathology of Best's macular dystrophy. *Arch Ophthalmol* 1982; **100**: 1108–14.

252 Weinstein JM, Kelman SE, Bresnick GH, Kornguth SE. Paraneoplastic retinopathy associated with antiretinal bipolar cell antibodies in cutaneous malignant melanoma. *Ophthalmology* 1994; **101**: 1236–43.

253 Weissgold DJ, Budenz DL, Hood I, Rorke LB. Ruptured vascular malformation masquerading as battered/shaken baby syndrome: a nearly tragic mistake. *Surv Ophthalmol* 1995; **39**: 509–12.

254 Welch RB. Von Hippel–Lindau disease: the recognition and treatment of early angiomatous retinae and the use of cryosurgery as an adjunct to therapy. *Trans Am Ophthalmol Soc* 1970; **68**: 367–424.

255 Wells J, Wroblewski J, Keen J *et al*. Mutations in the human retinal degeneration slow (RDS) gene can cause either retinitis pigmentosa or macular dystrophy. *Nat Genet* 1993; **3**: 213–18.

256 Whitcup SM, Vistica BP, Milam AH *et al*. Recoverin-associated retinopathy: a clinically and immunologically distinctive disease. *Am J Ophthalmol* 1998; **126**: 230–7.

257 White VA, Gascoyne RD, Paton KE. Use of the polymerase chain reaction to detect B- and T-cell gene rearrangements in vitreous specimens from patients with intraocular lymphoma. *Arch Ophthalmol* 1999; **117**: 761–5.

258 White VA, Rootman J. Orbital pathology. In: Albert DM, Jakobiec FA eds. *Principles and practice of ophthalmology* 2nd edn. Philadelphia, PA: WB Saunders, 2000: 3816–74.

259 Wilkinson WS, Han DP, Rappley MD, Owings CL. Retinal hemorrhage predicts neurologic injury in the shaken baby syndrome. *Arch Ophthalmol* 1989; **107**: 1472–4.

260 Wilson DJ, Weleber RG, Green WR. Ocular clinicopathologic study of gyrate atrophy. *Am J Ophthalmol* 1991; **111**: 24–33.

261 Winkler BS, Dang L, Malinoski C, Easter SSJ. An assessment of rat photoreceptor sensitivity to mitochondrial blockade. *Invest Ophthalmol Vis Sci* 1997; **38**: 1569–77.

262 Wolter JR. Ectopic meningioma of the superior orbital rim. *Arch Ophthalmol* 1976; **94**: 1920–1922.

263 Wright JE, McNab AA, McDonald WI. Primary optic nerve sheath meningioma. *Br J Ophthalmol* 1989; **73**: 960–6.

264 Yi X, Mai LC, Uyama M, Yew DT. Time-course expression of vascular endothelial growth factor as related to the development of the retinochoroidal vasculature in rats. *Exp Brain Res* 1998; **118**: 155–60.

265 Yokota T, Shiojiri T, Gotoda T *et al*. Friedreich-like ataxia with retinitis pigmentosa caused by the His101Gln mutation of the alpha-tocopherol transfer protein gene. *Ann Neurol* 1997; **41**: 826–32.

266 Zack DJ, Dean M, Molday RS *et al*. What can we learn about age-related macular degeneration from other retinal diseases? *Mol Vis* 1999 (Nov 3); **5**: 30.

267 Zhang Y, Stone J. Role of astrocytes in the control of developing retinal vessels. *Invest Ophthalmol Vis Sci* 1997; **38**: 1653–66.

17

Hypothalamus and pituitary

EVA HORVATH, BERND W. SCHEITHAUER, KALMAN KOVACS AND RICARDO V. LLOYD

INTRODUCTION

In a remarkably integrated manner, the hypothalamus and the pituitary gland secrete a number of hormones, the role of which is the regulation of endocrine and metabolic functions as well as the maintenance of homoeostasis. Whereas distinctly hypothalamic lesions are uncommon, abnormalities of the pituitary are not rare. Some represent incidental autopsy findings whilst others cause characteristic syndromes, some mild, others severe or even life threatening. Given its close anatomical and functional relationship to the hypothalamus, diseases of the pituitary gland have traditionally fallen under the purview of neuropathology.

With advances in ultrastructural, immunochemical and molecular biological methods, unprecedented progress has been made. Of particular importance have been the ultrastructural identification of the various adenohypophyseal cell types, the characterization of pituitary as well as hypothalamic releasing hormones, and the development of specific antisera to these substances. These have simplified the diagnosis and classification of hypothalamic and of pituitary diseases, and provided insight into their pathogenesis, thus developing logical approaches to therapy. Despite impressive progress, numerous issues remain unresolved to pose major challenges to basic scientists, endocrinologists, neurosurgeons and pathologists alike.

In view of the complex anatomical and physiological relationships that exist between the hypothalamus and the pituitary, as well as the wide variety of lesions that affect these structures (Table 17.1), the concise treatment of this subject represents a challenge. The task is complicated by the need to correlate pathobiology with the intricate structure and function relationships that characterize this region. Considering the constraints of space, this chapter will focus upon common lesions that lend themselves to clinicopathological correlation, particularly with regard to hypothalamic lesions.

MORPHOLOGY AND HORMONES OF THE NORMAL HYPOTHALAMUS AND PITUITARY

Embryology

The hypothalamus originates near to the anterior neuropore. The embryological basis of its structural and functional relationships is poorly understood, but some events in its development have been identified. The constituents of the hypothalamus are derived from primordial cells of the ventricular zone. Essential landmarks, including its nuclei, are discernible during the third month of gestation. Among the first structures to appear is the mamillary complex (32 days). The development of its nuclei parallels the development of fibre tracts, including the mamillotegmental and mamillothalamic tracts, as well as the median forebrain bundle. The rostral hypothalamus develops during the third month, well after the mamillary complex. Its nuclei become apparent as protuberances beneath the ventricular surface. The supraoptic, paraventricular and ventromedial nuclei are formed during the ninth and tenth weeks. Hypothalamic development continues beyond birth, as evidenced by increasing size of nuclei, neuronal processes and myelination of fibre tracts. The degree to which postnatal events influence hypothalamic development and 'chemical differentiation' remains to be determined.[298,385]

The human pituitary can be divided into two parts. The first to develop is the adenohypophysis, which arises from

Table 17.1 *Functional disorders and lesions of the hypothalamus and the sellar region*

Hyperfunctional	Hypofunctional
Medical diseases	
Precocious puberty	Hypothalamic dwarfism
McCune–Albright syndrome	Diencephalic syndrome
Cushing's disease due to corticotrophic hyperplasia	Kallmann's syndrome
	Diabetes insipidus
Ectopic hypothalamic hormone production	Wolfram's (DIDMOAD) syndrome
Tumoral	
Gangliocytomas (see below)	
Syndromes of inappropriate antidiuretic hormone	
secretion (SIADH)	
Idiopathic	
Laurence–Moon syndrome	
Sotos' syndrome (cerebral gigantism)	
Prader–Willi syndrome	
Anorexia nervosa	
Idiopathic hypothalamic-releasing hormone deficiency	
Hyperprolactinaemia due to hypothalamic dopamine depletion (hypothyroidism,	
bromocryptine-treated parkinsonism, endurance athletes)	
Malformations and hamartomas	**Cysts and cystic neoplasms**
Anencephaly	Epidermoid cyst
Pituitary dystopia	Dermoid cyst
Ectopic anterior pituitary	Colloid cyst of the third ventricle
Septo-optic dysplasia	Rathke's cleft cyst
'Gangliocytomas'	Craniopharyngioma
Hypothalamic neuronal hamartoma	
Hypothalamic hamartoblastoma	
Adenohypophyseal neuronal choristoma	
Neoplasms	
Benign	*Malignant*
Granular cell tumour	Germ cell tumours
Pituitary adenoma	Chordoma
Meningioma	Gliomas
Glioma	Metastatic neoplasms
Pilocytic astrocytoma	Pituitary carcinoma
Ganglioglioma	Lymphoma, primary
Lipoma	Lymphoma, secondary
Neurilemmoma	Plasmacytoma
Haemangioblastoma	Leukaemia
Myxoma	Rhabdomyosarcoma
Paraganglioma	Haemangiopericytoma
Glomangioma	Postirradiation neoplasms
	Glioma
	Sarcoma
	Meningioma
Inflammatory disorders	**Infectious diseases**
Lymphocytic hypophysitis	Viral
Sarcoidosis	Bacterial
Giant cell granuloma	Whipple's disease
Histiocytosis X	Tuberculosis
	Syphilis
	Fungal abscess
	Toxoplasmosis
	Hydatid disease
	Cysticercosis

(Continued.)

Table 17.1 *(Continued)*

Hyperfunctional	Hypofunctional
Metabolic diseases Wernicke's encephalopathy Haemochromatosis (hypogonadism)	
	Degenerative diseases Alzheimer's disease Parkinson's disease Huntington's disease Infantile neuroaxonal dystrophy Familial dysautonomia (Riley–Day syndrome) Hypothalamic atrophy

Vascular lesions
Aneurysm
Pituitary infarction/haemorrhage
  Sheehan's syndrome
  'Respirator brain'
  Arteritis
  Subarachnoid haemorrhage
  Haematological disorders
  Petechial haemorrhage
Hypertension
	Physical injury
	Pituitary, stalk section
	Trauma
	Radiation injury
	Hydrocephalus

Table 17.2 *Autonomic functions of the hypothalamus: localization and pathology*

Function		Localization	Comments
Eating	Hunger[a] Satiety[a] or cessation of eating	Lateral hypothalamus, lateral to ventral medial nucleus, region of lower fornix Ventromedial nucleus	Lesions of the hypothalamus in general often result in hyperphagia and resultant obesity, e.g. Frölich's syndrome in children wherein obesity is associated with hypogenitalism. Selective lesions of the ventral medial nucleus have been reported to produce hyperphagia in humans, whereas lesions of the lateral hypothalamus have been reported to produce cachexia
Drinking	Thirst[a] Satiety (cessation of drinking)	Dorsomedial nucleus ?Supraoptic and paraventricular nuclei	Thirst after destruction of the supraoptic and paraventricular nuclei may be due to urinary water loss rather than the destruction of a putative 'thirst centre.'
Temperature	Heat conservation[a] (shivering, vasoconstriction) Heat loss[a] (pyrexia, sweating)	Dorsolateral or posterior hypothalamus Preoptic and anterior hypothalamic area Lower fornix (stimulation produces rage)	Third ventricular lesions in general have been associated with thermoregulatory defects, but few are sufficiently localized to permit anatomic–physiological correlation
Emotions	Rage Passivity	Ventromedial nucleus, dorsolateral region (destruction produces rage) Lateral hypothalamus (destruction produces passivity)	

[a]Destruction of these areas results in an opposite effect.

Rathke's pouch, an evagination of stomodeal ectoderm that makes its appearance at 26 days. It comes into contact with the diencephalon at 32 days. Thereafter, the neurohypophysis develops as a downward extension of the brain, the neurohypophyseal evagination (33 days). Their fusion results in the formation of the pituitary gland. Although the suggestion that the adenohypophysis is of neuroectodermal origin finds support in the quail-chick chimera model, there is no conclusive evidence for such an occurrence in mammalian embryos.[85,86]

Regional anatomy

HYPOTHALAMUS

Although the general anatomy of the hypothalamic–sellar region is well known (Fig. 17.1), our knowledge is mainly derived from animal studies. Owing to considerable species variation in both anatomy and physiology, investigative methods such as stimulation and ablation experiments were of limited value when their results were extrapolated to man. Being based in large part upon experimental studies and upon limited knowledge of the effects of localized lesions occurring in man, diagrammatic representations of nuclear groups (Fig. 17.2) are therefore crude. Sophisticated neurophysiological methods, the isolation and characterization of hypothalamic hormones, and the development of immunocytochemistry and *in situ* hybridization methods promise more precise correlations. The hypothalamus has an endocrine function in its association with the pituitary, and is also part of a complex neurohormonal circuit which interacts with other portions of the brain, including the cerebrum, diencephalic structures, the brainstem and even the spinal cord. Its functional repertoire is broad, including not only endocrine, but also autonomic and neuropsychiatric effects.

The anatomical limits of the hypothalamus are defined by its relation to surrounding structures (Figs 17.1, 17.2). A line through the anterior commissure, lamina terminalis and anterior optic chiasm define its anterior border, whereas the posterosuperior and posteroinferior boundaries are delimited by the midbrain tegmentum and the posterior aspect of the mamillary bodies, respectively. The lateral limits of the hypothalamus are demarcated by the substantia innominata, internal capsule, subthalamic nucleus and cerebral peduncle. The superior and inferior borders are the hypothalamic sulcus and the floor of the third ventricle, respectively. The tuber cinereum, the central portion of the third ventricular floor in continuity with the pituitary gland, consists of the infundibulum, the funnel-shaped upper portion of the neural stalk and the median eminence.

Whereas topographically discrete, somewhat functionally distinct cell clusters or 'nuclei' are present in lower species and in the developing human, they are far less

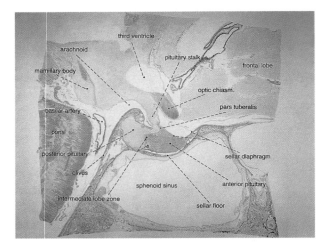

Figure 17.1 *Anatomy of the hypothalamic sellar region.*

evident in adults (Fig. 17.3). The delineation of structure–function relationships is further complicated by the fact that a given hormone is often produced in more than one nucleus, and that in some instances a single nucleus produces more than one hormone, e.g. the paraventricular nucleus. Such observations bring into question the functional significance of designating various nuclei as distinct entities. Relatively few hypothalamic nuclei or regions are truly individualized given their discrete nature or the physiological responses associated with their stimulation or ablation (Table 17.2).

At the level of the posterior chiasm, two magnocellular nuclei, the paraventricular and supraoptic nuclei, are encountered. Their fibres traverse the pituitary stalk to terminate in the posterior or neural lobe. Their anatomy and physiology are further discussed below. Among the principal nuclei of the tuberal region are the dorsomedial and ventromedial nuclei, which are visualized in sections through the mid- and posterior portions of the tuber cinereum. Whereas stimulation of the dorsomedial nuclei and destruction of the ventromedial nuclei produce rage in experimental animals, the ventromedial nuclei are thought to mediate the balance between hunger and satiety. These nuclei establish connections with both the orbital portion of the frontal lobe and the amygdaloid complex. Also in the tuberal region are the periventricular and arcuate nuclei (Fig. 17.4). Both are important components of the hypophysiotropic area which, by way of neural secretion, modulates anterior pituitary function. Also of interest is the subventricular nucleus, which lies within the floor of the third ventricle posterior to the arcuate nucleus. Its parvicellular neurons undergo hypertrophy in late pregnancy, the postmenopausal state, posthypophysectomy and in starvation.[129,380] The posterior hypothalamic nucleus lies within the mamillary region, being situated between the third ventricle and the mamillothalamic tract as well as superior to the mamillary bodies. It produces sympathetic effects when stimulated and is thought to play a role in temperature regulation. Situated within the preoptic region is a sexually dimorphic cell group, the suprachiasmatic nucleus, which lies dorsal to the optic chiasm and anterior to the supraoptic nucleus. Although its physiological function has not been fully characterized, this nucleus decreases in volume with age and is located in an area essential for gonadotropin release and for the control of sexual behaviour in lower animals.[404] Ontogenetically, the brain is female in nature and remains so if not exposed to male gonadal hormones at a certain stage in development. The suprachiasmatic nucleus may well be the neural substrate of this differentiation.[118]

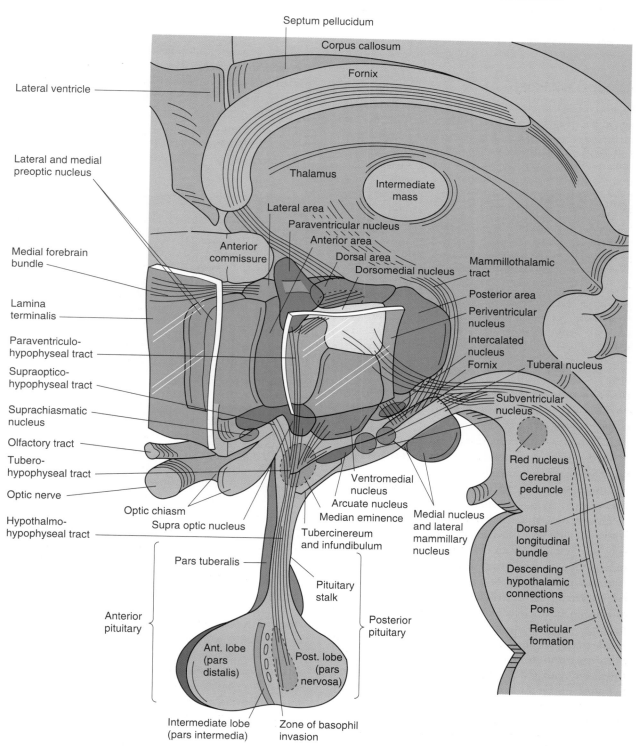

Figure 17.2 *Anatomy of the hypothalamic region and the pituitary (schematic representation).*

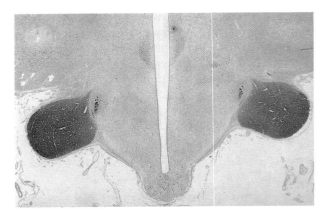

Figure 17.3 *Hypothalamus. Coronal section showing the location of the supraoptic nuclei above the optic tracts, the paraventricular nuclei in the opposing walls of the third ventricle and the arcuate nucleus within the infundibulum. (LFB/CV.)*

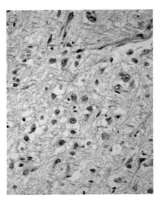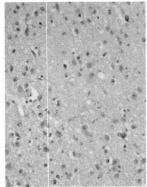

Figure 17.4 *Arcuate nucleus. Situated in the infundibulum, its parvicellular neurons are the site of growth hormone-releasing hormone production.*

The hypothalamus receives several distinct afferent pathways, originating from such diverse sites as the forebrain and limbic system, the visual system, the thalamus and the brainstem. It is unclear to what extent the neocortex communicates with the hypothalamus. Major afferent tracts include the median forebrain bundle, which provides limbic input to the hypothalamus, the hippocampal–hypothalamic tract, the amygdalohypothalamic tract and the retinohypothalamic tract, a pathway indirectly affecting the pineal gland and playing a role in the establishment of circadian rhythms. That the neocortex may have some input to the hypothalamus is suggested by the finding of small numbers of corticohypothalamic fibres originating from the orbital gyrus of the frontal lobe. Their physiological significance is uncertain. Efferent hypothalamic projections include the median forebrain bundle, which serves to integrate visceral and olfactory functions, the mamilothalamic and mamilotegmental tracts and, the hypothalamohypophyseal tract. The latter consists of the supraopticohypophyseal and the paraventriculohypophyseal tracts, which carry vasopressin and

oxytocin via the pituitary stalk to the posterior lobe. A minor component of the hypothalamohypophyseal tract is the tuberoinfundibular tract, which originates from neurosecretory neurons engaged in the production of hypophysiotropic substances (hypothalamic releasing and inhibiting hormones).

The median eminence, the specialized midportion of the tuber cinereum, represents the site of hypophysiotropic hormone release. Such hormones may be stimulatory or inhibitory. Nerve cell processes carrying these hormones converge upon the complex capillary plexus of the median eminence (Fig. 17.5). Architecturally, the median eminence consists of an internal zone composed of nerve fibres of the supraopticohypophyseal and paraventriculohypophyseal tracts, and an external zone consisting of axon terminals of the tuberohypophyseal system. The latter terminates upon capillaries comprising the primary plexus of the portal circulation (Fig. 17.5).

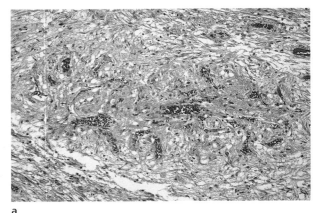

a

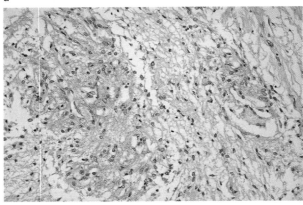

b

Figure 17.5 *Median eminence. The specialized, highly vascular region in the infundibulum and proximal pituitary stalk is the area wherein hypophysiotropic hormones are released from axonal terminations into the complex capillaries of the gomitoli. (a) The gomitoli are specialized vascular complexes consisting of a central arteriole giving off a spiral array of capillaries. (H&E.) (b) Muscular sphincters at the arteriolar–capillary junction control the flow of hypophysiotrophic factor-containing blood to the pituitary. Note perivascular immunoreactivity for corticotropin-releasing hormone. (ICC for CRH.)*

Ultrastructurally, the external zone consists of nerve terminals containing membrane-bound secretory granules, fenestrated capillaries surrounded by pericytes (the origin of the portal circulation) and a specialized variant of ependymal cells peculiar to the third ventricular region termed tanycytes. Secretion from nerve terminals is by granule exocytosis.

NEUROHYPOPHYSIS

Viewed in a functional context, the neurohypophysis represents part of a neurosecretory unit which begins with the paired supraoptic and paraventricular nuclei of the hypothalamus. The axons of these magnocellular nuclei form the bulk of the hypothalamohypophyseal tract. The supraoptic nuclei overlie the optic tract just behind the chiasm, whereas the flat, subependymally situated paraventricular nuclei are located superior and caudal to the supraoptic nuclei (Figs 17.6, 17.7). Both nuclei are highly vascular and well defined, and consist of approximately 30 000–50 000 neurons with large (20–35 nm) cell bodies. Their cells are characterized by eccentric nuclei, prominent nucleoli and abundant Nissl substance (Fig. 17.6). Architecturally, the paraventricular nuclei are more complex, with a medial parvicellular component (Fig. 17.7) engaged in hypophysiotropic hormone production, particularly corticotropin-releasing hormone (CRH). Vasopressin-producing cells are present in the highest number in the supraoptic nuclei. Both vasopressin and oxytocin, as well as their respective neurophysins, are encountered in separate cells (Fig. 17.8).

A major component of the neurohypophysis includes the pars nervosa (neural or posterior lobe), the infundibular process (pituitary stalk) and the pars infundibularis (infundibulum), the funnel-shaped downward extension of the hypothalamus (Fig. 17.2). The pituitary stalk and posterior lobe are composed of non-myelinated nerve fibres (Figs 17.8, 17.9), their processes and terminations containing neurosecretory substances including vasopressin and oxytocin, the two 'posterior

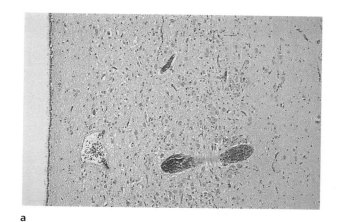

a

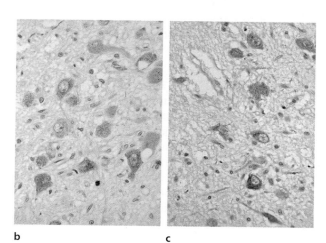

b   c

Figure 17.7 *Paraventricular nucleus. Unlike the supraoptic nuclei (a) these paired nuclei combine both magnocellular and parvicellular neurons. The magnocellular components are immunoreactive for:* **(b)** *vasopressin;* **(c)** *neurophysin. (ICC.)*

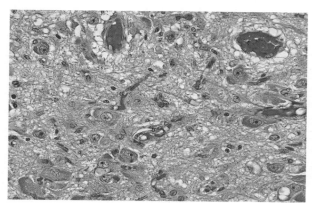

Figure 17.6 *Supraoptic nucleus. Characteristic of this nucleus are large numerous, crowded magnocellular neurons with prominent Nissl substance and numerous capillaries. The latter are intimately associated with neurons. (H&E.)*

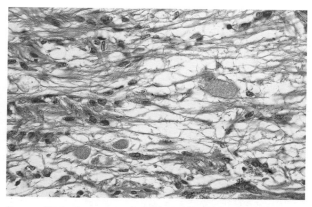

Figure 17.8 *Pituitary stalk. Longitudinal section illustrating normally occurring eosinophilic axonal swellings, some large and globular (herring bodies).*

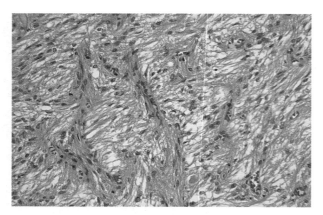

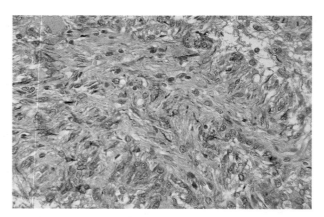

Figure 17.9 *Posterior pituitary. This consists in large part of axons of the hypothalamo-hypophyseal tract terminating upon vasculature. Most nuclei belong either to endothelial cells or to pituicytes, modified astrocytes with special vascular relations.*

Figure 17.11 *Posterior pituitary. Immunostained sections to demonstrate the relative frequency of 'pituicytes', specialized astrocytes thought to affect mechanically the release of vasopressin and oxytocin into the vasculature. (ICC for glial fibrillary acidic protein.)*

pituitary hormones' (Fig. 17.10). Also present are specialized glial cells of the neurohypophysis termed pituicytes (Fig. 17.11). The posterior lobe blood supply is independent from that of the anterior lobe (see below).

The nerve fibres of the supraopticohypophyseal and paraventriculohypophyseal tracts, comprising much of the posterior lobe, transport vasopressin and oxytocin to the posterior lobe by way of axonal flow. In transit as well as in storage within axonal dilations (Fig. 17.8) and their terminals (Fig. 17.12), the hormones are bound to their respective neurophysins, large protein carrier molecules. Oxytocin and vasopressin are stored in secretory granules (Fig. 17.12). Because of their chemical composition they can be demonstrated by histochemical stains such as chromalum haematoxylin or aldehyde thionin. More specific identification of these hormones is achieved by immunocytochemical staining, a method which also permits the localization of both forms of neurophysin. The anatomical and functional integrity of the neurohypophysis is dependent upon the integrity of its constituent axons. Not only does the posterior lobe undergo

marked atrophy after destruction of the hypothalamus and magnocellular nuclei or of the hypothalamohypophyseal tract, but neurons of the supraoptic and paraventricular nuclei undergo involution and atrophy if their axons are interrupted (see Mechanical injury, below).

ADENOHYPOPHYSIS

The pituitary lies within the sella turcica or hypophyseal fossa, a midline, saddle-shaped depression in the sphenoid bone (Fig. 17.1). The sella is lined by dura, which also forms the variably complete sellar diaphragm. The arachnoid membrane does not normally enter the sella. At the central part of the sellar diaphragm, a small opening is evident which admits the pituitary stalk and accompanying vasculature, both of which functionally connect the pituitary with the hypothalamus.

Grossly, the pituitary is bilaterally symmetrical, a bean-shaped organ which in the adult measures 13 mm transversely, 10 mm anteroposteriorly and 6 mm vertically. On average, the adult pituitary weighs 0.6 g; however, it enlarges during pregnancy and by the end of gestation may weigh in excess of 1.0 g. Although after pregnancy or lactation the gland decreases in size, its regression is incomplete. For example, in multiparous women, even years after the last pregnancy, the pituitary usually weighs 0.7–0.8 g. Senescence brings about a decrease in pituitary size; the reduction in its weight is mild to moderate and is more conspicuous in men than in women.

The adenohypophysis comprises approximately 80% of the entire pituitary. It consists of the pars distalis (pars anterior, anterior lobe), the pars intermedia (intermediate lobe, intermediate zone) and the pars tuberalis (pars infundibularis, pars proximalis). Of these, the pars distalis is the largest and, from the endocrine viewpoint, the most important part. In man the pars intermedia does not form an anatomically separate zone: after normal fetal devel-

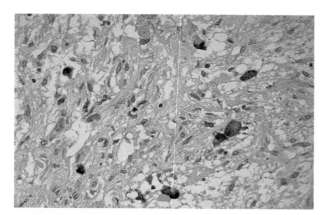

Figure 17.10 *Posterior pituitary. Section showing bulbous axonal terminations immunoreactive for neurophysin.*

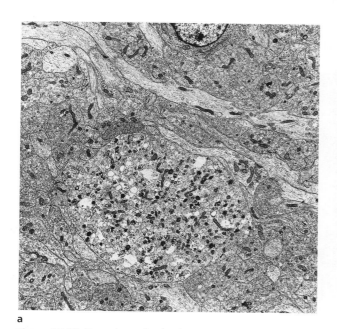

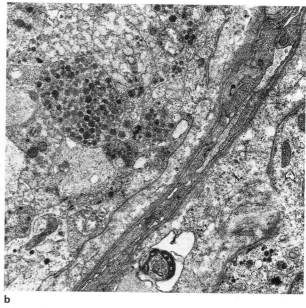

a   b

Figure 17.12 *Neurohypophysis. Electron micrographs showing: (**a**) neuronal processes, some dilated and filled with neurosecretory material; (**b**) neuronal processes abutting on a capillary with a fenestrated endothelium.*

opment its cells are incorporated within the anterior lobe around birth. The term pars distalis includes both anterior and intermediate lobes. The physiological function of pars intermedia is not known.[162] The pars tuberalis represents a proximal, upward extension of the pars distalis along the pituitary stalk. It is composed primarily of chromophobic cells and to a lesser extent acidophilic and basophilic cells. Immunocytochemistry demonstrates mainly follicle-stimulating hormone (FSH), luteinizing hormone (LH) and α-subunit within their cytoplasm. During adult life, cells of the pars tuberalis show a tendency to undergo squamous metaplasia, as evidenced by their immunoreactivity for cytokeratin. According to current views, the pars tuberalis does not play a significant role in adenohypophyseal function.

Adenohypophyseal cells may also be found outside the adenohypophysis. Accumulation of basophilic cells in the posterior lobe, known as basophil cell invasion, is discussed further below. Another extrapituitary site of adenohypophyseal cells is the pharyngeal pituitary. Typically less than 4 mm in diameter, it usually lies embedded in the sphenoid bone and consists of small clusters of chromophobic cells interspersed with a few acidophilic and basophilic cells. In contrast to the pars distalis, the pharyngeal pituitary appears richly innervated but has no portal blood supply in that blood circulating within it has no humoral contact with the hypothalamus. Thus, it does not contain any high concentrations of hypothalamic hormones.[232] Although immunocytochemistry demonstrates various adenohypophyseal hormones within the cytoplasm of its cells, the pharyngeal pituitary has no endocrine significance. It has been suggested but not proven that in cases of anterior pituitary hypofunction, such as occurs after hypophysectomy, the pharyngeal pitu-

itary assumes the endocrine function of the anterior pituitary. Ectopic pituitary adenomas rarely originate in the pharyngeal pituitary.[62,149,232]

Lastly, adenohypophyseal cells are rarely found as an adenoma in ovarian teratomas,[314] and may produce various adenohypophyseal hormones; it may cause endocrine hyperfunction, including hyperprolactinaemia or Cushing's syndrome. Resection of such teratomas is curative.

It should be noted that considerable differences exist among various species in the structural features of the pituitary. Thus, great caution is needed when trying to extrapolate from the pituitary of animal to the human gland.

BLOOD SUPPLY OF THE HYPOTHALAMUS AND PITUITARY

Knowledge of the circulation of the hypothalamus and pituitary is essential to understanding the functional relationship between these structures.[117] Since the hypothalamus plays a major role in regulating secretory activity of the anterior pituitary, use of the functional term 'hypothalamic–pituitary' axis is fully justified.

The blood supply of the hypothalamus is less complex than that of the pituitary (Fig. 17.13). It is derived from arteriolar branches of the circle of Willis as well as from the superior hypophyseal arteries. Most of this circulation, aside from that supplying the supraoptic and paraventricular nuclei, resembles the vasculature of other portions of the brain. The highly vascular magnocellular nuclei show their capillaries to be so intimately associated with neurosecretory cells (Fig. 17.6) that the capillaries appear to pass through their cytoplasm. Also highly spe-

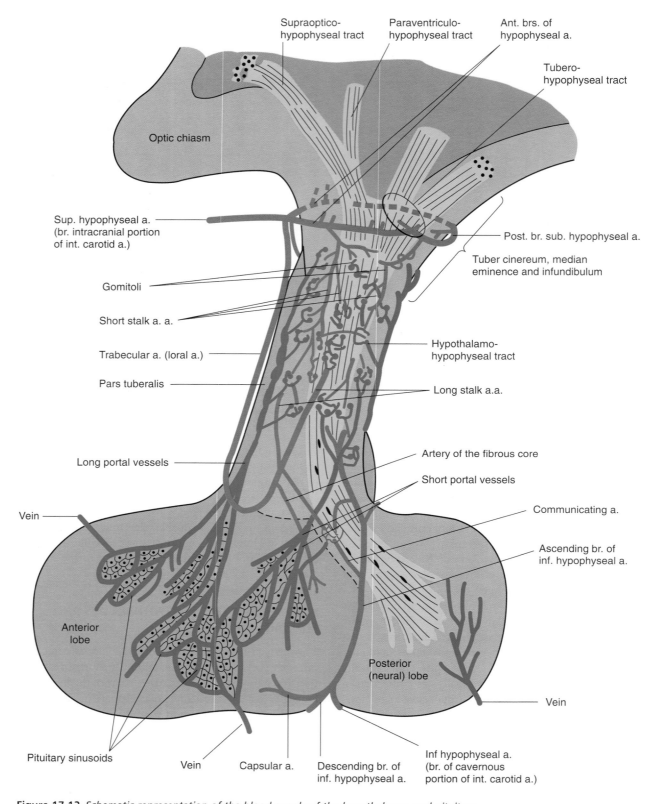

Figure 17.13 *Schematic representation of the blood supply of the hypothalamus and pituitary.*

cialized is the circulation of the median eminence, particularly that of the external zone, which is derived from the superior hypophyseal arteries. Its capillary bed is connected to that of the anterior pituitary via the portal vasculature. It is at the level of the external plexus of the median eminence that the contact between neurosecretory neurons and the blood supply of the pituitary is maximal (Fig. 17.5). This contact facilitates the transfer of hypothalamic releasing and inhibiting factors to the capillary bed of the anterior lobe. The pituitary receives its blood supply from the superior and inferior hypophyseal arteries (Fig. 17.13) with bilateral blood vessels arising from the internal carotid arteries.[155] Ascending branches of the two superior hypophyseal arteries penetrate the infundibulum, and terminate either in gomitoli or in their associated capillary networks. The former, present in large number in the infundibulum and proximal pituitary stalk, are complex vascular structures approximately 1–2 mm long and 0.1 mm wide. They consist of a central artery with a prominent muscular coat surrounded by a dense capillary plexus (Fig. 17.5). Although the precise function of the gomitoli is not known, they appear to regulate blood flow to the adenohypophysis, thereby affecting the entry of hypothalamic regulatory hormones into its circulation. As noted above, hypothalamic regulatory hormones, synthesized in neurons within various hypothalamic nuclei, flow downwards along the non-myelinated nerve fibres to the level of the infundibulum, wherein they are released into the bloodstream in the perigomitolar capillary plexus (Fig. 17.6). Large parallel veins, termed long portal vessels, originate from these capillaries and travel within the pituitary stalk to terminate in the capillaries of the adenohypophysis. These portal vessels transport high concentrations of hypothalamic hormones which regulate the endocrine activity of adenohypophyseal cells. In addition, short portal vessels arise in the distal pituitary stalk and neural lobe, these vessels being of importance in that they permit the passage of biologically active peptides and proteins from the neurohypophysis to the adenohypophysis. The portal circulation as a whole provides a direct neurohumoral link between the hypothalamus and adenohypophysis, thus explaining how the endocrine activity is ultimately regulated by the hypothalamus.

The adenohypophyseal blood supply is not derived exclusively from the portal circulation.[396] Studies indicate that between 70 and 90% of adenohypophyseal blood originates from the long and to a lesser extent the short portal vessels. Morphological investigations have provided direct evidence that a small proportion of adenohypophyseal blood flow is arterial in origin. The loral or trabecular artery, which delivers blood to the infundibulum and upper part of the stalk, gives rise to the artery of the fibrous core. In that the latter penetrates the pars distalis without passing through the infundibulum, it carries arterial, non-portal blood to adenohypophyseal cells. Arterial blood is also carried to the adenohypophysis by the capsular arteries, small blood vessels originating from the inferior hypophyseal arteries and carrying blood not only to the pituitary capsule but also to a thin zone of subcapsular adenohypophyseal cells. The inferior hypophyseal arteries also carry arterial, non-portal blood to the posterior pituitary. Venous blood exiting the pituitary enters peripituitary venous sinuses which are drained bilaterally to the internal jugular veins. It is of note that venous outflow from the adenohypophysis is smaller than that of blood reaching the pituitary, an observation suggesting that circulation of blood within the common neurohypophyseal vascular bed may be reversed. Thus, it appears that short portal vessels serve as both afferent and efferent channels and that blood from the pituitary may also flow to the hypothalamus, to affect there the regulatory function of the hypothalamus upon the anterior pituitary.[39] Ultrastructural studies have shown that adenohypophyseal capillaries are lined by fenestrated endothelium which overlies a subendothelial space and a distinct basal lamina. Hormones discharged from adenohypophyseal cells therefore must first pass through their own periacinar basal lamina and subsequently all layers of the capillary wall in order to enter the bloodstream. Since the hormone-containing secretory granules within adenohypophyseal cells become invisible upon their release into the extracellular space, the process of hormone transport between the secretory cells and the capillary lumen cannot be investigated by current morphological methods.

The blood supply of the posterior lobe of the pituitary is partly derived not from the portal vasculature but from the systemic circulation via the inferior hypophyseal arteries (Fig. 17.13). These vessels carry systemic blood devoid of high concentrations of the hypothalamic regulatory hormones. Quantitatively, the posterior lobe receives a greater blood supply than does the anterior lobe.

INNERVATION OF THE PITUITARY

With the exception of few sympathetic fibres which enter the anterior lobe along blood vessels, the adenohypophysis does not have a nerve supply. These perivascular nerve fibres may affect blood flow to the adenohypophysis, but they do not appear to play a role in the control of adenohypophyseal endocrine activity.

Normal morphological variations

BASOPHIL INVASION

The presence of basophilic, periodic acid–Schiff (PAS)-positive cells within the substance of the posterior pituitary (Fig. 17.14) is perceived as a normal variation, although it may represent pathology. The cells are immunoreactive for ACTH, but do not display Crooke's hyalinization in the clinical setting of hypercortisolism. Their accumulation greatly increases with age and they may extend deep into

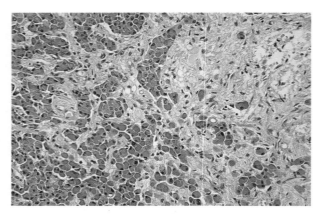

Figure 17.14 *Basophil invasion. The presence of corticotroph cells within the posterior lobe, which are physiologically different from those of the adenohypophysis, is a normal age-related process not associated with endocrinopathy.*

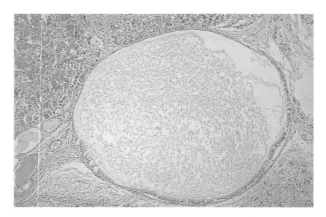

Figure 17.16 *Rathke's cleft cysts. Microscopic cysts are commonly encountered as incidental findings at autopsy. At the interface of the anterior and posterior lobes, these mucin-containing, epithelial-lined cysts represent derivatives of Rathke's pouch, the anlage of the anterior pituitary.*

the substance of the posterior lobe.[201] The ACTH-immunoreactive cells probably represent hyperplastic proliferation of pars intermedia derived cells, particularly frequent in pituitaries of elderly men.[162] Impressive numbers of such cells may occasionally mimic pituitary adenoma. Apparently non-functioning basophil adenomas have been observed within the posterior pituitary or the pituitary cleft, and the posterior lobe basophilic cell is probably the parent cell of the silent 'corticotroph' adenoma subtype 1 (see Silent adenomas).

SALIVARY GLAND REMNANTS

Given the origin of the anterior pituitary from stomodeum, the finding of ectopic salivary gland tissue, usually on the upper surface of the posterior pituitary, is not surprising.[369] Microscopically, most resemble serous acini (Fig. 17.15). Such remnants are the presumed origin of rare salivary gland tumours rising from the sellar region.

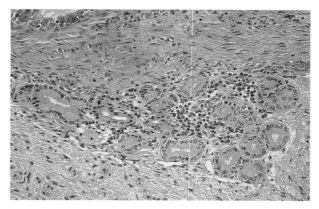

Figure 17.15 *Salivary gland rest. Typically serous in nature at the surface of the genu of the posterior lobe, they differ from Rathke's cleft remnants (see Fig. 17.16) and rarely give rise to salivary gland tumours of the sella.*

RATHKE'S CLEFT REMNANTS

Remnants of the anterior pituitary anlage are frequently encountered as glands and cleft-like spaces at the interface of the anterior and posterior pituitary lobes. Cells comprising such structures may be cuboidal, columnar, mucin-producing or ciliated, and are on occasion pituitary hormone-producing. Progressive accumulation of secretions within such cysts gives rise to Rathke's cleft cysts, which are common incidental autopsy findings[14] (Fig. 17.16).

INTRAVASCULAR HYALIN BODIES

The capillaries of the pituitary stalk are on occasion seen to contain eosinophilic, cylindrical, hyalin bodies which resemble intravascular thrombi.[45] Occurring in otherwise normal subjects, such structures appear to be without clinical significance.

Lymphocytic foci are seen in somewhat over 10% of normal subjects, and may be encountered in the region of the interlobar groove of the pituitary.[377] Histologically, such cells are readily distinguished from the widespread, destructive infiltrate of lymphocytes seen in lymphocytic hypophysitis (see below). Lymphocytic microfoci have no clinical importance.

Age-related changes in the pituitary and hypothalamus

Pituitary changes related to ageing are few.[359] In the hypothalamus the alterations accompanying sexual maturation and ageing are subtle and involve primarily changes in nuclear size and in cell population.[403] More obvious are clinically insignificant accumulations of corpora amylacea, especially in the region of the supraoptic nuclei. Nonetheless, magnocellular nuclei and their hormone content are relatively unaffected by age. The mamillary bodies diminish in volume with age, but neuronal loss is not evident. Lipofuscin accumulation, a common feature of ageing neurons, does not appear to affect the secretory neurons of the hypothalamus.

The weight of the anterior pituitary decreases in old age, especially in men. Probably related to diminishing blood flow, mild to moderate interstitial fibrosis may be noted. Deposition of amyloid and haemosiderin may occur occasionally. Among hormone-producing cells only the growth hormone (GH)-immunoreactive cells decrease in number. Incidental adenomas are fairly common findings. Nearly half of them are positive for prolactin (PRL); the rest appear to be clinically non-functioning. Other types are rare among incidental adenomas.

Functional cytomorphology of the normal adenohypophysis

The relatively recent development of precise, morphological definitions of the various pituitary cell types represents a major advance. The inflexible one cell–one hormone hypothesis coupled with light-microscopical observations led to the recognition of five functionally distinctive cell types.[152] It also influenced our thinking regarding the function and regulation of the pituitary gland, as well as the classification of pituitary lesions. Immunohistochemistry, which more specifically localized the different hormones in their corresponding cell types, at first strongly supported the one cell–one hormone theory. Later, the conclusion that plurihormonality, i.e. presence of more than one hormone in the same cell, was a common occurrence in adenomas, became inescapable.[360] Recognition of reversible transdifferentiation in the normal gland, i.e. transformation of one cell type into another upon functional demand, reaffirms the notion of plurihormonality.[107,398,429] In addition to their hormones, the various pituitary cells contain and probably produce a variety of other substances such as regulatory peptides, neurotransmitters, growth factors and cytokines, suggesting paracrine and autocrine influences.[16,81,327,408] As a result of recent data, a significant paradigm shift is taking place revealing the pituitary not as a static, but as a remarkably adaptable organ.

Accurate identification of pituitary cell types is crucial to diagnosis. Presently, the single most effective tool is electron microscopy, with its capacity of revealing distinctive features of numerous cells in a single specimen.[152] Alternative techniques, based on different principles and definitions, often provide different results. For instance, immunohistochemistry detects cytoplasmic hormone stores, a positive signal on *in situ* hybridization indicates the transcription of a specific gene,[233] and the cumbersome reverse haemolytic plaque assay, still an experimental technique, provides evidence of active hormone release.[108] In most instances, these methods detect only a portion

of the cell population under study. Even by electron microscopy, a varying percentage of cells may remain unidentified as a result of overlapping features. The possible existence of presently unidentified cell types (see Silent adenomas) further compounds the difficulties inherent in cell classification.

When studying the adenohypophysis in man, it has to be considered that the anatomical distribution of certain cell types differs within the gland, with corticotrophs being situated in the midline, and growth hormone and prolactin cells being most abundant in the lateral and posterolateral portions, respectively (Figs 17.17, 17.18). This circumstance, among others, makes the performance of cell counts on intact autopsy specimen a cumbersome activity. Moreover, it renders estimates of cell proportions in fragmented biopsy of non-tumorous pituitary tissue virtually useless in most instances.

GH cells or somatotrophs account for approximately 50% of the pituitary cell mass.[152,201] Somatotrophs are the

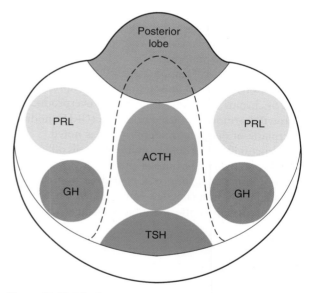

Figure 17.17 *Distribution of pituitary cell types within the anterior lobe.*

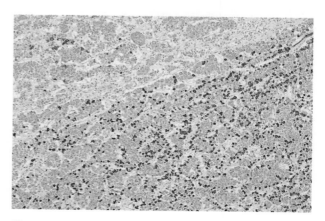

Figure 17.18 *Normal pituitary, junction of lateral wing and median wings. (ICC for growth hormone.)*

predominant component of the lateral wings, whereas the median wedge contains only scattered GH cells. Immunocytochemistry detects strong positivity for GH (Fig. 17.18). Immunogold double labelling at the ultrastructural level may detect other substances such as PRL and α-subunit, a finding suggesting that the somatotroph population is heterogeneous.[152] The variations in the ultrastructural appearance of GH cells are also consistent with the hypothesis that somatotrophs are not a uniform cell population but rather a mosaic.[152] The archetypical GH cell is a medium-sized, ovoid cell with a central nucleus, moderately developed, peripheral rough endoplasmic reticulum (RER), a globoid Golgi complex and numerous spherical, evenly dense secretory granules ranging in diameter from 150 to 500 nm (Fig. 17.19). Yet other GH cells are polyhedral with larger secretory granules, measuring up to 1000 nm, or more. These largest granules are not spherical but are typically elongate or irregular. At the other end of the spectrum are GH cells with small granules (150–200 nm); such cells are recognized as somatotrophs only with the aid of immunoelectron microscopy. A characteristic marker, infrequently seen in normal somatotrophs, is the crystallization of secretory material within granules resulting in distinctly geometrical forms.[152]

The morphological response of the GH cell to changing functional demand appears rather unimpressive. In cases of chronic stimulation, such as in overproduction of growth hormone-releasing hormone (GRH), nodular hyperplasia of deeply eosinophilic cells is noted.[152,157,414] Ultrastructurally, these densely granulated cells differ from 'normal' cells only in the unusual prominence of the Golgi complex. Functional suppression, such as by treatment with somatostatin analogues, causes either no obvious alterations or only subtle quantitative changes, including slightly increased size and volume density of secretory granules.[98]

PRL cells vary in frequency, representing 10–30% of adenohypophyseal cells, the lowest value being in men and the highest in multiparous women.[21] With the exception of the posterolateral rim of lateral wings, where PRL cells predominate, they lie randomly scattered throughout the remainder of the pars distalis.[152,201] They occur in two morphologically distinct forms, the more numerous, sparsely granulated or chromophobic variety and the uncommon, densely granulated form which is strongly acidophilic. Immunocytochemistry detects the former as small cells with long processes, with immunopositivity chiefly juxtanuclear in the Golgi apparatus. Cytoplasmic granules are scant and may not be discernible. The densely granulated form displays strong immunopositivity throughout the cytoplasm.

By electron microscopy, the sparsely granulated PRL cell is small and polyhedral, and occurs in groups of three to four cells within acini[152] (Fig. 17.20). Their slender cytoplasmic processes abut the basal lamina. Prominent nucleoli, well-organized RER, lucent cytoplasm, prominent Golgi complexes and small, sparse (150–300 nm) secretory granules are noted. Granule extrusion (exocytosis) is a prolactin cell marker in the human pars distalis; extrusions may be orthotopic, taking place at cell surface facing basal lamina, or 'misplaced', occurring at lateral cell membranes. The densely granulated type is ovoid or polyhedral with more numerous and larger (400–600 nm) opaque, greyish black granules.

Depending upon their functional state, PRL cells exhibit a wide range of ultrastructural appearances.[152] Sustained stimulation (loss of dopaminergic inhibition, oestrogen effect, neuroleptic drugs, etc.) results in pro-

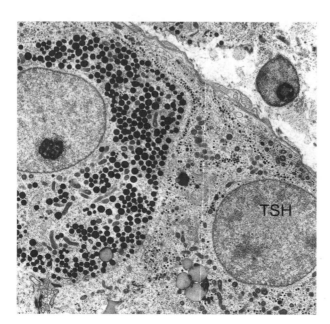

Figure 17.19 *Normal pituitary. Electron micrograph showing features of a growth hormone and thyroid-stimulating hormone cell.*

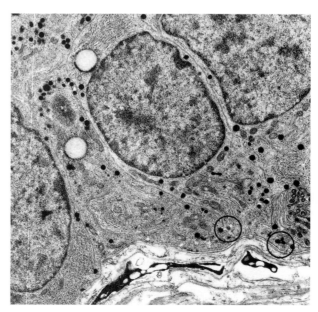

Figure 17.20 *Normal pituitary. Electron micrograph of a group of prolactin cells. Note granule extrusions (circles).*

gressive cytoplasmic expansion, an increase in RER and Golgi membranes, and diminution in secretory granules (Fig. 17.21). Prolactin cell hyperplasia accompanies pregnancy[366] (Fig. 17.22). It may occur in association with oestrogen treatment as well as any process compressing the pituitary stalk and thereby interfering with dopamine transport to the anterior lobe.[152,157] It may also accompany ACTH-producing tumours and thyroid-stimulating hormone (TSH) hyperplasia. Idiopathic PRL cell hyperplasia is very rare.[176] Suppression of PRL cell function (dopaminergic drugs and feedback effect of increased PRL levels) results in nucleolar heterochromasia and diminution of cytoplasmic volume due in large part to involution of RER and Golgi complexes[152] (Fig.

17.23). Markedly suppressed PRL cells resemble null cells in being small, lacking in markers of PRL differentiation and losing their contact with the basal lamina.

Corticotrophs or ACTH cells account for approximately 10% of adenohypophyseal cells, are basophilic and PAS positive, and reside chiefly within the median wedge of adenohypophysis.[152,201] Such medium-sized, ovoid cells stain strongly for 1-39 ACTH and other peptide derivatives of the pro-opiomelanocortin (POMC) precursor. Their ultrastructural appearance is fairly stable. They are ovoid or angular and abut the basal lamina. Corticotrophs possess dense cytoplasm, and numerous spherical, irregular or indented granules. Ranging in size up to 600 nm, most measure between 300 and 450 nm (Fig. 17.24). A specific marker of human corticotrophs is type 1 (cytokeratin) filaments which lie in bundles in the perinuclear region.[152] A large electron-lucent lysosome, visible even at the light-microscopic level, is often present.

Stimulation does not cause any noticeable change in corticotroph morphology. As primary stress responders, ACTH cells are probably always ready to discharge their hormones. Functional suppression (negative feedback effect of elevated cortisol levels) induces a unique, specific and largely unexplained reaction. Termed Crooke's hyalinization, it consists of a massive, perinuclear, ring-like accumulation of cytokeratin filaments[152,201] (Fig. 17.25). The effect appears to be reversible. Non-neoplastic proliferation of corticotrophs, usually nodular hyperplasia, is an uncommon cause of Cushing's disease. It may be idiopathic or induced by ectopically produced CRH.[157]

The thyrotrophs or TSH cells represent approximately 5% of adenohypophyseal cells.[152,201] Largely restricted to the anteromedial rim of the median wedge, they

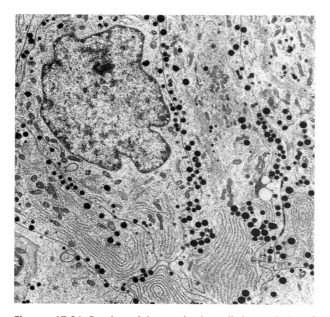

Figure 17.21 *Focal nodular prolactin cell hyperplasia of unknown aetiology in an otherwise normal anterior lobe. Note the abundant rough endoplasmic reticulum and prominent Golgi complex.*

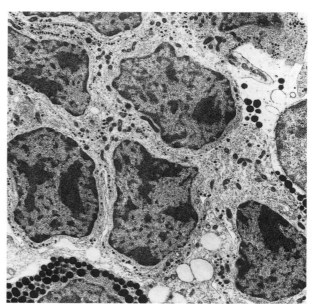

Figure 17.23 *Suppressed prolactin cells. Noted in the non-tumorous part of a pituitary harbouring PRL cell adenoma, they have features similar to those of null cells.*

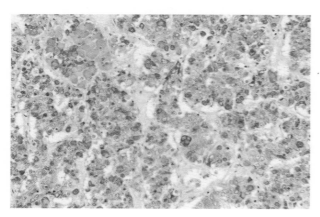

Figure 17.22 *Prolactin cell hyperplasia. Pronounced changes in the pituitary of a woman who died close to term. (ICC for PRL.)*

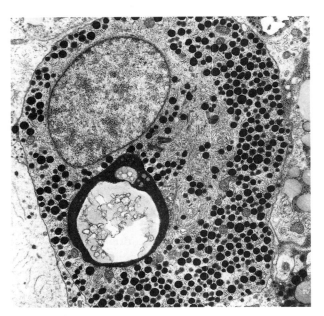

Figure 17.24 *Normal pituitary. Electron micrograph of a corti- cotroph cell. Note bundles of cytokeratin filaments and the prominent lysosome visible by light microscopy.*

are slightly basophilic, PAS positive and of varying size. Most are angular in configuration, their long processes being well demonstrated by intense immuno- reactivity for TSH (Fig. 17.26). On electron microscopy, thyrotrophs exhibit a significant interface with the basal lamina, some processes actually traversing the entire acinus to make contact with it. Thyrotrophs possess

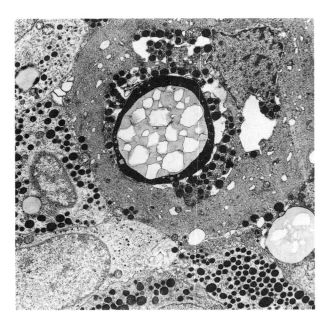

Figure 17.25 *Suppressed corticotrophs. Electron micrograph of Crooke's hyalinization which affects large parts of the cyto- plasm. The secretory granules are either entrapped within the Golgi region or displaced to the cell periphery by the accumu- lating masses of cytokeratin filaments.*

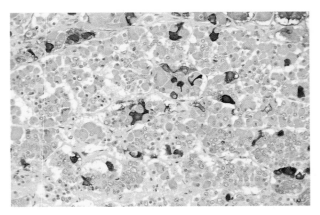

Figure 17.26 *Normal thyrotrophs in the pituitary. Section taken from an autopsy specimen. Note the characteristic angular shape of the cells. (ICC for thyroid-stimulating hormone.)*

euchromatic nuclei, moderately developed RER, globoid Golgi complexes and small, approximately 200-nm secretory granules (Figs 17.19, 17.27). Some thyrotrophs contain pleomorphic secretory granules; it is not clear whether such cells represent a morphological variant of thyrotroph, a specific physiological state or a separate clone.

Sustained thyrotrophin-releasing hormone (TRH) oversecretion due to untreated hypothyroidism results in stimulation of thyrotrophs which progresses from a dif- fuse increase in cell number to massive nodular hyper- plasia, which leads to enlargement of the gland and local symptoms.[152,157] Owing to associated hyperprolacti- naemia, the result of TRH elevation, the lesion may mimic PRL-producing adenoma. As a result, the patient, often a young female in the postpartum period, may be brought

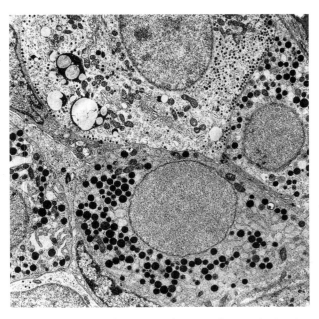

Figure 17.27 *Normal pituitary. Electron micrograph showing details of a thyrotroph and of three gonadotrophs.*

to surgery.[157] The stimulated TSH cells (thyroid deficiency or 'thyroidectomy' cells) are large and polyhedral, with pale cytoplasm and PAS-positive globules. Ultrastructurally, they are characterized by proliferation and dilation of RER[152,157] (Fig. 17.28). In some treated cases, TSH cell hyperplasia fails to regress, even when patients are rendered clinically euthyroid.

The morphology of suppressed thyrotrophs in the setting of hyperthyroidism has only been well studied by immunocytochemistry.[365] Ultrastructurally, non-tumorous thyrotrophs in pituitaries harbouring TSH adenoma causing hyperthyroidism often show remarkable involution. The cells still retain their angular shape, but RER and Golgi membranes are scanty, secretory granules are sparse and lysosomes of various sizes are apparent.

Gonadotrophs producing FSH and LH are ovoid, small to medium sized, and are randomly distributed throughout the anterior lobe.[152,201] These basophilic, strongly PAS-positive cells represent 15–20% of adenohypophyseal cells and show variable immunoreactivity for FSH and/or LH. Ultrastructurally, they are ovoid or elongate, some stretching across the entire acinus, and have a broad interface with the basal lamina. Gonadotroph cells have euchromatic nuclei, variably developed, slightly dilated RER, and large ring-like Golgi complex. Their secretory granules vary in electron density and morphology, with some having small (200 nm) or larger ones (300–600 nm) (Fig. 17.29). Gonadotrophs are often surrounded by PRL cells, an arrangement suggesting a paracrine relationship between the two cell types.[152]

As a response to deficiency of gonadal hormones, gonadotroph hormone-releasing hormone (GnRH)

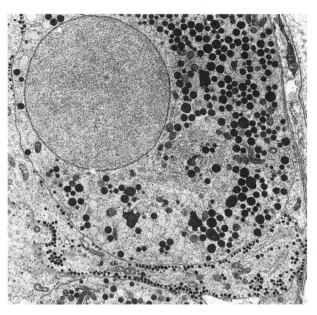

Figure 17.29 *Gonadotroph. Electron micrograph of a normal cell.*

stimulation induces and sustains the progressive development of gonadectomy or 'castration' cells.[152,201] As in the case of stimulated thyrotrophs, gonadotrophs also respond with proliferation and gradual dilation of RER which appears to be filled with proteinaceous substance. Although the degree of RER dilation is similar within any one cell, it varies considerably from one cell to another. In the extreme form, 'signet-ring' cells appear, in which a single, markedly distended RER profile occupies much of the cytoplasm. An unusually large ring of Golgi complexes may also be visible, even by light microscopy. Gonadectomy cells are seen in the pituitaries of postmenopausal women as well as of gonadectomized men and women, but true hyperplasia of FSH and LH cells is extremely rare.[157] Even the exceptional hyperplasia occurring in cases of primary hypogonadism (such as Klinefelter's syndrome) does not lead to noticeable enlargement of the gland.

Functional suppression of gonadotrophs is seen in hypogonadotrophic hypogonadism (Kallmann's syndrome)[207] and in the non-tumorous pituitary surrounding gonadotroph adenomas. These are small ovoid cells with heterochromatic nuclei, the cytoplasm of which is dominated by large lysosomes, leaving little space for the markedly involuted RER and Golgi membranes.

Folliculostellate cells are nearly or completely agranular, attached by terminal bars at their apical surfaces and extending long processes between the glandular cells. Chiefly *in vitro* studies ascribed a multitude of functions to the morphologically unassuming cells. Their contribution to the pathology of the adenohypophysis is uncertain, and therefore it will not be discussed here.[9,81,246]

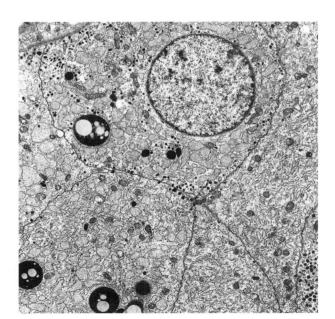

Figure 17.28 *Thyrotroph hyperplasia. The markedly stimulated thyroid deficiency cells are characterized by dilated profiles of proliferating rough endoplasmic reticulum.*

Table 17.3 *Major hypothalamic hormones: composition and localization*

Hormone	Composition	Hypothalamic sites	Extrahypothalamic sites
Growth hormone-releasing hormone (GRH, somatoliberin, somatocrinin)	40 and 44 amino acids	Arcuate nucleus	?
Thyrotropin-releasing hormone (TRH)	3 amino acids	Widely distributed in CNS with concentration in ventromedial, dorsal and paraventricular nuclei, particularly on the left	Brain and spinal cord, pancreatic islet cells, gut endocrine cells
Gonadotropin-releasing hormone (GnRH, gonadoliberin)	10 amino acids	Widespread distribution with concentration in the arcuate, ventromedial, dorsal and paraventricular nuclei	Brain (limbic system), breast (lactation), placenta
Corticotropin-releasing hormone (CRH, corticoliberin)	41 amino acids	Periventricular, medial paraventricular nuclei	Brain (cerebral cortex, limbic system, brainstem, spinal cord)
Somatostatin [somatotropin release inhibiting hormone (SRIH)]	14 amino acids	Periventricular nucleus, paraventricular nuclei (parvicellular neurons), arcuate nuclei	Brain, peripheral nervous system, pancreatic islet cells, gut endocrine cells, thyroid, placenta
Dopamine	Catecholamine	Arcuate nucleus	Brain, gastrointestinal tract
Vasopressin [antidiuretic hormone (ADH)]	9 amino acids	Paraventricular, supraoptic nuclei	Brain
Oxytocin (OT)	9 amino acids	Paraventricular, supraoptic nuclei	Brain

Hypothalamic hormones and their release

The principal hypothalamic efferent is the hypothalamo-hypophyseal tract: it consists not only of fibres carrying vasopressin and oxytocin from the magnocellular nuclei, but also tuberal infundibular efferents derived from hypothalamic nuclei engaged in the production of releasing and inhibiting hormones. Their composition, specific hypothalamic sites of origin and occasional extrahypothalamic sites of production are summarized in Table 17.3. The neurons forming these tracts are termed 'neurosecretory', being capable of releasing hormones into the circulation from a nerve terminal. The concept of neurosecretion was confirmed by studies of the production and release of antidiuretic hormone (ADH; vasopressin) by the supraoptic and paraventricular nuclei.[378] The process involves transfer of hormones from the nerve cell body to its terminal by a process of axoplasmic flow, a basic property of all neurons. In addition to vasopressin and oxytocin, a variety of hypophysiotropic hormones has been characterized. Of these, some have been identified at extrahypothalamic sites, an observation suggesting that they serve more than one specific function. Not only have hypothalamic hormones been found at systemic sites but other regulatory hormones encountered at systemic sites have been identified in the hypothalamus; these include

some associated with gastrointestinal function (motilin), vasoactive intestinal polypeptide (VIP), galanin and substance P. Their physiological roles in the hypothalamus have not been clarified.

The release of oxytocin and vasopressin takes place in the posterior or neural lobe of the pituitary where fibres of the supraopticohypophyseal and paraventriculohypophyseal tracts terminate upon specialized perivascular spaces (Fig. 17.12). Ultrastructurally, the nerve fibres contain secretory granules of varying electron density, multilamellar bodies and electron-lucent vesicles. A minority of vasopressin- and oxytocin-containing fibres originating in the paraventricular nuclei projects to the vasculature of the median eminence, thus explaining failure to produce diabetes insipidus by low-level stalk transection and also suggesting a regulatory role for vasopressin in anterior pituitary function, possibly the promotion of stress-related ACTH release. Additional fibres from the paraventricular nuclei project to extrahypothalamic sites.

Hypothalamic posterior lobe-associated hormones

Both vasopressin and oxytocin are nonapeptides and are characterized by a ring structure with a disulfide bond.

Minor chemical differences exists among the hormone products of different species. In man, arginine vasopressin is produced in the hypothalamus, whereas in some animal species lysine vasopressin is the main form.[359]

Vasopressin has a molecular weight of 1084. Its main effect is the retention of water by the kidney, its action being upon the renal tubules by reabsorbing water from the glomerular filtrate. In higher concentrations vasopressin contracts smooth muscle, raises blood pressure, and stimulates prostaglandin synthesis and hepatic glycogenolysis. By acting as a corticotropin-releasing factor, vasopressin is an important stimulator of ACTH release.

Oxytocin is a nonapeptide with a molecular weight of 1007. Its primary effect is upon the uterus, inducing contraction of smooth-muscle cells; thus, it plays a major role in uterine contraction during labour. Oxytocin also affects lactation by inducing contraction of myoepithelial cells surrounding mammary ducts. Contraction of these cells is important in the process of milk ejection. Lastly, oxytocin also has some natriuretic effect and is involved in the maintenance of sodium homoeostasis.

The regulation of vasopressin and oxytocin secretion is complex and depends a great deal upon neural stimuli and various stresses. Vasopressin is hypersecreted in patients with dehydration, increased plasma osmotic pressure and decreased blood volume. In contrast, suppression of vasopressin secretion occurs when the osmotic pressure of the plasma is low or when the extracellular space is expanded, as in subjects with overhydration. Nicotin stimulates, whereas ethanol inhibits vasopressin release.

Anterior pituitary hormones

The anterior pituitary produces several distinct hormones which affect practically every activity of the body. Thus, it is not surprising that the pituitary and its regulatory centre, the hypothalamus, are regarded as the conductors of the endocrine orchestra, their role being the maintenance of endocrine homoeostasis.[415]

GH (somatotropin) is a 191 amino acid polypeptide with a molecular weight of 21 500. It is produced by and released from a distinct adenohypophyseal cell, the GH cell or somatotroph. GH is derived from a large 28 000 molecular weight precursor molecule, a prehormone cosecreted with GH but being of no major physiological or pathological significance. The action of GH is mediated via insulin-like growth factor-1 (IGF-1; somatomedin-C), a substance produced mainly in the liver, and the blood level of which is elevated in patients with acromegaly or gigantism. The effect of GH is systemic; it promotes growth, increases protein synthesis, has a protein anabolic effect and decreases protein catabolism. It also mobilizes fat, decreases utilization of carbohydrates, inhibits glucose uptake into cells and causes insulin resistance, and in some

species may induce diabetes mellitus. Regulation of GH secretion is very complex. The most important regulators of GH secretion are GRH, which stimulates it, and somatostatin, or somatotropin release inhibiting factor (SRIF), which inhibits GH secretion. Both of these regulatory hormones are produced in the hypothalamus. Although many other factors affect growth hormone synthesis and/or release, their description is beyond the scope of this chapter.

PRL (lactotropin, mammotropin) is a polypeptide composed of 198 amino acids with a molecular weight of 22 000. Produced and released by a well-defined type of adenohypophyseal cell, the PRL cell (lactotrope, mammotrope) it originates from an ancestral molecule common to GH and human placental lactogen. This prohormone, with a molecular weight of 40 000–50 000, is cosecreted with PRL. Despite similarities in the evolution and amino acid composition of GH and PRL, the two molecules differ significantly and can be distinguished on chemical assays and by immunocytochemistry. The principal effect of PRL is the postpartum stimulation of lactation. Its documented effects upon gonadal function are less well understood. PRL may influence behaviour and may have effects similar to those of GH upon protein, carbohydrate and lipid metabolism. The secretion of PRL is regulated primarily by the hypothalamus. In contrast to other adenohypophyseal hormones, the hypothalamus inhibits PRL synthesis and discharge. The main PRL-inhibiting hormone is dopamine, a substance produced within hypothalamic nuclei and transported to the pituitary via the portal circulation. Other than dopamine, several compounds increase PRL secretion; these include VIP, galanin and TRH. Oestrogens are known not only to elevate blood PRL levels but also to evoke proliferation of PRL cells. Recently, a hypothalamic, apparently cell-specific PRL-releasing peptide has been identified. The effects of the new, presumed regulatory substance are not yet sufficiently documented.[144,448]

ACTH (adrenocorticotropin) is a 39 amino acid peptide with a molecular weight of 4500 which is produced and released by a specific adenohypophyseal cell type, the corticotrope or ACTH cell. Its prohormone, POMC, has a molecular weight of 28 500 and is cleaved to a large number of biologically active or inactive fragments. In addition to ACTH, the peptides include β-melanocyte-stimulating hormone (β-MSH), corticotropin-like intermediate lobe peptide (CLIP), the endorphins and enkephalins. All can be distinguished from ACTH by chemical assays and immunocytochemistry. Although cosecreted with ACTH, some of the peptides have different actions. Many are glycosylated, thus explaining the strong PAS positivity of the cytoplasm of corticotrophs.

The principal effect of ACTH is the stimulation of the adrenal cortex. In endogenous or exogenous ACTH excess the adrenal cortices undergo hyperplasia and secrete high quantities of adrenocortical hormones, mainly glucocorticoids; the principal product is cortisol. ACTH and the related peptides increase adrenal blood flow, and affect several metabolic activities, including protein, carbohydrate, lipid, mineral and water metabolism, as well as affecting blood pressure, behaviour and mental status. Hyperpigmentation of the skin results from overproduction of POMC peptides. ACTH secretion is stimulated by CRH, a 41 amino acid peptide produced in the hypothalamus. Adrenocortical hormones inhibit ACTH release. This negative feedback effect of peripheral hormones is important in the control of pituitary ACTH secretion.

FSH and LH (interstitial cell stimulating hormone in the male) are the two gonadotrope hormones. Both are produced in the same cell, the gonadotrope or FSH/LH cell. Chemically and biologically distinct, they are 29 000 molecular weight glycoprotein hormones composed of two subunits. The β-subunits are hormone specific, possess the biological activity, and can be demonstrated in the blood and tissues by chemical assays and immunocytochemistry. In contrast, the α-subunits appear biologically inactive and are similar or practically identical to that of TSH.

In women, FSH is responsible for the development and maturation of ovarian follicles. It also affects oestrogen secretion. In men, FSH stimulates growth of the testicle, affects spermatogenesis and increases the production of androgen-binding globulin by Sertoli cells. As well as having a luteinizing effect upon the ovaries, LH stimulates ovulation and the subsequent formation, maturation and maintenance of the corpus luteum. In addition, LH stimulates the secretion of the ovarian hormones, oestrogen and progesterone. In men, LH stimulates Leydig cells (interstitial cells), the result being their hyperplasia and increased testosterone secretion. Spermatogenesis is also affected by LH. Secretion of FSH and LH is stimulated by GnRH (or LRH, LHRH, luteinizing hormone-stimulating-hormone), a decapeptide produced by the hypothalamus. The gonadal hormones exert a negative feedback effect on FSH/LH secretion.

TSH (thyrotropin) is a 28 000 molecular weight glycoprotein which, like the gonadotropins, is composed of two chemically different subunits. The β-subunit underlies the biological activity of TSH, whereas the α-subunit is inactive and is chemically similar to the α-subunits of FSH and LH and as well as human chorionic gonadotropin (hCG). Synthesized separately, the two subunits then combine to acquire a carbohydrate component which renders them PAS positive.

The principal effect of TSH is stimulation of the thyroid gland, an increase in thyroid blood flow, and enhanced secretion of thyroid hormones, including thyroxin (T_4) and triiodothyronin (T_3). Protracted stimulation results in enlargement of the thyroid (goitre). Secretion of TSH is regulated primarily by hypothalamic TRH, a tripeptide that stimulates TSH secretion and causes pituitary thyrotroph hyperplasia. The negative feedback effect of thyroid hormones exerts significant inhibition upon TSH secretion. Several other factors, including somatostatin, glucocorticoid hormones and neural influences, also play a role in the regulation of TSH secretion.

PATHOLOGY OF THE HYPOTHALAMUS AND PITUITARY

Disorders of hypothalamic and posterior pituitary hyperfunction

PRECOCIOUS PUBERTY

Demonstrable hypothalamic pathology is seen in less than 10% of cases of precocious puberty. Most are idiopathic or are attributable to androgen- or oestrogen-producing neoplasms (precocious pseudopuberty). Defined as the premature development of secondary sexual characteristics as well as of a postpubertal endocrine profile, precocious puberty is associated with elevated blood levels of GnRH, FSH and LH, as well as sex steroids.

Despite the absence of a demonstrable lesion, idiopathic precocious puberty is presumably hypothalamic in origin. It is sporadic and is a prominent feature of the McCune–Albright syndrome, a disorder not associated with a demonstrable hypothalamic lesion.[204] 'Neurogenic precocious puberty' can be divided into two major groups. The first includes lesions that elaborate GnRH, e.g. hypothalamic neuronal hamartoma (see below)[146,182] and the second includes endocrine inactive lesions that nonspecifically affect hypothalamic centres engaged in the control of sexual maturation. The latter usually affect the posterior hypothalamus and include a variety of lesions, e.g. germ-cell tumours, gliomas, infection, hydrocephalus and after head injury. Also implicated is craniopharyngioma, the tumour most often associated with pubertal delay.

ECTOPIC PRODUCTION OF HYPOTHALAMIC HORMONES

A variety of tumours, the majority neuroendocrine in nature, is known to produce hormones which, both biochemically and in terms of their endocrine effects, are indistinguishable from releasing hormones of hypothalamic origin. Of these, ectopic GRH and CRH production are best documented. ADH (vasopressin) is the principal posterior lobe-related hormone to be ectopically produced. Less obviously 'ectopic' in origin are tumour-associated hypersecretion of VIP, substance P or somatostatin.

Extrahypothalamic production of GRH occurs in a significant minority of neuroendocrine tumours, primarily pancreatic islet cell and bronchial carcinoid tumours.[20] Biochemical evidence of its production is noted in association with nearly half of GRH-containing carcinoid tumours.[290] Although GRH production has

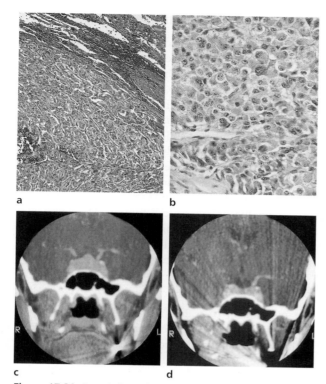

Figure 17.30 *Ectopic hypothalamic hormone secretion. Ectopic production of growth hormone-releasing hormone (GHRH): (a) by a bronchial carcinoid tumour. (H&E.) (b) Immunoreactivity for GRH. (ICC for GHRH.) (c) In such situations the pituitary shows marked enlargement due to GH cell hyperplasia, which (d) remits after resection of the tumour. (CT scans with contrast.)*

also been demonstrated in thymic carcinoid tumours, medullary carcinoma of the thyroid, phaeochromocytoma and small cell carcinoma of the lung, clinical acromegaly due to tumoral GRH production is very uncommon[352] (Fig. 17.30).

Ectopic production of CRH must be considered in the differential diagnosis of Cushing's disease.[370] The finding of simultaneous tumoral production of CRH and ACTH suggests that a minority of such neoplasms may be autostimulatory.[447]

THE SYNDROME OF INAPPROPRIATE ANTIDIURETIC HORMONE (VASOPRESSIN) SECRETION (SIADH)

This not uncommon disorder may be due to a variety of conditions (Table 17.4), some of which include congestive heart failure, cirrhosis and renal disease, and the brain injury may actually represent normal physiological increases in ADH rather than pathological hyperfunction. Unlike diabetes insipidus, the anatomical basis of which is usually obvious, that of SIADH is poorly understood. Whereas stimulatory osmoreceptors lie close to the ADH-producing magnocellular nuclei, inhibitory pathways are diffuse, their centres lying as far afield as the brainstem.[424] As a result, lesions remote from the hypothalamus and posterior pituitary may result in ADH

Table 17.4 *Disorders associated with an excess of antidiuretic hormone*

Neoplasia
Carcinoma of the lung ('oat cell' and adenocarcinoma), duodenum, pancreas, ureter and prostate
Lymphoma, leukaemia and Hodgkin's disease
Mesothelioma
Ewing's sarcoma
Esthesioneuroblastoma

Central nervous system disease
Trauma, neurosurgery
Infection: meningitis (tuberculous), encephalitis, brain abscess, malaria
Mass lesions
Tumours (glioma, etc.)
Medical diseases: hydrocephalus, delirium tremens, Guillain–Barré syndrome
Vascular: subarachnoid haemorrhage, subdural haematoma, stroke

Pulmonary disease
Tuberculosis
Cavitary aspergillosis[a]
Pneumonia (viral, bacterial or fungal)[a]
Positive-pressure ventilation[a]

Endocrine diseases
Addison's disease, myxoedema, hypopituitarism, acute intermittent porphyria

Miscellaneous
Cirrhosis with ascites[a]
Myocardial infarction[a]
Congestive heart failure[a]
Postoperative state[a]

Drugs
Vasopressin, oxytocin, chlorpropamide, chlorothiazide, Atromid-S, Tegretol, nicotine, phenothiazines, cyclophosphamide, morphine, barbiturates

[a]Disorders that may induce 'appropriate' ADH hypersecretion (SAADH).

release. Ectopic ADH production is most often associated with pulmonary malignancy or infection, particularly tuberculosis.[432] Acute, rapidly evolving forms of SIADH may produce cerebral oedema. The treatment of ADH excess consists of water restriction and slow re-establishment of sodium balance; too rapid an elevation may result in central pontine myelinolysis.[286]

Hypothalamic and posterior pituitary hypofunction

HYPOTHALAMIC HYPOGONADISM

This disorder may result from decreased GnRH production or from its non-pulsatile secretion. For instance, isolated deficiency of GnRH characterizes Kallmann's syndrome, an inherited disorder associated with anosmia.[417] In one fully studied case the hypothalamus showed marked hypoplasia of the lateral tuberal nuclei as well as an increase in neurons in the subventricular nucleus, the latter perhaps being due to chronic steroid deficiency. The anterior pituitary demonstrated a marked decrease in gonadotroph cells[207] (Fig. 17.31). Kallmann's syndrome is treatable; administration of GnRH results in normalization of gonadotropin levels.

A variety of midline malformations may also be associated with GnRH deficiency. As noted previously, hypogonadism is regularly associated with hypothalamic lesions due to sarcoidosis, Langerhans' histiocytosis and a variety of neoplasms. Hypogonadism associated with haemochromatosis is not due to hypothalamic dysfunction but rather to iron deposition in gonadotroph cells of the anterior pituitary.[36]

HYPOTHALAMIC DWARFISM

In addition to pituitary disease or end-organ resistance to GH, dwarfism may result from hypothalamic dysfunction. In many instances, as a result of their proximity and shared circulation, the hypothalamus and pituitary are simultaneously involved by inflammatory, infectious, neoplastic, congenital or neonatal diseases associated with growth retardation. Underlying causes include bacterial meningitis, granulomatous disease, Langerhans' histiocytosis, hypothalamic neuronal hamartoma and neoplasms, particularly craniopharyngioma and germ-cell tumours.

Aside from the more often idiopathic nature of hypothalamic growth retardation in early childhood, it may also be due to disorders of gestation, labour and delivery, or of the neonatal period.[69] Midline developmental defects such as septo-optic dysplasia may also be responsible.[13,268] Of particular interest is an autosomal recessive form of hypothalamic dwarfism, one associated with failure to produce GRH. In such instances, GH cells of the pituitary appear structurally normal and are engaged in GH production.[331]

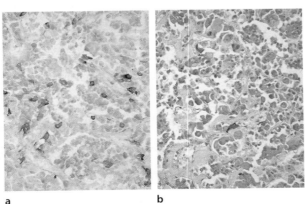

Figure 17.31 *Kallmann's syndrome. (a) Normal gonadotroph density; (b) marked reduction of follicle-stimulating hormone (FSH) immunoreactive gonadotrophs; the effect of diminished hypothalamic stimulation. (ICC for FSH.)*

DIENCEPHALIC SYNDROME

This well-recognized syndrome of emaciation in infancy[54,183,309] is typified by severe weight loss despite normal linear growth, ophthalmological abnormalities including late optic atrophy, and signs of hypothalamic dysfunction including euphoria, hyperkinesis, hypertension and hypoglycaemia. Hydrocephalus is of late occurrence. A number of endocrine abnormalities may be seen, including abnormal dynamics and increased GH levels as well as abnormalities of ACTH regulation.

In almost all instances, the syndrome is due to a neoplasm, such as fibrillary or pilocytic astrocytoma, craniopharyngioma or a germ-cell tumour. Developmental cysts or inflammatory lesions are less often the cause. Some cases are congenital. Involvement of the anterior hypothalamus is the common feature.[309]

DIABETES INSIPIDUS

The mechanism of water balance is dependent upon functioning hypothalamic osmoreceptors, the capacity of the hypothalamus to produce vasopressin, the structural and functional integrity of the pituitary stalk and posterior lobe, the presence of renal vasopressin receptors and a normal response to thirst. Diabetes insipidus may therefore be central, i.e. neurogenic or pituitary in origin, or may be nephrogenic. Central diabetes insipidus may be idiopathic or due to a variety of lesions (Table 17.5).

The spectrum of lesions causing central diabetes insipidus has dramatically changed over time. Early in the twentieth century principal causes included primary and secondary neoplasia (64%), syphilis (13%), head injury (10%), inflammatory lesions (8%) and tuberculosis[105] (5%). A more recent series showed different frequencies: surgical trauma (29%), tumours (26%; the vast majority primary), Langerhans' histiocytosis (10%), head injury (5%) and tuberculosis (2%).[91] Given the variety of causes of diabetes insipidus, ranging from focal to diffusely destructive processes, the prognosis varies considerably. Resultant diabetes insipidus may be transient or permanent depending upon the level of the lesion and its degree of tissue destruction. Although selective ablation of the supraoptic nuclei in the dog produces permanent diabetes insipidus,[106] such limited lesions occur only rarely in humans. In most cases of hypothalamic involvement, both supraoptic and paraventricular nuclei are affected; in addition, other signs of hypothalamic disease are commonly seen. A destructive lesion proximal in the neurosecretory system, such as the upper portion of the pituitary stalk, produces permanent diabetes insipidus due to retrograde axonal degeneration and atrophy of the magnocellular nuclei[230] (Fig. 17.32) (see Physical injury, below).

Neuronal loss must be extensive to produce permanent deficits; in the dog model, loss of 90% of magnocellular neurons is required.[136] In man, destructive lesions producing permanent diabetes insipidus must be high,

Table 17.5 *Diabetes insipidus: variants and causes*

Central diabetes insipidus
Primary
  Idiopathic–autoimmune disease (?)
  Hereditary–autosomal-dominant
  Sex-linked recessive
    Wolfram's (DIDMOAD) syndrome
Secondary
  Hypothalamic disease
    Trauma (surgical trauma and 'stalk section', head
    injury, etc.
  Neoplasia
    Primary (craniopharyngioma, glioma, germ cell tumour)
    Metastatic carcinoma, e.g. lung or breast, leukaemia
Infection
  Encephalitis or meningitis (mycobacteria, bacteria, fungi)
Vascular
  Hypoxic tissue injury
  Postpartum pituitary necrosis
  Intraventricular haemorrhage
Systemic disease
  Sarcoidosis, Langerhans' histiocytosis
  Extramedullary haemopoesis

Nephrogenic diabetes insipidus
Primary
  Hereditary (X-linked): vasopressin unresponsive
  Renal tubules
Secondary
  Electrolyte disturbance (hypokalaemia, hypercalcaemia)
  Chronic renal disease
  Drugs

DIDMOAD, diabetes insipidus, diabetes mellitus, optic atrophy, neural deafness.

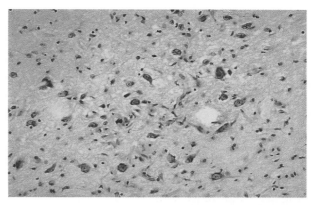

Figure 17.32 *Familial central diabetes insipidus. Marked reduction in the size and number of secretory neurons. The patient, a 70-year-old male with life-long diabetes insipidus and several affected family members, had a serum vasopressin level of 1.5 pg/ml which did not rise with dehydration. (CV.) (Courtesy of Dr C Bergeron, University of Toronto, Toronto, Ontario, Canada.)*

insipidus',[121] of which a significant number is thought to be autoimmune.[367] In occasional cases, magnocellular nuclei appeared morphologically normal but lack vasopressin immunoreactivity.[273] Hereditary diabetes insipidus may also be seen in Wolfram's syndrome,[84] a disorder characterized by atrophy of hypothalamic nuclei, degeneration of the optic nerves, chiasm and tract, as well as degeneration of the pons and cerebellum.[59] Inherited diabetes insipidus also occurs in experimental animals. The Brattleboro rat, despite normal appearing magnocellular neurons, is incapable of vasopressin production,[425] whereas in the Wistar rat, supraoptic neurons are enlarged but the posterior pituitary lacks vasopressin.[393]

involving the infundibular region or median eminence. Low stalk lesions or destruction of the posterior pituitary produces only temporary diabetes insipidus in that a small proportion of axons originating in the supraoptic nucleus terminates at high levels in the median eminence and is consequently spared. Furthermore, destruction of the stalk at the low level permits axonal regeneration to occur.[73] Although approximately 30% of cases are considered to be idiopathic, it should be noted that diabetes insipidus may be an early sign of a hypothalamic disease which only becomes apparent over time.

Hereditary diabetes insipidus is exceedingly rare, representing only 1% of central diabetes insipidus.[26] Several clinical variants occur in man, most being autosomal dominant or sex-linked recessive disorders. From a therapeutic point of view, all are vasopressin responsive. As a group, these are degenerative diseases of magnocellular neurons of both the supraoptic and paraventricular nuclei.[185,247] Affected patients show little response to osmotic stimuli. Autopsy studies are few but demonstrate striking neuronal loss and gliosis[38,51,121] (Fig. 17.33). Similar changes have been described in 'idiopathic diabetes

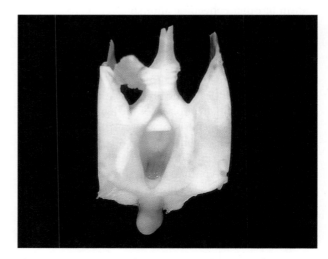

Figure 17.33 *Pituitary dystopia. Coronal section of hypothalamus showing a short pituitary stalk and a rudimentary neural lobe devoid of association with anterior lobe tissue. Incidental finding at autopsy in apparent endocrine-normal elderly female patient.*

Malformations and hamartomas of the pituitary and hypothalamus

ANENCEPHALY

Anencephaly is associated with absence not only of the hypothalamus but also of posterior pituitary tissue. The resulting lack of neurohumoral control is thought to affect the adenohypophysis, which is hypoplastic or absent in half the cases. This does not explain the uniform presence of a pharyngeal pituitary in anencephalics.[149] Nonetheless, the division of anencephaly into premature examples with subnormal body weight and full-term examples of normal body weight is a reflection of the absence or presence of functioning anterior pituitary tissue.[272] Yet unexplained is the frequent paucity of gonadotrophs[315] and absence of corticotrophic cells despite the representation of other functional cell types,[300] an observation suggesting that stimulatory effects of the hypothalamus are not essential for the development of most adenohypophyseal cell types. Ultrastructural degenerative changes have been noted in corticotrophic cells.[131] Lack of a fetal cortex in the adrenal of anencephalics suggests that adrenal hypoplasia in this disorder is pituitary dependent. The gonads and the thyroid gland are usually normal.

PITUITARY DYSTOPIA

This rare anomaly consists of failure of union of the anterior and posterior lobes.[222,358] The posterior lobe remains extrasellar, appears as a nodule on a foreshortened pituitary stalk (Fig. 17.33), and may be either unattached or tenuously associated with the anterior lobe. Pituitary dystopia is usually without clinical significance and represents an incidental autopsy finding. In some instances it may be associated with growth retardation, hypogonadism or other congenital anomalies.

SEPTO-OPTIC DYSPLASIA (DE MORSIER'S SYNDROME)

The features of this rare malformative process include midline abnormalities of the brain, such as aplasia of the septum pellucidum, hypoplasia of the hypothalamus and visual apparatus, agenesis of the corpus callosum, or microcephaly. The syndrome is often incompletely expressed.[268] Endocrinopathy associated with septo-optic dysplasia includes hypothalamic dysfunction (precocious puberty, secondary hypopituitarism) and diabetes insipidus. Pituitary function may occasionally be normal.[68,376] Two immmunocytochemical studies showed no abnormalities of the adenohypophysis.[68,336]

RATHKE'S CLEFT CYST

This non-neoplastic lesion is derived from remnants of Rathke's pouch, the anlage of the adenohypophysis. The pouch arises as an evagination of the stomodeum. In forming the pituitary gland, it comes to fuse with the developing neural lobe. During this process, remnants of the pouch form cleft-like or microcystic spaces at the interface of the anterior and posterior lobes. The vast majority remains examples of asymptomatic microscopic findings (Fig. 17.16), although larger examples are not uncommon (Fig. 17.34).

The slow accumulation of colloid secretion within the lumen occasionally results in the formation of symptomatic cysts. Such lesions typically measure at least 1 cm in diameter and produce not only endocrine but also neurological symptoms, which develop over protracted periods. Approximately 100 cases have been reported.[340,418] Of these, half are intrasellar, 15% are suprasellar and the

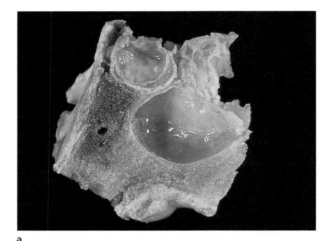

a

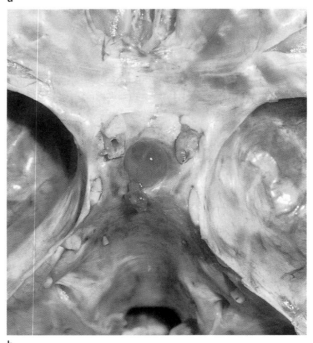

b

Figure 17.34 *Rathke's cleft cysts. Grossly, they may be:* **(a)** *within the sella, or* **(b)** *partly or entirely suprasellar. These thin-walled cysts contain clear to turbid serous to viscid fluid. Unlike craniopharyngioma, calcification is lacking.*

remainder involve both locations.[25] One rare example was reported to reside in the sphenoid bone.[116] Most frequently symptoms include visual disturbance, hypofunction of the gonadal, thyroid or adrenal axis, growth retardation and diabetes insipidus. The latter is evident at presentation in approximately 15% of cases, but may also result from overambitious cyst resection. Hyperprolactinaemia is commonly observed and is a reflection of pituitary stalk compression. On occasion hydrocephalus, aseptic meningitis due to leakage of cyst contents,[399] or superimposed infection with abscess formation[83] is seen. On neuroimaging, the cysts are frequently non-enhancing and lack calcification. Unlike craniopharyngiomas, Rathke's cleft cysts are filled with mucoid, opalescent fluid. Their single-layered epithelium resembles that of the incidental cysts in being columnar and both mucin producing and ciliated (Fig. 17.35). The proportion of these epithelial types varies. On rare occasions, scattered pituitary secretory cells may be seen. Squamous metaplasia is an uncommon finding (Fig. 17.36), as is xanthomatous reaction.[337,439] Cyst rupture may also engender a granulomatous reaction.[337] In occasional cysts, small numbers of neuroendocrine cells may be seen (Fig. 17.37) and immunocytochemistry reveals pituitary hormones. The ultrastructure of Rathke's cleft cyst has been well characterized.[213] Cytological methods may be useful in the intraoperative assessment of sellar region cysts.[392]

In view of the frequent occurrence of incidental pituitary adenomas,[251] it is not a surprise that occasional Rathke's cleft cysts are found in association with pituitary adenoma.[283] Their close association may be the basis of what has been termed a 'transitional tumour'.[187] Abscess formation superimposed upon Rathke's cleft cyst is a rare complication (see Infectious disease, below). A significant minority of cysts recurs,[271] thus, excision, rather than marsupialization, as well as long-term follow-up, are necessary.

The differential diagnosis of Rathke's cleft cyst includes primarily the two variants of craniopharyngioma. They differ from the adamantinomatous variant in that nearly all Rathke's cleft cysts lack calcification, machine-oil content rich in macrophages and cholesterol, complex epithelial patterns, 'wet keratin' and an irregular interface with brain parenchyma. Rathke's cleft cysts differ from the papillary variant of craniopharyngioma in being thin rather than thick walled, in their lack of papillata and abundance of squamous epithelium, and in the frequency of ciliated and mucinous epithelium, which is a very focal feature, at best, in a papillary craniopharyngioma.[71] Lastly, an animal model of Rathke's cleft cyst has recently been developed.[5]

ARACHNOID CYST

Although very infrequent, arachnoid cysts occur within the sella, where they are associated with headache and visual symptoms, and with signs of anterior and pituitary dysfunction.[257]

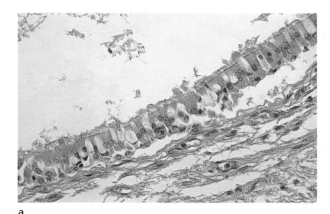
a

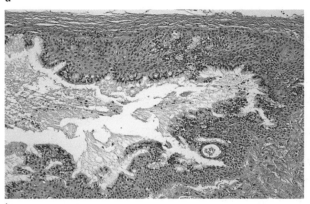
b

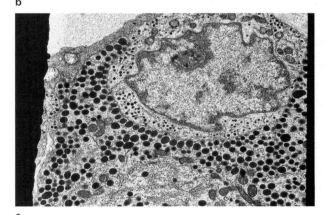
c

Figure 17.35 *Rathke's cleft cysts. Morphologically, they consist of: (a) mucus-producing and ciliated epithelium. (H&E.) (b) Squamoid metaplasia is an uncommon feature. (H&E.) (c) Occasionally, adenohydophyseal secretory cells are seen in keeping with an origin from the pituitary anlage. (Electron micrograph.)*

HYPOTHALAMIC NEURONAL HAMARTOMA

Asymptomatic, usually microscopic, ectopias composed of nearly normal hypothalamic tissue are encountered in approximately 20% of random autopsies. Their statistical association with an increased frequency of endocrinopathy and neoplasia remains unexplained.[381] Occasional examples can be seen with the naked eye (Figs 17.36, 17.37).

Symptomatic hypothalamic hamartomas are rare malformations, the natural history of which is not fully

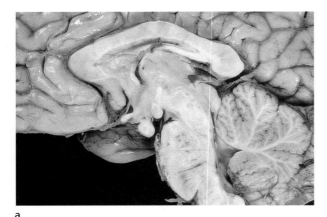

a

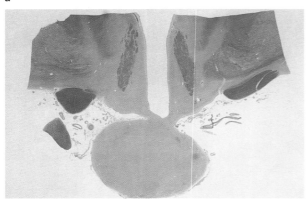

b

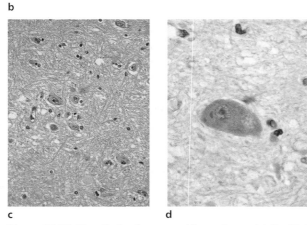

c   d

Figure 17.36 *Hypothalamic neuronal hamartoma. (a) Sagittal section of the whole brain shows a pedunculated lesion suspended from the floor of the third ventricle and lying within the suprasellar space. (Courtesy of Dr PC Burger, Johns Hopkins Medical Institution, Baltimore, MD.) (b) Similar to (a), an incidental finding at autopsy in an adult without an associated endocrinopathy. (LFB/CV.) (c) Histologically, such hamartomas resemble normal hypothalamic tissue and immunostains for releasing hormone. (H&E.) (d) Hormones.*

understood.[243] They vary in size as well as in their relationship to the hypothalamus. Whereas some develop within the hypothalamus, others may occupy the suprasellar region. Occasional examples lie within the interpeduncular fossa, attached only to basilar blood vessels. Most hypothalamic hamartomas occur in young patients.

Symptoms include primarily headache and visual disturbance. Precocious puberty, the most frequent endocrine disturbance, is in some instances due to lesional production of GnRH.[243] One case of acromegaly resulting from production of GRH has also been reported.[22,363] Hypothalamic hamartomas may occasionally be associated with other malformations of the central nervous system (CNS).[139]

Microscopically, hypothalamic hamartomas closely resemble normal hypothalamic tissue wherein mature neurons often lie disposed in clusters within abundant neuropil. Particularly in those hamartomas connected to the hypothalamus by a pedicle, axonal processes are disposed within ill-defined tracts. Immunocytochemical stains show a variety of hypothalamic-releasing hormones within the cytoplasm of neurons (Fig. 17.36). The distinction between hypothalamic hamartoma and gangliocytoma is not well defined (Fig. 17.37). As a rule, glial cells in both lesions are normal appearing. In gangliocytoma, the cellularity exceeds that of normal hypothalamic tis-

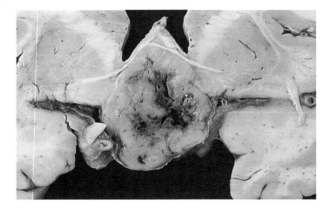

a

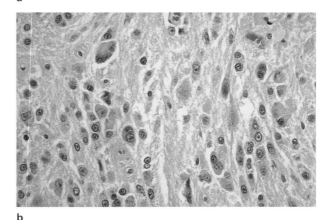

b

Figure 17.37 *Gangliocytoma of the hypothalamus. This rare lesion produced growth hormone-releasing hormone that resulted in acromegaly and was associated with a growth hormone cell adenoma (for clinical details see Ref. 363). (a) Coronal section through the hypothalamic region. (b) Histologically the lesion resembles a hypothalamic hamartoma but is more cellular and shows greater cytological variation. (H&E.)*

sue and the neurons are relatively greater in number, but they exhibit normal cytological and ultrastructural features.[363] Resection, when technically feasible, is curative. In those instances wherein hamartomas are intimately associated with functioning hypothalamic tissue, resection is necessarily subtotal; residual hamartoma tissue grows only slowly if at all.

HYPOTHALAMIC HAMARTOBLASTOMA

Associated with the Pallister–Hall syndrome, a complex, usually lethal condition characterized by pituitary agenesis, hypopituitarism, dwarfism, facial dysformation, postaxial polydactyly, anorectal atresia, renal, pulmonary and cardiac anomalies, the hypothalamic hamartoblastoma differs from the hamartoma described above. Hamartoblastomas are more cellular and they are composed of primitive-appearing, immature neurons lacking atypia or mitotic activity.[61,126] Several familial cases have been reported;[209,386] the mode of inheritance has yet to be determined, but in one instance an unbalanced chromosome translocation was identified.[209] Endocrine evaluation has demonstrated hypothalamic deficiency and pituitary deficits.[386]

Neoplasms and related lesions of the hypothalamus, posterior pituitary and sellar region

A variety of benign and malignant neoplasms affects the hypothalamus and posterior pituitary. Principal among these are craniopharyngioma of both the adamantinomatous and papillary type, meningioma, germ-cell tumours, granular cell tumours, pituicytoma and metastatic tumours. Even salivary gland tumours occur in the sellar region, where they mimic pituitary adenoma.[113]

CRANIOPHARYNGIOMA

In recent years it has become apparent that craniopharyngiomas occur in two clinicopathologically distinct forms.[406] Their clinicopathological and surgical characteristics are the subject of a recent, large series review.[88] Both are thought to be derived from the pituitary anlage from Rathke's pouch. The squamous nests frequently encountered in the pars tuberalis of the pituitary represent an age-related metaplastic change. It occurs primarily in gonadotrophs and ACTH cells[19] and is not a precursor lesion of craniopharyngioma.

Adamantinomatous craniopharyngioma

Representing 5% of intracranial neoplasms in the paediatric age group, this variant of craniopharyngioma shows a peak incidence in the first decade.

Occasional examples have been described in the neonatal period or in senescence. Clinical features include visual disturbance, anterior pituitary dysfunction,

growth retardation, pubertal delay and diabetes insipidus. Increased intracranial pressure is often noted in paediatric patients. The vast majority is suprasellar and nearly half have an intrasellar component (Fig. 17.38). Fully 15% are apparently entirely ectopic examples involving the optic chiasm, sphenoid bone, pharynx and cerebellopontine angle.[120,271,358]

Most craniopharyngiomas are to some extent cystic and calcified. Many exhibit an irregular interface with the brain as well as occasional firm attachment to vascular structures at the base of the brain. Craniopharyngiomas consist of squamous epithelium exhibiting varied, highly characteristic histological patterns (Fig. 17.38). The constituent cells are squamous and include peripherally situated columnar or polygonal cells, and an internal layer of loose-textured element termed 'stellate reticulum'. In some instances, partial simplification of the cyst lining results in the formation of flattened epithelium somewhat resembling that of epidermoid cyst (Fig. 17.38). Diagnostic, even in the absence of the highly typical epithelial element, is a finding of wet keratin, which is entirely different from the flaky keratin of epidermoid cyst (Fig. 17.38). Nodules of wet keratin often show a tendency to dystrophic calcification. The finding of cholesterol-rich, machine oil-like cyst content is strongly suggestive of adamantinomatous craniopharyngioma, as is the finding of calcification, fibrosis or a chronic inflammation, particularly a histiocytic reaction (Fig. 17.38). Intraoperative cytological examination may be diagnostic.[392] Abundant acute inflammation suggests superimposed abscess formation, which is a rare event (see Infectious disease, below). On occasion, cyst fluid and cerebrospinal fluid are found to contain elevations of hCG.[147] The irregular interface of the tumours with brain parenchyma is characterized by intense, fibrillary gliosis, rich in Rosenthal fibres, which in a small biopsy simulates pilocytic astrocytoma (Fig. 17.38). Recurrence after gross total removal is approximately 10–20%. Regrowth of craniopharyngiomas due to operative implantation of tumour remote from the site of the primary tumour is uncommon.[324] Malignant transformation of craniopharyngioma is rare.[278] The focal finding of oestrogen receptor staining in a majority of cases is of uncertain significance.[412]

Papillary craniopharyngioma

In clinical, radiological, and microscopic terms, this only recently characterized variant of craniopharyngioma differs significantly from the adamantinomatous type.[71] It occurs almost exclusively in adults, often involves the third ventricle (Fig. 17.39) and, unlike adamantinomatous tumours, lacks calcification and machine-oil content. Solid portions often have an arborizing appearance, the fibrovascular papillae and cyst surfaces being lined by architecturally simple squamous epithelium (Fig. 17.39). Keratin formation is lacking (Fig. 17.39). Cilia my be seen

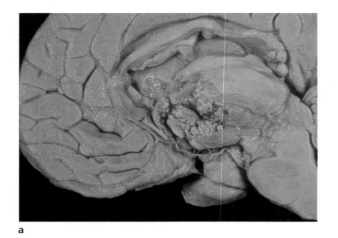

a

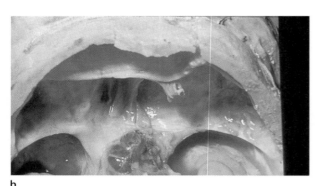

b

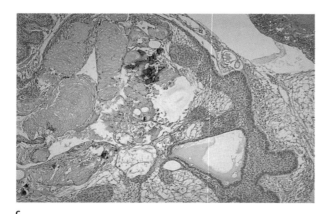

c

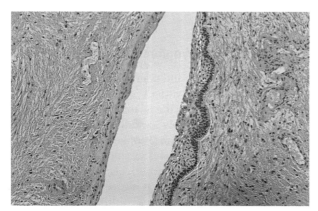

d

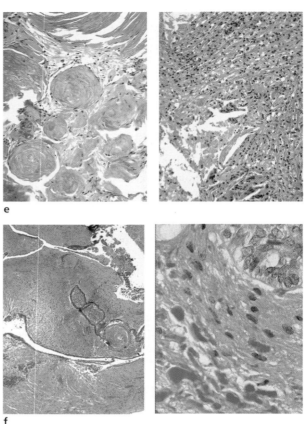

e

f

Figure 17.38 *Adamantinomatous craniopharyngioma. (a) Mid-sagittal cut through brain of a child to reveal a mass in the suprasellar region. (b) Less commonly they are found in the sella. Most present as a thick-walled variably calcified and cystic tumour containing cholesterol-rich debris and thick, brown fluid grossly resembling 'machine oil'. (c) Craniopharyngiomas are histologically complex epithelial tumours. Note the peripheral palisading of nuclei, loose 'stellate reticulum' and the production of 'wet keratin', which frequently undergoes dystrophic calcification. 'Wet keratin' and cholesterol-containing, histocyte-rich debris are typically encountered in the degenerate contents of cranio-pharyngioma. (d) A minority of tumours partly consists of simple squamous epithelium. (H&E.) (e) The finding of 'wet keratin', which differs from the dry, flaky keratin of epidermoid cysts, is diagnostic of carniopharyngioma even in the absence of epithe-lium. (H&E.) (f) The irregular, somewhat infiltrating interface of adamantinomatous tumours with the surrounding brain is associated with intense gliosis, wherein Rosenthal fibres may be sufficiently numerous to mimic pilocytic astrocytoma. (H&E.)*

in occasional examples. Intraoperative cytological exam-ination of the cyst wall may provide an intraoperative diagnosis.[392] The interface of papillary craniopharyngioma with brain parenchyma is often smooth, thus permitting a more ready gross total removal than is the case in adamantinomatous tumours. Although only less than 10% of papillary craniopharyngiomas recur, there are no significant differences in survival between the two variants.[2,71]

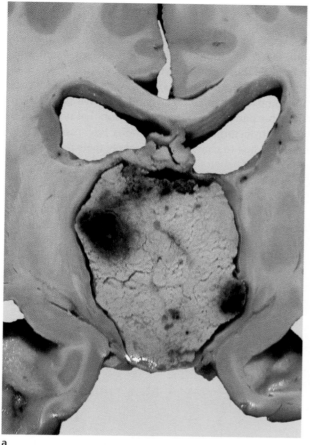

a

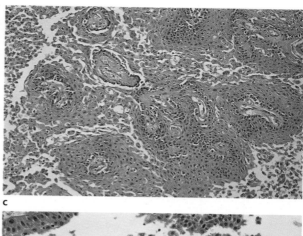

c

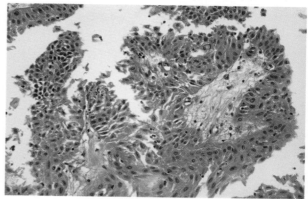

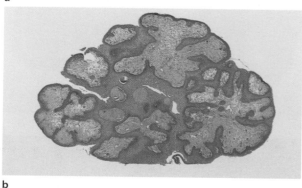

b

Figure 17.39 *Papillary craniopharyngioma. (**a**) Coronal section of the brain through the hypothalamus revealing a highly distinctive lesion that differs from the more common adamantinomatous variant in affecting older patients, more often involving the third ventricle. (**b**, **c**) Microscopically, it has a papillary architecture or (**d**) a simple squamous epithelium. In addition, the papillary variant lacks calcification, keratin production and 'machine-oil' fluid content. (H&E.)*

MENINGIOMA

Approximately 15% of intracranial neoplasms are meningiomas; the majority occurs in adult females in their reproductive years. In the chiasmal and sellar region, approximately 10% of neoplasms are meningiomas.[191,394] Of particular interest are examples arising from the sellar diaphragm (Fig. 17.40) and the tuberculum sellae. Most effectively mimicking pituitary adenomas are meningiomas arising from the inferior leaf of the sellar diaphragm. Such tumours produce primarily temporal hemianopia and hypopituitarism. Sellar region meningiomas, including rare examples arising in the sella[287] or even the pituitary stalk,[133] also have a tendency to produce hyperprolactinaemia by

mechanical effects upon the pituitary stalk. As a result, these endocrinologically non-functioning neoplasms may mimic prolactinoma. The clinical distinction of pituitary adenoma from meningioma is aided by neuro-imaging. Meningiomas demonstrate uniform, bright enhancement on magnetic resonance imaging (MRI), a tumour 'blush' on angiography and a blood supply originating from the ophthalmic segment of the internal carotid artery. The histological spectrum of meningiomas is broad[192] and is discussed elsewhere (see Volume II, Chapter 11). Of importance is the distinction of meningioma variants, be they typical or atypical, from dural haemangiopericytoma, a malignant, non-meningothelial neoplasm. The latter shows a marked tendency to recurrence

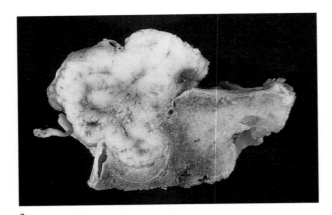

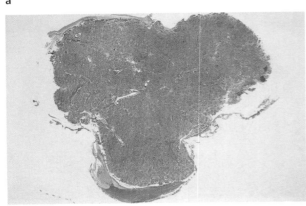

Figure 17.40 *Meningioma of the sellar diaphragm. (a) Sagittal section. Whereas the supra-sellar component results in brain displacement the intrasellar element is seen to compress the pituitary. (b) The relationship between the tumour and the displaced pituitary is best seen on the corresponding whole-mount section. (H&E.)*

and late metastasis.[124] Rare intrasellar examples of haemangiopericytoma have also been reported.[245]

Despite their central location, one recent large series of suprasellar meningiomas reported low perioperative mortality (2%) and morbidity (6%), recurrence (4%) and progression of residual tumour (10%).[322] In contrast, meningiomas of the cavernous sinus are often unresectable owing to invasion of the trigeminal ganglion, carotid artery and pituitary gland.[374]

GLIOMA

Of gliomas affecting the hypothalamus and third ventricular region, the majority is astrocytomas or diffusely infiltrative, low grade fibrillary gliomas. The majority of pilocytic astrocytomas arises within the visual system, particularly the optic chiasm, or the brain parenchyma surrounding the third ventricle. Associated hypothalamic involvement may produce the diencephalic syndrome.[6] Extension of such astrocytomas to involve the pituitary stalk is uncommon and involvement of the neural lobe is rare. Anaplastic transformation or the occurrence of cerebrospinal seeding is rare.[284]

A special subtype of low-grade astrocytoma, arising within and often limited to the posterior pituitary and its stalk, has been termed 'pituicytoma' or 'infundibuloma'.[50,170,339] Although their clinical features somewhat resemble those of pilocytic astrocytoma, their morphological spectrum varies. Of reported cases, most lack the compact and microcystic patterns as well as the Rosenthal fibre and granular body formation that typifies pilocytic astrocytomas.[170] Too few bona fide examples have been studied to characterize precisely their pathology or behaviour. Diabetes insipidus may develop.

Fibrillary astrocytomas more often arise within the cerebral hemispheres or basal ganglia and less frequently involve the hypothalamic region. Widely invasive and prone to high-grade transformation, such tumours are associated with a poor prognosis (see Volume II, Chapter 11). Extension into the pituitary stalk or posterior lobe is rare (Fig. 17.41). As a consequence of radiotherapy for pituitary adenoma or craniopharyngioma, astrocytomas may on occasion arise within the hypothalamic region.[421,423,446] The majority is high grade. The latency period between therapy and the presentation of the

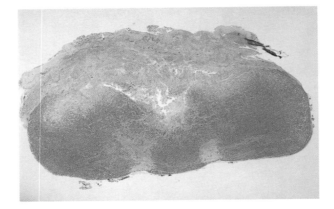

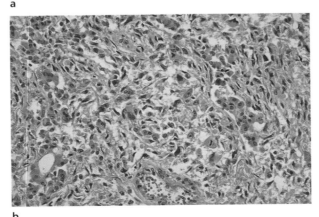

Figure 17.41 *Anaplastic astrocytoma with secondary pituitary involvement. This tumour arose in the parietal lobe of a 35-year-old man, underwent recurrence and spread downwards to involve the hypothalamus. Descent within the pituitary stalk resulted in infiltration of (a) the posterior lobe and (b) the anterior lobe. (H&E.)*

glioma is usually around 10 years. Postirradiation ependymoma[130] and oligodendroglioma[169] are rare.

GRANULAR CELL TUMOURS

Clinically insignificant clusters and minute nodules of granular cells are commonly found in the normal posterior pituitary and stalk, particularly in adults. Termed 'tumourlets,' the nodules occur singly or in multiple form in approximately 15% of autopsy pituitaries[242] (Fig. 17.42). In contrast, symptomatic granular cell tumours are rare.[148,231] Although clinically and radiologically they mimic pituitary adenoma, unlike the latter, granular cell tumours are usually associated with diabetes insipidus. Most are circumscribed lesions, but occasional examples infiltrate surrounding structures. Granular cell tumours consist of sheets and lobules of polygonal to oval cells devoid of mitotic activity. Their cytoplasmic eosinophil-ia and granularity result from the accumulation of PAS-positive lysosomes (Fig. 17.42). Immunocytochemistry demonstrates S-100 protein and CD68 immunoreactivi-ty,[211] as well as α_1-antitrypsin, α_1-antichymotrypsin and cathepsin B.[285] Unlike peripheral granular cell tumours, neurohypophyseal examples lack neuron-specific enolase, myelin basic protein and vimentin staining.[285] Although GFAP immunoreactivity has been demonstrated ultra-structurally,[430] it is generally lacking on light microscopy. Ultrastructurally, the cells contain abundant pleomorphic lysosomes, some engaged in autophagocytosis (Fig. 17.42). Intraoperative bleeding is a common complication. As a rule, gross total resection is curative any recurrences are infrequent. Since these distinctive neoplasms are thought to derive from pituicytes, modified astrocytes normally occurring in the posterior pituitary and its stalk, granular cell tumours may also be considered to be a form of glioma.[53]

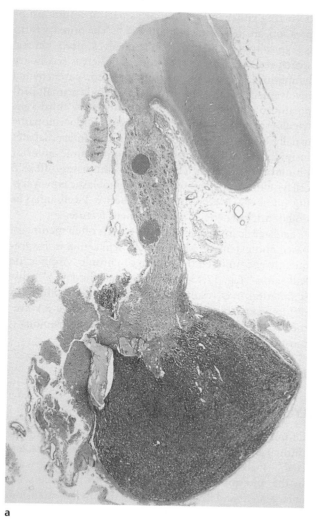

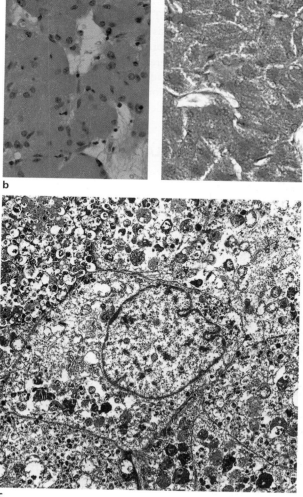

Figure 17.42 *Granular cell tumourlets and tumour.* (**a**) *Mid-sagittal section through the optic chiasm and pituitary showing two granular cell tumourlets within the pituitary stalk. Such incidental autopsy findings are common and are of no clinical significance. (H&E.)* (**b**) *Both asymptomatic and symptomatic granular cell tumours consist of plump eosinophilic cells with granular cytoplasm and often eccentric nuclei (left). (H&E.) Owing to cytoplasmic accumulation of lysosomes, PAS stains (right) are strongly positive.* (**c**) *Electron micrograph showing abundant lysosomes within the cytoplasm of the tumour cells.*

PITUITARY ADENOMA

Whereas macroadenomas with a suprasellar extension often come in contact with the optic chiasm to produce bitemporal hemianopia or compress the pituitary stalk with resultant prolactinaemia, significant hypothalamic dysfunction is uncommon and is generally limited to large examples which displace the hypothalamus and indent the third ventricle. It is of note that diabetes insipidus is rarely a complication of pituitary adenoma. A variety of sellar region tumours may mimic adenoma.[357]

LIPOMA

CNS lipomas, lesions sharing some features of both malformation and neoplasia, are rare. The majority comprises incidental post-mortem findings, some associated with developmental abnormalities. In the hypothalamic region, they are usually encountered between the tuber cinereum and the mamillary bodies.[95] Most consist entirely of adipose tissue, which is readily identified on computed tomographic (CT) scan, whereas others contain other elements such as fibrous tissue, cartilage or bone.[109] Osteolipomas comprise approximately 40% of all suprasellar lipomas.[390] Whereas some lipomas are so intimately associated with the adjacent brain parenchyma as to preclude their total resection, others are suspended from the tuber cinereum by a delicate pedicle. Lipomas are benign.

POSTIRRADIATION NEOPLASIA

Of postirradiation gliomas, most are high-grade astrocytomas;[446] oligodendrogliomas and ependymomas rarely develop. Radiation doses vary greatly. The latency between treatment, often of pituitary adenoma or craniopharyngioma, and the appearance of the induced neoplasm is generally 10 years; the patients are generally young, and the tumours are high grade and involve the temporal lobe.[389]

As a rule, postirradiation neoplasms of the sella and skull base are sarcomas; these include fibrosarcoma, osteosarcoma and unclassifiable, poorly differentiated sarcomas. In many instances, the primary lesion was a pituitary adenoma or retinoblastoma. Fibrosarcomas complicating the treatment of pituitary adenomas are of particular interest in that the sarcoma is often intimately associated with a residual adenoma[313,382] and is locally aggressive rather than metastasizing. Radiation doses responsible for sarcomas are generally greater than 20 Gy. The latency period averages 10 years. Survival after diagnosis is generally 1 year.

METASTATIC NEOPLASMS

Tumours secondarily involving the hypothalamus and posterior pituitary are chiefly carcinomas and haemopoetic tumours (Fig. 17.43). The vast majority is part of disseminated disease. Sarcomas are rare. Symptoms include cranial nerve deficits (70%) and pituitary dysfunction (30%), more often referable to the posterior than to the anterior lobe.

Secondary extension to the pituitary from nearby deposits of metastatic carcinoma or simple compression of these structures is more frequently seen than is direct metastasis (Fig. 17.43). Diabetes insipidus usually results from involvement of the posterior lobe. In rare instances of hormone-producing metastases, such as of neuroendocrine carcinoma, specific forms of endocrinopathy may result from stimulation of the pituitary.[57,87] Selective involvement of the hypothalamus, particularly of the median eminence or of the posterior pituitary or its stalk is uncommon (Fig. 17.43). On rare occasions, pituitary metastases simulate a pituitary adenoma.[49] Most are adenocarcinomas, with breast and renal primaries being frequent. Haemorrhage within the substance of a metastatic deposit may also mimic pituitary apoplexy.

Systemic as well as the primary CNS lymphomas, occurring either in isolation or as part of immunosuppression, are increasing in frequency.[297] The primary form is typically parenchymal and involves deep central structures, such as the basal ganglia, whereas secondary lymphoma is typically meningeal based, parenchymal involvement being a secondary event. Only a small proportion of lymphomas primarily affects the third ventricular region or the hypothalamus. Endocrinopathy usually occurs late in the course and includes diabetes insipidus as well as measurable hypothalamic–anterior pituitary dysfunction. The majority comprises diffuse B cell lymphomas of large-cell or immunoblastic type. Varying numbers of accompanying reactive T-cells may be noted. Angiocentricity is a prominent feature.

Leukaemic involvement of the CNS is often meningeal based and extensive. Myelogenous leukaemia is less frequently encountered than acute or chronic lymphocytic leukaemia (Fig. 17.43). Cerebrospinal fluid (CSF) dissemination may result in the formation of nodular or diffuse ventricular deposits. Although selective involvement of the hypothalamus is rare, diabetes insipidus is most frequently observed.[177,323]

Inflammatory lesions

LYMPHOCYTIC HYPOPHYSITIS

Of non-infectious, inflammatory processes affecting the pituitary, lymphocytic hypophysitis is the best characterized.[413] It consists of a diffuse lymphocytic infiltrate within the anterior lobe, often sufficient to produce sellar enlargement and in some instances suprasellar extension. Clinically and radiologically, the features of lymphocytic hypophysitis closely resemble those of pituitary adenoma. Furthermore, in that prolactin elevation due to pituitary stalk compression is a common accompaniment, the mimicry of prolactinomas is complete and often prompts surgical intervention. In all but a few instances,

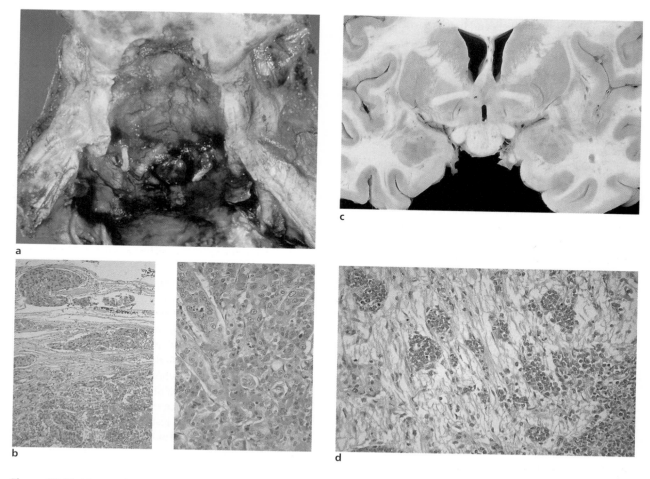

Figure 17.43 *Metastasis to the hypothalamus and sellar region. Metastasis to the sella may, on occasion, mimic pituitary adenoma. (a) The same is true of primary sellar region tumours, such as this plasmacytoma in an elderly patient. (b) Sellar metastases from epithelial tumours such as breast carcinoma typically involve the pituitary and dural investment by direct extension from bone. Involvement of the meninges (left) and infiltration of the anterior pituitary capillary anterior (right) may occur. (H&E.) (c) Metastatic breast carcinoma in a patient with diabetes insipidus. Metastases directly to the hypothalamus are uncommon. (d) Leukaemic involvement of the pituitary, such as this example of myelogenous leukaemia, typically manifests as intravascular and perivascular deposits, seen here in the pituitary stalk. (H&E.)*

lymphocytic hypophysitis affects females, usually late in pregnancy or in the postpartum period. Males are rarely affected.[329] Whereas females average 30 years of age at diagnosis, male patients are somewhat older.

Endocrine abnormalities, including oligomenorrhoea or amenorrhoea in females and impotence in males, are the principal findings. As a rule, variable pituitary hormone deficiencies also result. Diabetes insipidus is very uncommon.[66] On occasion, lymphocytic hypophysitis leads to an isolated hormone deficiency rather than panhypopituitarism.[178] Approximately a quarter of cases were diagnosed at autopsy, a fact that underscores the potentially lethal nature of untreated lymphocytic hypophysitis.

Microscopically, biopsy specimens demonstrate widespread lymphocytic infiltration of the anterior lobe (Fig. 17.44), often punctuated by lymphoid follicle formation. Plasma cells in small number are commonly seen. Fibrosis supervenes in chronic cases and is

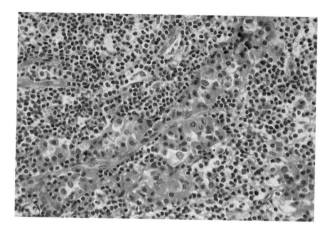

Figure 17.44 *Lymphocytic hypophysitis. A large portion of adenohypophyseal tissue is replaced by large cellular infiltrate consisting of lymphocytes, plasma cells and macrophages. (H&E.)*

occasionally massive. Both T- and B-cells participate in the process. Antipituitary antibodies, usually directed towards PRL cells, may also be detectable. Although most cases of lymphocytic hypophysitis are unassociated with systemic autoimmune disorders, similar inflammatory infiltrates are occasionally noted in either or both the thyroid and adrenal glands. Parathyroid involvement is rare. A rare case of lymphocytic hypophysitis has been reported in association with pulmonary sarcoidosis.[132]

The differential diagnosis of lymphocytic hypophysitis includes primary fungal or mycobacterial infection. By definition, special stains for organisms as well as cultures are negative. Although occasional cases feature scattered or clustered histiocytes, the process cannot be confused with giant cell granuloma of the pituitary, a lesion in which the anterior lobe is largely replaced by numerous sarcoid-like granulomas.

The relationship between lymphocytic hypophysitis and histologically similar infiltrates involving not only the anterior lobe but the posterior lobe, hypothalamus or cavernous sinus,[198,288,305] or ones limited to the neurohypophysis and hypothalamus,[172,434] is unclear.

GIANT CELL GRANULOMA

This rare condition,[173,383] unlike sarcoidosis, selectively affects the anterior pituitary. Involvement of the neurohypophysis is infrequent and of the hypothalamus is rare. Giant cell granuloma affects adults over a wide range of age and shows a definite predilection for females. Unlike lymphocytic hypophysitis, however, no association with pregnancy has been noted. The clinical presentation is one of anterior pituitary failure and/or diabetes insipidus. Giant cell granulomas typically mimic pituitary adenoma with suprasellar extension. Histologically, they consist of non-caseating granulomatous inflammation resembling that of sarcoidosis. Giant cells containing occasional Schaumann bodies, epithelioid macrophages and small numbers of lymphocytes are present (Fig. 17.45). Special stains as well as cultures are, by definition, negative

for fungi and tubercle bacilli. Careful scrutiny of other endocrine organs, such as the thyroid, adrenals or testes, may occasionally reveal scattered giant cells. The pathogenesis of giant cell granuloma is uncertain but is likely to be autoimmune in nature. Panhypopituitarism due to granulomatous inflammation of the sella has been described in association with Crohn's disease.[76]

SARCOIDOSIS

In systemic sarcoidosis, clinical signs of CNS involvement are apparent in approximately 5% of patients. By contrast, pituitary disease is observed in less than 1%[400] and is only rarely the presenting lesion.[218] Neurosarcoidosis demonstrates a female predilection and affects primarily adults. The basal and posterior fossa leptomeninges, the floor of the third ventricle, the infundibulum and the optic system are chiefly affected (Fig. 17.46). Less frequently, ependymal or choroid plexus involvement is evident.

The frequency of hypothalamic involvement approaches 50%. Mass lesions are uncommon and most often affect the temporal lobe. Although half of the patients show no clinical signs of systemic disease, sarcoidosis confined to the CNS is rare. Signs of hypothalamic and pituitary disease are evident in 15–30% of cases and include obesity, hypothermia, somnolence and diabetes insipidus. Sophisticated endocrine testing shows hypothalamic involvement to be reflected as often in adenohypophyseal dysfunction as in diabetes insipidus.[438] Gonadotropic, thyrotropic and adrenocorticotropic functions are usually affected. Not surprisingly, hyperprolactinaemia is common, as a result of pituitary stalk compression. Both on neuroimaging and on gross examination, the process appears to undergo downward extension from the hypothalamus to the infundibulum, pituitary stalk and posterior pituitary. The anterior lobe is rarely extensively affected. As a result, sellar enlargement is uncommon. Isolated involvement of the supraoptic and paraventricular nuclei is a highly unusual but distinctive pattern of disease. The infiltrates of sarcoidosis result in enlargement of the affected structures to form a firm, yellow-appearing lesion rich in non-caseating granulomas. The latter are frequently perivascular. A lymphocytic infiltrate is often seen concentrated around the granulomas. Multinucleated giant cells vary considerably in number, and occasional Schaumann bodies may be seen (Fig. 17.46). The granulomas of sarcoidosis may demonstrate central fibrinoid change which should not be confused with necrosis.[427] Sarcoidal granulomas are also reticulin-rich compared with infectious granulomas of similar size. By definition, special stains are negative for fungi and tubercle bacilli as are cultures. Electron microscopy does not play a role in diagnosis.

Histologically, the infiltrate varies over time. Granulomas and giant cells tend to diminish, whereas fibrosis and calcification become more apparent later (Fig. 17.46). In end-stage disease, only a fibrous scar containing the occa-

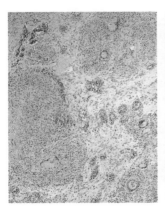
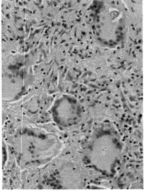

Figure 17.45 *Giant cell granuloma. The adenohypophysis is replaced by granuloma tissue containing several multinucleated giant cells. (H&E.)*

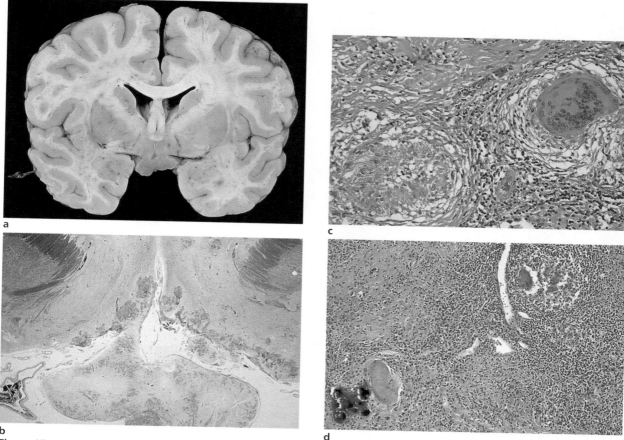

Figure 17.46 *Sarcoidosis. (a) Coronal section showing that the hypothalamus, optic chiasm and posterior pituitary are preferentially affected. (b) The infiltrate typically centres upon the leptomeninges and perivascular spaces. (LFB/CV.) (c) Sarcoidosis shows histological evolution over time, ranging from non-caseating granulomatous inflammation in the early phase to (d) a predominance of chronic inflammation, fibrosis and calcification in advanced disease. (H&E.)*

sional histiocyte may be seen. The diagnosis of neurosarcoidosis therefore depends heavily upon clinical, neuroradiological and microbiological correlation. CSF studies often show mild lymphocytic pleocytosis, moderate elevations of protein as well as immunoglobulins, and a decrease in glucose level. Normal cerebrospinal fluid parameters do not exclude the diagnosis, nor do normal neuroimaging studies.[142]

LANGERHANS' HISTIOCYTOSIS

CNS involvement by Langerhans' histiocytosis is seen in approximately 25% of patients with systemic disease.[227] It occurs almost entirely in association with multifocal osseous lesions,[93,227] but in occasional cases pituitary–hypothalamic involvement precedes systemic disease.[368] Isolated brain involvement is rare[122] and includes hypothalamic and pituitary lesions.[282,289] The most common manifestation is diabetes insipidus, its cause being compression of the pituitary stalk and neurohypophysis by bone disease, extension of infiltrate from bone to pituitary, or lesions of the pituitary and the hypothalamus proper. Associated signs of hypothalamic dysfunction include obesity, hypogo-

nadism and growth retardation. The pituitary stalk and posterior lobe are most severely affected, but involvement of the hypothalamus and occasionally the nearby optic nerves may also be seen (Fig. 17.47). The anterior lobe is typically unaffected. CNS lesions are often multifocal and may arise in a synchronous or metachronous fashion. Neuroimaging typically shows single or multiple foci of contrast enhancement surrounded by limited oedema. The terms Gagel's granuloma, Ayala's disease and hypothalamic granuloma have all been applied to localized Langerhans' histiocytosis of the brain. Its features have been well characterized.[188] Unlike classic histiocytosis X, Letterer–Siwe disease, a rare aggressive variant of Langerhans' histiocytosis, is a diffuse process with prominent meningeal involvement.[94] As part of a multiorgan disease, the diagnosis of Langerhans' histiocytosis does not pose a problem, but atypical presentations such as involvement of the CNS alone may present a diagnostic challenge.[341] Like sarcoidosis, histiocytosis demonstrates morphological variation (Fig. 17.47) and evolution over time. The microscopic spectrum is particularly broad. Active lesions are characterized by histiocytes with foamy cytoplasm accompanied by giant cells, lymphocytes, plasma cells,

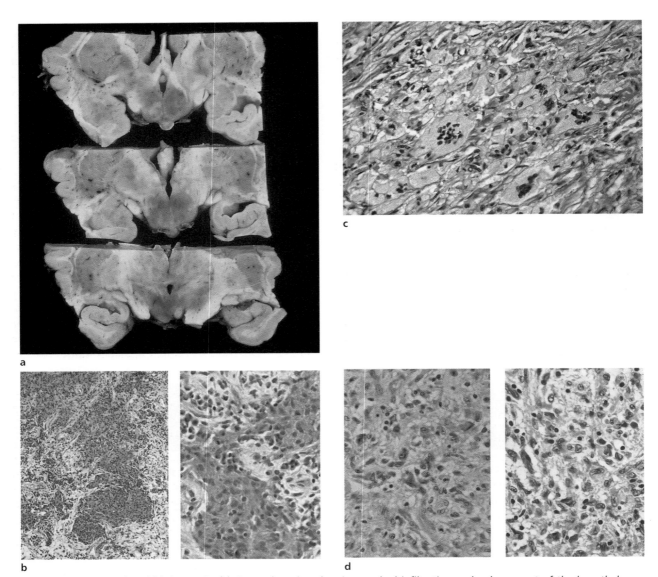

Figure 17.47 *Langerhans' histiocytosis. (a) Coronal section showing marked infiltration and enlargement of the hypothalamus and infundibulum. The patient was a 17-year-old girl with an onset of diabetes insipidus at the age of 4 years. At 16 years there was growth retardation, delayed puberty, diminished visual acuity, panhypopituitarism and emotional lability. At autopsy there was involvement of the skull, lungs and thymus. The cerebellar white matter and dentate nuclei were also affected. (b) The histology is variable, ranging from cohesive carcinoma-like clusters of epitheloid cells (H&E) through (c) sheets of heavily lipidizid and often multinucleate cells (H&E) to (d) loose aggregates of typical Langerhans' cells with folded nuclei (right). (Blue stain.) Their S-100 protein immunoreaction is a helpful diagnostic feature. (ICC for S-100.)*

eosinophils and microglia. Such lesions, given their tendency to perivascular orientation, may suggest encephalitis or a lymphoreticular malignancy. More typical Langerhans' histiocytes demonstrate folded nuclei and stronger cytoplasmic S-100 protein immunoreactivity (Fig. 17.47). Unfortunately, classic Langerhans' cells are not always evident, particularly in largely lipidized lesions. Infiltrates composed of clusters and sheaths of epithelioid histiocytes are less common but may mimic an epithelial neoplasm. Ultrastructural studies may not demonstrate diagnostic Birbeck granules in all cases. (Birbeck granules, the diagnostic markers of both normal and abnormal Langerhans' cells, are 34-nm-wide rod-shaped tubular intracytoplasmic structures with a zipper-like central core.[94]) Often accompanying the infiltrates of histiocytosis X is remarkable gliosis which, when selectively sampled, may be mistaken for astrocytoma. Late-stage disease is accompanied by progressive fibrosis, a finding most apparent in patients who have received radiotherapy.

MISCELLANEOUS

Ostensibly non-infectious examples of chronic, necrotizing infundibulohypophysitis[4] have recently been described; their nature is not known. Diabetes insipidus has also been reported in association with Wegener's granulomatosis.[333,338] Plasma cell granuloma also affects the sellar region.[221]

Infectious disease

Various infectious processes affect the hypothalamus and pituitary gland. These include bacteria, mycobacteria, spirochetes, fungi, and protozoa. Although a complete discussion of the spectrum and their associated tissue reactions is the subject of Chapters 1–3 in Volume II, clinicopathological relationships pertinent to infections of the hypothalamus and pituitary will be addressed.

Viral infections of the hypothalamus occur almost always in association with encephalitis. Endocrine abnormalities are late manifestations and may be transient or permanent. Documented examples include encephalitis lethargica, the hypothalamus being somewhat preferentially affected, polio,[24] coxsackie,[125] influenza A,[210] varicella,[229] and herpes simplex viruses[210,402] (Fig. 17.48).

Bacterial infection, most often meningitis, only rarely results in hypothalamic dysfunction, usually diabetes insipidus. In most cases, the resulting surface fibrosis of the tuber cinereum does not produce endocrine abnormalities. Abscesses may occur in the setting of sepsis or septic embolism. The hypothalamus may also be infected by direct extension of the infectious process from nearby tissues, usually accessory sinuses.[262] Organisms implicated include β-haemolytic streptococcus, pneumococcus and, in the neonate, *Listeria monocytogenes*.

Whereas the hypothalamus is rather infrequently involved by bacterial infection, pituitary abscess is not as rare. Posterior lobe microabscesses are a common preterminal complication. Such lesions are clinically insignificant and are found incidentally at autopsy. In contrast, abscesses centring upon the anterior lobe are of clinical importance.[373] Associated morbidity and mortality are high. They simulate pituitary adenoma, from which they differ by the frequent association with diabetes insipidus. Symptoms of infection are lacking unless meningitis or nearby infection accompanies the abscess. Although the source of infection may not be apparent, some are asso-

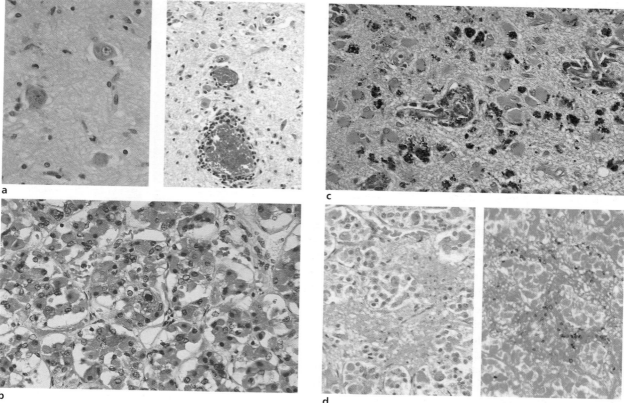

Figure 17.48 *Infections. (a) With few exceptions viral infections are asymptomatic. The fatal case of rabies infection demonstrates cytoplasmic Negri bodies within neurosecretory neurons of the hypothalamus. (H&E.) Courtesy of Dr I Felix, Hospital Zo de Nov, ISSTE, Mexico City, Mexico. (b) Cytomegalovirus in a patient with AIDS may affect pituitary secretory cells. (H&E.) With permission from Dr MH Oelbaum. (c) Whipple's disease. The infiltrate consists of histiocytes with a distinct tendency for perivascular accumulation. The cells contain strongly PAS-positive bacilli. Scattered extracellular organisms are also seen. (PAS.) (d) Rarely in patients with AIDS there may be pneumocystis infection of the pituitary. (Left: H&E; right: silver-strained.) With permission from Dr MH Oelbaum.*

ciated with sinusitis, meningitis or cavernous sinus thrombophlebitis. Occasional cases represent postoperative complications of adenomectomy.[334] Pituitary abscess may also arise within or complicate sellar region cysts and neoplasms.[48,83,279,291] Pituitary abscess rarely presents with apoplexy. Since infarction of a pituitary adenoma may in some instances be associated with polymorphonuclear leukocyte infiltration, it enters into the differential diagnosis of pituitary abscess.[43]

Primary Whipple's disease of the CNS is rare;[1] brain involvement almost always occurs as part of multisystem infection. It includes hypothalamic dysfunction evidenced by hypersomnia, hyperphagia, and endocrinopathy.[306] Whipple's disease in the CNS affects primarily the grey matter to produce indistinct, yellow, granular-appearing lesions, necrosis, microglial proliferation and astrocytosis. Sites of predilection include the basal ganglia, the temporal lobe and the cerebellum. The organism has been classified as *Tropheryma whippelii*, a PAS-positive, rod-shaped bacterium which in affected tissues is seen to accumulate in large numbers within macrophages. The latter are most numerous in perivascular spaces (Fig. 17.48). Free bacteria lack strong PAS reactivity (see also Volume II, Chapter 3).

Mycobacterial infection of the hypothalamus and sellar region, a now uncommon problem, was usually secondary to tuberculous meningitis[304] (Fig. 17.48). Isolated pituitary or hypothalamic involvement is rare.[79,310] Secondary arteritis is a frequent accompaniment that results in microinfarcts of the hypothalamus and pituitary stalk. Diabetes insipidus is a far more frequent complication than is anterior pituitary dysfunction. Massive necrotizing granulomas (tuberculomas) may also been seen (Fig. 17.49). Intrasellar examples mimic pituitary adenoma.[325] The diagnosis of acute tuberculosis is easily made. In contrast, chronic tuberculosis poses a diagnostic problem (Fig. 17.49); most often the lesions consist of encapsulated intrasellar masses with central necrosis, cholesterol deposits, chronic inflammation and calcification. Although such an end-stage lesion typically results from organization of a tuberculoma, it may be mimicked by syphilitic gumma[34,293] and by rare examples of craniopharyngioma showing similar involutional changes. Associated pituitary destruction may be extensive.

Fungal abscesses of the pituitary are very uncommon, most being due to *Aspergillus* or *Mucor* species. *Candida albicans* is rarely implicated, particularly in the absence of immunodeficiency.[135] Infections associated with immunosuppression are also increasing in frequency owing primarily to the increased use of immunosuppressive drugs and the spread of the acquired immunodeficiency syndrome (AIDS).[354] Associated infections include fungal lesions such as cryptococcosis or even pneumocystis (Fig. 17.49). Parasitic infections such as toxoplasmosis[258,277] or cysticercosis[46] may also affect the sellar region. Infectious diseases and other lesions involving the pituitary in the setting of AIDS have been documented.[269,354]

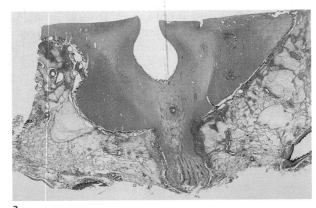

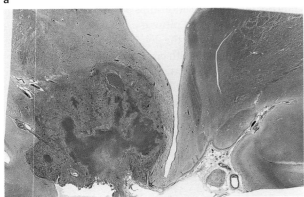

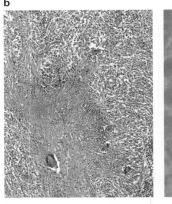
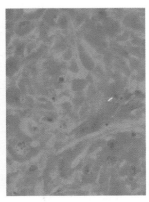

Figure 17.49 *Tuberculosis. (a) Preferentially involves the base of the brain and may manifest as a diffuse leptomeningeal infiltrate which eventuates as a dense fibrous scar. (H&E.) (b) May present as a mass ('tuberculoma') often associated with leptomeninges. Specimen from a 42-year-old man with a 1-year history of neurological symptoms. (LFB/CV.) (c) Organisms within the typically necrotizing granuloma may be difficult to demonstrate. (Left: H&E; right: auramine rhodamine preparation.)*

Metabolic disorders

WERNICKE'S ENCEPHALOPATHY

Thiamine deficiency is the best known nutritional disorder affecting the CNS.[328] Its clinical manifestations are in

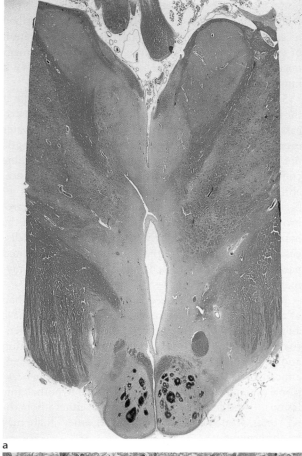

a

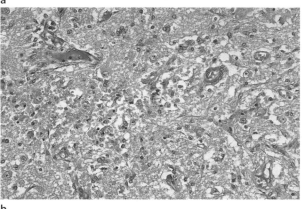

b

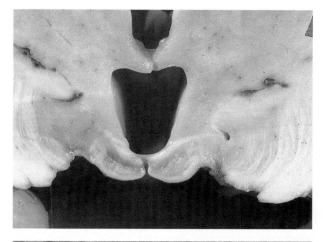

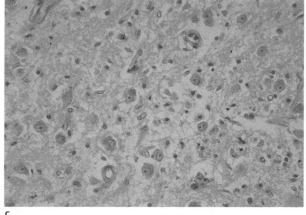

c

Figure 17.50 *Wernicke's encephalopathy: acute and chronic. (a) Early features include hyperaemia and petechial haemorrhage, as seen in the coronal whole-mount section. (LFB/CV.) (b) Histologically, there is capillary proliferation, red blood cell extravasation and infiltration by histiocytes. (H&E.) (c) In the chronic phase, the mamillary bodies contract (top), and there is neuronal loss, gliosis and siderosis (bottom). (LFB/CV.)*

large part ophthalmological (Wernicke's encephalopathy) or psychiatric (Korsakoff's syndrome). Their neuropathological basis has been characterized.[128,419,428] Although the changes in Wernicke's encephalopathy occur primarily in association with chronic alcoholism, they have also been noted in patients with uraemia, requiring dialysis and parenteral nutrition, and with gastrointestinal disease (see p. 610). The clinical and morphological severity of the disorder varies greatly. The anatomical distribution and morphology of the lesions resemble those induced in chronic experimental alcohol administration.[223] Primarily affected are the mamillary

bodies, hypothalamic nuclei surrounding the third ventricle, periventricular portions of the thalamus, the periaqueductal region, the colliculi, fornices and the inferior olives. Grossly, the lesions of Wernicke's encephalopathy vary in appearance depending upon disease stage. Acute, phase lesions are often more widespread than chronic lesions. Acute-lesions are characterized by haemorrhage, whereas chronic ones demonstrate tissue shrinkage and brown discoloration (Fig. 17.50). Histological features (Fig. 17.51) show striking prominence of the microvasculature, axonal and myelin loss in excess of neuronal dropout, as well as oedema. The abnormal capillaries

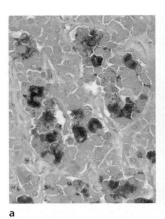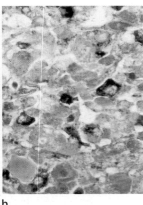

a   b

Figure 17.51 *Haemochromatosis. In systemic iron overload there may be selective deposition of iron in the pituitary gonadotrophs. (a) Prussian blue iron reaction. (b) Double staining for iron and ICC for LH.*

demonstrate endothelial hyperplasia and the accumulation of adventitial macrophages. Perivascular interstitial haemorrhage underlies the petechial haemorrhages. As vascular changes and oedema diminish in chronic disease, only cystic changes, neuronal loss, gliosis and haemosiderin deposition remain (Fig. 17.52). The anatomical basis of Korsakoff's syndrome, although not always apparent, has been related to morphologically similar lesions affecting the dorsomedial thalamus.[244]

Thiamine deficiency appears to be the basis of the lesions of Wernicke's encephalopathy, but the distribution of the lesions has been linked to that of serotoninergic neurons[318] as well as to the high level of transketolase, a thiamine-requiring enzyme, within neurons in these regions.[44] Whether due to a low intake, poor absorption, rapid utilization or increased excretion, deficiency of thiamine results in lesions the topography of which is reflected in decreased glucose utilization (see also Chapter 10, this Volume).

Haemochromatosis

As noted previously, iron overload states result in siderosis of gonadotrophs, which in some instances result in hypogonadism of the anterior pituitary rather than of hypothalamic origin.[36] In one series, half of the patients with haemochromatosis had hypogonadism and other endocrine impairments were also noted[137] (Fig. 17.53). Reversal of hypogonadism may follow iron depletion.[110]

Degenerative diseases

Neurofibrillary tangles and senile plaques are observed in approximately 75% of cases of Alzheimer's disease. Involved structures include the mamillary bodies as well as the tuberal, posterior and suprachiasmatic nuclei.[276,356,405] The cytoskeletal changes within the hypothalami of Alzheimer's patients have been described recently.[426] The degree to which the content and secretion of vasopressin as well as neuron numbers within magnocellular nuclei are affected by Alzheimer's disease is not known (see Volume II, Chapter 4).

Several endocrine abnormalities, most apparent only at the biochemical level, have been noted in Parkinson's disease. These include disturbed circadian control of water excretion and blood pressure related to supraoptic nucleus pathology,[12] diminished hypothalamic dopamine content, dysautonomia and temperature intolerance, abnormal GH dynamics, abnormal serum levels of β-endorphin and somatostatin, and abnormalities of cerebrospinal fluid MSH levels.[349] Lewy bodies occur in the hypothalamic nuclei in nearly all cases of Parkinson's disease.[217] This is also true of the dopaminergic arcuate and paraventricular nuclei, which do not show any loss of pigmented cells[250] (see Volume II, Chapter 5).

In Huntington's disease, affected individuals and half of asymptomatic first-degree relatives are found to have an abnormality of prolactin secretion.[134] In infantile neuroaxonal dystrophy, rare patients may exhibit emaciation and endocrine abnormalities related to severe hypothalamic involvement.[274] In the Riley-Day syndrome, an occasional patient may have extensive bilateral hypothalamic lesions,[299] and in hypothalamic atrophy, either idiopathic[138] or associated with Wolfram's syndrome,[59] there may be abnormalities.

Vascular diseases

With the exception of localized processes such as saccular aneurysm, vascular lesions of the hypothalamus usually arise as part of diffuse cerebrovascular disease,[186] intracerebral or subarachnoid haemorrhage, hypotensive shock, increased intracranial pressure or trauma. In most instances, their effects upon the hypothalamus are irreversible.

Saccular aneurysms, particularly those of the cavernous sinus segment of the internal carotid artery, may mimic pituitary adenoma (Fig. 17.52). Hypopituitarism results in most cases and, despite surgical intervention, is irreversible.[435] Such aneurysms have been described as a complication of yttrium-90 implantation for pituitary adenoma.[252] Aneurysms of the circle of Willis may also mimic pituitary adenoma with suprasellar extension. Some deeply indent the third ventricle. By compressing either the pituitary stalk or its vasculature, such lesions produce pituitary dysfunction. The hypothalamus may be secondarily affected by ischaemic necrosis, most lesions being less than 5 mm in size. Some 60% of ruptured intracranial saccular aneurysms are associated with hypothalamic haemorrhage or ischaemic necrosis.[70] Seemingly selective petechial haemorrhage may affect the supraoptic nuclei; it is uncertain whether this is due to reflex motor disturbances accompanying aneurysm rupture or to venous back-pressure produced by haemorrhage in the chiasmatic cistern.[70] In any case, destruction of these nuclei is uncommon. Although saccular aneurysms are usually identified by radiological methods, their thrombosis may frustrate an angiographic diagnosis. Limited biopsies of such lesions typically show degenerative chronic inflammatory changes within the aneurysm wall and its surroundings, thus precluding definitive diagnosis (Fig. 17.52). False aneurysm of the cavernous carotid artery has been described as a complication of transsphenoidal surgery.[326]

The best known and most thoroughly studied effect of hypovolaemic shock on pituitary and hypothalamic function is postpartum pituitary necrosis (Fig. 17.53). The direct effects of hypovolaemic shock include primarily spasm of arterioles of the tuber cinereum and pituitary stalk, followed by thrombosis of portal blood vessels and anterior pituitary capillaries. Although the anterior lobe of the pituitary is most severely affected,[379] posterior lobe involvement may also be seen.[3] Involvement of the

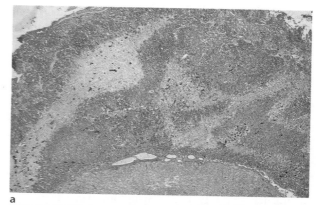

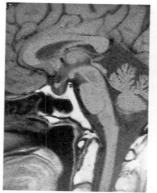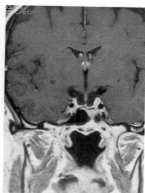

Figure 17.53 *Acute Sheehan's syndrome. (a) There is extensive confluent necrosis of the adenohypophysis. (b) MRI sagittal section of the pituitary shows marked atrophy of both the anterior lobe and posterior lobe: S, pituitary stalk. There is virtual absence of the pituitary gland and apparent elongation of its stalk in a chronic case. Reproduced with permission from Treip CS. The hypothalamus and pituitary gland. In: Blackwood W, Corsellus JAN eds. Greenfield's Neuropathology. London: Edward Arnold, 1976.*

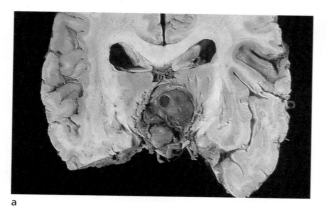

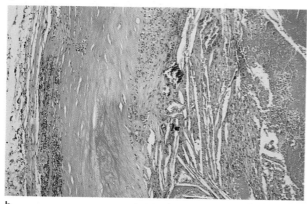

Figure 17.52 *Saccular aneurysm. (a) Arising from the basilar artery in a 48-year-old woman, the aneurysm displaced the hypothalamus and extended into the third ventricle. (b) A biopsy of such an aneurysm, particularly when thrombosed due to the fibrous nature of its wall and cholesterol-rich content, may be confused with other cystic or necrotic lesions. (H&E.) Courtesy of Dr PC Burger, Johns Hopkins University, Baltimore, MD, USA.*

supraopticohypophyseal and paraventriculohypophyseal tracts results in magnocellular nuclear atrophy.

Infarction of the anterior pituitary is a recognized complication of increased intracranial pressure;[74] the posterior lobe is least frequently affected. As an idiopathic lesion, isolated posterior lobe necrosis is rare.[266]

In approximately 90% of cases, subarachnoid haemorrhage is accompanied by ischaemic lesions of the hypothalamus. It is thought that arterial spasm, mediated by dysfunction of the autonomic hypothalamus, underlies these lesions.[437] Thrombotic or septic emboli as well as fat emboli rarely produce hypothalamic infarction.

Whereas hypothalamic infarction is a rare complication of temporal arteritis,[96] lesions have been described in moyamoya disease.[295] Haemorrhagic necrosis may be seen in disseminated intravascular coagulation[119] as well as thrombotic thrombocytopenic purpura.[259]

Although petechiae within the posterior lobe of the pituitary are a common autopsy artefact, petechial haemorrhage in the hypothalamus, particularly when associated with microglial and astrocytic reaction, may explain the occurrence of hypothalamic–pituitary coma.[436] Primary haematoma of the sella is rare.[346]

Studies of the hypothalamus in hypertension suggest the occurrence of hypertrophy of supraoptic and paraventricular neurons, a change which may correlate with increased vasopressin secretion.[320]

PITUITARY APOPLEXY

Massive haemorrhage with or without accompanying infarction of a pituitary adenoma represents a surgical emergency[41,90,261] (Fig. 17.54). Symptoms typically include headache (95%), vomiting (69%) and predominantly visual disturbance due to chiasmal compression.[41] The process may be either clinically apparent or abrupt or may be a subclinical event evidenced by the finding of focal organizing necrosis or fibrosis associated with haemosiderin deposition, or of cysts within an adenoma. Such changes may be seen in 10–20% of adenomas. Children are rarely affected.

Although pituitary apoplexy occurs most often in large, non-functioning adenomas, all immunotypes may be affected.[90] Even apoplexy in a small tumour may be clinically catastrophic. Both non-treated and previously radiated tumours are subject to haemorrhage. On occasion, apoplexy results in cure of a microadenoma. Specimens typically consist of blood and necrotic tumour, the latter being difficult to identify without the application of special stains, such as a reticulin preparation, which shows the underlying vascular pattern of adenoma (Fig. 17.54). Immunostaining is generally not worthwhile since non-specific reactivities are the rule. The basis for haemorrhage into adenomas is unclear. Although the principal factor appears to be tumour size, mechanical effects such as compression or traction upon blood vessels may play a role. Inherent abnormalities in the structure of adenoma blood vessels may also be implicated.[145,202] The recent demonstration of tissue factor in pituitary adenomas, a substance implicated in systemic coagulopathy in cancer patients and in proliferative and invasive activities of tumour cells, suggests that it may contribute to vascular events such as infarction and haemorrhagic infarction in pituitary adenomas.[281] On rare occasions apoplexy occurs in an ectopic adenoma,[292] a pituitary metastasis,[228] or a sellar abscess,[220] and may be precipitated by endocrine stimulation testing.[296]

Physical injury

THERAPEUTIC STALK SECTION

Transection of the pituitary stalk, a surgical procedure once undertaken to inhibit hypothalamic stimulation of the anterior pituitary, is no longer performed. The result was highly variable anterior pituitary necrosis as well as characteristic alterations in the neural lobe, pituitary stalk and magnocellular nuclei. Whereas anterior pituitary changes are rapid, those affecting the hypothalamo-hypophyseal tract undergo sequential development over time.[73] The posterior lobe and distal pituitary stalk undergo marked atrophy due to the loss of continuity of nerve fibres. Changes in the proximal stalk, after an initial phase of localized venous infarction and necrosis of the nerve fibres, consist of an attempt to reform a rudimentary neural lobe at the proximal margin, a feature also noted to occur in experimental animals.[82] Changes in the hypothalamus are notable at 1 month and consist of retrograde degeneration and a 50% loss of neurons within the supraoptic nuclei. Given their mixed composition, the paraventricular nuclei are less obviously affected. Although no appreciable loss of neurosecretory substances is apparent, loss of magnocellular neurons may approach 90% at 6 months (Fig. 17.32). Neuronal hormone content becomes significantly reduced by 2 years. Changes similar to those of therapeutic stalk section are noted after hypophysectomy. The effect of stalk transection upon the anterior pituitary is hypopituitarism, endocrine abnormalities being most apparent in gonadal, adrenal and

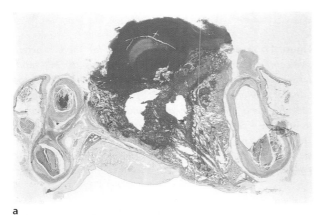

a

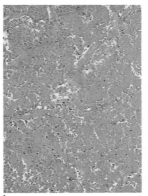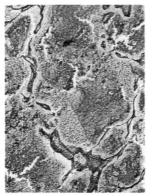

b

Figure 17.54 *Pituitary apoplexy. (a) Whole-mount coronal section through the sella showing acute massive haemorrhaging within a macroadenoma. (H&E.) (b) Left: microscopy revealing blood and tumour necrosis. (H&E.) Right: silver stains serve to highlight the stromal architecture of the adenoma and aid in diagnosis. (Reticulin.)*

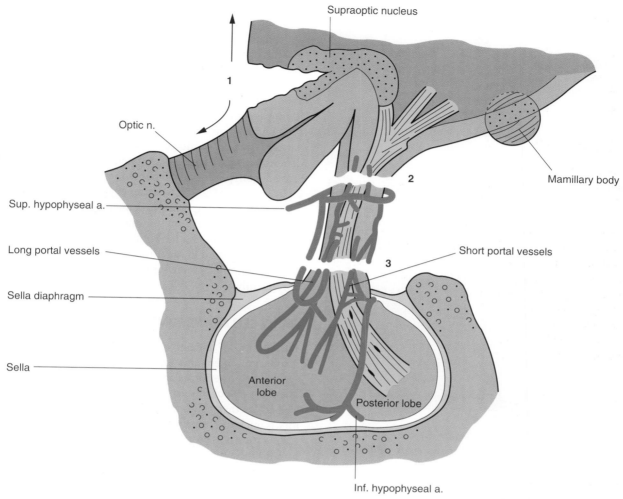

Figure 17.55 *Mechanisms of hypothalamic–pituitary damage in head injury. There are three principal patterns: (a) Tearing of the supraoptic nucleus in deceleration injury is due in part to firm anchoring of the optic nerve at its foramen. (b) High stalk disruption with accompanying injury to the hypophysial anterior ring and its branches results in inferior hypothalamic infarction, with surviving patients often magnifying diabetes insipidus. (c) Low stalk disruption results in damage to long portal blood vessels with resultant infarction of much of the anterior lobe as well as atrophy of the posterior lobe, the hypothalamus being spared. Modified from Treip CS. The hypothalamus and pituitary gland, In: Blackwood W, Corsellis JAN eds.* Greenfield's neuropathology. *London: Edward Arnold, 1976.*

thyroid function. Although GH secretion is less affected, traumatic stalk transection at birth may underlie some cases of pituitary dwarfism.[189] PRL levels are either unaffected or elevated after pituitary stalk section and the resultant loss of dopamine delivery. Diabetes insipidus is permanent.

TRAUMA

The effects of head injury upon the hypothalamus and pituitary are varied in both nature and extent. Haemorrhage and ischaemia may be focal or diffuse and may affect the hypothalamus, pituitary stalk, neural lobe, anterior pituitary or a combination of sites[75,197] (Fig. 17.55). Most frequently seen are anterior lobe infarction and posterior lobe haemorrhage, ischaemia and haemorrhage in the anterior hypothalamus, and destruction of the pituitary stalk. Avulsion of the pituitary stalk with resultant interruption of pituitary blood supply is more often seen than is direct pituitary injury. The features of post-traumatic hypopituitarism are similar to those of surgical stalk transection.[92] Although post-traumatic haemorrhage into the neural lobe occurs with some frequency, extensive infarction is uncommon.[197] At autopsy, careful examination of the brain is required to reveal underlying lesions that may be obscured by accompanying haemorrhage. Since neural lobe damage is usually limited, post-traumatic diabetes insipidus is typically transient. Permanent post-traumatic diabetes insipidus indicates damage at a higher level than the pituitary stalk, either to the infundibulum or to the hypothalamus. In instances of post-traumatic hypothalamic injury, disruption and

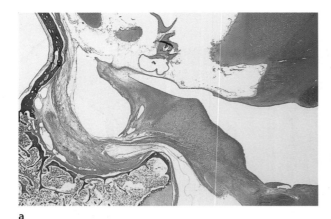

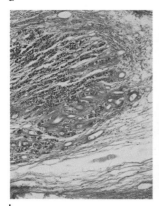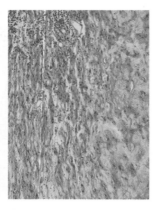

Figure 17.56 *Irradiation. (a) Sagittal whole-mount section showing diffuse atrophy of the hypothalamus, pituitary stalk and pituitary. (LFB/H&E.) (b) Left: The anterior lobe shows striking loss of secretory cells and fibrosis; right: the pituitary stalk shows loss of nerve fibres and extensive gliosis. (H&E.) Courtesy of Dr PC Burger, Johns Hopkins Medical Institution, Baltimore, MD, USA.*

haemorrhage in the supraoptic nuclei and the optic tracts may develop. This pattern of hypothalamic–visual system injury is a reflection of the proximity of these structures and the fact that the visual system, tethered at the optic nerve, is exposed to shearing stresses during deceleration injury. Only a few reports of acute and chronic endocrine effects after head injury have been published.[33,80,92,190] Their relation to prognosis has also been studied.[78] Direct injury to the pituitary, as by bullet wound, is rarely seen; the clinicopathological features of eight cases have been documented[241] (see also Chapter 14, this Volume).

RADIATION INJURY

In the course of treatment of extracranial, brain or sellar region neoplasms, the hypothalamus may be exposed to high doses of radiation. This is particularly true in the case of pituitary adenoma, craniopharyngioma or glioma. Effects include both direct tissue injury and the induction of postirradiation neoplasms.

The degree to which the hypothalamus or the hypothalamic–pituitary axis is affected varies depending upon the distribution of radiation and its dose. Abnormalities may affect multiple functions or may be relatively limited. Examples of the latter include growth retardation,[375] and the development of subtle biochemical abnormalities. The latter may be apparent on dynamic testing as soon as 1 year after irradiation.[214] The frequency of endocrinopathy appears to be dose related: 80% of patients treated to doses exceeding 40 Gy developed deficits between 2 and 3 years later.[348] Atrophy of neural and adenohypophyseal tissues is the principal morphological finding (Fig. 17.56). Parenchymal radionecrosis is an uncommon complication, being seen most often after radiation for sellar region tumours, particularly pituitary adenomas. Although the optic nerves and chiasm are frequently exposed to radiation, particularly in the treatment of pituitary adenoma, they are injured only infrequently.

EMPTY SELLA SYNDROME

The finding of a relatively empty sella, with the sellar diaphragm open and the flattened pituitary pressed against the posterior sellar floor, is not uncommon; its frequency is 5% of unselected autopsies. The nature of the lesion, whether malformative or due to mechanical factors, is unclear. The primary form of empty sella syndrome results from the protrusion of an arachnoidal diverticulum into the sella through a defective sellar diaphragm. Chronic compression of the pituitary gland results in its flattening and inferoposterior displacement. Rhythmic pulsations of CSF presumably contribute to the effect. No aetiological role has specifically been attributed to increased intracranial pressure (Fig. 17.57). The primary empty sella is seen most often in middle-aged females who may be hypertensive and obese. Headache is a common symptom. As a rule, no endocrinopathy is apparent. Endocrine hypofunction and hyperprolactinaemia due to traction on the pituitary stalk are uncommon.[181] Children are infrequently affected; they exhibit a higher incidence of secondary empty sella (15%) and of endocrine (66%) and visual (47%) abnormalities.[67] Owing to the relative frequency of incidental pituitary adenomas, it is not surprising that an occasional example may be associated with adenoma.[112] Rarely, visual disturbance may result from intrasellar prolapse of the optic chiasm. Histology shows compression of the gland but the full spectrum of immunoreactive adenohypophyseal cells is still evident.[37]

A secondary form of empty sella syndrome most often occurs postoperatively or after radiation therapy of a pituitary adenoma, when the intracranial subarachnoidal space extends into the sella to occupy dead space. Secondary empty sella may also occur after spontaneous infarction or involution of a pituitary adenoma.

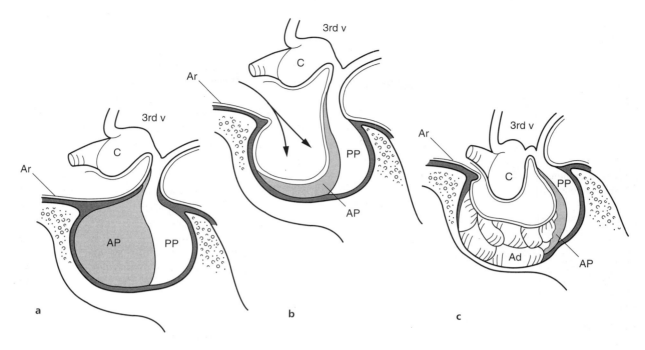

Figure 17.57 *Empty sella syndrome. Schematic representation of (a) the normal relationship of the subarachnoid space relative to the sella and its contents, (b) the primary empty sella wherein an arachnoid diverticulum enters the sella to compress the gland posteroinferiorly, and (c) the secondary empty sella wherein sellar contents, either normal or neoplastic, undergo destruction to vacate the sella.*

HYDROCEPHALUS

Chronic hydrocephalus may result in dysfunction of the hypothalamic–pituitary axis, specifically precocious puberty, amenorrhoea,[265] abnormalities of temperature control,[123] diabetes insipidus, and abnormalities of autonomic regulation and biological rhythms.[302] Effects of chronic hydrocephalus include enlargement of the third ventricle with resultant compression of surrounding parenchyma. With time, the basal hypothalamus may be transformed into a thin membrane, and histologically there is loss of nuclear architecture, gliosis and occasional loss of neurons. The latter may be the result of vascular compression and chronic ischaemia.

Pituitary adenomas

Benign adenomas represent the overwhelming majority of adenohypophyseal lesions. They are common, and small, incidental adenomas occur in up to 20% of pituitary glands removed at autopsy.[55,251,263] Based on neuroimaging data grade I adenomas are intrapituitary 'microadenomas' with a diameter of less than 10 mm. Grade II adenomas are larger than 10 mm, but are still contained within the intact sella. Grade III adenomas cause focal sellar erosion, whereas grade IV tumours may invade any parasellar structure including the brain.[201]

Every cell type gives rise to one or more histological types of adenoma.[206] The reason for the existence of different phenotypes with the same hormonal function is not clear. It may be the result of variations in genetic programming, receptor status and regulatory influences within the same cell population.

Adenomas display a limited number of histological patterns, none of which is specific or unique to a particular histological type.[201] The staining characteristics of adenoma cells (acidophil, basophil, chromophobe) are still used in the descriptive morphology but their relevance to hormonal function is limited.

Although the hormonal immunostaining patterns of pituitary adenomas are well known,[360] only a single study has systematically assessed the general immunophenotype of pituitary adenomas.[240] All were synaptophysin and neuron-specific enolase positive; other reactivities included chromogranin (70%) low molecular weight keratin (83%), Leu-7 (35%) and S-100 protein (13%). Thus, despite their relative histological similarity at the light-microscopic level, no single generic immunotype is diagnostic of pituitary adenoma. Therefore, the demonstration of even focal staining for pituitary hormones remains the simplest diagnostic method, particularly in a clinically non-functioning adenoma.

The functional classification, developed on the basis of immunocytochemical and ultrastructural features, disclosed differences in the biological behaviour and the natural history of various tumour types. Some of the characteristics of pituitary adenomas are summarized in Table 17.6.

Table 17.6 *Chief characteristics of pituitary adenoma types based on the unselected surgical material of 2091 biopsies, collected during the period 1971–1994*

Adenoma type	Frequency (%)	M:F Ratio	Immunohisto-chemical marker(s)	Ultrastructural marker(s)	Miscellaneous
Densely granulated GH cell adenoma	7.1	1:0.7	GH, α-subunit (PRL, TSH LH, FSH)[a]	Numerous, predominantly spherical secretory granules (up to 600 nm)	Rarely endocrine amyloid
Sparsely granulated GH cell adenoma	6.2	1:1.16	GH (Golgi pattern) (PRL, α-subunit)	Fibrous body, SER, super-numerary centriole, scanty secretory granules (<250 nm)	Rarely endocrine amyloid
Densely granulated PRL cell adenoma	0.4	–	PRL	Numerous (chiefly 300–450 nm) secretory granules, exocytosis (orthotopic and misplaced)	–
Sparsely granulated PRL cell adenoma	27.0	1:2.5	PRL (Golgi pattern)	Abundant RER, large Golgi apparatus with pleomorphic granules, sparse secretory granules (<300 nm), exocytosis (orthotopic and misplaced)	Calcification, endocrine amyloid
Mixed (GH cell-PRL cell) adenoma	3.5	1:1.1	GH, PRL (α-subunit, TSH)	Two distinct cell types (mostly) densely granulated GH and sparsely granulated PRL cells)	Calcification, endocrine amyloid
Mammosomato-troph cell adenoma	1.2	1:1.1	GH, PRL (α-subunit, TSH)	Large (up to 200 nm) often irregular secretory granules, secretory granules with mottled content, exocytosis (orthotopic and misplaced)	–
Acidophil stem cell adenoma	1.6	1:1.5	PRL, GH	Oncocytic change, giant mitochondria, exocytosis (chiefly orthotopic), fibrous body/SER, sparse secretory granules (<200 nm)	–
Corticotroph cell adenoma	9.6	1:5.4	ACTH (LH, α-subunit)	Numerous (chiefly 300–350 nm) spherical, dented or heart shaped secretory granules, type 1 (cytokeratin) filaments	Excessive deposition of cytokeratin filaments (Crooke's hyaline change)
Thyrotroph cell adenoma	1.1	1:1.3	TSH (GH, PRL, α-subunit)	Nuclear pleomorphism, small (up to 250 nm) peripherally disposed secretory granules	Fibrosis, rarely calcification, may appear non-functioning
Gonadotroph cell adenoma	9.8	1:0.8	FSH, LH α-subunit (ACTH)	Polarity of cells, unevenly distributed secretory granules follicle formation, light bodies. Tumours of females: honeycomb Golgi complex	May appear clinically non-functioning
Silent 'corticotroph' adenoma, subtype 1	1.5	1:1.7	ACTH	Same as for corticotroph cell adenoma	High propensity for haemorrhage within adenoma
Silent 'cortico-troph' adenoma subtype 2	2.0	1:0.2	β-Endorphin, ACTH	Drop-shaped or irregular secretory granules (mostly) 250–350 nm)	–
Silent adenoma subtype 3	1.4	1:1.1	No known specific marker (any pituitary hormone)	Nuclear inclusions, large cells, abundant RER, SER, tortuous Golgi apparatus, complex interdigitations between cell membranes	Mimics PRL cell adenoma in women

(Continued.)

Table 17.6 *(Continued)*

Adenoma type	Frequency (%)	M:F Ratio	Immunohisto-chemical marker(s)	Ultrastructural marker(s)	Miscellaneous
Null cell adenoma	12.4	1:0.7	(FSH, LH, TSH, α-subunit)	Only markers of endocrine differentiation	–
Oncocytoma	13.4	1:0.5	(FSH, LH, TSH, α-subunit)	Major or generalized oncocytic change	–
Unclassified	1.8	NA	NA	NA	NA

ᵃMinor immunoreactivities possibly due to plurihormonal differentiation. M, male: F, Female; GH, growth hormone; PRL, prolactin; TSH, thyroid-stimulating hormone; LH, luteinizing hormone; FSH, follicle-stimulating hormone; ACTH, adrenocorticotrophic hormone; NA, not applicable; SER, smooth endoplasmic reticulum; RER, rough endoplasmic reticulum.

GH-PRODUCING ADENOMAS

The two clinical syndromes resulting from GH over-production, acromegaly and the much less frequently occurring gigantism, may be caused by five distinct morphological types of acidophil cell line tumour.[200,256] Of these, two are monomorphous GH cell adenomas, composed of either densely or sparsely granulated GH cells. These two equally frequent tumour types account for approximately 15% of surgically removed pituitary adenomas. The slow-growing, densely granulated tumour results in enlargement or ballooning of the sella, is equally prevalent in both sexes and most often comes to surgery in the sixth decade. The more aggressive, sparsely granulated tumour peaks earlier, has a higher incidence in women, and is likely to present as a diffuse, invasive macroadenoma at surgery.[151] The densely granulated GH cell adenoma displays a diffuse or trabecular growth pattern and shows varying degrees of cytoplasmic acidophilia. Immunocytochemistry demonstrates strong immunoreactivity for GH throughout the cytoplasm (Fig. 17.58). This subtype frequently shows a plurihormonal immunophenotype, and an overwhelming majority exhibits scattered staining for PRL as well as varying degrees of glycoprotein hormone reactivity for TSH, rarely LH and FSH and most frequently α-subunit.[200,201,301]

Scattered TSH immunoreactivity is not exceptional in densely granulated GH adenomas.[360] Nonetheless, hyperthyroidism rarely complicates acromegaly. When it does, it is invariably associated with the densely granulated GH component. Although adenomas causing both acromegaly and hyperthyroidism are likely to be bimorphous, consisting of densely granulated GH cells and TSH-like cells, the two hormones may rarely be produced by a single phenotype.

Electron microscopy demonstrates the tumour cells to be similar to normal somatotrophs[155–157,200,201] (Fig. 17.59). The polyhedral or rounded cells have fairly uniform, centrally placed nuclei, peripherally disposed slender cisternae of RER and a spherical Golgi complex associated with immature granules. Secretory granules are numerous and of high electron density, and occur in a wide range of sizes (150–1000 nm), although most measure 300–450 nm. Whereas small granules are round, those larger than 600 nm are often ovoid or irregular. In some instances varying numbers of secretory granules are markedly elongate, or are rhomboid or other shapes. Crystal formation of secretory material is specific for densely granulated GH-producing cells.

The sparsely granulated GH adenoma consistently exhibits a diffuse pattern. Its cells are chromophobic or only slightly acidophilic. Varying degrees of nuclear and cellular pleomorphism are the norm and the unstained image of a spherical intracytoplasmic structure (fibrous body) is often seen. Loss of intercellular cohesion and subsequent spherulation of adenoma cells is common. This finding is considered a fixation artefact apparently correlating with the presence and size of the fibrous body. Immunoreactivity for GH is typically variable, being scattered in cells, often limited to the Golgi region.[200,201] Although minor PRL positivity may be observed without ultrastructural signs of PRL differentiation, the extensive plurihormonality observed in the densely granulated variant is not evident.[360] The intense dot-like cytokeratin immunoreactivity of the fibrous bodies serves as an excellent marker.[355]

Electron microscopy shows this tumour to consist of a cell type not known to occur in the normal gland.[155–157,200,201] The spherical or irregular cells often possess either eccentric flattened to crescentic nuclei or peripherally disposed multiple or lobulated nuclei. The RER is more likely to form randomly scattered short profiles than parallel cisternae or concentric whorls. The Golgi zone is often occupied by the fibrous body (Fig. 17.60), a diagnostic marker composed of a spherical aggregate of cytokeratin filaments and/or tubular smooth endoplasmic reticulum (SER).[150] The latter is always present, at least at the periphery of fibrous bodies. Golgi cisternae are either enmeshed within the filamentous mass or are displaced by it. Secretory granules are sparse and randomly distributed, and usually do not exceed 250 nm. Supernumerary centrioles may be located nearby or within the fibrous body.

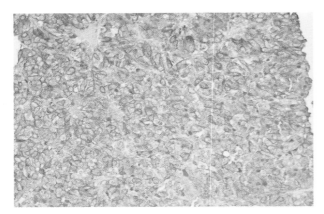

Figure 17.58 *Densely granulated growth hormone cell adenoma, showing generalized immunoreactivity. (ICC for GH.)*

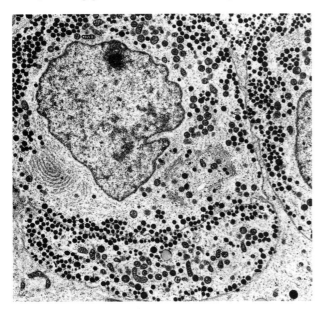

Figure 17.59 *Electron micrograph showing characteristic numerous, chiefly spherical secretory granules, most often in the 300–500 nm range.*

Ancillary features and variants

Amyloid deposition: Production and extracellular deposition of stellate masses of endocrine amyloid may be observed in all types of GH producing adenomas (Fig. 17.61). The change is often focal and not detectable by histological methods. Massive amyloid deposits are rare.[156,216]

Pituitary adenoma–neuronal choristoma (PANCH) is an infrequent variant invariably has features of a GH cell adenoma of sparsely granulated type associated with a neuronal component consisting of ganglion-like cells and neuropil (Fig. 17.62). Microscopically, therefore, such lesions are composite, consisting of an adenoma and ganglion cells. The neuronal element has variably been referred to as a intrasellar gangliocytoma, ganglioneuroma, and neuronal hamartoma or choristoma, terms which reflect the cytogenetic mechanisms thought to underlie

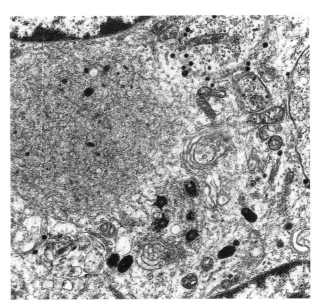

Figure 17.60 *Sparsely granulated growth hormone cell adenoma. Electron micrograph showing a fibrous body consisting of type II cytokeratin filaments and tubular smooth endoplasmic reticulum. Supernumery centrioles may be present. The secretory granules are sparse and small.*

their development. Recent morphological evidence suggests that the unusual association is the result of neuronal metaplasia of the epithelial cells comprising the adenoma.[165] Such transdifferentiation is known to occur in other neuroendocrine neoplasms.

The notion that the lesion results from ganglion cell production of hypothalamic releasing hormones[15] still has its proponents.[344] It is of note that one such lesion has been reported to be associated with a lipomatous component.[391]

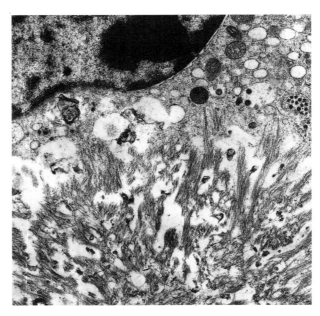

Figure 17.61 *Growth hormone adenoma, with an extracellular stellate mass of fibrillar endocrine amyloid.*

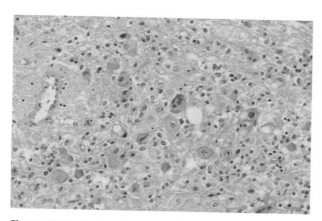

Figure 17.62 *Pituitary adenoma–neuronal choristoma (PANCH). The association of chromophobic adenoma, neuron-like cells and usually neuropil is usually accompanied by acromegaly. (H&E.)*

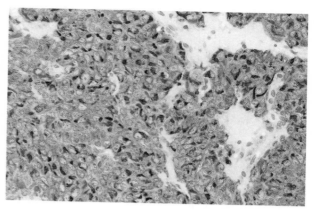

Figure 17.63 *Sparsely granulated prolactin cell adenoma. Strong immunoreactivity is seen, chiefly visualizing the prominent Golgi region. (ICC for PRL.)*

PRL CELL ADENOMA

This common type of pituitary adenoma is among the most frequent causes of hyperprolactinaemia.[154] The latter results in the amenorrhoea–galactorrhoea syndrome as well as in infertility in women of reproductive age; endocrine symptoms are less conspicuous in postmenopausal females. In men, infertility, diminished libido and impotence result, signs that are often overlooked until local mass effect or invasion makes its appearance. PRL cell adenomas occur in all age groups. Although few arise in childhood they, together with ACTH-producing adenomas, are the most frequent paediatric adenomas.[89,308] In surgical series, the majority of patients comprises young adults; women outnumber men in a ratio of 2:1. Male PRL cell adenomas occur primarily in adults and are more uniformly distributed by age.[151] At diagnosis, young women of child-bearing age often have microadenomas, whereas the tumours of postmenopausal women as well as men have frequently spread beyond the sella. Small, incidental PRL cell adenomas found at autopsy, usually in older individuals, show the same high frequency (45%) in both sexes.[251] The wide range of biological behaviour exhibited by PRL cell adenomas is usually not reflected in their morphology.[154,155,201] However, the proliferation rate, as shown by the MIB-1 nuclear labelling index, is higher in the macroadenomas of men and postmenopausal women than in the tumours of younger females.[56]

The vast majority of PRL cell adenomas is chromophobic or slightly acidophilic but, by virtue of their high RER content, some may display a basophilic hue. Strong acidophilia is exhibited only by the rare densely granulated variant.[154] Three histological patterns are recognized, the common diffuse pattern, the papillary form, one seen primarily among the incidental autopsy microadenomas and one containing large amounts of hyalinized connective tissue stroma. Strong, often globular PRL immunoreactivity seen throughout these tumours represents the prohormone-filled profiles of large Golgi complexes (Golgi pattern), since cytoplasmic secretory granules are otherwise scant and do not contribute significantly to immunopositivity (Fig. 17.63). As a rule, most PRL cell adenomas are monohormonal,[154,201,360] only a small minority show scattered positivity for α-subunit.

The ultrastructural appearance of untreated, sparsely granulated PRL cell adenoma is highly characteristic[154–156,201] (Fig. 17.64). The predominantly euchromatic nucleus may be spherical or irregular, and a large, dense nucleolus is often seen. No adenoma type contains more abundant RER, which appears as arrays of parallel cisternae or concentric whirls (Nebenkern). The prominent, elaborate Golgi apparatus contains numerous maturing secretory granules which are usually spherical but, as a result of fusion, may be pleomorphic. This unusual feature renders the Golgi complex a good marker of PRL cell adenoma.[150] The most distinctive hallmark of PRL production in the human pituitary is granule exocytosis. Such extrusion of secretory granules may be either orthotopic or misplaced, i.e. it takes place on the lateral cell membrane distant from the basal lamina. Although its frequency within any one tumour is highly variable, granule extrusion is a uniform feature in PRL cell adenoma.

The densely granulated PRL cell adenoma is a rare variant. Its polyhedral or ovoid cells, smaller than those of sparsely granulated tumours, contain considerably less RER and a small Golgi apparatus. The numerous 400–450-nm secretory granules, which range in size up to 700 nm, endow the cells with an appearance similar to that of densely granulated GH adenoma. Again, the distinguishing marker of PRL cell differentiation is the presence of granule extrusions. Occasional granules, especially those undergoing extrusion, may exhibit uneven electron density, a feature also seen only in PRL cells.

Ancillary features

With the exception of PRL cell adenoma, calcification is rare in pituitary adenomas.[154,155,201,330] Ranging from

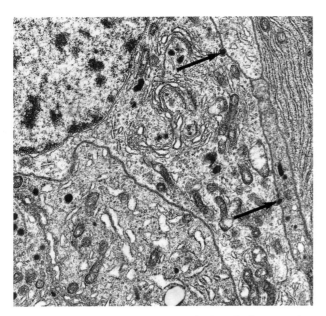

Figure 17.64 *Sparsely granulated prolactin cell adenoma. Electron micrograph wherein there were irregular granules within the Golgi apparatus and two granule extrusions ('misplaced exocytosis', arrows).*

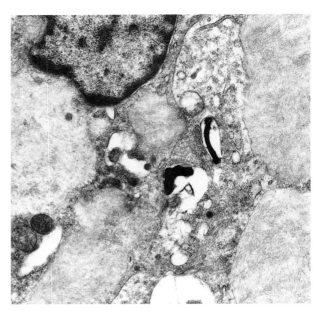

Figure 17.65 *Prolactin cell adenoma. Electron micrograph of intracellular membrane-bound aggregates of endocrine amyloid.*

scattered calcified foci to massive formation of calcospherites, it is observed in an estimated 15–20% of tumours, but the reason for this propensity is unclear.

Endocrine amyloid production occurs in almost 5% of PRL cell adenomas.[154,156,201,216] In most instances the deposition of this fibrillar protein is focal and detectable only by electron microcopy. Two forms are distinguished: intracellular and extracellular. In the former, early stage amyloid production takes the form of intracytoplasmic membrane-bound aggregates (Fig. 17.65). Extensive accumulation may lead to cell death, thus rendering the filamentous mass extracellular. The other form of endocrine amyloid, similar to that seen in GH cell adenomas, is not detected within adenoma cells. Instead, it appears that polymerization of the fibrillar protein takes place in the extracellular space (Fig. 17.66). In PRL cell adenomas, this form of amyloid may be associated with formation of sizeable microcysts, that gradually fill up with amyloid discharged by adjacent tumour cells. The massive formation of spherical deposits conspicuous at light microscopy is rare. In a tumour showing massive deposition, the spherical form of amyloid was found to represent a 4000 molecular weight peptide having the amino acid sequence of the N-terminal 1–34 fragment of the prolactin molecule.[143]

GH- AND PRL-PRODUCING ADENOMAS

Three tumour types, each representing a well-defined ultrastructural entity, are known to synthesize both GH and PRL within one or more cell population.[200] They may also show immunoreactivity for the α-subunit. Since they lack distinctive histological features and exhibit overlapping immunohistochemical profiles, electron microscopy is indispensable in diagnosis.

Mixed GH cell–PRL cell adenoma

This is the most common of these subtypes.[65,362] Clinically it is associated with acromegaly or gigantism as well as varying degrees of hyperprolactinaemia. A minority of such mixed adenomas is aggressive and difficult to treat.

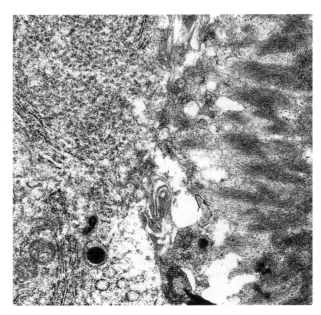

Figure 17.66 *Prolactin cell adenoma. Electron micrographs of extracellular fibrillar endocrine amyloid which fills a lumen formed by adenoma cells.*

In most cases, histology shows the tumour to be composed of both acidophilic and chromophobic cells distributed in a patchy or an intermingled pattern. Immunohistochemically, the acidophils usually represent GH cells, whereas the chromophobic cells are PRL positive.

Electron microscopy reveals a bimorphous tumour composed primarily of densely granulated GH cells and sparsely granulated PRL cells[155,156,200,362] (Fig. 17.67). Sparsely granulated GH cell components and especially densely granulated PRL cells are rarely encountered.

Mammosomatotroph adenoma

This is similarly associated with acromegaly or gigantism and variable, usually mild hyperprolactinaemia.[104,161] In that most are slow-growing tumours, the biological behaviour of which is similar to that of densely granulated GH cell adenoma, the distinction of these two tumours is not of clinical significance.

Mammosomatotroph adenomas exhibit a diffuse pattern of growth and varying degrees of acidophilia. Immunoreactivity for GH is always seen, whereas PRL staining is variable. Their ultrastructural appearance is similar to that of densely granulated GH cell adenomas. In some instances, the secretory granules include ovoid and irregular forms, their size ranging up to 1000–1500 nm. The ultrastructural markers include scattered secretory granules with uneven, mottled cores, extrusion of secretory granules and persistence of extruded secretory material in the extracellular space[156,161,201] (Fig. 17.68).

Acidophil stem cell adenoma

This is an infrequent, often invasive tumour that mainly produces PRL. Typically, the degree of hyperprolacti-

naemia is disproportionate compared with the size of the tumour. Physical stigmata of acromegaly, either with or without elevations of serum GH, are uncommonly associated with this adenoma.[155,156,167,201]

Histologically, acidophil stem cell adenomas are predominantly chromophobe and exhibit a diffuse growth pattern. Clear cytoplasmic vacuoles are often present, but are not a reliable diagnostic feature. Immunocytochemistry demonstrates greatly variable PRL staining. GH immunoreactivity is usually weak, scattered or even absent. Few tumours exhibit GH reactivity comparable to that of PRL.

Electron microscopy demonstrates a monomorphous adenoma composed of cells showing signs of both PRL and GH differentiation; these include secretory granule exocytosis as well as fibrous body formation and/or SER accumulation[155,156,167,201] (Fig. 17.69). In the majority of instances PRL cell features dominate; only occasional adenomas resemble sparsely granulated GH cell adenoma with exocytoses. Both RER and Golgi complexes are less prominent than in PRL cell adenomas and the sparse, spherical secretory granules rarely exceed 200 nm. The majority of acidophil stem cell adenomas is endowed with another distinctive feature, the presence of generalized oncocytic change with the development of giant mitochondria. The latter may attain the size of the nucleus, and with their lack of cristae, and granular substance, may contain electron-dense tubular structures. The giant mitochondria represent the ultrastructural equivalent of the clear cytoplasmic vacuoles observed by histology.

Although clinically the acidophil stem cell adenoma blends into the spectrum of other PRL- and GH-pro-

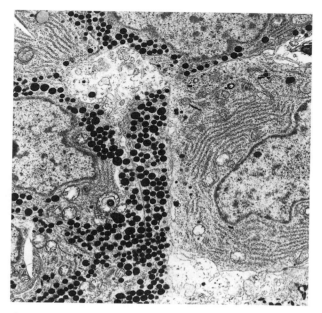

Figure 17.67 *Mixed adenoma. Electron micrograph of densely granulated growth hormone cell adenoma (left) and sparsely granulated prolactin cells (right).*

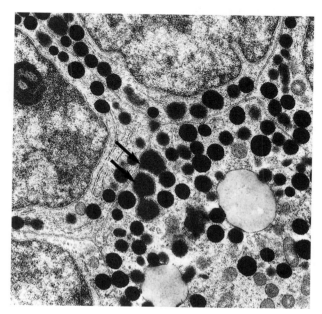

Figure 17.68 *Mammosomatotroph adenoma. The electron micrograph appearance is similar to that of densely granulated growth hormone adenoma, except for the large, somewhat fuzzy granules undergoing exocytosis (arrows).*

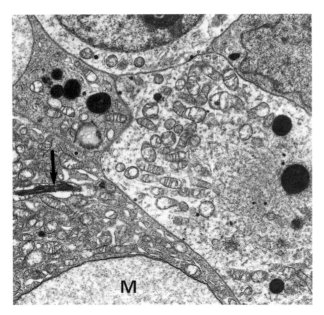

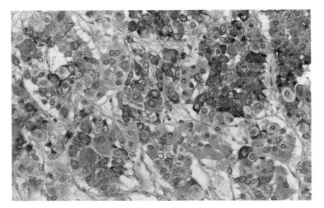

Figure 17.70 *Normal anterior pituitary. Localization of growth hormone mRNA in formalin-fixed paraffin-embedded tissue sections with a digoxigenin-labelled oligonucleotide probe. The positive cells have blue cytoplasmic staining. [Nitroblue tetrazolium (MBT) 5-bromo-4-chloro-3-indolylphosphate (BCIP) reaction.]*

Figure 17.69 *Acidophilic stem cell adenoma. Electron micrograph demonstrating entrapment by the fibrous body of a few small secretory granules, the oncocytic change, the electron-dense tubular structures within enlarged mitochondrion (arrow) and part of a giant mitochondrion (M).*

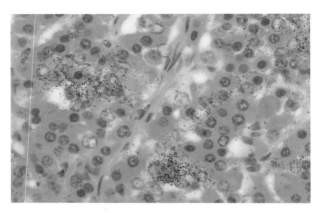

Figure 17.71 *Normal anterior pituitary. Localization of prolactin mRNA. The positive cells have silver grains over the cytoplasm and nucleus. (³⁵S-Labelled oligonucleotide probe.)*

ducing tumours, its unique ultrastructure makes it a distinct morphological entity. Some features associated with PRL cell adenoma, such as calcification and endocrine amyloid formation, have not been encountered so far in acidophil stem cell adenoma.

HYBRIDIZATION STUDIES OF GH- AND PRL-PRODUCING ADENOMAS

Most *in situ* hybridization studies of human pituitaries have examined GH- and PRL-secreting tumours (Figs 17.70–17.74). This may be related to the relative abundance of these tumour types in surgically excised pituitary neoplasms. In one of the early studies of pituitary tumours in man by *in situ* hybridization, Pixley and co-workers[317] analysed dissociated cells from GH-producing pituitary tumours using a complementing DNA (cDNA) probe. They noted a decrease in the percentage of cells expressing growth hormone messenger RNA (mRNA) in the cells that were cultured for 2–3 days. Various investigators have used formalin-fixed paraffin-embedded tissue sections to examine gene expression in the pituitary. Lloyd *et al.*[234] showed that most GH-secreting pituitary tumours expressed both GH and PRL mRNA. PRL-producing cells and tumours commonly express only PRL but not GH message, supporting the concept that PRL-producing cells and tumours are terminally differentiated. Levy and Lightman[226] examined the effects of GRH and somatostatin on GH gene expression in human pituitary tumours by quantitative *in situ* hybridization. When two GH adenomas were studied in culture, GRH and hydro-

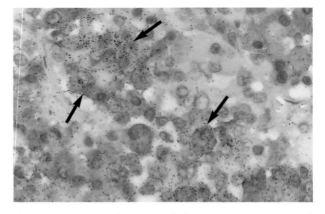

Figure 17.72 *Normal anterior pituitary. Mammosomatotroph (MS) detected in situ followed by immunostaining for growth hormone (GH) protein. The MS cells have silver grains over the cytoplasm and a brown DAB-peroxidase reaction product (arrows). Cells with only prolactin (PRL) mRNA have silver grains over the cytoplasm, while the GH cells have a brown reaction product in the cytoplasm. (In situ for PRL mRNA; ICC for GH.)*

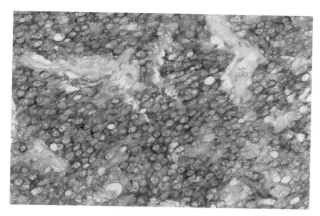

Figure 17.73 *Prolactinoma. There is considerable expression of prolactin mRNA digoxigenin-labelled probe.*

cortisone did not change GH mRNA level expression, although the GH mRNA transcript could be readily detected in the tumours. Kovacs *et al.*[205] examined GH-secreting tumours using *in situ* hybridization immunohistochemistry and electron microscopy. They showed that the GH gene and protein products were expressed in the tumour cells, although the patients did not have acromegaly. The functions of the GH message and proteins in patients with silent GH tumours is currently unknown. Saeger *et al.*[345] studied 40 pituitary adenomas from patients with acromegaly and compared immunohistochemistry and *in situ* hybridization. They found 100% correlation for GH and 60% for PRL of the hybridization signal and the hormone content. Their finding that 87% of the GH tumours express PRL mRNA is in agreement with earlier studies by Lloyd *et al.*[234] Stefaneanu *et al.*[398] studied pituitaries from pregnant and lactating women. GH cells express PRL mRNA during pregnancy, arising in pituitary of pregnant and lactating women.[398] These important observations suggested that there was a transformation of cell types with the development of mammosomatotroph cells expressing both PRL and GH in this altered physiological state. Kovacs *et al.*[208] studied the effects of bromocriptine treatment on PRL-secreting pituitary adenomas by *in situ* hybridization and observed that PRL mRNA was decreased by bromocriptine in a population of small cells, indicating that these cells responded to the drug with decreased cytoplasmic volume. However, a subpopulation of larger PRL cells expressed significant amounts of PRL mRNA, in spite of bromocriptine therapy indicating a resistance to this dopamine agonist.

CORTICOTROPH CELL ADENOMA

Among the various forms of pituitary adenoma, the corticotropin-producing tumour poses the most frequent problems in neuroimaging, laboratory diagnosis, surgery and morphological assessment. Pituitary-dependent Cushing's disease is associated with typical signs and symptoms of cortisol excess, including moon-like facies, hirsutism, truncal obesity, abdominal striae, easy bruising, mood changes, hypertension and muscle weakness. Corticotroph cell adenomas exhibit a marked (5:1) female preponderance.[151] The severity of clinical symptoms does not correlate well with tumour size. Indeed, florid Cushing's disease is often caused by a minute microadenoma, whereas some diffuse or invasive macroadenomas may be accompanied by only subtle signs of disease. The substantial majority of corticotropic tumours is not large enough to alter the sellar configuration. Indeed, many may not even be conclusively demonstrated on CT and MRI scans. It is increasingly more common for surgeons to proceed with partial or total hypophysectomy if no distinct tumour mass is detected at surgery. In a few cases, the pathologist may not find the adenoma. However, serial sectioning may uncover the tumour, thus underscoring the importance of collecting and processing all available tissues. Negative results may mean that the adenoma had not been removed, the tumour was lost during surgery, or that no tumour was present. In this last case the clinical syndrome is caused either by corticotroph cell hyperplasia, an uncommon and controversial lesion, or by an extrapituitary source of ACTH. Non-tumorous adenohypophysis is often sampled in pituitary specimens of patients with Cushing's disease or syndrome. In such instances, non-tumorous corticotrophs display Crooke's hyalinization, an alteration previously described in detail.[152,201] It should be noted that this alteration is not specific for corticotroph adenomas, but rather for hypercortisolism regardless of its aetiology.

Most corticotroph cell adenomas are strongly basophilic and PAS-positive microadenomas with a sinusoidal growth pattern[155,156,201,332] (Fig. 17.74). Macroadenomas usually exhibit a diffuse pattern and are less basophilic; occasional examples are partly or entirely chromophobic. Immunostains for 1-39 ACTH and other peptides of POMC show variable reactivity (Fig. 17.74). Whereas plurihormonality is very uncommon in small ACTH-producing tumours, weak or focal reactivity for LH and/or α-subunit may be seen in macroadenomas, particularly in recurrent tumours.[35,353] Cytokeratin reactivity reflects the presence of type 1 filaments.[280]

By electron microscopy, the basophilic variety of corticotroph cell adenoma consists of polyhedral, often elongated cells with rather electron-dense cytoplasm.[156,201,332] The RER is moderately developed and may show focal, uneven dilation. The roughly spherical Golgi apparatus contains maturing granules, some of which may have an asymmetrical core. Secretory granules are numerous; although the majority measure 300–350 nm, their range is 200–450 nm, similar to that seen in densely granulated GH cell adenoma. What sets apart the two entities is the distinctive morphology of corticotroph granules. They include not only spherical but indented, teardrop and heart-shaped examples of variable electron density. In cases in which secretory granules are less numerous, they

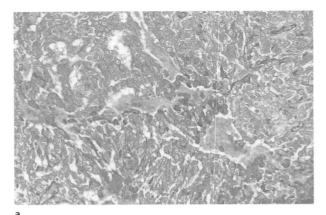

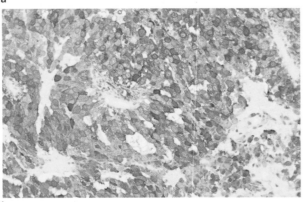

a

b

Figure 17.74 *Corticotroph cell adenoma. (a) Strong PAS positivity. (b) Immunostaining for adrenocorticotropic hormone.*

tend to line up along the cell membrane, thus explaining the frame-like pattern of immunoreactivity delineating cell contours. Another morphological marker of corticotropic differentiation is the presence of type 1 cytokeratin filaments forming elongated perinuclear bundles (Fig. 17.75). Adenomas associated with Nelson's syndrome have similar ultrastructure, but contain few, if any, cytokeratin filaments.

Morphological variants and associated features

Very infrequently, corticotroph adenomas show minimal or no basophilia or PAS positivity and only scanty ACTH immunoreactivity.[156,201] Macroadenomas may be associated with a relatively mild form of Cushing's disease. At the ultrastructural level they exhibit lesser degrees of functional differentiation, having sparse cytoplasm, poorly developed membranous organelles, sparse, smaller (200–300 nm) secretory granules of uncharacteristic morphology and few type 1 filaments.

Given that corticotroph cell adenomas are autonomous and that Crooke's hyalinization is indicative of the negative feedback effect of elevated cortisol levels, Crooke's change is expected to occur only in suppressed, non-tumorous corticotrophs. In reality, the cells of some corticotroph tumours display excessive, ring-like accumulation of Crooke's hyalin[103,156,158,201] (Fig. 17.76). Such tumours, termed Crooke's cell adenomas, exhibit considerable variations in cellularity and functional differentiation. Neither the presence nor the degree of hyalin formation correlates with the clinical severity of Cushing's disease.[158]

HYBRIDIZATION STUDIES OF CORTICOTROPH CELL ADENOMAS

In situ hybridization of ACTH-secreting tumours has been done by several groups (Figs 17.77, 17.78). Lloyd *et al.*[238] analysed a series of ACTH-immunoreactive pituitary tumours for POMC mRNA expression and found that most of the non-functional tumours classified as type 1 silent adenomas, and which were morphologically similar to functional pituitary tumours in patients with Cushing's disease, expressed POMC mRNA. Only a few of the type 2 and 3 tumours had detectable levels of POMC mRNA.

These studies strongly suggested that the morphological features of corticotroph tumours may be related to POMC production in functional and in subtype 1 silent adenomas. Nagaya *et al.*[275] reported that the size of the POMC transcript in a case of a silent ACTH tumour was similar to that in functional ACTH adenomas when analysed by Northern hybridization. This observation suggests that in silent tumours the mRNA may not be an abnormal molecule, unlike the longer POMC mRNA transcript present in some neuroendocrine tumours.[77] McNicol *et al.*[255] used digoxigenin-labelled oligonucleotide probes to show that the mRNA for POMC as well as for PRL and GH could be readily detected with this

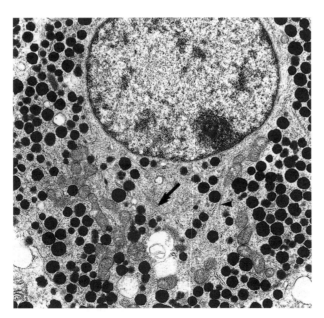

Figure 17.75 *Corticotroph cell adenoma. In an adenoma associated with Cushing's disease, the electron micrograph shows some dented, irregular or heart-shaped secretory granules. A few fine bundles of cytokeratin filaments are also seen (arrows).*

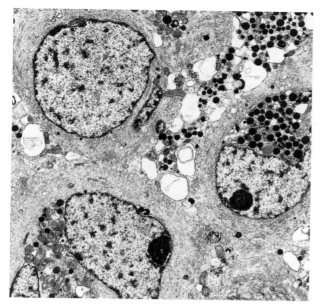

Figure 17.76 *Corticotroph cell adenoma. Electron micrograph showing massive ring-like accumulation of cytokeratin filaments (Crooke's hyaline material). The absence of a continuous plasma membrane is a common artefact in advanced Crooke's change, probably due to swelling and regression of the filmentous mass during fixation and dehydration.*

non-isotopic technique in pituitary tumours in man. Pituitaries from 16 patients with Cushing's disease and 10 patients with Nelson's syndrome, analysed by *in situ* hybridization with digoxigenin-labelled probes, showed that the signal was significantly greater in Nelson's syndrome than in Cushing's disease, suggesting differences in POMC transcript expression in these two conditions.[102]

THYROTROPH CELL ADENOMA

This tumour accounts for no more than 1% of resected adenomas. Owing to its rarity, only a small number of cases has been studied in detail. Nonetheless, several aspects of

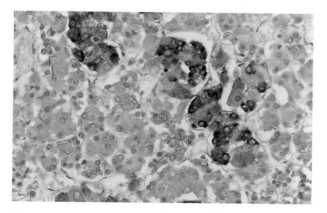

Figure 17.77 *Normal pituitary. Localization of a pro-opiomelanocortin (POMC) mRNA digoxigenin-labelled oligonucleotide probe.*

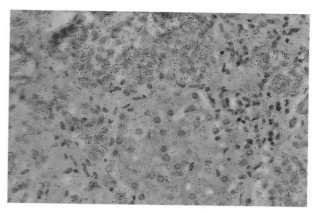

Figure 17.78 *Adrenocorticotropin-producing carcinoma. The patient presented with Nelson's syndrome. The pituitary carcinoma cells in the liver metastasis are strongly positive for pro-opiomelanocortin (POMC) mRNA, as indicated by the silver grains.*

these tumours remain unexplored. Thyrotroph cell adenomas occur in both sexes and at any age. Some produce hyperthyroidism associated with inappropriate TSH production, whereas others occur in the setting of prolonged hypothyroidism, arising from pre-existing hyperplasia of thyrotroph cells.[29,30,441] Inexplicably, tumours with the morphological attributes of TSH adenoma may also occur in euthyroid subjects. At surgery, most thyrotroph adenomas are macroadenomas displaying invasive growth. Their morphological variations show no correlations with clinical signs and symptoms.[115,212,441]

Thyrotroph cell adenomas are predominantly chromophobic and rarely show sufficient granulation to provide basophilia or PAS positivity. Their histological pattern is often sinusoidal with associated perivascular pseudorosette formation. A minority is diffuse, possibly with focal nuclear pleomorphism. For no known reason, varying degrees of primarily perivascular fibrosis may be seen (Fig. 17.79). Immunoreactivity for TSH is highly variable and shows no close correlation with hormonal function. Lesser or focal immunostaining for α-subunit and GH is often present.[351,360,441]

Ultrastructurally, the most frequently occurring well-differentiated TSH adenomas consist of polar cells which simulate the normal thyrotrophs.[115,156,201] Their nuclei are uniform and chiefly euchromatic. Cisternae of the prominent RER are slightly dilated, and the globoid Golgi apparatus contains a number of immature granules. The small (150–250 nm) and usually sparse secretory granules are prone to be singly aligned beneath the cell membrane, thus outlining cell borders (Fig. 17.80). Secretory granules are greatest in number within cell processes. Variable functional differentiation, even within the same lesion, as evidenced by patchy immunostaining, is also reflected in the quantity and appearance of RER and Golgi membranes. In less differentiated areas, cytoplasmic organization resembles that of null cell adenoma, regardless of hormonal activity.

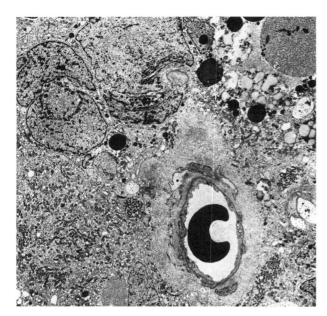

Figure 17.79 *Thyrotroph cell adenoma. Electron micrograph in which there is some nuclear pleomorphism and perivascular fibrosis.*

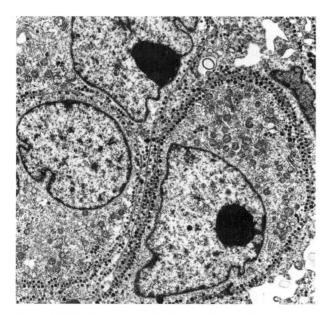

Figure 17.80 *Thyrotroph cell adenoma. The patient manifested hyperthyroidism. Electron micrograph showing small secretory granules aggregated along the plasmalemma in a single layer outlining the cell contours.*

GONADOTROPH CELL ADENOMA

More common than previously thought, gonadotroph cell adenomas form 10% of adenomas in unselected surgical series, a figure much higher than in clinical studies. The reason for the discrepancy is that a considerable number of adenomas, exhibiting gonadotrophic differentiation by immunocytochemistry and electron microscopy, clinically appears to be hormonally inactive. Alternatively, tumours associated with elevated FSH and/or LH levels, usually in male patients, may possess morphological features resembling null cell adenoma.[153]

Gonadotroph cell adenomas are chromophobic or, when oncocytic change is present, may show variable acidophilia.[153,201,420] The histological pattern may be sinusoidal, diffuse or, rarely, papillary (Fig. 17.81). Occasional PAS-positive follicles may be seen.[153] Adenomas in men are likely to show immunoreactivity for FSH and/or LH, the staining being variable and most often unevenly distributed, a feature suggesting varying degrees of functional differentiation. With the exception of the uncommon densely granulated and strongly immunoreactive form of gonadotroph cell adenomas, most tumours in women are poorly immuno-reactive,[153,155] displaying only scant or, in some cases, no staining for FSH or LH. α-Subunit, the increased secretion of which is a good clinical indicator of glycoprotein hormone producing-adenomas, is not a reliable marker.

Gonadotroph cell adenomas are the only known neoplasms exhibiting a sex-linked ultrastructural dichotomy.[153,195,201] The well-differentiated tumours of males consist of somewhat polar cells with well-developed RER and a prominent Golgi apparatus. Secretory granules measure 150–250 nm and are less frequent in the nuclear pole than in cytoplasmic processes, an arrangement that serves as an excellent marker of glycoprotein hormone differentiation (Fig. 17.82). However, the often focal finding of null cell-like features underscore the need for multiple sampling. Oncocytic change, a common feature of gonadotroph cell adenomas of men, is evident in approximately 50% of such tumours.[195]

The ultrastructure of gonadotroph adenomas is less variable in women, wherein 70% of tumours are highly differentiated composed of polar cells with long, attenu-

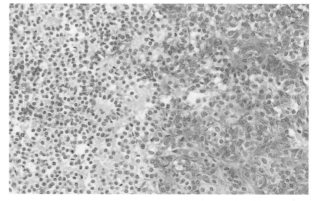

Figure 17.81 *Gonadotroph adenoma. There are variable degrees of hormonal differentiation. One part comprised elongated polar cells and was strongly positive for follicle-stimulating hormone, while an adjacent area consisting of smaller, polyhedral cells was positive only for α-subunit (not shown). (ICC for FSH.)*

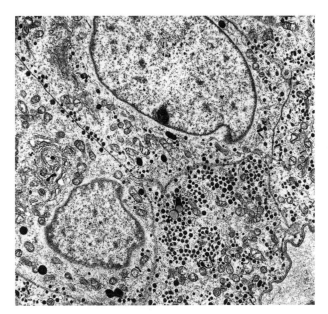

Figure 17.82 *Gonadotroph adenoma. Male patient. Electron micrograph in which the majority of small secretory granules accumulate in cell processes.*

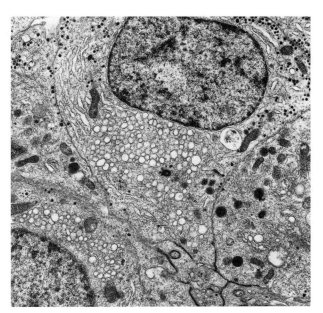

Figure 17.84 *Gonadotroph adenoma. Female patient. Electron micrograph with features of a honeycomb Golgi complex present in three tumour cells.*

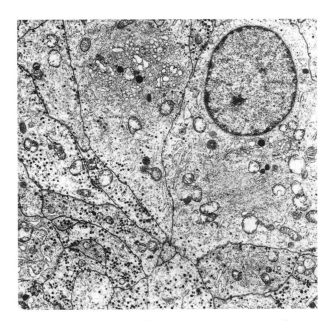

Figure 17.83 *Gonadotroph adenoma. Female patient. Electron micrograph in which strikingly polar cells contain few secretory granules within the nuclear pole, whereas numerous granules collect within the slender cell processes. Note the honeycomb Golgi complex.*

ated processes (Fig. 17.83). The ultrastructural marker is the vacuolar or honeycomb transformation of their prominent Golgi apparatus, the result being clusters of uniform spheres filled with a low-density proteinaceous substance harbouring only occasional, if any, maturing secretory granules[153,156,195] (Fig. 17.84). The overwhelming majority of granules within such cells is minute

(100–150 nm) and accumulates in the cell processes, leaving the nuclear pole nearly devoid of granules. Oncocytic change is not frequent in this subtype. A minority of gonadotroph tumours in females shows highly differentiated features alternating with a null cell-like component; in these cases the honeycomb transformation of Golgi is less pronounced or lacking. Although the cause of vesicular transformation is unclear, the near total absence of immature secretory granules in this unique structure suggests that packaging of secretory material is defective or lacking. This, in turn, may result in the loss of their highly soluble secretory product during processing, accounting for the poor FSH and LH immunoreactivity often seen in these tumours.

Morphological variants and associated features

For reasons unknown, the secretory granules of most gonadotroph adenomas are much smaller than those of normal gonadotrophs. There are, however, a few tumours, occurring chiefly in postmenopausal women, composed of polyhedral cells, variable quantities of RER, conventional Golgi complexes and numerous randomly distributed, variably electron-dense secretory granules measuring up to 500 nm. Their appearance is similar to that of normal gonadotrophs.[153,195]

A few ultrastructural markers occur with sufficient frequency to aid in the recognition of gonadotroph adenomas. These include the formation of follicles (Fig. 17.85) and the presence of light bodies.[150] The PAS-positive content of follicles is already apparent on histological examination. Follicles occur most commonly in the adenomas of men.

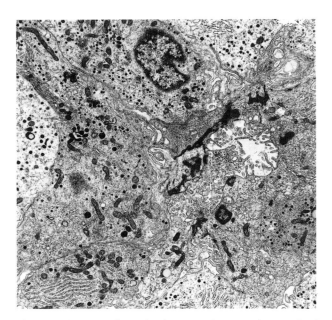

Figure 17.85 *Gonadotroph adenoma. Electron micrograph of follicle formation, which is fairly common.*

The light bodies are infrequent 800–3000-nm cytoplasmic bodies, with a tubular–granular internal structure, and bound by a single, ruffled membrane. Although their origin and significance are unknown, they appear to denote gonadotroph differentiation.[150]

HYBRIDIZATION STUDIES OF GONADOTROPH ADENOMAS

There have only been a few studies of *in situ* hybridization analyses of gonadotrophic, null-cell and oncocytic adenomas (Fig. 17.86). α-Subunits of glycoprotein hormones, β-FSH and/or β-LH mRNA were seen in most gonadotroph and null-cell tumours but in very few oncocytomas.[237] These findings led these investigators to postulate that gonadotroph and null-cell tumours are probably closely related and the oncocytomas may represent a dedifferentiated tumour related to null-cell

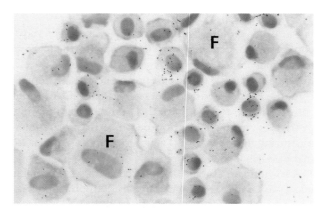

Figure 17.86 *Null-cell adenoma. Culture in serum-free media expresses follicle stimulating hormone-β mRNA in many of the pituitary cells, while the fibroblasts (F) are negative.*

adenomas. About one-third of 40 clinical and non-functional pituitary tumours expressed β-hCG or β-LH; a few also expressed PRL or GH mRNA.[27]

SILENT ADENOMAS

The designation 'silent adenoma' should not be confused with the more frequently occurring clinically non-functioning adenomas of the null cell adenoma–oncocytoma group. The three tumour types that are the subject of this section are well-differentiated, ultrastructurally distinctive adenomas, unassociated with a specific hypersecretory syndrome or biochemical abnormality. Their characteristic features notwithstanding, silent adenomas cannot be linked to any of the known adenohypophyseal cell types. It is reasonable to assume that silent corticotroph subtype 1 and 2 tumours originate in POMC cells derived from the pars intermedia,[162] whereas the parent cell of silent adenoma subtype 3 is matter for conjecture. At present, electron microscopy is required for their conclusive identification.[155,156,160,201]

Silent corticotroph adenoma, subtype 1

This type has the same histological, immunocytochemical and ultrastructural features as do well-differentiated, basophilic, corticotroph cell adenomas causing Cushing's disease,[160] but showing only moderate female preponderance (Fig. 17.87). Nevertheless, it is not associated with signs and symptoms of hypercortisolism. Most are macroadenomas at the time of clinical diagnosis. Silent corticotroph adenomas, subtype 1, also display a distinct tendency to spontaneous haemorrhage, a feature which brings them to clinical attention in 40% of cases.

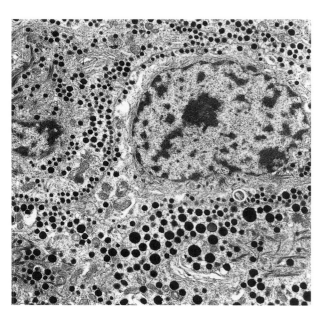

Figure 17.87 *Silent 'corticotroph' adenoma subtype 1. Electron micrograph that is indistinguishable from that of adrenocorticotropic cell adenoma.*

Silent corticotroph cell adenoma, subtype 2

This tumour, which affects primarily males, is unassociated with endocrine symptoms of hyperfunction.[160] Since the tumours grow undetected, they are typically macroadenomas at the time of diagnosis. Histologically, they are chromophobic, slightly PAS positive and display distinct, although rarely widespread immunoreactivity for ACTH and for β-endorphin in particular. Ultrastructurally, the polyhedral adenoma cells have a central nucleus with irregular contours, moderately developed RER, Golgi complexes and mitochondria, as well as randomly distributed 200–400-nm secretory granules, which are often teardrop shaped or indented and of varying electron density. No cytokeratin filaments are detectable (Fig. 17.88).

Silent adenoma, subtype 3

This uncommon but unique tumour shows no sex predilection but its occurrence is strikingly age related. Most women come to surgery between 20 and 35 years, whereas in men no such predilection is apparent.[168] Whereas in men nearly all silent adenomas of subtype 3 are macroadenomas, in women they produce mild to moderate hyperprolactinaemia detected at an early, microadenoma stage. The basis for PRL elevation, apparently from the non-adenomatous pituitary, is not adequately explained by stalk compression. It is not surprising that in women this adenoma type is often mistaken for PRL cell adenoma. Dopamine agonist treatment in this setting normalizes serum PRL levels, but tumour growth remains unimpeded.[168]

Histologically, this adenoma exhibits a diffuse or lobular pattern and often consists of large, chromophobic or slightly acidophilic cells with mild nuclear pleomorphism and fine PAS-positive granules.[160,168] Since the normal counterpart of its constituent cells is unknown, immunohistochemistry is not helpful in diagnosis. Indeed, it can even be misleading. Most tumours display minor immunopositivity for any or any combination of known pituitary hormones. A minority of silent subtype 3 adenomas are entirely immunonegative for pituitary hormones.

In sharp contrast, electron microscopy consistently reveals a highly differentiated adenoma with characteristics resembling those of a glycoprotein hormone-producing tumour.[156,160,168,201] The often large, somewhat pleomorphic nuclei may contain conspicuous, even multiple spheridia. The ample cytoplasm is filled with abundant RER, varying quantities of SER, an elaborate, often tortuous Golgi apparatus and a fair number of mitochondria which lie in clusters displaced by the proliferating endoplasmic reticulum (Fig. 17.89). Secretory granules are sparse and most often measure 200 nm. In some tumours adjacent cell membranes form conspicuous interdigitation. Tumours with less abundant membranous organelles show a strong resemblance to thyrotroph adenoma.

Immunoreactivity for GH is common in silent subtype 3 adenomas which are typically plurihormonal in differentiation. Nonetheless, clinical acromegaly is rare, having been occasionally noted in male patients.

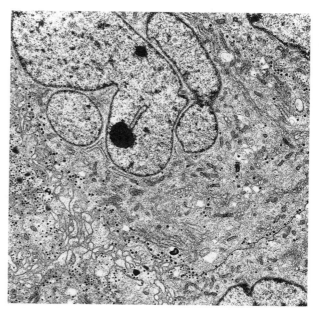

Figure 17.89 *Silent adenoma subtype 3. Electron micrograph of a large cell with an irregular nucleus with spheridia, well-developed smooth and rough endoplasmic reticulum, elaborate Golgi apparatus and small, sparse secretory granules. Note the multiple interdigitations between adjacent cell membranes.*

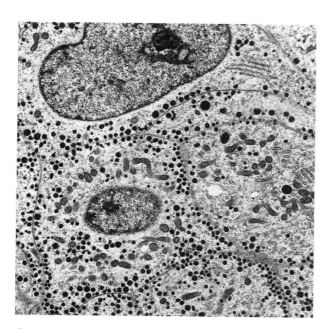

Figure 17.88 *Silent 'corticotroph' adenoma subtype 2. Electron micrograph in which there are spherical as well as drop-shaped secretory granules. There are no cytokeratin filaments.*

Clinically non-functioning adenomas

These slow-growing neoplasms account for 25% of surgically resected pituitary tumours and as many as 50% of incidental adenomas encountered at autopsy.[14,155,157,201] Most occur in older patients, particularly in men.[151] Aside from mild hyperprolactinaemia, which is probably the result of stalk compression, null-cell adenomas are unassociated with signs or symptoms of hormonal hypersecretion. Some are discovered incidentally, but the majority, owing to their large size, are symptomatic, causing headache, visual disturbances and cranial nerve palsies. Varying degrees of hypopituitarism may be clinically evident. Based upon the mitochondrial content, clinically non-functioning tumours are divided into non-oncocytic (null cell) adenoma and oncocytoma.

NULL-CELL ADENOMA

The term signifies the lack or paucity of morphological, especially ultrastructural markers that would indicate their cell of origin or direction of differentiation.[199,203] Histologically, these tumours are predominantly chromophobe, exhibiting a diffuse pattern often punctuated by perivascular pseudorosettes. Immunocytochemistry often detects minimal immunoreactivity for pituitary hormones, usually FSH, LH and their α-subunit, and rarely for other hormones.[14,155,157,201,203,342]

Electron microscopy reveals small cells with irregularly outlined nuclei, paucity of RER and a small Golgi complex (Fig. 17.90). Spherical or infrequently rod-shaped, randomly distributed secretory granules are also very scant. Although the mitochondria appear normal, a small minority of tumour cells may exhibit the oncocytic change. If more differentiated cells are seen, they usually exhibit characteristics of glycoprotein hormone-producing cells; these include cell polarity and uneven distribution of secretory granules.[156,199,201,203]

PITUITARY ONCOCYTOMAS

The cells of oncocytomas are somewhat larger than null cells and often show varying degrees of coarse, granular acidophilia owing to the accumulation of mitochondria.[155,157,201] The latter bind acid dyes and are phosphotungstic acid–haematoxylin reactive. The histological pattern is always diffuse. Immunocytochemical findings are similar to those seen in the null-cell variant.[155,199,201,203,342]

Ultrastructurally, the salient feature is the mitochondrial abundance in the majority of adenoma cells (Fig. 17.91); the remaining morphological details are those of null-cell adenoma.[155,156,201] In oncocytes, the cytoplasmic volume density of mitochondria varies from 15 to 50%, as opposed to the 8–10% observed in normal adenohypophyseal cells.[442] Oncocytes may be of the 'dark' type when filled with rod-shaped mitochondria having numerous cristae and an electron-dense matrix, or 'light' when rich in round to oval mitochondria showing signs of swelling and loss of cristae. The former appear acidophilic, while the latter are chromophobe on light microscopy.[156,201]

Whether considered from the histological, immunocytochemical or ultrastructural point of view, there exists an apparent overlap between the null-cell adenoma–oncocytoma group and the well-differentiated

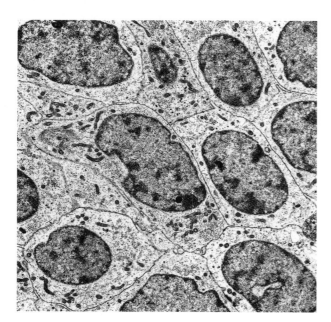

Figure 17.90 *Null cell adenoma. Electron micrograph of small cells with undeveloped cytoplasm with only a few minute secretory granules but no other markers that would indicate their derivation or differentiation.*

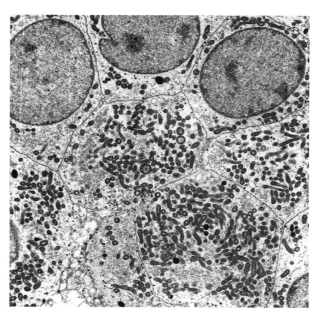

Figure 17.91 *Pituitary oncocytoma. Electron micrograph showing an oncocytic form of null cell adenoma.*

glycoprotein hormone-producing tumours, particularly gonadotroph cell adenomas. The problem is compounded by the uneven, clonal pattern of differentiation, so often seen in immunocytochemical preparation or on ultrastructure. This finding underlies the importance of examining large or multiple tissue samples. Although a majority of tumours in the null-cell adenoma/oncocytoma group appears to be related to the glycoprotein hormone-producing cell line,[14,18,175,196,199,203,342,442] this general group of non-functioning adenomas is not homogeneous. For instance, where pituitary adenomas are assessed by clinical or light microscopical criteria alone, i.e. without the benefit of ultrastructural study, the group of clinically non-functioning adenomas will include some of the silent (subtypes 1–3) adenomas as well as silent forms of other adenoma types, e.g. silent GH adenoma,[249,253,347,443] thus further expanding this nosologically already heterogeneous group.

Plurihormonality in pituitary adenomas

Broadly interpreted, the term plurihormonal is applied to neoplasms that are capable of producing more than one hormone. Such tumours may consist of one or more morphologically distinctive cell types, i.e. monomorphous versus plurimorphous adenomas. Plurihormonality, although widespread among endocrine tumours should not be overdiagnosed. The increasing sensitivity of immunocytochemical techniques permits its detection in the majority of pituitary adenomas. Since the genetic basis and functional significance of plurihormonality is as yet unclear, a certain amount of caution is necessary, particularly since adenomas may incorporate surrounding normal pituitary cells. Plurihormonality does not appear to be a random phenomenon; various tumour types are associated with certain patterns of plurihormonality.

GH–PRL–GLYCOPROTEIN HORMONE

The most common hormonal association is that of GH and PRL, the result being the three morphologically distinct adenoma types previously discussed. In addition to PRL, densely granulated GH adenomas nearly always express some immunoreactivity for α-subunit,[301,360] less frequently for TSH, and rarely for LH and FSH.[155,360] In contrast, the sparsely granulated variant of GH adenoma is likely either to be monohormonal or to contain a few PRL and/or α-subunit-immunoreactive cells. Another commonly occurring pattern is any combination of glycoprotein hormones and their α-subunit with or without minor GH and/or PRL immunoreactivity; such tumours most often show ultrastructural features of gonadotroph differentiation.[199,360] Tumours exhibiting GH, PRL and glycoprotein reactivity may be monomorphous, bimorphous or trimorphous. The last actually consist of cells with ultrastructural features of GH, PRL or mamosomatotrophic and glycoprotein cells.[166]

GH–TSH

As a result of thyrotroph differentiation within GH-producing adenomas, hyperthyroidism may rarely develop in the course of the acromegaly.[31,58] The syndrome is invariably associated with the densely granulated variant of GH adenoma. With rare exceptions, most adenomas in acromegaly–hyperthyroidism are ultrastructurally bimorphous. The development of acromegaly due to somatotrophic differentiation in a thyrotroph cell adenoma initially causing only hyperthyroidism is exceedingly rare; only one unpublished case was observed in the authors' large surgical experience.

ACTH–GLYCOPROTEIN HORMONE

Two infrequent patterns of plurihormonality are associated with corticotroph and gonadotroph adenomas, respectively. As a rule, corticotroph adenomas express POMC and its cleaved products, particularly ACTH. Rare, usually recurrent or aggressively growing macroadenomas, display scattered positivity for LH and/or α-subunit.[35,155] The opposite may also be seen, i.e. the presence of variable (usually light, scattered) ACTH immunoreactivity in rare examples of primarily female-type gonadotroph adenomas.[155] Given the often sparse, weak FSH–LH immunoreactivity exhibited by the latter, examples showing appreciable immunoreactivity for ACTH will inevitably be misdiagnosed unless an ultrastructural study is performed. There is a single report documenting Cushing's disease associated with this variant of gonadotroph adenoma.[171]

As a rule, multiple immunoreactivities represent only a facet of tumour morphology in that plurihormonality infrequently results in multihormone endocrine dysfunction. The diagnosis of 'plurihormonal adenoma' is made only if the tumour is associated with multiple hormonal functions and/or consists of more than one morphological cell type. In most cases, the designation of adenoma type is followed by a list of the immunoreactivities that have been documented.

MISCELLANEOUS PLURIHORMONAL ADENOMAS

The few reported examples of ACTH–PRL, FSH–PRL, TSH–LH and others suggest that all combinations are possible. Such plurihormonal adenomas are rare and some of them represent 'one of a kind' lesion.

In the 1990s three examples of a previously unrecognized bizarre, yet well-defined entity occurring in adolescents were reported.[7,63,294] The tumours of unknown aetiology presented as macroadenomas that had caused delayed growth and development. Morphologically, they consist of PAS-positive and ACTH- and β-endorphin-immunoreactive cells (probably of pars intermedia origin) and of stimulated steroid hormone-producing cells. The existence of prominent junctions between the two components suggests functional interaction.

MORPHOLOGICAL ASPECTS OF MEDICAL THERAPY OF PITUITARY ADENOMAS

The ergot derivative bromocriptine, introduced in the early 1970s for the management of hyperprolactinaemia, remains the most important and widely used compound.[264] A dopamine agonist, the drug reduces serum PRL levels through stimulation of D_2 dopamine receptors. A large percentage of PRL producing adenomas responds to bromocriptine, the degree of response being largely dependent upon their D_2 dopamine receptor status. The most responsive adenomas display a marked reduction in size due chiefly to diminution of the cytoplasmic volume of tumour cells.[159,343,416] Histologically, this produces a remarkable increase in cellularity, the result being a lymphoma-like appearance. Ultrastructurally, the most conspicuous finding is striking irregularity of the heterochromatic nucleus, a change signalling suppression at the level of transcription. The cytoplasm, reduced to a narrow perinuclear rim, contains only scant profiles of RER, a few mitochondria, and rare, if any, Golgi membranes (Fig. 17.92). Secretory granules are sparse and small (less than 200 nm), but exocytoses are still seen. Chronic administration of bromocriptine may lead to fibrosis and calcification. It appears that endocrine amyloid deposition also occurs with increased frequency. Prolactin cell adenomas less amenable to dopamine agonist treatment display similar changes, albeit to a lesser degree.[159] A small minority of tumours responds only with an increase in the number and size of secretory granules as well as lysosomal activation; these effects are considered to be post-translational. Although uneven or mixed responses may be seen, few tumours are unresponsive.[159]

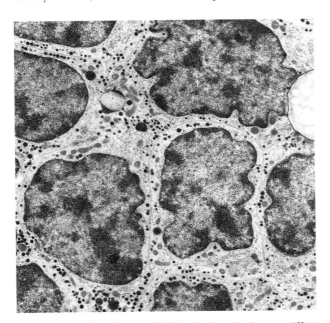

Figure 17.92 *Sparsely granulated prolactin cell adenoma. Effect of bromocriptine treatment. Electron micrograph showing irregular heterochromatic nucleus as well as marked involution of rough endoplasmic reticulum and Golgi complex, signifying functional suppression of adenoma cells.*

In theory, cessation of bromocriptine treatment should enable adenoma cells to regain their original function and structure. Although many do, morphological studies of PRL cell tumours in patients having undergone remote dopamine agonist treatment show that groups of adenoma cells or even larger portions of some tumours exhibit morphological features indicating profound suppression.[159] Such observations suggest that dopamine agonist therapy may elicit a permanent change in the function and probably in the D_2 receptor status of selected subpopulations of tumour cells.

In addition to oral bromocriptine, an injectable long-acting form of the drug is available. As a result of continuous functional suppression, the effects of this preparation are even more pronounced. While haemorrhage and necrosis are uncommon during oral bromocriptine treatment, such changes are likely to be seen when the long-acting agent is administered. In tumours exhibiting significant cell loss, cytoplasmic involution may be so extreme that affected cells may be incapable of even basic housekeeping functions. In recent years new dopamine agonist drugs (cabergoline, quinagolide) have become available,[40,384] but no detailed studies are available on their morphological effects.

Although bromocriptine and other dopamine agonists may be used in the clinical management of acromegaly, their morphological effects have not been sufficiently studied. In the authors' limited experience, lysosomal activation was the only obvious, albeit inconsistent, alteration.

Another compound that revolutionized the medical management of various endocrine tumours, especially of GH- and TSH-producing pituitary adenomas, is the long-acting somatostatin analogue octreotide.[32,98,319,384,410] In-depth clinicopathological studies have shown that the morphological effects of octreotide on GH-producing tumours are less pronounced and less consistent than those of bromocriptine.[32,98,319] Indeed, some tumours show no morphological effects. Yet others demonstrate varying degrees of perivascular and interstitial fibrosis in addition to an increase in the size and number of secretory granules, as well as an increased lysosomal activity with crinophagy. Tumour shrinkage with associated marked nuclear changes and significant reduction in the cytoplasmic volume of cells are infrequent. Deposition of endocrine amyloid may be more common in GH adenomas exposed to octreotide.

Other pharmacological agents such as luteinizing hormone-releasing hormone (LHRH) analogues in the treatment of gonadotroph adenoma have not gained wide acceptance and their morphological effects have not been sufficiently studied.[64]

ECTOPIC PITUITARY ADENOMA

Pituitary adenomas rarely arise outside the sella. Their location, be it in the sphenoid sinus,[62,235] the suprasellar region,[248] the third ventricle[193] or the cavernous sinus,[350] is a reflection of their origin in a developmental rest. Rare adenomas arise in teratomas.[307]

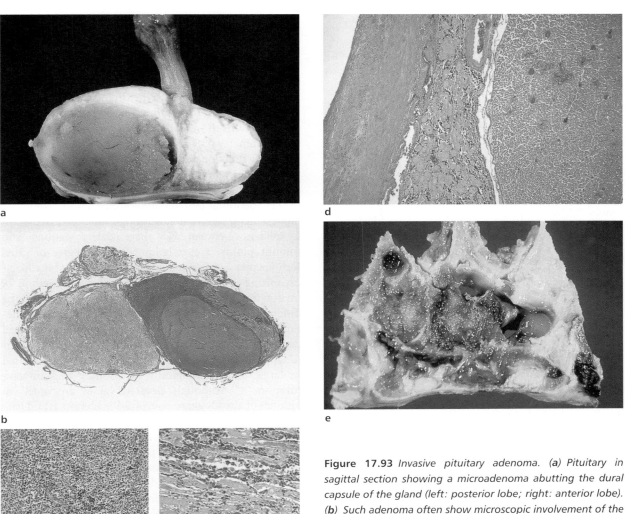

Figure 17.93 *Invasive pituitary adenoma. (a) Pituitary in sagittal section showing a microadenoma abutting the dural capsule of the gland (left: posterior lobe; right: anterior lobe). (b) Such adenoma often show microscopic involvement of the dura. (H&E.) (c) Left: Many adenomas smoothly abut the dural capsule of the gland; right: others infiltrate to involve surrounding structures such as the sinus submucosa. (H&E.) (d) In addition to diffuse spread, some tumours infiltrate between tissue planes, as in this example, wherein a tongue of tumour separates vasculature of the cavernous sinus and cranial nerve. (H&E.) (e) Extensive invasion may be fatal. (H&E.)*

INVASIVE PITUITARY ADENOMAS

Pituitary adenomas are usually slow-growing tumours and most commonly are within the substance of the gland. Although grossly well demarcated, adenomas are not surrounded by a fibrous capsule. Histologically, their interface with the non-tumorous pituitary varies from a distinct border composed of compressed acini and their surrounding reticulin-rich stroma to an ill-defined zone in which tumour intermingles with normal adenohypophyseal cells. Immunostained sections may mimic a mixed or plurihormonal adenoma.

In optimally orientated autopsy specimens, even small adenomas are occasionally seen to invade the pituitary capsule (Fig. 17.93). Only purposeful sampling of dura

adjacent to an adenoma provides the pathologist with evidence of something other than infiltration of pituitary parenchyma. This is uncommon in routine surgical practice in which the capsule is only occasionally sampled. The frequency of dural invasion in microadenomas, macroadenomas and macroadenoma with suprasellar extension was 66, 87 and 94%, respectively.[372] The study not only showed a direct relationship between tumour size and dural invasion but also emphasized the high frequency with which even microadenomas were invasive. This being the case, the occasional finding of microscopic infiltration of a dural fragment is thought to be of little prognostic significance. Rather, it has become practice to consider 'significant' invasion as that grossly evident at surgery. As defined, invasion is seen in 35% of all adenomas. Its

Table 17.7 *Frequency of invasion by pituitary adenomas*

Adenoma cell type	No. of cases	Invasion (%)
GH	23	50
PRL	24	52
GH-PRL	35	31
ACTH (Cushing)	60	15
ACTH (Nelson)	20	50
ACTH (silent)	11	82
FSH/LH	32	21
TSH	4	75
Null	93	42
Plurihormonal	63	52
Total	365	35 (mean)

GH, growth hormone; PRL, prolactin; ACTH, adrenocorticotropic hormone; FSH, follicle-stimulating hormone; LH, luteinizing hormone; TSH, thyroid-stimulating hormone.

frequency varies considerably, not only being higher in endocrinologically functional than in 'non-functioning tumours' but also differing significantly in relation to tumour immunotype[361] (Table 17.7).

Although macroadenomas are more frequently invasive than microadenomas, the latter are also capable of invading adjacent structures. It is customary not to consider invasion by pituitary adenomas as evidence of malignant behaviour. Like meningiomas, pituitary adenomas show a distinct tendency to invade bone and soft tissue (Fig. 17.93). They tend more often to displace or surround blood vessels and cranial nerves, including the optic nerve and chiasm, than to infiltrate these structures (Fig. 17.93). Displacement of brain is also much more common than is actual brain invasion.

Gross invasion by pituitary adenomas takes several forms, some with characteristic clinical manifestations; common examples include cavernous sinus involvement with cranial neuropathies, and direct extension through bone to invade the sphenoid sinus. Invasive adenomas, particularly macroadenomas, may result in a variety of abnormalities, including cranial nerve palsies, visual disturbances, signs and symptoms of increased intracranial pressure, or various degrees of hypopituitarism. If not treated, they may ultimately lead to the death of the patient (Fig. 17.93). The development of diabetes insipidus in association with pituitary adenomas, even with widely invasive tumour, is extremely rare.

It would be of practical importance to predict the invasive potential of pituitary adenomas. Unfortunately, methods presently available do not provide entirely reliable criteria. Although cytological features such as cellular and nuclear pleomorphism are not closely correlated with invasiveness, brisk mitotic activity is generally associated with aggressive growth. The behaviour of pituitary adenomas, particularly invasion, has been studied in terms of DNA content as well as flow cytometry, cytochemical and immunocytochemical proliferation-associated mark-

ers. Aneuploidy has been reported in nearly 50% of pituitary adenomas, its frequency varying among tumours with different functional types.[11]

A recent correlative DNA ploidy study of the full spectrum of adenoma types also found non-diploid patterns, particularly triploidy and hyperdiploidy and to a lesser extent aneuploidy, to be more common in male patients, particularly in those with PRL cell adenomas (65%).[219] Flow cytometry or S-phase studies also show variation in indices by functional tumour type. Although in one study values were highest in acromegaly associated tumours,[11] a recent study of a larger series found male prolactinomas, ACTH adenomas and aneuploid tumours to exhibit the highest %S-phase values. Although no close association is evident between %S-phase determinations and tumour ploidy, a correlation with frequency of gross tumour invasion is evident. The assessment of nucleolar organizing regions provides an inexpensive method of identifying aggressive neoplasms in some tissues, but the differences observed between expansive and invasive adenomas are not significant.[397] The immunocytochemical demonstration of proliferation markers, particularly Ki-67, appears to be more promising.[422] Indices are elevated in large, endocrinologically functioning and invasive tumours.[52,194] Although elevated values are noted in biopsies of already aggressive, invasive adenomas and particularly in carcinomas,[409] the long-term prognostic significance of such studies remains to be established. Immunoreactivity for p53 protein, although present in nearly all pituitary carcinomas and a minority of invasive adenomas, is lacking in non-invasive tumours;[411] p53 gene mutations are nonetheless rarely seen.[224] Preliminary studies suggest that yet other biological markers such as interleukin-6 and heat shock p27Kip1 may also be of value in the identification of aggressive pituitary adenomas.[111,239]

Pituitary carcinomas

Primary pituitary carcinomas are epithelial neoplasms composed of adenohypophyseal cells.[270,312] Usually, cerebrospinal or extracranial metastases are the necessary feature to distinguish pituitary carcinoma from invasive adenoma. Although brain invasion is considered to be synonymous with malignancy, there are no reliable radiological indicators distinguishing brain displacement from invasion, nor is the brain sampled at the time of pituitary surgery, even in cases of obviously aggressive adenoma. As a result, brain invasion is, with rare exceptions, an autopsy finding rather than a factor in the diagnosis of biopsies (Fig. 17.94). Pituitary carcinomas are extremely rare; to date, approximately 50 metastasizing examples have been reported.[312]

The majority of pituitary carcinomas (75%) are clinically hormone producing. Most produce either PRL or ACTH.[114,311] GH cell carcinoma is least common[401] and only one TSH-producing and one gonadotroph

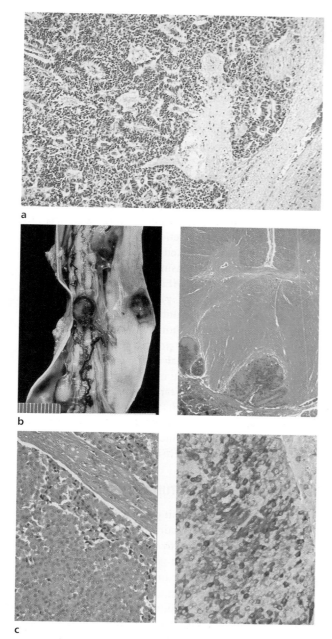

Figure 17.94 *Pituitary carcinoma. (a) Although frank brain invasion is indicative of malignancy it is rarely seen in surgical specimens. Therefore, it is not used as a criterion of pituitary carcinoma in life. (H&E.) (b) More often seen in the clinical setting is craniospinal dissemination. (H&E.) (c) Systemic metastasis may also occur. (H&E.) (b) and (c) are examples from patients with Nelson's syndrome.*

carcinoma have been reported.[28,260] Only a minority appears to be endocrinologically inactive. Carcinomas secreting hormones in excess are not only accompanied by clinically obvious endocrine abnormalities but often associated with exceedingly high blood hormone levels.

Secondary deposits arising from pituitary carcinomas may involve various parts of the brain and spinal cord (Fig. 17.94). Metastases outside the CNS are less frequent

and show a tendency to involve lymph nodes (Fig. 17.94), bones, the lungs and the liver. It is unclear why extracranial metastases are so uncommon. It may relate to the fact that the cells of pituitary carcinomas may infiltrate the adventitia but do not exhibit transmural blood vessel invasion. An alternative, albeit less likely explanation, is that, with rare exception, metastatic tumour cells are unable to colonize other tissues.

As in the case of invasive adenomas, histological features generally cannot be relied upon to predict biological behaviour. At present there are no available immunocytochemical or molecular biological methods that reliably predict which tumours will recur, invade or metastasize. Morphologically, pituitary carcinomas show variable cellular and nuclear pleomorphism, nucleolar prominence and mitotic activity. Despite their rapid growth rate and limited capacity for promoting angiogenesis, focal necrosis is only occasionally seen. As a rule, however, a firm diagnosis of carcinoma cannot be made on the basis of histology alone. Electron microscopy may demonstrate a marked lack or loss of differentiation of tumour cells. Although in some instances the latter may be so marked as to preclude the identification of the cell type, secretory granules are always observed. Preliminary studies suggest that across the spectrum of pituitary neoplasms, proliferation markers[409] and the immunocytochemical demonstration of p53 gene expression[312,411] may be indicators of aggressive behaviour.

At present, the question of whether carcinomas arise *de novo* by transformation of normal adenohypophyseal cells or whether they originate in gradual transition from pre-existing adenomas has not been resolved. In the authors' experience with 15 pituitary carcinomas, all of which occurred in adults with sex predilection, each had been considered a pituitary adenoma at initial resection. All were invasive tumours. The interval between diagnosis of invasive adenoma and carcinoma ranged from months to many years (mean 7 years). Histologically, the carcinomas showed a greater frequency or degree of cellular pleomorphism, nuclear atypia, nucleolar prominence, mitotic activity and aneuploidy than did the primary tumours. Necrosis was infrequent. Immunoreactivity for p53 protein was noted in all metastases but in only a minority of primary tumours.

OTHER MOLECULAR BIOLOGICAL ANALYSIS OF PITUITARY ADENOMAS

Various investigators have used clonal analysis to examine pituitary adenomas. Herman *et al.*[141] analysed various pituitary adenomas and found that somatotroph adenomas (three cases), lactotroph adenomas (four cases) and corticotroph adenomas (three of four cases) and one gonadotroph adenoma were all monoclonal, while normal pituitary tissue was polyclonal. These data suggested that somatic cell mutations occurred before clonal expansion of the neoplasm. A similar study by Jacoby *et al.*[174]

revealed similar findings in a study of 12 adenomas from selected female patients. In this analysis three pituitary adenomas were informative for the clonal analysis and these included one mixed PRL–GH adenoma, one gonadotroph adenoma and one non-functional adenoma. Other investigators found monoclonal inactivation in six clinically non-functional pituitary tumours. Not all clonal analysis of pituitary tumours have found monoclonal populations.[8] In the study by Schulte et al.,[371] six tumours from patients with Cushing's disease, including four with macroadenomas and two microadenomas, showed monoclonal populations. There were three additional pituitary adenomas, including one microadenoma and two macroadenomas which showed a polyclonal pattern of X chromosome inactivation. The latter findings and occasional reports of polyclonal tumours in other studies suggest that some corticotroph adenomas may arise from a single cell or possibly from more than one cell.

Polymerase chain reaction (PCR) analyses have been used extensively in the study of pituitary disorders. Landis et al.[215] and Spada et al.[395] analysed GH-secreting adenomas and observed mutations of the α-gene of the guanine nucleotide binding protein, G_s, which stabilizes the protein active conformation by inhibiting the intrinsic guanosine triphosphatase activity. GH tumours with this mutation had increased secretory activity; ultrastructural studies showed densely granulated cells with prominent RER and Golgi regions. The mutated GH tumours were smaller than other GH tumours without the G_s mutation and were more sensitive to inhibitory agents such as somatostatin and dopamine. PCR techniques characterized the G mutant proteins at two critical sites, namely arginine-201 and glycine-227. This G_s mutation was present in approximately 40% of patients with GH-secreting tumours. Patients with PRL, TSH, ACTH and non-functional tumours did not have this mutation. These findings suggested that G_s mutations in pituitary GH tumours may arise from a yet to be characterized specific oncogene. Yoshimoto et al.[444] found G_s α-mutations in four of 53 pituitary tumours, in a small percentage of thyroid neoplasms as well as adrenocortical adenomas. In contrast, other endocrine tumours including parathyroid, pancreatic endocrine and phaeochromocytomas did not have a G_s mutation, indicating that specific subsets of endocrine tumours have G_s mutations.

Techniques involving PCR have been used to analyse other types of mutations in pituitary tumours. Alvaro et al.[10] recently found that there was a point mutation in position 294 of the protein in the B3 region of the protein kinase C (PKC) α-isoform which resulted in overexpression of the PKC α-isoform in pituitary tumours in man. This mutation was seen more commonly in invasive tumours than in non-invasive tumours.

Hypothalamic releasing hormones have been detected in the pituitary gland by PCR in recent years. Pagesy et al.[303] detected GnRH mRNA in the anterior pituitary of the rat. Other studies have detected GRH mRNA in human pituitary tumours using PCR techniques,[433] and it was localized by Levy and Lightman,[225] by in situ hybridization in human pituitary tumours. PCR techniques have also been helpful in analysing molecular heterogeneity in pituitary hormone genes. Kamijo and Phillips[184] studied isolated GH deficiency type 1A, which is caused by deletion in GH-1 genes. A recent study of GH deficiency by PCR[431] detected GH type 1A deficiency in subjects with severe growth retardation. In a cohort of seven Chinese subjects with severe growth retardation they identified two patients with isolated GH deficiency type 1A. They concluded that this approach could be used to detect this type of GH deficiency in children with severe GH deficiency of early onset.

Many recent studies of cell-cycle proteins in the pituitary have shown the increasing importance of genes and proteins such as p27, p53 MEN1 and p16 in the development and progression of pituitary tumours.[17,101] The cyclin-dependent kinase inhibitor p16 is hypermethylated in some pituitary tumours[440] and another cyclin-dependent kinase inhibitor protein p27 decreases during progression from normal to neoplastic pituitary tumour.[180] The MEN1 gene may also be involved in the pathogenesis of some pituitary tumours, although these findings are controversial.[321,449] Recent studies have shown that chromosome 13q is a frequent target for gene deletion in pituitary tumours, although the exact target does not appear to be the RB1 gene.[388]

GROWTH FACTORS IN PITUITARY ADENOMAS

The role of growth factors in pituitary tumour proliferation and differentiation is currently under intense investigation. A variety of growth factors has been examined in human pituitary cells in vitro.[99,387] These polypeptide molecules can stimulate or inhibit cell proliferation and modulate cell differentiation. Growth factors that have been identified in the pituitary include epidermal growth factor (EGF), transforming growth factor (TGF)-α and -β, insulin-like growth factors (IGF-1 and IGF-2), nerve growth factor (NGF) and fibroblast growth factor (FGF).[127,179] Receptors for many of these growth factors have also been identified in the pituitary. EGF receptors have been found in normal human pituitary cells[42] using biochemical assays. While EGF binding was readily detected in normal human pituitary tissues obtained from post-mortem specimens, it was not detected in any of the 22 pituitary adenomas studied. One possible explanation was the possibility of an altered c-erb-B proto-oncogene which normally encodes the wild-type EGF receptor. Basic fibroblast growth factor (bFGF) and angiogenic and mitogenic factors in many cells have been found in bovine and human pituitary gland tissues. Silverlight et al.[387] observed that bFGF was more abundant in normal human pituitaries than in pituitary adenoma, as evaluated by immunocytochemistry, which suggests that reduction in the levels of this growth factor in many pituitary tumours may favour the stimulation of pituitary growth. Other growth factors including IGF have been analysed in human pituitaries using molecular and cell biological techniques. The IGFs are homologous to pro-insulin and share metabolic properties with insulin, growth stimulation and metabolic effects. IGF-1 and somatostatin-C have been found in normal and neoplastic rat pituitary tissues. IGF may be under the control of GH and probably participates in the endocrine and paracrine pathways in the regulation of GH synthesis and secretion.[100]

In vitro studies have shown that various growth factors can stimulate differentiation in cultured pituitary cells.[60] Atkin *et al.*[23] showed that IGF-1 in cultured gonadotroph pituitary adenomas stimulated FSH secretion as well as the number of glycoprotein-secreting cells entering into the S-phase of the proliferation cycle. This is one of the few examples in which growth factors stimulated cell proliferation in human pituitary tumours.

CYTOGENETIC ABNORMALITIES AND ONCOGENES IN PITUITARY ADENOMAS

Cytogenetic analyses of pituitary tumours have contributed to our knowledge of these neoplasms. Rock *et al.*[335] examined the karyotypes of 18 resected pituitary tumours and found abnormalities associated with chromosomes 1, 4, 7 and 19 in some tumours. Thakker *et al.*[407] observed lesions involving 11q13 in four of 12 sporadic GH-producing pituitary tumours. The 11q13 region of chromosome 11 is associated with tumour development with multiple endocrine neoplasia type 1 including tumours of the pituitary, parathyroid and pancreas. In a subsequent study, Boggild *et al.*[47] analysed pituitary tumours from 88 patients and found activating dominant mutations of $G_s \alpha$ by PCR in 36% of the tumours. They found deletions of chromosome 11 in 16 tumours (18%). These deletions were found in all four major subtypes of pituitary tumours, including GH, PRL, ACTH and non-functional tumours. Deletions on other autosomal chromosomes were found in less than 6% of the tumours. In addition, they found multiple autosomal losses in two aggressive adenomas and suggested that there may be a multistep progression in the development of these more aggressive neoplasms. They did not find amplification or rearrangement of various cellular oncogenes examined, including N-*ras*, *myc* and *fos* in the adenomas.

A new cytogenetic technique, comparative genomic hybridization (CGH), which scans the entire human genome and localizes genetic alterations to specific chromosomal regions, has been used in the study of pituitary tumours. Preliminary studies have detected DNA abnormalities in various regions, including chromosome 13q and in other regions in non-functional adenomas.[72] Another study observed that sites of chromosomal copy gains were more common in functioning adenomas than

in non-functioning tumours and that the most frequently deleted region was in chromosome 13q14, suggesting that a putative tumour suppressor gene in this region may be important in the development of pituitary adenomas.[140]

This overview of the molecular analysis of pituitary disorders highlights the tremendous progress that has been made during the 1990s in understanding the molecular basis of pituitary diseases. Based on the accelerated pace of knowledge accrued in molecular biology an ever-increasing amount of information about the molecular basis of pituitary disease can be anticipated.

Pituitary hyperplasia

Non-neoplastic proliferation of various pituitary cell types rarely causes endocrine hypersecretory disorders.[163] Morphologically, such lesions may be difficult to diagnose in surgical specimens, given that: (1) adenohypophyseal cells are normally unevenly distributed; (2) abnormal proliferations are occasionally focal in nature; (3) fragmentation of transsphenoidal specimens interferes with their assessment, particularly the determination of the precise anatomical site of the biopsy; and (4) mechanical and freezing artefacts are a frequent occurrence. The rarity of pituitary hyperplasia, as well as a lack of experience on the part of pathologists, further make diagnosis difficult.

Morphologically, two basic forms of hyperplasia may be encountered, either singly or in combination. Diffuse hyperplasia refers to a mild to moderate increase in the number of any cell type and does not result in noticeable distortion of acinar architecture. This form of hyperplasia may be difficult to detect in fragmented specimens. In contrast, sustained stimulation of a cell type may result in nodular hyperplasia, i.e. significant, often multifocal proliferation and hypertrophy of adenohypophyseal cells resulting in enlargement and confluence of acini (Figs 17.95, 17.96). The latter is evidenced by expansion and

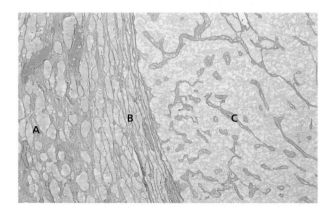

Figure 17.95 *Adenoma and adjacent anterior pituitary. (A) Normal acinar architecture of the non-tumorous pars distalis; (B) the compressed layer of adenohypophyseal tissue, termed the pseudocapsule, around the adenoma; and (C) complete break-up within an adenoma. (Reticulin stain.)*

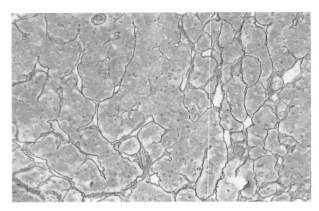

Figure 17.96 *Nodular hyperplasia. Expansion and confluence of acini, leading to major distortion of the normal pattern. (Reticulin stain.)*

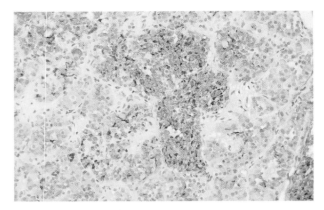

Figure 17.97 *Focal nodular hyperplasia of prolactin cells. (ICC for PRL.)*

early disruption of the acinar reticulin pattern. Only the nodular form of hyperplasia can occasionally be recognized in small fragmented specimens. Supervening adenoma formation is primarily, albeit infrequently, associated with the nodular form. A lesion intermediate between hyperplasia and adenoma, the 'tumourlet', bears resemblance to pulmonary neuroendocrine proliferations of the same name.

GH CELL OR MAMMOSOMATOTROPH CELL HYPERPLASIA

This may cause acromegaly with or without hyperprolactinaemia, as described in the rare McCune–Albright syndrome[204] and in occasional cases of gigantism beginning in infancy or early childhood.[267,450] These hyperplastic lesions display variable eosinophilic granularity and may be ultrastructurally atypical, exhibiting both GH and PRL cell differentiation. Practically all cases of acromegaly not caused by an autonomous GH cell adenoma are induced by ectopic overproduction of GRH. Although the production of GRH by endocrine neoplasms, such as pancreatic islet cell tumour, bronchial carcinoid tumour or phaeochromocytoma, is not particularly rare,[352] only a small fraction elicits GH cell hyperplasia and acromegaly.[97] Nodular GH cell hyperplasia is an acidophilic lesion composed of heavily granulated cells which, aside from their unusually prominent Golgi apparatus, exhibit otherwise typical ultrastructural features of GH cells.[152,157,414] Adenoma formation may rarely be seen to arise in the hyperplasia accompanying ectopic GRH production.

PRL CELL HYPERPLASIA

This is more common than GH cell hyperplasia. It is well known that hyperprolactinaemia may occur in association with any process compressing the pituitary stalk and thereby compromising dopamine transport. If the lesion persists, PRL cell hyperplasia ensues.[152,157] Approximately 10% of non-PRL-producing adenomas elicit significant

hyperprolactinaemia. Among non-tumorous conditions, various cysts, lymphocytic hypophysitis and granulomas are common causes of the stalk effect.

Although primary pituitary disorders such as corticotroph adenoma may infrequently be accompanied by nodular PRL hyperplasia, the association is more common with thyrotroph hyperplasia.[316] Hyperplasia of PRL cells in such cases results from associated TRH excess and has important clinical implications. The resulting hyperprolactinaemia modifies the clinical presentation, often diverting attention from the underlying hypothyroidism and leading to unwarranted pituitary surgery.

In contrast to the diffuse form of physiological PRL cell hyperplasia that accompanies pregnancy and lactation, hyperplasia secondary to various pathological processes is most often multifocal and nodular (Fig. 17.97). An example is long-term oestrogen administration.[364] Histologically, the lesion is chromophobe. At the ultrastructural level the voluminous cells exhibit masses of RER and an extensive Golgi apparatus, whereas most of the secretory granules are restricted to the Golgi region. An idiopathic form of nodular PRL cell hyperplasia is exceptionally rare.[176]

CORTICOTROPH CELL HYPERPLASIA

This is an uncommon cause of pituitary-dependent Cushing's disease.[236,254] The idiopathic form is thought to be due to hypothalamic dysfunction. Given the often nodular disposition of ACTH-immunoreactive cells in the normal pituitary, it is notoriously difficult to diagnose in fragmented specimens. In some glands, morphological heterogeneity of corticotrophs may be evident. Foci of normally distributed ACTH cells display Crooke's hyalinization, whereas the hyperplastic corticotrophs within enlarged acini are smaller and show no signs of excess hyaline accumulation. Transition from nodular hyperplasia to ACTH cell adenoma may occur.[445]

Ectopic production of CRH is also capable of inducing corticotroph hyperplasia.[57]

THYROTROPH HYPERPLASIA

This well-known condition, resulting from protracted primary hypothyroidism, is often but not invariably reversible by adequate thyroid hormone replacement. One would not expect to encounter this lesion in surgical material, yet several cases have been reported.[164,316] In hypothyroidism, TRH stimulation of thyrotrophs may progress from a moderate generalized increase in TSH cells (diffuse hyperplasia) to massive nodular hyperplasia with resultant enlargement of the gland and the production of symptoms due to local mass effects. In some cases, hypothyroidism has previously been diagnosed and treated, but the thyrotroph hyperplasia failed to regress despite clinical euthyroidism. In such instances the patient's pituitary enlargement appears unrelated to hypothyroidism. It is in patients of this kind that the frequently associated hyperprolactinaemia may occur (see above) and the lesion may mimic a PRL-producing adenoma. As a result, a young female patient may undergo pituitary surgery.

Thyrotroph hyperplasia is a lesion of chromophobes consisting of large, often polar cells with pale, vacuolated cytoplasm crowded within and filling markedly enlarged acini (Fig. 17.98). The presence of coarse PAS-positive cytoplasmic globules representing lysosomes is characteristic of thyroid deficiency cells. A small number of other adenohypophyseal cells always lies intermingled. The hyperplastic cells display variable immunoreactivity for TSH. By electron microscopy, the marker of these thyroid deficiency or 'thyroidectomy' cells is abundance of RER, dilated profiles of which are filled with a flaky or granular proteinaceous substance of low density. Secretory granules may be sparse, thus explaining the often weak TSH immunopositivity of some cells. In instances in which the patient has received preoperative thyroid hormone replacement therapy, the persisting hyperplastic TSH cells are smaller, slightly basophilic, PAS positive and strongly immunoreactive for TSH, and contain more abundant secretory granules.[152,157,164,316]

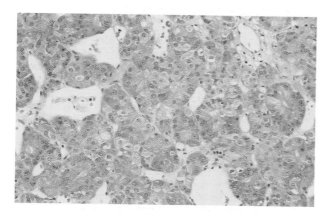

Figure 17.98 *Nodular thyrotroph cell hyperplasia in long-standing hypothyroidism. (H&E.)*

GONADOTROPH HYPERPLASIA

This is probably the least frequent form of pituitary hyperplasia.[157] Massive, nodular hyperplasia causing enlargement of the entire gland and evoking local symptoms is not seen in surgical material. Significant gonadotroph hyperplasia may, however, be seen at autopsy in cases of life-long primary hypogonadism, e.g. Klinefelter's syndrome. Although the development of gonadotroph adenoma in a few patients with long-standing hypogonadism suggests a role for target organ deficiency in adenoma genesis, such tumours may be purely coincidental considering the prevalence of gonadotroph adenoma in older patients.

In the postgonadectomy state in either sex or in postmenopausal females, gonadotrophs appear numerous but are unassociated with a change in pituitary architecture. Unfortunately, reliable cell counts establishing limits of normal gonadotroph number in various age groups, particularly prepubertal and adult males as well as prepubertal, cycling and postmenopausal females, are not available. Thus, unless the increase in gonadotroph cell number is marked, a diagnosis of diffuse gonadotroph hyperplasia cannot be made.

REFERENCES

1 Adams M, Rhyner PA, Day J et al. Whipple's disease confined to the central nervous system. *Ann Neurol* 1987; **21**: 104–8.

2 Adamson TE, Wiestler OD, Kleihues P, Yasargil MG. Correlation of clinical and pathological features in surgically treated craniopharyngiomas. *J Neurosurg* 1990; **73**: 12–17.

3 Aguilo F Jr, Vega LA, Haddock L, Rodriguez O Jr. Diabetes insipidus syndrome in hypopituitarism of pregnancy. Case report and a critical review of the literature. *Acta Endocrinol* 1969; **60** (Suppl 137): 1–32.

4 Ahmed SR, Aiello DP, Page R et al. Necrotizing infundibulo-hypophysitis: a unique syndrome of diabetes insipidus and hypopituitarism. *J Clin Endocrinol Metab* 1993; **76**: 1499–504.

5 Akita S, Readhead C, Stefaneanu L et al. Pituitary-directed leukemia inhibitory factor transgene forms Rathke's cleft cysts and impairs adult pituitary function. A model for human pituitary Rathke's cysts. *J Clin Invest* 1997; **99**: 2462–9.

6 Albright AL, Price RA, Guthkelch AM. Diencephalic gliomas of children. A clinicopathologic study. *Cancer* 1985; **55**: 2789–93.

7 Albuquerque FC, Weiss MH, Kovacs K et al. A functioning composite 'corticotroph' pituitary adenoma with interspersed adrenocortical cells. *Pituitary* 1999; **1**: 279–84.

8 Alexander JM, Biller BM, Bikkal H et al. Clinically nonfunctioning pituitary tumors are monoclonal in origin. *J Clin Invest* 1990; **86**: 336–40.

9 Allaerts W, Carmeliet P, Denef C. New perspectives in the function of pituitary folliculo-stellate cells. *Mol Cell Endocrinol* 1990; **71**: 73–81.

10 Alvaro V, Levy L, Dubray C et al. Invasive human pituitary tumors express a point-mutated α-protein kinase-C. *J Clin Endocrinol Metab* 1993; **77**: 1125–9.

11 Anniko M, Tribukait B, Wersall J. DNA ploidy and cell phase in human pituitary tumors. *Cancer* 1984; **53**: 1708–13.

12 Ansorge O, Daniel SE, Pearce RK. Neuronal loss and plasticity in the supraoptic nucleus in Parkinson's disease. *Neurology* 1997; **49**: 610–13.

13 Arslanian SA, Rothfus WE, Foley TP Jr, Becker DJ. Hormonal, metabolic, and neuroradiologic abnormalities associated with septo-optic dysplasia. *Acta Endocrinol (Copenh)* 1984; **107**: 282–8.

14 Asa SL. Tumors of the pituitary gland. *Atlas of tumor pathology*. Third Series, Fascicle 22. Washington, DC: Armed Forces Institute of Pathology, 1998: 1–210.

15 Asa SL, Bilbao JM, Kovacs K, Linfoot JA. Hypothalamic neuronal hamartoma associated with pituitary growth hormone cell adenoma and acromegaly. *Acta Neuropathol (Berl)* 1980; **52**: 231–4.

16 Asa SL, Ezzat S. Molecular determinants of pituitary cytodifferentiation. *Pituitary* 1999; **1**: 159–68.

17 Asa SL, Ezzat S. The cytogenesis and pathogenesis of pituitary adenomas. *Endocr Rev* 1998; **19**: 798–827.

18 Asa SL, Gerrie BM, Singer W *et al*. Gonadotropin secretion *in vitro* by human pituitary null cell adenomas and oncocytomas. *J Clin Endocrinol Metab* 1986; **62**: 1011–19.

19 Asa SL, Kovacs K, Bilbao JM. The pars tuberalis of the human pituitary: a histologic, immunohistochemical, ultrastructural and immunoelectron microscopic analysis. *Virchows Arch Pathol Anat* 1983; **399**: 49–59.

20 Asa SL, Kovacs K, Thorner MO *et al*. Immunohistological localization of growth hormone-releasing hormone in human tumors. *J Clin Endocrinol Metab* 1985; **60**: 423–7.

21 Asa SL, Penz G, Kovacs K, Ezrin C. Prolactin cells in the human pituitary: a quantitative immunocytochemical analysis. *Arch Pathol Lab Med* 1982; **106**: 360–3.

22 Asa SL, Scheithauer BW, Bilbao JM *et al*. A case for hypothalamic acromegaly: a clinicopathologic study of six patients with hypothalamic gangliocytomas producing growth hormone-releasing factor. *J Clin Endocrinol Metab* 1984; **58**: 796–803.

23 Atkin SL, Landolt AM, Jeffreys RV *et al*. Differential effects of insulin-like growth factor 1 on the hormonal product and proliferation of glycoprotein secreting human pituitary adenomas. *J Clin Endocrinol Metab* 1993; **77**: 1059–66.

24 Baker AB, Cornwell S, Brown IA. Poliomyelitis. VI. The hypothalamus. *Arch Neurol Psychiatry* 1952; **68**: 16–36.

25 Barrow DL, Spector RH, Takei Y, Tindall GT. Symptomatic Rathke's cleft cyst located entirely in the suprasellar region: review of diagnosis, management, and pathogenesis. *Neurosurgery* 1985; **16**: 766–72.

26 Baylis PH, Robertson GL. Vasopressin function in familial cranial diabetes insipidus. *Postgrad Med J* 1981; **57**: 36–40.

27 Baz E, Saeger W, Uhlig H *et al*. HGH, PRL and βHCG/βLH gene expression in clinically inactive pituitary adenomas detected by *in situ* hybridization. *Virchows Arch Pathol Anat* 1991; **418**: 405–10.

28 Beauchesne P, Trouillas J, Barral F, Brunon J. Gonadotropic pituitary carcinoma: a case report. *Neurosurgery* 1995; **37**: 810–16.

29 Beck-Peccoz P, Brucker-Davis F, Persani L *et al*. Thyrotropin-secreting pituitary tumors. *Endocr Rev* 1996; **17**: 610–38.

30 Beck-Peccoz P, Persani L, Asteria C *et al*. Thyrotropin-secreting pituitary tumors in hyper and hypothyroidism. *Acta Med Aust* 1996; **23**: 41–6.

31 Beck-Peccoz P, Piscitelli G, Amr S *et al*. Endocrine biochemical and morphological studies of a pituitary adenoma secreting growth hormone, thyrotropin (TSH), and α-subunit: evidence for secretion of TSH with increased bioactivity. *J Clin Endocrinol Metab* 1986; **62**: 704–11.

32 Beckers A, Stevenaert A, Kovacs K *et al*. The treatment of acromegaly with SMS 201–995. *Adv Biosci* 1988; **69**: 227–8.

33 Benvenga S, Lo Giudice F, Campenni A *et al*. Post-traumatic selective hypogonadotropic hypogonadism. *J Endocrinol Invest* 1997; **20**: 675–80.

34 Benzick AE, Wirthwein DP, Weinberg A *et al*. Pituitary gland gumma in congenital syphilis after failed maternal treatment: a case report. *Pediatrics* 1999; **104**: e4.

35 Berg KK, Scheithauer BW, Felix I *et al*. Pituitary adenomas that produce adrenocorticotropic hormone and α-subunit: clinicopathological, immunohistochemical, ultrastructural and immunoelectron microscopic studies in nine cases. *Neurosurgery* 1990; **26**: 397–401.

36 Bergeron C, Kovacs K. Pituitary siderosis: a histologic, immunocytologic, and ultrastructural study. *Am J Pathol* 1978; **93**: 295–309.

37 Bergeron C, Kovacs K, Bilbao JM. Primary empty sella: a histologic and immunocytologic study. *Arch Intern Med* 1979; **139**: 248–9.

38 Bergeron C, Kovacs K, Ezrin C, Mizzen C. Hereditary diabetes insipidus: an immunohistochemical study of the hypothalamus and pituitary gland. *Acta Neuropathol* 1991; **81**: 345–8.

39 Bergland RM, Page RB. Pituitary–brain vascular relations: a new paradigm. *Science* 1979; **204**: 18–24.

40 Biller BM, Molitch ME, Vance ML *et al*. Treatment of prolactin-secreting macroadenomas with the once-weekly dopamine agonist cabergoline. *J Clin Endocrinol Metab* 1996; **81**: 2338–43.

41 Bills DC, Meyer FB, Laws ER Jr *et al*. A retrospective analysis of pituitary apoplexy. *Neurosurgery* 1993; **33**: 602–9.

42 Birman P, Michard M, Li JY *et al*. Epidermal growth factor-binding sites, present in normal human and rat pituitaries, are absent in human pituitary adenomas. *J Clin Endocrinol Metab* 1987; **65**: 275–81.

43 Bjerre P, Riishede J, Lindholm J. Pituitary abscess. *Acta Neurochir (Wien)* 1983; **68**: 187–93.

44 Blass JP, Gibson BE. Abnormality of a thiamine-requiring enzyme in patients with Wernicke–Korsakoff syndrome. *N Engl J Med* 1977; **297**: 1367–70.

45 Blotner H. Primary or idiopathic diabetes insipidus – a system disease. *Metabolism* 1958; **7**: 191–200.

46 Boecher-Schwarz HG, Hey O, Higer HP, Perneczky A. Intrasellar cysticercosis mimicking a pituitary adenoma. *Br J Neurosurg* 1991; **5**: 405–7.

47 Boggild MD, Jenkinson S, Pistorellio M *et al*. Molecular genetic studies of sporadic pituitary tumors. *J Clin Endocrinol Metab* 1994; **78**: 387–92.

48 Bognar L, Szeifert GT, Fedorcsak I, Pasztor E. Abscess formation in Rathke's cleft cyst. *Acta Neurochir (Wien)* 1992; **117**: 70–2.

49 Branch CL Jr, Laws ER Jr. Metastatic tumors of the sella turcica masquerading as primary pituitary tumors. *J Clin Endocrinol Metab* 1987; **65**: 469–74.

50 Brat DJ, Scheithauer BW, Staugaitis SM *et al*. Pituicytoma. A distinctive low-grade glioma of the neurohypophysis. *Am J Surg Pathol* 2000; **24**: 362–8.

51 Braverman LE, Mancini JP, McGoldrick DM. Hereditary idiopathic diabetes insipidus: a case report with autopsy findings. *Ann Intern Med* 1965; **63**: 503–8.

52 Buchfelder M, Falbusch R, Adams EF *et al*. Invasive pituitary adenomas: frequency and proliferation. *Endocr Pathol* 1992; **3** (Suppl 1): S5.

53 Burger PC, Scheithauer BW. *Tumors of the central nervous system*. Third Series, Fascicle 10. Washington, DC: Armed Forces Institute of Pathology, 1994: 1–452.

54 Burr IM, Slonim AE, Danish RK *et al*. Diencephalic syndrome revisited. *J Pediatr* 1976; **88**: 439–44.

55 Burrow GN, Wortzman G, Rewcastle NB et al. Microade-nomas of the pituitary and abnormal sellar tomograms in an unselected autopsy series. N Engl J Med 1981; **304**: 156–8.

56 Calle-Rodrigue R, Giannini C, Scheithauer BW. Prolactino-mas in males and females: a comparative clinicopathologic study. Mayo Clin Proc 1998; **73**: 1046–52.

57 Carey RM, Varma SK, Drake CR et al. Ectopic secretion of corticotropin-releasing factor as a cause of Cushing's syn-drome: a clinical, morphologic, and biochemical study. N Engl J Med 1984; **311**: 13–20.

58 Carlson HE, Linfoot JA, Braunstein GD et al. Hyperthy-roidism and acromegaly due to a TSH and GH-secreting pituitary tumor: lack of hormonal response to bromocrip-tine. Am J Med 1983; **74**: 915–23.

59 Carson MJ, Slager UT, Steinberg RM. Simultaneous occur-rence of diabetes mellitus, diabetes insipidus, and optic atrophy in a brother and sister. Am J Dis Child 1977; **131**: 1382–5.

60 Chaidrun SS, Eggo M, Stewart PM et al. Role of growth fac-tors and estrogen as modulators of growth, differentiation and expression of gonadotropin subunit genes in primary cultured sheep pituitary cells. Endocrinology 1994; **134**: 935–44.

61 Clarren SK, Alvord EC Jr, Hall JC. Congenital hypothalamic hamartoblastoma, hypopituitarism, imperforate anus, and postaxial polydactyly – a new syndrome? Part 2: neu-ropathologic considerations. Am J Med Genet 1980; **7**: 75–83.

62 Coire CI, Horvath E, Kovacs K et al. Cushing's syndrome from an ectopic pituitary adenoma with peliosis. Histo-logical, immunohistochemical and ultrastructural study and review of the literature. Endocr Pathol 1997; **8**: 65–74.

63 Coire CI, Horvath E, Kovacs K et al. A composite silent 'cor-ticotroph' pituitary adenoma with interspersed adreno-cortical cells. Neurosurgery 1998; **42**: 650–4.

64 Colombo P, Ambrosi B, Saccomanno K et al. Effects of long-term treatment with the gonadotropin-releasing hormone analog nafarelin in patients with non-functioning pituitary adenomas. Eur J Endocrinol 1994; **130**: 339–45.

65 Corenblum B, Sirek AM, Horvath E et al. Human mixed somatotrophic and lactotrophic pituitary adenomas. J Clin Endocrinol Metab 1976; **42**: 857–63.

66 Cosman F, Post KD, Holub DA, Wardlaw SL. Lymphocytic hypophysitis: report of 3 new cases and review of the lit-erature. Medicine 1989; **68**: 240–56.

67 Costigan DC, Daneman D, Harwood-Nash D, Holland FJ. The 'empty sella' in childhood. Clin Pediatr 1984; **23**: 437–40.

68 Coulter CL, Leech RW, Schaefer GB et al. Midline cerebral dysgenesis, dysfunction of the hypothalamic-pituitary axis, and fetal alcohol effects. Arch Neurol 1993; **50**: 771–5.

69 Craft WH, Underwood LE, Van Wyk JJ. High incidence of perinatal insult in children with idiopathic hypopituitarism. J Pediatr 1980; **96**: 397–402.

70 Crompton MR. Hypothalamic lesions following the rupture of cerebral berry aneurysms. Brain 1963; **86**: 301–14.

71 Crotty TB, Scheithauer BW, Young WF Jr et al. Papillary cran-iophyaryngioma. A clinico-pathologic study of 48 cases. J Neurosurg 1995; **83**: 206–14.

72 Daniel M, Aviram A, Adams EF et al. Comparative geno-mic hybridization analysis of nonfunctioning pituitary tumors. J Clin Endocrinol Metab 1998; **83**: 1801–5.

73 Daniel PM, Prichard MML. Studies of the hypothalamus and the pituitary gland: with special reference to the effects of transection of the pituitary stalk. Acta Endocrinol Suppl (Copenh) 1975; **201**: 1–216.

74 Daniel PM, Spicer EJ, Treip CS. Pituitary necrosis in patients maintained on mechanical respirators. J Pathol 1973; **111**: 135–8.

75 Daniel PM, Treip CS. Lesions of the pituitary gland associ-ated with head injuries. In: Harris GW, Donovan BT eds. The pituitary gland. Berkeley, CA: University of California Press, 1966: 519–34.

76 de Bruin WI, van't Verlaat JW, Graamans K, de Bruin TW. Sellar granulomatous mass in a pregnant woman with active Crohn's disease. Neth J Med 1991; **39**: 136–41.

77 de Keyzer Y, Bertagna X, Luton JP, Kahn A. Variable modes of proopiomelanocortin gene transcription in human tumors. Mol Endocrinol 1989; **3**: 215–23.

78 Della Corte F, Mancini A, Valle D et al. Provocative hypo-thalamopituitary axis tests in severe head injury: correla-tions with severity and prognosis. Crit Care Med 1998; **26**: 1419–26.

79 Delsedime M, Aguggia M, Cantello R et al. Isolated hypophyseal tuberculoma: case report. Clin Neuropathol 1988; **7**: 311–13.

80 DeMarinis L, Mancini A, Valle D et al. Hypothalamic derangement in traumatized patients: growth hormone (GH) and prolactin response to thyrotropin-releasing hor-mone and GH-releasing hormone. Clin Endocrinol 1999; **50**: 741–7.

81 Denef C. Paracrine mechanisms in the pituitary. In: Imura H ed. The pituitary gland 2nd edn. New York: Raven Press, 1994: 351–78.

82 Dierickx K. Regeneration of the neural lobe of the hypophysis after extirpation of the median eminence in Rana temporaria. Acta Anat (Basel) 1965; **60**: 181–6.

83 Domingue JN, Wilson CB. Pituitary abscesses: report of seven cases and review of the literature. J Neurosurg 1977; **46**: 601–8.

84 Dreyer M, Rudiger HW, Bujara K et al. The syndrome of dia-betes insipidus, diabetes mellitus, optic atrophy, deafness, and other abnormalities (DIDMOAD-syndrome): two affected sibs and a short review of the literature (98 cases). Klin Wochenschr 1982; **60**: 471–5.

85 Dubois PM, ElAmraoui A. Embryology of the pituitary gland. Trends Endocrinol Metab 1995; **6**: 1–7.

86 Dubois PM, ElAmraoui A, Heritier AG. Development and dif-ferentiation of pituitary cells. Microsc Res Techn 1997; **39**: 98–113.

87 Duchen LW. Metastatic carcinoma in the pituitary gland and hypothalamus. J Pathol Bacteriol 1966; **91**: 347–55.

88 Duff JM, Meyer FB, Ilstrup DM et al. Long-term outcomes for surgically resected craniopharyngiomas. Neurosurgery 2000; **46**: 291–305.

89 Dyer EH, Civit T, Visot A et al. Transsphenoidal surgery for pituitary adenomas in children. Neurosurgery 1994; **34**: 207–12.

90 Ebersold MJ, Laws ER Jr, Scheithauer BW, Randall RV. Pitu-itary apoplexy treated by transsphenoidal surgery: a clini-copathology and immunocytochemical study. J Neurosurg 1983; **58**: 315–20.

91 Edwards CRW. Diabetes insipidus. In: Lant AF ed. Advanced medicine (Symposium 11). London: Pittman Medical, 1975: 276–88.

92 Edwards OM, Clark JD. Post-traumatic hypopituitarism. Six cases and a review of the literature (Review). Medicine (Bal-timore) 1986; **65**: 281–90.

93 Enriquez P, Dahlin DC, Hayles AB, Henderson ED. Histiocy-tosis X: a clinical study. Mayo Clin Proc 1967; **42**: 88–99.

94 Erlandson RA. Diagnostic transmission electron microscopy of tumors. New York: Raven Press, 1994: 149.

95 Esposito S, Nardi P. Lipoma of the infundibulum, case report. J Neurosurg 1987; **67**: 304–6.

96 Everett GD, Amatruda JM, Woolf PD. Hypothalamic–hypopituitarism due to temporal arteritis. *Arch Intern Med* 1979; **139**: 474–5.

97 Ezzat S, Asa SL, Stefaneanu L *et al*. Somatotroph hyperplasia without pituitary adenoma associated with a longstanding growth hormone-releasing hormone-producing bronchial carcinoid. *J Clin Endocrinol Metab* 1994; **78**: 555–60.

98 Ezzat S, Horvath E, Harris AG, Kovacs K. Morphological effects of octreotide on growth hormone-producing pituitary adenomas. *J Clin Endocrinol Metab* 1994; **79**: 113–18.

99 Ezzat S, Melmed S. The role of growth factors in the pituitary. *J Endocrinol Invest* 1990; **13**: 691–8.

100 Fagin JA, Pixley S, Slanina S *et al*. Insulin-like growth factor I gene expression in GH3 rat pituitary cells: messenger ribonucleic acid content, immunocytochemistry and secretion. *Endocrinology* 1987; **120**: 2037–43.

101 Farrell WE, Clayton RN. Molecular biology of human pituitary adenomas. *Ann Mol* 1998; **30**: 192–8.

102 Fehn M, Farquharson MA, Sautner P *et al*. Demonstration of pro-opiomelanocortin mRNA in pituitary adenomas and paraadenomatous gland in Cushing's disease and Nelson's syndrome. *J Pathol* 1993; **169**: 335–9.

103 Felix IA, Horvath E, Kovacs K. Massive Crooke's hyalinization in corticotroph cell adenoma of the human pituitary. A histological, immunocytological, and electron microscopic study of three cases. *Acta Neurochir (Wien)* 1982; **58**: 235–43.

104 Felix IA, Horvath E, Kovacs K *et al*. Mammosomatotroph adenoma of the pituitary associated with gigantism and hyperprolactinemia. A morphological study including immunoelectron microscopy. *Acta Neuropathol (Berl)* 1986; **71**: 76–82.

105 Fink EB. Diabetes insipidus: a clinical review and analysis of necropsy reports. *Arch Pathol* 1928; **6**: 102–20.

106 Fisher C, Ingram WR, Ranson SW. *Diabetes insipidus and the neuro-hormonal control of water balance: a contribution to the structure and function of the hypothalamico-hypophyseal system*. Ann Arbor, MI: Edwards Brothers, 1938.

107 Frawley LS, Boockfor FR. Mammosomatotropes: presence and functions in normal and neoplastic pituitary tissue. *Endocr Rev* 1991; **12**: 337–55.

108 Frawley LS, Boockfor FR, Hoeffler JP. Identification by plaque assays of a pituitary cell type that secretes both growth hormone and prolactin. *Endocrinology* 1985; **116**: 734–7.

109 Friede RL. Osteolipomas of the tuber cinereum. *Arch Pathol Lab Med* 1977; **101**: 369–72.

110 Gama R, Smith MJ, Wright J, Marks V. Hypopituitarism in primary haemochromatosis: recovery after iron depletion. *Postgrad Med J* 1995; **71**: 297–8.

111 Gandour-Edwards R, Kapadia SB, Janecka IP *et al*. Biologic markers of invasive pituitary adenomas involving the sphenoid sinus. *Mod Pathol* 1995; **8**: 160–4.

112 Gharib H, Frey HM, Laws ER Jr *et al*. Coexistent primary empty sella syndrome and hyperprolactinemia: report of 11 cases. *Arch Intern Med* 1983; **143**: 1383–6.

113 Gilcrease MZ, Delgado R, Albores-Saavedra J. Intrasellar adenoid cystic carcinoma and papillary mucinous adenocarcinoma: two previously undescribed primary neoplasms at this site. *Ann Diagn Pathol* 1999; **3**: 141–7.

114 Giordana MT, Cavalla P, Allegranza A, Pollo B. Intracranial dissemination of pituitary adenoma. Case report and review of the literature. *Ital J Neurol Sci* 1994; **15**: 195–200.

115 Girod C, Trouillas J, Claustrat B. The human thyrotropic adenoma: pathologic diagnosis in five cases and critical review of the literature. *Semin Diagn Pathol* 1986; **3**: 58–68.

116 Giuffre R, Gagliardi FM. Unusual hypophyseal tumour of Rathke's cleft origin. *Neurochirurgia (Stuttg)* 1968; **11**: 81–9.

117 Gorczyca W, Hardy J. Arterial supply of the human anterior pituitary gland. *Neurosurgery* 1987; **20**: 369–78.

118 Gorski RA. Sexual differentiation of the brain. *Hosp Pract* 1978; **13**: 55–62.

119 Graus F, Rogers LR, Posner JB. Cerebrovascular complications in patients with cancer. *Medicine* 1985; **64**: 16–35.

120 Graziani N, Donnet A, N'jee Bugha T *et al*. Ectopic basisphenoidal craniopharyngioma: case report and review of the literature. *Neurosurgery* 1994; **34**: 346–9.

121 Green JR, Buchan GC, Alvord EC Jr, Swanson AG. Hereditary and idiopathic types of diabetes insipidus. *Brain* 1967; **90**: 707–14.

122 Greenwood SM, Martin JS, Towfighi J. Unifocal eosinophilic granuloma of the temporal lobe. *Surg Neurol* 1982; **17**: 441–4.

123 Gubbay SS. Derangement of temperature control in hydrocephalus. *Dev Med Child Neurol* 1967; **Suppl 13**: 125–32.

124 Guthrie BL, Ebersold MJ, Scheithauer BW, Shaw EG. Meningeal hemangiopericytoma: histopathological features, treatment and long-term follow-up of 44 cases. *Neurosurg* 1989; **25**: 514–22.

125 Hagg E, Astrom L, Steen L. Persistent hypothalamic–pituitary insufficiency following acute meningoencephalitis. A report of two cases. *Acta Med Scand* 1978; **203**: 231–5.

126 Hall JG, Pallister PD, Clarren SK *et al*. Congenital hypothalamic hamartoblastoma, hypopituitarism, imperforate anus, and postaxial polydactyly – a new syndrome? Part 1: clinical, causal, and pathogenetic considerations. *Am J Med Genet* 1980; **7**: 47–74.

127 Halper J, Parnell PG, Carter BJ *et al*. Presence of growth factors in human pituitary. *Lab Invest* 1992; **66**: 639–45.

128 Harper C. Wernicke's encephalopathy: a more common disease than realized. A neuropathological study of 51 cases. *J Neurol Neurosurg Psychiatry* 1979; **42**: 226–31.

129 Hart MN. Hypertrophy of human subventricular hypothalamic nucleus in starvation. *Arch Pathol* 1971; **91**: 493–6.

130 Haselow RE, Nesbit M, Dehner LP *et al*. Second neoplasms following megavoltage radiation in a pediatric population. *Cancer* 1978; **42**: 1185–91.

131 Hatakeyama S. Electron microscopic study of the anencephalic adenohypophysis with reference to the adrenocorticotrophs and their correlation with the functional differentiation of the hypothalamus during the foetal life. *Endocrinol Jpn* 1969; **16**: 187–203.

132 Hayashi H, Yamada K, Kuroki T *et al*. Lymphocytic hypophysitis and pulmonary sarcoidosis. Report of a case (Review). *Am J Clin Pathol* 1991; **95**: 506–11.

133 Hayashi Y, Hamada Y, Oki H, Yamashita J. Pituitary stalk meningioma: case report. *Neuroradiology* 1997; **39**: 351–3.

134 Hayden MR, Vinik AI, Paul M, Beighton P. Impaired prolactin release in Huntington's chorea. Evidence for dopaminergic excess. *Lancet* 1977; **2**: 423–6.

135 Heary RF, Maniker AH, Wolansky LJ. Candidal pituitary abscess – case report. *Neurosurgery* 1995; **36**: 1009–12.

136 Heinbecker P, White HL. Hypothalamico-hypophysial system and its relation to water balance in the dog. *Am J Physiol* 1941; **133**: 582–93.

137 Hempenius LM, VanDam PS, Marx JJ, Koppeschaar HP. Mineralocorticoid status and endocrine dysfunction in severe hemochromatosis. *J Endocrinol Invest* 1999; **22**: 369–76.

138 Hendricks SA, Lippe BM, Kaplan SA, Bentson JR. Hypothalamic atrophy with progressive hypopituitarism in an adolescent girl. *J Clin Endocrinol Metab* 1981; **52**: 562–4.

139 Hennekam RC, Beemer FA, Van Merrienboer F et al. Congenital hypothalamic hamartoma associated with severe midline defect: a developmental field defect report of a case. Am J Med Genet Suppl 1986; 2: 45–52.

140 Herada K, Nishizaki T, Ozaki S et al. Cytogenetic alterations in pituitary adenomas detected by comparative genomic hybridization. Cancer Genet Cytogenet 1999; 112: 38–41.

141 Herman V, Fagin J, Gonsky R et al. Clonal origin of pituitary adenomas. J Clin Endocrinol Metab 1990; 71: 1427–33.

142 Herring AB, Urich H. Sarcoidosis of the central nervous system. J Neurol Sci 1969; 9: 405–22.

143 Hinton DR, Polk RK, Linse KD et al. Characterization of spherical amyloid protein from a prolactin-producing pituitary adenoma. Acta Neuropathol 1997; 93: 43–9.

144 Hinuma S, Habata Y, Fuji R. A prolactin-releasing peptide in the brain. Nature 1998; 393: 272–6.

145 Hirano A, Tomiyasu U, Zimmerman HM. The fine structure of blood vessels in chromophobe adenoma. Acta Neuropathol (Berl) 1972; 22: 200–7.

146 Hochman HI, Judge DM, Reichlin S. Precocious puberty and hypothalamic hamartoma. Pediatrics 1981; 67: 236–44.

147 Honegger J, Mann K, Thierauf P et al. Human chorionic gonadotrophin immunoactivity in cystic intracranial tumours. Clin Endocrinol (Oxf) 1995; 42: 235–41.

148 Hori A, Altsmansberger M, Spoerri O, Beuche W. Granular cell tumor in the third ventricle. Case report with histological, electron-microscopic, immunohistochemical, and necropsy findings. Acta Neurochir (Wien) 1985; 74: 49–52.

149 Hori A, Schmidt D, Rickels E. Pharyngeal pituitary: development, malformation, and tumorigenesis. Acta Neuropathol 1999; 98: 262–72.

150 Horvath E. Ultrastructural markers in the pathologic diagnosis of pituitary adenomas. Ultrastruct Pathol 1994; 18: 171–9.

151 Horvath E, Kovacs K. Age-related occurrence of various types of pituitary adenoma in surgical material. In: Hiroshige T, Fujimoto S, Honma K eds. Endocrine chronobiology. Sapporo: Hokkaido University Press, 1992: 185–93.

152 Horvath E, Kovacs K. Fine structural cytology of the adenohypophysis in rat and man. J Electron Microsc Tech 1988; 8: 401–32.

153 Horvath E, Kovacs K. Gonadotroph adenomas of the human pituitary: sex-related fine structural dichotomy. A histologic, immunohistochemical, and electron microscopic study of 30 tumors. Am J Pathol 1984; 117: 429–40.

154 Horvath E, Kovacs K. Pathology of prolactin cell adenomas of the human pituitary. Semin Diagn Pathol 1986; 3: 4–17.

155 Horvath E, Kovacs K. The adenohypophysis. In: Kovacs K, Asa SL eds. Functional endocrine pathology 2nd edn. Malden: Blackwell Science, 1998: 247–81.

156 Horvath E, Kovacs K. Ultrastructural diagnosis of human pituitary adenomas. Microsc Res Tech 1992; 20: 107–35.

157 Horvath E, Kovacs K. Ultrastructural diagnosis of pituitary adenomas and hyperplasias. In: Lloyd RV ed. Major problems in pathology Vol. 27, Surgical pathology of the pituitary gland. Philadelphia, PA: Saunders, 1993: 52–84.

158 Horvath E, Kovacs K, Josse R. Pituitary corticotroph cell adenoma with marked abundance of microfilaments. Ultrastruct Pathol 1983; 5: 249–55.

159 Horvath E, Kovacs K, Killinger DW et al. Diverse ultrastructural response to dopamine agonist medication in human pituitary prolactin cell adenoma. In: Hoshino K ed. Prolactin gene family and its receptors; molecular biology to clinical problems. International Congress Series 819. Amsterdam: Elsevier, Excerpta Medica, 1988: 307–11.

160 Horvath E, Kovacs K, Killinger DW et al. Silent corticotropic adenomas of the human pituitary gland: a histologic, immunocytologic and ultrastructural study. Am J Pathol 1980; 98: 617–38.

161 Horvath E, Kovacs K, Killinger DW et al. Mammosomatotroph cell adenoma of the human pituitary: a morphologic entity. Virchows Arch Pathol Anat 1983; 398: 277–89.

162 Horvath E, Kovacs K, Lloyd RV. Pars intermedia of the human pituitary revisited: morphologic aspects and frequency of hyperplasia of POMC-peptide immunoreactive cells. Endocr Pathol 1999; 10: 55–64.

163 Horvath E, Kovacs K, Scheithauer BW. Pituitary hyperplasia. Pituitary 1999; 1: 169–80.

164 Horvath E, Kovacs K, Scheithauer BW. Surgical pathology of pituitary thyrotroph hyperplasia: an oxymoron? Endocr Pathol 1992; 3 (Suppl 1): S14–15.

165 Horvath E, Kovacs K, Scheithauer BW, Lloyd RV, Smyth HS. Pituitary adenoma with neuronal choristoma (PANCH): composite lesion or lineage infidelity? Ultrastruct Pathol 1994; 18: 565–74.

166 Horvath E, Kovacs K, Scheithauer BW et al. Pituitary adenomas producing growth hormone, prolactin, and one or more glycoprotein hormones: a histologic, immunohistochemical, and ultrastructural study of four surgically removed tumors. Ultrastruct Pathol 1983; 5: 171–83.

167 Horvath E, Kovacs K, Singer W et al. Acidophil stem cell adenoma of the human pituitary: clinico-pathological analysis of 15 cases. Cancer 1981; 47: 761–71.

168 Horvath E, Kovacs K, Smyth HS et al. A novel type of pituitary adenoma: morphological features and clinical correlations. J Clin Endocrinol Metab 1988; 66: 1111–18.

169 Huang CI, Chiou WH, Ho DM. Oligodendroglioma occurring after radiation therapy for pituitary adenoma. J Neurol Neurosurg Psychiatry 1987; 50: 1619–24.

170 Hurley TR, D'Angelo CM, Clasen RA et al. Magnetic resonance imaging and pathological analysis of a pituicytoma: case report. Neurosurgery 1994; 35: 314–17.

171 Ikeda H, Yoshimoto T, Kovacs K, Horvath E. Cushing's disease due to female gonadotroph adenoma of the pituitary. Clin Endocrinol 1995; 43: 383–6.

172 Imura H, Nakao K, Shimatsu A et al. Lymphocytic infundibuloneurohypophysitis as a cause of central diabetes insipidus. N Engl J Med 1993; 329: 683–9.

173 Inoue T, Kaneko Y, Mannoji H, Fukui M. Giant cell granulomatous hypophysitis manifesting as an intrasellar mass with unilateral ophthalmoplegia – case report. Neurol Med Chir 1997; 37: 766–70.

174 Jacoby LB, Hedley-Whyte T, Pulaski K et al. Clonal origin of pituitary adenomas. J Neurosurg 1990; 73: 731–5.

175 Jameson JL, Klibanski A, Black PMcL et al. Glycoprotein hormone genes are expressed in clinically nonfunctioning pituitary adenomas. J Clin Invest 1987; 80: 1472–8.

176 Jay V, Kovacs K, Horvath E et al. Idiopathic prolactin cell hyperplasia of the pituitary mimicking prolactin cell adenoma: a morphological study including immunocytochemistry, electron microscopy and in situ hybridization. Acta Neuropathol (Berl) 1991; 82: 147–51.

177 Jellinger K, Radaskiewicz TH, Slowik F. Primary malignant lymphomas of the central nervous system in man. Acta Neuropathol Suppl (Berl) 1975; 6: 95–102.

178 Jensen MD, Handwerger BS, Scheithauer BW et al. Lymphocytic hypophysitis with isolated corticotropin deficiency. Ann Intern Med 1986; 105: 200–3.

179 Jin L, Chandler WF, Lloyd RV. Localization of basic fibroblast growth factor (bFGF) protein and mRNA in human pituitaries: regulation of bFGF mRNA by gonadotropin releasing hormone. Endocr Pathol 1994; 5: 27–34.

180 Jin L, Qian X, Kulig E et al. Transforming growth factor β, transforming growth factor β receptor II, and p27 expression in non-tumorous and neoplastic human pituitaries. Am J Pathol 1997; **151**: 509–19.

181 Jordan RM, Kendall JW, Kerber CW. The primary empty sella syndrome: analysis of the clinical characteristics, radiographic features, pituitary function, and cerebrospinal fluid adenohypophyseal hormone concentrations. Am J Med 1977; **62**: 569–80.

182 Judge DM, Kulin HE, Page R et al. Hypothalamic hamartoma: a source of luteinizing-hormone-releasing factor in precocious puberty. N Engl J Med 1977; **296**: 7–10.

183 Kalsbeck JE. Diencephalic syndrome. In: Wilkins RH, Rengachary SS eds. Neurosurgery Vol. 1. New York: McGraw-Hill, 1985: 925–7.

184 Kamijo T, Phillips JA III. Detection of molecular heterogeneity in GH-1 gene deletions by analysis of polymerase chain reaction amplification products. J Clin Endocrinol Metab 1992; **74**: 786–9.

185 Kaplowitz PB, D'Ercole AJ, Robertson GL. Radioimmunoassay of vasopressin in familial central diabetes insipidus. J Pediatr 1982; **100**: 76–81.

186 Kelemen J, Becus T. Histopathologic changes of the human hypothalamus in systemic atherosclerosis (a clinicopathological study). Neurol Psychiatr (Bucur) 1977; **15**: 65–72.

187 Kepes JJ. Transitional cell tumor of the pituitary gland developing from a Rathke's cleft cyst. Cancer 1978; **41**: 337–43.

188 Kepes JJ, Kepes M. Predominantly cerebral forms of histiocytosis X. A reappraisal of 'Gagel's hypothalamic granuloma,' granuloma infiltrans of the hypothalamus and 'Ayala's disease' with a report of four cases. Acta Neuropathol (Berl) 1969; **14**: 77–98.

189 Kikuchi K, Fujisawa I, Momoi T et al. Hypothalamic–pituitary function in growth hormone-deficient patients with pituitary stalk transection. J Clin Endocrinol Metab 1988; **67**: 817–23.

190 King LR, Knowles HC Jr, McLaurin RL et al. Pituitary hormone response to head injury. Neurosurgery 1981; **9**: 229–35.

191 Kinjo T, Al-Mefty O, Ciric I. Diaphragma sellae meningiomas. Neurosurgery 1995; **36**: 1082–92.

192 Kleihues P, Burger PC, Scheithauer BW. Histological typing of tumors of the central nervous system 2nd edn. Berlin: Springer, 1993.

193 Kleinschmidt-DeMasters BK, Winston KR, Rubinstein D, Samuels MH. Ectopic pituitary adenoma of the third ventricle. Case report. J Neurosurg 1990; **72**: 139–42.

194 Knosp E, Kitz K. Pituitary adenomas with high proliferation rates: measurement by monoclonal antibody Ki-67. Endocr Pathol 1992; **3** (Suppl 1): S19.

195 Kontogeorgos G, Horvath E, Kovacs K. Sex-linked ultrastructural dichotomy of gonadotroph adenomas of the human pituitary: an electron microscopic analysis of 145 tumors. Ultrastruct Pathol 1990; **14**: 475–82.

196 Kontogeorgos G, Kovacs K, Horvath E, Scheithauer BW. Null cell adenomas, oncocytomas, and gonadotroph adenomas of the human pituitary: an immunocytochemical and ultrastructural analysis of 300 cases. Endocr Pathol 1993; **4**: 20–7.

197 Kornblum RN, Fisher RS. Pituitary lesions in craniocerebral injuries. Arch Pathol 1969; **88**: 242–8.

198 Koshiyama H, Sato H, Yorita S et al. Lymphocytic hypophysitis presenting with diabetes insipidus: case report and literature review (Review). Endocr J 1994; **41**: 93–7.

199 Kovacs K, Asa SL, Horvath E et al. Null cell adenomas of the pituitary : attempts to resolve their cytogenesis. In: Lechago J, Kameya T eds. Endocrine pathology update. Philadelphia, PA: Field and Wood, 1990: 17–31.

200 Kovacs K, Horvath E. Pathology of growth hormone-producing tumors of the human pituitary. Semin Diagn Pathol 1986; **3**: 18–33.

201 Kovacs K, Horvath E. Tumors of the pituitary gland. In: Atlas of tumor pathology. Second Series, Fascicle 21. Washington, DC: Armed Forces Institute of Pathology, 1986: 1–264.

202 Kovacs K, Horvath E. Vascular alterations in adenomas of human pituitary gland. An electron microscopic study. Angiologica 1973; **10**: 299–309.

203 Kovacs K, Horvath E, Ryan N, Ezrin C. Null cell adenoma of the human pituitary. Virchows Arch Pathol Anat 1980; **387**: 165–74.

204 Kovacs K, Horvath E, Thorner MO, Rogol AD. Mammosomatotroph hyperplasia associated with acromegaly and hyperprolactinemia in a patient with the McCune–Albright syndrome: a histologic, immunocytologic and ultrastructural study of the surgically-removed adenohypophysis. Virchows Arch Pathol Anat 1984; **403**: 77–86.

205 Kovacs K, Lloyd RV, Horvath E et al. Silent somatotroph adenomas of the human pituitary. A morphologic study of three cases including immunocytochemistry, electron microscopy, in vitro examination, and in situ hybridization. Am J Pathol 1989; **134**: 345–53.

206 Kovacs K, Scheithauer BW, Horvath E, Lloyd RV. The World Health Organization classification of adeno-hypophysial neoplasms. A proposed five-tier scheme. Cancer 1996; **78**: 502–10.

207 Kovacs K, Sheehan HL. Pituitary changes in Kallmann's syndrome: a histologic, immunocytologic, ultrastructural, and immunoelectron microscopic study. Fertil Steril 1982; **37**: 83–9.

208 Kovacs K, Stefaneanu L, Horvath E et al. Effect of dopamine agonist medication on prolactin producing pituitary adenomas. A morphological study including immunocytochemistry, electron microscopy and in situ hybridization. Virchows Arch Pathol Anat 1991; **418**: 439–46.

209 Kuller JA, Cox VA, Schonberg SA, Golabi M. Pallister–Hall syndrome associated with an unbalanced chromosome translocation. Am J Med Genet 1992; **43**: 647–50.

210 Kupari M, Pelkonen R, Valtonen V. Postencephalitic hypothalamic–pituitary insufficiency. Acta Endocrinol (Copenh) 1980; **94**: 433–8.

211 Kurtin PJ, Bonin DM. Immunohistochemical demonstration of lysosome-associated glycoprotein CD68 (KP-1) in granular cell tumors and schwannomas. Hum Pathol 1994; **25**: 1172–8.

212 Kuzuya N, Inoue K, Ishibashi M et al. Endocrine and immunohistochemical studies on thyrotropin (TSH)-secreting pituitary adenomas: responses of TSH, α-subunit, and growth hormone to hypothalamic releasing hormones and their distribution in adenoma cells. J Clin Endocrinol Metab 1990; **71**: 1103–11.

213 Lach B, Scheithauer BW, Gregor A, Wick MR. Colloid cyst of the third ventricle. A comparative immunohistochemical study of neuraxis cysts and choroid plexus epithelium. J Neurosurg 1993; **78**: 101–11.

214 Lam KS, Tse VK, Wang C et al. Early effects of cranial irradiation on hypothalamic-pituitary function. J Clin Endocrinol Metab 1987; **64**: 418–24.

215 Landis C, Masters SB, Spada A et al. GTPase inhibiting mutations activate the α chain of Gs and stimulate adenylyl cyclase in human pituitary tumors. Nature 1989; **340**: 692–6.

216 Landolt AM, Kleihues P, Heitz PU. Amyloid deposits in pituitary adenomas. Differentiation of two types. Arch Pathol Lab Med 1987; **111**: 453–8.

217 Langston JW, Forno LS. The hypothalamus in Parkinson disease. Ann Neurol 1978; **3**: 129–33.

218 Lara Capellan JI, Cuellar Olmedo L, Martinez Martin J et al. Intrasellar mass with hypopituitarism as a manifestation of sarcoidosis. Case report. J Neurosurg 1990; **73**: 283–6.

219 Leech R, Scheithauer BW, Blick K et al. Pituitary adenoma: a DNA ploidy study of 157 operated tumors with correlation of clinical parameters, tumor size, invasiveness, and immunotypes (Abstract). Patologia 1994; **25**: 205–6.

220 Leech RW, Goodkin D, Obert G, Scheithauer B. Etiology of pituitary apoplexy: review and case presentation. Clin Neuropathol 1987; **6**: 7–11.

221 LeMarc'hadour F, Fransen P, Labat-Moleur F et al. Intracranial plasma cell granuloma – a report of four cases. Surg Neurol 1994; **42**: 481–8.

222 Lennox B, Russell DS. Dystopia of the neurohypophysis: two cases. J Path Bact 1951; **63**: 485–90.

223 Lescaudron L, Beracochea D, Verna A, Jaffard R. Chronic ethanol consumption induces neuronal loss in mammillary bodies of the mouse: a quantitative analysis. Neurosci Lett 1984; **50**: 151–5.

224 Levy A, Hall L, Yendall WA, Lightman SL. P53 gene mutations in pituitary adenomas – rare events. Clin Endocrinol (Oxf) 1994; **41**: 809–14.

225 Levy A, Lightman SL. Growth hormone releasing hormone transcripts in human pituitary adenomas. J Clin Endocrinol Metab 1992; **74**: 1474–6.

226 Levy A, Lightman SL. Quantitative in situ hybridization histochemistry studies on growth hormone (GH) gene expression in acromegalic somatotrophs: effects of somatostatin, GH-releasing factor and cortisol. J Mol Endocrinol 1988; **1**: 19–26.

227 Lieberman PH, Jones CR, Dargeon HWK, Begg CF. A reappraisal of eosinophilic granuloma of bone. Hand–chuller–Christian syndrome and Letterer–Siwe syndrome. Medicine 1969; **48**: 375–400.

228 Lieschke GJ, Tress B, Chambers D. Endometrial adenocarcinoma presenting as pituitary apoplexy. Aust NZ J Med 1990; **20**: 81–4.

229 Lipsett MB, Dreifuss FE, Thomas LB. Hypothalamic syndrome following varicella. Am J Med 1962; **32**: 471–5.

230 Lipsett MB, Maclean JP, West CD et al. An analysis of the polyuria induced by hypophysectomy in man. J Clin Endocrinol Metab 1956; **16**: 183–95.

231 Liwnicz BH, Liwnicz RG, Huff JS et al. Giant granular cell tumor of the suprasellar area: immunocytochemical and electron microscopic studies. Neurosurgery 1984; **15**: 246–51.

232 Lloyd RV. Ectopic pituitary adenomas. In: Lloyd RV ed. Surgical pathology of the pituitary gland. Philadelphia, PA: WB Saunders, 1993: 116–20.

233 Lloyd RV. Molecular biological analysis of pituitary disorders. In: Lloyd RV ed. Major problems in pathology Vol. 27, Surgical pathology of the pituitary gland. Philadelphia, PA: WB Saunders, 1993: 85–93.

234 Lloyd RV, Cano M, Chandler WF et al. Human growth hormone and prolactin secreting pituitary adenomas analyzed by in situ hybridization. Am J Pathol 1989; **134**: 605–13.

235 Lloyd RV, Chandler WF, Kovacs K, Ryan N. Ectopic pituitary adenomas with normal anterior pituitary glands. Am J Surg Pathol 1986; **10**: 546–52.

236 Lloyd RV, Chandler WF, McKeever PE, Schteingart DE. The spectrum of ACTH-producing pituitary lesions. Am J Surg Pathol 1986; **10**: 618–26.

237 Lloyd RV, Fields K, Chandler WF et al. Analysis of pituitary hormones and chromogranin A mRNAs in null cell adenomas, oncocytomas and gonadotroph adenomas by in situ hybridization. Am J Pathol 1991; **139**: 553–64.

238 Lloyd RV, Fields K, Jin L et al. Analysis of endocrine active and clinically silent corticotropic adenomas by in situ hybridization. Am J Pathol 1990; **137**: 479–88.

239 Lloyd RV, Jin L, Qian X, Kulig E. Aberrant p27Kip1 expression in endocrine and other tumors. Am J Pathol 1997; **150**: 401–7.

240 Lloyd RV, Scheithauer BW, Kovacs K, Roche P. The immunophenotype of pituitary adenomas. Endocr Pathol 1996; **7**: 145–50.

241 Lo Iudice, D'Alessandro B, Esposito V et al. Hypopituitarism following a direct bullet injury to the pituitary. A case report (Review). Minerva Endocrinol 1989; **14**: 251–4.

242 Luse SA, Kernohan JW. Granular-cell tumors of the stalk and posterior lobe of the pituitary gland. Cancer 1955; **8**: 616–22.

243 Mahachoklertwattana P, Kaplan SL, Grumbach MM. The luteinizing hormone-releasing hormone-secreting hypothalamic hamartoma is a congenital malformation: natural history. J Clin Endocr Metab 1993; **77**: 118–24.

244 Mair WG, Warrington EK, Weiskrantz L. Memory disorder in Korsakoff's psychosis: a neuropathological and neuropsychological investigation of two cases. Brain 1979; **102**: 749–83.

245 Mangiardi JR, Flamm ES, Cravioto H, Fisher B. Hemangiopericytoma of the pituitary fossa: case report. Neurosurgery 1983; **13**: 58–62.

246 Marin F, Stefaneanu L, Kovacs K. Folliculo-stellate cells of the pituitary. Endocr Pathol 1991; **2**: 180–92.

247 Martin FIR. Familial diabetes insipidus. Q J Med 1959; **28**: 573–82.

248 Matsumura A, Meguro K, Doi M et al. Suprasellar ectopic pituitary adenoma: case report and review of the literature (Review). Neurosurgery 1990; **26**: 681–5.

249 Matsuno A, Teramoto A, Takekoshi S et al. HGH, PRL and ACTH gene expression in clinically nonfunctioning adenomas detected with nonisotopic in situ hybridization method. Endocr Pathol 1995; **6**: 13–20.

250 Matzuk MM, Saper CB. Preservation of hypothalamic dopaminergic neurons in Parkinson's disease. Ann Neurol 1985; **18**: 552–5.

251 McComb DJ, Ryan N, Horvath E, Kovacs K. Subclinical adenomas of the human pituitary. New light on old problems. Arch Pathol Lab Med 1983; **107**: 488–91.

252 McConachie NS, Jacobson I. Bilateral aneurysms of the cavernous internal carotid arteries following yttrium-90 implantation. Neuroradiology 1994; **36**: 611–13.

253 McConnon JK, Smyth HS, Horvath E. A case of sparsely granulated growth hormone cell adenoma associated with lymphocytic hypophysitis. J Endocrinol Invest 1991; **14**: 691–6.

254 McNicol AM. Patterns of corticotropic cells in the adult human pituitary in Cushing's disease. Diagn Histopathol 1981; **4**: 335–41.

255 McNicol AM, Farquharson MA, Walker E. Non-isotopic in situ hybridization with digoxigenin and alkaline phosphatase labeled oligodeoxynucleotide probes. Applications in pituitary gland. Pathol Res Pract 1991; **187**: 556–8.

256 Melmed S. Acromegaly. In: Melmed S ed. The pituitary. Cambridge: Blackwell Science, 1995: 413–42.

257 Meyer FB, Carpenter SM, Laws ER Jr. Intrasellar arachnoid cysts. Surg Neurol 1987; **28**: 105–10.

258 Milligan SA, Katz MS, Craven PC et al. Toxoplasmosis presenting as panhypopituitarism in a patient with the acquired immune deficiency syndrome. Am J Med 1984; **77**: 760–4.

259 Mishra SK. Thrombotic thrombocytopenic purpura. Semin Neurol 1985; **5**: 317–20.

260 Mixson AJ, Friedman TC, Katz DA et al. Thyrotropin secreting pituitary carcinoma. J Clin Endocrinol Metab 1993; **76**: 529–33.

261 Mohr G, Hardy J. Hemorrhage, necrosis, and apoplexy in pituitary adenomas. *Surg Neurol* 1982; **18**: 181–9.

262 Mohr PD. Hypothalamic–pituitary abscess. *Postgrad Med J* 1975; **51**: 468–71.

263 Molitch ME. Incidental pituitary adenomas. *Am J Med Sci* 1993; **306**: 262–4.

264 Molitch ME, Elton RL, Blackwell RE et al. Bromocriptine as a primary therapy for prolactin-secreting macroadenoma: results of a prospective multicenter study. *J Clin Endocrinol Metab* 1985; **60**: 698–705.

265 Molitch ME, Reichlin S. Hypothalamic hyperprolactinemia: neuroendocrine regulation in man. In: MacLeod RM, Thorner MO, Scapagnini U eds. *Prolactin*. Berlin: Springer, 1985: 709–19.

266 Mooney EE, Toner M, Farrell MA. Selective necrosis of the posterior pituitary gland – case report. *Clin Neuropathol* 1995; **14**: 42–4.

267 Moran A, Asa SL, Kovacs K et al. Gigantism due to pituitary mammosomatotroph hyperplasia. *N Engl J Med* 1990; **323**: 322–6.

268 Morishima A, Arannoff GS. Syndrome of septo-optic pituitary dysplasia: the clinical spectrum. *Brain Dev* 1986; **8**: 233–9.

269 Mosca L, Costanzi G, Antonacci C et al. Hypophyseal pathology in AIDS. *Histol Histopathol* 1992; **7**: 291–300.

270 Mountcastle RB, Roof BS, Mayfield RK et al. Case report: pituitary adenocarcinoma in an acromegalic patient: response to bromocriptine and pituitary testing: a review of the literature on 36 cases of pituitary carcinoma. *Am J Med Sci* 1989; **298**: 109–18.

271 Mukherjee JJ, Islam N, Kaltsas G et al. Clinical, radiological and pathological features of patients with Rathke's cleft cysts: tumors that may recur. *J Clin Endocrinol Metab* 1997; **82**: 2357–62.

272 Naeye RL, Blanc WA. Organ and body growth in anencephaly: a quantitative, morphological study. *Arch Pathol* 1971; **91**: 140–7.

273 Nagai I, Li CH, Hsieh SM et al. Two cases of hereditary diabetes insipidus, with an autopsy finding in one. *Acta Endocrinol (Copenh)* 1984; **105**: 318–23.

274 Nagashima K, Suzuki S, Ichikawa E et al. Infantile neuroaxonal dystrophy: perinatal onset with symptoms of diencephalic syndrome. *Neurology* 1985; **35**: 735–8.

275 Nagaya T, Seo H, Kuwayama A et al. Proopiomelanocortin gene expression in silent corticotroph cell adenoma and Cushing's disease. *J Neurosurg* 1990; **72**: 262–7.

276 Nakamura S, Takemura M, Ohnishi K et al. Loss of large neurons and occurrence of neurofibrillary tangles in the tuberomammillary nucleus of patients with Alzheimer's disease. *Neurosci Lett* 1993; **151**: 196–9.

277 Navia BA, Petito CK, Gold JW et al. Cerebral toxoplasmosis complicating the acquired immune deficiency syndrome: clinical and neuropathological findings in 27 patients. *Ann Neurol* 1986; **19**: 224–38.

278 Nelson GA, Bastian FO, Schlitt M, White RL. Malignant transformation in craniopharyngioma. *Neurosurgery* 1988; **22**: 427–9.

279 Nelson PB, Haverkos H, Martinez AJ, Robinson AG. Abscess formation within pituitary tumors. *Neurosurgery* 1983; **12**: 331–3.

280 Neumann PE, Horoupian DS, Goldman JE, Hess MA. Cytoplasmic filaments of Crooke's hyaline change belong to the cytokeratin class. An immunocytochemical and ultrastructural study. *Am J Pathol* 1984; **116**: 214–22.

281 Nishi T, Goto T, Takeshima H et al. Tissue factor expressed in pituitary adenoma cells contributes to the development of vascular events in pituitary adenomas. *Cancer* 1999; **86**: 1354–61.

282 Nishio S, Mizuno J, Barrow DL et al. Isolated histiocytosis X of the pituitary gland: case report. *Neurosurgery* 1987; **21**: 718–21.

283 Nishio S, Mizuno J, Barrow DL et al. Pituitary tumors composed of adenohypophysial adenoma and Rathke's cleft cyst elements: a clinicopathological study. *Neurosurgery* 1987; **21**: 371–7.

284 Nishio S, Takeshita I, Fukui M et al. Anaplastic evolution of childhood optico-hypothalamic pilocytic astrocytoma: report of an autopsy case. *Clin Neuropathol* 1988; **7**: 254–8.

285 Nishioka H, Li K, Llena JF, Hirano A. Immunohistochemical study of granular cell tumors of the neurohypophysis. *Virchows Arch Cell Pathol* 1991; **60**: 413–17.

286. Norenberg MD, Leslie KO, Robertson AS. Association between rise in serum sodium and central pontine myelinolysis. *Ann Neurol* 1983; **11**: 128–35.

287 Nozaki K, Nagata I, Yashida K, Kikuchi H. Intrasellar meningioma: case report and review of the literature. *Surg Neurol* 1997; **47**: 447–52.

288 Nussbaum CE, Okawara SH, Jacobs LS. Lymphocytic hypophysitis with involvement of the cavernous sinus and hypothalamus (Review). *Neurosurgery* 1991; **28**: 440–4.

289 Ober KP, Alexander E Jr, Challa VR et al. Histiocytosis X of the hypothalamus. *Neurosurgery* 1989; **24**: 93–5.

290 Oberg K, Norheim I, Wide L. Serum growth hormone in patients with carcinoid tumours; basal levels and response to glucose and thyrotrophin releasing hormone. *Acta Endocrinol (Cophenh)* 1985; **109**: 13–18.

291 Obrador S, Blazquez MG. Pituitary abscess in a craniopharyngioma: case report. *J Neurosurg* 1972; **36**: 785–9.

292 O'Connor G, Dinn J, Farrell M et al. Pituitary apoplexy in an ectopic pituitary tumour. *Eur J Ophthalmol* 1991; **1**: 33–8.

293 Oelbaum MH. Hypopituitarism in male subjects due to syphilis with a discussion of androgen treatment. *Q J Med* 1952; **21**: 249–64.

294 Oka H, Kameya T, Sasano H et al. Pituitary choristoma composed of corticotrophs and adrenocortical cells in the sella turcica. *Virchows Arch* 1996; **427**: 613–17.

295 Oka K, Yamashita M, Sadoshima S, Tanaka K. Cerebral haemorrhage in moyamoya disease at autopsy. *Virchows Arch Pathol Anat* 1981; **392**: 247–61.

296 Okuda O, Umezawa H, Miyaoka M. Pituitary apoplexy caused by endocrine stimulation tests – a case report. *Surg Neurol* 1994; **42**: 19–22.

297 O'Neill BP, Tomlinson FH, Kurtin PJ et al. Primary malignant non-Hodgkin's lymphoma of the brain: a clinicopathologic study of 89 cases. *J Neuropathol Exp Neurol* 1993; **52**: 268.

298 O'Rahilly R, Muller F, Hutchins GM, Moore GW. Computer ranking of the sequence of appearance of 100 features of the brain and related structures in staged human embryos in the first five weeks of development. *Am J Anat* 1984; **171**: 243–57.

299 Orbeck H, Oftedal G. Familial dysautonomia in a non-Jewish child. *Acta Paediatr Scand* 1977; **66**: 777–81.

300 Osamura RY. Functional prenatal development of anencephalic and normal anterior pituitary glands – in human and experimental animals studied by peroxidase-labeled antibody method. *Acta Pathol Jpn* 1977; **27**: 495–509.

301 Osamura RY. Immunoelectron microscopic studies of GH and α-subunit in GH secreting pituitary adenomas. *Pathol Res Pract* 1988; **183**: 569–71.

302 Page RB, Galicich JH, Grunt JA. Alteration of circadian temperature rhythm with third ventricular obstruction. *J Neurosurg* 1973; **38**: 309–19.

303 Pagesy P, Li JY, Berthet M, Peillon F. Evidence of gonadotropin-releasing hormone mRNA in the rat anterior pituitary. *Mol Endocrinol* 1992; **6**: 523–8.

304 Pai KG, Rubin HM, Wedemeyer PP, Linarelli LG. Hypothalamic–pituitary dysfunction following group B beta hemolytic streptococcal meningitis in a neonate. *J Pediatr* 1976; **88**: 289–91.

305 Paja M, Estrada J, Ojeda A et al. Lymphocytic hypophysitis causing hypopituitarism and diabetes insipidus, and associated with autoimmune thyroiditis, in a non-pregnant woman. *Postgrad Med J* 1994; **70**: 220–4.

306 Pallis CA, Lewis PD. The neurology of gastrointestinal disease. *Major Probl Neurol* 1974; **3**: 1–262.

307 Palmer PE, Bogojavlensky S, Bhan AK, Scully RE. Prolactinoma in wall of ovarian dermoid cyst with hyperprolactinemia. *Obstet Gynecol* 1990; **75**: 540–3.

308 Partington MD, Davis DH, Laws ER Jr, Scheithauer BW. Pituitary adenomas in childhood and adolescence. *J Neurosurg* 1994; **80**: 209–16.

309 Pelc D. The diencephalic syndrome in infants. A review in relation to optic nerve glioma. *Eur Neurol* 1972; **7**: 321–34.

310 Pereira J, Vaz R, Carvalho D, Cruz C. Thickening of the pituitary stalk: a finding suggestive of intrasellar tuberculoma. Case report. *Neurosurgery* 1995; **36**: 1013–16.

311 Pernicone PJ, Scheithauer BW. Invasive pituitary adenomas and pituitary carcinomas. In: Lloyd RV ed. Major problems in pathology Vol. 2 *Surgical pathology of the pituitary gland*. Philadelphia, PA: Saunders, 1993; 121–36.

312 Pernicone PJ, Scheithauer BW, Sebo TJ et al. Pituitary carcinoma: a clinicopathologic study of fifteen cases (Abstract). *J Neuropath Exp Neurol* 1995; **54**: 456.

313 Pieterse S, Dinning TA, Blumbergs PC. Postirradiation sarcomatous transformation of pituitary adenoma: a combined pituitary tumor. Case report. *J Neurosurg* 1982; **56**: 283–6.

314 Pilavdzic D, Chiu B, Kovacs K et al. Adenohypophysial tissue in immature teratoma of the human ovary. *Endocr Pathol* 1993; **4**: 48–52.

315 Pilavdzic D, Kovacs K, Asa SL. Pituitary morphology in anencephalic human fetuses. *Neuroendocrinology* 1997; **65**: 164–72.

316 Pioro EP, Scheithauer BW, Laws ER Jr et al. Combined thyrotroph and lactotroph cell hyperplasia simulating prolactin-secreting pituitary adenoma in long-standing primary hypothyroidism. *Surg Neurol* 1988; **29**: 218–26.

317 Pixley S, Weiss M, Melmed S. Identification of human growth hormone messenger ribonucleic acid in pituitary adenoma cells by *in situ* hybridization. *Clin Endocrinol Metab* 1987; **65**: 575–80.

318 Plaitakis A, Hwang EC, Woert MH et al. Effect of thiamin deficiency on brain neurotransmitter systems. *Ann NY Acad Sci* 1982; **378**: 367–81.

319 Plockinger U, Reichel M, Fett U et al. Preoperative octreotide treatment of growth hormone-secreting and clinically nonfunctioning pituitary macroadenomas: effect on tumor volume and lack of correlation with immunohistochemistry and somatostatin receptor scintigraphy. *J Clin Endocrinol Metab* 1994; **79**: 1416–23.

320 Postnov Yu V, Strakhov EV, Glukhovets BI, Gorkova SI. Hypothalamic neurosecretory nuclei and nucleus habenularis of epithalamus in essential hypertension. *Virchows Arch Pathol Anat* 1974; **364**: 275–83.

321 Prezant JR, Levine J, Melmed S. Molecular characterization of the MEN1 tumor suppressor gene in sporadic pituitary tumors. *J Clin Endocrinol Metab* 1998; **83**: 1338–91.

322 Puchner MJ, Fischer-Lampsatis RC, Hermann HD, Freckmann N. Suprasellar meningiomas – neurological and visual outcome at long-term follow-up in a homogeneous series of patients treated microsurgically. *Acta Neurochir* 1998; **140**: 1231–8.

323 Puolakka K, Korhonen T, Lahtinen R. Diabetes insipidus in preleukaemic phase of acute myeloid leukaemia in two patients with empty sella turcica. A report of two cases. *Scand J Haematol* 1984; **32**: 364–6.

324 Ragoowansi AT, Piepgras DG. Postoperative ectopic craniopharyngioma. Case report. *J Neurosurg* 1991; **74**: 653–5.

325 Ranjan A, Chandy MJ. Intrasellar tuberculoma. *Br J Neurosurg* 1994; **8**: 179–85.

326 Reddy K, Lesiuk H, West M, Fewer D. False aneurysms of the cavernous carotid artery: a complication of transsphenoidal surgery. *Surg Neurol* 1990; **33**: 142–5.

327 Renner U, Pagotto U, Arzt E, Stalla GK. Autocrine and paracrine roles of polypeptide growth factors, cytokines, and vasogenic substances in normal and tumorous pituitary function and growth: a review. *Eur J Endocrinol* 1996; **135**: 515–32.

328 Reuler JB, Girard DE, Cooney TG. Current concepts. Wernicke's encephalopathy. *N Engl J Med* 1985; **312**: 1035–9.

329 Riedl M, Czech T, Slootweg J et al. Lymphocytic hypophysitis presenting as a pituitary tumor in a 63-year-old man. *Endocr Pathol* 1995; **6**: 159–66.

330 Rilliet B, Mohr G, Robert R, Hardy J. Calcification in pituitary adenomas. *Surg Neurol* 1981; **15**: 249–55.

331 Rimoin DL, Schechter JE. Histological and ultrastructural studies in isolated growth hormone deficiency. *J Clin Endocrinol Metab* 1973; **37**: 725–35.

332 Robert F, Hardy J. Human corticotroph cell adenomas. *Semin Diagn Pathol* 1986; **3**: 34–41.

333 Roberts GA, Eren E, Sinclair H et al. Two cases of Wegener's granulomatosis involving the pituitary. *Clin Endocrinol* 1995; **42**: 323–8.

334 Robinson B. Intrasellar abscess after transsphenoidal pituitary adenomectomy. *Neurosurgery* 1983; **12**: 684–6.

335 Rock JP, Babu VR, Drumheller T, Chason J. Cytogenetic findings in pituitary adenoma: results of a pilot study. *Surg Neurol* 1993; **40**: 224–9.

336 Roessmann U, Velasco ME, Small EJ, Hori A. Neuropathology of 'septo-optic dysplasia' (de Morsier syndrome) with immunohistochemical studies of the hypothalamus and pituitary gland. *J Neuropathol Exp Neurol* 1987; **46**: 597–608.

337 Roncaroli F, Bacci A, Frank G, Calbucci F. Granulomatous hypophysitis caused by ruptured Rathke's cleft cyst: report of a case and review of the literature. *Neurosurgery* 1998; **43**: 146–9.

338 Rosete A, Cabral AR, Kraus A, Alarcon-Segovia D. Diabetes insipidus secondary to Wegener's granulomatosis: report and review of the literature. *J Rheumatol* 1991; **18**: 761–5.

339 Rossi ML, Bevan JS, Esiri MM et al. Pituicytoma (pilocytic astrocytoma). Case report. *J Neurosurg* 1987; **67**: 768–72.

340 Roux FX, Constans JP, Monsaingeon V, Meder JF. Symptomatic Rathke's cleft cysts: clinical and therapeutic data. *Neurochirurgia* 1988; **31**: 18–20.

341 Rube J, De La Pava S, Pickren JW. Histiocytosis X with involvement of brain. *Cancer* 1967; **20**: 486–92.

342 Saeger W, Gunzl H, Meyer M et al. Immunohistological studies on clinically silent pituitary adenomas. *Endocr Pathol* 1990; **1**: 37–44.

343 Saeger W, Mohr K, Caselitz J, Ludecke DK. Light and electron microscopical morphometry of pituitary adenomas in hyperprolactinemia. *Path Res Pract* 1986; **181**: 544–50.

344 Saeger W, Puchner MJ, Ludecke DK. Combined sellar gangliocytoma and pituitary adenoma in acromegaly or Cushing's disease. *Virchows Arch Pathol Anat* 1994; **425**: 93–9.

345 Saeger W, Uhlig H, Baz E et al. In situ hybridization for different mRNA in GH-secreting and in inactive pituitary adenomas. *Pathol Res Pract* 1991; **187**: 559–63.

346 Saito K, Takayasu M, Akabane A et al. Primary chronic intrasellar haematoma: a case report. *Acta Neurochir (Wien)* 1992; **114**: 147–50.

347 Sakurai T, Seoh H, Yamamoto N et al. Detection of mRNA of prolactin and ACTH in clinically nonfunctioning adenomas. *J Neurosurg* 1988; **69**: 653–9.

348 Samaan NA. Hypopituitarism after external irradiations of nasopharyngeal cancer. In: Linfoot JA. *Recent advances in the diagnosis and treatment of pituitary tumors*. New York: Raven Press, 1979: 315–30.

349 Sandyk R, Iacono RP, Bamford CR. The hypothalamus in Parkinson disease. *Ital J Neurol Sci* 1987; **8**: 227–34.

350 Sanno N, Tahara S, Yoshida Y et al. Ectopic corticotroph adenoma in the cavernous sinus: case report. *Neurosurgery* 1999; **45**: 914–18.

351 Sanno N, Teramoto A, Matsuno A et al. Clinical and immunohistochemical studies on TSH-secreting pituitary adenoma: its multihormonality and expression of Pit-1. *Mod Pathol* 1994; **7**: 893–9.

352 Sano T, Asa SL, Kovacs K. Growth hormone-releasing hormone-producing tumors: clinical, biochemical and morphologic manifestations. *Endocr Rev* 1988; **9**: 357–73.

353 Sano T, Kovacs K, Asa SL, Smyth HS. Immunoreactive luteinizing hormone in functioning corticotroph adenomas of the pituitary. Immunohistochemical and tissue culture studies of two cases. *Virchows Arch (A)* 1990; **417**: 361–7.

354 Sano T, Kovacs K, Scheithauer BW et al. Pituitary pathology in acquired immunodeficiency syndrome. *Arch Pathol Lab Med* 1989; **113**: 1066–70.

355 Sano T, Ohshima T, Yamada S. Expression of glycoprotein hormones and intracytoplasmic distribution of cytokeratin in growth hormone-producing pituitary adenomas. *Pathol Res Pract* 1991; **187**: 530–3.

356 Saper CB, German DC. Hypothalamic pathology in Alzheimer's disease. *Neurosci Lett* 1987; **74**: 364–70.

357 Sautner D, Saeger W, Ludecke DK. Tumors of the sellar region mimicking pituitary adenomas. *Exp Clin Endocrinol* 1993; **101**: 283–9.

358 Scheithauer BW. Pathology of the pituitary and sellar region: exclusive of pituitary adenoma. *Pathol Annu* 1985; **20**(Part 1): 67–155.

359 Scheithauer BW. The hypothalamus and posterior pituitary. In: Kovacs K, Asa S eds. *Functional endocrine pathology* 2nd edn. Malden: Blackwell Science, 1998: 171–246.

360 Scheithauer BW, Horvath E, Kovacs K et al. Plurihormonal pituitary adenomas. *Semin Diagn Pathol* 1986; **3**: 69–82.

361 Scheithauer BW, Kovacs KT, Laws ER Jr, Randall RV. Pathology of invasive pituitary tumors with special reference to functional classification. *J Neurosurg* 1986; **65**: 733–44.

362 Scheithauer BW, Kovacs K, Randall RV et al. Pathology of excessive production of growth hormone. *Clin Endocrinol Metab* 1986; **15**: 655–81.

363 Scheithauer BW, Kovacs K, Randall RV et al. Hypothalamic neuronal hamartoma and adenohypophyseal neuronal choristoma: their association with growth hormone adenoma of the pituitary gland. *J Neuropathol Exp Neurol* 1983; **43**: 648–63.

364 Scheithauer BW, Kovacs KT, Randall RV, Ryan N. Effects of estrogen upon the human pituitary: a clinicopathologic study. *Mayo Clin Proc* 1989; **64**: 1077–84.

365 Scheithauer BW, Kovacs K, Young WF Jr, Randall RV. The pituitary gland in hyperthyroidism. *Mayo Clin Proc* 1992; **67**: 22–6.

366 Scheithauer BW, Sano T, Kovacs K et al. The pituitary gland in pregnancy: a clinicopathologic and immunohistochemical study of 69 cases. *Mayo Clin Proc* 1990; **65**: 461–74.

367 Scherbaum WA, Bottazzo GF. Autoantibodies to vasopressin cells in idiopathic diabetes insipidus: evidence for an autoimmune variant. *Lancet* 1983; **1**: 897–901.

368 Schmitt S, Wichmann W, Martin E et al. Pituitary stalk thickening with diabetes insipidus preceding typical manifestations of Langerhans cell histiocytosis in children. *Eur J Pediatr* 1993; **152**: 399–401.

369 Schochet SS Jr, McCormick WF, Halmi NS. Salivary gland rests in the human pituitary. Light and electron microscopical study. *Arch Pathol* 1974; **98**: 193–200.

370 Schteingart DE, Lloyd RV, Akil H et al. Cushing's syndrome secondary to ectopic corticotropin-releasing hormone–adrenocorticotropin secretion. *J Clin Endocrinol Metab* 1986; **63**: 770–5.

371 Schulte HM, Oldfield EH, Allolio B et al. Clonal composition of pituitary adenomas in patients with Cushing's disease: determination by X-chromosome inactivation analysis. *J Clin Endocrinol Metab* 1991; **73**: 1302–8.

372 Selman WR, Laws ER Jr, Scheithauer BW, Carpenter SM. The occurrence of dural invasion in pituitary adenomas. *J Neurosurg* 1986; **64**: 402–7.

373 Selosse P, Mahler C, Klaes RL. Pituitary abscess. Case report. *J Neurosurg* 1980; **53**: 851–2.

374 Sen C, Hague K. Meningiomas involving the cavernous sinus: histological factors affecting the degree of resection. *J Neurosurg* 1997; **87**: 535–43.

375 Shalet SM. Iatrogenic hypothalamic–pituitary disease. In: Beardwell C, Robertson GL eds. *Clinical endocrinology* Vol. 1, *The pituitary*. Boston, MA: Butterworths, 1981: 175–210.

376 Shammas NW, Brown JD, Foreman BW et al. Septo-optic dysplasia associated with polyendocrine dysfunction. *J Med* 1993; **24**: 67–74.

377 Shanklin WM. Lymphocytes and lymphoid tissue in the human pituitary. *Anat Rec* 1951; **111**: 177–91.

378 Sharrer E, Scharrer B. Secretory cells within the hypothalamus. *Res Publ Assoc Res Nerv Ment Dis* 1940; **20**: 170–94.

379 Sheehan HL, Davis JC. *Post-partum hypopituitarism*. Springfield, IL: Charles C Thomas, 1982.

380 Sheehan HL, Kovacs K. Neurohypophysis and hypothalamus. In: Bloodworth JMB Jr ed. *Endocrine pathology: general and surgical*. Baltimore, MD: Williams & Wilkins, 1982: 55–7.

381 Sherwin RP, Grassi JE, Sommers SC. Hamartomatous malformation of the posterolateral hypothalamus. *Lab Invest* 1962; **11**: 89–97.

382 Shi T, Farrell MA, Kaufmann JC. Fibrosarcoma complicating irradiated pituitary adenoma. *Surg Neurol* 1984; **22**: 277–84.

383 Shimizu C, Kubo M, Kijima H et al. Giant cell granulomatous hypophysitis with remarkable uptake on Gallium-67 scintigraphy. *Clin Endocrinol* 1998; **49**: 131–4.

384 Shimon I, Melmed S. Management of pituitary tumors. *Ann Intern Med* 1998; **129**: 472–83.

385 Sidman RL, Rakic P. Development of the human central nervous system. Chapter 1. In: Haymaker W, Adams RD eds. *Histology and histopathology of the nervous system* Vol. 1. Springfield, IL: Charles C Thomas, 1982: 3–145.

386 Sills IN, Rapaport R, Robinson LP et al. Familial Pallister–Hall syndrome: case report and hormonal evaluation. *Am J Med Genet* 1993; **47**: 321–5.

387 Silverlight JJ, Prysor-Jones RA, Jenkins JS. Basic fibroblast growth factor in human pituitary tumors. *Clin Endocrinol (Oxf)* 1990; **32**: 669–76.

388 Simpson DJ, Magnay J, Bicknell JG et al. Chromosome 13q deletion mapping in pituitary tumors: infrequent loss of the retinoblastoma susceptibility gene (RB1) locus despite loss of RB1 protein product in somatotrophinomas. Cancer Res 1999; 59: 1562–6.

389 Simmons NE, Laws ER Jr. Glioma occurrence after sellar irradiation: case report and review. Neurosurgery 1998; 42: 172–8.

390 Sinson G, Gennarelli TA, Wells GB. Suprasellar osteolipoma: case report. Surg Neurol 1998; 50: 457–60.

391 Slowik F, Fazekas I, Balint K et al. Intrasellar hamartoma associated with pituitary adenoma. Acta Neuropathol 1990; 80: 328–33.

392 Smith AR, Elsheikh TM, Silvermen JF. Intraoperative cytologic diagnosis of suprasellar and sellar cystic lesions. Diagn Cytopathol 1999; 20: 137–47.

393 Sokol HW, Valtin H. Morphology of the neurosecretory system in rats homozygous and heterozygous for hypothalamic diabetes insipidus (Brattleboro strain). Endocrinology 1965; 77: 692–700.

394 Solero CL, Giombini S, Morello G. Suprasellar and olfactory meningiomas. Report on a series of 153 personal cases. Acta Neurochir (Wien) 1983; 67: 181–94.

395 Spada A, Arosio M, Bochicchio D et al. Clinical, biochemical and morphological correlates in patients bearing growth hormone-secreting pituitary tumors with or without constitutively active adenylyl cyclase. J Clin Endocrinol Metab 1990; 71: 1421–6.

396 Stanfield JP. The blood supply of the human pituitary gland. J Anat 1960; 94: 257–73.

397 Stefaneanu L, Kovacs K, Horvath E et al. Adenohypophyseal changes in mice transgenic for human growth hormone-releasing factor: a histologic, immunocytochemical and electron microscopic investigation. Endocrinology 1989; 125: 2710–18.

398 Stefaneanu L, Kovacs K, Lloyd RV et al. Pituitary lactotrophs and somatotrophs in pregnancy: a correlative in situ hybridization and immunocyto chemical study. Virchows Arch B Cell Pathol 1992; 62: 291–6.

399 Steinberg GK, Koenig GH, Golden JB. Symptomatic Rathke's cleft cysts. Report of two cases. J Neurosurg 1982; 56: 290–5.

400 Stern BJ, Krumholz A, Johns C et al. Sarcoidosis and its neurological manifestations. Arch Neurol 1985; 42: 909–17.

401 Stewart PM, Carey MP, Graham CT et al. Growth hormone secreting pituitary carcinoma: a case report and literature review. Clin Endocrinol 1992; 37: 189–95.

402 Sung JH, Hayano M, Mastri AR, Okagaki T. A case of human rabies and ultrastructure of the Negri body. J Neuropathol Exp Neurol 1976; 35: 541–59.

404 Swaab DF, Fliers E. A sexually dimorphic nucleus in the human brain. Science 1985; 228: 1112–15.

403 Swaab DF. Ageing of the human hypothalamus. Horm Res 1995; 43: 8–11.

405 Swaab DF, Fliers E, Partiman TS. The suprachiasmatic nucleus of the human brain in relation to sex, age, and senile dementia. Brain Res 1985; 342: 37–44.

406 Szeifert GT, Sipos L, Horvath M et al. Pathological characteristics of surgically removed craniopharyngiomas: analysis of 131 cases. Acta Neurochir (Wien) 1993; 124: 139–43.

407 Thakker RV, Pook MA, Wooding C et al. Association of somatotrophinomas with loss of alleles on chromosome 11 and with gsp mutations. J Clin Invest 1993; 91: 2815–21.

408 Thapar K, Kovacs K, Laws ER Jr, Muller PJ. Pituitary adenomas: current concepts in classification, histopathology, and molecular biology. Endocrinologist 1993; 3: 39–57.

409 Thapar K, Kovacs K, Scheithauer BW et al. Proliferative activity and invasiveness in pituitary adenomas and carcinomas: an analysis using the MIB-1 antibody. Neurosurgery 1996; 38: 99–107.

410 Thapar K, Kovacs K, Stefaneanu L et al. Antiproliferative effect of the somatostatin analog octreotide on growth hormone producing pituitary tumors. Results of a multi center trial. Mayo Clin Proc 1997; 72: 893–900.

411 Thapar K, Scheithauer BW, Kovacs K et al. P53 expression in pituitary adenomas and carcinomas: correlation with invasiveness and tumor growth fractions. Neurosurgery 1996; 38: 763–70.

412 Thapar K, Stefaneanu L, Kovacs K et al. Estrogen receptor gene expression in craniopharyngiomas – an in situ hybridization study. Neurosurgery 1994; 35: 1012–17.

413 Thodou E, Asa SL, Kontogeorgos G et al. Clinical case seminar: lymphocytic hypophysitis: clinico-pathological findings. J Clin Endocrinol Metab 1995; 80: 2302–11.

414 Thorner MO, Perryman RL, Cronin MJ et al. Somatotroph hyperplasia. J Clin Invest 1982; 70: 965–77.

415 Thorner MO, Vance ML, Laws ER Jr et al. The anterior pituitary. In: Wilson JD, Foster DW, Kronenberg HM, Larson PR eds. Williams textbook of endocrinology, 9th edn, Chapter 9. Philadelphia, PA: WB Saunders, 1998: 249–340.

416 Tindall GT, Kovacs K, Horvath E, Thorner MO. Human prolactin-producing adenomas and bromocriptine: a histological, immunocytochemical, ultrastructural and morphometric study. J Clin Endocrinol Metab 1982; 55: 1178–83.

417 Toledo SP, Luthold W, Mattar E. Familial idiopathic gonadotropin deficiency: a hypothalamic form of hypogonadism. Am J Med Genet 1983; 15: 405–16.

418 Tomlinson FH, Scheithauer BW, Young WF Jr et al. Rathke's cleft cyst – a clinicopathologic study of 31 cases. Brain Pathol 1994; 4: 453.

419 Torvik A. Topographic distribution and severity of brain lesions in Wernicke's encephalopathy. Clin Neuropathol 1987; 6: 25–9.

420 Trouillas J, Girod C, Sassolas G, Claustrat B. The human gonadotropic adenoma: pathologic diagnosis and hormonal correlations in 26 tumors. Semin Diagn Pathol 1986; 3: 42–57.

421 Tsang RW, Laperriere NJ, Simpson WJ et al. Glioma arising after radiation therapy for pituitary adenoma. A report of four patients and estimation of risk. Cancer 1993; 72: 2227–33.

422 Turner HE, Wass JAH. Are markers of proliferation valuable in the histological assessment of pituitary tumours? Pituitary 1999; 1: 147–51.

423 Ushio Y, Arita N, Yoshimine T et al. Glioblastoma after radiotherapy for craniopharyngioma: case report. Neurosurgery 1987; 21: 33–8.

424 Valiquette G. The neurohypophysis. Neurol Clin 1987; 5: 291–331.

425 Valtin H. Hereditary hypothalamic diabetes insipidus in rats (Brattleboro strain). A useful experimental model. Am J Med 1967; 42: 814–27.

426 van de Nes JA, Kamphorst W, Ravid R, Swaab DF. Comparison of beta-protein/A4 deposits and Alz-50-stained cytoskeletal changes in the hypothalamus and adjoining areas of Alzheimer's disease patients: amorphic plaques and cytoskeletal changes occur independently. Acta Neuropathol 1998; 96: 129–38.

427 van Maarsseveen AC, Veldhuizen RW, Stam J et al. A quantitative histomorphologic analysis of lymph node granulomas in sarcoidosis in relation to radiological stage I and II. J Pathol 1983; 139: 441–53.

428 Victor M, Adams RD, Collins GH. The Wernicke–Korsakoff syndrome. A clinical and pathological study of 245 patients, 82 with post-mortem examinations. Contemp Neurol Ser 1971; 7: 1–206.

429 Vidal S, Horvath E, Kovacs K et al. Transdifferentiation of somatotrophs to tyrotrophs in the pituitary of patients with protracted primary hypothyroidism. Virchows Arch 2000; 436: 43–51.

430 Vinores SA. Demonstration of glial fibrillary acidic (GFA) protein by electron immunocytochemistry in the granular cells of a choristoma of the neurohypophysis. Histochemistry 1991; 96: 265–9.

431 Vnencak-Jones CL, Phillips JA, Wang DF. Use of polymerase chain reaction in detection of growth hormone gene deletions. J Clin Endocrinol Metab 1990; 70: 1550–3.

432 Vorherr H, Massry SG, Fallet R et al. Antidiuretic principle in tuberculous lung tissue of a patient with pulmonary tuberculosis and hyponatremia. Ann Intern Med 1970; 72: 383–7.

433 Wakabayashi I, Inokuchi K, Hasegawa O et al. Expression of growth hormone (GH)-releasing factor gene in GH-producing pituitary adenoma. J Clin Endocrinol Metab 1992; 74: 357–61.

434 Watanabe A, Ishii R, Hirano K et al. Central diabetes insipidus caused by nonspecific chronic inflammation of the hypothalamus: case report. Surg Neurol 1994; 42: 70–3.

435 White JC, Ballantine HT Jr. Intrasellar aneurysms simulating hypophyseal tumours. J Neurosurg 1961; 18: 34–50.

436 Whitehead R. The hypothalamus in post-partum hypopituitarism. J Pathol Bacteriol 1963; 86: 55–67.

437 Wilkins RH. Hypothalamic dysfunction and intracranial arterial spasms (Review). Surg Neurol 1975; 4: 472–80.

438 Winnacker JL, Becker KL, Katz S. Endocrine aspects of sarcoidosis (concluded). N Engl J Med 1968; 278: 483–92.

439 Wolfsohn AL, Lach B, Benoit BG. Suprasellar xanthomatous Rathke's cleft cyst. Surg Neurol 1992; 38: 106–9.

440 Woloshak M, Yu A, Post KD. Frequent inactivation of the p16 gene in human pituitary tumors by gene methylation. Mol Carcinogenesis 1997; 19: 221–4.

441 Wynne AG, Gharib H, Scheithauer BW et al. Hyperthyroidism due to inappropriate secretion of thyrotropin in 10 patients. Am J Med 1992; 92: 15–24.

442 Yamada S, Asa SL, Kovacs K. Oncocytomas and null cell adenomas of the human pituitary: morphometric and in vitro functional comparison. Virchows Arch Pathol Anat 1988; 413: 333–9.

443 Yamada S, Sano T, Stefaneanu L et al. Endocrine and morphological study of a clinically silent somatotroph adenoma of the human pituitary. J Clin Endocrinol Metab 1993; 76: 352–6.

444 Yoshimoto K, Iwahana H, Fukuda A et al. Rare mutations of the Gs alpha subunit gene in human endocrine tumors. Mutation detection by polymerase chain reaction-primer-introduced restriction analysis. Cancer 1993; 72: 1386–93.

445 Young WF Jr, Scheithauer BW, Gharib H et al. Cushing's syndrome due to primary multinodular corticotrope hyperplasia. Mayo Clin Proc 1988; 63: 256–62.

446 Zampieri P, Zorat PL, Mingrino S, Soattin GB. Radiation-associated cerebral gliomas: a report of two cases and review of the literature. J Neurosurg Sci 1989; 33: 271–9.

447 Zarate A, Kovacs K, Flores M et al. ACTH and CRF-producing bronchial carcinoid associated with Cushing's syndrome. Clin Endocrinol (Oxf) 1986; 24: 523–9.

448 Zhang X, Danila DC, Katai M et al. Expression of prolactin-releasing peptide and its receptor messenger ribonucleic acid in normal human pituitary and pituitary adenomas. J Clin Endocrinol 1999; 84: 4652–5.

449 Zhang Z, Ezzat SZ, Vortmeyer AO et al. Mutation of the MEN1 tumor suppressor gene in pituitary tumors. Cancer Res 1997; 57: 5446–51.

450 Zimmerman D, Young WF Jr, Ebersold MJ et al. Congenital gigantism due to growth hormone-releasing hormone excess and pituitary hyperplasia with adenomatous transformation. J Clin Endocrinol Metab 1993; 76: 216–22.

18

Regional neuropathology: diseases of the spinal cord and vertebral column

UMBERTO DE GIROLAMI, MATTHEW P. FROSCH AND CHARLES H. TATOR

VASCULAR DISEASE OF THE SPINAL CORD

Normal anatomy of the blood supply of the spinal cord

The arterial blood supply of the spinal cord is divisible into three vascular territories: superior, intermediate and inferior[198] (Fig. 18.1). The superior region, from the first cervical to the uppermost thoracic segments (T1 and T2), is supplied by branches of the vertebral arteries, which in turn are branches of the subclavian arteries. Just before their junction to form the basilar artery at the level of the foramen magnum, the two vertebral arteries typically give off medially directed twigs which unite in the midline on the anterior aspect of the uppermost cervical cord to form the anterior spinal artery. The anterior spinal artery forms a continuous vascular trunk along the length of the spinal cord, with resupply at several levels. The initial portion of the anterior spinal artery nourishes the first four cervical segments; below this, the superior arterial territory is supplied by two to four large radicular arteries coming from the vertebral arteries as it passes through the foramina transversaria of the cervical spinal column, or from cervical branches of the subclavian artery.[151,324] Below the upper thoracic region, the spinal cord receives its blood supply directly from the paired segmental intercostal and lumbar branches of the aorta. During embryological development each of these segmental arteries gives off a spinal branch which, on entering the dura, divides into anterior and posterior radicular arteries that accompany the spinal roots and, on reaching the spinal cord, form the posterior spinal arteries and replenish the anterior spinal artery.[111] Initially, these radicular arteries are of generally equal size and importance; however, as fetal development continues some of these radicular arteries fail to grow, or involute, while others become enlarged and form the definitive arterial supply of the cord.[149]

Several distinct larger radicular branches resupply the superior arterial territory of the spinal cord. The intermediate territory, comprising general cord segments T3–T8, receives blood from a branch called the dorsal radicular artery, which accompanies the fifth, sixth or seventh thoracic anterior root. The remainder of the spinal cord (the inferior arterial territory, from about T8 through all of the lumbosacral segments) is supplied by a single large radicular artery, the arteria radicularis magna, first described by Adamkiewicz[3,4] and now often called the artery of Adamkiewicz.

The subdivision of the arterial blood supply of the spinal cord into individual vascular territories means that the region of the cord between any two of these territories is relatively remote from the main source of blood supply through the segmental and radicular arteries. These border-zone regions correspond therefore to a territory that is vulnerable to decreases in arterial perfusion pressure, which can be of pathophysiological importance.[359]

The intrinsic blood supply of the spinal cord comes from the anterior spinal artery, the posterior spinal arteries, and an irregular anastomosing plexus of small arter-

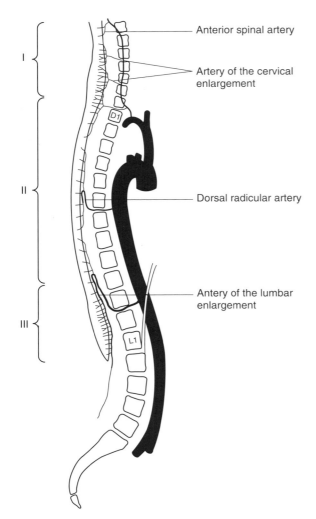

Anterior spinal artery

Artery of the cervical enlargement

Dorsal radicular artery

Antery of the lumbar enlargement

Figure 18.1 *The arterial blood supply of the spinal cord (according to Ref. 198).*

ies that interconnect the anterior and posterior spinal arteries (Fig. 18.2). The anterior spinal artery sends off centrally directed branches, the central, or sulcal, arteries, which enter the cord from the depths of the anterior median sulcus and extend, alternating from one side to the other, into the anterior grey matter and the adjacent white matter. Other branches of the anterior spinal artery are laterally directed and ramify on the surface of the cord, sending radially directed penetrating arteries into the anterior and lateral parts of the white matter. Similar radially directed branches of the posterior spinal arteries supply the posterior horns of the grey matter and the posterior columns of the white matter. The posterior spinal arteries and their branches are more slender and irregular in their distribution than are the anterior spinal arteries. The distribution of the arteries forming the intrinsic blood supply of the spinal cord is such that within the cord there are border-zone territories of relatively marginal blood supply, which can also have pathophysiological significance[2,3,111,168,169,272,309,312,324] (Fig. 18.3). For example, the

intrinsic blood supply of the spinal cord appears to influence the distribution and severity of the damage after trauma.[319]

The venous drainage of the cord has not been as extensively studied as the arterial supply; a good description is provided by Gillilan.[112] The venous architecture is considerably more variable than the corresponding arterial distribution, and the blood vessels are more tortuous. There tends to be a prominent midline vein that in general follows the course of the posterior median sulcus.[3,138,169,311,324] Otherwise the veins follow the same pattern as the intrinsic, radicular and segmental arteries (Fig. 18.3a).

Occlusive vascular disease: ischaemic myelopathy

INTRINSIC VASCULAR DISEASE OF THE SPINAL CORD

Obstruction of the blood supply of the spinal cord, and consequent ischaemic injury to the cord, is relatively rare compared with occlusive intracranial vascular disease. Review of the general experience with ischaemic myelopathy resulting from interruption of the arterial supply indicates that, in most cases, the vascular occlusion is the result of emboli arising from a more proximal site in the arterial system, rather than locally developing thrombosis secondary to a pathological process in the walls of blood vessels. The spinal cord is vulnerable to emboli of two kinds: (1) fragments of thrombi or of atheromatous plaques, and (2) fibrocartilaginous emboli. Unlike the intracranial arteries, the intrinsic arteries of the spinal cord do not often develop atheromatous lesions.[162,218] The presence of atheromatous material, often including evidence of cholesterol crystals, within the spinal arteries can safely be interpreted as indicating embolization.[153,156,195,258,297,343,356,357] Ischaemic lesions of the spinal cord due to atheromatous (often referred to as cholesterol) embolism are, on the whole, a rare occurrence. One study, based on a series of 1000 autopsies, indicated that of 28 patients representing a high-risk group (evidence of atheromatous embolization of abdominal viscera and history of aortic graft emplacement for arteriosclerotic aneurysm), atheromatous emboli were found in arteries of the spinal cord in 12 with infarction of the cord in only one.[297] These findings suggest that ischaemic myelopathy from atheromatous emboli is much less frequent than asymptomatic embolism. Some of the reported atheromatous emboli have occluded major spinal arteries, both the anterior spinal artery[195,297,357] and the posterior spinal arterial system.[120,258,341] These occlusions resulted in infarction of the cord in the affected territories of arterial supply. Occasionally, emboli most probably originating from atheromatous aortic plaques lead to multiple irregular foci of infarction in the cord.[83,156,343,356]

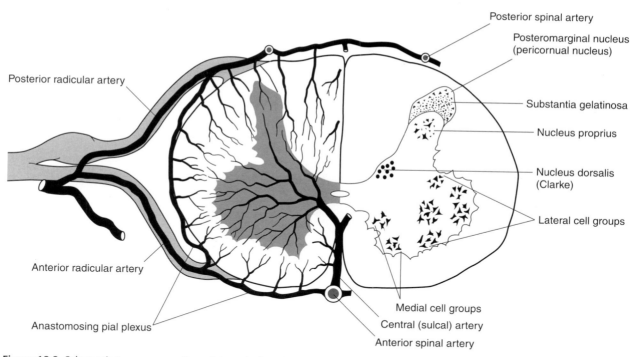

Figure 18.2 *Schematic transverse section of the spinal cord. Note segmental arterial supply (left) and distribution of major neuronal groups (right) (according to Ref. 129).*

In other cases, ischaemic lesions of the cord have been found to be associated with organized, perhaps recanalized, thrombi in the corresponding spinal arteries, indicating that the thrombi have been present for some time. In such cases, the arterial wall is normal.[64,135,334] Under these circumstances, embolization seems a probable explanation for the vascular obstruction, although this possibility must remain speculative.

Arrest of the circulation through the main intrinsic arteries of the spinal cord produces necrosis of the cord in distributions that are relatively constant from case to case. Of these, the most frequent localization is in the territory of supply of the anterior spinal artery (Fig. 18.4). In this lesion both anterior horns of the grey matter are largely destroyed, together with the medially situated anterior funiculi of the white matter.[64,135,195,297] In some cases the necrosis extends to involve the entire ventral half of the cord, sparing the posterior horns of the grey matter, the adjacent portion of the lateral corticospinal tracts, the dorsal spinocerebellar tracts and the posterior columns.[357] The vertical extent of the lesion is generally about four segments, but in one case it extended from C6 to T10[357] and in another it involved the entire length of the cord.[297] There is a slight preponderance of cases of lumbosacral infarction, but localization to the cervical or cervicothoracic segments also occurs.

Infarction of the spinal cord secondary to fibrocartilaginous embolization of intrinsic blood vessels has been documented in 36 clinicopathological studies.[26,28,39,40,47,58,66,74,101,124,142,147,148,167,180,181,196,212,231,237,242,256,271,280,301,325,354]

In these reports the patients have been women about twice as often as men, ranging in age from young adulthood to late middle age, in whom a rapidly evolving tetraparesis and paraparesis developed, generally with an associated sensory level below the site of the lesion. In some patients the myelopathy followed trauma to the spine (e.g. fall on the buttocks or back, forced bending of the neck, heavy lifting), but in others it occurred with only a relatively minor insult or no identifiable antecedent. Death from respiratory failure or sepsis, usually without a precise clinical diagnosis, followed days or months after the onset of symptoms. Post-mortem examination in these cases has shown multifocal infarction predominantly in the territory of distribution of the anterior spinal artery, involving most often the mid- to low-cervical and upper thoracic spinal cord, less frequently the thoracic and lumbosacral cord, and rarely the medulla oblongata[174] (Fig. 18.5), associated with secondary long-tract ascending/descending degeneration in long-standing survivors. These infarcts have been accompanied by fibrocartilaginous embolic material (well demonstrated with the Alcian blue stain; Fig. 18.5e) within subarachnoid and intrinsic arterioles and venules. Clinical, radiological and autopsy examinations of the spine have been unrevealing but systematic studies are lacking. The pathogenesis of this remarkable clinicopathological syndrome is not understood, but there is speculation that fibrocartilaginous material from the vertebral bodies and intervertebral discs becomes forcibly injected into the sinusoidal veins of the intravertebral bone marrow and then makes its way into the

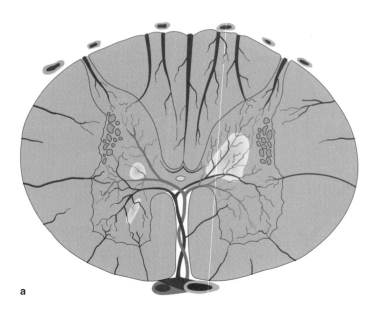

a

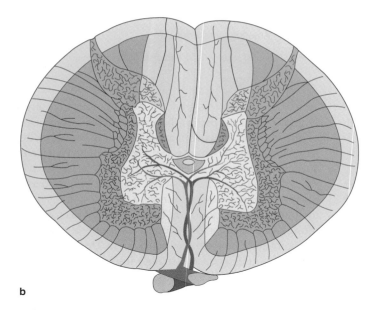

b

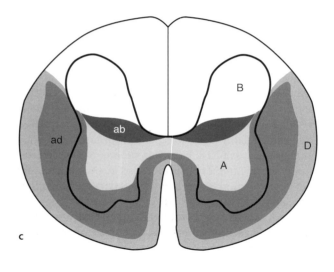

c

Figure 18.3 *Diagrams illustrating the distribution of the intrinsic arteries and veins of the spinal cord. (**a**) anterior and posterior spinal arteries (red) and anterior spinal vein (blue).[2] (**b**[2] and **c**[111]) comparison of topographic distribution of intrinsic arteries: (i) A, areas of distribution of the central artery (pink); (ii) D, the penetrating arteries from the lateral and ventral pial plexus (light green); (iii) ad, the areas which may be supplied by either the central or lateral and ventral penetrating arteries (darker green); (iv) B, the regions served by the penetrating arteries from the posterior plexus (yellow–green); (v) ab, the areas which may be served by either the central or by the posterior penetrating arteries (orange); area of posterior columns supplied by separate set of posterior arterial plexus (chartreuse; not separately designated by Ref. 111).*

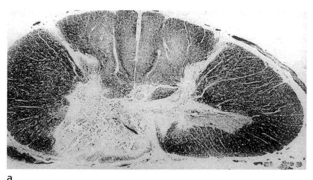

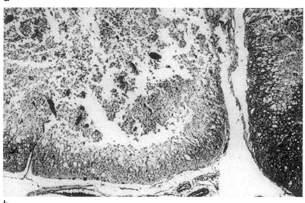

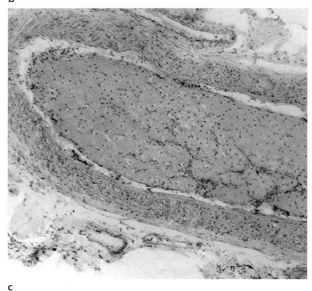

c

Figure 18.4 *Anterior spinal artery thromboembolism. (a) Transverse section of spinal cord at C7 segmental level. An irregular area of infarction affects the anterior grey horns, the commissure and one anterior white column, this last-mentioned area corresponding to the supply of a laterally directed sulcal artery. (Weil for myelin.) (b) Anterior white column at C3 segmental level. Note the partial preservation of the most outer part of the spinal cord supplied by the centripetal part of the arterial supply. (c) Anterior spinal artery occluded by thromboembolism in a separate case. (a) and (b) courtesy of Hughes.[149]*

arterial and venous systems, thereby causing embolic infarction of the spinal cord.[301] Other authors, recognizing that in many cases the calibre of the occluding embolus is of a size that would be unlikely to move through the capillary microcirculation, postulate retrograde arterial migration of fibrocartilaginous tissue into spinal branches of intercostal arteries[355] followed by anterograde embolization into the anterior and posterior radicular arteries of the spinal cord.[326] Shunting of embolic material into intraosseous arteriovenous fistulae, particularly under circumstances of nucleus pulposus injury and reactive neovascularization, has also been hypothesized.[325]

Infectious and non-infectious vasculitides can affect the blood vessels of the spinal cord along with those of other regions of the nervous system; these vascular lesions are discussed elsewhere (see Chapter 6, this Volume). When single or multiple spinal leptomeningeal blood vessels or intraspinal blood vessels become occluded, the resulting infarcts may be located in the territories of distribution of the anterior and posterior spinal arteries, or involve patches of grey and white matter throughout the length of the cord.[7,62,134,350]

SPINAL CORD DISEASE WITH HYPOTENSION AND HYPOPERFUSION

Several studies have drawn attention to the neuropathological findings in the spinal cord of adults and children in low blood-flow states, especially after cardiac arrest, but also occurring with prolonged and severe hypotension in a variety of other related clinical settings. Histopathological examination has disclosed total necrosis of anterior grey matter and surrounding white matter in severely affected cases, usually sparing the dorsal-most parts of the posterior horns (Fig. 18.6). Selective necrosis of grey matter restricted to multifocal neuronal dropout with scattered astrocytic and microglial proliferation was seen in less severely involved regions at the rostral and caudal edges of the major destructive lesion; it also was found as the principal lesion in other patients who had suffered a less severe hypotensive insult. The distribution of the lesions was almost invariably lumbosacral, sometimes extending into the posterior aspect of the lower thoracic anterior horns.[20,21,27,38,106,109,120,136,273,278,284,295] Autopsy studies of adults with a clinical syndrome of progressive amyotrophy without a clearly documented hypotensive episode have also shown a similar segmental pattern of grey matter involvement affecting multiple cord levels, particularly the regions of the upper thoracic and low cervical cord.[107,166]

These cases are particularly remarkable because the selective involvement of the grey matter does not conform to the vascular territory of the anterior or posterior spinal arteries but rather to the border zone between these two circulations. This observation suggests that the pathogenesis of the lesion is related to selective vulnerability of the affected regions based on low blood flow and

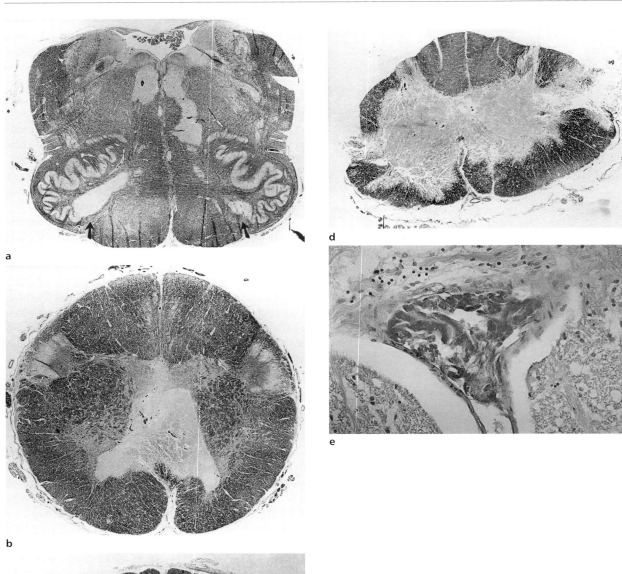

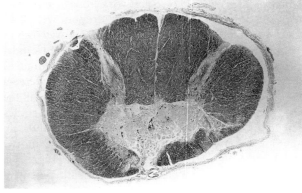

Figure 18.5 *Fibrocartilaginous embolization of the anterior spinal artery, showing infarction of the medulla and anterior territory of the cervical spinal cord. (a–d) Sequential rostrocaudal transverse sections showing the distribution of lesions shown as an area of pallor of myelin staining. (Heidenhahn–Woelke.) (e) Artery occluded by fibrocartilaginous embolism. (Alcian blue.) Dr C Kase, Department of Neurology, Boston University Medical Center.[174]*

undoubtedly other contributing factors, including the relatively high metabolic demand of the spinal cord grey matter compared with the white matter.

Selective grey matter necrosis of the cord has also been observed in the border zones of the vascular territories between the vertebral, intercostal and lumbar arterial branches, which form the anterior and posterior spinal arteries and supply, respectively, the cervical, thoracic and lumbar cord. Time-honoured anatomical and clinical studies have indicated that the most susceptible region to low-flow states is at T4 for the anterior circulation: it extends between three and four midthoracic segments in the posterior circulation.[198,359,360] However, these studies, along with several subsequent reports,[67,108,166,197,203] have emphasized that the precise segmental level of this border zone is variable. Of related interest is a largely clin-

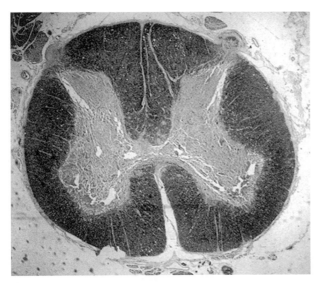

Figure 18.6 *Necrosis of the grey matter. Section from the upper lumbar cord in a case of dissecting aortic aneurysm showing good preservation of the white matter. The grey matter at this power appears fragmented and granular. The necrotic changes in the grey matter involve both the anterior and posterior horns entirely.[179] (Weil–Weigert.)*

ical study of 44 patients with ischaemic insults of the spinal cord in a wide range of medical settings, which reported a statistical mean of T8 (range C2–S2) for the observed spinal level of sensory deficit.[71] There is also a less vulnerable border zone in the lowest thoracic to upper lumbar segments.

EXPERIMENTAL STUDIES

Experimental animal studies have closely duplicated the histopathological characteristics and the distribution of the spinal cord lesion as described above in man[82] (Fig. 18.7). In these studies, mainly with rabbits and dogs, the abdominal aorta just below the renal arteries was temporarily occluded by external compression, or ligation, as originally described by Steno (Stensen) in 1667.[304] These experiments showed that the longitudinal segmental distribution of the lesion (low thoracic to sacral), and its transverse extent from the central portions of the anterior horns, are directly related to the duration of interruption of aortic blood flow.

SPINAL CORD ISCHAEMIA WITH AORTIC DISEASE

As discussed above, atherosclerosis involving the aorta does not ordinarily give rise to embolic occlusion of blood vessels supplying the spinal cord. Vascular insufficiency of the spinal cord has, however, been recognized in three types of aortic disease: aortic dissection, coarctation of the aorta and occlusion of the abdominal aorta, especially in relation to surgical intervention.

Aortic dissection occurs principally in the setting of two risk factors: hypertension and connective tissue disorders

such as Marfan's syndrome. Rarely, it may occur as an iatrogenic complication of arterial cannulation. Aortic dissection occurs at the site of a tear in the intima, usually in the arch of the aorta, through which arterial blood from the lumen penetrates into the media and extends rostrally or caudally, forcibly splitting the aortic wall. The intercostal and lumbar arteries which supply the spinal cord may thus become compromised. In such cases the clinical neurological manifestations reflecting spinal cord ischaemia are characterized by a sudden onset of paraparesis with a sensory level (usually at or below T6), often associated with bladder and bowel dysfunction.[140,328,339] There are a few detailed reports on the pathology of the spinal cord in patients with aortic dissection in whom neurological deficits developed.[139,180,236,267,289,323,339] For the most part the lesions of the spinal cord in these cases have been characterized by selective necrosis of the grey matter, involving the thoracolumbar cord. Intraparenchymal and subarachnoid haemorrhage may develop and cord infarction can occur in the territory of distribution of the anterior spinal artery.[290] The neurological and pathological manifestations of 16 cases of non-traumatic aortic dissection indicate that hypotension, and intermittent obstruction of aortic branches or their complete occlusion through propagation of the dissection, are important contributing factors and may explain the somewhat variable patterns of ischaemic necrosis found in the nervous system of these patients.[69]

A body of literature from the mid-twentieth century describes the clinical experience with the neurological manifestations before and after surgical treatment of coarctation of the aorta and patent ductus arteriosus.[6,55,93,330] Before surgery, the most commonly observed signs and symptoms of spinal cord vascular insufficiency are cramps, weakness and sensory disturbances, mainly involving the lower extremities. Paraplegia, sphincteric disturbances and a sensory level at T8 developed following cross-clamping of the aorta for 58 min during a surgical repair of an aortic coarctation; the patient improved somewhat during the course of a 13-year follow-up.[85] In the case studied by Beattie *et al.*, clamping of the aortic arch for 38 min during surgical repair of coarctation was followed immediately by bilateral leg paralysis; the patient died of pulmonary oedema 5 days later, and autopsy showed acute ischaemic changes (neuronal cytoplasmic vacuolization and nuclear pyknosis), and acute haemorrhages in the anterior horns of the lower lumbar and upper sacral cord.[29]

Occlusion of the abdominal aorta consequent upon thrombosis of an atherosclerotic aneurysm, surgical clamping or insertion of replacement grafts may be associated with reversible or irreversible neurological symptoms referable to the lumbosacral cord (weakness evolving to flaccid paralysis, sphincter disturbances, variable sensory manifestations).[207] Pathological studies have been described in relatively few instances, beginning with the early report of Helbing, whose patient developed

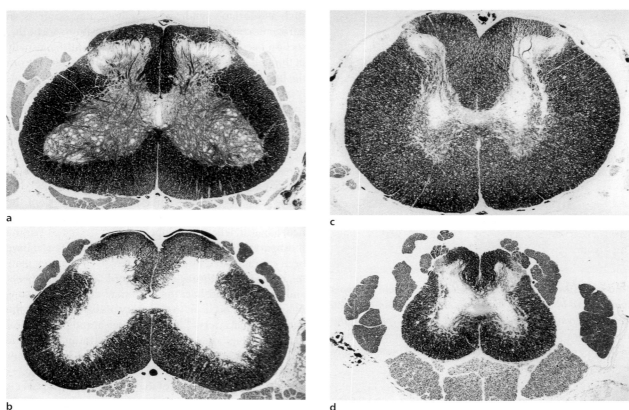

Figure 18.7 *Ischaemic necrosis of the spinal cord: transverse sections through the spinal cord of a rabbit 1 week after a 1-h occlusion of the aorta. (a) Mid-lumbar level in a control animal. Note the fine myelinated fibres coursing through the grey matter of the anterior and posterior horns. (b) Mid-lumbar level in an experimental animal. There is necrosis of the grey matter, some preservation of myelinated fibres in the dorsal root entry zone, tract of Lissauer and substantia gelatinosa, preservation of long white matter tracts and secondary degeneration of anterior roots. (c) Rostral extent of the lesion at the low thoracic level. Note that the necrotic lesion is confined to the central portions of the anterior horns, entirely sparing the posterior horns. (d) Caudal extent of the lesion at the sacral level. Note necrosis of the central portions of the anterior horns and secondary degeneration of the anterior roots.[82] (Celloidin section, Loyez.)*

paralysis of both legs and gangrene of the right lower leg and buttock following a saddle embolus to the aortic bifurcation, and in whom 'degenerative' changes were found in the grey and white matter and roots of the lumbar cord.[131]

Postoperative paraplegia after resection of abdominal aortic aneurysm has long been recognized clinically, and early autopsy studies demonstrated that the neurological deficit was due to infarction of the spinal cord.[106,227] In a case reported by Hogan and Romanul, an elderly man became abruptly hypotensive and was found to have a ruptured abdominal aortic aneurysm, which was resected during cross-clamping of the aorta for 3 h just below the renal arteries.[143] Postoperatively, he lived for 3 weeks, paraplegic and doubly incontinent. Autopsy examination showed infarction of the central portion of the spinal cord from T12 to S2 and a normal artery of Adamkiewicz, although the artery was believed to have been transiently occluded by the clamp. In another patient with an abdominal aortic aneurysm, who developed sudden paralysis of the legs and bowel and bladder incontinence,

post-mortem examination showed multifocal centrally distributed infarcts from T12 to S3 which were due to cholesterol emboli apparently from atheromatous plaques of the aneurysm.[139] A different distribution of spinal cord infarction was noted in the cases reported by Anderson and Willoughby, who described five patients with a cauda equina syndrome following temporary occlusion of the aorta by an intra-aortic balloon pump inserted to maintain effective arterial blood pressure, or by other surgical manipulations on the distal aorta.[14] In the one case studied post-mortem there was patchy necrosis of the L5 and sacral segments of the conus medullaris.

VENOUS INFARCTION OF THE SPINAL CORD

Pathologically documented examples of acute infarction of the spinal cord due to occlusion of intraspinal or subarachnoid draining veins have been infrequent.[150,152, 183,259,265,349] The clinical features of the cases with an acute course are not easily distinguishable from those observed with arterial occlusion. The underlying clinical setting has been septicaemia or of leptomeningitis, or obstruction to venous return. Pathological findings have been difficult to interpret in the older cases traditionally included as bona fide instances of venous infarction of the cord. More recent reports describe patients with carcinoma (pancreas and breast) in whom extensive intramedullary venous thrombosis was associated with haemorrhagic infarction involving the posterior and central portions of the cord at multiple segmental levels, not regularly confined to a particular region.[150,265] Non-haemorrhagic cord infarction associated with venous occlusion has also been reported in a remarkable case of a 71-year-old man with positive serological tests for syphilis who developed a transverse myelopathy and at autopsy was found to have extensive necrosis of the lumbar cord in association with occluded and recanalized veins.[183]

FOIX–ALAJOUANINE SYNDROME (ANGIODYSGENETIC NECROTIZING MYELOPATHY)

There is an additional category of necrotizing myelopathy resulting from faulty blood supply, with features that are so distinctive as to require separate consideration. The classic description is that of Foix and Alajouanine[103] who, on the basis of two case reports, recorded the major attributes that are unique to this syndrome. Their patients were men (aged 31 and 37 years) in whom a progressive, initially spastic then flaccid, areflexic paralysis of the lower limbs gradually evolved over 1–3 years, leading to death from terminal sepsis. Post-mortem studies of the spinal cord showed centrally located necrosis of the lumbosacral segments, affecting grey matter structures more severely than the white matter, in combination with enlarged, tortuous veins with thickened walls overlying the surface of the cord, and apparently increased numbers of small blood vessels with greatly thickened fibrotic walls within the affected segments of the cord. Foix and Alajouanine attributed the remarkable appearance of these blood vessels to an inflammatory alteration resulting from infection. Subsequently, about 40 similar cases have been reported in which clinical and post-mortem neuropathological studies have been undertaken.[9,13,19,23,56,65,102,103,117,122,165,186,187,204,206,217,219,249,252,266,287,288]

From these observations, it is reasonable to conclude that the disorder described by Foix and Alajouanine represents a distinct clinicopathological entity. Clinically, it is characterized by intermittently progressive, often asymmetrical, paraparesis, variably spastic or areflexic–amyotrophic, accompanied by varying degrees of pain and sensory disturbance in the lower limbs and, usually, derangement of bladder, bowel and sexual functions. The syndrome occurs most frequently in men of middle to late adult years, and typically evolves over a period of months to years. The pathological features consist of clusters or masses of enlarged, engorged tortuous subarachnoid veins, most prominent over the posterior aspects of the cord; patchy necrosis of the spinal-cord tissue,

involving the lower thoracic and lumbosacral segments in most instances; and the presence, within the affected segments of the cord, of enlarged, apparently proliferated small blood vessels (of capillary to arteriolar or venular size) with thickened collagenous walls and lack of features defining them clearly as either arteries or veins (Fig. 18.8).

The necrotic lesions in the spinal cord tend, on the whole, to be characterized by coagulative necrosis, in which the intrinsic tissue elements present an amorphous, homogeneous appearance, without evidence of phagocytosis or gliosis. At the margins of these foci of coagulative necrosis, bordering upon the more intact tissue, lipid-laden macrophages and gliosis can be seen. The posterior aspects of the cord are more severely affected than the anterior regions, and the central parts more than the peripheral, but the anterior horns are involved, to varying degrees, in most cases. In some patients, the entire cross-section of the cord is destroyed, with the possible exception of a narrow encircling, or anterior peripheral, rim of better preserved tissue.[9,19,102,186,187,287,288] An invariable accompaniment of the lesions in the lower part of the cord, when looked for, is ascending (wallerian) degeneration of the fasciculus gracilis and of the dorsal spinocerebellar tracts. In nearly all cases of the Foix–Alajouanine syndrome the necrosis is confined to the lower thoracic and lumbosacral segments of the cord. Isolated cervical localization is extremely rare, although occasional examples have been described.[65,102]

The major distinguishing features of the Foix–Alajouanine syndrome are the alterations in the blood vessels. The abnormal vessels in the subarachnoid space are characterized both by enlargement and, often, by thickened walls that are made up of fibroblasts and a few smooth-muscle cells, without an internal elastic lamina; they have accordingly been identified as veins. The extrinsic arteries of the spinal cord, meanwhile, are unremarkable. Within the spinal cord, the segments that are affected by the necrotizing process show a striking prominence of the small blood vessels throughout the entire cross-section of the cord. This prominence is due to a remarkable thickening and tortuosity of the walls of these blood vessels both within and outside the necrotic regions. Most of these blood vessels appear to be veins or capillaries. Arteries seem to be relatively spared,[217] but in general the pathological changes in the walls make it impossible to identify individual vessels as arteries or veins. In the more intact parts of the cord, the blood vessel walls are composed of densely packed, concentrically arranged collagen fibres with a few fibroblast nuclei among them; the endothelial lining is intact, but the lumen is often narrowed. In the necrotic zones, the blood-vessel walls are homogeneous in appearance (hyalinized) and relatively acellular, and some show fibrinoid necrosis or proteinaceous exudation.[164,186,287,288] Often, a few lymphocytes surround some of the intramedullary blood vessels, but they are not sufficiently numerous, or constant, to

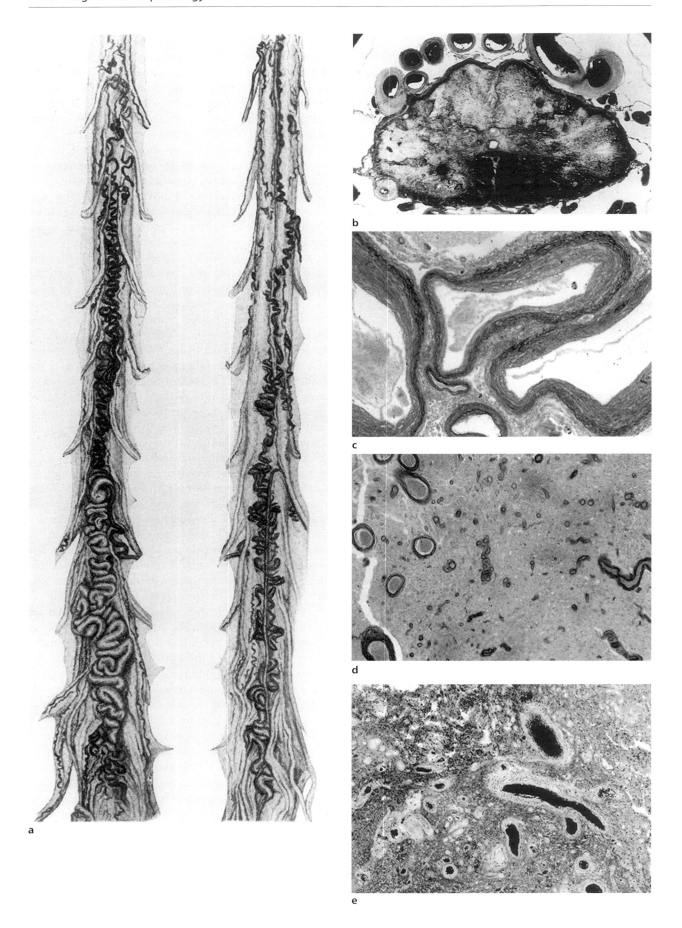

a

b

c

d

e

suggest a primary inflammatory reaction. The overall appearance of the vasculature in these affected parts of the cord suggests that the vessels are increased in number, and this suggestion receives support from the frequent presence of scattered groups or clusters of these thickened blood vessels in a random distribution throughout the cross-section of the cord. In the portions of the cord beyond the zones of necrosis, the blood vessels in general are normal but, as is evident in a case studied by the present authors, intact segments of the cord close to the necrotic regions can show extensive thickening of the small intramedullary blood vessels.

Foix and Alajouanine[103] and most subsequent observers of this form of myelopathy have considered that the abnormalities in the blood vessels are the primary cause of the lesions in the spinal cord. Wyburn-Mason[347] and others have thought that the engorged tortuous blood vessels ramifying over the surface of the cord represented a variety of developmental vascular anomaly of the veins that they classified as angioma racemosum venosum. The concept of a congenital basis for the vascular abnormalities also finds expression in the term introduced by Scholz and Manuelidis[287] and appearing repeatedly in the subsequent literature: angiodysgenetic necrotizing myelopathy (or, in the terminology of Bodechtel and Erbslöh[41] in their review, angiodysgenetic myelomalacia).

The development of radiographic techniques for the *in vivo* demonstration of the vasculature of the spinal cord has resulted in a change of point of view regarding the myelopathy of Foix–Alajouanine type. To an increasing degree it has been shown that the engorged veins overlying the cord are associated with a dural, arteriovenous shunt (generally within or near a root-sleeve) resulting in a reflux of arterial blood, via an arterialized vein, into the venous drainage of the spinal cord.[43,78,119,157,177,229,232,310] It has been surmised that these arteriovenous fistulae are acquired lesions, rather than congenitally derived angiomas, but their pathogenesis remains unknown. The fistulous connection between the dural arterial system and the venous plexus of the cord is thought to result in increased venous pressure in the draining veins of the cord

Figure 18.8 Shown opposite. *Foix–Alajouanine syndrome. (a) Drawing of the dorsal (left) and ventral (right) surfaces of the spinal cord showing dilated and tortuous blood vessels.[206] (b) Low-power micrograph of the lower thoracic cord showing ischaemic necrosis of the posterior and lateral funiculi and many large, thick-walled blood vessels (veins) over the posterior and anterior surfaces of the cord.[8] (c) Thick-walled subarachnoid veins under higher magnification. The adventitia contains numerous interspersed elastic fibres. A small artery of wholly normal appearance is included (bottom, centre). (Elastic tissue – Van Gieson.) (d) Multiple thick-walled small blood vessels, some in clusters, the lateral funiculus. (Haematoxylin–Van Gieson.) (e) Necrosis of cord tissue, and abundant thickened blood vessels. (Weil stain for myelin.)*

and, subsequently, ischaemic injury to the cord. The lower end of the cord appears to be especially susceptible, but it has been shown that intracranial arteriovenous fistulae can be associated with cervical myelopathy.[222,255,346]

NON-TRAUMATIC HAEMORRHAGE INTO THE SPINAL CORD (HAEMATOMYELIA) AND SPINAL CANAL (HAEMATORRHACHIS)

Intraspinal haemorrhage can occur in any of the three extramedullary compartments (subarachnoid, subdural or epidural) – haematorrhachis – or within the substance of the spinal cord – haematomyelia. It most often is induced by trauma, as will be discussed later. Recognized causes of non-traumatic causes of intraspinal haemorrhage include iatrogenic procedures such as lumbar puncture or spinal surgery, vascular lesions such as vascular malformations, haemorrhage related to tumours, and bleeding diatheses (due to either therapeutic anticoagulation or disease-related coagulopathy).

General experience indicates that, when the spinal cord of clinically asymptomatic patients is studied microscopically as part of a complete post-mortem examination, scattered small foci of acute petechial haemorrhage involving the grey and white matter are regularly encountered. The pathogenesis of these lesions has remained obscure. Clinically apparent non-traumatic intramedullary haemorrhage, in the absence of concomitant infarction, is infrequent and not ordinarily associated with the commonly observed causes of spontaneous intracranial haemorrhage (i.e. hypertension, amyloid angiopathy, vasculitis); rather, it is usually traceable to vascular malformations (discussed above), a haemorrhagic diathesis or the administration of anticoagulant drugs. Some individuals have developed sudden onset of sensory and motor symptoms referable to the long tracts of the spinal cord associated with the demonstration of blood and xanthochromia of the cerebrospinal fluid. Pathologically documented cases of haematomyelia are rare.[200,218]

Spontaneous or non-traumatic epidural haematomas are the most common type of spontaneous intraspinal haemorrhage and have been associated with coagulopathy, haematoma of a vertebral body, vascular anomalies and arthropathies such as Paget's disease and ankylosing spondylitis. Most of the epidural haematomas lie dorsal to the cord and can occur at any level in the spine. Magnetic resonance imaging (MRI) is currently the best method for diagnosing these lesions, and prompt treatment, usually by laminectomy, is required to relieve spinal cord compression.

COMPRESSION OF THE SPINAL CORD

Compression of the cord by encroachment on its space is of major importance as a cause of injury to its tissues. In many cases, the compression occurs acutely as a consequence of abrupt mechanical displacement of the structures of the spinal column induced by trauma; the pathological effects on the cord are discussed elsewhere (see Non-penetrating injuries, below).

Progressively evolving or chronic compression results from intrinsic diseases of bone that involve the vertebral column (see Diseases of the vertebral column affecting the spinal cord, below), as well as from neoplasms (Chapter 11, Volume II) and infections (Chapters 1–3, Volume II). To a considerable extent the deleterious effects of compression are produced by impairment of the intrinsic circulation. As indicated by Hughes[149] in his review, mechanical pressure on the cord tends to compress the veins more than the arteries, leading to venous stasis and oedema. The chief effects at the early stages are suffered by the myelin sheaths, which become swollen, imparting a vacuolated appearance to the white matter, initially in the posterior part of the lateral columns. With advance of the compressive process, more and more of the cord becomes affected, leading to necrosis and cavitation, particularly in the centre of the cord. The end result is a gliotic scar involving both grey and white matter, with preservation of some of the axons. Interruptions of the ascending and descending fibre tracts result in secondary (wallerian) degeneration at all levels distal to the lesion (see Chapter 3, this Volume). Thus, above the lesion there is fibre loss in the posterior columns (fasciculus gracilis and, to a varying extent, the fasciculus cuneatus, depending on whether the interruption is above, at or below the cervical enlargement) and in the spinothalamic and spinocerebellar tracts, while below the lesion the corticospinal (indirect and direct pyramidal) tracts degenerate.

DISEASES OF THE VERTEBRAL COLUMN AFFECTING THE SPINAL CORD

Intervertebral disc disease and spondylosis

Early descriptions of the anatomy of the intervertebral disc are given in the writings of Vesalius.[332] Mention of sciatica and of the neurological symptoms now recognized as characteristic of nerve root involvement by protrusion of an intervertebral disc can be found in a number of historical documents dating back 3000 years.[91,126] The first monograph on 'sciatica' is that of Cotugno in 1764.[76] Contemporary understanding of the clinical, radiological and surgical manifestations of degenerative disease of the intervertebral disc and spondylosis and the postulated pathophysiological mechanisms involved is summarized in several reviews and monographs.[61,79,84,125,161,192,249,344]

NORMAL ANATOMY

Complete descriptions of the embryology, anatomy and pathology of the intervertebral disc date to the work of Keyes and Compere[182] and DePalma and Rothman.[84] The intervertebral disc is a flattened, cylindrical structure which is directly continuous with the thin plate of hyaline cartilage that forms the inferior and superior surfaces of the vertebral body. Transverse section through the midportion of the disc demonstrates a densely packed skein of circumferentially arranged connective tissue fibres and fibrocartilage that form a ring encircling the outer two-thirds of the disc (annulus fibrosus). The central and somewhat posteriorly directed part of the adult disc, the nucleus pulposus, is a gelatinous matrix containing cartilage cells, loose connective tissue containing proteoglycan molecules, physaliphorous cells and remnants of notochordal tissue. In man the notochordal elements, which represent a prominent component of the nucleus pulposus in embryonic life and are more evident in the high cervical and lumbosacral regions than in the thoracic region, progressively disappear early in the first decade of life as they are replaced, first by cartilage ingrowth and then, in late adult life, by dense fibrous connective tissue.[182] The adult disc is devoid of blood vessels and nerve fibres. The disc is bounded anteriorly by the anterior longitudinal ligament and posteriorly by thin posterior longitudinal ligaments, the fibres of which fuse with those of the annulus fibrosus. The posteriorly directed pedicles arising from the vertebral bodies join with the vertebral laminae to form the neural arch which encloses the meninges, spinal cord and nerve roots within the spinal (vertebral) canal. The ligamentum flavum is a paired structure which runs longitudinally along the inner surface of the laminar arches; its high content of elastin allows for the considerable flexibility of the vertebral column. Adjacent vertebral arches articulate at the superior and inferior articular facet processes (zygapophyseal joints). From the neural arch emerge two lateral transverse processes and a posteriorly directed spinous process that serve as attachments for the tendons and muscles of the neck and back. The nerve roots emerge laterally from the spinal canal through the intervertebral foramina, openings between adjacent vertebrae just posteriolateral to the posterior surface of the annulus fibrosus.

DEGENERATION AND PROTRUSION OF THE INTERVERTEBRAL DISC

Perhaps as a consequence of remote traumatic injury, but ordinarily for reasons that are not understood, nucleus pulposus tissue may be pushed rostrally or caudally through a crack in the cartilaginous plate into the vertebral body. These Schmorl's nodes[283] can be seen on radiological studies in about one-third of normal adults, especially when secondary sclerosis of the spongiosa of the vertebral body around the extruded fragment has taken place. Luschka is credited as being the first to recognize intervertebral disc protrusion.[211] They may also be found in the context of acute trauma.[97] It was later established, early in the twentieth century, that degenerative disorders of the intervertebral disc cause neurological manifestations when there is posterolateral protrusion and herniation of the nucleus pulposus and compromise of neighbouring neural structures: the spinal cord and roots in the cervical (and, rarely, the thoracic) spine and the cauda equina in the lumbar spine.[113,230,234,283,308] In addition to the degenerative changes that develop in intervertebral discs with age,[15,262] a variety of factors has been demonstrated to contribute to the development of symptomatic disc displacement. Traumatic injury, when superimposed on discs which show degenerative changes, can lead to the onset of neurological dysfunction from spinal cord or nerve root compromise.[321] A prominent risk factor for displacement of intervertebral discs has been shown to be the load carried by the vertebral column, as reflected through height and weight.[46,132] Epidemiological studies have not strongly supported the popular association of symptomatic intervertebral disc disease and lifting. While some studies have demonstrated an association between occupation, lifting and risk,[210,238,239] others point towards other activities, such as prolonged motor vehicle driving.[176,210,333]

Detailed histopathological studies of degenerative disc disease have been carried out.[114,182,191] The nucleus pulposus is eccentrically situated towards the posterior end of the intervertebral disc and the annulus fibrosus is therefore narrower, and the disc somewhat thinner, posteriorly. Degenerated disc material most commonly bulges posteriorly, through rents in the annulus fibrosus and, usually, posterolateral to the most peripheral strands of the posterior longitudinal ligament. Fraying of the fibres of the posterior longitudinal ligament may also occur, especially in the cervical region, with posteromedial disc protrusion. This shift of nucleus pulposus material and the associated fibrosis create an outward swelling ('hard disc') on the posterior surface of the disc, which is visible radiologically and to the naked eye at surgery or autopsy. In time, further tearing of the fibres of the posterior annulus connective tissue results in escape of degenerated nucleus pulposus material ('disc herniation') into the spinal canal, which may impinge upon the spinal cord or a root in the intervertebral foramen as it exits the dural sac.

Disc degeneration, not necessarily associated with nucleus pulposus protrusion, occurs normally with advancing age. The nucleus pulposus zone is gradually taken over by annulus and fibrous tissue and the disc becomes thinned. Any pathological process which damages the nucleus pulposus will severely affect the cushioning function of the disc. In time, this leads to narrowing of the disc space and a shift of the vertically directed forces on to the anterior and lateral portions of the vertebral body with forward and lateral bending movements, thus contributing to the bony outgrowths from the ventral aspect of the lower thoracic and lumbar vertebral bodies (osteophyte and spur formation, or 'lipping') and misaligning of the intervertebral facet joints characteristic of spondylosis, as seen in middle-aged and older individuals.

While collagen I is the predominant component of the annulus fibrosis, and collagen II is present in the nucleus pulposus, other proteins are present in intervertebral discs.[251] Among these, collagen IX is a minor component but has been associated with several diseases including those of the spine.[77] Some mutations in collagen IX subunits have been linked to the syndrome of multiple epiphyseal dysplasia (EDM2),[42,144,240] as well as causing degenerative disease of cartilage in mouse models.[159] Of particular interest for degenerative disease of the spine, an allele of the gene encoding the alpha 2(IX) subunit has been linked to intervertebral disc disease.[16] While this observation remains to be confirmed in other populations, it represents a possible explanation for the genetic component[276,292] of this clearly multifactorial disease process.

SPONDYLOSIS

Spondylosis is a generic term which includes several related degenerative diseases of the spinal column that involve the vertebrae, intervertebral joints, ligaments and intervertebral discs.

Cervical spondylosis and cervical disc disease

This is a disease primarily affecting middle-aged men (about three times more often than women), with characteristic clinical and radiological findings.[51–53,73,114,118,340] The most common radiological findings in patients with cervical spondylosis are: (1) narrowing of the intervertebral disc spaces due to thinning and posteriolateral bulging or frank herniation of portions of the intervertebral disc (often affecting multiple discs), with reversal of the normal curvature of the spine; (2) osteophyte formation and fusion forming a bony ridge on the posterior margins of the vertebral bodies; (3) degenerative joint disease of the intervertebral facet joints with partial subluxation of the vertebrae; and (4) hypertrophy of the dorsal longitudinal ligament and redundancy ('buckling') of the ligamentum flavum, especially during neck extension. These changes reduce the cervical spinal canal to less than 11 mm (normal width being about 17 mm), or to 7 mm with neck extension, and narrow intervertebral foramina, resulting in compromise of the spinal cord and spinal root function, respectively. Encroachment of the spinal canal, as shown radiographically, is said to occur with hyperextension and hyperflexion of the neck because the posterior longitudinal ligament (which is somewhat more lax in the cervical region) or the ligamentum flavum are prone to infold, buckle and press upon the cord. Neurological manifestations occur in a relatively small proportion of patients with radiographical evidence of cervical

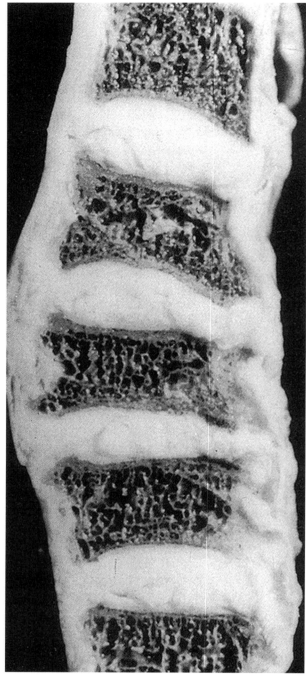

a

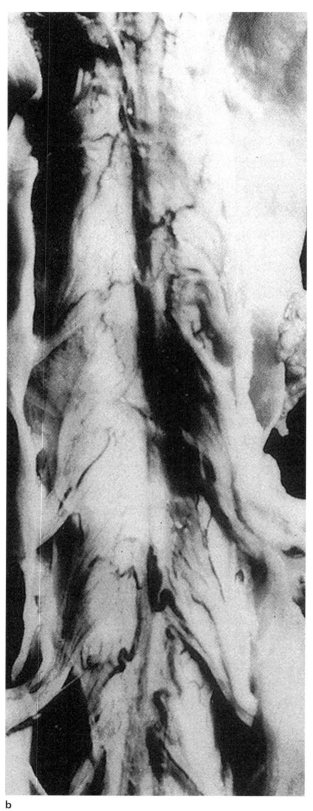

b

Figure 18.9 *Cervical spondylosis. (a) Right half of sagittally sawn upper spine from C4 to T1 vertebral bodies. Severe spondylosis affects the C4/C5, C5/C6 and C6/C7 disc spaces and has caused a huge posterior protrusion from C5 to C7, seen to the left of the picture. (b) The spinal cord viewed from the anterior aspect. Note the deep indentation of the cord at C6/C7 corresponding to the cervical spondylosis seen in the spine in (a). (c) Posterior aspect of the cord seen in (b). Note the dilatation of the posterior spinal veins.*[149]

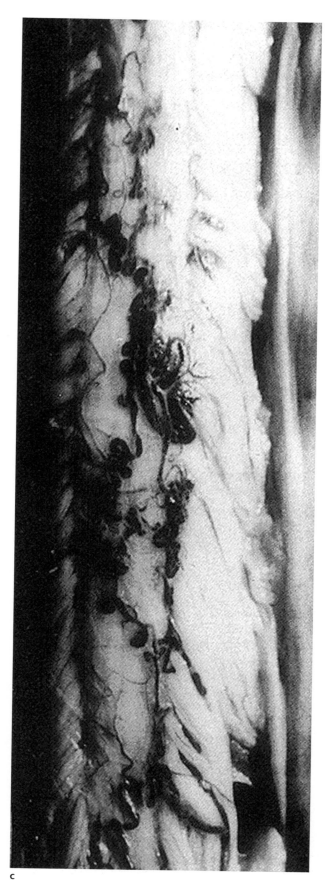

spondylosis, possibly in the setting of a congenitally small vertebral canal. The most commonly observed symptoms of myeloradiculopathy due to cervical spondylosis are neck and shoulder pain in the early stages of the disease, followed later by radicular arm pain and weakness in the C5 or C6 (or, less often, C6–C7) distribution due to involvement of the fifth or sixth intervertebral disc. Compromise of the spinal cord leads to variable symptoms, including a gradually progressive spastic hemiparesis or paraparesis with prominent ataxia of gait. Sensory manifestations in all four limbs may ensue, sometimes with a sensory level. Bowel and bladder dysfunction are infrequent and only observed in severely affected individuals. Antecedent trauma to the most mobile neck vertebrae is an important aetiological factor for the development of either myelopathy in young individuals or spondylosis with disc degeneration in the elderly.

Careful neuropathological studies of the spine, spinal cord and roots in neurologically affected patients with cervical spondylosis with or without disc protrusion have been carried out in a few instances.[30,53,114,146,216,340]

Macroscopically, lesions of the spinal cord consist of transverse indentations, generally on the anterolateral surface of the cord underlying the bony protrusions of the vertebral bodies (Fig. 18.9). The shape of the cord is altered, being flatter than normal and sometimes of reduced total volume.[30,114,340] At the site of the bony lesions, sections of the underlying cord demonstrate ill-defined pallor of myelin staining in the lateral funiculi and in the ventral parts of the dorsal columns, either unilaterally or bilaterally, often associated with axonal damage and gliosis (Fig. 18.10). There is variable loss of anterior horn neurons either at the level of the spondylotic lesions or some distance away. Both subarachnoid and intrinsic blood vessels of the microcirculation may be thickened, but frank vascular occlusion with tissue infarction has not been a feature of the disease in cases with a chronic clinical course. The meninges are often thickened, with fibrous adhesions between the dura and the posterior longitudinal ligament, and fibrosis of the leptomeninges around the roots. Cord infarction, especially involving the central grey regions, was noted when the spinal cord was examined at autopsy immediately or long after a clinical episode of acute spinal cord compression;[53,146] in a unique case, there was thrombosis of the anterior spinal artery with necrosis of the spinal cord in the territory of distribution of the blood vessel.[155] Some secondary ascending and descending wallerian degeneration of long tracts is regularly observed either in cases of clear-cut destructive lesions at the site of the greatest bony deformity, or in patients without cord necrosis in whom a presumed compressive force on the dorsal roots and spinal cord is believed to have taken place during life. In chronic cases, the posterior and anterior nerve roots are abnormally adherent to thickened meninges, and there is a loss of axons with evidence of regenerative sprouting and neuroma formation in the ventral roots.

c

Figure 18.9 *(Continued).*

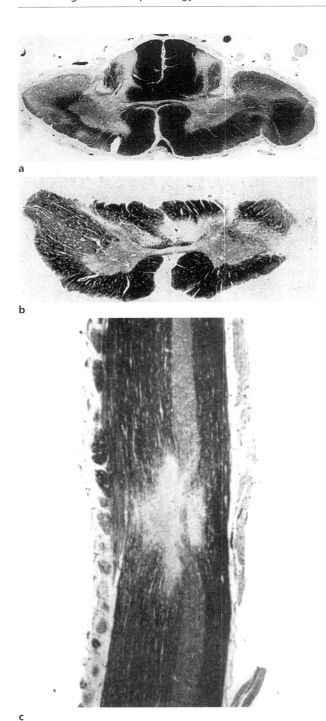

a

b

c

Figure 18.10 *Cervical disc protrusion. (a) Section of the cord at the level of C4–C5 from a case with multiple disc protrusions involving chiefly the intervertebral foramina at the lower cervical level. The cord is flattened anteroposteriorly and shows degeneration in the dorsal columns due to lesions of the lower cervical nerve roots. (Myelin stain.) (b) Section of the cord at the level a disc protrusion (C6–C7) showing degeneration in the region of attachment of the ligamentum denticulatum on one side and degeneration in the ventral part of the dorsal columns chiefly on the same side. (Myelin stain.) (c) Longitudinal section of the cervical cord from a case with 18 years' history of slight paraplegia due to degeneration of disc between C7 and T1. (Myelin stain.)*[115]

The pathogenesis of the spinal cord lesions seen most commonly has been the subject of considerable speculation.[5,52,201,248,320,340] The long-tract lesions in the white matter do not conform to a clear-cut vascular territory and have somewhat unsatisfactorily been attributed to 'mechanical compression'; the older hypothesis that damage to the long tracts is due to 'tethering' of the cervical cord by the denticulate ligament[114,171] has received little notice recently. Secondary degeneration in the fasciculus cuneatus of the posterior columns may be related in some cases to compression of posterior roots by cartilaginous overgrowth and osteophytes of the intervertebral canals; in other cases, the degeneration is confined to a small part of the posterior columns and is therefore not explained by this mechanism. The flattened shape and small size of the cord in the regions of most severe spondylosis argue in favour of compression of the cord due to a reduction in the size of the spinal canal and form the basis for the somewhat controversial current surgical management of these patients.[274]

Redundancy with buckling of the ligamentum flavum during extension of the neck and ligament mineralization of the ligamentum flavum and other longitudinally directed ligaments are believed to be contributing compression factors.[241,303,307,337] The regular occurrence of neuronal loss in anterior horn cells and elsewhere lends some support to the suggestion that vascular insufficiency (on an unknown basis, but supposedly due to compression) and ischaemic injury gives rise to a low blood-flow state in the terminal territory of the anterior spinal artery or, alternatively, to venous stasis.

Lumbar and thoracic disc disease

Lumbar disc disease is most common in young middle-aged men. It is, at times, related to direct trauma to the lumbosacral spine or to heavy physical strain, but commonly it develops without a definite antecedent event.[125,234] Protrusion of the lumbar intervertebral discs is most common at the L5–S1 interspace; it also occurs, in decreasing order of frequency, at the L4–L5, L3–L4 and L2–L3 interspaces, and only rarely affects the Ll–L2 disc. At these levels, the cord is not damaged but the neurological effects are borne by the roots of the cauda equina.[205] The disc most often herniates posterolaterally to the posterior longitudinal ligament and may produce symptoms when it lodges in the intervertebral canal or foramen.

In the thoracic region, the ribs and intercostal muscles limit the flexion of the spine, thereby reducing the possibility of injury to the vertebrae and intervertebral discs; thoracic disc disease is therefore relatively rare, occurring in less than 5% of all cases in most series. In the unusual cases in which degenerative thoracic disc disease occurs, the T6–T7 and T5–T6 interspaces are the most affected. Lumbar stenosis is a clinicoradiological entity, often occurring in combination with cervical spondylosis. It is characterized by a reduction in the size of the lumbar vertebral canal, and by neurological manifestations indicative of persistent compression of the cauda equina roots. It may be due to congenital stenosis of the vertebral canal or spondylosis with superimposed degenerative disc disease, or both. Clinically, lumbar stenosis is characterized by pain, paraesthesiae and weakness in the back and legs, caused by entrapment of lumbosacral roots due to the narrowing of the vertebral canal and the intervertebral foramina. In children, lumbar spinal stenosis is most often due to skeletal dysplasias and dysraphias. There have been no detailed pathological studies of this process.

Bony abnormalities of the region of the foramen magnum

The articulation at the atlas and axis is the most mobile part of the vertebral column, permitting both rotational and flexion–extension movements. The atlas is a unique vertebra, having a ring-like structure and no vertebral body. It has a synovial articulation rostrally with the occipital condyles of the skull and caudally with the odontoid process (dens) of the axis. The odontoid process is bounded anteriorly by the anterior arch of the atlas and posteriorly by the transverse atlantal ligament, and it is attached to the skull by means of the lateral alar ligaments and the midline apical ligament. There is also articulation of the first and second vertebrae at the inferior articular facet of the atlas and the superior articular facet of the axis.

The high cervical spinal cord may be compromised under circumstances in which there are abnormalities of the floor of the posterior cranial fossa or of the atlas and the axis.[226] Three main abnormalities give rise to neurological symptoms:

- Congenital fusion of the atlas and foramen magnum (occipitalization of the atlas), where there is partial or complete fusion of the atlas with the occipital bone at the foramen magnum: this was found in 28 of 100 cases with bony abnormalities at the craniocervical junction in one series.[226] Neurological abnormalities were detected when the anteroposterior diameter of the spinal canal behind the dens was less than 19 mm.
- Platybasia and basilar invagination: these are conditions in which high cervical cord compression may occur because of a congenital or acquired (as in Paget's disease, osteogenesis imperfecta, rickets or rheumatoid arthritis) change in the craniocervical angle and in the normal position of the first two cervical vertebrae. Platybasia refers to a flattening of the angle formed by the intersection of the clivus and the floor of the anterior fossa to more than 135°. Basilar invagination (or impression) refers to upward displacement of the occipital condyles above the plane of the foramen magnum, and radiological demonstration of protrusion of the tip of the dens above a line drawn in a lateral skull projection between the floor of the hard palate and the posterior edge of the foramen magnum (Chamberlain's line).

- Atlantoaxial dislocation: this is a congenital or trauma-related condition wherein the odontoid process of the axis becomes partly or totally separated from the atlas. It results in neurological abnormalities that can be acute or chronic.

Rheumatoid arthritis and ankylosing spondylitis

Rheumatoid arthritis may involve the small joints of the cervical spine and the atlantoaxial joint of Cl–C2.[95] Anterior subluxation of C2 on Cl has been detected in patients with rheumatoid arthritis with a frequency ranging from 25 to 43%.[75,257] It may lead to impingement of the odontoid process on the spinal cord (Fig. 18.11). Similar atlantoaxial subluxation can complicate other forms of arthritis, including psoriatic arthritis,[32] ankylosing spondylitis,[264] systemic lupus erythematosus[22] and, rarely, osteoarthritis.[80] While the relationship between the degree of subluxation and neurological symptoms remains variable, measurements of alteration in cord diameter have been correlated with severity of symptoms. Specifically, the ratio of the anteroposterior dimension of the cord to its lateral width at the level of greatest compression as well as the ratio of the transverse diameter of the cord at the point of maximal compression to the comparable diameter at the lower margin of the body of the axis were both found to predict neurological deficits.[243] Rheumatoid disease of subaxial cervical vertebrae may also lead to partial subluxations and compression of roots and cord.[105,133] Although involvement of the cervical spine is a relatively common manifestation of rheumatoid arthritis, neurological complications are infrequent and related to either chronic compression of the

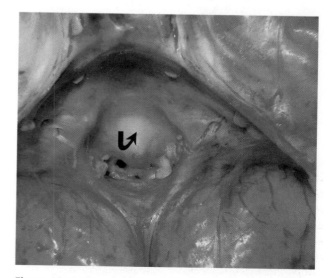

Figure 18.11 *Rheumatoid arthritis. Base of the skull, showing the foramen magnum from above. There is upward dislocation of the odontoid process of the axis, which is seen in the foramen magnum as a bony protuberance (arrow) pushing the medulla and spinal cord backwards.*

spinal cord with sensory disturbances referable to involvement of the posterior columns[133] or an acute deterioration with central cord infarction.[244] Subsequent to a report describing acute cord compression causing death in a patient with rheumatoid arthritis,[81] it has become clear that sudden neurological deterioration can be seen in as many as 10% of patients with rheumatoid arthritis.[228]

Ankylosing spondylitis is an inflammatory disease of unknown cause which affects primarily the joints of the axial skeleton, thereby leading, in the late stages of the disease, to ossification of the intervertebral joints and fusion of the vertebrae (Fig. 18.12). Affected individuals are at increased risk of cervical spine fractures, sometimes after relatively minor trauma, and increased mortality rates.[104] Epidural haematoma may be found in association with the vertebral fracture or may also occur in the absence of a fracture.[141] Atlantoaxial subluxations also occur in these patients, but at a lower frequency than that observed in individuals with rheumatoid arthritis.[264,298] Well-defined nerve root lesions appear to be a relatively infrequent neurological component of the disease, although pain is common in the active stages of the disorder.[224,322] A cauda equina syndrome has been described as a late form of neurological involvement in ankylosing spondylitis, often after the disease has become otherwise quiescent.[48] The few autopsy studies of the spinal cord in these patients have described increased fibrous tissue around nerve roots with little inflammation,[127] dural diverticula extending into the laminae and spinous processes of the lumbar vertebrae and the roof of the sacral canal,[224] and spinal cord compression in cases with vertebral fractures. An association has been reported between ankylosing spondylitis and multiple sclerosis[63,224] although direct pathological evidence for the concurrence of the two disorders is lacking in most cases.[88]

Other diseases of bone with spinal cord involvement

Paget's disease is occasionally a cause of spinal cord compression with vertebral involvement. This results from a

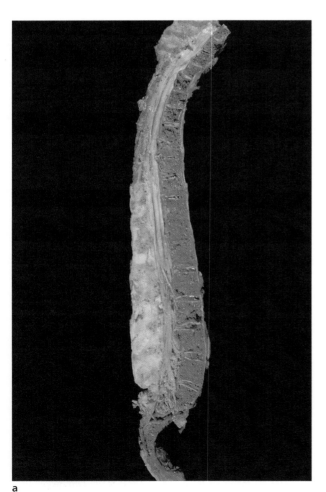

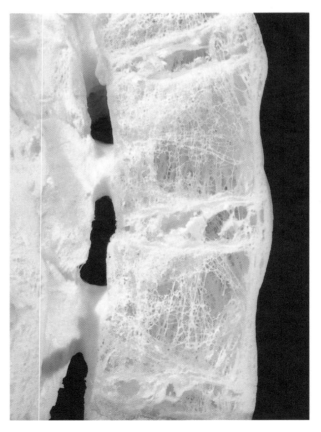

a
b

Figure 18.12 *Ankylosing spondylitis. (a) Longitudinal section of the spinal column with the spinal cord in situ in the spinal canal showing fusion of vertebral bodies and some narrowing of caudal portions of the spinal canal. (b) Close-up view of a macerated section of the spinal column showing fusion of vertebrae through the ossification of intervertebral discs.*

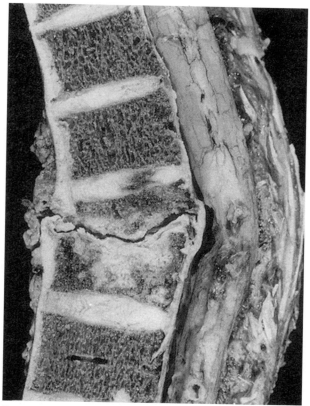
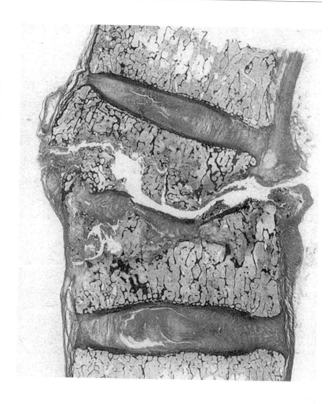

a   b

Figure 18.13 *Pott's paraplegia. (a) Right half of the sagittally sawn specimen of the thoracic spine. There is collapse of T7 and T8 vertebral bodies due to a tuberculous osteitis which has involved the T7/T8 intervertebral disc. The anterior aspect of the spinal cord is compressed by the gibbosity of the kyphosis. There is, incidentally, a Schmorl's node in the lower part of T9 vertebral body. (b) Section of the decalcified spine seen in (a), of which the histological appearances are mirror images.[151] (Haematoxylin–Van Gieson.)*

combination of flattening of vertebral bodies, thickening of the neural arches and extension of partially mineralized osteoid masses into the vertebral canal; less commonly it can ensue upon vertebral fractures or subluxations.[282,329,348] In addition, the hypermetabolic state of pagetoid bone may result in a 'vascular steal' phenomenon, leading to spinal cord ischaemia, which has been reported to be rapidly reversible with medical therapy.[70,351] In patients with evidence of spinal cord involvement, Paget's disease typically involves multiple contiguous vertebrae, especially in the thoracic spine where the vertebral canal is narrowest. Clinical manifestations are often characterized by progressive numbness with weakness and pain is a frequent complaint. Early autopsy studies describe focal posterior column degeneration; however, there is insufficient description of the spinal column to be confident that the long tract findings are directly related to Paget's disease.[110,202] Paget's disease may also encroach upon the spinal roots, and when it involves the base of the skull it can cause basilar impression and lower cranial nerve palsies.

Compressive cord syndromes have also been observed in clinicoradiological case studies in a wide range of conditions affecting the vertebral column, including osteopetrosis, achondroplasia, mucopolysaccharidoses, osteogenesis imperfecta and kyphoscoliosis. The most often reported neurological manifestations of osteopetrosis are cranial nerve deficits;[160,185] clinical evidence of myelopathy has been related to involvement of the cervical vertebrae.[225] In achondroplasia the spinal canal and intervertebral foramina are narrowed, with ensuing progressive myeloradiculopathies.[37,299] Cervical cord compression syndromes are observed in several of the mucopolysaccharidoses.[178,352]

Infectious and other disease of the spine with spinal cord involvement

Only a few aspects of this broad topic as it relates to spinal cord compression will be discussed briefly here, since infectious diseases and tumours are covered elsewhere in this text.

Involvement of the spine by *Mycobacterium tuberculosis* (Pott's disease) may result in vertebral body collapse (Fig. 18.13), most commonly at the thoracic and lumbar levels, epidural abscess and reactive changes with compression of the spinal cord directly or interference with its blood supply.[149] Spinal epidural abscess secondary to pyogenic bacteria (mainly *Staphylococcus aureus*, streptococci and Gram-negative bacilli) causing osteomyelitis or septicaemia was found to be an important cause of surgically treatable cord compression in a series of 39 patients, who developed acute or gradually evolving paraplegia.[24] Post-mortem examination was carried out in eight patients and in the majority of cases the abscess was located in the adipose tissue of the posterior thoracic or lumbar epidural space. Destructive lesions were found in the adjacent spinal cord, sometimes extending well beyond the site of compression, suggesting compromised venous return as a contributing pathogenetic factor. Subsequent series accumulated during the 1990s have found that *S. aureus* remains the most common organism[215,268] and have emphasized the current role of MRI in the early detection of epidural abscesses.

One of the unique structural aspects of the spinal cord and its covering, which differ from those of the brain and skull, is the presence of a true physiological epidural space. Increases in the volume of epidural fat, normally present in this space, can result in compression of the spinal cord. This syndrome of spinal epidural lipomatosis is most commonly associated with Cushing's syndrome (including iatrogenic hypercortisolism associated with systemic steroid administration or local therapy).[68,130,173,275,294,358] It can also occur without evidence of excess glucocorticoids; in these cases, obesity appears to be a major determinant.[31,45,123,193,263,270,302,305] While they can respond to weight reduction, decompression may be needed for more immediate relief.[270] These cases show a strong male predominance and are roughly evenly distributed between thoracic and lumbar levels.[270]

Another process which alters the normally stable relationship between the spinal cord and the dura is termed idiopathic spinal cord herniation. This syndrome, which affects the spinal cord in the thoracic region of middle-aged individuals, involves the displacement, or prolapse, of a short segment of spinal cord through a dural defect.[1,44,57,128,158,194,220,221,223,233,235,245,250,293,327,331,345] Similar spinal cord herniation through a traumatic disruption of the dura with development of the Brown–Séquard syndrome has been reported.[199] In these idiopathic cases, however, the defect in the dura can be associated with an arachnoid cyst, although in the majority of cases there is no clear basis for the alteration in dural integrity. These patients typically present with a Brown–Séquard syndrome or a spastic paraparesis which has developed over months. With surgical reduction of the cord from its prolapsed location, recovery is expected, even in cases in which the deficits were present for a long period.

The ligaments surrounding the dural sac may become thickened and ossified, thereby resulting in spinal cord compression. The most common form of this lesion is ossification of the posterior longitudinal ligament (OPLL); ossification of the ligamentum flavum also occurs, although it is much less common. The aetiology of these conditions is unknown, but their occasional concurrence with other diseases, such as diffuse idiopathic skeletal hyperostosis, suggests that they may at times be a manifestation of a systemic disorder. OPLL is frequently associated with cervical spondylosis. It is much more commonly observed in patients from Japan and in other Asian peoples than in individuals of European descent. The cervical spine is the most common site of involvement, although the disease can occur at all levels of the spine and several vertebral levels are often ultimately involved. The ossification frequently affects the dura as well. The ossified ligament is easily detected by computerized resonance imaging techniques. The clinical manifestation consequent to spinal cord compression and the treatment options are comparable to those in the cervical myelopathy associated with cervical spondylosis.

TRAUMA

General remarks, epidemiology and clinical manifestations of spinal cord trauma

Spinal cord injury (SCI) occurs with an incidence of 15–40 cases per million population per year in most countries; approximately 85% of cases are males. The causes of SCI vary among countries. In most industrialized nations up to 50% are due to motor vehicle and traffic mishaps involving principally drivers, pedestrians and bicyclists; 20% are sports related or incurred during recreational activities (e.g. diving, motor sports, team sports); other cases are due to falls occurring at work and 15% at home, especially in the elderly.[317] In some urban regions there is an alarmingly high incidence of SCI resulting from violence involving shooting, stabbing or suicide attempts.

The overall mortality rate for all SCI is probably as high as 50%; it is approximately 15% for those patients who are able to reach the hospital alive.[317] The dramatic difference in the mortality rate between these two groups is due to the implementation of first-aid resuscitation, the pharmacological control of infection (mainly affecting the respiratory and urinary tracts), and measures designed to prevent the development of leg thrombophlebitis and pulmonary embolism.

The clinical manifestations, prognosis and seriousness of the injuries depend largely on the age of the patient, the presence of associated injuries, the degree of neurological deficit (completeness of the injury), the level of the injury along the vertebral column, and the extent of the lesion in the anteroposterior and rostrocaudal planes. Approximately 60% of injuries occur in the cervical region, and approximately 60% are incomplete injuries with some preservation of sensory and/or motor function below the level of the injury.[314] A complete injury occurs when there is major damage to the entire cross section of the spinal cord which causes loss of function in all ascending and descending tracts and the grey matter. The rostrocaudal extent of the lesion is variable and may extend from a few millimetres to several centimetres. Indeed, the American Spinal Injury Association (ASIA)/ IMSOP[12] classification of spinal cord injuries recognizes the tendency for complete (ASIA A) lesions to have a considerable rostrocaudal dimension. In some of these individuals partial neurological function may be preserved in the region of injury when there is some sparing of spinal cord tissue; this spared region is termed the zone of partial preservation. The injured zone is often fusiform or spindle-shaped rostrocaudally and tends to affect the central grey matter and the adjacent white matter, especially the white matter commissures and the adjacent ventral aspect of the dorsal columns. In more severe injuries, this fusiform zone of damaged cord consists of haemorrhagic necrosis which ultimately may become cavitated.

Several syndromes of incomplete neurological deficit are recognized. These are classified as ASIA grades B, C or D: in ASIA B there is always some preservation of sensory function in the lowest sacral dermatomes, S4 and S5; and in addition in ASIA C or D there is some distal motor function. These syndromes are found in patients with spinal cord lesions which involve the cervicomedullary junction, the central region of the cord, the anterior cord, the posterior cord, half of the cord (Brown–Séquard lesion) and the conus medullaris. Complete and incomplete cauda equina clinicopathological syndromes are also recognized.[316]

In general, the incomplete syndromes are classified according to the presumed location and extent of the injury in the transverse plane of the spinal cord, which can often be related to the mechanism of injury. In the anterior cord syndrome, the anterior aspect of the spine is damaged, usually from a ruptured disc or burst fracture, in which case there may be preservation of the dorsal columns with preserved touch, position and vibration sense, but loss of all motor function and pain and temperature sensation. Patients with the central cord syndrome develop a distinctive set of clinical manifestations consisting of a motor deficit with weakness greater in the upper than the lower extremities; this syndrome is associated with damage to the central portions of the spinal cord and extends to the corticospinal tracts. The very rare posterior cord syndrome involves injury to the posterior aspect of the spinal cord. It occurs with trauma from bone fragments from a fractured lamina. Clinical manifestations of the posterior cord syndrome include retained spinothalamic function but loss of movement and proprioception due to damage to the lateral and posterior columns, respectively. The Brown–Séquard syndrome occurs in association with penetrating and non-penetrating injuries of the cord which result in damage to one lateral half of the spinal cord. It is characterized by loss of ipsilateral motor and proprioceptive function and contralateral pain and temperature sensation. The cervicomedullary syndrome, also known as Bell's cruciate

paralysis, is caused by injuries which damage the spinal cord just below the level of the foramen magnum, such as occur from C1–C2 dislocations. The clinical expression of this syndrome consists of a motor deficit similar to that observed in the central cord syndrome, that is, manifesting greater upper than lower extremity weakness. The conus medullaris syndrome occurs in patients who have suffered spinal injuries from T11–T12 to L1–L2 and is characterized by a combination of upper and lower motor neuron deficits due to damage to the long tracts and the grey matter in the conus. The prognosis for recovery in the conus medullaris syndrome is not as good as that observed in the cauda equina syndromes in which the nerve roots of the cauda equina are injured at the L2 spinal level, or below.

There are also several reversible or transient spinal cord injury syndromes, such as spinal cord concussion wherein the patient shows complete recovery of neurological function usually within minutes and always within hours. The pathophysiological basis for the clinical manifestations of spinal cord concussion is unknown, but leakage of potassium from the intracellular to the extracellular space may be an important contributing factor.

Pathophysiology of experimental and human acute spinal cord injury

Spinal cord damage in man occurs in a variety of circumstances involving diverse forms of injury including compression, contusion, stretch and laceration. Our knowledge of the pathophysiology of human injuries[145,342] has been enhanced by a number of experimental animal models which attempt to simulate the conditions of injury that occur in man. Several of the different experimental models of SCI show quite comparable pathological findings, which in turn are similar to those observed in man. Many of the pathophysiological mechanisms believed to be operative in SCI are also believed to play a role in brain injury, cerebral ischaemia and subarachnoid haemorrhage.

PRIMARY INJURY MECHANISMS

After experimental or clinical SCI, the pathological appearance of the lesion changes dramatically over the course of the first few days. This evolving process is believed to be based on a number of factors which are conceptually subdivided into primary and secondary mechanisms of injury. In man, the most common primary injury mechanism is a combination of rapid impact plus persisting compression of the cord which occurs in burst fractures, fracture–dislocations, missile injuries and ruptured discs. Impact alone, without persisting compression, occurs in hyperextension of the spine in cervical spondylosis in which the cord is momentarily compressed between an anterior bulging disc or osteocartilaginous bar and a posterior infolded ligamentum flavum. Hyperflexion is a common mechanism of injury throughout the spine which can lead to unilateral or bilateral facet dislocation or reversal in the cervical or thoracolumbar region or to fracture–dislocation in any region. Axial loading is also a common mechanism of injury in which the forces are transmitted in an axial direction through the spine, such as when a helmeted hockey player strikes the boards head first, following which the vertebral body sustains a burst fracture: the spinal cord is crushed by fragments of the telescoped vertebral body which protrude posteriorly into the spinal canal to crush the spinal cord, after which there is usually persisting compression. Excessive stretching of the spinal column and spinal cord can occur during hyperflexion, especially in children with lax ligaments and undeveloped paraspinal musculature, and can produce the syndrome of spinal cord injury without radiological abnormality (SCIWORA).[253] More common in adults, especially in patients with cervical spondylosis, is the syndrome of spinal cord injury without radiological evidence of trauma (SCIWORET).[279,316] Laceration of the cord, with or without dural laceration, can occur from sharp bone fragments or severe stretching. Missile injuries can produce a combination of laceration, compression and concussion.[145] Cord lacerations can occur to varying degrees up to total transection.

Experimental models can simulate most of these mechanisms of human cord injury.[99,313] The most frequently used model has been the weight-drop model introduced by Allen,[10,11] which causes impact alone without significant persisting compression since the weight is usually removed quickly. Other models, such as the acute extradural clip compression technique,[269] cause acute impact plus persisting compression.

SECONDARY INJURY MECHANISMS

The concept of the secondary mechanisms of injury was first postulated by Allen[10,11] when he found that myelotomy and removal of post-traumatic haematomyelia in the central portion of the injured canine cord resulted in improvement of neurological function after weight-drop injury. He theorized that there was a noxious agent present in the haemorrhagic necrotic material which caused further damage to the cord. This autodestructive process has been reviewed elsewhere[121,318] and only a brief description is provided here.

Vascular damage: systemic and local

SCI can cause neurogenic shock, especially with complete cervical injury in which the bradycardia and hypotension may be profound initially, and then prolonged for days to months. It is due to a combination of decreased sympathetic tone, unopposed cardiac vagotonia and possible secondary changes in the heart.[121,184] The hypotension may contribute to the vascular injury of the cord.

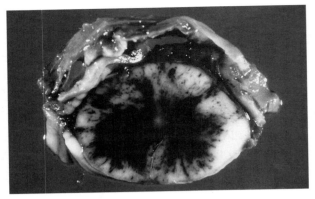

Figure 18.14 *Human spinal cord injury: cervical cord. The patient died on the day of injury. The ventral dura was removed at autopsy. Almost the entire grey matter is haemorrhagic, including the dorsal and ventral horns. The haemorrhages have also extended into the white matter.*[315]

One of the main features of the pathology of SCI common to all experimental models and cord injury in man is the early onset and subsequent spread of haemorrhages beginning in the central region of the injured cord, especially in the grey matter (Figs 18.14, 18.15). These haemorrhages are due to mechanical disruption of capillaries, venules and some arterioles by the primary mechanisms of injury.[86] In severe experimental injury, the haemorrhages may be progressive and continue for up to 2 h. The large blood vessels of the cord, such as the anterior spinal artery and the anterior sulcal arteries, usually remain patent, as shown by angiographic studies in man and microangiographic studies experimentally.[188–190,313,319] However, there is a major loss of the microcirculation due to damage to the capillaries and venules, not only at the injury site, but also spreading for a considerable distance rostrally and caudally (Fig. 18.16). Post-traumatic ischaemia worsens over time, as demonstrated by serial measurements of spinal cord blood flow in a variety of injury models in various species.[313,318] The haemorrhagic and ischaemic zones are in similar locations, possibly owing to an injurious 'biochemical irritation' unleashed from the haemorrhagic necrotic zone, as suggested by Allen.[10] Vasospasm of sulcal arteries was demonstrated in experimental SCI in the laboratory both by scanning[188,189] and by transmission electron microscopy,[18] and may be initiated by the mechanical injury or by one or more vasoconstrictor substances released at the injury site, such as catecholamines, glutamate and prostaglandins.[313,318] Intravascular thrombosis, which may contribute to post-traumatic ischaemia, has been observed with the light[247] and electron microscope[18] after experimental and human SCI.

Biochemical and electrolyte changes

Trauma causes an early intracellular accumulation of sodium, producing cytotoxic oedema and a concomitant

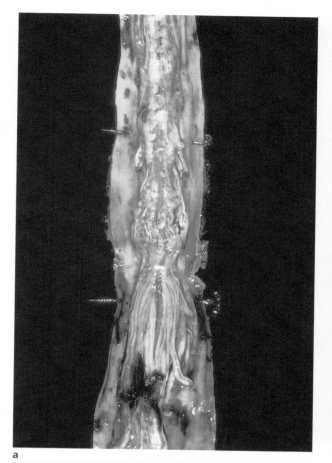

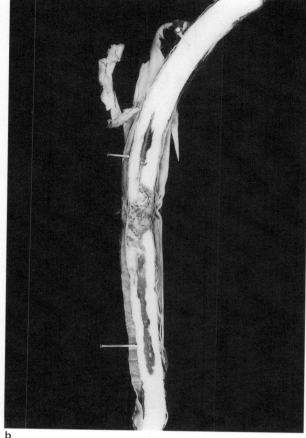

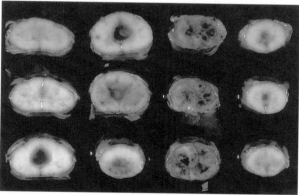

Figure 18.15 *Traumatic spinal cord injury. (**a**) Posterior view of the spinal cord in a case of fracture–dislocation at the junction of T12 and L1 with crushing of the lumbar cord. Haemorrhage can be seen around some roots of the cauda equina. (**b**) Longitudinal section of the spinal cord showing the site of direct cord trauma and rostral and caudal haemorrhagic extension. (**c**) Twelve transverse sections through the cervical and thoracic cord. The three blocks in the third row from the left show almost complete haemorrhagic necrosis. Haemorrhages can be seen in the grey matter in the other blocks above and below for several centimetres. (**a**) and (**c**) courtesy of RD Adams, Massachusetts General Hospital, Boston, MA, USA.[8]*

elevation of intracellular calcium.[306,353] Raised levels of intracellular calcium can, in turn, activate calcium-dependent proteases such as protein kinase C or lipases such as phospholipase C that cause further damage owing to breakdown of cytoskeletal components, including neurofilaments and microtubules, and dissolution of cell membranes. Intracellular influx of calcium has been termed the 'final common pathway of toxic cell death' in the nervous system.[72,281] After trauma, calcium can shift into neurons in a variety of ways, including through disrupted cell membranes, by depolarization and entry through voltage-sensitive calcium channels, or through receptor-mediated calcium channels activated by the excitatory amino acid neurotransmitter glutamate.[96,254] Ischaemia can also increase intracellular calcium through glutamate release. The successful use of steroids in human SCI[50] is strong evidence of the importance of secondary mechanisms of injury, especially those related to lipid peroxidation and the production of oxygen-free radicals. The excess production of arachidonic acid and eicosanoids such as prostaglandins may be related to lipid peroxidation and oxygen-free radicals and may, in turn, cause tissue damage by inducing vasospasm and post-traumatic ischaemia.

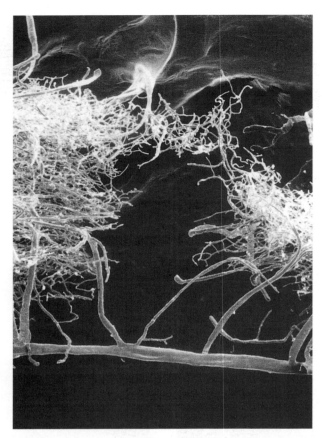

Figure 18.16 *Experimental spinal cord injury. Parasagittal view of the rat spinal cord 15 min after acute clip compression as demonstrated by the vascular corrosion cast technique and scanning electron microscopy. The ventral aspect of the spinal cord is towards the bottom and shows the patent anterior spinal artery. The anterior sulcal arteries extend obliquely upwards from the anterior spinal artery, and are displaced away from the site of injury and narrowed. The site of injury is the large avascular zone in the centre in which the microcirculation is no longer patent.[315]*

Oedema

Significant and progressive oedema can follow SCI[335] but it is not known whether the oedema is injurious in itself or whether it is an epiphenomenon of another injury mechanism such as ischaemia or glutamate toxicity. For example, as noted above, the latter causes sodium to enter neurons with resulting cytotoxic oedema. Oedema can spread in the cord from the site of injury for a considerable distance rostrally and caudally in both experimental models and clinical cases.[145,342]

Conduction block in spinal cord injury

In the acute phase of SCI axonal conduction block may be due to biochemical changes, especially electrolyte shifts. For example, as noted above, increased extracellular potassium may cause excessive depolarization and account for

spinal neurogenic shock[92] and spinal cord concussion. More severe mechanical axonal injuries with membrane disruption cause persisting failure of conduction. The demonstration in man that conduction can be restored in some clinically complete injuries by the potassium channel antagonist 4-aminopyridine emphasizes the role of increased extracellular potassium on the demyelinated axons present in the chronic phase of cord injury.[35]

PATHOLOGY OF SPINAL CORD INJURY

Our knowledge of the pathological features of acute SCI is based on a relatively small number of clinical studies supplemented by a much larger number of experimental studies.

Central zone of injury

As noted above, the central region of the cord at the injury site comprising the grey matter and the immediately adjacent white matter is more severely affected than the more peripheral white matter, especially in acute compression injuries such as those due to burst fracture or fracture–dislocation (Figs 18.14, 18.15). Hypothetical reasons for the propensity of this lesion to centre on the grey matter include the softer consistency of the grey matter relative to other structures of the cord and its greater vascularity.[342] In the early stage of severe injury, numerous petechial haemorrhages due to diapedesis from small blood vessels are seen, together with a coalescence of these haemorrhages into larger pools of blood, especially in the grey matter. The bleeding is usually from capillaries, venules and arterioles, and almost never from arteries such as the anterior spinal artery, and can continue at the injury site for about 2 h.[314] Central haematomyelia, defined as a large space-occupying haemorrhage with distension of the cord, is very rare.[145,172,342] Remote haemorrhages occur at considerable distances rostral and caudal to the injury site, especially at the base of the dorsal columns at the junction of the dorsal white commissure and grey matter.[145,342] These types of haemorrhage have been shown in experimental studies to be venous in origin.[190]

There is worsening of the pathological changes over time.[89,342] At 12–24 h, structures in the central region of the cord begin to lose their definition and appear as central haemorrhagic necrosis with the haemorrhagic zones becoming more confluent. The definition of grey and white matter becomes blurred (Fig. 18.17) and, as noted above, progressive ischaemia can lead to post-traumatic infarction. Indeed, many of the pathological features of non-traumatic arterial or venous infarction of the cord described above in this chapter resemble the features seen after trauma.

Subarachnoid haemorrhage is very common with contusions or lacerations, but subdural or extradural

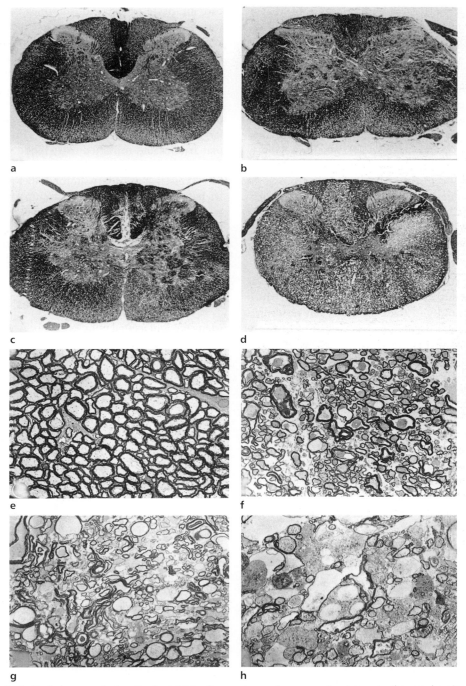

Figure 18.17 *Pathological changes during the first 24 h after acute cord compression injury in the rat showing the progression of changes. (**a, e**) Normal cord; (**b, f**) 15 min after injury; (**c, g**) 2 h after injury; (**d, h**) 24 h after injury: there is gradual worsening of the gross and microscopic changes. (**e–h**) are from the dorsolateral white matter and show progressive damage to the myelinated axons. There is a marked decline in the number of intact axons with increasing time. The myelin sheaths become very thin, and some giant axons appear at 24 h.[315]*

haematomas are very rare,[189,342] although the latter can occur in ankylosing spondylitis. During the first 24 h, there is gross swelling and softening of the spinal cord at the injury site which spreads rostrally and caudally for a considerable distance, depending on the severity of the injury.[145,338,342]

Degree of transection

It has been generally accepted that even after severe clinically complete injury a portion of the spinal cord at the injury site usually remains in continuity.[172] Bunge *et al.*[59] examined at post-mortem 22 cases of human SCI and found that in only 62% was there evidence of 'central neural tissue continuity through the epicentre of the lesion'. They excluded from statistical analysis cases where only non-central nervous tissue such as nerve roots or meninges remained in continuity. In patients with clinically complete injuries only 50% showed 'some parenchymal continuity across the epicentre of the lesion', including 'nerve fibres transversing the lesion site.' Thus, the incidence of neural continuity in clinically complete cases was found to be lower than previously thought. These findings also provide some pathological confirmation of the 'discomplete' injury, a term used to describe those clinically complete cases in whom sensory- or motor-evoked potentials or other neurophysiological tests show signals traversing the injury site. Bunge's group[59] also classified the lesions in man into four pathological types:

- Contusion cyst, present in 23% of their cases, was believed to be due to moderate contusion forces which leave the continuity of the cord intact but result in a centrally located haematomyelia which evolves to become a stable cyst.
- Cord maceration due to massive compression, present in 32%, was characterized by severe destruction of most or all nervous tissue, breaching of the pia and subsequent connective tissue scarring. Surprisingly, in a minority of cases there was a 'fragment of remaining CNS parenchyma'.
- Cord laceration due to open injuries such as gunshot wounds, present in 27%, was characterized by torn cord parenchyma and ingrowth of dense scar tissue.
- Solid cord injury, in which the overall form of the cord was retained without central haematomyelia or cyst, was found in 18% of cases.

In the latter, the damage was largely confined to the white matter, especially the dorsal part of the lateral funiculi in the region of the corticospinal tract where there was diffuse axonal disruption, particularly of the large diameter axons. Surprisingly, the grey matter was not affected, and all four patients in this group had the central cord syndrome which previously was thought to involve primarily central haematomyelia with spreading oedema.[286]

Only those types 2 and 3 involving cord maceration or laceration, where the pia was breached, showed connective tissue scarring. Even in cases with extensive scarring, the role that scar tissue may play in preventing recovery by blocking axonal regeneration is poorly understood.[98]

The question of large blood vessel occlusion

Schneider[285] suggested that some SCIs, especially those with the anterior cervical cord syndrome, were due to thrombosis of, or impaired circulation in the territory irrigated by, the anterior spinal artery. His studies also raised the possibility that the lesion in some cases of thoracic cord injuries, especially those in which the T4 border zone was affected, may have been due to a remote event which caused traumatic or compressive interruption of a major artery supplying the spinal cord, a radicular artery or the anterior spinal artery.[286] However, Wolman's series of 95 fatal spinal cord injuries contained only three cases with demonstrable thrombosis of the anterior spinal artery in the thoracic cord, none of which showed thrombosis of large vessels in the cervical cord.[342] Thrombosis of small pial arteries and intramedullary blood vessels was often present in these cases. Holmes[145] observed thrombosis of blood vessels at the injury site, but other more recent studies have found no evidence of trauma-related occlusion of the major arteries supplying the spinal cord.[49,163] Experimental studies have supported the latter findings. Indeed, even after extremely severe cord injury in the rat, the anterior spinal artery always remained patent[188–190] (Fig. 18.16).

Axonal and myelin sheath injuries

Many types of axonal injuries have been described in clinical and experimental studies of acute SCI. The electron-microscopic studies by Dohrmann et al.[87] Bresnahan,[54] Balentine[25] and Anthes et al.[17,18] have shown significant axonal changes within 15 min of injury which then progress markedly during the next 24 h (Figs 18.17, 18.18). The axonal changes include axonal transection, rupture of the axolemma with spillage of organelles into the extracellular space, granular degeneration of the axoplasm, axonal swelling including the development of giant axons, and excess accumulation of organelles such as mitochondria within the axoplasm around a neurofilamentous core. Changes in the myelin sheaths also progress rapidly during the first few hours and include rupture of the myelin sheaths, separation of the myelin from the axons with the development of large periaxonal spaces and vesicular myelin[17] (Figs 18.17, 18.18). Some of these early axonal and myelin changes have also been observed at the light-microscopic level in man.[145,342]

The relationship between the remaining number of axons in the spinal cord and persisting neurological function after injury has been examined in both experimental[100] and clinical studies.[170] It appears that only 5–10% of axons remaining in the corticospinal tract are necessary for voluntary motor function of grade 2–3 (movement against gravity).

Inflammatory and glial responses

There is an intense initial acute inflammatory response during the first 3 days after SCI which then gives way to intense microglial activation. The inflammatory response includes large numbers of macrophages of both local and systemic origin with phagocytic properties which peak at 3–7 days,[246,261,285] and T-cells are present at these times. There is also a major accumulation of macrophages and other inflammatory cells at considerable rostrocaudal dis-

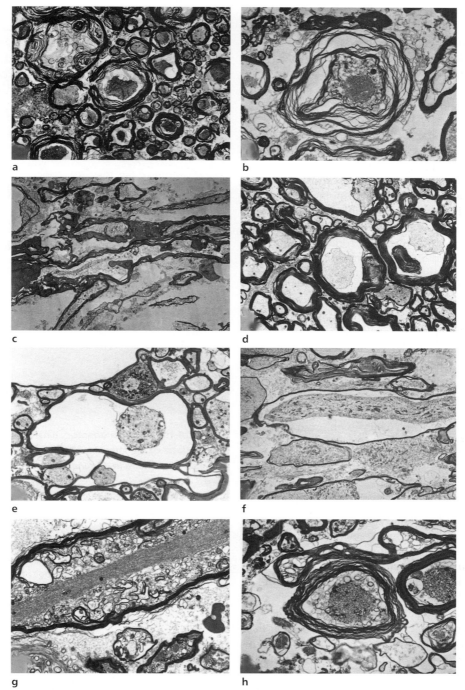

Figure 18.18 *Experimental spinal cord injury: pathological changes in the axons after acute clip compression injury in the rat. (a) Rupture of the myelin sheaths around two axons in the centre. (b) Vesicular myelin change with separation of the myelin lamellae. (c, d) Examples of myelin invagination within the periaxonal space in a longitudinal section (c) and a transverse section (d). (d, f) Marked enlargement of the periaxonal space between the axon and myelin sheath. (g, h) Central accumulation of axoplasmic organelles around a neurofilamentous core.*[315]

tances from the injury site in both grey and white matter. Reactive astrocytes are present in the first few days, and then become more prominent during the first 4 weeks, especially rostral and caudal to the injury site. The glial scar also contains oligodendrocytes. Trauma induces the proliferation and migration of a population of cells considered to be oligodendrocyte precursors which express two surface antigens, the NG2 proteoglycan and the alpha-receptor for platelet-derived growth factor (PDGF aR). These NG2/PDGF aR-positive cells show an early response to trauma and peak at about 7 days, but remain in the region for several weeks.[98]

Apoptosis

Apoptosis, a form of programmed cell death, occurs in SCI and is distinguished from necrotic cell death on the basis of morphological and biochemical criteria. Apoptosis is characterized by cell shrinkage, chromatin aggregation with genomic fragmentation and nuclear pyknosis. Apoptosis has been seen in both human and experimental spinal cord injury,[94] and especially affects oligodendrocytes adjacent to the site of injury and also rostrocaudally in the white matter in association with wallerian degeneration. It may also involve neurons adjacent to the injury site in the early stages, and microglial cells. Apoptotic cells can be identified within a few hours of injury, and continue to be seen for weeks to months. Apoptosis is considered to be an additional mechanism of secondary injury, and the delayed and continuing development of apoptosis following SCI has prompted at least one successful therapeutic trial which reduced its occurrence and enhanced recovery.[208]

Subacute and chronic phases

Within days of the acute injury, a large number of reparative, degenerative and regenerative processes begins to occur at the injury site as well as rostrally and caudally, and then continues for months or years in severe cases. As the polymorphonuclear leukocytes diminish in number, there follows a marked increase in macrophages derived from resident microglial cells and from the circulating blood. The macrophages phagocytose debris, especially myelin and red blood cells. The role of these inflammatory changes is of current major interest since macrophages secrete cytokines such as interleukin-1 and other agents which may stimulate angiogenesis.[36] There is also evidence that inflammation and macrophages may play a role in causing secondary injury.[34]

In severe injuries, small and large cavities develop within the spinal cord at the injury site (Fig. 18.19) which may communicate with the ependymal-lined central canal. In up to 20% of cord injuries,[90,300] the small cavities at the injury site coalesce to form a larger cavity which can increase in size and extend for a considerable distance rostrally and caudally, producing the syndrome of post-traumatic syringomyelia (Fig. 18.20). In some animal models there is a 30% incidence in cavitation of the cord which extends above or below the level of the post-traumatic lesion.[336] The tissue surrounding the spinal cord cavities in these animal experiments shows gliosis; the cavities are often multiloculated and separated from each other by septae of gliovascular tissue. The mechanism whereby the post-traumatic cavity gradually extends into previously uninvolved spinal cord tissue is uncertain, although arachnoiditis and blockage of the subarachnoid space may be contributing factors. Another recognized form of post-traumatic degeneration of the central portions of the spinal cord, occurring in the absence of

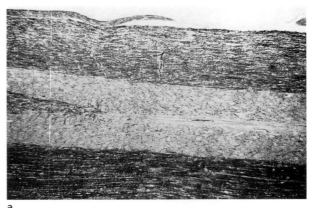

a

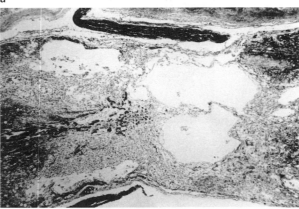

b

Figure 18.19 *Normal rat thoracic spinal cord. (**a**) Normal white matter tracts of the lateral columns above and below and the grey matter centrally. (**b**) Coronal section of a rat thoracic spinal cord 8 weeks after clip compression injury, showing marked cavitation at the injury site with major necrosis and demyelination. In this rat there was ascending post-traumatic syringomyelia which extended for several segments above the injury site. There was also extensive arachnoiditis and ependymal cell proliferation centrally (seen in the centre of the section as small islands of darkly staining cells). The nerve root at the top of the section survived the injury reasonably well in comparison with the cord, although both the root and the cord were compressed by the clip.[315] (Luxol fast blue/H&E.)*

syringomyelia, is microcystic myelomalacia[300] or 'marshy cord syndrome'.[213] Arachnoiditis has been associated with this condition.

In clinical and experimental studies of severe SCI, any persisting axons at the injury site are almost always located subpially (Fig. 18.21). This subpial rim of axons may extend around the entire perimeter of the cord or may localized to one side only.[33] These axons are often demyelinated or have thinner myelin sheaths than normal axons, and also show a shift towards a smaller calibre compared with uninjured axons. Possible explanations for the persisting subpial rim include continuing perfusion from the centripetal pial plexus, and altered glutamate metabolism in subpial astrocytes which protects axons.

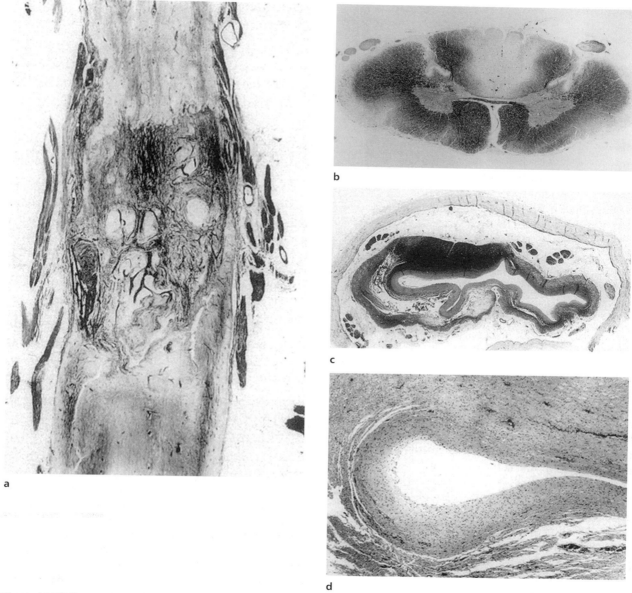

Figure 18.20 *Traumatic spinal cord injury and post-traumatic syringomyelia. (a) Spinal cord 16 years after injury: longitudinal histological section through the post-traumatic scar. The injured spinal cord segments are telescoped and three occupy the space of one. The centre of the scar is connective tissue which is invaded by regenerating fibres from the posterior roots.*[151] *(b) Cervical spinal cord above a complete transverse traumatic lesion incurred many years previously, showing ascending degeneration in the posterior columns and spinocerebellar and spinothalamic tracts. (c) Transverse section at T2 segmental level from a case in which cavitation ascended from an injury centred on T11 spinal cord segment. (Myelin.) (d) Detail of part of the syrinx. Note the thick astrocytic glial lining of the cavity. (Haematoxylin–van Gieson.)*

Sharply circumscribed areas of necrosis with the appearance of infarcts are frequent in the chronic stage. These necrotic foci may occur at a considerable distance from the injury site, and have been identified in both experimental[277] and clinical material.[145,342] Some of these lesions conform to the distribution of anterior sulcal arteries,[188–190] while others do not conform to arterial zones and may be venous in origin. The exact pathophysiology of these lesions is unknown. They are clinically important because they help to explain clinical deficits from lesions remote from the principal site of injury.

Intramedullary scarring occurs to a variable extent, even in major injuries. As noted above, extensive scarring with collagen in the cord, or bridging to the arachnoid and dura, frequently occurs as a sequela to lacerations of the dura. In the absence of a dural laceration, intramedullary collagenous scarring is usually minimal. Similarly, the degree of astrocytic scarring or gliosis is variable, and often is minimal.[60]

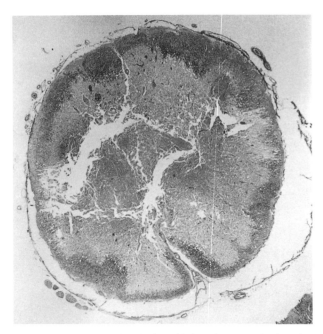

Figure 18.21 *Traumatic spinal cord injury: human spinal cord at C1–C2 18 days after injury. The central portion of the cord is entirely necrotic but there is a preserved peripheral rim of myelinated axons. The anterior spinal artery at the ventral aspect of the anterior median sulcus is patent. (Luxol fast blue/H&E.)*

Wallerian degeneration involving axonal degeneration and demyelination can be detected in the afferent tracts such as the dorsal columns and spinothalamic tracts rostral to the lesion, and in the efferent tracts such as the lateral corticospinal tract caudal to the lesion. As a result, the spinal cord in the chronic stage is atrophic not only at the injury site, but also rostrally and caudally.

A range of regenerative changes can also be seen in the chronic stage. The most marked change is ingrowth of

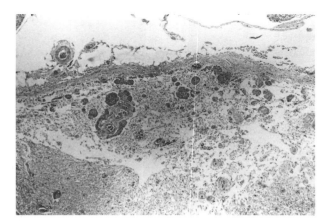

Figure 18.22 *Traumatic spinal cord injury. The dorsal columns of the human spinal cord near the injury site at C1–C2 9 months after an acute spinal cord injury show infiltration of the necrotic white matter by proliferating Schwann cells forming small neuromatous knots. There is also severe arachnoiditis surrounding the cord with virtually complete obliteration of the subarachnoid space.[315]*

Schwann cells and associated peripheral axons and peripheral myelin from both the dorsal and ventral roots (Fig. 18.22). The proliferation of Schwann cells may be extensive, giving the appearance of an intramedullary neuroma.[154] There may also be a proliferation of small blood vessels,[36] and ependymal cells proliferate, especially during the first 7–14 days after trauma, and then migrate for a considerable distance from the central canal.[246,315]

Chronic adhesive spinal arachnoiditis

A chronic inflammatory response of the spinal arachnoid and pial membranes may be aetiologically related to trauma, persistent infection, repeated surgical procedures on the spine or the introduction of a toxic substance into the subarachnoid space for diagnostic, anaesthetic or therapeutic purposes. Most often the cause of the chronic meningitis is unknown. A typical clinical picture in many patients is that of an intermittently progressive or persistent pain syndrome developing in the lower back and legs after multiple myelograms or surgical procedures for intervertebral disc rupture.[214,291] At surgery or autopsy, the exposed cord and roots are encircled by tenacious leptomeningeal fibrous tissue, usually containing loculated

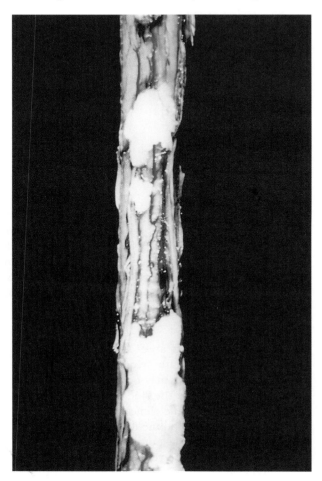

Figure 18.23 *Eggshell plaques.*

cysts, and so tightly adherent as to be impossible to dissect off the underlying structures. In some studies the spinal cord has been found to be damaged by cleft-like ('syringomyelic') spaces.[192,209,214] In a series of cases of arachnoiditis believed to be related to a contaminant in solutions used for spinal anaesthesia, the walls of subarachnoid arteries and veins were found to be thickened and their lumen was narrowed; these changes were thought to be the cause of nearby infarcts of the lower cord.[116]

Mention should be made of calcified and ossified plaques of the arachnoid membrane ('eggshell' plaques). These are flat, plate-like deposits on the outer surface of the arachnoid overlying the dorsal aspect of the cord; they are visible radiologically, at surgery or at autopsy[137,260,296] (Fig. 18.23). When looked for, they are present in as many as three-quarters of autopsy cases, according to some studies. Microscopically, they consist of a thin, calcified or ossified layer abutting the cap-cell layer of the arachnoid. They are generally believed to be age related, but there is really no satisfactory explanation for their occurrence. In general, they are of no clinical significance, but one study identified a particularly aggressive form, termed arachnoiditis ossificans, which gave rise to a myelopathy.[175]

Additional diseases of the spinal cord discussed elsewhere

A. Developmental abnormalities (Chapter 7, this Volume):
  1. dysraphic states (spina bifida, meningomyelocele, etc.)
  2. syringomyelia, hydromyelia
  3. diastematomyelia
  4. diplomyelia
  5. neurenteric canal cyst.
B. Infectious diseases (Chapter 3, Volume II):
  1. bacterial infections:
     (a) pyogenic infections: meningitis; epidural and intramedullary abscess
     (b) tuberculosis
     (c) neurosyphilis
     (d) neuroborreliosis (Lyme disease)
  2. viral infections (Chapter 1, Volume II):
     (a) poliomyelitis
     (b) herpes zoster
     (c) HIV (AIDS and related conditions)
     (d) HTILV-1 (tropical spastic paraparesis)
     (e) rabies
     (f) cytomegalovirus
  3. fungal and parasitic infections (Chapter 2, Volume II).
C. Demyelinating diseases (Chapter 8, Volume II):
  1. multiple sclerosis
  2. acute disseminated (postinfectious) encephalomyelitis
  3. acute necrotizing myelitis.

D. Degenerative diseases (Chapter 6, Volume II):
  1. motor neuron disease:
     (a) spinal muscular atrophies
     (b) amyotrophic lateral sclerosis
     (c) primary lateral sclerosis
  2. Friedreich's ataxia
  3. familial spastic paraparesis.
E. Metabolic diseases (Chapters 10, 11, 12, this Volume):
  1. inborn errors of metabolism
  2. acquired metabolic diseases.
F. Intoxications (Chapter 13, this Volume):
G. Tumours (Chapter 11, Volume II):
  1. intramedullary tumours:
     (a) astrocytoma
     (b) ependymoma
  2. filum terminal tumours:
     (a) myxopapillary ependymoma
  3. nerve sheath tumours:
     (a) schwannoma
     (b) neurofibroma
     (c) neurothekeoma
  4. metastatic lesions
  5. leukaemia/lymphoma.

Acknowledgements

The authors wish to express their gratitude to Dr JG Greenfield, JT Hughes and EP Richardson Jr, who contributed text and illustrations for this chapter in previous editions of this book.

REFERENCES

1 Abe M, Komori H, Yamaura I, Kayano T. Spinal cord herniation into an extensive extradural meningeal cyst: postoperative analysis of intracystic flow by phase-contrast cine MRI. *J Orthoped Sci* 1999; **4**: 450–6.
2 Adamkiewicz A. Die Blutgefässe des menschlichen Rückenmarkes. I. Die Gefässe der Rückenmarkssubstanz. *Sitzungberichte der Kaiserlichen Akademie der Wissenschaften in Wien* 1881; **84**: 469–502.
3 Adamkiewicz A. Die Blutgefässe des menschlichen Rückenmarkes. II. Die Gefässe der Rückenmarksoberfläche. *Sitzungberichte der Kaiserlichen Akademie der Wissenschaften in Wien* 1882; **85**: 101–30.
4 Adamkiewicz A. Die Kreislaufsstörungen in den Organen des Centralnervensystems. Berlin: Köllner, 1899.
5 Adams C. Cervical spondylotic radiculopathy and myelopathy. In: Vinken P, Bruyn G eds. *Handbook of clinical neurology* Vol. 26. Amsterdam: Elsevier, 1976: 97–112.
6 Adams HD, van Geertruyden HH. Neurologic complications of aortic surgery. *Ann Surg* 1956; **144**: 574–609.
7 Adams RD, Merritt AH. Meningeal and vascular syphilis of the spinal cord. *Medicine* 1944; **23**: 181–214.
8 Adams RD, Sidman RL. *Introduction to neuropathology*. New York: McGraw-Hill, 1948.
9 Alexandrov SV, Morgunov VA, Adarcheva LS. Angiodisgenetick nekrotick mielopathia (syndrom Foix–Alajouanine). *Arkh Patol* 1991; **53**: 55–9.

10 Allen AR. Remarks on the histopathological changes in the spinal cord due to impact. An experimental study. *J Nerv Ment Dis* 1914; **41**: 141–7.

11 Allen AR. Surgery of experimental lesions of the spinal cord equivalent to crush injury of fracture dislocation of the spinal column. A preliminary report. *JAMA* 1919; **57**: 878–80.

12 American Spinal Injury Association. *Standards for neurological and functional classification of spinal cord injury.* Chicago, IL: American Spinal Injury Association, 1992.

13 Aminoff MJ, Barnard RO, Logue V. The pathophysiology of spinal vascular malformations. *J Neurol Sci* 1974; **23**: 255–63.

14 Anderson NE, Willoughby EW. Infarction of the conus medullaris. *Ann Neurol* 1987; **21**: 470–4.

15 Andersson G. What are the age-related changes in the spine? *Ballieres Clin Rheumatol* 1998; **12**: 161–73.

16 Annunen S, Paassilta P, Lohiniva J et al. An allele of COL9A2 associated with intervertebral disc disease. *Science* 1999; **285**: 409–12.

17 Anthes DL, Theriault E, Tator CH. Characterization of axonal ultrastructural pathology following experimental spinal cord compression injury. *Brain Res* 1995; **702**: 1–16.

18 Anthes DL, Theriault E, Tator CH. Ultrastructural evidence for arteriolar vasospasm after spinal cord trauma. *Neurosurgery* 1996; **39**: 804–14.

19 Antoni N. Spinal vascular malformations (angiomas) and myelomalacia. *Neurology* 1962; **12**: 795–804.

20 Antoni N, Lindgren E. Steno's experiment in man as a complication of lumbar aortography. *Acta Chir Scand* 1949; **98**: 230–47.

21 Azzarelli B, Roessmann V. Diffuse 'anoxic' myelopathy. *Neurology* 1977; **27**: 1049–52.

22 Babini SM, Maldonado Cocco JA, Babini JC et al. Atlantoaxial subluxation in systemic lupus erythematosus: further evidence of tendinous alterations. *J Rheumatol* 1990; **17**: 173–7.

23 Badejo L, Sangalang VE. Vascular malformations of the spinal cord (angiodysgenetic myelomalacia): a critique on its pathogenesis. *Surgl Neurol* 1979; **11**: 101–6.

24 Baker AS, Ojemann RG, Swartz MN, Richardson EP Jr. Spinal epidural abscess. *N Engl J Med* 1975; **283**: 463–8.

25 Balentine JD. Pathology of experimental spinal cord trauma. II. Ultrastructure of axons and myelin. *Lab Invest* 1978; **39**: 254–66.

26 Banerjee AK, Deodhar SD. Embolism of spinal cord (Letter). *J Neurol Neurosurg Psychiatry* 1989; **52**: 1021–2.

27 Bartsch W, Hopf HC. Neue Beobachtungen über die Beziehungen zwischen Herzleistung und Rückenmarkskreislauf. *Dtsch Z Nerven* 1963; **184**: 288–307.

28 Barz H, Hackebeil C. Knorpelgewebsembolie als Ursache einer Myelomalazie. Kausuistik und Literaturübersicht. *Pathologe* 1989; **10**: 300–5.

29 Beattie EJ, Nolan J, Howe JS. Paralysis following surgical correction of coarctation of the aorta. *Surgery* 1953; **33**: 754–60.

30 Bedford PD, Bosanquet FD, Russell WR. Degeneration of the spinal cord associated with cervical spondylosis. *Lancet* 1952; **263**: 55–9.

31 Bednar DA, Esses SI, Kucharczyk W. Symptomatic lumbar epidural lipomatosis in a normal male. A unique case report. *Spine* 1990; **15**: 52–3.

32 Blau RH, Kaufman RL. Erosive and subluxing cervical spine disease in patients with psoriatic arthritis. *J Rheumatol* 1987; **14**: 111–17.

33 Blight AR. Cellular morphology of chronic spinal cord injury in the cat: analysis of myelinated axons by line-sampling. *Neuroscience* 1983; **10**: 521–43.

34 Blight AR. Delayed demyelination and macrophage invasion: a candidate for secondary cell damage in spinal cord injury. *Cent Nerv Syst Trauma* 1985; **2**: 299–315.

35 Blight AR. Effect of 4-aminopyridine on axonal conduction-block in chronic spinal cord injury. *Brain Res Bull* 1989; **22**: 47–52.

36 Blight AR. Remyelination, revascularization, and recovery of function in experimental spinal cord injury. *Adv Neurol* 1993; **59**: 91–104.

37 Blondeau M, Brunet D, Blanche JM et al. Compression de la moelle cervicale dans l'achondroplasie. *Semaine Hópitaux Paris* 1984; **60**: 771–5.

38 Blumbergs PC, Byrne E. Hypotensive central infarction of the spinal cord. *J Neurol Neurosurg Psychiatry* 1980; **43**: 751–3.

39 Bocknek WL, Bach JR, Alba AS, Cravioto HM. Fibrocartilaginous emboli to the spinal cord: a case report. *Arch Phys Med Rehabil* 1990; **71**: 754–7.

40 Bodechtel G. Über differentialdiagnostische Schwierigkeiten auf den Grenzgebieten der inneren Medizin zur Neurologie. *Münchner Med Wochenschr* 1968; **110**: 969–80.

41 Bodechtel G, Erbslöh F. Die Foix–Alajounaninesche Krankheit ('Myélite nécrotique subaigue' – Angiodysgenetische Myelomalacie). In: Lubarsch O, Henke F, Rössle R eds. *Handbuch der speziellen pathologischen Anatomie und Histologie* Vol. 13 (1A) Berlin: Springer, 1957: 1576–99.

42 Bonnemann CG, Cox GF, Shapiro F et al. A mutation in the alpha 3 chain of type IX collagen causes autosomal dominant multiple epiphyseal dysplasia with mild myopathy. *Proc Nat Acad Sci USA* 2000; **97**: 1212–17.

43 Borden JA, Wa JK, Shucart WA. A proposed classification for spinal and cranial dural arteriovenous fistulous malformations and implications for therapy. *J Neurosurg* 1995; **82**: 166–79.

44 Borges LF, Zervas NT, Lehrich JR. Idiopathic spinal cord herniation: a treatable cause of the Brown–Sequard syndrome – case report. *Neurosurgery* 1995; **36**: 1028–32; Discussion 1032–3.

45 Borstlap AC, van Rooij WJ, Sluzewski M et al. Reversibility of lumbar epidural lipomatosis in obese patients after weight-reduction diet. *Neuroradiology* 1995; **37**: 670–3.

46 Bostman OM. Body mass index and height in patients requiring surgery for lumbar intervertebral disc herniation. *Spine* 1993; **18**: 851–4.

47 Bots GTAM, Wattendorff AR, Buruma OJS et al. Acute myelopathy caused by fibrocartilaginous emboli. *Neurology* 1981; **31**: 1251–6.

48 Bowie EA, Glasgow GL. Cauda equina lesions associated with ankylosing spondylitis: report of three cases. *BMJ* 1961; **ii**: 24–7.

49 Braakman R, Penning L. Injuries of the cervical spine. In: Vinken PJ, Bruyn GW eds. *Handbook of clinical neurology* Vol. 25. Amsterdam: North-Holland, 1976: 227–380.

50 Bracken MB, Shepard MJ, Collins WF et al. A randomized, controlled trial of methylprednisolone or naloxone in the treatment of acute spinal cord injury. Results of the Second National Acute Spinal Cord Injury Study. *N Engl J Med* 1990; **322**: 1405–11.

51 Bradshaw P. Some aspects of cervical spondylosis. *Q J Med* 1957; **50**: 177–208.

52 Brain WR. Discussion on rupture of the intervertebral disc in the cervical region. *Proc R Soc Med* 1948; **41**: 509–16.

53 Brain WR, Northfield D, Wilkinson M. The neurological manifestations of cervical spondylosis. *Brain* 1952; **75**: 187–227.

54 Bresnahan JC. An electron-microscopic analysis of axonal alterations following blunt contusion of the spinal cord of

the rhesus monkey (*Macaca mulatta*). *J Neurol Sci* 1978; **37**: 59–82.

55 Brewer LA, Fosburg RG, Mulder GA, Verska JJ. Spinal cord complications following surgery for coarctation of the aorta. *J Thorac Cardiovasc Surg* 1972; **64**: 368–81.

56 Brion S, Netzky MG, Zimmerman HM. Vascular malformations of the spinal cord. *Arch Neurol Psychiatry* 1952; **68**: 339–61.

57 Brugieres P, Malapert D, Adle-Biassette H *et al.* Idiopathic spinal cord herniation: value of MR phase-contrast imaging. *Am J Neuroradiol* 1999; **20**: 935–9.

58 Budka H, Perneczky A, Pusch S. Bandscheibengewebsembolien in Spinalgefässen als Ursache von Myelomalazien vorwiegend in Spinalis-posterior-Versorgungsgebieten. *Wien Klin Wochenschr* 1979; **91**: 578–82.

59 Bunge RP, Puckett WR, Becerra JL *et al.* Observations on the pathology of human spinal cord injury: a review and classification of 22 new cases with details from a case of chronic cord compression with extensive focal demyelination. In: Seil FJ ed. *Advances in neurology.* New York: Raven, 1993: 75–89.

60 Bunge RP, Puckett WR, Hiester ED. Observations on the pathology of several types of human spinal cord injury, with emphasis on the astrocyte response to penetrating injuries. *Adv Neurol* 1997; **72**: 305–15.

61 Byrne TH, Waxman SG. *Spinal cord compression.* Philadelphia, PA: Davis, 1990.

62 Caccamo DV, Garcia JH, Ho K-L. Isolated granulomatous angiitis of the spinal cord. *Ann Neurol* 1992; **32**: 580–2.

63 Calin A. Is there an association between ankylosing spondylitis and multiple sclerosis? *Ann Rheum Dis* 1989; **48**: 971–2.

64 Case Records of Massachusetts General Hospital. Case 38012. *N Engl J Med* 1952; **246**: 30–4.

65 Case Records of the Massachusetts General Hospital. Case 44191. *N Engl J Med* 1958; **258**: 949–54.

66 Case Records of the Massachusetts General Hospital. Case 5-1991. *N Engl J Med* 1991; **324**: 322–32.

67 Castro-Moure F, Kupsky W, Goshgarian HG. Pathophysiological classification of human spinal cord ischemia. *J Spinal Cord Med* 1997; **20**: 74–87.

68 Chapman PH, Martuza RL, Poletti CE, Karchmer AW. Symptomatic spinal epidural lipomatosis associated with Cushing's syndrome. *Neurosurgery* 1981; **8**: 724–7.

69 Chase TN, Rosman NP, Price DL. The cerebral syndromes associated with dissecting aneurysm of the aorta. A clinicopathological study. *Brain* 1968; **91**: 173–90.

70 Chen J-R, Rhee RC, Wallach S *et al.* Neurologic disturbances in Paget disease of bone: response to calcitonin. *Neurology* 1979; **29**: 448–57.

71 Cheshire WP, Santos CC, Massey WW, Howard JF. Spinal cord infarction: etiology and outcome. *Neurology* 1996; **47**: 321–30.

72 Cheung JY, Bonventre JV, Malis CD *et al.* Calcium and ischemic injury. *N Engl J Med* 1986; **314**: 1670–6.

73 Clarke E, Robinson PK. Cervical myelopathy: a complication of cervical spondylosis. *Brain* 1956; **79**: 483–510.

74 Clinicopathologic Conference of the Beekman–Downtown Hospital New York City. Sudden onset of severe chest pain and paralysis. *N Y State J Med* 1969; **69**: 446–54.

75 Conlon PW, Isdale IC, Rose BS. Rheumatoid arthritis of the cervical spine: an analysis of 333 cases. *Ann Rheum Dis* 1966; **25**: 120–6.

76 Cotugno D. *De Ischiade Nervosa Commentarius.* Neapoli: Apud Fratres Simonios, 1764.

77 Cremer MA, Rosloniec EF, Kang AH. The cartilage collagens: a review of their structure, organization and role in the pathogenesis of experimental arthritis in animals and in human rheumatic disease. *J Mol Med* 1998; **76**: 275–88.

78 Criscuolo GR, Oldfield H, Doppman JL. Reversible acute and subacute myelopathy in patients with dural arteriovenous fistulas. *J Neurosurg* 1989; **70**: 354–9.

79 Critchley E, Eisen A. *Diseases of the spinal cord.* London: Springer, 1992.

80 Daumen-Legre V, Lafforgue P, Champsaur P *et al.* Anteroposterior atlantoaxial subluxation in cervical spine osteoarthritis: case reports and review of the literature. *J Rheumatol* 1999; **26**: 687–91.

81 Davis FWJ, Markley HE. Rheumatoid arthritis with death from medullary compression. *Ann Intern Med* 1951; **35**: 451–4.

82 De Girolami U, Zivin J. Neuropathology of experimental spinal cord ischemia in the rabbit. *J Neuropathol Exp Neurol* 1982; **41**: 129–49.

83 Demange É. Scléroses médullaires d'origine vasculaire. *Rev Méd* 1884; **4**: 753–66.

84 DePalma AF, Rothman RH. *The intervertebral disc.* Philadelphia, PA: Saunders, 1970.

85 Dodson WE, Landau WM. Motor neuron loss due to aortic clamping in repair of coarctation. *Neurology* 1973; **23**: 539–42.

86 Dohrmann GJ, Wagner FC Jr, Bucy PC. The microvasculature in transitory traumatic paraplegia. An electron microscopic study in the monkey. *J Neurosurg* 1971; **35**: 263–71.

87 Dohrmann GJ, Wagner FC Jr, Bucy PC. Transitory traumatic paraplegia: electron microscopy of early alterations in myelinated nerve fibers. *J Neurosurg* 1972; **36**: 407–15.

88 Dolan AL, Gibson T. Intrinsic spinal cord lesions in 2 patients with ankylosing spondylitis. *J Rheumatol* 1994; **21**: 1160–1.

89 Ducker TB, Kindt GW, Kempf LG. Pathological findings in acute experimental spinal cord trauma. *J Neurosurg* 1971; **35**: 700–8.

90 Edgar R, Quai P. Progressive post-traumatic cystic and non-cystic myelopathy. *Br J Neurosurg* 1994; **8**: 7–22.

91 Edmonson JM. Historical perspective on sciatica. In: Hardy RW ed. *Lumbar disc disease.* New York: Raven, 1993: 1–4.

92 Eidelberg E, Sullivan J, Brigham A. Immediate consequences of spinal cord injury: possible role of potassium in axonal conduction block. *Surg Neurol* 1975; **3**: 317–21.

93 Ekström G. The surgical treatment of patent ductus arteriosus. *Acta Neurol Scand Suppl* 1952; **169**: 153–7.

94 Emery E, Aldana P, Bunge MB *et al.* Apoptosis after traumatic human spinal cord injury. *J Neurosurg* 1998; **89**: 911–20.

95 Eulderink F, Meijers KAE. Pathology of the cervical spine in rheumatoid arthritis: a controlled study of 44 spines. *J Pathol* 1976; **120**: 91–108.

96 Faden AI, Simon RP. A potential role for excitotoxins in the pathophysiology of spinal cord injury. *Ann Neurol* 1988; **23**: 623–6.

97 Fahey V, Opeskin K, Silberstein M *et al.* The pathogenesis of Schmorl's nodes in relation to acute trauma. An autopsy study. *Spine* 1988; **23**: 2272–5.

98 Fawcett JW, Asher RA. The glial scar and central nervous system repair. *Brain Res Bulletin* 1999; **49**: 377–91.

99 Fehlings MG, Tator CH. A review of experimental models of acute spinal cord injury. In: Illis LS ed. *Spinal cord dysfunction: assessment.* Oxford: Oxford University Press, 1988: 3–4.

100 Fehlings MG, Tator CH. The relationship among the severity of spinal cord injury, residual neurological function, axon counts, and counts of retrogradely labeled neurons after experimental spinal cord injury. *Exp Neurol* 1995; **132**: 220–8.

101 Feigin I, Popoff N, Adachi M. Fibrocartilagenous venous emboli to the spinal cord with necrotic myelopathy. *J Neuropathol Exp Neurol* 1965; **24**: 63–74.

102. Flament J, Vicente AN, Coërs C, Guazzi G. La myélopathie angiodysgénétique (Foix–Alajouanine) et sa différenciation des nécroses spinales sur angiomatose intra-médullaire. *Rev Neurol (Paris)* 1960; **103**: 12–29.

103 Foix C, Alajouanine T. La myélite nécrotique subaigue. *Rev Neurol (Paris)* 1926; **46**: 1–42.

104 Foo D, Sarkarati M, Marcelino V. Cervical spinal cord injury complicating ankylosing spondylitis. *Paraplegia* 1985; **23**: 358–63.

105 Fujiwara K, Fujimoto M, Yonenobu K, Ochi T. A clinicopathological study of cervical myelopathy in rheumatoid arthritis: post-mortem analysis of two cases. *Eur Spine J* 1999; **8**: 46–53.

106 Garcin R, Godlewski S, Rondot P. Étude clinique des médullopathies d'origine vasculaire. *Rev Neurol (Paris)* 1962; **106**: 592–631.

107 Garcin R, Grunner J. Nécrose cavitaire des cornes antérieures de la moelle au cours d'un syndrome realisant une forme pseudo-polynévritique de sclerose latérale amyotrophique. *Presse Méd* 1953; **61**: 1723–4.

108 Garcin R, Zülch KJ, Lazorthes G, Gruner J. *Pathologie vasculaire de la moelle*. Paris: Masson, 1962.

109 Gilles FH. Vulnerability of the human spinal cord in transient cardiac arrest. *Neurol* 1971; **21**: 833–9.

110 Gilles de la Tourette G, Marinesco G. La lésion médullaire de l'ostéite déformante de Paget. *Nouvelle Iconographie de la Salpétriére* 1895; **8**: 205–13.

111 Gillilan LA. The arterial blood supply of the human spinal cord. *J Comp Neurol* 1958; **110**: 75–103.

112 Gillilan LA. Veins of the spinal cord. *Neurology* 1970; **20**: 860–8.

113 Goldthwait J. The lumbo-sacral articulation. An explanation of many cases of 'lumbago', 'sciatica' and paraplegia. *Boston Med Surg J* 1911; **164**: 365–72.

114 Greenfield JG. Malformations et dégénerescences des disques intervértebraux de la région cervicale. *Rev Méd Suisse Romande* 1953; **73**: 227–50.

115 Greenfield JG. Lesions of the nervous system associated with diseases or malformations of the cranium and spinal column. In: Blackwood W, McMenemey WH, Meyer A *et al*. eds. *Greenfield's neuropathology*. Baltimore, MD: Williams and Wilkins, 1963: 650–65.

116 Greenfield JG, Rickards AG, Manning GB. The pathology of paraplegia occurring as a delayed sequela of spinal anaesthesia, with special reference to the vascular change. *J Pathol Bacteriol* 1955; **69**: 95–107.

117 Greenfield JG, Turner JWA. Acute and subacute necrotic myelitis. *Brain* 1939; **62**: 227–52.

118 Gregorius FG, Estrin T, Crandall PH. Cervical spondylotic radiculopathy and myelopathy. *Arch Neurol* 1976; **33**: 618–25.

119 Grote EH, Voigt K. Clinical syndromes, natural history, and pathophysiology of vascular lesions of the spinal cord. *Neurosurg Clin North Am* 1999; **10**: 17–45.

120 Gruner J, Lapresle J. Étude anatomo-pathologique des médullopathies d'origine vasculaire. *Rev Neurol (Paris)* 1962; **106**: 592–631.

121 Guha A, Tator CH. Acute cardiovascular effects of experimental spinal cord injury. *J Trauma* 1988; **28**: 481–90.

122 Haberland K. Über ein spinales Angioma racemosum venosum. *Arch Psychiat Z Neurol* 1950; **184**: 417–25.

123 Haddad SF, Hitchon PW, Godersky JC. Idiopathic and glucocorticoid-induced spinal epidural lipomatosis. *J Neurosurg* 1991; **74**: 38–42.

124 Hanski W, Rydzewska M, Fundowicz R. Zatory naczyn rdzenia kregowego tkanka jadra miazdzystego. *Neuropatol Polska* 1977; **15**: 479–90.

125 Hardy RW. *Lumbar disc disease*. New York: Raven, 1993.

126 Harrington TR. Sciatica and the history of surgical treatment of lumbar disk disease. *Barrow Neurol Inst Q* 1988; **4**: 24–9.

127 Hauge T. Chronic rheumatoid polyarthritis and spondylarthritis associated with neurological symptoms and signs occasionally simulating an intraspinal expansive process. *Acta Chir Scand* 1961; **120**: 395–401.

128 Hausmann ON, Moseley IF. Idiopathic dural herniation of the thoracic spinal cord. *Neuroradiology* 1996; **38**: 503–10.

129 Haymaker W. *Bing's local diagnosis in neurological diseases*. St Louis, MO: CV Mosby, 1956.

130 Heirholzer J, Benndorf G, Lehmann T *et al*. Epidural lipomatosis: case report and literature review. *Neuroradiology* 1996; **38**: 343–8.

131 Helbing C. Zur Kenntniss der Rückenmarksveränderungen beim Menschen nach Thrombose der Aorta abdominalis. *Dtsch Med Wochenschr* 1896; **22**: 672–4.

132 Heliovaara M. Body height, obesity and risk of herniated lumbar intervertebral disc. *Spine* 1987; **12**: 469–72.

133 Henderson FC, Geddes JF, Crockard HA. Neuropathology of the brainstem and spinal cord in end stage rheumatoid arthritis: implications for treatment. *Ann Rheum Dis* 1993; **52**: 629–37.

134 Hénin D, Smith TW, De Girolami K *et al*. Neuropathology of the spinal cord in the acquired immunodeficiency syndrome. *Hum Pathol* 1992; **23**: 1106–14.

135 Henneaux J. Nécrose médullaire par thrombose de l'artère spinale antérieure. *Acta Neurol Psychiat Belg* 1956; **56**: 365–85.

136 Henson RA, Parsons M. Ischemic lesions of the spinal cord: an illustrated review. *Q J Med* 1967; **142**: 205–22.

137 Herren RY. Occurrence and distribution of calcified plaques in the spinal arachnoid in man. *Arch Neurol Psychiatry* 1939; **41**: 1180–6.

138 Herren RY, Alexander L. Sulcal and intrinsic blood vessels of the human spinal cord. *Arch Neurol Psychiatry* 1939; **41**: 679–87.

139 Herrick MK, Mills PE. Infarction of the spinal cord. Two cases of selective gray matter involvement secondary of asymptomatic aortic disease. *Arch Neurol* 1971; **24**: 228–41.

140 Hill SC, Jasquez JM. Massive infarction of spinal cord and vertebral bodies as a complication of dissecting aneurysm of the aorta. *Circulation* 1962; **25**: 997–1000.

141 Hissa E, Boumphrey F, Bay J. Spinal epidural hematoma and ankylosing spondylitis. *Clin Orthop Res* 1986; **208**: 225–7.

142 Ho K-L, Gorell JM, Hayden MT. Fatal spinal cord infarction caused by fibrocartilaginous embolization of the anterior spinal artery. *Hum Pathol* 1980; **5**: 471–5.

143 Hogan EL, Romanul FCA. Spinal cord infarction occurring during insertion of aortic graft. *Neurology* 1966; **16**: 67–74.

144 Holden P, Canty EG, Mortier GR *et al*. Identification of novel pro-alpha2(IX) collagen gene mutations in two families with distinctive oligo-epiphyseal forms of multiple epiphyseal dysplasia. *Am J Hum Genet* 1999; **65**: 31–8.

145 Holmes G. The Goulstonian lectures on spinal injuries of warfare. 1. The pathology of acute spinal injuries. *BMJ* 1915; **ii**: 769–74.

146 Höök O, Lidvall H, Åström K-E. Cervical disk protrusion with compression of the spinal cord. Report of a case. *Neurology* 1960; **10**: 834–41.

147 Hubert J-P, Ectors M, Ketrlbant-Balasse P, Flament-Durand J. Fibrocartilaginous venous and arterial emboli from the nucleus pulposus in the anterior spinal system. *Eur Neurol* 1974; **11**: 164–71.

148 Hubert J-P, Retif J, Brihaye J, Flament-Durand J. Infarctus médullaire par emboles de noyau pulpeux. Nouvelle observation anatomo-clinique. *Acta Neurol Belg* 1974; **74**: 297–303.

149 Hughes J. Disorders of the spine and spinal cord. In: Adams JH, Duchen LW eds. *Greenfield's neuropathology*. New York: Oxford University Press, 1992: 1083–115.

150 Hughes JT. Venous infarction of the spinal cord. *Neurology* 1971; **21**: 794–800.

151 Hughes JT. *Pathology of the spinal cord*. Philadelphia, PA: Saunders, 1978.

152 Hughes JT. Vascular disorders of the spinal cord. In: Vinken PJ, Bruyn GW, Klawans HL eds. *Handbook of clinical neurology* Vol. 55. Amsterdam: Elsevier, 1989: 95–106.

153 Hughes JT. Neuropathology of the spinal cord. *Neurol Clin* 1991; **9**: 551–71.

154 Hughes JT, Brownell B. Aberrant nerve fibers within the spinal cord. *J Neurol Neurosurg Psychiatry* 1963; **26**: 528–34.

155 Hughes JT, Brownell B. Cervical spondylosis complicated by anterior spinal artery thrombosis. *Neurology* 1964; **14**: 1073–7.

156 Hughes JT, Brownell B. Spinal cord ischemia due to arteriosclerosis. *Arch Neurol* 1966; **15**: 189–202.

157 Hurst RW, Kenyon LC, Lavi E et al. Spinal dural arteriovenous fistula: the pathology of venous hypertensive myelopathy. *Neurology* 1995; **45**: 1309–13.

158 Isu T, Iizuka T, Iwasaki Y et al. Spinal cord herniation associated with an intradural spinal arachnoid cyst diagnosed by magnetic resonance imaging. *Neurosurgery* 1991; **29**: 137–9.

159 Jacenko O, Olsen BR. Transgenic mouse models in the studies of skeletal disorders. *J Rheumatol* 1995; **43** (Suppl): 39–41.

160 Jacques S. Osteopetrosis (Albers–Schönberg disease). In: Vinken PJ, Bruyn GW eds. *Handbook of clinical neurology* Vol. 38. Amsterdam: North-Holland, 1979: 371–80.

161 Jeffries E. *Disorders of the cervical spine*. Oxford: Butterworth-Heinemann, 1993.

162 Jellinger K. Spinal cord arteriosclerosis and progressive vascular myelopathy. *J Neurol Neurosurg Psychiatry* 1967; **30**: 195–206.

163 Jellinger K. Neuropathology of cord injuries. In: Vinken PJ, Bruyn GW eds. *Handbook of clinical neurology* Vol. 25. New York: Elsevier, 1976; 43–121.

164 Jellinger K. Pathology of spinal vascular malformations and vascular tumors. In: Pia H, Djindjian R eds. *Spinal angiomas*. Springer-Verlag: Berlin, 1977: 18–44.

165 Jellinger K, Minauf M, Garzuly F, Neumayer E. Angiodysgenetische nekrotisierende Myelopathie. *Arch Psychiat Nervenkrank* 1968; **211**: 377–404.

166 Jellinger K, Neumayer E. Myélopathie progressive d'origine vasculaire. Contribution anatomoclinique aux syndromes d'une hypovascularisation chronique de a moelle. *Acta Neurol Psychiat Belg* 1962; **62**: 944–56.

167 Jurovic I, Eiben E. Fatal myelomalacia caused by massive fibrocartilagenous venous emboli from nucleus pulposus. *Acta Neuropathol* 1970; **15**: 284–7.

168 Kadyi H. Über die Blutgefässe des menschlichen Rückenmarkes. *Anat Anz* 1886; **1**: 304–14.

169 Kadyi H. *Über die Blutgefässe des menschlichen Rückenmarkes*. Lemberg: Gubrynowicz & Schmidt, 1889.

170 Kaelan C, Jacobsen P, Morling P, Kakulas BA. A quantitative study of motorneurons and cortico-spinal fibres relat-

ed to function in human spinal cord injury (SCI). *Paraplegia* 1989; **27**: 148–9.

171 Kahn EA. The rôle of the dentate ligaments in spinal cord compression and the syndrome of lateral sclerosis. *J Neurosurg* 1947; **4**: 191–9.

172 Kakulas BA. Pathology of spinal injuries. *Cent Nerv Syst Trauma* 1984; **1**: 117–29.

173 Kaplan JG, Barasch E, Hirshfeld A et al. Spinal epidural lipomatosis: a serious complication of iatrogenic Cushing's syndrome. *Neurology* 1989; **39**: 1031–4.

174 Kase CS, Varakis JN, Stafford JR, Mohr JP. Medial medullary infarction from fibrocartilaginous embolism to the anterior spinal artery. *Stroke* 1983; **14**: 413–18.

175 Kaufman AB, Dunsmore RH. Clinicopathological considerations in spinal meningeal calcification and ossification. *Neurology* 1971; **21**: 1243–8.

176 Kelsey JL. An epidemiological study of the relationship between occupations and acute herniated lumbar intervertebral discs. *Int J Epidemiol* 1975; **4**: 197–205.

177 Kendall BE, Logue V. Spinal epidural angiomatous malformations draining into intrathecal veins. *Neuroradiology* 1977; **13**: 181–9.

178 Kennedy P, Swasch M, Dean MF. Cervical cord compression in mucopolysaccharidosis. *Dev Med Child Neurol* 1973; **15**: 194–9.

179 Kepes JJ. Selective necrosis of the spinal cord gray matter. A complication of dissecting aneurysm of the aorta. *Acta Neuropathol* 1965; **4**: 293–8.

180 Kepes JJ, Reynard JD. Infarction of the spinal cord and medulla oblongata caused by fibrocartilaginous emboli. Report of case. *Virchows Arch A Pathol Anat Histopathol* 1973; **361**: 185–93.

181 Kestle JR, Resch L, Tator CH, Kucharczyk W. Intervertebral disc embolization resulting in spinal cord infarction; case report. *J Neurosurg* 1989; **71**: 938–41.

182 Keyes DC, Compere EL. The normal and pathological physiology of the nucleus pulposus of the intervertebral disc. *J Bone Joint Surg* 1932; **14**: 897–938.

183 Kim RC, Smith HR, Henbest ML, Choi BH. Nonhemorrhagic venous infarction of the spinal cord. *Ann Neurol* 1984; **15**: 379–85.

184 Kiss ZHT, Tator CH. Neurogenic shock. In: Geller ER ed. *Shock and resuscitation*. New York: McGraw-Hill, 1993: 421–40.

185 Klintworth GK. The neurologic manifestations of osteopetrosis (Albers–Schönberg's disease). *Neurology* 1963; **13**: 512–19.

186 Koeppen AH, Barron KD, Cox JF. Foix–Alajouanine syndrome. *Acta Neuropathol* 1974; **29**: 187–97.

187 König P-A. Die Gefässprozesse bei Myelitis necroticans. *Virchows Arch Pathol Anat* 1955; **327**: 737–53.

188 Koyanagi I, Tator CH, Lea PJ. Three-dimensional analysis of the vascular system in the rat spinal cord with scanning electron microscopy of vascular corrosion casts. Part 1: Normal spinal cord. *Neurosurgery* 1993; **33**: 277–84.

189 Koyanagi I, Tator CH, Lea PJ. Three-dimensional analysis of the vascular system in the rat spinal cord with scanning electron microscopy of vascular corrosion casts. Part 2: Acute spinal cord injury. *Neurosurgery* 1993; **33**: 285–92.

190 Koyanagi I, Tator CH, Theriault E. Silicone rubber microangiography of acute spinal cord injury in the rat. *Neurosurgery* 1993; **32**: 260–8.

191 Krämer J. *Intervertebral disc diseases. Causes, diagnosis, treatment and prophylaxis*. New York: Thieme, 1990.

192 Kramer W. Multilocular myelomalacia following adhesive arachnoiditis. *Neurology* 1956; **6**: 594–600.

193 Kumar K, Nath RK, Nair CPV, Tchang SP. Symptomatic epidural lipomatosis secondary to obesity. Case report. *J Neurosurg* 1996; **85**: 348–50.

194 Kumar R, Taha J, Greiner AL. Herniation of the spinal cord. Case report. *J Neurosurg* 1995; **82**: 131–6.

195 Laguna J, Cravioto H. Spinal cord infarction secondary to occlusion of the anterior spinal artery. *Arch Neurol* 1973; **28**: 134–6.

196 Laterre EC. Syndrome spinal antérieur par embolies multiples du tissu fibro-cartilagineux. *Rev Neurol (Paris)* 1962; **106**: 685–90.

197 Lazorthes G, Gouaze A, Zadeh JO et al. Arterial vascularization of the spinal cord. Recent studies of the anastomotic substitution pathways. *J Neurosurg* 1971; **35**: 253–62.

198 Lazorthes G, Poulhes J, Bastide G et al. La vascularisation artérielle de la moelle. Recherches anatomiques et applications à la pathologie médullaire et à la pathologie aortique. *Neurochirurgie* 1958; **4**: 3–19.

199 Lee ST, Lui TN, Jeng CM. Spinal cord herniation after stabbing injury. *Br J Neurosurg* 1997; **11**: 84–6.

200 Leech RW, Pitha JV, Brumbach RA. Spontaneous haematomyelia: a necropsy study. *J Neurol Neurosurg Psychiatry* 1991; **54**: 172–4.

201 Lestini WF, Wiesel SW. The pathogenesis of cervical spondylosis. *Clin Orthop* 1989; **239**: 69–93.

202 Lévy L. Un cas d'ostéite déformante de Paget. Interprétation des lésions de la moelle épinière. *Nouvelle Iconographie de la Salpétriére* 1897; **10**: 113–23.

203 Lhermitte F, Corbin JL. La circulation artérielle de la moelle et ses troubles en pathologie. *Rev Practicien* 1960; **10**: 2921–34.

204 Lhermitte J, Fribourg-Blanc A, Kyriaco N. La gliose angéiohypertrophique de la moelle épinière (Myélite nécrotique de Foix–Alajouanine). *Rev Neurol (Paris)* 1931; **56**: 37–53.

205 Lindbolm K, Rexed B. Spinal nerve injury in dorso-lateral protrusions of lumbar disks. *J Neurosurg* 1948; **5**: 413–32.

206 Lindemann A. Varicenbildung der Gefässe der Pia mater spinalis und des Rückenmarks als Ursache einer totalen Querschnittläsion. *Z Gesamte Neurol Psychiat* 1912; **12**: 522–9.

207 Lintott P, Hafez HM, Stansby G. Spinal cord complications of thoracoabdominal aneurysm surgery. *Br J Surg* 1998; **85**: 5–15.

208 Liu XZ, Xu XM, Hu R. Neuronal and glial apoptosis after traumatic cord injury. *J Neurosci* 1997; **17**: 5395–406.

209 Lubin AJ. Adhesive spinal arachnoiditis as a cause of intramedullary cavitation. *Arch Neurol Psychiatry* 1940; **44**: 409–20.

210 Luoma K, Riihimaki H, Raininko R et al. Lumbar disc degeneration in relation to occupation. *Scand J Work Environ Health* 1998; **24**: 358–66.

211 Luschka H. *Die Halbgelenke des Menschlichen Körpers.* Berlin: Reimer, 1858.

212 Lvovsky AM. Embolia sosudov spinnogo mozga tkaniu mezhpozvonkovo diska (Embolism of the spinal vessels by tissues of the intervertebral discs). *Zh Nevropatol Psikhiatrii Korsakov* 1969; **69**: 1151–7.

213 MacDonald RL, Findlay JM, Tator CH. Microcystic spinal cord degeneration causing post-traumatic myelopathy. Report of two cases. *J Neurosurg* 1988; **68**: 466–71.

214 Mackay RP. Chronic adhesive spinal arachnoiditis. *JAMA* 1939; **112**: 802–8.

215 Mackenzie AR, Laing RB, Smith C et al. Spinal epidural abscess: the importance of early diagnosis and treatment. *J Neurol Neurosurg Psychiatry* 1998; **65**: 209–12.

216 Mair WGP, Druckman R. The pathology of spinal cord lesions and their relation to the clinical features in protrusion of the cervical intervertebral discs. *Brain* 1953; **76**: 70–91.

217 Mair WGP, Folkerts JF. Necrosis of the spinal cord due to thrombophlebitis (subacute necrotic myelitis). *Brain* 1953; **76**: 563–75.

218 Mannen T. Vascular lesions in the spinal cord in the aged. *Geriatrics* 1966; **21**: 151–60.

219 Markiewicz T. Zur Frage der 'kolloiden' Degeneration und ähnlicher Vorgänge im Zentralnervensystem. *Z Gesamte Neurol Psychiat* 1937; **159**: 60–74.

220 Marshman LA, Hardwidge C, Ford-Dunn SC, Olney JS. Idiopathic spinal cord herniation: case report and review of the literature. *Neurosurgery* 1999; **44**: 1129–33.

221 Masuzawa H, Nakayama H, Shitara N, Suzuki T. Spinal cord herniation into a congenital extradural arachnoid cyst causing Brown–Sequard syndrome. Case report. *J Neurosurg* 1981; **55**: 983–6.

222 Matsko DE, Panuntsev VS, Ivanova NE et al. Arteriovenous malformation of the cervical spinal cord with unusual drainage into the cranial cavity. *Pathol Res Pract* 1996; **192**: 942–7.

223 Matsumura T, Takahashi MP, Nozaki S, Kang J. A case of idiopathic spinal cord herniation. *Rinsho Shinkeigaku* 1996; **36**: 566–70.

224 Matthews WB. The neurological complications of ankylosing spondylitis. *J Neurol Sci* 1968; **6**: 561–73.

225 McCleary L, Rovit RL, Murali R. Case report: Myelopathy secondary to congenital osteopetrosis of the cervical spine. *Neurosurgery* 1987; **20**: 487–9.

226 McRae DL. Bony abnormalities in the region of the foramen magnum: correlation of anatomic and neurologic findings. *Acta Radiol* 1952; **40**: 335–54.

227 Mehrez IO, Nabseth DC, Hogan EL, Deterling RA. Paraplegia following resection of abdominal aortic aneurysm. *Ann Surg* 1962; **156**: 890–7.

228 Meijers KAE, van Beusekom GT, Luyendijk W, Duijfjes F. Dislocation of the cervical spine with cord compression in rheumatoid arthritis. *J Bone Joint Surg* 1974; **56B**: 668–80.

229 Merland JJ, Riche MC, Chiras J. Les fistules artério-veineuses intra-canalaires, extra-médullaires à drainage veineux médullaire. *J Neuroradiol* 1980; **7**: 271–320.

230 Middleton GS, Teacher JH. Injury of the spinal cord due to rupture of an intervertebral disc during muscular effort. *Glasgow Med J* 1911; **76**: 1–6.

231 Mikulis DJ, Ogilvy CS, Mckee A et al. Spinal cord infarction and fibrocartilagenous emboli. *Am J Neuroradiol* 1992; **13**: 155–60.

232 Mirich DR, Kucharczyk W, Keller MA, Deck J. Subacute necrotizing myelopathy: MR imaging in four pathologically proved cases. *Am J Neuroradiol* 1992; **12**: 1077–83.

233 Miura Y, Mimatsu K, Matsuyama Y et al. Idiopathic spinal cord herniation. *Neuroradiology* 1996; **38**: 155–6.

234 Mixter WJ, Barr JS. Rupture of the intervertebral disc with involvement of the spinal canal. *N Engl J Med* 1934; **211**: 210–15.

235 Miyake S, Tamaki N, Nagashima T et al. Idiopathic spinal cord herniation. Report of two cases and review of the literature. *J Neurosurg* 1998; **88**: 331–5.

236 Moersch FP, Sayre GP. Neurologic manifestations associated with dissecting aneurysm of the aorta. *JAMA* 1950; **144**: 1141–8.

237 Moorhouse DF, Burke M, Keohane C, Farrell MA. Spinal cord infarction caused by cartilage embolus to the anterior spinal artery. *Surg Neurol* 1992; **37**: 448–52.

238 Mundt DJ, Kelsey JL, Golden AL et al. An epidemiologic study of sports and weight lifting as possible risk factors for herniated lumbar and cervical discs. The Northeast Collaborative Group on Low Back Pain. *Am J Sports Med* 1993; **21**: 854–60.

239 Mundt DJ, Kelsey JL, Golden AL *et al*. An epidemiologic study of non-occupational lifting as a risk factor for herniated lumbar intervertebral disc. The Northeast Collaborative Group on Low Back Pain. *Spine* 1993; **18**: 595–602.

240 Muragaki Y, Mariman EC, van Beersum SE *et al*. A mutation in the gene encoding the alpha 2 chain of the fibril-associated collagen IX, COL9A2, causes multiple epiphyseal dysplasia (EMD2). *Nat Genet* 1995; **12**: 103–5.

241 Nagashima C. Cervical myelopathy due to ossification of the posterior longitudinal ligament. *J Neurosurg* 1972; **37**: 653–60.

242 Naiman JL, Donohue WL, Prichard JS. Fatal nucleus pulposus embolism of spinal cord after trauma. *Neurology* 1961; **11**: 83–7.

243 Nakajima K, Onomura T, Tanida Y, Ishibashi I. Factors related to the severity of myelopathy in atlantoaxial instability. *Spine* 1996; **21**: 1440–5.

244 Nakano KK, Schoene WC, Baker RA, Dawson DM. The cervical myelopathy associated with rheumatoid arthritis: analysis of 32 patients, with 2 postmortem cases. *Ann Neurol* 1978; **3**: 144–51.

245 Nakazawa H, Toyama Y, Satomi K *et al*. Idiopathic spinal cord herniation. Report of two cases and review of the literature. *Spine* 1993; **18**: 2138–41.

246 Namiki J, Tator CH. Cell proliferation and nestin expression in the ependyma of the adult rat spinal cord after injury. *J Neuropathol Exp Neurol* 1999; **58**: 489–98.

247 Nemecek S. Morphological evidence of microcirculatory disturbances in experimental spinal cord trauma. *Adv Neurol* 1978; **20**: 395–405.

248 Nurick S. The pathogenesis of the spinal cord disorder associated with cervical spondylosis. *Brain* 1972; **95**: 87–100.

249 Nussbaum ES, Rengachary SS. Cervical disc disease and spondylosis. In: Rengachary S, Wilkins R eds. *Principles of neurosurgery*. London: Wolfe, 1993: 44.1–16.

250 Oe T, Hoshino Y, Kurokawa T. A case of idiopathic herniation of the spinal cord associated with duplicated dura mater and with an arachnoid cyst. *Nippon Seikeigeka Gakkai Zasshi* 1990; **64**: 43–9.

251 Olsen BR. Collagen IX. *Int J Biochem Cell Biol* 1997; **29**: 555–8.

252 Osterland G. Ein morphologischer Beitrag zur Kenntnis der Foix–Alajouanineschen Krankheit (phlebodysgenetische Myelomalacie). *Arch Psychiatrie Z Gesamte Neurol* 1960; **200**: 123–45.

253 Pang D, Wilberger JE Jr. Spinal cord injury without radiographic abnormalities in children. *J Neurosurg* 1982; **57**: 114–29.

254 Panter SS, Yum SW, Faden AI. Alteration in extracellular amino acids after traumatic spinal cord injury. *Ann Neurol* 1990; **27**: 96–9.

255 Partington MD, Rüfenacht DA, Marsch WR, Piepgras G. Cranial and sacral dural arteriovenous fistulas as a cause of myelopathy. *J Neurosurg* 1992; **76**: 615–22.

256 Peiffer J, Wenig C, Mäusle E. Akutes Querschnittssyndrom durch Embolien von Nucleus-pulposus-Gewebe. *Dtsche Med Wochenschr* 1976; **101**: 583–6.

257 Pellicci PM, Ranawat CS, Tsairis P, Bryan WJ. A prospective study of the progression of rheumatoid arthritis of the cervical spine. *J Bone Joint Surg* 1981; **63A**: 342–50.

258 Périer O, Demanet J-C, Hennaux J, Nunès Vicente A. Existe-t-il un syndrome des artères spinales postérieures? A propos de deux observations anatomo-cliniques. *Rev Neurol (Paris)* 1960; **103**: 346–409.

259 Petrén K. Ein Fall von akuter Infektionskrankheit mit Thrombosen in den pialen Gefässen des Rückenmarks. *Nord Med Ark* 1898; **9**: 1–48.

260 Pomerance A. Spinal arachnoiditis ossificans. *J Pathol* 1964; **87**: 421–3.

261 Popovich PG, Wei P, Stokes BT. Cellular inflammatory response after spinal cord injury in Sprague–Dawley and Lewis rats. *J Comp Neurol* 1997; **377**: 443–64.

262 Prescher A. Anatomy and pathology of the aging spine. *Eur J Radiol* 1998; **27**: 181–95.

263 Qasho R, Ramundo OE, Maraglino C *et al*. Epidural lipomatosis with lumbar radiculopathy in one obese patient. Case report and review of the literature. *Neurosurg Rev* 1997; **20**: 206–9.

264 Ramos-Remus C, Gomez-Vargas A, Guzman-Guzman L *et al*. Frequency of atlantoaxial subluxation and neurologic involvement in patients with ankylosing spondylitis. *J Rheumatol* 1995; **22**: 2120–5.

265 Rao KR, Donnenfeld H, Chusid JG, Valdez S. Acute myelopathy secondary to spinal venous thrombosis. *J Neurol Sci* 1982; **56**: 107–13.

266 Reinisch H. Über das Wesen der Foix–Alajouanineschen Krankheit. Angiodysgenetische myelomalacie. *Virchows Arch Pathol Anat* 1963; **336**: 570–9.

267 Reitter K. Aneurysma dissecans und Paraplegie, zugleich ein Beitrag zur Pathologie der Blutzirkulation im Rückenmark. *Dtsch Arch Klin Med* 1916; **119**: 561–74.

268 Rigamonti D, Liem L, Sampath S *et al*. Spinal epidural abscess: contemporary trends in etiology, evaluation and management. *Surg Neurol* 1999; **52**: 189–96.

269 Rivlin AS, Tator CH. Effect of duration of acute spinal cord compression in a new acute spinal cord injury model in the rat. *Surg Neurol* 1978; **10**: 38–43.

270 Robertson SC, Traynelis VC, Follett KA, Menezes AH. Idiopathic spinal epidural lipomatosis. *Neurosurgery* 1997; **41**: 68–75.

271 Roitzsch E. Die Faserknorpelembolie der Rückenmarksgefässe – eine seltene Ursache der Myelomalazie. *Zentralbl Allgemeine Pathol Pathol Anat* 1975; **119**: 100–3.

272 Romanes GJ. The arterial blood supply of the human spinal cord. *Paraplegia* 1965; **2**: 199–207.

273 Rousseau S, Metral S, Lacroix C *et al*. Anterior spinal artery syndrome mimicking infantile spinal muscular atrophy. *J Perinatol* 1993; **10**: 316–18.

274 Rowland LP. Surgical treatment of cervical spondylotic myelopathy. *Neurology* 1992; **42**: 5–13.

275 Roy-Camille R, Mazel C, Husson JL, Saillant G. Symptomatic spinal epidural lipomatosis induced by a long-term steroid treatment. Review of the literature and report of two additional cases. *Spine* 1991; **16**: 1365–71.

276 Sambrook PN, MacGregor A, Spector TD. Genetic influences on cervical and lumbar disc degeneration: a magnetic resonance imaging study in twins. *Arthritis Rheum* 1999; **42**: 366–72.

277 Sandler AN, Tator CH. Effect of acute spinal cord compression injury on regional spinal cord blood flow in primates. *J Neurosurg* 1976; **45**: 660–76.

278 Sandson TA, Friedman JH. Spinal cord infarction. Report of 8 cases and review of the literature. *Medicine* 1989; **68**: 282–92.

279 Saruhashi Y, Hukuda S, Katsuura A *et al*. Clinical outcomes of cervical cord injuries without radiological evidence of trauma. *Spinal Cord* 1998; **36**: 567–73.

280 Schairer E, von Albert H-H. Aufsteigende Querschnittssymptomatik bei embolischem Verschluss der Rückenmarksarterien durch Bandscheibengewebe. *Münchner Med Wochenschr* 1977; **119**: 1433–6.

281 Schanne FAX, Kane AB, Young EE *et al*. Calcium dependence of toxic cell death: a final common pathway. *Science* 1979; **206**: 700–2.

282 Schmidek HH. Neurologic and neurosurgical sequelae of Paget's disease of bone. *Clin Orthop* 1977; **127**: 70–7.

283 Schmorl G. Zur pathologischen Anatomie der Wirbelsäule. *Klin Wochenschr* 1929; **8**: 1243–9.

284 Schneider H, Drally J, Ebhardt G. Läsionen des Rückenmarks nach temporärem Kreislaufstillstand. *Z Neurol* 1973; **204**: 165–78.

285 Schneider RC. The syndrome of acute anterior spinal cord injury. *J Neurosurg* 1955; **12**: 95–122.

286 Schneider RC, Crosby EC, Russo RH *et al.* Traumatic spinal cord syndromes and their management. *Clin Neurosurg* 1973; **20**: 424–92.

287 Scholz W, Manuelidis EE. Myélite nécrotique (Foix–Alajouanine) – Angiodysgenetische nekrotisierende Myelopathie. *Dtsch Z Nervenheil* 1951; **165**: 56–71.

288 Scholz W, Wechsler W. Ein weiterer Beitrag zur angiodysgenetischen nekrotisierende Myelopathie (Foix–Alajouaninesche Krankheit). *Arch Psychiatrie Z Gesamte Neurol* 1959; **1959**: 609–29.

289 Schwarz GA, Shorey WK, Anderson NS. Myelomalacia secondary to dissecting aneurysm of the aorta. *Arch Neurol Psychiatry* 1950; **64**: 401–16.

290 Scott RW, Sancetta SM. Dissecting aneurysm of aorta with hemorrhagic infarction of the spinal cord and complete paraplegia. *Am Heart J* 1949; **38**: 747–56.

291 Shaw MDM, Russell JA, Grossart KW. The changing pattern of spinal arachnoiditis. *J Neurol Neurosurg Psychiatry* 1978; **41**: 97–107.

292 Simmons EDJ, Guntupalli M, Kowalski JM *et al.* Familial predisposition for degenerative disc disease. A case–control study. *Spine* 1996; **21**: 1527–9.

293 Sioutos P, Arbit E, Tsairis P, Gargan R. Spontaneous thoracic spinal cord herniation. A case report. *Spine* 1996; **21**: 1710–13.

294 Sivakumar K, Sheinart K, Lidov M, Cohen B. Symptomatic spinal epidural lipomatosis in a patient with Cushing's disease. *Neurology* 1995; **45**: 2281–3.

295 Sladky JT, Rorke LB. Perinatal hypoxic/ischemic spinal cord injury. *Pediatr Pathol* 1986; **6**: 87–101.

296 Slager UT. Arachnoiditis ossificans. *Arch Pathol* 1960; **70**: 322–7.

297 Slavin RE, Gonzalez-Vitale JC, Marin OSM. Atheromatous emboli to the lumbosacral spinal cord. *Stroke* 1975; **6**: 411–16.

298 Sorin S, Askari A, Moskowitz RW. Atlantoaxial subluxation as a complication of early ankylosing spondylitis: Two case reports and a review of the literature. *Arthritis Rheum* 1979; **22**: 273–6.

299 Spillane JD. Three cases of achondroplasia with neurological complications. *J Neurol Neurosurg Psychiatry* 1952; **15**: 246–52.

300 Squier MV, Lehr RP. Post-traumatic syringomyelia. *J Neurol Neurosurg Psychiatry* 1994; **57**: 1095–8.

301 Srigley JR, Lambert CD, Bilbao JM, Pritzker PH. Spinal cord infarction secondary to intervertebral disc embolism. *Ann Neurol* 1981; **9**: 296–301.

302 Stambough JL, Cheeks ML, Keiper GL. Nonglucocorticoid-induced lumbar epidural lipomatosis: a case report and review of literature. *J Spinal Disord* 1989; **2**: 201–7.

303 Stechison MT, Tator CH. Cervical myelopathy in diffuse idiopathic skeletal hyperostosis. Case report. *J Neurosurg* 1990; **73**: 279–82.

304 Steno N. *Elementorum Myologiæ Specimen, seu Muscululi descriptio Geometrica. Cui Accedunt Canis Carchariæ Dissectus Caput, et Dissectus Piscis Ex Canum Genere.* Florentiæ: Stellæ, 1667: 86.

305 Stern JD, Quint DJ, Sweasey TA, Hoff JT. Spinal epidural lipomatosis: two new idiopathic cases and a review of the literature. *J Spinal Dis* 1994; **7**: 343–9.

306 Stokes BT, Fox P, Hollinden G. Extracellular calcium activity in the injured spinal cord. *Exp Neurol* 1983; **80**: 561–72.

307 Stoltmann HF, Blackwood W. The role of the ligamenta flava in the pathogenesis of myelopathy in cervical spondylosis. *Brain* 1964; **164**: 45–50.

308 Stookey B. Compression of the spinal cord due to ventral extradural cervical chondromas. Diagnosis and treatment. *Arch Neurol Psychiatry* 1928; **20**: 275–91.

309 Suh TH, Alexander L. Vascular system of the human spinal cord. *Arch Neurol Psychiatry* 1939; **41**: 659–77.

310 Symon L, Kuyama H, Kendall B. Dural arteriovenous malformations of the spine. Clinical features and surgical results in 55 cases. *J Neurosurg* 1984; **60**: 238–45.

311 Tadié M, Hemet J, Freger P *et al.* Anatomie morphologique et circulatoire des veines de la moelle (Morphological and functional anatomy of spinal cord veins). *J Neuroradiol* 1985; **12**: 3–20.

312 Tanon L. Les artères de la moelle dorso-lombaire. Thèse pour le doctorat en médecine. Paris: Vigot Frères, 1908.

313 Tator CH. Review of experimental spinal cord injury with emphasis on the local and systemic circulatory effects. *Neurochirurgie* 1991; **37**: 291–302.

314 Tator CH. Clinical manifestations of acute spinal cord injury. In: Benzel EC, Tator CH eds. *Contemporary management of spinal cord injury*. Park Ridge, IL: American Association of Neurological Surgery: 1995: 15–26.

315 Tator CH. Pathophysiology and pathology of spinal cord injury. In: Wilkins RH, Rengachary SS eds. *Neurosurgery*. New York: McGraw-Hill, 1996: 2847–59.

316 Tator CH. Spinal cord syndromes with physiologic and anatomic correlations. In: Menezes A, Sonntag VKH eds. *Principles of spinal surgery*. New York: McGraw-Hill, 1996: 785–99.

317 Tator CH, Duncan EG, Edmonds VE *et al.* Changes in epidemiology of acute spinal cord injury from 1947 to 1981. *Surg Neurol* 1993; **40**: 207–15.

318 Tator CH, Fehlings MG. Review of the secondary injury theory of acute spinal cord trauma with special emphasis on vascular mechanisms. *J Neurosurg* 1991; **75**: 15–26.

319 Tator CH, Koyanagi I. Vascular mechanisms in the pathophysiology of human spinal cord injury. *J Neurosurg* 1997; **86**: 483–92.

320 Taylor AR. Vascular factors in the myelopathy associated with cervical spondylosis. *Neurology* 1964; **4**: 62–8.

321 Terhaag D, Frowein RA. Traumatic disc prolapses. *Neurosurg Rev* 1989; **12** (Suppl 1): 588–94.

322 Thomas DJ, Kendall MJ, Whitfield AGW. Nervous system involvement in ankylosing spondylitis. *BMJ* 1974; **i**: 148–50.

323 Thompson GB. Dissecting aortic aneurysm with infarction of the spinal cord. *Brain* 1956; **79**: 111–18.

324 Thron AK. *Vascular anatomy of the spinal cord*. New York: Springer, 1988.

325 Toro G, Roman GC, Narvarro-Roman L *et al.* Natural history of spinal cord infarction caused by nucleus pulposus embolism. *Spine* 1994; **19**: 360–5.

326 Tosi L, Rigoli G, Beltramello A. Fibrocartilaginous embolism of the spinal cord: a clinical and pathogenetic reconsideration. *J Neurol Neurosurg Psychiatry* 1996; **60**: 55–60.

327 Tronnier VM, Steinmetz A, Albert FK *et al.* Hernia of the spinal cord: case report and review of the literature. *Neurosurgery* 1991; **29**: 916–19.

328 Tuohy EL, Boman PG, Berdez GL. Spinal cord ischemia in dissecting aortic aneurysm. *Am Heart J* 1941; **22**: 305–13.

329 Turner JWA. The spinal complications of Paget's disease (Osteitis deformans). *Brain* 1940; **63**: 321–49.

330 Tyler HR, Clark DB. Neurologic complications in patients with coarctation of the aorta. *Neurology* 1958; **8**: 712–18.

331 Uchino A, Kato A, Momozaki N et al. Spinal cord herniation: report of two cases and review of the literature. *Eur Radiol* 1997; **7**: 289–92.

332 Vesalius A. *De Humani Corporis Fabrica Libri Septem*. Basileae: Oporini, 1555: 70–5.

333 Videman T, Battie MC. The influence of occupation on lumbar degeneration. *Spine* 1999; **24**: 1164–8.

334 Vogel P, Meyer H-H. Über eine akute Querlähmung des Rückenmarks und ihre anatomische Grundlage (Verschluss der vorderen Spinalarterie). *Dtsch Z Nervernheil* 1939; **143**: 217–28.

335 Wagner FC Jr, Stewart WB. Effect of trauma dose on spinal cord edema. *J Neurosurg* 1981; **54**: 802–6.

336 Wallace MC, Tator CH, Lewis AJ. Chronic regenerative changes in the spinal cord after cord compression injury in rats. *Surg Neurol* 1987; **27**: 209–19.

337 Waltz TA. Physical factors in the production of the myelopathy of cervical spondylosis. *Brain* 1967; **90**: 395–404.

338 Wang R, Ehara K, Tamaki N. Spinal cord edema following freezing injury in the rat: relationship between tissue water content and spinal cord blood flow. *Surg Neurol* 1993; **39**: 348–54.

339 Weisman AD, Adams RD. The neurological complications of dissecting aortic aneurysm. *Brain* 1994; **67**: 69–92.

340 Wilkinson M. The morbid anatomy of cervical spondylosis and myelopathy. *Brain* 1960; **83**: 589–617.

341 Williamson RT. Spinal softening limited to the parts supplied by the posterior arterial system of the cord. *Lancet* 1895; **ii**: 520–1.

342 Wolman L. The disturbance of circulation in traumatic paraplegia in acute and late stages: a pathological study. *Paraplegia* 1965; **2**: 213–26.

343 Wolman L, Bradshaw P. Spinal cord embolism. *J Neurol Neurosurg Psychiatry* 1967; **30**: 446–54.

344 Woolsey RM, Young RR eds. Disorders of the spinal cord. In: *Neurologic clinics* Vol. 9. Philadelphia, PA: Saunders, 1991.

345 Wortzman G, Tasker RR, Rewcastle NB et al. Spontaneous incarcerated herniation of the spinal cord into a vertebral body: a unique cause of paraplegia. Case report. *J Neurosurg* 1974; **41**: 631–5.

346 Wrobel CJ, Oldfield EH, Di Chiro G et al. Myelopathy due to intracranial dural arteriovenous fistulas draining intrathecally into the spinal medullary veins. *J Neurosurg* 1988; **69**: 934–9.

347 Wyburn-Mason R. *The vascular abnormalities and tumors of the spinal cord and its membranes*. London: Henry Kimpton, 1944.

348 Wyllie WG. The occurrence in osteitis deformans of lesions of the central nervous system with a report of four cases. *Brain* 1923; **46**: 336–51.

349 Wyss O. Weber acute hämorrhagische Myelitis. *Dtsch Med Wochenschr* 1898; **24**: 81.

350 Yoong M, Blumbergs PC, North B. Primary (granulomatous) angiitis of the central nervous system with multiple aneurysms of spinal arteries. *J Neurosurg* 1993; **79**: 603–7.

351 Yost JH, Spencer-Green G, Krant JD. Vascular steal mimicking compression myelopathy in Paget's disease of bone: rapid reversal with calcitonin and systemic steroids. *J Rheumatol* 1993; **20**: 1064–5.

352 Young R, Kleinman G, Ojemann RG et al. Compressive myelopathy in Maroteaux–Lamy syndrome: clinical and pathological findings. *Ann Neurol* 1980; **8**: 336–40.

353 Young W, Yen V, Blight A. Extracellular calcium ionic activity in experimental spinal cord contusion. *Brain Res* 1982; **253**: 105–13.

354 Yousef OM, Appenzeller P, Kornfeld M. Fibrocartilagenous embolism: an unusual cause of spinal cord infarction. *Am J Forensic Med Pathol* 1998; **19**: 395–9.

355 Yuh WTC, Marsh EE, Wang AK et al. MR imaging of spinal cord and vertebral body infarction. *Am J Neuroradiol* 1992; **13**: 145–54.

356 Yutani C, Imakita M, Ishibashi-Ueda H et al. Cerebro-spinal infarction caused by atheromatous emboli. *Acta Pathol Jpn* 1985; **35**: 789–801.

357 Zeitlin H, Lichtenstein BBW. Occlusion of the anterior spinal artery. Clinicopathologic report of a case and a review of the literature. *Arch Neurol Psychiatry* 1936; **36**: 96–111.

358 Zenter J, Buchbender K, Vahlensieck M. Spinal epidural lipomatosis as a complication of prolonged corticosteroid therapy. *J Neurosurg Sci* 1995; **39**: 81–5.

359 Zülch KJ. Mangeldurchblutung an der Grenzzone zweier Gefässgebiete als Ursache bisher ungeklärter Rückenmarksschädigungen. *Dtsch Z Nerven* 1954; **172**: 81–101.

360 Zülch KJ. Réflexions sur la physiopathologie des troubles vasculaires médullaires. *Rev Neurol (Paris)* 1962; **106**: 632–45.

Index

Entries appearing in Volume I are indicated by the numeral I; those in Volume II, by the numeral II.